U0273855

Rosen & Barkin's 5-Minute Emergency Medicine Consult

(6th Edition)

急诊科5分钟速查

主编 Jeffrey J. Schaider
Roger M. Barkin
Stephen R. Hayden
Richard E. Wolfe
Adam Z. Barkin
Philip Shayne

主译 林兆奋 李文放 童朝阳 潘曙明

Wolters Kluwer 上海科学技术出版社

图书在版编目（CIP）数据
急诊科5分钟速查 /（美）杰弗里·J.沙伊德等主编 ；
林兆奋等主译. -- 上海 ：上海科学技术出版社，2025.
1. --（5分钟速查）. -- ISBN 978-7-5478-5644-4
Ⅰ. R459.7
中国国家版本馆CIP数据核字第2024XA1225号

This is a translation of Rosen & Barkin's 5-Minute Emergency Medicine Consult，6th Edition by Jeffrey J. Schaider，Roger M. Barkin，Stephen R. Hayden，Richard E. Wolfe，Adam Z. Barkin，and Philip Shayne
ISBN：9781496392954

上海市版权局著作权合同登记号　图字：09－2021－0168号

急诊科5分钟速查

主编　Jeffrey J. Schaider
Roger M. Barkin
Stephen R. Hayden
Richard E. Wolfe
Adam Z. Barkin
Philip Shayne
主译　林兆奋　李文放　童朝阳　潘曙明

上海世纪出版(集团)有限公司
上海科学技术出版社　出版、发行
(上海市闵行区号景路159弄A座9F－10F)
邮政编码201101　www.sstp.cn
上海雅昌艺术印刷有限公司印刷
开本 889×1194　1/16　印张 73.75
字数：2100千字
2025年1月第1版　2025年1月第1次印刷
ISBN 978－7－5478－5644－4/R·2470
定价：498.00元

内容提要

Wolters Kluwer 出版公司的 5 分钟速查系列图书是广受欢迎的速查工具书，其编写颇有特色，采用词条式的编写方式，每个词条占用 2 页，阅读约需花 5 分钟，每个词条的内容从基本概念到临床再到延伸阅读，采用精要式的编写方法，词条范围涵盖了该学科几乎所有的内容，包括疾病、症状、治疗等。在词条的编排方面，通过目录与索引，读者既可以通过字典式的词序来查阅，也可以根据"话题"的类别和性质来查阅，方便读者快速建立关于词条的"知识地图"，有助于读者快速掌握问题的概貌，非常适合临床速查使用。

《急诊科 5 分钟速查》由美国权威的急诊科专家编写，由 600 多个词条组成，涵盖了急诊科临床实践中的各种紧急事件、检查流程、院前处理、急诊治疗和程序，每个词条还附有要点和误区，方便急诊科医师在"混乱"的临床环境中快速找到所需信息。本书特点：第一，内容全面、系统，600 多个词条几乎涵盖整个急诊临床领域；第二，由美国各大医院高级专家撰写，反映了目前世界先进水平；第三，独特的编写方式方便查阅与记忆，对提高急诊科医师的医疗水平有重要帮助。

本书是为繁忙的急诊科医师准备的一本大型速查类工具书，同时也可以作为年轻住院医师及医学生的学习用书。

献辞

Peter Rosen 博士是一位传奇人物，许多人将他视为“急诊医学之父”。他是我们的指导者、教师、灵感来源和朋友，也许最重要的是，他作为丈夫、父亲、祖父和叔叔，始终坚守对家庭的责任。在我们与他的每一次相遇中，他总能展现自己的魅力、热情和对生活的热爱。他因此成为一位楷模，这是我们之所以热爱急诊医学专业的根源所在。Peter 教我们如何照顾急诊科最危重的患者。

最初 Peter 在军队服役时接受的是普通外科医师的培训，后来他在怀俄明州执业，随后在芝加哥大学工作，在那里他开始了急诊科住院医师生涯。Peter 在丹佛担任急诊科主任直到 1989 年，在那里他创造了一个激励学习、有着优质临床实践和领导力的环境。得益于 Peter 的远见卓识，丹佛项目成为过去 30 年来许多急诊医学先驱的“家”。随后，Peter 受邀到加利福尼亚大学圣地亚哥分校工作，成为新一代急诊医学学生的导师和榜样。在临床工作之外，Peter 热爱滑雪、打网球、打高尔夫球和航海。

在 Peter 的职业生涯中，他曾担任许多世界领先的急诊医学教科书和期刊的编辑，也曾任职于许多学术协会，包括美国急诊医学委员会在其形成时期的董事会，并因杰出的贡献和领导能力而获得美国急诊医学院和美国急诊医学学会认可。

Peter 在急诊医学领域留下的印记对我们专业的发展及对急诊患者救治的进步起到了重要作用。

我们怀着对 Peter 无比的崇敬、尊重和爱撰写《急诊科 5 分钟速查》(*Rosen & Barkin's 5-Minute Emergency Medicine Consult*)。在最初构思本书时，Peter 为本书定下了基调，我们据此不断地完善它。

感谢 Peter 近 50 年来对同事、学生和患者的奉献。我们所有人都从 Peter 的智慧和洞察力中受益，并将永远感谢 Peter 在我们作为临床医师和教师的成长过程中给予的指导。

致　谢

感谢作者的奉献和读者的投入，它们是这本书的基础。在整个撰写过程中，Ashley Wolters Kluwe 出版社的 Fischer 一直帮助我们。

感谢我的妻子安娜、儿子雅各布和艾萨克，感谢你们不断给予的支持和鼓励。感谢库克县的急诊医师和住院医师，他们在过去的 30 年里照顾了数百万需要帮助的患者，并为我提供了丰富多彩和具有挑战性的环境，让我成长为一名临床医师。我永远感激所有人。

Jeffrey J. Schaider

我非常感激家人给我的支持。Suzanne Barkin 博士一直是临床医师的典范，也是她所培训的住院医师的楷模。Adam、Jill、Jacob、Eli 和 Michael 每日提醒我们作为临床医师的重要性，使我们追求卓越的承诺日益坚定。必须感谢我们的同事，他们不断地让我们获益，希望这本书对他们的实践有帮助。

Roger M. Barkin

致我的妻子 Marina，以及我的孩子 Connor、Maia 和 Kenny，没有他们的支持和理解，我不可能从事急诊医学学术工作，以及完成这本书的编写。致我现在的住院医师和过去的毕业生，我希望这本书中的信息有助于他们的临床决策，并使他们始终保持求知心。

Stephen R. Hayden

感谢我的妻子 Alice，她不懈的支持、耐心和幽默为我的努力提供了支持。感谢哈佛大学医学院 BIDMC 医学中心的教职员工，他们提供了本书努力实现的愿景和高标准。敬 Peter，他是我一生的导师和榜样。

Richard E. Wolfe

致 Jill、Jacob 和 Eli，他们给我们带来了如此多的快乐、支持、欢笑和爱。

Adam Z. Barkin

感谢我的妻子 Helen，感谢她给予我无限的耐心、支持和指导，感谢她给了我创作这本书的自由。也要感谢 Dylan 和 David，他们让我明白什么才是最重要的。

Philip Shayne

译者名单

主　译

林兆奋　李文放　童朝阳　潘曙明

副主译

马林浩　王　虑

译　者

李　岩　王海嵘　宋振举　陆晓晔　彭　沪　庄育刚　徐　兵　许　磊　谭美春
姜　颢　万　健　单　怡　马林浩　朱　妍　吴　昊　王　虑　刘雪峰　陈奇通
何　超　王胜云　段立伟　伍力学　张　晟　常　亮　瞿金龙　郑金浩　何融冰
江伟伟　周秋香　袁晓伟　周　健　冯　伟　朱雨锋　斐　蕾　孙立柱

总校对

李文放　单　怡　马林浩　何　超　王胜云　王　虑

编写者名单

主 编

Jeffrey J. Schaider, MD
Professor, Department of Emergency Medicine
Rush Medical College
Chairman, Department of Emergency Medicine
Cook County Health
Chicago, Illinois

Roger M. Barkin, MD, MPH
Clinical Professor of Emergency Medicine and Pediatrics
University of Colorado School of Medicine
Attending Physician (ret.)
Department of Emergency Medicine
Denver Health Medical Center
Denver, Colorado

Stephen R. Hayden, MD
Professor of Clinical Emergency Medicine
Faculty Mentoring Director
Department of Emergency Medicine
University of California
Editor-in-Chief, Journal of Emergency Medicine Medical Center
San Diego, California

Richard E. Wolfe, MD
Associate Professor
Department of Emergency Medicine
Harvard Medical School
Chief of Emergency Medicine
Beth Israel Deaconess Medical Center
Boston, Massachusetts

Adam Z. Barkin, MD, MPH
Assistant Clinical Professor
Department of Emergency Medicine
University of Colorado School of Medicine
Aurora, Colorado
Chairman and Medical Director
Emergency Services
Sky Ridge Medical Center
Lone Tree, Colorado

Philip Shayne, MD
Professor
Vice Chair for Education
Department of Emergency Medicine
Assistant Dean for Graduate Medical Education
Emory University School of Medicine
Atlanta, Georgia

编写者

Jamie L. Adler, MD
Attending Physician
Department of Emergency Medicine
Beth Israel Deaconess Medical Center
Harvard Medical Faculty Physicians
Boston, Massachusetts

Rami A. Ahmed, DO, MHPE, FACEP
Associate Professor, Emergency Medicine
Northeast Ohio Medical University
Simulation Fellowship Director
Summa Akron City Hospital
Akron, Ohio

Steven E. Aks, DO, FACMT, FACEP
Professor, Emergency Medicine
Rush Medical College
Director, Toxikon Consortium
Division of Toxicology, Emergency Medicine
Cook County Health
Chicago, Illinois

Dunya Nasrallah Alfaraj, MD
Fellow, Emergency Medicine
UC San Diego
California, San Diego
Emergency Medicine Consultant
Department of Emergency Medicine
Imam Abdulrahman Bin Faisal University
Dammam, Saudi Arabia

Walla A. Alfaraj, MD
Resident
Department of Emergency Medicine
Emory University School of Medicine
Atlanta, Georgia

Mohammad M. Alkhawajah, MD
Full-Time Student, Master of Advanced Study
UC San Diego Health Sciences
San Diego, California

Paul J. Allegretti, DO, FACOEP
Professor and Program Director, Emergency Medicine
Midwestern University/Chicago College of Osteopathic
Professor and Program Director, Emergency Medicine
Provident Hospital of Cook County
Chicago, Illinois

Mohannad F. Allehyani, MBBS
Teaching Assistant
Department of Emergency Medicine
Faculty of Medicine
King Abdulaziz University
Jeddah, Saudi Arabia

Bryant K. Allen, MD
Assistant Professor
Assistant Residency Program Director
Emergency Medicine Residency Program
Department of Emergency Medicine
Carolinas Medical Center
Charlotte, North Carolina

Kendra Amico, MD
Assistant Professor, Emergency Medicine
University of Central Florida
Emergency Medicine Attending
Dr. P. Phillips Hospital Orlando Health Emergency Medicine
Orlando, Florida

Dhara P. Amin*，MD
Assistant Professor，Emergency Medicine
Rush Medical College
Assistant Program Director
Department of Emergency Medicine
Cook County Health and Hospital System
Chicago，Illinois

Francisco Javier Andrade Jr.，MD
Resident Physician，Emergency Medicine
Carolinas Medical Center
Charlotte，North Carolina

Nathan Ansbaugh，MD，MPH
Chief Resident，Emergency Medicine
Hennepin County Medical Center
Minneapolis，Minnesota

L. Kristian Arnold，MD，MPH，FACEP，FACOEM
Chief Medical Officer
ArLac Health Services
Assistant Professor（ret.），Emergency Medicine
Boston University School of Medicine
Affiliate Staff，Occupational and Environmental Medicine
Boston Medical Center
Boston，Massachusetts

Stefani Ashby，MD
Pediatric Emergency Medicine Specialist
Wolfson Children's Hospital
Jacksonville，Florida

Hany Y. Atallah，MD，FACEP
Chief，Emergency Medicine
Grady Health System
Associate Professor
Department of Emergency Medicine
Emory University
Atlanta，Georgia

Veronique Au，MD，MMM
Chief of Staff
Department of Emergency Medicine
Novato Community Hospital
Novato，California

Christine A. Babcock，MD，MSc
Associate Professor
Residency Program Director
Section of Emergency Medicine
University of Chicago
Chicago，Illinois

Matthew R. Babineau，MD
Assistant Professor
Geisel School of Medicine
Department of Emergency Medicine
Dartmouth-Hitchcock Medical Center
Lebanon，NH

Anika Backster*，MD，MSCR
Associate Professor，Emergency Medicine
Emory University School of Medicine
Atlanta，Georgia

Myung Bae，DO
Senior Resident，Emergency Medicine
Baystate Medical Center，University of Massachusetts Medical School
Springfield，Massachusetts

Japheth J. Baker，DO
EMS Medical Director
Department of Emergency Medicine
Magnolia Regional Health Center
Corinth，Mississippi

Ilona A. Barash，MD，PhD
Volunteer Clinical Professor
Department of Emergency Medicine
UC San Diego
Primary Care Sports Medicine
UCSD Student Health Services
San Diego，California
Physician
Scripps Torrey Pines Urgent Care
La Jolla，California

Kara E. Barker，DO
Fellow
Department of Emergency Medicine
Baystate Medical Center
Springfield，Massachusetts

Adam Z. Barkin，MD，MPH
Assistant Clinical Professor
Department of Emergency Medicine
University of Colorado School of Medicine
Aurora，Colorado
Chairman and Medical Director
Emergency Services
Sky Ridge Medical Center
Lone Tree，Colorado

Suzanne Z. Barkin，MD
Associate Professor（retired），Radiology
University of Colorado School of Medicine
Aurora，Colorado

David Barlas，MD
Associate Professor
Ronald O. Perelman Department of Emergency Medicine
New York University School of Medicine
New York，New York

Todd Baumbacher，MD，MS
Emergency Physician
Department of Emergency Medicine
Sharp Grossmont Hospital
San Diego，California
Associate Clinical Professor
University of California Riverside School of Medicine
Riverside，California

Jamil D. Bayram*，MD，MPH，EMDM，MEd，PhDc
Associate Professor
Department of Emergency Medicine
Johns Hopkins University
Baltimore，Maryland

Sierra Beck，MD
Senior Lecturer
Department of Medicine
University of Otago
Emergency Medicine Consultant
Dunedin Hospital
Southern District Health Board
Dunedin，New Zealand

Ioan Belovarski，MD，MPH
Resident
Department of Emergency Medicine
UC San Diego
San Diego，California

W. Bryson Bendall，MD
Resident
Department of Emergency Medicine
University of Arizona-University Campus
Tucson，Arizona

Scott Bentz，MD，FAAEM
Medical Director，Emergency
Medical Staff Past-President
Presbyterian/St Luke's Medical Center
Denver，Colorado

Cristiana Benucci*，MD
Clinical Assistant
Anna Meyer Children's Hospital
Florence，Italy
General Pediatrics
Department of Pediatrics
Meyer Children's Hospital
Florence，Italy

Ross P. Berkeley，MD
Professor
Interim Chair and Program Director
Director of Quality and Education
Department of Emergency Medicine
University of Nevada，Las Vegas School of Medicine
University Medical Center of Southern Nevada
Las Vegas，Nevada

Matthew R. Berkman*，MD，FACEP
Clinical Professor，Emergency Medicine
The University of Arizona
Banner University Medical Center
Tucson，Arizona

Tyler J. Berliner，MD
Resident，Emergency Medicine
Denver Health and Hospital Authority
Denver，Colorado

Ajay Bhatt，MD
Assistant Professor
Department of Surgery
John A. Burns School of Medicine
University of Hawaii
Honolulu，Hawaii

Leslie A. Bilello，MD
Associate Program Director
Harvard-Affiliated Emergency Medicine Residency
Clinical Instructor，Emergency Medicine
Beth Israel Deaconess Medical Center
Boston，Massachusetts

Matthew D. Bitner，MD，MEd，FACEP
Chair
Department of Emergency Medicine
Greenville Health System
Associate Professor
University of South Carolina School of Medicine
Columbia，South Carolina
Associate Chief
Medical Staff Affairs
Baptist Easley Hospital
Easley，South Carolina
Clinical Associate Professor
Clemson University School of Health Research
Greenville，South Carolina

Elizabeth Black，MD
Toxicology Fellow，Toxikon Consortium
University of Illinois Chicago
Fellow
Department of Emergency Medicine
John H. Stroger Hospital of Cook Country

* 本书所表达的观点均为作者的意见，不反映陆军部、海军部、国防部、空军部或美国政府的官方政策。

University of Illinois Chicago Hospital
Chicago, Illinois

Paul Blackburn, DO
Clinical Associate Professor
Department of Emergency Medicine
University of Arizona College of Medicine
Associate Professor, Affiliate Faculty
Department of Emergency Medicine
Creighton University School of Medicine
Phoenix, Arizona

Chelsea C. Bonfiglio, MD
Department of Emergency Medicine
Creighton University School of Medicine/Maricopa Medical Center
Phoenix, Arizona

Michael J. Bono*, MD
Vice Chair, Medical Student Clerkship Director
Department of Emergency Medicine
Eastern Virginia Medical School
Norfolk, Virginia

Vincent Bounes, MD, PhD
Professor
Rangueil Medical Faculty
Toulouse University
Chief
Prehospital Medical
University Hospital of Toulouse
Toulouse, France

Karen J. Bowers, MD, MS, Med
Resident
Department of Emergency Medicine
Emory University School of Medicine
Atlanta, Georgia

Steven H. Bowman, MD
Associate Professor
Department of Emergency Medicine
Rush Medical College
Program Director
Department of Emergency Medicine
Cook County Health and Hospital System
Chicago, Illinois

Heather E. Boynton, MD
Chief Resident, Emergency Medicine
UC San Diego
San Diego, California

James P. Brewer, MD
Emergency Physician
CarePoint Healthcare
Associate Medical Director
Rose Medical Center
Denver, Colorado

Nicholle D. Bromley, MD
Attending Physician
Emergency Medicine
Palomar Medical Center
Escondido, California

David F.M. Brown, MD
Trustees Endowed Professor and Chair
Department of Emergency Medicine
Massachusetts General Hospital
Harvard Medical School
Boston, Massachusetts

Joseph R. Brown, MD
Resident Physician
Department of Emergency Medicine
University of California
San Diego, California

Brian J. Browne, MD
Professor and Chairman
Department of Emergency Medicine
University of Maryland School of Medicine
Baltimore, Maryland

Gary Bubly, MD, MHCI, FACEP
Clinical Professor, Emergency Medicine and Medicine
Vice Chair, Clinical Integration and Innovation
Department of Emergency Medicine
The Miriam Hospital/Alpert Medical School of Brown University
Providence, Rhode Island

Michael D. Burg, MD
Associate Clinical Professor, Emergency
UCSF/Fresno
Attending Physician, Emergency
Communism Regional Medical Centre
Fresno, California

Brian R. Bush, MD
Resident Physician, Emergency Medicine
University of Chicago Medical Center
Chicago, Illinois

Sean M. Bryant, MD
Associate Professor, Emergency Medicine
Rush Medical College
Attending Physician, Emergency Medicine
Cook County Health
Chicago, Illinois

Alexa Camarena-Michel, MD
Resident, Emergency Medicine
Denver Health Residency in Emergency Medicine
Denver Health and Hospital Authority
Denver, Colorado

Martine Lory Camille, MD
Resident
Department of Emergency Medicine
Emory University School of Medicine
Atlanta, Georgia

Colleen J. Campbell, MD, RDMS
Professor
Department of Emergency Medicine
UC San Diego
Director, Emergency Ultrasound
UCSD Medical Center
San Diego, California

Jesse B. Cannon, MD
Attending Emergency Physician
Department of Emergency Medicine
Northside Hospital
Atlanta, Georgia

Aubri S. Carman, MD
Chief Resident
Maricopa Emergency Medicine Residency
Creighton University School of Medicine
Phoenix, Arizona

Stephen M. Carroll, DO, MEd
Assistant Professor, Emergency Medicine
Emory University School of Medicine
Atlanta, Georgia

Wallace A. Carter, MD
Associate Professor, Emergency Medicine
Weill Cornell Medicine
Vagelos College of Physicians and Surgeons
Program Director
Emergency Medicine Residency
New York Presbyterian
New York, New York

Brittany L. Catanach, MD
Denver Health Residency in Emergency Medicine
Denver Health Medical Center
Denver, Colorado

Zachary A. Certa, MD
Chief Resident
Thomas Jefferson University Hospital
Philadelphia, Pennsylvania

Austen-Kum Chai, MD
Assistant Professor
Department of Emergency Medicine
Rush Medical College
Attending Physician
Department of Emergency Medicine
Cook County Health and Hospital System
Chicago, Illinois

Theodore C. Chan, MD
Professor and Chair, Emergency Medicine
University of California San Diego
San Diego, California

Shruti Chandra, MD
Assistant Professor
Associate Clerkship Director
Associate Director for Education and Curricula
Department of Emergency Medicine
Thomas Jefferson University
Philadelphia, Pennsylvania

Andrew K. Chang, MD, MS
Vincent P. Verdile, MD, '84 Endowed Chair for Emergency Medicine
Attending Physician
Vice Chair of Research and Academic Affairs
Professor, Emergency Medicine
Albany Medical College
Attending Physician
Department of Emergency Medicine
Albany Medical Center
Albany, New York

Navneet Cheema, MD
Assistant Professor
Assistant Residency Program Director, Emergency Medicine
University of Chicago Medical Center
Chicago, Illinois

Juliana H. Chen, MD
Staff Psychiatrist
Massachusetts General Hospital & Newton-Wellesley Hospital
Part-time Instructor
Department of Psychiatry
Harvard Medical School
Boston, Massachusetts

Douglas W. Chesson, MD
Assistant Professor, Emergency Medicine
Emory University School of Medicine
Atlanta, Georgia

Michele M. Chetham, MD, FAAP
Pediatric Emergency Physician
Carepoint Health
Rocky Mountain Hospital for Children
Denver, Colorado

Gordon S. Chew, MD
Chief, Emergency Department
Kaiser Permanente Vallejo Medical Center
Vallejo, California

Richard Childers, MD
Staff Physician, Emergency Medicine
University of California, San Diego Health
San Diego, California

David T. Chiu, MD, MPH
Instructor, Emergency Medicine
Harvard Medical School
Director, Operations
Beth Israel Deaconess Medical Center
Boston, Massachusetts

Yi-Mei Chng, MD, MPH
Clinical Instructor
Department of Emergency Medicine
Stanford University School of Medicine
Senior Physician
Department of Emergency Medicine
Kaiser Permanente Santa Clara Medical Center
Santa Clara, California

Erika Phindile Chowa*, MD
Assistant Professor
Department of Emergency Medicine
Emory University School of Medicine
Atlanta, Georgia

Ryan Circh, MD, FAWM
Attending Physician, Emergency Medicine
The Medical Center of Aurora
Aurora, Colorado

Galeta C. Clayton, MD
Assistant Professor, Emergency Medicine
Rush Medical College
Attending Physician, Emergency Medicine
Rush University Medical Center
Chicago, Illinois

Michael N. Cocchi, MD
Assistant Professor, Emergency Medicine
Harvard Medical School
Director, Critical Care Quality Department of Health Care Quality
Beth Israel Deaconess Medical Center
Boston, Massachusetts

Christanne H. Coffey, MD, FACEP, FAWM
Assistant Professor, Emergency Medicine
Director, Wilderness Medicine Fellowship
Department of Emergency Medicine
UC San Diego
San Diego, California

Alberto Cohen-Abbo, MD, FAAP
Assistant Professor, Pediatrics
University of Connecticut
Attending Physician, Pediatric Infectious Diseases
CT Children's in Hartford
Attending Physician, General Pediatrics
CT Pediatrics at CHC
Hartford, Connecticut

Connor A. Cohick, MD
Resident
Department of Emergency Medicine
Prisma Health — Upstate
Greenville, South Carolina

Lotiffa Colibao, MD
Resident Physician
Department of Emergency Medicine
Cook County Health
Chicago, Illinois

Kevin P. Collins*, MD, PhD
Assistant Professor
Albany Medical College
Attending Physician
Department of Emergency Medicine
Albany Medical Center
Albany, New York

Andrew Connor*, DO
Department of Emergency Medicine
Greenville Health System
Greenville, South Carolina

Matthew D. Cook, DO
Chief, Division of Medical Toxicology
Department of Emergency Medicine
Lehigh Valley Health Network
Allentown, Pennsylvania

Megan Bevis Core*, MD
Assistant Professor
College of Medicine
University of Central Florida
Emergency Medicine Physician
Department of Emergency Medicine
Orlando Veterans Affairs Medical Center
Orlando, Florida

Matthew Correia, MD
Resident Physician
Department of Emergency Medicine
University of California San Diego
San Diego, California

Brian N. Corwell, MD
Assistant Professor/Attending Physician
Department of Emergency Medicine
Department of Orthopaedics
University of Maryland School of Medicine
Team Physician, University of Maryland
College Park, Maryland

Conor Cosgrave, MB, BCh, BAO
Registrar
Department of Emergency Medicine
Dunedin Public Hospital
Otago, New Zealand

Francis L. Counselman, MD
Chidester Endowed Chair of Emergency Medicine
Professor and Chairman
Department of Emergency Medicine
Eastern Virginia Medical School
Emergency Physicians of Tidewater
Norfolk, Virginia

Linda C. Cowell*, MD
Neurological Consultant
Medical Department
Lincoln Financial Group
Hartford, Connecticut

Dalton Cox*, MD
Clinical Faculty
Department of Emergency Medicine
Carolinas Medical Center at Atrium Health
Charlotte, North Carolina
Assistant Professor, Emergency Medicine
Department of Emergency Medicine
Carolinas Medical Center at Atrium Health
Charlotte, North Carolina

Christopher J. Coyne, MD, MPH
Assistant Professor, Emergency Medicine
UC San Diego Health System
San Diego, California

Kirk L. Cumpston, DO
Associate Professor, Emergency Medicine
Virginia Commonwealth University
Medical Director of the Virginia Poison Center
Division of Clinical Toxicology
Virginia Commonwealth University Medical Center
Richmond, Virginia

Alison Sisitsky Curcio, MD
Clinical Assistant Professor, Emergency Medicine
Newton Wellesley Hospital
Tufts University School of Medicine
Newton, Massachusetts

Liesl A. Curtis*, MD
Assistant Professor
Department of Emergency Medicine
Medstar Georgetown University Hospital
Washington, DC

Christian Dameff, MD, MS
Assistant Professor, Emergency Medicine
UC San Diego
San Diego, California

Mark Darocki, DO
Attending Physician
Department of Emergency Medicine
Ocean Medical Center
Brick, New Jersey

Joanna W. Davidson, MD
Clerkship Site Director
Attending Physician, Emergency Medicine
University of Chicago
NorthShore University Health System
Evanston, Illinois

Natalie L. Davis, MD
Assistant Professor/Attending Physician, Pediatrics
University of Maryland School of Medicine
Baltimore, Maryland

Betty B. Dean, MD
Emergency Medicine
Denver, Colorado

Sandra A. Deane, MD, FACEP
Associate Professor, Emergency Medicine
Department of Emergency Medicine
Eastern Virginia Medical School
Norfolk, Virginia

David Della-Giustina, MD
Professor
Chief, Education Section
Residency Program Director
Department of Emergency Medicine
Yale School of Medicine
New Haven, Connecticut

Karen Della-Giustina, MD
Pediatrician, Children's Emergency Center
Department of Emergency Medicine
Bridgeport Hospital
Bridgeport, Connecticut

Brenna Derksen, MD
Fellow, Undersea and Hyperbaric Medicine
Department of Emergency Medicine
UC San Diego

San Diego, California

Paul H. Desan, MD, PhD
Assistant Professor, Psychiatry
Yale School of Medicine
Director, Psychiatric Consultation Service
Yale New Haven Hospital
New Haven, Connecticut

Ashley L. Deutsch, MD
Director, Quality and Patient Safety
Assistant Professor, Emergency Medicine
Department of Emergency Medicine
Baystate Medical Center
University of Massachusetts Medical School
Springfield, Massachusetts

Eric Deutsch, MD
Clinical Instructor, Emergency Medicine
Eastern Virginia Medical School
Norfolk, Virginia

Sean Devanney, MD
Fellow, Wilderness Medicine
Department of Emergency Medicine
University of Massachusetts Medical School — Baystate Health
Springfield, Massachusetts

Jason Devgun, MD
Clinical Instructor
Attending Physician
University of Illinois Hospital and Health Sciences System
Chicago, Illinois

Kelly K. DiLorenzo, MD
Resident Physician, PGY-3
Department of Emergency Medicine
UC San Diego Health
San Diego, California

Vinodinee L. Dissanayake, MD
Associate Professor, Emergency Medicine
Rush University Medical Center
Chicago, Illinois

Aaran B. Drake, MD
Assistant Professor, Emergency Medicine
George Washington University
Washington, DC

Jeremy N. Driscoll, MD
Resident Physician
Department of Emergency Medicine
Carolinas Medical Center
Charlotte, North Carolina

Jeffrey Druck, MD
Assistant Dean for Student Affairs
Co-Director, Office of Professional Excellence
Associate Professor
Department of Emergency Medicine
University of Colorado School of Medicine
Aurora, Colorado

Susan E. Dufel, MD, FACEP
Associate Professor, Emergency Medicine
University of Connecticut School of Medicine
Farmington, Connecticut

Christopher J. Dudley, MD
Assistant Professor, Emergency Physician
Department of Emergency Medicine
Emory University School of Medicine
Grady Memorial Hospital
Atlanta, Georgia

Luke J. Duncan, MD
Assistant Professor
Albany Medical College
Attending Physician
Department of Emergency Medicine, Department of Surgery, Division of Surgical Critical Care
Albany Medical Center
Albany, New York

Elizabeth R. Dunn, MD, MS
Assistant Professor
Department of Psychiatry
Harvard Medical School
Director, Psychiatric Consultation Liaison Service
Beth Israel Deaconess Medical Center
Boston, Massachusetts

Sean P. Dyer, MD
Clinical Instructor, Emergency Medicine
Rush Medical College
Attending Physician
Department of Emergency Medicine
Cook County Health
Chicago, Illinois

Maxim Dzeba, MD
Toxicology Fellow
Toxicon Consortium
Department of Emergency Medicine
UIC Hospital
Stroger/Cook County Hospital
Chicago, Illinois

Jonathan A. Edlow, MD, FACEP
Professor, Emergency Medicine
Harvard Medical School
Vice Chair, Emergency Medicine
Beth Israel Deaconess Medical Center
Boston, Massachusetts

Thomas W. Engel II*, MD
PGY-4
Department of Emergency Medicine
Cook County Health and Hospital System
Chicago, Illinois

Stephen K. Epstein, MD, MPP
Assistant Professor, Emergency Medicine
Harvard Medical School
Beth Israel Deaconess Medical Center
Boston, Massachusetts

Timothy B. Erickson, MD, FACEP, FACMT
Associate Professor of Emergency Medicine
Chief, Division of Medical Toxicology
Department of Emergency Medicine
Brigham and Women's Hospital
Harvard Medical School
Harvard Humanitarian Initiative
Boston, Massachusetts

Barnet Eskin, MD, PhD
Associate Professor, Emergency Medicine
Sidney Kimmel Medical College of Thomas Jefferson University
Assistant Research Director and Core Faculty
Morristown Medical Center Residency in Emergency Medicine
Morristown, New Jersey

Robyn R. Essendrop*, MD
Resident Physician
Department of Emergency Medicine
Madigan Army Medical Center
Tacoma, Washington

Brian D. Euerle, MD
Associate Professor, Emergency Medicine
University of Maryland School of Medicine
Baltimore, Maryland

Morgan P. Eutermoser, MD, DTMH
Medical Director
Denver Health NurseLine
Denver, Colorado
Attending Physician
Denver Health Emergency Medicine
Denver, Colorado
Assistant Professor
University of Colorado School of Medicine
Aurora, Colorado

Juliet Evans, MD
Attending Physician
Department of Emergency Medicine
Utah Valley Hospital/Intermountain Healthcare
Provo, Utah

Saleh Fares*, MD, MPH, FRCPC, FACEP, FAAEM
Consultant, Emergency Medicine, EMS, and Disaster Medicine
Zayed Military Hospital
Abu Dhabi, United Arab Emirates

Chad B. Farr, DO
Emergency Physician
Sunrise Hospital and Medical Center
Las Vegas, Nevada

Helen M. Farrell*, MD
Lecturer, Harvard Medical School
Department of Psychiatry
Beth Israel Deaconess Medical Center
Boston, Massachusetts

Robert J. Feldman, MD
Assistant Professor, Emergency Medicine
Rush Medical College
Emergency Management Director
Cook County Health
Chicago, Illinois

Ian Glen Ferguson, DO
Clinical Associate Professor
Department of Emergency medicine
Stanford University
Stanford, California
Director of Clinical Informatics
Department of Emergency Medicine
Watsonville Community Hospital
Watsonville, California

Jorge Fernandez, MD
Assistant Clinical Professor
Department of Emergency Medicine
University of California, San Diego Health
San Diego, California

Rosaura Fernández, MD
Associate Program Director of Cook County Emergency Medicine
Department of Emergency Medicine
Cook County Health and Hospital System
Assistant Professor, Emergency Medicine
Rush Medical College
Chicago, Illinois

Christopher M. Fischer, MD
Assistant Professor, Emergency Medicine
Harvard Medical School
Cambridge Health Alliance

Cambridge, Massachusetts

Jonathan Fisher, MD, MPH
Professor, Emergency Medicine
University of Arizona College of Medicine-Phoenix
Maricopa Emergency Medicine Residency
Creighton University School of Medicine
Phoenix, Arizona

Sarah K. Flaherty, MD
Emergency Physician
Department of Emergency Medicine
University of Pittsburgh Medical Center
Pittsburgh, Pennsylvania

Sean N. Fling, MD
Emergency Medicine Resident
Department of Emergency Medicine
Carolinas Medical Center/Atrium Health
Charlotte, North Carolina

Jonathan Florman, MD
Assistant Professor/Associate Director, Psychiatric Consultation Service
Department of Psychiatry
Harvard Medical School
Beth Israel Deaconess Medical Center
Boston, Massachusetts

Elizabeth M. Foley*, MD
Assistant Professor, Emergency Medicine
Hartford Hospital
University of Connecticut School of Medicine
Hartford, Connecticut

Christina O. Foreman, MD, MPH
Attending Physician
Department of Emergency Medicine
Franciscan Health
Michigan City, IN
Riverside Medical Center
Kankakee, IL

Alison Foster-Goldman, MD
Attending, Emergency Medicine
Honor Health Scottsdale
Scottsdale, Arizona

Nicole M. Franks, MD
Associate Professor, Emergency Medicine
Emory University School of Medicine
Chief Quality Officer
Emory University Hospital Midtown
Atlanta, Georgia

Jessica Freedman, MD
Emergency Physician
New York, NY

Andrew J. French, MD
Chief Medical Officer
St. Anthony's North Health Campus
Centura Health
Westminster, Colorado

Sam L. Frenkel, MD
Emergency Medicine Resident
Department of Emergency Medicine
UC San Diego
San Diego, California

Benjamin W. Friedman, MD, MS
Professor, Emergency Medicine
Albert Einstein College of Medicine
Montefiore Medical Center
Bronx, New York

Franklin D. Friedman, MD, MS
Assistant Professor
Director of Prehospital Care and Emergency Preparedness
Medical Director of Geriatric Emergency
Department of Emergency Medicine
Tufts University School of Medicine
Tufts Medical Center
Boston, Massachusetts

Rohn S. Friedman, MD
Associate Professor, Part-Time
Vice-Chairman
Department of Psychiatry
Harvard Medical School
Beth Israel Deaconess Medical Center
Boston, Massachusetts

Christie L. Fritz, MD, MS
Clinical Fellow
Beth Israel Deaconess Medical Center
Boston, Massachusetts

Rodney M. Fullmer, DO, MBS
Assistant Professor and Core EM Faculty, Emergency Medicine
Midwestern University/Chicago College of Osteopathic Medicine
Swedish Covenant Health
Chicago, Illinois

Brad D. Gable, MD, MS, FACEP
System Medical Director
OhioHealth Simulation
Site Director, Emergency Medicine
Riverside Methodist Hospital
Clinical Associate Professor, Emergency Medicine
Ohio University Heritage College of Osteopathic Medicine
Mid-Ohio Emergency Services
Columbus, Ohio

Richard Gabor, MD
Assistant Professor, Emergency Medicine
UMass Medical School
Pediatric Emergency Department — Baystate Health
Springfield, Massachusetts

Sophie W. Galson, MD
Global Health Fellow
Division of Emergency Medicine
Duke University Medical School
Durham, North Carolina

D. Taylor Gammons, MD
Resident Physician, Emergency Medicine
Eastern Virginia Medical School
Norfolk, Virginia

Michael Ganetsky, MD, FACEP, FACMT
Assistant Professor, Emergency Medicine
Harvard Medical School
Core Medical Toxicology Faculty
Harvard Medical Toxicology Fellowship
MA/RI Poison Control Center
Director, Division of Medical Toxicology
Department of Emergency Medicine
Beth Israel Deaconess Medical Center
Boston, Massachusetts

Christopher Gardner, MD
Emergency Medicine Resident
Department of Emergency Medicine
Carolinas Medical Center — Atrium Health
Charlotte, North Carolina

Gregory L. Gaskin, MD
Resident
Department of Emergency Medicine
University of Arizona
Banner University Medical Center — Tucson
Tucson, Arizona

Rajender K. Gattu, MD
Assistant Professor, Pediatrics
Division of Pediatric Emergency Medicine
University of Maryland School of Medicine
Baltimore, Maryland

Sean P. Geary, MD
Assistant Professor/Attending Physician
Department of Emergency Medicine and Department of Surgery Division of Surgical Critical Care
Albany Medical College
Albany, New York

Naomi George, MD, MPH
Assistant Professor, Emergency Medicine
Department of Critical Care, Emergency Medicine
University of New Mexico
Albuquerque, New Mexico

Delaram Ghadishah, MD
Physician, Emergency Medicine
Kaiser Permanente
Los Angeles, California

Tyler Giberson, MD
Resident Physician
Department of Emergency Medicine
Emory University Hospital/Grady Healthcare System
Atlanta, Georgia

Daniel B. Gingold, MD, MPH
Assistant Professor
Department of Emergency Medicine
University of Maryland School of Medicine
Baltimore, Maryland

Laura B. Glicksman, MS, DMD
Clinical Orthodontist, Private Practice
Glicksman Orthodontics
Needham, Massachusetts

Steven P. Gohsler, MD, FACEP
Clinical Assistant Professor, Emergency Medicine
Sidney Kimmel Medical College, Thomas Jefferson University
Philadelphia, Pennsylvania
Attending Physician
Assistant Program Director
Emergency Medicine
Morristown Medical Center
Morristown, New Jersey

Katja Goldflam, MD
Assistant Professor, Emergency Medicine
Associate Residency Program Director
Department of Emergency Medicine
Yale School of Medicine
New Haven, Connecticut

Stacy M. Gomez, MD
Attending
Department of Emergency Medicine
Pioneers Memorial Hospital
Brawley, California

Dolores Gonthier, MD
Consultant
Wexford, Pennsylvania

Matthew N. Graber, MD, PhD
Assistant Professor, Emergency Medicine
Midwestern University
Emergency Medicine Residency Program Director
Department of Emergency Medicine
Abrazo Health Network
Phoenix, Arizona

Charles S. Graffeo, MD, ABEM-UHM
Professor and Assistant Residency Director
Department of Emergency Medicine
Eastern Virginia Medical School
Norfolk, Virginia

Jeremy Graham, DO
Department of Emergency Medicine
Magnolia Regional Health Center
Corinth, Mississippi

Annette M. Grajny, MD, MS-HPeD
Assistant Professor
Department of Emergency Medicine
Albany Medical College
Albany, New York

Ashley L. Greiner, MD, MPH
Physician, Emergency Medicine
Atlanta Veterans Affairs Medical Center
Decatur, Georgia

Shamai A. Grossman, MD, MS
Associate Professor, Medicine and Emergency Medicine
Harvard Medical School
Vice Chair for Health Care Quality
Beth Israel Deaconess Medical Center
Department of Emergency Medicine
Boston, Massachusetts

Heather L. Groth, MD
Attending Physician
Department of Emergency Medicine
CarePoint Healthcare Presbyterian
St. Luke's and Sky Ridge Medical Center
Denver, Colorado

Casey A. Grover, MD
Chair
Division of Emergency Medicine
Community Hospital of the Monterey Peninsula
Monterey, California

Ian R. Grover, MD
Clinical Professor, Emergency Medicine
UCSD Medical Center
UC San Diego
San Diego, California

John A. Guisto, MD
Professor, Emergency Medicine
University of Arizona College of Medicine
Attending Physician, Emergency
Banner University Medical Center
Tucson, Arizona

Kama Z. Guluma*, MD
Professor, Emergency Medicine
UC San Diego School of Medicine
La Jolla, California
Attending Physician/Faculty Physician
Department of Emergency Medicine
UC San Diego Health System
San Diego, California

Atul Gupta, DO, FACEP
Attending Physician
Department of Emergency Medicine
Southern California Permanente Medical Group
Los Angeles, California

Kiersten L. Gurley, MD
Clinical Instructor
Harvard Medical School
Attending Physician
Assistant QI Director
Department of Emergency Medicine
Beth Israel Deaconess Medical Center
Boston, Massachusetts

Matthew M. Hall*, MD
Instructor
Department of Emergency Medicine
Harvard Medical School
Beth Israel Deaconess Medical Center
Boston, Massachusetts

Marilyn M. Hallock, MD, MS, FACEP
Assistant Professor, Emergency Medicine
Rush University Medical Center
Chicago, Illinois

Sarah M. Halstead, MD
Instructor
Department of Pediatric Emergency Medicine
Children's Hospital Colorado
Aurora, Colorado

Allan V. Hansen, MD
Medical Director, Emergency Department
Palomar Escondido and Poway
Palomar Health
Escondido, California

Susanne M. Hardy, MSHS, DO
Assistant Professor
Department of Emergency Medicine
Emory University/Emory Healthcare
Atlanta, Georgia

Benjamin S. Heavrin*, MD
Attending Physician
Emergency Department
Nashville General Hospital
Nashville, Tennessee

Tarlan Hedayati, MD, FACEP
Assistant Professor
Rush Medical College
Associate Program Director
Cook County Health
Chicago, Illinois

Brian Z. Hedges, MD
Resident Physician, Emergency Medicine
Carolinas Medical Center
Charlotte, North Carolina

Robin R. Hemphill, MD, MPH
Chief Quality and Safety Officer
Virginia Commonwealth University Health System
Associate Dean for Quality and Safety
Gene Peterson Professor of Quality, Safety, and Service
Clinical Professor, Emergency Medicine

Gregory W. Hendey, MD
Professor and Chair, Emergency Medicine
David Geffen School of Medicine at UCLA
Ronald Reagan UCLA Medical Center
Los Angeles, California

Sarah E. Herold, MD
Instructor, Psychiatry
Harvard Medical School
Staff Psychiatrist
Beth Israel Deaconess Medical Center
Boston, Massachusetts

Aaron Hexdall, MD
Associate Professor, Emergency Medicine
Global Health Fellowship Director
Department of Emergency Medicine
University of Massachusetts School of Medicine
Baystate Medical Center
Springfield, Massachusetts

Braden Hexom, MD
Associate Professor
Department of Emergency Medicine
Rush Medical College
Residency Program Director
Department of Emergency Medicine
Rush University Medical Center
Chicago, Illinois

Colleen N. Hickey, MD
Assistant Professor, Emergency Medicine
Northwestern University, Feinberg School of Medicine
Chicago, Illinois

Katherine Hiller, MD, MPH
Professor, Emergency Medicine
University of Arizona
Tucson, Arizona

J. Patrick Hoffman, MD
Simulation Faculty
Cook County Health and Hospital System
Chicago, Illinois
Department of Emergency Medicine
NorthShore University HealthSystem
Evanston, Illinois

Amanda Lamond Holden, MD
Board-Certified Emergency Physician
Palomar Health — Vituity Partnership
San Diego, California

Michael J. Holman*, MD
Emergency Physician
Department of Emergency Medicine
Sharp Chula Vista Medical Center
San Diego, California

Jeffrey A. Horenstein, MD, PhD
Clinician
Department of Emergency Medicine
Beth Israel Deaconess Medical Center
Boston, Massachusetts

Carl K. Hsu*, MD, FACEP
Attending Physician
Department of Emergency Medicine
Contra Costa Regional Medical Center
Martinez, California

Kate E. Hughes, DO
Clinical Assistant Professor, Emergency Medicine
University of Arizona
Faculty Physician, Emergency Medicine
Banner — University Medical Center Tucson
Tucson, Arizona

Patrick G. Hughes, DO, MEHP
Assistant Professor, Emergency Medicine
Integrated Medical Sciences

Charles E. Schmidt College of Medicine/Florida Atlantic University
Boca Raton, Florida

Nicholas B. Hurst, MD, MS, FAAEM
Assistant Professor, Emergency Medicine
Associate Program Director, University Campus Residency
Department of Emergency Medicine
Medical Toxicology Consultant
Arizona Poison and Drug Information Center
University of Arizona
Tucson, Arizona

Waleed Mohammed Hussein, MBBS
Emergency Medicine Physician
King Faisal Medical City for Southern Regions
Abha, Saudi Arabia
Emergency Ultrasound Fellow
Division of Emergency Ultrasound
Department of Emergency Medicine
LAC+USC Medical Center
Keck School of Medicine
Los Angeles, California

Lauren C. Hyde, MD
Chief Resident
Harvard-Affiliated Emergency Medicine Residency
Beth Israel Deaconess Medical Center
Boston, Massachusetts

Eric C. Hyder, MD
Senior Resident
Department of Emergency Medicine
Harvard-Affiliated Emergency Medicine
Beth Israel Deaconess Medical Center
Boston, Massachusetts

Annette M. Ilg, MD
Chief Resident
Department of Emergency Medicine
Harvard-Affiliated Emergency Medicine Residency
Beth Israel Deaconess Medical Center
Boston, Massachusetts

Jason C. Imperato, MD, MBA
Assistant Professor
Department of Emergency Medicine
Harvard Medical School
Associate Chair
Department of Emergency Medicine
Mount Auburn Hospital
Cambridge, Massachusetts

Paul Ishimine, MD
Clinical Professor, Emergency Medicine and Pediatrics
University of California, San Diego School of Medicine
La Jolla, California

Kenneth C. Jackimczyk, MD
Professor, Emergency Medicine
University of Arizona COM, Phoenix Campus
Associate Chair
Department of Emergency Medicine
Maricopa Medical Center
Phoenix, Arizona

Lisa A. Jacobson, MD
Assistant Professor, Surgery
John A. Burns School of Medicine
Honolulu, Hawaii
Medical Director, Emergency Department
Advents Health Castle Medical Centre
Kailua, Hawaii

Liudvikas Jagminas, MD, FACEP
Department of Emergency Medicine
Associated Physicians of Harvard Medical Faculty
Physician at Beth Israel Deaconess Medical Center

Gregory D. Jay, MD, PhD
Professor
Department of Emergency Medicine
Alpert School of Medical School of Brown University
Vice Chair for Research
Department of Emergency Medicine
Rhode Island Hospital
Providence, Rhode Island

Dorka M. Jiménez Almonte, MD
Pediatric Emergency Fellow
Department of Emergency Medicine
University of Massachusetts Medical School
Baystate Medical Center
Springfield, Massachusetts

Albert S. Jin, MD
Partner Physician
Department of Emergency Medicine
Kaiser Orange County
Orange County, California

Katharine Y. Joo*, MD
Staff Psychiatrist
California Medical Facility
California Department of Corrections and Rehabilitation
Vacaville, California

Joshua W. Joseph, MD, MS
Assistant Professor
Harvard Medical School
Attending Physician
Director of Operations Research
Department of Emergency Medicine
Beth Israel Deaconess Medical Center
Boston, Massachusetts

Madeline M. Joseph, MD, FAAP, FACEP
Associate Dean, Inclusion and Equity-College of Medicine Jacksonville
Professor, Emergency Medicine and Pediatrics
Assistant Chair, Pediatric Emergency Medicine Quality Improvement
Department of Emergency Medicine
University of Florida College of Medicine — Jacksonville
Jacksonville, Florida

Joseph H. Kahn, MD
Associate Professor, Emergency Medicine
Boston University School of Medicine
MD Advisor
Boston Medicine Centre
Boston, Massachusetts

Mohamad Kanso, MD, MSc
Resident
Department of Emergency Medicine
American University of Beirut Medical Center
Beirut, Lebanon

Bonnie Kaplan, MD, MA
Assistant Professor, Emergency Medicine
University of Colorado Hospital
Denver Health Medical Center
Denver, Colorado

Adam S. Kaye, MD
Resident, Emergency Medicine
Harvard Medical School
Beth Israel Deaconess Medical Center Academic Institution
Boston, Massachusetts

Amin Antoine Kazzi, MD, FAAEM, MAAEM
Professor, Clinical Emergency Medicine
Department of Emergency Medicine
American University of Beirut
Beirut, Lebanon

Matthew T. Keadey*, MD
Assistant Professor
Chief, Emergency Medicine
Department of Emergency Medicine
Emory University Hospital
Atlanta, Georgia

Samuel M. Keim, MD, MS
Professor and Chair
Department of Emergency Medicine
University of Arizona College of Medicine, Tucson
Tucson, Arizona

Adam Kellogg, MD
Associate Professor, Emergency Medicine
University of Massachusetts Medical School — Baystate Health
Springfield, Massachusetts

Maura Kennedy, MD, MPH
Assistant Professor, Emergency Medicine
Harvard Medical School
Division Chief, Geriatric Emergency Medicine
Massachusetts General Hospital
Boston, Massachusetts

Kathleen A. Kerrigan, MD
Assistant Professor
Department of Emergency Medicine
University of Massachusetts Medical School, Baystate
Director of Simulation
Department of Emergency Medicine
Baystate Medical Center
Springfield, Massachusetts

James Killeen, MD
Clinical Professor, Emergency Medicine
Departments of Emergency Medicine, Biomedical Informatics
UC San Diego Health System/UC San Diego School of Medicine
San Diego, California

Daewon Kim, MD
Chief Resident, Emergency Medicine
University of Arizona College of Medicine
Tucson, Arizona

Theresa Kim, MD
Emergency Physician
Department of Emergency Medicine
NorthShore University HealthSystem
Evanston, Illinois

Reneé A. King, MD, MPH
Department of Emergency Medicine
Emergency Medicine Director
Miners Colfax Medical Center
Raton, NM

Richard S. Klasco, MD, FACEP
Assistant Professor, Emergency Medicine
University of Colorado School of Medicine
Aurora, Colorado

Martin D. Klinkhammer, MD, MPH
Assistant Professor
Department of Emergency Medicine
Eastern Virginia Medical School
Staff Physician
Department of Emergency Medicine
Sentara Norfolk General Hospital
Norfolk, Virginia

Barry J. Knapp, MD
Professor
Department of Emergency Medicine
Eastern Virginia Medical School
Norfolk, Virginia
Distinguished Professor, Emergency Medicine
Department of Emergency Medicine
Eastern Virginia Medical School
Norfolk, Virginia

Thomas L. Knorr, MD
Attending Physician
Department of Emergency Medicine
Beth Israel Deaconess Medical Center
Boston, Massachusetts

Paul Kolecki*, MD, FACEP
Associate Professor
Department of Emergency Medicine
Sidney Kimmel Medical College
Thomas Jefferson University Hospital
Philadelphia, Pennsylvania

Amy V. Kontrick, MD
Assistant Professor, Emergency Medicine
Northwestern University, Feinberg School of Medicine
Chicago, Illinois

Jason A. Kopec, MD
Resident Physician
Section of Emergency Medicine
University of Chicago
Chicago, Illinois

Matthew C. Kostura, MD, FAAEM
Associate Staff
Cleveland Clinic Emergency Services Institute
Clinical Assistant Professor
Cleveland Clinic Lerner College of Medicine
Cleveland, Ohio

Richard S. Krause, MD
Assistant Professor, Emergency Medicine
Department of Emergency Medicine
Jacobs School of Medicine and Biomedical Sciences
Buffalo, New York

Joel Kravitz, MDCM, FACEP
Physician, Emergency Medicine
Capital Health System
Trenton, New Jersey

Johanna E. Kreafle, MD
Resident Physician
Department of Emergency Medicine
Carolinas Medical Center
Charlotte, North Carolina

Ryan M. Kring*, MD
Chief Resident
Harvard-Affiliated Emergency Medicine Residency
Beth Israel Deaconess Medical Center
Boston, Massachusetts

Allyson A. Kreshak, MD, FACEP, FACMT
Associate Clinical Professor
Associate Medical Director
Department of Emergency Medicine
UC San Diego Health
San Diego, California

Lara K. Kulchycki, MD, MPH
Department of Emergency Medicine
Marin General Hospital
Greenbrae, California

Alan M. Kumar, MD, FACHE
System Chief Medical Officer
Community Healthcare System
Munster, Indiana

Craig J. Kutz, MD, PhD
Resident Physician, Emergency Medicine
University of California
San Diego, California

Rashid F. Kysia, MD, MPH
Attending Physician
Department of Emergency Medicine
Cook County Health
Assistant Professor
Rush Medical School
Chicago, Illinois

Andrew T. LaFree, MD
Clinical Faculty
Department of Emergency Medicine
UC San Diego
San Diego, California

Michelle D. Lall, MD, MHS, FACEP
Assistant Professor
Associate Residency Director
Department of Emergency Medicine
Emory University School of Medicine
Atlanta, Georgia

Patrick M. Lank, MD, MS, FACEP
Assistant Professor
Attending Physician
Department of Emergency Medicine
Northwestern University, Feinberg School of Medicine
Chicago, Illinois

Erica Lash, MD
Resident Physician, Emergency Medicine
The Warren Alpert Medical School/Brown University/Rhode Island Hospital
Providence, Rhode Island

Daniel R. Lasoff, MD
Associate Clinical Professor
Associate Physician
Department of Emergency Medicine
University of California, San Diego Medical Center
San Diego, California

Robert Kregg Laundon
Resident Physician, PGY-2
Department of Emergency Medicine
Carolinas Medical Center at Atrium Health
Charlotte, North Carolina

Minh V. Le, MD
Clinical Instructor
Department of Family Medicine
University of California San Diego
Physician
Department of Emergency Medicine
Mission Hospital Regional Medical Center
Mission Viejo, California

Paul A. Leccese, MD
Resident Physician
Denver Health Residency in Emergency Medicine
Denver, Colorado

Moon O. Lee, MD, MPH
Assistant Professor
Department of Emergency Medicine
Stanford University School of Medicine
Stanford, California

Terrence T. Lee, MD, MPH
Clinical Instructor
Department of Emergency Medicine
Harvard Medical School
Attending Physician
Department of Emergency Medicine
Beth Israel Deaconess Medical Center
Boston, Massachusetts

Donald J. Lefkowits, MD
Medical Director, Emeritus, Emergency Department
Rose Medical Center
Denver, Colorado

Eric Legome, MD, FACEP
Site Chair
Department of Emergency Medicine
Mount Sinai West & Mount Sinai St. Luke's Hospitals
Department of Emergency Medicine
Icahn Mount Sinai School of Medicine
New York, New York

Daniel F. Leiva, DO, MS
Senior Resident, Emergency Medicine
Baystate Medical Center, University of Massachusetts Medical School
Springfield, Massachusetts

Steven Lelyveld, MD
Associate Professor
Section of Emergency Medicine, Department of Medicine
Pritzker School of Medicine
University of Chicago
Chicago, Illinois

William J. Lewander, MD
Professor
Departments of Emergency Medicine and Pediatrics
Warren Alpert Medical School
Brown University
Vice Chair, Pediatric Emergency Medicine
Hasbro Children's Hospital
Providence, Rhode Island

Trevor Lewis, MD
Associate Professor
Department of Emergency Medicine
Rush Medical College
Medical Director, Emergency Department
Cook County Health and Hospital System
Chicago, Illinois

Lazaro Lezcano, MD
Assistant Professor
Department of Pediatrics
Albert Einstein College of Medicine
Director
Division of Neonatology
SBH Health System
Bronx, New York

Richard Lichenstein, MD
Professor
Department of Pediatrics

University of Maryland School of Medicine
Director, Pediatric Emergency Medicine Research
University of Maryland Children's Hospital
Baltimore, Maryland

Ashley M. Licursi, PAC, MMS, MS
Instructor, Emergency Medicine
University of Colorado Hospital/University of Colorado
Aurora, Colorado

Christopher S. Lim, MD
Associate Physician
Department of Emergency Medicine
Kaiser Permanente San Jose Medical Center
San Jose, California

Alexander T. Limkakeng, Jr., MD, MHSc, FACEP
Associate Professor and Vice Chief of Research
Department of Emergency Medicine
Duke University/Duke University Medical Center
Durham, North Carolina

Margaret J. Lin, MD
Assistant Clinical Professor, Emergency Medicine and Pediatrics
Attending Physician, Emergency Medicine
UCSF Benioff Children's Hospital, Mission Bay
Zuckerberg San Francisco General Hospital and Trauma Center
San Francisco, California

Jamie L. Linker, MD, MBE
Attending Physician, Emergency Department
Sky Ridge Medical Center
Lone Tree, Colorado

Benjamin I. Liotta, MD
Resident Physician, Emergency Medicine
UC San Diego
San Diego, California

Rodolfo Loureiro, MD
Resident Physician, Emergency Medicine
Beth Israel Deaconess Medical Center/Harvard Medical School
Boston, Massachusetts

Frank LoVecchio, DO, MPH, FACEP, ABMT
Professor, Emergency Medicine, Pharmacology and Medicine
University of Arizona College of Medicine
Maricopa and Banner Medical Centers
Phoenix, Arizona

Lisa G. Lowe Hiller, MD, MPH, FACEP
Emergency Physician and Clinical Instructor
Departments of Emergency Medicine, Emergency Ultrasound
UCSD Health Systems
Sharp Memorial Hospital
San Diego, California

Joshua W. Loyd, MD, NRP
Medical Director, Med Flight
Medical Director, Critical Care Transport
Novant Health
Charlotte, North Carolina

Jenny J. Lu, MD, MS
Assistant Professor
Department of Emergency Medicine, Division of Medical Toxicology
Rush Medical College
Cook County Health and Hospital System
Chicago, Illinois

Daniella C. Lucas, MD
Emergency Medicine Resident
Department of Emergency Medicine
Cook County Health and Hospital System
Chicago, Illinois

Nicole L. Lunceford, DO
Physician, Emergency Medicine
Scripps Mercy Chula Vista
Chula Vista, California

Binh T. Ly, MD, FACMT
Professor, Emergency Medicine
Vice Chair, Division of Medical Toxicology
Department of Emergency Medicine
UC San Diego Health System
San Diego, California

Timothy K. Lynch, MD
Resident
Department of Emergency Medicine
Beth Israel Deaconess Medical Center
Harvard-Affiliated Emergency Medicine Residency
Boston, Massachusetts

Gene Ma, MD
Assistant Clinical Professor, Medicine; Voluntary
Department of Emergency Medicine
UC San Diego
San Diego, California

Tracy MacIntosh, MD, MPH
Assistant Professor, Emergency medicine
University of Central Florida
Orlando, Florida
Attending Physician, Emergency medicine
Osceola Regional Medical Centre
Kissimmee, Florida

Rene Mack, MD, RDMS, FACEP
Assistant Professor, Emergency Medicine
University of Central Florida College of Medicine
Lake Nona, Florida

Fraser C. Mackay, MD
Assistant Professor, Medicine
Divisions of Emergency Medicine, Pulmonary and Critical Care Medicine
Beth Israel Lahey Health System
Tufts School of Medicine
Burlington, Massachusetts

Laura J. Macnow[*], MD
Assistant Professor
Department of Emergency Medicine
Harvard Medical School
Attending Physician
Department of Emergency Medicine
Beth Israel Deaconess Medical Center
Boston, Massachusetts

Bo E. Madsen[*], MD, MPH
Assistant Professor, Emergency Medicine
Mayo Clinic College of Medicine and Science
Rochester, Minnesota

Christian D. Magallanes, MD
Senior Resident
Department of Emergency Medicine
Denver Health Medical Center
Denver, Colorado

John Mahoney, MD
Professor
Department of Emergency Medicine
University of Pittsburgh School of Medicine
Pittsburgh, Pennsylvania
Associate Dean for Medical Education
University of Pittsburgh School of Medicine
Pittsburgh, Pennsylvania

Nathaniel Mann, MD
Assistant
Department of Emergency Medicine
Massachusetts General Hospital
Clinical Fellow
Harvard Medical School
Boston, Massachusetts

Francesco Mannelli, MD
Chief (ret.)
Pediatric Emergency Department
Anna Meyer Children's Hospital
Florence, Italy

William Manning, MD
Department of Emergency Medicine
Greenville Health System
Greenville, South Carolina

Alexandra Mannix, MD
Assistant Professor
Department of Emergency Medicine
University of Florida College of Medicine-Jacksonville
Jacksonville, Florida

Armando Marquez, Jr., MD, FACEP, FAAEM
Assistant Clinical Professor (ret.), Emergency Medicine
The University of Illinois at Chicago, College of Medicine
Attending Physician
Swedish American Medical Center @ Belvidere
Chicago, Illinois

Taraneh Matin, DO, MA
Intern Resident, Medicine
Larkin Community Hospital
Miami, Florida

C. Hunter Matthews, MD
Resident Physician
Department of Emergency Medicine
Prisma Health Upstate
Greenville, South Carolina

Benjamin B. Mattingly, MD, FAWM
Assistant Professor
Department of Emergency Medicine
University of Massachusetts Medical School
Director, Wilderness Medicine Fellowship
Baystate Medical Center
Springfield, Massachusetts

Suzan S. Mazor, MD
Associate Professor, Pediatric Emergency Medicine, Toxicology, Pediatrics
Seattle Children's Hospital/University of Washington School of Medicine
Seattle, Washington

Christopher J. McCabe, MD, MPH
Chief Resident
Maricopa Emergency Medicine Residency
Creighton University School of Medicine
Phoenix, Arizona

Robert F. McCormack, MD
Professor and Chair
Department of Emergency Medicine
Jacobs School of Medicine and Biomedical Sciences

University at Buffalo
Buffalo General Hospital
Buffalo, New York

Taylor McCormick, MD, MS
Assistant Professor
Department of Emergency Medicine
Denver Health Medicine Center
University of Colorado School of Medicine
Denver, Colorado

Samantha E.M. McGlone, MD
Resident
Department of Emergency Medicine
UC San Diego
San Diego, California

Kevin J. McGurk, MD
Resident Physician
Department of Emergency Medicine
Cook County Health and Hospital System
Chicago, Illinois

Michele R. McKee, MD, MS
Associate Professor
Department of Pediatrics
Section of Emergency Medicine
Medical Director, Pediatric Emergency Medicine
UCMC Medical Director for Emergency Preparedness
Comer Director for Emergency Services and Disaster Preparedness
University of Chicago
Comer Children's Hospital
Chicago, Illinois

Garth D. Meckler*, MD, MSHS
Associate Professor
Departments of Pediatrics and Emergency Medicine
University of British Columbia
Division Head
Pediatric Emergency Medicine
BC Children's Hospital
Vancouver, British Columbia

Anthony J. Medak, MD, FACEP
Clinical Professor, Emergency Medicine
UC San Diego Health System
San Diego, California

Sar Medoff, MD, MPP
Attending Physician
Department of Emergency Medicine
Emory Decatur Hospital
Decatur, Georgia

Timothy J. Meehan*, MD, MPH, FACEP
Associate Clinical Professor
Department of Emergency Medicine
Division of Medical Toxicology
University of Illinois at Chicago College of Medicine
Chicago, Illinois

Patrick G. Meloy, MD, FACEP
Assistant Professor
Department of Emergency Medicine
Emory University School of Medicine
Residency Site Director
Emory University Hospital Midtown
Atlanta, Georgia

Sarah H. Michael, DO, MS
Assistant Professor, Emergency Medicine
University of Colorado School of Medicine
Aurora, Colorado

Alexander D. Miller*, MD, MBA
Assistant Professor, Military/Emergency Medicine
Vice Chairman, Emergency Medicine
Naval Medical Center
San Diego/Uniformed Services University of Health Sciences
San Diego, California

Scott A. Miller, MD
Attending Physician
Department of Emergency Medicine
San Antonio Regional Hospital
Upland, California

Emily M. Mills, MD
Assistant Program Director
Department of Emergency Medicine
University of Michigan/St. Joseph Mercy Hospital
Ann Arbor, Michigan

Christy Rosa Mohler, MD
Attending Physician
Department of Emergency Medicine
Scripps Mercy Hospital Chula Vista
San Diego, California

Aaron J. Monseau, MD
Associate Professor, Emergency Medicine
Department of Emergency Medicine
West Virginia University
Morgantown, West Virginia

Nicolas M. Monte, MD
Resident Physician
Department of Emergency Medicine
University of Massachusetts Medical School — Baystate
Baystate Medical Center
Springfield, Massachusetts

Brooks L. Moore, MD
Assistant Professor
Department of Emergency Medicine
Emory University School of Medicine
Associate Medical Director
Department of Emergency Medicine
Grady Memorial Hospital
Atlanta, Georgia

Kristen G. Moore, MD, Med
Assistant Professor
Department of Emergency Medicine
Emory University
Creator and National Director
Foundations of Emergency Medicine

Maria E. Moreira, MD
Medical Director of Continuing Education and Simulation
Denver Health and Hospital Authority
Denver, Colorado
Associate Professor, Emergency Medicine
University of Colorado School of Medicine
Aurora, Colorado

Daniel F. Morris, MD
Senior Emergency Physician
Department of Emergency Medicine
Kaiser Permanente Napa/Solano
Vacaville, California

Kirsten L. Morrissey*, MD
Assistant Professor, Pediatric Emergency Medicine
Department of Emergency Medicine
Albany Medical College/Albany Medical Center
Albany, New York

Jarrod M. Mosier, MD
Associate Professor, Emergency Medicine and Medicine
Department of Emergency Medicine
Department of Medicine, Division of Pulmonary, Allergy, Critical Care, and Sleep
University of Arizona College of Medicine
Banner University Medical Center
Tucson, Arizona

Jordan Moskoff, MD
Assistant Professor
Department of Emergency Medicine
Rush Medical College
Associate Medical Director AES
Department of Emergency Medicine
Cook County Health
Chicago, Illinois

Maia Alexandra Mosse*
Medical Student
Stanford University
Stanford, California

Ivette Motola, MD, MPH
Associate Director, Gordon Center for Simulation and Innovation in Medical Education
Associate Professor, Emergency Medicine
University of Miami Miller School of Medicine
Attending Physician and Residency Core Faculty
Department of Emergency Medicine
Jackson Memorial Hospital
Miami, Florida

Linda Mueller, MD
Attending Physician, Emergency Medicine
Director of Quality for ED
Edward-Elmhurst Hospital
Naperville, Illinois

David W. Munter, MD, MBA
President, The DESA Consulting Group
Chesapeake, Virginia

Michael S. Murphy MD
Assistant Professor, Emergency Medicine
Tufts University School of Medicine
Emergency Medicine Physician
Tufts Medical Center
Boston, Massachusetts

Mark B. Mycyk, MD
Associate Professor
Department of Emergency Medicine
Northwestern University, Feinberg School of Medicine
Attending Physician
Department of Emergency Medicine
Cook County Health
Chicago, Illinois

Isam F. Nasr, MD
Assistant Professor
Department of Emergency Medicine
Rush Medical College
Attending Physician
Cook County Health and Hospital System
Chicago, Illinois

Erin Nasrallah, MD
Physician, Emergency Medicine
Lutheran General Hospital
Park Ridge, Illinois

Sean-Xavier Neath, MD, PhD
Associate Professor, Clinical Emergency Medicine

UC San Diego
San Diego, California

James A. Nelson, MD
Assistant Clinical Professor
Department of Emergency Medicine
University of California
San Diego, California
Attending Physician
Department of Emergency Medicine
Pioneers Memorial Hospital
Brawley, California

Michael E. Nelson, MD, MS
Associate Clinical Professor
Department of Emergency Medicine
University of Chicago
Chicago, Illinois
Attending Physician, Emergency Medicine, Medical Toxicology, Addiction Medicine
NorthShore University Health System
Evanston, Illinois
Assistant Clinical Professor
Department of Emergency Medicine
Rush University
Attending Physician, Emergency Medicine, Medical Toxicology
Cook County Health
Chicago, Illinois

Rahul V. Nene, MD, PhD
Resident Department of Emergency Medicine
UC San Diego School of Medicine
San Diego, California

Natalie R. Neumann, MD
Resident Physician
Section of Emergency Medicine
University of Chicago
Chicago, Illinois

Edward Newton, MD, FACEP
Professor, Emergency Medicine
Keck School of Medicine
LAC+USC Medical Center
Los Angeles, California

Thien H. Nguyen, MD
Resident Physician
Department of Emergency Medicine
University of California
San Diego, California

Kahra Nix*, MD
Associate Professor
Department of Emergency Medicine
Emory University School of Medicine
Atlanta, Georgia

Matthew Michael Nolan, MD
Emergency Medicine Resident
Department of Emergency Medicine
UC San Diego
San Diego, California

Jessica M. Noonan, MD, FACEP
Assistant Professor
Assistant Residency Program Director
Department of Emergency Medicine
Albany Medical Center
Albany, New York

Sean Patrick Nordt, MD, PharmD, DABAT, FAACT, FAAEM, FACMT
Associate Dean, Academic Affairs
Chief Medical Officer
Gavin Herbert Endowed Professor of Pharmacy
Chapman University School of Pharmacy
Crean College of Health and Behavioral Sciences
Chapman University
Irvine, California
Adjunct Associate Professor, Emergency Medicine
University of California
Orange, California

Charles W. O'Connell, MD
Clinical Instructor
Department of Emergency Medicine
Division of Medical Toxicology
UC San Diego
San Diego, California

Neal P. O'Connor, MD, FACEP
Chief Medical Officer
CarePoint Healthcare
Greenwood Village, Colorado

Yasuharu Okuda, MD
Professor, Emergency Medicine
University of South Florida Health
Executive Director
Center for Advanced Medical Learning and Simulation
University of South Florida Health
Tampa, Florida

Jonathan S. Olshaker*, MD
Professor and Chairman
Department of Emergency Medicine
Boston University School of Medicine
Chief, Department of Emergency Medicine
Boston Medical Center
Boston, Massachusetts

Benjamin W. Osborne, MD
Associate Professor
Department of Emergency Medicine
UMMS-Baystate
Springfield, Massachusetts

Jessica L. Osterman, MS, MD
Assistant Professor, Clinical Emergency Medicine
Assistant Residency Program Director
Department of Emergency Medicine
LAC+USC Medical Center
Los Angeles, California

Elizabeth A. Owen, MD
Department of Emergency Medicine
Kaiser Permanente, San Diego Medical Center
San Diego, California

Leslie C. Oyama, MD, FACEP
Clinical Professor
Residency Program Director
Department of Emergency Medicine
UC San Diego
San Diego, California

Lynne M. Palmisciano, MD
Assistant Professor
Department of Emergency Medicine and Pediatrics
Clinical Educator
The Warren Alpert Medical School
Department of Emergency Medicine
Hasbro Children's Hospital
Providence, Rhode Island

Joseph S. Palter*, MD
Assistant Professor
Department of Emergency Medicine
Rush University Medical Center
Attending Physician
Department of Emergency Medicine
Cook County Health Chicago
Chicago, Illinois

Patricia De Melo Panakos, MD
Assistant Program Director
Attending Physician
Jackson Health System/University of Miami Miller School of Medicine Emergency Medicine Residency Program
Assistant Professor, Emergency Medicine
Jackson Memorial Hospital
Miami, Florida

Konstantina A. Papathomas, MD
Resident Physician
Department of Emergency Medicine
Thomas Jefferson University Hospital, Jefferson Health
Philadelphia, Pennsylvania

Catherine D. Parker, MD
Assistant Professor
Department of Emergency Medicine
University of Missouri
Columbia, Missouri

Vishnu Parthasarathy*, MD, MS
Resident Physician, PGY-4, Emergency Medicine
UC San Diego
San Diego, California

Robert A. Partridge MD, MPH, FACEP
Adjunct Associate Professor, Emergency Medicine
Department of Emergency Medicine
Warren Alpert Medical School of Brown University
Rhode Island Hospital
Providence, Rhode Island
Department of Emergency Medicine
Emerson Hospital
Concord, Massachusetts

Céline Y. Pascheles, MD
Harvard-Affiliated Emergency Medicine Residency
Beth Israel Deaconess Medical Center
Boston, Massachusetts

Hiren Patel, MD
Clinical Instructor
Department of Emergency Medicine
Massachusetts General Hospital
Associate Fellowship Director
Division of Global Health and Human Rights
Department of Emergency Medicine
Massachusetts General Hospital
Boston, Massachusetts

Ketan Patel, MD
Associate Professor and Associate Program Director
Department of Emergency Medicine
University of Nevada, Las Vegas School of Medicine
Las Vegas, Nevada

David A. Peak, MD
Assistant Professor, Emergency Medicine
Massachusetts General Hospital
Harvard Medical School
Boston, Massachusetts

David A. Pearson, MD, MS, MBA
Professor, Emergency Medicine
Carolinas Medical Center/Atrium Health
Charlotte, North Carolina

Bradley Peckler, MD, FACEP, FACEM
Simulation Clinical Lead

Emergency Medicine Consultant
Wellington Hospital
Wellington, New Zealand

David A. Perlstein, MD, MBA
Professor, Pediatrics
CUNY School of Medicine
President and CEO
SBH Health System
Bronx, New York

Marie-France Petchy, MD
Instructor
Department of Medicine
Universite des Antilles
Attending Physician
Department of Emergency Medicine
Centre Hospitalier de la Basse-Terre
University Hospital of Guadeloupe, FWI
Guadeloupe, France

Andrew P. Pirotte, MD
Clinical Assistant Professor
Department of Emergency Medicine
University of Kansas Hospital/University of Kansas School of Medicine
Kansas City, Kansas

Matthew J. Pirotte, MD, FACEP
Assistant Professor
Assistant Residency Director
Department of Emergency Medicine
Northwestern Memorial Hospital
Chicago, Illinois

Charles V. Pollack, Jr., MA, MD, FACEP, FAAEM, FAHA, FESC, FCPP
Associate Provost for Innovation in Education
Thomas Jefferson University
Associate Dean for CME and Strategic Partner Alliances
Thomas Jefferson University
Professor and Senior Advisor for Interdisciplinary Research and Clinical Trials
Department of Emergency Medicine
Sidney Kimmel Medical College of Thomas Jefferson University
Philadelphia, Pennsylvania

Daniel A. Popa, MD, PhD
Clinical Instructor
Department of Emergency Medicine
Clinical Instructor and Clerkship Director
Division of Undersea and Hyperbaric Medicine
University of California San Diego
San Diego, California

William A. Porcaro, MD, MPH
Instructor
Department of Emergency Medicine
Harvard Medical School
Attending Physician
Department of Emergency Medicine
Mount Auburn Hospital
Cambridge, Massachusetts

Yanina A. Purim-Shem-Tov, MD, MS, FACEP
Associate Professor
Department of Emergency Medicine
Rush University Medical Center
Vice Chair of Faculty Development and Research
Department of Emergency Medicine
Rush University Medical Center
Chicago, Illinois

Arkady Rasin*, MD
Fellow, Toxikon Consortium
Visiting Clinical Instructor
Department of Emergency Medicine
University of Illinois at Chicago
Chicago, Illinois

Neha Raukar, MD, MS, FACEP
CAQ Primary Care Sports Medicine
Mayo Clinic
Associate Professor
Department of Emergency Medicine
Rochester, Minnesota

Lee A. Replogle, MD
Resident Physician
Department of Emergency Medicine
Harvard Medical School
Beth Israel Deaconess Medical Center
Boston, Massachusetts

Lindsey M. Retterath, MD
Resident Physician
Emergency Medicine, Pediatrics
The University of Arizona
Tucson, Arizona

James W. Rhee, MD, FACMT, FACEP, FAAEM
Assistant Clinical Professor
School of Medicine
University of California, Riverside
Temecula, California
Regional Medical Director
Envision Physician Services
Emergency Services
Cedars-Sinai — Marina del Rey Hospital
Temecula, California

Christopher T. Richards, MD, MS, FAEMS, FACEP
Assistant Professor
Attending Physician
Department of Emergency Medicine
Northwestern University, Feinberg School of Medicine
Chicago, Illinois

Jaime B. Rivas*, MD
Department of Emergency Medicine
Palomar Health
Regional Director, Vituity
San Diego, California

Keri Robertson, DO, FACOEP
Associate Clinical Professor and Chair of Emergency Medicine
Chicago College of Osteopathic Medicine and Swedish Covenant Hospital
Chicago, Illinois

Matthew T. Robinson, MD, FACEP
Associate Professor
Department of Emergency Medicine
University of Missouri-Columbia Health System
Chairman
Department of Emergency Medicine
Columbia, Missouri

Kristine Knuti Rodrigues, MD, MPH
Assistant Professor
Department of Pediatrics
University of Colorado School of Medicine
Pediatric Attending Physician
Pediatric Emergency Department and Urgent Care
Denver Health Medical Center
Denver, Colorado

Kyle Roedersheimer, MD
Resident Physician, Emergency Medicine
Carolinas Medical Center
Charlotte, North Carolina

Jennifer A. Rogers*, MD
Associate Professor, Emergency Medicine
Rush University Medical College
Attending Physician, Emergency Medicine
Stroger Hospital of Cook County
Chicago, Illinois

Steven C. Rogers, MD, MS-CTR
Attending Physician
Division of Emergency Medicine
Director
Emergency Mental Health Services
Connecticut Children's Medical Center
Research Scientist
Connecticut Children's Injury Prevention Center
Associate Professor
University of Connecticut School of Medicine
Hartford, Connecticut

Genie E. Roosevelt, MD, MPH
Professor Director, Pediatric Emergency Department and Urgent Care
Department of Emergency Medicine
University of Colorado School of Medicine
Denver Health Medical Center
Aurora, Colorado

Carlo L. Rosen, MD
Associate Professor, Emergency Medicine
Harvard Medical School
Program Director
Emergency Medicine
Beth Israel Deaconess Medical Center
Boston, Massachusetts

Lawrence S. Rosenthal, PhD, MD
Professor, Medicine
Division of Cardiology
UMTSS Memorial Medical Center
Chief
Section of Electrophysiology and Pacing
UMTSS Memorial Medical Center
Worcester, Massachusetts

Joanne C. Routsolias, PharmD, RN
Clinical Pharmacist, Emergency Medicine/Toxicology
Adjunct Clinical Assistant Professor
Department of Emergency Medicine/Pharmacy
University of Illinois College of Pharmacy
Cook County Health
Chicago, Illinois

David H. Rubin, MD
Chairman
Department of Pediatrics
St. Barnabas Hospital
Professor, Pediatrics
Albert Einstein College of Medicine
Bronx, New York

Alexander J.M. Ruby, MD, MSc
Resident Physician
Department of Emergency Medicine
Cook County Health and Hospitals System
Chicago, Ilinois

Brandon T. Ruderman, MD
Resident Physician
Division of Emergency Medicine
Duke University Medical Center
Durham, North Carolina

Frances E. Rudolf, MD
Medical Education Fellow
Department of Emergency Medicine
University of California, San Diego
San Diego, California

Gary S. Sachs, MD
Associate Clinical Professor, Psychiatry
Harvard Medical School
Massachusetts General Hospital
Boston, Massachusetts

Charlotte A. Sadler, MD
Assistant Professor, Emergency Medicine and Hyperbaric Medicine
Fellowship Director, Undersea and Hyperbaric Medicine
University of California, San Diego
San Diego, California

Roxanna A. Sadri, MD, FACEM
Consultant
Department of Emergency Medicine
Christchurch Hospital
Clinical Senior Lecturer
University of Otago
Christchurch, New Zealand

Anthony C. Salazar, MD
Emergency Medicine
Kaiser Permanente
San Diego, California

Rama A. Salhi, MD, MHS
Resident Physician
Department of Emergency Medicine
University of Michigan/St. Joseph Mercy Hospital
Ann Arbor, Michigan

Woodrow J. Sams, MD
Resident, Emergency Medicine
University of Michigan
Ann Arbor, Michigan

Czarina E. Sánchez*, MD
Emergency Medicine Staff
Department of Emergency Medicine
Northwest Medical Center
Bentonville, Arkansas

Arthur B. Sanders, MD, MHA
Professor, Emergency Medicine
University of Arizona College of Medicine
Tucson, Arizona

John P. Santamaria, MD, FAAP, FACEP, FAAHPM
Medical Director
Community PedsCare
Community Hospice of NE Florida
Associate Professor, Pediatrics
University of Florida School of Medicine
Jacksonville, Florida

Sally A. Santen, MD, PhD
Senior Associate Dean and Professor, Emergency Medicine
Virginia Commonwealth University Health System
Richmond, Virginia

Elaine M. Sapiro, MD, MPH
Assistant Clinical Professor
Attending Physician (Hospital)
Department of Emergency Medicine
UC San Diego Health System
San Diego, California

Uziel Sauceda, MD, CAQ Sports Medicine
CAQ Sports Medicine
Assistant Clinical Professor
Department of Family Medicine
University of California Riverside
Riverside University Health System
Riverside, California

Mary Saunders, MD
Clinical Instructor
Department of Pediatrics, Section of Emergency Medicine
University of Colorado School of Medicine, Children's Hospital
Littleton, Colorado

Assaad J. Sayah*, MD
SVP and CMO
Cambridge Health Alliance
Assistant Professor, Emergency Medicine
Harvard Medical School
Cambridge, Massachusetts

Timothy M. Scarella, MD
Instructor, Psychiatry
Harvard Medical School
Staff Psychiatrist
Beth Israel Deaconess Medical Center
Boston, Massachusetts

Shari Schabowski, MD
Assistant Professor
Department of Emergency Medicine
Rush Medical College
Attending Physician
Department of Emergency Medicine
Cook County Health and Hospital System
Chicago, Illinois

Jeffrey I. Schneider, MD
Associate Professor, Assistant Dean for GME
Department of Emergency Medicine
Boston University School of Medicine
Designated Institutional Official for ACGME
Department of Emergency Medicine, Office of Graduate Medical Education
Boston Medical Center
Boston, Massachusetts

David W. Schoenfeld, MD, MPH
Director, Division of EMS
Department of Emergency Medicine
Beth Israel Deaconess Medical Center
Boston, Massachusetts

Suzanne Schuh, MD, FRCP(C), FAAP, ABPEM
Staff Pediatrician, Division of Pediatric Emergency Medicine
Senior Associate Scientist, Research Institute, Hospital for Sick Children
Professor, Pediatrics
University of Toronto
Toronto, Canada

Nicholas M.V. Schulack, DO
Senior Resident
Department of Emergency Medicine
University of Nevada, Las Vegas School of Medicine
University Medical Center of Southern Nevada
Las Vegas, Nevada

James Scott, MD
Professor, Emergency Medicine and Health Policy and Management
George Washington University
Washington, DC

Sarah Tolford Selby, DO
Assistant Professor
Department of Emergency Medicine
University of Colorado School of Medicine
Clinical Faculty
Department of Emergency Medicine
University of Colorado Hospital
Aurora, Colorado

Michelle J. Sergel, MD
Assistant Professor, Emergency Medicine
Cook County Health and Hospitals System
Chicago, Illinois

Fred A. Severyn, MD, FACEP, FAEMS
Associate Professor
Department of Emergency Medicine
University of Colorado School of Medicine
Aurora, Colorado

Nathan I. Shapiro, MD, MPH
Professor, Emergency Medicine
Harvard Medical School and Beth Israel Deaconess Medical Center
Boston, Massachusetts

Siri Shastry, MD
Instructor
Department of Emergency Medicine
Fellow, Clinician Scientist Research Training Program (T32) in Emergency Care Research
Icahn School of Medicine at Mount Sinai
New York, New York

Erica B. Shaver, MD, FACEP
Vice Chair of Education and Training/Residency Program Director
Associate Professor, Emergency Medicine
West Virginia University School of Medicine
Morgantown, West Virginia

Philip Shayne, MD
Professor
Vice Chair for Education
Department of Emergency Medicine
Assistant Dean for Graduate Medical Education
Emory University School of Medicine
Atlanta, Georgia

Scott C. Sherman, MD
Associate Professor
Department of Emergency Medicine
Rush Medical College
Associate Residency Director
Department of Emergency Medicine
Cook County (Stroger) Hospital
Chicago, Illinois

Chester D. Shermer, MD
Professor, Emergency Medicine
University of Mississippi Medical Centre
Jackson, Mississippi

Christopher J. Shestak, MD
Associate Physician of Harvard Medical Faculty Physicians
Beth Israel Deaconess Medical Center
Department of Emergency Medicine
Boston, Massachusetts

Robert D. Sidman, MD, FACEP
Vice President of Medical Affairs
Hartford HealthCare
Norwich, Connecticut

Christine Tsien Silvers, MD, PhD
Chief Medical Officer
HealthReveal, Inc.
New York, New York

Anumeha Singh, MD
Assistant Professor
Department of Emergency Medicine
Hartford Hospital/UConn
Hartford, Connecticut

Terry Singhapricha, MD
Senior Associate
Division of Ultrasound
Department of Emergency Medicine
Emory University School of Medicine
Atlanta, Georgia

Emma K. Sizemore, MD, MPH
Instructor, Emergency Medicine
Emory University School of Medicine
Atlanta, Georgia

Carl G. Skinner*, MD
Chief, Emergency Medicine
Madigan Army Medical Center
Tacoma, Washington

Christian M. Sloane*, MD
Clinical Professor
Department of Emergency Medicine
UCSD School of Medicine
La Jolla, California
Director, Quality and Performance Improvement
UCSD Medical Center
San Diego, California

Lauren M. Smith, MD, MBA
Assistant Professor
Department of Emergency Medicine
Rush Medical College
Chair, Division of Quality and Observation
Department of Emergency Medicine
Cook County Health
Chicago, Illinois

Rebecca Smith-Coggins, MD
Professor, Emergency Medicine and Associate Dean for Medical Student Life Advising
Stanford University
Co-Director of Faculty Affairs, Emergency Medicine
Stanford Medical Center
Stanford, California

Cameron S. Smyres*, MD
Fellow, Emergency Medicine Ultrasound
Department of Emergency Medicine
UC San Diego Health System
San Diego, California

Brian K. Snyder, MD
Clinical Professor
Department of Emergency Medicine
UC San Diego
San Diego, California

Peter H.D. Solomon, MD
Resident Physician
Emergency Medicine
University of California, San Diego
San Diego, California

Sarah K. Sommerkamp, MD, RDMS
Assistant Professor
Department of Emergency Medicine
University of Maryland School of Medicine
Director of Emergency Ultrasound
University of Maryland Midtown Campus
Baltimore, Maryland

Julia H. Sone, MD
Physician
Department of General Surgery
Mid-Atlantic Permanente Medical Group
Virginia Hospital Center in Arlington
Springfield, Virginia

Dale W. Steele, MD, MS
Professor
Departments of Emergency Medicine, Pediatrics, Health Services Policy & Practice
Brown University, Alpert Medical School and School of Public Health
Attending Physician, Pediatric Emergency Medicine
Hasbro Children's Hospital
Providence, Rhode Island

Peter L. Steinwald, MS
MD Candidate, Class of 2020
Tulane University School of Medicine
New Orleans, Louisiana

Lori A. Stolz, MD
Associate Professor
Director, Emergency Ultrasound
Department of Emergency Medicine
University of Cincinnati
Cincinnati, Ohio

John R. Storey, MD, JD
Emergency Medicine Resident
UCSD Health System
San Diego, California

Helen Straus, MD, MS
Assistant Professor
Department of Emergency Medicine
Rush Medical College
Attending Physician
Cook County Health and Hospital System
Chicago, Illinois

Ryan A. Stroder, DO, FACEP
Assistant Professor
Department of Emergency Medicine
Texas Christian University and University of North Texas Health Science Center School of Medicine
Fort Worth, Texas
Clinical Assistant Professor
Department of Emergency Medicine
Parkland Memorial Hospital
Dallas, Texas

John E. Sullivan, MD
Assistant Clinical Professor (Voluntary), Emergency Medicine
Charles E. Schmidt College of Medicine
Florida Atlantic University
Attending Physician, Emergency Medicine
Boca Raton Regional Hospital
Boca Raton, Florida

Radhika Sundararajan, MD PhD
Assistant Professor
Department of Emergency Medicine
NY-Presbyterian/Weill Cornell Medicine
New York, New York

Patrick H. Sweet III*, MD
Clinical Professor, Assistant Health Sciences
UCSD School of Medicine
Medical Director of Mountain Health & Community Services
Commander, Medical Corps, US Navy
Mountain Health & Community Services
San Diego, California

Paul A. Szucs, MD
Clinical Assistant Professor, Emergency Medicine
Sidney Kimmel Medical College
Thomas Jefferson University
Residency Program Director
Department of Emergency Medicine
Morristown Medical Center — Atlantic Health System
Morristown, New Jersey

Allison Tadros, MD, FACEP
Faculty Physician/Clerkship Director
Professor, Emergency Medicine
West Virginia University School of Medicine
Morgantown, West Virginia

Jamal J. Taha, MD
Third-Year Resident
Department of Emergency Medicine
Denver Health Medical Center
Denver, Colorado

Taku Taira, MD
Assistant Professor, Clinical Emergency Medicine
Department of Emergency Medicine
LAC＋USC
Los Angeles, California

David A. Tanen, MD
Professor, Emergency Medicine
Harbor-UCLA Medical Center
Torrance, California

Lindsay Taylor, MD, RDMS, RDCS, RVT
Assistant Professor, Emergency Medicine
Virginia Commonwealth University Health System
Richmond, Virginia

Todd A. Taylor, MD
Assistant Professor
Department of Emergency Medicine
Emory University School of Medicine
Atlanta, Georgia

Christopher M. Tedeschi, MD, MA
Associate Professor, Emergency Medicine
Columbia University Medical Center
New York, New York

Brigham R. Temple, MD, FACEP, FAAEM
Clinical Assistant Professor, Emergency Medicine
Pritzker School of Medicine, University of Chicago
Medical Director of Immediate Care Medicine
Medical Director of Emergency Preparedness
NorthShore University HealthSystem
Evanston, Illinois

Trevonne M. Thompson, MD
Associate Professor, Emergency Medicine and Medical Toxicology
University of Illinois College of Medicine
Attending Physician
Department of Emergency Medicine
University of Illinois Hospital & Health Sciences System
Chicago, Illinois

Robyn P. Thom, MD
Resident
Harvard Longwood Psychiatry Residency
Brigham and Women's Hospital

Beth Israel Deaconess Medical Center
Boston，Massachusetts

Stephen L. Thornton，MD
Associate Professor
Department of Emergency Medicine
University of Kansas Health System
Kansas City，Missouri

Carrie D. Tibbles，MD
Director of Graduate Medical Education
Designated Institutional Official
Beth Israel Deaconess Medical Center
Boston，Massachusetts

Aleksandr M. Tichter，MD，MS
Assistant Professor，Emergency Medicine
Columbia University Medical Center
Columbia University College of Physicians and Surgeons
New York，New York

Vaishal M. Tolia，MD，MPH，FACEP
Associate Clinical Professor，Emergency Medicine
UC San Diego Health
San Diego，California

Daniel J. Tonellato，MD
Resident Physician，Emergency Medicine
Massachusetts General Hospital
Boston，Massachusetts

Susan P. Torrey，MD
Associate Professor，Emergency Medicine
UMass Medical Center
Baystate Medical Center
Springfield，Massachusetts

Jason A. Tracy，MD
Chair
Department of Emergency Medicine
South Shore Health
South Weymouth，Massachusetts

Megan Tresenriter，MD
Emergency Medicine Resident
Department of Emergency Medicine
UC San Diego
San Diego，California

James M. Tsahakis，MD
Emergency Medicine Physician
Saint Joseph Hospital
Denver，Colorado

Alina Tsyrulnik*，MD
Assistant Professor
Department of Emergency Medicine
Yale University School of Medicine
Associate Program Director
Emergency Medicine Residency Program
Department of Emergency Medicine
Yale University School of Medicine
New Haven，CT

Sami H. Uwaydat，MD
Associate Professor
Department of Ophthalmology
University of Arkansas for Medical Sciences
Little Rock，Arkansas

Bernardino Vaccaro，MD
Assistant Professor (part time)，Psychiatry
Harvard Medical School
Department of Psychiatry
Beth Israel Deaconess Medical Center
Boston，Massachusetts

Carla C. Valentine，MD
Attending Physician
Department of Emergency Medicine
Santa Barbara Cottage Hospital
Santa Barbara，California

Karen B. Van Hoesen，MD
Clinical Professor
Department of Emergency Medicine
Co-Director San Diego Center of Excellence in Diving
UC San Diego Health Sciences
San Diego，California

Gary M. Vilke，MD
Professor，Clinical Emergency Medicine
University of California，San Diego Health
San Diego，California
Vice Chair，Clinical Operations
Department of Emergency Medicine
UCSD Health
San Diego，California

Jody A. Vogel，MD，MSc
Assistant Professor
Department of Emergency Medicine
University of Colorado School of Medicine
Denver Health Medical Center
Denver，Colorado

Kathryn A. Volz，MD
Associate Chair and Director of Clinical Operations
Department of Emergency Medicine
St. Joseph Mercy Health System
Ann Arbor，Michigan

Stevan A. Vuckovic，DO，FACOEP，FACEP
Clinical Assistant Professor，Emergency Medicine
Midwestern University
Downers Grove，Illinois
Regional Medical Director-EMS
Northern Indiana
Envision Healthcare
Medical Director
Department of Emergency Medicine
Franciscan Health Rensselaer
Rensselaer，Indiana

Gina T. Waight，MD
Assistant Professor，Emergency Medicine
Department of Emergency Medicine
NewYork-Presbyterian/Columbia University Medical Center/Columbia University
Vagelos College of Physicians and Surgeons
New York，New York

Michael S. Wahl，MD
Senior Clinician Educator
Division of Emergency Medicine
University of Chicago
Medical Director
Illinois Poison Center
Illinois Health and Hospital Association
Chicago，Illinois

Daniel Beslin Walk，MD
Instructor，Emergency Medicine
Harvard Medical School
Resident Physician
Department of Emergency Medicine
Beth Israel Deaconess Medical Center
Boston，Massachusetts

Sulynn Walker，MD
Resident
Department of Emergency Medicine
UMMS-Baystate Medical Center
Springfield，Massachusetts

Bradley A. Wallace，MD
Assistant Professor
Department of Emergency Medicine
Emory University School of Medicine
Atlanta，Georgia

Claire T. Wang，MD
Emergency Medicine
UCSD Medical Center
San Diego，California

Gabriel Wardi，MD，MPH
Assistant Clinical Professor
Department of Emergency Medicine
Division of Pulmonary，Critical Care，and Sleep Medicine
UC San Diego
San Diego，California

Anna L. Waterbrook，MD
Professor，Emergency Medicine
The University of Arizona
Tucson，Arizona

Sarah A. Watkins，DO
Clinical Instructor，Emergency Medicine
Department of Emergency Medicine
Chief Fellow，Medical Toxicology
Arizona Poison and Drug Information Center
The University of Arizona
Tucson，Arizona

Christopher James Watson，MD
Resident Physician
Department of Emergency Medicine
Beth Israel Deaconess Medical Center
Boston，Massachusetts

Kevin R. Weaver，DO，FACOEP
Associate Professor
Morsani School of Medicine
University of South Florida
Vice Chairman — Education
Emergency Medicine Residency Program Director
Department of Emergency Medicine
Lehigh Valley Health Network
Allentown，Pennsylvania

Bruce Webster，MD，PhD
Department of Emergency Medicine
Swedish Medical Center
Seattle，Washington

Kathryn West，MD，MS
Assistant Professor，Emergency Medicine
Department of Emergency Medicine
Carolinas Medical Center/Atrium Health
Charlotte，North Carolina

Melissa H. White，MD，MPH
Associate Professor，Emergency Medicine
Emory University School of Medicine
Atlanta，Georgia

Patrick M. Whiteley，MD
Senior Physician，Emergency Medicine/Medical Toxicology
Kaiser Permanente
San Jose，California

Denise A. Whitfield，MD，MBA
Assistant Professor，Clinical Medicine
Department of Emergency Medicine

David Geffen School of Medicine at UCLA
Los Angeles, California
Clinical Faculty
Department of Emergency Medicine
Harbor-UCLA Medical Center
Torrance, California

Herbert Neil Wigder, MD
Visiting Clinical Associate Professor
Department of Emergency Medicine
University of Illinois Chicago College of Medicine
Chicago, Illinois
Vice Chair, Emeritus
Department of Emergency Medicine
Advocate Lutheran General Hospital
Park Ridge, Illinois

Darin S. Williams, MD
Carrollton Emergency Physicians
Carrollton, Georgia

James Willis, MD
Assistant Professor, Emergency Medicine
SUNY Downstate
Associate Residency Director
Emergency Medicine
Kings County Hospital Center
Brooklyn, New York

Daniel A. Willner, MD, MPH
Assistant Professor
Physician, Emergency Medicine
Department of Emergency Medicine
University of Colorado School of Medicine
Aurora, Colorado

Duncan K. Wilson*, MD
Captain, US Air Force
Emergency Services Physician
Joint Base Andrews, Maryland

Michael P. Wilson, MD, PhD, FAAEM, FACEP
Assistant Professor, Departments of Emergency Medicine and Psychiatry
Emergency Medicine, Psychiatry
University of Arkansas for Medical Sciences
Little Rock, Arkansas

Ashlea Winfield-Dial, MD, MSPH
Resident Physician
Department of Emergency Medicine
Cook County Health and Hospital System
Chicago, Illinois

Peter Witucki*, MD
Associate Professor, Emergency Medicine
UC San Diego
San Diego, California

Richard E. Wolfe, MD
Associate Professor
Department of Emergency Medicine
Harvard Medical School
Chief of Emergency Medicine
Beth Israel Deaconess Medical Center
Boston, Massachusetts

Matthew L. Wong, MD, MPH
Instructor
Department of Emergency Medicine
Harvard Medical School
Attending
Department of Emergency Medicine
Beth Israel Deaconess Medical Center
Boston, Massachusetts

Stella C. Wong, DO
Assistant Professor
Department of Emergency Medicine
Emory University School of Medicine
Atlanta GA, USA

Daniel T. Wu, MD
Associate Professor, Emergency Medicine
Emory University School of Medicine
Atlanta, Georgia

Peggy A. Wu, MD, MPH
Associate Professor
Department of Dermatology
University of California, Davis
Sacramento, California

Ryan H. Wyatt, MD
Resident
Department of Emergency Medicine
John Peter Smith Hospital
Fort Worth, Texas

Jennifer Yee, DO, FAAEM
Clinical Assistant Professor
Emergency Medicine Simulation Director
Department of Emergency Medicine
The Ohio State University
Columbus, Ohio

Kenneth Young, MD
Medical Director
Grainger Center for Simulation and Innovation
Section of Emergency Medicine
Northshore University Health System
Evanston, Illinois

Chao Annie Yuan, MD, FACEP
Physician
Department of Emergency Medicine
Marin General Hospital
Marin, California
Good Samaritan Hospital
Los Gatos, California

Michele Zell-Kanter, PharmD
Clinical Assistant Professor, Medical Toxicology
Department of Emergency Medicine
University of Illinois
Coordinator, Toxikon Consortium
Department of Emergency Medicine
Cook County Hospital
Chicago, Illinois

Julie A. Zeller, MD
Emergency Medicine Attending
Emerson Hospital
Concord, Massachusetts

Andrew B. Ziller, MD
Medical Director
Emergency Department
Rose Medical Center
Denver, Colorado

Gary D. Zimmer, MD, FACEP
Adjunct Assistant Professor
Philadelphia College of Osteopathic Medicine
Principal HedDI, LLC
Bryn Mawr, Philadelphia

Karen P. Zimmer*, MD, MPH, FAAP
Medical Executive, Health IT, Patient Safety, and Quality Consulting
Associate Professor
Thomas Jefferson University
Instructor
Jefferson College of Population Health
Philadelphia, Pennsylvania

致谢第五版作者

第六版主编和作者十分感谢下列为第五版做出贡献的作者：

Jennifer Audi
Amer Aldeen
Beverly Bauman
Kenneth R.L. Bernard
Carli Blomquist
Kyle R. Brown
Melissa P. Bui
Christopher S. Cambell
Ingrid Carter
Jeremy Chou
Ryan E. Christensen
Chris Colwell
Christopher B. Colwell
Rita K. Cydulka
Jamila Danishwar
Daniel Davis
Arunachalam Einstein
Robyn Heister-Girard
Daniel J. Henning
Adam Herringhaus
Doodnauth Hiraman
Eva Tovar Hirashima
Austin Hopper
Maureen L. Joyner
Elicia Sinor Kennedy
Jennifer L. Kolodchak
Ruth L. Lamm
Emi M. Latham
Denise S. Lawe
Calvin A. Lee
Moses S. Lee
John Lemos
Steven Lindsay
Douglas W. Lowery
Douglas Lowery-North's
Christopher McCarthy
Richard McCormick
Daniel C. McGillicuddy
Sheila McMorrow
Matthew B. Mostof
Scott Murray
Celeste N. Nadal
Carolyn Maher Overman
Peter J. Park
Jennifer De la Pena
Niels K. Rathlev
Colleen M. Rivers
Lucas Roseire
Mark Sagarin
Leon D. Sánchez
Davut J. Savaser
Emily S. Sbiroli
Michael Schmidt
Virag Shah
Patricia Shipley
Jeffrey N. Siegelman
Sandra E. Sincular
Joshua J. Solano
Shannon Straszewski
Marie Carmelle Tabuteau
Joseph P. Tagliaferro
William D. Timbers
Edward Ullman
Chad M. Valderrama
Catherine M. Visintainer
Jonathan B. Walker
Cameron R. Wangsgard
Joseph M. Weber
Tammy L. Weitner
Marian Xu
David N. Zull

中文版序言

急诊科患者的疾病特点决定了急诊科医师需要在极为有限的时间内根据患者症状、体征和有限的临床资料快速做出诊疗决策，这就需要急诊科医师具备极为高效的诊疗思维和极为高超的处理能力。在我国这样一个大型医院里急诊就诊人数居高不下的大背景下，这些“苛刻”的要求体现得更加明显。急诊科医师往往需要在很短的时间内首先识别出最可能危及生命的重要病情，及时给予处理；同时还需要尽可能高效地在后续诊疗过程中找到所有可能的致病病因，避免漏诊与误诊。这无疑是具有相当难度的挑战，急诊科医师需要经过反复多年的经验积累和培训学习，才有可能将临床所学转化到急诊医学诊疗活动与实践之中。

《急诊科 5 分钟速查》就是基于以上急诊临床工作需要而编写、出版的。它是由美国 500 余位急诊科医师共同编写的一本实用性极强的工具书。从本书的目录就可以看出，内容涵盖了急诊科几乎所有的具体疾病类型。与同类图书不同的地方在于，本书目录中包含了急诊科所有常见的主诉症状。通过对每一种主诉症状进行抽丝剥茧的分析，明确每一种可能的病因并提出相应的处置措施，从而最大限度地提高急诊科医师的临床工作效率。除了病因诊断和纷繁复杂的鉴别诊断，对于急危重症的识别和处理也同样重要。本书的设计，既体现了急诊科医师在诊断方面需要考虑的全面性，避免漏诊、误诊，同时也以提纲、条块式的结构，重点突出了诊断明确后，急诊科医师需要进行的处置，特别是重症监护病房内的综合处理措施。这也再一次体现出国际上对急危重症患者连贯一体化的诊疗过程的运行惯例，因为这一诊疗模式毫无疑问更容易使急危重症患者从中受益。

《急诊科 5 分钟速查》内容体量很大。为了能够准确反映图书内容，主译专家组织了上海多家医院数十位急诊和重症医学同道，花费了近 2 年时间才完成本书的翻译工作。在这一过程中，各位参与翻译工作的专家和同道，花费了大量的时间和心血，认真翻译并且反复修改,旨在为急诊科医师提供一本高质量的临床实用工具书。在此,对各位专家、同道的辛勤付出表示衷心感谢!

相信这本书一定能够为急诊医师的临床诊疗提供极大的帮助,也欢迎大家在后续的临床实践中,针对本书多提宝贵意见!

杨兴易

上海长征医院急诊、重症医学科

2024 年 7 月 10 日

中文版前言

急诊医学作为一门独立学科(二级学科),在我国已经走过了 40 余载的春秋。现代急诊医学主要以应对各种突发性疾病、创伤及突发公共卫生事件,迅速评估患者、做出临床诊疗决策为根本目的。其中涉及至少两个层面的内容,包括积极救治并稳定生命体征,以及诊断与鉴别诊断、确定病因。这其实是并不矛盾的两个层面要求,在急诊诊疗过程中,需要相辅相成、完美衔接,才能妥善地处理好各种患者,特别是急危重症患者。在急诊诊疗实践中,我们往往面对的是各种急性症状、体征甚至是一些检查结果,而不是已经确诊的疾病;在接诊患者的很短时间内确定恰当的诊疗处置方案并加以实施,对于各级急诊科医师来说都是难度不小的挑战。在这一过程中,我们当然不能过于追求精确诊断,而应该首先排除致命性急症或并发症,并且尽快采取稳定病情的初步措施;紧接着,在寻找病因的同时,更应该关注患者的急性病理生理学改变,如循环衰竭、呼吸衰竭、肾衰竭等,掌握快速稳定生命体征、实施器官功能支持的方法和手段。而这些措施往往也是为急危重症患者争取到最终明确诊断的时间创造条件。由此可以看出,急诊医学的工作特点决定了,急诊科医师需要在最短的时间内首先识别出最可能危及生命的重要病情与症状,并给予及时处置;同时在器官功能支持和保护的过程中查找可能的致病病因,避免漏诊与误诊。

《急诊科 5 分钟速查》的内容设计很好地契合了上述需求。它是由美国 500 余位急诊科专家共同编写的一本实用性极强的工具书。其内容不仅涵盖了急诊科几乎所有的疾病类型,也包含了急诊科所有就诊主诉症状,其中针对同一症状,还区别了成人和儿童不同的疾病特点及不同的诊疗需求。通过辞书式的编排设计,可以使临床医师在有需要的时候,迅速查找,快速定位,获取有帮助的诊疗建议。在诊疗内容方面,不仅有具体的需要优先安排的重要检验和检查,也包括了临床治疗中的具体处置措施、药物名称和剂量等,以便于临床医师参考。

由于急诊医学涉及的知识面很广，这本书内容丰富、体量较大，翻译工作着实是一项巨大挑战，但翻译团队有决心、有毅力完成这样一本优秀工具书的翻译工作，为国内广大的急诊同道提供有益的诊疗参考。在图书翻译过程中，我们团结了上海多家医院的急诊同道们，大家不辞辛苦，花费了工作之余的时间，精心翻译，仔细修改，力保译文准确。在此，对各位参编专家的辛勤付出表示由衷的感谢！同时，也对在图书翻译过程中多次给予关怀和指导的杨兴易教授及后期参与校对的各位专家、同道，一并表示最诚挚的谢意！

期待本书的出版能够给各位急诊同道的临床工作带来帮助，也欢迎各位同道在使用本书的过程中，多多提出宝贵的意见和建议。

《急诊科 5 分钟速查》翻译组

2024 年 6 月

英文版前言

《急诊科5分钟速查》能反映出急诊医学实践的特质。急诊工作导致临床医师要面临各种挑战，包括临床情况的复杂多变、急性病的时间限制、环境因素、繁忙的急诊科后勤需求等。时间至关重要！这本书是为了满足在急诊环境工作的临床医师的需要而编写的。为了寻找诊断，临床医师必须认真思考，而急诊科工作的特点是没有足够的时间给医师深思熟虑。然而，我们必须形成这样一种认知：要考虑统计学上罕见但临床上严重的情况，而不是仅仅去考虑统计学上可能但不危及生命的诊断。

本书简洁的格式使得忙碌的急诊科医师能对每个患者进行适当的处理，这意味着它应随手可得、经常被用于急诊科的“战壕”中。本书由执业临床医师为同行们编写，格式紧凑的内容中包含了大量信息，启发临床医师进行分析和后续的评估。

我们力图将作者们的专业知识、经验和基础知识整合入本书。本书并非要提供诊断工具，而是要提供一个地方，当医生在得出由临床判断和患者呈现出的主观、客观证据所支持的诊断时，该诊断可以在此得到证实。作者们为读者提供了精确的、与临床高度相关的总结，这些总结对治疗患者很有帮助，同时也为医学生和住院医师提供了处理具体疾病的知识结构。感谢作者们对这项工作所做的贡献。

编写本书时，我们希望它能方便地应用于临床实践，而不是希望它是决定性的和包罗万象的。与过去版本一样，本版包含了临床处理的信息和方法，同时也反映了我们所面临的新挑战。

我们希望本书对急诊医学的新手和有经验的临床医师都有用。本书所反映的信息和采用的编排设计，其目的是便于读者在“混乱”的临床环境中使用。

临床的敏锐性、判断和经验是我们临床实践的基础。我们希望本书能服务于急诊科医师、护士、医师助理、急救医务人员和学生，成为他们随时可用的资源。在提升急诊医学专业水平的同时，为患者提供优质的护理，将永远是我们努力的重点。

Jeffrey J. Schaider
Roger M. Barkin
Stephen R. Hayden
Richard E. Wolfe
Adam Z. Barkin
Philip Shayne

目录 1

1 5-羟色胺综合征(药物诱导) Serotonin Syndrome (Drug-Induced)
2 Brugada 综合征 Brugada Syndrome
3 HELLP 综合征 HELLP Syndrome
5 QT 间期延长综合征 QT Syndrome, Prolonged
7 β受体阻滞剂中毒 Beta-Blocker Poisoning
9 γ-羟基丁酸中毒 GHB Poisoning

A

11 阿米巴病 Amebiasis
13 阿片类药物中毒 Opiate Poisoning
14 埃立克体病 Ehrlichiosis

B

17 巴贝虫病 Babesiosis
19 巴比妥中毒 Barbiturates Poisoning
20 白细胞增多症 Leukocytosis
22 白血病 Leukemia
23 百日咳 Pertussis
25 包茎 Phimosis
26 包皮嵌顿 Paraphimosis
27 孢子丝菌病 Sporotrichosis
29 暴力管理 Violence, Management of
31 爆裂性骨折 Blow-Out Fracture
33 爆震伤 Blast Injuries
34 贝尔麻痹 Bell's Palsy
35 背痛 Back Pain
38 贲门黏膜撕裂综合征 Mallory-Weiss Syndrome
39 苯丙胺中毒 Amphetamine Poisoning
41 苯二氮䓬类药物中毒 Benzodiazepine Poisoning
43 苯环己哌啶中毒 Phencyclidine Poisoning
44 苯妥英中毒 Phenytoin Poisoning
45 鼻出血 Epistaxis
47 鼻窦炎 Sinusitis
49 鼻骨骨折 Nasal Fractures
51 鼻腔异物 Foreign Body, Nasal
53 闭经 Amenorrhea
54 扁桃体周脓肿 Peritonsillar Abscess
56 便秘 Constipation
58 髌骨损伤 Patellar Injuries
59 病态窦房结综合征 Sick Sinus Syndrome
61 玻璃体出血 Vitreous Hemorrhage
62 布尔哈夫综合征 Boerhaave Syndrome

C

64 茶碱中毒 Theophylline Poisoning
65 产后出血 Postpartum Hemorrhage
67 产后感染 Postpartum Infection
69 肠梗阻(小肠和大肠) Bowel Obstruction(Small and Large)
71 肠扭转 Volvulus
73 肠旋转不良 Malrotation
74 肠套叠 Intussusception
76 肠系膜缺血 Mesenteric Ischemia
78 肠易激综合征 Irritable Bowel Syndrome
79 成骨不全症 Osteogenesis Imperfecta
80 痴呆 Dementia
83 出血热 Hemorrhagic Fevers
85 川崎病 Kawasaki Disease
87 传染性红斑 Erythema Infectiosum
88 传染性软疣 Molluscum Contagiosum

90 喘鸣 Stridor
91 创伤(多部位) Trauma, Multiple
93 创伤(儿童) Pediatric Trauma
95 创伤(老年人) Geriatric Trauma
97 创伤后应激障碍 Post-Traumatic Stress Disorder(PTSD)
98 创伤性断肢/再植 Traumatic Amputation/Replantation
100 创伤性主动脉破裂 Aortic Rupture, Traumatic(TAI)
102 刺激性气体暴露 Irritant Gas Exposure
104 丛集性头痛 Headache, Cluster

D

106 大麻素和合成大麻素中毒 Cannabinoids and Synthetic Cannabinoids Poisoning
107 带状疱疹 Herpes Zoster
109 丹毒 Erysipelas
111 单胺氧化酶抑制药中毒 Monoamine Oxidase Inhibitor Poisoning
113 单纯疱疹 Herpes Simplex
115 单关节性关节炎 Arthritis, Monoarticular
118 单核细胞增多症 Mononucleosis
119 胆管炎 Cholangitis
121 胆结石 Cholelithiasis
122 胆囊炎 Cholecystitis
124 胆石性肠梗阻 Gallstone Ileus
125 登革热 Dengue Fever
126 低钙血症 Hypocalcemia
129 低钾血症 Hypokalemia
130 低钠血症 Hyponatremia
132 低血糖 Hypoglycemia
134 骶骨骨折 Sacral Fracture
135 地高辛中毒 Digoxin, Poisoning
137 癫痫发作(成人) Seizure, Adult
139 癫痫发作(儿童) Seizure, Pediatric
141 电击伤 Electrical Injury
144 动脉导管未闭 Patent Ductus Arteriosus
145 动脉气体栓塞 Arterial Gas Embolism(AGE)
146 动物咬伤 Bite, Animal
148 动眼神经麻痹 Oculomotor Nerve Palsy
150 冻伤 Frostbite
152 毒蕈中毒 Mushroom Poisoning
154 短暂性脑缺血发作 Transient Ischemic Attack
157 短暂性全面性遗忘症 Transient Global Amnesia
158 对乙酰氨基酚中毒 Acetaminophen Poisoning
160 多发性骨髓瘤 Multiple Myeloma
162 多发性神经病 Polyneuropathy
163 多发性硬化 Multiple Sclerosis
165 多形红斑 Erythema Multiforme

E

167 呃逆 Hiccups
168 儿科复苏 Resuscitation, Pediatric
170 耳外伤 Otologic Trauma
172 二尖瓣脱垂 Mitral Valve Prolapse

F

174 发绀 Cyanosis
176 发热(成人) Fever, Adult
178 发热(儿童) Fever, Pediatric
180 发热性癫痫(高热惊厥) Seizure, Febrile
182 反应性关节炎 Reactive Arthritis
183 房室传导阻滞 Atrioventricular Blocks
184 非心源性肺水肿 Noncardiogenic Pulmonary Edema
186 非甾体抗炎药中毒 Nonsteroidal Anti-Inflammatory Poisoning
187 肥厚型心肌病 Cardiomyopathy, Hypertrophic
189 肺孢子虫病 Pneumocystis Pneumonia
190 肺挫伤 Pulmonary Contusion
191 肺栓塞 Pulmonary Embolism
193 肺水肿 Pulmonary Edema
196 肺炎(成人) Pneumonia, Adult
198 肺炎(儿童) Pneumonia, Pediatric
200 肺源性心脏病 Cor Pulmonale
202 分娩(无并发症) Delivery, Uncomplicated
203 分娩(早产和胎膜早破) Labor
205 风湿热 Rheumatic Fever
206 风湿性关节炎 Arthritis, Rheumatoid
208 风疹 Rubella
209 蜂窝织炎 Cellulitis
212 辐射损伤 Radiation injury
214 腐蚀性化学物中毒 Caustic Ingestion
216 附睾炎和睾丸炎 Epididymitis/Orchitis
218 复视 Diplopia
219 富尼埃坏疽 Fournier Gangrene
221 腹部穿透性创伤 Abdominal Trauma, Penetrating
222 腹部创伤影像 Abdominal Trauma, Imaging
224 腹部钝性创伤 Abdominal Trauma, Blunt

225 腹腔积液 Ascites
227 腹痛 Abdominal Pain
230 腹泻(成人) Diarrhea, Adult
231 腹泻(儿童) Diarrhea, Pediatric
234 腹主动脉瘤 Abdominal Aortic Aneurysm

G

236 钙通道阻滞剂中毒 Calcium Channel Blocker Poisoning
237 肝肾综合征 Hepatorenal Syndrome
239 肝损伤 Hepatic Injury
240 肝性脑病 Hepatic Encephalopathy
242 肝炎 Hepatitis
244 肝硬化 Cirrhosis
247 肛裂 Anal Fissure
248 高钙血症 Hypercalcemia
250 高钾血症 Hyperkalemia
251 高钠血症 Hypernatremia
253 高黏滞综合征 Hyperviscosity Syndrome
254 高渗综合征 Hyperosmolar Syndrome
256 高铁血红蛋白血症 Methemoglobinemia
258 高血压急症 Hypertensive Emergencies
260 高压氧治疗 Hyperbaric Oxygen Therapy
261 高原病 High-Altitude Illness
263 睾丸扭转 Testicular Torsion
265 膈肌外伤 Diaphragmatic Trauma
266 弓形虫病 Toxoplasmosis
268 肱骨骨折 Humerus Fracture
270 汞中毒 Mercury Poisoning
272 共济失调 Ataxia
274 股骨干滑脱 Slipped Capital Femoral Epiphysis
275 股骨骨折 Femur Fracture
277 股骨头骨骺炎 Legg-Calvé-Perthes Disease
278 骨骺骨折 Epiphyseal Injuries
279 骨盆骨折 Pelvic Fracture
281 骨髓炎 Osteomyelitis
283 骨折(儿童) Fractures, Pediatric
285 骨质疏松症 Osteoporosis
287 鼓膜穿孔 Tympanic Membrane Perforation
288 关节损伤 Knee Injury
290 管饲并发症 Feeding Tube Complications
292 过度通气综合征 Hyperventilation Syndrome
294 过敏 Anaphylaxis
295 过敏性紫癜 Henoch-Schönlein Purpura

H

298 海绵窦血栓 Cavernous Sinus Thrombosis
299 海洋生物蜇伤 Marine Envenomation
301 横纹肌溶解 Rhabdomyolysis
303 红细胞增多症 Polycythemia
305 红眼 Red Eye
308 虹膜炎 Iritis
310 喉骨折 Larynx Fracture
311 喉头炎 Croup
313 喉炎 Laryngitis
314 呼吸机管理 Ventilator Management
317 呼吸窘迫 Respiratory Distress
319 呼吸困难 Dyspnea
321 呼吸暂停(儿童) Apnea, Pediatric
323 华法林的并发症 Warfarin Complications
325 滑囊炎 Bursitis
327 化学武器中毒 Chemical Weapons Poisoning
329 踝关节骨折/脱位 Ankle Fracture/Dislocation
331 踝关节扭伤 Ankle Sprain
332 坏疽 Gangrene
333 坏死溃疡性龈炎 Necrotizing Ulcerative Gingivitis
334 坏死性软组织感染 Necrotizing Soft Tissue Infections
337 环/束带移除损伤 Ring/Constricting Band Removal
338 缓慢性心律失常 Bradyarrhythmias
341 幻觉 Hallucinations
343 黄疸 Jaundice
345 会厌炎(成人) Epiglottitis, Adult
347 会厌炎(儿童) Epiglottitis, Pediatric
348 昏迷 Coma
350 霍纳综合征 Horner Syndrome

J

352 机会性感染 Opportunistic Infections
354 肌腱撕裂伤 Tendon Laceration
355 肌腱炎 Tendonitis
357 肌萎缩侧索硬化症 Amyotrophic Lateral Sclerosis
359 肌张力障碍反应 Dystonic Reaction
360 吉兰-巴雷综合征 Guillain-Barr'e Syndrome
362 急性冠脉综合征：冠状动脉血管痉挛 Acute Coronary Syndrome: Coronary Vasospasm
364 急性冠脉综合征：无 Q 波(非 ST 段抬高)心肌梗死 Acute Coronary Syndrome: Non-Q-Wave (Non-ST-Elevation) MI

366 急性冠脉综合征：心肌梗死 Acute Coronary Syndrome：Myocardial Infarction
368 急性冠脉综合征：心绞痛 Acute Coronary Syndrome：Angina
370 急性精神病 Psychosis，Acute
372 急性肾损伤 Kidney Injury，Acute
374 脊髓灰质炎 Polio
376 脊髓综合征 Spinal Cord Syndromes
377 脊椎滑脱和脊椎前移 Spondylolysis/Spondylolisthesis
379 脊椎损伤(成人，颈部) Spine Injury：Cervical，Adult
381 脊椎损伤(儿童，颈部) Spine Injury：Cervical，Pediatric
382 脊椎损伤(尾骨) Spine Injury：Coccyx
383 脊椎损伤(胸部) Spine Injury：Thoracic
385 脊椎损伤(腰部) Spine Injury：Lumbar
387 家庭暴力 Domestic Violence
388 甲苯中毒 Toluene Poisoning
390 甲醇中毒 Methanol Poisoning
392 甲沟炎 Paronychia
393 甲状旁腺功能减退症 Hypoparathyroidism
395 甲状旁腺功能亢进症 Hyperparathyroidism
397 甲状腺功能减退症 Hypothyroidism
399 甲状腺功能亢进症 Hyperthyroidism
402 贾第虫病 Giardiasis
404 间室综合征 Compartment Syndrome
405 肩关节脱位 Shoulder Dislocation
406 肩锁关节损伤 Acromioclavicular Joint Injury
408 减压病 Decompression Sickness
409 睑腺炎和睑板腺囊肿 Hordeolum and Chalazion
411 碱中毒 Alkalosis
413 腱鞘炎 Tenosynovitis
415 降糖药中毒 Hypoglycemic Agent Poisoning
417 焦虑症 Agitation
419 角膜擦伤 Corneal Abrasion
420 角膜异物 Corneal Foreign Body
422 角膜灼伤 Corneal Burn
424 接触性皮炎 Contact Dermatitis
426 结肠损伤 Colon Trauma
427 结核 Tuberculosis
429 结节病 Sarcoidosis
431 结节性红斑 Erythema Nodosum
432 结膜炎 Conjunctivitis
434 疥疮 Scabies
436 紧急剖宫产 Cesarean Section，Emergency
438 进食障碍 Eating Disorders
440 惊恐发作 Panic Attack
442 精神分裂症 Schizophrenia
444 精神症状的躯体因素和精神因素 Psychosis，Medical vs. Psychiatric
446 精神状态改变 Altered Mental Status
448 颈部绞窄伤和悬吊伤 Neck Injury by Strangulation/Hanging
450 颈部腺炎 Cervical Adenitis
452 颈前部穿透伤 Neck Trauma，Penetrating，Anterior
453 颈前部钝性创伤 Neck Trauma，Blunt，Anterior
455 胫骨粗隆骨软骨病 Osgood-Schlatter Disease
456 胫骨和腓骨骨折 Tibial/Fibular Shaft Fracture
458 胫骨平台骨折 Tibial Plateau Fracture
460 静脉功能不全 Venous Insufficiency
462 静脉曲张 Varices
464 酒精戒断 Withdrawal，Alcohol
465 酒精性酮症酸中毒 Alcoholic Ketoacidosis
467 酒精中毒 Alcohol Poisoning
469 巨细胞动脉炎 Giant Cell Arteritis

K

471 卡马西平中毒 Carbamazepine Poisoning
472 咯血 Hemoptysis
475 开放性骨折 Fracture，Open
476 抗胆碱能药中毒 Anticholinergic Poisoning
477 抗利尿素分泌异常症 Syndrome of Inappropriate Antidiuretic Hormone Secretion(SIADH)
479 抗抑郁药中毒 Antidepressant Poisoning
481 咳嗽 Cough
483 可卡因中毒 Cocaine Poisoning
485 口腔溃疡 Aphthous Ulcers
487 口腔念珠菌病 Candidiasis，Oral
488 库欣综合征 Cushing Syndrome
490 快速节律障碍 Tachydysrhythmias
493 髋部损伤 Hip Injury
495 狂犬病 Rabies
496 眶后血肿 Retro-Orbital Hematoma
498 眶周和眼眶蜂窝织炎 Periorbital and Orbital Cellulitis

L

500 莱姆病 Lyme Disease
501 阑尾炎 Appendicitis

504 滥用大麻 Marijuana Abuse
506 肋骨骨折 Rib Fracture
508 泪囊炎和泪腺炎 Dacryocystitis and Dacryoadenitis
510 锂中毒 Lithium Poisoning
511 粒细胞减少症 Granulocytopenia
514 连枷胸 Flail Chest
516 镰状细胞病 Sickle Cell Disease
518 链球菌病 Streptococcal Disease
519 淋巴管炎 Lymphangitis
521 淋巴结炎 Lymphadenitis
523 淋病 Gonococcal Disease
525 流感 Influenza
527 颅脑穿透伤 Head Trauma，Penetrating
529 卵巢囊肿/扭转 Ovarian Cyst/Torsion
530 落基山斑疹热 Rocky Mountain Spotted Fever

M

533 麻疹 Measles
534 马尾综合征 Cauda Equina Syndrome
535 慢性阻塞性肺疾病 Chronic Obstructive Pulmonary Disease
537 毛滴虫病 Trichomonas
538 毛细支气管炎 Bronchiolitis
540 玫瑰糠疹 Pityriasis Rosea
541 玫瑰疹 Roseola
542 梅毒 Syphilis
544 梅克尔憩室 Meckel Diverticulum
546 梅尼埃病 Ménière Disease
548 孟乔森综合征做作性障碍 Munchausen Syndrome (Factitious Disorder)
549 弥散性血管内凝血 Disseminated Intravascular Coagulation
551 蜜蜂蜇伤 Sting，Bee
553 免疫 Immunizations
554 免疫抑制 Immunosuppression
556 面部骨折 Facial Fractures
558 拇指骨折 Thumb Fracture

N

560 囊性纤维化 Cystic Fibrosis
562 脑出血 Intracerebral Hemorrhage
564 脑动脉瘤 Cerebral Aneurysm
566 脑积水 Hydrocephalus
567 脑膜炎 Meningitis
570 脑膜炎球菌血症 Meningococcemia
572 脑室腹膜分流 Ventricular Peritoneal Shunts
573 脑血管意外 Cerebral Vascular Accident
576 脑炎 Encephalitis
577 脑再灌注治疗 Reperfusion Therapy，Cerebral
580 内耳迷路炎 Labyrinthitis
582 内脏穿孔 Perforated Viscous
583 拟交感神经药中毒 Sympathomimetic Poisoning
586 溺水 Drowning
587 尿崩症 Diabetes Insipidus
589 尿布疹 Diaper Rash
591 尿道创伤 Urethral Trauma
592 尿道瘘 Urinary Tract Fistula
593 尿道炎 Urethritis
595 尿路感染（成人） Urinary Tract Infections，Adult
597 尿路感染（儿童） Urinary Tract Infections，Pediatric
599 尿潴留 Urinary Retention
601 颞下颌关节损伤/综合征 Temporal-Mandibular Joint Injury/Syndrome
602 凝血病逆转（非华法林药物所致） Coagulopathy Reversal（Nonwarfarin Agents）
605 脓毒性关节炎 Arthritis，Septic
607 脓毒症 Sepsis
609 脓疱病 Impetigo
610 疟疾 Malaria
613 虐待（儿童，非意外性创伤） Abuse，Pediatric （Nonaccidental Trauma，NAT）
615 虐待（老年人） Abuse，Elder

O

617 呕吐（成人） Vomiting，Adult
619 呕吐（儿童） Vomiting，Pediatric

P

621 帕金森病 Parkinson Disease
622 膀胱损伤 Bladder Injury
623 佩吉特病 Paget Disease
625 盆腔炎 Pelvic Inflammatory Disease
627 皮肤或软组织脓肿 Abscess，Skin/Soft Tissue
629 皮肤癣 Tinea Infections，Cutaneous
631 皮肌炎和多肌炎 Dermatomyositis/Polymyositis
632 皮疹 Rash

635 疲乏 Fatigue
636 脾脏损伤 Splenic Injury
638 蜱咬伤 Tick Bite
639 偏头痛 Headache, Migraine
640 贫血 Anemia
643 破伤风 Tetanus
645 葡萄球菌烫伤样皮肤综合征 Staphylococcal Scalded Skin Syndrome
646 葡萄胎 Hydatidiform Mole

Q

649 气喘 Wheezing
650 气道辅助装置 Airway Adjuncts
652 气道管理 Airway Management
654 气胸 Pneumothorax
656 气压伤 Barotrauma
657 憩室病 Diverticulosis
659 憩室炎 Diverticulitis
661 铅中毒 Lead Poisoning
663 前臂骨干/远端骨折 Forearm Fracture, Shaft/Distal
664 前房积血 Hyphema
666 前列腺炎 Prostatitis
667 前庭大腺脓肿 Bartholin Abscess
669 前置胎盘 Placenta Previa
670 强直性脊柱炎 Ankylosing Spondylitis
672 鞘膜积液 Hydrocele
673 青光眼 Glaucoma
675 氰化物中毒 Cyanide Poisoning

R

678 桡骨小头半脱位(保姆肘) Nursemaid's Elbow
679 人类免疫缺陷病毒/获得性免疫缺陷综合征 HIV/AIDS
681 妊娠(无并发症) Pregnancy, Uncomplicated
682 妊娠剧吐 Hyperemesis Gravidarum
684 妊娠期阴道出血 Vaginal Bleeding In Pregnancy
686 肉毒中毒 Botulism
688 乳突炎 Mastoiditis
690 乳腺炎 Mastitis
691 软下疳 Chancroid
692 瑞氏综合征 Reye Syndrome

S

695 腮腺炎 Mumps
696 三叉神经痛 Trigeminal Neuralgia
697 三环类抗抑郁药中毒 Tricyclic Antidepressant Poisoning
699 瘙痒 Pruritus
701 闪电击伤 Lightning Injuries
703 疝 Hernias
705 烧伤 Burns
707 蛇毒液螫伤 Snake Envenomation
709 社区获得性耐甲氧西林金黄色葡萄球菌感染 MRSA, Community Acquired
710 砷中毒 Arsenic Poisoning
712 深静脉血栓形成 Deep Vein Thrombosis
714 神经阻滞剂恶性综合征 Neuroleptic Malignant Syndrome
716 肾病综合征 Nephrotic Syndrome
718 肾结石 Renal Calculus
720 肾上腺功能减退症 Adrenal Insufficiency
722 肾损伤 Renal Injury
724 肾小球肾炎 Glomerulonephritis
726 肾炎综合征 Nephritic Syndrome
728 肾盂肾炎 Pyelonephritis
730 生物武器 Biologic Weapons
732 生长发育滞缓 Failure to Thrive
734 生殖器疱疹 Herpes, Genital
736 失血性休克 Hemorrhagic Shock
738 虱病 Pediculosis
740 湿疹/特应性皮炎 Eczema/Atopic Dermatitis
741 史-约综合征 Stevens-Johnson Syndrome
743 十二指肠损伤 Duodenal Trauma
745 食管创伤 Esophageal Trauma
747 食管异物 Foreign Body, Esophageal
749 视觉丧失 Visual Loss
751 视神经炎 Optic Neuritis
753 视网膜脱离 Retinal Detachment
754 视网膜中央动脉阻塞 Central Retinal Artery Occlusion
755 视网膜中央静脉阻塞 Central Retinal Vein Occlusion
756 室上性心动过速 Supraventricular Tachycardia
758 室性心动过速 Ventricular Tachycardia
761 嗜铬细胞瘤 Pheochromocytoma
763 手部感染 Hand Infection
765 手指骨损伤 Phalangeal Injuries, Hand
767 输血并发症 Transfusion Complications
769 束支传导阻滞 Bundle Branch Blocks
770 双硫仑样反应 Disulfiram Reaction
772 双相障碍 Bipolar Disorder

774 水痘 Varicella
776 水杨酸盐中毒 Salicylate Poisoning
778 水肿 Edema
779 睡眠呼吸暂停 Sleep Apnea
781 撕裂伤处理 Laceration Management
783 四肢穿透伤 Extremity Trauma，Penetrating
784 酸中毒 Acidosis
786 锁骨骨折 Clavicle Fracture

T

788 胎盘早剥 Placental Abruption
789 糖尿病(青少年) Diabetes Mellitus，Juvenile
791 糖尿病酮症酸中毒 Diabetic Ketoacidosis
793 泰瑟枪损伤 Taser Injuries
794 特发性颅内高压 Idiopathic Intracranial Hypertension
796 特发性血小板减少性紫癜 Idiopathic Thrombocytopenic Purpura
798 疼痛（原则、药物、舒适护理） Pain（Principles/Meds/Comfort Care）
800 体温过低 Hypothermia
802 体温过高 Hyperthermia
804 天疱疮 Pemphigus
806 铁中毒 Iron Poisoning
808 烃类物质中毒 Hydrocarbon Poisoning
809 痛风和假性痛风 Gout/Pseudogout
811 头部钝性伤 Head Trauma，Blunt
813 头痛 Headache
816 头晕/眩晕 Dizziness/Vertigo
818 透析并发症 Dialysis Complications
820 兔热病 Tularemia
822 退行性关节炎 Arthritis，Degenerative
823 吞咽困难 Dysphagia

W

826 外耳道炎 Otitis Externa
827 外耳道异物 Foreign Body，Ear
829 外耳软骨炎/脓肿 External Ear Chondritis/Abscess
830 腕骨骨折 Carpal Fractures
832 腕管综合征 Carpal Tunnel Syndrome
833 危险物暴露所致损伤 Hazmat
835 围生期心肌病 Cardiomyopathy，Peripartum
837 胃肠出血 Gastrointestinal Bleeding
839 胃肠炎 Gastroenteritis
841 胃出口梗阻 Gastric Outlet Obstruction
842 胃食管反流病 Gastroesophageal Reflux Disease
844 胃炎 Gastritis
846 喂养问题(儿童) Feeding Problems，Pediatric
848 蚊媒疾病：登革热、基孔肯亚病和西尼罗病毒感染 Mosquito-Borne Diseases：Dengue，Chikungunya，and West Nile Virus
850 无创呼吸机管理 Ventilation Management，Noninvasive
852 无力 Weakness

X

855 膝关节脱位 Knee Dislocation
856 系统性红斑狼疮 Systemic Lupus Erythematosus
858 细菌性气管炎 Bacterial Tracheitis
860 下颌骨骨折 Mandibular Fractures
861 先天性代谢缺陷 Inborn Errors of Metabolism
863 先天性巨结肠 Hirschsprung Disease
864 先天性心脏病(发绀型) Congenital Heart Disease，Cyanotic
867 先天性心脏病(无发绀型) Congenital Heart Disease，Acyanotic
868 纤维肌痛 Fibromyalgia
870 纤维囊性乳腺病 Fibrocystic Breast Changes
871 消化性溃疡 Peptic Ulcer
873 小肠损伤 Small-Bowel Injury
875 哮喘(成人) Asthma，Adult
877 哮喘(儿童) Asthma，Pediatric
879 蝎蜇伤 Sting，Scorpion
881 斜颈 Torticollis
882 心包积液/心脏压塞 Pericardial Effusion/Tamponade
884 心包炎 Pericarditis
886 心房颤动 Atrial Fibrillation
888 心房扑动 Atrial Flutter
891 心肌病 Cardiomyopathy
893 心肌挫伤 Myocardial Contusion
895 心肌炎 Myocarditis
897 心力衰竭 Heart Failure
900 心内膜炎 Endocarditis
902 心室颤动 Ventricular Fibrillation
904 心室停搏 Asystole
905 心源性休克 Cardiogenic Shock
906 心脏瓣膜病 Valvular Heart Disease
908 心脏检查 Cardiac Testing

911 心脏起搏器 Cardiac Pacemakers
912 心脏停搏 Cardiac Arrest
915 心脏移植术后并发症
Cardiac Transplantation Complications
917 心脏杂音 Heart Murmur
919 心脏再灌注治疗 Reperfusion Therapy, Cardiac
921 新生儿复苏 Resusicitation, Neonate
923 新生儿黄疸 Neonatal Jaundice
925 新生儿脓毒症 Neonatal Sepsis
927 新型口服抗凝剂并发症
Novel Oral Anticoagulant Complications
928 性病淋巴肉芽肿 Lymphogranuloma Venereum
929 性侵犯 Sexual Assault
932 胸廓出口综合征 Thoracic Outlet Syndrome
933 胸腔积液 Pleural Effusion
935 胸锁关节损伤 Sternoclavicular Joint Injury
937 胸痛 Chest Pain
939 胸外伤,穿通伤 Chest Trauma, Penetrating
941 胸外伤,钝器伤 Chest Trauma, Blunt
943 胸主动脉夹层 Aortic Dissection, Thoracic
945 休克 Shock
947 悬雍垂炎 Uvulitis
949 血管性水肿 Angioedema
951 血管性血友病 Von Willebrand Disease
953 血管炎 Vasculitis
955 血尿和蛋白尿 Hematuria/Proteinuria
957 血清病 Serum Sickness
958 血栓性血小板减少性紫癜
Thrombotic Thrombocytopenic Purpura
960 血胸 Hemothorax
962 血友病 Hemophilia
964 荨麻疹 Urticaria

Y

966 牙痛 Toothache
967 牙外伤 Dental Trauma
970 牙周脓肿 Periodontal Abscess
971 咽后脓肿 Retropharyngeal
973 咽峡炎 Ludwig Angina
975 咽炎 Pharyngitis
977 烟雾吸入 Smoke Inhalation
978 炎症性肠病 Inflammatory Bowel Disease
981 眼球破裂 Globe Rupture
982 摇头丸中毒 MDMA Poisoning
983 咬伤(人) Bite, Human
985 药物戒断 Withdrawal, Drug
986 一氧化碳中毒 Carbon Monoxide Poisoning
988 胰腺创伤 Pancreatic Trauma
989 胰腺炎 Pancreatitis
991 移植排斥 Transplant Rejection
994 乙烯乙二醇中毒 Ethylene Glycol Poisoning
996 异丙醇中毒 Isopropanol Poisoning
997 异常子宫出血 Uterine Bleeding, Abnormal
999 异位妊娠 Ectopic Pregnancy
1001 异烟肼中毒 Isoniazid Poisoning
1002 抑郁症 Depression
1004 阴道出血 Vaginal Bleeding
1006 阴道分泌物/阴道炎 Vaginal Discharge/Vaginitis
1008 阴茎持续勃起 Priapism
1010 阴茎折断 Penile Shaft Fracture
1011 银屑病 Psoriasis
1013 婴儿猝死 Sudden Infant Death Syndrome(SIDS)
1015 婴儿烦躁 Irritable Infant
1016 硬膜外脓肿 Epidural Abscess
1018 硬膜外血肿 Epidural Hematoma
1019 硬膜下血肿 Subdural Hematoma
1021 幽门狭窄 Pyloric Stenosis
1023 疣 Warts
1025 有机磷中毒 Organophosphate Poisoning
1027 幼儿皮疹 Rash, Pediatric
1029 幼年型特发性关节炎 Arthritis, Juvenile Idiopathic
1031 浴盐——合成卡西酮中毒
Bath Salts — Synthetic Cathinones Poisoning
1032 预激综合征 Wolff-Parkinson-White (WPW) Syndrome
1034 月骨脱位 Lunate Dislocation
1035 月骨周围脱位 Perilunate Dislocation
1036 晕厥 Syncope
1038 孕妇外伤 Pregnancy, Trauma In

Z

1041 谵妄 Delirium
1043 掌骨损伤 Metacarpal Injuries
1043 针刺伤 Needlestick
1045 镇静药中毒 Neuroleptic Poisoning
1047 支气管炎 Bronchitis
1049 脂溢性皮炎 Seborrheic Dermatitis

1051 蜘蛛咬伤(黑寡妇) Spider Bite, Black Widow
1053 蜘蛛咬伤(棕色隐士) Spider Bite, Brown Recluse
1055 直肠创伤 Rectal Trauma
1057 直肠脱垂 Rectal Prolapse
1058 直肠异物 Foreign Body, Rectal
1059 直肠周围脓肿 Perirectal Abscess
1060 植入式除颤器 Defibrillators, Implantable
1063 植物中毒 Plant Poisoning
1065 致幻剂中毒 Hallucinogen Poisoning
1066 痔 Hemorrhoid
1068 中毒 Poisoning
1070 中毒性表皮坏死松解症 Toxic Epidermal Necrolysis
1071 中毒性滑膜炎 Synovitis, Toxic
1073 中毒性休克综合征 Toxic Shock Syndrome
1075 中毒与解毒 Poisoning, Antidotes
1078 中毒与洗胃 Poisoning, Gastric Decontamination
1079 中毒与中毒综合征 Poisoning, Toxidromes
1081 中耳炎 Otitis Media
1083 肿瘤压迫综合征 Tumor Compression Syndromes
1085 重症肌无力 Myasthenia Gravis
1087 舟状骨骨折 Scaphoid Fracture
1088 周期性呕吐综合征 Vomiting, Cyclic
1089 周期性瘫痪 Periodic Paralysis
1092 周围神经疾病 Peripheral Neuropathy
1093 周围血管疾病 Peripheral Vascular Disease
1095 肘部损伤 Elbow Injuries
1097 蛛网膜下腔出血 Subarachnoid Hemorrhage
1099 主动脉闭塞 Arterial Occlusion
1101 椎基底动脉供血不足 Vertebrobasilar Insufficiency
1103 子宫内膜异位症 Endometriosis
1104 子痫前期和子痫 Preeclampsia/Eclampsia
1106 紫癜 Purpura
1108 紫外线角膜炎 Ultraviolet Keratitis
1109 自发性细菌性腹膜炎 Spontaneous Bacterial Peritonitis
1111 自然流产 Abortion, Spontaneous
1113 自杀,危险评估 Suicide, Risk Evaluation
1115 纵隔气肿 Pneumomediastinum
1117 足部骨折 Foot Fracture
1118 足趾骨受伤 Phalangeal Injuries, Foot
1119 左心室装置急诊 Left Ventricular Device Emergencies
1121 坐骨神经痛/椎间盘突出 Sciatica/Herniated Disc

1123 **附录**
1123 急诊用药
1126 快速序列插管(RSI)
1126 镇静和诱导剂
1127 儿科生命体征和复苏设备尺寸
1127 温度换算：摄氏度↔华氏度
1128 重量换算：磅(lb)↔千克(kg)

目录 2

症状和体征

35 背痛 Back Pain
45 鼻出血 Epistaxis
90 喘鸣 Stridor
115 单关节性关节炎 Arthritis，Monoarticular
167 呃逆 Hiccups
321 儿童呼吸暂停 Apnea，Pediatric
174 发绀 Cyanosis
176 发热(成人) Fever，Adult
178 发热(儿童) Fever，Pediatric
182 反应性关节炎 Reactive Arthritis
206 风湿性关节炎 Arthritis，Rheumatoid
227 腹痛 Abdominal Pain
272 共济失调 Ataxia
292 过度通气综合征 Hyperventilation Syndrome
294 过敏 Anaphylaxis
305 红眼 Red Eye
317 呼吸窘迫 Respiratory Distress
319 呼吸困难 Dyspnea
341 幻觉 Hallucinations
343 黄疸 Jaundice
348 昏迷 Coma
417 焦虑症 Agitation
446 精神状态改变 Altered Mental Status
481 咳嗽 Cough
472 咯血 Hemoptysis
605 脓毒性关节炎 Arthritis，Septic
607 脓毒症 Sepsis
617 呕吐(成人) Vomiting，Adult
619 呕吐(儿童) Vomiting，Pediatric
635 疲乏 Fatigue
649 气喘 Wheezing
650 气道辅助装置 Airway Adjuncts
652 气道管理 Airway Management
964 荨麻疹 Urticaria
699 瘙痒 Pruritus
736 失血性休克 Hemorrhagic Shock
749 视觉丧失 Visual Loss
778 水肿 Edema
798 疼痛(原则/药物/舒适护理) Pain (Principles/Meds/Comfort Care)
813 头痛 Headache
816 头晕/眩晕 Dizziness/Vertigo
822 退行性关节炎 Arthritis，Degenerative
823 吞咽困难 Dysphagia
852 无力 Weakness
912 心脏停搏 Cardiac Arrest
937 胸痛 Chest Pain
945 休克 Shock
949 血管性水肿 Angioedema
1006 阴道分泌物/阴道炎 Vaginal Discharge/Vaginitis
1015 婴儿烦躁 Irritable Infant
1029 幼年型特发性关节炎 Arthritis，Juvenile Idiopathic
1036 晕厥 Syncope
1088 周期性呕吐综合征 Vomiting，Cyclic
1106 紫癜 Purpura

心脏急症

2 Brugada 综合征 Brugada Syndrome

5 QT 间期延长综合征 QT Syndrome，Prolonged
59 病态窦房结综合征 Sick Sinus Syndrome
144 动脉导管未闭 Patent Ductus Arteriosus
172 二尖瓣脱垂 Mitral Valve Prolapse
183 房室传导阻滞 Atrioventricular Blocks
187 肥厚型心肌病 Cardiomyopathy，Hypertrophic
200 肺源性心脏病 Cor Pulmonale
205 风湿热 Rheumatic Fever
258 高血压急症 Hypertensive Emergencies
338 缓慢性心律失常 Bradyarrhythmias
362 急性冠脉综合征：冠状动脉血管痉挛 Acute Coronary Syndrome：Coronary Vasospasm
364 急性冠脉综合征：无 Q 波(非 ST 段抬高)心肌梗死 Acute Coronary Syndrome：Non-Q-Wave(Non-ST-Elevation) MI
366 急性冠脉综合征：心肌梗死 Acute Coronary Syndrome：Myocardial Infarction
368 急性冠脉综合征：心绞痛 Acute Coronary Syndrome：Angina
490 快速节律障碍 Tachydysrhythmias
577 脑再灌注治疗 Reperfusion Therapy，Cerebral
756 室上性心动过速 Supraventricular Tachycardia
758 室性心动过速 Ventricular Tachycardia
769 束支传导阻滞 Bundle Branch Blocks
835 围生期心肌病 Cardiomyopathy，Peripartum
864 先天性心脏病(发绀型) Congenital Heart Disease，Cyanotic
867 先天性心脏病(无发绀型) Congenital Heart Disease，Acyanotic
882 心包积液/心脏压塞 Pericardial Effusion/Tamponade
884 心包炎 Pericarditis
886 心房颤动 Atrial Fibrillation
888 心房扑动 Atrial Flutter
891 心肌病 Cardiomyopathy
895 心肌炎 Myocarditis
897 心力衰竭 Heart Failure
900 心内膜炎 Endocarditis
902 心室颤动 Ventricular Fibrillation
904 心室停搏 Asystole
905 心源性休克 Cardiogenic Shock
906 心脏瓣膜病 Valvular Heart Disease
908 心脏检查 Cardiac Testing
911 心脏起搏器 Cardiac Pacemakers
912 心脏停搏 Cardiac Arrest
915 心脏移植术后并发症 Cardiac Transplantation Complications
917 心脏杂音 Heart Murmur
919 心脏再灌注治疗 Reperfusion Therapy，Cardiac
937 胸痛 Chest Pain
1032 预激综合征 Wolff-Parkinson-White (WPW) Syndrome
1060 植入式除颤器 Defibrillators，Implantable
1119 左心室装置(急诊) Left Ventricular Device Emergencies

皮肤、软组织急症

87 传染性红斑 Erythema Infectiosum
88 传染性软疣 Molluscum Contagiosum
107 带状疱疹 Herpes Zoster
109 丹毒 Erysipelas
113 单纯疱疹 Herpes Simplex
165 多形红斑 Erythema Multiforme
209 蜂窝织炎 Cellulitis
219 富尼埃坏疽 Fournier Gangrene
332 坏疽 Gangrene
334 坏死性软组织感染 Necrotizing Soft Tissue Infections
392 甲沟炎 Paronychia
424 接触性皮炎 Contact Dermatitis
431 结节性红斑 Erythema Nodosum
434 疥疮 Scabies
487 口腔念珠菌病 Candidiasis，Oral
519 淋巴管炎 Lymphangitis
521 淋巴结炎 Lymphadenitis
540 玫瑰糠疹 Pityriasis Rosea
589 尿布疹 Diaper Rash
609 脓疱病 Impetigo
627 皮肤或软组织脓肿 Abscess，Skin/Soft Tissue
629 皮肤癣 Tinea Infections，Cutaneous
632 皮疹 Rash
645 葡萄球菌烫伤样皮肤综合征 Staphylococcal Scalded Skin Syndrome
964 荨麻疹 Urticaria
690 乳腺炎 Mastitis
641 软下疳 Chancroid
699 瘙痒 Pruritus
734 生殖器疱疹 Herpes，Genital
738 虱病 Pediculosis
740 湿疹/特应性皮炎 Eczema/Atopic Dermatitis
741 史-约综合征 Stevens-Johnson Syndrome
763 手部感染 Hand Infection

781 撕裂伤处理 Laceration Management
804 天疱疮 Pemphigus
829 外耳软骨炎/脓肿 External Ear Chondritis/Abscess
870 纤维囊性乳腺病 Fibrocystic Breast Changes
928 性病淋巴肉芽肿 Lymphogranuloma Venereum
1011 银屑病 Psoriasis
1023 疣 Warts
1027 幼儿皮疹 Rash, Pediatric
1043 针刺伤 Needlestick
1049 脂溢性皮炎 Seborrheic Dermatitis
1070 中毒性表皮坏死松解症 Toxic Epidermal Necrolysis

内分泌急症

393 甲状旁腺功能减退症 Hypoparathyroidism
395 甲状旁腺功能亢进症 Hyperparathyroidism
397 甲状腺功能减退症 Hypothyroidism
399 甲状腺功能亢进症 Hyperthyroidism
477 抗利尿素分泌异常症 Syndrome of Inappropriate Antidiuretic Hormone Secretion (SIADH)
488 库欣综合征 Cushing Syndrome
587 尿崩症 Diabetes Insipidus
720 肾上腺功能减退症 Adrenal Insufficiency
761 嗜铬细胞瘤 Pheochromocytoma
789 糖尿病(青少年) Diabetes Mellitus, Juvenile
791 糖尿病酮症酸中毒 Diabetic Ketoacidosis
1089 周期性瘫痪 Periodic Paralysis

环境突发情况

141 电击伤 Electrical Injury
145 动脉气体栓塞 Arterial Gas Embolism (AGE)
146 动物咬伤 Bite, Animal
150 冻伤 Frostbite
212 辐射损伤 Radiation Injury
260 高压氧治疗 Hyperbaric Oxygen Therapy
261 高原病 High-Altitude Illness
299 海洋生物蜇伤 Marine Envenomation
408 减压病 Decompression Sickness
551 蜜蜂蜇伤 Sting, Bee
589 溺水 Drowning
656 气压伤 Barotrauma
701 闪电击伤 Lightning Injuries
707 蛇毒液螫伤 Snake Envenomation
800 体温过低 Hypothermia
802 体温过高 Hyperthermia
833 危险物暴露所致损伤 Hazmat
879 蝎蜇伤 Sting, Scorpion
977 烟雾吸入 Smoke Inhalation
983 咬伤(人) Bite, Human
1051 蜘蛛咬伤,黑寡妇 Spider Bite, Black Widow
1053 蜘蛛咬伤,棕色隐士 Spider Bite, Brown Recluse

胃肠道急症

38 贲门黏膜撕裂综合征 Mallory-Weiss Syndrome
56 便秘 Constipation
62 布尔哈夫综合征 Boerhaave Syndrome
69 肠梗阻(小肠和大肠) Bowel Obstruction (Small and Large)
71 肠扭转 Volvulus
74 肠套叠 Intussusception
76 肠系膜缺血 Mesenteric Ischemia
73 肠旋转不良 Malrotation
78 肠易激综合征 Irritable Bowel Syndrome
119 胆管炎 Cholangitis
121 胆结石 Cholelithiasis
122 胆囊炎 Cholecystitis
124 胆石性肠梗阻 Gallstone Ileus
214 腐蚀性化学物中毒 Caustic Ingestion
225 腹腔积液 Ascites
230 腹泻(成人) Diarrhea, Adult
231 腹泻(儿童) Diarrhea, Pediatric
237 肝肾综合征 Hepatorenal Syndrome
240 肝性脑病 Hepatic Encephalopathy
243 肝炎 Hepatitis
244 肝硬化 Cirrhosis
247 肛裂 Anal Fissure
290 管饲并发症 Feeding Tube Complications
462 静脉曲张 Varices
501 阑尾炎 Appendicitis
544 梅克尔憩室 Meckel Diverticulum
582 内脏穿孔 Perforated Viscous
617 呕吐(成人) Vomiting, Adult
619 呕吐(儿童) Vomiting, Pediatric
657 憩室病 Diverticulosis
659 憩室炎 Diverticulitis
703 疝 Hernias
747 食管异物 Foreign Body, Esophageal

823 吞咽困难 Dysphagia
837 胃肠出血 Gastrointestinal Bleeding
839 胃肠炎 Gastroenteritis
841 胃出口梗阻 Gastric Outlet Obstruction
842 胃食管反流病 Gastroesophageal Reflux Disease
844 胃炎 Gastritis
863 先天性巨结肠 Hirschsprung Disease
871 消化性溃疡 Peptic Ulcer
978 炎症性肠病 Inflammatory Bowel Disease
989 胰腺炎 Pancreatitis
1057 直肠脱垂 Rectal Prolapse
1058 直肠异物 Foreign Body, Rectal
1059 直肠周围脓肿 Perirectal Abscess
1066 痔 Hemorrhoid
1088 周期性呕吐综合征 Vomiting, Cyclic
1109 自发性细菌性腹膜炎 Spontaneous Bacterial Peritonitis

泌尿生殖系统急症

25 包茎 Phimosis
26 包皮嵌顿 Paraphimosis
216 附睾炎和睾丸炎 Epididymitis/Orchitis
219 富尼埃坏疽 Fournier Gangrene
263 睾丸扭转 Testicular Torsion
542 梅毒 Syphilis
591 尿道创伤 Urethral Trauma
592 尿道瘘 Urinary Tract Fistula
593 尿道炎 Urethritis
595 尿路感染(成人) Urinary Tract Infections, Adult
597 尿路感染(儿童) Urinary Tract Infections, Pediatric
599 尿潴留 Urinary Retention
666 前列腺炎 Prostatitis
672 鞘膜积液 Hydrocele
691 软下疳 Chancroid
734 生殖器疱疹 Herpes, Genital
928 性病淋巴肉芽肿 Lymphogranuloma Venereum
955 血尿和蛋白尿 Hematuria/Proteinuria
1008 阴茎持续勃起 Priapism
1010 阴茎折断 Penile Shaft Fracture

妇科急症

53 闭经 Amenorrhea
523 淋病 Gonococcal Disease
529 卵巢囊肿/扭转 Ovarian Cyst/Torsion
537 毛滴虫病 Trichomonas
625 盆腔炎 Pelvic Inflammatory Disease
667 前庭大腺脓肿 Bartholin Abscess
684 妊娠期阴道出血 Vaginal Bleeding in Pregnancy
690 乳腺炎 Mastitis
734 生殖器疱疹 Herpes, Genital
810 纤维囊性乳腺病 Fibrocystic Breast Changes
929 性侵犯 Sexual Assault
997 异常子宫出血 Uterine Bleeding, Abnormal
1004 阴道出血 Vaginal Bleeding
1006 阴道分泌物/阴道炎 Vaginal Discharge/Vaginitis
1103 子宫内膜异位症 Endometriosis

头颈部急症

31 爆裂性骨折 Blow-Out Fracture
34 贝尔麻痹 Bell's Palsy
45 鼻出血 Epistaxis
47 鼻窦炎 Sinusitis
49 鼻骨骨折 Nasal Fractures
51 鼻腔异物 Foreign Body, Nasal
54 扁桃体周脓肿 Peritonsillar Abscess
170 耳外伤 Otologic Trauma
287 鼓膜穿孔 Tympanic Membrane Perforation
298 海绵窦血栓 Cavernous Sinus Thrombosis
313 喉炎 Laryngitis
345 会厌炎(成人) Epiglottitis, Adult
347 会厌炎(儿童) Epiglottitis, Pediatric
450 颈部腺炎 Cervical Adenitis
485 口腔溃疡 Aphthous Ulcers
527 颅脑穿透伤 Head Trauma, Penetrating
546 梅尼埃病 Ménière Disease
556 面部骨折 Facial Fractures
580 内耳迷路炎 Labyrinthitis
601 颞下颌关节损伤/综合征
Temporal-Mandibular Joint Injury/Syndrome
688 乳突炎 Mastoiditis
811 头部钝性伤 Head Trauma, Blunt
826 外耳道炎 Otitis Externa
827 外耳道异物 Foreign Body, Ear
829 外耳软骨炎/脓肿 External Ear Chondritis/Abscess
860 下颌骨骨折 Mandibular Fractures
881 斜颈 Torticollis
947 悬雍垂炎 Uvulitis

949 血管性水肿 Angioedema
966 牙痛 Toothache
967 牙外伤 Dental Trauma
970 牙周脓肿 Periodontal Abscess
971 咽后脓肿 Retropharyngeal Abscess
973 咽峡炎 Ludwig Angina
975 咽炎 Pharyngitis
1081 中耳炎 Otitis Media

血液科急症

20 白细胞增多症 Leukocytosis
3 HELLP 综合征 HELLP Syndrome
303 红细胞增多症 Polycythemia
516 镰状细胞病 Sickle Cell Disease
549 弥散性血管内凝血 Disseminated Intravascular Coagulation
602 凝血病逆转(非华法林药物所致)
Coagulopathy Reversal (Nonwarfarin Agents)
640 贫血 Anemia
767 输血并发症 Transfusion Complications
796 特发性血小板减少性紫癜
Idiopathic Thrombocytopenic Purpura
951 血管性血友病 Von Willebrand Disease
958 血栓性血小板减少性紫癜
Thrombotic Thrombocytopenic Purpura
962 血友病 Hemophilia

免疫系统急症

294 过敏 Anaphylaxis
352 机会性感染 Opportunistic Infections
511 粒细胞减少症 Granulocytopenia
554 免疫抑制 Immunosuppression
679 人类免疫缺陷病毒/获得性免疫缺陷综合征 HIV/AIDS
699 瘙痒 Pruritus
796 特发性血小板减少性紫癜
Idiopathic Thrombocytopenic Purpura
856 系统性红斑狼疮 Systemic Lupus Erythematosus
949 血管性水肿 Angioedema
953 血管炎 Vasculitis
957 血清病 Serum Sickness
991 移植排斥 Transplant Rejection

传染病急症

11 阿米巴病 Amebiasis
14 埃立克体病 Ehrlichiosis
17 巴贝西虫病 Babesiosis
20 白细胞增多症 Leukocytosis
23 百日咳 Pertussis
27 孢子丝菌病 Sporotrichosis
47 鼻窦炎 Sinusitis
83 出血热 Hemorrhagic Fevers
85 川崎病 Kawasaki Disease
107 带状疱疹 Herpes Zoster
113 单纯疱疹 Herpes Simplex
118 单核细胞增多症 Mononucleosis
125 登革热 Dengue Fever
189 肺孢子虫病 Pneumocystis Pneumonia
196 肺炎(成人) Pneumonia, Adult
198 肺炎(儿童) Pneumonia, Pediatric
205 风湿热 Rheumatic Fever
208 风疹 Rubella
209 蜂窝织炎 Cellulitis
216 附睾炎和睾丸炎 Epididymitis/Orchitis
219 富尼埃坏疽 Fournier Gangrene
266 弓形虫病 Toxoplasmosis
281 骨髓炎 Osteomyelitis
333 坏死溃疡性龈炎 Necrotizing Ulcerative Gingivitis
334 坏死性软组织感染 Necrotizing Soft Tissue Infections
345 会厌炎(成人) Epiglottitis, Adult
347 会厌炎(儿童) Epiglottitis, Pediatric
374 脊髓灰质炎 Polio
402 贾第虫病 Giardiasis
427 结核 Tuberculosis
450 颈部腺炎 Cervical Adenitis
495 狂犬病 Rabies
498 眶周和眼眶蜂窝织炎 Periorbital and Orbital Cellulitis
500 莱姆病 Lyme Disease
518 链球菌病 Streptococcal Disease
519 淋巴管炎 Lymphangitis
521 淋巴结炎 Lymphadenitis
523 淋病 Gonococcal Disease
525 流感 Influenza
530 落基山斑疹热 Rocky Mountain Spotted Fever
533 麻疹 Measles
537 毛滴虫病 Trichomonas
541 玫瑰疹 Roseola
542 梅毒 Syphilis

553 免疫 Immunizations
567 脑膜炎 Meningitis
570 脑膜炎球菌血症 Meningococcemia
576 脑炎 Encephalitis
593 尿道炎 Urethritis
595 尿路感染(成人) Urinary Tract Infections, Adult
597 尿路感染(儿童) Urinary Tract Infections, Pediatric
607 脓毒症 Sepsis
609 脓疱病 Impetigo
610 疟疾 Malaria
625 盆腔炎 Pelvic Inflammatory Disease
627 皮肤或软组织脓肿 Abscess, Skin/Soft Tissue
629 皮肤癣 Tinea Infections, Cutaneous
632 皮疹 Rash
638 蜱咬伤 Tick Bite
643 破伤风 Tetanus
645 葡萄球菌烫伤样皮肤综合征 Staphylococcal Scalded Skin Syndrome
666 前列腺炎 Prostatitis
686 肉毒中毒 Botulism
688 乳突炎 Mastoiditis
690 乳腺炎 Mastitis
691 软下疳 Chancroid
695 腮腺炎 Mumps
709 社区获得性耐甲氧西林金黄色葡萄球菌感染 MRSA, Community Acquired
734 生殖器疱疹 Herpes, Genital
741 史-约综合征 Stevens-Johnson Syndrome
763 手部感染 Hand Infection
774 水痘 Varicella
820 兔热病 Tularemia
848 蚊媒疾病:登革热、基孔肯亚病和西尼罗病毒感染 Mosquito-Borne Diseases: Dengue, Chikungunya, and West Nile Virus
895 心肌炎 Myocarditis
900 心内膜炎 Endocarditis
928 性病淋巴肉芽肿 Lymphogranuloma Venereum
975 咽炎 Pharyngitis
1043 针刺伤 Needlestick
1070 中毒性表皮坏死松解症 Toxic Epidermal Necrolysis
1073 中毒性休克综合征 Toxic Shock Syndrome

代谢急症

126 低钙血症 Hypocalcemia
129 低钾血症 Hypokalemia
130 低钠血症 Hyponatremia
132 低血糖 Hypoglycemia
248 高钙血症 Hypercalcemia
250 高钾血症 Hyperkalemia
251 高钠血症 Hypernatremia
254 高渗综合征 Hyperosmolar Syndrome
411 碱中毒 Alkalosis
465 酒精性酮症酸中毒 Alcoholic Ketoacidosis
784 酸中毒 Acidosis
791 糖尿病酮症酸中毒 Diabetic Ketoacidosis

神经系统急症

34 贝尔麻痹 Bell's Palsy
80 痴呆 Dementia
104 丛集性头痛 Headache, Cluster
137 癫痫发作(成人) Seizure, Adult
139 癫痫发作(儿童) Seizure, Pediatric
148 动眼神经麻痹 Oculomotor Nerve Palsy
154 短暂性脑缺血发作 Transient Ischemic Attack
157 短暂性全面性遗忘症 Transient Global Amnesia
162 多发性神经病 Polyneuropathy
163 多发性硬化 Multiple Sclerosis
180 发热性癫痫(高热惊厥) Seizure, Febrile
218 复视 Diplopia
298 海绵窦血栓 Cavernous Sinus Thrombosis
348 昏迷 Coma
350 霍纳综合征 Horner Syndrome
357 肌萎缩侧索硬化症 Amyotrophic Lateral Sclerosis
359 肌张力障碍反应 Dystonic Reaction
360 吉兰-巴雷综合征 Guillain-Barr'e Syndrome
376 脊髓综合征 Spinal Cord Syndromes
469 巨细胞动脉炎 Giant Cell Arteritis
534 马尾综合征 Cauda Equina Syndrome
562 脑出血 Intracerebral Hemorrhage
564 脑动脉瘤 Cerebral Aneurysm
566 脑积水 Hydrocephalus
572 脑室腹膜分流 Ventricular Peritoneal Shunts
573 脑血管意外 Cerebral Vascular Accident
576 脑炎 Encephalitis
577 脑再灌注治疗 Reperfusion Therapy, Cerebral
621 帕金森病 Parkinson Disease
639 偏头痛 Headache, Migraine

696 三叉神经痛 Trigeminal Neuralgia
714 神经阻滞剂恶性综合征 Neuroleptic Malignant Syndrome
794 特发性颅内高压 Idiopathic Intracranial Hypertension
813 头痛 Headache
852 无力 Weakness
1016 硬膜外脓肿 Epidural Abscess
1018 硬膜外血肿 Epidural Hematoma
1041 谵妄 Delirium
1085 重症肌无力 Myasthenia Gravis
1089 周期性瘫痪 Periodic Paralysis
1092 周围神经疾病 Peripheral Neuropathy
1097 蛛网膜下腔出血 Subarachnoid Hemorrhage
1101 椎基底动脉供血不足 Vertebrobasilar Insufficiency

非创伤性肌肉骨骼急症

35 背痛 Back Pain
79 成骨不全症 Osteogenesis Imperfecta
115 单关节性关节炎 Arthritis，Monoarticular
182 反应性关节炎 Reactive Arthritis
206 风湿性关节炎 Arthritis，Rheumatoid
274 股骨干滑脱 Slipped Capital Femoral Epiphysis
277 股骨头骨骺炎 Legg-Calvé-Perthes Disease
281 骨髓炎 Osteomyelitis
285 骨质疏松症 Osteoporosis
301 横纹肌溶解 Rhabdomyolysis
325 滑囊炎 Bursitis
337 环/束带移除损伤 Ring/Constricting Band Removal
355 肌腱炎 Tendonitis
377 脊椎滑脱和脊椎前移 Spondylolysis/Spondylolisthesis
392 甲沟炎 Paronychia
413 腱鞘炎 Tenosynovitis
455 胫骨粗隆骨软骨病 Osgood-Schlatter Disease
605 脓毒性关节炎 Arthritis，Septic
623 佩吉特病 Paget Disease
631 皮肌炎和多肌炎 Dermatomyositis/Polymyositis
670 强直性脊柱炎 Ankylosing Spondylitis
809 痛风和假性痛风 Gout/Pseudogout
822 退行性关节炎 Arthritis，Degenerative
832 腕管综合征 Carpal Tunnel Syndrome
868 纤维肌痛 Fibromyalgia
1029 幼年型特发性关节炎 Arthritis，Juvenile Idiopathic
1071 中毒性滑膜炎 Synovitis，Toxic
1121 坐骨神经痛/椎间盘突出 Sciatica/Herniated Disc

产科急症

3 HELLP 综合征 HELLP Syndrome
65 产后出血 Postpartum Hemorrhage
67 产后感染 Postpartum Infection
202 分娩(无并发症) Delivery，Uncomplicated
203 分娩(早产和胎膜早破) Labor
436 紧急剖宫产 Cesarean Section，Emergency
646 葡萄胎 Hydatidiform Mole
669 前置胎盘 Placenta Previa
681 妊娠(无并发症) Pregnancy，Uncomplicated
682 妊娠剧吐 Hyperemesis Gravidarum
684 妊娠期阴道出血 Vaginal Bleeding in Pregnancy
788 胎盘早剥 Placental Abruption
835 围生期心肌病 Cardiomyopathy，Peripartum
999 异位妊娠 Ectopic Pregnancy
1038 孕妇外伤 Pregnancy，Trauma In
1104 子痫前期和子痫 Preeclampsia/Eclampsia
1111 自然流产 Abortion，Spontaneous

肿瘤急症

22 白血病 Leukemia
160 多发性骨髓瘤 Multiple Myeloma
253 高黏滞综合征 Hyperviscosity Syndrome
1083 肿瘤压迫综合征 Tumor Compression Syndromes

眼科急症

61 玻璃体出血 Vitreous Hemorrhage
218 复视 Diplopia
305 红眼 Red Eye
308 虹膜炎 Iritis
409 睑腺炎和睑板腺囊肿 Hordeolum and Chalazion
419 角膜擦伤 Corneal Abrasion
420 角膜异物 Corneal Foreign Body
422 角膜灼伤 Corneal Burn
432 结膜炎 Conjunctivitis
496 眶后血肿 Retro-Orbital Hematoma
498 眶周和眼眶蜂窝织炎 Periorbital and Orbital Cellulitis
508 泪囊炎和泪腺炎 Dacryocystitis and Dacryoadenitis
664 前房积血 Hyphema
673 青光眼 Glaucoma
749 视觉丧失 Visual Loss
751 视神经炎 Optic Neuritis

753 视网膜脱离 Retinal Detachment
754 视网膜中央动脉阻塞 Central Retinal Artery Occlusion
755 视网膜中央静脉阻塞 Central Retinal Vein Occlusion
947 悬雍垂炎 Uvulitis
981 眼球破裂 Globe Rupture
1108 紫外线角膜炎 Ultraviolet Keratitis

骨伤

58 髌骨损伤 Patellar Injuries
98 创伤性断肢/再植 Traumatic Amputation/Replantation
134 骶骨骨折 Sacral Fracture
182 反应性关节炎 Reactive Arthritis
268 肱骨骨折 Humerus Fracture
275 股骨骨折 Femur Fracture
278 骨骺骨折 Epiphyseal Injuries
279 骨盆骨折 Pelvic Fracture
288 关节损伤 Knee Injury
329 踝关节骨折/脱位 Ankle Fracture/Dislocation
331 踝关节扭伤 Ankle Sprain
379 脊椎损伤(成人,颈部) Spine Injury: Cervical, Adult
381 脊椎损伤(儿童,颈部) Spine Injury: Cervical, Pediatric
382 脊椎损伤(尾骨) Spine Injury: Coccyx
383 脊椎损伤(胸部) Spine Injury: Thoracic
385 脊椎损伤(腰部) Spine Injury: Lumbar
405 肩关节脱位 Shoulder Dislocation
406 肩锁关节损伤 Acromioclavicular Joint Injury
456 胫骨和腓骨骨折 Tibial/Fibular Shaft Fracture
458 胫骨平台骨折 Tibial Plateau Fracture
475 开放性骨折 Fracture, Open
493 髋部损伤 Hip Injury
558 拇指骨折 Thumb Fracture
663 前臂骨干/远端骨折 Forearm Fracture, Shaft/Distal
678 桡骨小头半脱位(保姆肘) Nursemaid's Elbow
763 手部感染 Hand Infection
765 手指骨损伤 Phalangeal Injuries, Hand
786 锁骨骨折 Clavicle Fracture
830 腕骨骨折 Carpal Fractures
855 膝关节脱位 Knee Dislocation
935 胸锁关节损伤 Sternoclavicular Joint Injury
1034 月骨脱位 Lunate Dislocation
1035 月骨周围脱位 Perilunate Dislocation
1043 掌骨损伤 Metacarpal Injuries
1087 舟状骨骨折 Scaphoid Fracture
1095 肘部损伤 Elbow Injuries
1117 足部骨折 Foot Fracture
1118 足趾骨受伤 Phalangeal Injuries, Foot

小儿急症

23 百日咳 Pertussis
73 肠旋转不良 Malrotation
74 肠套叠 Intussusception
85 川崎病 Kawasaki Disease
93 创伤(儿童) Pediatric Trauma
139 癫痫发作(儿童) Seizure, Pediatric
144 动脉导管未闭 Patent Ductus Arteriosus
168 儿科复苏 Resusicitation, Pediatric
178 发热(儿童) Fever, Pediatric
180 发热性癫痫(高热惊厥) Seizure, Febrile
196 腹泻(成人) Diarrhea, Adult
198 肺炎(儿童) Pneumonia, Pediatric
278 骨骺骨折 Epiphyseal Injuries
283 骨折(儿童) Fractures, Pediatric
295 过敏性紫癜 Henoch-Schönlein Purpura
311 喉头炎 Croup
321 呼吸暂停(儿童) Apnea, Pediatric
347 会厌炎(儿童) Epiglottitis, Pediatric
381 脊椎损伤(儿童,颈部) Spine Injury: Cervical, Pediatric
560 囊性纤维化 Cystic Fibrosis
589 尿布疹 Diaper Rash
579 尿路感染(儿童) Urinary Tract Infections, Pediatric
613 虐待(儿童,非意外性创伤)
Abuse, Pediatric (Nonaccidental Trauma, NAT)
619 呕吐(儿童) Vomiting, Pediatric
645 葡萄球菌烫伤样皮肤综合征
Staphylococcal Scalded Skin Syndrome
672 鞘膜积液 Hydrocele
678 桡骨小头半脱位(保姆肘) Nursemaid's Elbow
692 瑞氏综合征 Reye Syndrome
732 生长发育滞缓 Failure to Thrive
789 糖尿病(青少年) Diabetes Mellitus, Juvenile
846 喂养问题(儿童) Feeding Problems, Pediatric
858 细菌性气管炎 Bacterial Tracheitis
861 先天性代谢缺陷 Inborn Errors of Metabolism
863 先天性巨结肠 Hirschsprung Disease
877 哮喘(儿童) Asthma, Pediatric
921 新生儿复苏 Resusicitation, Neonate

923 新生儿黄疸 Neonatal Jaundice
925 新生儿脓毒症 Neonatal Sepsis
1013 婴儿猝死 Sudden Infant Death Syndrome (SIDS)
1015 婴儿烦躁 Irritable Infant
1021 幽门狭窄 Pyloric Stenosis
1027 幼儿皮疹 Rash, Pediatric
1047 支气管炎 Bronchitis

心理行为急症

29 暴力管理 Violence, Management of
97 创伤后应激障碍 Post-Traumatic Stress Disorder (PTSD)
341 幻觉 Hallucinations
359 肌张力障碍反应 Dystonic Reaction
370 急性精神病 Psychosis, Acute
387 家庭暴力 Domestic Violence
417 焦虑症 Agitation
438 进食障碍 Eating Disorders
440 惊恐发作 Panic Attack
442 精神分裂症 Schizophrenia
444 精神症状的躯体因素和精神因素 Psychosis, Medical vs. Psychiatric
464 酒精戒断 Withdrawal, Alcohol
548 孟乔森综合征(做作性障碍) Munchausen Syndrome (Factitious Disorder)
613 虐待(儿童,非意外性创伤) Abuse, Pediatric (Nonaccidental Trauma, NAT)
615 虐待(老年人) Abuse, Elder
772 双相障碍 Bipolar Disorder
985 药物戒断 Withdrawal, Drug
1002 抑郁症 Depression
1041 谵妄 Delirium
1113 自杀,危险评估 Suicide, Risk Evaluation

胸肺部急症

184 非心源性肺水肿 Noncardiogenic Pulmonary Edema
189 肺孢子虫病 Pneumocystis Pneumonia
191 肺栓塞 Pulmonary Embolism
193 肺水肿 Pulmonary Edema
196 肺炎(成人) Pneumonia, Adult
198 肺炎(儿童) Pneumonia, Pediatric
200 肺源性心脏病 Cor Pulmonale
311 喉头炎 Croup
314 呼吸机管理 Ventilator Management
319 呼吸困难 Dyspnea
427 结核 Tuberculosis
429 结节病 Sarcoidosis
535 慢性阻塞性肺疾病 Chronic Obstructive Pulmonary Disease
538 毛细支气管炎 Bronchiolitis
560 囊性纤维化 Cystic Fibrosis
650 气道辅助装置 Airway Adjuncts
652 气道管理 Airway Management
654 气胸 Pneumothorax
779 睡眠呼吸暂停 Sleep Apnea
850 无创呼吸机管理 Ventilation Management, Noninvasive
858 细菌性气管炎 Bacterial Tracheitis
875 哮喘(成人) Asthma, Adult
877 哮喘(儿童) Asthma, Pediatric
932 胸廓出口综合征 Thoracic Outlet Syndrome
933 胸腔积液 Pleural Effusion
1047 支气管炎 Bronchitis
1115 纵隔气肿 Pneumomediastinum

肾脏科急症

301 横纹肌溶解 Rhabdomyolysis
372 急性肾损伤 Kidney Injury, Acute
716 肾病综合征 Nephrotic Syndrome
718 肾结石 Renal Calculus
724 肾小球肾炎 Glomerulonephritis
726 肾炎综合征 Nephritic Syndrome
728 肾盂肾炎 Pyelonephritis
818 透析并发症 Dialysis Complications
955 血尿和蛋白尿 Hematuria/Proteinuria

毒理学相关急症

1 5-羟色胺综合征(药物诱导) Serotonin Syndrome (Drug-Induced)
13 阿片类药物中毒 Opiate Poisoning
19 巴比妥中毒 Barbiturates Poisoning
39 苯丙胺中毒 Amphetamine Poisoning
41 苯二氮䓬类药物中毒 Benzodiazepine Poisoning
43 苯环己哌啶中毒 Phencyclidine Poisoning
44 苯妥英中毒 Phenytoin Poisoning
64 茶碱中毒 Theophyline Poisoning
102 刺激性气体暴露 Irritant Gas Exposure
106 大麻素和合成大麻素中毒 Cannabinoids and Synthetic Cannabinoids Poisoning

111 单胺氧化酶抑制药中毒 Monoamine Oxidase Inhibitor Poisoning
135 地高辛中毒 Digoxin, Poisoning
152 毒蕈中毒 Mushroom Poisoning
158 对乙酰氨基酚中毒 Acetaminophen Poisoning
186 非甾体抗炎药中毒 Nonsteroidal Anti-Inflammatory Poisoning
214 腐蚀性化学物中毒 Caustic Ingestion
236 钙通道阻滞剂中毒 Calcium Channel Blocker Poisoning
256 高铁血红蛋白血症 Methemoglobinemia
270 汞中毒 Mercury Poisoning
323 华法林的并发症 Warfarin Complications
327 化学武器中毒 Chemical Weapons Poisoning
388 甲苯中毒 Toluene Poisoning
390 甲醇中毒 Methanol Poisoning
415 降糖药中毒 Hypoglycemic Agent Poisoning
467 酒精中毒 Alcohol Poisoning
471 卡马西平中毒 Carbamazepine Poisoning
476 抗胆碱能药中毒 Anticholinergic Poisoning
479 抗抑郁药中毒 Antidepressant Poisoning
483 可卡因中毒 Cocaine Poisoning
504 滥用大麻 Marijuana Abuse
510 锂中毒 Lithium Poisoning
551 蜜蜂蜇伤 Sting, Bee
583 拟交感神经药中毒 Sympathomimetic Poisoning
661 铅中毒 Lead Poisoning
9 γ-羟基丁酸中毒 GHB Poisoning
675 氰化物中毒 Cyanide Poisoning
697 三环类抗抑郁药中毒 Tricyclic Antidepressant Poisoning
707 蛇毒液螫伤 Snake Envenomation
710 砷中毒 Arsenic Poisoning
730 生物武器 Biologic Weapons
7 β受体阻滞剂中毒 Beta-Blocker Poisoning
770 双硫仑样反应 Disulfiram Reaction
776 水杨酸盐中毒 Salicylate Poisoning
806 铁中毒 Iron Poisoning
808 烃类物质中毒 Hydrocarbon Poisoning
833 危险物暴露所致损伤 Hazmat
879 蝎蜇伤 Sting, Scorpion
927 新型口服抗凝剂并发症 Novel Oral Anticoagulant Complications
977 烟雾吸入 Smoke Inhalation
982 摇头丸中毒 MDMA Poisoning
986 一氧化碳中毒 Carbon Monoxide Poisoning
994 乙烯乙二醇中毒 Ethylene Glycol Poisoning
996 异丙醇中毒 Isopropanol Poisoning
1003 异烟肼中毒 Isoniazid Poisoning
1025 有机磷中毒 Organophosphate Poisoning
1031 浴盐——合成卡西酮中毒 Bath Salts — Synthetic Cathinones Poisoning
1045 镇静药中毒 Neuroleptic Poisoning
1051 蜘蛛咬伤(黑寡妇) Spider Bite, Black Widow
1053 蜘蛛咬伤(棕色隐士) Spider Bite, Brown Recluse
1063 植物中毒 Plant Poisoning
1065 致幻剂中毒 Hallucinogen Poisoning
1068 中毒 Poisoning
1075 中毒与解毒 Poisoning, Antidotes
1078 中毒与洗胃 Poisoning, Gastric Decontamination
1079 中毒与中毒综合征 Poisoning, Toxidromes

外伤

622 膀胱损伤 Bladder Injury
31 爆裂性骨折 Blow-Out Fracture
33 爆震伤 Blast Injuries
49 鼻骨骨折 Nasal Fractures
91 创伤(多部位) Trauma, Multiple
93 创伤(儿童) Pediatric Trauma
95 创伤(老年人) Geriatric Trauma
146 动物咬伤 Bite, Animal
170 耳外伤 Otologic Trauma
190 肺挫伤 Pulmonary Contusion
221 腹部穿透性创伤 Abdominal Trauma, Penetrating
222 腹部创伤影像学 Abdominal Trauma, Imaging
224 腹部钝性创伤 Abdominal Trauma, Blunt
239 肝损伤 Hepatic Injury
265 膈肌外伤 Diaphragmatic Trauma
310 喉骨折 Larynx Fracture
354 肌腱撕裂伤 Tendon Laceration
376 脊髓综合征 Spinal Cord Syndromes
387 家庭暴力 Domestic Violence
404 间室综合征 Compartment Syndrome
426 结肠损伤 Colon Trauma
448 颈部绞窄伤和悬吊伤 Neck Injury by Strangulation/Hanging
452 颈前部穿透伤 Neck Trauma, Penetrating, Anterior
453 颈前部钝性创伤 Neck Trauma, Blunt, Anterior
496 眶后血肿 Retro-Orbital Hematoma

506 肋骨骨折 Rib Fracture
514 连枷胸 Flail Chest
527 颅脑穿透伤 Head Trauma，Penetrating
556 面部骨折 Facial Fractures
562 脑出血 Intracerebral Hemorrhage
586 溺水 Drowning
591 尿道创伤 Urethral Trauma
613 虐待(儿童,非意外性创伤)
Abuse，Pediatric (Nonaccidental Trauma，NAT)
615 虐待(老年人) Abuse，Elder
636 脾脏损伤 Splenic Injury
654 气胸 Pneumothorax
701 闪电击伤 Lightning Injuries
705 烧伤 Burns
722 肾损伤 Renal Injury
743 十二指肠损伤 Duodenal Trauma
745 食管创伤 Esophageal Trauma
781 撕裂伤处理 Laceration Management
783 四肢穿透伤 Extremity Trauma，Penetrating
793 泰瑟枪损伤 Taser Injuries
811 头部钝性伤 Head Trauma，Blunt
873 小肠损伤 Small-Bowel Injury
893 心肌挫伤 Myocardial Contusion
939 胸外伤,穿通伤 Chest Trauma，Penetrating
941 胸外伤,钝器伤 Chest Trauma，Blunt
960 血胸 Hemothorax
967 牙外伤 Dental Trauma
983 咬伤(人) Bite，Human
988 胰腺创伤 Pancreatic Trauma
1010 阴茎折断 Penile Shaft Fracture
1018 硬膜外血肿 Epidural Hematoma
1019 硬膜下血肿 Subdural Hematoma
1038 孕妇外伤 Pregnancy，Trauma In
1055 直肠创伤 Rectal Trauma
1097 蛛网膜下腔出血 Subarachnoid Hemorrhage

血管相关急症

76 肠系膜缺血 Mesenteric Ischemia
100 创伤性主动脉破裂 Aortic Rupture，Traumatic (TAI)
234 腹主动脉瘤 Abdominal Aortic Aneurysm
298 海绵窦血栓 Cavernous Sinus Thrombosis
332 坏疽 Gangrene
460 静脉功能不全 Venous Insufficiency
469 巨细胞动脉炎 Giant Cell Arteritis
564 脑动脉瘤 Cerebral Aneurysm
712 深静脉血栓形成 Deep Vein Thrombosis
943 胸主动脉夹层 Aortic Dissection，Thoracic
1093 周围血管疾病 Peripheral Vascular Disease
1099 主动脉闭塞 Arterial Occlusion

5-羟色胺综合征(药物诱导) Serotonin Syndrome (Drug-Induced)

Jenny J. Lu 周健 潘曙明 译

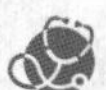

基础知识

描述

• 过度刺激中枢和外周5-羟色胺(5-HT)受体导致的体征和症状。
• 症状的范围可能从轻微的和微妙的表现到严重的,有时是致命的毒性。
• 单独使用5-羟色胺能药物,或与其他5-羟色胺能药物联合使用(可能是治疗性的、故意过量的、娱乐性的、药物相互作用)的结果。
• 典型三联症:
- 自主神经功能障碍:体温过高、心动过速、高血压。
- 认知变化:意识错乱、不安、幻觉、反应能力下降。
- 神经肌肉兴奋性:反射亢进、肌阵挛、震颤。

流行病学

发病率和患病率估计

• 选择性再摄取抑制剂(SSRI)最常涉及,单独或与其他药物合用。
• 女性发病率较高,但男性死亡率较高。
• 19~39岁人群发病率最高。
• 大多数死于药物作用、药物相互作用或娱乐性滥用。

病因

• L-色氨酸代谢产生的血清素(5-羟色胺)。
• 对5-羟色胺受体产生作用,这些受体中,有7种作用于中枢和外周神经系统:
- 影响睡眠和体温调节、情感行为、食物摄取、偏头痛、呕吐、性行为、痛觉、运动张力、胃肠动力、血管张力。
• 广泛性5-羟色胺能药物,精神药物[SSRI、5-羟色胺-去甲肾上腺素再摄取抑制剂(SNRI)]最为常见:
- 例如:西酞普兰、地文拉法辛、度洛西汀、依西酞普兰、氟西汀、氟伏沙明、帕罗西汀、舍曲林、曲唑酮、文拉法辛。
• 其他5-羟色胺能药物(并非全部):
- 布吡酮、可卡因、右美沙芬、芬太尼、锂、单胺氧化酶抑制剂(MAOI)、摇头丸(MDMA)、哌替啶、美沙酮、甲氧氯普胺、昂丹司琼、丙炔苯丙胺、圣约翰草(St. John's wort)、三环类、曲马多、曲普坦类(有争议)。

诊断

症状和体征

病史

• 可能很难获得:
- 家人、朋友、院前急救医疗服务(EMS)人员可能提供其他信息。
• 患者用药清单:处方药、非处方药、草药及补品。
• 发病情况:
- 癫痫发作、偏头痛、注意缺陷多动障碍、帕金森病、最近的疾病发作史。
• 精神病史。
• 非法药物滥用史。
• 出现症状:
- 心理状态或行为变化、体温变化、肌肉僵硬或阵挛。

体格检查

• 生命体征:
- 体温过高。
- 窦性心动过速。
- 高血压或低血压(可发展为明显休克和心血管性虚脱)。
• 皮肤:出汗,颜色正常。
• 胃肠道:腹泻,肠鸣音亢进。
• 精神状态和神经系统:
- 激越。
- 精神状态改变。
- 眼球阵挛。
- 幻觉。
- 谵妄或谵语。
• 肌肉骨骼:
- 肌肉抽搐:诊断中最有帮助的发现,下肢更严重。
- 高张力和韧性,下肢更严重。
- 反射亢进,下肢更严重。

基本检查

仔细进行病史和体格检查。
• Hunter标准:最敏感(84%)和最具特异性(97%)的诊断标准。需要服用或一直服用5-羟色胺能药物,并有下列1种表现:
- 自发的阵挛。
- 诱导阵挛+激越或出汗。
- 眼阵挛+激越或出汗。
- 震动+反射亢进。
- 张力亢进+体温>38℃+眼阵挛或诱导阵挛。
• 考虑其他病因,如败血症、咳嗽变异性哮喘(CVA)等。

诊断检查与说明

实验室检查

血液生化、电解质、肾功能检查。
• 尿液和血清毒理学筛查可以检测出共摄取物。
• 乳酸、pH。
• 总肌酸激酶(CK)。
• 怀疑感染时测细胞计数,做血液或尿液培养。

影像学检查

• 酌情考虑头颅CT(创伤、感染)。
• 心电图:
- 评估QRS、QT间期、心律失常。

鉴别诊断

• 其他中毒,如可卡因、苯丙胺、抗胆碱能药、摇头丸、苯己哌啶(苯环利定):
- 抗神经病药恶性综合征。
- 拟交感神经毒性。
- 恶性高热。
- 抗胆碱能毒性。
- 感染过程(脑膜炎、脑炎)。
- 戒断综合征(ETOH)。

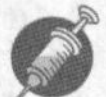

治疗

院前

• 稳定气道。
• 监测生命体征。
• 建立静脉通路。
• 监测末梢血糖。
• 必要时给予吸氧。

初步稳定/治疗

• 稳定气道,建立静脉通道,持续监测心脏功能和体温。
• 住院期间避免使用额外的5-羟色胺能药物(谨慎使用芬太尼、利奈唑利、哌替啶、右美沙芬)。
• 支持性护理是治疗的基础,尤其是积极的降温措施。

- 如果出现高热，积极采取降温措施尤为重要。

■ **急诊治疗/程序**

• 苯二氮䓬类药物是一线药物：
• 劳拉西泮(氯羟去甲安定)、地西泮。
• 积极降温：
- 冰袋、冷却毯、凉雾或风扇。
- 体温升高可能源于肌肉僵硬，通常对退热药没有反应。
• 症状严重(如无法控制的高体温)时可能需要插管：
- 可能需要使用麻痹剂来控制肌肉僵硬和体温过高。
• 赛庚啶：
- 对于严重的病例，可考虑使用5-羟色胺2A拮抗剂活性的非特异性抗组胺药，但其疗效尚未确定。
- 口服(必须压碎并通过口胃管或鼻胃管给予)。
• 参考中毒控制中心指南。

随访

■ **进一步处理**

入院指征

• 所有怀疑有5-羟色胺中毒的患者，即使看上去不太严重，也应该予以监测和治疗。
• 严重症状包括无法控制的高血压、精神状态改变、心血管疾病不稳定、体温过高需要重症监护。

出院指征

• 所有症状消失时可考虑出院。
• 对出院带药的仔细评估和患者教育至关重要。
• 建议使用中毒控制中心指南。

■ **随访建议**

出院后进行初级护理。

要点和误区

• 5-羟色胺综合征的表现可能从轻微到严重。轻微病例的诊断常常难以确定，易漏诊。
• 精神状态变化、体温升高、下肢的肌肉抽搐是重要的发现。
• 高体温症是由于肌肉僵硬，应积极控制，对退热药不起反应。
• 尚未明确环庚啶是有益的，但在严重的情况下可考虑。
• 细心的支持性护理和避免5-羟色胺能药物是治疗的主要内容。

Brugada综合征 Brugada Syndrome

Richard E. Wolfe 黄聪华 译

基础知识

■ **描述**

• 钠通道改变引起的突发性心脏病，但无心脏结构的改变。
• 大部分因心室纤颤突然死亡。
• 2年死亡率在30%。
• 以前认为的特发性心室颤动中，40%～60%可能为Brugada综合征。
• 东南亚发病率最高，可在发生在各个年龄、性别及种族。

■ **病因**

• 遗传：
- 50%为常染色体显性遗传。
- 不完全外显。
• 钠通道改变：
- >70%为基因突变。
- 不完全外显。
- *SCN5A*基因突变占20%。

诊断

■ **症状和体征**

• 一般表现为突发死亡(因心室颤动)、晕厥或多形性室性心动过速导致的自限的眩晕。

病史

• 现病史：
- 晕厥或眩晕。
- 心悸。
- 心搏骤停。
- 伴随疾病：发热、代谢疾病、电解质紊乱。
- 使用可卡因。
- 三环类抗抑郁药(TCA)和精神药物。
- 夜间濒死感。
• 家族史：
- 因晕厥溺水或在水下出现心律失常。
- 突发或接近突发的心源性猝死。
- 亲戚有Brugada综合征病史。

体格检查

• 完善体格检查，注意有无其他导致晕厥和心律失常的原因：
- 心脏杂音。
- 漏斗胸(心电图正常变异)。
- 运动员。
- 心脏起搏器。

■ **基本检查**

• 12导联心电图。
• 详细的既往史及家族史。
• 病理学筛查。

■ **临床诊断及心电图表现**

• 基本表现：
- 右束支传导阻滞或完全性右束支传导阻滞伴右心前区导联ST段抬高。
• V_1～V_3 QRS-T形态：
- ST段改变。
- 有时只有V_1导联改变，V_3很不明显。
• Ⅰ型下斜型：
- ST段起始太高≥2 mm，并缓慢下降。
- 负向T波。
- 没有清晰的r′波。
- V_1～V_6 QRS波群持续时间不匹配。
• Ⅱ型马鞍型：
- 高R′波抬高≥2 mm。
- 伴有ST段突起。
- V_1～V_6 QRS波群持续时间不匹配。

实验室检查

• 血液检查：
- 生化检查，排除电解质紊乱导致心律失常或晕厥。
- 心肌梗死标志物肌钙蛋白(TNI)、肌酸激酶同工酶(CK-MB)。
- D-二聚体，部分人群(威尔士人及法国人)需排除肺栓塞。
- 血常规，评估晕厥原因。

影像学检查

• X 线平片：

- 评估心脏大小。

• 胸部 CT：

- 如果怀疑肺栓塞。

诊断程序/外科

• 电生理检查：

- 钠通道阻滞剂行药物激发试验（1a 和 1c 型）。

• 埋藏式自动电复律除颤器（AICD）安置：

- 死亡率可将至 0。

鉴别诊断

• 晕厥：

- 原发性心源性。
- 血管迷走性。
- 神经源性。
- 低血容量。
- 妊娠。

• 心律失常：

- 阵发性心房颤动。
- 心房颤动伴快速心室率。
- 预激综合征（WPW 综合征）。
- Lown-Ganong-Lerine 综合征（LGL 综合征）。
- 室性心动过速。
- 多发性房性心动过速。
- 自发终止的心室颤动。
- 有症状的心动过缓。
- 高度房室传导阻滞。
- QT 间期延长综合征。
- 过量 TCA。

• 心电图：

- 完全性右束支传导阻滞。
- 运动员。
- 室间隔肥厚。
- 漏斗胸。
- 致心律失常性右心室发育不良。
- ST 段抬高型心肌梗死。

• 其他全身性疾病：

- 电解质紊乱。
- 心包炎。
- 心肌炎。
- 心肌心包炎。

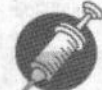

治疗

院前

• 气道、呼吸和循环管理（ABC 管理）。

• 高级心脏生命支持（ACLS）。

初步稳定/治疗

• ABC 管理。

• 开始或继续 ACLS。

急诊治疗/程序

• 全程心电监测。

• 心脏病史询问：

- 电生理学评估。
- 除颤和起搏。

• 纠正潜在疾病：

- 补充电解质。
- 纠正代谢紊乱。
- 无症状患者的处理仍有争议，目前的共识是行电生理学（EP）评估，但文献不支持。

药物治疗

• ACLS 协议药物。

• 抗心律失常药通常没有帮助。

儿科注意事项

• 儿科高级生命支持（PALS）和除颤。

• 根据基础体重调整药物和能量。

随访

进一步处理

入院指征

• 临床发现有 Brugada 综合征的心电图表现。

• 不明原因的晕厥。

• 无法快速获得心脏病学随访。

• 持续的心律失常，即使自发终止。

出院指征

• 血流动力学稳定。

• 无症状。

• 排除心脏病。

• 发病后植入 AICD：

- AICD 植入后。

随访建议

• 有心电图改变及相关病史的患者应该额外进行 EP 评估。

• 避免使用Ⅰ类抗心律失常药物，以及酒精和可卡因。

要点和误区

• 重视任何一个突发性心源性猝死或晕厥，特别是家族中有相同病史的。

• 心电图诊断显示右束支传导阻滞或完全性右束支传导阻滞，伴有右胸导联 ST 段抬高。

• 警惕有类似心电图表现的患者，$V_1 \sim V_6$ 常有一致的 QRS 波群，而 Brugada 综合征患者 QRS 群改变仅在 $V_1 \sim V_3$。

• 对高死亡风险的患者进行低门槛的心脏病咨询。

• AICD 植入是彻底治疗，几乎消除了心源性猝死的风险。

• 没有发现抗心律失常药物有帮助。

• Brugada 模式可能在全身性疾病中被"显现"，尤其是伴有发热的情况，即使心电图恢复正常，患者仍应进行电生理检查的后续随访。

HELLP 综合征 HELLP Syndrome

Michael J. Bono 刘雪峰 译

基础知识

描述

• HELLP 综合征（溶血性肝功能异常血小板减少综合征）：

- 溶血。
- 肝酶升高。
- 血小板减少。

• 没有普遍接受的 HELLP 定义。

• 多与严重的子痫相关，大多数患者有妊娠期高血压疾病。

• 肝脏病变是其特点：

- 其他器官也可涉及（如脑、肾、肺）。

• 多数孕妇死亡病例发生在 1 级。

• 死亡率与肝出血、中枢神经系统损害、心肺肾血管损伤相关。

• 孕妇的发病率约为 0.2%。
• 12%～18%的患者血压正常。
• 伴有重度子痫的孕妇发病率在 20%。
• 诊断方面：52%发生在妊娠期，18%发生在足月分娩时，32%发生在产后。

危险因素

高龄多胎妊娠的白种人产妇。

儿科注意事项

发作 HELLP 综合征的母体所产的婴儿死亡率非常高。

病因

• 尚不清楚，但与有 4 种病因的先兆子痫的病因学有关：
- 子宫血管滋养层异常侵犯。
- 对母亲、父亲和胎儿组织的免疫反应。
- 孕妇对妊娠期心血管或炎症变化的反应。
- 遗传因素。

• HELLP 可能的机制：
- 胎盘碎屑释放到母体循环中，引起全身炎症反应。
- 血管收缩导致血液流动阻力增加和高血压。
- 血管痉挛可能会直接损害血管。
- 内皮细胞受损，导致内皮细胞间渗漏。

• 毛细血管渗漏：
- 血小板和纤维蛋白原在血管内皮下层堆积。
- 严重病例可见纤维素沉积。

• 血管损伤和局部组织缺氧造成出血、坏死及终末器官损害。

诊断

症状和体征

病史

• 询问病史和体格检查，需要留意腹痛、恶心、呕吐、头痛等症状与体征。
• 孕产史：
- 产次。
- 分娩。
- 妊娠期高血压的病史。
- 估算孕周。
- 产前检查。

• 可有类似流感症状，如疲倦、乏力、不适。
• 恶心，常常伴有呕吐。
• 上腹和右上腹疼痛：
- 疼痛程度与疾病轻重相关。

• 头痛，常伴视力改变。
• 下列症状提示预后不良：呼吸困难和/或液体过量提示心源性或非心源性肺水肿：
- 呼吸困难常与肺栓塞有关。
- 胸痛提示心肌缺血。
- 意识障碍，癫痫：
  ◦ 高血压脑病。
  ◦ 脑水肿。
  ◦ 出血性脑血管意外。
- 外周性水肿。
- 腹水。
- 血尿。
- 尿量减少。

> **注意**
>
> 测定孕周和胎儿的体外存活能力在 HELLP 综合征中非常重要。

体格检查

• 注意血压的生命体征，正常血压＜140/90 mmHg。
• 血压通常在妊娠中期和晚期早期下降。
• 监测生命体征，注意血压。
• 可能不伴有收缩期或舒张期高血压。
• 许多患者存在右上腹疼痛，关注是否存在肝包膜下血肿。
• 液体超量的征象。
• 仔细的神经系统体征检查。
• 胎心音。

基本检查

• 血细胞与血小板计数和涂片、肌酐、尿素氮、肝功能、凝血功能、血清镁浓度。
• 尿蛋白分析、尿路感染筛查。
• 记录患者的体重变化。

诊断检查与说明

实验室检查

• 全血细胞检查：
- 贫血。
- 血小板减少症。
- 外周血涂片观察溶血性贫血（锯齿状和裂片红细胞）。
- 其他溶血表现：乳酸脱氢酶（LDH）、胆红素、网织红细胞升高。

• 血小板计数与涂片：
- 血小板（PLT）＜100 000/μl（1×10^9/L＝1 000/μl）。

• 弥散性血管内凝血（DIC）筛查。
• 凝血功能：
- 凝血酶原时间（PT）。
- 活化部分凝血活酶时间（APTT）。

• 尿素氮、肌酐、血清镁浓度。
• 肝功能检查评估溶血及肝功能损害状况：
- 天冬氨酸转氨酶＞40 IU/L。
- 丙氨酸转氨酶＞40 IU/L。
- LDH＞600 IU/L。
- 血清胆红素＞1.2 mg/dl（1 mg/dl＝17 μmol/L）。

影像学检查

• 胸部 X 线片：
- 怀疑肺水肿。

• 头颅 CT：
- 意识障碍或局限性神经定位体征。

• 盆腔超声（经腹部或经阴道）：
- 胎儿与胎盘状况评估。

鉴别诊断

• 消化系统疾病：
- 胆囊炎。
- 胆石症。
- 胆绞痛。
- 胰腺炎。
- 肝炎。
- 溃疡。
- 急性妊娠性脂肪肝。
- 急性胃炎。
- 食管裂孔疝。
- 重度胃食管反流。

• 血液系统：
- 子痫相关性血小板减少。
- 妊娠期血小板减少。
- 特发性血小板减少性紫癜。
- 血小板减少性紫癜。
- 溶血性尿毒症综合征。

• 神经系统：
- 癫痫。
- 脑炎。
- 脑膜炎。
- 脑病。
- 颅脑肿瘤。
- 颅内出血。

• 其他：
- 药物滥用。
- 肾盂肾炎。
- 脓毒症。

治疗

院前

提醒：

• 左侧卧位转运患者，预防下腔静脉综合征。

• 对可能癫痫发作的患者建立静脉通道。

• 日常癫痫管理(推荐硫酸镁)。

注意

转运至能提供处理高风险产科保健的医疗单位。

初步稳定/治疗

• 急救 ABC 管理。

• 患者取左侧卧位，预防下腔静脉综合征。

• 经面罩高流量吸氧。

• 母体监测：

- 心电监测。
- 指脉氧饱和度。
- 宫缩描记。
- 胎儿监测。

急诊治疗/程序

• 使用药物控制高血压(详见药物)：

- 避免血管紧张素转换酶抑制剂(ACEI)类药物对胎儿的副作用。

• 应避免使用肝素以防出血性并发症。

• 使用硫酸镁控制先兆子痫和子痫：

- 硫酸镁不适用于治疗高血压。

• 配血筛查以防患者可能需要输血。

• 产科急会诊，可申请新生儿科会诊：

- 可考虑紧急分娩、终止妊娠。
- 对于合并严重疾病的产后患者，早期血浆置换有益处。

• 与会诊医师商定糖皮质激素的使用：

- 有争议，所以与会诊医师讨论。
- 帮助胎儿肺成熟。
- 静脉注射地塞米松比肌内注射倍他米松更加有效。
- 取决于胎儿的胎龄。
- 不能减轻疾病的严重程度或缩短病程，但可以提高血小板计数。

• 进行限制性液体管理，除非有脱水的临床表现：

- 过量输液可加重毛细血管渗漏。
- 乳酸林格液或生理盐水以 60 ml/h 的速度输注，不可超过 125 ml/h。
- 通过导尿记录尿量。

• 在没有活动性出血的情况下，如孕妇血小板计数＜20 000/μl 时亦可输注血小板，以避免产后出血。

• PLT＞40 000/μl 时认为经阴道分娩时安全的。

• 如果计划剖宫产，需要提升 PLT＞50 000/μl。

• 如果存在凝血功能障碍，与产科商讨后可输注新鲜冰冻血浆、洗涤红细胞。

• 血红蛋白＜100 g/L 时输注洗涤红细胞。

药物治疗

一线药物

• 肼屈嗪：2.5 mg，静脉滴注，然后 5～10 mg/(15～20)min。

- 直至 40 mg 总剂量，保持舒张压＜110 mmHg。
- 静脉滴注，滴速 5～10 mg/h。

• 拉贝洛尔(柳胺苄心定)：10 mg，静脉滴注，然后 20～80 mg/10 min。

- 累计至 300 mg。
- 静脉滴注，滴速 1～2 mg/min。

• 硝苯地平：初始剂量 10 mg，必要时 30 min 内重复。

- 不要服舌下剂量。

二线用药

• 硝普钠：0.25 μg/(kg·min)，静脉滴注。

- 每 5 min 增加 0.25 μg/(kg·min)。
- 仅在患者对一线药物无反应时使用。

• 硫酸镁：负荷剂量：4～6 g 加入 100 ml 液体静脉注射，持续 15～20 min 或以上。

- 维持剂量，起始滴速 2 g/h。
- 滴速取决于临床效果。
- 观察毒性反应(葡萄糖酸钙作为解毒剂，10 ml，静脉注射，持续时间＞3 min)。
- 4～6 h 测定血清镁浓度；调整滴速，使镁浓度达到 4～7 mmol/L。

随访

进一步处理

入院指征

• 所有需要连续监护母体和胎儿的患者。

• ICU 收治标准：

- 肺水肿。
- 呼吸衰竭。
- 脑水肿。
- 血流动力学不稳定的消化道出血。

出院指征

HELLP 综合征患者均应收治入院，出院需要产科医师决定。

转诊问题

急诊治疗稳定后，除非即将临产，否则都应转送至能够处理复杂高风险产科问题的医院。

随访建议

患者应由产科医师密切随访：产后 48 h 内部分患者可发生 HELLP 综合征。

要点和误区

• 合并有腹痛、肝功能异常、血小板减少的妊娠期高血压疾病患者需要急诊治疗，并请产科会诊。

• HELLP 综合征患者血压可正常。

• 稳定后应转入能够处理这类复杂情况的医疗机构。

QT 间期延长综合征 Long QT Syndrome, Prolonged

Jason A. Tracy 郑金浩 毛恩强 译

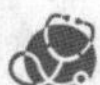

基础知识

描述

以心肌复极障碍为特点，在心电图上表现为 QT 间期延长的疾病。

• 病理生理学复杂且不完全清楚：

- 心脏钠、钾或钙离子流的改变。
- 心脏交感神经支配失衡。

• 心室复极延长，导致心电图上 QT 间期延长的表现：

- “暂停依赖”延长归因于短-长-短序列，一个窦性心搏后紧跟着一个期前收缩(短)，然后是期前收缩后的暂停(长),以室性期前收缩结束(短)。

-“肾上腺素依赖”的暂停可于先天性病例中发现。

• 症状发生前常有剧烈运动、情绪紧张或噪声。

• 夜间心动过缓可延长 QT 间期,引起睡眠相关症状。

• 恢复节律可导致尖端扭转型室性心动过速、室性心动过速和心室颤动。

• 心律失常导致的血流动力学紊乱可导致晕厥或死亡。

• 心源性猝死的独立危险因素。

危险因素

遗传学

• 有 10 种基因与长 QT 间期综合征相关:

- 与耳聋相关的常染色体隐性遗传(Jervell-Lange-Nielsen 综合征)。

- 与耳聋不相关的常染色体显性遗传(Romano-Ward 综合征)。

- 肾上腺素刺激(恐惧、劳累、震颤性谵妄、较强的听觉刺激)在某些基因型可促进心律失常,而睡眠相关症状则在其他基因型中被发现。

• 10%~15%的基因携带者 QT 间期基线正常。

• 每年未经治疗的患者有 1%~2%发生死亡:

- 药物导致的 QT 间期延长可能同样具有遗传背景。

- 先天性的发生率为 1/(3 000~5 000),40 岁之前的死亡率为 6%。

儿科注意事项

• 疑似有晕厥、心搏骤停或猝死的儿童。

• 情绪紧张或剧烈运动后晕厥。

• 10%的儿科患者死亡前无先兆症状。

病因

• 药物:

- 完整列表见 www. crediblemeds. org。

- Ⅰa 类抗心律失常药:奎尼丁、普鲁卡因胺、双异丙吡胺。

- Ⅲ类抗心律失常药:索他洛尔、伊布利特、胺碘酮。

- 抗生素:红霉素、戊烷脒、氯喹、甲氧苄啶-磺胺甲噁唑。

- 抗真菌药:酮康唑、伊曲康唑。

- 精神类药物:吩噻嗪、氟哌啶醇、利培酮、三氯醋酸钠。

- 西沙必利。

- 抗组胺药。

- 有机磷农药。

- 麻醉药:美沙酮。

• 电解质异常:

- 低钾血症。

- 低镁血症。

- 低钙血症。

• 心脏:

- 缓慢性心律失常。

- 动静脉阻断。

- 二尖瓣脱垂。

- 心肌炎。

- 心肌缺血。

• 中枢神经系统:

- 蛛网膜下腔出血。

- 脑卒中。

• 先天性(特发性)。

• 其他:

- 禁食时蛋白质缺乏。

- 神经性厌食症。

- 甲状腺功能减退症。

- 低温。

诊断

症状和体征

• 心悸。

• 眩晕。

• 头晕。

病史

• 晕厥。

• 近期晕厥史。

• 癫痫发作。

• 晕厥或猝死家族史。

• 先天性耳聋。

• 用药史。

基本检查

心电监测。

• 心电图。

• 男性 QTc(心率校正后的 QT 间期)>0.44 s,女性>0.46 s。

• QT 间期的测量是从随机信号的开始至 T 波结束:

- 测量最好在肢体导联,应取 3~5 次心率的平均值。

- 对于心率校正(QTc)公式尚没有专家共识。

- 目前最常用的是 Bazett 公式(QT 间期除以 RR 间期的平方根)。

- QT 间期变异性增加。

• T 波异常(T 波交替,双相)。

• U 波出现。

• 室性心动过速。

• 心室颤动。

• 尖端扭转型室性心动过速。

诊断检查与说明

实验室检查

• 全套电解质,包括钙和镁。

• 毒理学筛查。

影像学检查

超声心动图排除其他心脏原因。

诊断步骤/外科

• 心电图负荷试验可在疑似患者中诱发 QT 间期延长。

• 动态心电图监测 QTc。

• 疑似先天性的患者行遗传咨询或检测。

• 家族性心电监测。

鉴别诊断

• 心肌梗死。

• 肥厚型心肌病。

• 心脏瓣膜缺损。

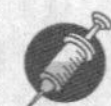

治疗

院前

• 辅助供氧。

• 建立静脉通路。

• 心电监测。

注意

• QT 间期延长的稳定患者转运途中未干预。

• 为确诊尖端扭转型室性心动过速的不稳定患者进行复律。

• 确诊尖端扭转型室性心动过速的稳定患者给予硫酸镁治疗。

初始稳定/治疗

• 建立静脉通路。

• 心电监测。

• 确定血流动力学稳定。

• 不稳定患者需要立即电复律。

急诊治疗/程序

• 尖端扭转型室性心动过速患者经静脉给予硫酸镁。

• 静脉补钾使血清钾水平维持在 4.5~5 mg/L。

• 经硫酸镁治疗复发的难治性尖端扭转型室性心动过速(QT间期缩短)给予临时心脏起搏器(起搏心率为100～120次/分)。

• 难治性患者或血流动力学不稳定的获得性长QT间期的患者(对先天性患者无效)对静脉起搏无反应,可静脉给予异丙肾上腺素。

• 停用任何可导致该病的药物,纠正代谢紊乱。

• 对于有症状的长QT间期患者使用最大剂量的β受体阻滞剂,需咨询心脏病学专家。

• 对于那些怀疑先天性长QT间期而无晕厥史、心源性猝死家族史和室性心律失常的患者无需急诊治疗(咨询心脏病学专家)。

• 对于高风险的患者,无论有无颈胸段星状神经节切除(减少肾上腺素刺激),可能都需要植入心脏起搏器或除颤器。

• 对于先天性患者,使用β受体阻滞剂可预防70%的心血管事件。

药物治疗

一线用药

• 硫酸镁:2 g(25～50 mg/kg),静脉注射,超过2～3 min;随后2～4 mg/min,静脉滴注。

• 异丙肾上腺素:1 μg/min(0.05～0.1 μg/kg),静脉持续滴注,根据效果调整滴速,最大剂量为10 μg/min。

二线用药

普萘洛尔:2～3 mg/(kg·d),口服(咨询心脏病学专家)。

随访

进一步处理

入院指征

• 有症状的长QT间期患者。

• 晕厥。

• 心律失常。

• 可能的心血管或缺血事件。

• 代谢紊乱。

出院指征

无症状的长QT间期患者在咨询心脏病学专家后决定。

随访建议

建议所有新诊断的长QT间期的患者随访。

要点和误区

• 晕厥的患者需考虑QT间期延长。

• QT间期延长是心源性猝死的独立危险因素。

• 纠正电解质紊乱并停用导致QT间期延长的药物。

• 尖端扭转型室性心动过速患者硫酸镁治疗后予以起搏治疗。

β受体阻滞剂中毒 Beta Blocker Poisoning

Maxim Dzeba · Steven E. Aks 宋振举 童朝阳 译

基础知识

描述

人体生理学

• 心血管系统:β受体至少存在3种不同类型。$β_1$受体主要分布在心肌组织,激活此类受体会增加心率,增强心肌收缩力和房室传导,并且减少房室结不应性;$β_2$受体存在于心肌组织,但在支气管和外周血管的平滑肌中分布更广,激活此类受体会引起血管舒张和支气管舒张;$β_3$受体存在于脂肪组织和心脏,激活此类受体可能介导儿茶酚胺诱导的产热作用,并且可能会降低心肌收缩力。

- 通过刺激β受体,腺苷三磷酸(ATP)被腺苷酸环酶转化为环磷酸腺苷(cAMP)。
- cAMP激活蛋白激酶后,蛋白激酶磷酸化肌质网蛋白。
- 肌质网释放钙离子。
- 发生兴奋-收缩耦联。

• β受体阻滞剂的作用:

- 心血管系统:
  - 减少兴奋/收缩。
  - 膜的稳定性。
  - 钠通道阻滞导致QRS波群的延长(某些药物)。
  - 延长QTc间期,导致室性心律失常(与某些药物)。
  - 内在交感神经活动。
  - 部分激动剂性质(与某些药物)。
- 神经系统:
  - 中枢神经系统效应与亲脂剂(普萘洛尔、美托洛尔、拉贝洛尔)。

诊断

症状和体征

• 心血管:
- 低血压。
- 心动过缓。
- 心脏传导迟滞。
- 心脏传导阻滞。
- 心力衰竭。
- 电-机械分离。
- 药物过量使得选择性β受体阻滞剂丧失其选择性。

• 神经系统:
- 昏迷。
- 癫痫发作。

• 肺:
- 支气管痉挛。
- 肺水肿。

• 代谢:
- 低血糖。

病史

• 询问并评估药物使用错误的风险。

• 询问使用过的β受体阻滞剂的种类(普萘洛尔或美托洛尔)。

• 了解自杀意念的风险与意图。

• 询问与儿科患者可能接触的药物。

体格检查

• 低血压。

• 心动过缓。

• 心律失常。

• 精神状态的变化。

基本检查

• 不明原因摄入:伴随心动过缓、低血压的可疑β受体阻滞剂中毒。

• 心电图：
- 传导延迟。
- 一度、二度、三度心脏传导阻滞。
- 心动过缓。

诊断检查与说明

• 全血细胞计数。
• 电解质、血尿素氮、肌酐、血糖。
• 毒理学筛查。

鉴别诊断

• 钙通道阻滞剂中毒。
• 氯尼定中毒。
• 洋地黄中毒。
• 急性心肌梗死伴心脏传导阻滞。
• 心源性休克。

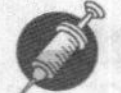

治疗

院前

当怀疑过量服用药物时，保存并转移药物和药盒。

初步稳定/治疗

• ABC管理：
- 根据精神状态选择气道保护措施。
- 必要时吸氧。
- 生理盐水静脉滴注。
- 血流动力学监测。
• 如果精神状态改变则使用纳洛酮和维生素 B_1(硫胺素)。
• 床旁血糖的测定，用50%葡萄糖溶液治疗低血糖。
• 使用苯二氮䓬类药物治疗长期发作的癫痫。

急诊治疗/程序

目标

• 心率>60次/分。
• 收缩压>90 mmHg。
• 充足的尿量。
• 意识水平的提高。

胃肠道净化

• 吐根糖浆：在院前和急诊设置禁止使用。
• 如果在1h内摄入，可以考虑使用Ewald管灌洗。
• 普萘洛尔可能导致食管痉挛，对胃引流管的放置和拔除造成阻碍。
• 活性炭对人体有帮助，特别是在有吸收剂的情况下。

心动过缓和低血压

• 阿托品：
- 首选药物。
- 低成功率。
• 胰高血糖素：
- 对于β受体阻滞剂引起的血流动力学不稳定是首选药物。
- 在阿托品不能提高心率的情况下使用。
- 通过刺激β受体以外的受体位点来促进cAMP的产生。
- 可能会导致恶心和呕吐。
- 同生理盐水或5%葡萄糖溶液混合使用。
• 液体管理：
- 在低血压患者中谨慎使用。
- 通过Swan-Ganz导管或监测中心静脉压(CVP)。
• 氨力农：
- 选择性磷酸二酯酶抑制剂。
- 间接增加cAMP提高心肌收缩力。
- 和胰高血糖素共同使用来治疗有症状的持续性心动过缓。
• 血管加压药：
- 当使用阿托品、胰高血糖素后仍存在有症状的低血压、心动过缓时开始使用。
- 应用有创监测技术以协助治疗。
- 由于β受体阻滞的关系，药物使用效果可能有限：
◦ 可能需要更大的剂量。
- 异丙肾上腺素(非选择性β受体激动剂)：
◦ 用于血压和心率的滴定。
- 肾上腺素(强效α和β受体激动剂)：
◦ 血压上升，由于直接刺激心肌，加快心率、血管收缩。
◦ 使用异丙肾上腺素时血压无改善。
- 高剂量多巴胺。
• 碳酸氢钠：
- 理论上而言，如果有证据表明QRS波群延长>100 ms，由于某些β受体阻滞剂导致，同时也会使钠通道阻滞导致QRS波群的延长。
- 并不是常规在所有的β受体阻滞剂中毒时使用。
• 电起搏：当其他治疗方案失败时。

实验性治疗方案

• 咨询当地毒物研究中心。
• 高剂量胰岛素：
- 促进更有效的心肌代谢。
- 低血糖常见于过量使用β受体阻滞剂的情况中，需要经常监测葡萄糖浓度。
- 与当地毒物研究中心进行协商。
• 静脉滴注脂肪乳剂(20%脂肪乳剂)。

强化清除

• 血液透析有助于水溶性β受体阻滞剂：
- 纳多洛尔。
- 阿替洛尔。
- 索他洛尔。
• 静脉滴注脂肪乳剂(20%脂肪乳剂)：
- 未来可能的治疗手段。

药物治疗

• 活性炭：1 g/kg，口服。
• 氨力农：负荷剂量0.75 mg/kg；维持剂量2～20 μg/(kg·min)，滴定以获效果。
• 阿托品：0.5 mg(儿童：0.02 mg/kg)，静脉注射；重复0.5～1 mg，静脉注射(儿童：0.04 mg/kg)。
• 多巴胺：2～20 μg/(kg·min)，静脉注射。
• 右旋糖酐：50% 1安瓿(50 ml或25 g；儿童：25% 2～4 ml/kg)，静脉注射。
• 肾上腺素：2 μg/min[儿童：0.01 mg/kg(0.1 ml/kg 1∶10000)]，滴定以获效果。
• 胰高血糖素：3～5 mg，静脉注射，1～2 min注完(儿童：0.03～0.1 mg/kg)。
• 胰岛素(常规胰岛素)：1 U/kg，静脉注射，然后0.5～1 U/(kg·h)滴定到临床反应(一定要补充葡萄糖)。
• 异丙肾上腺素：5 μg/min，静脉注射，滴定至改变心率。
• 去甲肾上腺素：开始2～4 μg/min，静脉注射，滴定至1～2 μg/(kg·min)，静脉注射。
• 碳酸氢钠：1 mEq/kg，静脉推注。

一线治疗

• 静脉输液。
• 胰高血糖素。
• 血管加压素。

二线治疗

• 碳酸氢钠。
• 血液透析。

随访

进一步处理

入院指征

• 因神志不清或血流动力学不稳定(心动过缓、传导延迟、低血压)入住ICU。
• 观察和监测24 h的长效或缓释制剂，原因是潜在的延迟症状。

出院指征

在服用短效或速效释放制剂后无症状8～

10 h。

■ 随访建议

• 对所有自杀患者进行精神状况评估。

• 对儿童误食的父母进行预防中毒指导。

要点和误区

• 对低血压和心动过缓的患者要考虑β受体阻滞剂。

• 宽大畸形的QRS型心律失常患者应该用碳酸氢钠来治疗。

γ-羟基丁酸中毒

Amy V. Kontrick · Mark B. Mycyk　祝各亮 译

基础知识

■ 描述

• γ-氨基丁酸(GABA)的天然类似物。
• 可以用于治疗嗜睡症。
• 非医学用途：
- 健身。
- 致欣快。
• γ-羟基丁酸(GHB)的前体[γ-丁内酯(GBL)、1,4-丁二醇(1,4-BD)、γ-羟基戊酸酯(GHV)和γ-戊内酯(GVL)]与GHB具有相同的效果。
• 起效时间：服用后15～30 min。
• 持续时间：2～6 h。

■ 病因

故意或意外摄入GHB。

诊断

■ 症状和体征

• 中枢神经系统：
- 中枢神经系统抑制。
- 共济失调或头晕。
- 判断力减弱。
- 攻击行为。
- 四肢阵挛性运动。
- 昏迷。
- 癫痫发作。
• 肺：
- 呼吸抑制。
- 呼吸暂停。
- 喉痉挛(罕见)。
• 消化道：
- 恶心。
- 呕吐。
• 心血管：
- 心动过缓。
- 房室传导阻滞。
- 低血压。
• 其他：
- 眼球震颤。
- 低温。
• 切断症状：
- 高血压。
- 心动过速。
- 发热。
- 兴奋。
- 发汗。
- 震颤。
- 恶心、呕吐和腹部绞痛。
- 幻觉、妄想和精神疾病。

■ 基本检查

• 根据临床表现和病史做出诊断。
• 如果症状和体征与GHB中毒不一致，应当检查其他的摄入物。

■ 诊断检查与说明

实验室检查

• 针对GHB中毒的筛查通常需要外送到专门的机构，不能影响急诊室的诊疗措施。
• 通过尿液毒性筛查排除其他的摄入物。
• 血清酒精(乙醇)水平。
• 如果患者存在长期抑制或兴奋，怀疑横纹肌溶解，应检测尿液和血清肌酸激酶(CK)。

影像学检查

• 心电图：
- 窦性心动过缓。
- 房室传导阻滞。
• 胸部X线片(胸片)：
- 吸入性肺炎。
• 怀疑头颅损伤行头颅CT检查。

■ 鉴别诊断

• 酒精中毒。
• 巴比妥酸盐过量。
• 苯二氮䓬类药物过量。
• 抗精神病药物过量。
• 阿片类药物过量。
• 切断症状：
- 酒精戒断。
- 镇静催眠药戒断。

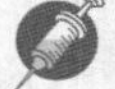

治疗

■ 院前

将涉及药物过量的所有片剂、药瓶和用具全部送至急诊室进行鉴别。

■ 初步稳定/治疗

• 心肺复苏：
- 气道控制。
- 吸氧。
- 有指征时及时插管。
• 对于精神抑制状态的患者，补充硫胺素、葡萄糖和纳洛酮。

■ 急诊治疗/程序

• 支持治疗。
• 心动过缓：
- 阿托品。
- 临时起搏。
• 低血压：
- 静脉补充生理盐水。
- 调节体位。
- 多巴胺升压。
• 癫痫发作：
- 苯二氮䓬类进行初始治疗。
- 苯巴比妥治疗难治性癫痫。
• 戒断症状：
- 用苯二氮䓬类进行积极治疗。
- 如果大剂量苯二氮䓬类治疗无效果，则改用苯巴比妥或异丙酚(丙泊酚)。

■ 药物治疗

• 葡萄糖：50～100 ml 5%葡萄糖(儿童：

2 ml/kg 2.5%葡萄糖，超过 1 min)；静脉推注，必要时可重复。

• 地西泮：5～10 mg(儿童：0.2～0.5 mg/kg)，静脉推注，q10～15 min。

• 多巴胺：2～20 μg/(kg · min)，静脉滴注。

• 劳拉西泮：2～4 mg(儿童：0.03～0.05 mg/kg)，静脉推注，q10～15 min。

• 纳洛酮：0.4～2 mg(儿童：0.1 mg/kg；新生儿：10～30 μg/kg)，静脉推注或肌内注射。

• 苯巴比妥：10～20 mg/kg，静脉推注(负荷剂量)，需监测是否发生呼吸抑制。

• 丙泊酚：0.5～1 mg/kg，静脉推注(负荷剂量)，后 5～50 μg/(kg · min)(维持剂量)。

• 硫胺素：100 mg(儿童：50 mg)，静脉推注或肌内注射。

随访

进一步处理

入院指征

• 气管插管的患者。

• 低体温或其他血流动力学不稳定的患者。

• 摄入物延长了中毒的持续时间。

出院指征

• 6 h 观察后无症状。

• 无戒断症状的临床表现。

注意

GHB 的戒断症状严重时会致命，其表现类似于酒精戒断症状。可以适当延长该类患者的住院治疗时间。

随访建议

• 对于有毒瘾的患者使用脱毒药物替代治疗。

• 意外中毒的患者需要对其进行预防教育。

• 故意中毒(如自杀)的患者需要对其进行精神状态评估。

要点和误区

• 需考虑非毒性原因造成的长期精神状态改变。

• 医院常规药品检验不能够明确 GHB 或其他常见毒品的滥用。

阿米巴病 Amebiasis

Benjamin W. Osborne · Nicolas M. Monte 马林浩 林兆奋 译

 基础知识

描述

- 侵袭性寄生虫感染伴有肠道和肠外表现。
- 在世界范围内流行，特别是卫生条件差的地区。
- 风险人群：
  - 来自流行地区（印度、非洲、墨西哥、中美洲和南美洲地区）的旅行者、移居者和当地居民。
  - 相关机构的人。
  - 口-肛门性活动者。
  - 男男性接触者（MSM）。
  - 人类免疫缺陷病毒（HIV）感染者。
- 疾病和并发症严重程度增加的风险因素：
  - 免疫功能低下：使用皮质类固醇、HIV 感染、营养不良、恶性肿瘤。
  - 高龄。

病因

- 溶组织内阿米巴，一种厌氧、无鞭毛的原生动物。
- 粪口传播：
  - 人类是唯一的传染源。
- 摄入的生物会引起侵袭性结肠炎。
- 肠外扩散是血源性的。

诊断

症状和体征

- 肠道疾病：
  - 暴露后 1 周到 1 个月开始。
  - 急性腹泻（非痢疾性结肠炎）：
    - 80％的病例。
    - 发热。
    - 便血。
    - 腹部检查结果良性。
  - 经典痢疾：
    - 血性黏液性腹泻。
    - 腹痛、腹部检查结果显示良性。
    - 里急后重。
    - 体重降低（50％）。
    - 发热（30％）。
  - 暴发性结肠炎：
    - 罕见，0.5％的病例。
    - 患者中毒表现。
    - 腹部硬（25％）。
    - 发热。
    - 严重的血性腹泻。
    - 快速进展至肠穿孔和明显腹膜炎。
    - >40％的死亡率。
  - 中毒性巨结肠：
    - 患者中毒表现。
    - 大量腹泻（每日 10 次大便）。
    - 发热。
    - 腹胀、气腹、腹膜炎体征。
    - 与皮质类固醇有关。
    - 死亡率高。
  - 阿米巴瘤：
    - 腔内颗粒状肿块。
    - 查体可触及。
  - 阿米巴性狭窄：
    - 由于慢性炎症、瘢痕。
    - 腹部疼痛。
    - 恶心与呕吐（可能不稳定）。
    - 部分或完全肠梗阻。
  - 慢性阿米巴结肠炎：
    - 轻度腹泻、腹部绞痛和里急后重的轻度反复发作。
    - 可能会持续多年。
- 肠外疾病：
  - 阿米巴肝脓肿：
    - 最常见的肠外表现（3％～9％）。
    - 右叶单脓肿（50％～80％）。
    - 可能在暴露后数月至数年（中位数为 3 个月）。
    - 发热。
    - 右上腹疼痛。
    - 肝大，轻度压痛。
    - 右肺底有啰音。
    - 并发腹泻（20％～33％）。
    - 并发症：胸膜腔破裂（10％～20％），腹膜或心包（罕见）。
    - 如果直径>5 cm 或位于左叶位置，破裂的风险会增加。
  - 肝脏阿米巴脓肿：
    - 脑。
    - 肺。
    - 肾周。
    - 脾。
    - 阴道、子宫颈和子宫。
  - 皮肤阿米巴病：
    - 会阴和生殖器。
    - 疼痛、形状不规则的溃疡。
    - 脓性渗出物。
    - 可能引起直肠阴道瘘。

儿科注意事项

暴发性结肠炎的可能性更大。

妊娠注意事项

暴发性结肠炎的可能性更大。

病史

- 可能的暴露源。
- 成为高风险组。
- 前往流行地区>1 个月。

体格检查

- 确定腹膜炎、败血症或休克的证据。
- 腹部肿块需要对肝脓肿或阿米巴瘤进行检查。
- >70％的患者直肠指诊显示血液中有大量或隐匿性血液。

诊断检查与说明

实验室检查

- 全血细胞计数（CBC）：
  - 阿米巴肝脓肿和腹膜炎中的白细胞增多症。
- 碱性磷酸酶和丙氨酸氨基转移酶（ALT）：
  - 在阿米巴肝脓肿中升高。
- 血清电解质、BUN/肌酐改变，长期腹泻或有脱水的证据。
- 粪便聚合酶链反应（PCR）是诊断金标准：
  - 100％敏感且特异性高。
- 溶组织内阿米巴特异性抗原的粪便酶联免疫吸附试验（ELISA）：敏感性为 74％～95％，特异性为 93％～100％。
- 抗组织溶解性抗体：
  - 如果怀疑肝脓肿，必须行该检查，这些患者很少在粪便中排出寄生虫，阿米巴肝脓肿敏感性为 90％～100％，阿米巴结肠炎敏感性为 70％～90％。
- 粪便显微镜检测的灵敏度<60％，不再是首选的检查。
- 粪便白细胞和培养物：
  - 规定感染肠道侵袭性细菌。
  - 阿米巴阴性。

影像学检查

- 腹部超声：对肝脓肿的敏感性为 58％～90％：

A

- 灵敏度受尺寸和位置的影响。
- 评估脓肿增加破裂的风险(>5 cm 或位于左叶)。

• 腹部 CT 或 MRI:
- 与超声相同,用于检查肝脓肿。
- 优于超声检查其他器官的脓肿。

• 头部 CT 或 MRI:
- 如果已知阿米巴病的患者的精神状态改变或局灶性神经系统表现,则应观察阿米巴脑脓肿。
- 不规则的非增强性病变。

• 胸部 X 线检查(CXR):
- 在肝脓肿中右侧膈肌抬高和/或右侧胸腔积液。

诊断步骤/外科

• 结肠镜检查和活组织检查提供阿米巴痢疾、结肠炎、阿米巴瘤和阿米巴病肠腔狭窄的明确诊断。

• 如果非诊断性血清学或抗疟疾治疗失败,经皮细针肝穿刺排除细菌性脓肿。
- 不适用于肝脓肿的初级治疗。

鉴别诊断

• 肠道阿米巴病:
- 侵袭性细菌感染(葡萄球菌、大肠埃希菌、志贺菌、沙门菌、耶尔森菌、弯曲杆菌)。
- 炎症性肠病。
- 缺血性结肠炎。
- 动静脉畸形。
- 腹主动脉瘤。
- 十二指肠溃疡穿孔。
- 脓毒症和憩室炎。
- 胰腺炎。
- 直肠癌。
- 阑尾炎。

• 阿米巴脓肿:
- 细菌性脓肿。
- 结核腔。
- 棘球蚴囊肿。
- 恶性肿瘤。
- 胆囊炎。

• 皮肤阿米巴病:
- 癌。
- STD(尖锐湿疣、软下疳、梅毒)。

治疗

初步稳定/治疗

• ABC 管理。

• 如果出现明显休克的迹象,给予生理盐水静脉补液。

急诊治疗/程序

• 如果轻微,口服补液。如果中度、严重脱水,给予生理盐水静脉补液。

• 避免使用止泻药。

• 纠正血清电解质紊乱。

• 用于溶组织内阿米巴 PCR 或 ELISA 的粪便样品,以及用于抗溶组织内阿米巴血清学抗体。

• 如果粪便或血清对溶组织内阿米巴呈阳性:
- 甲硝唑或替硝唑是治疗全身性阿米巴病的一线药物(治愈率为 90%)。
- 氯喹是一种替代的全身用药。
- 始终使用腔内药物进行全身治疗以根除肠道定植(红霉素、双碘喹啉、硝唑尼特、巴龙霉素或四环素)。
- 不要单独腔内用药。

• 如果粪便或血清对溶组织内阿米巴呈阴性:
- 请胃肠病学家会诊进行结肠镜检查和活组织检查。
- 7 日内重复血清学检查。
- 如果高度怀疑阿米巴病和患者病情严重,考虑甲硝唑的经验疗程。

• 如果有腹膜炎或败血症的证据:
- 添加针对厌氧和革兰阴性细菌的抗生素静脉给药。
- 如果有毒性巨结肠或穿孔、手术。

• 如果怀疑肝脓肿:
- 肝胆系统超声或 CT,并阿米巴血清学检查。
- 如果成像显示脓肿但血清学阴性,用抗阿米巴治疗,并在 7 日内重复血清学检查。
- 结合非杀菌治疗,由外科医师或介入放射科医师行脓肿引流。
- 如果在经验性杀菌治疗 5~7 日后症状没有改善,可考虑细针穿刺以排除细菌性脓肿或肝细胞瘤。
- 考虑由外科医师或介入放射科医师结合杀菌剂进行脓肿引流。

妊娠注意事项

• 在妊娠早期慎用甲硝唑,但如果患者患有暴发性结肠炎或阿米巴脓肿,不要有所保留。

• 使用红霉素或硝唑尼特和甲硝唑合用。

• 红霉素或硝唑尼特可单独用于妊娠早期的轻度痢疾。

• 氯喹、双碘喹啉、巴龙霉素、四环素和替硝唑是禁忌的。

药物治疗

一线用药

• 甲硝唑:500~750 mg[儿童:30~50 mg/(kg·24 h)],口服/静脉,q8 h,持续 5~10 日。

• 替硝唑:2 g/日[儿童:50~60 mg/(kg·d)],口服,持续 3~6 日,适用于 3 岁以上的儿童。

二线用药

• 氯喹:1 000 mg/d,口服,持续 2 日,500 mg/d,口服,持续 14 日;或 200 mg,肌内注射,持续 10~12 日。

• 红霉素:250~500 mg[儿童:30~50 mg/(kg·24 h)],口服,q6 h,持续 10~14 日。

• 双碘喹啉:650 mg,口服,q8 h,持续 20 日。

• 硝唑尼特:500 mg,口服,q12 h。对于>12 岁的儿童,持续 3 日(如果存在肝脓肿则为 1 日)。

• 巴龙霉素:500 mg[儿童:25~30 mg/(kg·24 h)],口服,q8 h,持续 5~10 日。

• 四环素:250~500 mg[儿童>12 岁:25~50 mg/(kg·24 h)],口服,q6 h,持续 10 日。

儿科注意事项

• 四环素禁用于 8 岁以下的儿童。

• 长时间高剂量使用于儿童时,双碘喹啉可能引起更严重的不良反应。

妊娠注意事项

• 妊娠早期谨慎使用。

• 使用红霉素或硝唑尼特。

随访

进一步处理

入院指征

• 休克、败血症或腹膜炎。

• 低血压或心动过速对静脉输液无反应。

• 脱水>10%的儿童。

• 严重的电解质紊乱。

• 饮水无法补充足够的水分:
- 年龄,认知障碍,合并重大疾病。

• 暴发性结肠炎或中毒性巨结肠。

• 肠梗阻。

• 肠外脓肿。

• 门诊治疗失败。

出院指征

• 急性或慢性痢疾无中毒表现。

• 能够保持足够的口服补液和药物依从性。

• 脱水对静脉补充液体有反应。

转诊问题

如果有腹膜炎、中毒性巨结肠、结肠穿孔或肝脓肿的证据，考虑手术。

随访建议

- 胃肠病学和传染病随访 7 日，重复血清学和可能的内镜评估。
- 14 日内进行体格检查，以评估治疗效果和并发症或肠外疾病的发展。

要点和误区

- 避免止泻药。
- 除非有禁忌证，否则应始终使用全身性无阿米巴(甲硝唑、替硝唑或氯喹)和肠道抗菌药(红霉素、双碘喹啉、硝唑尼特、巴龙霉素或四环素)进行联合治疗。
- 始终保持警惕高死亡率的并发症，如暴发性结肠炎或肠外疾病。

A

阿片类药物中毒

Poisoning

Amy V. Kontrick · Mark B. Mycyk　朱妍 译

 基础知识

描述

- 与中枢和外周神经系统(PNS)的 μ、κ 和 δ 阿片受体结合。
- 躯体和精神依赖性。
- 血浆峰值水平：
  - 经口：1～2 h。
  - 肌内注射：0.5～1 h。
  - 静脉或经鼻给予：数秒至数分钟。

病因

- 中重度疼痛过度使用或滥用口服止痛药(处方药)。
- 街头使用的阿片类药物可能含有掺杂物：
  - 可卡因。
  - 双氯醇胺。
  - 苯环己哌啶。
  - 士的宁。
  - 右美沙芬。
  - 奎宁。
  - 莨菪碱。

诊断

症状和体征

- 中枢神经系统：
  - 中枢抑制。
  - 昏迷。
  - 癫痫。
- 胃肠道：
  - 恶心。
  - 呕吐。
  - 便秘。
- 心血管：
  - 低血压。
  - 心动过缓。
  - 心悸。
- 呼吸：
  - 呼吸抑制。
  - 气管痉挛。
  - 肺水肿。
  - 呼吸暂停。
- 其他：
  - 瞳孔缩小。
  - 低体温。
- 戒断症状：
  - 高血压。
  - 心动过速。
  - 呼吸急促。
  - 腹部痉挛。
  - 腹泻。
  - 寒战。
  - 打哈欠。

儿科注意事项

- 新生儿戒断症状：
  - 药物依赖母亲生下的孩子。
  - 发病：出生后 12～72 h。
  - 兴奋、震颤、喂食情况差、脱水。
- 地芬诺酯(止泻宁)：比起成人，毒性在小儿中更严重，甚至致命。

基本检查

明确暴露史后，监测生命体征和呼吸状况：

- 血脉氧或动脉血气。
- 如果持续低氧血症或可能误吸，需行胸部 X 线检查。
- 如果怀疑体内藏毒，行腹部放射检查。
- 行全身检查寻找隐藏的贴剂(如芬太尼)。

诊断检查与说明

实验室检查

- 血浆阿片类药物水平临床不实用：
  - 治疗基于临床表现而不是阿片类药物水平。
- 行尿毒物筛查阿片类药物不能识别一些合成阿片类(如美沙酮)。
- 过度使用或滥用口服止痛药(处方药)行对乙酰氨基酚水平检查。

鉴别诊断

- 可乐定过量。
- 巴比妥过量。
- 苯二氮䓬过量。
- γ-羟基丁酸盐(GHB)过量。
- 地西泮(安定)过量。
- 隐匿性脑损伤。

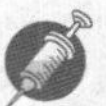 治疗

院前

- 将所有有关过量使用的药片或药瓶带至急诊室，便于确诊。
- 提供呼吸支持。
- 使用纳洛酮。

初步稳定/治疗

- ABC 管理：
  - 气道管理是根本。
  - 吸氧治疗。
- 应用纳洛酮：
  - 阿片类药物过量中逆转呼吸抑制和昏迷。
  - 如果纳洛酮不能逆转呼吸抑制则行气管插管。

急诊治疗/程序

- 使用纳洛酮：
  - 阿片类药物依赖患者从小剂量开始。
  - 逆转丙氧酚、美沙酮和芬太尼的影响需使用高剂量(10 mg)。

- 应用重复剂量逆转症状，每 20～60 min 按需给药。
- 对长效阿片类药物，考虑每小时注射 2/3 所需剂量逆转症状。

• 清除毒物：
- 应用活性炭清除经口摄入。
- 应用聚乙二醇全肠道灌洗避免无症状的身体藏毒者。

• 使用可乐定或美沙酮治疗阿片类药物戒断。

• 低血压：
- 生理盐水大量静脉输注。
- Trendelenburg 测试。
- 初始使用多巴胺纠正低血压。

• 癫痫：
- 初始治疗使用地西泮。
- 癫痫持续状态使用苯巴比妥。

药物治疗

• 活性炭：1～2 g/kg，口服。

• 可乐定：0.1～0.3 mg，口服，每日 2 次，连续 10 日；0.1～0.2 mg/(kg · d) 透皮贴剂。

• 地西泮：5～10 mg，静脉注射（儿童：0.2～0.5 mg/kg，静脉注射），q10～15 min。

• 多巴胺：2～20 μg/(kg · min)，静脉滴注至起效。

• 美沙酮：15～40 mg/d。

• 纳洛酮：0.4～2 mg（儿童：0.1 mg/kg；新生儿剂量与儿童相同，除非怀疑新生儿戒断使用 0.001 mg/kg，静脉注射），静脉注射、肌内注射或雾化。

• 苯巴比妥：10～20 mg/kg 静脉注射（负荷剂量），监测呼吸抑制。

• 聚乙二醇：2 L/h 直至清除直肠毒物和/或肠内容物。

注意

阿片类贴剂可通过不同途径滥用（经皮、经口、吸入、注射），甚至大剂量使用药物的同时仍使用贴剂。

非药物芬太尼、U-47700 和其他高效合成阿片类药物可能会污染市售的海洛因，导致更严重的呼吸抑制，并且在标准的医院毒理学筛查中没有发现。

随访

进一步处理

入院指征

• 口服过量后有症状者。

• 需重复使用或注射纳洛酮逆转症状。

• <5 岁的儿童摄取地芬诺酯后应观察 24 h。

• 阿片类药物身体藏毒者。

• 伴随毒物暴露导致的持续症状（如双氯醇胺）。

出院指征

• 口服过量 6 h 后症状消失者。

• 应用纳洛酮 4 h 后症状消失者。

• 完全清除阿片类药物。

随访建议

• 药物滥用参照患者滥用口服阿片类药物。

• 非故意（偶然）的中毒患者需要毒物预防咨询。

• 故意中毒患者（如自杀）需精神病评估。

要点和误区

• 慢性阿片类药物口服滥用的患者应考虑隐性对乙酰氨基酚中毒。

• 丁丙诺啡在儿科患者中可引起延长的镇静作用。

• 半合成和合成阿片类药物不能提供医院毒物筛查阿片类药物的阳性结果。

• 建议患者参加药物滥用治疗计划（如 SBIRT）。

• 考虑在出院时开纳洛酮或丁丙诺啡诱导药。

埃立克体病 Ehrlichiosis

Roger M. Barkin · Jonathan A. Edlow　姜颢 译

基础知识

描述

• 人感染蜱传播病表现为非特异性的发热性疾病。

• 存在数种埃立克体病，在北美占主导地位的有 2 种：
- 人单核细胞埃立克体病（HME），首次记述于 20 世纪 80 年代晚期：
  ◦ 媒介蜱：美洲花蜱（孤星蜱）。
  ◦ 地理范围：美国中部、南部和中大西洋地区，范围扩大到新英格兰部分地区。
- 人粒细胞埃立克体病（HGE）或人粒细胞无形体病（HGA），首次记述于 1994 年：
  ◦ 媒介蜱：肩胛硬蜱（鹿蜱）。
  ◦ 地理范围：美国东海岸地区、中部各州、西北太平洋地区（同莱姆病分布区域相同，但莱姆病更常见）。
- 1999 年发现由伊氏埃立克体导致的第三种类型。

• 都是蜱传播，但有不同的媒介和地理范围。已报道其他种类，但目前 HME 和 HGE 仍是重要的人类埃立克体病原体。

病因

• 2 种不同种类的专性细胞内生物。

• 近年来随着越来越多的 DNA 和核糖体 RNA 数据变得可用，这些病原体的分类发生了改变。

• HME 是由查非埃立克体这一生物体引起的。

• HGE/HGA 是由嗜粒细胞无形体（2002 年的新名称）引起的。

• 落基山斑疹热（RMSF）发现的血管炎通常是不存在的。

• 第三种类型也可能遇到，由伊氏埃立克体引起，它有孤星蜱的蜱载体，临床表现与 HME 相似。

• 与 RMSF 相比，老年人通常易受影响，年龄一般大于 40 岁。

诊断

症状和体征

• HME 的症状与体征和 HGE/HGA 相似。

• 许多感染者发生无症状血清转换。

• 报道的范围可能会过多地呈现受影响更

严重的患者。

• 无论患者感染任何蜱传播病，同一蜱叮咬可合并感染 1 种以上病原体：
- 可能有 2 种不同疾病的复杂表现。
• 1/4 的儿童有严重疾病。

病史

• 季节和其他流行病学因素对诊断蜱传疾病很重要：
- 最常见于 4—10 月。
- 可能随年份和不同地区气候模式的变化而变化。
• 症状发生于继蜱叮咬后 1～2 周(平均 9～10 日)：
- 相对于较小的鹿蜱，患者更容易回忆起被较大孤星蜱叮咬的场所。
• 突然出现：
- 发热。
- 寒战。
- 头痛。
- 肌痛。
- 乏力。
• 皮疹：
- HME(35%～60%的病例)。
- HGE 或 HGA(5%～10%的病例)。
- 经常延迟，可能是多变的。
• 症状可能与埃立克体病的并发症有关，如：
- 急性呼吸窘迫综合征。
- 肾衰竭。
- 低血压和休克。
- 横纹肌溶解。
- 胃肠功能紊乱。
- 中枢神经系统或外周神经系统受损，如脑病、脑膜炎及癫痫发作。
- DIC。
- 免疫功能不全的患者有更严重的并发症。

体格检查

• 发热。
• 皮疹：
- 可能是斑疹、斑丘疹或瘀点。
- 在疾病的第 1 周可能缺如。
• 通常累及躯干，手和足不受损。
• 淋巴结大。
• 肝脾大。
• 神经系统检查：
- 异常心理状态。
- 脑膜刺激征。
- 眼球震颤。
• 肺部表现(湿啰音、干啰音)取决于肺部并发症。

儿科注意事项

• 48%存在发热、头痛、皮疹。
• 45%有淋巴结肿大。

> **注意**
>
> • 埃立克体病是一种潜在的致命性蜱传播疾病，通常被临床诊断。
>
> • 所有的非特异性发热性疾病患者都应考虑该诊断，特别是在 1 年中的温暖月份，如有蜱叮咬史则肯定要考虑。
>
> • 疾病预防控制中心(CDC)定义该病为发热和 1 个或多个以下表现：头痛、肌痛、贫血、白细胞减少、血小板减少或血清转氨酶升高；＋血清学证据：通过免疫荧光试验测定的 IgG 特异抗体 4 倍变化，或通过 PCR 分析测定特异性指标，活检或尸检样本的证明，或细胞培养生物的分离。

诊断检查与说明

实验室检查

• 全血细胞计数：
- 白细胞减少症。
- 血小板减少症。
- 贫血。
• 肝转氨酶：
- 通常高于正常值 2～6 倍。
• 间接免疫荧光抗体检测，为 HME 和 HGA 的特异检测：
- 可用的常规检测。
- 一个阳性实验阈值通常由个体的实验室血清检测决定。
- 从发病起超过 14 日时获得的第二个样本有 94%～99%的敏感性。
• 外周血瑞特染色：
- 可以看到桑椹胚：
  ◦ 小的胞质内埃立克体 DNA 包涵体。
  ◦ 特征性的。
  ◦ 看到桑椹胚的敏感性取决于观察的人、时间长短及患者的免疫能力。
  ◦ HGE/HGA(50%)较 HME(10%～15%)更常见。
• HGA 和 HGA 培养及 PCR 检测：
- 不常规使用。
• 抗体滴度测试：
- 不可实时使用。
• 腰椎穿刺：
- 淋巴细胞增多和总蛋白增加。

影像学检查

• 脑病者行头颅 CT。
• 发热、呼吸困难者行胸部 X 线检查。

鉴别诊断

• 多数蜱传疾病：
- 蜱传热。
- 莱姆病。
- 巴贝虫病。
• 许多病毒和细菌感染，以及许多其他传染性疾病，尤其是在病程早期，可首先表现为与埃立克体病相似的非特异性发热性疾病。
• 单核细胞增多症。
• 血栓性血小板减少性紫癜。
• 血液恶性肿瘤。
• 胆管炎。
• 肺炎。

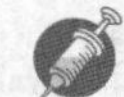

治疗

初步稳定/治疗

常规治疗。

急诊治疗/程序

• 开始抗生素治疗：
- 多西环素：
  ◦ 药物选择。
  ◦ 感染的儿童也应该接受多西环素。治疗 14 日并不引起恒牙明显变色。对于 9 岁以下的儿童，应该与父母专门讨论风险和获益。
  ◦ 治疗应在退热过后持续至少 3 日，以达至少 7 日的总疗程。严重或复杂的疾病需要更长的疗程。
- 利福平：
  ◦ 妊娠患者。
  ◦ 多西环素过敏。
  ◦ 9 岁以下的儿童轻度感染。
  ◦ 妊娠患者，对多西环素过敏；轻度感染者，可予以 7～10 日利福平。
• 开始治疗其他可能共同传播的蜱传疾病。

药物治疗

多西环素：

• 成人：100 mg，静推/口服，q12 h，持续 10 日或退热后 3～5 日。
• 儿童(严重感染)：4.4 mg/(kg · 24 h)分 2 次给药，静脉或口服，到成人最大剂量；较大儿童可用成人剂量。

儿科注意事项

尽管多西环素一般是禁用于 9 岁以下的

患者，但它是埃立克体病严重影响儿童的首选药物，因为短疗程应用出现牙齿变色的风险相对较低。利福平已被成功用于感染较轻的儿童。

妊娠注意事项

利福平可用于治疗合并埃立克体病的孕妇。当存在威胁生命的疾病时，可考虑多西环素。

随访

进一步处理

入院指征

- 重大并发症、严重感染。
- 不能口服抗生素。
- 免疫低下患者。
- HME 具有高达 3%的病死率。

出院指征

- 外观健康。
- 症状通常持续 1～2 周，恢复时未出现后遗症。
- 有报道过长期神经系统并发症。

转诊问题

严重疾病或存在并发症。

巴贝虫病

Jonathan A. Edlow 吴增斌 潘曙明 译

B

基础知识

描述

• 蜱传播的传染病由寄生于红细胞内的原生动物巴贝虫属致病，其感染大部分的脊椎动物，导致寄生的红细胞溶解。

• 无症状或严重或危及生命的感染取决于巴贝虫的种类和患者的免疫状况：

- 无症状感染：
  ◦ 25%的被感染儿童和25%的被感染成人是没有症状的。
- 轻中度感染：
  ◦ 通常是免疫力较好的患者。
  ◦ 感染是自限性的，或者经抗感染治疗能治愈。
  ◦ 死亡率<5%。
- 严重感染：
  ◦ 定义住院超过2周，住ICU大于2日，或者死亡的患者为严重感染患者。
  ◦ 与免疫抑制疾病相关：脾切除术后、癌症、HIV感染、血红蛋白病，以及慢性心、肺、肝疾病。
  ◦ 其他有严重感染高风险的人群：新生儿、年龄>50岁、服用免疫抑制药(利妥昔单抗、抗白血病治疗药物——依那西普、单克隆抗体)。
  ◦ 免疫抑制患者被感染后死亡率能高达21%。

• 并发症发生于大约一半的住院患者：

- 急性呼吸窘迫综合征(ARDS)、DIC最常见。
- 慢性心力衰竭、昏迷、肝功能衰竭、肾衰竭、脾破裂也可以见到。

• 在下列情况下，有些地区会出现该感染与其他蜱传播疾病共存的情况：

- 莱姆病(伯氏疏螺旋体)，伴皮疹。
- 人嗜粒细胞无形体病(嗜噬细胞)，延迟性白细胞减少。

• 罹患重症的危险因素：

- 脾切除术后。
- 恶性肿瘤。
- HIV感染。
- 免疫抑制药物。
- 年龄>50岁。
- 碱性磷酸酶升高。
- 白细胞计数升高。
- 男性。

病因

• 巴贝虫：

- 对人致病的种类：
  ◦ *Babesia microti*：美国北部和中西部(美国最常见的致病原)。
  ◦ *Babesia divergens*：欧洲。
  ◦ *Babesia duncani*：美国北部太平洋沿岸。
- 亚洲、非洲、澳大利亚、南美洲报道过的巴贝虫病。
- 以动物为寄主：
  ◦ *B. microti*：白足鼠、白尾鹿。
  ◦ *B. divergens*：牛、鼠。

• 通过携带病菌的蜱虫传播：

- 最常见的传播人巴贝虫病的携带者。
- 蜱虫需要通过在脊椎动物吸血，传给生命周期的各个阶段(幼虫、幼体、成虫)：
  ◦ 很多病例是因在晚春和早夏被幼体蜱虫叮咬致病，成虫叮咬也可以传播疾病。

• 致病原的生命周期及发病机制：

- 原生动物经蜱幼虫腺体分泌到哺乳动物的血液中，再到红细胞内成熟，分裂。
- 成熟的原虫离开红细胞，破坏细胞膜，使红细胞溶解，从而导致溶血性贫血和血红蛋白尿。
- 破坏的红细胞变形能力差，加快脾对其的清除。但是无脾患者清除被感染红细胞的能力下降，导致感染加重。
- 受损的红细胞使微循环障碍，引起继发的肝、脾、心、肾和脑缺血损害。

• 通过输红细胞、血小板传播：

- 1975年后发生过150多例，其中75%发生于2000年后。
- *B. microti* 是此类传播常见的病原体。
- 血中寄生虫数量少时，并不能在捐献者的血涂片中发现，但能传播疾病。
- 存在免疫抑制或伴严重疾病的受者经常病情严重。

儿科注意事项

传播可以发生在子宫或经分娩传播。

诊断

症状和体征

蜱虫叮咬1～4周后，或者输过被污染的血制品1～9周后，逐渐开始不安和疲乏，伴发热，可达40.6℃。

• 常见症状：寒战、冷汗、头痛、厌食、干咳、关节痛和恶心。

• 较不常见症状：呕吐、咽喉痛、腹痛、结膜充血、畏光、体重减轻、情绪不稳定、消沉和感觉过敏。

病史

• 在下列患者中出现发热、流感样的症状：

- 在过去的2个月内住在或旅行去过传染病流行地区(特别是在春夏季节)。
- 在过去的6个月内有输血史。

• 有上述病史的患者出现休克或脓毒血症，特别提示病情严重。

体格检查

• 发热(最常见)。

• 肝脾大。

• 咽喉斑疹。

• 黄疸。

• 视网膜病变伴破裂出血。

• 视网膜血管梗死。

• 皮疹可见：

- 瘀点、瘀斑。
- 迁移游走性斑疹(提示并发莱姆病)。

• 严重疾病：

- 呼吸急促。
- 低氧血症。
- 低血压。
- 精神状态变化。

基本检查

• 薄血涂片革兰染色或瑞特染色后显微镜下证实有巴贝虫病原体。

• 如果血涂片结果阴性，可用PCR分析验证。

• 如果显微镜下和PCR试验均阴性，间接抗体免疫荧光试验也能被用来证明巴贝虫病原体感染。

诊断检查与说明

• 显微镜下：

- 红细胞内的寄生虫可以是圆形、椭圆形和梨形的。
- 寄生虫在出芽四分体形成(马耳他十字形状)是明确诊断巴贝虫的依据，但不常见到。
- 最常见的发现是红细胞内有圆形或椭圆形环，环内有淡蓝色的细胞质和红染的染色体。

- 寄生虫血浓度高时可见到细胞外的寄生虫。
- 寄生虫血浓度一般在 1%～10%，也可以高到 80%。小于 1%可能是疾病的早期。
- 环形结构与恶性疟原虫（疟疾）结构类似。巴贝虫没有色素沉着（疟原虫色素），色素沉着常见于疟疾。

• PCR：
- 巴贝虫 18 sRNA 放大扩增后比镜检更灵敏。
- 结果能在 24 h 内出来。
- 适用于寄生虫血浓度低时。

• 血清学：
- 镜检和 PCR 试验均阴性时，间接抗体免疫荧光试验可用。
- IgM 抗体能在发病 2 周后检出。
- IgG 滴度≥1∶256 提示活动性感染或正在被感染；IgM 滴度≥1∶64 提示急性感染。

• 在巴贝虫病可见到常规实验室检查的异常：
- 轻中度溶血性贫血（低血细胞比容/血红蛋白，低结合珠蛋白，网织红细胞数、乳酸脱氢酶、总胆红素升高）。
- 血小板减少常见。
- 肝功能检查（碱性磷酸酶、转氨酶、乳酸脱氢酶、胆红素升高）。
- 尿常规（血红蛋白尿、蛋白尿）。
- 尿素氮、血肌酐升高提示肾功能不全。
- 高钾血症可能是大量溶血引起的。

■ 鉴别诊断

• 疟疾。
• 其他蜱虫传播疾病：
- 莱姆病。
- 人嗜粒细胞无形体病。
- 埃立克体病。
- 落基山斑疹热。
- Q 型流感。
- 野兔病。
- 回归热。
• 伤寒热。
• 急性溶血性贫血。

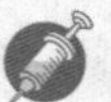

治疗

■ 院前

• 保证呼吸窘迫患者的气道通畅。
• 必要时给予氧气和辅助通气。
• 患者休克，建立静脉通道，给予快速静滴 500 ml 0.9%氯化钠（儿童：20 ml/kg）。

■ 初始稳定/治疗

• 急性呼吸衰竭患者吸氧，辅助通气。
• 有危重指征或危险因素的患者需建立静脉通道。
• 休克患者补液和升压药维持。
• 心电监测：重危患者可能发展为心肌梗死、心律失常。

■ 急诊治疗/程序

• 发热时用退热药。
• 有显微镜下和 PCR 证据的有症状患者开始抗生素治疗。
• 轻中度感染：
- 口服阿托诺酮＋阿奇霉素 7～10 日是基本方案。
- 克林霉素＋奎宁是一种有效的另一个方案，但有并发症（耳鸣、眩晕、胃肠炎）时可能需要减少剂量，1/3 的患者需要停止服药。
• 严重感染：
- 克林霉素静滴＋奎宁口服是一种治疗方案（奎宁静滴也可以用，但有可能会造成心室心律不常，需要监测 QT 间期）。
- 寄生虫血浓度＞10%，血红蛋白＜10 g/dl（100 g/L）提示输血。
- 反复或持续感染见于免疫抑制患者，这类患者需要接受至少 6 周的抗生素治疗，血涂片转阴后还需持续 2 周，可采取标准联合用药。
• 无症状感染：
- 不需要抗生素治疗，除非寄生虫病血涂片阳性已持续 3 个月。

■ 药物治疗

• 对乙酰氨基酚：500 mg（儿童：10～15 mg/kg，24 h 内不要超过 5 次），口服，q4～6 h，24 h 不超过 4 g。
• 阿托诺酮：第 1 日 750 mg（儿童：20 mg/kg；最大剂量：500 mg），口服，接下来每日 250 mg（儿童：5 mg/kg；最大剂量：250 mg），口服，6 日。
• 克林霉素：300～600 mg（儿童：7～10 mg/kg，q6～8 h），静脉滴注，q6 h；600 mg（儿童：7～10 mg/kg，q6～8 h），口服，7～10 日。
• 布洛芬：400 mg[儿童：20～40 mg/(kg·d)]，口服，q6～8 h，必要时。
• 奎宁：650 mg[儿童：25 mg/(kg·d)]，口服，q8 h，7～10 日。

随访

■ 进一步处理

入院指征

• 寄生虫血浓度＞4%，重度贫血（血红蛋白＜100 g/L），症状显著或并发症明显、需要输血的患者需要随访：
- 呼吸衰竭。
- 低血压或休克。
- 新发肾功能不全或肝功能衰竭。
- 精神状态不稳定。
- 严重溶血（黄疸、血尿）：
◦ 脾切除术后的患者。
◦ 恶性肿瘤。

出院指征

• 无症状、轻中度感染患者。
• 寄生虫血浓度＜4%。
• 脾完整、免疫正常。
• 能耐受口服药物。

转诊问题

• 免疫抑制的患者在首要治疗后容易持续或反复感染，应该被转到感染中心治疗。
• 有红细胞置换适应证的患者可能需要转移到能够进行红细胞置换的机构。

■ 随访建议

诊断为巴贝虫病的患者，有症状或无症状但持续血涂片阳性 3 个月的患者，在抗生素治疗完成后应该继续联系主治医师或感染病专科医师监测寄生虫血浓度。

要点和误区

• 巴贝虫病在无脾患者是有生命威胁的。
• 患者有去疫区旅游史，发生呼吸衰竭、休克，巴贝虫病可以考虑为一个潜在因素。
• 疾病早期，寄生虫血浓度低时，显微镜下可能发现不了。
• 该病患者合并感染莱姆病很常见，抗感染治疗需兼顾考虑这一因素。

巴比妥中毒 Barbiturate Poisoning

Denise A. Whitfield · David A. Tanen 宋振举 童朝阳 译

基础知识

描述

- 诱导药物类：镇静催眠药。
- 巴比妥酸衍生物。
- 机制：
- 提高 γ-氨基丁酸(GABA)活性。
- 浓度高时，直接打开 GABA-A 相关氯化物通道。
- 抑制血管平滑肌收缩。
- 可能会导致直接的心肌收缩减弱。

病因

巴比妥剂量过大。

- 有意或无意。

诊断

症状和体征

- 神经系统：
- 嗜睡。
- 言语模糊。
- 肢体不调。
- 共济失调。
- 昏迷(可能有脑死亡征象)。
- 反射消失。
- 心血管系统：
- 高血压。
- 心动过缓。
- 视觉系统：
- 瞳孔缩小(通常伴有深昏迷)。
- 眼球震颤。
- 不良共轭凝视。
- 其他：
- 呼吸抑制。
- 体温降低。
- 水疱或大水疱。
- 呼吸骤停、循环衰竭导致死亡。

病史

- 确定是否存在有意过量情况：
- 查看药瓶。
- 是否有抑郁病史或自杀倾向。
- 确定是否存在药物错用：
- 患者是否服用其他药物。
- 近期剂量是否有所改变。
- 估算患者无应答状态的持续时间。

体格检查

- 神经系统异常：
- 共济失调至昏迷。
- 呼吸抑制。
- 心血管系统：
- 心动过缓或高血压。
- 视觉系统：
- 瞳孔缩小(通常伴有深昏迷)。
- 眼球震颤。
- 不良共振凝视。
- 低体温。
- 水疱或大水疱。

基本检查

- 指尖采血测血糖。
- 氧饱和度监测。
- 血压监测。

> **注意**
> 巴比妥中毒可能会有脑死亡征象。
> • 在排除巴比妥中毒前提下才能判定脑死亡。

诊断检查与说明

实验室检查

- 电解质、尿素氮(BUN)、血肌酐及血糖：
- 计算阴离子间隙。
- 评估肾衰竭。
- 尿液检查：
- 肌红蛋白检测。
- 尿结晶体(扑米酮)检测。
- 检测磷酸肌酸判定是否有横纹肌溶解。
- 尿毒理学筛查。
- 获取血苯巴比妥钠水平(若疑似)。
- 若怀疑自杀，检测对乙酰氨基酚和水杨酸。
- 甲状腺功能检查。

影像学检查

- 头部 CT：检查精神状态，检查是否有变化。
- 胸部 X 线：检查是否有误吸。

诊断步骤/外科

- 头部非增强 CT。
- 腰椎穿刺。

鉴别诊断

- 诱导性镇静催眠药物中毒(包括 GHB 及其前体)。
- 一氧化碳中毒。
- 神经系统感染。
- 颅脑占位损伤。
- 低血糖。
- 尿毒症。
- 电解质紊乱(高镁血症)。
- 迟发型癫痫。
- 甲状腺功能减退症。
- 肝衰竭。
- 精神疾病。

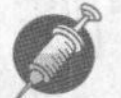

治疗

院前

- 需要专业护理人员转运患者以中和中毒情况。
- 可能存在呼吸抑制与窒息，患者通常需要插管。
- 开放静脉并给氧：
- 为纠正低血压采取静脉补液。

初步稳定/治疗

- 急救：
- 给氧。
- 严重中毒时通常需要气管插管。
- 生理盐水：
- 低血压患者需要至少 1～2 L 的静脉补液复苏。
- 以升压药纠正顽固性低血压。
- 活性炭吸附巴比妥可以降低系统吸收率。

急诊治疗/程序

- 应用 1 个剂量活性炭：
- 如果在服药 1 h 内给予，则用最大剂量。
- 保证患者在应用活性炭前清醒并有警觉(或保护气道)。
- (只要有肠鸣音)可考虑通过每 2～4 h 给予 1 次活性炭(无山梨糖醇)进行“肠道透析”。
- 如果体温过低，给予患者体温复苏(参见“低体温”)。
- 使用血管升压药(多巴胺、去甲肾上腺素、肾上腺素)治疗对静脉补液无反应的低血压。
- 用钙、碳酸氢钠、胰岛素和葡萄糖和/或钾结合剂治疗高钾血症(肌肉分解导致的)。
- 在 2～4 h 复查苯巴比妥水平以确定水平是否正在增加。

- 如果患者存在肾功能受损或肾衰竭，考虑进行血液透析：
- 长期昏迷。
- 血清苯巴比妥水平＞100 mg/dl。
- 难治性低血压。
- 碱化尿液没有作用。

■ 药物治疗

一线用药

- 活性炭：1 g/kg 口服。
- 多巴胺：5～10 μg/(kg·min)滴定至所需效果，最大剂量为 20 μg/(kg·min)。
- 去甲肾上腺素：2～4 μg/min 滴定至所需效果，最大剂量为 10 μg/min。

二线用药

肾上腺素：0.1 μg/(kg·min)滴定至所需的效果，最大剂量为 1 μg/(kg·min)。

随访

■ 进一步处理

入院指征

收入 ICU：

- 昏迷。
- 呼吸抑制。
- 低血压。
- 低体温。
- 横纹肌溶解。

出院指征

在出院前至少观察 6 h 无症状，并连续 2 次检测到苯巴比妥水平低于毒性水平。

■ 随访建议

- 如果故意过量服用，将需要精神科评估。
- 对于无意的过量服用，推荐调整药量。

■ 随访建议

对于无意的过量服用，可能需要转诊以调整药量或将药物改为具有更大治疗窗口的药物。

要点和误区

- 体温过低的诊断可能被误诊：
- 测量准确的核心温度。
- 针对横纹肌溶解进行检查，因为患者可能已经瘫痪了一段时间。
- 巴比妥类中毒会导致长时间的昏迷：
- 做出脑死亡的诊断之前确保巴比妥药效已经得到缓解。

白细胞增多症

Sierra Beck · Conor Cosgrave 王胜云 段立伟 译

基础知识

■ 描述

- 白细胞总数大于正常值。
- 白细胞数正常值(1×10^9/L＝1 000/mm^3)：
- 成人：4 500～11 000/mm^3。
- 儿童：
  - 1 周以内婴儿：5 000～21 000/mm^3。
  - 1～4 岁儿童：6 000～17 500/mm^3。
  - 4 岁以上儿童：5 500～15 500/mm^3。
- 孕妇：
  - 妊娠 3 个月以内：5 000～14 000/mm^3。
  - 妊娠 3～6 个月：5 000～15 000/mm^3。
  - 妊娠 6～9 个月：5 000～17 000/mm^3。
- 正常范围受以下因素影响：
- 运动。
- 女性。
- 吸烟。
- 日间时间。
- 应根据临床具体情况确定正常范围。
- 中性粒细胞：
- 绝对值＞7 500/mm^3。
- 半数中性粒细胞黏附于血管壁上，遇急性刺激时可快速释放，能使白血病数量翻倍。
- 另外一些中性粒细胞、未成熟晚幼粒细胞存在于骨髓中，在感染、炎性反应刺激下可快速释放，未成熟细胞的释放可以造成核左移现象。
- 淋巴细胞：
- 绝对值＞4 000/mm^3。
- 主要存在于脾、淋巴管、胸腺和骨髓中，遇外源性抗原和病毒感染时可释放。
- 白细胞增多(＞100 000/mm^3)：
- 主要在恶性血液病中常见。

■ 流行病学

- 全血细胞计数是急诊最普通的检测项目。
- 白细胞增多是检验科最常见的检测异常指标。
- 接受全血细胞计数检查的急诊患者中有17%白细胞增多。

■ 病因

- 中性粒细胞数量增多：
- 应激反应：
  - 应激。
  - 运动。
  - 手术。
  - 癫痫。
  - 创伤。
  - 缺氧。
  - 疼痛。
  - 呕吐。
- 炎症反应：
  - 风湿性关节炎。
  - 痛风。
  - 炎症性肠病。
  - 血管炎。
- 细菌感染。
- 实验室误差。
- 分娩。
- 类白血病反应。
- 药物：
  - β受体激动剂(肾上腺素、可卡因等)。
  - 激素。
  - 锂盐。
  - 粒细胞集落刺激因子。
- 代谢性疾病：
  - 糖尿病酮症酸中毒。
  - 甲状腺功能亢进症。
  - 尿毒症。
- 恶性肿瘤。
- 骨髓增殖性疾病：
  - 慢性粒细胞性白血病。
  - 真性红细胞增多症。
- 妊娠。
- 出血、溶血。
- 组织坏死：

◦ 肿瘤。
◦ 烧伤。
◦ 骨折。
• 淋巴细胞增多：
- 病毒感染：
◦ 单核细胞增多症。
◦ 带状疱疹病毒感染。
◦ 巨细胞病毒感染。
◦ 病毒性肝炎。
- 特殊细菌感染：
◦ 百日咳。
◦ 肺结核。
◦ 梅毒。
◦ 立克次体感染。
◦ 巴贝虫感染。
◦ 巴尔通体病。
- 甲状腺功能减退症。
- 免疫反应：
◦ 免疫接种。
◦ 自身免疫性疾病。
◦ 移植排异反应。
- 淋巴增生性疾病：
◦ 急性淋巴细胞性白血病。
◦ 慢性淋巴细胞性白血病。
◦ 非霍奇金淋巴瘤。
- 脾切除。
• 单核细胞增多症：
- 感染：
◦ EB 病毒。
◦ 真菌。
◦ 原生生物。
- 自身免疫性/风湿性疾病。
- 脾切除术后。
• 嗜酸性粒细胞增多症：
- 感染，主要是寄生虫和真菌。
- 过敏性疾病：
◦ 过敏性鼻炎。
◦ 哮喘。
◦ 药物过敏。
- 血液恶性肿瘤。
- 结缔组织病。
• 嗜碱性粒细胞增多症：
- 过敏性疾病。
- 血液恶性肿瘤。

诊断

症状和体征

• 与现病史有关。
• 感染相关症状：
- 咳嗽。
- 发热。
- 皮疹。
- 呕吐、腹泻。
- 排尿困难，尿频。
• 慢性炎症相关症状：
◦ 关节疼痛。
◦ 皮疹。
• 恶性肿瘤相关症状：
◦ 体重减轻。
◦ 易疲劳。
◦ 盗汗。

体格检查

• 根据现病史。
• 局部感染症状：
- 局部脓肿/蜂窝织炎。
- 耳炎。
- 咽炎。
- 肺炎。
• 恶性肿瘤症状：
- 肝脾大。
- 淋巴结肿大。
- 面色苍白。
- 出血。
• 慢性炎症症状：
- 关节疼痛、肿胀。
- 皮疹。

诊断检查与说明

• 白细胞增多：
- 白细胞增多具有高度非特异性。
- 白细胞升高的时间：
◦ 数小时至数日：很可能是急性事件（感染、急性白血病）。
◦ 数月至数年：慢性感染阶段或恶性白血病（风湿性关节炎、实体器官肿瘤、慢性白血病、淋巴瘤）。
• 细胞数量及分类：
- 如果其他类型细胞数量太少，白细胞数量增多可能是假象。
- 核左移现象可能提示为急性感染或恶性肿瘤。
- 细胞数量的差异不能有效区分细菌和病毒感染。
• 手工分类或外周血涂片：
- 考虑有实验室仪器自动检测误差时。
• 红细胞及血小板计数：
- 数量减低考虑恶性肿瘤或骨髓浸润可能。
• 儿童：
- 发热儿童的评估：
◦ 白细胞数量＞15 000/mm^3 应考虑严重感染可能，可给予抗生素治疗，留取血培养并进一步住院治疗。
◦ 白细胞升高＞25 000/mm^3 并不意味着更严重的疾病。

基本检查

• 取决于患者的临床情况。
• 病原学不清楚、血液恶性肿瘤不能除外的情况下，细胞数量分类可能对明确诊断起作用。
• 患者怀疑血液系统恶性肿瘤可行外周血涂片及骨髓穿刺活检。

鉴别诊断

主要从病因及临床表现进行鉴别。

治疗

• 主要基于潜在考虑的疾病进行治疗。
• 恶性肿瘤所导致的白细胞极度升高应采取以下措施：
- 开通静脉输液。
- 输血。
- 别嘌醇。
- 羟基脲。
- 血液科会诊。

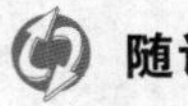

随访

进一步处理

主要根据患者的临床症状对症处理，全面综合考虑，避免仅根据患者白细胞情况做出错误判断。

要点和误区

• 医务人员的诊疗判断会受白细胞增多症的影响。
• 入院率增加。
• 检测项目花费会增加。
• 多种原因都可以导致白细胞增多。
• 对判断病情严重程度缺乏敏感性和特异性。
• 血液恶性肿瘤患者出现极度白细胞升高可能会危及生命，应接受紧急治疗。

白血病 Leukemia

Linda Mueller 王胜云 段立伟 译

基础知识

描述

- 白细胞向恶性肿瘤细胞方向分化。
- 白细胞数量增多：
  - 白细胞总数>100 000/mm³。
  - 主要导致肺部或脑部的小血管闭塞。
  - 可有神志不清、呼吸急促等表现。

慢性粒细胞性白血病

- 粒细胞过度增生。
- 中性粒细胞功能下降。
- 血小板下降。
- 嗜碱性粒细胞增多。
- 骨髓中 Ph 染色体>95%。

慢性淋巴细胞性白血病

- 多见于成年患者。
- 淋巴细胞过度增生。
- 细胞主要分布于淋巴结、骨髓、肝和脾。
- 容易并发疱疹病毒感染。

急性白血病

- 未成熟细胞（幼稚细胞）数量增多：
  - 急性粒细胞白血病（AML）：未成熟髓性细胞。
  - 急性淋巴细胞白血病（ALL）：未成熟淋巴细胞。
- 病情进展迅速。

病因

- 由多种基因突变引起，这些突变允许细胞不受限制地增殖和异常成熟。
- 慢性淋巴细胞白血病(CLL)可见家族发病。
- 电离辐射可以导致急性淋巴细胞白血病、急性粒细胞白血病及慢性粒细胞白血病(CML)发病率增加。

儿科注意事项

- 通常为急性淋巴细胞性白血病，最常见的儿童血液肿瘤。
- 60%～80%的患者经治疗可缓解。
- >1 岁的儿童预后更好。
- 可能在较低水平发展为白细胞淤滞。
- >30%伴有骨或脊柱疼痛。
- 可能胸腺增大。
- 别嘌醇的剂量为 3 mg/kg。
- 头孢他啶的剂量为 50 g/kg。

妊娠注意事项

- 90%的患者为急性粒细胞白血病或急性淋巴细胞白血病。
- 粒细胞白血病更常见。
- 孕妇中慢性淋巴细胞白血病非常罕见。
- 化疗可能会导致早产及婴儿先天畸形。
- 预后与非孕妇一致，因此勿推迟治疗。
- 相较非孕妇应尽早输血，使血红蛋白保持 98 g/L 以上。

老年注意事项

主要表现为慢性粒细胞白血病和慢性淋巴细胞白血病。

诊断

症状和体征

慢性粒细胞白血病

- 可无症状。
- 易疲劳。
- 体重减轻。
- 左上腹轻压痛。
- 腹部饱胀感。
- 脾大(最常见)。
- 晚期症状：
  - 头痛。
  - 骨痛。
  - 关节痛。
  - 发热。
  - 白细胞性症状：
    - 呼吸困难。
    - 嗜睡。
    - 意识错乱。

慢性淋巴细胞白血病

- 可无症状。
- 易疲劳。
- 体重减轻。
- 淋巴结肿大。
- 嗜睡。
- 脾大。
- 肝大。

急性粒细胞白血病

- 发热。
- 易疲劳。
- 面色苍白。
- 头痛。
- 心绞痛。
- 充血性心力衰竭、劳力性呼吸困难。
- 骨痛。
- 盗汗。
- 粒细胞肉瘤。
- 出血倾向：
  - 皮肤瘀点。
  - 瘀斑。
  - 鼻出血。
  - 其他脏器出血。
- 感染（粒细胞减少性）。
- 进展性急性淋巴细胞性白血病累及器官：
  - 淋巴结病。
  - 脾大。
  - 白血病性脑膜炎：
    - 头痛。
    - 恶心。
    - 癫痫发作。

病史

- 电离辐射暴露。
- 烷化剂暴露。
- 近期病毒感染，尤其是 EB 病毒。

体格检查

- 出血倾向（瘀点、瘀斑）。
- 肝脾大。
- 面色苍白。
- 腊肠样出血性视网膜静脉。
- 牙龈增生。
- 皮肤白血病：可见的皮损。

基本检查

- 全血细胞计数/血小板：
  - 慢性粒细胞性白血病：
    - 白细胞数范围 10 000～1 000 000/mm³。
    - 以中性粒细胞为主。
    - 50%的患者出现血小板增多。
  - 急性粒细胞性白血病：
    - 淋巴细胞计数>5 000/mm³。
    - 白细胞数范围 40 000～150 000/mm³。
  - 急性白血病：
    - 贫血程度。
    - 血小板减少情况。
    - 白细胞数的升高或下降。

诊断检查与说明

实验室检查

- 电解质、尿素氮、肌酐、血糖、钙水平。
- 尿酸水平：
  - 常见升高，尤其在急性淋巴细胞白细胞中。
- 乳酸脱氢酶：

- 急性白血病常见升高。
- 凝血检查：
- PT/APTT、纤维蛋白原、纤维蛋白原降解产物。
- 弥散性出血应怀疑血管内凝血。
- 发热时行血尿标本培养。
- 动脉血气分析/血氧饱和度监测，观察呼吸情况。

影像学检查

合并感染患者拍摄胸部X线片。

诊断步骤/外科

- 骨髓穿刺活检：
- 需明确诊断。
- 慢性粒细胞白血病：髓细胞异常增生。
- 慢性淋巴细胞白血病：淋巴细胞增生(30%～100%)。
- 急性白血病：替代正常髓细胞的幼稚细胞增生。
- 白细胞碱性磷酸酶检测：
- 慢性粒细胞白血病见中性粒细胞减少。
- 慢性粒细胞白血病可见Ph1染色体。

鉴别诊断

- 慢性粒细胞白血病：
- 淋巴细胞白血病。
- 骨髓增生综合征。
- 全身性红斑狼疮。
- 感染：细菌、真菌、分枝杆菌。
- 慢性淋巴细胞白血病：
- 百日咳。
- 传染性淋巴细胞增多症。
- 巨细胞病毒。
- EB病毒/单核细胞增多症。
- 肝炎。
- 风疹。
- 急性白血病：
- 再生障碍性贫血。
- 类白血病反应。
- 淋巴母细胞性淋巴瘤。

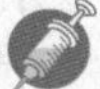

治疗

初步稳定/治疗

- 缺氧、呼吸急促者吸氧。
- 建立静脉通道。
- 血小板减少引起的严重出血，予以输注血小板。
- 对发热和粒细胞减少患者给予广谱抗生素治疗。
- 治疗DIC。

急诊治疗/程序

- 治疗白细胞减低：
- 生理盐水静脉水化(500 ml，20 ml/kg)。
- 乙酰唑胺碱化尿液。
- 早期使用别嘌醇。
- 白细胞洗脱。
- 使用地塞米松。
- 慢性粒细胞白血病患者使用羟基脲(20～30 ml/kg，每日剂量)。
- 贫血患者给予输血：
- 可能需要。
- 后期治疗：
- 慢性粒细胞白血病：
- 化疗。
- 血小板减少患者给予泼尼松冲击治疗。
- 局部肿块的放疗。
- 慢性淋巴细胞白血病：
- 干扰素治疗。
- 化疗。
- 骨髓移植。
- 急性淋巴细胞白血病：
- 化疗。
- 鞘内注射甲氨蝶呤/放疗。
- 骨髓移植。
- 急性粒巴细胞白血病：
- 化疗。
- 骨髓移植。

药物治疗

一线用药

- 积极地静脉补液，从生理盐水开始，随后碱化。
- 根据需要补充红细胞和血小板。

二线用药

- 发热：头孢他啶。
- 如果有肿瘤溶解的风险，使用别嘌醇或拉布立酶和利尿剂。

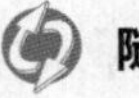

随访

进一步处理

入院指征

- 新近诊断白血病患者有以下情况者：
- 贫血。
- 白细胞>30 000/mm³。
- 血小板减少。
- 合并出血、DIC等生命体征不平稳者收入ICU治疗。

出院指征

症状消失、实验室检查无异常。

随访建议

新发白血病患者定期复查血常规。

要点和误区

- 注意肿瘤细胞溶解导致的高钾血症。
- 白细胞增多可以表现为呼吸衰竭和出血。

百日咳 Pertussis

Adam Z. Barkin · Roger M. Barkin 马林浩 译

基础知识

描述

- 急性呼吸道感染，由小的呼吸道飞沫传播。
- 细菌(菌毛)接触呼吸道上皮细胞并且在其上增殖，产生毒素：
- 纤毛功能紊乱、细胞碎片累积、呼吸道黏液的形成增加，淋巴细胞和粒细胞浸润。
- 细支气管充血、阻塞及坏死。
- 由于黏液栓形成的气道阻塞，导致缺氧和肺换气不足。
- 胸腔内或颅内压力增加。
- 继发细菌性感染可能导致呼吸窘迫或衰竭恶化。
- 由脑炎、颅内压增加和/或缺氧引起的中枢神经系统损伤。
- 简单病例持续6～10周，有一半病例持续<6周。
- 死亡率：
- 在<1岁的群体中死亡率最高。
- 在<1个月的病患中死亡率为1.3%。

- 在2～11个月的儿童中死亡率为0.3%。
- 90%的死亡继发于细菌性肺炎。
- 传染病：
- 潜伏期为6～20日，通常是7～10日。
- 大多数发于年轻儿童，有24%是发生于<6个月的儿童。
- 青少年的发生率逐年增加。
- 成人是病原储存体。
- 高峰发生期在夏末或秋季。
- 用破伤风-白喉-百日咳(Tdap)混合疫苗可以预防。

病因

百日咳波氏杆菌：
- 一种复杂的、革兰阴性、多形性的芽孢杆菌。

诊断

症状和体征

- 大体分为3个可识别的阶段：
- 对婴儿来说可能各阶段模糊不清。
- 黏膜期：
- 持续1～2周。
- 鼻漏。
- 轻咳。
- 低热。
- 阵发期：
- 持续1～6周。
- 典型的哮喘性咳嗽，严重程度在增加：
  - 咳嗽痉挛，以突然吸入空气结束——有喘息声；不间断发作。
- 黄萎病，伴有呼吸窘迫或衰竭。
- 呼吸暂停(发生于<6个月的婴儿)。
- 继发于缺氧或脑炎的精神状态变化。
- 恢复期：
- 持续2～12周。
- 咳嗽减弱。
- 呼吸状况改善。
- 非典型描述：
- <6个月的儿童中常常是非典型表现。
- 部分免疫的儿童病情较轻。
- 成人临床表现常常为只有流涕、咽喉痛、持续性咳嗽，常常发生在家庭成员当中。

病史

- 黏膜期：
- 心神不安。
- 低热。
- 鼻漏。
- 咽喉痛。
- 阵发期：
- 哮喘性咳嗽。
- 咳嗽阵发期的黄萎病。
- 咳嗽阵发期的呕吐。
- 阵发期有哮喘声。
- 黏膜期：
- 持续性咳嗽。

体格检查

- 黏膜期：
- 低热。
- 鼻漏。
- 流泪。
- 干咳(晚期)。
- 结膜炎。
- 阵发期：
- 哮喘性咳嗽。
- 恢复期：
- 偶尔阵发性咳嗽。

基本检查

- 应该基于患者临床表现做出急诊诊断。
- 尝试了解患者的接触史。
- 观察患者的阵发性咳嗽，是否有特征性的哮喘声。
- 使用相关的辅助性研究来进一步支持临床诊断，并排除并发症。

诊断检查与说明

实验室检查

- PCR：
- 高敏感性和特异性。
- 高敏感性导致更多的假阳性。
- PCR测试的最好做法：
  - 只测试有相关症状的。
  - 在咳嗽4周后或使用抗生素后进行测试，会增加假阳性概率。
  - 通过针吸或后鼻咽拭子取样，最大化回收DNA片段。
- 使用该测试应结合细胞培养。
- 对鼻咽黏液进行直接免疫荧光抗体试验：
- 高假阳性率。
- 在补体结合中间物上进行鼻咽培养或咳碟培养：
- 需要7～12日。
- 高特异性。
- 低敏感性：
  - 仍然是金标准试验。
- 血清学：
- 在后期诊断中有用。
- 在咳嗽发作2～8周后执行。
- 白细胞计数：
- 白细胞增多(2万～5万个/L)并带有显著的淋巴细胞增多。
- 恢复期的标准测试。
- 白细胞增多及淋巴细胞增多对应咳嗽的严重程度增加。
- 通过荧光免疫检验和酶免疫检测来排除呼吸道合胞体病毒。
- 对鼻腔冲洗液或鼻咽拭子(涤纶)进行相关检查。

影像学检查

胸部X线检查：
- 最常见的常态检查。
- 肺门浸润。
- 肺不张。
- 偶尔出现特征性的右心室边界蓬松。
- 继发性的细菌性肺炎。

鉴别诊断

- 感染：
- 由副百日咳博德特菌、沙眼衣原体、衣原体肺炎、支气管炎博德特菌或腺病毒引起的类似百日咳综合征。
- 肺炎：
  - 细菌性。
  - 支原体。
  - 分枝杆菌。
- 细支气管炎：
  - 呼吸道合胞体病毒。
  - 流行性感冒。
  - 其他病毒。
- 反应性呼吸道疾病。
- 异物。
- 囊胞性纤维症。

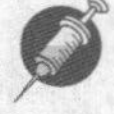

治疗

院前

- 给氧。
- 呼吸道管理。
- 抽吸。

初步稳定/治疗

- 给氧及通气支持。
- 抽吸黏液栓。

急诊治疗/程序

- 全面性防护措施：
- 疾病特异性要求在开始抗菌疗法5日后进行飞沫预防。
- 保持适当补液。

- 在疾病发作期间进行监测氧合功能,给氧。
- 在更年轻的儿童群体中,呼吸道管理可能起到救生作用。
- 抗生素:
  - 在黏膜期很有效。
  - 在阵发期预防进一步传播。
  - 阿奇霉素是首选药剂。
  - 优选地,可以用克拉霉素、红霉素或复方新诺明(甲氧苄啶-磺胺甲噁唑,TMP-SMX),但是功效未经证明;红霉素如果不产生耐药就是有用的。
- 皮质类固醇和舒喘宁可能减少咳嗽阵发,但是需要进一步研究。
- 百日咳在青少年和成人中的发病率在增加,急诊医师可以通过在接种破伤风疫苗的时候接种百日咳疫苗来降低百日咳发病率:
  - 破伤风类毒素,减量的白喉类毒素,无细胞百日咳菌苗(百白破联合疫苗,Tdap)。

药物治疗

支气管扩张剂和类固醇一般不建议用于百日咳治疗。

一线用药

- 阿奇霉素(成人用量):第 1 日口服用量 500 mg,然后连续 4 日口服用量 250 mg,每日 1 次。
- 阿奇霉素(不满 5 个月的婴儿的用量):按体重用药,每日 10 mg/kg,服用 5 日。
- 阿奇霉素(5 个月以上的婴儿至成人用量):按体重用药,第 1 日口服用量 10 mg/kg(最大剂量 500 mg),然后连续 4 日每日口服用量为 5 mg/kg(每日最大量 250 mg)。
- Tdap:0.5 ml 肌内注射:
  - Adacel 疫苗:批准在 11 岁及以上使用。
  - Boostrix 疫苗:批准在 10 岁及以上使用。

妊娠注意事项

- 免疫接种咨询委员会(ACIP)推荐孕妇患者在妊娠内使用 Tdap。
- 可以再任何时间用药,但倾向于在妊娠 27~36 周使用。

二线用药

- 克拉霉素:按体重日用量为 15 mg/(kg·d),每日 2 次,服用 7 日(最大用量 1 g/d)。
- 红霉素:按体重日用量为 40~50 mg/(kg·d),每日 4 次,服用 14 日(最大用量 2 g/d)。在执行用药的前 2 周与幽门狭窄的风险有关。
- 甲氧苄啶-磺胺甲噁唑:按体重用量为 0.2 mg/(kg·d),每日 2 次,服用 14 日(最大用量 0.2 mg/d):
  - 不可对不满 2 个月的婴儿用药。

随访

进一步处理

入院指征

- 不满 1 岁的患者。
- 呼吸暂停。
- 咳嗽阵发期的黄萎病。
- 显著的相关性肺炎。
- 脑炎。

出院指征

- 儿童没有出现呼吸暂停、呼吸系统损害、精神状态变化或并发症和呼吸窘迫症。
- 通过热饮可缓解咳嗽痉挛。
- 对婴儿群体,通过球吸可清除厚厚的分泌物。
- 补液良好。
- 避免接触咳嗽引发因素:烟气、污染物、香水。
- 建议对所有近距离接触的人员[在有症状的人 3 ft(1 ft=30.48 cm)以内的接触]采取暴露后预防措施:
  - 建议使用和疾病携带者相同的抗生素。
  - 有症状的儿童应该从学校或工作场所隔离,百日咳患者应该在全疗程治疗后 5 日进行复查。

随访建议

出院儿童需要严密随访,监测补液状态和呼吸系统损害。

> **注意**
> 法律要求内科医师应向国家健康部门报告百日咳病例。

并发症

- 头部、眼部、耳部、颈部及喉部:
  - 鼻出血。
  - 结膜下出血。
- 呼吸系统:
  - 急性呼吸停止。
  - 由继发性感染引起的肺炎。
  - 气胸。
  - 带有捻发音的皮下或纵隔气肿。
  - 支气管扩张。
- 胃肠道:
  - 白线疝:腹股沟或腹部。
  - 直肠脱垂。
- 神经病学:
  - 癫痫。
  - 脑炎。
  - 昏迷。
  - 颅内出血。
  - 脊髓硬脑膜外出血。

> **注意**
> 患有百日咳的儿童可能有显著的呼吸窘迫或呼吸暂停。

要点和误区

- <1 岁的百日咳患儿要入院治疗。
- Tdap 注射应该给那些符合条件的需要破伤风预防的患者。
- 在有效的抗菌治疗后,执行 5 日的飞沫预防。
- 建议对所有的家庭接触进行化学物质预防,无论年龄和免疫状态。

包茎 Phimosis

Nicole M. Franks 瞿金龙 译

基础知识

描述

- 真性包茎是由于瘢痕导致的包皮不能翻上去将阴茎头露出。
- 平时不能将阴茎头露出来不一定是真性包茎。
- 出生时由于包皮内层和阴茎头正常的粘连,包皮很少翻上去。
- 到 3 岁时 90% 的包皮可以翻上去;17 岁时当包皮垢脱落,99% 的包皮可以正常翻上去。

• 患者不能过度外翻包皮。

病因

引起真性包皮的原因包括：

• 创伤导致的包皮过度收缩。

• 尿布皮炎反复发作。

• 龟头包皮炎反复发作。

• 个人卫生差。

• 包皮环割切手术不当。

• 先天异常。

诊断

症状和体征

• 排尿困难、血尿。

• 尿流过细。

• 包皮口发白、狭窄。

• 包皮水肿、发红、压痛。

• 龟头包皮炎。

• 少数患者排尿时包皮囊形成。

体格检查

检查必须包括潜在并发症的评估：

• 嵌顿包茎。

• 发生在极个别的患者。

基本检查

• 大部分患者不需要特别的检查。

• 在部分严重狭窄的患者，可能发生尿路梗阻的并发症，可能需要进一步检查：

- 肾功能评估，包括肌酐和尿素氮。

- 肾脏超声。

• 继发于龟头包皮炎的包茎，需做糖尿病方面的检测：

- 尿液分析、血清糖、糖化血红蛋白（HbA_{1c}）。

鉴别诊断

• 在年轻人，包皮粘连很常见。

• 龟头包皮炎没有包茎。

治疗

院前

• 院前个人和家庭成员在医师评估前不能试图翻包皮。

• 不当的处理可能将一个受损伤的正常的包皮变成严重的包皮嵌顿。

初步稳定/治疗

大部分患者无需特别处理。

急诊治疗/程序

• 通过导尿解决尿路梗阻。

• 龟头的血供被阻断时，需紧急切开包皮的背侧：

- 形成龟头的血供（龟头嵌顿部分有详细步骤）。

- 在包茎中很少需要。

• 类固醇类药物减少包茎的发生：

- 0.05%～0.1%二丙酸倍他米松：包皮口外用每日 2 次，使用 4～6 周。

儿科注意事项

儿科处理时必要时，可予以镇静处理。

药物治疗

必要时可以使用控制疼痛的药物。

随访

进一步处理

入院指征

• 梗阻发生。

• 严重的龟头包皮炎合并缺血或坏死。

出院指征

• 有能力排尿。

• 有方便的泌尿外科随访。

转诊问题

类固醇类药物治疗需门诊随访，包皮开放手术后进行必要的包皮扩张。

随访建议

生理性包茎可等年龄大了在随访确定需不需要处理，其间保持包皮的个人卫生。

要点和误区

• 新生儿期到 3 岁，包皮有时候很难翻起。

• 在 3～17 岁，不需要特别去翻起包皮，因为这时段的包茎可能是生理性的。

• 必要时需要做背侧切开来防止龟头缺血坏死。

包皮嵌顿

Nicole M. Franks　王忠 译

基础知识

描述

• 阴茎龟头周围包皮环形收缩。

• 致淋巴管和静脉回流受阻，进而影响龟头的动脉血供。

• 包皮嵌顿是泌尿外科的急症。

病因

• 以下的一些情况可能导致包皮嵌顿：

- 包皮过长。

- 炎症反应。

- 创伤。

- 性知识缺乏，未在性交前将过长的包皮缩短。

• 医源性的原因也很常见，如检查后包皮复位不当、导管插入或清洁龟头。

诊断

症状和体征

• 包皮收缩。

• 疼痛。

• 龟头肿胀水肿。

• 局部蜂窝织炎。

• 未治疗的患者出现过龟头坏死。

体格检查

检查生殖器时需检查收缩的异物或收缩带。

注意事项

• 包皮嵌顿是个临床诊断，是在先前的临床检查中发现并描述的。

• 治疗要尽早，不能因为实验室或影像学检查而耽误。

诊断检查与说明

影像学检查

如果病史提示阴茎有外来异物影响，需在血管压迫减轻的情况下立即行影像学检查。

■ 鉴别诊断

• 阴茎被外力压缩会产生类包皮嵌顿的效果,包括:
- 止血带。
- 性虐待时使用的线、绳和其他东西。
• 龟头包皮炎。
• 创伤(拉链伤)。
• 急性自发性龟头水肿。

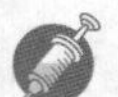

治疗

■ 院前

• 患者应尽早转运,不要尝试在原地复位。
• 院前急救人员可以在充分保护皮肤的前提下,予以冰块冷敷阴茎。
• 控制疼痛。

■ 初步稳定/治疗

• 准备将包皮归纳时可以用冰块冰敷阴茎:
- 用橡胶手套拇指端装冰进行冰敷。
• 嵌顿的包皮应尽快将其复位松解以防止阴茎缺血坏死。
• 实行包皮归纳术,术中疼痛需联合镇静、镇痛和局部麻醉共同处理。

■ 急诊治疗/程序

• 包皮嵌顿的治疗包括安抚患者,减轻包皮水肿,并将包皮恢复到原来的位置和状态。
• 治疗的步骤需按照下面的顺序进行:
- 在包皮上进行牵引的同时,通常可以使用阴茎阻滞和手动压缩龟头来减少包皮异常症。
- 阴茎阻滞麻醉使用 5 ml 不含肾上腺素的 1%利多卡因皮下浸润,作用于耻骨联合下支角之间:
◦ 再用另外 5 ml 沿阴茎 1 圈皮下浸润注射。
◦ 5 min 后产生阻滞麻醉的效果。
- 成功的复位需要稳定远端水肿部位周边压力,同时人工复位包皮。
- 对于儿童,镇静常常是十分必要的。
- 如果手法复位不成功,那么多重穿刺术将会帮助复位:
◦ 用 26G 清洁针头在水肿包皮周围扎 20 个孔,可以让水肿液流出,再行手法复位。
- 如果上述方法还是无法使包皮回到原来位置,那就需要消毒后将缩窄环背侧的包皮切开:
◦ 如果切口过长则需要在复位后用 3.0 可吸收线做间断缝合。
• 如果包皮嵌顿的治疗因为某些情况被推迟了,可以用 50%葡萄糖将纱布片浸湿敷于水肿处,利用渗透的原理减轻水肿利于包皮复位。
• 如果患者不愿行包皮环切术治疗,那么类固醇药物可以减轻纤维环。泌尿外科医师建议:
- 0.1%氟羟氢化泼尼松乳膏涂患处持续 6 周。
- 如果效果不佳,仍需行包皮环切术。

■ 药物治疗

• 适度的镇痛和麻醉是需要的。
• 一般无需使用抗生素,除非合并蜂窝织炎或龟头包皮炎。

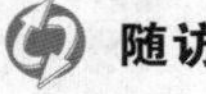

随访

■ 进一步处理

入院指征

阴茎坏死或蜂窝织炎。

出院指征

• 成功复位症状缓解。
• 泌尿外科医师密切随访。

转诊问题

• 需要泌尿外科医师的会诊。
• 是否行包皮环切术以防止嵌顿复发,在医学界仍有争议,但历史经验上该手术常会执行。

■ 随访建议

• 重点教育患者复位后包皮的替代。
• 重点注意包皮卫生清洁。

要点和误区

• 治疗目标是减轻包皮水肿以使包皮复位覆盖龟头。
• 一般来说,无创性的手法复位 2～3 次都能取得成功;背侧纵切复位一般用于嵌顿十分严重的患者。

孢子丝菌病

Sean Devanney · Adam Kellogg 江伟伟 李文放 译

基础知识

■ 描述

• 皮肤淋巴管:
- 最常见的形式。
- 将真菌(申克孢子丝菌)接种到皮肤或软组织中。
- 用土壤或植物材料进行创伤性接种后伴有或不伴有血行播散。
- 继发于动物叮咬/划痕,特别是来自猫的创伤。
- 高风险:农民、园艺工作者、景观设计师、林业工作者。
• 肺:
- 吸入从土壤、植物产生的分生孢子。
- 高风险:酒精中毒、糖尿病、慢性阻塞性肺疾病、长期使用激素的患者。
• 多发性皮肤外:
- 皮肤接种和血液传播。
- 高风险:HIV 感染/使用免疫抑制剂患者。

■ 病因

• 申克孢子丝菌引起的真菌感染。
• 二相性真菌。
• 发生在温带和热带环境中腐烂的植被、苔藓和土壤上。
• 动物载体,特别是猫和犰狳。
• 常见环境暴露:玫瑰丛、干草包、泥炭藓、针叶树幼苗。

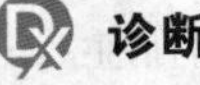

诊断

■ 症状和体征

• 几种临床表现/综合征。
• 由接种方式和宿主因素决定。
• 皮肤淋巴管型:
- 接种后几日至几周出现初始病变。
- 开始为丘疹,变成结节性,经常溃烂:

B

◦ 更常见的是累及远端肢体。
◦ 大小：数毫米至 4 cm。
◦ 轻微疼痛或不痛。
◦ 非脓性积液。
- 全身症状通常不存在。
- 继发性结节性病变沿淋巴管发展。
- 如果未经处理，可能会常年反复复发。
• 固定型表现：
- 在接种部位（通常是面部和四肢）的斑块或疣状病变。
- 常见溃疡。
- 不表现出淋巴管扩张。
- 常见于南美洲的流行地区。
• 皮肤黏膜型：
- 骨关节：
◦ 继发于局部或血液学接种。
◦ 化脓性关节炎比骨髓炎更常见。
◦ 关节炎、积液和疼痛。
◦ 四肢的单肢或多关节受累：膝关节、肘关节、腕关节、踝关节。
◦ 无痛发作，全身症状少。
◦ 腱鞘炎、化脓性关节炎、滑囊炎、神经卡压综合征。
◦ 由于延误诊断，通常预后不佳。
• 肺型：
- 类似于分枝杆菌感染（TB）。
- 发热，体重减轻，疲劳，盗汗。
- 咳嗽，咯血，呼吸困难。
- 如果未经处理，死亡率高。
• 多发性皮肤外（播散型）：
- 低热，体重减轻。
- 皮肤损伤。
- 关节炎、溶骨性病变、脑实质受累。
- 慢性淋巴细胞性脑膜炎。
- 眼附属器，眼内炎。
- 泌尿生殖器，鼻窦。
- 未经处理可能致命。
- 常见于免疫力低下患者。

病史

• 暴露于流行地区的土壤、苔藓、有机物质或猫抓伤。
• 固定型或皮肤淋巴管型：健康的宿主。
• 播散型或皮肤黏膜型：糖尿病、慢性阻塞性肺疾病、HIV/获得性免疫缺陷综合征（AIDS）。

体格检查

• 固定型和皮肤淋巴管型：检查时发现病变。
• 播散型：非特异性病变。

■ 基本检查

诊断依赖于感染部位分离申克孢子丝菌：
• 病原学培养是诊断的金标准。
• 从抽吸材料、组织活检或痰液中留取培养标本。

■ 诊断检查与说明

实验室检查

• 血液检查对皮肤疾病的意义不大。
• 皮肤黏膜型行痰液、滑液、脑脊液、血液培养。
• 没有可靠的血清学分析。

影像学检查

• 肺型：
- X 线片显示空洞病变。
• 皮肤黏膜型或播散型：
- 免疫功能缺陷患者行骨扫描。

诊断步骤/外科

• 皮肤淋巴管型或固定型：
- 活检显示肉芽肿性炎症，3～5 mm 雪茄形状酵母。
• 肺型：
- 痰液的革兰染色可能产生酵母，痰培养往往是阳性的。
• 皮肤黏膜型或播散型：
- 脑脊液显示淋巴细胞性脑膜炎，蛋白质增加/葡萄糖降低。

■ 鉴别诊断

• 皮肤淋巴管型：
- 利什曼病。
- 诺卡菌病。
- 海洋分枝杆菌。
- 兔热病。
• 固定型：
- 细菌脓皮病。
- 异物肉芽肿。
- 炎症性皮肤癣菌感染。
- 芽生菌病。
- 分枝杆菌。
• 骨关节：
- 类风湿关节炎。
- 痛风。
- 结核。
- 细菌性关节炎。
- 色素绒毛结节性滑膜炎。
• 肺和脑膜炎：
- 杆菌感染。
- 组织胞浆菌病。
- 球孢子菌病。
- 隐球菌病。
- 结节病。

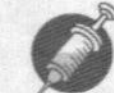 治疗

■ 初步稳定/治疗

严重皮肤外临床表现的患者气道管理及维持血流动力学稳定。

■ 急诊治疗/程序

• 皮肤淋巴管型和固定型：
- 伊曲康唑（首选药物）：有效但价格昂贵，有潜在的肝毒性，与许多药物有相互作用，引起心力衰竭。
- 特比萘芬：用于伊曲康唑无效时，是便宜的替代品，仅用于皮肤疾病。
- 碘化钾饱和溶液（SSKI）：价格便宜，但苦味，有副作用（厌食、恶心、腹泻、发热、唾液腺肿胀），患者不易接受。
- 对皮肤疾病（>35 ℃）局部热疗可抑制真菌生长，用于妊娠患者或其他无法耐受药物治疗的患者，疗程可能需要 3～6 个月。
• 肺型：
- 伊曲康唑或两性霉素 B 在疾病早期 30% 的病例有效。
- 更严重的疾病往往需要加两性霉素 B。
• 骨关节型：
- 伊曲康唑：一线治疗超过 1 年，效果不佳可使用两性霉素 B。
• 播散型：
- 首选两性霉素 B。
- 伊曲康唑在稳定、免疫功能正常的患者。
- HIV 感染和孢子丝菌病：初次感染后推荐使用伊曲康唑治疗。

■ 药物治疗

• 两性霉素 B：脂质体形式每日 3～5 mg/kg（优选，尤其是在妊娠和儿童中）；脱氧胆酸盐形式（无肾功能损害风险）每日 0.7～1 mg/kg，并输注 2 h 以上。
• 伊曲康唑：皮肤淋巴管型：100～200 mg（儿童：6～10 mg/kg，最多 400 mg），口服，每日 3 次，用 3 日；然后 100～200 mg/d，2～4 周；肺型和骨关节型整合：200 mg，口服，每日 3 次，用 3 日；然后每日 2 次，用 12 个月。
• SSKI：5 滴（儿童：1 滴）滴于水或果汁每日 3 次；每周每剂量增加 5 滴直到最大。可耐受 40～50 滴每日 3 次（儿童：最大剂量 1

滴/kg),持续 6～12 周或直至病灶消退。

• 特比萘芬：皮肤淋巴管型 250～500 mg,口服,每日 1 次,治疗 2～4 周后病变愈合。

随访

进一步处理

入院指征

• 全身症状和体征。

• 肺、中枢神经系统、多系统疾病。

• 免疫抑制宿主伴有播散性疾病。

出院指征

皮肤淋巴管型/固定型,无毒。

转诊问题

传染科会诊。

随访建议

传染科、皮肤科、骨科、神经内科随访。

要点和误区

固定型、肺型、皮肤淋巴管型、播散型继发于申克孢子丝菌感染：

• 接触土壤、苔藓或有机物质(皮肤破损或吸入)。

• 与猫接触。

• 固定型和皮肤淋巴管型多见于正常人,皮肤黏膜型和播散型多见于免疫缺陷的人。

• 弥漫性疾病表现为非特异性症状,常常导致诊断延误和预后不良。

• 口服伊曲康唑是一线治疗,播散型最初使用两性霉素 B。

B

暴力管理

Katherine Y. Joo · Elizabeth R. Dunn　吴昊　李文放 译

基础知识

描述

• 急诊室和候诊室是暴力事件的高发地区,从语言攻击到枪击事件。

• 较繁忙的急诊室的风险较高(>260 000 人次/年),还有市区创伤中心。

• 护士在急诊室经历暴力的风险最高。

• 实施暴力的个体可能是患者的家庭成员、朋友或访客,而不是患者本人。

• 暴力不仅可能针对医护人员,也可能针对患者或来访者。

• 关于急诊室肢体暴力的危险因素,没有很好的描述。

病因

• 尚不清楚,但通常是多因素的。

• 急性精神病问题：

- 常见的精神病。

• 慢性精神病问题：

- "B组"人格障碍：反社会、自恋、边缘化。

• 物质中毒和戒断。

• 急性基本医疗问题：

- 感染。
- 新陈代谢。
- 毒理学。
- 神经学。

• 慢性原发性医疗问题：

- 痴呆。
- 智力损伤。
- 创伤性脑损伤。

• 犯罪行为或精神病。

诊断

症状和体征

• 暴力的一般风险因素：

- 既往有暴力史或是暴力/虐待受害者。
- 药物滥用史或中毒史。
- 冲动控制不佳。
- 教育程度低。
- 失业。
- 社会支持有限。
- 男性。
- 年龄<35 岁。
- 参与帮派。
- 反社会人格障碍或精神病。
- 活跃的、未经治疗的躁狂症/精神病+愤怒。

• 即将发生暴力风险的警告信号：

- 凝视、攻击性眼神接触或避免眼神接触。
- 身体激动或紧张(踱步、握紧拳头、眼神闪烁)。
- 挑衅性或辱骂性语言。
- 提出不合理的要求,无法应对限制性设置。
- 忽视物理环境或个人边界。

病史

• 风险评估/既往史：

- 暴力行为史。
- 自残行为史。
- 医疗和精神病史。
- 药物使用史。
- 法律或犯罪史。

• 现病史：

- 问一些常规问题,以引起精神状态改变和/或激动的医学原因。
- 询问最近的药物使用情况。
- 评估是否存在妄想症和/或迫害妄想症。
- 评估他杀倾向或对特定个体的强烈愤怒。

体格检查

• 体格检查信号提示精神状态改变的医学原因：

- 生命体征异常。
- 局灶性神经系统表现。
- 活动性癫痫。
- 没有酒精或药物滥用证据的语言或步态缺陷。

基本检查

• 识别早期警告标志。

• 在神经和精神状态检查期间仔细观察发现并注意生命体征。

• 如果安全需要,可以在患者受约束的情况下进行检查。

诊断检查与说明

• 遵循临床指标进一步测试,但如果计划以精神病人院,则行实验室和影像学检查。

• 基本的实验室检查和心电图可能有助于评估和监测与化学物质使用相关的风险。

实验室检查

• 进行临床指示性实验室检查项目,如果怀疑是由医学原因引起的谵妄/精神状态改变。

• 检查是否有摄入或使用药物的嫌疑。

影像学检查

如果怀疑出血或脑卒中，可以考虑头部CT。

诊断步骤/外科

如果使用化学物质抑制剂，要做心电图检查。

B

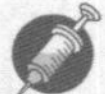

治疗

注意

• 如果患者持有致命武器，联系警察和保安人员。

• 医疗检查和治疗是重要的，但在紧急情况下，你可能首先需要稳定潜在的暴力患者，以减少伤害自己或他人的风险。

院前

• 如有必要，从身体上限制暴力患者并寻求帮助。

• 如果运送的是暴力患者，通知接收医院。

• 将武器和其他危险物品(尖锐物体、药物、绳索等)放在患者不能触及的地方。

初步稳定/治疗

• 预防：

– 将危险物品放在患者够不到的地方，考虑分离式ID线。

– 控制进入急诊的通道：安全门、限制入口和监控入口。

– 考虑使用金属探测器、自动锁定系统、中心员工区周围用玻璃隔断。

– 可见的保安人员。

– 张贴明显的标语，声明禁止使用武器，并对暴力行为采取不容忍政策。

– 检查室出口无障碍物。

• 程序：

– 急诊室暴力史患者给予在线提醒。

– 在分诊时识别和筛选高危患者。

– 在分诊后对患者进行搜身/脱衣；如果迫在眉睫的风险和需求，确保重新记录风险和提供者的理由。

– 培训所有临床人员识别和处理潜在的暴力情况。

– 清晰的急诊暴力协议管理和记录干预措施。

– 考虑使用指定的危机管理团队。

– 安装紧急按钮或密码短语，以指示其他人呼叫安全。

– 警察或保安的直接电话线。

– 减少急诊等待时间。

– 迅速解决舒适和痛苦的需求。

• 接近潜在的暴力患者：

– 确保你在其他员工或保安的视线范围内。

– 为患者和工作人员保持开放式出口。

– 取下你自己身边可能用作武器的个人物品(领带、珠宝、外伤剪等)。

– 在你和患者之间保持两臂的距离，保持开放的姿势。

– 自我介绍并尽快解决患者的顾虑。

– 如果有公开的暴力威胁或可能出现迫在眉睫的暴力事件，立即离开并开始封闭或限制。

急诊治疗/程序

• 尽可能遵循创伤知情护理原则。

• 环境改造：

– 将患者转移到一个平静、安静但不孤立的环境中。

– 如有可能，房间内不应存放容易投掷或用作武器的物品(如椅子、静脉输液杆)。

• 用语言平息：

– 最好选用与患者沟通最融洽的人员进行沟通。

– 如果无法与患者保持冷静，请听从团队其他成员的意见。

– 尝试澄清和确认患者的主要顾虑。

– 以直接但非正面的方式处理暴力行为或升级。

– 总是认真对待患者的威胁。

– 避免说谎(甚至为了安抚)、打断或批评患者。

– 冷静地解释如果暴力行为降级不成功，可能需要限制。

– 为患者提供可能的干预措施(例如，口服药与肌内注射药物、抗精神病药物类型)的选择，但必须在患者有机会表达他们的需求之后。

– 若患者有认知障碍、精神错乱或精神症状，语言平息可能不太成功。

• 隔离：

– 如果有合适的房间，这就不需要拘束了。

• 身体限制：

– 遵循协议规定，必须记录适当的限制原因，试图以口头形式平息，并制定适当的监督和重新评估计划。

– 请注意，在某些情况下，强制干预可能会使暴力行为升级。

– 只要有可能，治疗医师不应该成为约束团队的一员。

– 为好斗的患者使用皮革保护装置，对那些不太友好或试图逃跑的患者进行限制。

– 如果患者需要检查，仰卧位；如果误吸风险很大，则需要侧位。

– 在少数情况下，当暴力患者妊娠状态并需要身体约束时，使用左侧卧位。

• 药物限制：

– 给暴躁患者提供口服或静脉镇静药物。

– 对已被限制患者避免使用口服药物，以免咬伤。

– 药物的选择应该取决于潜在的原因，苯二氮䓬类或神经松弛药或两者都可能是合适的：

◦ 如果激动导致其他医疗状况恶化，则首先尝试治疗潜在的病因。

◦ 考虑苯二氮䓬类药物用于暴躁(包括可卡因)状态，或者作为抗精神病药物。

◦ 对于大多数主要的医疗或精神病学原因、镇静药中毒或主要的行为原因可考虑使用神经松弛药。

◦ 通常联合使用。

– 神经松弛药禁忌证：

◦ 了解或怀疑帕金森病、路易体痴呆或额颞叶痴呆。

◦ 神经阻滞剂恶性综合征、肌张力障碍反应或紧张症。

◦ 延长QT间期。

◦ 抗胆碱能过量。

– 潜在的不利影响：

◦ 肌张力障碍：肌内注射苯托品1 mg或肌内注射苯海拉明50 mg。

◦ QTc间期延长和/或尖端扭转型室性心动过速(罕见)。

◦ 神经阻滞剂恶性综合征(罕见)：停止所有抗精神病药物，开始密切监测和支持治疗。

注意

有内科疾病、神经系统疾病或认知障碍的老年患者，更容易受到不良反应的影响，并且可能对较低剂量药物出现药物反应。

药物治疗

一线用药

• 氟哌啶醇：5～10 mg，静脉注射、肌内注射或口服。

– 如果第一剂肌内注射氟哌啶醇无效，可在30～60 min后重复。

– 劳拉西泮：1～2 mg，静脉注射、肌内注射或口服。

二线用药

• 氟哌利多：2.5～5 mg，静脉注射或肌内注射，监测 QTc 间期。

• 奥氮平：5～10 mg，肌内注射或口服，如果肌内注射，由于存在呼吸抑制风险，不要给予肌内注射或静脉注射。

• 利培酮：1～2.5 mg，口服。

• 齐拉西酮：每 10 mg，肌内注射，每日不超过 40 mg。

随访

进一步处理

入院指征

• 在急诊中暂时或可逆转的医疗条件下住院。

• 如果需要进一步的检查，而急诊设置不是最佳的。

• 如果患者有适合住院治疗的精神疾病，可在精神科住院。

• 根据美国各州法律规定的标准，可能需要非自愿的安全保护。

出院指征

• 基础疾病或精神病因已稳定。

• 适合固定地点随访。

• 已经评估了武器的使用情况。

• 如果中毒在出院前进行清醒状态下的重新评估。

• 如果仍然没有精神病或医疗问题，警方拘留可能适用。

• 如果患者潜逃，必须考虑对自己或他人的迫在眉睫的危险，如果风险高或安全评估未完成需通知警察。

• 警告或保护第三方免受伤害风险的责任：美国各州之间的“Tarasoff”法律各不相同，需要知晓。

转诊问题

• 急诊中的精神科咨询可能会有所帮助，特别是怀疑有主要精神疾病时。

• 其他咨询可以基于潜在的病因来指示。

随访建议

• 精神病患者应该跟随社区心理健康服务提供者。

• 使用毒品的患者应提供咨询和/或戒毒。

要点和误区

• 暴力行为通常是多因素的，很少仅仅是由于精神疾病。

• 适当监控受限制的患者，包括定期的护理检查和静脉注射；如果需要化学物质限制，考虑实验室检查和心电图。

• 文件要求各不相同：根据医院协议记录约束需求；根据医院/州政策填写事故报告和/或联系当地执法部门。

• 教育部的工作场所暴力发生率很高，而且可能报告不足。

• 在急诊室经历暴力的后遗症包括轻微/重大身体伤害、精神/情感创伤和员工倦怠。

爆裂性骨折 Blow-Out Fracture

Shari Schabowski · Ashlea Winfield-Dial 宋振举 童朝阳 译

基础知识

描述

• 定义为眼眶底骨折，由眼球突然钝性损伤引起：

- 经典的致病因素是由大于半个拳头大小的弹射的力量引起。
- 外力通过眼球的不可压缩结构传递到最薄弱的结构点，即眼眶底，使其“爆裂”。

• 眶底作为上颌窦和筛窦充满空气的顶：

- 间隙间的联通导致眼眶气肿。

• 不同部位的气体挤压导致眼眶气肿：

- 眶内的脂肪组织可固定眼球位置。
- 眶底骨折可能会导致眼眶下表面的脂肪嵌入上颌窦或筛窦。
- 因眼眶容积减小和鼻窦充血导致眼球内陷，水肿和出血可能继发积液。

• 眶下神经在眶下 3 mm 处穿出骨性通道：

- 损伤可能导致同侧面颊和上唇的感觉减退。
- 为了区分面部感觉减退是由于局部肿胀还是神经损伤，在眶下神经分布范围内的同侧齿龈上进行感觉测试。

• 下直肌和下斜肌沿眶底走行：

- 由于骨折、挫伤或脑神经功能障碍，可能会导致眼外肌活动受限。
- 通常表现为向上凝视时复视。
- 在体格检查时不能正常上抬患侧眼球。

• 内直肌位于筛窦上方：

- 嵌顿少见。
- 同侧凝视时复视。

病因

由抛射物撞击眼球所致。力由眼球周围的刚性结构传导至结构最薄弱处：眶底，从而导致爆裂性骨折。

儿科注意事项

• 眼眶顶部骨折伴中枢神经损伤在儿童中更为常见。

• 眶底骨折：7 岁之前较为少见：

- 因儿童鼻旁窦并不含气，其眶底并不是眼眶的薄弱部位。

• 不幸的是，骨折仍可能发生于儿童，并且可能导致难以鉴别的直肌肌肉嵌顿，被定义为“白眼”骨折。不易被发现，可能很少有相关的软组织损伤：

- 这些儿童可能会出现明显的恶心、呕吐、头痛和易激惹的症状，提示头部损伤，而这些通常会影响正确的诊断。

诊断

症状和体征

• 眶周压痛、肿胀和瘀斑。

• 眼球活动受限或复视：

- 由于下直肌嵌顿导致的向上凝视受限。
- 由于中直肌嵌顿导致的同侧凝视受限。

• 眶下感觉异常：

- 由眶下神经的压迫/挫伤导致。
- 可能延伸到上唇。

• 眼球内陷：

- 由于骨折使眶内脂肪移位导致眼球向后移位。

• 眶周气肿：

- 从筛窦或上颌窦。

• 鼻出血。

• 视力正常：

- 如果情况并非如此，考虑更广泛的损伤。

• 没有眶缘下移。

B

相关严重损伤

• 眼部损伤。

- 眼球破裂:

◦ 在爆裂性骨折中发生率高达 30%。

◦ 眼科急诊。

- 球后出血。

- 气肿性视神经受压。

• 颈椎或颅内损伤。

• 常见的相关损伤:

- 结膜下出血。

- 角膜擦伤、撕裂伤。

- 眼前房出血。

- 创伤性瞳孔放大。

- 创伤性虹膜炎(葡萄膜炎)。

• 较少见:

- 虹膜根部离断。

- 视网膜剥脱。

- 玻璃体出血。

- 视神经损伤。

• 相应骨折:

- 鼻骨骨折。

- 颧弓骨折。

- Le Fort 骨折。

• 晚期并发症:

- 鼻窦炎。

- 眼眶感染。

- 眼外肌运动永久性受限。

- 眼球内陷。

病史

被投掷物击中眼睛,如彩弹、手球、壁球、棒球、石头,也可能是拳头。大尺寸的投掷物很可能会被眶缘挡住。常见于车祸之后,这也是造成颌面部创伤的最常见原因。

体格检查

• 彻底的眼科检查:

- 触诊眶周的骨性结构以寻找眼球向后移位的证据。

- 排除眼球破裂前,注意不要对眼球施加压力:

◦ 当眼睑肿胀时可以用 Desmarres 眼睑拉钩来评估患眼情况。

• 记录瞳孔反应。

• 视力(应不受影响):

- 手持式视力 Rosenbeaum 卡适用于损伤。

• 非共轭凝视和复视时应检查眼外肌运动。

• 测试眶下神经分布部位的感觉情况。

• 检查眼睑和相应结构:

- 可能存在眶内气肿。

• 使用裂隙灯和眼底检查来发现相应损伤。

• 进行全身体检来发现相关损伤和神经损害。

诊断检查与说明

实验室检查

• 术前实验室检查。

• 放射性检查前需排除妊娠。

影像学检查

• 如果无法使用 CT 或存在禁忌证,X 线平片可提供重要信息:

- 面部底片。

- 眼眶。

- 沃特斯视图和扩大沃特斯视图:

◦ 经典的"泪滴征"提示眶内物嵌入同侧上颌窦内。

◦ 在上颌窦内出现不透明化或气液平(较不明确)。

◦ 眶底骨折。

◦ 和眶内气肿相一致的眶内透亮影。

• CT 优先考虑的情况:

- 明确相关解剖关系。

- 行轴位及冠状位扫描,层厚 1.5 mm:

◦ 不建议行冠状位重建,除非无法定位。

诊断步骤/外科

被动牵拉试验。

• 鉴别神经功能障碍与嵌顿。

• 对侧结膜局部麻醉,将眼球从怀疑嵌顿处牵拉,如果眼球不移动,则试验阳性——定义为物理性嵌顿。

儿科注意事项

• 眼周 CT:首选。

- X 线平片帮助较小。

• 发现早期嵌顿十分必要,诊断不及时很可能会影响长期的预后:

- 早期对嵌顿进行手术干预可以大幅提高预后。

鉴别诊断

• 脑神经麻痹。

• 眼窝蜂窝织炎。

• 眶周蜂窝织炎。

• 眶周挫伤、瘀斑。

• 球后出血。

• 眼球破裂。

治疗

院前

• 如果怀疑眼球损伤尽可能用金属保护眼罩。

• 呈仰卧位。

初步稳定/治疗

初始方法和紧急处理。

• 评估相关的颅内或颈椎损伤。

• 排除眼球破裂。

• 视力测试:

- 如视力下降,提示更为广泛的损伤。

急诊治疗/程序

• 在排除眼球破裂后,在第一个 24~48 h 使用冷敷,以最大限度减轻肿胀,逆转嵌顿和避免手术干预。

• 避免 Valsalva 动作和擤鼻,防止加重眶内气肿。

• 预防性抗生素应用抗感染。

• 如果没有禁忌,使用鼻解充血剂。

• 必要时使用镇痛药。

• 预防性注射破伤风。

药物治疗

• 建议预防性应用抗生素预防鼻窦炎和眼蜂窝织炎:

- 头孢氨苄 250 mg, q6 h,持续 10 日。

• 推荐使用全身皮质激素加速水肿吸收,以便更准确地评估肌肉是否嵌顿和眼眶损害程度:

- 泼尼松(60~80 mg/d)在 48 h 内使用,持续 5 日。

• 排除禁忌情况下,可使用鼻减充血剂:

- 苯肾上腺素鼻喷雾剂:2~4 日。

随访

进一步处理

入院指征

• 很少需要。

• 85%的处理方案不需要手术干预。

• 请颌面部整形外科会诊并在以下情况考虑入院:

- 50%以上面积的眶底骨折。

- 已经确诊的复视或嵌顿。

- 儿童。

- 眼球内陷≥2 mm。

出院指征

在大多数情况下,观察 10~14 日,直到肿胀消退,然后颌面部整形外科医师随访以确定是否需要外科干预。

随访建议

症状随时间改善。

• 患者任何时候出现肿胀、压痛、发红或眼周疼痛，须回急诊再次评估。

• 出现任何视觉障碍、视力损失或眼球疼痛加重，须回急诊再次评估。

要点和误区

• 在检查瞳孔反应和视力时要保持高度警惕：
- 出现异常可能是严重并发症的首要信号：
  ◦ 眼球破裂。
  ◦ 眶内气肿或球后压迫可能导致视神经损伤。

• 仔细评估是否存在嵌顿：
- 对所有人，尤其是儿童，排除"白眼"眶底爆裂性骨折和长期并发症十分必要。

• 眼心反射(Aschner 反射)可能与此损伤有关，表现为与眼外肌和/或眼球压迫相关的脉率下降：
- 在儿童中更常见。
- 减压治疗，在某些情况下可能需要阿托品。

B

爆震伤 Blast Injury

John R. Storey · Vaishal M. Tolia　黄昊　伍力学 译

基础知识

描述

爆炸造成的急性压力变化所导致的组织损伤：

• 可分成四类：
- 原发性损伤：由爆炸的冲击波直接导致的损伤。
- 继发性损伤：爆炸产生的碎片翼中所致的损伤，与致伤物的速度相关。
- 三发性损伤：受害者被冲击波投掷到固定物体上所致的损伤，与被投掷速度有关。
- 其他附带损伤：爆炸中与有害物质接触(如化学品、灰尘、毒素)或烧伤(直接热损伤或爆炸引起的火灾)。

• 依据牛顿经典力学[外力(F) = 质量(m)× 加速度(a)]，冲击波通过可以相对较小的力能使质量很轻的气体产生较大的加速度。

• 爆炸有四种能量来源：
- 机械：压缩容器的结构裂解后释放的液压力。
- 电：电弧产生的热量会造成压力的骤增。
- 核：核裂变或聚变产生热量。
- 化学物质：化学反应物可以扩散(可燃气体或微粒物质)并与空气混合以产生能量，也可以凝结(如液体或固体)，化学反应物通常分为低阶或高阶两类。

• 最常见的意外或故意爆炸伤害的原因是化学爆炸。固体/液体爆炸物被点燃后时变成气体，压力和温度骤增，压力会产生 6～8 km/s 的冲击波，形成超过环境压力的超压峰值，这种峰值通常非常短暂和强烈。

• 空气中冲击波的峰值压力与爆炸距离成反比，如必须产生 8 倍于峰值压力的冲击波，才能造成 2 倍的破坏。

• 冲击波通过密度越大的材料传播，超压峰值越大，持续时间越短，传播速度越快。

• 冲击波在封闭空间中的反射会造成更高的超压、更长的持续时间和更多的原发性爆炸伤害。

• 通过组织传播的冲击波主要在不同密度区的交界处造成原发性损伤，如肺、肠、鼓膜等。损伤潜力与超压峰值的持续时间和高度直接相关，利用压力-持续曲线可预测临床结局。

流行病学

• 继发性和附带损伤虽然更为常见，但原发爆炸伤害才是爆炸伤所特有的。恐怖主义炸弹袭击的受害者多为浅表继发性爆炸伤，较严重的伤害一般发生在距爆炸源 10～15 m 的范围。

• 最常见的原发性冲击性损伤是鼓膜下部线状撕裂。在压力只有 2～5 psi 的情况下可以发生。耳蜗的损伤也很常见，通常可导致耳鸣和感音神经性听力损害。

• 第二常见的原发性爆炸伤是肺部弥漫性肺挫伤和肺泡出血，发生在 15～50 psi(1 psi= 6.895 kPa)的峰值超压。全身性空气栓子可通过肺泡和肺静脉之间的裂隙发生；当受害者有异常的神经系统表现，发生猝死或爆炸伤后心搏骤停时，应怀疑这一原因。

• 原发性肠爆震损伤需要高峰值超压，在冲击波通过水传播时更为常见。可发生浆膜撕裂、肠壁内出血和穿孔。

• 颅脑损伤(TBI)可由血管内压力的增加引起，特别是当冲击波到达胸腔时，甚至在没有直接头部损伤的情况下即可出现。

诊断

症状和体征

• 呼吸困难，胸痛，咯血。

• 胸部爆炸伤后可观察到低血压和心动过缓。

• 听力下降，外耳道出血。

• 脑震荡，局灶性神经表现。

• 腹痛，恶心，呕吐，里急后重。

体格检查

• 评估每个器官系统，优先评估气道、呼吸、循环系统。

• 一定要检查鼓膜。

• 评估化学物质和热烧伤。

诊断检查与说明

采集病史和检查中发现的特殊损伤将决定需要进行哪些诊断性检查。

基本检查

• 保持呼吸和循环稳定。

• 积极查找原发性损伤，通常继发性和三发性损伤表现更为明显。

• 识别动脉栓塞。

实验室检查和影像学检查

• 胸部 X 线检查。

• 实验室检查，强烈推荐动脉血气分析(ABG)作为判读有无肺损伤的早期指标。

诊断步骤/外科

如果怀疑有筋膜室综合征，必须测量筋膜室压力。

鉴别诊断

• 压力波的伤害通常很明显。

• 穿透性损伤。

• 烧伤。

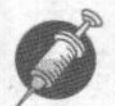

治疗

院前

• 保证环境安全。

B

• 准确地分类伤情。

初步稳定/治疗

• 高流量吸氧。

• 谨慎使用液体输注(有肺水肿风险)。

急诊治疗/程序

• 胸部X线检查、血气分析。

• 气管插管(必要时)。

• 谨慎使用正压通气,考虑低呼吸末正压通气(PEEP)以避免进一步气压损伤和全身空气栓塞。

• 严重肺损伤者: 应用低潮气量和允许性高碳酸血症的容量控制(VC)/同步间歇指令通气(SIMV)通气策略已被证明是有益的。

• 避免全身麻醉,宜采用局部麻醉。

• 腹部冲击性损伤的处理与钝性创伤相似。

• 继发性损伤: 如果为小爆炸,可以用最小的探查法处理;如果伤口较大,应彻底探查并尽可能多地清除碎片,保持伤口敞开,以便延迟一期缝合。

• 鼓膜破裂: 有自然愈合的可能,如果大而中央可以用膜片修补。

• 鼓膜穿孔可在受伤10个月后行鼓膜成形术。

随访

进一步处理

• 多发伤: 转创伤中心。

• 全身性空气栓塞: 高压氧治疗(HBO)。

• 钝性损伤与鼓膜破裂: 观察24 h。

• 门诊随访。

入院指征

• 闭合性损伤或骨性损伤。

• 伴随有基础疾病的恶化者。

• 胸部影像学提示急性异常改变。

出院指征

• 取决于具体病情,类似于其他创伤。

• 经观察无病情恶化征象者。

• 重点关注肺部情况。

• 回家后相关防范措施严格到位。

• 基层医疗机构可实现密切门诊随访。

转诊问题

如果需要空运往高压氧舱治疗,建议加压或使用低空飞行器,以防止进一步的空气栓子和气胸。

随访建议

• 取决于确定的具体伤情况。

• 鼓膜或内耳损伤应由耳鼻喉科医师随访。

• 骨折和其他骨科损伤应由骨科专家随访。

• 其他创伤应由创伤外科医师或急诊外科医师随访。

• 化学物质或热烧伤应继续与烧伤专科医师联系。

要点和误区

• 在现场进行准确的检伤和分类至关重要。

• 不要遗漏提示系统性空气栓塞的征象(例如,神经功能改变、循环改变或可能提示心肌缺血的疼痛症状)或创伤性颅脑损伤(TBI)。

• 插管后无创正压通气(NIPPV)或压力预设性(PPV)通气模式可能会加重空气栓塞或气胸。

贝尔麻痹 Bell's Palsy

Robert F. Mccormack · Richard S. Krause 宋振举 童朝阳 译

基础知识

描述

• 急性、特发性外周第7对脑神经(面神经,CN Ⅶ)麻痹。

• 85%的病例未经治疗完全康复。

• 病变程度与预后相关:

- 完全性病变预后最差。
- 部分病变往往预后较好。

• 恢复通常在2周内开始(通常味觉最先恢复),并在2~3周完成:

- 高龄和恢复缓慢是不良预后因素。

• 男女受累程度均等。

• 3~5岁好发(但可能发生在任何年龄段)。

• 糖尿病和妊娠增加风险。

• 发病率为每年(15~40)/10万。

病因

• 特发性,可能为病毒性原因(特别是单纯性疱疹)。

• 莱姆病、传染性单核细胞增多症(EB病毒感染)、水痘-带状疱疹感染等可能导致第7对脑神经瘫痪。

• 机制: 乳突孔内水肿和神经退变。

• 额头两侧的神经支配来自两个运动皮质:

- 单侧皮质过程不会完全破坏前额的运动活动。
- 只有外周或脑干病变才能中断前额一侧的运动功能。

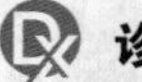

诊断

症状和体征

病史

突然发生的单侧面部下垂,不完全的眼睑闭合,额头肌肉张力丧失:

• 几乎所有病例的5日内达到最大损伤症状(50%为2日)。

• 流泪(68%)或眼睛干涩(16%),患侧眨眼次数减少。

• 患侧的麻木感。

• 味觉异常,流涎。

• 音觉过敏(对高音敏感)。

• 乳突后胀感或疼痛。

• 常有报道称患者存在病毒前驱症状。

体格检查

• 单侧面部麻痹,包括额头。

• 如果前额肌肉张力没有丧失,强烈暗示为中枢性病灶(即排除贝尔麻痹)。

• 仅限于第7对脑神经分布的运动神经衰弱:

- 累及面部上半部分和下半部分。

• 否则进行常规神经系统检查,包括所有的脑神经和肢体运动功能。

• 可能看到贝尔征(患者闭眼时双眼球向外上方转动)。

基本检查

基于病史和体格检查,临床性诊断。

B

■ 诊断检查与说明

实验室检查

• 对贝尔麻痹的诊断没有帮助。

• 怀疑莱姆病或有疫区接触史时，莱姆滴度很有用。

• 怀疑 EB 病毒感染时，行单核细胞增多症(CBC，传染性单核细胞增多症检测试剂盒)检测。

影像学检查

除非怀疑腮腺肿瘤、乳突炎等，否则对贝尔麻痹的诊断没有帮助。

■ 鉴别诊断

• 影响第 7 对脑神经的脑干事件(肿块、出血、梗死)几乎总是涉及第 6 对脑神经(异常 EOM)并可能影响长时程运动区域：

- 病例报道(罕见)单纯性脑干瘫痪的第 7 对脑神经麻痹。

• 莱姆病：蜱虫叮咬、迁徙性红斑疹或疫区接触史。

• 带状疱疹(Ramsay Hunt 综合征)：有无疱疹囊泡，询问有无耳鸣或眩晕。

• 传染性单核细胞增多症：有无咽炎、后颈部腺病。

• 肿瘤：腮腺、骨或转移性肿块，听神经瘤(耳聋)。

• 外伤：颅骨骨折或穿透性面部损伤可能会损伤第 7 对脑神经。

• 中耳或乳突手术或感染、胆脂瘤。

• 脑膜感染。

• 急性炎症性脱髓鞘性多发性神经病(吉兰-巴雷综合征，又称格林-巴利综合征)：存在其他神经功能缺陷[如上行性肌无力或深反射减弱(DTR)]。

• 基底动脉动脉瘤，应存在其他神经功能缺损。

• 双侧外周第 7 对脑神经麻痹：考虑多发性硬化、结节病、白血病和吉兰-巴雷综合征。罕见病例中特发性(贝尔)麻痹可能是双侧的。

• 早期 HIV 感染。

• 贝尔麻痹可能复发，这种情况下治疗不变。

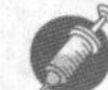 治疗

■ 院前

无。

■ 初步稳定/治疗

单纯的外周第 7 对脑神经麻痹患者病情往往是稳定的。

■ 急诊治疗/流程

• 眼睑闭合不全可能导致角膜损伤：

- 通常需要使用眼科制剂润滑和保湿。

- 在夜间进行眼部修补。

• 起病 1 周(最好 72 h)内开始口服类固醇，可能促进康复：

- 治疗并发症很少见。

• 抗病毒治疗(阿昔洛韦或伐昔洛韦)与类固醇可能对改善功能性神经恢复有效：

- 起病 72 h 内启动。

- 没有被证明有效获益。

- 可能适用于严重麻痹。

• 疑似莱姆病应该用多西环素或阿莫西林治疗。

• 手术减压可能适用于无法改善症状的完全性病变，然而这尚存在争议。

■ 药物治疗

一线用药

• Lacri-Lube 或人造眼泪：睡前或必要时使用，解决受累眼干燥/刺激(或等同物)。

• 泼尼松：30～40 mg，口服，每日 2 次[剂量：2 mg/(kg · d)，口服，最大剂量 60 mg]。

二线用药

伐昔洛韦 1 g，口服，每日 3 次，持续 7 日(剂量：20 mg/kg，每日 3 次)可能对严重病例有用。

 随访

■ 进一步处理

入院指征

单纯的外周第 7 对脑神经麻痹无需住院。

出院指征

单纯的外周第 7 对脑神经麻痹可以在门诊治疗。

■ 随访建议

1 周内随访。

要点和误区

• 孤立于第 7 对神经分布的运动神经衰弱：

- 涉及上半面部和下半面部。

- 如果前额没有失去支配，就不是贝尔麻痹。

• 上述条件不符合时，应进行常规神经系统检查，包括所有脑神经和肢体运动功能。

• 保护眼睛。

• 类固醇有益，而抗病毒药物存在争议。

背痛 Back Pain

James Willis · Eric Legome 王海嵘 潘曙明 译

 基础知识

■ 描述

• 腰痛：

- 下肋骨与臀沟之间的疼痛，常放射至大腿。

• 坐骨神经痛：

- 下腰椎根分布区域疼痛。

- 可能伴有神经感觉和运动障碍。

• 疼痛分类：

- 急性：<6 周。

- 亚急性：6～12 周。

- 慢性：>12 周。

■ 病因

• 非特异性肌肉韧带来源(占大多数)(如肌肉、韧带、筋膜)。

• 髓核突出。

• 骨关节或软骨层退行性变。

• 脊髓狭窄。

• 解剖异常，尤其是脊柱滑脱。

• 由于创伤和骨质疏松引起的骨折。

• 潜在的系统性疾病(占少数)：

- 肿瘤。

- 感染。

- 血管病变(夹层、颅内动脉瘤和血栓)。

- 肾脏病变。

- 胃肠道病变。

- 盆腔脏器病变。

诊断

症状和体征

• 肌肉韧带：
- 背部、臀部隐痛，局限性差，不伴有膝上方的放射。
- 常没有客观的神经系统体征。
- 背部肌肉痉挛，多变，重复性差。

• 坐骨神经痛：
- 剧痛，局限性好。
- 腿部症状常比背部症状明显。
- 可能伴随：
  ◦ 腱反射不对称。
  ◦ 皮区分布的感觉减退。
  ◦ 乏力。

• 中央椎间盘突出(马尾)：
- 会阴感觉减弱。
- 充盈性尿失禁。
- 大便失禁。

• 感染：
- 发热。
- 椎体局部叩击痛。

• 骨损伤：
- 疼痛持续，不随休息改变。
- 全身症状。

• 血管性疾病：
- 严重，常为“撕裂样”疼痛。
- 可能与寒冷或者无感觉的四肢有关。

病史

• 能帮助集中和缩小鉴别诊断，帮助排除疼痛的原因：
- 强度。
- 性质。
- 位置及放射。
- 发作的情况。
- 加重或缓解的因素。
- 社会或心理因素。
- 对先前治疗的反应。

• 严重疾病的危险因素：
- 发热。
- 全身症状。
- 创伤。
- 年龄＞60 岁。
- 肿瘤病史：
  ◦ 特别是骨转移的肿瘤。
- 长期使用类固醇药物。
- 静脉吸毒。
- 近期进行器械操作或发生菌血症。
- 夜晚疼痛。症状持续大于 6 周。

体格检查

• 发热。

• 痉挛或软组织触痛，重复性差：
- 椎体压痛灵敏但对于感染非特异。

• 直腿抬高-仰卧时腿抬高，腿伸直抬高超过 35%：
- 同时出现坐骨神经症状。
- 同侧抬高，灵敏度高，但没有特异性。
- 交叉腿抬高，极其非特异性，灵敏度不高。

• 踝关节和踇趾背屈和足底屈曲(L_5、S_1 神经根)。

• 踝关节深反射(S_1)。

• 皮肤感觉检查：
- 鞍区感觉缺失评估。

• 直肠括约肌紧张。

基本检查

• 全面了解病史和体格检查，包括详细的神经和血管检查。

• 对于无合并症的肌肉韧带或坐骨神经疼痛进行非特异性检查。

• 快速诊断性试验和关于主动脉病变的血管会诊。

诊断检查与说明

• 怀疑是以下情况时进行尿液分析：
- 尿路感染、肾盂肾炎。
- 前列腺炎。

• 红细胞沉降率(ESR)：
- 高度灵敏，但对于炎症或者炎症非特异。
- 用于排除疾病的筛查。

影像学检查

• 在院前急救中，非特异性背痛不推荐进行常规影像检查。

• 腰骶部 X 线片：
- 明显的创伤。
- 年龄在 50～60 岁或以上。
- 肿瘤的病史或症状与体征。
- 发热。
- 静脉吸毒者。
- 休息时疼痛。
- 怀疑炎症性疾病。
- 疼痛 4 周后没有改善。

• 床旁超声：
- 膀胱充盈提示尿潴留。
- 腹主动脉瘤(AAA)。
- 患者情况稳定可行腹部 CT。

• MRI：
- 怀疑脓肿：
  ◦ 发热、免疫低下、静脉吸毒者、菌血症病史。
- 怀疑转移瘤：
  ◦ 全身性恶性肿瘤、体重减轻。
- 怀疑血肿：
  ◦ 抗凝治疗，近期进行脊髓麻醉。
- 迅速进展的神经症状。
- 与背痛相关的尿潴留或大便失禁。

• CT：
- 当 MRI 不能诊断脓肿、肿瘤或大块椎间盘突出的辅助诊断。
- X 线片提示潜在不稳定骨折的选择检查。
- 对病情稳定患者的血管评估有很高的灵敏度。

鉴别诊断

• 脊髓起源：发现绝大多数患者没有精确的解剖定位：
- 肌肉韧带(占绝大多数)。
- 椎间盘。
- 骨折。
- 脊椎前移。
- 强直性脊柱炎。
- 硬膜外脓肿、血肿。
- 肿瘤。

• 非脊髓原因：
- 腹主动脉瘤。
- 前列腺炎。
- 上尿路感染。
- 腹部肿瘤。
- 肾绞痛。
- 主动脉夹层。

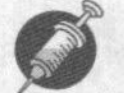

治疗

院前

• 对于非创伤性疼痛，通常不推荐固定。

• 对于血管问题，快速转运患者。

急诊治疗/程序

• 对患者进行宣教和宽慰：
- 帮助其建立对疼痛控制效果和康复过程的合理预期。

• 非甾体抗炎药(NSAIDs)：
- 肌肉韧带疼痛。
- 肾绞痛。
- 好处类似于对乙酰氨基酚(APAP)，但副作用不太理想。

• 对乙酰氨基酚：被认为是轻中度疼痛的一线治疗：
- 中等但相矛盾的证据表明 NSAIDs 和对

乙酰氨基酚联用对术后疼痛的个体有益。

- 对乙酰氨基酚和 NSAIDs 对坐骨神经痛没有效果。

• 肌松药：

- 环苯扎林、美索巴莫、卡立普多或替扎尼定。

- 副作用必须与益处平衡，主要是镇静、头晕和口干。

- 最近的证据表明，服用非甾体抗炎药对控制急性疼痛没有益处。

• 苯二氮䓬类：

- 与骨骼肌松药没有明显的区别。

- 成瘾的风险可能更高。

- 最近的证据表明，服用非甾体抗炎药对控制急性疼痛没有益处。

• 麻醉性止痛剂：

- 对于不能被抗感染药或对乙酰氨基酚缓解的剧烈疼痛可以给予合理的疗程（3～5日）治疗。对神经性疼痛有效。

- 应考虑并与患者讨论风险效益状况。

• 皮质醇类：

- 神经根性或非根性背痛无益处。

- 硬膜外注射治疗对神经根疼痛有效。

- 全身使用类固醇激素可以改善恶性肿瘤的症状和疼痛。

• 脊柱推拿术：

- 短疗程（<2 周）对无坐骨神经痛的急性腰痛可能有帮助。

• 理疗与运动：

- 对适应证没有明确的共识。

- 可能有助于缓解症状，预防进一步发作和指导患者。

- 早期转诊可改善急性疼痛和伤残的发生，减少处方药的使用。

- 包括社会心理干预在内的多学科方法已显示出益处。

• 针灸：

- 效果有争议，可能对慢性肌肉骨骼疼痛有益。

- 与其他方式相比没有明显的好处。

- 触发点治疗没有对慢性腰痛有益的证据，对于急性腰痛还未进行研究。

• 推拿：

- 结合锻炼和指导可能会有好处。

• 热疗与冷疗：

- 对于背部疼痛<3 个月的患者，有限的证据支持热敷疗法可能有助于减轻疼痛和残疾。可作为锻炼的辅助手段。

• 卧床休息：

- 无助于加速恢复，并可能阻碍病情改善。如果患者急需卧床休息或症状有改善，可以推荐 1～2 日。

• 背部锻炼：

- 在急性期不太可能有用，可能有助于预防今后的发作。

• 预期恢复到无痛状态：

- 相矛盾的数据，大部分在非急救室的环境。

- 约 33%在 1 周内。

- 约 90%在 6～8 周。

- 低社会地位、女性、残疾和慢性腰痛在 1～3 周预后明显差。

- 最新的急救室数据显示，50%的患者疼痛 3 个月内功能受到限制。

• 复发是常见的：约 40%。

■ 药物治疗

一线用药

• 对乙酰氨基酚：500 mg（儿童：10～15 mg/kg，不超过 5 倍剂量/24 h），口服，q4～6 h，不超过 4 g/24 h。

• 布洛芬：600～800 mg，口服，q6～8 h（儿童：10 mg/kg，q6 h）。

• 萘普生：250～500 mg，口服，q12 h。

二线用药

• 非甾体抗炎药和对乙酰氨基酚是否可以联用。

• 可以联合一线和二线治疗，但会增加副作用。

• 最新的证据表明这并不能改善急性的非特异性背痛。

• 环苯扎林：5～10 mg，口服，每日 3 次。注意患者可能出现嗜睡。

• 美索巴莫：500～1 500 mg，口服，q6 h。注意患者可能出现嗜睡。

• 地西泮（安定）：5～10 mg，口服，q8 h。

• 可以结合一线和二线药物治疗，但副作用将会增加。

三线用药

• 氢可酮/对乙酰氨基酚：5/500 mg，口服，q4～6 h。

• 对于对一线和二线治疗无效的顽固性疼痛，以及恶性肿瘤、感染和神经性疼痛等病因所致的严重的背痛，可考虑使用阿片类药物。

• 最近的证据表明急性疼痛对非特异性背痛没有改善。

随访

■ 进一步处理

入院指征

• 剧烈疼痛不能行走。

• 疼痛对急救室治疗无反应。

• 进行性神经功能障碍。

• 马尾神经综合征的症状。

• 感染、血管或肿瘤病因。

出院指征

能简单地控制疼痛和走动。

老年注意事项

• 对包括血管病因、肿瘤或感染在内的严重疾病保持高度怀疑。

• 对影像学检查或诊断性试验有较低的阈值。

• 更仔细地随访患者 NSAIDs 或阿片类药物治疗的并发症或不良事件。

儿科注意事项

• 背痛在儿科患者中是不常见的，但必须保持对传染性病因的高度怀疑。

• 对于肌肉韧带的疼痛，一个单独的试验发现布洛芬提供了副作用低的良好疼痛控制。

妊娠注意事项

有限的证据表明，加强和盆腔倾斜运动与常规产前护理相结合可能对治疗腰痛有帮助；不清楚它们是否能预防疼痛。

转诊问题

紧急神经外科或骨科会诊，明确诊断或高度怀疑脓肿或病变（椎间盘、肿瘤或其他），伴有快速进展的客观神经学发现。

■ 随访建议

• 单纯背痛：1～2 周到初级保健医师随访。

• 新的坐骨神经痛不伴神经学表现：7～10 日到初级保健医师或专科医师随访。

• 仅伴有感觉症状或轻微运动症状：24～48 h。

• 有明显或迅速进展的运动症状，或肠、膀胱表现，假如不能随访，需要在急诊室或转诊中进行专家咨询。

要点和误区

• 考虑 MRI 对静脉药物依赖者病史的影响来排除硬膜外脓肿或非骨性脊柱转移瘤的可能。

• 老年人有小创伤可发生持续性骨折。

• 老年人首先出现背痛，考虑血管原因。

• 告知患者，这通常是一个漫长的过程，他们不应该期望迅速解决。

• 阿片类药物应限于急救室内短期疗程使用。

B

贲门黏膜撕裂综合征 Mallory-Weiss Syndrome

Galeta C · Clayton 王胜云 段立伟 译

基础知识

描述

- 食管远端或胃近端的部分腔内纵向黏膜撕裂。
- 腹腔内和/或经胃压力突然增加导致：
  - 轻度至中度的黏膜下动脉和/或静脉出血：
    - 可能与潜在病理有关。
    - 内镜下可见，干呕期间不断膨胀的胃进入食管。
  - 8%～15%的上消化道出血由此所致。

病因

- 相关：
  - 用力咳嗽、大笑或干呕。
  - 举重。
  - 压力。
  - 腹部闭合性损伤。
  - 癫痫。
  - 分娩。
  - 心肺复苏术。
- 危险因素：
  - 酗酒：
    - 特别是最近狂欢之后。
  - 患者食管裂孔疝。
  - 妊娠剧吐。
  - 糖尿病酮症酸中毒。
  - 化疗。
- 更大的出血相关：
  - 门静脉高压。
  - 食管静脉曲张。
  - 凝血病。

诊断

症状和体征

病史

- 多次无血丝呕吐和/或紧随其后干呕：
  - 大部分出血很小同时溶解。
  - 会发生大规模危及生命的出血。
- 上腹部疼痛。
- 后背疼痛。
- 脱水：
  - 眩晕、头晕和晕厥。

体格检查

- 呕血。
- 黑粪症。
- 体位性低血压。
- 休克。

基本检查

- 全血细胞计数。
- 血型和抗体筛查。
- 放置鼻胃管检查是否有活动性出血。

诊断检查与说明

实验室检查

- PT、APTT、国际标准化比值(INR)。
- 电解质、血尿素氮、肌酸酐、葡萄糖、肝功能检查。
- 如果腹痛检查淀粉酶和脂肪酶。
- 类型和交叉配型：
  - 如果出血严重的话，至少 4 U 浓缩红细胞(PRBC)。

影像学检查

- 老年人或有心脏病史的做心电图。
- 从食管或胃穿孔的自由空气状态下直立位 X 线片。
- 胃镜检查(食管胃镜检查)：
  - 选择程序定位，识别，并且处理出血来源。

鉴别诊断

- 鼻咽出血。
- 咳血。
- 食管破裂(Boerhaave 综合征)。
- 食管炎。
- 胃炎。
- 肠胃炎。
- 十二指肠炎。
- 溃疡疾病。
- 静脉曲张。
- 癌。
- 血管肠瘘。
- 血管瘤。

治疗

院前

- 气道控制：
  - 如果没有反应或气道不通畅岌岌可危，100%的氧气或插管。
- 如果血流动力学上不稳定或大出血：
  - 启用 2 支大口径静脉导管。
  - 1 L 大丸剂(儿童：20 ml/kg)乳酸林格液或生理盐水。

初步稳定/治疗

- ABC 管理：
  - 输液方式：至少 1 支大口径导管，如果不稳定则需要更多。
  - 如果不稳定的话，放置中心静脉导管更高效地输液和监测中心静脉压。
  - 如果稳定的话，输生理盐水(或乳酸林格液)250 ml/h。如果血流动力学不稳定，放开补液速度。
  - 使用多巴胺改善持续低血压，刺激液体复苏。
- 置入鼻饲管检测活动性出血。
- 如果出现低血压并且对 2 L 晶体液没有反应，立即输入 O 型阴性红细胞。
- 大部分出血在保守治疗后会自发停止。

急诊治疗/程序

- 禁食。
- 如果出现不稳定或血细胞比容降低，伴随持续脑出血，输入蛋白质。
- 密切监测体液状况。
- 若有持续出血，立刻安排内镜检查：
  - 通过以下控制阻断出血：
    - 电凝法。
    - 注射疗法(肾上腺素)。
    - 套扎术。
    - 止血夹。
    - 凝血剂的应用。
  - 食管球囊填塞。
  - 动脉栓塞。
- 大量出血静脉使用血管加压素，不可行内镜检查。
- 如果内镜治疗无效或患者不适合手术，则考虑动脉栓塞血管造影。
- 手术是最后但最终确定的治疗方式，可能包括缝合出血或行胃切除术。
- 恶心和呕吐的止吐药。
- 抑制胃酸的质子泵抑制剂(PPI)。
- 避免使用三腔二囊管(特别是出现食管裂孔疝时)。

药物治疗

- 甲氧氯普胺：10 mg，肌内注射。
- 昂丹司琼：4 mg，静脉注射。

- 泮托拉唑：20～40 mg，静脉注射。
- 抗利尿激素（血管升压素）：0.1～0.5 U/min 借道静脉输液法，需要的话增加滴定至 0.9 U/min。

随访

进一步处理

入院指征

- 以下情况进入 ICU：
  - 持续或大出血。
  - 血流动力学不稳定。
  - 年龄极大。
  - 基本医疗条件落后。
  - 并发症。
  - 以下情况进入普通病房：
  - 清除后患者稳定出血量很小。
  - 有再出血风险因素的患者（门静脉高压、凝血病）。

出院指征

- 最小出血已经停止。
- 血流动力学稳定。
- 血细胞比容正常或稳定。
- 没有或微量阳性血红素粪便。
- 没有或微量胃液。

转诊问题

如果有严重的上消化道出血或怀疑需要紧急内镜检查，可请消化科会诊。

随访建议

如果临床指征稳定可以出院，进行门诊内镜检查和消化道随访。

要点和误区

- 对上消化道出血的患者置入 2 支大口径的静脉导管。
- 对大量的消化道出血，过早地启动了输血。
- 紧急内镜检查大量出血过早接触了消化道。
- 最初内镜检查时出血活跃，并且较低的初始血细胞比容和复杂的临床病程相关。
- 通常在 24 h 内会出现再出血，对有凝血病的患者来说极为常见。
- 出院的患者应该口服 PPI 2 周。

苯丙胺中毒 Amphetamine Poisoning

James W. Rhee　马林浩　林兆奋 译

基础知识

描述

- 去甲肾上腺素、多巴胺和血清素的释放增加。
- 儿茶酚胺再摄取减少。
- 对 α 受体和/或 β 受体直接作用。

病因

- 处方药：
  - 苯丙胺（benzedrine）。
  - 右旋苯丙胺（dexedrine）。
  - 二乙基丙酸（tenuate）。
  - 氟苯丙胺（pondimin）。
  - 甲基苯丙胺。
  - 哌甲酯（利他林）。
  - 苯甲吗啉（preludin）。
  - 芬特明。
- “非法药物”：
  - 非法药的变种。
  - 经常在地下实验室中合成。
  - “晶体”“冰”：
    - 结晶甲基苯丙胺盐酸盐。
    - 吸入，吹气或注射。
    - 起效快，持续几小时。
  - “曲柄”。
  - “摇头丸”（3,4-亚甲二氧基甲基苯丙胺、MDMA、XTQE）：
    - 经常用于舞会和/或狂欢派对。
    - 脱水可导致体温过高、低钠血症甚至死亡。
  - MDA（3,4-亚甲二氧基苯丙胺）。
  - 甲卡西酮（“cat”“Jelf”“mulka”）：
    - 常青树（Catha edulis）中发现的卡西酮的衍生物。
    - 在家庭实验室可以合成。
    - 不会在尿液毒理学筛查时查出来。
  - 甲氧麻黄酮：
    - 可能含在“浴盐”中。

诊断

症状和体征

- 中枢神经系统：
  - 激动。
  - 谵妄。
  - 多动。
  - 震颤。
  - 头晕。
  - 瞳孔散大。
  - 头痛。
  - 舞蹈症运动。
  - 反射亢进。
  - 脑血管意外。
  - 癫痫发作和癫痫持续状态。
  - 昏迷。
- 精神方面：
  - 兴奋。
  - 侵略性增加。
  - 焦虑。
  - 幻觉（视觉、触觉）。
  - 强制性重复动作。
- 心血管系统：
  - 心悸。
  - 高血压危象。
  - 心动过速或（反射）心动过缓。
  - 心律失常。
  - 心血管塌陷。
- 其他：
  - 横纹肌溶解综合征。
  - 肌红蛋白尿。
  - 急性肾衰竭。
  - 厌食。
  - 发汗。
  - DIC。

病史

- 确定苯丙胺暴露的类型、数量、时间和途径。
- 评估可能的合并症。
- 评估终末器官损伤的症状：
  - 胸痛。

- 呼吸急促。
- 头痛、意识混乱、呕吐。

体格检查

• 常见的发现包括：
- 激动。
- 心动过速。
- 发汗。
- 瞳孔散大。

• 严重中毒的特点是：
- 心动过速。
- 高血压。
- 发热。
- 谵妄。
- 癫痫。
- 发汗。

• 低血压和呼吸窘迫可能在心血管衰竭之前发生。

• 评估相关条件：
- 蜂窝织炎和软组织感染。
- 心脏舒张期或不等脉冲。
- 仔细检查创伤。
- 吸入性损伤引起的气胸。
- 局部神经功能缺损。

基本检查

• 生命体征：
- 温度：＞40℃。
  ◦ 必要时记录核心温度。
  ◦ 外周温度可能偏低。
  ◦ 提示紧急降温。
  ◦ 不祥的预后迹象。
- 血压：
  ◦ 严重的高血压可导致心脏和神经系统异常。
  ◦ 晚期，由于儿茶酚胺耗尽，低血压可能会随后发生。

• 心电图：
- 心肌缺血的迹象。
- 室性心律失常。
- 反应性心动过缓。

诊断检查与说明

实验室检查

• 尿液检查：
- 血尿。
- 肌红蛋白尿。

• 电解质、BUN/肌酐、葡萄糖：
- 低血糖可能导致精神状态改变。
- 酸中毒可伴有严重毒性。
- 横纹肌溶解可能导致肾衰竭。
- 急性肾衰竭导致的高血钾症危及生命。
- 高血钾。

• 用于监测潜在DIC的凝血功能：
- INR、PT、APTT、血小板。

• 肌酸磷酸激酶(CPK)：
- 横纹肌溶解明显加重。

• 尿毒理学检查：
- 其他具有类似效果的毒素(如可卡因)。
- 可能检测不到某些苯丙胺类物质(如甲基卡西酮)。

• 如果有自杀倾向，阿司匹林和对乙酰氨基酚水平可检测到。

• 动脉血气(ABG)。

影像学检查

• X线片：
- 成人呼吸窘迫综合征。
- 心源性肺水肿。

• 脑部CT：
- 严重的头痛。
- 意识状态改变。
- 局部神经系统体征。
- 用于蛛网膜下腔出血、脑出血。

诊断步骤/外科

腰椎穿刺：

• 疑似脑膜炎(头痛、精神状态改变、高热)。

• 疑似蛛网膜下腔出血和CT正常。

鉴别诊断

• 脓血症。

• 甲状腺危象。

• 5-羟色胺综合征。

• 抗精神病药恶性综合征。

• 嗜铬细胞瘤。

• 蛛网膜下腔出血。

• 引起谵妄的药物：
- 抗胆碱能：
  ◦ 颠茄生物碱。
  ◦ 抗组胺药。
- 三环类抗抑郁药。
- 可卡因。
- 乙醇戒断。
- 镇静/催眠戒断。
- 致幻剂。
- 苯环利定。

• 引起高血压和心动过速的药物：
- 拟交感神经药。
- 抗胆碱能药物。
- 乙醇戒断。
- 苯环利定。
- 咖啡因。
- 苯丙醇胺。

• 麻黄碱：
- 单胺氧化酶抑制剂。
- 茶碱。
- 尼古丁。

• 引起癫痫发作的药物：
- 一氧化碳。
- 卡马西平。
- 氰化物。
- 可卡因。
- Cholinergics(有机磷杀虫剂)。
- 樟脑。
- 氯化烃。
- 乙醇戒断。
- 镇静/催眠戒断。
- 异烟肼。
- 茶碱。
- 降糖药。
- 铅。
- 锂。
- 局部麻醉剂。
- 抗胆碱能药物。
- 苯环利定。
- 吩噻嗪。
- 苯妥英。
- 丙氧芬。
- 水杨酸。
- 士的宁。

治疗

院前

• 患者可能不合作或暴力。

• 安全的静脉通路。

• 防止自我创伤。

初步稳定/治疗

• ABC管理。

• 建立静脉通路，生理盐水补液。

• 心电监护。

• 如果神志改变，给予纳洛酮、右旋糖(或Accu-Chek)和硫胺素。

急诊治疗/程序

• 去除污染：
- 活性炭的应用。
- 聚乙二醇溶液的全肠灌洗。

• 高血压危象：
- 如果激动、烦躁，最初使用苯二氮䓬类药物。
- 酚妥拉明作为二线用药。

- 硝普钠治疗严重、无反应的高血压。
- 避免β受体阻滞剂，可能加剧高血压。
• 躁动，急性精神病：
- 给予苯二氮䓬类药物。
• 高热：
- 如果躁动，给予苯二氮䓬类药物。
- 温度＞40℃时主动降温：
◦ 温水薰蒸。
◦ 吹风扇。
- 麻痹：
◦ 肌肉僵硬和过度活动导致的持续性高热。
◦ 非去极化剂（如维库溴铵）。
◦ 避免使用琥珀胆碱。
◦ 插管，机械通气。
- 应用降温毯。
• 横纹肌溶解：
- 给予苯二氮䓬类药物。
- 含生理盐水的水合物。
- 保持尿量在1～2 ml/min。
- 血液透析治疗（急性肾衰竭和发生高钾血症）。
• 癫痫发作：
- 保持呼吸道通畅。
- 给予苯二氮䓬类药物。
- 如果对苯二氮䓬类药物无反应给苯巴比妥。
- 苯妥英类禁忌。
• 低血压：
- 由于儿茶酚胺耗尽，可能会发现晚。
- 初始用等渗晶体溶液推注。
- 如果没有反应，给予去甲肾上腺素。
- 多巴胺可能无效。

▪ 药物治疗

• 活性炭：1～2 g/kg 至 100 g，口服。
• 葡萄糖：D_{50}W 1 安瓿；50 ml 或 25 g（儿童：D_{25}W 2～4 ml/kg），静脉注射。
• 地西泮（苯二氮䓬类）：5～10 mg（儿童：0.2～0.5 mg/kg），静脉注射。
• 劳拉西泮（苯二氮䓬类）：2～6 mg（儿童：0.03～0.05 mg/kg），静脉注射。
• 硝普钠：1～8 μg/（kg · min），静脉注射（滴定至 BP）。
• 苯巴比妥：15～20 mg/kg，25～50 mg/min，直到癫痫发作停止。
• 酚妥拉明：5 min 内 1～5 mg，静脉注射（滴定至血压）。
• 维库溴铵：0.1 mg/kg，静脉推注。

随访

▪ 进一步处理

入院指征

• 过高热。
• 持续改变的精神状态。
• 高血压危象。
• 癫痫发作。
• 横纹肌溶解。
• 持续性心动过速。

出院指征

• 观察 6 h 后无症状。
• 缺少上述入院标准。

▪ 随访建议

患者可能需要转诊进行化学依赖性康复和排毒。

要点和误区

• 辨认患有严重或持续症状的患者。
• 监测核心温度：
- 高温＞40℃可能危及生命。
- 强效镇静和主动冷却治疗。
- 识别横纹肌溶解和高钾血症。
- 尽可能避免患者激动。
• 考虑相关的紧急情况：
- 患有胸痛的患者应评估急性冠状动脉综合征，并进行相应的治疗。
- 改变患有发热和静脉药物使用史的患者的感染。
- 与创伤性损伤有关的甲基苯丙胺滥用。
• 苯二氮䓬类药物是有症状的甲基苯丙胺中毒的一线治疗药物。
• 一些较新的刺激性滥用药物在化学结构上类似于苯丙胺。

苯二氮䓬类药物中毒 Benzodiazepine Poisoning

Michael E. Nelson 宋振举 童朝阳 译

基础知识

▪ 描述

• 通过与特定受体结合，增强γ-氨基丁酸（GABA，一种主要的抑制性神经递质）的活性。
• 可促进 GABA 与其特定受体结合。
• 造成氯离子内流、细胞膜超极化，以及抑制细胞兴奋。
- 苯二氮䓬类药物（BZD）增加氯离子通道开放的频率。
- 抑制脊髓反射及网状激活系统。
• 经胃肠道快速吸收。
- 血浆蛋白结合率高。
- 表观分布容积（Vd）大。
- 多数经肝脏代谢，部分代谢产物具有活性。
- 起效时间与药物脂溶性成反比，脂溶性高的药物（透过血脑屏障）进入中枢神经系统更快。
- 药效持续时间：劳拉西泮＞地西泮＞咪达唑仑。
- 与其他镇静安眠药物（如乙醇、巴比妥类药物、丙泊酚）同用，药效增强。

诊断

▪ 症状和体征

• 中枢神经系统：
- 镇静、嗜睡。
- 言语不清。
- 瞳孔中等大或缩小。
- 谵妄。
- 昏迷。
• 神经肌肉：
- 运动不协调。
- 自主运动变慢。
- 共济失调。
- 肌张力降低。
- 反射减弱/消失。
• 心血管系统：
- 轻度抑制。
- 罕见服用单药致死。
• 呼吸系统：
- 轻度抑制，但弱于巴比妥类。

- 短效药物和静脉用药抑制更甚。

• 胃肠道：

- 恶心、呕吐、腹泻。

• 其他：

- 低体温。

- 并发症可包括脑缺氧、横纹肌溶解和压迫性神经病变。

儿科注意事项

罕见反常性不安和躁动。

老年人注意事项

增加谵妄、跌倒、骨折和认知障碍的风险。

基本检查

诊断基于：

• 近期口服或注射史。

• 与中枢抑制相关的临床表现。

诊断检查与说明

实验室检查

• 指氧饱和度。

• 电解质、尿素氮、肌酐、血糖。

• 甲状腺功能。

• 若出现昏迷或长时间持续恶化则行尿常规查肌红蛋白。

• 血清磷酸肌酸激酶(CPK)持续降低。

• 动脉血气。

• 尿定性筛查：

- 可证实药物暴露，但不能提示或估计中毒程度，且与临床表现无关联性。

- 有假阴性结果的报道。

- 免疫法定性只能检出被代谢为奥沙西泮的 BZD。

- 尿定性筛查不能检出不经上一条代谢通路的药物(氯硝西泮、劳拉西泮、咪达唑仑、阿普唑仑)。

- 血药浓度无急诊指导意义。

- 临床体征和症状比理论的半数致死量(LD_{50})和血药浓度更为重要。

• 酒精浓度。

• 巴比妥类浓度(如苯巴比妥)。

• 对乙酰氨基酚和水杨酸盐浓度。

• 妊娠试验。

影像学检查

• 心电图。

• 胸部 X 线平片查吸入性肺炎。

• 考虑头部 CT。

诊断步骤/外科

核心体温。

鉴别诊断

• 导致意识水平下降的药物和毒物：

- 低血糖。

- 其他镇静安眠药物(巴比妥类、水合氯醛、γ-羟基丁酸、溴化物)。

- 抗抑郁药-抗精神病药。

- 毒品。

- 阿片类。

- 抗惊厥药。

- 一氧化碳/氰化物。

- 乙醇。

• 非中毒性疾病：

- 低氧血症。

- 低体温。

- 头部外伤(颅内出血)。

- 感染(脑膜炎或脑炎)。

- 电解质或代谢紊乱。

治疗

院前

• 注意气道和呼吸。

• 心电监测。

• 静脉通路。

• 快速血糖测定。

• 如怀疑药物过量应取得药瓶/药片。

初步治疗

• ABC 管理：

- 确保气道畅通并使用供氧装置辅助通气以防止低氧血症和休克。

- 静脉注射生理盐水。

- 心电监测。

• 如意识状态改变/昏迷，应用纳洛酮、硫胺素和葡萄糖。

急诊治疗/方法

• 摄入致死量 1 h 内应考虑洗胃，同时谨慎地做好气道保护。

• 如气道已保护，可予以活性炭口服/鼻胃管注入。

• 利尿剂、透析和碳血灌注没有作用。

• 氟马西尼(FZ)：

- 竞争性苯二氮草受体抑制剂。

- 快速逆转 BZD 导致的昏迷。

- 1～2 min 起效，6～10 min 达峰，持续 1～2 h(提示可重复使用)。

- 效果取决于被拮抗的 BZD 剂量及使用的氟马西尼剂量。

- 摄入药物未知或作为“昏迷鸡尾酒疗法”的一部分时，不得经验性使用本品。

- 可减少气管插管的需要，但不能持续逆转呼吸抑制。

- 有助于缩短住院时间及鉴别诊断。

- 适应证包括单独摄入 BZD 过量的非依赖性患者出现中枢抑制、心电图正常、生命体征平稳及神经系统查体阴性。

- 对逆转医源性中毒(清醒镇静)最为有效。

- 禁忌证包括：

◦ 同时服用可降低惊厥阈值的药物 TCA。

◦ 有癫痫病史或正在发作。

◦ 过敏。

◦ 神经肌肉阻滞。

◦ 低血压、低氧血症、心律失常或颅内压增高者禁用。

◦ 可导致包括惊厥在内的撤药反应，且不能再使用 BZD 治疗。

用药治疗

• 活性炭：1 g/kg 口服/鼻胃管注入(理想剂量：活性炭/摄入药物＝10/1)。

• 葡萄糖：若低血糖，给予 50％糖溶液 1 安瓿 50 ml 或 25 g(儿童：25％糖溶液 2～4 ml/kg)。

• 氟马西尼：

- 初始：30 s 内静脉注射 0.2 mg(成人)。

- 若无反应，30 s 后静脉注射 0.3 mg。

- 若仍然无反应，静脉注射 0.5 mg，每分钟重复一次，最大剂量为 3 mg。

- 若需重复剂量以维持反应则持续输注 0.1～1 mg/h。持续输注未经 FDA 批准。

- 小儿剂量：滴定最大值，累计剂量 0.05 mg/(kg · d)。曾有连续输注 0.005～0.01 mg/(kg · h)的报道。

- 因可导致惊厥或心律失常，只能用于特定患者(见上)。

- 使用后观察有无再镇静(使用后 20～120 min 发生)。

• 纳洛酮：静脉注射 0.4～2 mg(小儿：0.1 mg/kg)或初始剂量。

• 硫胺素：100 mg，静脉注射或肌内注射。

随访

进一步处理

入院指征

• 持续或严重的中枢抑制。

• 心血管或呼吸抑制。

• 摄入潜在的迟发性毒物。

出院指征

• 观察连续 4 h 无 BZD 中毒的症状或体征，可出院。

• 若使用氟马西尼，额外注意观察有无再镇静 2～4 h。

转诊问题

故意服药过量应接受精神科诊疗。

■ 随访建议

依赖性患者停药后可有 BZD 撤药反应。

• 自主神经失调、震颤、感觉异常、惊厥。

要点和误区

有些 BZD 的静脉注射剂（如劳拉西泮）可含有丙二醇溶剂，可导致高渗透压间隙和高阴离子间隙性代谢性酸中毒。

B

苯环己哌啶中毒 Phencyclidine Poisoning

Steven E. Aks　瞿金龙　林兆奋 译

基础知识

■ 描述

• 苯环己哌啶（PCP）是一种结构与氯胺酮相关的游离式麻醉剂：

- 会造成疼痛和躁动觉降低。

• 半衰期为 21～24 h，若用药过量可能会延长。

• 注意新的 PCP 类似物，如甲氧- PCP（3 - MeO - PCP、4 - MeD - PCP）的形式。

■ 病因

• 滥用药物：

- 经常遇到大麻掺杂物。

• 其他常用名称：

- 天使粉。
- Wicky 棍。
- Wicky 大麻。
- 古怪大麻。
- 湿粉。
- 伊利粉。
- 防腐液粉。
- 谢尔曼粉。

儿科注意事项

通过被动报道在幼童中曝光。

诊断

■ 症状和体征

• 中枢神经系统：

- 精神状态改变。
- 兴奋。
- 异乎寻常的行为或暴力行为表现。
- 好斗。
- 昏迷。
- 癫痫。
- 眼球震颤。

• 心血管：

- 高血压。
- 心动过速。

• 肌肉与骨骼：

- 外伤性损伤（疼痛知觉降低）。
- 横纹肌溶解（由于剧烈的肌肉收缩）。

• 重要症状：

- 体温过低。

病史

PCP 是如何成瘾的？

• 吸食大麻。

• 摄取。

体格检查

• 兴奋。

• 昏迷。

• 高血压。

• 心动过速。

• 发汗。

• 眼球震颤（垂直、水平或旋转）。

• 体温过高。

• 剧烈的肌肉收缩。

■ 基本检查

• 基于尿毒理学筛查报告的临床诊断：

- 美沙芬和氯胺酮可能导致假阳性。

• 仔细体格检查排除隐匿性创伤。

• 排除其他精神状态改变的原因。

■ 诊断检查与说明

实验室检查

• 全血细胞计数检查：

• 电解质、血尿氮、肌酸酐、葡萄糖。

• 尿液检查：

- 浸取肌红蛋白（横纹肌溶解）。

• 肌酸磷酸激酶：

- 如果尿液隐血呈阳性。

• 乙醇（酒精）水平。

影像学检查

• 对吸入性肺炎行胸部 X 线检查。

• 当有相关外伤对四肢及脊柱行 X 线检查。

• 当头部有外伤或精神状态改变时进行头部 CT 检查。

■ 鉴别诊断

• 滥用药物：

- 可卡因。
- 苯丙胺。
- 致幻药：
  ◦ 甲卡西酮（"喵喵"）。
  ◦ 摇头丸。
  ◦ 冰毒（甲基苯丙胺）。
- 酒精。
- 氯胺酮。
- 拟交感神经药。

• 引起眼球震颤的药物：

- 锂。
- 卡马西平。
- 镇静催眠药。
- 酒精。
- 吩噻嗪。
- 美沙芬。

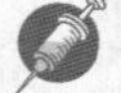

治疗

■ 院前

注意

使用限制措施或用额外的人员来控制住好斗的患者。

■ 初步稳定/治疗

• 基本体征。

• 静脉注射。

• 心脏监测仪。

• 如果精神状态改变，使用纳洛酮、硫胺素、葡萄糖（或 Accu-Chek）等药物。

• 保护患者和工作人员不受外伤。

急诊治疗/程序

• 保持患者在一个安静的地方，避免刺激。

• 对暴力的患者进行身体限制。

• 镇静：

- 苯二氮䓬类。
- 理论上丁酰苯类（氟哌啶醇）能降低癫痫发作阈值。

• 如果经口进食使用活性炭。

• 静脉注射生理盐水补液，注射碳酸氢钠-甘露醇来缓解横纹肌溶解。

药物治疗

一线用药

• 劳拉西泮：2 mg，静脉注射增量。

• 地西泮：5 mg，静脉注射增量。

二线用药

• 活性炭浆：1～2 g/kg 高至 90 g，口服。

• 右旋葡萄糖：$D_{50}W$ 1 安瓿：50 ml 或 25 g（儿童：$D_{25}W$ 2～4 ml/kg），静脉注射。

• 甘露醇：25～50 g，静脉注射。

• 纳洛酮（盐酸纳洛酮）：初次剂量 2 mg（儿童：0.1 mg/kg），静脉注射或肌内注射。

• 碳酸氢钠：2 安瓿（50 mEq/安瓿）稀释至 1 L D_5W，给药速度在 125～250 ml/h（对横纹肌溶解）直到尿的 pH 为 7。

• 硫胺素（维生素 B_1）：初次剂量 100 mg（儿童：50 mg），静脉注射或肌内注射。

随访

进一步处理

入院指征

• 长时间的精神状态的改变。

• 重大创伤。

• 横纹肌溶解。

• 体温过高。

出院指征

观察一段时间（6 h）后变得清醒。

随访建议

精神或社会工作转诊为自杀倾向或长期的药物依赖。

要点和误区

• PCP 中毒能导致致命的外伤性损伤。

• 需要用苯二氮䓬类药进行适当的化学限制来阻止过度的肌肉活动以防导致横纹肌溶解。

• 美沙芬是导致 PCP 尿液检查毒理学筛查呈假阳性的一个常见原因。

• 报道称曲马多会导致 PCP 筛查呈假阳性。

• 氯胺酮滥用可出现与 PCP 滥用相似的体征和症状。

苯妥英中毒 Phenytoin Poisoning

Michele Zell-Kanter　瞿金龙　林兆奋　译

基础知识

描述

• 苯妥英遵循零级药代动力学：

- 小剂量增加能导致在血浆中浓度的大幅增加。

• 过量用药半衰期延长，可能高达 70 h。

• 静脉注射给药产生的心血管毒性，可归因于稀释的丙二醇。

• 磷苯妥英，肠外给药的一种前药，可代谢产生苯妥英，也是磷苯妥英药物的活性成分。

病因

• 苯妥英中毒可发生于急性、慢性或慢加急性给药。

• 如果患者接受慢性苯妥英治疗而产生中毒的原因不清楚，考虑：

- 苯妥英生产商的变化。
- 剂量形式的变化。
- 药物的相互作用。
- 血清白蛋白的变化。

诊断

症状和体征

• 药物水平在 20～40 mg/L：

- 眼球震颤。
- 头昏、眼花。
- 共济失调。
- 嗜睡。
- 恶心或呕吐。
- 复视。
- 言语不清。

• 药物水平在 40～90 mg/L：

- 意识模糊。
- 定向障碍。

• 药物水平＞90 mg/L：

- 昏迷。
- 呼吸抑制。
- 反常痉挛。

• 快速静脉注射给药出现的低血压或心搏缓慢：

- 磷苯妥英注射不包含丙二醇。
- 磷苯妥英不可能造成低血压或节律障碍。

• 慢性给药伴随过敏性反应：

- 皮疹。
- 发热。
- 中性粒细胞减少症。
- 粒细胞缺乏症。
- 肝炎。
- 胆管炎。

基本检查

• 确定摄入的时间、使用途径和剂量。

• 苯妥英水平：

- 口服过量后，24 h 后或急性摄入才能达到血浆浓度顶峰。
- 吸收会随着各种口腔制剂和生产商的不同而变化。
- 每 4 h 重复一次，直到药物水平已经达到顶峰和继续稳步下降。
- 当药物水平开始下降，每 24 h 检查一次直到药物水平＜30 mg/L。
- 低白蛋白血症或代谢差的患者可能需要游离苯妥英水平。

诊断检查与说明

实验室检查

• 磷苯妥英水平：

- 按苯妥英来检测。
- 当磷苯妥英完全转换成苯妥英后进行检测(静脉输液后 2 h 或肌内注射后 4 h 检测)。
- 在完全转换成苯妥英之前,由于与磷苯妥英的交叉反应,免疫分析技术可能会高估血浆苯妥英浓度。

• 电解液、血尿氮、肌酸酐、葡萄糖:
- 检查由于静脉注射制剂中的丙二醇导致的共摄入物及癫痫产生的阴离子间隙代谢性酸中毒。
- 改变精神状态的葡萄糖。

■ **鉴别诊断**

• 其他中枢神经系统抑制剂的中毒。
• 吉兰-巴雷综合征。
• 肉毒杆菌中毒。
• 颅后窝肿瘤。
• 急性小脑炎。

治疗

■ **院前**

• 苯妥英诱导的分化改变精神状态远离其他潜在严重的因素:
- 头部外伤常见于癫痫人群。

• 收集或运输药瓶和药物有助于识别和量化摄入。

■ **初步稳定/治疗**

• 基本体征:
- 建立静脉通路。
- 心电监测(伴随静脉注射超剂量)。

• 对精神状态的改变:
- Accu-Chek。
- 使用所示的纳洛酮、葡萄糖和硫胺素。

• 通过静脉输液和头低足高位治疗低血压。
• 多巴胺治疗顽固性低血压。
• 地西泮治疗反常痉挛。

■ **急诊治疗/程序**

• 提供支持性护理。
• 活性炭:
- 使用单剂量。
- 多剂量活性炭可能会清除更多的苯妥英,与苯妥英中毒患者的临床改善无关。

■ **药物治疗**

• 活性炭浆:1~2 g/kg 高至 90 g,口服。
• 右旋葡萄糖:D_{50} W 1 安瓿 50 ml 或 25 g (儿童:D_{25} W 2~4 ml/kg),静脉注射。
• 多巴胺:2~20 μg/(kg·min),静脉注射,滴定至所要血压水平。
• 纳洛酮(盐酸纳洛酮):初次剂量 2 mg(儿童:0.1 mg/kg),静脉注射或肌内注射。
• 硫胺素(维生素 B_1):初次剂量 100 mg(儿童:50 mg),静脉注射或肌内注射。

随访

■ **进一步处理**

入院指征

• 精神状态的改变、严重共济失调、苯妥英水平的增加。
• 药物水平>25 μg/ml。
• 入院时使用苯妥英中毒。
• 预防跌倒。

出院指征

• 药物水平≤25 μg/ml。
• 可运动,无共济失调。

■ **随访建议**

• 对于故意摄入或企图自杀者要转诊精神科。
• 结束一级护理后检查苯妥英水平。
• 当生产商或制剂配方有任何变化时,要预期药物动力学和苯妥英水平的改变。

要点和误区

• 由于苯妥英遵循零级药代动力学,所以苯妥英剂量上小的增量能导致中毒。
• 每 4 h 检查一次苯妥英水平,直到下降。

鼻出血 Epistaxis

Richard E. Wolfe 单怡 译

基础知识

■ **描述**

• 鼻出血是一种急诊常见病,急诊就诊率约为 0.5%。
• 鼻出血通常是轻微的且具有自限性,但也可能是威胁生命的紧急症状:
- 终身发病率约为 60%:
  ◦ 双峰年龄分布,常见于年龄小于 10 岁的儿童和 70~79 岁的老年人。
  ◦ 老年人后鼻出血更常见。
  ◦ 男性多于女性。
  ◦ 需要外科干预的严重出血更常见于 50 岁以上的患者。
  ◦ 多发生于湿度较低的冬季、北方气候、高海拔地区。

• 鼻腔血管源于颈内动脉和颈外动脉。
• 出血的部位决定治疗方案:
- 前鼻出血(90%的病例):在前鼻腔可以直接观察到出血。
  ◦ 大多数常见出血位于克氏静脉丛,克氏静脉丛为前下鼻中隔的静脉吻合网。
  ◦ 少见的出血位于鼻腔或鼻中隔后部。
- 后鼻出血(10%的病例):不在直接可视化范围内的出血。
- 蝶腭动脉后外侧。

■ **病因**

• 先天原因:
- 鼻黏膜干燥(湿度低)。

• 鼻腔异物:
- 儿童、智能发育迟缓的患者、精神病患者。

• 感染:
- 鼻窦炎。
- 鼻白喉病。
- 鼻毛霉菌病。

• 过敏性鼻炎。
• 创伤:
- 挖鼻(常见于儿童)。
- 术后。
- 面部创伤。
- 气压伤。

• 环境刺激物:
- 氨。
- 汽油。
- 硫酸。
- 戊二醛。

• 鼻内瘤:乳头状瘤最常见。

• 凝血功能障碍：
- 血友病 A 或 B。
- 血管性血友病。
- 血小板减少症：肝脏疾病、白血病、化疗或自身免疫性疾病。
- 血小板功能异常：肾功能损害或慢性酒精滥用。
• 药物诱发：
- 水杨酸酯。
- 非甾体抗炎药。
- 抗凝药物。
• 遗传性出血性毛细血管扩张症（奥斯勒-韦伯-朗迪病）。
• 鼻血管动脉粥样硬化。
• 子宫内膜异位症。
• 医源性：
- 留置鼻胃管。
- 经鼻支气管镜插管。
- 留置经鼻气管插管。

诊断

症状和体征

病史

• 出血的偏侧。
• 鼻孔出血的量和程度。
• 反复鼻出血。
• 持续鼻阻塞。
• 呕吐或咳嗽。
• 已知肿瘤和凝血功能障碍。
• 异常出血或易擦伤，提示潜在凝血功能障碍。
• 存在缺血引起的系统性疾病（冠状动脉疾病、慢性阻塞性肺疾病）。

体格检查

• 评估失血性休克时的生命体征。
• 仔细检查凝血功能障碍的迹象：
- 擦伤。
- 瘀斑和紫癜。
• 鼻咽部检查：
- 将棉棒浸于麻醉药和血管活性药物后麻醉鼻咽腔。
• 尝试用鼻镜明确出血部位。
• 牙齿或口咽部出血。

基本检查

• 评估稳定性：气道顺应性，低血容量。
• 明确出血来源（前鼻/后鼻）。
• 考虑是否有潜在的凝血功能障碍。

诊断检查与说明

实验室检查

• 考虑严重出血或凝血功能障碍：
- 全血细胞计数、血型和交叉配血试验、凝血酶原时间/国际标准化比值、活化部分凝血活酶时间、血尿素氮。

诊断步骤/外科

用鼻内镜直接显示鼻黏膜：
• 局部血管收缩剂和麻醉预处理。
• 保证充足的照明（如前照灯）和负压吸力。

鉴别诊断

• 呕血。
• 咯血。

儿科注意事项

• 后鼻出血在儿童中是罕见的，考虑进一步检查出血倾向。
• 考虑鼻腔异物或肿瘤，如鼻咽纤维血管瘤、乳头状瘤。
• 外用抗菌药膏 4 周可降低复发出血率。

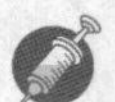

治疗

院前

• 稳定的患者：患者应腰部向前倾；捏鼻闭合鼻孔，吐出血而不是吞下。
• 不稳定的患者：
- 如果气道阻塞时应行气管插管。
- 建立静脉通路。
- 如果出现低血容量征象晶体液复苏。

初步稳定/治疗

• 确保无意识的，有面部外伤或存在梗阻、误吸风险的患者气道安全。
• 必要时，使用晶体液和血液制品纠正低血压，确保足够的静脉通路。
• 高血压治疗价值认识不足。

急诊治疗/程序

• 通常需预防血液/液体污染。
• 前鼻腔出血源：
- 患者直接捏鼻孔按压 15 min。这可能控制出血并看清鼻腔。
- 在检查前，让患者擤鼻涕排出血块。
- 如果出血持续，用止血钳将棉纱布浸泡在缩血管药和麻醉药物后放入鼻孔。
- 如果鼻腔有血看不清，让患者擤鼻涕或冲洗吸引鼻血。
- 用鼻镜观察出血点。
- 用硝酸银或电烙烧灼有限区域：
◦ 在烧灼前，使用浸有血管收缩剂和局麻剂的棉纱布，以确保鼻中隔干燥。
◦ 而后使用抗生素软膏和凡士林软膏。
• 前鼻腔填塞：
- 烧灼未能控制出血时采用。
- 可能存在明显的不适感、鼻窦炎和中毒性休克的感染风险。
- 前鼻气囊止血：
◦ 插入前检查气囊的完整性。
◦ 涂抹水润滑剂或黏性利多卡因。
◦ 插入装置并使其缓慢充气以避免不适。
◦ 如果该气囊在某处停留超过数小时，就要用盐水来进行膨胀。
- 预制鼻腔止血塞：
◦ 放置鼻塞前应保证鼻腔通道充分的麻醉。
◦ 用抗生素软膏润滑海绵塞尖部。
◦ 将它以 45°角插入鼻腔 1～2 cm。
◦ 旋转鼻塞的长轴至水平面，把它牢牢地推入鼻腔。
◦ 如果鼻塞在血液中没有充分扩张，可用生理盐水来完成扩张。
◦ 用束带将其固定在脸颊上。
- 液状石蜡（石蜡油）浸渍的纱布：
◦ 在纱布上涂抹抗生素软膏。
◦ 确保置入后纱布尾端仍然在鼻外。
◦ 从鼻平面开始，将纱布尽可能放入深部。
◦ 手风琴式铺纱布。
◦ 反复使用内镜固定纱布位置直到鼻腔完全填满。
- 前鼻腔填充完后，仍有新的持续性出血可能说明填塞不充分或鼻出血为后鼻腔来源。
- 如果单侧填充失效，则可能需要使用双侧填充来压迫止血。
- 常规使用浸有抗生素的鼻塞预防鼻窦炎，防止或限制金黄色葡萄球菌感染导致的中毒性休克综合征（TSS）。
• 后鼻腔出血源：
- 早期内镜观察和烧灼出血源可避免后鼻腔填塞的需要。
- 后鼻腔填塞可使用成品设备（如 Nasostat 或 Epistat）完成。
- 如果无法获取成品填塞设备，气囊管可直接进入后鼻咽直到口咽部可见。气囊充气直到气囊固定在后鼻咽时撤回导管。导管用钳夹住固定。
- 由于感染风险后鼻腔填塞不应超过 3 日。因有迷走神经反应的风险，患者应入院并监测。
• 鼻腔填塞的并发症：

- 压力过大致后咽部坏死(勿过量充气)。
- 鼻外伤。
- 鼻中隔穿孔。
- 鼻窦炎。
- 中毒性休克综合征。
- 迷走神经反射性心动过缓。
- 误吸。
- 缺氧。

• 如果患者在服用抗凝剂或有出血疾病,应根据具体情况使用拮抗剂或血液制品。

• 对于压迫止血不能控制的鼻出血,经耳鼻喉科会诊后可考虑以下选择:
- 血管结扎术。
- 鼻中隔手术。
- 内镜电灼术。
- 血管造影栓塞术。

▪ 药物治疗

• 血管活性药物:
- 4%可卡因。
- 2%丁卡因与肾上腺素(1∶1000)1∶1混合液。
- 0.05%羟甲唑啉与4%利多卡因溶液1∶1混合液。
- 0.5%~1%去氧肾上腺素。

• 抗生素:填塞时使用。
- 阿莫西林-克拉维酸钾:250 mg,口服,q8 h。
- 头孢氨苄:250 mg,口服,q6 h。
- 氯林可霉素:150 mg,口服,q6 h。
- 甲氧苄啶-磺胺甲噁唑:160/800 mg,口服,q12 h。

随访

▪ 进一步处理

入院指征

• 需要输血的大量失血。

• 严重的凝血功能障碍,患者存在进一步出血风险。

• 如果担心氧合或患者虚弱,则进行双侧填塞。

• 后鼻腔填塞:耳鼻咽喉科会诊和并住院监测,吸氧,必要时镇静和观察,可能需进一步手术干预(如动脉结扎或栓塞)。

• 前鼻腔填塞后48 h内不能随访的患者。

出院指征

稳定患者:

• 使用羟甲唑啉喷鼻2日。

• 抗生素软膏润滑鼻腔或使用洗鼻盐水,每日3~4次。

• 增加空气湿度。

• 避免鼻腔填塞。

• 所有鼻腔填塞过程中使用抗葡萄球菌抗生素(阿莫西林-克拉维酸、头孢氨苄、甲氧苄啶-磺胺甲噁唑)预防急性鼻窦炎和中毒性休克综合征的患者。

转诊问题

• 48 h内将鼻腔填塞患者交给专科医师处理。

• 未明确出血源,可疑病变,经常性同侧出血或鼻塞的患者应转至耳鼻喉科检查排除肿瘤或异物的可能。

▪ 随访建议

• 出现压力高出血无法控制、发热、呼吸困难或呕吐时再次急诊就诊。

• 出血停止后12 h内避免擤鼻涕。

• 避免挖鼻孔或放任何东西入鼻。

• 如果再次出血,坐起来,身体向前倾,紧紧捏鼻的柔软部分10 min避免流血。

• 避免提重物或马上做太多的工作。

• 如果鼻有没有填塞,向鼻内放少量凡士林或抗生素药膏,每日2次,持续4~5日。

• 在家中使用加湿器或喷雾器。

要点和误区

• 儿童、精神病患者和精神发育迟滞患者任何单侧鼻出血应怀疑有异物存在。

• 避免用抗生素软膏覆盖前鼻腔气囊,因为以石蜡油为基础的材料可能会导致气囊破裂。

• 避免鼻气囊过膨或填塞太紧,因为它会导致坏死或焦痂。

• 填塞的患者应接受预防性抗生素治疗。

鼻窦炎 Sinusitis

James M. Tsahakis · Maria E. Moreira 周健 潘曙明 译

基础知识

▪ 描述

• 鼻腔和鼻腔内壁黏膜发炎,窦腔内积液或不积液。

• 分类:
- 急性:<4周的症状和体征。
- 亚急性:4~8周的症状和体征。
- 慢性:尽管进行了抗生素治疗,但>8周的症状和体征。
- 周期性:每年3次或以上。

▪ 病因

• 急性鼻窦炎的病理生理:
- 病毒上呼吸道感染或过敏引起黏膜发炎。
- 发炎导致窦口阻塞,黏膜纤毛清除减少和分泌物增厚。
- 病毒是主要病因,但在细菌被感染并繁殖后,有0.5%~2.2%的细菌发展成细菌感染,从而导致化脓。
- 与鼻胃管和鼻气管相关的医院鼻窦炎。
- 免疫功能低下的患者患上鼻窦炎的风险更高。

• 亚急性和慢性鼻窦炎的病理生理:
- 多因素作用,细菌的作用仍然难以捉摸。
- 过敏性炎症导致狭窄的口孔和阻塞的引流。
- 免疫功能障碍导致感染风险增加。
- 睫状功能受损导致黏液清除率降低。
- 牙源性感染引起上颌窦炎。
- 真菌球。
- 解剖性阻塞或息肉阻塞窦口。

• 微生物学:
- 急性鼻窦炎:
  ◦ 非典型性流感嗜血杆菌。
  ◦ 肺炎链球菌。
  ◦ 卡他莫拉菌。
  ◦ 金黄色葡萄球菌。
  ◦ 厌氧菌。
  ◦ 病毒:副流感病毒、腺病毒、鼻病毒、流感病毒。
- 慢性鼻窦炎:
  ◦ 与急性细菌相同,通常是多微生物,厌氧菌和革兰阴性菌增多。

B

– 医院鼻窦炎：
◦ 金黄色葡萄球菌。
◦ 链球菌。
◦ 假单胞菌。
◦ 克雷伯菌。
◦ 曲霉。
◦ 毛霉。
– 免疫功能低下的鼻窦炎患者：
◦ 上述细菌。
◦ 真菌病原体。
◦ 曲霉。
◦ 毛霉。

儿科注意事项

• 非典型性流感嗜血杆菌比肺炎链球菌更常见于儿童急性细菌性鼻窦炎。
• 出生时即存在筛骨和上颌窦。
• 蝶窦在5岁时发育，额窦在7岁时发育。
• 鼻窦炎多见于儿童。
• 眶周/眼眶蜂窝织炎是儿童筛窦性鼻窦炎的常见并发症：
– 骨膜周围肿胀，凹陷；上睑下垂，眼球突出，以及眼外运动疼痛或减少。

诊断

症状和体征

• 面部及牙齿疼痛，头痛，口臭，咳嗽。
• 化脓性鼻涕和鼻后引流。
• 发热。
• 额窦炎：
– 下前额下部疼痛。
– 躺着时疼痛加剧。
– 直立时改善。
• 上颌窦炎：
– 颧骨面部疼痛。
– 上颌牙齿疼痛。
– 耳痛。
– 头部直立或向前弯曲会使疼痛加重，而向后倾斜可改善疼痛。
• 筛窦炎：
– 眼眶后痛。
– 眶周水肿。
• 蝶窦炎（非常罕见）：
– 枕骨或乳突疼痛。
– 仰卧或向前弯曲时疼痛更严重。

病史

• 急性病毒性鼻窦炎：
– 症状通常在7～10日解决。
• 需要抗生素治疗的急性细菌性鼻窦炎可以三种不同的方式出现：
– 出现方式1：持续的症状持续>10日而无改善。
– 出现方式2：严重症状：
◦ 发病初期温度>39℃，脓性鼻涕持续3～4日。
– 出现方式3：症状恶化：
◦ 上呼吸道感染持续5～6日后症状有所改善。
• 其他重要病史：
– 症状病史和时间过程。
– 过敏史。
– 最近的鼻胃管NG管或NT管放置。
– 免疫受损状态。

体格检查

• 生命体征，有毒/无毒外观。
• 鼻黏膜和鼻甲水肿。
• 鼻孔或咽后部化脓。
• 鼻窦发热、压痛或蜂窝织炎。
• 触诊时窦区压痛。
• 牙周水肿。
• 上颌窦透照显示不清：
– 通过味觉观察。
• 口腔科检查显示上颌牙脓肿或压痛。

基本检查

• 基于病史和体格检查的临床诊断。
• 确定患者是否适合使用抗生素治疗的急性细菌性鼻窦炎。

诊断检查与说明

实验室检查

• 实验室检查无助于诊断或治疗。
• 鼻咽培养几乎没有价值，不推荐。

影像学检查

• 在一般情况下无需成像。
• X线平片：
– 正常X线片不能排除细菌引起的感染。
– 沃特斯视图可能有用，但对上颌窦异常的诊断敏感性中等，对其他鼻窦病变的诊断敏感性较弱。
– 口腔科检查和Panorex胶片可能会漏掉牙源性上颌窦炎，但CT上明显表现为根尖透明性。
• CT：
– 如果需要成像则首选。
– 适用于复杂性鼻窦炎、严重头痛、癫痫发作、局灶性神经功能缺损、眼眶周围水肿或眼内肌功能异常的患者。
– 静脉使用造影剂，如果考虑骨髓炎或脓肿颅内延伸：
◦ 大脑静脉窦血栓形成。

诊断步骤/外科

• 鼻窦穿刺培养：
– 是进行微生物诊断的金标准，但未常规执行。
• 出院培养可能有好处，但尚未研究，通常不进行。
• 功能性内镜鼻窦手术（FESS）：
– 恢复生理性鼻窦引流。但一般只适用于药物治疗失败的情况。

儿科注意事项

• 对于药物治疗无效的慢性鼻窦炎患儿，根须切除术是首选。
• FESS对儿童是一种安全有效的治疗方法。

鉴别诊断

• 单纯性病毒性或过敏性鼻炎。
• 中耳炎。
• 泪囊炎。
• 偏头痛和丛集性头痛。
• 牙痛。
• 三叉神经痛。
• 颞下颌关节疾病。
• 巨细胞动脉炎/颞动脉炎。
• 药物鼻炎（减充血剂、β受体阻滞剂、降压药、避孕药）。
• 鼻息肉、肿瘤或异物。
• 中枢神经系统感染。
• 肉芽肿或睫状体疾病。
• 曲霉病。
• 毛霉病：
– 罕见的快速进行性真菌感染。
– 发生在糖尿病患者和免疫功能低下。
– 眼眶/面部疼痛与检查不一致。
– 全身性疾病患者的胸闷、头痛。
– 黑色焦痂或鼻黏膜上的苍白区域。

妊娠注意事项

• 妊娠期鼻炎：
– 雌激素对黏膜有胆碱能作用。
– 妊娠晚期更严重。
– 在产后2周内解决。

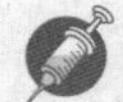

治疗

院前

没有特别考虑。

初步稳定/治疗

出现严重脓毒症的患者可能需要气道处

理和液体复苏。

■ 急诊治疗/程序

• 确定需要抗生素的鼻窦炎。

• 为症状持续时间少于 10 日的轻微症状的患者提供咨询和保证。

■ 药物治疗

• 非抗生素疗法：
- 疼痛控制。
- 盐水鼻腔冲洗可能有益。
- 口服皮质类固醇作为口服抗生素的辅助药是有效的，但数据有限。
- 鼻内类固醇被推荐作为抗生素的辅助药物，主要用于那些有过敏的人：
 ◦ 丙酸氟替卡松：每日每个鼻孔喷 2 次（没有证据表明一种类固醇比另一种更有效）。
- 抗组胺药物推荐给潜在的过敏患者。
 ◦ >3 日不推荐使用鼻或口服减充血剂，因为有反弹充血的风险（苯肾上腺素、伪麻黄碱、奥氧美唑啉）。
- 研究人员可能会有所帮助：
 ◦ 愈创甘油醚：
  ▪ 成人：口服，200～400 mg；不大于 2.4 g/24 h。
  ▪ 2～5 岁儿童：50～100 mg，口服；不大于 600 mg/24 h。
  ▪ 6～11 岁儿童：口服，100～200 mg；不大于 1.2 g/24 h。

• 抗生素：
- 阿莫西林-克拉维酸盐：875 mg，口服[儿童：45 mg/(kg·24 h)拆分口服，基于阿莫西林成分]。
- 如果高风险（日托，年龄<2 岁或>65 岁，出院时出现全身性热/发热>39 ℃，最近住院，上个月使用抗生素或免疫功能低下），则使用阿莫西林-克拉维酸：2 g 口服，每日 2 次[儿童：90 mg/(kg·d)，基于阿莫西林成分]。
- 强力霉素：100 mg，口服，每日 2 次（成人初始经验疗法的替代方案）。

• 由于肺炎患者的耐药性，不再推荐将第二代和第三代口服头孢菌素用于经验性单药治疗。可以使用以下组合：
- 头孢泊肟：200～400 mg，口服，每日 2 次[儿童：10 mg/(kg·d)，口服，每日 2 次]；或头孢呋辛：250～500 mg，口服，每日 2 次[儿童：15 mg/(kg·d)，口服，每日 2 次]+克林霉素：每 6 h 150～300 mg，口服[儿童：8～16 mg/(kg·d)，口服，拆分，q6～8 h，MRSA 怀疑使用 40 mg/(kg·d)，口服，拆分，q6～8 h]。

• 不推荐使用大环内酯类药物（克拉霉素和阿奇霉素），因为在肺炎链球菌（30%）耐药率很高。

• 不推荐使用甲氧苄啶-磺胺甲噁唑（TMP-SMX），因为肺炎链球菌和流感嗜血杆菌（30%～40%）的耐药率很高。

• 1 型青霉素过敏：
- 左氧氟沙星：每日最大 500 kg 以下的儿童每日服用 500 mg，口服（儿童：8 mg/kg）。剂量 250 mg/d。超过 50 kg 的儿童剂量 500 mg/d。
- 莫西沙星：每日（成人）400 mg，口服。

• 如果使用一种抗生素 3～5 日后症状仍未改善，请换用另一种抗生素。

• 建议的治疗时间：
- 急性：儿童 10～14 日；成人 5～7 日。
- 慢性：3～6 周疗程的抗生素（有争议的）。

一线用药

支持性治疗。

二线用药

抗生素类。

随访

■ 进一步处理

入院指征

• 感染扩散到窦腔或出现中毒患者以外的证据。

• 具有广泛感染的免疫功能低下或糖尿病患者。

• 多发性窦或额窦受累。

• 极端年龄。

• 严重合并症。

• 如果患者病情严重，免疫功能低下或患有全乳腺炎并出现不适，则进行 ENT 评估和抽吸。

出院指征

大多数无并发症的鼻窦炎病例可在门诊治疗。

转诊问题

• 急性感染并发症。

• 免疫功能低下的患者。

• 慢性鼻窦炎或鼻息肉。

• 有关骨髓炎、中枢神经系统感染或脓肿的问题。

• 急性鼻窦炎-曲霉病。

■ 随访建议

如果患者在初始治疗和非抗生素治疗后仍无缓解，请进行初级保健医师或耳鼻随访。

要点和误区

• 出现<10 日的轻度症状的患者应接受支持治疗。

• 出现>10 日症状，发热 4～5 日时出现严重症状或在最初改善后恶化的患者可以诊断为急性细菌性鼻窦炎，应使用抗生素治疗。

• 首选鼻窦炎，因为鼻窦发炎很少发生而没有鼻黏膜发炎。

鼻骨骨折 Nasal Fracture

David W. Munter 黄昊 译

基础知识

■ 描述

• 鼻骨是人体中最容易发生骨折的骨骼。

• 大多数鼻骨骨折由钝性损伤所致，常见于机动车事故、运动损伤和打斗损伤。

• 侧面受力相对于正面受力更易导致骨折移位。

• 以下表现提示有其他并发损伤：
- 有严重的外力致伤史。
- 意识丧失。
- 有面骨损伤。
- 额面部有骨摩擦音。
- 脑脊液漏。

■ 病因

• 绝大多数鼻骨骨折源于直接创伤。

• 成人鼻骨骨折中多数来源于打斗致伤。

• 直接撞击，尤其是运动伤，占儿童鼻骨骨折中的大多数。

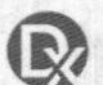

诊断

■ 症状和体征

• 鼻骨变形，不对称，肿胀或淤血。
• 鼻出血。
• 眶周淤血（"熊猫眼"）是由于筛骨动脉分支所致：
- 可能存在鼻额筛窦复合体损伤。
• 触摸时有骨摩擦音和异常活动。
• 可触及锋利的边缘，有压痛或其他不规则改变时，提示有鼻骨骨折。
• 鼻中隔血肿：
- 鼻中隔表面覆盖蓝色液性囊肿。
- 及时发现是关键，因为需要行引流处理。
- 引流失败可能导致鼻中隔坏死。
• 鼻骨根部扁平内眦距离增宽：
- 提示有严重的鼻额筛窦复合体损伤。
• 持续有清亮的鼻液溢出提示可能存在脑脊液漏：
- 鼻液溢出症状可能延迟发生。
• 有嗅觉丧失提示有明显损伤。
• 泪管损伤可有异常流泪症状。
• 眼部相关损伤：
- 结膜下出血。
- 眼前房出血。
- 视网膜脱落。

病史

• 被直接击打。
• 相关损伤和症状。
• 鼻出血。
• 视觉或味觉改变。

体格检查

• 视诊和触诊至关重要。
• 及时识别鼻中隔血肿很关键：
- 鼻中隔壁上可见青紫隆起包块。
• 鼻中隔移位。
• 鼻出血或鼻腔内撕裂伤。
• 仔细检查有无内眦增宽：
- 内眦宽度在 30～35 mm 或以上。
- 宽度超过一眼宽。
- 提示可能存在鼻额筛复合体骨折。
- 通常伴有鼻柱塌陷。
• 脑脊液鼻漏：
- 提示存在严重的深部面骨骨折或颅骨骨折。
- 将漏出的液体置于滤纸时如发现混有血液则应加倍警惕，但是这一症状并非 100% 可靠。

■ 基本检查

如考虑损伤不仅是简单鼻骨骨折者：
• 评估鼻泪管通畅性：
- 以荧光剂缓慢滴眼并观察下鼻甲下方的鼻咽部有无荧光剂流入。
- 未见荧光剂则提示鼻导管损伤。
• 睫毛牵引试验：
- 捏住睫毛并向侧方牵拉眼睑：
- 如眼睑边缘未绷紧呈弓弦状，则提示肌腱中间部分断裂。
- 这一试验可应用于上、下眼睑：
◦ 提示一部分肌腱出现选择性断裂。

■ 诊断检查与说明

实验室检查

出现不可控的鼻出血时，如患者正使用抗凝药物，则需检查凝血功能。

影像学检查

• 鼻部 X 线平片提示意义较小：
- 通常不会影响初始和后续处理方案。
- 鼻部肉眼观存在畸形者需转诊。
- 不伴畸形的骨折无论影像学是否有异常均可保守治疗。
- 如患者有面部骨骼畸形、骨摩擦音或压痛者需要行 X 线片。
• 超声可以用来检测骨折，并且像普通胶片一样敏感。
• 考虑面部骨折时，CT 检查可做备选，鼻额筛复合体或颅骨凹陷性骨折；如怀疑其他部位损伤时可减低 CT 适用门槛。

■ 鉴别诊断

• 其他面部损伤如眼眶、额窦、上颌窦或筛窦骨折。
• 鼻额筛骨复合体骨折。

治疗

■ 院前

• 优先畅通气道。
• 经鼻气管插管禁忌证。
• 如需建立确定型人工气道，可行经口气管插管或环甲膜切开。
• 颈部有相关损伤，应行预防性颈椎保护措施。
• 鼻出血通常可通过局部按压得到控制，同时挤压两侧鼻孔。

■ 初步稳定/治疗

• 经口气管插管或气管切开术，保持气道畅通：
- 经鼻气管插管是禁忌证。
• 颈椎预防性保护措施。
• 优先处理其他部位损伤。

■ 急诊治疗/程序

• 擦伤和撕裂伤：
- 适当的创面清洁至关重要。
- 撕裂伤需要缝合。
• 鼻出血如不能自行停止则需积极控制：
- 局部应用麻药、血管收缩药，如可卡因、利多卡因或新福林喷剂。
- 寻找出血点，必要时电凝止血。
- 以凡士林、浸湿的纱块等填塞鼻孔。
- 鼻腔深部很少需要填塞。
- 如果放置后填充物，可能需要预防性抗生素以防止鼻窦感染，大多数证据表明前填充物不需要它们：如阿莫西林、阿莫西林-克拉维酸钾、青霉素过敏者可用甲氧苄啶-磺胺甲噁唑或阿奇霉素。
- 骨折移位无须在急诊室复位，除非气道受压。
- 尽管有部分专家建议局麻下立即复位，但一般推荐骨折后 3～5 日，待水肿减轻后再行骨折复位术。
• 鼻中隔血肿需立即在急诊室行引流：
- 给予可卡因或利多卡因局部麻醉并用新福林收缩血管。
- 可尝试用 18～20 号针的 3 ml 注射器抽吸。
- 以棉签拭子在鼻中隔下部旋动可促进引流。
- 清除附着在软骨表面的黏膜以防止血液再次蓄积。
- 可以使用油纱作引流。
- 应同时压迫双侧鼻孔以确保有足够压力：
◦ 纱块留置 3～5 日直至耳鼻喉科再次随访。
- 预防性应用抗生素。

■ 治疗药物

• 阿莫西林：500 mg，口服，每日 3 次（儿童：40 mg/kg，分次口服，每日 3 次）。
• 阿莫西林-克拉维酸钾：500/125～875/125 mg，口服，每日 2 次[儿童：40 mg/(kg · d)，克拉维酸钾，口服，每日 2 次]。
• 阿奇霉素：首日 500 mg，口服；第 2～4 日，250 mg/d，口服（儿童：首日 10 mg/kg，

口服；第 2～4 日，5 mg/kg，口服）。

• 可卡因：4%，局部应用。

• 利多卡因：1%～2%，不加肾上腺素。

• 新福林喷鼻剂。

• 甲氧苄啶-磺胺甲噁唑：剂量加倍，口服，每日 2 次[儿童：磺胺甲噁唑 40 mg/(kg・d)，口服，每日 2 次]。

随访

进一步处理

入院指征

• 大部分鼻骨骨折无需住院治疗。

• 有鼻筛窦区或更多颅面部损伤者需收治入院。

出院指征

• 头、颈或其他部位无明显损伤者。

• 鼻出血已得到控制。

• 有可靠的陪护照顾者。

儿科注意事项

• 尽早请专科会诊，因为儿童的纤维组织将在 3～4 日开始愈合。

• 若怀疑患者属非意外损伤者，则应与儿童权益保护机构取得联系：

- 提供的病史与受伤情况不相符。
- 切记非意外损伤也是受伤的可能原因之一。

• 儿童骨折少见，儿童鼻骨骨折更多的是软骨骨质。

• 发生在儿童的严重损伤有时难以识别。

随访

随访建议

• 3～7 日至耳鼻喉科、整形或口腔颌面外科随访处理：

- 有鼻中隔血肿者须在引流后 24 h 内随访再评估。

• 有鼻漏、呼吸困难、发热或合并头部损伤者应随访。

要点和误区

• 每一例患者均应记录有无鼻中隔血肿的情况。

• 后鼻填塞出院的患者应使用抗葡萄球菌抗生素，单纯前鼻填塞的患者一般不需要抗生素。

• 鼻骨损伤后出现清亮鼻漏者应考虑筛板骨折可能。

• 怀疑其他部位有并发损伤或骨折者，应降低 CT 检查的应用门槛。

B

鼻腔异物 Foreign Body, Nasal

Jeremy N. Driscoll・David A. Pearson 万健 译

基础知识

描述

• 异物损害发生在鼻腔内。

• 鼻腔是儿童塞入异物最常见的部位。

• 异物类型受鼻孔限制。

• 可能会延迟几周或几个月才被诊断。

• 通常位于下鼻甲底部或中鼻甲前。

• 风险人群：

- 2～6 岁儿童最多见。
- 心智发育迟缓。
- 精神疾病。

• 导致损害加重和取出困难的因素：

- 遇湿膨胀的物质。
- 黏膜水肿不退。

• 并发症：

- 鼻窦炎。
- 异物移行到鼻窦内。
- 鼻中隔穿孔。
- 误吸。
- 钮扣电池具有并发症高风险：
  ◦ 黏膜缺血。
  ◦ 鼻甲或鼻中隔受损。
  ◦ 鞍鼻畸形。

病因

• 器质性或非器质性病变。

• 食物。

• 豆类。

• 种子。

• 珠子。

• 石子。

• 纸。

• 玩具碎片。

• 海绵碎片。

• 植物。

• 昆虫和活蠕虫。

• 钮扣电池：

- 相对其他异物来说有更高的并发症风险（组织坏死、鼻中隔穿孔、鞍鼻畸形），需尽快取出。
- 隔膜穿孔最短可在 4 h 内发生。

• 磁铁：

- 穿鼻妆。
- 常嵌入鼻黏膜内而取出困难。
- 一旦误吞可能发生肠穿孔，特别是新型的钕高能磁石。

• 玻璃碎片。

诊断

症状和体征

• 多数鼻腔异物没有症状。

• 单侧鼻腔阻塞。

• 鼻痛。

• 经鼻呼吸困难。

• 鼻腔有分泌物：

- 急性或慢性。
- 单侧的。
- 鼻腔异味。
- 口臭。

• 鼻窦部不适。

• 持续性鼻出血。

• 局部炎症。

• 鼻中隔穿孔。

• 异物摄入或嵌入史。

病史

• 有人目睹儿童将异物放入鼻腔。

• 父母或看护人发现儿童鼻腔异物。

• 许多儿童因为担心被成人责怪而不愿意承认将异物放入鼻腔史。

• 迟发性表现：

- 当没有目击者时，儿童鼻腔异物表现可能在数周后出现，如鼻腔有分泌物和出血。
- 常被误诊为鼻窦炎。
- 单侧、脓性、恶臭的鼻涕时保持高度警惕。

基本检查

• 鼻腔内检视以发现异物，应该双侧鼻孔都检查。

• 使用良好的照明（前照灯）和嗅探位置以

获得最佳视觉效果。

■ 诊断检查与说明

实验室检查不需要。

影像学检查

• 若鼻镜未能发现异物，应用纤维光镜检视。

• 病程较长或怀疑电池或磁铁时应摄鼻窦X线片：

- 虽然异物已被取出并使用了抗生素。

• 有异物摄入、误吸史者可能还需要胸部或腹部X线片。

■ 鉴别诊断

• 鼻窦炎。

• 下鼻甲肿胀：

- 有时会被误诊为粉色弹珠。

• 鼻炎。

• 鼻息肉。

• 鼻腔良性肿瘤：

- 血管瘤最多见。

• 恶性肿瘤：

- 淋巴瘤。

- 横纹肌肉瘤。

- 鼻咽癌。

- 鼻腔神经胶质瘤(也称嗅神经胶质瘤)。

• 先天性包块：

- 皮样囊肿。

- 脑膨出。

- 胶质瘤。

- 畸胎瘤。

• 咽后壁脓肿。

• 创伤性鼻骨移位或分离。

• 鼻畸形：

- 常与腭裂相关。

• 鼻咽腔病理性狭窄。

• 药物性鼻炎：

- 过度使用缩血管滴鼻剂引起鼻黏膜水肿似弹球。

治疗

■ 院前

• 注意：

- 异物位置变化：

◦ 避免后鼻腔的异物脱位引起窒息。

• 避免强行干预烦躁状态下的儿童：

- 哭闹时用力吸气的负压可能将异物吸入而发生窒息。

■ 急诊治疗/程序

• 表面缩血管滴鼻剂：

- 取异物时发现鼻黏膜水肿或出血。

- 肾上腺素喷剂。

- 可卡因：4%溶液。

- 羟甲唑林：0.05%溶液。

- 苯肾上腺素：0.125%～0.5%溶液。

- 不建议纽扣电池使用，因为可能会增加腐蚀性物质的泄漏。

• 正压法：

- 阻塞对侧鼻孔。

- 尽可能坐直。

- 向口内加压吹气(最好由父母来做)。

- 当患儿开始吸气时猛向其口内吹气。

- 父母可告诉患儿送其一个"大大的亲吻"。

- 或用4 cm×4 cm大小的纱布敷在吹气者的颊部。

- 异物可能喷到吹气者脸上或房间里。

- 必要时可重复进行上述动作。

- 可以面罩加压替代口对口吹气。

- 连接10～15 L/min氧气带储气袋面罩加压吹气。

- 连接10～15 L/min氧气管插入对侧鼻孔鼻加压吹气。

◦ 持续不断、不可调节的正压吹气可能引起气压伤。

• 带钩探针和鳄鱼嘴钳：

- 位于鼻前部易取的异物。

- 需戴额灯和鼻内镜。

- 有将异物推向更深处的风险。

• 吸引管：

- 可滚动、光滑的异物。

- 最好是可回拉的吸引管。

- 吸引管头端对准异物。

- 开大吸引力渐至100～140 mmHg。

- 靠吸引管将异物一并拉出鼻腔。

• 丙烯酸蓝组织胶(cyanoacrylate tissue glue)：

- 在一空心塑料探针尖端贴一片组织胶。

- 用探针将组织胶压在异物上60 s，然后回撤探针带出异物。

- 注意组织胶可能对组织有刺激。

• 充气球囊导管：

- 试用于常用方法失败后。

- 5F或6F Foley或Fogarty球囊导管，表面涂布2%利多卡因凝胶。

- 导管头端插到异物后方。

- 向球囊充气2～3 ml，轻轻回撤导管，带出异物。

• 用磁铁吸引取出了解清楚的金属异物，但仅限于有经验的医师。

• 套取术：

- 用血管钳将24G金属丝扭成一个环。

- 事先了解异物的大小更好。

- 将金属细丝滑过肿胀的组织直至异物后方，套住异物拉出。

■ 药物治疗

• 可卡因：4%溶液，2滴，患侧鼻孔。

• 利多卡因：4%溶液，2滴，患侧鼻孔。

• 羟甲唑林：0.05%溶液，2～3滴/喷，患侧鼻孔。

• 苯肾上腺素：0.125%～0.5%，2～3喷，患侧鼻孔。

• 必要时可予以镇静。

- 由于异物有可能后移和误吸，需要保持气道通畅。

随访

■ 进一步处理

入院指征

转诊到外科手术取异物：

• 急诊室内取异物失败或后移。

• 需要全身麻醉下进行。

出院指征

• 确认没有气道受压。

• 如有出血、感染(鼻腔流分泌物)需复诊。

• 如果为钮扣电池，取出后仍需门诊随访：

- 黏膜缺血。

- 鼻甲或鼻中隔损伤。

- 鞍鼻畸形。

转诊问题

• 有下列情形时请耳鼻喉专科会诊：

- 急诊室内取异物失败。

- 异物是纽扣电池或磁铁，考虑鼻黏膜损伤。

■ 随访建议

• 如果出现以下情况，立即回急诊科复诊：

- 咳嗽、头晕、耳鸣或呼吸困难。

- 恶心、憋气、窒息感、流涎、颈部或喉部疼痛、吞咽困难。

• 父母应密切观察患儿，一旦有以下情况立即送医院：

- 发热。

- 头痛或面颊痛。

- 持续鼻出血。

- 持续鼻腔流液。

要点和误区

• 对 2～6 岁儿童出现鼻窦炎表现时应想到鼻腔异物可能。

• 父母最适合对患儿采取正压法取异物，可避免其受到惊吓：

- 常能在不用或少用镇静的条件下获得成功。
- 即便失败，仍可以用其他方法获得成功。

• 40%～70%的开放性骨折患者合并其他创伤性损害。

• 4%利多卡因和羟甲唑林等量混合滴鼻。

闭经 Amenorrhea

Andrew J. French · Jamal J. Taha　马林浩　林兆奋 译

基础知识

描述

• 没有月经。

• 原发性闭经：

- 在乳房发育后 5 年或 16 年以内的自发性子宫出血，应在 13 岁时发生。

• 继发性闭经：

- 先前月经正常的女性出现 3 个月的子宫出血，或者对于先前有月经过少的女性出现 9 个月的出血。
- 比原发性闭经更常见。
- 妊娠是最常见的原因。

病因

• 原发性：

- 性腺功能衰竭。
- 下丘脑-垂体疾病。
- 染色体异常。
- 无孔的处女膜。
- 性腺发育不全如特纳综合征。

• 继发性：

- 妊娠、哺乳或产后。
- Asherman 综合征(宫腔粘连)。
- 下丘脑-垂体-卵巢轴的功能障碍。
- 多囊卵巢综合征(PCOS)。
- 内分泌疾病。
- 肥胖、饥饿、神经性厌食症或剧烈运动。
- 药物：
  ◦ 口服避孕药。
  ◦ 抗精神病药。
  ◦ 抗抑郁药。
  ◦ 钙通道阻滞剂。
  ◦ 化疗药物。
  ◦ 洋地黄。
  ◦ 大麻。
- 自身免疫性疾病。
- 卵巢衰竭。
- 绝经。

诊断

症状和体征

病史

• 月经和月经史。

• 性活动。

• 运动，减肥。

• 久病。

• 药物。

• 以前的中枢神经系统放疗或化疗。

• 家族史。

• 不孕不育。

• 避孕用药。

• 溢乳：

- 垂体瘤。

• 多毛症和痤疮：

- PCOS。
- 库欣综合征。
- 高雄激素血症。

• 非法使用毒品：

- 对催乳素的影响。

• 头痛或视力改变：

- 中枢神经系统肿瘤。

• 温度不耐受、心悸、皮肤变化、腹泻、震颤。

- 甲状腺功能。

体格检查

• 低雌激素：

- 萎缩性阴道黏膜。
- 情绪波动，烦躁。

• 高雄激素：

- 向心性肥胖。
- 多毛症。
- 粉刺。
- 男性型秃发。

• 甲状腺检查。

• 骨盆/生殖器检查。

• Tanner 分期。

基本检查

妊娠测试。

诊断检查与说明

实验室检查

• 如果妊娠测试结果为阴性，则不需要进一步的测试。

• 可送促甲状腺激素(TSH)、催乳素(PRL)、黄体生成素(LH)、卵泡刺激素(FSH)用于妇科或初级保健医师的随访。

影像学检查

除非关注异位妊娠或患者介绍的其他紧急情况，否则不需要紧急检查。

诊断步骤/外科

不需紧急进行。

鉴别诊断

• 妊娠。

• 苗勒管发育不全：

- 先天性生殖道畸形。
- 正常乳房发育，无初潮。
- 有关联的：
  ◦ 融合椎骨。
  ◦ 泌尿道缺陷。

• 阴道横隔。

• 处女膜穿孔。

• 完全性雄激素不敏感综合征。

• 阿什曼综合征(子宫腔粘连综合征)：

- 宫腔粘连。
- 妇科检查所致。

• 原发性卵巢功能不全。

• 下丘脑-垂体疾病。

• 先前的中枢神经系统感染、创伤或垂体自身免疫破坏。

• PCOS。

• 避孕药的使用。

• 甲状腺疾病：

- 甲状腺功能亢进症多于甲状腺功能减退症。

B

• 肾上腺疾病。

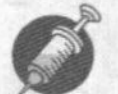

治疗

院前

如果因妊娠导致闭经，请根据妊娠情况稳定患者。

急诊治疗/程序

确保安全并转诊。

药物治疗

推迟至妇产科评估结束。

随访

进一步处理

入院指征

除非担心异位妊娠，否则无需入院。

出院指征

会诊后无异常可出院。

转诊问题

转诊到妇科。

随访建议

建议进行妇科随访。

要点和误区

• 妊娠是急诊科最常见的闭经病因。

- 尿妊娠试验（UPT）可能会出现尿液比重低的假阴性。

- UPT 对 β-HCG 水平的灵敏度可能因型号、制造商而异。由于妊娠引起的闭经应高度关注，特别是异位妊娠，可能需要进行定性血清妊娠试验。

• 神经性厌食症是闭经患者的一个重要考虑因素，特别是在青少年中。

• 使用抗精神病药引起的高泌乳素血症是精神病患者闭经的常见病因。

扁桃体周脓肿 Peritonsillar Abscess

Alexa Camarena-Michel · Maria E. Moreira　马林浩 译

基础知识

描述

• 扁桃体周脓肿（PTA）是化脓性扁桃体炎的并发症，感染由腭扁桃体与咽肌间的扁桃体囊向外扩散。

• 最常见的头颈部深度感染（每年发生率为 30/10 万）。

• 美国每年有 45 000 个新增病例。

• 发生在所有年龄段，在青年人群中更为常见（平均年龄为 20～40 岁）。

• 最常见的发病时节是 11—12 月和 4—5 月（与链球菌性咽炎在这些时节的最高发病率相符合）。

• 并发症：

- 呼吸道不畅（不常见）。
- 败血症（不常见）。
- 复发（概率在 12%～15%）。
- 症状扩展到侧颈或纵隔。
- 自发性穿孔和吸入性肺炎。
- 颈静脉血栓（Lemierre 综合征）。
- 链球菌感染后遗症（肾小球肾炎、风湿热）。
- 扩展性出血和颈动脉鞘糜烂。
- 重度脱水。
- 颅内扩散（脑膜炎、海绵窦血栓、脑脓肿）。
- 硬膜静脉窦血栓。

病因

• 有两个理论对扁桃体周脓肿的病因做出解释：

- 急性咽炎时细菌直接入侵至深层组织。
- 上扁桃体的小唾液腺（韦伯腺）发生急性梗阻和细菌感染。

• 吸烟是危险因素。

• 最常见病原体：

- A 群链球菌（化脓性链球菌）。
- 葡萄球菌，包括耐甲氧西林金黄色葡萄球菌（MRSA）。
- 厌氧菌（普氏菌、消化链球菌、梭菌）。
- 多种微生物。

诊断

症状和体征

病史

• 咽喉痛。

• 发热。

• 嗓音变化。

• 吞咽疼痛（吞咽困难）。

• 流涎。

• 头痛。

• 辐射至耳部的疼痛。

• 口服摄入量减少。

• 心神不安。

体格检查

• 发热。

• 张口困难。

• 嗓音发生变化。

• 扁桃体或软腭红肿。

• 扁桃体上极在患侧发生向下的医学性偏移。

• 小舌音偏离患侧。

• 口臭。

• 颈部淋巴腺炎。

• 同侧颈的颌角压痛。

基本检查

• 对扁桃体周脓肿之外的深度感染进行评估，辅助影像学检查或身体检查后可能需要住院或手术。

• 评估并确保呼吸道的通畅性：检查有无喘鸣、三脚架位或无力解决分泌物的问题。

• 确诊手段采用针吸或切开引流术，紧接着使用一个疗程的抗生素。

诊断检查与说明

• 通常是通过对口咽部视觉性的检查做出临床诊断。

• 患者严重的张口困难可能不便于检测。

实验室检查

• 咽培养和单滴试验（患有扁桃体周脓肿者发生单核细胞增多症的概率为 20%）。

• 某些情况下，血常规和脓肿细菌培养可能会用到。

• 对于出现进食减退和有临床脱水体征者，基础代谢功能检查试验可能会有用。

影像学检查

• 侧向口内超声检查：

- 使用带有协助识别和定位脓肿的润滑乳

胶盖的高频腔内超声仪。
- 如患者配合，可将超声仪放在最大压痛点的位置。
• 如果患者张口非常困难，选择经皮颈部超声的方法，使用腔内探头。
• 颈侧部软组织透射：
- 怀疑有会厌炎或者咽后脓肿时使用。
• 胸部 X 线检查：
- 有严重的呼吸困难症状或流脓时使用。
• 颈部 CT：
- 怀疑颈部存在其他深度感染时，可能要做 CT。
- 如果患者由于张口困难导致无法得到好的检查，推荐做 CT。
- 在针吸失败后，CT 可用来定位脓肿袋。
• MRI 可能对评估深度感染并发症有用（内颈静脉血栓或颈动脉鞘糜烂）。

诊断步骤/外科

• 针吸术是诊断性的且通常颇有疗效。
• 侧向切开引流术。

鉴别诊断

• 扁桃体周围蜂窝织炎。
• 会厌炎。
• 咽后脓肿。
• 咽周脓肿。
• 气管炎。
• 脑膜炎。
• 咽后出血。
• 颈骨髓炎。
• 颈淋巴结炎。
• 硬脑膜外脓肿。
• 传染性单核细胞增多症。
• 颈内动脉瘤。
• 淋巴瘤。
• 颈部异物。
• 颈部的其他深度感染。

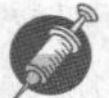

治疗

院前

很少与呼吸道紧急状况有关，但是病情诊断很可能会因为运输因素变得不确定，所以应在旁边备好抽吸和插管器材以防万一：
• 血氧饱和仪、辅助供氧设备。
• 心电监测。
• 快速静脉通路。

儿科注意事项

• 在已有扁桃体周脓肿病例中（每 10 万人中有 14 人发病），发于儿童（<18 岁）的占 25%～30%。
• 如果打算对脓肿实施切开引流术或针吸操作，年轻儿童可能需要镇静或全身麻醉。
• 对于有上呼吸道梗阻症状的年轻儿童，需要在口部检查前获取其颈侧软组织透射影像。

初步稳定/治疗

• 同院前注意事项。
• 呼吸道管理可能是必要的。
• 插管和环甲膜切开术器材应该可用。

急诊治疗/程序

• 合理使用抗生素。
• 对于脱水患者应该给予静脉输液。
• 控制疼痛很重要。
• 单次量的类固醇药物可能有利于改善症状。
• 在针吸或切开引流操作之前使用适当的麻醉比较重要：
- 苯唑卡因喷雾。
- 利多卡因，1% 的剂量与 1∶100 000 的肾上腺素一同使用。
• 没有一种排液技术明显优于另一种排液技术：
- 针式排液：
  ◦ 成功率为 87%～94%。
  ◦ 应该由有排液操作经验或熟练掌握高级呼吸道技术的人来执行。
  ◦ 疼痛越小，侵入性比切开引流术就要越小。
  ◦ 颈内动脉位于扁桃体后外侧～2.5 cm 处；谨慎包覆活检针，要防止针的介入小于 0.5 cm。
  ◦ 扁桃体上极是波动最大的最常见区域（其次是中极和下极）。
  ◦ 有 10% 的情况下需要进行重复的针吸排液。
- 切开引流术：
  ◦ 成功率为 90%～92%。
  ◦ 使用 11 或 15 号手术刀片的手术刀刺切扁桃体的波动性区域。
  ◦ 使用切边塑料鞘保护手术刀，留 1 cm 刀片外露。
  ◦ 切开深度避免超过 0.5 cm。
  ◦ 内侧和上极切口更能避免伤及颈动脉。
  ◦ 典型切口应高于软腭区域的扁桃体。如切到扁桃体会造成过度流血且可能漏掉位于软腭的扁桃体周软组织中的脓肿。
  ◦ 应该准备抽吸清除化脓的血水。
  ◦ 不得使用压紧操作。
- 扁桃体切除术（多适用于儿童）：
  ◦ 上呼吸道阻塞。
  ◦ 早前有严重复发性的咽炎或扁桃体周脓肿发作的病史。
  ◦ 使用其他排液技术处理脓肿失败。
  ◦ 能快速执行，或者在解决完急性感染之后。

药物治疗

• 抗生素治疗时间应该为 14 日（<10 日的疗程可能用来治疗病情复发）。
• 使用类固醇药物辅助治疗会改善症状。

静脉注射抗生素

• 氨苄西林-舒巴坦（优立新），每次用量 3 mg，q6 h。
• 青霉素，每次用量 1 000 万 U，q6 h。
• 如果病患对青霉素过敏，使用克林霉素，每次用量 900 mg，q8 h。

口服抗生素

• 阿莫西林-克拉维酸（沃格孟汀），每次服用量 875 mg，每日 2 次。
• 青霉素 V 钾与灭滴灵（甲硝唑）一起服用，两者服用量都是每次 500 mg，q6 h。
• 克林霉素，每次服用量 600 mg，每日 2 次；或者每次服用量 300 mg，q6 h。

类固醇药物

• 地塞米松，每次用量 10 mg，静脉注射、肌内注射或口服，每日单次用量。
- 儿童：按体重用量 0.6 mg/kg，总用量不得超过 10 mg。
• 甲泼尼龙，按体重用量 2 mg/kg，总用量不得超过 250 mg。

随访

进一步处理

入院指征

• 呼吸道不畅。
• 败血症。
• 精神状态改变。
• 脱水及口服摄入不当。
• 感染扩展至超过扁桃体周脓肿（如深度颈部感染）。

出院指征

• 大多数扁桃体周脓肿病患者在排掉脓肿液后都可以出院回家，口服抗生素。
• 必须能忍受充分的口服药物及抗生素摄入。

转诊问题

• 转诊到耳鼻喉科专家或外科医师处。

• 出现转诊，建议在脓肿治疗 6～8 周后进行扁桃体切除术。

随访建议

建议在 24～48 h 安排严密的随访：

• 治疗失败和复发相对常见。

要点和误区

• 在重度感染中，未能提前做好呼吸道保护。

• 未能识别较高级的深度颈部感染。

• 在执行针吸或侧向切开引流术前必须熟知相关解剖学。

• 在区分和识别扁桃体周脓肿和扁桃体周围蜂窝织炎的过程中，侧向超声是有用的辅助手段。

B

便秘 Constipation

Julia H. Sone 陈奇通 译

基础知识

描述

便秘诊断的罗马标准需要以下 2 个或以上症状，且持续至少 3 个月：

• 排便用力>25%的病程。

• 大便发硬>25%的病程。

• 排便不完全>25%的病程。

• 每周 2 次或更少的肠道活动。

儿科注意事项

• 3%的儿科门诊是因为排便异常。

• 脑瘫儿童常出现功能性便秘。

• 可被划分至亚组：

- 解剖性便秘(肛门狭窄、移位肛门、肛门闭塞、骶尾畸胎瘤)。
- 结肠神经肌肉疾病(Hirschsprung 病)。
- 排便异常(功能性便秘和非潴留性遗粪)。
- 功能性粪便潴留。

• 最常见的粪便潴留和遗粪的病因是功能性粪便潴留：

- 因排便异常相关的恐惧引起。
- 与易激惹性、腹部绞痛、食欲降低和早饱有关。

病因

• 代谢性和内分泌性：

- 糖尿病。
- 尿毒症。
- 卟啉症。
- 甲状腺功能减退症。
- 低钾血症(严重)。
- 低镁血症(严重)。
- 高钙血症。
- 嗜铬细胞瘤。
- 全垂体功能减退症。
- 妊娠。

• 功能性和特发性：

- 结肠型肠易激综合征。
- 憩室病。
- 结肠迟钝。
- 巨结肠。
- 骨盆肠套叠。
- 耻骨直肠肌失迟缓。
- 脱肛、乙状结肠下垂。
- 子宫切除后综合征。
- 会阴下垂。

• 药物性：

- 止痛药。
- 麻醉药。
- 抗酸药。
- 抗胆碱能药。
- 抗惊厥药。
- 抗抑郁药。
- 止吐药(昂丹司琼)。
- 抗组胺药。
- 抗高血压药。
- 钙通道阻滞剂。
- 利尿剂。
- 含铁药物。
- 通便药物滥用。
- MAOIs。
- 肌松药。
- 副交感神经阻滞剂。
- 硫代二苯胺。
- 治疗精神病药物。

• 精神性：

- 中枢性帕金森病。
- 多发性硬化。
- 脑血管意外。
- 脊髓病灶、损伤。
- 外周希尔施普龙病(Hirschsprung 病)。
- 美洲锥虫病(Chagas 病)。
- 多发性神经纤维瘤。
- 自主神经病变。

• 机械性梗阻：

- 新生物。
- 结肠、直肠或肛门的狭窄。
- 疝。
- 肠扭转。
- 肠假性梗阻。

诊断

症状和体征

• 便秘是症状而非疾病。

• 排出硬的粪便。

• 排便用力、困难。

• 肠道活动不频繁。

• 腹部扩张、膨胀。

• 肛门指检可及牢固的、硬的大便：

- 可能出现直肠内空虚。
- 腹泻(液体粪便从牢固粪便旁通过)。

病史

• 症状开始的年龄。

• 饮食和运动规律。

• 粪便大小、直径、连续性、频率和排便缓解情况。

• 医疗和手术病史：

- 药物能够减慢结肠内运送，比如 β 受体阻滞剂、高剂量钙通道阻滞剂和麻醉药物。

• 灌肠、泻药和手指处理以方便排便的使用史。

• 相关的骨盆平面的功能异常：

- 排尿症状。
- 脱肛。

体格检查

• 腹部检查可能发现粪便导致的包块。

- 直肠检查以评估排出道梗阻：
- 收缩和舒张括约肌的能力。
- 是否有脱肛或膀胱脱垂。
- 评估粪便的牢固性。

■ 基本检查

完整的病史和体格检查：

- 医疗、手术、精神性检查和起始时期。
- 注意腹部扩张、疝、压痛或包块。
- 完成肛门直肠检查，以寻找肛门狭窄、裂缝、新生物、括约肌张力、会阴下降、压痛和痉挛。

■ 诊断检查与说明

实验室检查

- 仅在考虑代谢性、内分泌性异常时是必要的。
- 如果是炎症或新生物来源则行全血计数。
- 有以下风险时，测电解质和钙：
- 低钾血症。
- 低钙血症。
- 患者有甲减表现时性甲状腺功能检查。

影像学检查

- 除非怀疑有潜在病因时使用，一般很少需要。
- 腹部摄片：
- 结肠内大量粪便。
- 扩张的结肠，需要减压。
- 腹痛、发热的老年便秘患者行腹部或骨盆CT检查以确诊/排除穿孔。
- 钡餐、泛影葡胺灌肠研究：
- 憩室病。
- 巨直肠。
- 巨结肠。
- 先天性巨结肠。
- 炎症或肿瘤引起的狭窄。

■ 鉴别诊断

- 见病因。
- 肠梗阻。

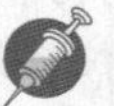

治疗

■ 院前

明显腹痛的患者需建立静脉通路。

■ 初步稳定/治疗

脱水/低血压患者给予静脉液体。

■ 急诊治疗/程序

- 清理结肠：
- 灌肠、塞剂。
- 硬的粪便则手工解除梗阻。
- 泻药。
- 维持肠道规律：
- 增加非咖啡因液体(每日8～10杯)。
- 增加饮食纤维摄入(20g/d)。
- 粪便软化剂。
- 锻炼。
- 更改导致便秘的药物。

■ 药物治疗

- 灌肠：
- 快速：120 ml(儿童：5～11岁：60～120 ml)，灌肠。
- 矿物油：60～150 ml(儿童：5～11岁，30～60 ml；大于12岁，60～150 ml)，灌肠每日。
- 自来水：100～500 ml，灌肠。
- 纤维素补充：
- 甲基纤维素：每日最多6 g，分剂量为0.45～3 g。
- 洋车前子：每日最多30 g，每次2.5～7.5 g剂量(儿童：6～11岁，每日最多15 g，每次2.5～3.75 g剂量)。
- 聚卡波非钙：每日1 250 mg 1～4次(儿童：6～12岁，625 mg每日1～4次；超过12岁，1 250 mg每日1～4次)。
- 小麦糊精：4 g混合于1杯水中(儿童：6～12岁，2 g混合于1杯水中；12岁以上：4 g混合于1杯水中)。
- 泻药(渗透性)：
- 乳果糖：15～30 ml(儿童：1 ml/kg)，口服，每日1～2次。
- 聚乙烯二醇：17 g[儿童：0.8 g/(kg·d)溶解到4～8盎司液体内]，溶解至液体，口服，每日1次。
- 镁奶：2 400～4 800 mg氢氧化镁口服(儿童6个月至1岁：40 mg/kg氢氧化镁；2～5岁：400～1 200 mg氢氧化镁；6～11岁：1 200～2 400 mg氢氧化镁；大于12岁：2 400～4 800 mg氢氧化镁)每日1次或必要时。
- 泻药(刺激性)：
- 比沙可啶：10～15 mg，口服，每日(儿童：小于3岁，5 mg，灌肠，每日1次；3～12岁，5～10 mg，口服/灌肠，每日1次；大于12岁，5～15 mg，口服，每日10 mg，或灌肠每日1次)。
- 番泻叶：每日0.5～2 g(儿童：2～6岁，每日0.15～0.6 g；6～12岁，每日0.25～1 g)。
- 粪便软化剂：
- 多库酯钠：100 mg[儿童：3～5 mg/(kg·d)，分次使用]，口服，每日1～2次。
- 矿物质油：15～45 ml(儿童：5～15 ml)，口服，每日1次。
- 栓剂：
- 甘油：2～3 g(儿童：2～6岁，1～1.2 g；>6岁，2 g)。

随访

■ 进一步处理

入院指征

- 有严重腹痛、恶心和呕吐的患者。
- 无法在急诊或家中清空肠道的神经损伤、老年、合并肥胖患者。
- 肠梗阻、腹膜炎。

出院指征

- 无需要住院的合并症。
- 无疼痛。
- 充分清空。

转诊问题

消化科医师随访以进一步评估和治疗。

■ 随访建议

负责医师或消化科医师随访持续便秘的患者。

要点和误区

- 建议患者进行合理饮食和生活方式改善以降低便秘发生。
- 进行全面的病史采集和体格检查以排除明显医疗或手术病因引起的便秘。

髌骨损伤 Patellar Injuries

Stacy M. Gomez · Stephen R. Hayden 王虑 译

基础知识

描述

脱臼

• 由于膝关节突然弯曲或过度旋转，同时股四头肌收缩造成。

• 由髌骨直接损伤造成的比较少见。

• 髌骨侧脱位最为常见，髌骨侧移位到股骨髁的位置。

• 不常见的脱位还有上脱位、中脱位和极少见的内脱位。

骨折

• 直接创伤：

- 最常见的原因。
- 直接撞击或摔倒，膝盖着地。
- 常造成粉碎性骨折、微小移位骨折或开放性骨折。

• 间接暴力：

- 突然摔倒减速造成的伸肌过大的张力引起（能造成髌骨肌腱断裂）。
- 突然收缩造成股四头肌腱撕裂伤。
- 常造成横向或移位性骨折（常两者都有）。

• 髌骨骨折的类型：

- 横断骨折：50%～80%（常见中低位）。
- 粉碎性骨折（或星形）：30%～35%。
- 纵向骨折：25%。
- 骨软骨骨折。

髌骨韧带断裂

• 常是膝关节在屈曲状态下遭外力作用股四头肌反常收缩所致（如跳起落地和举重）。

• 常发生在老运动员。

- 重复动作造成微小创伤。

髌骨腱炎

反复加速和减速所致过度使用综合征（跳起、落地）。

病因

脱位

• 髌骨脱位的危险因素：

- 膝外翻。
- 膝外屈。
- 浅股骨外侧髁。
- 股内侧肌缺失。
- 髌腱外侧嵌入术。
- 浅髌骨沟。
- 高位髌骨。
- 髌骨畸形。
- 扁平足。

• 运动员尤其是女运动员常见。

• 发生髌骨脱位年龄越轻，复发的风险越大。

骨折

• 男性和女性的比例为 2∶1。

• 最高发的年龄段在 20～50 岁。

髌骨韧带断裂

• 30～40 岁为最常见人群：

- 常见于运动员。

• 风险因素：

- 髌骨腱炎病史。
- 糖尿病史、糖皮质激素注射史、风湿性关节炎病史、痛风、系统性红斑狼疮。
- 曾行过膝关节手术。

髌骨腱炎

• 过度使用致韧带的微小撕裂。

• 最常见于跳高运动员、排球和篮球运动员、田径运动员。

诊断

症状和体征

脱臼

• 感觉膝盖"脱出"，有爆开、撕裂的感觉。

• 疼痛。

• 不能负重。

• 明显的髌骨侧位畸形。

• 轻中度肿胀。

• 常在到急诊室之前程度减轻。

• 髌骨触痛。

• 恐惧试验或费尔班克斯征：

- 尝试从侧面推髌骨引发患者恐惧。
- 尝试从中间推髌骨。

骨折

• 整个膝盖疼痛。

• 行走困难。

• 移动髌骨疼痛增加。

• 髌骨触痛肿胀。

• 困难或无法伸膝。

• 明显感觉膝关节处缺陷感、捻发音、关节腔红肿积液。

髌骨韧带断裂

• 突然出现的剧烈的疼痛。

• 负重力下降。

• 有时有关节积血。

• 最近的髌骨移位。

• 不完全伸肌功能障碍。

• 不能对抗外力伸膝。

髌骨腱炎

• 髌骨腱区域疼痛。

• 当从坐立站起时或上楼梯时疼痛加重。

• 髌骨远端或近端髌骨腱触痛。

基本检查

必需行 X 线摄片。

诊断检查与说明

影像学检查

• 膝关节前后位、侧位和应力位及复位前和复位后都需拍摄。

• 复位后摄片可以排除软骨骨折（髌骨脱臼病例）。

• 双侧髌骨（髌骨附件通过软骨连接为一整体）会被误诊为骨折：

- 不同角度摄片对比能帮助鉴别。

• 对怀疑髌骨韧带断裂患者摄片，可见高位髌骨（髌骨处于高于髁间凹陷的位置）。

• 对于髌骨腱炎，症状出现时间少于 6 个月的摄片无明显异常。

鉴别诊断

• 髌骨半脱位。

• 股骨和胫骨骨折。

• 创伤性黏液囊炎。

• 股四头肌腱断裂。

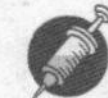

治疗

院前

需将患者置于仰卧位，膝关节放松伸直固定。

初步稳定/治疗

收集病史和体格检查以鉴别相关的伤情（如股骨骨折、髋骨骨折、髋关节后脱位）并评估伸肌的机制。

急诊治疗/程序

脱臼

• 对于简单的髌骨侧脱位，可通过将膝关节轻轻伸展到 180°复位：

- 压力同时从中间作用于髌骨的侧面。

• 其他类型的髌骨脱位（上脱位、内脱位、关节内脱位)不要尝试复位,请骨科医师会诊。

• 关节内出血情况复位困难时应该注意无菌技术。

• 如果有软骨骨折(28%～50%病例),参考骨科医师建议。

• 尽管复位比较容易成功,但程序化的镇静和注射止痛剂是必要的。

• 尽管非手术复位的患者有60%复发概率,但没有证据表明手术治疗适合所有脱位患者。

骨折

• 出现骨折后需参考骨科医师意见。

• 没有移位的骨折且伸展功能正常的应尝试非手术治疗。

• 最初的治疗包括长腿夹板固定和后期的手术治疗。

髌骨韧带断裂

骨科医师建议在2～6周行手术治疗。

髌骨腱炎

休息,避免剧烈运动,热敷和非甾体抗炎药。

■ **药物治疗**

• 枸橼酸芬太尼:0.5～1.5 μg/kg(儿童:0.5～1.0 μg/kg),静脉注射。

• 咪达唑仑:1～2.5 mg(儿童:0.05～0.1 mg/kg,最大剂量6 mg),静脉注射。

• 硫酸吗啡:2～5 mg/次(儿童:0.1～0.2 mg/kg),静脉注射。

• 哌替啶:50～150 mg(儿童:1.1～1.8 mg/kg),肌内注射,必要时每3～4 h一次。

• 酮洛酸:60 mg,肌内注射;30 mg,静脉注射(儿童:0.5～1 mg/kg,如果体重<50 kg最大剂量15 mg;如果体重>50 kg最大剂量30 mg,静脉注射)。

• 美索比妥:1～1.5 mg/kg(1 ml/5 s)(儿童:0.5～1 mg),静脉注射。

• 丙泊酚(异丙酚):1～2 mg/kg,静脉注射(20 mg,45 s内快速注射)推注要慢,避免血压下降(儿童:1 mg/kg,不超过40 mg)。

随访

■ **进一步处理**

入院指征

• 患有髌骨上脱位、内脱位、关节内脱位的患者和侧脱位不能复位的,需在急诊由骨科医师会诊,条件允许时入院治疗。

• 髌骨脱位合并骨折的(骨软骨或股骨外侧髁)需骨科医师会诊。

• 需要手术干预的:

- 骨折碎片移位>4 mm。
- 大腿无法伸起离开床。
- 关节下降>3 mm。

• 所有的开放性骨折需清创冲洗的患者需收入院。

• 髌骨韧带断裂的患者需骨科医师会诊。

出院指征

• 脱臼:髌骨侧脱位得到成功复位并且摄片示正常的患者,可以在膝关节制动拐协助及骨科医师随访的情况下出院。

• 骨折:移位<3 mm且关节伸展活动完全:

- 膝关节制动,或长腿夹板固定,膝关节能在拐杖辅助下完全或部分负重,骨科医师随访一段时间。

要点和误区

• 髌骨侧移位常能在患者到医院急诊前自行复位,但不能忽略患者的髌骨脱位病史。

• 对于髌骨韧带断裂的患者,韧带断裂常不被发现,但一段时间过后会出现关节的肿胀。

病态窦房结综合征

Nathaniel Mann 周健 潘曙明 译

基础知识

■ **描述**

• 描述窦房结自动性和冲动功能障碍的统称。

• 机制:

- 由窦房结(SA)固有功能的逐步退化引起。
- 以无法解释的窦房结功能障碍为特征,导致心律失常,通常没有适当的心房或交界性节律。

• 病态窦房结综合征(SSS)包括:

- 慢性SA淋巴结功能障碍。
- 经常失去起搏功能。
- 节内传导障碍。
- 直流电复律后SA活动缓慢。

• 适用于所有年龄段(平均年龄>65岁)。

• 男女比例为1∶1。

■ **病因**

• 内在原因:

- 最常见的原因:窦房结特发性变性纤维化。
- 冠状动脉或SA结动脉疾病。
- 心肌病。
- 离子通道突变/家族性SSS。
- 白血病和转移性疾病。
- 浸润性心脏或胶原血管疾病,包括淀粉样变性。
- 手术创伤。

• 炎性疾病:

- 类风湿性心脏病。
- 美洲锥虫病。
- 心包炎和心肌炎。

• 外部原因(不是真正的SSS,而是类似的表现):

- 药品:
  - β受体阻滞剂、钙通道阻滞剂、可乐定。
  - 地高辛、胺碘酮。
  - 锂、苯妥英。
- 自主介导综合征(胆碱酯酶缺乏症)。
- 高钾血症和低钾血症。
- 甲状腺功能减退症。
- 低体温。
- 低血糖。
- 败血症和感染。

儿科注意事项

与先天性异常和随后的手术修复及先天性SA结动脉缺乏症相关。

诊断

■ **症状和体征**

症状表现为心律不齐或传统的心血管表

B

现导致中枢神经系统灌注不足。

病史

• 无症状。
• 心悸、疲劳。
• 晕厥、晕厥前兆、头晕。
• 等效心绞痛(胸痛、稳定型心绞痛)。
• 活动无耐力。
• 猝死。

体格检查

• 心动过缓。
• 交替性心动过缓和房性心动过速。
• 精神状态改变。
• 紫癜。
• 短暂性脑缺血发作/脑卒中。

基本检查

• 确定病因。
• 12 导联心电图。
• 胸部 X 线检查。

诊断检查和说明

实验室检查

• 血清电解质(包括镁和钙)。
• 心脏标志物。
• 地高辛水平(如适用)。
• 甲状腺功能检查。

影像学检查

心电图:

• 最常见的发现:慢性不稳定的窦性心动过缓。
• SA 停搏或 SA 阻滞。
• 心房纤颤伴缓慢的心室反应。
• 心脏复律或颈动脉按摩后长时间停顿。
• 缓慢性心律失常可能伴有室上性心律失常。
• 心动过速综合征:阵发性心动过速与心动过缓。

诊断程序/外科

由于敏感性和特异性差,不再推荐大多数电生理研究。

鉴别诊断

• 其他心律失常。
• 其他快速性心律失常:尤其要小心,将 SSS 与心房颤动区别开来,因为如果 SA 节点功能异常并存,则直流电复律或在心房颤动中使用控制心率药物可能有害。
• 电解质紊乱。
• 药物毒性:β 受体阻滞剂、钙通道阻滞剂、可乐定、地高辛。
• 迷走神经紧张。

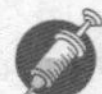

治疗

院前

• 生命体征稳定。
• 吸氧。
• 心电监护。
• 给予阿托品,如果心动过缓和血流动力学不稳定。
• 不稳定患者的经皮起搏。

初始稳定/治疗

• 给予阿托品,如果心律失常引起不稳定的体征/症状:心绞痛、精神错乱或低血压。
• 如果阿托品应用无效,则经皮起搏。
• 如果失败,紧急静脉起搏。

急诊治疗/程序

室上性心律失常伴心动过缓:

• 不稳定的患者:
- 心脏转复。
- 预期随后的严重心动过缓。
• 稳定的患者:
- 心电监测。
• 地高辛、地尔硫䓬、维拉帕米或镁剂可用于心律失常。
• 任何药物都可能导致严重的心动过缓。
• 心动过缓:
- 中止改变窦房结功能的药物。
- SA 可逆的条件:氧气,温度升高,葡萄糖。

> **注意**
> • 慢缓型心律失常患者应采用以温热为主的治疗。阿托品可引起这些患者心肌不稳定。
> • 抗凝治疗心房颤动和慢快综合征。

药物治疗

• 阿托品:0.5～1 mg,静脉或经气管给药:
- 根据需要重复 q5 min,最大剂量 0.04 mg/kg(儿童:0.02 mg/kg)。
• 地尔硫䓬:0.25 mg/kg 静脉输注 2 min。15 min 后以 0.35 mg/kg 静脉注射超过 2 min。
• 维拉帕米:超过 2 min 2.5～5 mg 静脉推注:
- 可重复 5～10 mg,最多 15～30 min。最大剂量 20 mg。
- 儿童<1 岁:2 min 内 0.1～0.2 mg/kg;重复 q30 min。1～15 岁:0.1～0.3 mg/kg,超过 2 min,最大值剂量 5 mg,可以重复一次。
• 地高辛:最初 0.5 mg 静脉注射,然后每 4 h 0.25 mg 静脉注射,直至达到预期效果(最大剂量 1 mg,静脉注射)。
• 异丙肾上腺素:2～3 μg/min 静脉滴定至目标心率/血压,最大 10 μg/min[儿童:0.1 μg/(kg·min)]。
- 不与肾上腺素合用,仅用于不稳定的患者。
• 肾上腺素:1 mg,静脉注射(儿童:0.01 mg/kg 静脉注射),用于心搏骤停。
• 胰高血糖素:0.05～0.15 mg/kg,静脉注射(儿童:0.05～0.10 mg/kg)。
• 肝素:负载 80 U/kg,静脉注射,以 18 U/(kg·h)输注。
• 镁:1～2 g,静脉注射。

一线用药

一线首选治疗是永久性起搏器,可为心律失常提供"基础":

• 患有快速性心律失常的患者将需要额外的控制心率药物。

二线用药

没有明确的证据区分一线和二线治疗。

随访

进一步处理

入院指征

• 新发。
• 症状:CHE 晕厥、胸痛、头晕。
• 持续性心律失常或心律失常。
• 高龄,>60 岁。
• 患者应接受心脏病学咨询后进入遥测层。
• 大多数人将需要永久起搏。

出院指征

• 无症状,否则健康的患者可以被评估为门诊患者。
• 动态心电图监测。

转诊问题

• 需要正式的心脏电生理评估。
• 需要永久性放置起搏器。

随访建议

老年人注意事项

• 患有基础疾病的病窦综合征患者中 CAD 的发生率很高,因此需要完整的心血管危险因素评估和预防。
• 心房颤动并有慢快综合征的患者需要长期抗凝治疗。
• 所有患者都需要心脏病学专家或电生理

学专家对永久性起搏器进行评估。

要点和误区

• 急诊无症状的患者可能具有正常的心电图。如果临床高度怀疑，可以考虑购买心律检查仪或动态心电图监护仪。

• 在 SSS 相关性心律失常患者中使用任何控制心率药物（如 β 受体阻滞剂、钙通道阻滞剂或地高辛）都可能导致 SA 阻滞或 SA 停搏，只有在准备经皮起搏时才应使用。

玻璃体出血 Vitreous Hemorrhage

Robyn R. Essendrop · Carl G. Skinner 吴昊 李文放 译

基础知识

描述

玻璃体出血是次要诊断，确定一个具体原因对于成功治疗是必要的：

• 玻璃体分离引起视网膜血管撕裂。
• 由于创伤导致血管突然撕裂。
• 新生血管性形成（如糖尿病）引起的自发性出血。

病因

• 钝挫伤或穿透伤。
• 视网膜破裂、撕裂、脱落。
• 任何增殖性视网膜病变。
• 糖尿病。
• 镰状细胞病。
• 视网膜静脉闭塞。
• 视网膜静脉周围炎。
• 年龄相关性黄斑变性。
• 视网膜血管瘤病。
• 视网膜毛细血管扩张。
• 外周葡萄膜炎。
• 蛛网膜下腔或硬膜下出血：
- 玻璃体积血综合征。
• 眼内肿瘤。

儿科注意事项

• 早产儿视网膜病变
• 先天性视网膜劈裂。
• 睫状体平坦部炎。
• 虐待儿童：
- 摇晃婴儿综合征。

诊断

症状和体征

• 突发的无痛的单侧丧失者视力下降。
• 视网膜上的黑斑（飞蚊症）、蜘蛛网或雾霾样的外观：
- 以上的研究结果有时伴随着闪烁感；飞蚊症随着头部动作而移动。
• 视力模糊，视力下降。
• 红光反射消失。
• 无法可视化眼底。
• 相对性传入瞳孔障碍。

病史

• 眼或全身性疾病。
• 外伤。

体格检查

• 眼底镜检查。
• 没有红光反射。
• 没有眼底的视野。
• 急性：
- 前玻璃体积血。
• 慢性：
- 血红蛋白分解，出现黄色外观。

基本检查

• 病史：特别关注已存在的系统性疾病和创伤。
• 完整的眼科检查包括：
- 裂隙灯。
- 眼压计。
- 散瞳眼底检查。

诊断检查与说明

实验室检查

• CBC。
• PT、APTT、INR（如果有的话）。
• 电解质、BUN、肌酸酐、葡萄糖。

影像学检查

• 当没有直接视网膜视图，用 B 超可以排除视网膜脱离或眼内肿瘤。
• 后房中有回声点、线状区域或漩涡。
• 不同的回声度取决于视敏度。
• 荧光血管造影确定原因。
• CT 扫描：前后/眶内膜排除眼内异物。

诊断步骤/外科

如果不是外伤性的，巩膜凹陷用间接检眼镜检查以加强视网膜检查。

鉴别诊断

• 玻璃体炎（玻璃体中的白细胞）：
- 可能包括前部或后部葡萄膜炎。
• 视网膜脱离不出血。
• 视网膜中央静脉阻塞（CRVO）。
• 中央视网膜闭塞症（CRVA）。

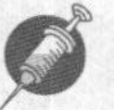

治疗

院前

保护眼睛免受创伤或压力：

• 监测血压。

初步稳定/治疗

• 卧床休息。
• 没有活动性，可用类似咽鼓管充气检查法的活动（举起、弯腰或沉重的运动）。
• 避免使用 NSAIDs 和其他抗凝剂。

急诊治疗/程序

基于出血原因需要在 24～48 h 紧急眼科咨询并治疗，并进行专科体检：

- 激光或冷冻治疗增殖性视网膜血管疾病。
- 视网膜脱离的修复。
• 手术玻璃体切除术需要：
- 时间不清的出血。
- 玻璃体出血来自视网膜脱离。
- 伴有新血管形成。
- 溶血性或幽门细胞性青光眼。

随访

进一步处理

入院指征

视网膜破裂或脱离。

出院指征

排除视网膜脱离或视网膜脱离为导致出

血的原因。

转诊建议

每日重新评估，持续 2～3 日；如果病因仍不清楚，每隔 1～3 周进行一次 B 超检查。

要点和误区

• 一定要考虑 CRVO 或 CRAO 的交替诊断。
• 排除 RD。
• 考虑视网膜脱离。
• 了解创伤史和使用血液稀释剂史。
• 即使轻微的出血也需要紧急的眼科咨询。
• 对任何疑似玻璃体出血和头部外伤，或疑似非意外外伤的儿童患者进行 CT 扫描。

B

布尔哈夫综合征 Boerhaave syndrome

Lauren M. Smith 杨伟强 译

基础知识

描述

• 也称为自发性食管破裂。
• 腹腔内压力的增加，胸腔内压力的减小，导致突发食管破裂：
- 完全性、全层的纵向食管撕裂。
• 食管无浆膜层(通常含有胶原蛋白和弹性纤维)：
- 薄弱结构容易穿孔和纵隔污染。
- 食管黏膜遭到破坏导致食管壁受损，如各种原因导致的食管炎。
• 大多数穿孔发生在食管下 1/3 段的左后外侧壁。
• 较高的治病率及死亡率(大多数消化道穿孔)：
- 撕裂伤本身造成的损伤。
- 食管内容物污染纵隔。
- 总体死亡率近 20%。
- 治疗延迟大于 24 h，导致死亡率加倍。
- 颈段食管破裂死亡率最低，其次分别为腹腔段及胸腔段食管。

> **注意**
> 谓之"自发"也许用词不当，因为它通常发生在呕吐之后。

病因

• 与以下因素相关：
- 呕吐和干呕(最常见)。
- 重体力活。
- 癫痫发作。
- 分娩。
- 钝性创伤。
- 催吐。
- 腐蚀。
- 大笑。
- Barrett 食管炎病史。
- 艾滋病病史。
- 药物性食管炎史。
- 食管癌史。
• 中老年人常见。
• 50%以上是由于医源性损伤导致的。

儿科注意事项

• 女性新生儿少见。
• 需考虑腐蚀性食管炎。

诊断

症状和体征

病史

• 症状无特异性。
• 常见的症状：
- 干呕或呕吐后出现的胸痛或食管疼痛。
• Mackler 三联征：
- 呕吐或干呕。
- 胸痛。
- 皮下气肿。
• 大多数患者出现胸骨后疼痛：
- 反复胸痛。
- 左肩反射痛。
- 吞咽困难。
• 吞咽痛。
• 食管狭窄段破裂的患者可能会出现：
- 颈部疼痛。
- 言语障碍。
- 吞咽困难。
• 吞咽可能会导致咳嗽。
• 有酗酒或大量饮酒史。

> **注意**
> 不典型的症状常导致治疗的延迟和较差的预后。

体格检查

• 呼吸困难。
• 多汗。
• 颈部及胸壁皮下气肿。
• 纵隔听诊异常爆裂音。
• 胸腔积液。
• 气促。
• 发热。
• 在严重病患中可出现休克。
• 假如治疗不及时，可出现纵隔脓肿。
• 出血不常见。

基本检查

• 最好是胸部后前位和侧位的立位 X 线片，用于评估：
- 纵隔气肿。
- 肺气肿。
- 胸腔积液。
- 气胸。
- 纵隔增宽。
- 液气胸。
- 脓胸。
- 腹腔游离气体。
- Naclerio V 征——射线通过心脏形成 V 形阴影(通气在左下纵隔)。
• 钡餐可见食管畸形：
- 用于术前评估。
- 水溶性造影剂或钡剂的使用存在争议。
- 如果水溶性造影剂发生渗漏进入纵隔，被认为具有较低毒性，吸入可导致坏死性肺炎和较高的假阴性率。
- 钡剂对诊断穿孔明显性更高，但是对纵隔更具有刺激性。
- 假如食管未受损，使用钡剂作为造影剂更加合适。

实验室检查

• 血常规。
• PT、APTT、INR。
• 血液培养。
• 乳酸。
• 胸腔积液检查：
- 淀粉酶含量。

- pH<6。
- 未经消化的食物残渣。
• 心电图。

影像学检查

• X线摄片。
• 内镜检查：
- 该项检查具有争议，有加重穿孔及纵隔气胸的风险。
• 胸部CT：
- 在证实游离气体、食管积液、纵隔增宽、胸腔积液、气胸时较为敏感。
- 显示食管。
- 评估其他胸腔结构。

■ 鉴别诊断

• 胆囊炎。
• 主动脉瘤。
• 肠梗阻。
• 肺脓肿。
• 肠系膜血管栓塞。
• 心肌梗死。
• 气胸。
• 心包炎。
• 肺炎。
• 胰腺炎。
• 肺栓塞。
• 腹腔脏器破裂。
• 自发性纵隔气肿(临床预后较好)。

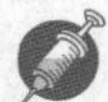

治疗

■ 院前

• 假如患者出现淡漠或潜在的气道危险，那么必须实施气道保护措施。
• 使用2个大口径的静脉导管滴注生理盐水治疗低血压。
• 阿片类药物会引起低血压等并发症，在急诊入院前避免使用。

■ 初步稳定/治疗

• ABC管理(心肺复苏)。
• 气道保护：对于淡漠或潜在气道危险的患者，给予100%纯氧吸入或气管插管。
• 建立静脉通路和治疗低血压：
- 快速静滴1 L(20 ml/kg)生理盐水或者乳酸林格液。
- 液体治疗无效时可使用多巴胺。
- 对于不稳定的患者，中心静脉导管可更加有限的实施液体治疗，并可以用于监测中心静脉压。

■ 急诊治疗/程序

• 禁食水(NPO)。
• 小心地放置鼻胃管，用于胃肠减压。
• 导尿管监测尿量。
• 早期诊断有助于减少治病率及死亡率。
• 及时外科干预。
• 相关治疗：
- 外科修复。
- 在适当的患者中实施鼻内镜检查。
- 穿孔的患者也可以选择保守治疗。
• 选择对口腔及胃肠道细菌具有针对性的广谱抗生素治疗：
- 氨苄西林-舒巴坦+庆大霉素。
- 亚胺培南-西司他丁。
- 替卡西林克拉维酸钾。
• 应用质子泵抑制剂：
- 泮托拉唑。
- 埃索美拉唑。

■ 药物治疗

• 氨苄西林-舒巴坦：3 g，静脉注射，q6 h。
• 多巴胺：2～20 μg/(kg·min)，静脉注射。
• 庆大霉素：负荷剂量2 mg/kg，然后1.7 mg/kg，静脉注射，q8 h；或者5～7 mg/kg，静脉注射，每日1次(肾功能正常的患者)。
• 亚胺培南-西司他丁：250～500 mg，静脉注射，q6 h。
• 埃索美拉唑：20 mg或40 mg，静脉注射。
• 去甲肾上腺素：0.01～0.03 μg/(kg·min)，静脉注射。
• 泮托拉唑：40 mg，静脉注射。
• 体重超过60 kg者，替卡西林-克拉维酸钾3.1 g，静脉注射，q4～6 h。

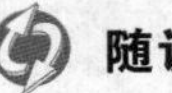

随访

■ 进一步处理

入院指征

所有布尔哈夫综合征患者必须进入外科ICU治疗。
• 颈部食管段穿孔仅需要引流治疗。
• 所有胸部及腹部食管穿孔需要外科介入治疗。

出院指征

无。

转诊问题

入院时需要胸外科或普外科医师会诊，可能需要手术干预。

■ 随访建议

参考外科医师的建议。

要点和误区

• X线片在损伤的早期可能是正常的。
• 左胸受累通常伴有远端食管穿孔。
• 右胸受累常与近端食管穿孔相关。
• 假如高度怀疑本病，但胸部X线检查阴性，可重复左侧、右侧卧位X线片检查。
• 外科治疗是本病治疗的关键。
• 诊断和治疗不及时明显增高患者死亡率。

茶碱中毒 Theophylline Poisoning

Brian R. Bush · Navneet Cheema 范浩浩 李文放 译

基础知识

描述

• 茶碱是一种甲基黄嘌呤，与咖啡碱和可可碱有关。
• 茶碱的临床应用包括：
- 治疗呼吸道疾病，包括：
◦ 支气管痉挛和哮喘。
◦ 慢性阻塞性肺疾病（COPD）。
- 新生儿呼吸暂停。
• 茶碱的作用机制：
- 刺激内源性儿茶酚胺的释放，从而刺激 β_1 和 β_2 受体。
- 腺苷受体拮抗剂。
- 磷酸二酯酶抑制剂（超治疗水平）：
◦ 增加细胞内 cAMP。
◦ cAMP 增强 β 受体激动。
• 有可速释剂和缓释剂两种剂型供选择。
• 吸收峰值时间：速释剂为 60～90 min，缓释制剂为 6～10 h。
• 半衰期是高度可变的：
- 在健康、不吸烟的成人中，半衰期通常为 4.5 h。
• 治疗血清浓度为 5～15 μg/ml。
• 急性过量：
- 之前没有使用过茶碱的患者 8 h 内间歇摄入。
• 慢性过量服药：
- 先前接受茶碱常规治疗剂量＞24 h 的患者单次过量使用。
• 慢性中毒：
- 接受常规治疗剂量＞24 h 的患者茶碱累计＞20 μg/ml，继发于：
◦ 药物与药物、药物与饮食或药物与疾病之间的相互作用。
- 连续使用过量。

病因

• 与慢性基础上的急性过量或慢性过量相比，急性中毒需要更大的浓度，以实现特定的毒性作用。
• 药物相互作用：
- 抑制茶碱代谢（同时使用时导致毒性）：
◦ H_2 受体拮抗剂。
◦ 大环内酯类抗生素。
◦ 氟喹诺酮类。
◦ 别嘌醇。
◦ 流感疫苗。
◦ 口服避孕药。
◦ 干扰素。
- 增强茶碱代谢（停用时导致的毒性）：
◦ 卡马西平。
◦ 巴比妥类。
◦ 吸烟。
◦ 利福平。
• 慢性茶碱积累：
- 不受控制的慢性心力衰竭。
- 肝脏疾病（肝硬化或重型肝炎）。
- 急性病毒感染。

诊断

症状和体征

• 心血管：
- 窦性、房性和室性心动过速：
◦ 多源性房性心动过速。
◦ 心房颤动。
◦ 室性期前收缩。
◦ 室性心动过速。
◦ 由于 β_1 受体体激动和腺苷拮抗引起。
- 低血压：
◦ 急性摄入和茶碱＞100 μg/ml 相关。
◦ 由于 β_2 受体激动诱导的血管舒张。
◦ 可能对扩容、体位和传统的血管加压药治疗反应差。
- 心肌缺血和急性心肌梗死。
• 中枢神经系统：
- 震颤。
- 心理状态改变。
- 癫痫：
◦ 14％的慢性中毒。
◦ 5％的急性中毒。
◦ 倾向于病情严重和反复发作。
◦ 通常对抗癫痫药物无效。
• 消化系统：
- 恶心和呕吐：
◦ 长期，常规剂量的止吐药可能不起作用。
◦ 75％的急性中毒。
◦ 30％的慢性中毒。
- 腹痛。
- 药物粪石：
◦ 由急性摄入大量缓释制剂的制备剂引起。
◦ 峰值浓度出现延迟。
• 代谢：
- 低钾血症：
◦ 通常会降低大约 3 mg/L。
◦ 由于 β 受体的激动。
- 高血糖症［＞11.2 mmol/L（200 mg/dl）］。
- 白细胞增多症。
- 低磷血症和低镁血症。
- 乳酸增高型的代谢性酸中毒。
- 刺激中枢神经系统的呼吸中枢，呼吸频率增加，进一步导致呼吸性碱中毒。

基本检查

• 血清茶碱浓度：
- 发现＞20 μg/ml 明确诊断。
- 当血清浓度在表现出严重症状：
◦ 90～100 μg/ml 或更高（急性中毒）。
◦ 40～60 μg/ml（慢性中毒）时。
• 心电图、肌钙蛋白和心电监测。
• 详细的病史来区分急性、慢性基础上的急性中毒和慢性中毒，关键点：
- 摄入茶碱的时间和量。
- 如果给患者开处方，注意茶碱的剂量。
- 医学并发症及状况。
- 当前用药。

诊断检查与说明

实验室检查

• 血清茶碱水平：
- 每 1～2 h 重复一次，直到下降，以确认吸收完成，峰值已经出现。
- 如果严重急性过量＞100 μg/ml，发病严重。
• 血常规。
• 血清电解质（尤其是钾）。
• 如果患者的肌肉张力增加、体温升高或全身反应，则应通过以下方法评估横纹肌溶解症：
- 血清 CK。
- 尿液分析。

鉴别诊断

• 咖啡因、β受体激动剂、支气管扩张剂过量。
• 苯丙胺。
• 拟交感神经药。
• 抗胆碱能药物。
• 戒断综合征。
• 嗜铬细胞瘤。
• 甲状腺功能亢进。

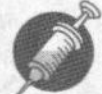

治疗

院前

怀疑药物过量时检查服用药物的药瓶和药丸样品。

初步稳定/治疗

- 检查气道、呼吸、循环：
- 心电监测。
- 低血压需等渗晶体复苏。
- 纳洛酮、硫胺素和右旋糖($D_{50}W$)适用于意识改变的患者。
- 心血管：
- 心电图评估心律失常，评估心脏缺血或急性心肌梗死。
- 应用β受体阻滞剂或钙通道阻滞剂控制室上性心动过速(SVT)的心室率。
- 腺苷被茶碱拮抗可能无法有效治疗SVT。
- 使用等渗晶体液进行低血压患者的液体复苏：
  - 治疗失败时，请考虑使用β受体阻滞剂逆转茶碱诱导$β_2$受体刺激的血管扩张。
  - 如果需要血管加压药，请选择非β受体激动剂血管加压药，如苯肾上腺素(去氧肾上腺素)。
- 常规治疗室性心律失常。
- 癫痫：
- 服用苯二氮䓬类药物。
- 苯妥英禁忌；在茶碱中毒时它通常是无效的，并可能使癫痫恶化。

急诊治疗/程序

净化治疗

- 应用活性炭，基础治疗。
- 大剂量活性炭：
- 特别是缓释剂型。
- 轻度至中度毒性。
- 25～50 g，q4～6 h，直至茶碱水平<20 μg/ml。
- 缓释剂型进行全肠灌洗：
- 使用聚乙二醇1～2 L/h直到直肠灌洗液无味无色或茶碱水平<20 μg/ml。
- 避免使用吐根糖浆催吐。

电解质紊乱

- 小心谨慎地治疗低钾血症：
- 由β受体介导的细胞外钾向细胞内移位造成相对低钾血症。
- 通常会在没有积极干预的情况下自发解决。
- 随着茶碱浓度的降低，积极纠正低血钾会导致潜在的高钾血症。
- 大多数电解质失衡对β受体阻滞剂治疗有效：
- 然而，通常不建议使用，因为没有相关的发病率，并且在肺疾病患者中，有β受体阻滞诱导阻塞性支气管痉挛的潜在风险。

呕吐

- 避免吩噻嗪类止吐药，因为它们可能降低癫痫发作的阈值：
- 用甲氧氯普胺或5-HT_3受体拮抗剂治疗持久性呕吐。

体外消除

开始血液透析或血液灌流时茶碱水平：

- ≥90～100 μg/ml，合并有急性摄取时的相关症状。
- ≥40 μg/ml，还有以下情况：
- 癫痫。
- 对静脉输液无反应的高血压。
- 室性心律失常。

药物治疗

- 活性炭：摄入量为1 g/kg，口服，如果摄入剂量已知，摄入10 g/1 g茶碱，最大剂量100 g。
- 大剂量活性炭25～50 g，4～6 h直到茶碱水平≤20 μg/ml。
- 地西泮：0.1 mg/kg，静脉注射，q5～10 min直至癫痫发作控制，最高30 mg。
- 地尔硫䓬：0.25 mg/kg，静脉推注；在有β受体阻滞剂禁忌的患者中可能需要15 min之后重复使用，然后输注5～15 mg/h，以控制心率。
- 艾司洛尔：500 mg/kg，静脉推注，随后50 μg/(kg·min)输注；50 μg/(kg·min)递增到最大剂量200 μg/(kg·min)。
- 甲氧氯普胺：10 mg，静滴推注；可以重复使用，最大剂量1 mg/kg。
- 昂丹司琼：0.15 mg/kg，静脉推注，最大剂量16 mg。
- 聚乙二醇(高分子量)：1～2 L/h，通过鼻胃管注入。

随访

进一步处理

入院指征

ICU：

- 急性过量血清茶碱浓度≥100 μg/ml。
- 慢性基础上的急性中毒或慢性中毒，血清浓度≥60 μg/ml的慢性茶碱或较低浓度的严重症状(癫痫、低血压)。
- 血管加压药和液体复苏难以控制的癫痫或低血压，且血清茶碱浓度>40 μg/ml。

出院指征

- 连续2次(间隔>2 h)血清茶碱浓度下降，最近的浓度<30 μg/ml。
- 轻度症状或无症状患者，符合以上标准并且没有自杀的迹象。

随访建议

- 医学毒理学家或初级保健医师随访。
- 如果患者长期服用茶碱，可能需要调整给药方案。

要点和误区

- 癫痫发作是一种主要的并发症，常规治疗通常难以奏效。
- 快速性心律失常在过量时很常见。
- 大剂量活性炭治疗茶碱过量有益。

产后出血 Postpartum Hemorrhage

Sarah H. Michael 瞿金龙 译

基础知识

描述

- 妊娠20周后产后出血(PPH)。
- 初期产后出血：分娩后24 h内出血。
- 又称早期产后出血。
- 后期产后出血：出血>24 h，但是<12周。
- 又称晚期产后出血。
- 定义：
- 顺产分娩后出血>500 ml。
- 剖宫产后出血>1 000 ml。
- 顺产发生率：4%。

• 剖宫产发生率：6%。
• 导致妊娠期死亡的主要原因：
- 25%：妊娠相关性死亡。
- 50%：产后死亡。
• 95%产后出血的原因：
- 50%～60%：子宫收缩乏力。
- 20%～30%：胎盘滞留。
- 10%：宫颈或阴道损伤。
• 并发症：
- 低血容量性休克。
- 输血。
- 急性呼吸窘迫综合征。
- 肝、肾衰竭。
- 希恩综合征(Sheehan 综合征)。
- 失去生育能力。
- DIC。

病因

• 4T：
- Tone，宫缩乏力。
- Tissue，组织残留。
- Trauma，创伤。
- Thrombin，凝血功能异常。
• 急性出血病因：
- 子宫收缩乏力。
- 会阴撕裂伤。
- 胎盘组织残留。
- 胎盘植入。
- 子宫破裂。
- 子宫转位。
- 产后血肿。
- 凝血病。
• 延迟性出血病因：
- 妊娠产物残留。
- 产后子宫内膜炎。
- 外源性雌激素停药。
- 产后血肿。
• 凝血病：
- 本已存在的特发性血小板减少性紫癜。
- 血栓型血小板减少性紫癜。
- 血管性血友病。
- 弥散性血管内凝血。
• 相关情况：
- 如果出血在其他部位也存在，应首先考虑凝血病。
• 高危因素：
- 早于产后出血的征象。
- 高龄孕妇。
- 妊娠期间的多种不良征象。
- 产程延长。
- 羊水过多。
- 器械助产。
- 死胎。
- 抗凝血治疗。
- 胎盘早剥。
- 子宫肌瘤。
- 催产素的超长使用。
- 剖宫产。
- 前置胎盘。
- 绒毛膜羊膜炎。
- 全身麻醉。

诊断

症状和体征

• 出血，常伴有疼痛。
• 严重的低血容量，导致：
- 心动过速。
- 呼吸急促。
- 脉搏细速。
- 尿量减少。
- 皮肤湿冷。
- 毛细血管灌注差。
- 体力改变。
• 心动过速和低血容量一般发生在出血量>1 500 ml 时。

病史

• 一般很快被产科医师发现。
• 延迟性产后出血，一般阴道内或会阴部见大量出血。
• 病史重要点：
- 分娩后的并发症
- 会阴切开。
- 产前凝血功能差的产妇。
• 低血容量的症状：
- 尿量减少。
- 头晕。
- 晕厥。
- 苍白皮肤。

体格检查

通过会阴部、阴道、子宫等检查。
• 体外视诊。
• 内镜检查。
• 双合诊。

基本检查

• 腹部和阴道检查，明确是否存在子宫收缩乏力、胎盘残留或其他解剖学异常。
• 血型鉴定和交叉配血。
• 快速的血红蛋白检测。

诊断检查与说明

诊断建立在临床怀疑和体格检查之上。

实验室检查

• 红细胞计数和血小板。
• PT、APTT。
• 纤维蛋白水平。
• 血型和交叉配血。

影像学检查

在迟发性出血中，超声用来评估子宫有无胎盘残留或判断是腹腔内出血还是子宫内出血。

诊断步骤/外科

超声检查之前可以用手检查。
• 敏感性高。
• 可以诊断和治疗。

鉴别诊断

• 注意有无合并症：会阴部的出血、直肠出血、下腹痛。
• 胎盘残留。

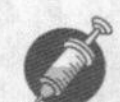

治疗

注意

• 产后出血的患者常常血流动力学不稳定。
• 静脉通路、有效的容量复苏非常重要，包括后续血细胞的输注。

院前

• 监测血流动力学。
• 有效的容量复苏，维持正常血压。

初步稳定/治疗

• 试图控制出血，稳定生命体征。
• 必要时开放气道和复苏治疗：
- 补氧。
- 心电监测。
• 静脉液体复苏。
• 导尿，记录尿量。

急诊治疗/程序

• 子宫收缩乏力：
- 催产素输注。
- 如果催产素失败，肌内注射甲基麦角新碱：
◦ 如果患者有高血压，尽量避免使用。
◦ 一般数分钟内起作用。
- 上述仍失败可予以 PGF_{2a} 肌内注射：
◦ 麻醉中禁忌。

- 内科保守治疗无效，可以进行手术治疗。
• 仔细观察有无阴道、子宫等损失：
- 如果损失≥2 cm，应手术修复。
- 使用2-0、3-0可吸收缝合线连续、锁边缝合。
• (急性)子宫扭转的处理：
- 通过Johnson或Harris操作法复位子宫：
◦ 左手放在腹壁上，稳定子宫底部。
◦ 右手手指通过阴道将子宫复位。
- 如果复位不成功，静脉推注特布他林或镁剂来松弛肌肉，从而来复位。
- 如果仍不成功，可以通过手术治疗亚急性或慢性的扭转。
• 对凝血功能异常患者的治疗：
- 新鲜冰冻血浆、血小板、凝血因子等。
- 维持正常的容量状态。
- 检测凝血变化。
- 积极对症治疗。
- 分娩后及时使用宫缩药物。
- 立即断脐带。
- 注意脐带和子宫的牵引(Brandt-Andrews方法)。
• 子宫填塞：
- 可以用于子宫收缩无力后的持续出血。
- 姑息性治疗措施。
- 压迫或填塞的方法止血。
- 可以使用导尿管，包括Foley导管、Rusch导管或Sengstaken-Blakemore尿管。
- 产科手术用硅树脂填塞：
◦ 特别是为产后出血设计的。

■ **药物治疗**

• 通过缩宫药收缩子宫来控制出血：
- 麦角新碱：0.2 mg，肌内注射，如果有高血压避免使用。
- 甲基麦角新碱：0.2 mg，肌内注射；0.2 mg口服，q6 h，如果有高血压避免使用。
- 欣母沛(15-甲基$PGF_{2\alpha}$)：0.25 mg，肌内注射；15～60 min可以重复使用。
- 催产素：10 U，肌内注射；或20～40 U，静脉滴注，刺激子宫收缩。
• 宫颈松弛可使子宫扭转更容易复位：
- 20%镁剂：2 g，肌内注射，10 min。
- 特布他林：0.25 mg，静脉注射，如果有高血压避免使用。

一线用药

• 缩宫素。
• 催产素输注。
• 甲基麦角新碱。

二线用药

• 手术治疗：
- 子宫切除术：1/1 000行手术治疗。
• 介入栓塞术。

随访

■ **进一步处理**

入院指征

• 所有怀疑产后出血的患者必须入院监测治疗。
• 产科会诊。
• 是否行手术治疗主要依据出血的原因。
• 如果血流动力学不平稳或有DIC倾向，必须收住ICU。
• 合并子宫内膜炎患者必须抗生素治疗。

出院指征

• 无明显活动性出血的延迟出血，并可以轻易控制。
• 非住院处理患者可口服甲基麦角新碱，0.2 mg q6 h，口服，前提是产科医师会诊和专科随访。

■ **随访建议**

• 产科密切随访。
• 出血复发，需紧急处理。

要点和误区

• 积极诊断和处理：
- 大部分死亡患者是由于未能及时诊断，以及液体或血制品复苏延迟。
• 缩宫素是可以最早应用的处理方法。
• 尽快使用液体和血制品进行液体复苏。
• 诊断流程必须明确。
• 尽快产科会诊。

C

产后感染 Postpartum Infection

Ashley M. Licursi · Sarah H. Michael 郑金浩 毛恩强 译

基础知识

■ **描述**

• 产后子宫内膜炎(PPE)：
- 早期产后子宫内膜炎：
◦ 产后48 h内发病。
◦ 大多数发生在剖宫产术后。
◦ 在普通经阴道分娩的发生率为1%～3%。
◦ 典型的临床表现：发热、下腹部子宫投影位置疼痛、刺鼻的恶露。
- 晚期子宫内膜炎：
◦ 在产后3日至6周发生。
◦ 一般发生在经阴道分娩后。
- 在高风险非选择的剖宫产人群，产后子宫内膜炎的发病率高达85%～95%。
• 产后子宫内膜炎的并发症：在剖宫产术后更常见。
- 盆腔血栓性静脉炎。
- 盆腔脓肿。
- 菌血症。
• 产后子宫内膜炎的危险因素：
- 剖宫产。
- 产程延长。
- 羊膜早破。
- 经阴道检查的次数。
- 使用侵入性胎儿监测技术。
• 脓毒症引起的血栓性静脉炎及另外两种产后肺栓塞不同的临床表现：
- 急性血栓：
◦ 大多数出现在右侧卵巢静脉。
◦ 急性血栓经常出现在48 h内，进而出现下腹部疼痛。
- 不明原因的发热：顽固性发热和心动过速。
• 脓毒症引起的流产：
- 在发展中国家不常见。
- 病原体经常是通过开放的宫颈口上行感染。
- 相关因素：
◦ 使用有菌仪器设备进行操作。
◦ 流产后滞留物的存留。
• 乳腺炎：
- 临床表现从局部的乳房红肿到全身发热、系统性疾病及脓肿。

- 比较常见(在产后人群有 1%～30%的发病率)。
- 常发生在产后 1～3 个月。
- 发病高峰在产后 2～3 周。
- 复发率为 4%～8%。

• 尿路感染与肾盂肾炎:
- 泌尿系统感染和乳腺炎占据了产后感染总数的 80%。

病因

• 产后子宫内膜炎:
- 大量的病原微生物从产道向上传播。
- 厌氧菌到达 80%,需氧菌约占 70%。
- 革兰阳性菌:
◦ A 型和 B 型链球菌。
◦ 肠球菌。
◦ 阴道加德纳菌。
- 革兰阴性菌:
◦ 大肠埃希菌。
◦ 肠杆菌。
- 厌氧菌:
◦ 脆弱杆菌。
◦ 消化链球菌。
- 其他常见的生殖器支原体一般出现在产后感染的后期:
◦ 解脲支原体。
◦ 人型支原体。
◦ 沙眼衣原体。

• 脓毒性流产:
- 通常合并多重感染。
- 大肠杆菌。
- 类杆菌属。
- 厌氧菌、革兰阴性杆菌。
- B 型链球菌。
- 葡萄球菌。
- 性传播疾病。

• 淋病:
- 沙眼衣原体。
- 阴道毛滴虫。

• 乳腺炎:
- 金黄色葡萄球菌。
- A 型和 B 型溶血性链球菌。
- 大肠杆菌。
- 类杆菌属。

诊断

症状和体征

病史

• 仔细询问分娩史:
- 剖宫产。
- 分娩的时长。
- 并发症。
- 性传播疾病的暴露史。
- B 型链球菌的检测/治疗。

• 先存在的免疫力低下或疾病。

• 子宫内膜炎:
- 寒战、发热。
- 腹痛。
- 恶露恶臭。

• 脓毒性流产:
- 和子宫内膜炎相似。
- 发热。
- 腹部疼痛。
- 可能有休克的临床表现:
◦ 呼吸困难(急性呼吸窘迫综合征、肺水肿)。
◦ 瘀斑、出血(DIC)。

• 乳腺炎:
- 发热。
- 乳房疼痛、充血、红肿。

• 其他来源的感染:
- 伤口感染:
◦ 红肿、疼痛。
- 泌尿系统感染和肾盂肾炎:
◦ 发热、尿频、排尿困难、肾区疼痛。

体格检查

• 腹部或子宫体表投影处压痛阳性。

• 恶露恶臭。

• 乳腺炎患者出现病变,乳房触痛,红肿。

• 检查外阴切口的感染情况。

• 检查耻骨弓上或肋脊角的压痛、反跳痛以排除泌尿系统的炎症或肾盂肾炎。

基本检查

• 腹部和盆腔检查。

• 子宫颈衣原体的培养。

• 子宫内膜刮取物的培养。

诊断检查与说明

实验室检查

• 血常规。

• 尿常规和培养。

• 血培养。

影像学检查

• CT 或 MRI 排查卵巢静脉血栓。

• 超声对于脓肿及产后滞留物敏感性强。

• X 线平片适用于脓毒性流产中的异物及游离气体。

鉴别诊断

• 其他原因引起的发热。

• 时间不超过 6 h:
- 早期链球菌感染。
- 输血反应。
- 移植排斥反应。
- 甲状腺危象。

• 48 h 以内:
- 肺不张。

• 72 h 以内:
- 尿路感染。
- 肺炎。

• 3～5 日:
- 乳腺炎。
- 乳房充血。
- 坏死性筋膜炎。

• 5～7 日:
- 乳腺炎。
- 脓毒性血栓性静脉炎。

• 7～14 日:
- 脓肿。

• ＞2 周:
- 乳腺炎。
- 肺栓塞。

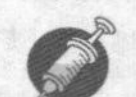

治疗

入院前

• ABC 管理。

• 如果有休克或濒临休克,建立静脉通路,补液。

初步稳定/治疗

• 管理气道和复苏。

• 立即评估呼吸和血流动力学的情况。

• 进行氧疗,必要时进行心电监护及指脉氧饱和度监测。

• 开通静脉通路,循环不稳定时使用晶体液补充血容量和使用升压药物维持血压。

急诊治疗/程序

• 使用抗生素并密切观察病情变化。

• 脓毒性流产常使用扩张刮宫,移除刺激性异物。

• 密切监测及早发现休克前期、循环衰竭、ARDS 及脓毒症。

• 如果高度怀疑存在血栓性静脉炎尽早使用肝素。

• 感染性伤口或脓肿需要敞开引流。

• 坏死性筋膜炎需要广泛清创,静脉使用抗生素并使用高压氧治疗。

• 腹膜炎需要进行影像学检查寻找病因。

■ 药物治疗

• 根据感染的情况,参考相应的抗感染章节有完整的抗感染药物具体内容(哺乳期要注意药物的安全性)。

子宫内膜炎

• 头孢西丁:2 g,静脉注射,q6 h。

• 头孢替坦:2 g,静脉注射,q12 h。

• 哌拉西林-他唑巴坦:3.375 g,静脉注射,q6~8 h。

• 氨苄西林-舒巴坦:1.5~3 g,静脉注射,q6 h。

• 克林霉素:600~900 mg,静脉注射,q8 h 联合。

• 庆大霉素:2 mg/kg 负荷剂量,然后 1~1.5 mg/kg 维持剂量,静脉注射,q8 h。

感染性流产

• 三联抗生素。

• 覆盖革兰阳性菌:

- 氨苄西林/舒巴坦:1.5~3 g,静脉注射,q6 h。

- 头孢西丁:2 g,静脉注射,q6 h。

- 头孢替坦:2 g,静脉注射,q12 h。

• 覆盖革兰阴性菌:

- 庆大霉素:2 mg/kg 负荷剂量,然后 1~1.5 mg/kg 维持剂量,静脉注射,q8 h。

• 覆盖厌氧菌:

- 克林霉素:600~900 mg,静脉注射,q8 h。

- 甲硝唑:500 mg,静脉注射。

乳腺炎

• 双氯西林:250 mg,q6 h,口服 10 日。

• 莫匹罗星:外用,每日 3 次。

• 头孢氨苄:500 mg,q6 h,口服 10 日。

• 克林霉素:300 mg,q6 h,口服 10 日。

• 红霉素:500 mg,q6 h,口服 10 日。

• MRSA 阳性:万古霉素 1 g,静脉注射,q12 h。

尿路感染及肾盂肾炎(住院患者)

• 环丙沙星:400 mg,静脉注射,q12 h。

• 哌拉西林-他唑巴坦:3.375 g,静脉注射,q6~8 h。

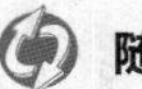

随访

■ 进一步处理

入院指征

• 患有子宫内膜炎或高度怀疑患有盆腔脓毒性血栓性静脉炎。

• 脓毒性流产。

出院指征

中毒表现消失,临床症状缓解可以考虑出院,产科需密切随访病情变化。

■ 随访建议

密切观察随访或主管医师评价治疗效果。

要点和误区

• 乳腺炎和尿路感染占产后感染的 80%。

• 剖宫产是产后子宫内膜炎的危险因素。

• 感染源不同其表现有很大的不同。

• 有早期使用广谱抗生素的指征。

C

肠梗阻(小肠和大肠) Bowel Obstruction(Small and Large)

Sean P. Dyer 李兰玉 译

基础知识

■ 描述

• 机械性或非机械性原因引起的正常肠道内容物流动受阻,可累及小肠或大肠。

• 可分为小肠梗阻(SBO)和大肠梗阻(LBO),也可分为非机械性和功能性梗阻。

• 也可分为部分梗阻、完全梗阻和闭袢性梗阻。

• 梗阻导致近端肠道扩张,由于吞入的空气和累积的肠道分泌物,导致肠腔内压力增加,引起呕吐。

• 肠壁逐渐水肿,额外的肠道分泌物造成肠道进一步的膨胀,第三间隙液体流入肠道内腔。

• 梗阻可能导致肠壁缺血(绞窄性梗阻),导致增加的需氧和厌氧菌感染,甲烷和氨气产生。随之而来的可能是腹膜炎、败血症及死亡。

• 闭袢梗阻:远端和近端肠管同时梗阻导致腔内压力快速增加和动静脉的充血及淤血,增加肠坏死风险。

• 未经治疗的绞窄性梗阻死亡率达 100%,如果 36 h 内进行手术治疗死亡率为 8%,但拖延到 36 h 后手术死亡率为 25%。

■ 病因

• 小肠梗阻:

- 20%为外科急腹症。

- 最主要的病因(60%)为粘连。

- 肿瘤。

- 疝。

- 炎性肠病引起的肠道狭窄。

- 外伤引起的肠壁血肿。

- 混杂病因(例如,蛔虫感染)。

• 大肠梗阻:

- 老年人常见。

- 60%为癌症。

- 20%为肠道憩室。

- 5%为肠扭转。

- 结肠炎(例如,缺血性、放射性)。

- 克罗恩病。

- 异物。

• 功能性,非机械性:

- 麻痹性肠梗阻(例如,电解质紊乱、损伤)。

- 假性梗阻[即 Ogilvie 综合征(如手术创伤和非手术创伤)占 11%]。

诊断

■ 症状和体征

病史

• 手术史、恶性肿瘤、疝、结肠镜检查史、明显的家族史。

• 腹痛:

- 早期为间歇性。

- 老年人或体质衰弱的患者中症状可能并不明显。

- 通常为绞窄性梗阻。

• 呕吐:

- 近端梗阻为胆汁样呕吐物。

- 远端梗阻为粪便样呕吐物。

• 顽固性便秘,大便不通畅,腹泻。

• 粪便形状改变,量减少。

体格检查

• 生命体征:

- 心动过速，伴严重容量不足的低血压。
- 绞窄或穿孔时有发热。
- 脓毒症时为低体温。
• 腹部体征：
- 腹胀。
- 柔韧性的改变，通常是弥漫性。
- 早期肠鸣音活跃，音调高亢；晚期肠鸣音减弱。
- 体征不明显的腹痛要考虑肠壁缺血或坏疽的可能。
- 腹膜炎征象提示肠道绞窄或穿孔。
• 疝(腹部、腹股沟、大腿根部)。
• 直肠指检：
- 直肠肿块。
- 便血，鲜血或隐血。

老年人注意事项

• 老年人腹痛疼痛性质多变，也可模糊不清。
• 恶心、呕吐和腹痛在老年急性心肌梗死患者中是常见症状：
- 腹胀、便秘、腹部绞痛提示病因为消化系统。

儿科注意事项

• 肠套叠：
- 婴儿肠梗阻的主要原因。
- 3～12个月龄最常见。
- 超声是选择的诊断检查。
• 腹股沟疝、脐疝。
• 肠扭转的旋转不良：
- 可早在3～7日龄发生。
- X线平片上的双泡征是由于十二指肠部分梗阻，导致空气聚集在胃和十二指肠第一段。
• 幽门狭窄：
- 渐进性，餐后喷射样呕吐。
- 男女比例：5∶1。
- 通常2～5周龄发病。
• 其他原因包括十二指肠闭锁、巨结肠、肛门闭锁。
• 当病因不考虑是肠套叠/阑尾炎时，CT是诊断梗阻的首选影像学检查。

基本检查

详细的病史和实验室检查。

诊断检查与说明

实验室检查

• 全血细胞计数：
- 白细胞增多常见。
• 电解质，血尿素氮/肌酐，血糖：
- 低钾血症。
- 低氯性代谢性碱中毒。
- 肾前性氮质血症。
• 乳酸。
• 淀粉酶、脂肪酶。
• 肝酶、肝功能排除肝胆管病变。
• 粪隐血检查。
• 尿液分析。
• 血型检查及交叉配血试验。
• 凝血功能检查。
• 有冠心病风险者行心电图检查。

影像学检查

• 胸部直立位X线片：
- 肺部病理学评估。
- 检查膈肌下游离气体。
• 腹部X线平片，仰卧位和直立位(敏感度75%；特异度53%)：
- 肠袢扩张(正常小肠直径<3 cm)。
- 扩张的结肠>13 cm提示潜在的穿孔。
- 液气平。
- 如果小肠内几乎完全充满液体会出现“串珠征”。
- 不利于区分绞窄性肠梗阻。
• 腹部CT扫描：
- 敏感性：小肠梗阻为90%；大肠梗阻为91%。
- 检测肿瘤来源和恶性肿瘤的分级。
- 有效确定阻塞的位置。
- 识别早期绞窄比X线平片更有效(通过静脉造影)。
- 排除其他偶然发现/原因。
- 减少使用肠道造影剂，使用方便。
• 磁共振成像：
- 敏感性与CT接近。
- 可用性变量。
• 超声检查：
- 比X线平片敏感、具体，但不如CT准确。
- 注意蠕动减少(“旋转”)和肠袢扩张>2.5 cm。
- 无创，可快速执行，但受患者体型限制。

诊断步骤/外科

上消化道钡剂灌肠/内镜：
• 如有可疑肿瘤或肿块。
• 减少CT的应用。
• 在体质衰弱的患者可能有痛苦或困难。

鉴别诊断

• 麻痹性肠梗阻。
• 假性肠梗阻(Ogilvie综合征)。
• 溃疡穿孔。
• 胰腺炎。
• 胆囊炎。
• 结肠炎。
• 肠系膜缺血。

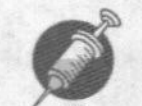

治疗

院前

脱水、呕吐或严重腹痛者建立静脉通道。

初步稳定/治疗

• 基础治疗。
• 严重容量缺失、绞窄或肠穿孔的患者静脉补充生理盐水或乳酸林格液：
- 成人：1 L，快速注射。
- 儿童：20 ml/kg，快速注射。
• 纠正电解质紊乱，尤其是低钾血症。

急诊治疗/程序

• 静脉输液(等渗盐水或乳酸林格液)。
• 留置胃管(NGT)。
• Foley导管检测尿量。
• 外科会诊。
• 可疑绞窄或肠穿孔的患者抗生素治疗：
- 抗生素选择应覆盖革兰阴性菌和厌氧菌。
• 止痛药。
• 止吐药。
• 针对病因治疗。

药物治疗

• 抗生素选择(广谱，怀疑肠缺血)：
- 联合治疗：
◦ 灭滴灵(甲硝唑)：1 g，静脉注射，然后500 mg，静脉注射，q6 h[儿童：7.5～30 mg/(kg·24 h)，分次静脉注射q6～8 h]。
◦ 环丙沙星：400 mg静脉注射，q12。
◦ 头孢曲松(头孢曲松钠)：1～2 g，静脉注射，q24 h[儿童：25～74 mg/(kg·d)，静脉注射，最大量2 g，分次注射，q12～24 h]。
- 单药治疗：
◦ 哌拉西林-他唑巴坦(哌拉西林钠-三唑巴坦钠注射剂)3.375 g[儿童：150～400 mg/(kg·24 h)，静脉注射，分次注射，q6～8 h]，静脉注射，q4～6 h。
◦ 氨苄西林-舒巴坦(优立新)：1.5 g～3 g[儿童：100～400 mg/(kg·24 h)，静脉注射，分次注射，q6 h]，静脉注射，q6 h。
◦ 美罗培南(美罗培南粉针剂)：1 g[儿童：60～120 mg/(kg·24 h)，静脉注射，q8 h]，静脉注射，q8 h。

◦ 亚胺培南-西司他丁液(普利马辛): 250～1 000 mg[儿童: 50～100 mg/(kg·24 h), 静脉注射 q6～12 h],静脉注射,q6～8 h。
• 止痛药:
- 吗啡: 2 ～ 10 mg/次(儿童: 0.1 ～ 0.2 mg/kg),静脉注射、肌内注射或皮下注射,q2～6 h,需要时用。
• 止吐药:
- 昂丹司琼(枢复宁): 4 mg[儿童: 0.1 mg/kg 静脉注射,分次注射,q8 h],静脉注射,q4～8 h,需要时用。
- 异丙嗪(二甲氨丙基吩噻嗪): 12.5～25 mg[儿童: >2 岁: 0.25～1 mg/(kg·d) 静脉注射、肌内注射或灌肠,分次注射,q4～6 h,需要时用],静脉注射、肌内注射或皮下注射,q4 h。

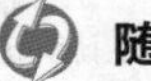

随访

进一步处理

入院指征

所有可疑或确诊为肠梗阻的患者都需要住院并接受早期外科干预。

出院指征

实验室检查或影像学结果正常,症状缓解,无进一步肠梗阻可能。

转诊问题

外科认为疑似肠梗阻。

随访建议

出院患者:
• 实验室和影像学检查正常。
• 及时再次评估。
• 详尽说明返回急诊室的症状和体征。

要点和误区

• 有呕吐病史的嵌顿性疝患者应详细检查。
• 漏诊绞窄性肠梗阻:
- 在老年人、婴儿及体质衰弱的患者症状模糊不清。
• 未能充分补足液体流失,纠正电解质紊乱。

C

肠扭转 Volvulus

Dhara P. Amin 吴昊 李文放 译

基础知识

描述

• 肠系膜周围胃肠道的一部分轴向扭曲,引起部分肠道完全性肠梗阻。
• 通常与其他消化道异常有关。
• 在儿科环境中,通常涉及婴儿:
- 胚胎发育异常。
• 可以通过结肠的病理性扩散而沉淀。
• 血液供应可能会受到静脉瘀血和最终动脉流入障碍的影响,导致肠和肠道梗死。

病因

• 结肠梗阻的第三大最常见原因(10%～15%)在肿瘤和憩室病之后。
• 流行病学:
- 0～1 年: 30%。
- 1～18 岁: 20%。
- 超过 18 岁: 50%。
• 常与其他胃肠道异常有关。
• 盲肠(52%):
- 在年轻人中比较常见,<50 岁。
- 由于肠系膜和腹膜后间隙先天性融合,导致盲肠在不同程度上自由移动。
- 伴随着增加的产气量(吸收和伪阻塞)。
- 可以在妊娠和结肠镜检查后看到。
• 乙状结肠(43%):
- 更常见于:
◦ 老年人。
◦ 住院患者。
◦ 慢性排便障碍(帕金森病)。
◦ 精神疾病(精神分裂症)。
- 由于冗长的肠系膜结肠肠系膜粘连。
- 与慢性便秘和通便药使用有关。
• 横结肠和脾弯曲(5%)。
• 胃扭转(罕见)与膈肌缺陷有关。

儿科注意事项

• 中肠扭转:
- 由于中肠在进入腹部时未能在子宫内正确旋转的先天性麻痹/旋转。
- 整个中肠从十二指肠下降到横结肠旋转围绕肠系膜,包括肠系膜上动脉。
- 常见新生儿(80%<1 个月,通常在第 1 周;6%～20%>1 岁)。
- 男性>女性,2∶1。
- 突发的胆汁性呕吐(97%)伴随腹部疼痛。
- 可能有以前的喂食问题、胆汁性呕吐。在 1 岁以上的儿童中,与发育迟缓、饮食不能耐受、慢性间歇性呕吐、血性腹泻有关。
- 便秘。
- 由于胃肠道阻塞较高,因此轻度呕吐。
- 根据局部缺血程度可能不会表现为中毒症状。

诊断

症状和体征

病史

• 婴儿: 呕吐 90%的食物:
- 可能为胆汁性。
• 年龄较大的儿童和成人: 易变且常常隐匿。
- 80%有慢性症状,几周到几个月甚至几年。
• 肠扭转继发肠梗阻:
- 绞痛,痉挛腹痛(90%)。
- 腹胀(80%)。
- 便秘(60%)。
- 恶心和呕吐(28%)。
• 盲肠扭转:
- 高度可变,间歇性发作突然发作的疼痛和膨胀。
• 乙状结肠扭转:
- 呕吐罕见。
- 更隐匿的发病。
- 腹痛和胀气、恶心和便秘。
• 胃扭转:
- Borchard 三联症: 严重的上腹胀、顽固性干呕、无法放置鼻胃管(30%的患者)。

体格检查

• 坏疽性肠道的存在:
- 增加疼痛。
- 腹膜体征: 肌卫,反跳痛,板状腹。
- 发热。
- 直肠指检带血。
- 心动过速和血容量不足。
• 盲肠扭转:
- 腹部膨隆。

- 通常在左上腹、中腹部可触及肿块。

儿科注意事项

• 在临床过程早期,体格检查可表现正常。

• 70%存在慢性症状。

• 40%的新生儿出现胆汁呕吐需要手术治疗。

• 便血、腹胀或疼痛,休克表示缺血或坏死。

基本检查

• CBC、BMP 和 UA。

• 腹部 X 线平片。

• 上消化道系列(儿童起初最佳检查)。

• 腹部和骨盆 CT 造影(最适合成人)。

• 钡灌肠。

• 超声。

诊断检查与说明

实验室检查

• 可能会提供坏疽肠道存在的线索,但正常的检查结果并不能排除疾病可能。

• 全血细胞计数:

- 白细胞增多症(>20 000/mm^3)表明患有感染/腹膜炎。

• 电解质、BUN、肌酸酐、葡萄糖:

- 由乳酸酸中毒引起的阴离子酸中毒。

- 由于脱水导致氮质血症。

• 尿液检查:

- 尿比重增加和酮。

影像学检查

• 腹部 X 线平片:

- 可提示但通常不确定。

- <70%的病例能通过检查发现。

- 乙状结肠扭转:由骨盆引起的倒 U 形结肠扩张结肠。

- 盲肠扭转扩张和移位:

◦ 盲肠在左腹部(肾形),通常伴有小肠扩张。

• CT 扫描:

- 盲肠"旋转"信号。

- 可能用于确定乙状结肠扭转阻塞程度。

• 上消化道系列(十二指肠最好,但需要看操作员水平):

- 突然出现的末端螺旋形的锥形(75%)。

- 细微的改变(25%)。

• 钡餐:

- "鸟喙"扭曲部位的畸形。

- 由于有穿孔风险,需谨慎行事。

- 注意由于婴儿没有固定的盲肠,担心假阳性结果。

• 超声(具体但不敏感):

- 肠系膜上静脉的异常位置(SMA 的左前)。

- 扭转的漩涡征:旋转的血管围绕着肠系膜的底部。

- 第三部分十二指肠不在正常位置(在肠系膜动脉和主动脉之间)。

儿科注意事项

• 中肠扭转的诊断:

- 十二指肠完全与 X 线平片上的脊椎相对。

- 双泡征是指立位片显示扩张性胃和近端十二指肠环。

- 上消化道吞咽试验:在右上象限盘旋的空肠。

- 在 20%的病例中出现平面正常。

注意

• 评估任何患有阻塞症状的儿童(包括呕吐和腹痛)肠扭转的迹象,即使他看起来没有腹膜炎。

• 延迟诊断 1~2 h 或以上会导致坏疽肠道,需要大量切除并永久胃肠外营养及伴随相关并发症。

诊断步骤/外科

• 腹腔镜检查:

- 对腹部 X 线平片正常的患者诊断有用。

- 可以区分先天性旋转和扭转。

鉴别诊断

• 阻塞性结肠肿瘤或憩室炎。

• 小肠梗阻。

• 肠梗阻。

• 肠套叠。

• 阑尾炎。

• 盆腔炎和输卵管炎,尤其是盲肠。

• 卵巢扭转。

• 内脏穿孔。

• 周期性呕吐综合征。

儿科注意事项

• 胎粪性肠梗阻。

• 先天性巨结肠。

• 十二指肠闭锁。

• 梅克尔憩室。

• 坏死性结肠炎(特别是早产儿)。

• 肠套叠。

• 阑尾炎。

• 其他:

- 肠绞痛。

- 过敏性紫癜。

- 先天性代谢异常。

- 外伤。

- 胃食管反流。

- 肾盂肾炎。

- 脑膜炎。

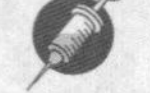

治疗

院前

• 建立静脉通道。

• NPO。

初步稳定/治疗

• 基本生命支持。

• 生理盐水推注 20 ml/kg(儿童)或 2 L 滴注(成人)行液体复苏。

• 糖耐量。

急诊治疗/程序

• 外科或消化科医师会诊。

• NPO。

• 纠正血容量不足和电解质紊乱。

• 如果怀疑脓毒症或穿孔,术前需使用广谱抗生素。

明确的治疗

乙状结肠扭转

• 一般情况好的患者:

- 用乙状结肠镜复位:

◦ 80%~95%成功。

◦ 60%复发(几小时到几周后)。

- 随后选择性乙状结肠切除和原发性吻合(<3%复发)。

• 有腹膜炎表现患者:

- 急诊切除乙状结肠和任何坏疽肠,并放置结肠造口术。

• 带直肠管放置的内镜减压术:

- 78%的乙状结肠扭转患者治疗成功,对盲肠扭转不太有效。

- 复发常见。

- 内镜下扭转后的选择性手术治疗。

盲肠扭转

• 紧急手术减压,然后进行结肠切除和初级吻合(首选),或者如果盲肠仍然存活(高度复发)。

儿科注意事项

• 在 1~2 h 剖腹手术以减少缺血的风险。

• 进行手术解除坏死性肠梗阻,腹腔镜预防复发性肠扭转。

药物治疗

• 氨苄西林-舒巴坦(unasyn):3 g[儿童:100~200 mg/(kg · 24 h)],静脉滴注,q6 h。

• 头孢西丁（mefoxin）：2 g［儿童：80～160 mg/(kg·24 h)］，静脉滴注，q6 h。

• 头孢曲松：1～2 g，静脉滴注，q12～24 h［儿童：50～75 mg/(kg·d)，q12～24 h］和灭滴灵 500 mg，静脉滴注，q8 h［儿童：30 mg/(kg·24)，q6 h］。

• 哌拉西林-他唑巴坦：3.375～4 g，静脉滴注，q4～6 h（儿童：200～300 mg/kg，哌拉西林组分，q6～8 h）。

随访

进一步处理

入院指征

所有外科医师怀疑可能患有肠扭转的患者。

出院指征

没有。

转诊问题

• 外科咨询不可或缺。

• 非典型的旋转：无症状或胃食管反流症状：

- 密切观察重复对比研究。
- 延期手术。

随访建议

随访手术后患者。

要点和误区

• 考虑任何1月龄以前呈现呕吐的儿童的肠扭转：

- 胆汁呕吐是由于机械性肠梗阻，直到另有证明。

• 延迟诊断导致发病率增加，成人比儿童常见：

- 70%成人直到最初有症状表现＞6个月才诊断出来，大多数出现慢性腹部症状。
- 如果坏疽存在，死亡率在25%～80%。

• 所有成年患者都可手术治疗。

• 上消化道对照是儿童最好的初始测试。

• 腹部和骨盆CT更适合成人。

肠旋转不良

Moon O. Lee 王胜云 段立伟 译

基础知识

描述

• 妊娠10周的期间内，胚胎形成期间从结肠外位置转变期间不完整的肠旋转和固定。

• 风险因素：

- 心脾综合征。

• 相关条件：

- 胃肠异常：
  - 十二指肠梗阻、闭锁。
  - 梅克尔憩室。
  - 肠套叠。
  - 胃食管反流。
  - 脐突出或腹裂。
  - 先天性膈疝。
  - 腹壁缺损。
  - 巨结肠。
- 代谢性酸中毒。
- 先天性心脏畸形，27%的患者出现肠旋转不良，增加发病率至61%。

病因

• 十二指肠与空肠交接处仍在中间偏右侧。

• 盲肠仍在腹部左上角，带有异常肠系膜附着物。

• 小肠绕着上肠系膜扭转到中肠时，肠扭结是肠扭转不良的并发症。

• 解剖结构异常易受阻碍物及其他条件的影响。

• 通常发现同时有其他先天性异常（70%）：心脏、食管、肛门。

• 27%的旋转异常的患者存在先天性心脏异常。

• 流行病：

- 活产婴：1/5000。
- 婴儿高死亡率：达到24%。
- 外科肠道坏死增加25倍的死亡率。
- 发病率：
  - 在新生儿中，男女比例为2∶1。
  - 75%在新生儿期被诊断。
  - 90%在1岁被诊断。
  - 会在成人期发病。

诊断

症状和体征

• 扭转发生前无症状。

• 新生儿：

- 呕吐物含胆汁。
- 腹部膨隆。
- 血便。
- 便秘和顽固便秘。
- 喂食困难。
- 体重增加缓慢。

• ＞1岁：呕吐物含胆汁，随后出现腹痛。

• 大一些的儿童及青少年：

- 慢性呕吐。
- 间歇性腹部绞痛。
- 腹泻。
- 咯血。
- 便秘。
- 无异常体征（50%～75%）。

• 成人：症状不典型。

• 一般情况：

- 脱水、酸中毒。
- 腹膜炎。
- 肠缺血。
- 败血症、休克。

病史

• 婴儿期呕吐是最常见的症状，可能含有或不含有胆汁。

• 幼儿早期小肠梗阻症状。

• 胆汁性呕吐与腹痛有关。

• 在年龄稍大的儿童及成人中，最常见的症状是腹痛。

• 其他相关病史——急性或慢性的腹痛、喂食情况差、嗜睡、吸收不良、慢性腹泻。

体格检查

• 腹部检查提示障碍性膨胀。

• 便血提示局部缺血。

• 评估先天异常。

基本检查

建议通过病史及体检进行诊断，并通过放

射线照相术的对比来确诊。

■ 诊断检查与说明

实验室检查

- 全血细胞计数。
- 动脉血气。
- 电解质、血尿素氮、肌酸酐和葡萄糖水平。
- 尿常规和尿培养。
- 血型鉴定和抗体筛选。
- PT、APTT、INR。
- 乳酸盐。

影像学检查

- 腹部 X 线平片：
  - 诊断＜30％。
  - 如果伴有以下症状，很可能是肠扭结：
    - 十二指肠梗阻。
    - 完全肠扭结下，胃胀带有少量管腔内气体在肠扭结远侧。
    - 小肠形态普遍膨胀。
    - 从引起胃部和十二指肠膨胀的局部十二指肠梗阻，双泡征可在直立影像中看到。
- 上消化道造影研究：
  - 诊断金标准：旋转不良的诊断敏感性为 93％～100％，肠扭转诊断的敏感性为 56％～79％。
  - 发现：
    - 缺少 Treitz 韧带或右腹部十二指肠错位。
    - 十二指肠近端膨胀，终端呈圆锥形或鸟嘴形。
    - 肠扭结的十二指肠呈现螺旋形。
    - 腹部右侧的近端空肠（在新生儿期很容易被取代）。
    - 小肠褶皱加厚。
- 肠道造影：
  - 对于不确定情况下盲肠的位置确定有帮助。
  - 评估在上腹中间或中间偏左的盲肠位置。
  - ＞20％假阴性结果。
- 超声：
  - 超声显示肠系膜上动脉与肠旋转不良的静脉的关系。
  - 肠系膜上动脉及静脉的多普勒超声波上漩涡征，扭转肠扭结中看到的肠系膜。
  - 正常的超声不会排除旋转不良的情况。
- CT：
  - 婴幼儿及儿童很少的益处。
  - 更可能用于成人诊断。

■ 鉴别诊断

- 早年：
  - 巨结肠。
  - 坏死性小肠结肠炎。
  - 肠套叠。
- 急性腹痛及腹膜症状的儿童：
  - 盲肠炎。
  - 肠套叠。
  - 脓毒症。
- 年长的儿童及成人带有腹部隐痛：
  - 肠易激综合征。
  - 消化性溃疡。
  - 胆道及胰腺疾病。
  - 精神疾病。

治疗

注意中肠旋转不良可能导致快速容量及电解质更换/补液的需要，以校正血容量过低及代谢性酸中毒。

■ 院前

快速转至急诊进行液体复苏。

■ 初步稳定/治疗

- ABC 管理。
- 生理盐水静推注（20 ml/kg）治疗休克、败血症或脱水。
- 考虑胃管。
- 2 条静脉通路和/或中心静脉导管。
- 应用广谱抗生素治疗败血症或腹膜炎。

■ 急诊治疗/程序

- 紧急外科诊治。
- 与中肠旋转不良有关时，可要求转运到带有儿外科技术的医疗单位，以实现：
  - 肠扭转矫正。
  - 肠道灌流恢复。
  - 明显坏死区域切除术。
- 饮食：
  - NPO。

■ 药物治疗

- 手术之前应用广谱抗生素。
- 保持液体及电解质平衡。
- 血管加压药。

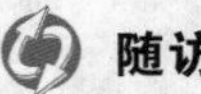

随访

■ 进一步处理

入院指征

- 急腹症。
- 手术治疗。
- 严重脱水。
- 酸中毒。
- 败血症。

出院指征

- 稳定无症状且偶然的没有相关症状和体征通常都会被承认。
- 出院前儿科手术评估。

转诊问题

诊断性评估经常要求在配有儿童外科及儿科放射性专业技术的三级儿科医院。

■ 随访建议

按照儿科服务要求。

要点和误区

- 儿童急腹症及时发现。
- 酸中毒及休克的及时治疗。
- 快速转移至适当医疗机构。

肠套叠 Intussusception

Roger M. Barkin　倪沁赟 译

基础知识

■ 描述

- 近端肠管内陷到远端肠管，导致梗阻和内陷肠管坏死：
  - 80％以上累及回盲部。
- 常发生于 2 岁以上儿童且有显著的病理特点：
  - 淋巴结肿大多发生于婴儿。
  - 2 岁以上儿童：1/3 的患者有特征性病理学表现。
  - 6 岁以上儿童：淋巴瘤是最常见的特点。

- 成人通常有特征性病理学表现。
• 在生命的第二个 2 年内肠梗阻的最常见原因。
• 美国流行病学：
- 最常见于 5～9 月龄的儿童。
- 发生率为 2.4/1000。
- 男女比例为 2∶1。
- 病死率<1%。
• 延误诊断会导致发病率增加。

注意

患者(特别是儿童患者)有肠梗阻的影像学表现，尤其是粪便隐血试验阳性或有精神状态改变，需要考虑肠套叠。

病因

• 大部分病例(85%)没有明显的基础病理表现。
• 导致肠管内陷的诱发因素，特别是年龄较大的儿童和成人：
- 肿块/肿瘤：
◦ 淋巴瘤。
◦ 脂肪瘤。
◦ 息肉。
◦ 淋巴结肿大。
◦ 梅克尔憩室。
- 感染：
◦ 腺病毒或轮状病毒感染。
◦ 寄生虫。
- 异物。
- 过敏性紫癜。
- 腹腔疾病和囊性纤维化(小肠肠套叠)。

诊断

症状和体征

病史

• 临床典型表现(存在于<50%的患者)：
- 腹痛。
- 呕吐，常见胆汁。
- 粪便带血和黏液(果浆样便)。
• 反复疼痛发作伴随面色苍白和双腿踢蹬，突然剧烈疼痛伴随尖叫和屈腿：
- 每间隔 5～20 min 发作。
• 精神状态改变：
- 易激惹。
- 嗜睡或者坐立不安，儿童可见跛行或洋娃娃外形。
- 可在腹部症状出现之前发病。
• 粪便指标：
- 隐血、血便或果浆样便。
• 腹痛发病前数日或数周的病兆：
- 腹泻。
- 病毒综合征。
- 亨诺-许兰紫癜。
• <10%的患者可出现复发性肠套叠。

体格检查

• 发热。
• 腹壁膨隆和肿胀：
- 右下腹可触及"腊肠样"包块。
- 右侧髂窝可触不到盲肠。
- 可见蠕动波。
- 直肠检查可见血便并可触及包块。
• 根据从发病到诊断之间的时间长短，可出现穿孔性腹膜炎及败血症。

基本检查

• 根据病史可诊断，影像学可进一步确诊。
• 便血可辅助诊断，尤其伴有嗜睡或坐立不安。

诊断检查与说明

实验室检查

• 全血细胞计数。
• 血清电解质、尿素氮。
• 血型和交叉配血。

影像学检查

• 腹部：
- 35%～40%的患者可见异常。
- 右侧结肠内气体和粪便减少。
- 腹部包块。
- 肠道充气显露出的肠套叠顶端。
- 小肠膨隆及继发于机械性肠梗阻的气液平。
- 可帮助排除肠穿孔。
• 灌肠：
- 通常为诊断性和治疗性。多数需重复操作：
◦ 肠套叠出现后 24 h 内成功率为 74%。
◦ 24 h 以后有效率为 32%。
◦ 肠套叠部位越远，影像学上的缓解率就越低。
◦ 复发性肠套叠(高达 10%)与初发性的缓解率相当。
- 并发症包括肠穿孔、坏死肠段切除、手术延迟的不完全性切除及最终的病理学检查。
- 内毒素和细胞因子引起的继发性低血容量性休克。
- 钡餐：
◦ 透视镜引导下使用。
◦ 水溶性造影诊断与治疗。
◦ 标志性的螺纹样改变。
- 充气或生理盐水：
◦ 透视镜引导下使用。
◦ 万一穿孔避免腹膜污染。
◦ 逐渐用于诊断和治疗。
- 禁忌证：
◦ 腹膜炎。
◦ 穿孔。
◦ 继发败血症或休克的危重患者。
• 超声检查十分精准并且可用于疾病筛查，与操作者相关：
- 主要表现为甜甜圈样靶征、螺纹征或牛眼样征象，中央呈高回声，边缘呈均匀性低回声。
- 诊断，不治疗。

诊断步骤/外科

如果灌肠无效，需要紧急行手术治疗。

鉴别诊断

• 感染：
- 急性胃肠炎。
- 传染性单核细胞增多症。
- 肺炎。
- A 组溶血性链球菌咽炎。
- 肾盂肾炎。
• 阑尾炎。
• 炎症性肠病。
• 疝气。
• 肠梗阻和腹膜炎。
• 绞窄性疝。
• 肠旋转不良和肠扭转。
• 先天性巨结肠。
• 创伤。
• 肠血管和出血性疾病。
• 肛裂和痔。
• 溃疡病。
• 血管畸形。
• 过敏性紫癜。
• 息肉。
• 蛋白质敏感的小肠结肠炎。牛奶过敏可能导致大便出血。
• 糖尿病。
• 凝血功能障碍。

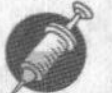

治疗

院前

• 建立静脉通道。

C

• 如果存在低血容量、腹胀、腹膜炎、脓毒症，静脉给予负荷剂量 20 ml/kg 生理盐水或乳酸林格液。
• 在院前，诊断很少明确。

■ 初步稳定/治疗

• 建立静脉通道，然后静脉给予负荷剂量 20 ml/kg 生理盐水或乳酸林格液。
• 留置鼻胃管。

■ 急诊治疗/程序

• 稳定患者的血流动力学。
• 外科会诊以发现潜在疾病。
• 腹部 X 线检查。
• 如果没有禁忌证，可行介入放射治疗来缓解症状：
- 灌肠对于复位有 75%～80%的成功率，反映该情况的持续时间。
- 复发可能降低介入放射治疗。
• 抗生素：
- 首先明确有无腹膜炎、穿孔或脓毒症的证据。
- 氨苄西林、克林霉素和庆大霉素。
- 氨苄西林-舒巴坦。
• 剖腹探查术：
- 适应证：
◦ 灌肠不成功。
◦ 灌肠有禁忌。
◦ 明确病理诊断。
◦ 多次复发。
- 过程：
◦ 操作时要轻柔。
◦ 完整切除不能成活的肠道。

■ 药物治疗

一线用药

• 氨苄西林：100～200 mg/(kg·d)，q4 h，静脉注射。
• 克林霉素：30～40 mg/(kg·d)，q6 h，静脉注射。
• 庆大霉素：5～7.5 mg/(kg·d)，q8 h，静脉注射。
• 氨苄西林-舒巴坦：100～200 mg/(kg·d)，q6 h，静脉注射。

随访

■ 进一步处理

入院指征

• 通过灌肠复位成功的患者入院观察是否存在并发症或复发。
• 接受手术治疗的患者。

出院指征

• 灌肠复位成功的患者经过一段长时间的观察后可考虑出院：
- 精神状态正常的稳定患者。
- 复位后腹痛症状缓解。
- 经过长时间的观察，家属知道如何观察潜在的复发。

转诊问题

外科医师注意患者潜在的肠套叠。

要点和误区

婴儿有阵发性腹痛、精神状态异常和血便通常需要考虑肠套叠。

肠系膜缺血 Mesenteric Ischemia

Rashid F. Kysia　段立伟 译

基础知识

■ 描述

• 肠系膜血管血流减少或阻塞导致肠局部缺血或梗死。
• 可分为动脉或静脉堵塞或低血流量状态 3 种情况。
• 入院率为 1/1 000。
• 所有入院患者腹痛发生率为 1%～2%：
- 多数病例年龄超过 50 岁。
- 死亡高达 60%～70%，特别是对于诊断/临床表现延迟到>24 h 的患者。

■ 病因

• 急性肠系膜动脉栓塞：
- 占急性肠系膜缺血的 50%。
- 平均年龄为 70 岁。
- 栓子最常来源于左心房或心室，由心律失常、瓣膜病变或先前的心肌梗死导致的心室血栓造成的。
- 通常情况下嵌顿在距离肠系膜上动脉(SMA)起源 3～10 cm 处。
◦ 保留近端小肠和大肠的血供。
- 危险因素包括：心律失常(尤其是心房颤动)、心脏瓣膜疾病、心肌梗死病史、主动脉瘤或主动脉夹层。
• 肠系膜动脉血栓：
- SMA 血栓占急性肠系膜缺血病例的 15%。
- 很少发生在其他血管。
- 由破裂的肠系膜动脉粥样硬化斑块发展而来。
- 50%～80%病例可能有长期的肠绞痛(慢性肠系膜缺血)。
- 危险因素包括：年龄、动脉粥样硬化疾病、高血压。
• 肠系膜静脉血栓形成：
- 占急性肠系膜缺血病例的 5%～15%。
- 亚急性或无痛性表现。
- 死亡率 20%～40%。
- 通常发生在有潜在高凝状态的年轻患者。
- 风险因素包括：
◦ 高凝状态(狼疮、蛋白 C 和蛋白 S 缺乏)。
◦ 镰状细胞病。
◦ 抗凝血酶Ⅲ缺乏。
◦ 恶性肿瘤(特别是侵犯到门静脉系统的肿瘤)。
◦ 妊娠。
◦ 脓血症。
◦ 肾衰竭需透析治疗患者。
◦ 雌激素治疗。
◦ 近期创伤或炎症状态。
• 非阻塞性肠系膜缺血：
- 占急性肠系膜缺血病例的 20%～30%。
- 低心排量导致肠系膜血流减少的情况下出现。
- 风险因素包括：充血性心力衰竭、脓毒症、低血压、低血容量、利尿剂的使用、近期手术(特别是心脏)或近期需要使用血管加压药物。
- 生存率低。
• 慢性肠系膜缺血：
- 肠绞痛：
◦ 进食约 1 h 后发生的弥漫性腹痛，持续

1～2 h。

◦ 患者可发展为厌食和少食多餐来避免疼痛。

• 不常见的病因：

- 自发性肠系膜动脉夹层。

- 正中弓状韧带综合征：膈肌弓形韧带压迫腹腔轴线或SMA。

- 肿瘤外源性压迫。

- 药物：

◦ 洋地黄。

◦ 麦角胺。

◦ 可卡因。

◦ 伪麻黄碱。

◦ 血管加压素。

诊断

症状和体征

• 突然发病，急性缺血时表现为严重的弥漫性腹痛：

- 疼痛与体征不成比例：

◦ 尽管患者腹痛剧烈，但体征较轻。

• 恶心。

• 呕吐。

• 腹泻。

• 隐匿性消化道出血。

• 老年患者可出现非特异表现，如精神状态改变、呼吸急促或心动过速。

• 后期表现：

- 不可逆肠管缺血导致的腹膜炎体征。

- 腹胀。

- 肠鸣音减弱。

病史

• 疼痛发作迅速。

• 风险因素，包括：

- 低血容量。

- 充血性心力衰竭。

- 心律失常。

- 瓣膜病变。

- 动脉粥样硬化。

- 腹部恶性肿瘤。

体格检查

急性期，腹痛症状与腹部体征不成比例。

基本检查

年龄＞50 岁的患者发生不明原因性腹痛时要高度怀疑。

诊断检查与说明

实验室检查

• 通常是非特异性的，不具有诊断性价值。

• 血常规：

- 白细胞计数升高（90%＞15 000/mm^3）。

• 生化检查：

- 大约 50%的患者有代谢性酸中毒。

• 淀粉酶：

- 50%的病例有高淀粉酶血症。

• 肌酸磷酸激酶（CPK）可能会升高。

• 乳酸：

- 90%的患者会升高。

- 提示晚期的组织损坏，在疾病早期可能不会升高。

- 乳酸高水平与高死亡率相关。

影像学检查

• 平卧和立位腹部 X 线片：

- 通常用于排除急性肠梗阻。

- 通常情况下正常。

- 后期表现：

◦ 由肠壁水肿和出血导致的拇纹征。

◦ 肠壁积气：肠壁内组织坏死产生的气体。

◦ 胆道积气是晚期表现，与不良结局相关。

• 腹部 CT 平扫：

- 可用于检测肠壁水肿和积气。

- 较新的螺旋多排 CT（MDCT）可以直接显示肠系膜血管解剖，并可以定位阻塞部位。

- MDCT 血管造影是更频繁使用的首选影像学检查方法。

• MRI：

- 可以很好地呈现肠系膜血管图像，尤其是磁共振血管造影。

- 采集时间和可用性限制了它的使用。

• 血管造影：

- 曾经是诊断的金标准，现已被 MDCT 取代。

- 可直视栓子，给予血管扩张剂或纤维蛋白溶解剂。

- 侵入性，费时，而且有潜在肾毒性。

• 多普勒超声：

- 可用以检测 SMA 血流量的减少，但在诊断慢性肠系膜缺血方面帮助更大。

- 患者最好在 8 h 内实行 NPO，限制了其在急诊室的应用。

鉴别诊断

• 肠梗阻。

• 肠扭转。

• 胃肠道恶性肿瘤。

• 憩室炎。

• 炎性肠病。

• 消化性溃疡。

• 内脏穿孔。

• 胆囊炎。

• 胆管炎。

• 胰腺炎。

• 阑尾炎。

• 腹主动脉瘤。

• 心肌梗死。

• 肾结石。

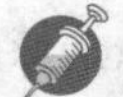

治疗

院前

为脱水或低血压患者启动液体治疗。

初步稳定/治疗

• ABC 管理，液体复苏。

• 警告：

- 早期诊断和治疗对于降低死亡率至关重要。

急诊治疗/程序

• 一般措施：

- 鼻胃管吸引，胃肠减压。

- NPO。

- 根据需要调整电解质溶液。

- 心电监护仪监测心律失常。

- 如果患者不稳定，考虑侵入性心脏监测。

- 监测尿量。

- 止痛药。

- 广谱抗生素，以覆盖肠道菌群（如果伴随肾衰竭，可能需要的调整剂量）。

◦ 哌拉西林-他唑巴坦。

◦ 氨苄西林-舒巴坦。

◦ 替卡西林-克拉维酸。

◦ 其他选择包括：亚胺培南、美罗培南、第三代头孢菌素加甲硝唑。

- 肝素抗凝。

- 外科会诊：有腹膜炎体征患者应该进行剖腹探查。

• 特殊治疗：

- 罂粟碱 30～60 mg/h，动脉内给药：

◦ 磷酸二酯酶抑制剂可使肠系膜血管扩张。

◦ 通过血管造影导管给药。

- 动脉内血栓溶解术可用于无腹膜炎或肠缺血的晚期症状。

- 外科血管成形术。

• 警告：

- 避免使用血管收缩的药物，因其可能会加重缺血。

◦ 如果需要使用血管加压药，应使用对肠系膜影响较小的药物，如多巴酚丁胺、小剂量多巴胺、米力农。

■ 药物治疗

• 氨苄西林-舒巴坦：3 g，静脉注射，q6 h[儿童：100～200 mg/(kg·d)]。

• 硫酸肝素：80 U/kg，静脉推注，随后 18 U/(kg·h)输注。

• 甲硝唑：首剂 1.0 g，静脉推注，随后 500 mg，静脉注射，q6 h(儿童：首剂 12 mg/kg 静脉推注，随后 7.5 mg/kg，静脉注射，q6 h)。

• 哌拉西林-他唑巴坦：3.375 g，静脉注射，q6 h[儿童：240～400 mg/(kg·d)]。

• 替卡西林-克拉维酸：3.1 g，静脉注射，q4～6 h。

 随访

■ 进一步处理

入院指征

所有肠系膜缺血患者均应入院治疗。

出院指征

无。

■ 随访建议

外科会诊。

要点和误区

• 必须积极地寻找病因，明确诊断。

• 症状出现 24 h 后仍未明确诊断者，死亡率高达 80%。

• 在进行急诊手术干预之前，必须进行早期手术评估。

C

肠易激综合征 Irritable Bowel Syndrome

Scott A. Miller 倪沁赟 译

基础知识

■ 描述

• 腹痛或腹部不适伴大便习惯改变，而无其他病理症状的一种综合征。

• 患病率估计为 10%～20%。

■ 病因

• 病理生理不确定，但有多种可能性存在。

• 胃肠动力改变：

- 肠道敏感性增加(内脏痛觉过敏)：

◦ 正常胃肠道生理的过度反应。

• 黏膜炎症：

- 感染后：

◦ 细菌性肠炎后，10%的患者持续存在肠易激综合征症状。

• 黏膜淋巴细胞浸润。

• 小肠或粪便菌群改变。

• 可能是对食物的敏感性，但并不能被证明。

• 心理障碍：

- 更多有焦虑、躯体形式障碍和滥用药物的患者寻求治疗。

- 没有证据表明没有寻求治疗的患者精神疾病增加。

 诊断

■ 症状和体征

• 腹部疼痛：

- 吃饭诱发。

- 排便后缓解。

• 粪便次数改变。

• 粪便稠度改变。

• 腹胀。

• 透明外观或白色黏液便。

• 里急外重。

注意

• 有以下"报警"症状存在考虑进一步诊断性检查：

- 发病>50 岁。

- 急性或进行性症状。

- 夜间症状。

- 体重下降。

- 缺铁性贫血。

- 便血。

- 发热。

病史

• ROME Ⅲ诊断标准：最近 3 个月内每周至少 1 日的复发性腹痛同时与≥2 个以下表现相关：

- 疼痛加剧(与排便有关)。

- 粪便次数的变化。

- 粪便形状(外观)的变化。

• 其他符合肠易激综合征的表现：

- 腹胀或胀气。

- 粪便带黏液。

- 粪便习惯改变(紧张、紧迫感或感觉不完全排空)。

• 女性>男性，寻求治疗的患者中发病率较高。

体格检查

• 通常情况下体格检查正常。

• 可能会紧张。

• 可能触及乙状结肠或见明显乙状结肠线。

■ 基本检查

临床诊断：仔细询问病史至关重要。

■ 诊断检查与说明

实验室检查

• 通常无异常发现。

• 考虑实验室检查(排除其他病理)：

- 全血细胞计数，C 反应蛋白筛查 IBD。

- 门诊腹腔血清学检查。

- 门诊粪便钙卫蛋白水平检查。

影像学检查

仅在排除急诊病理情况下需要。

诊断步骤/外科

行结肠镜或乙状结肠镜检查来选择患者(门诊)。

■ 鉴别诊断

• 腹腔疾病。

• 炎症性肠病：

- 溃疡性结肠炎和直肠炎。

- 克罗恩病。

• 感染性肠炎。

• 小肠细菌过度生长。

• 乳糖不耐受。

• 大肠癌。

• 憩室病。

• 胆道疾病。

• 糖尿病性胃轻瘫。

• 胰腺炎。

• 甲状腺功能异常。

• 梗阻。
• 消化性溃疡。
• 急性间歇性卟啉病。

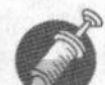

治疗

院前

无特殊治疗需要。

初步稳定/治疗

• 对症治疗。
• 疼痛控制。
• 如果脱水给予补液。

急诊治疗/程序

• 移情治疗方法：
- 医患关系是重要的。
• 锻炼：
- 改善胃排空和便秘。
• 饮食：
- 增加可溶性纤维(洋车前子、麸皮)。
- 经验上考虑排除面筋或乳糖饮食。
- 不包括产气食品。
- 低 FODMAP(核果、豆类、乳糖等中存在的可发酵糖)。
• 便秘症状：
- 高纤维饮食，补充纤维素。
- 渗透性泻药。
- 鲁比前列酮、利那洛特和普卡那肽增加肠道分泌，缩短存留时间。
• 腹泻症状：
- 止泻药(数据显示疗效有限)。
- 依洛沙多林受体。
- 阿洛司琼(严重 IBS－D 对初始治疗无反应)，可引起便秘和缺血性结肠炎。需要特殊的处方权。
• 腹痛和腹胀：
- 止痉药如山楂碱、双环胺甚至薄荷油可能在短期内有用。
- 利福昔明是一种最低限度吸收的抗生素，对 IBS 无便秘有一定疗效。
- 双歧杆菌和乳酸杆菌益生菌可能有好处。
- 抗抑郁药可能有帮助。TCA 具有抗胆碱能作用和缓慢的肠道转运。它们显示出了一些好处。包括 SSRI 在内的其他抗抑郁药的益处还不清楚。
• 心理疗法可能有效。

药物治疗

一线用药

• 双环胺：10～20 mg，口服，q6 h。
• 莨菪碱：0.125～0.25 mg，口服。
• 渗透性泻药。
• 止泻药。

二线用药

• 阿米替林：25 mg，口服，睡前。
• 利福昔明：550 mg，口服，每日 3 次，持续 14 日。
• 鲁比前列酮：8 μg，口服，每日 2 次。
• 利那洛肽：290 μg，口服，每日 1 次。
• 艾鲁沙多林：100 mg，每日 1 次。
• 双歧杆菌或乳酸菌益生菌。

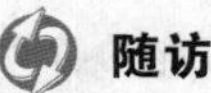

随访

进一步处理

入院指征

疑似但诊断不明显的急腹症。

出院指征

几乎所有患者都可以按门诊患者处理。

转诊问题

某些患者最好去胃肠道或精神科转诊。

随访建议

初级保健医师随访时建立一种治疗的医患关系更重要。

要点和误区

• 注意其他紧急病理表现。
• 肠易激综合征是常见的，所以很多腹部的基本检查都需要在急诊完成。

成骨不全症

Stephen R. Hayden 朱妍 译

基础知识

描述

• 前胶原氨基酸遗传序列异常。
• “脆性骨病”。
• 骨矿质不足和不完全骨化导致骨脆弱。
• 发病率为 1/20 000 活产儿。
• 异常骨胶原不同程度地影响所有结缔组织。
• 不同时期表现不同：
- 大多数病例在儿童期有骨折，在随后的青春期和成年早期不发病。

病因

• 前胶原缺陷导致骨质和结缔组织基质异常。
• 前胶原蛋白链上不同部位的缺陷导致更严重的表现。
• 缺陷有遗传性，不管是常染色体隐性遗传(一般较温和)还是常染色体显性遗传(更严重)。
• 致死病例涉及散发或新的基因突发。
• Ehlers-Danlos 综合征涉及同一前胶原蛋白在不同位置的突变。

儿科注意事项

• 大部分病例在儿童时期有病理性骨折。
• 多发性骨折开始经常被认为是非意外创伤，但也应该考虑病理性骨折的可能。

诊断

症状和体征

• 导致骨骼脆性的多发性遗传缺陷：
- 通常与其他结缔组织异常有关。
• 如果无明显诱因儿童发生疑似骨折或有多发性骨折史，应考虑此诊断。
• 注意社会因素，考虑非意外损伤的可能性。
• 骨骼：
- 多次复发性骨折(尤其是长骨)是本病的特征。
- 最常见的肱骨横断骨折。
- 骨折可能在出生时就存在或在老年复发。
- 缩短或弯曲的肢体、漏斗胸、弯曲的长骨、脊柱压缩性骨折、脊柱侧弯、脊柱后凸和颅骨变形。
- 所有骨骼都会受不同程度的影响(见影像学及特殊检查)。

• 眼睛：
- 蓝色巩膜是本病的另一特征。
- 未见报道合并视力下降。
• 耳：
- 听力减退通常开始于青春期。
- >90%的患者到 30 岁左右会出现不同程度的缺陷。
- 听力减退一般为感音神经性，但已证实可能有中耳畸形。
- 诊断难点是应该高度怀疑可能的听力障碍。
• 其他：
- 牙齿变色、脆弱和形态异常。
- 几个 Ehlers-Danlos 综合征的特征：
◦ 关节松动。
◦ 瓣膜问题。
◦ 血管异常。
• 甲状腺异常。
• 极端的病例可能导致新生儿死亡。

■ 基本检查

• 诊断通常需结合临床及影像学检查。
• 反复骨折史或有无明显原因的骨折。
• 彻底检查其他压痛点，评估眼睛、牙齿和关节对诊断有重要意义。
• 仔细检查骨折远端神经血管的状态。

■ 诊断检查与说明

实验室检查

• 评估是否存在代谢紊乱，如甲状旁腺功能亢进症、维生素 C 或维生素 D 的不足、钙/磷酸盐异常。
• 某些亚型可能有升高的血清碱性磷酸酶水平或高钙尿。
• DNA 检测适用于家族分析、产前检查和遗传咨询。
• 组织活检存在争议，但对鉴别肿瘤可能有帮助。

影像学检查

• 骨折部位的 X 线片：
- 可能显示骨质减少(通常较轻微)。
- 皱巴巴的长骨("手风琴股骨")。
- 变形部位的不完全骨化。
• 骨骼检查是必需的，尤其是儿童。
• 颅骨摄片可能显示不规则骨化的沃姆现象。
• 长骨两端爆米花样沉积是预后不良的表现。
• 老年患者有必要在门诊进行正规的听力测试。

■ 鉴别诊断

• 儿童非意外创伤。
• Ehlers-Danlos 综合征。
• 低磷酸酯酶症。
• 软骨发育不全。
• 坏血病(维生素 C 缺乏症)。
• 先天性梅毒。
• 腹腔疾病。

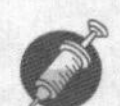

治疗

■ 院前

医务人员应取得关于能够指向病理性骨折还是非意外损伤的机制或社会因素信息。

■ 初步稳定/治疗

• 按指示进行气道管理和复苏。
• 骨折固定、夹板。

■ 急诊治疗/程序

• 具体骨折的处理由骨折类型和受伤部位决定。
• 需要牵引或手术固定者请骨科会诊。
• 目前对成骨发育不良无特殊治疗。
• 预防骨折的双膦酸盐治疗应由私人医生或顾问启动。

■ 药物治疗

• 按说明使用止痛药物。
• 老年妇女使用钙剂(1～1.5 g/d)或雌激素替代品(0.625 mg/d)可能会获益。

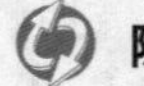

随访

■ 进一步处理

入院指征

• 多发伤或需要手术固定骨折者需入院治疗。
• 儿科患者可能需要入院检查非意外损伤的可能性。

出院指征

• 如果患者仅单部位骨折且能提供合适的家庭资源可在门诊治疗。
• 大部分患者出院后应该去骨科医师和家庭医师随访。

转诊问题

• 急性损伤促使患者到骨科复诊。
• 多部位或不同时间发生骨折，需考虑非意外损伤，应立即会诊或到当地医院就诊。

■ 随访建议

• 随访通常由急性外伤驱动。
• 家庭医师随访时应该制定鼓励治疗和监测疾病的方案。

要点和误区

• 照顾这些患者最大的挑战是辨别病理性骨折、成骨发育不良及非意外损伤。有任何疑问，应该立即在当地医院咨询或复诊。
• 儿童成骨发育不良的患者比其他患者疼痛较轻。
• 呼吸道感染的易感性。

C

痴呆 Dementia

Gabriel Wardi · Vaishal M. Tolia 许磊 译

基础知识

■ 描述

• 定义：涉及一个或多个认知领域(语言、记忆、复杂注意力、感知运动、社会认知)进行性恶化的临床综合征，由于大脑皮质功能的改变，严重到足以干扰日常生活活动和独立性。
• 慢性进行性器质性脑综合征。
• 超过 50 种不同的原因。
• 最常见的病因是阿尔茨海默病(60%～80%的病例)，其次是血管性痴呆、混合性痴呆、路易体痴呆。
• 年龄在 65～85 岁的人群中有 5%～16%的人罹患，85 岁以上的人群中有 30%～

40%的人罹患。

• 在过去的几十年里，痴呆的发病率有所下降，但全世界痴呆患者的绝对数有所上升。

• 以认知功能逐渐下降为特点的：

- 一般会在几年的时间里进展。
- 过程变化很大，持续时间从几个月到几年不等。
- 迅速下降表明其他原因，或罕见的快速发病的痴呆原因（朊病毒病、进行性核上性麻痹）。

• 可变遗传性：

- 阿尔茨海默病患者一级亲属患阿尔茨海默病的风险增加。
- 载脂蛋白 EA 是唯一患有晚发性阿尔茨海默病的成熟突变。

■ **病因**

• 原发性痴呆：

- 皮质（阿尔茨海默病、额颞老年痴呆症）。
- 皮质下（亨廷顿病、帕金森病、进行性核上性麻痹）。

• 继发性痴呆：

- 脑血管疾病（多发梗死性痴呆）。
- 毒性、新陈代谢、营养失调。
- 朊病毒病（克雅病或牛海绵状脑病及其变种）。
- 感染性因素（HIV 感染、梅毒、脑炎）。
- 血管炎（系统性红斑狼疮、血栓性血小板减少性紫癜）。
- 创伤性（慢性硬膜下血肿、拳击性痴呆、慢性创伤性脑病）。
- 器质性（常压性脑积水、脑肿块）。
- 宾斯旺格病。

• 可逆性原因（～15%）包括常压脑积水、药物、颅内肿块和酒精滥用综合征。

• 假性痴呆：

- 老年抑郁症可出现痴呆症样症状。
- 常见于轻度痴呆患者，查找症状持续时间短的精确事件。
- 一般有精神疾病史，重点在经历失败事件和残疾的人。

诊断

■ **症状和体征**

• 潜伏性发作，最初的主诉是焦虑、抑郁、沮丧、健忘增加。

• 通常在“轻度认知损害”之前，这是一种介于正常衰老和符合痴呆症标准的认知功能的中间状态。

• 可分为 3 类：

- 早期：注意力不集中，记忆障碍，困难复杂的任务，社交退缩。
- 中等：主要表现为记忆困难，日常生活活动时需要援助。
- 严重：说话或沟通能力极低，进食困难，精神运动技能丧失。

• 诊断标准（由美国精神病学协会，DSM-5）：

- 多种认知障碍发展，表现为两种：
  ◦ 记忆力减退。
  ◦ 一个（或更多）以下的认知障碍：失语、失用、失认、干扰执行功能。
- 认知缺失影响日常活动的自主性。
- 谵妄时不会发生认知缺陷。
- 认知缺陷不能用其他精神疾病解释。

病史

• 必须包括来自家人和朋友的供述。

• 药物的完整列表。

• 共患疾病。

• 类似的行为在此之前的病史。

• 发生和进展。

• 考虑使用蒙特利尔认知评估，心理状况短期测试（替代简易精神状态检查）。

体格检查

完全彻底的身体检查：

• 头部到足趾的评估，包括所有的器官系统。

• 细致的神经系统检查：

- 精神状态评估。
- 脑神经。
- 反射。
- 运动、感觉、小脑及步态。
- 重要的是找出“基线”情况并评估衰退情况。

■ **基本检查**

• 痴呆的诊断通常由急诊室外随访患者有一段时间的医师做出。

• 必须消除急性可逆或加重因素，如谵妄。

• 检查的程度与病史和疾病的过程相关：

- 对新诊断的广泛评估。
- 对于突然变化痴呆的直接评估。
- 对病情稳定的有限评估。

• 必须能够识别老年痴呆症可逆因素的症状和体征。

■ **诊断检查与说明**

实验室检查

• 评估的程度取决于患者病情和疑似病因。

• 新发痴呆或突然恶化应该及时评估应激事件或感染情况：

- CBC。
- ESR/CRP。
- CMP。
- 氨。
- 尿液分析。
- 毒理学检查。
- 甲状腺刺激激素。
- 维生素 B_{12} 水平。
- 梅毒血清学（RPR）。
- HIV。
- 血培养，如果存在发热。
- 尿培养，如果存在发热。
- 抗核抗体，如果怀疑 SLE。

• 确诊病情稳定：研究可以不需要。

影像学检查

• 已确诊的老年痴呆症患者发生突然加重的时候应考虑：

- X 线胸片，如果感染考虑。
- 头颅 CT，没有做静脉造影。
- 脑电图，如果怀疑癫痫。
- 脑 MRI/MRA 在选定的情况下。

• 确诊病情稳定：研究可以不需要。

诊断步骤/外科

• 腰椎穿刺和脑脊液分析，梅毒血清学，特别是年龄<55 岁患者。

• 脑电图，如果怀疑癫痫发作。

■ **鉴别诊断**

• 抑郁（最常需鉴别的疾病，常伴随痴呆）。

• 毒性，代谢，营养异常：

- 毒品，镇静剂，安眠药。
- 酒精（乙醇）。
- 重金属。
- 脱水。
- 电解质紊乱。

• 假性痴呆。

• 谵妄。

• 衰老的老化。

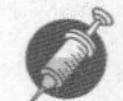

治疗

■ **院前**

• 从朋友、家人中获得病史。

• 提供患者和人员的安全。

• 控制焦虑。

• 专注于合并症。

• 治疗急性毒性和代谢性疾病：

- 低血糖。
- 低温。
- 热疗。

■ 初步稳定/治疗

- 确保有足够的空气流通。
- 输入氧气,如果缺氧。
- 确保生命体征正常。
- 建立静脉通路,如果需要。
- 对于烦躁的患者,保证患者和人员安全。

■ 急诊治疗/程序

- 在积极治疗之前,与患者、代理人及高级专家一起探讨治疗目标。
- 必须明确,如果患者出现急性精神状态的改变。
- 考虑全面的鉴别诊断,评估和正确对待:
- 治疗低血糖,口服或静脉补充葡萄糖。
- 如果低温给予复温。
- 如果高温给予退热。
- 静脉输液治疗脱水。
- 纠正电解质异常。
- 管理抗生素控制感染:
  ○ 尿路感染和肺炎最常见的隐匿性感染:寻找伤口和压疮。
- 治疗癫痫:
- 51%的痴呆患者表现出易怒的迹象,34%出现幻觉;在急诊科,躁动更常见,需要适当的治疗。
- 镇静激动:
- 开始用低剂量,并根据需要增加以获得满意的临床效果。
- 抗精神病药:氟哌啶醇、利培酮、喹硫平、奥氮平。
- 避免使用苯二氮䓬类。
- 如果化学镇静效果不佳实行软约束。
- 尝试限制药物的数量:
- 降低毒性的可能性。
- 减少药物与药物之间作用的可能性。
- 如果激动不是一个问题,杜绝一切镇静催眠药。
- 运用BEERS标准,在老年人中,尽量减少潜在副作用药物的使用。
- 治疗抑郁症。

■ 药物治疗

- 任何针对痴呆症的药物的开始或停止,都应与患者的初始治疗医师一起进行。
- 神经精神症状的控制应包括社会、环境和心理,一旦这些方法不能控制症状,就应使用药物。
- 常用到治疗阿尔茨海默病的药物:
- 多奈哌齐:5~10 mg,口服,在睡前。
- 卡巴拉汀:1.5~6 mg,口服,每日2次。
- 加兰他敏:4~12 mg,口服,每日2次。
- 以上3种抗胆碱能药物没有明确的剂量,注意监测副作用,包括恶、呕吐、腹泻。
- 美金刚(NMDA受体拮抗剂),对于那些抗胆碱能药物反应不佳的:5 mg(口服,每日4次)到10 mg(口服,每日2次)。
- 效果温和,最好一开始就服用,由主要提供者改变。
- 大量的临床试验显示不一致或负作用的抗炎剂、雌激素,他汀类药物对老年痴呆症较好。
- 抗抑郁药:先从最低剂量开始使用:
- 过度镇静的问题。
- 可能恶化老年痴呆症。
- 对无法入睡的患者有用。
- 镇静剂:始终以最低剂量开始。
- 氟哌啶醇:0.5~2 mg,口服,每日2次;先从最低剂量开始,0.5~2.5 mg,肌内注射或静脉给药,如果需要快速起效。
- 喹硫平:25~50 mg,口服,每日1次,如果需要可以加量。
- 奥氮平:2.5~5 mg,每日1次,可以肌内注射以快速控制谵妄。
- 利培酮:0.5~2 mg,口服,每日2次;从最低剂量开始。
- 纳洛酮:0.4~2 mg,静脉推注。

随访

■ 进一步处理

入院指征

- 生命体征不稳定。
- 重大合并症,需要肠外药物治疗:
- 肺炎。
- 尿路感染(UTI)。
- 脱水和严重电解质紊乱。
- 不确定的诊断需要评估和管理不适合门诊患者。
- 不充足家庭支持并且不能从急诊安排合适的位置。
- 关注老年人受虐待和忽视的情况。

出院指征

- 生命体征平稳。
- 没有显著不稳定合并症。
- 安全诊断或排除危及生命的器质性病变。
- 充足的家庭支持,尽力的监护。
- 可靠地获得后续治疗。

转诊问题

- 患者可能需要援助、交通、财务状况等。
- 患者有其他合并症需转诊到合适的专家。

■ 随访建议

- 初级卫生保健。
- 老年医学。
- 精神科医师。
- 神经病学专家。

要点和误区

- 痴呆症的主要特点是缓慢的,稳定进展的,而且很少在急诊室被诊断:
- 一定要和谵妄区分开来。
- 患者痴呆症样症状,需重点考虑抑郁症和药物的副作用,作为可逆的原因。
- 痴呆症状可以波动,作为疾病和合并症治疗的结果。
- 护理人员的倦怠和对精神病患者的忽视是真实存在的,如果考虑到这些因素应予以解决。
- 50%的晚期痴呆患者在死亡后2周内被诊断为肺炎。
- 90%的医疗保健代理人表明,晚期痴呆患者护理的首要目标是安慰。

出血热 Hemorrhagic Fever

Fraser C. Mackay 陈奇通 译

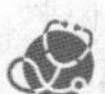

基础知识

描述

• 病毒性出血热(VHF)是由一组不同的病毒引起的。

• 初期阶段类似流感样疾病,而后期阶段(出血性阶段和恢复期)包括相当数量的危重患者。后期发展为多系统器官功能障碍、休克和死亡。大多数 VHF 在美国大部分地区不是地方病,没有快速诊断检查;诊断需要高度的怀疑指数和有针对性的详细病史。

病因

• 重要的高频诱因:

- 汉坦病毒科(HV):啮齿动物宿主、啮齿动物喷雾状排泄物(美国西南部):
  ◦ 肾综合征出血热。
  ◦ 汉坦病毒肺综合征。
- 丝状病毒:果蝠宿主,传播方式不明(撒哈拉以南非洲):
  ◦ 埃博拉病毒。
  ◦ 马尔堡出血热。
- 沙粒病毒:啮齿动物宿主、啮齿动物喷雾状排泄物(撒哈拉以南非洲):
  ◦ 拉沙热。
  ◦ 南美出血热。
- 黄病毒:人类宿主,通过蚊子(热带地区,越来越多地在全世界范围内出现)传播:
  ◦ 登革热(最常见病因)。
  ◦ 黄热病。
- 布尼亚病毒科:啮齿动物宿主,通过蜱或蚊子传播(欧洲、南亚、非洲)传播:
  ◦ 裂谷热。
  ◦ 克里米亚-刚果出血热(CCHF)。

• 在特定地理区域具有人畜共患生命周期的 RNA 病毒。

病理生理

• VHF 可以导致血管内皮损伤,增加血管通透性,出血,甚至休克。

• VHF 的休克阶段属于低血容量性和分布性休克,并且很难被逆转。低血压可以迅速发生与发展,一般这意味着高死亡率。

• 弥散性血管内凝血(DIC)可能是马尔堡出血热和 CCHF 的固定阶段,但很少出现在沙粒病毒感染病例中。

• 登革热是免疫介导的,通常是继发性感染的结果。这也是 VHF 最常见的原因。

• 短潜伏期(2～21 日)。

诊断

症状和体征

• 最普遍的症状(>50%):
- 急性发热。
- 乏力。
- 头痛。
- 恶心与呕吐。
- 面红。
- 腹泻(不含血)。
- 腹痛。
- 肌肉痛。

• 较少见症状(<30%):
- 牙龈出血。
- 结膜感染及出血。
- 瘀点。
- 呕血。
- 黑便。
- 鼻出血。
- 瘀斑。

• 出血性表现超过 3 日为疾病:
- 皮肤、静脉部位、牙龈、鼻、肺、胃肠道或子宫。
- 弥漫性肺泡出血或 ARDS。
- 在 CCHF、拉沙热、马尔堡出血热、埃博拉出血热、汉坦病毒肺综合征更常见。

• 皮疹:
- 马尔堡出血热和埃博拉出血热:在 5～7 日暴发非瘙痒的向心形丘疹、红斑,然后合并成为边界清楚的斑疹,一般考虑为出血热。
- 黄热病:黄疸。
- 登革热:轻压躯干的红色斑丘疹,可使颜色变白(经常处于下肢动脉)。

• 血流动力学衰竭,休克,惊厥,昏迷,死亡:
- 疾病的晚期,常为不可逆。

病史

• 曾到过疾病流行地区。

• 在密闭的生活空间/空气中接触禽畜或害虫。

• 曾接触相关疾病。

• 疾病聚集发生时应考虑生物武器攻击或者疾病暴发。

体格检查

• 对医疗工作者的保护:
- 普遍的血液和身体防护措施。

• 生命体征:监测血压,发热,心动过速。
- 脉压小(<20 mmHg)多提示即将发生心血管衰竭。

• 出血(见症状和体征)。

• 皮疹(见症状和体征)。

• 右上腹柔软或肝大:
- 肝炎。

• 不定肺音。

基本检查

• 对于旅行者,将检查重点放在与其他急性发热疾病的区别上。

• 重视肺部损害,因为它往往提示全身性疾病和较差预后。

• 当出现患者数量不同寻常时应考虑生物攻击的可能。

• 根据病史查明潜在的病原体:
- 包括最近的旅游、患病或其他暴露。
- 通常患者并没有意识到动物接触史。

诊断检查与说明

实验室检查

• 血液、痰、粪便、尿液培养。

• 疟疾涂片。

• CBC:
- 可能白细胞增多、白细胞减少、血小板减少或全血细胞减少。
- 血小板减少或全血细胞减少通常预示病程不良。
- 血液浓缩应提示汉坦病毒感染,可提示严重血容量不足。

• 电解质、尿素氮、肌酐及血糖水平:
- 急性肾损伤和急性肾小管坏死常见于重症。

• 肝功能检查:
- 肝脏受累较常见,但黄疸多在黄热病中出现。

• 血型鉴定和抗体筛查、凝血酶原时间、部分促凝血酶原时间及 D-二聚体试验:
- 凝血功能障碍和 DIC(多见于 CCHF、埃博拉出血热及马尔堡出血热)。

• 妊娠试验。

• 特殊实验室检查:

C

- 在一些专业实验室中(生物安全水平 4 级),明确的诊断需要根据病毒分离培养、RT-PCR 或者免疫组织化学结果。
- 与疾病预防控制中心协调。
- 厚薄涂片,帮助与疟疾区分。

影像学检查

胸部 X 线检查、头颅和腹部 CT:

- 患者隔离是至关重要的。CT 检查时考虑暴露风险。
- 检查肺部病变。
- 颅内和腹腔内出血。

诊断步骤/外科

在一些特殊实验室可对血清和唾液进行 RT-PCR 分析。

C

鉴别诊断

- 疟疾:
- 关注发热的旅行者。
- 登革热:
- 旅行中常见发热。
- 立克次体:
- 落基山斑疹热。
- 斑疹伤寒。
- 细菌性:
- 脑膜炎球菌血症。
- 脓毒血症。
- 肠出血性大肠杆菌(大肠埃希菌 O157:H7)。
- 系统性疾病:
- 白血病。
- 血栓性血小板减少性紫癜(TTP)、特发性血小板减少性紫癜(ITTP)。
- 蝮蛇咬伤。

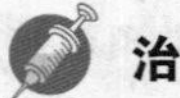

治疗

院前

- 早期发现 VHF(自然或生物攻击是控制疫情的关键)。向疾病预防控制中心及时报告。
- 大部分的病例来源于曾因旅游去过或与病毒流行区域的人接触过的患者。

初步稳定/治疗

- 支持治疗。
- 全面的血液和身体防护措施。
- 将患者隔离。
- 在进行吸气引液、导尿和伤口更换敷料时穿戴防护衣及 HEPA 材质口罩,从而减少在气溶胶中的暴露。
- 休克状态:
- 通常低血容量是继发性的大量胃肠道丢失。
- 分布性休克也经常发生。
- 失血性休克很少见。

急诊治疗/程序

- 经验性广谱抗生素治疗类似于脓毒症休克疗法和抗疟方案,直到获得明确诊断:
- 对严重疾病开始服用青蒿素。
- 经验性广谱抗生素治疗类似败血性休克的综合征。
- 出血通常较轻,威胁生命的大出血罕见:
- 结果表明,出血可以通过输注血液、血小板、凝血因子等方法控制。
- 扩容,液体支持:
- 口服补液盐是那些能够口服液体的首选。
- 乳酸林格液和晶体液是首选的静脉输入晶体液。
- 肺水肿。
- 重复注射 500~1000 ml 晶体液,而不是大量,在前 10~12 h 总剂量在 30~40 ml/kg 及以下。
- 缩血管药物:
- 去甲肾上腺素,肾上腺素首选用于难治性休克。
- 在出现症状的第 1 周内输血免疫血浆(恢复期血浆疗法)治疗南美出血热。
- 若怀疑程度高,可考虑早期传染病或危重症医学咨询。

药物治疗

- 利巴韦林(WHO 2006 年建议):
- 静脉输注负荷剂量 33 mg/kg,接着按 16 mg/kg, q6 h,治疗 4 日;然后 8 mg/kg 治疗 3 日。
- 预防用量为 500 mg,口服,q6 h,持续 1 周。
- 疫苗:
- 黄热病可广泛使用。
- 南美出血热、裂谷热、汉坦病毒、登革热、埃博拉出血热和马尔堡出血热正在开发中。
- 其他的药物治疗仍在调查研究:
- S-腺苷高半胱氨酸水解酶的核苷类似物抑制剂可以抑制 Ebola 在鼠体内的复制。
- Zidampidine:一种 AZT 的衍生物,可以提高被拉沙病毒感染鼠的存活率。

一线用药

- 血流动力学支持。
- 利巴韦林。
- 抗疟疾药物。

二线用药

在疫苗和抗病毒药物实验研究中出现职业暴露而导致的所有疑似病例,都应及时联系疾病预防控制中心。

随访

进一步处理

入院指征

VHF 的可疑病例,尤其是那些怀疑多系统损伤的病例。

- 隔离须知。
- 休克和有多器官功能衰竭的患者需收入 ICU。

出院指征

没有具体指征,如果怀疑 VHF,患者必须被隔离同时通知当地疾病预防控制中心。

随访建议

考虑员工与患者的接触过程中的职业暴露问题,包括疫苗和抗病毒药物。及时与当地疾病预防控制中心联系。

要点和误区

- 非常谨慎地对待容量复苏。
- 血液浓缩和肺部受累是危险信号。
- 当处理一名从疾病流行区域来的患者时,应考虑出血性热的可能。
- 建立全面的防护和隔离措施,从而减少疾病的传播。
- 任何可疑病例请及时与疾病预防控制中心联系。

川崎病 Kawasaki Disease

Adam Z. Barkin 何超 段立伟 译

 基础知识

描述

- 急性炎症累及多个器官。
- 发达国家儿童心脏病的主要病因。
- 引起中等关节的严重血管炎。
- 心脏后遗症：
  - 冠状动脉动脉瘤：治愈后会留有发绀的后遗症。
  - 巨大动脉瘤：可能会破裂。
  - 心肌病。
  - 心包炎。
- 阶段：
  - 急性(持续 1～2 周)：
    - 发热。
    - 口腔黏膜红斑。
    - 结膜炎。
    - 手足红斑或水肿。
    - 颈腺病。
    - 无菌性腹膜炎。
    - 肝功能障碍。
    - 腹泻。
    - 心肌病。
    - 心包积液(20%～40%)。
    - 超声心动图检查(ECHO)未检出动脉瘤。
  - 亚急性(发热、皮疹、淋巴结病持续 4 周)：
    - 神经性厌食。
    - 易怒。
    - 手足脱屑。
    - 血小板增多症。
    - 冠状动脉动脉瘤(未治疗患者中发生率在 20%)。
    - 猝死的危险最高。
  - 康复阶段(一般 6～8 周)：
    - 临床症状消失。
    - 红细胞沉降率恢复正常。
  - 流行病学：
    - 80%的病例发生在小于 4 岁的儿童中，高峰期在 1～2 岁，但是很少在 3 个月以下的儿童中发生。
    - 也有成人的病例被报道过。
    - 亚洲人高发。
    - 男性多于女性，1.5∶1。
- 遗传学：
  - 有遗传倾向。
- 对传统治疗方案无疗效的危险因素(发生率在 10%～15%)：
  - 分叶核计数增高。
  - 血清白蛋白水平低。
  - 超声检查发现异常回声。
- 发生冠状动脉动脉瘤的危险因素：
  - 极端的年龄。
  - 男性。
  - 治疗后出现持续高热。
  - 发热时间长。
  - 诊断发生延误。
  - 白细胞计数或分叶核计数增高。
  - 低血细胞比容。
  - 红细胞沉降率或 C 反应蛋白的显著增高。

病因

- 至今未知，一直认为是以感染为基础的一种疾病，流行病学发现在冬季或初春病例数目会增多。
- 目前的理论：
  - 由于感染所引发的免疫系统的激活。
  - 存在个体的遗传易感性。
  - 对于某些人种存在更高的发病率，如亚洲人对该病更易感。

诊断

- 传统诊断标准：
  - 持续 5 日的发热和以下 5 点中得 4 项：
    - 细菌性结膜感染。
    - 口腔黏膜的变化。
    - 多形性红斑皮疹。
    - 手足改变——肿胀、红斑、脱屑。
    - 颈部淋巴结病变大小>1.5 cm。
    - 如果符合以上≥4 个，以及合并发热 4 日，也可诊断为川崎病。
- 一些非典型性的病例可能不满足诊断标准：
  - 发热持续 5 日以上合并 2～3 项诊断标准并且红细胞沉降率>40 mm/h，C 反应蛋白>3 mg/L。
  - 婴儿发热≥7 日并且红细胞沉降率>40 mm/h，C 反应蛋白>3 mg/L。
  - 如果满足以下 3 项以上可诊断为不完全性川崎病：
    - 白蛋白<3 g/dl。
    - 贫血。
    - ALT 升高。
    - 白细胞计数>15 000/mm^3。
    - 尿检高倍视野下发现 10 个以上白细胞。
    - 7 日后检查血小板>45 000/mm^3。
    - 超声心动图提示阳性。

症状和体征

- 体温>38.5℃并且持续 5 日以上：
  - 突然出现并且持续 2 周以上。
- 心脏：
  - 呼吸短促。
  - 胸痛。
- 五官：
  - 眼睛：
    - 结膜炎。
    - 畏光。
  - 口腔：
    - 红斑。
    - 口唇干燥或裂缝。
- 皮肤红疹。
- 骨骼：
  - 关节痛或关节炎。
- 神经：
  - 四肢末端刺激感。
- 消化系统：
  - 腹泻。
  - 恶心。
  - 腹痛。

体格检查

- 心脏：
  - 充血性心力衰竭。
  - 心包炎证据。
    - 心包摩擦感。
  - 瓣膜病。
    - 心脏杂音。
- 五官：
  - 眼部：
    - 对称性的结膜炎和眼部渗出。
    - 球结膜比睑结膜更易受累。
    - 一般 2 日内出现高热并持续 1～2 周。
    - 畏光，刺激感，葡萄膜炎。
  - 口腔：
    - 红斑，口唇干燥、裂开，草莓舌，咽喉部红斑。
  - 淋巴：
    - 颈部淋巴结病(结节大小>1.5 cm)。
- 神经：
  - 脑膜刺激。

- 脑膜炎。
• 皮肤:
- 主要位于躯干部的红斑。
- 表现为斑丘疹、猩红热样斑疹或类似红皮病样的多形性红斑。
- 手足部的变化:红疹、肿胀(急性期),不愿负重。
- 疾病 2～3 周后在手指、足趾处出现的脱屑(亚急性期表现)。
• 泌尿系统:
- 尿道炎。
- 尿道口炎症。
• 消化系统:
- 胆囊积水。

C

基本检查

在发热合并皮肤红疹的儿童中要考虑此病。

诊断检查与说明

实验室检查

• 全血细胞计数:
- 白细胞一般会升高并且伴有急性期的核左移现象。
- 正细胞性贫血。
- 1 周后出现血小板增多症。
- 少见白细胞减少或血小板减少症。
◦ 一般出于感染的原因。
◦ 血小板减少症是发生冠状动脉疾病的危险因素。
• 尿液分析:
- 无菌性脓尿。
- 蛋白尿。
• 红细胞沉降率从初发第 1 日开始升高,一直持续 4～6 周。
• C 反应蛋白升高。
• 脑脊液细胞增多。
• 培养:血、尿、脑脊液、喉部的细菌性检查阴性。
• 转氨酶和胆红素升高。
• 低钠血症。
• 低蛋白血症。

影像学检查

• 超声评估冠状动脉动脉瘤:
- 以急性期的检查结果为标准。
- 2～3 周检查 1 次。
- 6～8 周检查 1 次。
• 胸部 X 线检查。

鉴别诊断

• 感染:
- 腺病毒。
- 肠病毒。
- 麻疹病毒。
- EB 病毒。
- 风疹病毒。
- 流感病毒
• 细菌感染:
- 猩红热(对青霉素的反应迅速,良好)。
- 葡萄球菌皮肤烫伤样综合征。
- 立克次体病,包括落基山斑疹热和细螺旋体病。
- 颈部淋巴腺炎。
• 免疫介导疾病:
- Stevens-Johnson 综合征。
- 多形性红斑。
- 血清病。
- 结缔组织病(如狼疮)。
- 其他形式的血管炎。

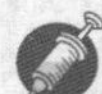

治疗

院前

• ABC 管理。
• 供氧。

初步稳定/治疗

心肺复苏要侧重心血管系统复苏。

急诊治疗/程序

• 静脉输注 γ 球蛋白和阿司匹林:
- 一般不需要监测体内水杨酸浓度,因为机体对于水杨酸的吸收减少而排除增多。
• 在病程的第一个 10 日内实施有效地治疗能够将心脏后遗症从 20%～25% 降低至 2%～4%。
• 心内科会诊。
• 在成人中要注意治疗心肌梗死。

药物治疗

一线用药

• 静脉注射用免疫球蛋白:2 g/kg 持续使用 10～12 h;针对病情持续(48～72 h 及以上)或复发性发热的患者治疗需适当延长时间。
- 需要进行密切的心电监护。
- 需要在病程的第一个 10 日内开始实施。
- 2 倍剂量后有 3%～4%的失败率。
• 阿司匹林:80～100 mg/kg 口服,每 6 h 给药一次直到病程的第 14 日或退热;若口服 3～5 mg/kg 剂量需要持续 6～8 周。24 h 剂量不要超过 4 g(儿童 24 h 剂量小于 120 mg)。
- 抗感染。
- 抗血小板。
- 加强静脉免疫球蛋白的作用。
- 在同时给予静脉免疫球蛋白的治疗下能后降低动脉瘤的发生率。
- 在急性期和亚急性期可以选择剂量 30 mg/kg。

二线用药

对 2 倍剂量的静脉注射用免疫球蛋白无效的情况下使用二线治疗方案。
• 糖皮质激素:
- 甲泼尼龙 30 mg/kg,持续 1～3 日。
- 与静脉注射用免疫球蛋白合用能够改善患者预后。
- 其他还可以考虑:
◦ 英夫利昔。
◦ 环孢素。
◦ 甲氨蝶呤。

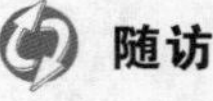

随访

进一步处理

入院指征

• 满足川崎病全部诊断标准的患者。
• 即使不完全满足川崎病诊断标准的患者但是中毒症状明显的患者。

出院指征

• 儿童的毒性症状消失,不再满足诊断标准。
• 出院后需要进行密切的随访。

随访建议

所有患者需要进行心内科随访。

要点和误区

• 使用合理地诊断和治疗后能够减少 95% 的动脉瘤的发生。
• 阿司匹林和静脉用免疫球蛋白是主要的治疗方案,如果在开始发热的 10 日内治疗,临床症状可以缓解 80%～90%。
• 对于因发热反复就诊的儿童患者应该考虑本病。
• 2 次静脉使用免疫球蛋白治疗失败的患者,需要进行严格的激素治疗。
• 有心肌梗死病史的年轻成人存在高患病率。

传染性红斑 Erythema infectiosum

Benjamin S. Heavrin 单怡 译

基础知识

描述

- 特征性病毒疹又称第五病：
  - 第五常见的儿童皮疹。
  - 麻疹(第一)、猩红热(第二)、风疹(第三)、杜克病(第四)、红疹(第六)。
- 常见症状：
  - 病毒性感冒。
  - 随后是面颊部皮疹。
  - 接下来出现弥漫性网状皮疹±关节病。
- 最常见于小于 14 岁的学龄儿童。
- 通常有自限性的持久免疫。
- 少数先天性贫血或免疫抑制的患者出现并发症和慢性病例。
- 妊娠合并感染时胎儿可能出现严重并发症。
- 可能与脑病、癫痫、脑膜炎、心肌炎、扩张型心肌病、自身免疫性肝炎、过敏性紫癜、特发性血小板减少性紫癜有关。

病因

- 由人类细小病毒 B19 引起，为小的单链 DNA 病毒：
  - 感染人红系祖细胞，抑制红细胞生成。
- 晚冬和春季最好发。
- 通过呼吸道飞沫和血液制品，以及母婴垂直传播。
- 潜伏期为 4～21 日。
- 大多在皮疹出现前即有传染性。
- 大多数成人有既往感染的血清学证据。

诊断

症状和体征

- 幼儿最常表现为“拍打性颊”。
- 发热。
- 全身不适。
- 迟发症状在 4～14 日后：
  - 弥散性，瘙痒，花边样皮疹(大多数成人没有)，四肢最明显。
  - 非对称性多关节病，中年妇女最常见：
    - 青少年和成人多侵犯小关节。
    - 儿童最常累及膝关节。
    - 继发免疫复合物沉积。
- 然而，大多数患者无症状或仅出现轻度非特异性病毒感染症状。

病史

- 轻微的全身症状(发热、头痛、鼻塞、恶心、咽喉痛)。
- 只有面部出现皮疹时才有传染性。

体格检查

- 第一期：
  - “拍打性颊”聚集性皮疹，局部发热，红斑，儿童水肿性丘疹伴口周苍白。
- 第二期：
  - 非特异性，弥散性，瘙痒，斑丘疹，网状暴发。
    - 出现于面部皮疹 4～21 日后，最多可持续 6 周。
    - 在四肢更明显。
    - 通常分布在手心和足心。
- 第三期：
  - 皮疹消退后阳光暴晒、紧张、运动、高温时会复发。
- 通常完全恢复不留瘢痕。

基本检查

临床诊断基于特征性的体征和症状。

诊断检查与说明

- 通常并不需要检查。
- 全血细胞计数和网织红细胞计数可帮助诊断再生障碍性危象。
- 免疫功能低下或妊娠的明确诊断：
  - 可用病毒 DNA PCR 检查。
  - IgM 抗体存在证实急性感染并持续 2～3 个月。
  - IgG 抗体存在与持久的免疫力有关。
- 在妊娠期间，超声可发现胎儿水肿。

鉴别诊断

- 过敏反应。
- 胶原血管病。
- 柯萨奇病毒感染。
- 药物疹。
- 肠道病毒感染。
- 丹毒。
- 传染性单核细胞增多症。
- 麻疹。
- 非特异性病毒性疾病。
- 类风湿关节炎。
- 红疹。
- 风疹。
- 猩红热。
- 晒伤。

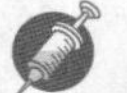

治疗

传染性红斑通常是自限性的，不需要治疗。

院前

对重症患者和中毒症状的患者行 ABC 管理。

初步稳定/治疗

- ABC 管理，应给予氧疗。
- 严重脱水时应给予液体复苏。
- 严重贫血可导致低血压和缺氧，一旦明确诊断应给予输注红细胞悬液。
- 对乙酰氨基酚及非甾体解热镇痛药控制疼痛，阿片类药物治疗严重的关节病。

急诊治疗/程序

- 没有可使用的特异性抗病毒治疗或疫苗。
- 重症患者行适合的实验室检查(全血细胞计数、网织红细胞抗体检测)。
- 必要时对症治疗：
  - 重度脱水时行液体复苏。
  - 若无潜在的肾功能障碍可用非甾体抗炎药治疗关节病。
  - 父母需注意孩子患急性高山反应的可能，可应用苯海拉明治疗瘙痒。
  - 发热时使用退热药。
- 严重贫血时输入人悬浮红细胞。
- 专家会诊：静脉用丙种球蛋白可能对免疫功能低下伴慢性症状和红细胞再生障碍性贫血的患者有益。
- 重症病例给予血液专科会诊。
- 再生障碍性危象的患者住院行呼吸道隔离。
- 妊娠即行产科会诊。

药物治疗

- 对乙酰氨基酚：500 mg(儿童：15 mg/kg 每剂)，口服，q6 h，发热必要时口服达 5 日。
  - 总剂量不超过 4 g/24 h。
- 苯海拉明：25 mg(儿童：1～2 mg/kg 每剂)，口服，q6 h，瘙痒必要时口服达 5 日。

• 布洛芬：400 mg（儿童：10 mg/kg 每剂），口服，q8 h，疼痛必要时口服达 5 日。

• 静脉用丙种球蛋白只在专家会诊后使用。

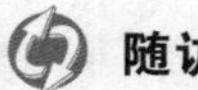

随访

进一步处理

入院指征

• 再生障碍性贫血或严重贫血。

• 严重的免疫功能低下。

• 胎儿水肿。

• 中毒表现。

• 严重关节炎。

出院指征

• 大多数患者可出院。

• 全血细胞计数正常，动脉血氧饱和度和血压正常。

• 患者出现面部皮疹后不再具有传染性，并可以回到日间病房、学校或工作场所。

转诊问题

• 所有无初始主治医师的患者必要时应转到全科医师处随访。

• 遗传性贫血患者应转入血液科随访 1～2 日。

• 所有的免疫功能低下的患者，需要及时专科随访。

• 妊娠合并新发感染的患者应至妇产科并借助超声进一步监测。

随访建议

• 孕妇细小病毒 B19 感染可能需要超声连续监测 10～12 周。

• 有再生障碍性贫血危象风险的患者应在出急诊室后重复检查全血细胞计数，专科随访 1～2 日。

患者教育

预防

• 没有可用的疫苗。

• 经常洗手有助于预防病毒传播。

• 不建议孩子不去上学，因为大多数孩子在诊断时已不具传染性。

• 妊娠的女性应选择远离疫情的工作场所，但目前没有正式的推荐意见。

并发症

• 患者出现再生障碍性危象的贫血：镰状细胞病、遗传性球形红细胞增多症、珠蛋白生成障碍性贫血（地中海贫血）、缺铁或其他红细胞寿命缩短的情况：

- 通常在 2 周内完全恢复。

• 持续感染伴严重贫血如免疫功能低下，无抗体反应，尤其是合并艾滋病时。

• 成人关节炎或过敏性皮肤炎：

- 可能有短暂的类风湿因子阳性，但没有真正的类风湿关节炎和关节破坏。

• 成人与丘疹紫癜性手套和袜子综合征有关：

- 对称性手和足疼痛的渐进性皮疹和水肿。
- 红斑进展为瘀斑、紫癜，偶尔出现大疱。
- 这种综合征也与许多其他病毒和药物相关。

• 极罕见：肝脾大、心力衰竭、脑卒中（中风）、血小板减少、白细胞减少症。

妊娠注意事项

• TORCH 感染：

- 弓形虫病。
- 其他。
  ◦ 梅毒。
  ◦ 水痘-带状疱疹。
  ◦ 细小病毒 B19。
- 风疹。
- 巨细胞病毒。
- 疱疹感染。

• 妊娠期间有胎儿水肿风险。

• 60%的孕妇容易遭到新发感染。

• 30%新发的母体感染有经胎盘传播的风险。

• 影响胎儿肝脏（制造红细胞的主要场所），导致贫血、充血性心力衰竭、心肌炎、胎儿宫内生长迟缓。

• 2%～6%胎儿死亡，在妊娠中期发生率最高。

要点和误区

• 细小病毒 B19 感染通常是自限性的、轻微的疾病。

• 常见的症状包括“拍打性颊”性皮疹及继发的花边样弥漫性皮疹和关节病。

• 当患者出现皮疹和再生障碍性危象时，不再具有传染性。

• 评估所有再生障碍性危象患者有无遗传性或缺铁性贫血的病史。

• 评估所有慢性感染伴持续贫血患者的免疫抑制病史。

• 所有妊娠患者应确诊。如果没有证实患者的免疫情况，注意监测胎儿并发症，并继续随访。

传染性软疣 Molluscum Contagiosum

Adam Z. Barkinl　段立伟 译

基础知识

描述

• 传染性软疣（MC）是一种良性的人类疾病，其特征为大量的小的无痛的珍珠样病变。

• 健康人通常在 6～9 个月自发消退。

• MC 出现在上皮表面，通过密切接触或自身接种传染。

• 定位于皮肤和黏膜。

• 5%～20%的 HIV 感染患者存在 MC 感染。

• 感染程度与 $CD4^+$ T 细胞计数呈负相关。

• 全世界范围内的发病率为 2%～8%，热带地区有较高分布。

病因

• MC 是由一种双链 DNA 痘病毒引起的。

• 儿童间的传播是通过直接的皮肤接触、非生物媒介、水池或浴缸里的水传播的。

• 通常通过皮肤上的一个破口进入人体。

• 成人间的传播通常是由性接触导致的，自身接种可见于任何年龄人群。

• 分娩时导致婴儿感染的病例很少有报道。

诊断

症状和体征

病史

• 潜伏期：14～50 日。

• 患者通常无症状，偶有瘙痒或压痛。

• 10%～25%的患者可以有围绕病变的湿疹反应。

• 对于免疫宿主，未经治疗的病变通常在数月之内缓解，但也可以持续长达5年。

体格检查

• 皮损表面平滑，紧实，球状丘疹，直径2～6 mm。

• 可为肉色，白色，半透明或淡黄色。

• 皮损存在蜡样凝乳状核心，它富含胶原脂质，其中含有大量的未成熟病毒。

• 25%的患者皮损可出现特征性的中央凹陷。

• 非典型表现包括：非凹陷性、持续性、弥散性或大块皮损，这些情况通常发生在免疫抑制的患者。

• 分布：

- 儿童：
  ◦ 面部。
  ◦ 躯干。
  ◦ 四肢。
- 健康成人：
  ◦ 生殖器。
  ◦ 下腹部。
  ◦ 偶尔出现在口周。
- 很少出现在手掌和足掌。

• MC在HIV感染患者中常见，可引起非典型的面部、颈部和躯干皮损，直径可达1.5 cm的渐进性病变，皮损可以在初次进行高效抗反转录病毒治疗时发生，它是免疫重建炎症综合征的一种表现。

• 高效抗逆转录病毒疗法（HAART）时也可能出现感染，这是免疫重建炎症综合征的一种表现。

• 偶尔有眼内或眼周受累，表现为沙眼或慢性滤泡性结膜炎。

基本检查

• 病史和仔细的皮肤检查。

• 皮肤活检以确诊。

• 成人患者存在皮损时要评估免疫状态。

• 儿童发生MC很少与免疫缺陷相关，不需要进一步检查。

诊断检查与说明

实验室检查

• 病因不明时应检查免疫状态：

- 血常规加分类计数。
- 如有提示，检查HIV。

• 如果病变位于肛周：

- 考虑HIV、梅毒、丙型肝炎检查。

诊断步骤/外科

皮肤活检以确诊。

鉴别诊断

• 基底细胞瘤。

• 组织细胞瘤。

• 角化棘皮瘤。

• 皮内痣。

• 毛囊角化病。

• 痣黄瘤内皮瘤。

• 汗管瘤。

• 上皮痣。

• 皮脂腺腺瘤。

• 特应性皮炎。

• 疱疹样皮炎。

• 蕈样肉芽肿。

• Jessner淋巴细胞浸润。

• 新型隐球菌。

治疗

院前

采取一般的预防措施。

初步稳定/治疗

一般情况下不需要。

急诊治疗/程序

• 干预并不是必要的：在具有免疫能力的患者中，是自限性的。

• 未经治疗的免疫功能低下的患者继发性炎症和细菌感染的风险更大。

• 治疗的目的是破坏或去除病毒感染的上皮细胞，以防止自身感染和传播。

• 如果有治疗必要，请转诊至皮肤科。

• 如果不能转诊至皮肤科，物理治疗一般是最有效的治疗方式：

- EMLA（低共熔混合物、利多卡因、丙胺卡因）或氯乙烷局部麻醉后刮出。
- 液氮冷冻治疗。
- 鬼臼树脂、三氯乙酸、斑蝥素、维A酸和西多福韦局部使用效果各异。
- 多次对皮损使用黏性胶带可以减轻表浅皮肤炎症。

• 口服灰黄霉素和美替沙腙对严重病例的疗效不一致。

• HAART可有效地降低HIV患者的发病率。

• 一些小型研究显示外用咪喹莫特有效。

• 检查性伴侣MC感染情况和其他性传播疾病：

- 患者应尽量避免接触性运动、游泳、共用浴室和毛巾、刮伤和剃须，直到病灶已经清除。

• 每2～4周重新检查治疗患者的复发状况，彻底清除病灶需2～4个疗程。

• 不建议抓挠病变皮损，因其可能会造成瘢痕或色素沉着改变。

药物治疗

• 0.9%斑蝥素和等份丙酮与火棉胶混合：外用，每7日1个疗程，用1～3个疗程，或直至缓解。

• 5%咪喹莫特：外用，连续应用3～5日，持续16周。

• 鬼臼树脂（普达非洛0.5%）：外用，q12 h，连续3日，停4日，再重复1周循环，最多循环4次，直到解决。

• 0.1%维A酸：外用，q12 h，连续10日或直到皮损清除。

• 三氯乙酸（50%～80%）：外用＋绷带覆盖5～6日。

• 口服西咪替丁[40 mg/(kg・d)]，分2次服用，持续2个月，曾用于治疗大范围皮损病例，然而其具体效果需研究证实。

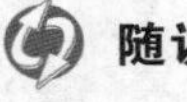

随访

进一步处理

入院指征

各种疾病重叠感染的免疫功能低下患者。

出院指征

可安全在门诊治疗的无重叠感染患者。

转诊问题

如有治疗和确诊的需要，应转诊皮肤科。

随访建议

每2～4周重新检查治疗患者的复发状况。

要点和误区

• 对于免疫功能正常患者，可采取不干预的态度。

• 如果患者免疫功能低下病因不明确，应积极寻找病因。

• 与药物治疗相比，物理疗法通常最有效。

喘鸣 Stridor

Saleh Fares 江伟伟 李文放 译

基础知识

描述

- 主要在吸气相可闻及哮鸣音。
- 上呼吸道梗阻。
- 喉气管阻塞。

病因

- 先天性：
  - 喉软骨软化病。
  - 喉网/环。
- 声带功能障碍：
  - 先天性。
  - 手术损伤。
  - 插管后创伤。
  - 甲状腺恶性肿瘤。
  - 纵隔肿物。
  - 神经异常（如脑膜脊膜囊肿、Arnold-Chiari 畸形）。
  - 反常声带运动。
- 声门下狭窄：
  - 术后瘢痕。
  - 放疗后。
  - 长期气管插管后。
- 声门下血管瘤。
- 感染：
  - 细菌性气管炎。
  - 会厌炎。
  - 病毒性腮腺炎。
  - 扁桃体脓肿。
  - 咽喉壁脓肿。
  - 声门上炎症。
  - 悬雍垂炎（如 Quincke 病）。
  - 咽峡炎。
  - 白喉。
  - 破伤风。
- 外源性压迫：
  - 外伤。
  - 血肿。
  - 血管异常（如环）。
- 气管内阻塞：
  - 异物。
  - 气管软化。
  - 囊肿。
  - 侵入性肿瘤。
  - 鳞状细胞。
  - 淋巴瘤。
  - 甲状腺肿块/癌。
  - 喉或气管乳头状瘤。
- 血管神经性水肿。

诊断

症状和体征

病史

- 呼吸困难。
- 可闻及哮鸣音（进食、哭泣和平躺时明显）。
- 成人声音嘶哑。
- 婴儿喂养困难（喂养量和胃食管反流反流量）。
- 呼吸暂停和发绀。
- 产前、围生期和出生时（如出生时复苏使用了气管插管）。
- 焦虑。
- 咳嗽。
- 流口水。
- 喉部疼痛。

体格检查

- 呼吸急促。
- 呼吸困难。
- 吞咽困难。
- 发热。
- 呼吸困难，激动时加重。
- 鼻翼扇动，肋间回缩，肋骨下凹。
- 异常膈肌运动（后期发现）。
- 哮鸣音（吸气/双相哮喘）。
- 发绀。
- 牙关紧闭：
  - 扁桃体周围脓肿、咽后脓肿、咽峡炎。

基本检查

- 上呼吸道的可视化：
  - 如果症状轻，进行影像学检查，不可掉以轻心。
- 在直接可视化下，外科医师行环甲软管切除术或气管切开术是最安全的方法。

诊断检查与说明

实验室检查

检查没有意义，不需检查，同时可能造成儿童不安。

影像学检查

颈部和胸部正侧位 X 线片：

- 不是必需的。
- 只在非常轻微的情况下或怀疑有异物吸入时才做。

诊断步骤/外科

- 纤维喉镜：
  - 为快速行气管插管，在纤维喉镜下进行。
- 直接喉镜：
  - 诊断的选择。
  - 快速气管插管下选择。

鉴别诊断

- 鼾声：
  - 这是一种由液体或组织的震动产生的低调、粗糙的爆裂样声响。
  - 提示上呼吸道有分泌物积聚。
- 支气管痉挛。
- 假病（患者呼吸闭合时呼吸）。

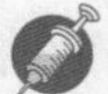

治疗

院前

- 如果可能，请妈妈让孩子保持平静。
- 吸氧。
- 保持气道通畅。
- 如果呼吸状态恶化，则使用面罩吸氧（BVM）。
- 如果 BVM 无效，则进行插管。
- 急诊通道快速运输。

初步稳定/治疗

- 儿童：避免激动，吸氧。
- 使用 100%非呼吸型面罩。
- 脉搏血氧测定法监测氧饱和度和监测生命体征。

儿科注意事项

- 避免儿童激动。
- 注意呼吸状态的迅速恶化。

急诊治疗/程序

- 气道管理：
  - 哮鸣音提示气道梗阻：
    - 插管前手术保障气道畅通。
    - 如果时间允许，与外科医师和儿科麻醉医师现场进行插管。
    - 插管比通常使用的小 1～2 in。
- 清醒插管：
  - 氯胺酮诱导。
  - 插管过程中，患者镇静，但有自主呼吸。

• 避免经鼻气管插管。
• 首选经口插管。经口插管后,换用相同管径的鼻导管。
• 如果插管失败或突然呼吸停止,则需手术开放气道。
• 在感染原因的情况下,插管前予以头孢曲松。
• 确保插管可靠后予以镇静药/肌松药。
• 当气管导管周围发生漏气时可尝试拔管,这可能发生在2~10日。
• 争议:
- 氦氧混合气疗法。
- 肾上腺素治疗。
- 早期插管。

■ 药物治疗

• 阿托品:0.02 mg/kg,静脉注射。
• 头孢曲松:1~2 g,静脉注射。
• 地西泮:2~10 mg,静脉注射(儿童:0.2~0.3 mg/kg)。
• 依托咪酯:0.3 mg/kg,静脉注射。
• 芬太尼:3 μg/kg,静脉注射。
• 氯胺酮:1~2 mg/kg,静脉注射;或4~7 mg/kg,肌内注射。
• 利多卡因:1.5 mg/kg,静脉注射。
• 咪达唑仑:1~5 mg,静脉注射(诱导0.07~0.3 mg/kg)。
• 维库溴铵:0.1 mg/kg,静脉注射。
• 雾化肾上腺素:用生理盐水将1 ml 1∶1000稀释至5 ml。
• 地塞米松:0.15 mg/kg,口服或静脉注射。

随访

■ 进一步处理

入院指征

在急诊科治疗期间,所有未能完全解决问题的患者要求入院。

出院指征

无哮鸣音或其他异常呼吸音。

转诊问题

在气道可视化之前,请耳鼻喉科医师或外科医师会诊。

要点和误区

• 对气道进行可视化前,而不进行紧急气管切开术的准备,是一个错误的认识。
• 喉部器官切除的结果决定了其他辅助检查的适应证,如钡剂吞咽、多导睡眠图、超声心动图、CT或颈部和胸部的磁共振扫描。
• 患者,特别是哮鸣音的患儿,常常伴有呼吸道异常,不仅要求喉镜进行内镜检查,还要求气管支气管检查。

C

创伤(多部位) Trauma, Multiple

Jorge Fernandez · Sam L. Frenkel · Peter L. Steinwald　张晟　林兆奋 译

基础知识

■ 描述

• ATLS为创伤提供了一种标准化的方法,包括快速评估和治疗。
• 危及生命的创伤必须首先稳定病情,然后才能进行初步检查。
• 每当患者病情恶化时,都应重复进行基础检查。

■ 病因

多种病因:
• 贯通伤。
• 机动车、摩托车事故。
• 高处坠落。
• 袭击(包括家暴)。
• 重大伤亡事故(包括恐怖行动)。
• 烧伤。
• 高危患者:高龄或幼儿、妊娠、出血性疾病(包括有效的抗血小板或抗凝剂使用)、格拉斯哥(GCS评分<14分)、生命体征异常、危险机制。

诊断

• 一般来说,严重受伤的患者(特别是生命体征不稳定的患者)如有可能需要紧急手术治疗,应立即送往最近的严重创伤中心。
• 根据EMS方案对主要创伤中心进行分诊。
• 基础检查应当场进行或在急救人员到达时完成。

■ 症状和体征

• 基础检查(ABCDE):
- 气道(同时保护颈椎):
◦ 在进入初步检查的下一步之前评估并保持气道通畅。
◦ 始终保护颈椎。
◦ 气道通畅的指标:清晰度语言或有效/静默的空气运动。
◦ 气道阻塞的指标:咯咯作响、刺耳、打鼾、窒息或无空气运动。
- 呼吸:
◦ 在进入初步检查的下一步之前评估并稳定呼吸。
◦ 胸廓对称起伏,两侧呼吸音相同,呼吸节律和氧饱和度正常的患者,提示有效通气。
◦ 胸廓起伏不对称,两侧呼吸音不同,呼吸节律不正常,氧饱和度降低,呼吸运动不良,反应迟钝的患者,提示通气不良。
◦ 单侧呼吸音减低,气管移位,过度扩张,叩诊过清音,皮下气肿,组织缺氧或血流动力学不稳定,应考虑张力性气胸。
◦ 呼吸音减低伴叩诊浊音提示血胸。
- 循环:
◦ 在进入初步检查的下一步之前评估并稳定循环。
◦ 基础评估包括血压、心率、脉搏性质、终末器官功能(如精神、尿量、毛细血管充盈)。
- 功能障碍:
◦ 在进入下一步初步检查前评估和稳定功能。
◦ 评估意识水平、粗大运动和感觉功能、瞳孔大小/反应性。
◦ 格拉斯哥昏迷量表最常用,评分低于8分提示严重头部损伤/昏迷。
◦ 脊髓损伤:粗略评估运动/感觉障碍的偏侧性。
◦ 通过瞳孔大小和对光反射评估脑干功能。
- 暴露:
◦ 完全脱掉衣服,然后被动取暖。
• 次要检查:
- 基础调查完成后实施。
- 完善详细体格检查。

- 身体各处都要检查到。

病史

• 主要特征：最初的临床表现、损伤机制、疑似损伤和治疗应从急救人员、家属和旁观者处得知。

• MVCS：记录所有车辆的大致速度、撞击点、车内患者的位置、安全带使用情况、乘客空间侵入、转向柱损坏或由EMS解救。

• 完整的病史：过敏、内科/外科问题、既往病史、最后一次口服药物、导致创伤的事件。(如果病情稳定，请讨论破伤风情况)。

体格检查

详见症状和体征。

初步评估稳定和基本检查一同进行。

C

基本检查

• 基础及次要检查。

• 重症患者：启动创伤小组，快速输液和实验室/影像学检查准备。

• 床旁即时检测(POC)超声检查(e-FAST)。

• 便携式X线片包括AP胸片、AP骨盆片和颈椎侧位片。

• CT：仅当血流动力学稳定或充分稳定时。

• 使用基于证据的临床决策标准(例如，Nexus标准、加拿大标准)以避免不必要的成像。

诊断检查与说明

实验室检查

• 失血性休克系列：即时血红蛋白。

• 精神状态改变：即时血糖。

• 重大创伤患者：血型、CBC、COAG、血气、乳酸、肾功能、脂肪酶、尿酸。

• 所有育龄女性：妊娠试验。

• 考虑对心脏损伤：心肌酶。

影像学检查

• 严重的胸部创伤需要通过e-FAST、CXR、CT、血管造影和/或开胸手术对肺、心脏和大血管进行客观评估。

• 钝性腹部创伤需要使用e-FAST进行客观评估，然后进行腹部CT或EXP检查：

- 如果e-FAST上有自由液体。
- 血流动力学稳定：CT静脉造影。
- 血流动力学不稳定：探索性栓塞。
  - 对于头部创伤，如果长期意识丧失、健忘、意识水平持续改变或严重的HA或呕吐，推荐使用CT。
  - 对于颈椎骨折：CT是高度敏感的。
  - 平扫CT(头部、颈部、胸部、腹部/骨盆一次通过静脉增强)漏诊率较低，但有明显的辐射照射。

• 疑似脊柱损伤(伴有神经缺损)：急诊MRI。

• 肢体损伤：

- X线可以识别大多数骨折(除了舟状骨、髋关节、胫骨平台、距骨等)。
- 怀疑血管损伤时需行血管造影或双重超声。

鉴别诊断

考虑导致创伤的医疗条件(例如，癫痫、心律失常和自杀未遂)。

治疗

初步稳定/治疗

• 初步检查：一旦发现任何严重创伤，立即稳定生命体征。

• 气道(同时颈椎保护)：

- 下颌推挤法，吸痰，口咽或鼻咽通气道，提供初始气道支持。

• 快速顺序插管是多发创伤患者气道管理的首选：考虑使用氯胺酮或依托咪酯来降低插管期低血压。

- 插管失败：声门外装置(如喉罩气道)或环甲切开术。
- 视频喉镜可以在对创伤性脑或不稳定颈椎损伤影响最小的情况下进行气管插管。

• 呼吸：

- 100%氧气及呼吸监测。
- 预氧合：8次深呼吸或3分钟潮气量。
- 临床诊断张力性气胸：紧急行胸腔穿刺置管紧急减压。
- 血胸：胸腔穿刺置管(28F)常规指征，如果大量血胸考虑术中自体输血和开胸。
- 开放性胸部创伤应用粘贴敷料覆盖并行胸腔闭式引流。
- 连枷段或肺挫伤引起的呼吸困难提示尽早正压机械通气插管(使用小潮气量+PEEP进行肺保护)。

• 循环：

- 心电监护。
- 建立静脉通道(理想情况下2个大口径外周静脉输液；替代方案包括骨髓腔穿刺、中心静脉置管或静脉切开术)。
- 用直接加压或止血带暂时控制活动性出血。
- 晶体液体滴注(10～20 ml/kg)是有争议的(例如，允许性低血压)。
- 用红细胞悬液、新鲜冰冻血浆、血小板比例为1∶1∶1的血制品代替失血。
- 骨盆外固定治疗不稳定骨盆骨折。
- 考虑给所有失血性休克患者用氨甲环酸(TXA)，作为大规模输血方案的一部分。
- 心脏压塞。
  - 稳定：急诊心包穿刺。
  - 不稳定：开胸手术。
- 有目击者确定为穿透性胸部创伤：考虑开胸手术(如果有外科医师的话)。

• 功能不全：

- 头部损伤且格拉斯哥昏迷量表评分低于8分时应启动降低颅内压的治疗，使用甘露醇或高渗盐水，快速序列插管，氧疗，并且将PCO_2控制在30～35 mmHg。抬高头部30°，保持脊柱制动治疗颅内高压。
- 颅内出血或脊髓损伤：请神经外科会诊；一般不推荐使用大剂量类固醇激素。

急诊治疗/程序

• 明确的治疗可能需要紧急手术或介入放射学。

• 及时稳定生命体征，早期认识手术干预的需求，最重要的是适当的创伤手术会诊。

• 重新评估是识别隐匿性/延迟性损伤的关键。

药物治疗

• 根据需要进行特定干预。

• 考虑对所有失血性休克患者给予氨甲环酸，作为大规模输血方案的一部分。

• 考虑使用短效、血流动力学中性的药物。

• 考虑在穿透伤中使用预防性抗生素。

• 确保必要的预防破伤风。

儿科注意事项

• 骨髓腔穿刺作为液体和药物静脉通道的备选。

• CT并不总是可靠地排除脊髓损伤的检查：需考虑MRI。

随访

进一步处理

入院指征

• 多数重大创伤患者应收入院观察，监测，进一步评估。

• 严重创伤或血流动力学不稳定的患者应收入ICU/手术室。

• 需要频繁评估的患者应收入ICU。

出院指征

微小创伤且无客观检查/影像学表现的患者可在观察一段时间后出院。

转诊问题

诸如创伤外科医师、神经外科医师、整形外科/手外科医师、耳鼻喉科医师、整形外科医师和烧伤专家小组的介入可能会显著影响发病率和死亡率。

随访建议

随访主要取决于损伤类型和所需的专科护理。

要点和误区

• 一般来说,有可能需要紧急手术治疗的重伤患者(特别是那些生命体征不稳定的患者)应该立即被送往最近的重大创伤中心。
• 创伤 ABCDE 评估仍然是对重大创伤进行初步评估和治疗的标准方法。
• 危及生命的损伤必须先把生命体征稳定下来,然后才能进行初步检查。
• 每当患者病情恶化时,都应该重复初步检查。
• 应保持对隐性损伤的高度怀疑,并保持低阈值的观察。
• 确保预防破伤风(必要时)。

C

创伤(儿童)

Taylor McCormick　王虑 译

基础知识

描述

• 儿童和成人在病理生理学和解剖上是相似的。
• 80%的小儿创伤是钝性伤,80%的多系统伤包括头部伤。
• 创伤是美国和欧洲>1 岁儿童致死和致残的原因。
• 大部分被虐儿童都<3 岁,其中 1/3 的儿童<6 个月。

病因

• 大部分小儿创伤是单系统的、小的钝性伤。
• 通常的致伤机制包括机动车碰撞或自行车事故,还有行人被交通工具撞、从高处坠落。
• 小儿穿刺伤比较少见。
• 风险因素包括成人监管不力、儿童去完成超过期能力范围的任务、对任务的注意力不够、冒风险承担任务、药物和酒精的风险。

诊断

症状和体征

病史

• 病史常直接由患儿、家长、目击者或急救人员提供。如果病史和伤情不太一致,可能存在虐待儿童。
• 受伤的机制对预测伤情的严重程度帮助不大,但能依此判断受伤的类型。
• 引起严重伤的可能性事件包括车把手伤、严重的行人空间被侵犯、机动车相撞时没有合适的防护、骑自行车或玩滑板时没戴头盔等。
• 翔实的病史资料还包括过敏史、药物治疗史、以往就医史、吃饭时间和一些导致伤害的事件。

体格检查

• 基本的检查:
- 所有受伤的儿童都需要按步骤对病情评估,包括气道的通畅、呼吸、循环、伤残和适当的暴露。
• 后续的检查:
- 一般情况:
  ◦ 创伤可能致不显性失水,增加低血压症的风险。
  ◦ 代偿机制会掩盖低血容量的一些体征。只有当血容量失去达到 20%~30%,失机制突然启动才会有异常表现。
  ◦ 全血容量比成人少(80 ml/kg)。
- 头:
  ◦ 囟门明显膨凸,头皮血肿,急性面容,耳鼻中隔血肿,裂伤,面部功能或面容受损,瞳孔异常。
  ◦ 囟门开放或颅骨多处骨折会使颅内压增高的症状和体征出现延迟。
  ◦ 当患者仰卧在成人背板上,头和枕骨致颈部屈曲。
- 眼、耳、鼻和咽喉检查:
  ◦ 检查有无出血、创伤、鼓室积血、眼充血和脑脊液外漏的证据。
  ◦ 舌过大或扁桃体肥大会堵塞气道。
- 颈:
  ◦ 气管移位和后颈部塌陷极少见于儿童。
  ◦ 气管短,气管插管进入左主支气管风险增加。
  ◦ 对于<8 岁的儿童环状软骨处是气道狭窄的地方。
  ◦ 但小孩受伤精神状态不稳定时,到急诊颈椎无法得到合适保护。这些小孩应带颈托保护。
  ◦ 假关节半脱位(C2、C3 关节向前脱位)的发生率为 20%。
  ◦ 脊髓损伤但放射影像学检查无异常(无骨折脱位脊髓损伤),在还没有磁共振检查时经常存在争议。
- 胸:
  ◦ 注意整体呼吸情况,有无咕噜声,双侧呼吸音是否对称,有无皮肤擦伤,有无胸廓畸形和捻发音。
  ◦ 儿童胸壁的弹性和顺应性较好,因此儿童肺挫伤比肋骨骨折常见。肋骨骨折常常是有虐待儿童的结果。
  ◦ 腹式呼吸。
- 腹部:
  ◦ 挫伤、擦伤和触痛。
  ◦ 腹部膨胀常是由于胃肠空气所致。
  ◦ 和成人比,儿童的肝脏和脾脏占身体比例更大。
  ◦ 胸腔包含腹部极少。
  ◦ <2 岁的儿童膀胱是在腹腔里的。
- 四肢:
  ◦ 通过触诊判断关节的稳定和柔和度。
  ◦ 触摸脉搏。
  ◦ 索尔特-哈里斯骨折分类。
  ◦ 儿童特有的青枝骨折。
- 神经系统:
  ◦ 符合不同年龄段的精神状态评估。
  ◦ 四肢活动度评估。
- 皮肤:
  ◦ 评估末梢循环和皮肤颜色苍白与否。
  ◦ 耳、足背和外阴的挫伤常提示受伤原因不是简单的意外事故。
- 受伤的模式:

◦ 车与行人：沃德尔三联征(股骨、躯干和头部伤)，不常见。
◦ 自行车车把伤可能刺伤儿童：胰腺或小肠损伤。
◦ 安全带综合征：腹部瘀斑和肠道伤，有的还会有腰椎骨折(钱斯骨折)。
◦ 小的创伤病史但伤很重：应考虑儿童虐待。

■ 基本检查

• 详细的病史和仔细的体格检查是对儿童伤情做出全面评估必需的工作。
• 放射学检查、实验室检查和创伤相关指标并不能作为诊断儿童伤情的确切证据。

C

■ 诊断检查与说明

实验室检查

• 实验室检查需个体化，需反映患者的临床表现。
• 最初血红蛋白和血细胞比容检查结果正常并不能排除严重的出血，能为后面的检查提供参考的参考值；心动过速可能是出血早期唯一的临床表现，但是这对出血量的判断没有特异性。
• 早期就做电解质检查没有什么必要。
• 常规淀粉酶和脂肪酶检查并不推荐，因为胰腺损伤很少见，假阳性结果比较常见。
• 肝功能异常不能作为决定患儿是否要行腹部CT检查的唯一因素。如果腹部创伤患儿谷草转氨酶大于200 U/L或谷丙转氨酶大于125 U/L且血流动力学稳定可以考虑CT检查。体格检查结果也能协助是否行影像学检查。
• 肉眼血尿(每高倍镜视野大于50个红细胞)考虑泌尿道损伤，但仅是镜下血尿不能认为就有泌尿道损伤。
• 血库样本筛选出合适的患者。
• 青少年女性需要验孕。
• 当有合适的影像学检查手段后，诊断性腹腔冲洗术就很少做了。

影像学检查

• 传统的脊柱、胸、骨盆全身扫描不再是普遍的做法，选择合适的部位检查更常用。
• 如果患儿清醒，警觉能配合的且颈部柔软没有疼痛，颈部运动试验也无疼痛可不考虑颈部影像血检查：
• 意识不清的颈部受伤患儿无法在急诊处理的，在入院前应行磁共振检查(CT更常见)。
• 胸部CT检查的情况包括发出咕噜声的呼吸、低氧血症、双侧呼吸音不对称、呼吸困难、捻发音、气管插管、胸腔闭式引流、颈内或锁骨下静脉置管等。
• 盆腔CT检查比较少见，当患儿表现为严重的盆腔疼痛和不稳定时可以同时行盆腔和腹部的CT检查。
• 头部CT检查的情况包括患儿精神状态异常、局灶性神经功能缺损、长时间的神志丧失、囟门膨胀、颅顶头皮血肿、颅骨压缩性骨折和不能控制的持续性呕吐。
• 腹部和盆腔CT检查典型的指征包括患儿精神状态的改变、肉眼血尿、髂骨以上腹部挫伤、把手伤、腹部触动伴有血流动力学改变。
• 超声还是有一定的局限性，其对腹腔积液(如血)的检查结果并不能一直作为剖腹探查的指征。腹部超声对于儿童创伤的有效性需要进一步研究。

■ 鉴别诊断

当伤情和所述病史不符时，需考虑非意外事故伤。

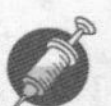

治疗

■ 院前

• 迅速转运至能处理小儿创伤的医疗机构。
• 首先需要处理的包括气道的通畅(由院前急救人员进行气管插管还有争议)呼吸和循环的稳定。
• 颈椎和四肢的固定。

■ 初步稳定/治疗

• 大部分创伤患儿在急诊病情就得到稳定。
• 稳定措施：
- 心肺和末梢血氧的监测。
- 早期氧气治疗。
- 2条静脉通路和积极晶体液复苏。
- 吗啡控制疼痛。
- 实验室和影像学检查。
- 如果2条静脉通路输注晶体液效果不佳可以输注浓缩红细胞。
- 气管内插管：
◦ 需在依托咪酯或氯胺酮和氯化琥珀胆碱药物配合下快速气管插管。
◦ 苯二氮䓬类药物或异丙酚镇静。
- 颈椎制动。
- 必要时行胸腔闭式引流。
- 插导尿管(尿道口有血液)。
- 鼻胃管或口胃管胃肠减压。

■ 急诊治疗/程序

• 根据病史和体格检查结果行风险评估。
• 普遍认为通过受伤的机制去评估伤情的严重程度有很大的局限性。
• 根据轻重缓急评估伤情，并根据病情变化多次再评估。
• 适当的镇静和止痛。
• 清创并骨折的固定。
• 病情需要予以破伤风抗毒素注射。
• 在复苏和治疗时允许父母在身边。

■ 药物治疗

• 正常生理盐水和林格液：20 ml/kg，静脉滴注。
• 浓缩红细胞：10 ml/kg，静脉滴注。
• 依托咪酯：0.3 mg/kg，静脉注射。
• 硫酸吗啡：0.1 mg/kg，静脉注射。
• 琥珀酰胆碱：1.5 mg/kg，静脉注射。
• 劳拉西泮(氯羟去甲安定)：0.1 mg/kg，静脉注射。
• 丙泊酚(异丙酚)：2 mg/kg，静脉注射。
• 氯胺酮：2 mg/kg，静脉注射(会增加眼内压和颅内压，当怀疑有头颅伤时不使用)。

随访

■ 进一步处理

入院指征

• 持续改变的精神状态、气管插管、胸腔闭式引流术、CT已明确的腹腔和颅内创伤、肺挫伤、需要手术的骨折、非意外事故创伤。
• 血流动力学不稳定。
• 需气道护理。
• 腹部CT检查没有阳性发现，但持续腹痛则有胰腺或肠道伤的可能。
• 没有家长照顾的患儿(如父母都受伤住院了)。

出院指征

• 受伤的患儿精神状态和影像学检查正常，可以在有可靠护理人的前提下予以出院回家。
• 伤后压力综合征会逐步发展，家长需听取专家的意见并注意病情发展。

■ 随访建议

• 与伤情相关的专家。
• 若有伤后压力综合征表现，需有精神科医师的建议。
• 神经科医师对脑震荡后综合征做出评估。

创伤(老年人)

Elizabeth A. Owen · Peter Witucki 祝各亮 译

基础知识

描述

• 老年创伤患者的注意事项和解决方法，一般年龄>65 岁。

• 应与公认的创伤标准联合使用。

• 高龄是创伤后不良后果的一个重要危险因素。

• 整体虚弱和共病会降低生理储备，导致较差的结果。

• 慢性病管理的进步使老年人的生活方式更加活跃，容易受伤。

病因

• 创伤是老年人死亡的第五大原因。

• 老年人更容易受到低能量机制的严重伤害。

最常见的发病机制：

• 跌倒最常见的原因，经常发生在平坦的表面上，并且经常在 1 年内频发。

• 机车碰撞：第二常见的病因，是最常见的致死病因。

• 人车碰撞：认知能力减弱，视力低下/听力障碍，步态障碍有助于增加发病率。

• 烧伤：在相同烧伤程度的情况下，老年人比年轻人有更高的致死率。

• 暴力：少于年轻人，如果存在的话需高度怀疑是否有虐待老年人的问题。

诊断

• 根据当地的协议，分流到主要的创伤中心。

• 受伤的患者具有外科、神经外科或骨科干预潜在需要的，应转移到主要的创伤中心。

• 对于老年人，现场分诊或转移到创伤中心的指征可放宽。

• 考虑为高危老年患者制定特定方案，包括老年医学咨询。

症状和体征

• 初步检查(ABCDE)和二次检查的模式与年轻患者一样。

• 正常的生命体征会导致安全的假象。

- 灌注不足常会被不恰当的生理反应、潜在的医学病理和药物作用所掩盖。
- 收缩压<110 mmHg 的患者死亡率较高。

• 气道，颈椎-通过固定颈椎建立和维持气道。

- 老年人的解剖变异会为气道维持带来困难(义齿、颈椎关节炎、颞颌关节炎)。
- 没有认识到早期气管插管的指征是一种常见的错误。

• 呼吸：保持充分有效的呼吸和通风。

- 呼吸肌减弱和胸壁退行性变，导致有效通气量减少。
- 对低氧、高碳酸血症和酸中毒反应迟钝会延迟症状的出现。
- 老年患者气管插管的指征可放宽。

• 循环：确保合适的灌注。

- 密切血流动力学监测。
- 心率、血压不总是与心输出量相关。
- 老年人通常对低血容量产生受损的变时性反应。
- 心血管反应可被心率控制药物(β受体阻滞剂、钙通道阻滞剂)减弱。
- 老年人很普遍的高血压，可以表现为相关性的低血压。
- 抗血小板和抗凝药物会加重出血。

• 残疾：对颅内和脊髓损伤情况进行快速神经系统评估。

- 脑萎缩会延迟压缩效应导致的症状。
- 潜在的痴呆或衰老会导致在判断精神状况时出现重大失误。

• 暴露：应当完全除去患者的衣物。

• 二次检查：

- 在初步检查完成之后进行。
- 确保任何方面的稳定。
- 从头到脚完整的体格检查。

病史

• 老年创伤患者应同时被视为伤员和患者。

• 老年患者可有明显的合并症，询问既往病史、用药史和过敏史是必不可少的。

• 其他的基础疾病会促成创伤事件的发生。

• 需考虑低血糖、晕厥、心律失常、脑卒中(中风)、心血管意外、泌尿道感染等。

• 需要向急救人员详细询问受伤机制、初始表现和处理情况。

体格检查

按照初步检查和二次检查进行。

诊断检查与说明

实验室检查

• 初步检查和二次检查。

• 头部、颈椎、胸部和腹部/盆腔的影像学检查应高度重视。

• 血常规、动脉血气和血型。

• 电解质、肾功能和血糖。

• 尿隐血，尿路损伤时可出现阳性。

• 凝血项目。

• 碱缺乏和乳酸可鉴别隐性休克。

• 乙醇水平和毒物检查。

影像学检查

• 由于老年人电离辐射致癌风险的降低，CT 可自由使用。

• 头部 CT 是老年闭合性脑外伤的首选方法。

• Nexus 标准已在年龄>65 岁的患者中得到验证；然而，老年外伤患者颈椎 CT 检查阈值较低。X 线平片显示不明显。

• 显著的钝性和穿透性胸部创伤需要进行心脏与大血管超声心动图、CT 扫描、血管造影的客观评估。

• 钝性腹部创伤需要客观的评估，方式取决于患者的病情。

- 血流动力学稳定的患者应该做一个腹部增强 CT。
- 如果临床状况允许，在造影剂负荷前考虑水合作用并评估基线肾功能。
- 不稳定的患者应进行快速检查或诊断性腹腔灌洗。

• 肢体损伤：

- X 线平片。
- 血管造影或双重超声检查可疑血管损伤。
- CT/MRI 对临床高度怀疑骨折但 X 线片阴性(即胫骨平台骨折)。

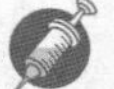

治疗

院前

重点应放在气道维持，控制外部出血和休克处理，并立即转移到适当的设施内。

初步稳定/治疗

• 气道：在建立气道时应考虑解剖变异。

• 呼吸：

- 连续脉搏血氧饱和度测定。
- 潮气末二氧化碳可能有帮助。
- 吸氧以维持血氧饱和度>95%。
- 连续 ABG 可早期了解呼吸功能和储备。
- 考虑通气功能受损患者的早期插管。
- 胸壁疼痛的充分镇痛是优化通气的关键。

• 循环：血流动力学不稳定的严重性常被临床医师低估。

- 连续补充 250~500 ml 单位的晶体液。
- 过于快速的容量置换会使老年患者出现失代偿。
- 考虑早期使用血液制品。
- 连续测定碱缺失和乳酸水平提供了休克初检的良好标准，并可指导急救措施。
- 老年人的肌酐清除率会下降。
- 肾脏更易受到低血容量、药物和肾毒性产品的损害。

• 残疾：

- 颅脑损伤：年龄是发病率和死亡率的一个独立危险因素。
- 年龄相关的萎缩和智力下降可影响精神状况的评估。
- 在抗凝治疗的钝性头部损伤患者中，如果最初的头部 CT 阴性，密切观察并及时复查 CT，因为延迟出血的风险增加。
- 立即开始治疗，如果有颅内压升高的症状或体征。

• 暴露：完全除去患者的衣物，但防止低温。

- 与年龄相关的生理变化和药物使老年人更易患低体温症。
- 低温不能全归因于休克或暴露，而更应关注脓毒症、内分泌失调或药物的摄入。

• 抗凝：

- 根据适应证，考虑凝血酶原复合物浓缩物、新鲜冰冻血浆、低温沉淀物和/或浓缩因子。
- 当心液体超载和逆转引起的血栓并发症。
- 在昏迷患者中确定新的抗凝剂的使用是很困难的，标准的创伤实验室没有揭示抗凝剂的使用或程度。

• 常见的损伤模式：

- 头部损伤：
  ◦ 不易发生硬膜外血肿。
  ◦ 硬膜下血肿的发生率较高。
- 颈椎损伤：
  ◦ 看似微小创伤也有可能造成颈椎损伤(站立或坐的高度落下)。
  ◦ 第 1 颈椎、第 2 颈椎和齿状突骨折在老年人中特别常见。
  ◦ 潜在的颈椎病变，如关节炎可能会诱发脊髓损伤。
  ◦ 过度拉伸造成的损伤，会增加中央脊髓综合征的风险。
- 脊椎损伤：
  ◦ 更容易骨折，尤其是前部的楔形压缩性骨折。
  ◦ 一个椎体水平骨折的患者需要对整个脊柱进行成像。
  ◦ 对于老年患者，考虑早期脊柱手术会诊。
- 胸部创伤：
  ◦ 肋骨骨折最为常见，对于老年患者，每增加一根肋骨骨折，都会增加患肺炎的风险和死亡率。
  ◦ 早期积极的疼痛控制包括局部神经阻滞或硬膜外麻醉。
  ◦ 刺激性肺活量测定法。
  ◦ 血气胸、连枷胸、肺挫伤和心脏挫伤可迅速导致失代偿。
- 腹部创伤：
  ◦ 与年轻人相似的损伤模式，但其死亡率是重伤的 5 倍。
  ◦ 早期发现血流动力学不稳定的迹象很重要。
  ◦ 血流动力学稳定的钝性肝脾损伤可非手术治疗。
  ◦ 下胸壁损伤的高怀疑腹腔内损伤。
- 骨创伤：由于骨量减少和骨质疏松，在老年人中更常见：
  ◦ 特别要考虑骨盆和髋部骨折。
  ◦ 侧压伤是老年创伤患者最常见的骨盆骨折类型。
  ◦ 老年盆腔外伤易导致出血增加，应考虑早期输血、手术和/或血管栓塞术。
  ◦ 骨创伤的目标是减少创面，明确流程，早期恢复功能。

▪ 急诊治疗/程序

• 早期建立肺和心血管系统的监测。

• 及时稳定生命体征，早期了解手术干预的需要。

• 老年患者会受益于积极救治和降低转移到创伤中心的标准，但事实上却很少能做到这一点。

• 护理必须包括医疗团队和家庭之间关于护理目标和预期生活质量的讨论。

• 寻找是否存在进一步的指示、生前预嘱或相关的法律文件。

• 社会因素：

- 建议老年医学专家尽早介入。
- 识别丧失独立性的高危患者，以帮助目标康复。
- 发展一个多学科的老年创伤团队，包括药房、病例管理人员、社会工作、物理治疗和职业治疗。

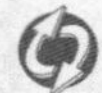 随访

▪ 进一步处理

入院指征

• 大部分的创伤患者应入院观察，监测，并进一步评估。

• 老年患者收治的门槛应降低。

• 老年患者有多发伤、明显的胸壁损伤、异常生命体征或灌注不足的表现的，都应该住进重症监护病房。

出院指征

创伤小、无需进行检查的患者可在急诊室观察数小时后出院。

转诊问题

根据创伤的类型后续治疗，进行持续和专业的护理。

▪ 随访建议

随访和转诊应取决于受伤类型所需的专业需求。

要点和误区

• 由于有限的生理储备、药物的影响及未表现出的低灌注，轻微的受伤机制可以产生严重的损伤和并发症。

• 药物的频繁使用，特别是β受体阻滞剂和抗凝血剂，使得评估和处理变得复杂。

• “正常”的血压和心率不代表容量也正常。

• 老年创伤患者必须同时作为伤员和患者进行处理。

创伤后应激障碍 Posttraumatic Stress Disorder (PTSD)

Bernardino Vaccaro 瞿金龙 林兆奋 译

基础知识

描述

• 由于受伤或严重的心理冲击而持续的精神和情绪压力的状态。

• 最近暴露在已知可能引发创伤后应激障碍(PTSD)事件中的患者。

• 已经患有创伤后应激障碍的个人:

- 暴力受害者。
- 性虐待。
- 医疗创伤。

• 这些患者在急诊介入治疗后可能会出现急性加重。

• 来自医学创伤或既往受害的未被识别的既往创伤后应激障碍,通常会使急诊室的表现和治疗复杂化。

流行病学

• 美国创伤后应激障碍的终身风险为8.7%。

• 美国12个月的患病率为3.5%。

• 风险因素:

- 强奸幸存者(最高比例)。
- 退伍军人:
  ◦ 战争。
  ◦ 囚禁。
- 急救人员。
- 医务人员。
- 家庭暴力。
- 出于政治或种族动机的拘留或种族灭绝风险。

病因

• 遗传易损性包括5-羟色胺转运蛋白变异的个体。

• 焦虑、敏感的人在发生创伤性事件时更容易患上创伤后应激障碍。

• 目前的观点认为,当个体的应对机制不堪重负时,创伤后应激障碍首先会出现过度唤醒和交感过度驱动的症状,然后在过度唤醒的情况下会通过激活迷走神经/副交感神经系统而发生分离。

• 在神经影像研究中,杏仁核的过度觉醒经常导致前额叶皮质的激活减少,这可以解释许多创伤中失去连贯的叙述感。

诊断

症状和体征

• 在检查患者之前获得许可,以免引发创伤反应。

• 详细记录过去的创伤、对压力的反应,以及通过急诊室的经历可以帮助患者保持冷静和彻底事情。

• 陈述过去的创伤史,以前对医疗干预的反应。

• 由于事件存在分离和可能的不良回忆,请彻底了解事件的可能工作和记录。

• 如果损伤机制使患者面临创伤风险,评估隐匿性创伤。

病史

• 暴露在创伤性事件中:

- 事件的亲身经历。
- 见证发生在他人身上的事件。
- 听到发生在亲密朋友或家人身上的事件。
- 反复接触事件的细节:
  ◦ 急救人员收集遗体。
  ◦ 警方讯问导致多次虐待细节曝光。

• 不由自主的噩梦。

• 侵扰性的想法或形象。

• 分离性发作。

• 对事件有强烈的生理或心理反应。

• 回避症状:

- 持续回避或试图回避记忆。
- 对与创伤有关的事件的思考。
- 努力避免外界对事件、人、事物的提醒,这些事情会让人想起创伤事件。

• 与创伤相关的认知和情绪的负面改变:

- 无法回忆起由于分离性健忘症造成的创伤的重要方面。
- 对自己的持续负面信念。
- 关于世界安全的原因或信念。
- 持续无法体验积极情绪。
- 持续的负面情绪状态(恐怖)。
- 对活动的兴趣明显减弱。
- 超然或疏远的感觉。

• 明显的易唤醒和多动程度:

- 易激动。
- 易愤怒暴发。
- 鲁莽或自毁行为。
- 高度警觉。
- 夸张的惊吓反应。
- 注意力和睡眠障碍问题。

体格检查

• 隐匿性创伤的评估。

• 神经学检查。

基本考虑事项

筛查药物使用和创伤性脑损伤、自我伤害史,考虑到它们是常见的并存疾病。

诊断检查与说明

实验室检查

尿液和血清毒理检测。

影像学检查

• 急性颅脑损伤的CT扫描。

• 弥漫性轴索损伤的MRI征象(如有指征)。

鉴别诊断

• 急性应激障碍。

• 妄想。

• 适应障碍混合特征。

• 物质使用障碍。

• 人格障碍。

• 焦虑障碍。

• 强迫症。

• 分离性障碍。

• 精神障碍。

• 外伤性脑损伤。

治疗

院前

• 创造安全环境。

• 离开危险或创伤区域。

• 消除创伤因素,倾向于受伤,开始管理疼痛。

初步稳定/治疗

创伤的治疗,适当的疼痛控制来控制一些由疼痛引起的急性觉醒,哌唑嗪或β受体阻滞剂也可能有助于破坏创伤性记忆的形成。

急救治疗/程序

• 患者教育:

- 关于最初反应的创伤和正常化。
- 关于未来几周的可能进程:
  ◦ 最初关注的是发生了什么。
  ◦ 睡眠困难。
  ◦ 提高了警觉性,这种警觉性可能会在接下来的几周里有所改善。

• SSRI有助于管理创伤后应激障碍的一些症状：

- 从治疗范围的低端开始，逐步滴定，直到达到预期的效果。

• 哌唑嗪：

- 可能对噩梦有帮助，根据噩梦减少的效果或低血压的副作用进行滴定。

- 要么是单一疗法，要么作为 SSRI 的辅助疗法。

• 在创伤后的最初阶段使用 β 受体阻滞剂可能有助于预防发展中的创伤后应激障碍。

• 长期使用苯二氮䓬类药物与病情恶化和难治性创伤后应激障碍有关。

• 教会以正念为基础的技能和膈膜呼吸可能有助于患者在早期调节过度警觉，并防止进一步的症状形成。

药物治疗

选择性血清素再吸收抑制剂：

• 帕罗西汀每日 5～10 mg 口服。

- 逐渐增加至 20～60 mg 口服。

• 舍曲林每日 12.5～25 mg 口服。

- 逐渐增加至 50～200 mg 口服。

• 氟伏沙明每日 25 mg 口服；或者 11.25 mg 口服每日 2 次；如果需要立即释放准备。

- 逐渐增加至 100～300 mg，口服。

• 西酞普兰：每日 10 mg，口服。

- 逐渐增加至 20～40 mg 口服。

• α 受体阻滞剂：

- 睡前服用哌唑嗪 1 mg 口服。

- 逐渐增加至 3～15 mg 口服。

• β 受体阻滞剂：

- 普萘洛尔(心得安)。

- 0.67 mg/kg 短效口服，2 h 后为 1 mg/kg 长效口服。

随访

■ 进一步处理

入院指征

• 急性中毒或戒酒风险。

• 自杀或杀人念头。

• 分离到不能照顾自己的程度的证据。

出院指征

• 生命体征稳定。

• 没有持续的精神状态变化。

• 提供心理教育。

• 回到安全的环境中。

转诊问题

尝试寻找创伤后应激障碍的专家将是有帮助的，因为通常不知情的创伤治疗可能会由于反复的过度唤醒而导致进一步的再创伤，而没有对这些症状进行适当的处理。

■ 随访建议

• 基于正念和基于暴露的治疗是护理的标准，包括认知处理治疗、长时间暴露治疗、眼动脱敏和再处理(EMDR)。

• 支持神经反馈、生物反馈、创伤信息瑜伽和虚拟现实再暴露疗法的新证据。

要点和误区

• 创伤后应激障碍(PTSD)在医学中经常被忽视。

• 有创伤后应激障碍病史的人，特别是暴力和性暴力、童年虐待的人，患药物使用障碍和不良医疗结果的风险更高。

• 退缩和行为失调可能是医疗过度刺激环境的触发和情绪泛滥的迹象。

• 冷静、尊重的态度，检查前征得许可，并询问在这些紧张的情况下什么是有帮助的，这可能会防止进一步的行为失调。

创伤性断肢/再植 Traumatic Amputation/Replantation

Mohammad M. Alkhawajahr · Charlotte A. Sadler 张晟 林兆奋 译

基础知识

■ 描述

• 部分断肢有连接远端和近端的组织，并接受血运重建治疗。

• 完全断肢没有连接组织，可以再植治疗。

• 从急诊的角度来看，上述两种情况的治疗都是相同的。

■ 病因

创伤性断肢可能是由机械、电动手动工具、家用电器、割草机、夹在物体之间、机动车碰撞、挤压伤、爆炸伤、枪伤、刀伤、手指脱套伤(环状撕裂)和动物咬伤引起的。

诊断

■ 症状和体征

病史

• 准确的损伤时间至关重要，因为缺血时间预示着再植的成功：

- 缺血 6 h 后出现不可逆转的肌肉坏死。

- 组织的温度和存在的肌肉的数量预测了可耐受的缺血时间。

- 断肢肌肉越少，耐受的缺血时间越长：

◦ 热缺血时间为 8～12 h。

◦ 冷缺血时间长达 24 h。

- 断肢肌肉质量越多，耐受的缺血时间越少：

◦ 热缺血时间为 4～6 h。

◦ 冷缺血时间为 10～12 h。

• 损伤机制：

- 切口整齐或“切纸机”截肢后再植的预后好于挤压或撕脱伤后再植。

• 阻碍再植成功的并存疾病：

- 糖尿病、外周血管疾病、风湿病、吸烟。

• 利手。

• 社会历史，包括职业和主要爱好。

体格检查

• 评估和记录受损肢体是至关重要的。

• 神经损害的症状：

- 感觉丧失和两点辨别能力丧失。

- 丧失主动活动范围。

• 部分截肢的血管损害迹象：

- 远端暗淡或发紫。

- 毛细血管再充盈延迟(>2 s)。

- 脉搏减弱或消失(多普勒或触诊)。

- 带状征象(截肢或肢体动脉扭曲)。

- 在手部损伤中使用 Allen 试验。

- 脉搏血氧饱和度测定可能对手部损伤有帮助。

• 软组织：评估皮肤、肌肉、肌腱和指甲床的完整性。

• 确定裸露的骨骼和骨折(肉眼畸形、压痛、龟裂)。

■ 急诊检查

急诊检查包括获得准确的病史和体格检查，稳定患者和受伤部分；如果可以选择再植，则会诊或转院。

诊断检查与说明

实验室检查

术前实验室检查，伤口培养。

影像学检查

断肢和残肢的 X 线片都很重要，但不应延误转运。

诊断程序/外科

由外科会诊决定的再植。

鉴别诊断

• 涉及神经、血管和软组织的完整性，以及再植/血运重建的可能性。

• 不要错过合并创伤的其他重大损伤。

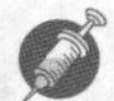

治疗

院前

• 收集所有断肢的部位，包括骨、组织和皮肤的碎片。

• 有关运输过程中截肢部位的护理，请参阅“初步稳定/治疗”。

• 将患者和断肢运送到最近的微血管再植中心，除非其他重大损伤需要运送到最近的创伤中心：

- 如果担心缺血时间，应考虑空运。

初步稳定/治疗

• 尽早咨询外科会诊。

• 建立静脉通路。

• 限制失血：

- 抬高受伤肢体。
- 如果无效则使用大体积的压力敷料或压力点直接施压。
- 如果上述方法不能起到理想的止血效果（袖带压＞收缩压 30 mmHg）。
- 部分断肢由于血管缺乏回缩和痉挛而出血更多。

• 避免对残肢或断肢部分造成进一步的损伤。

- 避免血管钳、烧灼术、血管结扎或清创术。
- 避免重复检查断肢或切除部分。

• 断肢部分的处理：

- 去除严重的污染/异物。
- 用生理盐水轻轻冲洗（避免使用消毒剂）。
- 用生理盐水湿润的纱布包裹。
- 放在干净、干燥的塑料袋或标本杯中。
- 将密封的袋子/杯子放在冰水中（半水半冰）或以 4 ℃冷藏。
- 切勿直接放在冰上或放入冰水中。
- 避免干冰以防止结冰。

• 护理残肢：

- 用生理盐水冲洗，用生理盐水湿纱布覆盖。
- 必要时夹板，保持截肢部位尽可能接近解剖位置。
- 保留所有组织碎片（即使看起来微不足道），因为它们可能用于皮肤、骨或神经移植。
- 肢体截肢时，如有必要，可以用 18G 插管插入近端动脉并用组织保存配方冲洗，这应由外科医师自行决定。

• 如有必要，可用静脉输液或血液制品维持正常血量。

急诊治疗/程序

• 预防性使用破伤风。

• 足够的静脉止痛。

• 患者 NPO。

• 如果组织失活、骨骼外露或受污染，预防性使用抗生素：

- 覆盖链球菌、金黄色葡萄球菌、产气荚膜梭菌。

• 所有患者都适合手术修复，除非专家另有决定。

• 限制截肢部位的缺血时间（即必要时尽早转移）。

• 决定再植时的患者考虑因素：

- 年龄（较年轻的患者更有可能再植）。
- 手指（拇指和长的手指更有可能再植，示指和小指不太可能再植）。
- 损伤程度（MCP 关节更有可能再植）。
- 职业/惯用手。
- 可用程度。
- 一般身体状况和基础疾病，特别是糖尿病、周围血管疾病。

• 再植适应证（无绝对适应证）：

- 拇指，任何水平（提供 40%的手功能）。
- 多指。
- 手掌和手腕远端截肢。
- 指浅屈肌肌腱止点远端和指间关节远端近端（DIP）。
- 一些单指环状撕脱伤。
- 前臂中段近端（如果严重或中度撕脱）。
- 几乎所有的儿童截肢（年轻患者成功率较低，但功能效果更好）。

• 再植成功：

- 一侧受伤（左侧更有可能存活）。
- 损伤区域（DIP 和 IP 关节更有可能存活，近端指骨可能性较小）。

• 再植禁忌证：

- 严重挤压或损毁部位。
- 多个平面的损伤。
- 故意自残的精神病患者。
- 指浅屈肌近端的单指截肢。
- 截肢部位肌腱从肌腱连接处撕脱。
- 下肢很少尝试，通常发生在儿童。
- 其他严重伤害或疾病继发的不稳定患者。
- 年龄较大或有全身麻醉禁忌证者。
- 缺血时间过长。

• 指尖截肢：最常见的上肢截肢类型，远端 DIP 关节：

- 治疗的主要目标：
  - 保持长度。
  - 良好的软组织覆盖。
  - 无痛指尖，皮肤耐用且敏感。
  - 指甲保存。
- 指尖背侧截肢比腹侧截肢预后更好。
- 如果没有暴露的指骨：
  - 用生理盐水冲洗，涂上凡士林浸泡的纱布，让它二次愈合（对于小于 1 cm^2 的伤口效果最好）。
- 少量暴露的指骨：
  - 用咬骨钳缩短骨，使其低于组织水平，达到一期愈合或二次愈合。
  - 任何剩余暴露的骨都需要额外的手术程序和会诊。
  - 出于美容或职业考虑（例如，音乐家），再植是一种选择。
- 如果指骨暴露，则考虑开放性骨折。因此，建议使用抗生素。
- 保留甲床和指甲以优化功能和美容。
- 治疗指甲下血肿。
- 夹板以防止指尖创伤愈合。
- 如果骨或软组织大量丢失，则需要会诊以进行可能的移植或皮瓣。

• 非肢体截肢（阴茎、耳、鼻）：截肢部位的护理应与上文类似，并紧急转诊专家再植：

- 阴茎截肢：最常继发于自残和精神疾病。
- 超过冷缺血 24 h 或热缺血 6 h 后不太可能成功再植。
- 耳截肢：应考虑由适当的专家进行再植。
- 鼻截肢：已成功再植，但结果参差不齐。

• 截肢并发症：

- 深静脉血栓形成。
- 残端血肿。
- 需要再次截肢。
- 幻肢疼痛。

- 屈曲挛缩。

儿科注意事项

• 所有儿童截肢手术都考虑再植。

• 指尖截肢手术通常会因二次意向而自行愈合：

- 即使指尖掌侧截肢的儿童也会自发再生指尖。

- 与成人不同的是，儿童指尖月状远端截肢可以成功移植。

老年人注意事项

高龄并不是再植的绝对禁忌证；然而，潜在的医疗问题往往使年长的患者不适合做手术。

药物治疗

• 一线用药：头孢唑林：0.5～1.5 g，静脉给药/肌内注射，q6～8 h[儿童：25～100 mg/(kg · d)，q8 h，最大剂量 6 g/d]。

• 二线用药：万古霉素 15～20 mg/kg，静脉给药，q12 h；或克林霉素：900 mg，静脉给药，q8 h。

• 如果担心梭菌感染，可考虑使用哌拉西林-他唑巴坦 80 mg/kg，静脉给药，q8 h。

随访

进一步处理

入院指征

所有接受再植或血运重建的患者均需住院。

出院指征

• 轻度指尖截肢或轻度脱套损伤，修复充分且血管系统稳定。

• 需要密切的外科或骨科随访。

转诊问题

• 了解确切的受伤机制和时间。

• 尽早转诊。

• 将影像资料和截肢部分与患者一起转移，储存在适当的介质中。

随访建议

出院但有明显皮肤脱落的患者应考虑植皮，术后随访密切。

要点和误区

• 应尽一切努力最大限度地减少缺血时间。

• 迅速就诊或转移到适当的外科医生和团队是至关重要的。

• 避免截肢部位与冰块直接接触。

• 进行彻底的 ATLS 检查，以避免遗漏其他不太明显但可能危及生命的损伤。

创伤性主动脉破裂 Aortic Rupture, Traumatic(TAI)

Craig J. Kutz · Charlotte A. Sadler　李岩　王瑞兰 译

基础知识

描述

• 创伤性主动脉破裂(也被称为创伤性主动脉损伤或 TAI)是大约 20%的致命性机动车碰撞的死因。

• 约 85%的创伤性主动脉破裂的患者在到达医院前死亡。

• 能存活到急诊的患者通常是限制性破裂，主动脉的血液被外膜包裹。

• 如果没有适当的治疗，只有 15%能活过疾病的初始阶段，49%在第一个 24 h 内死亡，90%在 4 个月内死亡。

• 主动脉破裂患者的平均年龄为 33 岁，70%为男性。

• 大多数撕裂是横向的，不是纵向的。

• 撕裂可以是部分或完全的一周。

病因

• 最常由＞30 mile/h(1 mile/h＝0.447 m/s)的机动车碰撞导致。

• 不系安全带的乘客、驾驶员(方向盘和仪表盘的伤害)，以及被弹出的乘客是最危险的。

• 其他机制：汽车与行人相撞、飞机坠毁、从大于 10 ft(1 ft＝30.48 cm)的高度坠落、挤压和爆炸伤害，直接打击到胸部。

• 主动脉损伤的机制：

- 与相对固定的降主动脉不相等的减速所产生的剪切力以及更多移动性弯曲。

- 主动脉峡部的弯曲应力可能会导致左主支气管和肺动脉上方的主动脉弓弯曲。

- 主动脉弓的弯曲明显地给它施加压力，并使它伸展。

- 当它们撞击脊柱时，骨性结构(例如，内侧锁骨、胸骨柄、第 1 肋骨)会挤压主动脉。

- 压力波引起主动脉瓣远端的主动脉爆裂。

诊断

症状和体征

> **注意**
>
> 不管损伤的严重性，经常出现复杂的共存伤的患者临床表现往往看似微小或不存在。1/3～1/2 的患者无胸部创伤的外部迹象。

病史

• 胸骨后疼痛是最常见的症状，但只存在于大约 25%的患者。

• 呼吸困难、声音嘶哑及喘鸣(扩张的血肿压迫气管)不常见。

体格检查

• 主动脉损伤的检查既不敏感，也无特异性。

• 广泛性高血压可能是由位于主动脉峡部的交感传入神经纤维的刺激引起的。

• 严重的心前区或肩胛间区收缩期杂音(见于 1/3 的患者)。

• 下肢缺血性疼痛，少尿/无尿，远离主动脉弓的降主动脉血流减少导致的截瘫。

• 颈部下方肿胀(血液外渗)。

• 急性主动脉综合征(1/3 的患者出现)：上肢高血压而下肢血压降低，是由主动脉周围血肿压迫主动脉管腔引起的。

基本检查

普通胸片是初步筛查工具，有大约 90%的敏感性，但特异性低。

诊断检查与说明

实验室检查

• CBC。

• 生化检查。

• 凝血酶原时间/部分凝血活酶时间。

• 血型和交叉配血(6～8 U 的 PRBC)。

影像学检查

• 普通 X 线胸片：

- 结果提示纵隔出血、血肿或相关的损伤：

◦ 主动脉弓水平的上纵隔增宽(定义为仰卧

位X线平片>8 cm，直立位>6 cm，或纵隔与胸部宽度比>0.25)是最敏感的征象。
◦ 主动脉弓处模糊不清也是一个敏感的征象。
◦ 更多特异的但不太敏感的迹象包括：主肺动脉窗模糊，鼻胃管向右位移，气管条影增宽，右椎旁交界面增宽。
- 正常纵隔X线片有7%～10%的假阴性率，一些发起人建议自主选用有快速的螺旋CT。
- 儿科患者：最常见的表现是左心尖帽、肺挫伤、主动脉影模糊、纵隔加宽。
• 螺旋CT血管造影：
- 是病情稳定患者首选的检查。
- 应用改良的CT技术，检测主动脉破裂的敏感性和特异性接近100%。
- 在很大程度上减少了主动脉造影的需要。
- 与主动脉X线片相比，优点包括：非侵入性造影，提供其他胸部结构的信息，更快速。
• 胸部CT平扫：
- 用于判定急性主动脉综合征和假阴性扫描高发率的次优工具。
• 主动脉造影：
- 仍被一些专家认为是诊断TAI的金标准。
- 为主动脉撕裂提供精确的解剖定位，对多于1个位点的主动脉损伤有用(15%～20%的病例)。
- 存在导管进一步损坏主动脉的风险。
- 随着CT成像质量的进步，这种方式的需求正在下降。
• 经食管超声(TEE)：
- 在急诊可以快速做完。
- 可以检测到相关的心脏损伤(挫伤、积液等)。
- 据报道有87%～100%的敏感性和98%～100%的特异性，因此需进一步研究TEE是否可靠。
- 禁用于颈部、上颌面或食管损伤的患者。
• MRI：
- 准确度高。
- 研究时间长和监测困难的患者限制使用。

儿科注意事项

大胸腺的存在可能使纵隔增宽的诊断变得困难。

鉴别诊断

• 仰卧位胸片可能导致假阳性的纵隔增宽，如果可能需做直立位PA片。
• 其他原因引起的纵隔血肿。
• 纵隔淋巴结肿大或肿瘤。
• 高血压导致主动脉迂曲。

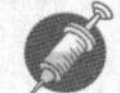

治疗

院前

在受伤现场搜集重要信息：
• 车速。
• 患者是在驾驶员座位，还是在乘客座位。
• 如果患者是司机，查看方向盘损坏程度。
• 弹出还是使用安全带。

初步稳定/治疗

• 遵循高级创伤生命支持原则。
• 危及生命的颅内、腹膜和腹膜后损伤优先治疗。

急诊治疗/程序

• 立即创伤外科会诊。
• 立即心胸外科或血管外科会诊。
• 避免可能导致主动脉样反应的操作(如窒息、紧张)。
• 最新的数据表明，积极的药物治疗血压和心率，延缓手术修复可能会改善结果。
• 药物治疗的目标是使目标心率达60±5次/分，收缩压100～120 mmHg，平均动脉压70～80 mmHg，以减少突然自发破裂和出血的风险：
- β受体阻滞剂如艾司洛尔、拉贝洛尔，是一线药物。
- 使用钙通道阻滞剂的患者禁用β受体阻滞剂(CHF、COPD、二度或三度房室传导阻滞)。
- 如果需要达到目标血压和心率，可添加血管扩张剂(硝普钠)。
- 在急性主动脉综合征中，抗高血压药物是相对禁忌。
• 对于严重低血压，开始快速扩容，包括血液。
• 升压药治疗顽固性低血压，去甲肾上腺素和肾上腺素是首选。
• 中心静脉和动脉导管。

> **注意**
> 只有使用负性肌力药后才使用血管扩张剂(β受体阻滞剂或钙通道阻滞剂)，因为血管扩张剂单独使用能引起完整的主动脉外膜的剪切力的增加。

药物治疗

• 艾司洛尔：500 μg/kg，静脉注射(儿童：100～500 μg/kg，静脉注射)，然后50～150 μg/(kg · min)，静脉输注[儿童：25～100 μg/(kg · min)，静脉注射]。
• 拉贝洛尔：20 mg，静脉注射，随后额外增加40 mg和80 mg(儿童：0.2～10 mg/kg，每次最大剂量20 mg)，q10～15 min，静脉注射，注射总量为300 mg；开始输液时2 mg/min，滴定至10 mg/min[儿童：0.4～3 mg/(kg · min)，静脉注射]。
• 地尔硫䓬：20 mg(0.25 mg/kg)，静脉注射，超过2 min；第二次25 mg(0.35 mg/kg)如果需要，在15 min内注射完；注射剂量5～15 mg/h。
• 去甲肾上腺素：开始时0.5～1 μg/min，滴定至产生所需的反应；8～30 μg/min为常用剂量[儿童：开始时0.05～0.1 μg/(kg · min)，最大剂量2 μg/(kg · min)]。
• 去氧肾上腺素：0.1～0.5 mg，静脉注射，q10～15 min，初始剂量不超过0.5 mg(儿童：5～20 μg/kg的剂量，q10～15 min)；100～180 μg/min或0.5 μg/(kg · min)滴定至预期效果[儿童：0.1～0.5 μg/(kg · min)，滴定至预期效果]。

随访

进一步处理

入院指征

所有主动脉损伤的患者，如果不直接进手术室，必须进入重症监护病房治疗。

随访建议

所有TAI患者均需住院。

要点和误区

• 对于从快速减速的机械装置中受伤的患者，必须保持高度怀疑TAI。
• 临床体征和症状可能是微小的或不存在的，需要依赖一些影像学资料来诊断。
• 应特别注意从创伤患者的胸部X线片上评估纵隔的情况。
• 当诊断确定后，早期药物控制血压和心脏率是最重要的。

C

刺激性气体暴露 Irritant Gas Exposure

Jason Devgun 何超 译

基础知识

描述

- 刺激性物质是指与呼吸道黏膜直接、长期或重复的接触后能够引起呼吸道局部的炎症反应的任何非侵蚀性的物质。
- 呼吸道刺激性物质可以气体、蒸气、小分子颗粒或液体溶胶的各种形式吸入。
- 吸入性刺激物质：
  - 对肺脏的毒性主要取决于物质的水溶性。
- 吸入的刺激性物质通常是刺激性气体和化学性窒息剂的混合物。
  - 一氧化碳。
  - 氰化氢。
  - 硫化氢。
  - 氮氧化合物。
  - 二氧化碳。
- 接触刺激性气体的潜在危险因素：
  - 职业性因素。
  - 蓄意策划的。
  - 意外发生的。
- 病理生理：
  - 刺激性物质在与呼吸道黏膜上的水分接触后产生酸性、碱性和自由基等物质，从而产生细胞毒性。

病因

- 环境：
  - 工业：化学性制造业、矿业、塑料制造和石油工业。
  - 家庭：化学性清洁剂的不合理的使用和储备。
  - 燃烧：燃烧农田所释放的毒性气体。
  - 社会暴动：防暴剂。
- 高水溶性刺激性气体或空气动力学直径>5 mm 的物质一旦与上呼吸道接触即可引发炎症反应。
  - 氨(肥料、制冷剂、染料、塑料品、合成纤维、清洁剂)。
    - 急性症状表现为轻度的水肿、红疹、皮肤全层烧伤及呼吸道梗阻症状。
  - 二氧化硫(生产过程使用的熏蒸消毒剂、漂白剂、制革、制酒酿造、烧煤、含硫化物矿石的冶炼)。
    - 一旦与水蒸气接触会形成硫酸。
  - 氯化氢(在聚氯乙烯等氯化烃的燃烧过程中形成)。
    - 与水结合后形成盐酸。
  - 氯胺(在氨与消毒剂混合过程中产生)。
    - 与湿润的物体表面接触后可形成次氯酸。
  - 丙烯醛(塑料制品的生产、制药、合成纤维、石油制品、纤维素、木材或纸质的燃烧)。
    - 通过与巯基的结合或产生自由基对蛋白质引起损伤。
  - 环氧乙烷(灭菌剂，乙二醇的生产过程中)：
    - 烷基化剂，可能过敏。
  - 甲醛(胶合板、刨花板、保温材料的生产过程中，煤炉或加热器燃烧过程中)。
    - 与水接触后形成甲酸或硫酸。
  - 氟化氢(氟化烃、石油和半导体工业的燃烧过程中)。
    - 消耗机体钙储备从而导致细胞死亡。
  - 防暴剂(辣椒素、氯乙酰苯)。
    - 催泪剂会造成短暂的眼部不适。
    - 高浓度和密闭空间可能会刺激呼吸道黏膜。
- 若刺激性气体水溶性较好或空气动力学直径在 1～5 mm，会在吸入后的数分钟到数小时内出现首发症状。
  - 氯(含氯化合物或漂白剂等物质)。
    - 一旦与水接触形成盐酸或次氯酸后会对上、下呼吸道形成损伤。
  - 硫化氢(污水/有机物衰变，石油工业)：
    - 低浓度(50～500 ppm)刺激物和高浓度(>500 ppm)化学窒息剂。
    - 与呼吸道分泌物反应形成硫化钠，一种腐蚀性物质，导致上下呼吸道损伤。
- 若刺激性气体的水溶性不佳或空气动力学直径<1 mm，会在 24 h 后出现首发症状。
  - 氮氧化合物的产生：
    - 染料或肥料工厂。
    - 电弧焊接。
    - 富含氮元素的饲料的发酵。
    - 硝酸纤维素和聚酰胺燃烧。
  - 光气(电弧焊接、杀虫剂、氯化烃及其溶剂的燃烧)。
  - 臭氧(电弧焊接过程中)。
  - 金属磷化物(与水反应生成磷化氢气体)。
  - 金属性肺炎：
    - 氧化镉(熔炼、焊接和电镀)可能延迟肺纤维增生。
    - 氧化锌(焊接、镀锌)金属烟雾热。
    - 汞蒸气(加热、抽真空)。

诊断

症状和体征

- 症状的轻重依赖于气体的水溶性。
- 水溶性高的气体：
  - 眼睛、鼻腔、喉部的烧伤。
  - 呼吸困难。
  - 喘息。
  - 咳嗽。
  - 声音嘶哑。
  - 喘鸣。
  - 气道梗阻。
- 水溶性一般的气体：
  - 上、下呼吸道受累。
  - 黏膜刺激性。
  - 气道痉挛。
  - 呼吸困难。
  - 喘息。
  - 咳嗽。
  - 啰音。
  - 可能会出现延迟性的肺水肿。
- 其他：
  - 皮肤的刺激。
  - 头痛。
  - 恶心。
  - 呕吐。
  - 痉挛。
  - 晕厥。

病史

- 已知暴露史。
- 化工业的类型。
- 急速出现的症状。
- 来自暴露地点的材料安全数据表。
- 物质的水溶性。

体格检查

- 五官：
  - 结膜充血。
  - 流泪。
  - 球结膜水肿。
- 呼吸道：
  - 喘鸣。
  - 声音的明显改变。
  - 呼吸困难。
  - 喘息。
  - 咳嗽。

• 消化系统：
- 口咽刺激。
- 呕吐。
• 皮肤：
- 皮肤红斑、皮疹或刺激性。
• 神经：
- 意识障碍。
- 发作性活动。

基本检查

老年患者，既往有心脏病病史或严重呼吸系统症状的患者需要进行心电图检查。

诊断检查与说明

以下患者做心电图：
• 老年人。
• 心脏病史。
• 明显肺部症状的证据。
• 接触氟化氢。

实验室检查

• 动脉血气：
- 氧饱和度。
- 通气状况。
- pH。
- 不能完全依赖指脉氧饱和度的检测。
• 吸入烟雾合并刺激性气体的患者需要检测一氧化碳水平：
• 若怀疑一氧化氮中毒，需测定高铁血红蛋白水平。
• 若怀疑氟化氢中毒，需要测定血清钙离子水平。
• 乳酸：可以提示一氧化碳或氰化物产生的细胞毒性。
• 对于育龄期妇女需要进行妊娠试验。
• 快速血糖测定。
• 若怀疑存在急性冠状动脉综合征的患者测定心肌酶谱。

影像学检查

胸部X线片。
• 初期出现症状的时期胸部X线片一般表现正常。
• 一般24 h之后才能发现肺水肿和弥漫性肺损伤的证据。

诊断步骤/外科

• 呼吸量测定法：
- 提供气道狭窄或支气管梗阻的诊断证据。
• 直视喉镜检查：
- 评估是否存在上呼吸水肿。
• 角膜荧光素检查：
- 评估角膜烧伤或损伤。

鉴别诊断

• 严重哮喘。
• 过敏性的刺激（如花粉）。
• 物理性刺激（冷空气）。
• 气管炎。
• 肺炎。
• 职业性哮喘。
• 过度敏感性肺炎。
• 充血性心力衰竭。

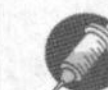

治疗

院前

施救者的目标就是使用必要的衣物或设备实现自我保护。

初始治疗

• ABC管理。
- 通过无复吸性面罩吸入100%全氧。
- 早期进行气管插管能够预防气道水肿。
- 机械通气。
- 必要时进行持续正压通气或呼气末正压通气能够提高氧合。
• 通过脱去污染的衣物和眼睛脱离污染物。

急诊治疗/程序

• 雾化吸入 β_2 受体激动剂（沙丁胺醇）治疗支气管狭窄。
• 吸入、静脉或口服糖皮质激素：倍氯米松、甲泼尼龙、泼尼松。
- 传统治疗方案。
- 尚无对照试验提示吸入刺激性气体后使用糖皮质激素类药物会给患者带来益处。
• 急性氯气中毒的患者可以雾化吸入碳酸钠（3.75%溶液）。
- 在许多个案报道中证明这样的做法能够提高氧合。
• 急性氟化氢吸入中毒的患者可以雾化吸入葡萄糖酸钙。
- 有所报道，但尚无实验证实对患者有益。
• 对怀疑氢氰酸中毒的患者使用羟钴胺素或氰化物解毒剂进行治疗。
• 对于一氧化碳中毒可以尝试氧疗或高压氧疗。

药物治疗

• 沙丁胺醇：0.5 ml（0.03～0.15 mg/kg）溶解于0.5%盐水进行雾化吸入。
• 倍氯米松：1～2喷（40～80 μ/喷），每日2次。
• 葡萄糖酸钙：0.15 g葡萄糖酸钙溶于6 ml生理盐水中，雾化吸入。
• 甲泼尼龙：静脉用药 80～125 mg（1～2 mg/kg）。
• 泼尼松：口服用药 40～80 mg（1～2 mg/kg）。
• 碳酸氢钠：3 ml 8.4%碳酸氢钠溶于2 ml生理盐水中，雾化吸入。

随访

进一步处理

入院指征

• ICU收入指征：
- 气管插管患者。
- 严重呼吸衰竭或存在上呼吸道梗阻风险的患者。
• 存在持续性的呼吸道痉挛。
• 暴露于影响周围气道的刺激性气体：
- 这样的患者可能会出现迟发性的肺水肿和呼吸衰竭。
• 对于儿童、老年人、孕妇及存在持续性慢性阻塞性肺疾病和冠状动脉疾病的患者需要进行保护性治疗策略。

出院指征

• 轻度刺激性气体中毒患者对于治疗反应良好，观察4～6 h不存在缺氧和气道痉挛症状。
• 出院之前，尤其是尚留存一定的临床症状或症状恶化的患者，需要进行影像学检查随访。

随访建议

• 对于职业性暴露于刺激性气体的患者需要提供医学职业指导。
• 对于反复暴露和症状复发的患者需要进行肺功能的随访。

要点和误区

• 需要警惕那些水溶性不佳的气体所引起的迟发症状，这种情况下一般需要观察23 h以上才会出现临床症状。
• 避免接触第一次暴露的患者并对其进行必要的消毒。

丛集性头痛

Andrew K. Chang · Kevin P. Collins 刘雪峰 译

基础知识

描述

- 难以忍受初发剧烈头痛：
  - 发病率低，约为 0.1%。
- 随着发作的时间逐渐减轻：
  - 发作持续 15～180 min，75%的患者发作时间<60 min。
- 男性多见，男女比例约为 3∶1。
- 初次发作多在 30～50 岁。
- 疼痛丛集性发作，持续数周至数月后缓解，缓解期>1 个月。
- 发作期大多持续 2～3 个月，每日发作 1～3 次。
- 常常每日固定时间发作。
- 常常每年固定时间发作：
  - 春秋季为高发季节。
- 慢性丛集性头痛：
  - 缓解期<1 个月。
  - 很多患者无明显缓解期。
  - 10%的患者可发展为慢性。
  - 通常由发作性丛集性头痛演变而来。
- 在临床表现和病理生理学方面与偏头痛有很多相似之处。
- 疼痛区域类似于三叉神经痛。

病因

- 完整反射弧：
  - 三叉神经血管反射通过正反馈机制和随后的下丘脑功能障碍增强三叉神经疼痛和丛集性头痛的颅自主神经特征。
  - 三叉神经血管周围传入神经释放 CGRP，导致三叉神经神经元的血管扩张/痛觉活动的调节，导致严重疼痛。

诊断

症状和体征

病史

- 单侧疼痛，发作期间的疼痛部位很少变化。
- 尖锐的穿透样刺痛。
- 突然发作，5～15 min 可达疼痛高峰。
- 突然停止。
- 发作导致患者疲惫不堪：
  - 部位：
    - 眼睛。
    - 太阳穴。
  - 疼痛放射至：
    - 耳。
    - 面颊。
    - 颌部。
    - 牙齿。
    - 鼻。
    - 同侧颈部。
- 多在夜间发作。
- 多与饮酒、服用硝酸甘油及含胺类物质有关。
- 多与压力、长时间紧张、过度劳累、烦躁情绪等相关。
- 没有前驱症状。

体格检查

- 情绪焦虑、烦躁不安。
- 与偏头痛患者喜欢安静休息不同，丛集性头痛患者喜欢站立或来回踱步。
- 伴随症状：
  - 疼痛同侧：
    - 鼻塞，流涕。
    - 结膜充血，流泪。
    - 面红。
    - 眼睑水肿。
    - Horner 征。
    - 面部、前额出汗。

基本检查

- 精确的病史和体格检查能够帮助明确诊断。
- 排除危及生命的问题。

诊断检查与说明

实验室检查

- 腰椎穿刺（鉴别脑膜炎或蛛网膜下腔出血）。
- 红细胞沉降率（鉴别颞动脉炎）。

影像学检查

CT/MRI（鉴别颅内出血、肿瘤）。

鉴别诊断

- 偏头痛。
- 三叉神经痛。
- 脑膜炎。
- 颞动脉炎。
- 颅内占位。
- 带状疱疹。
- 颅内出血。
- 口腔科疾病。
- 青光眼等眼及眼眶疾病。
- 颞颌关节综合征。

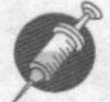

治疗

院前

- 识别危及生命的头痛病因。
- 面罩吸氧能够缓解症状。

初步稳定/治疗

- 排除危及生命的病因。
- 吸氧。

药物治疗

- 麦角碱：二氢埃托啡 0.5～1 mg，静脉注射，必要时可 1 h 重复给药。
- 芬太尼：2～3 μg/kg，静脉注射。
- 利多卡因：4%～10%喷 0.2 ml 经鼻同侧鼻孔，蝶腭神经节阻滞对难治性病例可能是有益的。
- 吗啡：2～4 mg，静脉注射或肌内注射，可 10 min 重复给药。
- 非甾体抗炎药：酮洛酸 15～30 mg，静脉注射或肌内注射。
- 氧气：面罩吸纯氧。
- 普鲁氯嗪：10 mg，静脉注射或肌内注射。
- 生长抑素：100 μg，皮下注射。
- 舒马曲坦：6 mg，皮下注射，1 h 内可重复给药 1 次，最大剂量为 12 mg/24 h。
- 速释型维拉帕米：可选择的预防药物，起始剂量 80 mg，每日 3 次。
- 佐米曲普坦：5～10 mg 滴鼻喷雾剂，单次使用于一个鼻孔。

一线药物

- 氧气：面罩吸氧，12 L/min，持续 15 min。
- 舒马曲坦。
- 二氢埃托啡。

二线药物

- 麻醉药物。
- 糖皮质激素。

 **随访**

■ 进一步处理

入院指征

- 常规治疗效果不佳。
- 诊断不明。

出院指征

- 诊断明确，神经系统查体无异常，疼痛缓解。
- 可家庭使用氧气和/或舒马曲坦。

转诊问题

安排神经科医师随访。

要点和误区

- 精确的病史对于诊断十分必要。
- 吸入纯氧是首选治疗。
- 剧烈的丛集性头痛可导致患者产生自杀倾向：
  - 对这部分患者的随访是必需的，可能持续数月。

C

大麻素和合成大麻素中毒 Cannabinoids and Synthetic Cannabinoids Poisoning

Elizabeth Black 陆晓烨 朱长青 译

基础知识

描述

• 大麻素是一种广泛的、结构上多样化的药物，通过与大麻素受体的结合和激动剂特性而结合。
• 大麻素是大麻的植物提取物：
- 可加工成：
◦ 压缩树脂(印度大麻，混合大麻)。
◦ 从树脂(哈希油)中提取的油，萃取到溶剂[丁烷哈希油(BHO)、710、dab、蜡、碎等]。
- 初级精神活性化合物是四氢大麻酚(THC)：
◦ THC含量在产品之间差异很大，提取物通常具有较高的百分比。
◦ 大麻酚和大麻二醇(CBD)有较少/轻微的精神活性，并且以不同的比例存在。
◦ 用于娱乐和医疗目的的法律允许程度在美国因州而异。
• 合成大麻素是大麻素受体激动剂中不断变化的群体，而这比起相似度的化学结构，其实与它们的营销策略更相关。
- 这一群体出现在2004年，作为草药香混合，与合成大麻素受体激动剂。
- 弓形虫更严重。
• 吸入或摄入：
- 当吸入时，在3～10 min达到峰值浓度。
- 当摄入时，发病可能需要3 h，峰值效应在2～6 h。

流行病学

预估发病率和流行率

• 大麻是美国最常用的非法异生物。
• 男性在其他方面使用的发生率较高。
• 一项2017年的调查报道了49.5%的受访者。>12岁的人一生中吸食过大麻，而在过去的1年里，19%的人吸食过大麻。
• 5.3%的12～17岁的受访者使用过大麻，12.4%在过去的1年，6.5%在过去的1个月。
• 大麻素剧吐综合征：
- 与长期大量吸食大麻有关。

诊断

症状和体征

病史

• 摄入方法有助于确定预期的摄入量。
• 症状的发作和持续时间。
• 可能确实有，也可能没有摄入。
• 有长期用药史的患者可能比首次使用患者更能耐受副作用。
• 在儿童摄入方面，仔细询问是否在家中接触到药物或其他物质。
• 患者可诉：
- 嗜睡/潮湿。
- 头晕。
- 视觉障碍。
- 心悸。
- 共济失调(儿童比较突出)。
- 精神状态改变。
- 焦虑/偏执。
• 大麻素剧吐综合征：
- 腹痛。
- 恶心。
- 高温淋浴/浴缸可以改善剧吐。
- 类阿片和抗吐药难治剧吐。

体格检查

• 可能会随着查体顺序的变化而变化。
• 合成大麻素的检查结果是可变的，并且不应期望与THC的包含物结果相似。

生命体征

• 心动过速和高血压：
- 在儿童及使用合成大麻素中更突出。
• 体位性低血压。

检查

• 呼吸功能不全/呼吸困难：
- 主要是儿童。
• 心动过缓或心动过速。
• 结膜注射。
• 嗜睡/潮湿。
• 协调性下降，共济失调。
• 妄想症，精神病特征。

合成大麻素的特征

• 极度激动。
• 癫痫发作。
• 心律失常或心动过缓。
• 胸痛，ACS。
• 呼吸衰竭。
• 急性肾衰竭。

基本检查

• 大麻/大麻衍生物/THC：
- 即时血糖水平。
- 全面体格检查。
• 合成大麻素：
- 电解质、BUN、肌酐、葡萄糖。
- 肌酐激酶。
- 肌钙蛋白。
- 尿检。

诊断检查与说明

实验室检查

• 尿液药物筛查：
- 对于儿科患者确认暴露，但由于无法确定暴露时间而受到限制。
• 任何出血的迹象或怀疑大麻素与溴鼠隆掺假进行凝血功能检查。

影像学检查

心电图用于诊断合成大麻素的摄入。

鉴别诊断

• 其他滥用药物：
- 卡西酮("浴盐")。
- 致幻剂：
◦ 迷幻药。
◦ 曼陀罗。
◦ 普斯普剂。
◦ 氯胺酮。
• 低血糖。
• 创伤性脑损伤。
• 精神疾病的基础。

治疗

院前

• 注意气道和呼吸。
• 心电监测。
• 建立静脉通路。
• 快速葡萄糖测定。
• 怀疑吸毒过量时要获得药丸瓶、药丸及胃内容物。

初始稳定/治疗

• ABC管理：
- 安全气道，并协助通气补充氧气，以防止低氧血症。
- 静脉补充生理盐水。
- 心脏功能监测。
• 使用纳洛酮、硫胺素和葡萄糖改变的精神状态/昏迷。

■ 急诊治疗/程序

• 大麻素中毒没有解药。
• 大麻的症状控制：
- 确认是否为大麻素中毒。
- 可用苯二氮䓬类药物。
• 合成大麻素：
- 苯二氮䓬类药物用于躁动、癫痫。
- 根据临床表现进行 AKI、ACS 治疗。
- 支持性护理。
• 儿科患者：
- 观察。
- 根据临床进行插管用于封闭或呼吸抑制。
• 大麻素剧吐综合征：
- 明确的治疗方法是停止使用大麻。
- 辣椒素奶油和氟哌啶醇在病例报道中改善症状，但这是超说明书用法。

凝血病

• 在 2018 年，合成大麻素的暴发。报道了与 brodifacoum（一种超华法林灭鼠剂，估计半衰期为 16～62 日）掺假的情况：
- 要求对使用合成大麻素和不明原因出血（血尿、鼻出血、牙龈出血等）的患者进行凝血功能检查。
- 通过控制任何危及生命的出血，纠正凝血功能障碍来治疗。
- 用口服维生素 K 治疗 INR 升高的稳定患者：
◦ 长期（周至月）门诊。监测凝血病和调整维生素 K 剂量所需的随访。

■ 药物治疗

• 葡萄糖：D_{50}W 1 安瓿 50 ml 或 25 g（儿童：D_{25}W 2～4 ml/kg），静脉注射，如果降糖。
• 地西泮：5～10 mg，静脉注射（儿童：0.2～0.5 mg/kg，静脉注射）。
• 氟哌啶醇（Haldol）：2.5～5 mg，静脉注射或肌内注射；不推荐给儿童。
• 劳拉西泮：1～4 mg，静脉注射或肌内注射（儿童：0.02～0.05 mg/kg，静脉注射或肌内注射），可根据需要重复。
• 纳洛酮（纳坎）：0.04～2 mg（儿童：0.1 mg/kg）初始剂量。
• 硫胺素（维生素 B_1）：100 mg，静脉注射或肌内注射。

 随访

■ 进一步处理

入院指征

• 持续改变的精神状态。
• 明确的摄入药物证据。
• 持续生命体征异常。
• 横纹肌溶解、凝血病的证据。

出院指征

• 正常精神状态/临床清醒。
• 正常的生命体征。

转诊问题

• 为滥用药物提供咨询。
• 儿童保护服务转介服务。
• 儿科暴露的情况。

■ 随访建议

儿科注意事项

就像任何药物一样，医用大麻应该远离儿童。

要点和误区

随着大麻被非刑罪化，商业的、可食用的产品增加了，这些产品在视觉上无法与良性食品和糖果区分开来。患者在不知情的情况下摄入巧克力或软糖等产品后出现大麻素中毒表现尤其严重，特别是在儿科患者中。

D

带状疱疹 Herpes Zoster

Daniel F. Leiva · Taraneh Matin · Aaron Hexdall 陈奇通 李文放 译

 基础知识

■ 描述

• 俗称带状疱疹（HZ）。
• 发病率为每 1 000 人中 3～5 人。60 岁或以上患者中，每年每 1 000 人有 6～8 人发病。
• 通常表现为单侧疼痛小疱的暴发，沿着单个皮肤节，但不典型的表现包括胶质瘤的形成。
• 免疫缺陷宿主的传播、并发症和死亡风险增加。
• 危险因素包括：
- 女性。
- 白种人。
- 家族史呈剂量依赖性。
- 自身免疫性疾病。
- 包括 CKD、DM、COPD 在内的共病情况。
- 哮喘、抑郁。
- 物理伤害。
- 他汀类药物使用。
• ＞50 岁年龄组带状疱疹引起的血管病变发生后 3～12 个月发生卒中和心肌梗死的风险增加。

■ 病因

• 由水痘-带状疱疹病毒（VZV）引起，属于疱疹病毒科家族中的一种 DNA 病毒。
• 背根神经节休眠病毒的再激活。
• 主要发生在以前患有水痘的个体中，很少发生在接种过疫苗的个体中。

妊娠注意事项

妊娠期带状疱疹与先天性水痘综合征风险增加无关。

儿科注意事项

可能发生在儿童时期，最常见于原发性水痘发生于子宫或出生后最初 6 个月。

 诊断

■ 症状和体征

• 单边皮区带状疱疹：
- 75%的患者有疼痛和感觉异常的前驱症状。
- 疼痛可能是尖锐的、钝的、刺痛的、烧灼的，或包括强烈的瘙痒。
- 也可能出现异位痛。
- 典型的皮疹是红斑基部的黄斑丘疹，然后形成小疱。
- 在 7～10 日进展结痂；每隔 2～3 周痂会脱落。
- 最常见的神经分布是胸、腰椎，其次是三叉神经和颈神经。
- 较少涉及多个相邻皮节或双侧皮节（不对

称时带状疱疹双侧皮节)。

- 无疹性带状疱疹：
  - 前驱期后未出现皮疹。
  - 对主诉神经根持续疼痛的患者增加怀疑。
- 眼带状疱疹(HZO)：
  - 三叉神经眼支受累。
  - Hutchinson 征-鼻窦病变。
  - 通常会导致角膜炎。
  - 可能导致点状角膜炎或角膜假性树突(溃疡性减轻，荧光素摄取少于 HSV 树突)。
  - 可导致以飞蚊症和疼痛性周边视力丧失为特征的急性视网膜坏死，或以无痛性视力丧失为特征的进行性外部视网膜坏死。
- 脑神经炎：
  - 表现取决于脑神经受累。
  - 例如，累及脑神经Ⅲ、Ⅳ和Ⅵ可表现为眼麻痹和上睑下垂。
  - 例如，Ramsay Hunt 综合征。
- Ramsay Hunt 综合征：
  - 脑神经Ⅶ和Ⅷ受累：外耳道病变、周围性面瘫、眩晕及前 2/3 舌麻痹。
  - 皮肤结痂形成过程超过 7～10 日，结痂在 2～3 周脱落；最常见的受累神经分布是胸部和腰部，其次是三叉神经和颈部。
- 播散性疾病可引起：脊髓炎、脑膜脑炎、周围神经病、肝炎、肺炎。
- 带状疱疹后神经痛(PHN)是带状疱疹的一种并发症：表现为皮肤病治愈后在带状疱疹病变部位持续 3 个月的疼痛；10%～70%的患者在病灶消退后会出现疼痛；发病率随年龄(大于 50 岁)增加，并伴有严重皮疹和严重疼痛。

基本检查

- 大多数患者的临床表现足以诊断。
- 实验室可能有助于非典型皮疹或播散性疾病患者的诊断。

诊断检查与说明

实验室检查

- VZV DNA PCR 是金标准：
  - 从囊泡刮擦血液、唾液、脑脊液或灌洗。
  - 可以区分 HSV 和 VZV。
  - 最敏感、最具特异性。
- Tzanck 涂片：廉价简易，刮无顶囊泡底部。
  - 在亚甲蓝、吉姆萨染色或瑞氏染色观察到核内包涵体的多核巨细胞。
  - 无法区分 VZV 和 HSV。
  - 低灵敏度。
- 血清学(IgM/IgG)：更难解读，敏感度和特异度低。
- 病毒培养：
  - 1～2 周出结果。
  - 特异性低，敏感性也低。

鉴别诊断

- 原发性水痘。
- 单纯疱疹病毒(HSV)。
- 角膜炎。
- 结膜炎(nonherpetic)。
- 三叉神经痛。
- 周围性眩晕。
- 偏头痛。
- 蜂窝织炎。
- 毒葛。
- 水疱脓疱病。
- 接触传染性软疣。
- 心绞痛。
- 胆绞痛和肾绞痛。
- 阑尾炎。
- 肌肉紧张。
- 神经根病。

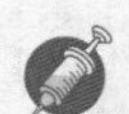

治疗

院前

带状疱疹具有传染性，可能导致非免疫医护人员出现水痘：病变应覆盖非结痂病变，保持常规预防措施。

急诊治疗/程序

- 自限性疾病。
- 治疗的目标是减少疼痛和病程，并预防 PHN。
- 非免疫缺陷者。
  - 抗病毒药物：普伐洛韦有最简单的剂量，似乎是最有效的；也可以使用阿昔洛韦(最便宜的选择)或泛昔洛韦；应该在出疹后 72 h 内开始使用，但一些专家建议如果仍有新的水疱出现，则应晚一点开始使用。
  - 镇痛药：柘台代理(轻度疾病)，长效阿片类药物。
  - 皮质类固醇激素(有争议)：一些研究显示皮肤愈合和急性神经炎略有改善，无助于预防 PHN；如果没有其他禁忌证，可以考虑给患有严重疾病或中枢神经系统受累的免疫缺陷患者使用。
- 免疫缺陷者：
  - 抗病毒治疗：静脉注射阿昔洛韦。
  - 镇痛药：如上。
  - 皮质类固醇激素：如上。
- 眼带状疱疹：眼科会诊的必要性；伐昔洛韦如上；静脉注射阿昔洛韦治疗免疫功能低下或脑神经受累；红霉素软膏治疗继发性细菌感染；虹膜炎相关的局部睫状肌麻痹；眼科医师可能推荐局部使用类固醇。
- PHN：未显示抗病毒药物，长效阿片类药物，三环类抗抑郁药是有效的，加巴喷丁和普瑞巴林也可能有帮助，局部利多卡因可短期缓解疼痛。
- 暴露后预防：
  - 对于以下患者，建议在暴露后 72 h 内使用 VariZIG：免疫功能低下的、妊娠的、妊娠<28 周的早产儿暴露的、妊娠>28 周的早产儿暴露于血清阴性母亲、母亲患有症状性水痘的新生儿在产前 5 日至产后 2 日内出生、在接种后续疫苗之前必须等待 5 个月。
- 疫苗：
  - Zostavax/ZVL(默克公司)是一种减毒活疫苗，推荐给所有>60 岁的患者，无论过去是否有带状疱疹病史：
    - 发现 60 岁以上的产品具有成本效益。
    - 禁用，如果免疫功能低下。
    - 功效随年龄增长而下降。
    - 无论如何，复发被发现不那么严重。
    - 效果随时间下降。
  - Shingrix/RZV(GlaxoSmithKline)是一种 2 剂量重组亚单位疫苗，最近已获得 FDA 批准，适用于 50 岁及 50 岁以上人群。
    - RZV 疫苗在预防 HZV 方面的有效性为 97%，并且比传统的 ZVL 疫苗持续时间更长。
    - RZV 尚未在免疫缺陷人群中进行调查。

妊娠注意事项

- 与免疫功能正常的患者相同的治疗。
- 妊娠期禁忌接种疫苗。

儿科注意事项

新生儿带状疱疹需要静脉注射阿昔洛韦治疗。

药物治疗

一线用药

- 口服抗病毒药物：
  - 缬阿昔洛韦：1 g，口服，q8 h，持续 7 日。
  - 阿昔洛韦：800 mg，口服，q4 h，持续 7～10 日。
- 静脉注射抗病毒药物：
  - 阿昔洛韦：10 mg/kg，静脉注射，q8 h，持续 7 日。
- 镇痛药：对乙酰氨基酚 500 mg，口服，

q6 h，不超过 4 g/d；布洛芬 600 mg，口服，q6 h；羟考酮铬 10 mg，口服，q12 h；阿米替林 25 mg，口服，qh，耐受增加至每日 100 mg；环戊醇眼药水 1%涂抹患眼 1 滴，q8 h。

• PHN 镇痛：
- 5%利多卡因贴片：在 24 h 内，最多使用 3 个贴片，最长 12 h。

• 泼尼松：
- 60 mg，口服，每日 1 次，持续 7 日；然后 30 mg，每日 1 次，持续 7 日；然后 15 mg，每日 1 次，持续 7 日。

• PEP：
- 水痘-带状疱疹免疫球蛋白(VariZIG)：每 10 kg 体重 125 U，肌内注射或静脉注射，最大剂量 625 U。

• 疫苗：
- Zostavax(默克)一次性皮下注射。

二线用药

• 阿昔洛韦耐药的免疫功能低下者：
- 膦甲酸：90 mg/kg，静脉注射，q12 h，输注 2 h(未经 FDA 批准)。
- 西多福韦：每周 5 mg/kg，连续 2 周，每隔 5 mg/kg(未获 FDA 批准)。

• 抗生素：
- 红霉素眼药膏 USP 0.5%：敷患眼，q4 h。

• 止痛剂：
- 加巴喷丁：100～300 mg，q8 h 时；或每小时增加 300 mg。100～300 mg 每 3 日 1 次，直到有充分的反应或最大剂量 3 600 mg/d。
- 普瑞巴林：75 mg 口服，q12 h；或 75 mg，每晚睡前；在耐受情况下，每 3 日增加 75 mg，每日 2 次，最大剂量 600 mg。
- 去甲替林：10～25 mg，每晚睡前；耐受时增加 10～25 mg×(3～7)日至最大 150 mg/d。

随访

进一步处理

入院指征

• 免疫功能低下。
• 播散性疾病。
• 脑神经受累的 HZO。
• 顽固性疼痛。
• 隔离：做好所有原发性水痘或播散性带状疱疹患者或带状疱疹免疫低下患者的空气传播隔离预防措施；患者在皮疹出现前 48 h 开始具有传染性，直到所有病灶结痂。

出院指征

• 大多数是门诊管理。
• 应告知患者，病变可能会因瘢痕愈合或留下脱色区域。
• 建议与孕妇或免疫缺陷者隔离，直到所有病灶结痂。
• PHN 可能需要长期随访和/或转介给疼痛专家。

妊娠注意事项

通常被视为门诊患者。

儿科注意事项

新生儿带状疱疹。

要点和误区

• 如果皮疹累及鼻尖(Hutchinson 征)，注意眼睛受累。
• 暴露每个胸痛患者的皮肤。
• 在没有皮疹的情况下不考虑诊断。
• 未能警告患者 PHN 的风险。

丹毒 Erysipelas

Kate E. Hughes 单怡 译

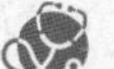

基础知识

描述

• 皮肤浅表性细菌感染伴浅表淋巴结受累。
• 常有白细胞计数增加。
• 3%～5%的血培养阳性。
• 涉及浅表淋巴管在内的真皮上层。
• 相反，蜂窝织炎损伤深层真皮和皮下脂肪。

病因

• A 组 β 溶血性链球菌为致病微生物(C 组和 G 组链球菌少见)。
• 侵入口：
- 皮肤溃疡。
- 局部创伤。
- 擦伤。
- 银屑病或湿疹样病变。
- 真菌感染。

儿科注意事项

• B 型流感嗜血杆菌(HIB)引起的面部蜂窝织炎患儿可能出现类似丹毒表现。
- 未接受免疫接种的儿童应考虑。
- 许多可能为菌血症，需要住院。
- 头孢呋辛或其他适当的流感嗜血杆菌的存在很重要。
- 由于 HIB 疫苗的广泛使用，H 型流感嗜血杆菌较少见。
• B 组链球菌可引起新生儿丹毒。
• 感染可来源于脐带残端。

妊娠注意事项

• 产褥期乳腺炎的乳腺红斑通常是由金黄色葡萄球菌引起的，因此应覆盖耐甲氧西林金黄色葡萄球菌(MRSA)抗感染治疗。
- 见分型。

诊断

症状和体征

• 最常见受累的部位是面部(5%～20%)、小腿(70%～80%)和耳。
• 皮肤呈现密集火红色，因此得名“圣安东尼热”。
• 脸部常双侧受累，但其他部位为单侧受累。
• 好发于婴儿、儿童和老人。
• 前驱的全身症状包括全身不适、发热、畏寒、恶心及呕吐；皮疹发生在前驱症状后 1～2 日。
• 不一定都能找到引起感染的原发皮肤损伤。
• 少数合并眶周蜂窝织炎或侵犯海绵窦。

病史

• 面部丹毒可能来源于鼻咽感染或创伤。
• 淋巴管阻塞的好发部位：
- 特别是在乳腺炎根治术后的上肢。
- 隐静脉制备或剥脱后发生频率增加。
- 可能是先前未确诊淋巴管阻塞或先天性淋巴水肿的患者(如 Milroy 病)的特征性表现。
• 3 年内复发率 30%，源于丹毒发作引起的淋巴管阻塞。

体格检查

• 受累皮肤：

- 水肿。
- 硬化。
- 疼痛。
- 边界清晰的斑块。

• 面部感染时脸颊和鼻上会出现典型的蝶形红斑。

• 严重感染时会出现水疱和大疱。

基本检查

• 临床诊断：

- 基于特征性的皮肤表现和临床诊断标准。

• 针吸伤口细菌培养阳性率较低，并不推荐。

诊断检查与说明

实验室检查

• 皮肤拭子培养并不推荐，因为只能显示皮肤表面生物菌群。

• 糖尿病和其他高危人群，或低血压患者和需要住院的患者应行全血细胞计数分类和血培养：

- 淋巴水肿患者血培养阳性率高。

• 糖尿病患者监测血糖，因为感染会影响血糖的控制。

• 尿常规：检查蛋白尿、血尿、红细胞管型。

- 有助于诊断链球菌感染后肾小球肾炎(PSGN)。
- 通常在皮肤感染 2 周后发病。

• 抗链球菌溶血素 O(ASL-O)、抗 DNA 酶 B 和链球菌溶血素抗体滴度变化可用于诊断链球菌感染后免疫疾病，如风湿热或肾小球肾炎。

- 不应过度应用于诊断和处理无并发症的丹毒。
- 不应常规应用，除非已经有并发症的表现。

影像学检查

• 典型的丹毒没有标准的影像学表现。

- 如果怀疑更深层次的感染如肌炎，手足 X 线平片或 CT 扫描可以用来评估气体存在。

• 如果怀疑丹毒超声可用于评估脓肿或下肢深静脉血栓。

鉴别诊断

• 脓肿。

• 急性细菌性鼻窦炎。

• 过敏性炎症。

• 蜂窝织炎。

• 接触性皮炎。

• 下肢深静脉血栓。

• 弥漫性炎性乳腺癌。

• 家族性地中海热。

• 带状疱疹，第Ⅴ脑神经第二支。

• 炎症性脓疱疮。

• 皮肤真菌病。

• 乳腺炎。

• 坏死性筋膜炎。

• 眶周蜂窝织炎。

• 系统性红斑狼疮(SLE)伴蝶形红斑。

• 链球菌或金黄色葡萄球菌中毒性休克综合征(晒伤样皮疹)。

• 静脉淤滞性皮炎。

• 病毒疹。

治疗

院前

接触患者前洗手戴手套，降低链球菌传播的风险。

初步稳定/治疗

患者可有中毒表现，需要静脉液体复苏或升压。

急诊治疗/程序

• 合理的抗生素治疗，治疗时间应为 10 日：

• 轻度：若无中毒症状，依从性好，并可保证密切随访的患者可口服治疗。

• 当症状符合丹毒诊断时，首选青霉素治疗。

• 如果难以和蜂窝织炎区别，应加用覆盖金黄色葡萄球菌的抗生素：

- 使用耐碳青霉烯类青霉素或第一代头孢菌素。
- 如果在 MRSA 高发地区，使用万古霉素或其他抗 MRSA 的抗生素。
- 传报对万古霉素耐药的葡萄球菌。

• 乙酰氨基酚类药物可治疗发热。

• 院内隔离。

- 感染性。

药物治疗

门诊：

• 青霉素Ⅴ：500 mg，口服，q6 h[儿童：25～50 mg/(kg·d)，q6～8 h]，连续应用 10 日。

• 阿莫西林：500 mg，口服，q8 h[儿童：50 mg/(kg·d)，每日 3 次]，连续应用 10 日。

• 氯洁霉素：300 mg，口服，每日 4 次[儿童：8～25 mg/(kg·d)，每日 3 次或每日 4 次]，连续应用 10 日。

• 双氯西林：500 mg，口服，q6 h[儿童：30～50 mg/(kg·d)，口服，q6 h]，连续应用 10 日。

• 红霉素：250～500 mg，口服，q6 h[儿童：40 mg/(kg·d)，口服，q6 h]，连续应用 10 日。

• 头孢氨苄：500 mg，口服，q6 h[儿童：40 mg/(kg·d)，口服，q8 h]，连续应用 10 日。

• 头孢呋辛：250～500 mg，口服，每日 2 次[儿童：30 mg/(kg·d)，口服，q12 h]，连续应用 10 日。

住院：

• 青霉素：200 万 U，q4 h，静脉注射(儿童：25 000 U/kg，静脉注射，q6 h)。

• 青霉素，普鲁卡因：60 万～120 万 U，q12 h，肌内注射。

• 氯洁霉素：600 mg，q8 h，静脉注射[儿童：20～40 mg/(kg·d)，静脉注射，q8 h]。

• 万古霉素：15 mg/kg，静脉注射，q12 h，超过 1.5～2 h 降低红人综合征死亡风险(儿童：10～15 mg/kg，静脉注射，q6 h)。

• 头孢曲松：1 g，静脉滴注，q24 h。

• 头孢唑林：1 g，静脉滴注，q8 h。

一线用药

• 口服或静脉注射：青霉素或第一代头孢菌素。

• 对青霉素过敏者使用克林霉素。

二线用药

口服：红霉素。

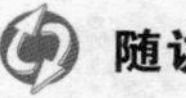

随访

进一步处理

入院指征

• 广泛受累、发热、有中毒表现的患者，或怀疑眼眶或眶周蜂窝织炎的患者。

• 潜在的免疫抑制性合并症(糖尿病、酒精中毒、免疫功能低下)。

• 独居或不能口服药物的患者，需住院静脉注射抗生素。

• 口服抗生素无效。

• 不能耐受口服抗生素。

• 儿童更常要求住院。

- 血培养。
- 未接受 HIB 疫苗免疫的患者应在初始治疗即静脉应用覆盖流感嗜血杆菌的抗生素。

出院指征

• 面部受累范围小。

- 无中毒表现。
- 无免疫功能低下。
- 能够接受和遵循口服治疗。
- 2～3 日充足的随访和监督。
- 诊断确定。

转诊问题

- 转入肾脏内科医师处评估和治疗链球菌感染后肾小球肾炎：
  - 血尿、蛋白尿、尿常规中测出红细胞。
  - 特别是 5～15 岁的儿童。
- 传染病医师会诊评估感染免疫功能低下患者感染不常见微生物的风险。

随访建议

- 用皮肤记号笔标记感染的边缘以监测感染。
- 下肢淋巴水肿患者使用弹力袜可降低复发率。
- 丹毒的腿部症状需随访，外用抗真菌霜或软膏治疗足癣。

要点和误区

- 难以恢复，或与疼痛不成比例的表现，提示更深层次的感染，需要进一步检查以排除坏死性筋膜炎，或混合需氧/厌氧菌坏死性蜂窝织炎。
- 治疗潜在的淋巴水肿可减少复发。
- 存在的小脓疱提示葡萄球菌感染/蜂窝织炎而不是丹毒，需要覆盖更广谱的抗生素。
- 皮肤有捻发音需要鉴别诊断。
- 由于感染很可能进入创伤破裂的皮肤，要记得检查破伤风免疫状态，必要时再次处理。
- 频繁复发的患者应做好预防。

单胺氧化酶抑制药中毒 Monoamine Oxidase Inhibitor Poisoning

James W. Rhee 伍力学 译

D

基础知识

描述

- 单胺氧化酶抑制药(MAOI)主要用于抗抑郁。
- 司来吉兰，有时被用于治疗帕金森，也可制成经皮贴剂。
- MAOI 的药理作用：
  - 破坏内生性单胺的合成和降解，从而导致：
    - 神经性去甲肾上腺水平升高。
    - 某些类型的受体水平下调。
  - 抑制不可逆(非竞争性)酶。
  - 抑制其他含维生素 B_6 的酶。
- 单胺氧化酶(MAO)：是神经活性胺类的最主要的灭活物。
  - MAO A：
    - 主要分布在肠道和肝脏。
    - 灭活与饮食相关的生物活性胺。
  - MAO B：
    - 主要存在于神经末梢和终板。
    - 灭活拟交感活性的胺类物质。

病因

- MAOI 过量：
  - 对该类药物的毒理学缺乏了解。
  - MAO 抑制剂：与苯丙胺化学结构相似。
    - 早期：间接的拟交感效应。
    - 晚期：阻滞交感反射(可引起低血压)。
- MAOI 高血压危象综合征：
  - 发病是由于去甲肾上腺素降解受阻，或一些间接或混合作用的拟交感药物所释放的去甲肾上腺素沉淀物的存在。
  - 常见的沉淀物有酪胺、可卡因、苯丙胺。
- 5-羟色胺综合征(SS)：
  - 常见病因一般为联合使用了影响 5-羟色胺代谢和作用的药物。
  - 5-羟色胺合成增加：色氨酸。
  - 5-羟色胺释放增多：
    - 间接和混合作用的拟交感药物及多巴胺受体激动剂。
  - 5-羟色胺重摄取减少：
    - 选择性 5-羟色胺重吸收抑制剂。
    - 三环类抗抑郁药。
    - 新型抗抑郁药：曲唑酮、奈法唑酮、文拉法新。
    - 阿片类药物：哌替啶、右美沙芬、曲马多、美沙酮、丙氧酚。
  - 直接 5-羟色胺受体激动剂：
    - 丁螺环酮、舒马曲坦、麦角酸、二乙基胺。
  - 5-羟色胺降解减少：
    - MAOI。
  - 非特异性 5-羟色胺活性增加：
    - 锂盐。

诊断

症状和体征

- MAOI 过量：
  - 起病时间在 6～12 h 以后。
  - 原发性高血压有头痛症状。
  - 肾上腺反应性增高。
    - 心动过速。
    - 血压升高。
    - 瞳孔扩大。
    - 烦躁不安。
  - 神经肌肉兴奋：
    - 眼球颤动。
    - 反射亢进。
    - 躯体颤动。
    - 肌阵挛。
    - 肌强直。
    - 癫痫发作。
  - 高热。
  - 相关并发症：
    - 横纹肌溶解。
    - 肾衰竭。
    - 弥散性血管内凝血(DIC)。
    - 急性呼吸窘迫综合征(ARDS)。
    - MAOI 高血压危象(MAOI 与药物或事物相互作用)：
  - 高血压。
  - 心动过速或心动过缓。
  - 高热。
  - 头痛，以枕部为多。
  - 情志改变。
  - 颅内出血。
  - 癫痫发作。
- 5-羟色胺综合征：
  - 神经肌肉反应性升高。
  - 腱反射增强：
    - 下肢比上肢更明显。
  - 肢体颤动。

- 肌阵挛。
- 自主神经反应性升高：
  - 高热。
- 中枢神经系统：
  - 烦躁不安。
  - 幻觉。
  - 精神错乱。
  - 昏迷。
- 腹泻。
- 5-羟色胺综合征与抗精神病药物恶性综合征(NMS)的鉴别：
  - 两者均可表现为中度到重度的临床症状及体征。
  - 起病时间：前者多在数小时内起病，后者多在数日内起病。
  - 胃肠道症状：前者可能有，后者则无。
  - 许多病例只能依靠用药史加以鉴别。

病史

- 询问服药时间。
- 让其提供相关药品的外包装。
- 询问是故意服药或意外服药。
- 询问是否同时服药其他药物。

体格检查

- 神经肌肉高反应性：
  - 肌阵挛。
  - 强直。
  - 震颤。
  - 反射亢进。
- 自主神经高反应性：
  - 心动过速或过缓。
  - 发热。
  - 出汗。
- 精神异常：
  - 烦躁、思维混乱、兴奋。

基本检查

- 服药史。
- 肛温监测。
- 血压及心电监护。

诊断检查与说明

实验室检查

- 尿液分析：
  - 血尿。
  - 肌红蛋白尿。
- 电解质、尿素/肌酐、葡萄糖：
  - 低血糖可能导致精神状态改变。
  - 酸中毒可能伴随严重中毒。
  - 横纹肌溶解可能导致肾衰竭。
  - 高血钾：急性肾衰竭所致的致命性后果。
- 凝血功能监测，防范潜在的DIC：
  - INR、凝血酶原时间、部分活化凝血活酶时间、血小板。
- 肌酸激酶：
  - 发生横纹肌溶解时显著升高。
- 尿毒物检测：
  - 考虑到一些MAOI类药物与苯丙胺化学结构相似，尿液检查可能提示苯丙胺阳性。
- 阿司匹林和对乙酰氨基酚水平在自杀病例中可能升高。
- 血气分析。

影像学检查

- X线胸片：
  - ARDS。
- 头颅CT检查可应用于有显著头痛、情志改变及神经系统定位体征者：
  - 蛛网膜下腔出血，颅内出血。

诊断步骤/外科

腰椎穿刺术：

- 可疑的脑膜炎(头痛、神志改变、高热)。
- 可疑的蛛网膜下腔出血和正常CT影像。

鉴别诊断

- 高热：
  - 感染。
  - 甲状腺功能亢进症。
  - 中暑。
  - 丘脑功能障碍。
  - NMS。
  - 恶性高热。
  - 恶性肌紧张。
  - 酒精或药物戒断反应。
  - 抗胆碱药中毒。
  - 拟交感药物过量。
  - 可卡因相关性谵妄及横纹肌溶解。
  - 水杨酸中毒。
  - 茶碱中毒。
  - 尼古丁中毒。
- 高血压：
  - 低血糖。
  - 类癌综合征。
  - 嗜铬细胞瘤。
  - 酒精或药物戒断反应。
  - 拟交感药物中毒。

治疗

院前

- 患者可能不配合，甚至有攻击性。
- 建立安全的静脉通路。
- 预防自伤。

初步稳定/治疗

- ABC管理。
- 如有低血压应给予静脉输液和液体复苏。
- 给氧。
- 心电监护。
- 如有神志改变可给予纳洛酮、硫胺素(维生素 B_1)并监测血糖。

急诊治疗/程序

- 胃肠道内毒物清除：
  - 服药时间在1h内者应考虑洗胃治疗。
  - 活性炭吸附治疗。
- 高热：
  - 苯二氮䓬类可用于有躁动患者。
  - 体温>40℃者要积极降温。
    - 给予喷雾降温。
    - 风扇促进蒸发降温。
  - 瘫痪：
    - 持续高热造成的肌强直和反射亢进。
    - 非去极化肌松药(如维溴库胺)。
    - 避免使用琥珀胆碱。
    - 气管插管；机械通气。
  - 应用对乙酰氨基酚。
  - 使用降温毯。
- 严重的恶性高血压：
  - 硝普钠(供MAOI过量者选用)。
  - 钙通道阻滞剂或酚妥拉明(供MAOI和食物有协同作用者选用)。
  - 应用短效静脉注射药物可快速控制病情。
- 低血压：
  - 首先使用大剂量等张晶体液。
  - 若无效，可使用去甲肾上腺素。
  - 但多巴胺效果较差。
- 心律失常(MAOI过量的发病前表现)。
  - 治疗可按心律失常治疗原则进行。
- 癫痫：
  - 苯二氮䓬类药物。
  - 巴比妥类药物(苯二氮䓬类无效时用)。
  - 维生素 B_6(难治性癫痫)。
- 肌强直：
  - 苯二氮䓬类。
  - 给予肌松药(维库溴铵)麻痹并行气管插管和机械通气。
- ARDS：
  - 氧疗。
  - 气管插管和适度的呼气末正压。
- DIC：
  - 新鲜冰冻血浆。

- 血小板。
- 输注全血。
• 横纹肌溶解：
- 静脉给予等张晶体液。
- 充分补液疗法并保持足够的尿量。
• 5-羟色胺综合征的特殊治疗：
- 主要措施：支持治疗，停用可能加重病情的药物。
- 非选择性 5-羟色胺受体拮抗剂：
◦ 赛庚啶。

> **注意**
> 酚妥拉明忌用于 MAOI 过量(会造成难逆的β受体激动作用)。

■ **药物治疗**

• 活性炭：1～2 g/kg，口服。
• 赛庚啶：4～8 mg，口服或鼻饲，q1～4 h，直到起效；每日最大剂量：0.5 mg/kg[儿童：0.25 mg/(kg·d)；最大剂量 12 mg/d，尚无 2 岁以下儿童的用药安全性数据]。
• 葡萄糖：50%葡萄糖 1～2 安瓿(相当于 50～100 ml 或 25～50 g)(儿童：25%葡萄糖 2～4 ml/kg)，静脉推注。
• 地西泮：5～10 mg(儿童：0.1 mg/kg 缓慢给药)，缓慢静脉推注。
• 劳拉西泮：1～2 mg，缓慢静脉推注。
• 硝普钠：0.3～10 μg/(kg·min)，静脉给药。
• 去甲肾上腺素：2～4 μg/(kg·min)[儿童 0.05～0.1 μg/(kg·min)]，静脉给药。
• 酚妥拉明：5 mg(儿童：0.05～0.2 mg/kg)，缓慢静脉推注。
• 碳酸氢钠：1～2 mEq/kg，静脉注射；成人输注：3 安瓿(1 安瓿相当于 50 mEq)碳酸氢钠钠溶于 1 000 ml 5%葡萄糖中以 2～3 ml/(kg·h)，静脉给药。
• 维库溴铵：0.1 mg/kg，静脉注射。

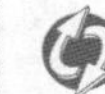

随访

■ **进一步处理**

> **注意**
> MAOI 中毒有迟发型，有必要延长临床观察时间。

入院指征

• 所有的 MAOI 过量患者均应收入监护病区观察 24 h 以上。
• 病情较重的应收入 ICU。

出院指征

高血压或 5-羟色胺综合征已基本缓解者，可在急诊室数小时后予以出院。

转诊问题

故意服药过量者应接受精神科随访以预防自杀。

■ **随访建议**

在出现明显 MAOI 中毒后，该类药物的应用方式应再评估以预防后续风险。

要点和误区

• 常在症状出现后 6～12 h 发病。
• 利奈唑胺和亚甲蓝是 MAOI。
• 酚妥拉明因禁忌用于绝对的β受体激动效应后的 MAOI 过量。
• 应注意不要服用任何其他具有 5-羟色胺特性的药物，因为这可能会加剧潜在的毒性。

D

单纯疱疹 Herpes Simplex

Aaron Hexdall · Myung Bae 陈奇通 译

基础知识

■ **描述**

• 多侵犯皮肤黏膜区，以反复发作的疼痛和水疱为特征。
• 常见于口唇、生殖器、直肠、手和眼。
• 感染分为两阶段：
- 第一阶段为原发性的感染，潜伏于神经节内。
- 第二阶段为同一部位疾病复发。
• 潜伏期一般为接触病毒后 0～4 日。
• 病毒在原发感染的 7～10 日消失，最长至 23 日。在复发感染时仅需要 3～4 日。
• 新生儿感染可发生于子宫内，常见于分娩时，产后也可发生。
- 每年美国有 1/3 500 的新生人口感染。
• 人和人之间传播。
• 单纯疱疹病毒 1 型(HSV-1)是美国脑炎最常见的病毒病因。
- 未经治疗的感染，死亡率>70%。
• HSV-1 通常从童年开始通过非性接触传播。
• 单纯疱疹病毒 2 型(HSV-2)几乎都是通过性传播的。
• 60%～90%的人口感染 HSV-1 和 HSV-2。
• 在年龄小于 40 岁的人群中，黑种人比白种人更常见。
• 女性多于男性。
• 单纯疱疹脑炎：经由嗅觉或三叉神经进入：
- 偏好内侧和下颞叶。

■ **病因**

• HSV-1 或 HSV-2 病毒是疱疹病毒科的 DNA 病毒。
• 病毒可能经由呼吸道飞沫、黏膜或破损的皮肤接触感染的分泌物进行传播：
- 单纯疱疹病毒复发性黏膜脱落可能传播病毒。
- 复发率随病毒类型和解剖部位的不同而不同。
• 两种病毒均能感染口腔或生殖器黏膜：
- 最常见的为 HSV-1 引起口腔感染和 HSV-2 引起的生殖器感染。

诊断

■ **症状和体征**

• 许多原发性感染不能被识别，只能用抗体滴度进行检测。
• 临床上可见红斑上有 1～2 mm 的水疱。
• 水疱内可出现清亮或浑浊的液体，或可能出现脓疱。

口腔颌面部感染

• 原发性感染：
- 龈口炎或咽炎：
◦ 累及牙龈和黏膜溃疡性皮疹。
◦ 发热，全身不适，烦躁，头痛，肌痛，颈淋巴结肿大。

◦ 原发性感染症状通常持续2～4周，愈合后不留瘢痕。
◦ 由于疼痛致使进食困难可能会导致脱水。
• 复发性感染：
- 常累及口唇、唇缘。
- 通常接触到阳光、热、压力、创伤(龟裂、擦伤)等因素，或处于免疫抑制状态。
- 患者会有瘙痒、刺痛、隐痛等症状，可见红斑、丘疹/囊，少有全身症状。
- 许多人抗体效价上升但是没有复发。
- HSV-1引起的口腔感染复发频率高于HSV-2引起的生殖器感染复发。HSV-2生殖器感染复发为HSV-1生殖器感染复发频率的6倍。

皮肤感染

• HSV-1或HSV-2暴露史。
• 突然出现发热、水肿、红斑和局部压痛。
• 疱疹性指头炎：
- HSV-2感染较HSV-1更常见，手指侧面出现单个或多个囊泡。
- 可能从口腔或生殖器感染或存在职业暴露。
- 持续3～4周。
- 可复发。
- 在年幼的孩子，吸吮拇指接触HSV-1可致龈口炎。
• 外伤性疱疹：
- 继发于手术、口腔处理后、阳光照射或烧伤。
- 运动员皮肤黏膜的感染常涉及胸部、面部及双手，尤其是摔跤运动员。
• 疱疹性湿疹：
- 与过敏性皮炎和HSV感染有关。
- 相比HSV-2，HSV-1引起的儿童和青年人的过敏性皮炎更为常见。
- 葡萄球菌二次感染常发生。
- 使用激素或感染艾滋病病毒风险较高。
- 水痘样疹可蔓延至周围皮肤。
- 发热，头痛，疲劳。
• HSV相关性多形性红斑：
- 通常见于手掌和足底。
- 持续2～3周。

眼睛

• 最常见的角膜致盲的原因。
• 通过面部感染扩散或直接感染而引起。
• 急性疼痛和畏光。
• 耳周淋巴结肿大，视力模糊，球结膜水肿，结膜炎。
• 单侧或双侧均有。
• 荧光检查可见角膜存在树突状病灶。
• 与水痘-带状疱疹的不同，不累及生皮层。
• 哈钦森征：
- 在鼻尖的囊泡通常表明眼部受累，累及鼻睫神经。

累及中枢神经系统/脑炎

• 是西方重症散发性脑炎最常见的原因。
• 通常为HSV-1感染所致。
• 在西方世界，严重散发性脑炎最常见的原因。
• 通常来自HSV-1再激活病。
• 标志性症状：急性发热和神经症状：
- 偏瘫，共济失调，局灶性癫痫，精神状态改变。
• HSV-2感染女性脑膜炎：
- 良性病程与脑炎比较。
- 有些可复发性淋巴细胞脑膜炎(Mollaret综合征)。

病史

有或没有HSV-1或HSV-2暴露史。

体格检查

在颜面部或会阴区皮肤黏膜病变。

儿科注意事项

• 60%～80%的HSV感染患儿的母亲无生殖器疱疹史。
• 初次检查时可有水疱性皮肤病变。
• 会阴区感染能够增加胎儿患病风险。
• 感染多发于童年，仅5%～10%的儿童有症状。
• 最常见的面部疾病为5岁以下小儿的龈口炎。
• 口腔疱疹的儿童吮吸手指可致甲沟炎或脓性指头炎。

基本检查

• 疱疹性脑炎：
- 疑有疱疹性脑炎应做腰椎穿刺检查。
• 眼部疱疹：
- 应进行荧光检查。

诊断检查与说明

• 面部：
- 通过病史和检查进行初步诊断。
- 确诊要素：
- PCR检测囊泡中的病毒(金标准)。
◦ 荧光抗体检测，血清抗体检测。
◦ Tzanck涂片或巴氏染色。
◦ 皮肤角化过度或苔藓样变的患者应进行皮肤活检。
• 眼睛：
- 荧光检查可见树突状角膜病变。
- 囊液病毒培养或荧光抗体检测。
• 中枢神经系统和脑炎：
- 腰椎穿刺检查可有脑脊液细胞增多，细菌抗体阴性。
- 脑脊液PCR检测。
- MRI和CT(可出现颞叶异常情况)。
- 脑电图显示颞叶尖峰电位异常。

实验室检查

• 皮损刮片进行培养或PCR检测。
• Tzanck涂片显示多核巨细胞、不典型角质细胞及巨大细胞核。
• 血清试验诊断力度有限。
• ELISA试验可检测HSV抗体，表明既往感染史。
• 血清学变化出现在2周到3个多月。

鉴别诊断

• 面部和皮肤：
- 细菌性咽炎。
- 肺炎支原体咽炎。
- 史-约综合征。
- 水痘。
- 带状疱疹。
- 天疱疮。
- 接触性皮炎或药物性皮炎。
- 脓疱病。
- 梅毒。
• 眼睛：
- 结膜炎：病毒性、细菌性或过敏性。
- 疱疹性眼炎。
- 闭角型青光眼。
- 角膜外伤。
• 神经：
- 急性播散性脑脊髓炎。
- 艾滋病脑炎。
- 复杂。
- 蛛网膜下腔出血。
- 细菌性脑膜炎。
- 偏头痛。
- 神经梅毒。
- 多种脑炎。
- 癫痫。

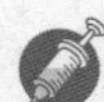

治疗

院前

• 对症支持综合治疗。
• 止痛。

初步稳定/治疗

昏迷患者和怀疑累及中枢的患者应进行

气道控制

■ 急诊治疗/程序

• 累及面部或口腔：
- 健康儿童原发性疾病一般不予以治疗。
- 轻度患者只需要对症支持治疗及镇痛。
- 重度患者或免疫功能低下的患者：静脉注射或口服阿昔洛韦、泛昔洛韦或伐昔洛韦。
- 口服用阿昔洛韦为治疗的一线药物。
- 复发如果有前驱症状或出现以下标志性病变，选择口服抗病毒药物较好：1～2 日症状减轻。
- 患者每年发作超过 6 次考虑预防；既往史有疱疹相关性多形性红斑或为运动员疱疹；即将有日光暴露或应激；口腔手术；面部治疗：
◦ 有效预防可减少口唇疱疹发生的频率和严重程度，有助于病毒的清除，从而降低传播风险。
◦ 无法治愈疾病。
◦ 预防停止后，大多数患者会有复发。
• 皮肤(非面部和会阴区)：
- 口服阿昔洛韦治疗。
- 如果继发细菌感染使用抗生素，不进行干预可能导致感染扩散。
• 眼睛：
- 口服阿昔洛韦，局部外用抗病毒治疗药物曲氟尿苷和阿糖腺苷。
- 儿童宜用用阿糖腺苷软膏。
- 激素可导致感染病毒扩散。
- 累及眼部应及时会诊。

妊娠注意事项
• 60%的孕妇 HSV-1 呈血清学阳性。
• 20%的孕妇 HSV-2 呈血清学阳性。
• 产妇在分娩时的原发性感染导致 60%的新生儿疱疹风险。
• 如果有生殖器疱疹病史，从 36 周开始进行抗病毒治疗直到分娩。
• 如有活动性病变，可选择剖宫产。

■ 药物治疗

• 阿昔洛韦：
- 面部和皮肤：400 mg，口服，每日 3 次，用 7～10 日，静脉注射(5～10 mg/kg)，8 h/次，连用 7～14 日。
- 儿童皮肤原发性感染：40～80 mg/kg，口服，分 3～4 次服用，连用 5～10 日；最大剂量 1 g/d。
- 眼部：400 mg，口服，2 次/日。
- 脑炎：60 mg/kg，静脉滴注，8 h/次，连用 14～21 日。
• 泛昔洛韦：
- 原发性面部疱疹：250 mg，3 次/日，连用 7～10 日(免疫功能正常)；500 mg，口服，连用 7～10 日(免疫功能抑制)。
• 曲氟尿苷：
- 成人和超过 6 岁的儿童：眼科会诊后，1 滴 1%眼膏眼，2 h/次(每日最多 9 滴)，至少 10 日，然后逐渐减量。
• 伐昔洛韦：
- 成人原发性皮肤黏膜病损：1 000 mg，口服，2 次/日，连用 7 日。
- 成人复发性皮肤黏膜：500 mg，口服，2 次/日，连用 3 日。
• 阿糖腺苷：
- 成人和 2 岁以上小儿：3%眼药膏外用，5 次/日。
• 复发性皮肤黏膜疱疹：
- 阿昔洛韦：400 mg，口服，3 次/日，连用 5 日。
- 泛昔洛韦：1 000 mg，口服，2 次/日，连用 1 日。
- valacydovir：500 mg，口服，2 次/日，连用 3 日。
• 长期预防：
- 阿昔洛韦：400 mg，口服，2 次/日。
- valacydovir：500 mg，口服，1 次/日。
- 泛昔洛韦：250 mg，口服，2 次/日。

注意
- 肾衰竭患者抗病毒药物的剂量可能需要调整。
- 局部抗病毒药物是可行的，但没有显示可以缩短症状的时间或减少复发。

随访

■ 进一步处理

入院指征
• 脑炎，浸润性疾病，脱水。
• 免疫低下患者出现局部或浸润性病变。
• 新生儿 HSV。
• 重症监护应进行气道支持。
• 眼部受累应进行眼科会诊。

出院指征
简单性局部病变。

转诊问题
• 抑制治疗。
• 孕妇感染。

■ 随访建议

皮肤和生殖器感染：与医师一起探讨治疗的风险和益处。

要点和误区

• 脑膜炎和脑炎的患者，难以考虑单纯疱疹病毒性脑炎。
• 患者出现眼部疼痛、视力下降和鼻部病变时应考虑眼部单纯疱疹。
• 疾病活动期以及预后的 1～2 周，应向患者告知传染风险。
• 疾病活动期应提醒患者避免接触病灶，以防止病变扩散到其他身体部位。

D

单关节性关节炎 Arthritis, Monoarticular

Mark Darocki · Binh T. Ly 汤璐佳 潘曙明 译

基础知识

■ 描述

• 局限于一个关节，非游走性。
• 病因可较多。
• 感染性关节炎：关节破坏迅速，可造成严重功能障碍。
- 连续扩展性炎症(蜂窝织炎、骨髓炎)、血源性播散、直接种植。
- 发病诱因：
◦ 局部因素(炎症性关节炎、创伤、人工关节)。
◦ 免疫抑制。
◦ 静脉使用药物。
• 结晶性关节炎：

- 痛风：尿酸过剩或过少，沉积在关节内或周围。
- 假性痛风：焦磷酸钙。
- 非炎症性因素：
- 骨关节炎、创伤（骨折、关节积血）、自身免疫疾病。
- 进行性关节破坏，功能损伤。
  - 骨骼反应性改变（骨刺）。
  - 软骨下骨侵蚀。

病因

- 感染（脓毒症）：
- 非淋菌性细菌多见。
  - 革兰阳性菌：链球菌、葡萄球菌（80%）。
- 非常见因素：
  - 金黄色葡萄球菌（创伤、静脉使用药物）。
  - 淋病奈瑟菌。
  - 沙门菌（镰状细胞）、链球菌及葡萄球菌亦可引起镰状细胞病。
  - 其他：真菌（慢性）、螺旋体（莱姆）、病毒（多关节型）、分枝杆菌（结核）。
- 结晶：
- 痛风：尿酸过剩或过少，沉积在关节内或周围。
- 痛风石：结晶反复沉积在同一位置，可增大，可形成溃疡，排除结晶。
- 反双折射结晶。
- 假性痛风：焦磷酸钙。
- 正双折射结晶。
- 肥胖手术：术后尿酸分泌常常明显增加，推荐使用预防性措施。
- 炎症：
- 应寻找可能的炎症因素：关节炎（风湿病、银屑病）、炎症性肠病、Reiter 综合征。
- 非炎症性因素：
- 骨关节炎或退行性关节病、关节使用过度、关节负荷过重（肥胖）。
- 创伤（骨折、关节积血）。
- 出血性疾病。
- 神经性疾病（夏科关节）。

儿童注意事项

- 感染性关节炎：
- 发病率低，死亡率高，脓毒症（8%）。
- 金黄色菌最常见，髋关节较膝关节常见，50%合并骨髓炎。
- 症状与成人类似：关节肿痛，活动时疼痛加剧；全身症状明显（发热、乏力）。
- 炎症因素：
- 排除感染性关节炎后诊断才可成立，诊断方法同成人。
- 非炎症因素：
- 骨科不应忽视。
- Salter-Harris 骨骺板骨折。
- 先天性髋关节发育不良。
- 股骨头骨骺滑脱。
- 肥胖青少年：
- 股骨头骨骺炎。
- 股骨头骨骺无菌坏死。
- 发病年龄为 4～9 岁：
- 出血性疾病。

诊断

早期准确诊断有利于及时治疗，尽早恢复功能便于日常活动，降低长期发病率。

症状和体征

- 局限于一个关节，非游走性。
- 急性红、肿、热、痛。
- 活动受限、不能负重（渗出、疼痛、骨髓炎）。
- 感染性关节炎：
- 持续发热、寒战，全身症状重。
- 大关节肿胀、活动受限。
- 膝关节＞髋关节＝肩关节＞踝关节＞腕关节。
- 淋病奈瑟菌：男性排尿痛，排脓尿。
- 莱姆病：
  - 伯氏疏螺旋体。
  - 鹿蜱（蓖籽硬蜱与达敏硬蜱）。
  - 中心性扩散，突发（慢性游走性红斑）。
  - 膝关节与肩关节多见。
- 结晶性：
- 突发剧痛，关节肿胀，红斑。
- 具有反复自限性。
- 痛风：趾关节肿大（痛风足）＞踝关节＞跗关节＞膝关节。
- 痛风石：关节上出现结晶性肉芽肿，溃疡，结晶排出。
- 假性痛风：膝关节＞腕关节＞踝关节＝肘关节。
- 炎症性：
- 症状不典型，常表现为全身症状。
- 可累及单一、多个、联合器官系统，如 Reiter 综合征：虹膜炎、尿道炎、关节炎。
- 非炎症性：
- 骨关节炎：晨僵，活动后好转，休息后复发。
- 创伤：近期或远期外伤，关节缓慢出现肿胀，疼痛症状同骨关节炎。
- 神经性疾病：夏科关节，关节疼痛不剧烈。
- 慢性神经性疾病。
- 出血性疾病。

病史

- 见“描述”“病因”“儿童注意事项”及“症状和体征”。
- 完整详细询问病史：关节累及情况（近期、远期）、全身系统症状（直接、间接）、免疫状态（HIV 感染、药物、疾病过程中）、淋病奈瑟菌（病史、接触史、治疗过程）、静脉用药史。

体格检查

见“描述”与“症状和体征”内容。

基本检查

- 详细询问病史，仔细进行体格检查。
- 相关诊断学因素。
- 关节穿刺抽取关节液进行分析是确诊手段之一。

诊断检查与说明

实验室检查

- 血液检查：从来都不是单关节炎首选的关键诊断研究，提供辅助性的确证、排除性的信息。
- 关节穿刺术进行滑液抽吸和分析：是确切的诊断程序和研究。
- 人工关节：关节穿刺前要咨询骨科医师。
- 滑膜液培养：是关于感染的明确的验证试验，但结果不是即时的。
- 如果可以对滑液进行 DNA 检测，可以考虑针对淋球菌和衣原体进行聚合酶链反应（PCR）检测。
- 液体外观：透明、浆液性、脓性、血性。
- 滑膜液中的白细胞（WBC）、多形核（PMN）占优势，提示有脓毒症相关病因。
- 白细胞＞50 000/mm^3 增加了脓性关节炎的可能性。＞100 000/mm^3 高度可疑。也有报道低至 20 000/mm^3 的化脓性关节炎。
- PMN＞75%会增加化脓性关节炎的可能性。
- 滑膜葡萄糖：与同时进行检测的血糖水平相比最有用。
- 滑膜葡萄糖低于血液值的一半，表明可能是脓毒症过程。
- 革兰染色（阳性）：指导最初的抗生素选

择,肠外给药。

- 革兰阳性球菌:万古霉素(20 mg/kg)。
- 革兰阴性球菌:头孢曲松(2 g)。
- 革兰阴性杆菌:头孢噻肟(1~2 g)。

• 革兰染色(阴性):临床怀疑为化脓性关节,经验性使用万古霉素+头孢噻肟。

• 怀疑是假单胞菌:头孢他啶+庆大霉素(1.5 mg/kg)。对头孢菌素过敏的则使用环丙沙星(400 mg)+庆大霉素。

• 青霉素过敏的患者:阿曲南(2 g)+庆大霉素。

• 晶体分析。偏振光显微镜检查双折射晶体:痛风(阴性),假性痛风(阳性)。

• 血性关节液中的脂肪球:怀疑骨折。

• 其他非急诊检查的考虑。

- 对可疑疾病进行风湿病学“筛查”。尿酸、C反应蛋白(CRP)、红细胞沉降率(ESR)、类风湿因子(RF)、抗环瓜氨酸肽(ACCP)。
- 对流行地区出现的单关节炎进行莱姆测试(抗伯氏疏螺旋体滴定或“莱姆滴定法”)。

影像学检查

• X线平片检查:

- 关节表面:软骨、软骨下侵蚀、关节边缘破坏或反应性骨形成(骨刺)、骨缺失、骨折。
- 感染:以上发现加软组织肿胀、关节腔变形。
- 结晶:以上发现加软组织钙化,痛风石常位于或接近于反复发作部位。

• 超声检查:可探查关节液、组织、血运、关节周围组织、异物(尤其是细小与组织密度类似的有机物)。

- 可为穿刺定位。

• MRI可发现骨坏死及细小骨折。

• 怀疑炎症性关节炎尤其是慢性炎症性关节炎患者不推荐进行骨扫描。

诊断步骤/外科

见上述“诊断检查与说明”内容。

• 关节腔穿刺抽液分析是确诊方法。

鉴别诊断

见“病因”“儿童注意事项”及“症状和体征”内容。

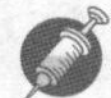

治疗

院前

随后的标题中包含所有相关内容。

初步稳定/治疗

• 关节固定,位置合适。

• 建立血管通路,以获得快速、可滴定、可预测的药物治疗效果。

• 症状控制。疼痛、恶心、呕吐、补液。

急诊治疗/程序

• 关节抽吸并进行液体分析。

• 肠外给药:革兰染色呈阳性。

- 革兰阳性球菌:万古霉素(20 mg/kg)。
- 革兰阴性球菌:头孢曲松(2 g)。
- 革兰阴性杆菌。头孢噻肟(1~2 g)。

• 革兰染色阴性,临床怀疑为化脓性关节。经验性使用万古霉素+头孢噻肟。

• 怀疑是假单胞菌:头孢他啶+庆大霉素(1.5 mg/kg)。

- 头孢类药物过敏:环丙沙星(400 mg)+庆大霉素。

• 青霉素过敏:阿曲南(2 g)+庆大霉素。

• 镰状细胞病:万古霉素+环丙沙星或亚胺培南(500 mg)。

• 骨科手术咨询,评估手术冲洗情况。

• 痛风:

- 非甾体抗炎药。禁忌:肾脏疾病、消化性溃疡(PUD)、心血管疾病、同时使用抗凝血剂。如果患者年龄大于60岁,则需谨慎用药。
- 秋水仙碱(口服):1.2 mg,1 h后再服0.6 mg。肝脏疾病、Cr<30,同时使用P-糖蛋白和/或CYP3A4抑制剂的患者应避免使用。如果Cr<45,请调整剂量。就消化道不良反应进行预防教育。
- 秋水仙碱(静脉注射)。由于剂量难以把握和不良反应常见,静脉注射秋水仙碱应谨慎使用,并咨询药剂师或风湿病学专家。
- 口服糖皮质激素。泼尼松每日30~40 mg,直到症状改善,然后在7日内逐渐减少胃肠道不良反应。
- 情绪变化、高血糖、液体潴留。
- 关节内糖皮质激素。只有在排除了感染和对口服治疗有禁忌的情况下才能使用。
- 其他注意事项。门诊随访,讨论预防/预防性治疗。

• 非炎症性:

- 镇痛剂。
- 物理治疗、康复。
- 骨科创伤:固定,控制疼痛,确保神经血管状态完整。
- 出血性原因。纠正因子水平,关节置换。

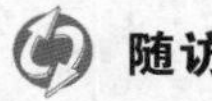

随访

进一步处理

入院指征

• 无法进行日常活动。

• 全身症状明显合并代谢紊乱(脓毒症、糖尿病酮症酸中毒)。

• 需要进行手术(包括冲洗术)。

• 难治性疼痛。

• 所有感染性关节炎:

- 常规医疗处理,普通病房床位。
- 如考虑脓毒症、代谢紊乱首选监护病房。

• 结晶性关节炎:

- 难治性恶心、呕吐、腹泻。
- 合并感染性关节炎。

出院指征

• 症状及并发症得到有效控制、体征稳定。

• 可以出院用药:可选择长期经济的药物并能够理解使用方法和剂量。

• 已安排随访。

转诊问题

感染病原体不明确、难治性疼痛、难以控制并发症、无法恢复日常活动时应及时会诊。

随访建议

• 应安排有经验的医师随访。

• 如无法安排合适的处置医师应及时送至急诊室。

要点和误区

• 关节腔穿刺抽液革兰染色是最重要、最直接的诊断方法,可为初步处置提供依据。

• 合并关节腔内类固醇注射治疗、糖尿病、吸毒、外伤、蜂窝织炎或关节外感染区域注射治疗患者应考虑感染性关节炎。

D

单核细胞增多症 Mononucleosis

Steven C. Rogers · Alberto Cohen-Abbo 伍力学 译

基础知识

描述

- 大多数病例为EB病毒(一种疱疹病毒)感染所致。
  - 非EB病毒所致的传染性单核细胞增多症(IM):
    - 巨细胞病毒(CMV)。
    - 腺病毒。
    - 甲型肝炎。
    - 疱疹病毒6型。
    - 人类免疫缺陷病毒(HIV)。
    - 风疹。
    - 弓形虫。
    - A组β溶血性链球菌。
- 超过90%的成人血清学检测提示既往存在EB病毒感染。
  - 多数人无法回忆是否存在特异性的IM感染症状。
- 传播途径为近距离或亲密接触,尤其是亲吻中有唾液接触者,可有或无症状。
  - 绰号"接吻病"。
  - 唾液中的病毒可终身存在。
  - 可发生在输血或器官移植后。
- 潜伏期:4~6周。
- 免疫反应:
  - T细胞反应:
    - T细胞反应是淋巴细胞绝对数升高及相关临床症状和并发症发生的原因。
    - T细胞亚型,细胞毒性CD8细胞(Downey细胞),内有偏心分布的分叶细胞核,细胞质有空泡:这种"异型淋巴细胞"易于区分。
  - B细胞反应:
    - EB病毒感染B细胞在其中复制。
    - B细胞随后转化成可分泌免疫球蛋白的浆细胞。
    - IgM抗体的分泌:该嗜异性抗体由红细胞抗原刺激性产生。
- 因IM致死的病例很少见,但下列并发症可能致死:
  - 气道水肿。
  - 神经系统并发症。
  - 继发细菌感染。
  - 脾破裂。
  - 肝衰竭。
  - 心肌炎。
- EB病毒感染与非洲Buikitt淋巴瘤和鼻咽癌的发生密切相关。

儿科注意事项

- <4岁的儿童,发生EB病毒感染时常无症状。
- 对于有症状的患儿,部分非典型症状具有倾向性:
  - 白细胞缺乏,肺炎和各型皮疹。
  - 肠系膜淋巴结炎和巨脾症使得该病患者有腹痛表现,易被误诊为阑尾炎。
  - 婴幼儿有时仅表现为易激惹和生长缓慢,无其他原因可以解释的,应考虑该病。

诊断

症状和体征

病史

- 典型者在潜伏数日至数周后突然起病。
- 乏力,精神不振,关节肌肉疼痛等为前驱症状,呈"盈-亏"消长二相表现。
- 明显而剧烈的咽痛、气道水肿或呼吸窘迫。
- 淋巴结肿大。
- 头痛。
- 明显的腹痛并不常见,一旦出现应考虑有无巨脾或脾破裂。
- 多型皮疹可见于18%~34%的儿童或青春期患者(与抗生素无关)。
- 对IM患者应用氨苄西林或阿莫西林可能诱发生皮疹。

体格检查

- 精神萎靡和/或乏力(90%~100%)。
- 咽炎(65%~85%)和扁桃体肿大。
- 发热(80%~95%)。
- 眼睑水肿(15%~35%)。
- 全身淋巴结肿大(100%)。
- 肝大(15%~25%)。
- 脾大(50%~60%)。
- 非特异性皮疹。
- 使用了氨苄西林或阿莫西林患者可出现麻疹样皮疹:
  - 典型者在抗生素治疗后5~9日出现(勿认为是青霉素过敏)。
- 皮肤或硬软腭移行处可出现瘀斑。
- 体检时注意以下并发症:
  - 气道水肿导致的梗阻(1%~5%)。
  - 剧烈腹痛可以是脾破裂的症状(疼痛可往肩部放射)。
  - 肝炎或肝衰竭所致的黄疸(5%):
    - 肝炎是最常见的并发症。
  - 神经系统伴随症状:
    - 脑炎或小脑炎。
    - 无菌性脑膜炎。
    - 吉兰-巴雷综合征。
    - 视神经炎。
    - 瘫痪。
- 贫血(面色苍白):可能源于溶血性贫血、血栓性血小板减少症、粒细胞缺乏、噬血性淋巴细胞增多症(HLH)。
- 睾丸炎。
- 疼痛所致的颈部僵直或活动受限:继发细菌性软组织感染,如咽后或扁桃体旁脓肿。
- 休克表现:由于脱水或继发性厌氧菌脓毒症诱发。

诊断检查与说明

实验室检查

- 白细胞改变:
  - 一般白细胞有中等程度的升高,达10 000~20 000,2周时达峰值但有时可高达30 000~50 000。一种罕见的情况是出现严重的粒细胞缺乏症,并伴有复发或持续发热,并在发病约1个月后再发展为颈腺疾病。
- 淋巴细胞计数有以下变化对诊断IM有提示意义。
  - 淋巴细胞比例>50%有鉴别意义。
  - 淋巴细胞绝对值>4 500。
  - 异性淋巴细胞比例>10%(超过90%的患者有这一特征)。
- 肝功能检测:
  - 80%~85%的患者在起病的前2周转氨酶高于正常值3倍以上。
  - 约5%的患者胆红素升高达可引起临床症状的界限。
- 特异性检测可发现嗜异性抗体存在:
  - 具有中等敏感性(85%)和高特异性(100%)。
  - 在CMV、白血病、淋巴瘤、风疹、肝炎、HIV或狼疮患者中,偶有假阳性。
  - 多数患者起病约1周后出现嗜异性抗体。
  - 少数患者始终无嗜异性抗体(<10%)。
  - 嗜异性抗体在2~5周达高峰并持续数月。
  - 效价>1:40为阳性。

- <4 岁的儿童结果可能为阴性。
• 目前有针对 EB 病毒的特异性抗体检测，但较昂贵且耗时，很少需要检测。
- 仅在非典型或病情严重的患者以及当 IM 特异性检测阴性但又需要明确诊断时采用。
- 由于 EB 病毒核抗原只出现在起病后 3～4 周的潜伏期内，因此没有针对 EB 病毒核抗原的抗体出现，而针对病毒衣壳抗原的抗体(IgG、IgM)阳性则可提示 EB 病毒的急性感染。
- EB 病毒核抗原阳性而 IgM 阴性则提示既往感染。

影像学检查

有明显腹痛者需行超声或腹部 CT 检查以明确有无脾脏破裂及阑尾炎征象。

鉴别诊断

可分为感染性疾病和非感染性疾病。
• 感染性疾病：
- 腺病毒感染。
- 巨细胞病毒感染。
- 链球菌性咽炎。
- HIV 感染。
- 风疹。
- 甲型、乙型、丙型肝炎。
- 见于非免疫人群的白喉。
- 腮腺炎。
- 弓形虫病。
• 非感染性疾病：
- 白血病。
- 淋巴瘤。
- 药物反应：苯妥英钠、磺胺类药物等。

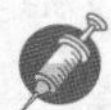

治疗

院前

注意
• 遵循国际通行的防范措施。
• ABC 管理。
• 若患者存在脱水，首先以普通生理盐水补液治疗。

初步稳定/治疗

• 按心肺复苏 ABC 模式处理。气道水肿需要及时干预。
• 尽量避免将该类患者与移植后和其他免疫缺陷患者置于同一区域。

急诊治疗/程序

• 支持治疗：
- 口服或静脉补液。
- 使用退热药物控制体温。
- 镇痛药缓解咽痛。
• 因咽/扁桃体存在水肿而有气道梗阻风险者，可应用皮质激素(甲泼尼龙、泼尼松或地塞米松)。注意是否有巨脾、心肌炎和溶血性贫血或 HLH。激素治疗目前仍存在争议，主要是可能增加继发感染或恶性疾病的风险。
• 目前无证据证明抗病毒治疗有助于缩短病程，但有新的研究认为可能有潜在的好处。
• 如考虑有继发细菌感染，可使用抗生素：
- 避免使用可能诱发皮疹的氨苄西林。
• 建议患者避免竞技性剧烈运动(详见随访建议)。

药物治疗

• 甲泼尼龙：125 mg，静脉推注(儿童：2 mg/kg，静脉推注，最大可达成人剂量)。
• 泼尼松：20～40 mg，口服，每日 1 次，共 7 日(儿童：1 mg/kg，最大可达成人剂量)，后续逐步减量。
• 地塞米松：12～16 mg，口服(儿童：0.3 mg/kg，最大可达成人剂量)。

随访

进一步处理

入院指征
• 有明显的气道水肿，有潜在气道梗阻可能者。
• 有神经系统或严重出血性、肝脏并发症者。
• 无法进食者。
• 疼痛难以控制者。

出院指征
• 无气道梗阻。
• 出血或肝炎不严重者。
• 能耐受口服补液。
• 发热多在 10 日内缓解，淋巴结肿大多在 4 周内好转；乏力症状可持续数周，部分可持续 2～3 个月。

转诊问题
• 在血清学未明确前有必要请感染科会诊。
• 有明显的并发症或症状持续不缓解者。

随访建议

• 在起病的 1～3 周，无论脾脏大小或症状如何，均应避免剧烈运动、体育课或其他激烈活动。
• 在病程 3 周后，患者应到门诊随访评估是否可以恢复正常活动。对于有包括巨脾等症状持续不缓解的患者需进一步检查(如超声)是否可以完全恢复正常活动。

要点和误区

• 尽管疾病常为自限性，但有可能出现严重并发症，需要会诊。
• 激素治疗有效，但有潜在的增加发生并发症的风险，目前仍存有争议。

D

胆管炎 Cholangitis

Jennifer A. Rogers 陈奇通 译

基础知识

描述

• 胆总管部分或完全梗阻导致胆管内压增高。
• 胆道的化脓性感染，由于细菌繁殖可能累及肝胆(GB)：
- 通常会导致菌血症和败血症。

病因

• 急性胆道梗阻(常为部分性而非完全性)。

- 胆总管结石(65%)。
- 恶性肿瘤所致狭窄(24%)。
- 良性狭窄(4%)。
- 硬化性胆管炎(3%)。
- Mirizzi 综合征：胆囊管或胆囊颈的胆囊结石对 CBD 的外源性压迫。

• 感染的细菌来源包括：
- 十二指肠源。
- 胆囊感染。
- 门静脉接种。
- 肝源性所致血行播散。
- 淋巴扩散。

• 细菌有机体包括：
- 厌氧菌(拟杆菌和梭菌属)。
- 肠道大肠杆菌(大肠杆菌、克雷伯杆菌)。
- 肠球菌。

• 获得性免疫缺陷综合征(艾滋病)硬化性胆管炎的特征：
- 乳头状狭窄或硬化性胆管炎导致肝外胆管梗阻。
- 巨细胞病毒(CMV)、隐孢子虫、微孢子虫分离，但因果作用尚未建立。

D

诊断

症状和体征

病史

• Charcot 三联征：
- 典型发热和寒战，50%～70%的患者存在右上象限(右上腹部)疼痛和黄疸。

• 休克和意识状态改变意味着更严重的胆源性脓毒症存在，我们称之为雷诺综合征(5%～7%的病例)。
• 大于 70%的患者存在右上腹疼痛。
• 艾滋病的硬化性胆管炎呈现类似的症状，但大多进展缓慢，血清胆红素水平也正常。

体格检查

• 90%的患者存在发热。
• 30%的患者存在腹膜症状。
• 40%的患者存在不明显的黄疸症状。

基本检查

• 冠心病患者的心电图检查。
• 血常规。
• 肝功能检测。
• 淀粉酶，脂肪酶。
• 尿液分析。
• 血培养。
• 腹部/骨盆 CT 增强扫描或胆囊造影。

诊断检查与说明

实验室检查

• 血常规。
- 免疫系统受损或严重脓毒症除外，白细胞数增多伴核左移。

• 肝功能试验符合胆汁淤积：
- 直接胆红素和碱性磷酸酶升高。

• 转氨酶略有升高(<200 U/ml)。
• 实验室检查滞后症状出现 24～48 h。
• 淀粉酶和脂肪酶正常或轻度升高。
• 胆红素尿检阳性。
• 75%的患者血液培养呈阳性。

影像学检查

• 腹部/骨盆 CT 静脉造影：
- 敏感性 85%～97%和特异性 88%～96%诊断 CBD 结石。
- 可鉴别肿块或其他并发症，如脓肿，通常漏诊。
- 有助于排除肠梗阻、穿孔或肺炎。
- 20%胆结石透视。

• 超声检测导管阻塞的程度和存在的胆石病因。
- CBD>7 mm 表示阻塞。
- 偶尔可以看到 CBD 的结石。

• 磁共振胰胆管造影(MRCP)对诊断胆道梗阻具有很高的准确性，但如果要行内镜逆行胰胆管造影(ERCP)则不必做该项检查。

诊断步骤/外科

在 12～24 h 对药物治疗效果不佳的患者，如果手术和经皮穿刺无法实施，可行急诊微创胆道造影和引流术。

鉴别诊断

• 急性胆囊炎。
• 肝炎或肝脓肿。
• 急性胰腺炎。
• 右肾盂肾炎。
• 右下叶肺炎或肺栓塞。
• 十二指肠溃疡穿孔。
• 阑尾炎。
• 非特异性肝功能异常所致脓毒症。
• Fitz-Hugh-Curtis 综合征。

治疗

院前

稳定脓毒症休克。

初步稳定/治疗

• 对脱水、血流动力学不稳定和脓毒症患者行快速静脉液体复苏。
• 在第一个 24 h 内 80%的患者对抗生素有反应。
• 对液体复苏后仍存在顽固性低血压患者予以升压药物(多巴胺)治疗。

急诊治疗/程序

• 广谱抗生素对大肠杆菌、厌氧菌、肠球菌等：
- 氨苄西林-舒巴坦＋氨基糖苷类(如庆大霉素)。
- 亚胺培南-西司他丁。
- 哌拉西林-他唑巴坦＋氨基糖苷类(如庆大霉素)。
- 对青霉素过敏：
  ◦ 成人使用左氧氟沙星(左氧氟沙星)和甲硝唑。
  ◦ 儿童使用克林霉素和甲硝唑。

• 肾功能不全患者氨基糖苷类替代氨曲南。
• 禁食。
• 持续呕吐及肠梗阻患者行胃肠引流。
• 静脉输注生理盐水补充容量及维持内环境稳定。
• 如果诊断明确，血流动力学稳定可予以麻醉镇痛。
• 立即手术和胃肠准备。
• 如果在 12～24 h 对药物治疗无反应，需行急诊微创胆道引流手术(手术、经皮或 ERCP)。

药物治疗

• 氨苄西林-舒巴坦：3 g[儿童：200 mg/(kg · 24 h)]，借道静脉输液(IVPB)，q6 h。
• 氨曲南：2 g[儿童：120 mg/(kg · 24 h)]，IVPB，q6 h。
• 克林霉素：600～900 mg[儿童：25～40 mg/(kg · 24 h)]，IVPB，q6～8 h。
• 庆大霉素：1.5～2 mg/kg[儿童 6～7 mg/(kg · 24 h)]，IVPB，q8 h。
• 亚胺培南-西司他丁：500 mg[儿童：60～100 mg/(kg · 24 h)]，q6 h。
• 左氧氟沙星：500 mg，q24 h，IVPB。
• 氢吗啡酮：0.5～2 mg(0.01～0.02 mg/kg)，静脉注射，滴定到疼痛。
• 甲硝唑：500 mg[儿童：30 mg/(kg · 24 h)]，IVPB，q6 h。
• 去甲肾上腺素：8～12 μg/min，静脉注射；滴定以维持血压。
• 哌拉西林-他唑巴坦：3.375 mg[儿童：300 mg/(kg · 24 h)]，IVPB，q6 h。

• 昂丹司琼：4～8 mg，静脉注射（0.15～0.3 mg/kg）（不超过 8 mg/每剂量），呕吐明显时根据需要 q4 h 使用。

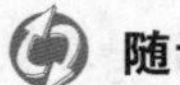

随访

进一步处理

入院指征

• 所有急性胆囊炎患者均应入选，行手术治疗和胃肠外科会诊。

• 对存在感染性休克患者需送入 ICU。

出院指征

无。

转诊问题

所有患者均需接受手术或消化内科会诊。

随访建议

入院接受静脉抗生素治疗和胆道减压手术（引流或 ERCP）。

要点和误区

• 过度的液体复苏。

• 早期应用广谱抗生素。

• CT 静脉造影优于超声。

• 立即进行消化科和外科会诊。

胆结石 Cholelithiasis

Jennifer A. Rogers　陈奇通 译

D

基础知识

描述

• 症状由胆囊管暂时性胆石阻塞引起。

• 胆道运动障碍产生的症状与非结石性胆绞痛相同。

• 胆总管结石，可能会导致长期疼痛、肝功能异常和胆红素升高，以及更多的并发症，如胆管炎或胰腺炎。

病因

• 胆固醇结石：

- 最常见的胆结石类型（在美国和欧洲 >90%）。
- 胆固醇代谢障碍形成。

• 色素性结石：

- 不常见。
- 由胆红素钙组成。
- 与溶血性疾病、肝硬化、囊性纤维化等导致未结合胆红素浓度升高的临床情况有关。

• 随着年龄的增长发病率增加，女性与男性发病率比例为 2∶1（生育期为 4∶1）。其他危险因素包括西班牙裔、肥胖、妊娠、体重迅速下降、药物诱导胆汁淤滞（如头孢曲松钠和口服避孕药）、胆结石家族史。

• 胆结石在儿童十分罕见，常见于镰状细胞病、遗传性球形红细胞增多症或导致色素结石形成的溶血性贫血。

• 胆泥：

- 非结石，晶状体，颗粒状基质。
- 常伴有体重快速减轻、妊娠、头孢曲松或奥曲肽治疗、器官移植。
- 可能发展到与胆石症及其并发症相似的症状。

• “瓷性胆囊”：由于胆管梗阻反复发作导致胆囊黏膜钙盐沉淀。

诊断

症状和体征

病史

• 上腹或右上腹（RUQ）钝痛：

- 起病时间超过 2～3 min，持续时间为 15 min 至 5 h。疼痛持续时间 >5 h 表明有复杂的胆结石。
- 疼痛通常是稳定的，而不是“胆绞痛”所指的间歇性疼痛。
- 可放射到右肩胛骨尖端、肩峰或胸椎。
- 常与大量脂肪膳食有关。

• 恶心与呕吐。

• 无发热。

• 发热和寒战提示胆囊炎或胆管炎。

体格检查

• 上腹部触痛，但无反跳痛。

• Murphy 征（RUQ 深触诊时吸气停顿），可能是在绞痛发作期间存在，但症状消失后会消失。

基本检查

• 心电图：可能因心肌缺血导致的疼痛。

• 全血细胞检查。

• 肝功能检查。

• 淀粉酶和脂肪酶。

• 尿液分析。

• 人绒毛膜促性腺激素（HCG）。

诊断检查与说明

实验室检查

• 全血细胞计数：

- 一般无白细胞升高。
- 白细胞升高提示胆囊炎或胆管炎。

• 肝功能检查：

- 在单纯性胆绞痛中通常是正常的。
- 升高提示胆总管梗阻、胆管炎、胆囊炎或肝炎。

• 淀粉酶/脂肪酶：

- 随着胆结石的推移正常或轻度升高。
- 在严重的持续性上腹痛情况下升高提示胰腺炎。

• 尿液分析：

- 排除肾结石或肾盂肾炎。
- 胆红素尿提示胆总管梗阻或肝炎。

影像学检查

• 超声：

- 检测胆结石的敏感性和特异性均 >95%。
- 正常胆总管直径：7 mm，扩张可提示梗阻，但急性梗阻可能是正常的。
- 胆囊壁增厚 >3 mm 或胆囊周围积液提示胆囊炎。
- 禁食患者（>6 h）时胆囊无收缩，准确性提高。
- 评估胆石症的床旁超声，如果症状消失，可以进行适当的手术随访。

• CT 扫描：

- 没有证据表明 CT 是评估胆绞痛的主要影像学检查方法。
- 检测胆结石敏感性低于超声。
  - 只有 20% 不透射线。
- 最有效的排除其他上腹部疼痛原因的方法，如主动脉瘤、肝周脓肿或胰腺假性囊肿。
- 排除罕见的并发症，如肺气肿、坏疽性或出血性胆囊炎、胆肠瘘或“瓷性胆囊”。

• 放射性核素扫描（HIDA）：

- 不能检测到胆结石，提供有关胆囊功能的信息。
- 对诊断急性胆囊炎（灵敏性 96%，特异性 90%）或胆管梗阻更有用。

鉴别诊断

- 心肌梗死。
- 腹主动脉瘤。
- 急性胆囊炎、胆管炎或胆总管结石。
- 肾绞痛或肾盂肾炎。
- 十二指肠球部溃疡穿孔。
- 急性胰腺炎。
- 肠梗阻。
- 消化性溃疡、胃炎或胃食管反流病。
- 右下叶肺炎、胸膜炎或肺梗死。
- 肝炎或肝脓肿。
- Fitz-Hugh-Curtis 综合征（盆腔感染合并肝周围炎）。

D

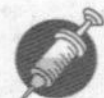

治疗

院前

对恶心、呕吐的患者建立静脉通路。

初步稳定/治疗

呕吐或低血压患者给予静脉快速补液。

急诊治疗/程序

- 如果呕吐，静脉输液用生理盐水。
- 禁食。
- 肠外的抗炎镇痛药（酮咯酸）可以减轻胆道痉挛，但可能加重消化性溃疡带来的疼痛。
- 麻醉镇痛药（吗啡）及止吐（昂丹司琼）：
- 一旦诊断确立即需处理顽固性疼痛。
- 硫酸吗啡可导致 Oddi 括约肌痉挛（临床意义尚不明确）。
- 抗胆碱能药物（格隆溴铵）对急性胆源性疼痛的疗效尚未证实。

药物治疗

- 酮咯酸：肌内注射 30 mg；或静脉推注 15 mg[儿童：初始剂量为 0.5 mg/kg，最大剂量为 1 mg/(kg · 24 h)]静脉推注，q6 h。
- 吗啡：静脉推注 0.5～2 mg（0.01～0.02 mg/kg），滴定至疼痛缓解。
- 昂丹司琼：静脉推注 4～8 mg（0.15～0.3 mg/kg）；呕吐时静脉推注（不超过为 8 mg/每剂），q4 h 需要时。

随访

进一步处理

入院指征

出现以下情况时入院、手术或胃肠科咨询：

- 急性胆囊炎。
- 急性胆管炎。
- 胆总管梗阻。
- 胆源性胰腺炎。

出院指征

- 缺乏临床、实验室或影像学证据提示胆囊炎、胆管炎、胆总管梗阻或胰腺炎。
- 所有的疼痛和压痛消失。
- 能够耐受口进食流质。

转诊问题

- 所有有症状的胆石症并有胆石症记录的病例或放射学发现“瓷性胆囊”（由于胆囊癌的风险增加）的需普通外科转诊。
- 急性外科会诊，适用于中度或重度胆绞痛或任何胆囊炎、胆石症、胆管炎或任何其他并发症的患者。

随访建议

- 建议对所有有症状的胆石症患者进行手术随访。
- 50%症状轻微的患者将继续进行选择性胆囊切除术。
- 选择性胆囊切除术通常在诊断后数周至数月内进行。

要点和误区

- 引起上腹部疼痛的其他原因可能错误地归于胆结石的偶然发现。
- 持续性疼痛需要进行急性手术评估，因为它可能指示其他并发症。
- 超声诊断比其他影像学检查更为灵敏，尤其是特异性胆石症。
- 放射性核素扫描（HIDA）不能看到结石，但它对胆囊管阻塞和胆囊炎有很高的诊断价值。
- 如果结石不透射线，CT 扫描可能漏诊胆结石。

胆囊炎 Cholecystitis

Jennifer A. Rogers　陈奇通 译

基础知识

描述

胆囊炎是由累及胆囊壁的炎症/感染过程引起的，在许多情况下是由于嵌顿性胆结石引起的。

病因

- 急性结石性胆囊炎：
- 继发于胆囊结石（见“胆石症”）嵌顿于胆囊颈部、胆囊管或胆总管，使得梗阻时间延长导致的胆汁淤积。
- 导致管腔内压升高和肠壁黏膜缺血。
- 释放的炎症介质导致腹胀、水肿和血供增加。
- 50%～58%的病例涉及细菌性炎症，通常是在病程后期发生的继发性事件。
- 非结石性胆囊炎：
- 20%的发生率。
- 潜在的疾病导致胆汁淤滞和黏膜缺血。
- 继发的黏膜炎症和感染。

儿科注意事项

- 小儿急性结石性胆囊炎极为罕见（参见“胆石症”）。
- 小儿非结石性胆囊炎比结石性胆囊炎更为常见：
- 伴有全身性细菌感染、猩红热、川崎病和寄生感染。

诊断

症状和体征

病史

- 急性结石性胆囊炎：
- 钝痛，疼痛，上腹或右上腹（RUQ）疼痛，可能辐射至右肩胛骨、肩峰或胸椎。
- 持续时间>5 h 更加提示胆囊炎而非单纯

性胆绞痛。

- 随着炎症的进展，壁层腹膜刺激导致尖锐的局部疼痛。
- 有恶心、呕吐、发热、寒战，但也有可能缺少上述症状。
- 10％的患者出现黄疸。
- 既往有胆绞痛或胆囊结石的病史有利于诊断。

• 非结石性胆囊炎：
- 发生于危重患者（烧伤、败血症、外伤、TPN或术后患者）。
- 往往表现为不明原因脓毒血症的症状。

体格检查

• 通常伴有低热。
• 局部壁层腹膜症状：
- 压痛。
- 随着病情的发展，反复的次数更多。
- 1/3患者可触及GB。

• Murphy征：
- 右上腹轻柔触诊时由于疼痛加重出现吸气停顿。
- 在所有体格检查中显示出阳性LR的结果最高。

■ 基本检查

• 心电图：有冠状动脉疾病风险的患者。
• 全血细胞计数。
• 肝功能检测。
• 淀粉酶和脂肪酶。
• 尿液分析。
• 人绒毛膜促性腺激素（HCG）。
• 胆囊超声或肝胆放射性核素扫描。

■ 诊断检查与说明

实验室检查

• CBC：
- 白细胞＞12 000/mm^3 支持诊断，但一半以上情况下也可以是正常的。

• 肝功能检查结果：
- 转氨酶、胆红素、淀粉酶、脂肪酶可以轻微升高，但一般都是正常的。
- 与转氨酶比较，直接胆红素和碱性磷酸酶升高不成比例，提示胆总管梗阻或胆管炎。

影像学检查

• 超声：
- 一般是首选对于胆结石诊断有高准确性的影像学检查。
- 阳性结果包括有炎症迹象的结石，包括：胆囊壁增厚（＞7 mm）和/或胆囊周围积液，敏感性为90％；特异性为80％。
- 患者禁食＞6 h后效果更佳。

• 放射性核素扫描（HIDA）：
- 当超声检查模棱两可或临床高度怀疑非结石性胆囊炎时有益于诊断。
- 造影剂显影见于小肠，而胆囊由于炎症没有正面显影。
- 急性胆囊炎敏感性＞95％；特异性为90％。
- 在非空腹状态下假阳性率增加，因此患者应禁食至少4 h。
- 静脉注射吗啡诱导Oddi括约肌收缩促进胆囊充盈从而减少假阳性结果。

• CT扫描：
- 有助于排除其他引起腹痛的原因，如肠穿孔或梗阻、主动脉瘤。
- 胆囊壁空气提示气肿性胆囊炎。
- 可能漏诊胆结石，只有20％的病例是不透光的。

■ 鉴别诊断

• 单纯性胆石症（胆绞痛）。
• 肝炎或肝脓肿。
• 胆管炎。
• 艾滋病硬化性胆管炎。
• 胰腺炎。
• 肠穿孔。
• 消化性溃疡，胃炎或称GERD。
• 十二指肠溃疡伴或不伴穿孔。
• 右下叶肺炎、胸膜炎或肺梗死。
• 心肌梗死。
• 腹主动脉瘤。
• 阑尾炎。
• Fitz-Hugh-Curtis综合征（盆腔感染合并肝周围炎）。
• 肾盂肾炎。

治疗

■ 院前

呕吐或剧烈疼痛的患者应建立静脉通路。

■ 初步稳定/治疗

• 开通静脉通路、吸氧、心电监测直到心肌缺血的可能被排除。
• 启动静脉输液治疗脱水、血流动力学不稳定或败血症。
• NPO。

■ 急诊治疗/程序

• 抗生素的使用是标准的，但是在计划行胆囊切除术的轻度疾病中可能使用有限。
• 广谱抗生素治疗大肠杆菌、厌氧菌和肠球菌：
- 头孢曲松加甲硝唑。
- 哌拉西林-他唑巴坦。
- 如果怀疑败血症或胆管炎添加氨基糖苷类（见"胆管炎"）。

• 青霉素过敏时更换抗生素：
- 成人：左氧氟沙星或环丙沙星、甲硝唑。
- 儿童：克林霉素和氨基糖苷类。

• 静脉补液和维持。
• 如果呕吐应用止吐药（昂丹司琼）。
• 难治性呕吐或肠梗阻进行鼻胃管负压吸引。
• 麻醉性镇痛药（吗啡）、止吐（昂丹司琼）：
- 一旦诊断确立即需处理顽固性疼痛。
- 硫酸吗啡可导致Oddi括约肌痉挛（临床意义尚不明确）。

• 抗胆碱能药物（格隆溴铵）是否对急性胆源性疼痛有益尚不确定。
• 外科会诊。

■ 药物治疗

• 头孢曲松：1～2 g，IVPB，q12～24 h。
• 环丙沙星：400 mg，IV，q12 h。
• 克林霉素：600～900 mg［儿童：25～40 mg/(kg·24 h)］，IVPB，q6～8 h。
• 庆大霉素：1.5～2 mg/kg［儿童：6～7 mg/(kg·24 h)］，IVPB，q8 h；逐级调整。
• 左氧氟沙星：500 mg，IVPB，q24 h；儿童禁忌。
• 吗啡：0.5～2 mg（001～0.02 mg/kg），IV，滴定至疼痛缓解。
• 甲硝唑：500 mg［儿童：30 mg/(kg·24 h)］，IVPB，q6 h。
• 哌拉西林-他唑巴坦：3.375 mg［儿童：300 mg/(kg·24 h)］，IVPB，q6 h。
• 昂丹司琼：4～8 mg（儿童：0.15～0.3 mg/kg），静脉注射（静推不超过8 mg），q4 h，呕吐时应用。

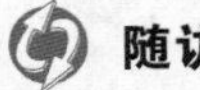

随访

■ 进一步处理

入院指征

• 所有胆囊炎患者均应收治：注射抗生素，止痛，补液，24～72 h进行胆囊切除术。
• 不稳定的患者（胆囊穿孔或败血症），需要立即手术治疗。

出院指征

无。

D

转诊问题

• 胆囊炎患者转诊普外科。

• 胆总管结石或怀疑胆管炎转诊胃肠外科。

■ 随访建议

住院患者入院进行外科评估和治疗，以及疼痛控制、液体置换和抗生素治疗。

要点和误区

• 超声是首选的。

• 当超声检查模棱两可或临床高度怀疑非结石性胆囊炎时，放射性核素扫描（HIDA）有益于诊断。

• 抗生素对更严重的疾病有帮助，但对那些没有器官损伤和轻度炎症的患者的有用性尚不清楚。如果将延迟胆囊切除术的最终治疗或患者有败血症的证据，则应使用。

胆石性肠梗阻

Joanna W. Davidson 祝各亮 译

基础知识

■ 描述

• 机械性肠梗阻继发于胆结石嵌入肠腔。

• 胆石直径通常＞2.5 cm。

• 占全部肠梗阻的1%～3%。

• 好发于65岁以上的老年人。

• 好发于女性，男女比例约为1∶5。

• 致死率为15%～18%。

■ 病因

• 慢性胆囊炎引起胆囊与邻近肠壁的粘连。

• 胆肠瘘形成导致胆石进入肠腔：

- 十二指肠是瘘管形成最多的部位，其次是结肠。

- 胃也可以是瘘管形成的部位，但发生率较低。

• 结石嵌顿部位：

- 终末回肠最为普遍（54%～65%）：

◦ 回盲瓣是小肠最为狭窄的部位。

- 空肠（27%）。

- 十二指肠（1%～3%）：

◦ 结石嵌顿于十二指肠导致胃出口梗阻称为 Bouveret 综合征。

- 大肠梗阻较为稀少。

诊断

■ 症状和体征

• 腹部不适：

- 随着结石埋入和离开肠壁而出现发作性腹部疼痛。

- 结石完全嵌顿会导致严重的、剧烈的腹部疼痛。

• 恶心。

• 呕吐：

- 可以是胆汁或不洁物。

• 顽固性便秘。

• 腹胀。

• 腹部压痛：

- 疾病过程晚期可出现腹膜刺激征。

• 肠鸣音异常。

病史

• 只有50%～60%的患者有胆绞痛或胆石症病史。

• 胆石性肠梗阻患者通常伴有心血管疾病、糖尿病和肥胖。

体格检查

• 腹部检查：

- 腹部膨隆或腹部压痛。

• 黄疸。

■ 基本检查

评估肠道梗阻情况。

■ 诊断检查与说明

实验室检查

• 患者饮食摄入减少及呕吐导致水电解质紊乱，需检测电解质、肌酐、血尿素氮及血糖。

• 肝功能指标及胆红素水平可能会升高。

• 淀粉酶：

- 梗阻晚期会升高。

• 血细胞计数/血细胞比容：

- 红细胞聚集继发于脱水。

- 非特异性的白细胞升高。

影像学检查

• 腹部立卧位X线片：

- 肠梗阻时可见肠管扩张及多个气液平。

- Rigler 三联征：出现2个以上症状的患者占30%～50%：

◦ 胆道积气。

◦ 部分或完全性肠梗阻。

◦ 在肠道内可以看见异位的结石。

• 胸部X线片：

- 气腹的评估。

• 腹部CT：

- 是选择性的检查。

- 可以直接看见并定位石头在肠腔中的位置。

• 腹部超声：

- 可以辨别胆道积气和胆结石，但不利于定位异位梗阻的结石。

■ 鉴别诊断

• 麻痹性肠梗阻。

• 肠道外梗阻：

- 肠粘连。

- 肠扭转。

- 肠疝。

- 肠套叠。

• 消化道恶性肿瘤。

• 憩室炎。

• 胃石症。

• 炎症性肠病。

• 假性肠梗阻。

• 胆囊炎。

• 上行性胆管炎。

• 胰腺炎。

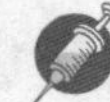

治疗

■ 院前

建立静脉通道。

■ 初始稳定/治疗

静脉补液。

■ 急诊治疗/程序

• 鼻胃管引流，胃肠减压。

• 禁食。

- 补充电解质。
- 记录尿量。
- 使用止痛剂。
- 使用覆盖肠道菌群的广谱抗生素：
  - 哌拉西林-他唑巴坦。
  - 氨苄西林-舒巴坦。
  - 替卡西林-克拉维酸。
  - 替代药物包括亚胺培南、美罗培南、第三代头孢菌素＋甲硝唑。
- 最终的治疗主要是外科手术。

药物

- 氨苄西林-舒巴坦：3 g[儿童：100～200 mg/(kg·24 h)]，q6 h，静脉注射。
- 哌拉西林-他唑巴坦：3.375 g[儿童：240～400 mg/(kg·24 h)]，q6 h，静脉注射。
- 替卡西林-克拉维酸：3.1 g，q4～6 h，静脉注射。

随访

进一步处理

入院指征

- 所有胆石性肠梗阻患者均有入院指征。
- 进行外科评估以明确是否需要紧急手术干预。

出院指征

无。

随访建议

外科随访以评估病情并及时手术干预。

要点和误区

- 胆石性肠梗阻是机械性的肠道阻塞而不是真正的肠梗阻。
- 需要急诊外科会诊以明确治疗方案。
- 诊断和对合并症处理的不及时往往会造成高致死率。
- 对于没有外科手术史但又出现肠道阻塞症状的老年患者，尤其是女性患者，需要高度怀疑胆石性肠梗阻的可能。
- 只有10%的异为结石可以在X线平片上看到，CT对于定位宫腔内的结石具有更高的敏感性和特异性。
- 只有1/2的患者之前有胆绞痛和胆石症病史。

D

登革热 Dengue Fever

Roger M. Barkin · Jessica Freedman 许磊 译

基础知识

描述

- 登革热继发于登革热病毒感染。
- 最常见的蚊子传播的病毒感染。
- 对引起登革出血热(DHF)和登革热休克综合征(DSS)的免疫病理反应知之甚少。
- DHF和DSS通常发生在既往暴露于登革热病毒的患者。
- 发热退热后出现出血。
- 血管通透性增加。
- 血浆外渗到血管外的空间，包括胸腔和腹腔。
- 出血倾向。
- 可能发生休克。
- 可能发生弥散性血管内凝血(DIC)。
- 登革热、DHF和DSS都是自限性的。
- 世界卫生组织诊断DHF的标准：
  - 发热。
  - 出血证明下列之一：止血带试验、瘀点、瘀斑、过敏性紫癜、胃肠道出血、注射部位出血。
  - 增加血管通透性和血浆泄漏就证明血细胞比容升高(＞20%)，后降低＞20%扩容或胸腔积液，腹水或低蛋白血症。
  - 血小板减少症(＜100 000/mm³)。
- 世界卫生组织诊断DSS标准：
  - 所有4个DHF的标准阳性。
  - 脉搏快而弱。
  - 窄脉冲压力或低血压年龄。
  - 冷，皮肤湿冷。
  - 躁动。
- 疫苗正在研制中。

病因

- 发生在热带和亚热带地区：亚洲、非洲、中美洲和南美洲，以及加勒比。
- 引起的登革热病毒血清型1～4。2013年发现了第五种血清型。
- 由蚊子传播：埃及伊蚊和白纹伊蚊。
- 潜伏期为3～14日。
- 只有短暂的和较差的交叉保护在4个血清型中。
- 每年发生高达3.9亿例感染，近1亿人致病。

诊断

症状和体征

- 症状通常比较轻微，常被误认为“流感”。
- 发热：
  - 突然发病上升到39℃以上。
  - 持续2～7日。
  - 双相(“马鞍”)曲线，2～7日之后基本返回正常。
  - 与额部或眼眶头痛。
- 皮疹：
  - 在50%的患者中全身性斑丘疹出现在发热上升期。可能在发热后2～5日出现。
  - 经过3～4日，皮疹变得广泛的红斑。
  - 褪色区出现。
  - 脱屑区域可能会出现。
  - 发热退热后，分散的瘀点可能发展到躯体、伸侧、四肢和腋下。
  - 手掌和足底幸免。
- 肌肉骨骼系统：
  - 开始发热后出现关节痛和肌痛。
  - 严重的腰部背部疼痛。
- 胃肠道：
  - 厌食症。
  - 恶心和呕吐。
  - 腹痛(有时严重)。
  - 味觉改变。
  - 肝大、腹水。
  - 胃肠道出血。
- 其他：
  - 鼻出血。
  - 出血倾向：牙龈出血。
  - 咯血。

- 弥散性血管内凝血。
- 低血压和循环衰竭，可能继而休克。
- 收窄脉压<20 mmHg。
- 眼眶痛。

■ 基本检查

• 主要临床诊断。
• 怀疑在流行地区。
• 怀疑在患者的旅行史。

■ 诊断检查与说明

实验室检查

• 全血细胞检查：
- 血小板减少。
- 中性粒细胞减少。
- 脱水引起血细胞比容升高。
• 电解质、尿素氮、肌酐：
- 升高的尿素氮。
- 低钠血症。
• 肝功能检查：
- 天门冬氨酸转氨酶（AST，或血清谷草转氨酶 SGOT）升高。
• 凝血功能：
- 长期 INR、PT 和 APTT。
- 低纤维蛋白原。
◦ D-二聚体。
- 病毒分离或检测登革热病毒特异性抗体（只有少数可用实验室检查），通过血凝抑制（HI）试验。

影像学检查

胸部 X 线检查：
• 胸腔积液。

诊断步骤/外科

止血带试验：
• 充气血压：袖带平均血压在患者的肢体。
• 测试为阳性，当 3 个或更多瘀点出现每平方厘米。

■ 鉴别诊断

病毒性疾病，非特异性。
• 流感。
• 风疹。
• 麻疹。
• 疟疾。
• 落基山斑疹热。
• 伤寒。
• 川崎病。
• 猩红热。
• 传染性红斑。
• 单核细胞增多。
• 玫瑰疹。
• 二期梅毒。
• 肠道病毒感染。
• 西尼罗病毒感染。
• 艾滋病。
• 钩端螺旋体病。
• 基孔肯亚出血热。
• 毒性休克综合征。
• 肝炎。
• 阑尾炎。
• 脑膜炎。

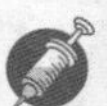

治疗

■ 院前

• 建立静脉通路。
• 静脉输注晶体溶液控制低血压。
• 给予氧气和监控不稳定的患者。

■ 急诊治疗/程序

• 治疗主要是支持性的。
• 对于休克和脱水患者予静脉输液。
• 对乙酰氨基酚：治疗发热。
- 止痛药：控制疼痛。
- 不超过 4 g/24 h。
• 血小板输血：用于严重的血小板减少。
• DIC 治疗，如有必要。

儿科注意事项

• 新生儿登革热的发生可通过垂直传播，如果受感染的母亲在分娩前 0～8 日：
- 婴儿可能发展 DHF 或 DSS 因母体被动免疫。
• DHF 和 DSS 最常见于 7～12 岁的小儿。

随访

■ 进一步处理

入院指征

• 入住 ICU：
- 低血压。
- DIC。
- 血小板减少。
- 血液浓缩。
• 定期检查：
• 15 岁的年龄或更年轻。
• 所有患者既往登革热接触。
• 任何患者，其中密切随访不可用。

出院指征

• 最小的明确的疾病。
• 密切随访。
• 可以口服用药。
• 疼痛得到控制。

要点和误区

• 考虑的登革热患者表现有发热和皮疹，最近去过流行地区。
• 可能被误诊为“流感”。
• 基孔肯亚出血热是一种新出现的传染病，也可见于旅游者，必须加以考虑。
- 在亚洲和非洲发现。

低钙血症 Hypocalcemia

Michelle J. Sergel · J. Patrick Hoffman 倪沁赟 译

基础知识

■ 描述

• 低钙血症的定义为血浆总钙水平<8.7 mg/dl：
- 离子钙可能在正常范围，但无特殊临床表现。
• 正常血清总钙浓度是 8.7～10.5 mg/dl。
• 正常的离子钙水平为 4.64～5.28 mg/dl。

■ 病因

• 低钙血症在总人群中的发病率为 0.6%。
• 发病机制：
- 从循环中丢失的钙增加或进入循环的钙

减少。
- 血管内的钙以 3 种方式循环：
◦ 与蛋白质结合（主要是白蛋白）：45%～50%。
◦ 与络合离子结合（柠檬酸、磷酸盐、碳酸盐）：5%～10%。
◦ 离子（自由）钙（具备生理活性）：45%～50%。
- 血清钙水平主要由 3 种激素控制：
◦ 甲状旁腺激素（PTH）。
◦ 血钙水平降低导致甲状旁腺激素分泌增加（增加骨质重吸收、肾脏吸收、肠道吸收、尿磷排泄）。
- 维生素 D[1,25-$(OH)_2$-D_3]：
◦ 血钙水平降低导致维生素 D 活化（增加骨质重吸收和肠道吸收）。
- 降钙素：
◦ 血钙水平增加直接抑制骨质重吸收。
• 低蛋白血症：最常见的病因：
- 血清白蛋白浓度每降低 1 g/dl，与蛋白质结合的血清钙浓度降低 0.8 mg/dl。
- 离子（自由）钙水平不变。

儿科注意事项

• 儿童正常血钙水平更高（9.2～11 mg/dl）。
• 新生儿低钙血症：血清总钙浓度<7.5 mg/dl 或血清离子钙水平<4 mg/dl。
• 婴儿低钙血症的临床表现：
- 多动，神经过敏。
- 呼吸急促。
- 呼吸暂停和发绀。
- 呕吐。

诊断

症状和体征

• 当血清离子钙水平<3.2 mg/dl 时出现。
• 与绝对的血钙浓度和血钙浓度的下降速度相关。
• 神经肌肉系统：
- 感觉异常。
- 反射亢进。
- 肌肉痉挛。
- 手足搐弱：
◦ 神经肌肉兴奋性增加。
◦ 罕见，除非血清离子钙浓度<4.3 mg/dl。
- 潜在性手足搐搦。
- Chvostek 征（轻扣外耳道前面神经引起面肌非随意收缩，口角抽搐即为阳性）。
- Trousseau 征（用血压计缚于前臂充气使手血供减少，促发腕痉挛）。
- 喉鸣。
- 癫痫。
- 舞蹈手足徐动症。
• 心血管系统：
- 心律失常：
◦ 尖端扭转型室性心动过速。
◦ 心脏传导阻滞。
- 低血压。
- 心肌收缩功能受损（心力衰竭）。
- 心电图改变：
◦ 心动过缓。
◦ QT 间期或 ST 段延长。
◦ T 波异常。
• 精神系统：
- 烦躁与焦虑。
- 精神错乱。
- 抑郁。
- 认知功能障碍。
- 妄想。
- 舞蹈症。
- 帕金森病。
• 眼睛：
- 视乳头水肿。
- 白内障。
- 主要发生在急性低钙血症患者。
• 内分泌。
- 胰岛素释放减少。

基本检查

血清离子钙水平。

诊断检查与说明

实验室检查

• 动脉血气分析：
- pH 每改变 0.1 U 相当于离子钙水平改变约 1.7 mg/dl。
• 血清白蛋白水平。
• 电解质、尿素氮/肌酐、血糖。
• 血镁水平。
• 磷酸盐：
- 磷酸盐浓度升高，提示甲状旁腺功能减退。
- 磷酸盐浓度降低，提示维生素 D 缺乏。
• 甲状旁腺激素：
- 甲状旁腺激素水平异常升高，提示假性甲状旁腺功能减退症。
- 甲状旁腺激素水平升高，提示维生素 D 缺乏。
- 甲状旁腺激素水平低，提示甲状旁腺功能减退。
• 血清骨化二醇或骨化三醇。

诊断步骤/外科

心电图：
• QT 间期延长。
• 心脏传导阻滞。

鉴别诊断

• 甲状旁腺激素活性或者分泌受损。
- 甲状旁腺或甲状腺手术或放射性颈部手术和/或头颈部肿瘤放射治疗。
- 自身免疫性疾病（通常发生在儿童时期）。
- 先天性甲状旁腺功能减退症。
- 新生儿继发与甲状旁腺功能亢进症的产妇。
- 假性甲状旁腺功能减退症（甲状旁腺激素抵抗）。
- 浸润性（淀粉样变性、结节病、转移性、铁超载）。
- 人类免疫缺陷病毒（HIV）感染。
• 维生素 D 合成或活性受损：
- 营养吸收不良或摄入不足。
- 肾脏疾病。
- 严重低磷血症。
• 感染或严重烧伤：
- 随着净离子离子钙进入细胞质，细胞功能紊乱。
- 甲状旁腺激素和骨化三醇分泌受损。
- 终末器官对甲状旁腺激素抵抗。
• 结合钙形成：
- 高磷血症。
- 乙二醇、乙二胺四乙酸（EDTA）和柠檬酸（输入性）。
- 胰腺炎、横纹肌溶解症。
- 横纹肌溶解（磷酸过载）。
- 碱中毒（即过度通气）。
• 低镁血症：
- 终末器官甲状旁腺激素抵抗引起。
- 甲状旁腺激素分泌下降。
- 慢性疾病和/或重症疾病。
- 必须通过补充镁离子来纠正低钙血症。
• 药物治疗：
- 光辉霉素、普卡霉素、磷酸盐、降钙素和二膦酸盐。
- 苯巴比妥和苯妥英。
- 顺铂。
- 镉和秋水仙碱。
- 氟化物、柠檬酸和质子泵抑制剂。
• 恶性肿瘤：
- 前列腺肿瘤。

D

- 乳腺癌。
- 肺癌。
- 软骨肉瘤。

• “骨饥饿综合征”：
- 甲状旁腺切除术后。
- 骨再矿化导致血钙水平的快速纠正。

• 急性呼吸性碱中毒：
- 增加钙与白蛋白的结合。
- 钙总量正常，但电离钙减少。

治疗

初步稳定/治疗

ABC 管理：

• 建立深静脉通道。

• 心电监护。

急诊治疗/程序

• 急性期管理。
- 有症状的低钙血症属临床急症，应通过静脉通道补钙。
- 静脉补钙负荷剂量：
  ◦ 葡萄糖酸钙 1～2 g 加入 5% 葡萄糖注射液 50 ml。
  ◦ 输注时间至少 20 min。
  ◦ 静脉输注速度过快会导致心律失常。
  ◦ 钙盐会刺激血管。
  ◦ 在静脉通道未建立的情况下肌内注射葡庚糖酸钙或葡萄糖酸钙。
  ◦ 静脉补钙给予负荷剂量增加离子钙水平持续时间仅 1～2 h，因此必须后续持续输注。
- 静脉补钙维持剂量：
  ◦ 维持静脉补钙速度：0.5～1.5 mg/(kg · h)。
  ◦ 禁止与碳酸氢盐或磷酸盐混合，导致盐沉淀物形成。
  ◦ 使用洋地黄的患者需要严格谨慎管理，可能会诱发或加剧洋地黄中毒。
- 治疗结果：
  ◦ 个体差异性。
  ◦ 治疗期间每 1～4 h 监测钙浓度的变化。
  ◦ 根据临床症状或心电图改变滴定治疗。
  ◦ 对补钙治疗无反应或失败需要考虑到低镁血症的存在：给予镁 2 g，10% 溶液纠正低镁血症。
  ◦ 如果存在酸中毒，首先纠正血钙水平。碱中毒会降低离子钙水平。
  ◦ 静脉补钙的副作用：恶心、呕吐、低血压和心律失常。

• 维持期管理。
- 口服钙剂的补充。
- 补钙剂量 1.5～2 g/d，分次补充。吸收不良患者可能会增加到 4 g/d。
- 维生素 D：
  ◦ 增加肠道吸收。
  ◦ 在补钙的基础上补充维生素 D，单独补充维生素 D 不足以恢复血钙水平。
  ◦ 19～50 岁补充 600 U。
  ◦ 51～70 岁补充 600 U。
  ◦ 71 岁以上补充 800 U。
  ◦ 复合维生素包含的维生素 D 量不固定。
- 维生素 D 准备：
  ◦ 钙化醇：125 μg/d。
  ◦ 二氢速甾醇：100～400 μg/d。
  ◦ 骨化二醇：50～200 μg/d。
  ◦ 骨化三醇：0.25～0.5 μg/d：快速起效。大部分的维生素活性代谢产物。

妊娠注意事项

妊娠末期需要 2～3 倍的骨化三醇需求量。

药物治疗

• 静脉补钙：
- 氯化钙：1 g/10 ml[1 g=360 mg(13.6 mEq)钙元素]。
- 葡萄糖酸钙（静脉或肌内注射）：1 g/5 ml[1 g=90 mg(4.5 mEq)钙元素]。
- 葡萄糖酸钙：1 g/10 ml[1 g = 90 mg(4.5 mEq)钙元素]。

• 口服补钙：
- 碳酸钙（片剂）：350～1 500 mg(1 g=400 mg)。
- 柠檬酸钙(片剂)：950 mg(1 g=211 mg 钙元素)。
- 葡乳醛酸钙（糖浆）：18 g/5 ml(1 g=65 mg 钙元素)。
- 葡萄糖酸钙（片剂）：500～1 000 mg(1 g=90 mg 钙元素)。
- 乳酸钙（片剂）：350～1 000 mg(1 g=130 mg 钙元素)。

儿科注意事项

• 给予 10% 葡萄糖酸钙负荷剂量应包含钙元素 9～18 mg/kg，早产儿 1～2 ml/kg，足月儿不超过 10 ml。

• 骨化三醇儿童剂量范围为 0.1～3 μg/d。

• 其他：
- 普通食物的钙含量：
  ◦ 牛奶或优格：8 oz(300 mg)。
  ◦ 切达芝士：1 oz(200 mg)。
  ◦ 高钙麦片：1 cup(300 mg)。
  ◦ 高钙橙汁：1 cup(270 mg)。
  ◦ 虾：3 oz(50 mg)。
  ◦ 花生：130 mg。
  ◦ 橘子：50 mg。

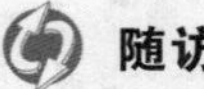

随访

进一步处理

入院指征

• 有临床症状或严重低钙血症（离子钙<3.2 mg/dl）。

• 需要持续静脉补钙维持血钙水平。

出院指征

• 无症状的低钙血症患者。

• 健康患者离子钙>3.2 mg/dl 且无其他伴随疾病。

• 可以用口服钙盐和饮食建议。

随访建议

甲状旁腺激素或维生素 D 活性受损或合成障碍的患者安排严密的内分泌科专家随访。

要点和误区

• 低钙血症的病因多。

• 治疗低钙血症因，根据病情的严重程度和基础原因调整。

• 有严重临床症状的患者需要通过静脉补钙快速纠正血钙水平。

• 为更有效地治疗伴有低镁血症的低钙血症，首先需要纠正血镁水平。

低钾血症 Hypokalemia

Stella C. Wong 倪沁赟 译

基础知识

描述

- 低钾血症的定义为血钾水平<3.5 mmol/L：
  - 轻度：3～3.5 mmol/L。
  - 中度：2.5～3 mmol/L。
  - 重度：<2.5 mmol/L。
- 体内98%的钾都在细胞内。
- 细胞钾梯度由 Na^+ - K^+ - ATP 酶维持细胞内和细胞外钾梯度的作用：
  - 静息细胞膜电位。
  - 心脏活动。
  - 肌肉和神经活动。

病因

肾脏丢失

- 钾流失最常见部位。
- 药物：利尿剂、青霉素及其衍生物、顺铂。
- 高醛甾酮症。
- 遗传性疾病：巴特综合征和吉特尔曼综合征。

胃肠道丢失

- NG 管引流。
- 造口术增加输出。
- 呕吐和腹泻。

摄入量不足(很少是唯一原因)

- 每日少于 1 g 钾。
- 慢性营养不良。
- 酗酒。

汗水

- 日常的 5%。

诊断

症状和体征

- 可能是无症状或下列任何一种：
  - 一般：全身无力、乏力、食欲或口服量下降。
  - 心脏：心悸。
  - 胃肠道：呕吐，腹泻。
  - 肾：泌尿系统症状的改变。

病史

- 药物治疗史。
- 最近的胃肠道疾病。
- 病史包括任何已知的遗传疾病。
- 甲苯暴露。

体格检查

- 可能是正常的，但也可能出现下列任何一种情况：
  - 生命体征：正常，高血压或低血压。
  - 一般：一般弱点。
  - 口腔：黏膜干燥。
  - 心血管：心动过速或心动过缓。
  - 皮肤：可怜的皮肤肿胀。
  - 神经：混乱，整体力量下降。

诊断检查与说明

实验室检查

- 电解质、尿素氮、肌酐、血糖：
  - 碳酸氢盐升高：利尿剂的使用、呕吐、巴特综合征、基特曼综合征。
  - 碳酸氢钠减少：腹泻、DKA、肾小管疾病。
- 尿钾/肌酐值更精确：
  - <13 mmol/L 或 1.5 mmol/mmol(非肾脏丢失)。
  - >13 mmol/L 或 1.5 mmol/mmol(肾脏丢失)。
- 甲状腺毒症有 TSH 和游离 T_4 症状。

心电图

- PR 延长。
- T 波低平。
- T 波倒置。
- ST 段压低。
- QT 间期延长(>500 ms 增加尖端扭转的风险)。
- U 型波(见于严重低钾血症)。
- 心律失常：室性早搏、心房纤颤、尖端扭转。

鉴别诊断

非常广泛，但不限于以下方面：

- 糖尿病的紧急情况。
- 病毒性疾病。
- 心肌梗死。
- 贫血。
- 脑血管意外。
- 神经肌肉接点功能障碍。
- 脊髓疾病。
- 心律失常(由潜在心脏病引起)。

治疗

院前

- 心电监护。
- 监测生命体征。
- 如果可能的话，建立静脉通路。
- 心电图。
- 如果患者病情不稳定或心电图异常，呼叫医师指导。
- 送往最近的急救室。

初步稳定/治疗

- ABC 管理。
- 心电监测。
- 心电图(即使心电图已做，也要重复)。
- 建立静脉输液通道。
- 如有需要，扩容复苏。
- 实验室检查。

急诊治疗/程序

- 停止药物导致损失钾。
- 口服补钾：轻度低钾血症患者，正常心电图，没有主动呕吐，生命体征稳定。
- 静脉补钾：中度到重度低钾血症患者，或低钾血症患者不能耐受口服摄入。
- 相应低镁血症治疗。
- 需要透析肾衰竭患者：如果 K^+ 在 3.5～3.9 mg/L，则不需要不补充钾。

药物治疗

- 注意：所有静脉输液都需要泵。通过外周线静脉滴钾的最大速度为 10 mmol/h。接受静脉注射钾的患者需要心电监测。氯化钾：20 mmol，口服，液体，一次，或氯化钾：10 mmol 100 ml，IVPB，q1 h，2 剂，注射 60 min 以上。
- 需要透析的肾衰竭患者：
  - K^+：3.0～3.4 mmol/L。
    - 配置氯化钾：20 mmol，口服，片剂，1 次。
    - 配置氯化钾：20 mmol，口服，液体，1 次。
    - 配置氯化钾：10 mmol 100 ml，IVPB，q1 h，2 剂，注射 60 min 以上。
  - K^+：<3.0 mmol/L。
    - 配置氯化钾：10 mmol 100 ml，IVPB，q1 h，2 剂，注射 60 min 以上。
- 年龄>70 岁或血清肌酐(SCr)>1.5：
  - K^+：3.5～3.9 mmol/L。
    - 配置氯化钾：20 mmol，口服，片剂，1 次。
    - 配置氯化钾：20 mmol，口服，液体，1 次。
    - 配置氯化钾：10 mmol 100 ml，IVPB，q1 h，2 剂，注射 60 min 以上。
  - K^+：3.0～3.4 mmol/L。

D

○ 配置氯化钾：40 mmol，口服，缓释剂型，1 次。
○ 配置氯化钾：40 mmol，口服，液体，1 次。
○ 配置氯化钾：40 mmol 500 ml，IVPB，1 次，注射 4 h 以上。
- K^+：<3.0 mmol/L。
○ 配置氯化钾：40 mmol 500 ml，IVPB，1 次，注射 4 h 以上。
• 年龄<70 岁，SCr>1.5。
- K^+：3.5～3.9 mmol/L。
○ 配置氯化钾：40 mmol，口服，缓释剂型，1 次。
○ 配置氯化钾：40 mmol，口服，液体，1 次。
○ 配置氯化钾：10 mmol 100 ml，IVPB，q1 h，2 剂，注射 60 min 以上。
- K^+：3.0～3.4 mmol/L。
○ 配置氯化钾：40 mmol，口服，缓释剂型，q4 h，2 剂。
○ 配置氯化钾：40 mmol，口服，液体，q4 h，2 剂。
○ 配置氯化钾：40 mmol 500 ml，IVPB，1 次，注射 4 h 以上。第一次服用后检查钾含量。如果低钾血症持续，相应给予第二次钾。
- K^+：<3.0 mmol/L。
○ 配置氯化钾：氯化钾：40 mmol 500 ml，IVPB，1 次，注射 4 h 以上。第一次服用后检查钾含量。如果低钾血症持续，相应给予第二次钾。

随访

进一步处理

入院指征

• 不稳定/异常生命体征。
• 心电图异常。
• 心脏节律障碍。
• 不能耐受口服，需要静脉补液和/或静脉补钾。
• 急救治疗后持续低钾血症。

出院指征

• 无症状/生命体征稳定。
• 正常心电图。
• 无心律失常。
• 通过口服补钾可以纠正。
• 急诊治疗后血清钾水平恢复正常。

转诊问题

• 患者应在出院后 1 周内与初级保健医师进行随访。没有初级保健医师的患者可能需要社会工作来帮助建立后续护理。

随访建议

停止服用引起低钾血症的药物，直到在出院后 1 周内与初级保健医师进一步讨论。增加从食物中口服钾的摄入量。

要点和误区

• 接受静脉注射钾的患者需要心脏监测。
• 严重低钾血症患者需住院。
• 检查低钾患者的镁水平，并相应地纠正低镁血症。
• 必须要做心电图。

低钠血症 Hyponatremia

Linda Mueller　倪沁赟 译

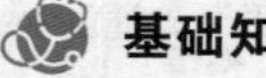

基础知识

描述

• 血钠<136 mmol/L。
• 最常见的电解质紊乱（住院患者发生率为 1%～4%）。

病因

假性低钠血症

• 血钠低但血浆渗透压正常。
• 继发于血清水钠的转移。
• 高脂血症或高蛋白血症。
• 实验室或血标本错误。
• 疾病：
- 多发性骨髓瘤。
- 高脂血症。

渗透压正常和容量过多时的低钠血症

• 不恰当的水潴留。
• 疾病：
- 充血性心力衰竭。
- 肝硬化。
- 肾衰竭。
- 肾病综合征。

渗透压正常和容量正常时的低钠血症

• 患者全身水量增加，但没有明显水肿。
• 单纯的稀释性低钠血症。
• 疾病：
- 内分泌异常：
○ 甲状腺功能减退症。
○ 应激。
○ 抗利尿激素分泌异常综合征(SIADH)。
- 可导致 SIADH 的疾病：
○ 肺脏疾病（肺结核、军团菌肺炎、肺曲霉病、慢性阻塞性肺疾病）。
○ 中枢神经系统疾病（恶性肿瘤、结节病、中枢感染）。
○ 癌症（小细胞性肺癌、胰腺癌、十二指肠癌）。
○ HIV 感染。
- 水中毒（3%～7%的住院精神疾病患者），也可发生于马拉松运动员。
- 盐皮质激素异常。
- 术后低钠血症（特别见于经尿道前列腺切除术后）。
- 大量饮酒。
- 摇头丸（迷幻药）。

渗透压正常和容量过低时的低钠血症

• 全身水及全身钠不足。
• 丢钠多于丢水。
• 可能的病因包括：
- 胃肠道丢失。
- 出汗。
- 脑盐耗综合征（发生于颅脑外伤或神经外科术后）。
- 烧伤。
- 囊性纤维化。
- 肾性盐耗。
- 利尿剂使用。

药物因素

• 药物可能刺激抗利尿激素分泌从而导致低钠血症：
- 胺碘酮。
- 巴比妥类药物。
- 溴隐亭。
- 卡马西平。
- 氯贝特。

- 环磷酰胺。
- 阿片类药物。
- 催产素。
- 长春新碱。

• 药物可能增加抗利尿激素敏感性从而导致低钠血症：
- 氯磺苯脲。
- 非甾体抗炎药(NSAIDs)。

• 药物可能刺激口渴中枢从而导致低钠血症：
- 阿米替林。
- 迷幻药。
- 氟西汀。
- 奋乃静。
- 氟哌啶醇。
- 盐酸舍曲林。
- 替沃噻吨。

高渗性低钠血症

• 因输注过多高渗透性物质。

• 可能的病因包括：
- 高血糖(低钠血症的常见原因)。
- 修正后的血钠浓度＝0.016×(所测血糖值－100)＋所测血钠值。
- 输注甘露醇。
- 麦芽糖和甘氨酸。

儿科注意事项

• 更容易发生水中毒。

• 医源性低钠血症的发生率高(补液浓度稀或仅补充水分)。

• 继发于糖尿病酮症酸中毒的低钠血症，因为对于儿童糖尿病酮症酸中毒推荐水化治疗。

• 年龄小于16岁和缺氧是医源性低钠血症的最大风险。

妊娠注意事项

考尼伐坦和托伐普坦对于妊娠患者为C级药物。

老年人注意事项

• 有更多的临床表现。

• 更多地继发于水排除障碍或低钠饮食。

诊断

症状和体征

• 轻度：Na^+＞120 mmol/L：
- 头痛。
- 恶心。
- 呕吐。
- 虚弱。
- 厌食症。
- 肌肉抽搐。
- 横纹肌溶解。

• 中度：110 mmol/L＜Na^+＜120 mmol/L：
- 对言语刺激反应受损。
- 对疼痛刺激反应下降。
- 视力与听力出现幻觉。
- 行为异常。
- 尿失禁。
- 过度换气。
- 步态异常。

• 重度：Na^+＜110 mmol/L：
- 脑疝。
- 去大脑强直。
- 心动过缓。
- 高血压。
- 体温调节点改变。
- 瞳孔扩大。
- 癫痫发作。
- 呼吸暂停。
- 昏迷/反应迟钝。

慢性低钠血症

可能无症状。

病史

回顾患者用药清单。

体格检查

• 评估患者容量状态包括皮肤肿胀、颈部血管、周围水肿情况和腹水情况。

• 完整的神经系统检查。

基本检查

血清钠水平：

• 即使复查已明确。

诊断检查与说明

实验室检查

• 电解质、尿素氮/肌酐。

• 血糖：
- 严重高血糖时需要纠正血钠值(血糖每升高100 mg/dl，血钠增加1.6)。

• 计算渗透压：
- 血浆渗透压＝[2×NA(mmol/L)＋血糖/18＋BUN/2.8]。

• 尿钠。

• 血、尿渗透压。

• 甲状腺功能检测。

• 肾上腺功能检测。

• 横纹肌溶解患者检测磷酸肌酸酶(CPK)。

影像学检查

• 胸部X线检查以排除充血性心力衰竭、感染和肿瘤。

• 如果患者有AMS，行头颅CT检查。

鉴别诊断

• 假性低钠血症：
- 高血糖。
- 高脂血症。
- 高蛋白血症。
- 使用造影剂，尤其是合并慢性肾功能不全的患者。

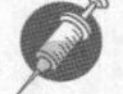

治疗

院前

• 建立静脉通道。

• 支持治疗。

初步稳定/治疗

• ABC管理。

• 静脉输注生理盐水。

• 有精神症状的患者给予纳洛酮、维生素B_1或50%葡萄糖注射液。

急诊治疗/程序

• 根据低钠血症的严重程度及慢性程度和基础病因。

• 慢性低钠血症应缓慢纠正，减少渗透性脱髓鞘综合征的发生。在24 h内血钠上升10～12 mmol/L。

• 急性低钠血症伴有神经系统症状：
- 静脉使用高渗盐水在4～6 h使血钠升高8～10 mmol/L或使血钠浓度＞120～125 mmol/L，当癫痫发作好转，减慢或暂停补充。
- 癫痫消退时缓慢或停止。
- 大部分成人在最初的2 h内需要输注3%盐水200～400 ml。

• 无急性神经症状的低钠血症：
- 计算钠摄入量：
  - ◦ Na^+逆差＝0.6(重量单位kg)(140－Na^+)。
  - ◦ 更换时间8～12 h，不超过要求的1/2。
  - ◦ 最大矫正率＝0.5 mmol/(L·h)。
- 低血容量性低钠血症：
  - ◦ 纠正根本原因。
  - ◦ 0.9%盐水静脉补液。
  - ◦ 恢复主要目标：
    - ▫ 细胞外液。
    - ▫ 心输出量。
    - ▫ 器官灌注。
- 血容量过多或等容量低钠血症：
  - ◦ 水限制到1 L/d，高盐摄入。

D

◦ 更快地校正钠：

▫ 给静脉注射 0.9% 盐水和袢利尿剂（呋塞米）。

■ 药物治疗

- 补钠：
  - 1 L 0.9%盐水＝154 mmol 钠。
  - 1 L 3%盐水＝513 mmol 钠。
  - 1 L LR＝130 mmol 钠。
  - 1 L 浆质体 140 mmol 钠。
- 呋塞米：20～40 mg，静脉推注。

一线用药

给予 500～1 000 ml 生理盐水进行液体复苏。如果钠含量没有变化或进一步降低，治疗 SIADH。

二线用药

- 考尼伐坦：精氨酸加压素拮抗剂。
- 在至少 30 min 内静脉给予 20 mg 负荷剂量，然后至少 24 h 给予 20 mg 持续静脉维持。
- 托伐普坦：选择性加压素 V_2 受体拮抗剂，给予 15 mg/d 口服，可以在 24 h 内加量至 30 mg。
- 考尼伐坦和托伐普坦仅用于治疗等容量性和高容量性低钠血症。

随访

■ 进一步处理

入院指征

- 有症状的低钠血症。
- 血钠＜120 mmol/L。
- 有合并因素的无症状性、轻度低钠血症（Na^+ 120～127 mmol/L）。

出院指征

- 血钠＞130 mmol/L，临床无明显症状。
- 有导致低钠血症的慢性病史，目前无急性改变。
- 无合并因素的无症状性、轻度低钠血症（Na^+ 120～129 mmol/L），但是必须严密随访。

■ 随访建议

1 周内复查血钠值，尤其是使用噻嗪类利尿剂的患者。

要点和误区

- 过快纠正血钠可能会导致渗透性脱髓鞘综合征。
- 女性、饮酒、营养不良、低钾血症及有肝移植病史是发生渗透性脱髓鞘综合征的危险因素。
- 治疗期间需要反复进行神经系统检查。
- 当血液丢失使用低渗液体静脉输液时警惕血钠的快速下降。
- 停用噻嗪类利尿剂治疗低钠血症仍可能持续约 2 周。
- 如果使用生理盐水监测高氯血症。

低血糖

Japheth J. Baker · Matthew N. Graber 倪沁赟 译

基础知识

■ 描述

- 抵抗激素缺乏（胰高血糖素、肾上腺素、皮质醇、生长激素）或胰岛素分泌增加。
- 血糖＜70 mg/dl。

■ 危险因素

- 胰岛素严格控制血糖。
- 既往有低血糖发作。
- 低血糖昏迷。
- 反调节作用下降。
- 年龄＜5 岁或老年人。
- 伴随疾病：
  - 肾脏疾病。
  - 营养不良。
  - 冠状动脉疾病。
  - 肝脏疾病。

遗传学

- 先天性代谢和内分泌疾病使糖异生能力下降（如遗传性果糖不耐症）。
- 先天性高胰岛素血症。
- 新生儿糖尿病（作用于 ATP 依赖的钾通道的突变）。

■ 病因

- 胰岛素水平增加：
  - 口服降糖药物或胰岛素过量。
  - 口服降糖药物（如 α-葡萄糖苷酶抑制剂、双胍类、噻唑烷二酮类），单独使用时没有出现低血糖，合并使用胰岛素或磺脲类药物时低血糖风险增加。
  - 脓毒血症。
  - 胰岛素瘤。
  - 自身免疫性低血糖。
  - 消化高胰岛素血症。
  - 肾衰竭（部分影响胰岛素代谢）。
  - 肝硬化（显著影响胰岛素代谢）。
- 葡萄糖生成减少：
  - 酒精（糖原储备和糖异生功能抑制）。
  - 药物。
  - 水杨酸。
  - β受体阻滞剂（包括滴眼液）。
  - 选择性 5-羟色胺再吸收抑制剂。
  - 某些抗生素（如磺脲类药物、喷他脒）。
  - 肾上腺皮质功能不全。
  - 营养不良。
  - 脱水。
- 脑水肿。
- 年龄过小或过大。
- 充血性心力衰竭。
- 反调节激素缺乏。
- 甲状腺功能减退症或甲状腺功能亢进症。

妊娠注意事项

- 妊娠第 3 个月的患者因相关底物缺乏导致低血糖的发生风险增加。
- 当母亲低血糖的发生继发于活性葡萄糖的胎盘转移时，胎儿很少发生低血糖：
  - 妊娠期间口服降糖药物可能会导致新生儿发生严重并长时间的低血糖。

儿科注意事项

最初 3 个月最常见的低血糖原因是婴儿持续高胰岛素血性低血糖（婴儿母亲患有糖尿病）。

诊断

■ 症状和体征

- 由过量反调节激素引起的肾上腺素释放（如肾上腺素）：
  - 发汗。
  - 焦虑。

- 心动过速或心悸。
- 饥饿。
- 感觉异常。
- 胸痛。
- 缺血性心电图改变。
• 神经低血糖：
- 脑血管意外表现。
- 功能性或有病灶的神经系统改变。
- 头晕。
- 困惑。
- 情绪改变。
- 行为极度活跃或出现精神异常。
- 口齿不清。
- 脑神经麻痹。
- 癫痫发作。
- 偏瘫。
- 去大脑强直。
• 新生儿表现：
- 无症状。
- 跛行。
- 心动过缓。
- 烦躁。
- 颤抖。
- 癫痫发作。
- 喂养困难。

注意

"未察觉的低血糖"患者降低了预警信号，没有意识到他们的血糖低，可能替代性地表现为癫痫发作、有病灶的神经功能改变、精神状态改变和昏迷。

病史

• 基础疾病或条件：糖尿病、肾衰竭、肝衰竭和饮酒史。
• 某些药物：长效胰岛素和口服降糖药物（影响更大）。
• 胰岛素或口服降糖药物过量。

体格检查

见症状和体征。

基本检查

• 诊断需要：
- 上述神经低血糖症状和体征。
- 低血糖的实验室证据。
- 葡萄糖输注后的症状改善。

诊断检查与说明

实验室检查

• 血气分析（最初的检查，同时在治疗之前进行）。
• 电解质、尿素氮、肌酐。
• 凝血酶原时间。
• 尿常规。
• 尿液及其他病原学培养，作为感染的依据。
• C肽（排除外源性胰岛素过量导致的低血糖）。

影像学检查

胸部X线检查：
• 低血糖期间可能有误吸的发生。
• 肺炎可能是感染的来源。

诊断步骤/外科

• 由于低血糖而出现心肌梗死/心肌缺血，或怀疑是低血糖发生的原因是行心电图检查。
• 低血糖可能会影响心脏电传导。

鉴别诊断

低血糖鉴别诊断范围较广：
• 神经系统：
- 脑血管意外或短暂性脑缺血发作。
- 癫痫发作。
• 药物或酒精中毒。
• 缺氧。
• 脓毒血症。
• 代谢紊乱。
• 内分泌紊乱。
• 环境因素。
• 精神病、抑郁或焦虑。

儿科注意事项

• 生长激素缺乏。
• 先天性代谢缺陷。
• 酮症性低血糖。
• 急性脑病综合征（Reye 综合征）。
• 摄入水杨酸。

治疗

院前

• 指尖血糖监测。
• 推荐静脉补充葡萄糖。
• 如果不能静脉补充葡萄糖，则口服含葡萄糖的液体。
• 如果不能静脉和口服葡萄糖，则使用胰高血糖素。

初步稳定/治疗

• 误吸和癫痫发作的预防。
• 葡萄糖：
- 静脉推注，情况允许的情况需持续给予。
- 没有静脉通道和误吸风险时，虚弱患者可给予口服葡萄糖。
- 无法建立静脉通道时可肌内注射胰高血糖素。

急诊治疗/程序

• 对意识水平下降的患者给予50%葡萄糖溶液50 ml：
- 可能需要2安瓿或3安瓿。
- 并发症包括容量过负荷和低钾血症。
• 奥曲肽使用：
- 如果患者存在难治性低血糖表现。
- 因使用磺脲类药物出现的低血糖。
- 静脉输注5%～20%葡萄糖溶液，轻度低血糖持续存在或患者无法进食。
• 胰高血糖素的使用：
- 如果患者存在难治性低血糖表现。
- 静脉通道尚未建立。
- 对酒精导致的低血糖和严重肝脏疾病无效。
- 需20～30 min重复使用。
- 对于肾上腺皮质功能不全的患者联合使用氢化可的松。
- 10～20 min有效。

老年人注意事项

老年患者临床低血糖征象不明显，常需要更多的时间进行鉴别，甚至会错过低血糖的合理治疗时间窗。

药物治疗

一线用药

• 50%葡萄糖溶液：50%葡萄糖溶液1～2安瓿（25 g）静脉推注。
- Zimmerman 原则：成人50%葡萄糖溶液1 ml/kg；儿童25%葡萄糖溶液2 ml/kg；婴儿10%葡萄糖溶液5 ml/kg。

二线用药

• 奥曲肽：50 μg静脉推注负荷量，然后50 μg/h静脉滴注；或者50 μg每12 h皮下注射或静脉推注。
• 胰高血糖素：0.5～2 mg，静脉推注、肌内注射或皮下注射。
- 儿童：0.03～0.1 mg/kg，静脉推注、肌内注射或皮下注射。
- 婴儿：0.3 mg/kg，静脉推注、肌内注射或皮下注射。
- 4 h内可能需要重复给药。
• 氢化可的松：100 mg（儿童：1～2 mg/kg），静脉推注。

• 口服葡萄糖：20 g，口服，相当于 12 oz 果汁，14 oz 可乐。
- 首选不含脂肪和蛋白质的碳水化合物(糖类)。
• 其他可能的解决方案：
- SSRI 药物。
- 选择性肾上腺素能拮抗剂。
- 阿片拮抗剂。
- 果糖。
- 选择性 ATP 敏感的钾通道激动剂。

随访

进一步处理

入院指征

• 过量使用长效口服降糖药物(如磺脲类药物)或长效胰岛素至少观察 24 h。
• 使用葡萄糖治疗后低血糖神经系统方面的症状无明显改善。
• 在急诊室低血糖复发。
• 患者无法耐受口服治疗。
• 有自杀倾向。
• 严重或时间较长的低血糖老年患者可能需要几日完全恢复正常。

出院指征

• 出院时使用小剂量胰岛素维持正常血糖或不需要口服摄入热量维持正常血糖，临床症状恢复，耐受口服治疗。
• 反复发作低血糖患者的家属会肌内注射葡萄糖。
• 出院之前至少血糖监测每 3 h 1 次。

转诊问题

如果患者低血糖症状反复发作，建议找上级医师指导药物或饮食的调整。

随访建议

由私人医师在 48 h 内对药物效果进行再评估。

要点和误区

• 口服葡萄糖或食物早期可能会使血糖水平更加降低，在情况允许的情况下推荐静脉使用葡萄糖。
• 常需要较多的 50%葡萄糖注射液。
• 不要过度依赖 10% 和 20% 葡萄糖注射液。
• 低血糖症状应该与所有神经和精神表现区分。
• 反复低血糖发作的患者神经系统功能恢复常常需要数小时至数日的时间。
• 反复出现的严重低血糖可能会导致长期的认知障碍，并刺激痴呆的发展，因此密切的随访旨在预防这一点是至关重要的。
• 低血糖可导致创伤，所有原因不明的创伤都应加以区分。

骶骨骨折 Sacral Fractures

Allan V. Hansen · Jaime B. Rivas 何融冰 译

基础知识

描述

• 发生在 45% 的骨盆骨折中，很少单独发生。
• 根据骨折线的定位来定义。
• 机制：
- 轴向压力。
- 直接后部创伤。
- 大面积挤压伤。
- 年长和骨折质疏松患者发生功能不全性骨折。

骨折分类

横断面
• S_4 以上：
- 神经系统损伤常见。
- 可发生马尾综合征(CES)。
• S_4 以下：
- 与直肠撕裂伤相关。
- 神经系统损伤少见。

垂直方向
• 骶孔外侧：
- 坐骨神经痛。
- L_5 神经根损伤。
- 神经缺损不常见。
• 骶孔(2 区)：
- 肠/膀胱功能障碍。
- 性功能障碍。
- L_5、S_1 神经根损伤。
- 神经功能障碍常见(>50%)。

病因

• 横向损伤：高处坠落、屈曲损伤、直接打击。
• 竖直方向损伤：通常高能量机制。

老年人注意事项

有严重背痛的老年人应考虑功能减退性骶骨骨折。

诊断

症状和体征

• 臀部、直肠周围和大腿后部的疼痛。
• 骶骨隆起部位的肿胀和瘀斑。
• 可能造成骶神经功能障碍。
- 肛门括约肌张力消失或减弱是一个重要表现。
- 肠或膀胱失禁。

基本检查

• 病史和体格检查注意肛门括约肌张力消失、会阴感觉、肠道及膀胱括约肌控制力。
• 骶骨骨折很少单独发生，检查联合伤。
• 直肠检查可引发骶骨疼痛；直肠中有血提示开放性骨折。

诊断检查与说明

影像学检查

• 只有 30% 的骶骨骨折可在 X 线平片上发现。
• CT 可提供更佳的影像来明确骶骨骨折。
• 当出现神经功能障碍时应行 MRI 检查。

鉴别诊断

• 挫伤。
• 腰椎骨折。
• 骨盆骨折。

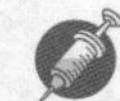

治疗

院前

• 骶骨骨折经常合并其他脊椎或腹腔内损伤。
• 用硬板和颈椎套圈制动。

■ 初步稳定/治疗

- 如需则行 ABC 管理。
- 不稳定骨盆和脊柱骨折需早期制动。
- 使用 NSAIDs 或麻醉镇痛药控制疼痛。

■ 急诊治疗/程序

- 竖直型不稳定骨折需要对威胁生命的损伤进行快速彻底的评估，同时请骨科医师会诊（见“骨盆骨折”）。
- 无移位的单发横向骶骨骨折可根据症状向受影响的部位施加向下的重量并尽早请骨科医师会诊。
- 波及神经损伤的骨折需要手术治疗。

■ 药物治疗

一线用药

如果需要则进行镇痛。

随访

■ 进一步处理

入院指征

- 有不稳定骨盆骨折的严重创伤患者。
- 神经损伤需骨科会诊。

出院指征

- 单独的非移位性骶骨骨折。
- 考虑间接或辅助治疗的老年人。

■ 随访建议

- 只有非移位的横形骨折适合院外随访。
- 移位骨折需迅速外科手术评估。

要点和误区

- 骶骨骨折很少单独发生，考虑合并骨盆骨折。
- 评估合并的骶神经根损伤需要进行仔细的神经学检查，包括肛门括约肌张力和会阴感觉。
- Foley 导尿管可能掩盖骶神经根损伤患者的排尿问题。

地高辛中毒 Digoxin

Kirk L. Cumpston 谭美春 译

基础知识

■ 描述

- 急性洋地黄效应（儿童药物含量过高和故意过量）：
  - 抑制细胞膜 Na^+ - K^+ - ATP 酶。
  - 细胞内钙增加。
  - 增加细胞外 K^+。
  - 提高迷走神经张力。
  - 减慢房室结（AV）的传导（迷走神经过敏）。
  - 增加自主收缩和传导系统不应期。
  - 缓慢性心律失常。
- 慢性洋地黄效应（老年患者治疗剂量至中毒量）：
  - 抑制细胞膜 Na^+ - K^+ - ATP 酶。
  - 增加细胞内钙离子浓度。
  - 增加迷走神经张力。
  - 增强自主收缩。
  - 低钾血症通常继发于使用利尿剂。
  - 心动过速。

■ 病因

- 地高辛/洋地黄毒苷药物。
- 含有强心苷类的动物和植物：
  - 毛地黄。
  - 夹竹桃（白色和黄色）。
  - 铃兰。
  - 红海葱。
  - 甘蔗蟾蜍、科罗拉多河蟾蜍。

诊断

■ 症状和体征

- 毒性发作：口服后 2 h 以内，静脉用药 15 min 以内。
- 毒性：
  - 使用正常剂量的地高辛时出现（慢性）。
  - 可能地高辛浓度的升高（急性）。
- 心血管：
  - 心律失常：
    - 阵发性房性心动过速（PAT）与房室传导阻滞。
    - 典型病征：双向性室性心动过速（VT）。
    - 最常见：室性期前收缩（室早）。
    - 非阵发性加速交界性心动过速。
    - 双向性室性心动过速。
    - 心室颤动。
    - 心房颤动、扑动。
    - 二联律。
    - 心动过缓。
    - 非阵发性房性心动过速。
    - 房室传导阻滞。
    - 窦性心律失常。
    - 期前收缩。
  - 充血性心力衰竭加重。
  - 低血压。
  - 休克。
  - 心血管性虚脱。
  - 晕厥。
- 中枢神经系统：
  - 精神状态的改变：
    - 焦虑。
    - 嗜睡。
    - 精神病。
- 视觉感知：
  - 模糊。
  - 盲点。
  - 绿色到黄色晕圈。
  - 畏光。
  - 色觉变化。
- 胃肠道：
  - 厌食、恶心、呕吐、腹痛。

病史

- 在已知剂量下成人或儿童的意外过量。
- 未长期服用地高辛的患者发生故意急性过量。
- 长期服用地高辛的患者发生故意急性或慢性过量。
- 在肾脏清除率降低或长期增量的情况下非故意的长期摄入地高辛。
- 近期使用抗生素（尤其是大环内酯类）能改变胃肠菌群，主要是通过减少迟缓真杆菌，增加药物吸收导致意外中毒。

体格检查

- 精神状态改变。
- 心动过缓。

- 心动过速。
- 心律不齐。
- 低血压。

基本检查

- 心电图：
  - 针对心律失常。
- 地高辛浓度：
  - 正常范围：0.5～2 ng/ml。
  - 口服用药 6 h 后才能全身分布，因此＞6 h 的血药浓度水平是最准确的稳态浓度。
  - 假性升高可能与使用螺内酯、妊娠、高胆红素血症、慢性肾衰竭、肝功能衰竭、充血性心力衰竭有关。
  - 给予地高辛特定 Fab 片段后可能假性升高。

D

诊断检查与说明

实验室检查

- 电解质、尿素氮、肌酐、葡萄糖：
  - 低钾血症将促进洋地黄中毒。
  - 高钾血症可见于急性中毒，其与急性洋地黄中毒死亡的相关性比地高辛血清药物浓度更优。
  - 随着 K^+ 浓度连续变化。
- 钙和镁。

> **注意**
>
> 不应该在使用地高辛特异性抗体的 Fab 片段之后检测血清地高辛浓度（SDC），因为将导致检验结果不准确。地高辛特异性 Fab 片段前后的游离地高辛血清浓度将保持准确。

鉴别诊断

- 过量：
  - 钙通道阻滞剂。
  - β受体阻滞剂。
  - 奎尼丁、普鲁卡因胺。
  - 可乐定。
  - 有机磷农药。
  - 抗心律失常药。
  - 其他抗高血压药。
- 原发性心律失常。
- 急性胃肠炎。

治疗

院前

- 建立静脉通路。
- 连续心电监护。
- 为潜在的心脏复律申请应用垫。

> **注意**
>
> - 如果心动过速有必要进行电复律，使用低功率(50 J)。
> - 可用于转复难治性心动过速。

初步稳定/治疗

基础治疗 ABC 管理：

- 静脉用药，给予氧气，监护：
  - 如果低血容量则静脉补液。
- 精神状态改变使用纳洛酮、硫胺素、葡萄糖。

急诊治疗/程序

- 心搏骤停复苏：
  - 除颤：心室颤动，无脉性室性心动过速。
  - 标准高级心脏生命支持（ACLS）协议。
  - 使用地高辛特异性抗体 Fab 片段（Digibind），最高达 5～20 小瓶静脉推注（IVP）。
  - 硫酸镁 2 g 静脉推注。
  - 使用地高辛特异性抗体 Fab 片段后继续复苏 30 min。
- 一般的措施：
  - 如果急性摄入用活性炭。
  - 及时补充镁剂。
  - 治疗高钾血症：胰岛素、葡萄糖、碳酸氢盐、聚苯乙烯磺酸钠。
  - 如果心律失常与高钾血症的影响一致，钙可用于治疗高钾血症。在地高辛急性或慢性中毒的情况下，高钾血症可能是由肾功能恶化引起的。
    - 如果患者因地高辛毒性而出现高钾血症，首先应使用地高辛特异性 Fab 片段进行治疗

心律失常的治疗

- 第一选择：地高辛特异性抗体 Fab 片段（Digibind，DigiFab）。
  - 适应证：
    - 在任何时间 SDC＞15 ng/ml，或稳定状态时＞10 ng/ml(6 h)。
    - 摄入量：成人＞10 mg，儿童＞0.2 mg/kg 或 4 mg。
    - 高钾血症＞5～5.5 mEq/L。
    - 血流动力学不稳定或危及生命的心律失常。
    - 室性心动过速。
    - 房性心动过速。
    - 易变的房室传导阻滞。
    - 对阿托品无反应性心动过缓。
    - 低血压。
  - 发病：20～30 min。
  - 由于 Fab 地高辛复合物和药物重新分布，治疗后地高辛的血药浓度会增加、减少或保持在治疗范围。
  - 药物抗体复合物的肾脏清除：
    - 药物浓度过大通过透析去除。
  - 如果毒性反弹，则进行第二次。
  - 地高辛特异性 Fab 片段的并发症：
    - 充血性心力衰竭加重。
    - 心房颤动伴快速心室率。
- 如果地高辛特异性抗体 Fab 片段没有立即起效则启动以下治疗：
  - 利多卡因：
    - 无房室传导阻滞的室性心律失常。
    - 非特效，但非有害。
  - 对于缓慢性心律失常：
    - 阿托品。
  - 起搏治疗：有症状的缓慢性心律失常。
  - 硫酸镁治疗：室性心律失常与尖端扭转型室性心动过速。
  - 奎尼丁、普鲁卡因酰胺禁忌使用。
- 心脏电复律作为严重情况、危及生命的快速心律失常的最后处理：
  - 开始用低功率 10～50 J，如果效果不佳再调大功率。
  - 如果地高辛浓度＜2 ng/ml 被视为安全情况。
- 如果地高辛特异性抗体 Fab 片段没有治疗作用，经皮或经静脉起搏可用于治疗心动过缓。

药物治疗

- 活性炭浆：
  - 如果在 1 h 内，1 g/kg。
- 地高辛特异性抗体 Fab 片段：
  - 40 mg 小瓶和 0.5 mg 地高辛。
  - 如果摄入量已知：
    - 用于治疗的小瓶数量＝[总摄入量(mg)/0.5(mg/瓶)]。
  - 如果稳态血药浓度已知：
    - 小瓶需要量＝[SDC(ng/ml)×体重(kg)]/100。
  - 如果摄入量及血药浓度均不知道：
    - 急性毒性：成人或儿童 5～10 小瓶。
    - 慢性毒性：成人或儿童 1～2 小瓶。

- 心搏骤停用地高辛特异性抗体 Fab 片段丸剂。
- 根据需要增加剂量。
• 标准治疗高钾血症和心动过缓,钙应该用于治疗高钾血症引起的心律失常。

老年人注意事项

• 剂量是根据体重和血清浓度确定的,肾、肝功能不全者剂量无须调整。
• 已有关于伴随肾衰竭患者毒性复发的报道。地高辛特异性抗体 Fab 片段再次使用时应被注明。

妊娠注意事项

地高辛特定 Fab 片段是妊娠 C 类药物。

 随访

■ 进一步处理

入院指征

• ICU:
- 急性或慢性中毒,心血管状态不稳定的患者。
• 遥感自动测量记录:
- 无症状或仅有轻度症状的心律失常。
- 毒性发作风险较高的患者。

出院指征

急慢性摄入:
• 地高辛浓度<2 ng/ml。
• 6 h 无症状,无心电图异常。

■ 随访建议

病情稳定的自杀患者精神科随访。

要点和误区

• 当用钙治疗地高辛中毒引起的高钾血症时,不再担心引起"石心"。在高钾血症诱导心律失常的情况下,钙可稳定心肌膜。
• 急性或慢性肾损伤通常会导致高钾血症,在治疗慢性地高辛毒性时,1～2 小瓶地高辛特异性抗体 Fab 片段是安全的选择,以避免慢性疾病的过度纠正和恶化。
• 地高辛特异性抗体 Fab 片段是地高辛毒性危及生命的体征和症状的最终解决方案。

D

癫痫发作(成人) Seizures, Adult

Daewon Kim · John A. Guisto 张溢叟 伍力学 译

 基础知识

■ 描述

• 广义癫痫:
- 双侧大脑半球的异常神经电活动。
- 典型的强直-痉挛(癫痫大发作):意识丧失,肌强直,有节奏的抽搐(阵挛)。
- 失神发作(小发作):意识改变,但无明显姿势变化;可有短暂的抽搐(肌阵挛)。
• 局灶型(部分)癫痫发作:
- 通常一侧大脑半球存有意识,可蔓延至双侧大脑半球并引起感觉中枢异常。
- 很可能继发于局灶性脑损害。
- 不再被划分为简单型(如杰克逊症)和复杂型(意识或心理状态受影响)局灶癫痫发作。
• 癫痫持续状态:
- 发作持续时间大于 5 min(经典定义为至少 30 min)或反复发作且两次发作之间的状态从未回复到基线水平者。
- 非惊厥性癫痫状态可能存在于>9%的住院患者且伴有长期精神状态下降。
- 如果发作持续时间>1 h,则致命性急症的发生率和病死率将达 30%。
- 至少有一半因癫痫发作被送入急诊的患者没有癫痫病史。
• 特殊人群的鉴别诊断:
- HIV 感染者:占位病变、脑病、带状疱疹、弓形虫病、隐球菌脑炎、神经梅毒、脑膜炎。
- 脑囊虫病:带状绦虫感染,发展中国家多见。
- 妊娠超过 20 周:子痫(高血压、水肿、蛋白尿、癫痫)。
- 酒精戒断性癫痫:在末次喝酒后 24 h 达到高峰,很少发生癫痫持续状态。
• 生命周期中发生症状性癫痫的风险为 8%～10%。
- 曾发作过癫痫的一次癫痫的患者 5 年内再次发作的风险为 35%。
• 2011 年的数据:
- 因癫痫到急诊就诊的人数为 160 万。
- 其中约 40 万为新发癫痫。

儿科注意事项

单纯发热惊厥(呈自限性和良性特征)。
• 发病年龄在 6 个月至 6 年。
• 全身性抽搐症状。
• 一般持续<15 min。
• 24 h 内不复发。
• 无中枢神经系统感染或其他神经系统疾病。

■ 病因

• 缺氧。
• 高血压脑病。
• 子痫。
• 感染性:
- 脑膜炎。
- 脑脓肿。
- 脑炎。
• 血管性:
- 缺血性脑卒中。
- 出血性脑卒中。
- 硬膜下血肿。
- 硬膜外血肿。
- 蛛网膜下腔出血。
- 动静脉畸形。
• 结构性:
- 原发性或转移性肿瘤。
- 退行性疾病(如多发性硬化症)。
- 既往创伤性损害。
• 代谢:
- 电解质。
- 高钠血症。
- 低钠血症。
- 低钙血症。
- 低血糖或高血糖。
- 尿毒症。
• 毒物和药物:
- 利多卡因。
- 三环类抗抑郁药。
- 水杨酸盐。
- 异烟肼。
- 可卡因。
- 酒精戒断。

- 苯二氮䓬戒断。
- 先天性异常。
- 特发性。
- 创伤。

诊断

■ 症状和体征

- 意识水平的改变。
- 非随意重复性肌肉运动：
- 强直性姿势或阵挛性抽搐。
- 突发癫痫发作：
- 先兆期可表现为局灶性癫痫。
- 持续时间通常为 90～120 s：
- 损害对事件的记忆。
- 发作后的状态是思维混乱和嗜睡。
- 近期癫痫发作的依据：
- 思维混乱或嗜睡。
- 急性口腔内损伤。
- 尿失禁。
- 后肩脱位。
- 托德瘫痪(癫痫发作后出现暂时性瘫痪，多在 48 h 内缓解)。
- 其他可能提示癫痫的病因的表现：
- 发热和颈部僵硬(中枢神经系统感染)。

蜘蛛痣：肝脏疾病引起的皮肤变化(药物性及酒精性)。

- 任何中毒综合征。
- 头部外伤：
- 视神经乳头水肿(颅内压增加)。
- 截断性肌力下降、感觉丧失或反射不对称。

病史

- 癫痫病史：
- 药物依从性。
- 近期疾病史。
- 头部外伤。
- 头痛。
- 抗凝治疗。
- 发热。
- 颈部僵硬。

体格检查

- 完整的神经病学检查：
- 托德瘫痪。
- 完善继发性和三发性病因排查，以评估有无导致癫痫发作的创伤或癫痫发作的潜在原因。

■ 基本检查

- 详细的病史是最重要的部分：
- 目击者问询。
- 先前癫痫发作史。
- 是否存在急性疾病史。
- 既往疾病史。
- 药物应用史。
- 其他特殊物质应用史。
- 患有慢性癫痫和典型癫痫的患者可能只需要检测血糖和抗惊厥药物的血药浓度。
- 新发癫痫发作则需要检测以下项目：
- 电解质包括钙、磷。
- 头颅 CT。
- 毒理学筛查。
- 育龄妇女妊娠试验。
- 下列情况需要行腰椎穿刺：
- 新发癫痫伴发热。
- 剧烈头痛。
- 免疫抑制状态。
- 持续的精神异常：
- 排查有无特殊的潜在病因。
- 依据患者的病情和随访条件决定是否需要在急诊室完成上述所有这些检查。

儿科注意事项

- 发热惊厥患者应根据临床情况接受发热筛查，但单纯发热惊厥患者不必行所有癫痫检查。
- 需要获取发热惊厥相关的家族史。
- 存在下列情形的发热惊厥应考虑行腰椎穿刺：
- 年龄＜1 岁。
- 有疾病表现(如嗜睡或喂养不良)。
- 未按时接种 Hib/PCV 疫苗。
- 存在脑膜刺激征象或检查困难。
- 无法确保有效随访。

■ 诊断检查与说明

实验室检查

- 血清抗惊厥药物浓度。
- 检测血液酒精浓度和毒物筛查。
- 毒理学检测。
- 白细胞水平常升高。
- 血生化检测：
- 碳酸氢根常较低。
- 乳酸和催乳素可能升高。
- 脑脊液：
- 白细胞水平可能短暂升高至 20/μl。

影像学检查

- 头颅 CT 平扫：
- 精神状态持续性或渐进性改变。
- 局灶性神经功能缺陷。
- 与创伤相关的癫痫。
- HIV 阳性患者应进行增强 CT 扫描，排除弓形虫病。
- MRI 对低级别肿瘤、小血管病变、早期炎症和早期脑梗死较敏感。
- 在新发癫痫中要合理选用。

诊断步骤/外科

- 脑电图可在门诊与神经病学检查一并安排。
- 如怀疑无惊厥性癫痫持续状态，可在急诊室中进行床边脑电图检查。
- 如果需要与晕厥、急性冠脉综合征、心律失常、中毒等鉴别，则需要做心电图。

■ 鉴别诊断

- 晕厥(可能还有尿失禁、抽搐和抽搐)。
- TIA、CVA、ICH、短暂性全面性遗忘。
- 颅内占位。
- 脑膜炎、脑炎、颅内脓肿。
- 运动障碍。
- 偏头痛。
- 后部可逆性脑病综合征。
- 睡眠障碍。
- 代谢紊乱。
- 心因性非癫痫性发作(PNES)。
- 惊恐发作或其他精神疾病。
- 震颤性谵妄。
- 破伤风。
- 甲状腺毒症。
- 药物或毒素(例如，抗精神病药所致的锥体外系症状)。
- 酒精中毒或戒断。

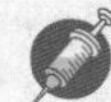

治疗

■ 院前

抗惊厥药物的使用参照当地相关流程。

■ 初步稳定/治疗

- 呼吸道管理。
- 出现癫痫持续状态、发绀、缺氧等情形强烈建议行快速气管插管。
- 脉搏血氧仪，吸氧，供氧，静脉通路：
- 颈椎预防性保护措施。
- 如果患者不能保证气道畅通或有缺氧或头部外伤，应行快速气管插管。
- 快速测定血清葡萄糖：
- 如果出现低血糖，给予静脉注射葡萄糖 25 g。
- 劳拉西泮、地西泮或咪达唑仑可用于癫痫发作。
- 如果考虑麻醉剂过量，给予纳洛酮。

急诊治疗/程序

- 首次癫痫发作：
- CT或MRI提示头部存在结构性损伤：
◦ 在咨询神经专科医师后开始应用抗癫痫药物。
- 复发性癫痫未使用抗癫痫药物者。
- 在咨询神经专科医师后开始应用抗癫痫药物。
- 复发性癫痫且使用了低于治疗剂量的抗癫痫药物者。
- 静脉注射或口服负荷剂量的速效抗癫痫药物。
- 复发性癫痫且使用了治疗剂量的抗癫痫药物者。
- 需要咨询评估癫痫的病因，有无新发损害等。
◦ 在咨询神经专科医师后调整或加量使用抗癫痫药物。
- 孕妇癫痫发作：
- 评估方式同癫痫患者。
- 处于孕20周至产后6周之间者，高度考虑子痫惊厥。
- 产科会诊，安排剖宫产。
- 硫酸镁是一线治疗药物。
- 酒精相关性癫痫：
- 确定癫痫发作是否由戒断(通常是末次饮酒后6～48 h)或其他原因引起。
- 苯二氮䓬类药物是一线治疗药物。

儿科注意事项

- 使用对乙酰氨基酚和布洛芬控制体温。
- 高热惊厥无需使用抗惊厥药。
- 使用抗惊厥药时应咨询神经专科医师。

药物治疗

一线用药

- 地西泮：10 mg(静脉注射)或10～20 mg(灌肠)，必要时；0.15～0.2 mg/kg，静脉注射(最大可用10 mg)；0.2～0.5 mg/kg，灌肠，必要时可增加至2 mg，5 min后可重复使用。
- 劳拉西泮：4 mg，静脉注射至少维持2 min；0.1 mg/kg，静脉注射或肌内注射(体重<40 kg者，最多可增至2 mg；其他可增至4 mg)，10 min后可重复使用。
- 咪达唑仑：10 mg，静脉注射、肌内注射、椎管内注射或口服；0.2 mg/kg，静脉注射、肌内注射或椎管内注射(体重<40 kg者，最大可增加至5 mg，其他可增至10 mg)；0.5 mg/kg，口服；10 min后可重复使用。

二线用药

- 磷苯妥英：20 mg苯妥英溶液当量(PF)/kg，静脉注射/肌内注射(输注<150 mg/min)。
- 戊巴比妥：首剂5～15 mg/kg，快速推注，0.5～5 mg/(kg · h)维持；须行气管插管。
- 苯巴比妥：15～20 mg/kg，静脉注射；可能需要行气管插管。
- 苯妥英：20 mg/kg，以1 mg/(kg · min)的速度给药。
- 异丙酚：首剂1～2 mg/kg，快速推注，然后20～200 μg/(kg · min)输注；须行气管插管。
- 丙戊酸钠溶液：20～40 mg/kg，静脉注射[最大可增至60 mg/(kg · d)]，以5 mg/(kg · min)速度输注。

特殊人群用药

- 右旋糖酐：25 g，静脉注射，D_{50}W(0～1月龄：2 ml/kg，静脉注射，D_{10}W；1月龄～2岁：2 ml/kg，静脉注射，D_{25}W；大于2岁：2 ml/kg D_{25}W)；成人最大剂量50 ml D_{50}W。
- 硫酸镁：首剂6 g静脉注射，至少维持15 min，然后以2 g/h维持；该药为子痫首选药物。
- 纳洛酮：0.4～2 mg，静脉注射、肌内注射、皮下注射、椎管内注射(儿童：0.1 mg/kg，静脉注射、肌内注射、皮下注射)。
- 吡哆醇：服用异烟肼患者，吡哆醛按与异烟肼等剂量给药(最大剂量5 g)，按0.5 g/min速度输注，直到癫痫发作被控制。

随访

进一步处理

入院指征

- 癫痫持续状态患者应入住ICU。
- 对继发于潜在疾病的癫痫患者(如脑膜炎、颅内病变)必须收治入院进行恰当的治疗和监测。
- 控制不良的反复发作患者应入院接受监护。
- 震颤性谵妄。

出院指征

- 相关检查结果恢复正常，精神状态恢复至正常水平，神经系统体检正常，后续能有恰当的神经病学随访。
- 无并发症的慢性癫痫患者。
- 可逆性原因诱发的癫痫：
- 低血糖诱发癫痫者，血糖稳定后。
- 酒精戒断性癫痫精神状态恢复正常且无癫痫进展者。
- 单纯发热惊厥。

转诊问题

- 应考虑行早期的神经病学随访。
- 抗惊厥药物血药浓度监测。

随访建议

在癫痫得到良好控制之前切勿进行驾驶车辆、游泳和其他潜在威胁活动。

要点和误区

- 苯二氮䓬类药物是治疗癫痫发作的一线药物。
- 大多数癫痫复发的常见原因是抗惊厥药物浓度不达标。
- 如果可识别的话，处理潜在的病因。
- 持续时间超过5～10 min的癫痫发作应按癫痫持续状态处理。
- 如果类似全身抽搐的运动症表现或局灶性癫痫伴意识清楚者，应考虑心因性非癫痫性发作。

癫痫发作(儿童) Seizure, Pediatric

John P. Santamaria · Stefani Ashby 张溢熤 伍力学 译

基础知识

描述

这是一种由于神经元突然异常放电而导致的行为或功能改变。

病因

- 发热性癫痫发作。
- 感染。
- 特发性。
- 创伤。
- 药物毒理：

- 药物摄取。
- 药物作用。
- 撤药戒断症状。
• 代谢：
- 低血糖
- 低钙血症。
- 先天性代谢缺陷。
• 围产期缺氧。
• 颅内出血。
• 中枢神经系统结构异常或畸形。
• 退行性疾病。
• 心因性。
• 脑缺血。
• 大面积脑损害。

诊断

■ 症状和体征

新生儿

• 细微的重复性运动异常：
- 面部动作。
- 斜视。
- 眼睑颤动。
- 嘴唇抖动和吸吮动作。
• 呼吸变化。
• 呼吸暂停。
• 癫痫活动：
- 局灶性或全身性强直。
- 局灶性或多灶性阵挛发作。
- 肌肉的阵挛性运动。
• 全身性疾病因素(代谢、感染等)可能伴随局灶性癫痫。

较年长的婴幼儿

• 全身性癫痫：
- 强直-痉挛。
- 强直。
- 痉挛。
- 肌阵挛。
- 肌张力突然消失("跌倒")。
- 失神发作。
• 部分或局灶性癫痫：
- 单纯性癫痫：
◦ 意识存在。
- 单纯性局部癫痫：
◦ 运动、感觉和/或认知症状。
◦ 局部异常运动：部分或一侧肢体。
◦ 感觉异常，幻视或幻听。
- 复杂性癫痫：
◦ 意识受损。
◦ 复杂的局部癫痫。
- 单纯性局部癫痫伴意识损害：
◦ 先兆意识改变，幻听、幻嗅和幻视。
◦ 可能出现全身症状。
• 癫痫持续状态：
- 定义是持续发作>30 min。当癫痫发作持续>5 min 没有恢复，即应开始治疗。
- 全身性发作最常见。
- 也可以是持续局部发作。
- 失神发作性痉挛抽搐。
- 持续的意识混乱，发作后状态。

病史

• 确定癫痫发作是发热性或非发热性。
• 确定发作的类型：
- 局部或全身性。
- 出现眼球异常运动、先兆症状、运动异常和发绀。
- 持续时间。
- 意识状态，发作后状态。
- 诱发条件、病史、家族史(带有遗传因素的综合征)。

体格检查

• 生命体征，包括体温。
• 仔细的神经系统检查，包括意识状态。
• 眼部，包括眼底镜检查。
• 皮肤检查，以确定神经皮肤疾病，如结节性硬化症。

■ 诊断检查与说明

实验室检查

• 床边血糖检测。
• 更全面的检测主要用于幼儿以及癫痫持续状态和其他有病史和体征者。
- 电解质。
- BUN。
- 肌酐。
- 葡萄糖。
- 钙。
- 镁。
- CBC。
- 毒理学检测。
• 正接受抗惊厥治疗者：
- 血药浓度水平。
• 癫痫伴发热：
- 如果怀疑有严重的潜在细菌感染，完善实验室检查。
• 脑脊液检查：
- 如果怀疑是脑膜炎或脑炎。
- 如果怀疑颅内压升高，应首先行 CT 检查。

影像学检查

• 头颅 CT：
- 局灶性发作。
- 新的局灶性神经异常。
- 疑似颅内出血或占位病变。
- 病因不明的新发癫痫持续。
- 不具常规征象首发癫痫。
• MRI：
- 癫痫发作很少需要行急诊 MRI。
• 脑电图：
- 急性发作时该检查意义不大。
- 通常用于癫痫发作的儿童作为复发风险的预测指标，以及用于对癫痫类型/癫痫综合征进行分类。
- 癫痫发作后 24～48 h 观察到的发作后迟缓，可能是暂时性的；如果可能的话，暂缓脑电图检查。
- 在急性情况下很少有用。

■ 鉴别诊断

• 新生儿：
- 其他原因引起的呼吸暂停。
- 睡眠肌阵挛。
- 焦躁或震颤。
- 胃食管反流。
• 婴幼儿：
- 屏气发作。
- 夜间惊恐。
• 儿童和青少年：
- 偏头痛。
- 晕厥。
- 假性癫痫发作。
- 转化症。

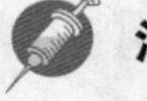

治疗

■ 院前

提醒：
• 许多情况可能被误认为是癫痫发作(见下列鉴别诊断)。
• 气道保护。
• 氧疗。
• 必要时给予呼吸支持措施。
• 如果怀疑有外伤，请颈椎制动。
• 测末梢血糖或酌情使用葡萄糖。

■ 初步稳定/治疗

• 检测血细胞计数。
• 气道：
- 给氧，监测血氧饱和度。
- 必要时，经鼻人工气道优于经口人工气道。

- 如果通气不足或持续缺氧，可给予呼吸球囊面罩辅助通气。
- 给予球囊面罩通气后仍无法逆转癫痫发作状态，应考虑气管插管。
- 将患者侧向一边，吸痰，避免误吸。
- 建立静脉通路：
- 如果低血糖，给葡萄糖。
- 如果怀疑有外伤，保持脊椎保护措施在位。

注意

在处理癫痫的同时，务必保持气道通畅和呼吸平稳。

注意

及早干预癫痫持续状态对降低潜在的发病率，包括脑损伤至关重要。

急诊治疗/程序

癫痫持续状态

- 立即处理各类代谢异常。
- 处理疑似或明确的药物过量。
- 逐步进行药物治疗：
- 苯二氮䓬：
  - 由于地西泮作用时间较长，因此静脉注射劳拉西泮是一线用药。
  - 也可以选择静脉注射地西泮。
  - 如果没有建立静脉通路：
  - 地西泮可直肠给药。
  - 劳拉西泮或咪达唑仑可经鼻给药。
  - 含服或肌内注射咪达唑仑(最方便)。
  - 如果癫痫发作为停止，可给予第二剂苯二氮䓬。
- 左乙拉西坦。
- 磷苯妥英：
  - 如果是毒物诱发的癫痫，使用苯巴比妥。
- 苯巴比妥：
  - 可使用丙戊酸替代。
  - 推荐用于茶碱类药物诱发的癫痫。
- 持续输注。
  - 咪达唑仑、异丙酚或戊巴比妥。
  - 需要行气管插管和持续心电监护。
- 新生儿：
- 苯巴比妥是一线用药。
- 也可选用磷苯妥英。

注意

二线、三线用药的有效率小于10%。持续的癫痫状态可导致永久性神经损害。癫痫失常时间越长，越不可能自行终止。

药物治疗

- D_{10}：5 ml/kg，静脉注射，适用于新生儿。
- D_{25}：2 ml/kg，静脉注射，适用于儿童。
- 地西泮(安定)：0.2 mg/kg，静脉注射或骨髓腔输注(IO)，(最大剂量 8 mg)；0.5 mg/kg PR(极量 20 mg)。
- 磷苯妥英：20 mg/kg，静脉注射，维持至少20 min。
- 劳拉西泮：0.1 mg/kg，静脉注射、椎管内注射或骨髓腔输注(极量 4 mg)。
- 咪达唑仑：0.15 mg/kg，静脉注射；0.2 mg/kg，含服或肌内注射(极量 10 mg)；0.3 mg，椎管内注射(极量 10 mg)。
- 戊巴比妥钠：首剂 10 mg/kg，静脉注射，维持 30～60 min；维持剂量 1～3 mg/(kg · h)，静脉注射；监测呼吸情况。
- 苯巴比妥：20 mg/kg，静脉注射或骨髓腔输注(极量 1 g)，维持 15～30 min；监测呼吸情况。
- 苯妥英：20 mg/kg，静脉注射，缓慢维持 30～45 min。
- 丙戊酸：20～40 mg/kg，维持 10～15 min。

随访

进一步处理

入院指征

- ICU：
- 活动期的癫痫、有气管插管或持续存在精神状态改变者。
- 短时间内反复发作的癫痫。
- 住院病房：
- 在急诊处理后已缓解的癫痫。
- 有潜在病因的癫痫病情未缓解、未控制或情况不明者。
- 颅内出血。
- 大面积损害。
- 脑膜炎和脑炎。
- 药物相关。
- 摄入毒物。

出院指征

- 患儿精神状态正常，神经系统检查正常。
- 没有需要住院治疗的潜在病因证据者。
- 有可靠的父母或看护者。

转诊问题

反应迟钝或癫痫反复发作。

随访建议

- 提供癫痫预防和护理指导。
- 初级保健医师或儿科神经学家随访。

要点和误区

- 对于没有静脉通路的患者，可考虑经口、经鼻或经直肠给予苯二氮䓬类药物。
- 请记住，用于治疗癫痫发作的药物本身可能会导致呼吸暂停、低通气或低血压。
- 大部分急性癫痫患儿会存在轻到中度血糖升高，无需特殊处理。

电击伤 Electrical Injury

Marilyn M. Hallock　单怡 译

基础知识

描述

- 电流是电子通过导体从高到低的跨梯度浓度的流动。
- 电击伤的性质和严重程度取决于电压、电流强度和类型、阻力和接触时间。
- 欧姆定律：电压(V) = 电流(I) × 电阻(R)：
- 电压和电流成正比，和电阻成反比。
- 高压电(>600 V)和低压电电源：
  - 电话线：65 V。
  - 家庭普通线路：110 V。
  - 吹风机：220 V。
  - 家用电线：220 V。
  - 机车的输电轨：600 V。
  - 住宅干线：7 620 V。
  - 工业电线：100 000 V。

- 家庭设备里的变压器，可以将低电压的设备转换成高压电流：
  - 微波炉、电视和计算机。
- 电阻取决于电流经过人体内的途径：
  - 神经、肌肉、血液的电阻比较低，比骨骼、腱、脂肪具有更好的导电性。
  - 皮肤上的水和汗可以减少电阻，皮肤较硬可增加电阻。
  - 电阻越大意味着电流越小，并且更多地转换成热量。
- 电流用安培计量，是对流经一个物体时的能量总量的测量。
  - "容许"电流是所能承受的最大电流。指人能够在肌肉强直触电前接收并释放的电流大小。
  - 家庭普通线路：15～30 A。
  - 刺痛感：0.2～2 mA。
  - 疼痛：1～4 mA。
  - 普通儿童的容许电流：3～5 mA。
  - 成人的容许电流：6～9 mA，男性高于女性。
  - 骨骼肌强直电流：16～20 mA。
  - 呼吸肌麻痹电流：20～50 mA。
  - 心室颤动：50～120 mA。

• 交流电：
- 电流有节奏地向相反方向流动：
  - 美国的家庭和办公室使用标准的 60 Hz。
- 长时间的接触能造成持续性的肌肉强直性收缩，肌肉自控能力下降。
- 比直流电更危险。
- 在家庭电流的水平中，更容易导致心室纤颤。
  - 刺激能够持续整个心动周期中的 T 波间期。

• 直流电：
- 电子在一个方向持续流动：
  - 除颤器、起搏器、工业电源。
- 大块的单个肌肉抽搐有助于触电者脱离接触源。
  - 增加了钝性创伤性损伤的风险。
  - 暴露时间更短。

• 电击伤的三峰分布：
- 幼儿(家用插座和电线)。
- 青少年(冒险行为)。
- 成人(工作相关性损伤)。

■ 病因

电击伤的分类：

• 直接接触导致组织损伤：
- 电击烧伤可以造成皮肤或深部组织的凝固性坏死。
- 深部组织广泛性损伤或许会因为伤口损伤不明显而误诊。
- 损伤位置是辨别接触电源及其范围的要点。

• 火焰：
- 被烧着的衣服或者其他物品烧伤。

• 直接接触电弧：
- 电流通过空气引起高压电弧的热力灼伤。
- 或许会造成热量和火焰的灼烧。
- 电弧灼烧通常造成皮肤的Ⅱ度烧伤。

• 主要电击伤的表现：
- 心律失常。
- 肌肉收缩和强直。

• 继发性损伤：
- 病理性的肌肉收缩。
- 跌倒或被抛出。

诊断

■ 症状和体征

• 头部、颈部、耳、鼻、喉：
- 高压电损伤的常见入口：
  - 面部和角膜的灼烧。
  - 骨膜穿孔。
  - 当时或 4～6 个月后出现白内障或视神经萎缩。
  - 眼内出血、葡萄膜炎。
  - 颈椎损伤。

• 心血管：
- 心搏骤停、心电静止和心室纤颤是首位死因。
- 其他心律失常和心电图表现：窦性心动过速、心房颤动、室性期前收缩(早搏)、心肌梗死、短暂 ST 段抬高、可逆的 QT 间期延长：
  - 有时延迟 12 h 出现。
  - 通常自行消失。
- 较少发生心肌损伤：
  - 通常是心外膜，而不是透壁性。
  - 损伤不随着冠状动脉分布。
  - 心电图不显示标准的损伤模式。

• 呼吸道：
- 脑损伤引起呼吸中枢抑制。
- 胸壁、膈肌强直性收缩与瘫痪。
  - 可能会造成呼吸暂停。
- 心搏骤停后呼吸骤停。
- 创伤性肺损伤。
- 肺组织可因含气能对抗电击伤。

• 神经系统：
- 呼吸骤停。
- 遗忘、一过性的意识障碍。
- 意识丧失、精神状态改变、癫痫、昏迷。
- 脊髓损伤：
  - 可因钝性创伤或直流电导致(电流从一端到另一端)。
  - 局部瘫痪，甚至四肢麻痹。
- 长期的神经系统并发症：
  - 癫痫、周围神经损伤、脊髓损伤综合征、精神问题。

• 血管：
- 肌肉坏死和筋膜室综合征。
- 静脉系统血流缓慢形成血栓。
- 血流速度快的动脉内膜损伤，可导致急性或慢性的动脉疾病。

• 肌红蛋白尿和/或血容量减少导致血浆外渗引起继发性肾衰竭：

• 骨骼系统与整形外科：
- 电刺激导致病理性的肌肉强制性收缩。
- 损伤的经典描述：
  - 脊柱骨折。
  - 肩关节后脱位。
  - 股骨颈骨折。

• 皮肤病：
- 接触部位伤口：手、足和头是最常见和最严重的损伤部位。
- "接吻式"的灼伤在屈肌表面有电流的出口和再入口。

儿科注意事项

咬合伤通常发生在<4 岁的孩子，吸吮或咬家用电器：

• 焦痂分离后可出现口唇血管的迟发型出血(3～5 日)。

• 生长中的牙齿有损坏的风险。

妊娠注意事项

婴儿较母亲对电击阻力小：

• 所有孕妇，无论有无症状，均应咨询或转入产科。
- 胎盘分离或先兆流产的风险。
- 胎儿>20 周需做监测。

既往史

• 确定接触电压的高低、接触的时间和地点以及并发的创伤。

• 如果患者无目击者发生呼吸骤停或室颤，应考虑电击伤。

体格检查

• 气道、呼吸、循环状况评估。

• 评估心率和脉搏情况。

• 寻找皮肤屈肌处或关节折痕处有无烧伤、

水疱、贯通伤、吻痕或弓形伤。

• 评估意识状况、瞳孔反射、感觉及运动情况。

• 眼部检查评估视敏度。

• 评估听力及鼓膜情况。

• 检查脊柱及四肢骨有无骨折或骨筋膜室综合征。

■ **基本检查**

• 尿肌红蛋白。

• 高压电击伤及低压电击伤患者主诉心脏和呼吸症状时，查心电图和心肌酶。

• 心电监护的适应证：

- 心脏停搏。
- 意识丧失。
- 胸痛。
- 低氧血症。
- 心电图异常。
- 院前有或急诊室发生过心律失常。
- 既往心脏病史。
- 存在冠心病高危因素。
- 怀疑有导电损伤。
- 合并损伤严重需要监护。

• 心电图正常，无心脏节律异常，接触电压＜240 V 的无症状患者不需要长时间的心电监护。

■ **诊断检查与说明**

实验室检查

• 大多数接触家用电的患者不需要检查：

- 靠近胸部和头部的低电压灼伤也可引起心律失常、癫痫及其他并发症。

• 肌红蛋白尿。

• 肌酸激酶、电解质、BUN 与肌酸：

- 尿肌红蛋白阳性和/或高压电接触史。
- 基础肾功能，可能出现高钾血症和代谢性酸中毒。

• 心肌标志物：

- 心电图异常或心律失常。
- 接触高压电源或接触低压电源患者主诉心脏和呼吸症状。

影像学检查

有临床指征时检查。

■ **鉴别诊断**

• 电弧所致的热力烧伤和深部电热伤。

• 不稳定的创伤性损伤和电烧伤。

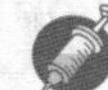

治疗

■ **院前**

• 现场：关闭高压电源。

• 假如患者有不稳定性损伤或意识丧失：

- 脊髓制动。

• 标准基础生命支持、高级心血管生命支持。

• 电击后早期 CPR 有助于心脏复跳。

• 用夹板固定骨折和移位。

• 用干净、干燥的衣服覆盖烧伤部位。

> **注意**
> 救治必须在保证救助者不接触活动性电源的地方进行。

■ **基本治疗**

• ABC 管理。

• 热力烧伤患者的局部伤口处理。

• 制动、减少骨折和移位。

■ **急诊治疗/程序**

• 静脉输液复苏。

- 由于肌肉组织损伤，大量液体积聚在第三间隙，因此需要输注大量补液。
- 快速体液复苏使尿量达到 1 ml/(kg·h)。
- 导尿。

• 监测肌红蛋白尿和避免肾衰竭：

- 维持足够的尿量。
- 静注碳酸氢钠增加尿中溶解的肌红蛋白。
- 呋塞米、甘露醇利尿。
- 监测肾功能。

• 预防破伤风。

• 需要时镇痛。

■ **药物治疗**

• 碳酸氢钠：1 支(50 mEq)，静脉注射，另外加 2 支到 5%葡萄糖水静滴维持尿 pH＞7.45。

• 呋塞米 0.5 mg/kg，静脉注射。

• 甘露醇：25 g(0.25～0.5 mg/kg)，静脉注射，接着 12.5 mg/(kg·h)静脉滴注维持尿量＞1 ml/(kg·h)。

随访

■ **进一步处理**

入院指征

• 有意识丧失病史。

• 心律失常、心电图异常或有心肌损伤证据。

• 怀疑深部组织损伤。

• 肌红蛋白尿或酸中毒。

• 烧伤已达到转入烧伤中心的标准。

• 创伤达到入院标准。

• 孕妇妊娠＞20 周。

出院指征

• 轻微的低压电击伤(＜240 V)，无合并伤，体格检查正常，无症状。

• 皮肤烧伤或有轻度症状，但心电图正常，无血红蛋白尿。

• 在监护室观察后病情稳定。

• 排除早期妊娠先兆流产。

• 儿科患者有口腔烧伤，需要成人照顾。

转诊问题

• 烧伤伤口的处理。

• 当前症状持续不缓解，或新出现迟发性症状：

- 神经系统的迟发性无力、感觉异常。

• 妊娠者需要产科处理。

• 小儿口腔烧伤需口腔科或牙齿整形外科手术。

■ **随访建议**

严重电击伤可发生迟发型白内障。

要点和误区

• 心电图正常，无心律失常，接触电压＜240 V 的无症状患者并不需要持续心电监护。

• 电烧伤严重患者，给予足够的静脉输液维持适当的尿量和稳定的生命体征：

- 第三间隙的扩张。

动脉导管未闭 Patent Ductus Arteriosus

Steven Lelyveld · Michele R. McKee 王虑 译

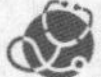 基础知识

■ 描述

• 动脉导管是胚胎时期连接心脏和肺动脉干末端的管道。
• 出生后不久，动脉导管正常收缩，关闭，萎缩：
- 局部氧分压迅速增加。
- 血管活性的类花生酸合成和代谢发生变化。
• 对于早产儿，导管持续的开放，是机体自救的正常反应。
• 动脉导管常常有正常的解剖结构。
• 导管开放的原因是缺氧和发育不成熟。
• 对于足月儿，导管未闭属于先天性畸形。
• 缺乏黏液细胞层和肌层。
• 随着肺血管阻力下降，动脉血分流进入肺动脉。
• 分流的大小取决于导管的口径和肺血管的系统阻抗。
• 左心室输出的 70%经动脉导管分流至肺循环。
• 危险因素：
- 早产儿。
- 并存的心脏异常。
- 低氧。
- 高海拔。
- 母亲风疹病毒感染。
- 男女比例为 3∶1。

■ 病因

• 早产儿。
• 先天畸形。
• 低氧。
• 前列腺素。

诊断

■ 症状和体征

病史

• 独立的动脉导管未闭，意外事件。
• 动脉导管未闭作为先天性心脏病的一种，需要通过妊娠期超声做出诊断。

体格检查

• 动脉导管未闭孔较小没有症状，但是会有些阳性的体征。
• 刚出生第 1 日，常表现为充血性心力衰竭。
• 脉压大。
• 心尖波动明显。
• 震颤。
• 心脏收缩持续性杂音。
• 听起来像陀螺声或滚雷声。
• 杂音在每轮心音开始时出现，在收缩末期达到高峰，在舒张末期衰减。
• 杂音局限于左肋第 2 肋间，或向下发散到胸骨左缘或左侧锁骨处。
• 反复发作的肺部感染。
• 生长发育迟缓。

■ 基本检查

• 在影像学基础上做出诊断。
• 排除并发症，如心力衰竭和心内膜炎。

■ 诊断检查与说明

对诊断该病没有帮助。

影像学检查

• 胸部 X 线片：
- 婴儿期摄片结果常正常：
- 小孩和成人：
◦ 肺内标志物增加。
◦ 钙化。
◦ 左心室和右心房扩大。
◦ 升主动脉扩张。
◦ 肺动脉扩张。
• 心电图：
- 如果导管口径大心电图变现异常：
◦ 左心室高电压。
◦ 如果右心室高电压则表明病情十分严重。
• 超声心动图：
- 如果导管口径小则超声心动图表现正常。
- 左心房扩大。
- 从胸骨上切迹处扫描可以确定导管口径的大小。
- 多普勒超声可以分析舒张期大动脉到肺动脉的血流。
• 心导管检查：
- 右侧肺压力增高或正常。
- 肺动脉的氧合血能判定血流左向右分流。
- 升主动脉注射造影剂可以看见不透明的肺动脉。

■ 鉴别诊断

• 静脉杂音：
- 不典型的杂音。
- 在颈部和胸前听到。
- 在收缩期和舒张期都能听到轻轻的嗡嗡声。
- 轻轻压迫颈静脉，杂音声响变小。
• 异常的肺静脉连接无名静脉：
- 持续的嗡嗡声像静脉哼鸣。
• 主动脉-肺动脉间隔缺损。
- 嗡嗡常仅发生在收缩期。
- 胸骨左侧可听见杂音。
• 主动脉窦破裂。
• 冠状动静脉瘘管。
• 异常起源于肺动脉的左冠状动脉。
• 肺动脉窦闭锁或缺失。
• 大动脉功能不全伴室间隔缺损。
• 次级肺动脉狭窄。
• 动脉干。

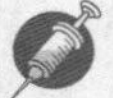 治疗

注意

慢性心功能不全时予以供氧。

■ 院前

监测和供氧。

■ 初步稳定/治疗

• 小的无症状的分流不需要关闭。
• 呼吸支持。
• 供氧。

■ 急诊治疗/程序

• 限制水钠。
• 纠正贫血将血细胞比容增加到>45%。
• 使用抗生素预防心内膜炎。
• 早产儿：
- 常自行关闭。
- 呼吸窘迫综合征的严重程度取决于分流血流量的大小。
- 在出生后 2～7 日使用对抗前列腺素合成的吲哚美辛(消炎痛)。
• 足月儿和儿童：

- 手术治疗封闭缺口很有必要的，即使是无症状患儿，因为自行封闭缺口还是比较少见的。
- 分离结扎。
- 经股动脉导管技术使用泡沫塑料塞或封堵伞进行。

■ 药物治疗

吲哚美辛：0.2～0.25 mg/kg，负荷剂量，静脉注射；基于新生儿学专家或在儿科心脏病学家指导下重复注射 0.1～0.2 mg/kg，q12～24 h，3～5 剂。

随访

■ 进一步处理

入院指征

• 心力衰竭。
• 心内膜炎。
• 肺动脉高压。

出院指征

• 无症状。
• 预防用抗生素。

转诊问题

儿科的心脏病学专家和新生儿学专家需共同参加有心力衰竭症状的患儿的诊治，特别是已经使用药物干预的情况下。

要点和误区

• 慢性心力衰竭会致肾小球滤过率下降，尿量减少。
• 吲哚美辛会致消化道出血。

动脉气体栓塞 Arterial Gas Embolism(AGE)

Nicole L. Lunceford 李岩 王瑞兰 译

D

基础知识

■ 描述

• 肺泡破裂气体进入肺静脉，然后通过全身的脉管系统进行传播。
- 临床表现取决于气泡在全身脉管系统中的位置。
• 也被称为减压性空气栓塞或脑空气栓塞。
• 由肺组织过度受压产生，造成胸膜撕裂，空气进入血液循环。
- 气泡趋于上升，进入脑血管，并在那里堵塞血流。
- 波义耳定律：温度恒定时，压力(P)与体积(V)是呈负相关的。
◦ $PV = K$(常数) 或 $P_1V_1 = P_2V_2$。
- 随着压力的增加/减少，体积减小/增大。

■ 病因

• 肺动脉房室(AV)分流，或作为通过未闭卵圆孔的反常性栓塞(在成人中在高达30%)。
• 在上升过程中屏住呼吸：
- 症状由一串气泡和多个血管受累引起。
• 中心静脉导管放置、心胸外科手术、血液透析过程中产生医源的损伤。
• 心脏穿通伤，急诊修补心脏创伤。

诊断

■ 症状和体征

• 脑：
- 起病急：
◦ 几乎所有 AGE 病例都在第一次上浮 5 min 内，但最常见的症状是在第一次上浮 2 min 内。
- 潜水相关性卒中。
- 潜水相关性死亡的第二要因(位于溺水之后)。
- 两个主要表现：
◦ 呼吸暂停和完全的心跳呼吸骤停。
◦ 各种神经症状。
- 表现取决于气体栓塞在动脉中的分布：
◦ 意识状态改变(40%)。
◦ 感觉丧失(20%)。
◦ 运动缺陷(20%)。
◦ 截瘫(10%)。
◦ 癫痫发作(4%)。
◦ 视觉改变。
◦ 失语。
◦ 皮肤感觉异常。
- 可能在发生最初的缺陷几分钟之后自发改善：
◦ 复发率高。
◦ 改善可能与影响流向大脑的气泡分布的姿态变化短暂相关。
• 肺：
- 呼吸急促。
- 血性泡沫痰。
- 气胸。
• 心脏：
- 冠状动脉内的空气导致心肌梗死。
- 由于空气被困在心室，心输出量减少。
- 阿曼征：在心脏听及捻发音。
• 肾：
- 空气栓塞导致的肾梗死。

病史

追问症状发作时间与潜水浮出水面的关系。

体格检查

神经系统表现的多样性，所以要做详细的神经系统检查。

■ 基本检查

• 临床诊断：识别危险因素及多种临床表现。
• 询问在上升过程中遇到的异常情况：
- 屏住呼吸。
- 恐慌，缺氧状况。
• 彻底的神经系统检查必须仔细记录运动、感觉、小脑和脑神经的缺损程度。

■ 诊断检查与说明

实验室检查

• 血清肌酐激酶活性：
- 脑 AGE 严重程度的标志。
• CBC。
• 电解质、尿素氮、肌酐、葡萄糖。
• 当呼吸道症状存在时进行动脉血气分析。

影像学检查

• 胸部 X 线片：
- 寻找气胸或纵隔气肿的证据。
• 胸部 CT：
- 对于可疑的肺栓塞，局部肺损伤或出血。
• 心电图。
• 超声：
- 寻找卵圆孔未闭的证据。

• 头部 CT：
- 精神状态改变时。
- 当临床高度怀疑 AGE 时，要及时做加压 CT。

■ 鉴别诊断

• 与气体栓塞无关的脑血管意外（CVA）。
• 由于减压病导致的神经功能障碍。

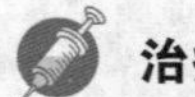

治疗

■ 院前

• 注意：
- 神经功能突然恢复的患者，可能随着气泡位置的变化快速复发。
- 将 AGE 作为潜在的诊断。
• 从压缩空气潜水中浮出水面 10 min 内，发生精神状态改变。
• 随着中心线的移位出现突然的神经功能失代偿。
• 争议：
- 头低足高位患者对于疑似 AGE 是无效的：
◦ 假设抬高腿部可能会导致气泡从脑循环中移出，脑内静水压增加会使气泡收缩。
◦ 头低足高位实际上可能通过增加脑内的压力而加重损伤。

■ 初步稳定/治疗

ABC 管理：
• 使用紧密贴合面罩给予 100%氧气。
• 根据气道通气/保护的需求进行气管插管。
• 建立静脉通路。

■ 急诊治疗/程序

• 高压氧加压治疗（见高压氧治疗）：
- 适用于所有年龄。
- 安排运送到最近的高压氧设备。
- 在飞机上可将座舱气压控制在 1 000 ft 的气压以下，最适合转运。
- 预防性胸腔置管用于单纯性气胸来预防再压缩过程中转变为张力性气胸。
- 用水或盐水填充气管和导尿管球囊，以避免再压缩过程中的收缩/损坏。
• 寻求潜水员急救网络（DAN）援助：

随访

■ 进一步处理

入院指征

观察和复查后的所有高压氧治疗均需收入院。

出院指征

AGE 患者不宜从急诊出院。

■ 随访建议

动脉栓塞患者需高压氧转诊治疗。

要点和误区

• 症状发生在上升过程中或到达地面 10 min 内。
• 神经功能突然恢复的患者，可能随着气泡的位置的变化快速复发。
• 用水或盐水填充气管和导尿管球囊，以避免再压缩过程中的收缩/损坏。

动物咬伤 Bite, Animal

Daniel T. Wu 宋振举 童朝阳 译

基础知识

■ 描述

• 动物咬伤很常见，占急诊患者的 1%左右。
• 大多数咬伤来自被激惹的动物。
• 犬咬伤：
- 大型犬可以造成严重的创伤（比特犬咬伤是人类意外死亡的原因）。
- 大多数意外死亡发生在儿童（70%），面部和颈部是咬伤的主要部位。
- 咬伤多来自家庭和朋友饲养的犬。
• 猫咬伤：
- 咬伤多来受伤者饲养的宠物猫。
- 就诊患者中感染的发生率为 50%。
- 穿刺伤多为锋利的牙齿引起的深部细菌感染。
• 猫抓病性淋巴结炎（catscratch disease，CSD）：
- 符合下述 4 条诊断标准的 3 条：
◦ 有猫接触史，有皮肤、眼睛、黏膜猫抓伤或接种病变。
◦ CSD 皮肤试验阳性。
◦ 典型的组织病理学。
◦ 实验室检查排除其他淋巴结病。
• 鼠咬伤：
- 发生在实验室人员或低收入阶层的儿童。
- 鼠咬热，美国发生率低，但病死率高。
- 狂犬病发生率低，不需常规预防。

■ 病因

• 犬咬伤和猫咬伤：
- 多杀巴斯德杆菌是主要的病原体：
◦ 猫咬伤的发生率是犬咬伤的 2 倍。
◦ 革兰阴性需氧菌的感染占猫咬伤感染的 80%。
◦ 感染发生在 24 h 内。
- 葡萄球菌属或链球菌属感染：
◦ 感染发生在 24 h 后。
- 其他病原体包括厌氧菌和二氧化碳嗜纤维菌（犬咬伤）。
• 猫抓病性淋巴结炎：
- 由韩瑟勒巴通菌（*Bartonella henselae*）引起。
• 鼠咬伤：
- 小螺菌或念珠状链杆菌引起的鼠咬热。

诊断

■ 症状和体征

• 哺乳动物咬伤的分布：
- 犬咬伤占 80%～90%。
- 猫咬伤占 5%～15%。
- 人咬伤占 2%～5%（见“人咬伤”）。
- 鼠咬伤占 2%～3%。
• 犬咬伤：
- 外观：
◦ 挤压伤（最常见）、撕裂伤、穿刺伤和划痕伤。
◦ 相对于人和猫咬伤，犬咬伤的感染率低。
- 感染往往伴随。
◦ 蜂窝织炎。

◦ 恶臭气体排出。
◦ 发热。
◦ 淋巴结病。
• 猫咬伤：
- 外观：
◦ 穿刺伤(最常见)。
◦ 擦伤。
◦ 撕裂伤。
- 由于是感染部位深的穿刺伤，感染发生率高(30%～50%)。
• CSD：
- 由猫、犬和猴导致的咬伤或抓伤。
- 小的斑点或水疱发展成丘疹。
◦ 接种 3～10 日后发病。
◦ 数日到数周缓解。
◦ 接种 3 周后出现局部淋巴结病。
◦ 质软。
◦ 非化脓性。
◦ 2～4 个月缓解。
◦ 低热，不适，头痛。
• 鼠咬热：
- 咬伤或抓伤。
- 念珠状链杆菌。
◦ 接触 2～10 日后发病。
◦ 主要发生在美国。
◦ 发热、寒战、迁移性多关节痛、头痛、恶心和呕吐。
- 小螺菌。
◦ 潜伏期 1～3 周。
◦ 亚洲常见。
◦ 关节炎少见。

病史

• 动物的行为、挑衅行为、位置和主人。
• 受到攻击至就诊的时间。
• 既往史：免疫功能缺陷状态、过敏史、破伤风史。

体格检查

• 记录损伤的位置和范围。
• 记录所有的肿胀、挤压伤或失活的组织。
• 记录被攻击部位的运动功能。
• 记录肌腱和神经功能。
• 记录可能感染征象，包括局部淋巴结肿大。
• 记录受累的关节和骨骼。

诊断检查与说明

实验室检查

• 对感染伤口进行需氧和厌氧培养。
• 不推荐对没有感染的伤口进行培养。
• 猫抓病性淋巴结炎。
- 亨氏罗卡利马体菌抗体效价升高，或者
- 抓伤抗原(cat-scratch antigen，CSA)反应阳性：
◦ 肌内注射 0.1 ml CSA。
◦ 硬结超过 48～72 h 或超过 5 mm 为阳性。

影像学检查

普通 X 线平片：
• 骨折。
• 怀疑异物(如牙齿)。
• 骨髓炎侵犯骨或关节的基线。
• 感染接近骨或关节部位。

鉴别诊断

• 人咬伤多引起挤压伤，而动物牙齿咬伤多引起穿刺伤和撕裂伤。
• 其他动物咬伤。
• CSD 引起的淋巴结病。
- 反应性淋巴结增生(16 岁以下儿童淋巴结病的主要原因)。
- 感染、慢性淋巴结炎、药物反应、恶性肿瘤、先天性淋巴结肿大。

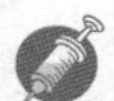

治疗

院前

压迫止血。

初步稳定/治疗

• 完成止血目标。
• 保护呼吸道通畅(如果咬伤发生在面部或颈部)。

急诊治疗/程序

• 伤口冲洗。
- 18G 的塑料针头，大量的生理盐水冲洗伤口。
- 不要因过高的冲洗压力将生理盐水冲入损伤的组织。
• 清创术。
- 去除异物、坏死的皮赘或失活的组织。
- 不要对穿刺伤进行清创。
- 清除结痂，冲洗结痂下面的脓液。
• 关闭伤口。
- 关闭伤口可能增加感染的风险，需要权衡一期愈合还是开放伤口二期愈合。
- 不要缝合感染的伤口或感染大于 24 h 的伤口。
- 创口修复时间超过 8 h(有争论的)。
- 关闭面部伤口(告知患者感染风险)。
- 感染伤口超过 24 h(咬伤时间起)和手部深部伤口需开放。
- 必要时，无菌切口胶布覆盖伤口，延期缝合伤口。
• 抗生素指征。
- 感染伤口。
- 猫咬伤。
- 手部伤口。
- 严重伤口伴挤压伤。
- 穿刺伤。
- 手部、面部和下肢贯穿伤。
- 需要手术清创的伤口。
- 伤口累及关节、肌腱、韧带或撕裂伤。
- 免疫功能不全的患者。
- 伤口超过 8 h(咬伤时间起)。
• 抬高受伤的肢体。
• 预防破伤风。
• 狂犬病免疫球蛋白。
- 啮齿类动物(松鼠、仓鼠、大鼠和小鼠)和兔子很少传播该疾病。
- 臭鼬、浣熊、蝙蝠和狐狸是狂犬病的主要宿主。
- 参见“狂犬病”章节的治疗指南。
• 抓伤疾病。
- 镇痛药。
- 局部受影响淋巴结热敷。
- 避免伤及淋巴结。
- 疾病通常为自限性。
- 抗生素使用有争议，严重咬伤或免疫功能缺陷的受害者可以使用。
• 鼠咬热。
- 高死亡率(10%)。
- 静脉使用青霉素或强力霉素。

药物治疗

一线用药

• 阿莫西林-克拉维酸(augmentin)：500/125 mg[儿童，40 mg/(kg · 24 h)]，q8 h，口服。
• 氨苄西林-舒巴坦(unasyn)：3 g，q6 h，静脉注射。
• 青霉素 100 万～200 万 U，q6 h，静脉注射[儿童：20 000～50 000 U/(kg · d)，q4 h，静脉注射]。
• 哌拉西林-他唑巴坦(zosyn)：4.5 g，q8 h，静脉注射。
• 替卡西林-克拉维酸(timentin)：3.1 g，q4 h，静脉注射。
• 头孢曲松(rocephin)：1 g/d，加用甲硝唑 500 mg，q8 h，静脉注射。

二线用药

- 两药治疗方案：下面一种药物+厌氧菌覆盖：
- 复方磺胺甲噁唑(septra DS)：1 片，q12 h(儿童：8 mg/kg 甲氧苄啶和 40 mg/kg 磺胺甲噁唑，分为 2 日用)，口服。
- 青霉素(青霉素 VK)：500 mg[50 mg/(kg·24 h)]，口服，q6 h。

  强力霉素：100 mg，口服，每日 2 次。
- +厌氧菌覆盖：
- 克林霉素(cleocin)：150～450 mg[儿童：8～20 mg/(kg·24 h)]，口服，q6 h；或 600～900 mg[儿童：20～40 mg/(kg·24 h)]，静脉注射，q8 h。
- 甲硝唑(flagyl)：500 mg，口服，每日 3 次(儿童：10 mg/kg，每日 3 次)。

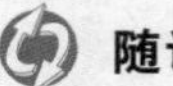

随访

进一步处理

入院指征

- 所用咬伤：
- 出现大面积感染伤口。
- 严重或进展的蜂窝织炎和淋巴管炎。
- 全身感染的征象。
- 感染伤口，门诊不便使用抗生素。
- 抓伤疾病：
- 持续发热，全身症状和/或明显的淋巴结病。

出院指征

- 健康的患者伴有局部伤口感染：带抗生素出院，并随访 24 h。
- 非感染伤口：
- 随访 48 h。

随访建议

- 手外伤专家接收转诊或随访手外伤感染的患者。
- 健康的患者伴有局部伤口感染：带抗生素出院，并随访 24 h。
- 非感染伤口，随访 48 h。

要点和误区

动物咬伤在许多地区需要向主管部门报告。

D

动眼神经麻痹 Oculomotor Nerve Palsy

Sarah Tolford Selby　朱妍 译

基础知识

描述

- 由 3 条脑神经(CN)支配的 6 块肌肉控制眼球运动：
- 动眼神经支配 6 块眼肌中的 4 块，也支配眼睑和瞳孔：
  - 内直肌：
    - 内收：向内侧鼻侧(内收)移动眼球。
  - 上直肌：
    - 仰角：向上移动眼球。
    - 扭转：使眼顶部转向鼻侧。
    - 轻度内收。
  - 下直肌：
    - 俯角：向下移动眼球。
    - 外旋：使眼顶部转离鼻侧。
    - 轻度内收。
  - 下斜肌：
    - 外旋：使眼顶部转离鼻侧。
    - 轻度上抬和外展。
  - 提上睑肌：
    - 提上眼睑。
  - 虹膜括约肌、瞳孔和睫状肌：
    - 瞳孔收缩(瞳孔缩小)。
    - 由 CN Ⅲ 的副交感神经支配。
- 第四脑神经支配上斜肌：
  - 外旋：使眼顶部转离鼻侧。
  - 凹陷和轻微外展(横向旋转)。
- 第Ⅳ脑神经支配外直肌：
  - 使眼球向外侧移动(外展)。
- 动眼神经麻痹是由于 CN Ⅲ 或其分支受损导致眼睛异常运动，眼睑下垂和/或瞳孔改变所致：
- 完全性动眼神经麻痹：
  - 眼睛“上下”，下垂，瞳孔散大。
  - 最常由压迫性病变引起。
    - 95%～97%的压迫性病变累及瞳孔。
    - 副交感神经纤维位于周围 CN Ⅲ。
    - 瞳孔散大通常是压迫的第一症状。
  - 保留瞳孔的完全性动眼神经麻痹：
    - 由于潜在的糖尿病、高血压和/或高脂血症引起的微血管疾病几乎总是缺血性的。
    - 缺血性损伤常常使瞳孔幸免于难，因为外副交感神经不受影响。
  - 经常良性，并在 3 个月内完全消退。
- 不完全性动眼神经麻痹(更常见)：
  - CⅢ功能部分丧失。
  - 最常见的原因是血管缺血。
- 动眼神经麻痹的病理生理学研究：
- 动眼神经核的中脑病变导致双侧 CN Ⅲ 瘫痪(基底动脉缺血)。
- 离开 CN Ⅲ 核的病变通常与其他神经系统表现有关，如偏瘫或共济失调(韦伯综合征、贝内迪克特综合征)。
- 蛛网膜下腔的病变导致完全瘫痪，并伴有瞳孔受累(压缩性动脉瘤)或完全瘫痪并保留瞳孔(由于危险因素造成的缺血)。
- 海绵窦和眶上裂的病变可导致孤立的 CN Ⅲ 麻痹，但通常与 CN Ⅳ、CN Ⅵ 和 CN Ⅴ 的上颌分区功能障碍有关。
- 眼眶内的病变与视力丧失(CN Ⅱ)、眼肌麻痹(CN Ⅲ、Ⅳ、Ⅵ)和眼球突出有关，并由创伤、肿块、炎症引起。
  - 不完全性 CN Ⅲ 麻痹起源于此，因为神经分为上、下两个分支。

病因

- 获得性病因：
- 血管疾病：
  - 糖尿病(DM)。
  - 高血压和心脏病。
  - 动脉粥样硬化。
  - 动脉瘤(特别是后交通动脉)。
  - 动静脉畸形(AVM)。
  - 颅内出血(非动脉瘤)。
  - 脑血管意外。
  - 海绵窦血栓形成。
- 传染性：
  - 脑膜炎。
  - 梅毒。
  - 带状疱疹。
- 炎症：
  - 结节病。

        - 巨细胞动脉炎、血管炎。
        - 系统性红斑狼疮。
    - 肿瘤：
        - 颅内肿瘤。
        - 垂体瘤。
        - 眼眶肿瘤。
        - 白血病。
    - 退化的：
        - 重症肌无力。
        - 吉兰-巴雷综合征。
    - 创伤：头部受伤，近期或偏远。
    - 偏头痛。
    - 医源性：
        - 化疗。
        - 放射治疗。
    - 特发性：
        - 特发性颅内高压(IIH)。
    - 先天性病因通常是未知的，但有些具有家族倾向。

儿科注意事项

- 外伤是获得性动眼神经麻痹的最常见原因。
    - 包括出生时创伤。
- 在神经纤维瘤病、眼科偏头痛伴复发性 CN Ⅲ麻痹和自发性颅内低血压中也可以看到。

诊断

症状和体征

动眼神经麻痹是一种临床诊断。

病史

- 最常见的症状：
    - 复视(复视)。
    - 眼睑下垂(下垂)。
    - 如果瞳孔受累：
        - 瞳孔散大(瞳孔散大)。
        - 视力模糊(住宿环境不佳)。
        - 光敏性(畏光)。
- 相关症状包括：
    - 头痛。
    - 眼痛。
- 可能还有其他神经系统症状：
    - 偏瘫。
    - 共济失调，震颤。
    - 精神状态改变。
- 病史：
    - DM。
    - 高血压。
    - 血管炎。
    - 创伤。
    - 感染。
    - 肿瘤。
    - 抽烟。

体格检查

- 眼科检查：
    - 视力：
        - 正常或轻微模糊。
    - 视野：
        - 正常。
    - 眼睛的位置和对准：
        - 眼球突出如果眼眶肿瘤。
    - 检查眼皮：
        - 上睑下垂。
    - 结膜和巩膜：
        - 正常。
    - 角膜、晶状体和瞳孔：
        - 伴有患眼散瞳的不等角视。
        - 瞳孔对光的反应迟钝。
        - 畏光。
    - 眼外运动：
        - 双眼复视。
        - 受影响的眼睛“向下和向外”。
        - 无法抬高，压低或加重眼睛。
    - 眼底检查：
        - 视乳头水肿。
    - 裂隙灯检查：
        - 观察虹膜或前房的结构异常。
- 神经系统检查应包括所有 CN，并进行详细的运动、感觉和步态检查，以寻找：
    - 其他颅神经功能障碍(尤其是 CN Ⅵ)。
    - 四肢无力。
    - 构音障碍。
    - 协调性改变。
- 完全性动眼神经麻痹：
    - 眼睛“向下并向外”。
    - 上睑下垂。
    - 散瞳眼球不对称。
- 不完全性动眼神经麻痹：
    - 可能累及 1 个或多个眼外肌，并且可能或可能不累及瞳孔。

基本检查

- 脑、眶及鼻窦的 CT 或 MRI 检查。
    - 排除压缩性动脉瘤或肿块。

诊断检查与说明

实验室检查

根据病史和体格检查考虑此病时需要：

- 血常规：用于鉴别。
- CMP。
- 红细胞沉降率(血沉)。
- 血脂。
- 抗核抗体、类风湿因子评估血管炎。
- 腰椎穿刺以评估感染或 IIH。

影像学检查

- 特别是当涉及瞳孔时，行脑及脑血管 MRI/MRA 检查。
- CT 血管造影如果考虑动脉瘤。
- 脑血管造影：风险与神经疾病的发病率和死亡率相关。
- 动静脉畸形、脑膜窦血栓时行多普勒超声成像。

诊断步骤/外科

眼压测量，排除青光眼的眼压。

鉴别诊断

- 颅内感染。
- 恶性肿瘤。
- 血管炎，巨细胞性动脉炎。
- 动脉瘤。
- 重症肌无力。
- 肉毒中毒。
- 眶内感染。
- 创伤。
- 晶状体病变。
- 视网膜病变。
- 青光眼。
- 多发性硬化。
- 甲状腺相关眼病。

儿科注意事项

考虑先天性动眼神经麻痹。

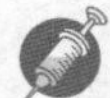

治疗

院前

如果无创伤，不需特殊院前措施。

初步稳定/治疗

- 创伤患者的初治治疗应关注潜在的损伤。
- 有证据表明脑疝的患者应实施以下步骤控制颅内压：
    - 插管后使用高频通气，控制呼吸使 PCO_2 控制在 35～40 mmHg。
    - 床头抬高 30°。
    - 甘露醇静滴。
- 戴眼罩缓解复视不适。

■ 急诊治疗/程序

治疗最初包括在手术干预之前对全身易感因素和降低压力的保守措施进行医疗管理：

- 区分完全性和不完全性，以及涉及和不涉及瞳孔的动眼神经麻痹，是指导急诊室治疗的关键。
- 所有<50 岁的动眼神经麻痹患者应考虑压迫性损伤（动脉瘤或肿块）。
- 如果涉及瞳孔，应行神经影像学检查及会诊以确定病因。
- 如果不涉及瞳孔，且患者有糖尿病或其他缺血性第三脑神经损伤的高危因素，嘱出院后门诊随访。
  - 如果部分涉及瞳孔或患者无以上危险因素，应会诊和神经影像学检查。
- 病因确定治疗原则：
  - 压迫性病变（动脉瘤、颅内肿瘤）：
    - 控制严重高血压。
    - 降低颅内压。
    - 控制通气。
    - 抬高头部。
    - 使用甘露醇。
    - 静脉注射类固醇。
  - 脑膜炎：
    - 迅速静脉使用抗生素。
    - 静脉用类固醇药物可有效减轻炎症反应和水肿。
  - IIH：
    - 乙酰唑胺。
  - 血管炎和胶原血管病：
    - 静脉使用类固醇药物降低炎性细胞浸润。
  - 重症肌无力：
    - 氯化埃德罗芬铵试验。
  - 有症状的眼球不均匀伴畏光。
    - 毛果芸香碱。
- 适时神经外科会诊。

儿科注意事项

MRI/MRA 适用于所有获得性动眼神经麻痹的患儿。

■ 药物治疗

- 头孢曲松：1～2 g（儿童：50～100 mg/kg），静脉注射。
- 地塞米松：10 mg，静脉注射（儿童：0.15～0.5 mg/kg，静脉注射，急诊室内单次剂量）。
- 依酚氯胺：5～8 mg，静脉注射（儿童：0.15 mg/kg，静脉注射；先给 1/10 的测试剂量）。
- 甘露醇：1 g/kg，静脉注射（儿童：不常规推荐）。
- 乙酰唑胺：500 mg，口服或静脉注射，每日 2 次[儿童：25 mg/(kg · d)，口服或静脉注射，q6～8 h]。
- 1%毛果芸香碱：1 gtt 受累眼，1 次（儿童：不建议常规使用）。

随访

■ 进一步处理

入院指征

- 任何原因的完全性动眼神经麻痹应收入院，急诊行神经外科评估。
- 伴有 CT、MRI 结果异常，实验室检查异常或其他神经系统定位病灶或原发性症状的不完全性动眼神经麻痹，应迅速予以神经科会诊和影像学检查。

出院指征

- 不完全动眼神经麻痹患者，如 CT、MRI 检查阴性，实验室检查正常，无其他症状，可急诊进行神经科评估。
- 完全性不涉及瞳孔动眼神经麻痹，有微血管疾病的高危因素（如糖尿病），可接受门诊神经科诊治。

■ 随访建议

如果患者将出院，建议定期进行神经科和眼科随访。

要点和误区

- 完全性损伤应立即评估。
- <50 岁的患者有不同程度的第三脑神经麻痹应评估压迫性损伤。
- 如果涉及瞳孔，病因常为压迫性损伤，应立即行 CTA、MRI 或 MRA。

冻伤 Frostbite

Christina O. Foreman　万健 译

基础知识

■ 描述

- 组织由于暴露于低温环境而损伤。
- 机制：
  - 组织损伤的原因：
    - 直接的细胞损伤：细胞内冰晶形成。
    - 间接的细胞损伤：细胞外冰晶形成引起细胞内脱水和酶的破坏。
    - 再灌注损伤：发生于复温时。
    - 由损伤的内皮渗出的大量炎性介质（前列腺素和血栓素）促进血管收缩和血小板聚集。
    - 细胞外渗液形成清水疱。
    - 深部的皮下血管破坏时出现血性水疱，提示更严重的组织损伤。
    - 后果是动脉血栓形成、局部缺血，最终坏死。
  - 坏死组织的界定随着损伤发展需历时超过数周甚至数月，因此有“一月份冻伤，七月份截肢”的说法。

■ 病因

- 寒冷暴露：持续暴露于寒风、潮湿的环境，穿着湿冷的衣物均增加冻伤的风险。
- 诱发因素：
  - 高龄。
  - 精神状态的改变（中毒或精神疾病）。
  - 恶化的循环状况。

诊断

■ 症状和体征

- 四肢手足（手指、足趾）和头部（耳、鼻）最常受累。
- 冻伤复温后的分类：然而初始的分类往往不能提供准确的预后，且不改变早期的处理。
- 浅表冻伤：
  - 仅仅累及皮肤，深部组织不受累。
  - 1 度：红斑和水肿，刺痛，阵痛，无水疱和坏死。

- 2 度：水肿明显，出现清水疱，麻木感。
- 深度冻伤：
- 组织损伤不可避免。
- 3 度：包括皮下组织。
- 由于皮下静脉丛损伤形成出血性水疱。
  ◦ 最初无感觉，随着复温损伤进展出现痛感。
- 4 度：累及肌肉、肌腱和骨组织，出现深红色斑或发绀。
- 不良预后的指标：出血性水疱、持续发绀、麻木感及复温后活动减少。
- 坏死组织的界定随着损伤发展需历时超过数周甚至数月，直至皮肤坏死和干黑状结痂形成。

基本检查

- 诊断依靠临床表现，伤口的描述应包括皮肤颜色、温度、水疱的性状和软组织质地。
- 神经系统和血管的检查应当包括脉搏（必要时依据多普勒）、毛细血管再充盈试验和 2 点识别。
- 寻找相关冷暴露的因素及并发症。
- 低体温。
- 创伤。
- 低血糖。
- 心脏或神经系统问题。
- 中毒或药物过量。
- 骨筋膜室综合征。

诊断检查与说明

实验室检查

- 轻症病例无处理。
- 深度冻伤：
- 血常规。
- 电解质、尿素氮/肌酐、血糖。
- 尿液分析/肌酸激酶，排除肌红蛋白尿。
- 对怀疑感染的部位进行培养和革兰染色。

影像学检查

^{99}Tc 闪烁扫描或者 MRA：
- 有助于早期鉴别具有抢救价值的组织。
- 对截肢进行早期决断。

诊断步骤/外科

设法在急救部创建温水浴室：
- Whirlpool（惠而浦）水疗，然而大部分医院急救都不具备。
- 在大水盆内混合热水和冷水。
- 将水温控制在 40～42 ℃。
- 水会很快变冷：间歇地往水盆里加入温水以确保水温在合适的范围。
- 较高的温度能导致热损伤，然而较冷的温度会延迟复温并降低组织复苏。

鉴别诊断

- 冻僵：
- 浅表的，冰晶形成是可逆的，不伴有组织损伤。
- 干性复温后出现短暂性麻痹和感觉异常。
- 壕沟（浸泡）足：
- 长期暴露于湿冷环境中。
- 神经血管损伤不伴有冰晶形成。
- 苍白，斑驳，感觉异常，无脉，麻痹麻木。
- 较难和冻伤鉴别。
- 干性复温需维持 6 周。
- 冻疮：
- 慢性反复发作于干冷环境下。
- 局部红斑，发绀，青紫，斑块，水疱。
- 血管炎患者易复发性发作。
- 对症治疗，干复温。

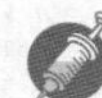

治疗

院前

- 在转运途中注意保护和固定冻伤部位。
- 去除湿冷的衣物。
- 在转运途中可能出现再次冻伤的情况下避免对冻伤肢体行干性复温。
- 在转运可能延迟但具有适当的设备情况下，可予以温水（40～42 ℃）复温。
- 禁忌摩擦冻伤的肢体。

> **注意**
> - 低体温症。
> - 常见于冻伤受害者。
> - 对严重低体温的患者需加强管理，预防发生心律失常的风险。

初步稳定/治疗

- ABC 管理。
- 鉴别并纠正低体温症。
- 予以生理盐水对重度冻伤患者进行扩容。
- 在治疗过程中注意保护冻伤的肢体。

急诊治疗/程序

- 若冻伤时间<24 h 且未复温：
- 尽快用 40～42 ℃的温水复温 15～30 min。
- 当肢体转暖、变红、变柔软时可停止复温。
- 注意严控水温避免烫伤。
- 镇痛：静脉注射吗啡。
- NSAIDs（如布洛芬）阻抗前列腺素对皮肤坏死的影响。
- 芦荟乳膏：
- 适用于所有类型的水疱。
- 阻抗花生四烯酸的反应。
- 避免使用酒精（乙醇）、水杨酸之类可影响芦荟的作用的药物。
- 水疱清创术或吸引术。
- 清水疱：
  ◦ 清除血栓素（凝血噁烷）和前列腺素。
- 血性水疱处理的禁忌：
  ◦ 暴露深部组织后出现脱水并感染。
- 预防破伤风。
- 预防使用抗生素：
- 考虑在严重冻伤区的充血复苏阶段使用（至少 2～3 日）。
- 抗链球菌、葡萄球菌、假单胞菌感染（头孢菌素、青霉素、喹诺酮）。
- 局部并用抗生素和芦荟乳膏被认为是二线方法。
- 抬高和夹板固定冻伤部位。
- 每日换药 2～4 次。
- 避免血管收缩药物（包括烟草）。
- 辅助治疗包括：
- 溶栓治疗（<24 h 的冷暴露）：
  ◦ 动脉内和全身使用 rt-PA 均可提高救治成功率。
  ◦ 在治疗前请整形科/烧伤科会诊。
- 输血管药物治疗：
  ◦ 己酮可可碱：临床数据有限。
  ◦ 伊洛前列素：临床数据和疗效有限。

药物治疗

- 芦荟汁：局部使用乳膏（70%），q6 h。
- 头孢氨苄（头孢菌素类）：500 mg[儿童：25～50 mg/(kg・24 h)，q6 h]，口服，每日 4 次。
- 环丙沙星（喹诺酮类）：500 mg，口服，每日 2 次。
- 双氯青霉素（青霉素类）：500 mg[儿童：12.5～25 mg/(kg・24 h)，q6 h]，口服，每日 4 次。
- 布洛芬（NSAIDs）：800 mg[儿童：40 mg/(kg・24 h)，q6～8 h]，口服，每日 3 次。
- 硫酸吗啡：0.1～0.2 mg/kg(儿童：0.1 mg/kg)，静脉注射或肌内注射，PRN（根据患者反应滴定）。

随访

进一步处理

入院指征

- 除了浅表冻伤的患者外其他均应收入院。

D

• 降低准入门槛将存在再次冻伤的风险。

• 浸泡足患者只有在能获得适当的治疗的环境下方可不入院。

出院指征

大部分好转，剩余小的浅表伤。

转诊问题

普外科、烧伤科、整形科、手外科均应包括在内。

随访建议

所有未入院的患者均应到普外科、烧伤科、整形科、手外科就诊。

要点和误区

• 出现冷冻、暖和、冷冻的不良循环。

• 在复温过程中未将水温控制在 40～42℃。

• 未发现低体温症或其他的系统疾病。

• 当肢体末端的脉搏搏动减弱时未考虑到筋膜室综合征。

毒蕈中毒 Mushroom Poisoning

Michael E. Nelson · Timothy B. Erickson　段立伟 译

D

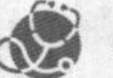

基础知识

描述

• 鹅膏毒素或鬼笔环肽：
- 种类：
  ◦ 暗色鹅膏蕈（"死亡之帽"）。
  ◦ 鳞柄白毒伞或外生菌根菌白毒伞（"毁灭天使"）。
  ◦ 纹缘盔孢伞、毒盔孢伞。
- 机制：
  ◦ 环肽毒素抑制 RNA 聚合酶 2，从而杀死胃肠上皮、肝细胞和肾细胞。

• 鹿花毒素：
- 种类：
  ◦ 鹿花菌（类羊肚菌）。
  ◦ 其他鹿花菌属。
- 机制：
  ◦ 鹿花毒素水解为一甲基肼。
  ◦ 抑制吡哆醛磷酸盐。
  ◦ 导致 GABA 生成减少。
  ◦ 毁坏红细胞、肝细胞、神经元。

• 毒蝇碱：
- 种类：
  ◦ 丝盖伞属（多种种类）。
  ◦ 杯伞属（多种种类）。
  ◦ 牛肝菌。
  ◦ 近圆孢牛肝菌。
- 机制：
  ◦ 拟副交感（神经）效应。

• 墨盖蘑菇氨酸：
- 种类：
  ◦ 墨汁鬼伞（"墨汁伞"）。
- 机制：
  ◦ 抑制乙醛脱氢酶。
  ◦ 若与酒类混合会产生类似戒酒硫样反应。

• 鹅膏蕈氨酸或蝇蕈醇：
- 种类：
  ◦ 瓢蕈（美洲豹）。
  ◦ 蛤蟆蕈（捕蝇蕈）。
- 机制：
  ◦ 鹅膏蕈氨酸是谷氨酸的衍生物。
  ◦ GABA 激动剂。

• 脱磷酸裸盖菇素或裸盖菇素：
- 种类：
  ◦ 裸盖菇属和豹亚科属及其他属。
  ◦ 柄在处理时可能会变成蓝色，但不是特有的。
- 机制：
  ◦ 与麦角酸酰二乙胺结构类似，影响 5-羟色胺受体。

• 胃部刺激毒素：
- 多种多样的蘑菇，包括那些一般认为可食用的。

• 奥莱毒素：
- 种类：
  ◦ 丝膜菌属（多种种类）。
- 机制：
  ◦ 直接毒害肾脏。

• 神经血管毒素：
- 种类：
  ◦ 毒矮生竹杯伞属蘑菇（毒芥子蘑菇）。
  ◦ 红斑性肢痛症相关性杯伞属。
- 机制：
  ◦ 丙烯酸 A-E、红藻氨酸类似物、外周谷氨酸受体。

• 洋地黄毒苷：
- 种类：
  ◦ "黄骑士"。
  ◦ 机制未知，导致横纹肌溶解。

诊断

症状和体征

• 鹅膏蕈碱或鬼笔环肽：
- 恶心。
- 呕吐。
- 腹部绞痛。
- 血性腹泻。
- 病程：
  ◦ 服用 6～36 h 后起病，以胃肠道症状首发。
  ◦ 潜伏期较短，持续 2 日左右（无疼痛和其他症状）。
  ◦ 可在 2～6 日发展成肝肾衰竭而死亡。
  ◦ 是毒性最强的蕈毒。

• 鹿花蕈素：
- 第 1 个 5～10 h：
  ◦ 腹部绞痛。
  ◦ 恶心、呕吐。
  ◦ 水样腹泻。
- 后期症状：
  ◦ 疲乏。
  ◦ 发绀。
  ◦ 意识不清。
  ◦ 癫痫。
  ◦ 昏迷。

• 毒蝇碱：
- 胆碱能神经症状：
  ◦ 瞳孔缩小。
  ◦ 流涎。
  ◦ 流泪。
  ◦ 出汗。
  ◦ 腹泻。
  ◦ 皮肤潮红。
  ◦ 恶心。

◦ 心动过缓。
◦ 气道痉挛。
- 多在 1 h 内发病(也可延迟)。
• 墨盖蘑菇氨酸：
- 如同时饮酒者可在数分钟至数小时内出现双硫仑样反应：
◦ 皮肤潮红。
◦ 出汗。
◦ 恶心、呕吐。
◦ 心悸。
• 鹅膏蕈氨酸或蝇蕈醇：
- 起病相对较快，30～120 min。
- GABA 激动效应：
◦ 幻觉。
◦ 构音障碍。
◦ 共济失调。
◦ 嗜睡或昏迷。
- 谷氨酸能神经效应(主要见于儿童)：
◦ 癫痫。
◦ 过激行为。
◦ 肌肉痉挛或肌阵挛运动。
• 脱磷酸裸盖菇素或裸盖菇素：
- 快速起病，一般在 6～12 h。
- 幻视。
- 情志改变。
- 瞳孔扩大。
- 心动过速。
- 儿童可有发热和癫痫。
• 胃肠道刺激毒素：
- 可致恶心、呕吐、肠痉挛和水样腹泻的一组毒素。
- 起病时间为 30 min 到 3 h，常在 6～12 h 后缓解。
• 奥莱毒素、史密斯鹅膏毒素：
- 恶心、呕吐。
- 头痛。
- 出汗。
- 寒战。
- 下背部疼痛。
- 烦渴。
- 病程：
◦ 可进展成少尿和急性肾衰竭。
◦ 起病时间较晚(2～14 日后)。
• 神经血管毒素类：
- 红斑性肢痛症：四肢远端红斑、肿胀、疼痛。
- 临床病程：
◦ 食用后 24 h 出现症状。
◦ 指端感觉异常，灼热性疼痛。
◦ 手足发红或肿胀。
◦ 温度变化和改变体位会加重疼痛。
◦ 可以持续几周到数个月。
- 肌电图：伴有感觉和运动纤维损害的多发性神经病。
• 肌毒素/马曲霉(T. equestre)：
- 急性横纹肌溶解：
◦ 肌痛、关节痛。
◦ 血尿、酱油色尿。
◦ 尿量减少。
- 脱水。
- 心肌炎、心律失常。

病史

• 食用时间。
• 发病时间。
• 食用数量。
• 毒蕈被食用时的状态：生食或熟食。
• 来源：野外采摘还是市场购买。
• 有无同时食用其他蕈类。
• 饮酒或用药史。
• 同食的其他家庭成员、朋友有无症状。

体格检查

• 生命体征。
• 神志变化。
• 瞳孔反射。
• 心肺检查。
• 腹部检查。
• 神经系统检查。

■ 基本检查

• 毒蕈描述：
- 蕈伞(帽)，边缘形状。
- 蕈柄(干)。
- 蕈褶(伞下栉片)。
- 蕈环(环形)。
- 蕈托。
• 将蕈类装入避光纸袋待后期进一步识别：
- 仅不到 3%的样本需进一步准确辨识。
- 拍摄图片并传往毒物中心或请真菌学家协助。

■ 诊断检查与说明

实验室检查

• 血常规。
• PT、APTT。
• 电解质、尿素氮、肌酐、血糖。
• 尿常规。
• 肝功能、肌酸激酶。
• 影像学检查。
• 孢子印：真菌学家需要行真菌种属鉴定。

■ 鉴别诊断

• 需鉴别的疾病谱较广泛。
• 胃肠炎。
• 肝炎、对乙酰氨基酚肝损害。
• 急性肾衰竭(多种病因)。
• 横纹肌溶解(多种病因)。
• 胆碱能综合征(如有机磷中毒)。
• 抗胆碱综合征。
• 癫痫(多种病因)。
• 血管炎。

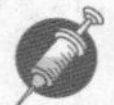

治疗

■ 院前

携带不明确种类的蕈类或蕈类碎片往医院以协助诊断：
• 如有可能，将蕈类标本装入深色纸袋避光冷藏保存。

■ 初步稳定/治疗

• ABC 管理。
• 建立静脉通路，生理盐水静脉滴注。
• 心电监护。
• 予以纳洛酮、50%高糖(并检测末梢血糖)和维生素 B_1 改善神志状况。

■ 急诊治疗/程序

一般措施

• 清除毒物：
- 活性炭(50～100 g)。
- 摄入时间不长或有以下情形者予以洗胃：
◦ 未曾呕吐。
◦ 神志和呼吸状况正常。
◦ 未出现过幻觉。
• 根据需要给予充分补液及补充电解质达到置换目的。
• 联系当地毒物鉴定中心及真菌学专家，传送图片等电子资料以资鉴别。

蕈类中毒特异性治疗

• 鹅膏蕈碱或鬼笔环肽：
- 口服活性炭，q2～4 h。
- 低血糖和 PT 延长：
◦ 肝功能衰竭征象。
◦ 有活动性出现者予以补充新鲜冰冻血浆和维生素 K 以纠正凝血功能异常。
- 有低钙者予以补钙。
- 严重肝坏死者行肝移植。
- 有条件可使用乙酰半胱氨酸、大剂量青霉素或水飞蓟素(使用硫辛酸有争议)。

D

• 鹿花毒素：

- 应用苯二氮䓬类药物控制癫痫。

◦ 症状严重的患者可用吡哆醛(维生素 B_6)。

- 处理肝功能不全方法同鹅膏毒碱或鬼笔环肽。

- 针对肾衰竭行透析治疗。

• 毒蝇碱：

- 严重者使用阿托品。

• 墨盖蘑菇氨酸：

- 为自限性毒素：可予以支持治疗。

- 避免使用含糖(或含酒精)的催吐剂。

- 有心律失常者可使用β受体阻滞剂。

• 鹅膏蕈氨酸或蝇蕈醇：

- 常表现为自限性。

- 可给予支持治疗。

- 监测有无低血压。

- 对一般性症状给予苯二氮䓬类药物，如有严重的抗胆碱症状，可予以扁豆毒碱治疗。

• 脱磷酸裸盖菇素或裸盖菇素：

- 自限性毒素。

- 出院后选择黑暗、安静的环境休息。

- 苯二氮䓬类药物镇静。

- 儿童患者需要时予以物理降温。

• 胃肠道刺激毒素：

- 若已明确为上述毒物类型，可予以补液并应用止吐药。

- 给予支持治疗。

• 奥莱毒素或史密斯鹅膏毒素(A. smthiana)：

- 密切监测尿素氮、血肌酐、电解质和尿量。

- 忌用呋塞米利尿。

- 若出现横纹肌溶解表现，则予以碳酸氢钠碱化尿液。

- 可能需要血液透析或肾移植。

• 红斑性肢痛症：

- 将有症状的肢体放在冷水中。

- 止痛药和支持治疗。

- 可以考虑使用烟酸(尚有争议)。

• 油口蘑菌("man on horse")：

- 补液水化。

- 监测肌酸磷酸激酶(CPK)。

- 监测尿量。

药物治疗

• 活性炭悬浮液：1～2 g/kg 至 100 g，口服。

• 阿托品：0.5 mg，静脉推注(儿童：0.02 mg/kg)，q10 min，如分泌物反复增多，儿童最大剂量 1 mg/kg，成人最大剂量 2 mg/kg。

• 葡萄糖：50%高糖 1 安瓿：50 ml 或 25 g (儿童：25%高糖 2～4 mg/kg)，静脉推注。

• 地西泮(苯二氮䓬类)：5～10 mg(儿童：0.2～0.5 mg/kg)，静脉推注。

• 劳拉西泮(苯二氮䓬类)：2～6 mg(儿童：0.03～0.05 mg/kg)，静脉推注。

• N-乙酰半胱氨酸：150 mg/kg，超过 1 h，然后 12.5 mg/(kg·h)，持续 4 h，然后 6.25 mg/kg，直到肝损伤消失。

• 纳洛酮：2 mg(儿童：0.1 mg/kg)，首剂静脉推注或肌内注射。

• 烟酸：20～100 mg/d×7 日，静脉滴注 1 h 以上；100 mg/d，口服 3 个月以上，逐渐减量。

• 毒扁豆碱：0.5～2 mg，肌内注射或静脉推注(成人)。

• 多黏菌素 B：1.5～2.5 mg/(kg·d)，分 2 次，静脉滴注 1 h。

• 普萘洛尔：1 mg(儿童：0.01～0.1 mg/kg)，静脉推注。

• 吡哆醛：25 mg/kg，缓慢静脉推注不少于 30 min。

• 水飞蓟：5 mg/kg，静脉推注不少于 1 h，然后 20 mg/(kg·d)，持续 3 日。

• 硫胺素(维生素 B_1)：100 mg(儿童：50 mg)，静脉推注或肌内注射。

随访

进一步处理

入院指征

• 所有有症状的患者：

- 迟发性呕吐、脱水、肝脏或肾脏毒性或癫痫。

• 早期有肾脏或肝脏衰竭者可转往三级医院。

• 有毒蕈接触史且有症状的婴幼儿：

- 有误食可能。

• 已知有鹅膏毒碱摄入史者应收入 ICU。

- 及早请肝脏专科会诊。

出院指征

观察 6～8 h 无症状者，可出院，但需 24 h 不间断居家观察病情和密切随访。

随访建议

休养期间给予以药物解毒治疗。

要点和误区

• 采蕈者有的老练，有的鲁莽，但老练的采蕈者绝不会鲁莽大意。

• 症状为迟发性(>6 h)多提示为致命性毒物。

• 识别真菌的方法有限。

• 必要时及时给予器官替代治疗或器官移植。

短暂性脑缺血发作 Transient Ischemic Attack

Casey Grorer · Rebecca Smith-Coggins 张晟 林兆奋 译

基础知识

描述

• 短暂性脑缺血发作(TIA)是由于流向中枢神经系统(CNS)某一区域的血液暂时减少而导致的可逆性神经功能障碍。

• 经典描述中症状持续<24 h，多数在 1 h 内缓解。

• 一些患者有短暂的神经症状，但在影像学上会有梗死表现称为"伴有短暂症状的脑卒中"。

• 脑卒中的预兆，12%～30%的脑卒中由 TIA 发展而来。

病因

• 中枢神经系统部分区域的灌注短暂减少，可能由以下原因引起：

- 动脉粥样硬化的大中动脉血栓形成(25%)。

- 颅内小血管病变(20%)。

- 心源性栓塞(20%)。

- 其他原因：包括动脉夹层、血管炎、高凝状态(5%)。

- 为发现明确血管性易感原因(25%)。

诊断

症状和体征

- 症状由受影响的血管分布部位决定。
- 大血管 TIA 症状。
  - 大脑前动脉：腿＞臂的单侧感觉/运动丧失，去抑制。
  - 大脑中动脉：面部/手臂＞腿部单侧运动/感觉丧失，如果优势半球，则是失语症，如果是非优势半球病变时（可能无语言障碍），同侧偏盲。
  - 大脑后动脉：同侧偏盲，可能有失读症，面孔失认症。
  - 小脑前下动脉：单侧耳聋，眩晕，耳鸣，呕吐，同侧面部乏力，肢体共济失调，对侧痛温觉减弱。
  - 小脑后下动脉：单侧腭无力，单侧肢体共济失调，单侧 Horner 征，对侧痛温觉减弱。
    - Wallenberg 征。
  - 椎-基底动脉：共济失调，动眼神经麻痹，面部麻痹，意识丧失，四肢瘫痪。
  - 颈动脉：面部、腿部、手臂的单侧运动/感觉丧失，如果是优势半球，则是失语症；如果是非优势半球，则忽略，同侧偏盲。
  - 颈内动脉狭窄“肢体颤抖”TIA：对侧肢体节律性抽搐。
- 小血管 TIA 症状：
  - 黑矇：颈内动脉眼支阻塞引起短暂性单眼失明。
  - 腔隙性脑梗死：脑深穿支动脉阻塞。
    - 常引起单纯运动功能障碍或感觉障碍。
    - 内囊：非利手偏瘫或构音障碍。
    - 放射冠：偏瘫。
    - 脑桥：非利手构音障碍。
    - 丘脑：一侧身体感觉丧失。

病史

- 提示有 TIA 的病史特点。
  - 突然发作。
  - 持续时间短（60%以上短于 1 h）。
  - 阴性症状：中枢神经系统灌注不足，因此无功能，故 TIA 的症状逐渐引起神经系统功能缺失——即无力或失语症。
  - 症状是局灶性的，与特定区域血运有关。
- 提示非 TIA 的病史特点。
  - 逐渐发病。
  - 全脑灌注不足的表现：晕厥、意识丧失、神志不清。
  - 阳性症状：特定区域的神经功能增强，如抽搐、刺痛或抽搐，提示与偏头痛或癫痫发作一样，中枢神经系统活动增强（“肢体颤抖”TIA 除外，如上所述）。

体格检查

- 详尽的体格检查：肌力、感觉、协调、步态、命名/言语、视野等。
- 持续性神经系统功能缺失提示急性脑卒中而非 TIA。
- NIHSS 是可靠且易重复的神经系统检查。

基本检查

- 快速的病史询问和体格检查，包括细致的神经系统检查。
- 指尖血糖：低血糖症可引起局部神经功能障碍。
- 头部 CT 平扫：排除出血。
- 如果患者表现为持续的缺血，获得 STAT 神经系统会诊，则考虑急性脑卒中而非 TIA。

诊断检查与说明

实验室检查

- 血糖。
- 电解质：检测钠离子、肾功能。
- CBC：贫血，多核细胞增多症。
- 肌钙蛋白：排除伴随性 ACS 或缺血。
- 监测患者的糖化血红蛋白和空腹血脂。

影像学检查

- CT：
  - 到达急诊室后，立即进行头颅 CT 平扫，以排除中枢神经系统出血或肿块。
- MRI：
  - 临床上有短暂性脑缺血发作的患者中，30%～50%的患者在 MRI 上会有梗死的证据。
    - 需在 24 h 内行 MRI。
    - 弥散加权成像（DWI）是检测组织梗死最敏感的检查方法。
- 血管造影：
  - 可在初次检查或住院后处理中行头颈部血管造影。
    - 可以识别哪些患者将从血运重建中受益，从而降低脑卒中风险。
  - 颈动脉多普勒超声可用于发现颈动脉狭窄。
  - CT 血管造影：
    - 可在初始 CT 平扫时进行。
    - 可用于发现颅内或颅外血管狭窄。
    - 要求对比。
  - MR 血管造影：
    - 可用于发现颅内或颅外血管狭窄。
    - TOF 序列可提供无需造影剂的血管造影图像。

诊断步骤/外科

- 心电图/遥测心电监护仪：评估（容易导致）血栓形成的节律如心房颤动。
- 无其他造成 TIA 的病因的患者行超声心动图：排除现有的血栓和异常的室壁运动或导致血栓的动脉瘤。

鉴别诊断

- 低血糖症。
- 癫痫。
- 癫痫后瘫痪。
- 不典型偏头痛。
- 精神性疾病。
- 脑卒中。
- 系统性感染。
- 高血压性脑病。
- 代谢紊乱（如低钠血症）。
- 周围性眩晕。
- CNS 肿瘤或转移。
- 硬膜下出血。
- 硬膜内出血。
- 多发性硬化。
- 脑出血。
- 空气栓塞。
- 血管炎。
- 动脉夹层。

儿科注意事项

- 先天性心脏病。
- 血管炎。
- 动脑夹层。
- 镰状细胞贫血。
- 神经皮肤综合征。
- 血管畸形。
- 脑膜炎。

治疗

院前

- 快速评估神经功能缺陷。
- 若功能缺陷持续，有条件时考虑转运至脑卒中中心。

初步稳定/治疗

- 建立静脉通道。
- 心电监护。
- 缺氧时予以氧疗。
- 评估患者是否有提示脑卒中的持续性神经缺陷-如果有，如果合适，迅速进行脑卒中

D

检查和溶栓。

急救治疗/程序

• 治疗 TIA 的主要目的。
- 改善缺血部位灌注。
- 防止发展为脑卒中。

• 控制血压。
- 除非达到 220/120 mmHg 以上，否则不应大幅度降低血压。
- 发生 TIA 的高血压患者在发病 24 h 后，如果血压稳定，则应降压。
- 患者情况是能否出院的关键。
- 一线：HCTZ 或 ACE 抑制剂。

• 抗血小板治疗。
- 所有无禁忌证的患者，都需要抗血小板治疗以预防脑卒中。
- 一线：阿司匹林(ASA)。
◦ 安全，经济，有效。
- ASA 过敏：氯吡格雷，噻氯匹定。
- ASA/双嘧达莫也许比 ASA 单独使用有效。

• 抗凝治疗。
- 表明存在新发房颤或未使用抗凝剂现有房颤。
- 可选择肝素或低分子肝素过渡到华法林或达比加群。
- 抗凝非紧急决定，需与内科医师会诊。

• 颈动脉内膜切除术 CEA。
- 颈动脉狭窄>70%时，TIA 患者 2 周内行 CEA 可减少 10%～15%的脑卒中风险。

• 脂质疗法。
- AHA 指南要求 TIA 患者运用他汀类药物治疗，LDH 低于 70 mg/dl。

• 患者情况是能否出院的关键。

药物治疗

• 抗血小板治疗：
- ASA：160～325 mg，每日 1 次。
- ASA-双嘧达莫：25 mg/200 mg，每日 1 次。
- 氯吡格雷：首剂 300 mg，75 mg 每日 1 次。

• 抗凝治疗：
- 肝素：5 000～7 500 U 静脉推注，随后 1 000 U 输液或 80 U/kg 静脉推注然后 18 U/(kg · h)。
- 华法林：剂量取决于年龄和体重，但心房颤动的目标 INR 应为 2～3。
- 达比加群：150 mg，每日 1 次(肾功能正常)。
- 利伐沙班：每日 20 mg。
- 阿派沙班：每日 2.5～5 mg。

• 紧急血压管理：
- 拉贝洛尔：20 mg 静脉推注，随后每 10 min 20～80 mg 静脉注射；累计剂量不超过 300 mg。
- 尼卡地平：5 mg/h 注射，每 5～15 min 增加 2.5 mg/h；最大剂量为 15 mg/h。

随访

进一步处理

入院指征

• 出院和入院无明确指标。

• TIA 患者有脑卒中的短期风险。

• 收入院的目的是防止高风险患者出现脑卒中。

• 心栓性 TIA 是继续卒中的高风险。

• 高危特征值得入院。
- 反复/言语不清的 TIA。
- 尽管接受了最大限度的药物治疗仍发 TIA。
- 存在人工瓣膜。
- 新的颈动脉杂音、心脏杂音。
- 新发房颤。
- 妊娠。
- 确认 TIA 是心脏栓塞源。
- 暂性脑缺血发作(TIA)急诊评估中神经症状的复发。
- 影像学上可见的梗死。
- 大血管狭窄或夹层。
- 无法进行门诊检查的患者，否则风险较低。

• 评分系统已经被开发用来预测脑卒中的短期风险，然而，已经证明它们在预测脑卒中风险方面具有可变的准确性，不再被推荐单独用于脑卒中风险评估。

• 最常用 ABCD2 评分：
- 年龄>60：1 分。
- 血压>140/90 mmHg：1 分。
- 临床特点：
◦ 单侧无力：2 分。
◦ 言语表达障碍：1 分。
- 持续时间：
◦ >60 min：2 分。
◦ 10～59 min：1 分。
◦ <10 min：0 分。
- 糖尿病：1 分。

• ABCD2 评分 0～3 分：低脑卒中风险(7 日内约 1%)。

• ABCD2 评分 4～5 分：中等脑卒中风险(7 日内 6%)。

• ABCD2 评分 6～7 分：高脑卒中风险(7 日内约 12%)。

• 没有高危特征的患者，如上所述，也可以考虑在以急诊为基础的观察单元进行快速评估，包括 MRI、24 h 动态心电图、± 回声、糖化血红蛋白和脂质治疗。

儿科注意事项

所有 TIA 小儿患者都应收入院进行神经系统观察，且认真考虑 ICU 级别的护理。

出院指征

• 无明确出院标准：
- 低短期脑卒中风险，随访良好。

转诊问题

• TIA 后脑卒中风险在 2 日内最高。

• 出院患者需在 24～48 h 进行神经系统护理。

• 考虑安排 24 h 动态心电图评估心律失常。

随访建议

• 基础护理/神经系统：管理大脑血管疾病的风险(高血压、糖尿病等)。

• 血管手术：颈动脉狭窄。1 周内随访，2 周内计划可能的 CEA。

• 心脏科：有心脏因素的脑卒中患者，如房颤或心肌病。

要点和误区

• 要点：
- 心源性 TIA 是卒中的高危因素，应该予以收入院。
- 颈动脉狭窄的患者需要迅速行血管手术随访。

• 误区：
- 未能进行全面的神经学检查以排除细微的脑卒中综合征。
- 局灶性神经功能缺损患者未能快速检查血糖。
- 达不到密切门诊随访的短暂性脑缺血发作患者出院。

短暂性全面性遗忘症 Transient Global Amnesia

Kama Z. Guluma 张晟 林兆奋 译

基础知识

描述

• 短暂性全面性遗忘症(TGA)有以下特点：
- 突然发病的遗忘症。
- 无局部神经症状或体征。
- 短暂、严重、顺行性遗忘症。
◦ 急性新记忆形成障碍。
◦ 发作后永久性记忆间隙。
- 暂时性短程逆行性遗忘症：
◦ 越是近期记忆风险越大。
◦ 此前编码的记忆暂时性不可获得。
- 逐渐缓解直到顺行性遗忘症造成的记忆间隙成为仅剩的记忆亏损。
◦ 有些逆行损失可能是永久性的。
- 平均症状持续时间：4～6 h。
◦ 多数问题在 8 h 内解决
• 发病率为每 100 000 人中 3～8 人：
- 75%发生于 50～70 岁人群中。
- 10%发生在 50 岁以下的患者中。
- 40 岁以下罕见。

病因

• 多模态磁共振、SPECT、PET 显示选择性易损的海马结构区域的血流异常。
• TGA 的病因尚不明确，发病机制仍有争议。
- 过度通气导致血管收缩。
◦ 心因性过度通气与年龄相关的脑血管自动调节障碍。
- Valsalva 致海马静脉阻塞。
◦ 超声检查显示颈内静脉功能不全患病率增加。
◦ 未见颅内静脉反流。
- 偏头痛(年轻患者)。
◦ 谷氨酸释放导致海马 CA1 区不稳定。
◦ TGA 患者偏头痛病史的增加。
◦ 偏头痛患者 TGA 频率无增加。
• TGA 和血栓栓塞性脑血管病之间并无相关性。
- 事实上，短暂性全面性遗忘症患者比短暂性脑缺血发作患者未来发生脑血管事件的风险更低。

诊断

症状和体征

诊断标准：
• 发病需有目击者。
• 急性发病的顺行性遗忘症。
• 意识方面无变化。
• 除遗忘症外无认知损伤。
• 无个人信息缺失(如年龄、生日、地址等)。
• 无局灶性神经症状。
• 无癫痫特征。
• 72 h 内无头部外伤史。
• 无癫痫病史。
• 24 h 内发病缓解。
• 排除遗忘症的其他病因。

病史

• 常由急性生理应激造成。
- 咳嗽，瓦氏试验。
- 体力消耗。
- 性交。
- 极度惊吓或打击。
- 强烈高温或低温。
• 患者可能自觉异样。
- 可能询问"我如何到这里来的"。
- 可能重复提问。
- 逐渐感知到发病。
• 发病时可能有短暂微妙的症状，如头痛、头晕、恶心等。
• 有助于排除其他诊断的病史特点。
- 发病可被察觉，没有癫痫活动或癫痫样特征。
- 2 个月内无癫痫病史。
- 近期无创伤性脑损伤史。
- 急性顺行性遗忘症伴有远程记忆的保留。

体格检查

• 显著的顺行性遗忘症。
- TGA 患者会忘记事实和事件(陈述性记忆)。
- TGA 患者不会忘记如何执行运动任务(程序记忆)。
• 多数病例(90%以上)有重复提问行为。
• 全身及神经系统检查均正常。
• TGA 患者无以下表现：
- 昏昏欲睡。
- 注意力不集中。
- 完全混乱。
- 虚构。
• TGA 患者有以下表现：
- 面向姓名、生日、地址、电话、日期等。
- 能够完成复杂任务，服从复杂指令。
• 失语症、失用症和失认症与 TGA 的发现不一致。
• 急诊要考虑的认知和评估。
- 测试及时记忆与延迟记忆：
◦ 让患者回忆一个数字范围，重复一系列数字，或者立即记住 3 个单词，然后延迟(5 min 后)。
◦ 即时记忆保持完好，而延迟记忆受损。
- 评估注意力持续时间。
◦ 让患者做序列 7 或反向拼写单词"world"。
◦ 在 TGA 期间保持不变。
- 测试程序记忆：
◦ 让患者做一项任务(例如，做一架纸飞机)。
◦ 在 TGA 期间保持不变。
- 测试认知功能：
◦ 失读症测试(无阅读能力)。
◦ 测试异常(无法命名对象)。
◦ 失用症测试(空间关系丧失：患者画个钟)。
◦ 在 TGA 期间保持不变。

基本检查

• 详尽病史和体格检查即可确诊 TGA。
• 若已确诊，则不需要其他基本检查。
• 对于无目击症状的发作，建议进行神经成像(MRI)检查。

诊断检查与说明

只有在诊断不明确时检测才有指导作用。

实验室检查

• CBC、综合生化检验：包括血糖、LET、NH_3、甲状腺检查、有机代谢中的 UA，与病因是密切相关的。
• 毒物测试，怀疑酒精水平为中毒病因。

影像学检查

• 必要时考虑 MRI。
- TGA 时，MRI 可能显示 DWI 或 T_2 海马局部区域缺血。
◦ 发病后 48～72 h 开始。

D

◦ 最长可见7～10日。

- 35%的TGA在MRI上没有发现。

• 必要时行头颅CT观察颅内肿块。

- 在真正的TGA中，头部CT将不会显示。

诊断步骤/外科

• 如果TGA的健忘持续时间异常短（<1 h）怀疑为癫痫或非惊厥性时行脑电图。

• 怀疑为脑炎时行腰椎穿刺及脑脊液检验。

鉴别诊断

• 其他病症可与TGA有相似表现，但可能有病史或体格检查表现，可与TGA鉴别。

- 短暂性癫痫健忘症（TEA，来自成人起病的颞叶内侧癫痫）。

◦ 顺行性或逆行性纯健忘症（TGA为顺行性）。

◦ 持续时间短（通常<1 h，TGA持续数小时）。

◦ 不完全性顺行健忘症（能够记住与TGA不能记忆不同）。

◦ 颞叶特征（例如，茫然的凝视、自动感、打嘴唇、嗅觉/味觉幻觉）。

◦ 在醒来后频繁快速复发。

- 脉络膜前动脉、大脑后动脉短暂性脑缺血发作：

◦ 其他神经系统症状如偏盲。

- 急性意识模糊状态、Korsakoff综合征、代谢紊乱。

◦ 酒精、药物治疗或毒素摄入。

◦ 注意力减退或脑病的其他表现。

◦ 连续减7实验，或倒序拼写“world”。

◦ 若时间允许可形成新记忆。

- 药物效应，如咪吡坦、苯二氮䓬类药物或大麻：

◦ 药物或毒品摄取的证据。

- 心因性健忘症。

◦ 有已知精神应激源的年轻患者。

◦ 显著的逆行性健忘症。

◦ 对个人身份、姓名、出生日期等的心因性记忆丧失等。

- 颞叶脑病变或脑炎影响颞叶。

◦ 有其他相关的神经系统症状（如视野切断、迷惑）。

◦ 进行性永久性遗忘症。

- 先前未确认的阿尔茨海默症。

◦ 有关个人信息的记忆丢失（如日期、电话、地址）。

◦ 整体认知功能障碍的症状。

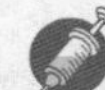

治疗

院前

• 筛查患者是否有脑卒中或癫痫的迹象。

• 收集所用药物的完整列表。

• 从目击者、朋友或家人那里收集确凿的病史。

• 如果可行，与患者的家人一起运送。

初步稳定/治疗

目前针对TGA无有效的治疗。

急诊治疗/程序

• TGA具有自限性，是相对良性的疾病。

• 观察患者病情进展。

• 如诊断为TGA，除了患者和家属知情外，没有任何急诊治疗措施。

药物治疗

一线用药

无。

二线用药

无。

随访

进一步处理

入院指征

• 处置时无显著缓解的患者应收入院进行进一步观察。

• 未明确诊断的患者。

• 有发病趋势而无良好家庭支持的患者。

出院指征

• 明确TGA的诊断。

• 失忆症已恢复或正在恢复。

• 良好社会支持。

转诊建议

• TGA的复发率为8%。

• 推荐有TGA复发风险的患者至神经病学专家处。

- 癫痫治疗中的动态心电图可能有益。

随访建议

考虑到TGA患者的中值年龄为60岁，全身心血管危险因素的基础预防可能有益。

• TGA目前无特殊后续建议。

• 为存在TGA复发风险的患者参见转诊问题。

要点和误区

• TGA为相对良性且显著的病症。

- 孤立性顺行性遗忘症急性发作。

- 脑病认知障碍。

- 有细微的神经系统症状或TIA。

• 如果对诊断存在疑问，多模MRI和脑电图是最有价值的检查。

对乙酰氨基酚中毒

Mark B. Mycyk　马林浩　林兆奋 译

基础知识

描述

• 对乙酰氨基酚（APAP）可单独使用，与阿片类药物口服的联合使用，以及>200 OTC感冒药：

- 涉及故意和无意中毒的最常见药物。

- 美国肝移植的首要原因。

• 当APAP被细胞色素P450代谢时产生N-乙酰基-对苯醌亚胺（NAPQI）：

- NAPQI通常被谷胱甘肽分解。

- 如过NAPQI过量，谷胱甘肽很快被耗尽，导致肝损伤。

- N-乙酰半胱氨酸（NAC）补充肝脏的谷胱甘肽储备。

• 毒性风险增加：

- 营养不良的患者谷胱甘肽储存量减少。

• 药代动力学：

- APAP的半衰期：

◦ 非过量服用需2.5～4 h。

◦ 过量服用需4 h。

- 急性毒性剂量>150 mg/kg。
- 摄入后 4 h 的毒性水平为 140 μg/ml(参见图 1 急性中毒的列线图)。
- 治疗血浆浓度为 5～20 μg/ml。

诊断

体征和症状

急性过量：

- 第 1 阶段：摄取后 0.5～24 h：
  - 恶心、呕吐、不适。
  - 服药过量。
  - 可能不是较小的毒性剂量。
- 第 2 阶段：摄取后 24～72 h：
  - 胃肠道症状减轻。
  - 正在发生肝脏损害。
  - 右上腹疼痛、压痛。
  - 肝酶、PT/INR、胆红素的升高。
  - 少尿。
  - 延长(>4 h)APAP 半衰期意味着肝毒性。
- 第 3 阶段：摄入后 72～96 h：
  - 预后的关键时期。
  - 肝功能异常。
  - 发生肝性脑病。
  - 如果 PT/INR 持续升高和/或肾功能不全发生在摄取后第 3 日，则患者很可能需要肝移植。
- 第 4 阶段：摄取后 96 h 至 10 日：
  - 肝损伤的恢复或进展为肝衰竭。

基本检查

- 所有含有 APAP 的产品的摄取历史记录。
- 摄入时间。
- APAP 水平：
  - 如果在摄取后>4 h，在摄取后 4 h 或在出现后立即获得。
  - 使用 Rumack-Matthew 列线图作为单次急性过量的治疗指南(图 1)。
  - 在慢性或非常晚期摄入(>24 h)，不要使用 Rumack-Matthew 列线图作为治疗指导。
- 呼叫毒物中心或毒理学家。

诊断检查与说明

实验室检查

- APAP 水平。
- 电解质、BUN、肌酐和葡萄糖。
- 肝酶。
  - 首次检测 AST 升高。
  - AST/ALT 水平在第 3 阶段可能升高，>10 000。
  - 胆红素。
- PT/INR。
- 妊娠检查。
- 毒理学筛查。

鉴别诊断

- 怀疑 APAP 与其他药物合用过量。
- 急性发作的肝损伤的原因。
  - 传染性肝炎。
  - 急性脑病综合征。
  - 毒蘑菇中毒。
  - 草药和膳食补充剂。
  - 酗酒。
  - 其他药物摄入。

治疗

院前

- 携带所有过量服用的药瓶或药丸，以便在急诊科进行鉴定。
- OTC 感冒药通常含有 APAP。

初步稳定/治疗

- ABC 管理。
- 吸氧。
- 服用纳洛酮、硫胺素、D_{50}(或 Accu-Chek)以改善精神状态。

急诊治疗/程序

- 支持治疗：
  - 静脉输液。
  - 止吐。
- 洗胃。
  - 如果最近摄入，服用单剂量活性炭。

NAC 防治管理

- 按照 Rumack-Matthew 图定义的毒性水平进行管理。

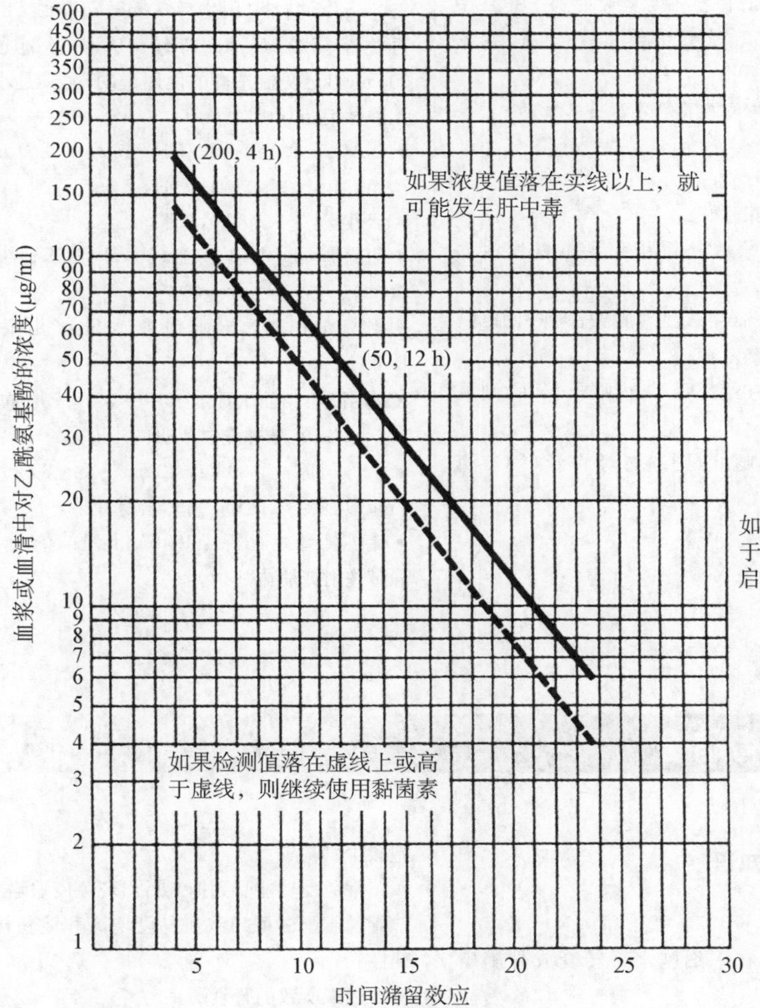

图 1

Rumack-Matthew 列线图(经许可引自 Rumack BH，Matthew H. Acetaminophen poisoning and toxicity. *Pediatrics*，1975；55：871－876)

• 如果在急性过量服用的 8 h 内，NAC 几乎100%对肝脏有保护作用。

• NAC 以口服或静脉滴入进入体内。

• <8 h：

- 检查 APAP 水平。
- 如果在摄入后 8 h 内无法获得 APAP 水平且怀疑有毒摄取，则启动 NAC。
- 如果 APAP 水平显示未中毒，停止使用 NAC。

• ≥8 h。

- 如果怀疑有毒摄入，立即启动 NAC。
- 检查 APAP 水平。
- 如果 APAP 水平显示未中毒，停止使用 NAC。

• >24 h 或慢性重复 APAP 摄入。

- 如果出现以下情况，请启动 NAC：
  ◦ 摄取>150 mg/kg APAP。
  ◦ 有症状。
  ◦ 肝功能筛查异常。
  ◦ 如果 APAP 降至不可检测的水平并且在摄取后 36 h 没有发生 AST 升高，则停止 NAC。
  ◦ 致电毒物中心或毒理学家寻求帮助。

NAC 准备

• 口服 NAC：

- 味道和气味不好：
  ◦ 用果汁或软饮料稀释至 5%，以增加适口性。
- 使用止吐药（甲氧氯普胺或昂丹司琼）以促进口服给药。
- 如果患者在给药后 1 h 内呕吐 NAC，则重复给药。
- 如果继续呕吐，则通过鼻胃管（NG）滴注 NAC。
- q4 h。

• 静脉滴注 NAC：

- 乙酰丙酮（acetadote）按照制造商的说明使用：
  ◦ 急性过量使用时给药需维持超过 21 h。
  ◦ 若异常输注或中毒晚期表现，可能需要充分延长用药时间；咨询中毒中心或毒理专家。
  ◦ 由于呕吐，口服形式不能耐受。

妊娠注意事项

• NAC 无致畸性。

• NAC 可有效保护胎儿肝脏：

- 妊娠 14 周后胎儿肝脏代谢 APAP 至毒性 NAPQI。

> **注意**
>
> 小儿 NAC 静滴需要谨慎计算剂量避免出错。

药物治疗

• 乙酰丙酮：21 h 持续静脉输入：150 mg/kg 持续 1 h，之后 50 mg/kg 持续 4 h，再之后 100 mg/kg 持续 16 h，总剂量 300 mg/kg（见制造商的使用说明，尤其是小儿静脉用药）。

• NAC：140 mg/kg，口服（成人和儿童），70 mg/kg，q4 h，再加 17 剂。

• 活性炭：1～2 g/kg，口服。

• 葡萄糖：$D_{50}W$ 1 安瓿（50 ml 或 25 g；儿童：$D_{25}W$ 2～4 ml/kg）。

• 甲氧多巴胺：起始剂量 10 mg（儿童：1 mg/kg）。

• 纳洛酮：起始剂量 0.4～2 mg（儿童：0.1 mg/kg），静脉注射或肌内注射。

• 昂丹司琼：>80 kg，12 mg；45～80 kg，8 mg（儿童：0.15 mg/kg），静脉注射。

• 硫胺素（维生素 B_1）：100 mg（儿童：50 mg），静脉注射或肌内注射。

妊娠注意事项

• 治疗母亲使胎儿得到最大程度的治疗。

• NAC 可以穿过胎盘，口服或静脉注射均被认为是安全的。

随访

进一步处理

入院指征

• APAP 肝毒性中毒水平需要全程 NAC 治疗（参见“治疗”）。

• 慢性摄入或晚期表现：肝功能检查（LFT）异常。

• 有自杀企图者需要精神病治疗。

出院指征

无症状的无毒物吸入患者不需要接受全疗程的 NAC 治疗。

转诊问题

有证据表明存在明显的肝毒性时需要通过肝胆专科和/或移植服务进行早期评估。

随访建议

• 滥用药物的患者要考虑其滥用口服阿片类制剂。

• 意外中毒的患者需要中毒预防咨询。

• 故意中毒患者如自杀，需要医师评估。

要点和误区

• 评估口服滥用阿片类药物患者的隐匿性 APAP 中毒。

• 对于长期摄入或晚期的患者不要使用 Rumack-Matthew 列线图。

• 在检测不到 APAP 水平和实验室和临床肝毒性证据的改善（或解决）之前，不要停止 NAC 治疗。

多发性骨髓瘤 Multiple Myeloma

Nicole M. Franks　伍力学　段立伟 译

基础知识

描述

• 正常细胞在干细胞水平转变成骨髓瘤细胞。

• 病理异常：

- 骨髓内的肿瘤细胞造成骨质破坏和血细胞减少。
- 正常免疫功能受到抑制后出现免疫缺陷。
- 骨髓瘤蛋白可导致血黏度增高和淀粉样变性。
- 多因素所致的肾衰竭。

• 浆细胞的分泌物激活破骨细胞而导致以下变化：

- 骨质溶解、病理性骨折和神经损害。
- 高钙血症（肾功能受损时更明显）。

• 骨髓浸润和肾功能不全所致的贫血。

• 免疫功能低下：

- 正常免疫球蛋白数量减少。
- T 细胞和 B 细胞亚群中数量和质量上均存在缺陷。

- 粒细胞缺乏。
- 细胞介导的免疫功能缺陷。
• 继发于蛋白质的蓄积的血黏度增高。
- 诱发高输出量性充血性心力衰竭。
• 骨髓瘤轻链在肾上皮细胞中累积并损害整个肾单元。
• 临床上表现为贫血、肾功能不全或溶骨性损害。
• 并发症：
- 病理性骨折。
- 高钙血症。
- 肾功能不全。
- 反复感染。
- 贫血。
- 脊髓压迫，可出现在10%的多发性骨髓瘤(MM)患者中。

■ 病因学

• 发病率：占人群的4/10万：
- 占恶性肿瘤患者的1%。
- 占所有造血细胞恶性肿瘤的10%。
- 死亡人数约10000人/年。
• 确诊时的平均年龄为66岁。
• 男性和非洲裔美国人发病率稍高(原因不明)。

儿科注意事项
• 儿童中罕见。
• 40岁以下的患者仅占不足2%。

诊断

■ 症状和体征

• 以骨痛为主要症状(可继发骨功能丧失或神经性后遗症)：
- 肋骨与胸骨。
- 脊柱。
- 锁骨。
- 颅骨。
- 肩胛骨。
- 坐骨。
• 全身症状：
- 贫血。
- 乏力。
- 易疲劳。
- 反复感染。
- 体重下降。
• 无症状(占20%)：
- MM是在随访或常规血液检验中发现的。
• 反复出现产荚膜细菌所导致的脓毒症(肺炎链球菌、流感嗜血杆菌、葡萄球菌)。

■ 基本检查

• 血常规、红细胞沉降率(ESR)、电解质、尿素氮、血肌酐、尿常规。
• 疼痛部位的骨X线平片：
- 骨骼评估：颅骨侧位片、前后位/侧位脊柱平片、前后位骨盆平片、肱骨和股骨平片。
• 骨骼X线平片未见异常但有持续性骨痛者行CT和MRI检查。
• 确诊：
- 血浆和尿蛋白电泳。
- 血浆和尿蛋白免疫固定电泳(电泳正常或无特异性时可资诊断)。
- 维生素D水平。
- 骨髓活检。

■ 诊断检查与说明

实验室检查
• CBC：
- 正细胞正色素性贫血。
- 血小板减少。
- 白细胞增多。
- 外周血红细胞呈缗钱状(堆叠排列)。
• 电解质、尿素氮、血肌酐、血糖：
- 肾功能不全。
• 血钙：
- 骨质重吸收引起高血钙。
• 尿常规：
- 筛查白蛋白和非轻链蛋白尿。
- 本周蛋白假阳性在尿检中很常见。
• 红细胞沉降率升高。
• 尿液和血清电泳显示单克隆蛋白峰。
• 轻链的定量检测有诊断意义。

影像学检查
• X线片：
- 溶骨性损害。
- 病理性损害。
• CT：
- 对小的损害灶更敏感。
- 在未行MRI检查时可与良性脊柱压缩性骨折鉴别。
• MRI：
- 更有助于发现及时压迫和软组织浆细胞瘤。
• PET-CT比PET/MRI能发现更多的病变，并能区分旧骨折和新骨折。怀疑脊椎骨折时首选。用于监测治疗反应。
• PET/MRI对弥漫性骨髓浸润的检出优于PET-CT。
• 锝-焦磷酸骨扫描：
- 可凸显骨沉积病灶。
- 对存在溶骨损害的MM病例行骨扫描时常出现假阴性，因为无法区分骨吸收和骨沉积病灶，而锝-焦磷酸骨扫描则能将这两种病灶区分开来。
• 骨髓活检：浆细胞数目增加。
• 细胞遗传学检查：可能有助于判断预后。

■ 鉴别诊断

• 单克隆丙种球蛋白病(临床意义不明)。
• 淀粉样变性。
• 慢性淋巴细胞白血病。
• 非霍奇金淋巴瘤。
• 巨球蛋白血症。
• 骨髓浆细胞疾病：包括胶原血管疾病、肝硬化、免疫复合物疾病、病毒行疾病和丘疹样黏蛋白病。

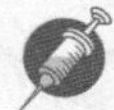

治疗

■ 院前

对有背部疼痛和神经系统症状的MM患者给予合适的固定措施。
• 注意防范可能发生的病理性脊柱骨折。

■ 初步稳定/治疗

• 识别和处理：
- 高钙血症。
- 肾衰竭。
- 脓毒症。
- 脊髓压迫。
- 贫血。

■ 急诊治疗/程序

• 阿片类镇痛药是急诊治疗的主要药物。
• 对病理性骨折部位行外固定，病理性骨折脊柱制动。
• 对高钙血症给予二膦酸盐治疗并配合足量的生理盐水进行水化。
• 对有症状的贫血予以输血和促红细胞生成素治疗。
• 血液科、肿瘤科会诊制定化疗方案，根据自体干细胞移植(ASCT)确定的方案：
- 早期或无症状者不需要化疗。
- 符合ASCT条件的：来那度胺和小剂量地塞米松(RD)，需要抗血栓预防性治疗；硼替佐米-地塞米松方案：沙利度胺(VTD)，来那度胺(VRD)，环磷酰胺(VCD)。
- 不符合ASCT：RD和VCD；由于干细胞损伤、继发性骨髓增生异常综合征和白血

D

病，马法兰方案已不使用。

- 每个患者都应该考虑 ASCT。早期、晚期或与化疗方案同时进行可提高总体存活率。

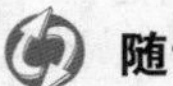

随访

进一步处理

入院指征

• 难治性疼痛需要全身镇痛药物者。

• 出现威胁生命的并发症，包括急性肾衰竭、高钙血症、脓毒症、脊髓压迫、血黏度增高、粒细胞减少和心脏压塞。

出院指征

疼痛可通过口服药物控制者。

转诊问题

• 无论疾病发现时处于哪一阶段均可转肿瘤科。

• 有持续性脊柱疼痛可能需要行经皮椎体成形术者可转往神经外科或骨科。

要点和误区

• 感染相关的并发症是导致死亡的主要原因，有发热者应针对常见的呼吸道和泌尿道感染给予经验性治疗。

• 对于有持续性疼痛等神经系统症状而病因不明者，应与多发性骨髓瘤鉴别诊断。

多发性神经病

Sandra A. Deane　瞿金龙 译

D

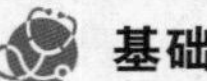

基础知识

描述

在身体多个功能神经同时出现周围神经功能障碍。

• 急性多发性神经病病因：

- 感染（细菌、病毒等）。
- 自身免疫（吉兰-巴雷综合征，又称急性炎症性脱髓鞘性多发性神经病）。
- 中毒（严重的精神障碍）：
  ◦ 铅。
  ◦ 水银（汞）。
- 药物：
  ◦ 抗惊厥类药物（苯妥英）。
  ◦ 抗生素（氯霉素、呋喃妥因、磺胺类）。
  ◦ 化疗药物（长春碱、长春新碱）。
  ◦ 镇静药。
- 肿瘤（多发性肌瘤）。

• 慢性多发性神经病病因：

- 糖尿病。
- 酗酒。
- 营养缺陷（维生素 B_{12}）。
- 甲状腺功能低下。
- 肝衰竭。
- 肾衰竭。
- 肺癌。
- 慢性炎症性脱髓鞘病变。

流行病学

发病率和流行病学分析

• 在美国，总的发生率不足人口的 2%。

• 超过 8%的 55 岁以上人发病。

• 美国大部分人因糖尿病引起，进行胰岛素治疗的糖尿病患者中不到 50%发病。

病因

• 髓鞘功能障碍：

- 在周围神经系统下抗原触发的引起类感染的交叉免疫反应。
  ◦ 包膜性细菌。
  ◦ 病毒。
  ◦ 疫苗。
- 吉兰-巴雷综合征：
  ◦ 髓鞘功能障碍急性表现。
  ◦ 进展快，很快发生呼吸衰竭。
- 慢性炎症性脱髓鞘病变：
  ◦ 髓鞘脂功能障碍急性表现。
  ◦ 症状可能发生到进展需要数月或数年。

• 血管神经引起：

- 血管供给障碍导致神经功能梗死形成。
- 病因：
  ◦ 慢性动脉粥样硬化。
  ◦ 脉管炎。
  ◦ 感染。
  ◦ 高凝状态。
  ◦ 轴突病。
- 轴突基本功能障碍。
- 毒物-代谢异常：
  ◦ 糖尿病。
  ◦ 营养不良。
  ◦ 药物或化学物质。

诊断

症状和体征

• 可能急性或慢性。

• 可能以感觉、运动、感觉-运动，或者自主神经功能障碍为主。

病史

• 常常下肢先于上肢发生，并且远端开始。

• 典型主诉：

- 感觉迟钝-麻木、灼烧感或肢体麻刺感。
- 肢体肌力减弱。
- 行走困难。
- 自主神经症状：
  ◦ 便秘。
  ◦ 大便失禁或小便失禁。
  ◦ 性功能障碍。
  ◦ 直立性头晕。
  ◦ 皮肤干燥。
  ◦ 出汗减少。

体格检查

• 典型体征是双侧，手套、袜子部位分布。

• 典型的阳性体征：

- 感觉减弱。
- 触觉和位置觉减弱。
- 运动功能减弱。
- 反射减弱。
- 肌肉萎缩。
- 肌束震颤。
- 麻痹。

• 特殊类型多发性神经病的阳性体征：

- 髓鞘功能障碍（急慢性）：
  ◦ 肌力减弱比肌肉萎缩看起来更严重。
  ◦ 感觉异常。
  ◦ 神经反射减弱。
  ◦ 离心性症状。
- 缺血性神经损伤（动脉硬化、脉管炎等）。
  ◦ 痛觉异常、灼烧感。
  ◦ 温痛觉减弱。
  ◦ 肌力减弱，肌肉萎缩。
  ◦ 反射亢进。

◦ 近端感觉多余。
◦ 脑神经较少有阳性体征。
- 原发性轴突功能障碍：
◦ 非上述原因引起的体征。
◦ 疼痛。
◦ 远心端，对称性。
◦ 手套、袜子部位分布。
◦ 远端发生较早。

▪ **基本检查**

• 在既往病史和体格检查指导下检查。
• 初始实验室检查：
- 全血细胞检查。
- 电解质。
- 血糖。
- 肝肾功能。
- 促甲状腺激素（TSH）。
- 红细胞沉降率。
- ANA。
- 维生素 B_{12}。
- 叶酸。
- 快速血浆反应素试验（RPR）。
- 人类免疫缺陷病毒（HIV）。
- 乙型肝炎和丙型肝炎。
- 莱姆病。
- 肌酸磷酸激酶（CPK）。
- 血浆蛋白电泳。
• 根据病史的实验室检查。
- 重金属水平（病史和暴露史）。
- 遗传性神经病的基因检查。
- 免疫介导神经病的血清抗体检测。

实验室检查

在病史和体格检查指导下。

诊断步骤/外科

• 肌电图。
• 神经传导速度检查。
• 脑脊液检查：
- 脑脊液蛋白水平。
- 吉兰-巴雷综合征和慢性多发性神经病。
• 皮肤神经活检。

▪ **鉴别诊断**

• 区分多发性神经病的病因：
- 内分泌疾病（糖尿病）。
- 感染（吉兰-巴雷综合征、莱姆病、HIV、梅毒）。
- 维生素缺乏。
- 肿瘤/类癌。
- 中毒。
- 肝脏疾病。
- 肾衰竭。
- 遗传疾病。
- 淀粉样变。
• 其他有类似表现的疾病：
- 小儿脊髓灰质炎。
- 卟啉症。
- 脊髓肌肉萎缩症。
- 儿茶酚胺分泌障碍。
- 心理精神异常。

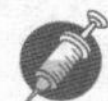

治疗

▪ **院前**

如需要基本的心肺复苏。

▪ **初步稳定/治疗**

• 必要时心肺复苏。
• 呼吸衰竭时呼吸支持。

▪ **急诊治疗/程序**

• 疼痛控制：
- 口服或不经口服都可以。
- 三环类抗抑郁药（阿米替林）。
- 抗惊厥（加巴喷丁）。
• 急性髓鞘功能障碍患者可以行血浆置换或免疫球蛋白。
• 慢性髓鞘功能障碍可以皮质类固醇激素或抗代谢类药物治疗。
• 自主神经功能障碍予以支持治疗。
• 监测呼吸肌力量。

随访

▪ **进一步处理**

入院指征

已经出现症状，并且需要快速诊断的患者。
• 呼吸衰竭。
• 血压不稳定。
• 不能行走或照顾自己。
• 需要药物控制疼痛。
• 隐藏性疾病没有控制。
• 进展快。

出院指征

• 潜在的临床症状已经稳定得到控制。
• 没有呼吸衰竭、自主神经不稳定的证据和高危因素。
• 能自己照顾自己。
• 得到控制的疼痛。
• 可以在门诊得到随访和进一步检查与治疗。

转诊问题

所有的患者需要内科和神经科医师检查与处理治疗。

▪ **随访建议**

• 初级保健医师。
• 神经科医师。
• 内科治疗。

要点和误区

• 潜在的病因是复杂的，但是病因诊断对治疗有很大帮助。
• 认识到有些病因是呼吸衰竭和自主神经功能障碍的高危因素。
• 很多病因，治疗主要是基于控制潜在的疾病发展。

D

多发性硬化 Multiple Sclerosis

Richard S. Krause 伍力学 段立伟 译

基础知识

▪ **描述**

• 病理生理：反复发作的中枢神经系统脱髓鞘病变。
- 症状和体征取决于损害部位和脱髓鞘病变的发生时间。
• 多发性硬化（multiple sclerosis，MS）可按疾病的进展特征分型：
- 循环复发型 MS：有 2 次或以上的发作，每次持续＞24 h，且间隔＞1 个月。
- 原发进展型 MS：起病后即缓慢进展超过

6 个月。

- 继发进展型 MS：首次发作后缓解，继以缓慢进展超过 6 个月。

- 稳定性 MS：无进展（未治疗情况下）达 18 个月以上。

▪ 病因

• MS 是一种中枢神经系统慢性脱髓鞘病变。

• 病因未明。

• 目前认为可能是一种 T 细胞介导的自身免疫疾病。

• 有证据证明该病由病毒感染所诱发。

• 病变发生在白质：

- 可见特征性的 T 细胞和巨噬细胞浸润灶。

• 在美国，北欧裔人群最易受累。

• 发病率分布从赤道地区向高纬度地区逐渐增高。

诊断

▪ 症状和体征

• 首发症状多为单发病灶（占 85%），起病突然，具有特征性（按发生频率从高到低排列如下）：

- 视神经炎：
  ◦ 眼痛逐渐加重甚至失明。
- 单侧肢体感觉异常（或感觉减退）。
- 肢体无力（以下肢多见）。
- 复视：
  ◦ 由内侧纵束病变引起的核性眼肌麻痹。
  ◦ 单侧或双侧内直肌麻痹导致眼球水平凝视。
- 三叉神经痛：
- 尿潴留。
- 眩晕。
- 横贯性脊髓炎：
  ◦ 特定脊髓平面出现急性的运动和感觉障碍。
  ◦ 常伴随大小便失禁。
  ◦ 可作为 MS 的早期表现。
  ◦ 常见的首发表现包括精神病、失语等。
  ◦ 首发症状可能较轻微，往往只在回溯时才被识别出来。

• 典型的症状常突然发生（在数分钟到数小时内），并持续 6～8 周。

• 最常见于北欧的年轻女性：

- 第一代后裔的发病风险明显增加。
- 发病高峰：30 岁。
- 男女比例为 1∶2。

• 急性疼痛不是 MS 的常见症状：

- 三叉神经痛和早期视神经炎引起的疼痛除外。

体格检查

体格检查：重点放在“困难的”神经系统检查。

• 局灶性神经病变。

• 瞳孔传入障碍。

• 核间性眼肌瘫痪。

• 感觉平面异常或括约肌功能失调（横断性脊髓炎）。

▪ 基本检查

• 依据病史和体格检查考虑是否存在 MS。

• 在诊治早期一般难以确诊。

- 需要继续观察病情并完善与确诊的相关检测。

> **注意**
>
> 感染，尤其是有发热者，是 MS 恶化的常见原因。

▪ 诊断检查与说明

实验室检查

脑脊液检测：

• 脑脊液凝胶电泳可显示血清中无法检出的寡克隆带。

- 临床诊断的 MS 患者中有 95%存在寡克隆带。

影像学检查

MRI 是最有意义的影像学检查：

• 大脑白质或脊髓中的病灶在 T_2 加权像呈现高信号。

• 斑块在 T_2 加权像上呈高信号，在 T_1 加权像上呈低信号。

• 几乎所有临床诊断 MS 的患者均有异常影像学表现。

• 麦克唐纳诊断标准中包括特异性影像学表现。

• 在 CT 中也可能看到病灶（敏感性较低）。

• MRI 可以区分活动性病变和慢性病变。

诊断步骤/外科

感觉诱发电位测试：

• 非急诊检测项目。

• 腰椎穿刺寡克隆带（在急诊通常不做）。

▪ 鉴别诊断

• MS 的症状和体征多呈局灶性：

- 一些易混淆疾病症状（如癫痫、晕厥和痴呆等）在 MS 患者中很少发生。

• 脑血管意外和短暂性脑缺血发作（TIA）：

- 常发生在有动脉粥样硬化或心房颤动的高危因素的老年患者。

• 系统性红斑狼疮：

- 中枢神经系统受累症状的发生可归因于已知的疾病且症状为非局灶性。

• 肉瘤：

- 中枢神经系统的临床表现一般有可溯的已知疾病并伴随肺损害。

• 莱姆病：

- 与 MS 很相似。
- 回溯病史，有无高危地区的蜱虫暴露史和皮疹。
- 莱姆抗体滴度测定有助于鉴别。

• 排除精神疾病诊断。

• 感染或免疫和脱髓鞘病变与 MS 较为相似，尤其在儿童患者。

• 吉兰-巴雷综合征的症状常为上升性和对称性且会在数小时到数日内逐步进展。

• 下列患者不考虑 MS 诊断：

- 神经系统检查正常者。
- 突发偏瘫。
- 突发失语。
- 明显的疼痛。
- 非常短暂的症状（数秒到数分钟）。
- <10 岁或>50 岁的患者。

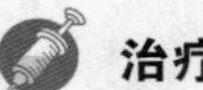

治疗

▪ 初步稳定/治疗

MS 所致的发热应予以积极处理，否则可加重 MS 的症状。

▪ 急诊治疗/程序

• 急性视神经炎的处理：

- 大剂量外用激素。
- 口服激素属于相对禁忌（有报道显示可增加复发风险）。

• 病情进展恶化的处理：

- 大剂量甲泼尼龙（可达 1 g/d）或其他外周的皮质激素。
- 大剂量口服激素（视神经炎者除外）。
- 血浆置换：通常用于对大剂量类固醇激素无反应的严重急性加重的患者。

• 全身用药：

- 强直：巴氯芬、替扎尼定。
- 震颤：氯硝西泮。
- 泌尿系统症状：
  ◦ 诊治尿路感染。
  ◦ 留置尿管。
  ◦ 奥普布宁：可缓解尿道刺激症状。

- 三叉神经痛：卡马西平。
- 疲劳和乏力症状：可选择金刚烷胺、哌甲酯和莫达非尼。
- 抑郁症状：5-羟色胺再摄取抑制剂(SSRI)有效。
- Ocrelizumab 最近已被批准用于治疗原发性进展性多发性硬化症。
  ◦ 通常不用于急诊治疗。

■ **药物治疗**

• 金刚烷胺：100 g，口服，每日 2 次。
• 巴氯芬：初始剂量 10 mg，每日 3 次，口服；可增加至 25 mg，每日 3 次，口服。
• 卡马西平：0.5 mg/d，口服；可逐增至 0.5 mg，每日 3 次，口服。
• 氯硝西泮：0.5 mg/d，口服，按 0.5 mg 递增，直至达每日 3 次。
• 甲泼尼龙：1 g/d，静脉用药(一线治疗)。
• 莫达非尼：100～200 mg/d，晨服。
• 奥昔布宁：5 mg，每日 2～3 次，口服。
• 替扎尼定：2～8 mg，每日 3 次，口服。

随访

■ **进一步处理**

入院指征

• 急性加重需要静脉用药者。
• 患者因病情危重不能自理者。
• 其他院外无法处理而需要住院治疗的情况。

出院指征

• 疑诊 MS 的患者：此类患者如一般情况允许并排除了其他需要住院观察的情况后，可在院外继续观察评估。
• 需要治疗并发症的 MS 患者：如门诊有条件治疗并发症并控制疾病进展的，可门诊治疗。

■ **随访建议**

疑诊 MS 的患者应转诊到社区医师或神经科医师处进一步观察评估。

要点和误区

• MS 的症状和体征呈局灶性。
• 弥漫性症状很少见。
• 口服激素存在相对禁忌。
• 发热应予以积极处理。

多形红斑 Erythema Multiforme

Gregory W. Hendey　单怡 译

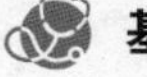

基础知识

■ **描述**

• 由过敏反应引起的皮疹：
- 可发生于各种药物、感染或其他疾病的反应。
• 轻型多形红斑(EM)：
- 典型靶形病变。
- 水肿性丘疹。
- 通常分布于外周。
- 良性、自限性皮疹一般不伴有急性、严重的疾病。
• 重型多形红斑：
- 靶形病变。
- 水肿性丘疹。
- 也分布于外周。
- 累及一个或更多的黏膜。
- <10%体表面积的表皮脱落。
• 区别：
- 史蒂文斯-约翰逊综合征(SJS)：
  ◦ 同样有<10%体表面积的表皮脱离。
  ◦ 鼻和面部常有广泛水疱。
  ◦ 累及黏膜。
- 中毒性表皮坏死松解症(TEN)：
  ◦ 30%体表面积的表皮脱离。
- EM 被认为完全不同于 SJS 和 TEM。
• 最常发生于儿童和年轻人(50%以上患者>20 岁)。
• 男性多于女性。

■ **病因**

• 过敏反应，可能是暂时性的自身免疫缺陷。
• 单纯疱疹病毒(HSV)是最常见的诱因(>70%)。
• 其他原因包括：
- 感染。
  ◦ 支原体感染。
  ◦ 艾滋病。
  ◦ 巨细胞病毒。
- 丙型肝炎。
  ◦ 磺胺药。
  ◦ 抗痉挛药物。
  ◦ 抗生素。
- 疫苗。
  ◦ 白喉破伤风疫苗。
  ◦ 乙型肝炎疫苗。
  ◦ 天花疫苗。
- 恶性肿瘤。
- 特发性疾病。

诊断

■ **症状和体征**

病史

• 前驱症状：常见的全身症状(低热、不适)，大多数病例中有前驱的单纯疱疹病毒感染(3 周内)。
• 通常不伴有严重的全身性疾病。

体格检查

特征性皮疹：
• 病变：
- 对称的暗红色斑丘疹。
- 演化成圆形、界限清楚中央空白的病灶。
- 轻型多形红斑无表皮坏死。
• 多形性是指不同阶段不同时间皮疹的演变。
• 分布：
- 四肢。
- 手背和足背。
- 伸肌表面。
- 肘部和膝盖。
• 这些皮疹中一个可能累及手掌和足掌。
• 扩散：从四肢向躯干扩散。
• 黏膜受累：轻微起泡或黏膜表面糜烂(唇、口)。
• 持续时间：通常 4 周，但也可呈慢性或复发性。

■ **基本检查**

完整的病史和体格检查，特别注意皮肤、泌尿生殖系统、近日的感染症状、近日使用的药物。

D

诊断检查与说明

实验室检查

无特殊实验室检查。

影像学检查

无特殊的有助于诊断的影像学检查。

诊断步骤/外科

• 皮肤活检显示真皮血管周围炎细胞浸润，无白细胞破碎性血管炎和坏死的表皮角质形成细胞。

• 大多数情况并无必要活检。

鉴别诊断

• 混合性药疹。
• 玫瑰糠疹。
• 二期梅毒。
• 游走性红斑。
• 荨麻疹。
• 史蒂文斯-约翰逊综合征(SJS)。
• 中毒性表皮坏死松解症(TEN)。
• 血管炎。
• 病毒疹。

D

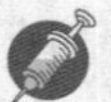

治疗

院前

没有传染性，不需要隔离或对暴露人员进行预防。

初步稳定/治疗

一般为良性和自限性，不需要初始的稳定治疗。

急诊治疗/程序

• 确定、治疗或去除潜在的病因和诱因。
• 对症治疗：冷敷，止痒。

药物治疗

• 抗病毒药物：
- 阿昔洛韦：400 mg，口服，每日 2 次。
- 发病 48 h 内治疗。
- 不影响临床病程。
• 止痒剂：
- 西替利嗪（仙特明）：10 mg/d（儿童：2.5～5 mg），口服。
- 苯海拉明：25～50 mg[儿童：5 mg/(kg・24 h)]，口服，q6～8 h。
- 羟嗪：25 mg，口服，q6～8 h[儿童：2 mg/(kg・24 h)，q6～8 h]。
• 中效局部糖皮质激素：
- 1%曲安奈德：每日 2～4 次。
- 不要用于面部或眼睑。
• 短效局部糖皮质激素。
- 用于面部或擦烂的部位。
- 1%氢化可的松，每日 2～4 次。
• 口腔病变的麻醉剂：
- 神奇漱口水。
• 口服糖皮质激素：
- 残留的严重黏膜病变。
- 泼尼松：40～60 mg，口服，每日 1 次，用药超过 2 周。
• 预防性用药：
- 阿昔洛韦：400 mg，口服，每日 2 次。
- 伐昔洛韦：500 mg，口服，每日 2 次。
- 泛昔洛韦：250 mg，口服，每日 2 次。

一线药物

• 抗病毒药。
• 止痒剂。
• 外用皮质类固醇(低至中效)。

二线药物

• 口服糖皮质激素。

随访

进一步处理

入院指征

• 继发的黏膜病变无法口服药物。
• 一般无需住院。

出院指征

多形红斑通常是一种良性疾病，不需要入院。

转诊问题

• 如果诊断不明确或皮疹不典型或病情严重，患者应转入皮肤科。
• 如果眼部受累应立即转入眼科。

随访建议

• 随访的主治医师 1 周内评估：
- 进一步评估潜在的病因(感染、药物、恶性肿瘤等)。
- 皮疹的进展或演变。
• 如果诊断不确定的，1 周内皮肤科医师随访。

要点和误区

• 患者有严重的全身性疾病，应考虑更严重的诊断，如 SJS 或 TEN。
• 大多数多形红斑患者有潜在的单纯疱疹病毒感染。
• 二期梅毒可在手掌和足掌产生类似的病变。
• 安抚患者多形红斑的皮疹是良性和自限性。

呃逆 Hiccups

Jeffrey A. Horenstein • Carrie D. Tibbies 陈奇通 译

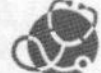

基础知识

描述

• 膈肌的突然间不随意收缩(通常单侧)和其他吸气肌因声门突然关闭而终止。
• 医学术语：Singultus。
• 通常发生频率为 4～60 次/分。
• 由于刺激打嗝反射弧而产生：
- 刺激迷走神经和膈神经。
- 打嗝中枢位于上脊髓或脑干。
• 分级：
- 呃逆：打嗝时间＜48 h。
- 持续呃逆：打嗝时间超过 48 h，甚至达 1 个月。
- 顽固性呃逆：打嗝时间超过 1 个月。
• 男性＞女性(4∶1)。

病因

• 胃肠道：
- 胃：胀气、暴饮暴食、进食过快。
- 食管：胃食管反流、贲门失弛缓症、念珠菌食管炎、食管癌。
- 胃：胃溃疡、胃癌。
- 肝：肝炎、肝癌。
- 胰腺：胰腺炎、假性囊肿、胰腺癌。
- 肠梗阻。
- 炎症性肠病。
- 胆石症和胆囊炎。
- 阑尾炎。
- 腹主动脉瘤。
- 手术后患者，腹部手术。
• 横膈刺激：
- 食管裂孔疝。
- 腹部肿块。
- 心包炎。
- 腹脏突出。
- 脾大和肝大。
- 腹膜炎。
• 中枢神经系统：
- 血管性疾病：缺血性/出血性脑卒中、头部外伤、脑动静脉畸形。
- 传染性疾病：脑炎、流行性脑炎、脓肿。
- 结构上的：癌症、帕金森病、多发性硬化症、脑积水。
- 脑室-腹腔分流术。
• 胸部：
- 传染性疾病：肺炎、肺结核。
- 心脏性疾病：心肌梗死、心包炎。
- 主动脉瘤。
- 癌症。
- 纵隔淋巴结增大。
• 头和颈：
- 异物刺激鼓膜。
- 咽炎。
- 喉炎。
- 甲状腺肿大。
- 咽后壁、扁桃体周围脓肿。
- 颈部包块。
• 代谢障碍：
- 尿毒症。
- 低钠血症。
- 低钙血症。
- 痛风。
- 糖尿病。
• 毒物/药物：
- 酒精。
- 烟草。
- α-甲基多巴。
- 苯二氮䓬类药物。
- 甾醇类。
- 巴比妥类。
- 麻醉药。
- 化疗药物。
- 抗生素。
- 全身麻醉。
• 心理性原因：
- 压力/兴奋。
- 悲伤。
- 诈病。
- 转换障碍。
• 特发性。

诊断

症状和体征

• 特征性的声音是突然以用力吸气终止呼吸动作。
• 通常呃逆之间间隔较短，持续几秒或几分钟。
• 当呃逆持续＞48 h 或者睡眠时仍持续，表明需考虑器官病因。

病史

• 通过针对性的病史询问和系统回顾，可以发现潜在病因的可能性：
- 当前发生的严重程度和持续时间。
- 以往的发病历史和治疗的尝试。

体格检查

• 仔细的体格检查以寻找根本原因，重点检查：
- 头部和颈部。
- 胸部。
- 腹部。
- 神经病学。

基本检查

对于持续或顽固性呃逆，详尽地了解病史和全面的体格检查有助于进一步的诊断试验。

诊断检查与说明

实验室检查

• 血常规。
• 电解质、尿素氮与肌酐。

影像学检查

• 胸部 X 线检查。
• 对于临床怀疑的特殊病因，进一步行影像学检查，有助于疾病诊断。这通常可以在门诊进行。

鉴别诊断

打嗝(嗳气)。

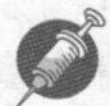

治疗

急诊治疗/程序

• 针对特殊原因行治疗：
- 取出耳内异物。
- 通过胃管减轻胃胀气。
• 非药物治疗：
- 导管刺激咽后壁。
- 使用棉签直接刺激悬雍垂。
- 眶上压迫。
- 按摩颈动脉窦。
- 直肠指诊。
- 枕骨放松。
  ◦ 轻柔地牵引与压迫颈后部，拉伸枕下肌肉与筋膜。
• 药物治疗：
- 一线，只有 FDA 批准的治疗呃逆药物：氯丙嗪。
• 其他药物：

- 加巴喷丁。
- 甲氧氯普胺。
- 氯苯氨丁酸。
- 氟哌啶醇。
- 利多卡因雾化吸入。
- 阿米替林。
- 苯妥英钠。

■ 药物治疗

• 阿米替林：10 mg，口服，每日 3 次。
• 氯苯氨丁酸：10 mg，口服，每日 3 次。
• 氯丙嗪：25～50 mg，静脉注射或肌内注射，25～50 mg，口服，每日 2～3 次。
• 加巴喷丁：100 mg，口服，每日 3～4 次。
• 氟哌啶醇：2～5 mg，肌内注射。
• 利多卡因(4%)：3 ml，雾化吸入，必要时可重复。
• 甲氧氯普胺：10 mg，静脉注射或肌内注射，10～20 mg，口服，每日 3 次。
• 苯妥英钠：200 mg，静脉注射。

随访

■ 进一步处理

入院指征

如果呃逆影响正常生活，导致营养和液体摄入减少、失眠、伤口裂开等需住院治疗。

出院指征

• 呃逆持续时间<48 h。
• 诊断检查与潜在器质性病因不一致。

转诊问题

对难治性的呃逆，查明潜在的原因和更多明确的治疗措施：
• 膈神经阻滞，挤压或者横断。
• 催眠。
• 行为矫正。
• 针灸。
• 心理干预。

■ 随访建议

家庭治疗针对可能复发：
• 吞下一匙糖。
• 吮吸硬糖或者吞服花生酱。
• 屏息或 Valsalva 动作。
• 咬一个柠檬。
• 舌牵引。
• 用冰匙托起悬雍垂。
• 从玻璃杯的远侧饮用。
• 惊吓。
• 伤害性刺激。
• 对着纸袋呼吸。

要点和误区

持久的呃逆预示着潜在的器质性疾病。

E

儿科复苏 Resuscitation, Pediatric

Taylor McCormick　袁晓伟　童朝阳 译

基础知识

■ 描述

• 儿童的呼吸衰竭、休克和心肺骤停需要及时干预。
• 休克：一种代谢供需的生理不匹配导致组织缺氧和多系统器官衰竭。
• 早期发现和治疗呼吸功能不全和休克可防止进展为心肺骤停。

■ 病因

• 呼吸衰竭导致无脉电活动(PEA)，然后心搏停止是儿童心肺骤停最常见的原因，尽管心脏和创伤的原因并不少见。
• 心室颤动和心动过速是罕见的，主要发生在青少年和儿童先天性心脏病。
• 休克可以细分为 4 种类型：
- 血容量不足：循环容量不足(如出血或摄入/排出异常)。
- 分布性：全身血管阻力降低，导致外周血分布不当(如脓毒症)。
- 心源性：心肌功能受损(如心肌炎)。
- 梗阻性：心脏充盈和排血受阻(如肺栓塞)。
• 脓毒性休克患儿可表现为“暖性休克”(高心排血量，低全身血管阻力)或“冷性休克”(低心排血量，高全身血管阻力)。
• 当通过心率增加、血管阻力、肌力收缩和静脉张力维持正常血压时，就会发生代偿性休克。如果干预不及时、不积极，这可能发展为晚期的、失补偿的休克。
• 低血压休克可迅速发展为心肺衰竭/骤停。

诊断

■ 症状和体征

病史

• 获得病史不应延误对儿童处于危重症或心肺停止的初步评估。
• 在适当的情况下，从护理人员和院前救护者处获取病史，包括患者的病史、手术史、手术史、饮食史、月经史和排气史。

体格检查

• 心肺骤停：无脉搏(婴儿股/臂)、呼吸困难和反应：启动 CPR 并遵循儿科高级生命支持/美国心脏协会(PALS/AHA)方法(见治疗)。
• 儿科三角评估法(PAT)：
- 快速识别呼吸或循环障碍。
- 外观(语气、互动、安慰、眼神/凝视、说话/哭泣)。
- 呼吸运动(气道音、定位、辅助肌肉使用)。
- 循环(面色苍白、发绀、末梢充盈情况、皮肤湿冷)。
- 如 PAT 异常，应同时进行原发性评估(ABCDE)和治疗。
- 如果 PAT 正常，进行二次/从头到脚的评估。
• 初步评估(ABCDE)和治疗应同时进行：
- 气道：
◦ 评估分泌物淤积，阻塞，说话或哭泣的能力。
◦ 如临床所示，可采用提颏、推颚、吸引、放置鼻咽或口咽气道。
◦ 如果矫正措施不成功，则进行气管插管。
- 呼吸：
◦ 评估呼吸频率、呼吸功、体位、呼吸音、呼噜声、鼻翼扇动、收缩、喘鸣、氧饱和度，考虑 $EtCO_2$ 监测。
◦ 对于饱和度<95%或即将发生的呼吸衰竭，通过鼻插管或无呼吸面罩吸氧，使用袋式阀面罩通气进行通气支持，针/管胸腔造口术治疗气胸，沙丁胺醇治疗支气管痉挛，吸入肾上腺素治疗可疑 Croup 综合征。如果干预不成功，进行气管插管。
- 循环：
◦ 评估低血压和休克的证据：毛细血管充盈延迟、苍白、四肢冰冷或斑驳、外周脉搏减少、低血压(<70 岁以上年龄×2)、心动过速或心动过缓；建立静脉通道。

◦ 床旁超声可迅速发现心包积液/填塞、大量腹腔内游离液、气胸、下腔萎陷、右心色斑或心脏结构性异常，协助处理。
◦ 如有需要，用 20 ml/kg 晶体液，必要时重复（如果未分化或对心脏病因学有任何顾虑，10 ml/kg），如果怀疑出血性休克，使用 pRBC 10 ml/kg，如果是液体难治性，则使用血管加压药，化学或电复律治疗心律失常。
- 后遗症：
◦ 使用儿童 GCS 或 AVPU 评估意识水平、瞳孔大小和反应性、癫痫样活动、肢体运动和语气；检查手指末梢葡萄糖水平。
◦ 针对疑似颅内压增高/即将发生的疝，床头抬高 30°，并给予高渗盐水或甘露醇，暂时过度通气，避免低血压和缺氧；纠正低血糖；用苯二氮草类药物治疗持续性癫痫发作。
- 暴露/环境：
◦ 完全暴露进行评估，然后遮盖保持正常体温。
• 二次评估：全面的全身检查。

基本检查

• 获得患儿体重以获取适当的设备尺寸和剂量重量（千克）；如果实际体重测量或父母估计不可能，使用基于长度或年龄的估计。
• 频繁的生命体征和心肺监测。
• 指尖末梢血糖。
• 少女妊娠测试。
• 通过彻底的病史、体格检查和鉴别诊断来确定进一步的实验室和放射学检查。

诊断检查与说明

实验室检查

• 实验室评估应由临床表现决定，可能包括：
- CBC、电解质、肝功能检查，病危时做静脉血气检查。
- 需要输血的患者的血型以及筛选/交叉匹配。
- 败血症评估包括乳酸、血液培养、尿液分析和尿液培养、脑脊液细胞计数/革兰染色和培养，如果需要还包括粪便检查（血液、白细胞计数、特异性病原体测试）。
- 凝血检查只有在患者服用抗凝剂、有已知凝血病变或有 DIC 担忧时才有必要。
- 如果缺血行 BNP 和肌钙蛋白检查，这可能与心肌炎或充血性心力衰竭有关。
- 送额外的红管血（如果担心代谢紊乱、先天异常）或第四根脑脊液管，以备将来的检测。
- 如果需要的话，进行毒理测试。

影像学检查

• 影像学和辅助测试应由临床表现决定，可能包括：
- CXR 检查感染、气胸和心脏大小。
- 颈椎和外伤的检查。
- CT 检查头部出血或肿块。
- 腹部、骨盆 CT 检查出血或腹腔内感染。

诊断步骤/外科

• 心电图检查：心动过速、慢缓性心律失常或结构性心脏病的证据。
• 脑电图：是否与癫痫持续状态有关。
• 超声心动图：检查结构型心脏病。

鉴别诊断

• 呼吸：
- 上呼吸道梗阻：哮吼、会厌炎、扁桃体周围或咽后脓肿、FB、气管炎、先天畸形。
- 下呼吸道梗阻：哮喘、肺炎、支气管炎、FB、肺泡纤维化、胸部创伤、溺水。
• 休克：
- 血容量不足：出血、腹泻、摄入不足、渗透性利尿/DKA、第三间隙、烧伤。
- 分布性：脓毒症、过敏反应，神经源性休克。
- 心源性：心肌炎、先天性心脏病、心肌病、药物毒性、心律失常、败血症。
- 梗阻性：心脏压塞、张力性气胸、PE、先天性心脏病。
- 休克的种类经常重叠，特别是在败血症、代谢紊乱和内分泌紊乱的情况下。
- 中枢神经系统疾病、SIDS、SUID、BRUE、ALTE、ASSB、过量等。
- 病史与疾病、受伤类型不符时，怀疑儿童受虐待。

治疗

急诊治疗/程序

• 心肺骤停：启动 CPR 并遵循 PALS/AHA 方案。
- 按压-气道-呼吸。
◦ 在急诊单纯按压和先按压的 CPR 是有争议的，按压和通气应同时进行。
◦ 婴儿和青春期前儿童的压缩通气比 15∶2，直到高级气道就位。
◦ 在坚固的表面上每分钟压缩 100～120 次。
◦ 幼儿：双手环绕胸部，用两个拇指压住胸骨下部（深度 1.5 in，约 3.8 cm）；儿童：传统双手技巧（深度 2 in，约 5 cm）。
◦ 在气管插管可行之前，应使用气囊面罩或声门上气道通气，如果气管插管不成功，则应继续使用，以避免长时间的按压中断。
- 除颤：
◦ 快速识别无脉性室性心动过速或室颤（VT/VF）。
◦ 进行高质量的按压，直到除颤器正确连接和充电，尽快进行电击，不要因建立气道而推迟。
◦ 8 岁以下儿童可使用儿童垫。
◦ 如果使用成人垫，前后位和前外侧位是等效的，以避免垫之间的接触。
◦ 第一次为 2 J/kg，第二次为 4 J/kg，第三次及以后为 10 J/kg。
- 药物（请参阅药物剂量）。
◦ 肾上腺素适用于所有复苏节律。
◦ 胺碘酮或利多卡因用于 VT/VF。
◦ 尖端扭转性心动过速用镁剂。
◦ 葡萄糖对低血糖。
◦ 考虑用碳酸氢钠治疗高钾血症或三环类抗抑郁药物中毒。
◦ 考虑使用氯化钙治疗高钾血症、低钙血症或钙通道阻滞剂过量。
- 复苏后治疗。
◦ 用去甲肾上腺素避免低血压；加多巴酚丁胺治疗疑似心源性休克。
◦ 优化呼吸机设置，以达到正常氧饱和度（目标 94%）和二氧化碳水平（目标 $PaCO_2$ 35～45 mmHg）。
◦ 避免高热；目标温度：33 ℃或 36 ℃。
◦ 在孩子的复苏过程中，应该选择让家属在场。
• 儿科三角评估（呼吸或循环功能不全）异常：上面列出了在初步评估期间要执行的救生和保肢干预措施。
- 初步的管理步骤应包括获得实际或估计的体重（kg），心肺监测，基本的气道机动/辅助设备，针对缺氧或即将呼吸衰竭者氧疗，建立静脉通道；如果有需要，补液。
- 呼吸衰竭：适当对患者进行湿化、加热、高流量鼻插管氧或持续气道正压试验；如果不成功或不适合，继续进行气管插管。
◦ 运用依托咪酯、氯胺酮、琥珀酰胆碱或罗库溴铵快速进行顺序插管。
◦ 阿托品预处理不必预防喉镜下的迷走神经反应；对于已有或围手术期的心动过缓，应给予阿托品预处理。
◦ 气管内插管（ETT）尺寸：年龄/4＋3.5（带套囊），年龄/4＋4（未套囊）；带套囊 ETT（cETT）适用于所有年龄段，未带套囊 ETT（uETT）适用于 1 岁以下。

◦ Miller/Mac 1 适用 0～2 年，Miller/Mac 2 适用 2～8 年，Miller/Mac 3 适用 8 年以上。
◦ 插入深度：3×uETT 大小(cm)。
◦ 如果气管插管不成功，继续袋阀面罩通气并放置声门上气道装置。
◦ 如无法插管或通气，可行环甲状针切开术。
– 休克：
◦ 分配：20 ml/kg NS/LR 液体推注×(2～3)，如果液体复苏效果不佳，开始去甲肾上腺素治疗"热休克"，使用肾上腺素如果液体难治"冷休克"，氢化可的松用于已知或疑似肾上腺功能不全，肾上腺素用于过敏反应。
◦ 心源性：启动去甲肾上腺素，如果需要，加入多巴酚丁胺进行离子支持，同步复律(0.5～2 J/kg)治疗不稳定的心动过速，肾上腺素和起搏治疗不稳定的心动过缓。
◦ 阻塞性：张力性气胸针减压术，心包穿刺填塞，肺栓塞溶栓。
◦ 低血容量：用 20 ml/kg 的 NS/LR 或 10 ml/kg 的 pRBC 丸进行体积扩张，并根据需要重复。

E

■ 药物治疗

• 给予静脉注射或骨髓腔注射，除非另有说明。
– 腺苷：0.1 mg/kg(最大剂量 6 mg)静脉注射快速推注；第二次剂量 0.2 mg/kg(最大剂量 12 mg)(骨髓腔注射无效)。
– 胺碘酮：5 mg/kg 静脉注射，最大剂量 300 mg，针对无脉性 VF/VT 快速推注；SVT/VT 在 30 min 输注。
– 阿托品 0.02 mg/kg(最小剂量 0.1 mg，最大剂量 0.5 mg)，静脉注射。
– 氯化钙 20 mg/kg(最大剂量 1 mg)。
– 心脏复律，同步 0.5～2 J/kg。
– 除颤 2 J/kg，然后 4～10 J/kg。
– 葡萄糖：1 ml/kg D_{50}；2 ml/kg D_{25}；5 ml/kg D_{10}。
– 多巴胺：5～20 μg/(kg · min)。
– 多巴酚丁胺：5～20 μg/(kg · min)。
– 肾上腺素：0.01 mg/kg 1∶10 000(最大剂量 1 mg)q3～5 min；如果没有静脉/静脉注射通道，通过 ETT 可以给 0.1 mg/kg(1∶1 000)；过敏反应 0.01 mg/kg 肌内注射 1∶1 000(最大剂量 0.5 mg)。
– 肾上腺素：0.1～1 μg/(kg · min)。
– 依托咪酯：0.3 mg/kg。
– 氢化可的松：25 mg(针对 CAH)。
– 氨胺酮：2 mg/kg，4 mg/kg 肌内注射。
– 利多卡因：1 mg/kg(最大剂量 150 mg)。
– 镁剂：50 mg/kg(最大剂量 2 g)。
– 甘露醇：0.5～1 g/kg。
– 米力农：50 μg/kg 负载 30 min 以上，维持剂量 0.25～0.75 μg/(kg · min)。
– 纳洛酮：0.1 mg/kg。
– 去甲肾上腺素：0.05～2 μg/(kg · min)。
– 生理盐水/乳酸林格液：20 mg/kg。
– pRBC：10 ml/kg。
– 前列腺素 E_1：0.1 μg/(kg · min)。
– 普鲁卡因胺：15 mg/kg(最大剂量 1 g，超过 30 min)。
– 异丙酚：2 mg/kg。
– 罗库溴铵：1.2 mg/kg。
– 碳酸氢钠：1 mmol/kg。
– 3% NaCl：5 ml/kg。
– 琥珀酰胆碱：1.5 mg/kg。

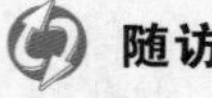

随访

■ 进一步处理

入院指征

• 心肺骤停的幸存者、呼吸衰竭或呼吸功能不全的儿童以及持续性休克的儿童应接受儿科重症监护临床医生的管理。如果需要，进行转移。

出院指征

• 肺或循环系统损害原因迅速解决且无生命危险且预计不会复发(如低血容量或过敏反应)的患者可考虑在长时间观察后出院。

■ 随访建议

• 出院的患者应立即进行初级保健随访，所有家庭都需要支持。
• 为护理人员提供心肺复苏培训资源。
• 对患者和/或护理人员进行自我肾上腺素过敏反应的教育。

要点和误区

• 通过早期识别呼吸衰竭和休克预防心肺骤停。
• 使用基于体重的药物剂量和设备尺寸的参考，以减轻认知负担。
• 让家人有机会为他们的孩子复苏。
• 如果病史不一致或与检查相矛盾，考虑非意外外伤。

耳外伤 Otologic Trauma

Brian Z. Hedges · David A. Pearson 王虑 译

基础知识

■ 描述

耳郭

• 耳软骨没有血供，主要靠软骨膜提供营养。
• 耳郭的血肿常常会影响骨膜和软骨。
– 会导致：
◦ 缺血。
◦ 软骨膜炎。
◦ 坏死。
◦ 菜花耳。
• 刺伤或咬伤可能导致耳软骨感染。

中耳

• 气腔由听小骨组成，易受中耳压力影响(爆炸、潜水)。
• 以颅窝为边界(包括颞骨和乳突)：
• 外伤性骨折可能导致脑脊液漏(耳漏、涕)。
– 会影响到前庭系统。
• 面神经从中耳腔经过，损伤后有可能导致外周神经麻痹。

■ 病因

• 钝器伤：最常见的机动车撞车或打架、接触性运动(摔跤、拳击)。
• 鼓膜被棉拭子或发夹穿破导致的戳伤。
• 动物或人的咬伤。
• 气压伤。
• 雷击伤：
– 鼓膜和听小骨有 50% 可能受雷击的伤害。
• 化学暴露伤。
• 烫伤。
• 潜水伤。
– 内耳气压伤。
– 鼓膜破裂。

儿童注意事项

考虑非偶然性的创伤。

诊断

症状和体征

• 剧烈的耳痛。
• 流血。
• 耳畸形。
- 水肿。
- 血肿。
◦ 淤青、波动感或耳郭块状肿胀。
- 裂开。
- 离断。
- 耳轮廓消失。
• 中耳创伤体征。
- 听力下降。
◦ 若部分听力下降考虑鼓膜破裂。
◦ 完全性听力丧失提示听小骨或内耳受损。
- 耳鸣。
- 中耳有液体流出。
- 外周神经麻痹。
- 前庭症状，如眼球震颤或呕吐。
◦ 内耳损伤也可能出现上述体征。
• 颅底骨折体征。
- 鼓室积血或大量液体流出。
- 耳后血肿。
- 耳漏或鼻液漏。
- 外周神经麻痹。

病史

• 发病机制。
• 外伤史。
• 耳疾病史。
• 药物治疗和过敏史。
• 破伤风状况。

体格检查

• 头痛。
• 脑神经(尤指 CN Ⅶ)。
• 血管结构。
• 耳郭。
• 外耳道。
• 鼓膜。
• 听力。
• 对于鼓膜破裂或穿孔患者可以考虑做韦伯和林纳测试以评估听力：
- 林纳试验：将振动的音叉柄置于患者乳突，直到听不到声音时再将音叉放到耳边：
◦ 正常：患者还能听见音叉的声音；气导大于骨导。
◦ 异常：听不见声音；气导小于骨导，提示传导性听力缺失。
- 韦伯试验：将振动的音叉柄置于患者前额。
◦ 正常：两侧声音大小相同。
◦ 因神经感觉缺失导致听力异常：患耳侧声音小。
◦ 因骨传导缺失导致听力异常：患耳侧声音大。

诊断检查与说明

实验室检查

如果有感染迹象，可以考虑伤口培养；如果有化脓性耳漏，可以考虑液体培养。

影像学检查

• 头面部 CT 平扫评估颅内伤或骨折。
• 若有严重中耳损伤征象，可做颞骨 CT 平扫。

鉴别诊断

• 感染。
• 血管瘤。
• 耳异物。

治疗

院前

若耳离断了，用湿纱布包裹放入塑料袋中，将袋子放在冰块上(切勿将冰块直接敷在截肢的四肢上)。

初步稳定/治疗

• 检查生命体征，对伤情做全面评估，必要时进行复苏。
• 无菌敷料覆盖伤口。

急诊治疗/程序

• 所有受伤的情况：
- 麻醉：
◦ 局部神经阻滞麻醉可以用 1%利多卡因或 0.25%布比卡因阻断下颌神经的耳颞分支、枕小神经、耳大神经和迷走神经耳支。
◦ 另外也可做环形局部浸润麻醉。
- 修复或切开引流后加压敷料：
◦ 将凡士林纱布填满耳郭的缝隙。
◦ 将纱布放在耳郭前后。
◦ 用柔软的纱布紧紧缠绕头部使其固定到位。
- 必要时预防性注射破伤风抗毒素。
• 特殊伤情。
- 耳血肿：
◦ 软骨膜重新贴近软骨以防止软骨坏死的引流势在必行。
◦ 可在受伤后 7 日内(在肉芽组织形成之前)进行。
◦ 吸引：
- 如果还没有形成血块，最好使用 18～20G 针头抽吸。
- 快速抽出血肿直到完全排出；加压敷料。
◦ 切开引流：对大血肿或凝结的血肿效果更好，用 15 号手术刀片沿耳缘做弧线切割，引流；在切口上加压敷料或缝合牙辊。
◦ 如果再次出现血肿是由于再积聚，则应再次抽出血肿并放置灯芯引流。
• 撕裂伤：
- 预防性使用抗生素还有争议，若是动物或人咬伤需用阿莫西林-克拉维酸抗感染。
- 清洁伤口，清除失活组织。
- 浅表伤：清洁伤口，抗生素药膏涂抹。
- 简单撕裂伤：可用单丝尼龙线或聚丙烯线缝合，然后加压包扎；也可用可吸收线缝合，以避免日后为拆线不得不将耳弯曲。
- 耳软骨暴露：仔细将伤口边缘修剪整齐，软骨要完全覆盖以防止软骨膜炎，可以去除一些小软骨以使皮肤可以连接，将近端软骨用可吸收线固定在骨性标志物上。
- 撕脱伤：
◦ <2 cm 的撕脱：可以通过移植存活。
◦ >2 cm 的撕脱：需紧急求助耳鼻喉科医师或整形科医师。
- TM 穿孔：
◦ 通常不需要手术治疗，因为大多数是自发愈合的。
◦ 可提供环丙沙星-地塞米松，如果受到污染(例如，如果发生在水中)。
◦ 避免让水进入耳道直到痊愈。
◦ 请参考耳鼻喉科进行重新评估，以确保愈合并考虑"打补丁"。

药物治疗

• 阿莫西林-克拉维酸：成人：875/125 mg，口服，每日 2 次[儿童：40 mg/(kg·d)，口服，每日 2 次]。
• 双氯西林：250～500 mg，口服，每日 4 次[儿童：30～50 mg/(kg·d)，口服，q6 h]。
• 环丙沙星-地塞米松耳用：4 滴，每日 2 次，连用 7～10 日。

随访

进一步处理

入院指征

• 不能接受口服抗生素治疗。
• 需要静脉用抗生素。
• 免疫缺陷的患者同时伴有严重感染、软骨膜炎或软骨炎。

E

出院指征

- 能口服抗生素。
- 便于安排随访。

随访建议

- 缝合后 5 日要随访。
- 血肿处理 24 h 后要随访，以评估再发的风险。

二尖瓣脱垂 Mitral Valve Prolapse

Liudvikas Jagminas 段立伟 译

基础知识

描述

- 二尖瓣的一个或多种病变导致的临床综合征。
- 当二尖瓣小叶边缘不闭合时发生。
- 通常是由于二尖瓣一个瓣叶在收缩期的异常的拉伸导致的：
  - 瓣叶的松质层黏液瘤增生引起纤维层的局部中断。
  - 腱索的过度伸展，牵引乳头肌。
- 胸痛的理论机制：
  - 小叶之间的角处的血小板聚集和纤维蛋白沉积导致冠状动脉微栓塞使心肌局灶性缺血。
  - 冠状动脉痉挛。
- 一些患者可发生二尖瓣反流。
- 发病年龄为 10～16 岁。
- 女性＞男性(3∶1)。
- 年轻女性通常为良性，而对于＞50 岁的男性，易发生严重的结局，往往因为大量反流需要手术治疗。
- 超声心动图检查可发现 2%～4%普通人群存在二尖瓣脱垂，尸体解剖检出率为 7%。
- 一些患者可发生多种神经内分泌和自主神经紊乱。
- 遗传学：
  - 强遗传背景。
  - 有时呈现外显率差异的常染色体显性遗传。

病因

- 马方综合征。
- 复发性多软骨炎。
- Ehlers-Danlos 综合征(如Ⅰ、Ⅱ、Ⅳ型)。
- 成骨不全症。
- 弹性假黄色瘤。
- 斯蒂克勒综合征。
- 系统性红斑狼疮。
- 多动脉炎结节。
- 多囊肾。
- 冯维勒布兰德综合征。
- 杜氏肌营养不良症。

诊断

症状和体征

分为 3 类：

- 与自主功能失调的相关症状。
- 与二尖瓣反流进展相关的症状。
- 相关并发症导致的症状(如脑卒中、心内膜炎或心律失常)。

病史

- 心悸的发生率高达 40%：
  - 通常为室性期前收缩或阵发性室上性心动过速。
  - 高达 40%的患者有自主神经功能异常症状。
- 胸痛的发生率为 10%：
  - 尖锐、局部、持续时间变异和非劳累性。
- 很少可能对硝酸甘油有反应。
- 惊恐发作。
- 焦急。
- 疲倦。
- 抑郁症高达 70%。
- 神经质。
- 偏头痛。
- 肠易激。
- 晕厥：
  - 发生率为 0.9%。
- 立位晕厥。
- 呼吸困难和疲劳比较少见。

体格检查

- 心尖部收缩中晚期喀喇音：
  - 站立或 Valsalva 动作时喀喇音接近第一心音。
  - 当脱垂在收缩早期出现时可加重第一心音。
  - 蹲踞动作时喀喇音接近第二心音。
- 晚收缩期杂音。
- 2/3 的患者可观察到骨骼异常：
  - 高度与重量比大于正常。
  - 臂展大于身高(细长指)。
  - 脊柱侧弯。
  - 漏斗胸。
  - 蜘蛛足样指。
  - 关节过度活动度。
- 乳腺过小。
- 巨腭。

基本检查

- 病史和心脏收缩中期喀喇音有利于诊断。
- 临床证据不足时，心脏超声有利于确诊。

诊断检查与说明

实验室检查

对确定诊断无意义。

影像学检查

- 心电图：
  - 通常是正常的。
  - 偶尔会在Ⅲ和 aVF 导联出现 ST-T 段压低和反转。
  - QT 间期延迟和永久性 Q 波。
  - 过早的心房和心室收缩。
- 胸片：
  - 通常正常。
  - 如果二尖瓣反流存在，可能会显示左心房和左心室扩大。
  - 马方综合征患者会出现二尖瓣环钙化。
- 心脏超声：
  - 典型二尖瓣脱垂：胸骨旁长轴观显示：收缩期二尖瓣小叶上移至左心房＞2 mm，瓣叶厚度＜5 mm。
  - 非典型二尖瓣脱垂：移位＞2 mm，最大瓣叶厚度＜5 mm。
  - 其他可作为诊断标准的超声心动图发现：瓣叶增厚，冗余，环形扩张，脊索延伸。
  - 次要标准：
    - 收缩期孤立的轻、中度二尖瓣后叶上移。
    - 收缩期两个瓣叶的中度上移。

诊断步骤/外科

当患者存在原因不明的胸痛时可行手术诊断。

鉴别诊断

- 心肌梗死与缺血。
- 肥厚型心肌病梗阻。
- 特发性肥厚性主动脉瓣下狭窄。
- 快速性心律失常。
- 心房颤动与扑动。
- 室间隔缺损。
- 乳头肌功能不全。
- 低钾血症。
- 低镁血症。
- 心脏瓣膜病。
- 嗜铬细胞瘤。
- 贫血。
- 甲状腺毒症。
- 妊娠。
- 可卡因、苯丙胺或其他拟交感神经药中毒。
- 室性心动过速。
- 预激综合征。
- 风湿性心内膜炎。
- 焦虑与恐慌症。
- 应激。
- 更年期。

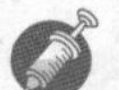

治疗

院前

- ABC 管理。
- 静脉通路。
- 补充氧气。
- 心电监测。
- 脉搏血氧监测。

初步稳定/治疗

- 心电监测。
- 吸氧。
- 静脉导管放置。

急诊治疗/程序

- 一般不需药物治疗，心悸严重时可给予β受体阻滞剂。
- 当患者出现短暂性缺血或脑卒中症状时，可给予抗血小板药物（阿司匹林、阿司匹林和缓释双嘧达莫、氯吡格雷）。
- 存在直立性低血压或晕厥前期症状时，应给予氯化钠片剂。如果治疗无效，可给予氟氢可的松。
- 补充镁剂：可改善典型二尖瓣脱垂患者症状。
- 对于存在高血压的患者，使用 ACEI 可以改善二尖瓣关闭不全症状。
- β受体阻滞剂：
  - 心动过速或严重胸部疼痛的患者使用。
- 地高辛：可用来治疗室上性心动过速和防止胸部疼痛和疲劳。
- 抗生素预防：
  - 需外科手术时（如被污染的创面修复、脓肿切开引流）。
  - 以下也情况提示可用：
    - 存在杂音。
    - 超声心动图显示二尖瓣关闭不全严重。
    - 男性>45 岁伴有瓣膜增厚。
  - 对只存在喀喇音而没有杂音，超声心动图显示无二尖瓣关闭不全证据或没有感染性心内膜炎的患者不建议预防性用药。

药物治疗

一线药物

- 阿莫西林：手术前 1 h 2 g 口服（儿童：手术前 1 h 50 mg/kg，口服）。
- 氨苄西林：手术前 30 min 2 g，静脉或肌内注射（儿童：手术前 30 min 50 mg/kg，静脉或肌内注射）。
- 克林霉素：手术前 1 h 600 mg，口服（儿童：手术前 1 h 20 mg/kg，口服，不超过 600 mg）。
- 普萘洛尔：1～3 mg，静脉滴注；1 mg/min，80～640 mg/d，口服[儿童：1～4 mg/(kg・d)，口服，2 次/日或 4 次/日]。
- 异丙肾上腺素：0.02～0.06 mg，静脉注射 1 次；0.01～0.02 mg，静脉注射或 2～20 mg/min 滴注。
- 阿替洛尔：0.3～2 mg/(kg・d)，口服，最大剂量 2 mg/(kg・d)。

二线药物

- 地高辛：0.5～1 mg，静脉或肌内注射。先给予 50%剂量，然后 25%分 2 次给予（q6～12 h）；或 0.125～0.5 mg/d，口服。
- 氟氢可的松：0.05～0.10 mg/d，口服。

随访

进一步处理

入院指征

- 重度二尖瓣关闭不全。
- 剧烈胸痛、缺血症状。
- 晕厥或近似晕厥。
- 危及生命的心律失常。
- 脑缺血事件，包括短暂性脑缺血发作。

出院指征

- 无症状。
- 没有实验室检查异常。
- 没有显著二尖瓣关闭不全或心律失常。

转诊问题

- 心脏科会诊以预防心室心律失常或猝死，以及严重的二尖瓣关闭不全的症状出现。
- 对于考虑瓣叶置换或修复的患者推荐心胸外科进一步治疗。
  - 有症状患者。
  - 心房颤动。
  - 射血分数<50%～60%。
  - 左心室收缩末期内径>45～50 mm。
  - 肺动脉压>50～60 mmHg。
- 瓣叶修复因不需后续抗凝治疗要优先于瓣叶置换。
- 飞行员伴有二尖瓣脱垂时，在正向 G 压力下可发展为二尖瓣反流（MR），并存在心律失常或晕厥的风险。

儿科注意事项

心律失常、猝死和感染性心内膜炎有过报道。

老年人注意事项

- 多呈现为非典型类型：
  - 多可能有全收缩期杂音和更严重的二尖瓣关闭不全。
- 但出现腱索断裂时可出现心力衰竭等相关的复杂症状。

妊娠注意事项

二尖瓣脱垂促成妊娠期任何风险的加重。

随访建议

- 3～5 年评估一次，以评估疾病进展。
- 二尖瓣脱垂和二尖瓣关闭不全的患者进行风险手术时，推荐使用抗生素预防感染性心内膜炎。
- 患者运动时发生胸痛时应排除冠状动脉异常。
- 当存在以下情况时，二尖瓣脱垂和存在心脏杂音患者应避免高强度的竞技运动。
  - 心律失常相关的晕厥。
  - 二尖瓣脱垂相关的猝死家族史。
  - 显著的室上性或室性心律失常。
  - 中度到重度二尖瓣关闭不全。

要点和误区

- 二尖瓣脱垂的诊断不应该是终止进一步诊断性评估患者胸痛、心悸、呼吸困难或晕厥症状的理由。
- 二尖瓣脱垂是导致运动员猝死的第三常见病因。

E

发绀 Cyanosis

Michael S. Murphy 陈奇通 译

基础知识

描述

皮肤或黏膜的异常的蓝紫色改变。

- 由毛细血管中去氧血红蛋白或血红蛋白衍生物异常增多造成：
  - 去氧血红蛋白>5 g/dl。
  - 高铁血红蛋白>1.5 g/dl。
  - 硫化血红蛋白>0.5 g/dl。
- 去氧血红蛋白的绝对含量致使形成蓝色斑点。
  - 氧合血红蛋白的含量不影响血液颜色。
  - 发绀在红细胞增多症的患者中较贫血患者更为常见。
- 发绀可随皮肤厚度和肤色呈现不同变化。
- 去氧血红蛋白的累积可产生全身性的中心性发绀或局限性的周围性发绀。
  - 中心性发绀：
    - 血氧不足。
    - 解剖学上由右向左分流。
    - 异常的血红蛋白衍生物。
  - 周围性发绀：
    - 组织从血液中摄取高于正常量的氧。
    - 低灌注。
    - 冷空气或冷水致使血管收缩。
    - 动脉供血不足。
    - 静脉功能不全。
    - 手足发绀：发病原因尚不明确的无痛的、对称的肢体末端发绀。

病因

中心性发绀

- 上呼吸道阻塞原因。
- 肺功能受损：
  - 通气不足：
    - 肺炎。
    - 慢性阻塞性肺病。
    - 肺水肿。
  - 通气血流灌注比值失调：
    - 哮喘。
    - 肺栓塞。
  - 弥散问题：
    - 间质性肺病。
    - 解剖分流。
  - 肺动静脉瘘：
    - 遗传性出血性毛细血管扩张症。
  - 16 000 ft 高海拔与降低大气压力相关。
  - 减少吸入氧气房火灾/毒气。
- 右向左分流型心脏异常：
  - 艾森门格综合征：
    - 肺动脉高压。
    - 长期存在的心内分流（室间隔缺损、动脉导管未闭、房间隔缺损）。
    - 肺动脉压超过阈值时导致的血流逆转。
- 异常血红蛋白：
  - 低氧亲和力血红蛋白突变体：
    - Kansas 血红蛋白。
    - Beth Israel 血红蛋白。
    - St. Mande 血红蛋白。
  - 先天性高铁血红蛋白症：
    - 细胞色素 B5 还原酶缺乏。
    - 血红蛋白 M 病。
  - 获得性高铁血红蛋白症：
    - 苯胺染料。
    - 氯喹、伯氨喹。
    - 氨苯砜。
    - 局麻药物如利多卡因。
    - 高剂量亚甲基蓝。
    - 萘。
    - 亚硝酸盐、硝酸甘油。
    - 磺胺类药物。
    - 蚕豆。
  - 硫化血红蛋白：
    - 一般良性。
    - 不可逆的血红蛋白改变。
    - 多种药物均可引起。
    - 二甲基亚砜。
    - 油漆。
    - 非那西汀。
    - 非那吡啶。
    - 对苯二胺。
    - 苯基羟胺。
    - 磺胺。
    - 磺胺吡啶。
    - 磺胺噻唑。
    - 硫化物。

外周性发绀

- 休克。
- 过度寒冷。
- 动脉供血不足。
- 静脉功能不全。
- 雷诺现象。
- 手足发绀。

儿科注意事项

- 心脏：
  - 先天性发绀：
    - 法洛四联症。
    - 大血管错位。
    - 动脉干。
    - 三尖瓣闭锁。
    - 三尖瓣下移畸形。
    - 假缩窄。
    - 动脉管未闭。
  - 肺静脉回流异常。
- 肺动脉狭窄：
  - 任何右向左分流。
- 呼吸系统：
  - 上呼吸道疾病：
    - 哮喘。
    - 细菌性气管炎。
    - 会厌炎。
    - 咽后脓肿。
    - 异物。
  - 下呼吸道疾病：
    - 哮喘。
    - 细支气管炎。
    - 肺炎。
    - 囊性纤维化。
    - 肺水肿、心力衰竭。
    - 肺栓塞。
- 神经系统：
  - 屏住呼吸。

诊断

症状和体征

- 皮肤和黏膜的蓝变色，按压可以变白：
  - 巧克力色：
    - 高铁血红蛋白症。
  - 石灰色：
    - 高铁血红蛋白症，硫血红蛋白。
  - 红蓝色：
    - 静脉淤滞。

病史

- 发绀出现的时间。
- 相关症状：
  - 疼痛。
  - 呼吸困难。
  - 疲劳。
  - 头痛。

F

- 精神状态改变。
- 用药清单。
- 职业暴露或化学药物的使用。

体格检查

- 休克和呼吸窘迫时的一般状况和重要生命体征。
- 按压是否可以变色？
  - 与异常的皮肤色素沉着鉴别。
- 变色的位置。
  - 四肢和黏膜对称性分布。
    - 中心性发绀。
  - 头、颈及上肢。
    - 上腔静脉综合征。
  - 下肢与上肢不受影响。
    - 差异性发绀。
    - 假性狭窄和动脉导管未闭。
    - 下腔静脉综合征。
  - 单侧肢体。
    - 动脉和静脉不全。
  - 对称的，疼痛的，累及四肢的。
    - 雷诺症。
  - 对称的，无痛的，累及四肢的且面部多汗。
    - 手足发绀。
- 杵状指。
  - 慢性缺氧。
- 肺部检查。
- 心脏检查。
- 四肢水肿状态、脉冲和体温。

基本检查

- 评估气道通气是首要的：
  - 稳定气道并提供足够的通气。
- 调查低氧的原因：
  - 心血管和呼吸系统问题常见。
  - 考虑高铁血红蛋白血症。

诊断检查与说明

实验室检查

- 脉搏血氧饱和度：
  - 不评估通气。
  - 下述情况可能结果不准确：
    - 异常的血红蛋白。
    - 指甲油。
    - 皮肤色素沉着。
    - 低灌注。
    - 使用某些重要的染料。
- 动脉血气：
  - 氧分压。
  - 测量血氧饱和度。
  - 氧分压正常的发绀，考虑高铁血红蛋白血症。
  - 高铁血红蛋白血症时血液呈巧克力色。
  - 高铁血红蛋白水平。
- 全血化学：
  - 检测血红蛋白。
- 新生儿先天性发绀进行高氧试验：
  - 吸 100% O_2 后 PO_2 未增至 100 mmHg，怀疑先天性心脏病。

影像学检查

- 胸部X线片检测呼吸或心脏病理：
  - 检查吸气/呼气视图是否有异物。
  - 疑似隐匿性气胸的呼气视图检测。
- 颈部X线摄片检测上呼吸道疾病：
  - 异物。
  - 尖塔影(哮喘)。
  - 椎前肿胀(咽后脓肿)。
  - 会厌肿胀。
- 心电图：
  - 心律失常、损伤或缺血。
- 超声：
  - 如果间隔缺损、疑似分流则做气泡研究。
  - 室壁运动、心脏瓣膜异常。
  - 心包积液。

鉴别诊断

- 异常的皮肤色素沉着(按压不能消退)：
  - 胺碘酮。
  - 米诺环素。
  - 长期大剂量氯丙嗪。
  - 银中毒(银沉积)。
  - 砷。
  - 尿黑酸尿症。
  - 金质沉着病(继发于胃肠道给药途径的金盐)。
  - 文身。
- 色汗症：
  - 罕见的分泌带颜色的汗液。

治疗

院前

- 评估并建立气道。
- 纠正呼吸道阻塞。
- 识别气管插管移位。
- 100%氧气使用无重复吸入装置。
- 确保充足的通气。
- 识别需要建立明确的气道。
- 迅速纠正张力性气胸。
- 如果怀疑有创伤应保护颈椎。
- 静脉通道，监测脉搏血氧饱和度。
- 支气管痉挛时用沙丁胺醇喷雾。
- 严重的哮喘使用外消旋肾上腺素雾化器。
- 肺水肿治疗方案的管理。

初步稳定/治疗

- 100%无重复吸入装置供给氧气。
- 立即评估并处理呼吸道问题。

一般治疗措施

- 识别并处理心肺异常。
- 高铁血红蛋白血超标30%使用亚甲蓝。
  - 患者有G-6-PD缺乏症时不能使用。

药物治疗

- 沙丁胺醇雾化吸入：0.03 ml/kg(5 mg/ml)。
- 地塞米松：(对于哮吼)0.75～9 mg/d 分次，q6～12 h。
- 呋塞米：0.5 mg/kg，静脉注射，超过1～2 min。如果效果不佳1 h后可用加倍剂量。
- 镁制剂：2 g，静脉注射，超过10 min (40 mg/kg，静脉注射，超过20 min)。
- 亚甲蓝：1～2 mg/kg，静脉注射，1%溶液超过5 min。
- 甲泼尼龙：1～2 mg/kg，静脉注射，q6 h。
- 吗啡：2～4 mg，静脉注射(0.05～0.1 mg/kg，静脉注射，q2 h，PRN)。
- 硝酸甘油：使用非PVC输液管5 μg/min，滴注5 μg/min每3～5 min直到达到预期效果。
- 前列腺素 E_1：0.05～0.1 μg/(kg·min)，静脉注射；最大量为0.4 μg/(kg·min)。
- 外消旋肾上腺素雾化：0.25～0.75 ml 2.25%外消旋肾上腺素加入2 ml生理盐水中稀释吸入。

随访

进一步处理

入院指征

- 最受影响的患者应当被送至医院。
- 不稳定的发绀患者需要ICU监护。

出院指征

缺氧病因已被逆转：

- 反应性呼吸道疾病对β受体激动剂有反应。
- 充血性心力衰竭患者有肺水肿但无明显可疑的心肌损伤和多尿。

要点和误区

- 首先假设为低氧血症，并立即评估气道和呼吸功能。
- 积极给氧后仍为巧克力色血液或氧饱和度不变：考虑高铁血红蛋白症。

F

发热(成人)

Matthew L. Wong · Timothy K. Lynch 万健 译

基础知识

描述

• 发热是由于体内体温调节点升高而引起核心体温的升高。

• 下丘脑前体合成前列腺素 E_2(PGE₂)控制体温调节器，达到退热目的。

• 核心体温波动于 37±2 ℃。

• 下丘脑自主放电可通过寒战和皮肤血管收缩升高核心体温。

• 核心体温的正常生理节律变化在凌晨最小，午后最大。

• 外源性和因源性的因素都能升高体温调定点：

– 内源性致热源包括 PGE_2、IL－1、IL－6、TNF、IFN－γ。

– 外源性致热源包括内毒素脂多糖(LPS)和其他 TLR 配体、中毒性休克综合征毒素(TSST－1)和其他 MHCⅡ配体。

• 体温最高＞41.5 ℃。

– 最常见的原因是中枢神经系统出血。

– 由于局部创伤、出血、肿瘤或内在的下丘脑功能不全，下丘脑设定值可能会升高到极端水平。

• 接受抗细胞因子药物或糖皮质激素治疗者发热的反应受损。

• 不明原因发热(FUO)：

– 发热＞38.3 ℃，门诊至少 3 周或住院 3 日，或门诊就诊 3 次以上未能确定病因。

病因

• 感染进程：

– 中枢神经系统、胸部和肺、胃肠道、泌尿生殖系统、皮肤、软组织和骨骼、血管和心脏。

– 医源性：导管、植入物、硬物、近期的外科感染灶。

• 中枢神经系统进展，如脑血管意外、创伤、癫痫。

• 肿瘤性发热。

• 药物热：

– 大多数药物可通过各种广泛的机制引起体温上调。

– 中毒综合征(如肾上腺素能药物、抗胆碱能药物、多巴胺、水杨酸过量、血清毒素)。

– 超敏反应：

◦ 过敏反应。

◦ 血清病。

– Jarisch-Herxheimer 反应。

– 刺激性药物引起局部静脉炎。

• 撤药反应：

– 酒精(乙醇)。

– 苯二氮䓬类药物。

• 系统性风湿性和炎症疾病(如家族性地中海发热、风湿性关节炎、结节病、系统性红斑狼疮、脉管炎)。

• 内分泌：

– 甲亢、嗜铬细胞瘤。

• 其他原因：

– 酒精性肝硬化。

– 金属烟雾热：

◦ 急性吸入暴露。

◦ 当某些金属被加热时暴露在烟雾中。

◦ 焊工通常暴露在外。

◦ 主要是氧化锌、氧化铝或氧化镁。

– 棉花热：

◦ 静脉药物依赖者使用受污染的棉花消毒注射后引起的发热。

– 镰状细胞病。

– 溶血性贫血。

– 肺栓塞。

• 不明来源发热的常见病因：

– 感染性：

◦ 腹腔和骨盆肿块。

◦ 心源性(心内膜炎、心包炎)。

◦ 猫抓病。

◦ 巨细胞病毒感染。

◦ EB 病毒感染。

◦ 结核(粟粒样、肾或脑结核)。

◦ 肠伤寒。

◦ 黑热病。

– 肿瘤性：

◦ 结肠腺癌。

◦ 肝癌和肝转移癌。

◦ 骨髓增生异常。

◦ 白血病和淋巴瘤。

◦ 肾细胞癌。

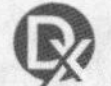

诊断

症状和体征

病史

• 寒战：

– 提示菌血症。

• 体重下降：

– 提示肿瘤、慢性感染或内分泌异常。

• 夜间盗汗：

– 提示肿瘤、慢性炎症性疾病或结核。

• 特殊热型：

– 日间体温升高。

◦ 粟粒性结核、伤寒热、结节性多动脉炎。

– 回归热：发热期和无热期相互间隔：

◦ 可见于疟疾、伯氏疏螺旋体感染、鼠咬热和淋巴瘤。

– 弛张热：体温有所下降，但未降至正常。

◦ 见于结核和病毒性疾病。

– 间歇热：昼夜节律变化增大。

◦ 见于全身性感染、肿瘤和药物热。

– 双峰热：

◦ 24 h 内通常有 2 个体温高峰。

◦ 不明原因发热，考虑粟粒性结核、黑热病和疟疾。

• 发热的高危因素：

– 抗细胞因子治疗(如 TNF－α 单克隆抗体、磷酸酶抑制剂)。

– 使用糖皮质激素。

– 免疫抑制状态。

– 疫苗接种不完全。

– 静脉应用药物。

– 妊娠和围生期患者。

– 皮疹。

– 近期的化疗史。

– 近期的旅游史。

– 脾切除术。

体格检查

• 核心体温升高：

– 直肠温度＞38 ℃(100.4 ℉)或口腔温度＞37.5 ℃(99.5 ℉)。

– 年龄超过 65 岁时体温阈值下降，因此发热反应不强。

• 出汗：

– 严重高热而不出汗提示抗胆碱能药物中毒或热休克。

• 心动过速：

– 体温升高 1 ℉，脉率增快 10 次/分。

– 相对心动过缓(Faget 征)：

◦ 可见于疟疾、伤寒热、中枢神经系统异常、淋巴瘤、药物热、布鲁菌病、鸟疫、军团菌病、莱姆病和人工性发热。

• 肌肉强直、抽搐和反射亢进：
- 可见于特殊的中毒综合征和药物性状态。
• 精神状态改变：
- 中毒：代谢性脑病和中枢神经系统异常。
• 皮疹：
- 皮损类型、分布和进展情况可为诊断提供线索。
- 涉及瘀斑、紫癜、水疱、黏膜或手掌和足底时需要特殊的注意。
• 甲亢的症状：
- 甲状腺肿。
- 突眼。

基本检查

• 测定直肠温度判断核心体温最为准确。
- 非血管性：直肠、食管或膀胱。
- 血管性：肺动脉导管(金标准)。
• 当精确测量体温会影响临床决策时，不应使用外周温度计(鼓膜、颞动脉、腋窝或口腔温度计)。
• 详细的询问病史和体格检查可确定是否需要进一步的诊断性检查。
- 应询问相关病史，包括接触患者、既往感染史、职业暴露、近期旅行、药物、动物或蜱类接触史和免疫状态。

诊断检查与说明

实验室检查

• 全血细胞计数：
- 有高危因素的患者诊断中性粒细胞减少症的重要检查。
- 中性粒细胞增多和杆状核粒细胞增多提示细菌感染。
- 淋巴细胞增多提示伤寒、结核、布鲁菌病和病毒感染性疾病。
- 非典型的淋巴细胞增多可见于单核细胞增多症、巨细胞病毒感染、人类免疫缺陷病毒感染、风疹、水痘、麻疹和病毒性肝炎。
- 单核细胞增多提示结核、布鲁菌病、病毒感染性疾病和淋巴瘤。
• 乳酸：
- 反复测定乳酸有助于监测脓毒症、危险分层和决定治疗策略。
• 尿常规和尿培养。
• 血培养：
- 所有全身疾病和有菌血症风险的患者需行血培养。
• 有寄生虫感染和红细胞内感染风险的患者行厚层和薄层血涂片和疟疾抗原检测。
• 可疑患者行粪便培养和难辨梭状杆菌检查。
• 部分患者选择性的嗜异性抗体检测。
• 红细胞沉降率(血沉)和 C 反应蛋白检查通常并无帮助：
- 红细胞沉降率明显增高提示心内膜炎、骨髓炎、结核和风湿性疾病。

老年人注意事项

免疫活性下降、全身播散的风险增加、暴露于卫生保健机构的机会增加，可能有共存疾病。

影像学检查

• 胸部 X 线检查：
- 体格检查发现心肺疾病及不明原因发热的患者需行胸片检查。
• 如考虑需行腰椎穿刺和有骨髓炎可能时，建议 CT 或 MRI 检查。

鉴别诊断

• 热疗：
- 体温调节正常的温度升高。
- 内生热过多或内生热量超过机体散热能力所致。
- 不涉及致热分子，特征是对退热药无反应。
- 见热疗。

治疗

院前

• 不需要特殊的干预。
• 不稳定的或精神状态改变的患者应予以监测并建立静脉通路。

初步稳定/治疗

• 不稳定的患者行 ABC 管理。
• 疑似脓毒症或生命体征不稳定的患者，尤其是严重细菌感染的高危患者，开始给予早期广谱抗生素治疗。

急诊治疗/程序

• 退热：
- 一般给予对乙酰氨基酚或非甾体抗炎药。
◦ 抑制环氧化酶，从而阻断前列腺素的合成。
• 中性白细胞减少的患者给予经验性抗生素治疗：
- 联合用药：
◦ 广谱 β-内酰胺类(头孢他啶、哌拉西林)联合氨基糖苷类抗生素。
- 单药：
◦ 头孢噻肟。
◦ 头孢他啶。
◦ 丙米嗪。
• 经验性抗生素治疗脾切除术后患者包膜性细菌感染。
• 经验性抗病毒治疗脑炎和可能有弥散性病毒感染的患者(如近期器官或骨髓移植的患者、获得性免疫缺陷综合征患者)。
• 不建议体外降温。

药物治疗

• 退热药物：
- 对乙酰氨基酚：650～1 000 mg，口服/灌肠，q4～6 h，24 h 不超过 4 g。
- 阿司匹林：650 mg，口服，q4 h，24 h 不超过 4 g。
- 布洛芬：800 mg，口服，q6 h。
• 抗生素：
- 头孢噻肟：2 g，静脉注射，q12 h。
- 头孢他啶：2 g，静脉注射，q8 h。
- 庆大霉素或妥布霉素：2 mg/kg，静脉注射负荷量，1.7 mg/kg，q8 h 加哌拉西林-他唑巴坦 3.375 g，静脉注射，q4 h；或替卡西林-克拉维酸 3.1 g，静脉注射，q4 h。
- 亚胺培南-西司他丁：500～1000 mg，静脉注射，q8 h。
- 美罗培南：1 g，静脉注射，q8 h。
- 环丙沙星：750 mg，口服，每日 2 次加阿莫西林-克拉维酸 875 mg，口服，每日 2 次。
• 抗病毒：
- 单纯疱疹病毒和水痘-带状疱疹病毒。
- 阿昔洛韦：10～15 mg/kg，静脉注射，q8 h。
- A 型和 B 型流感病毒。
- 奥司他韦：75 mg，口服，q12 h。

随访

进一步处理

入院指征

• 生命体征不稳定需要收入 ICU 的患者。
• 当发热来源确定后根据病情决定处置方案。
• 某些发热原因不明的高危人群：
- 中性白细胞减少的患者。
- 免疫抑制或免疫功能低下的患者。
- 脾切除术后的患者。

F

- 静脉药物依赖者。

• 年龄>60 岁或糖尿病患者入院标准有所降低。

出院指征

免疫功能低下的患者生命体征稳定后，发热原因明确的患者或怀疑非危及生命的感染的患者，出院是安全的。

转诊问题

发热的病因决定应转诊给初级保健医师或专科医师治疗。

随访注意

合理的门诊治疗和随访可协助进一步评估病因。

要点和误区

• 脓毒症需要监测乳酸。

• 早期、经验性、广谱抗生素治疗脓毒症。

• 需考虑所有感染的可能原因。

• 对于免疫抑制、高龄和静脉毒品使用者需严密诊治。

发热(儿童) Fever, Pediatric

Daniel J. Tonellato · David A. Peak　万健 译

基础知识

描述

• 发热定义为直肠温度 38℃(100.4℉)。

- 一般口温和耳温低 0.6～1℃。

• 6 个月以内婴儿耳温值不准确。当测量外耳后部和上部时，在螺旋顶端和小叶下缘之间的中点。

• 腋窝温度一般不可靠。

• 有可靠发热病史的无发热的儿童应认为有发热。

• 在急诊室就诊的儿童中，占 20%以上。目前的挑战是确定那些有明显潜在感染的儿童。

病因

• 概述：

- 菌血症。

- ≤90 日的婴儿：大肠杆菌和 B 组链球菌。

- 较大婴儿：肺炎链球菌。B 型流感嗜血杆菌在广泛的免疫接种中不常见。

- 病毒性疾病，常伴有皮疹(水痘、玫瑰疹、风疹)、柯萨奇病毒(手足口病)。

- B 型流感病毒疫苗和肺炎疫苗可减少嗜血杆菌和肺炎的发病率。

• 中枢神经系统：脑膜炎、脑炎。

• 头、眼、耳、鼻和喉部疾病：中耳炎、面部蜂窝织炎、眶下/眶周蜂窝织炎、咽炎(A 组溶血性链球菌、疱疹性咽峡炎、腺病毒咽结合膜热)、病毒性龈口炎(疱疹和柯萨奇病毒)、颈淋巴结炎、鼻窦炎、结膜炎、扁桃体周围/咽后壁脓肿。

• 呼吸系统：格鲁布感染(副黏病毒感染)、会厌炎、毛细支气管炎(呼吸道合胞病毒感染)、肺炎、脓胸、流感。

• 心血管系统：化脓性心包炎、心内膜炎、心肌炎。

• 泌尿生殖系统：膀胱炎、肾盂肾炎。

• 消化系统：细菌性腹泻、肠套叠、阑尾炎、肝炎。

• 四肢疾病：脊髓炎、化脓性关节炎、蜂窝织炎。

• 其他疾病：新生儿单纯疱疹感染、川崎病、疫苗接种反应、热惊厥/热休克、人为因素、家族性自主神经功能异常、甲亢、结缔组织病、脉管炎、风湿热、恶性肿瘤、药物热、新生儿脱水热(不常见，去除绑布后 15 min 再次评估)。

• 隐匿性菌血症与许多临床实体有关。高危人群为≤24 个月，发热≥39.4℃，白细胞数为 15 000 个细胞/mm^3。

• 高热，温度>41℃(105.8℉)，通常与严重感染有关。温度>42℃通常是非感染性原因，如高热、头部损伤、药物摄入、恶性高热。

诊断

症状和体征

• 必须评估临床表现。气道、呼吸和循环需要专门评估(特别是有无灌注不足、皮肤颜色改变的脱水特征)。

• 早期服用退热药有助于评估。

• 中毒症状表现为嗜睡、毛细血管充盈时间延长、通气不足或过度通气、哭声无力、进食减少；紫癜或瘀斑和/或肌张力减退。最初的观察是评估的关键。

• 心动过速或呼吸急促可能仅见于病情严重的患儿。

• 体温超过 38℃，每升高 1℃患儿心率增快 10 次/分。

• <24 个月的患儿体温超过 40℃，菌血症的概率明显升高。

• 意识状态的改变：

- 嗜睡提示意识水平降低。

- 抽搐。

- 对周围环境、父母、医师、玩具的反应降低。

- 行为观察对于大于 60 日儿童可能有帮助。

◦ 孩子看着临床医师，集中注意力，自发地探索房间。

◦ 孩子们自发地发出声音或以好玩的方式说话。

◦ 孩子玩耍并伸手去拿东西。

◦ 孩子微笑着与父母或临床医师互动。

◦ 孩子很容易安静下来，与父母或临床医师互动。

• 行体格检查寻找病因。

• 呼吸急促和低氧血症是肺炎最敏感的体征。其他有意义的体征为啰音、低氧血症、咳嗽超过 10 日及发热超过 5 日。

• 反复尿路感染的高危因素包括女孩、包皮过长的男孩、不明原因发热及体温超过 39℃。

• 发热和瘀点可能与病毒性疾病、落基山斑疹热或侵袭性细菌感染有关，最常见的是脑膜炎奈瑟菌。

• 不明原因发热(FUO)是指持续 14 日或更长时间的无明确病因的发热性疾病。病因可能是感染性、胶原血管、恶性肿瘤等。

• 癫痫发作(简单与复杂)。

• 体温超过 42℃通常由非感染性疾病引起。

• 重症感染可能不发热。

• 有潜在恶性肿瘤、中心静脉导管或室-腹腔分流术的患者除了发热外，可能很少有发现。

• 降温药物只控制症状不解决病因。可能

影响患者的评估,尤其是意识状态的评估。

• 约 20%的发热患儿在询问病史和体格检查后找不到明确的病因。

• 严重的细菌感染在患有 ALTE 的婴儿中并不常见。

基本检查

• 血氧饱和度可视为第 5 项生命体征。

• 必要时给予液体复苏。

• 确定疾病的时长、程度、发热的热型、降温药物使用史、既往用药史、药物过敏史、既往和现在的免疫状态、近期用药/抗生素使用史、6 个月以内患儿询问生产史、特殊接触史、喂养情况、活动情况、排尿/排便习惯、旅游史和相关系统问题。

• 寻找相关病因。

• 给予降温治疗。

诊断检查与说明

实验室检查

• 全血细胞计数。

• 所有 6 个月以内男性患儿、12 个月以内包皮过长的男性患儿和 2 岁以内的女性患儿均行尿常规和培养。尿培养标本应通过导尿管或耻骨上穿刺留取。

• 血培养:

- 自动血培养系统可以更快速地检测到病原。

• 有中枢感染症状的患儿及 1～28 日或 30 日的患儿行脑脊液细胞计数、革兰染色、培养、蛋白质和糖原检测。没有感染表现的 28～90 日及更年长的患儿同样需要排除脑炎。

• 有腹泻表现和提示细菌感染的患儿行粪便白细胞计数和培养。

• C 反应蛋白升高通常与提示感染。红细胞沉降率是另一项辅助检测指标。

• 降钙素原在某些情况下也可辅助确诊感染。血清浓度≤0.3 ng/ml 可能有助于作为一项附加测试,以确定小于 91 日的发热婴儿的死亡风险。

• 疑似 HSV 的新生儿应进行血液和脑脊液的 HSV - PCR 检测和皮损检测。

• 病毒检测(PCR)有助于对严重细菌感染进行风险分层。

影像学检查

• 呼吸急促或低氧血症的患儿行胸部 X 线检查排除肺炎。

• 其他检查用于评估感染病因。

鉴别诊断

见病因。

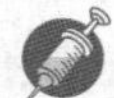

治疗

院前

• 必要时液体复苏。

• 使用解热镇痛药物退热。

初步稳定/治疗

• 处理危及生命的情况。

• 解热镇痛药物治疗。

• 蒸发散热法,如擦浴法,降温作用较小。

急诊治疗/程序

• 局部感染的评估和治疗。

• 小儿中毒症状明显者需立即清除感染灶并应用合适的抗生素治疗。

• 在处理常见急性症状前必须排除全部潜在的危及生命的情况。

• 0～28 日的患儿发热需行白细胞计数、尿常规、培养(血、尿、脑脊液)、腰椎穿刺检查排除脓毒症。怀疑肺炎时行胸部 X 线检查:

- 抗生素:氨苄西林、庆大霉素或头孢噻肟;单纯疱疹病毒感染风险的患儿给予阿昔洛韦治疗。

- 有癫痫、嗜睡、中毒症状、水疱病变、脑脊液多细胞增多或肝酶异常的新生儿应重点考虑 HSV 感染,经验性使用阿昔洛韦抗病毒。

- 住院治疗。

• 29～90 日的患儿应给予必要的检查、选择性应用抗生素(头孢曲松),并在 24 h 内再次评估病情:

- 广泛接种疫苗后 B 型流感病毒和肺炎的发病率明显降低。

- 目前低危患者(见“出院指征”部分的定义)行白细胞计数、尿常规、血培养、尿培养、选择性腰椎穿刺检查及头孢曲松肌内注射,并在 24 h 内再次评估是有益的。

- 尽管在这种情况下腰椎穿刺是选择性的检查,但不做腰椎穿刺仅经验性的抗生素治疗(头孢曲松)是再评估后的折中选择。

- 支气管炎、流感或其他病毒感染在这个年龄组减少,但并不降低细菌感染和脑炎的风险,而且尿路感染的风险也较高。

• 3 个月至 3 岁的患儿有选择性地评估病情,除非有中毒症状,仅出现病毒感染综合征(格鲁布感染、口腔炎、水痘、毛细支气管炎)的患儿一般不需要特殊检查;根据感染指征和培养结果个体化应用抗生素。

- 无相关临床表现、体温超过 39 ℃且无明确感染的患儿,6 个月以内的男性患儿、12 个月以内包皮过长的男性患儿和 2 岁以内的女性患儿均行尿常规和培养。尿培养标本应通过导尿管或耻骨上穿刺留取。

- 6 个月到 3 岁患儿应给予血液检查或腰椎穿刺检查。仅有发热表现就强制性的行腰椎穿刺检查成本效率较低,因此并不常规推荐。

- 3～6 个月免疫功能不完善、白细胞计数超过 15 000/mm^3 且无明确感染的患儿细菌感染的可能性大,在培养结果未报告前给予经验性的抗生素治疗是有益的。

- 3 岁以上的儿童需要对具体发现进行仔细的重点评估。虽然病毒性疾病占主导地位,但像 A 组链球菌、支原体和 EB 病毒这样的生物是常见的。

• 免疫抑制的患儿需要积极评估,发热合并瘀斑、紫癜或镰状细胞疾病的患儿也需要积极的评估。

• 如有耐甲氧西林金黄色葡萄球菌感染的可能,应用克林霉素或复方磺胺甲噁唑可能有效。

• 有恶性肿瘤、深静脉置管或脑室腹腔分流可能的患者除发热外可能有其他新发的问题。

药物治疗

一线用药

• 阿昔洛韦:60 mg/(kg · d),静脉注射,q8 h,持续 14～21 日,视培养物而定。

• 头孢噻肟:100～150 mg/(kg · d),静脉注射,q8 h。

• 头孢曲松:50～100 mg/(kg · d),静脉注射或肌内注射,q12 h。

• 万古霉素:如怀疑肺炎链球菌,40～60 mg/(kg · d),静脉注射,q6～8 h,直到药物敏感试验结果回报。

• 氨苄西林:150 mg/(kg · d),静脉注射,q4～6 h。

• 庆大霉素:5 mg/(kg · d),静脉注射,q8～12 h。

二线用药

• 对乙酰氨基酚:15 mg/kg,口服或灌肠,q4～6 h,24 h 不超过 5 个剂量。

F

• 布洛芬：10 mg/kg，口服，q6～8 h。
• 待定的情况选用特殊的抗生素。

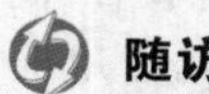

随访

进一步处理

入院指征

• 有中毒症状的患儿。
• 体温超过 38 ℃的 0～28 日的患儿。
• 无中毒症状、体温超过 38 ℃的 29～90 日的患儿，评分达不到低风险组标准者(低风险标准见出院指征)。
• 有发热、瘀斑、紫癜的患儿一般需要住院，除非有不危及生命的明确病因。
• 免疫功能低下的患儿。
• 依从性差或不能行随访的患儿。
• 需要入院治疗的儿童一般应在转院前服用抗生素。

出院指征

• 29～90 日患儿达到以下低风险标准：
- 无住院史、无慢性疾病、无需抗生素治疗、非早产儿。
- 家长可靠、有责任感，家中有电话可随时联系，能及时就诊，家中有体温计，家距离急诊室较近。
- 无明显局部感染的表现(除中耳炎外)、无中毒症状、活动正常、灌注良好、无脱水表现、生命体征平稳。
- 白细胞计数正常(5～15 000/mm^3)，尿常规正常(革兰染色或白细胞脂酶阴性，白细胞计数＜5 个/高倍视野)，粪常规正常(白细胞计数＜5 个/高倍视野)，脑脊液常规正常(白细胞计数＜8/mm^3、革兰染色阴性)。
• 既往体健的 3～36 个月的患儿中毒症状消失，并有良好随访条件者：
- 有退热药。
• 12～24 h 电话随访，24～48 h 根据父母叙述病情，重新评估病情变化，如病情发展或加重就需重新入院。

转诊问题

• 复杂传染病。
• 血液学/肿瘤学，用于免疫功能低下或发热和中性粒细胞减少症患者。

随访建议

• 出院时仍有发热的患儿需要密切的随访，当症状和体征变化或加重时，通常保健医师能给予及时治疗建议。
• 对乙酰氨基酚或布洛芬控制发热。

要点和误区

• 发热是儿童最常见的临床表现。发热可能反映了危及生命的病情。
• 28 日以内的患儿在培养结果回报前通常给予经验性抗感染治疗。
• 年长的患儿需要密切的随访及详细的出院医嘱。
• 细微的临床表现如心动过速、呼吸急促或意识变化都提示感染。

F

发热性癫痫(高热惊厥) Seizure, Febrile

John P. Santamaria · Stefani Ashby 张溢熤 伍力学 译

基础知识

描述

• 该病发生在 6 个月至 5 岁的婴幼儿，与发热相关：
- 没有颅内感染或其他确定的中枢神经系统原发病因。
- 平均发病年龄为 18～22 月龄。
- 曾有非发热性癫痫史的儿童应除外。
• 最常见的小儿痉挛性神经功能障碍：
- 2%～4%的美国儿童受累。
• 可发生在患有全身性病毒感染疾病的正常儿童身上。
• 高风险的患儿：
- 直系亲属的发热史。
- 神经发育迟缓。
- 男性。
• 亚组：
- 单纯性高热惊厥：
◦ 短暂性，自限性，持续时间 10～15 min 及以下，可自行缓解。
◦ 一般无任何局灶症状。
- 复杂性高热惊厥。
◦ 持续时间＞15 min。
◦ 局灶症状。
◦ 24 小时内发作超过 1 次。
• 复发风险：
- 约 1/3 病例存在复发。
- 幼龄首发，一级亲属有高热惊厥史及初始发作时体温＜40 ℃者，复发风险较大。
• 后续进展为癫痫风险：
- 存在神经发育异常基础且伴首次发作(＞15 min)、局灶性发作或有高热惊厥家族史者，风险最高。
- 若首发为单纯性高热惊厥且神经功能发育正常者，且风险仅略高于一般人群。

> **注意**
>
> 鉴于该病呈自限性，气道管理、呼吸支持及癫痫管理措施应予个体化考虑。

病因

常见的儿童感染：
• 上呼吸道疾病。
• 中耳炎。
• 红疹。
• 胃肠道感染。
• 志贺杆菌胃肠炎。

诊断

症状和体征

• 发热。
• 癫痫可与发热同时发生。
• 癫痫发作。
• 全身性强直-阵挛发作较常见：
- 强直阶段：
◦ 肌肉僵硬。
◦ 呼吸暂停和失禁。
◦ 自限性的，仅持续几分钟。
- 其他发作类型：
◦ 凝视。
◦ 疲软。
◦ 非强直性抽搐。

病史

• 仔细的病史和体格检查有助于确诊和排除其他病因。
• 传染病的症状和证据。
• 持续时间和热型。

- 药物和毒物暴露史。
- 近期免疫接种史。
- 外伤史。
- 成长环境和发育水平。
- 癫痫家族史。
- 完整描述癫痫表现。

体格检查

- 降低体温可能对评估有用,早期给予退热药。
- 传染性疾病的证据——皮疹、耳感染、呼吸道感染、腹泻等。
- 细致的神经系统检查,包括精神状况。
- 存在假性脑膜炎、囟门膨隆、颈项强直等。
- 局灶性神经缺陷或颅内压(ICP)增加的证据。

诊断检查与说明

实验室检查

- 常规实验室检查无提示意义。
- 如果怀疑有严重细菌感染,应评估发热来源:
  - 白细胞。
  - 尿酸。
  - 血液和尿液检查。
- 腰椎穿刺:
  - 虽然对于有中枢神经系统感染迹象的12月龄以下儿童,行腰椎穿刺检查的门槛应进一步降低,但该检查仍不常规推荐。
  - 12~18个月幼儿的腰椎穿刺适应证:
    - 易激惹、进食减少,昏睡。
    - 如果未行流感嗜血杆菌和肺炎链球菌免疫接种者应予以接种。
    - 存在脑膜炎/单纯疱疹病毒脑膜炎的体征或病史与脑膜炎/脑炎一致。
    - 复杂性癫痫。
    - 持续的癫痫发作后状态。
    - 用过抗生素者,临床表现可能有改变。
    - 癫痫发作后部分缓解后出现精神改变。
  - 大于18月龄的幼儿的腰椎穿刺指征:
    - 出现中枢神经系统感染的症状和体征。
- 有呕吐和腹泻症状的婴幼儿需要检查电解质和床旁血糖。
- 脑电图:
  - 对评估初发的高热惊厥没有帮助。
  - 对存在发育迟缓、有潜在的神经系统异常或局灶性癫痫者,可能会有提示意义。
  - 无助于预测癫痫的复发或后续癫痫发作风险。
- 正在使用抗惊厥药物者,应检测血药浓度水平。
- 如果病史和体格检查有相关提示,应完善血液和尿液的毒物监测。

影像学检查

- 胸部X线片仅适用于有明显呼吸道症状或体格检查发现有相关临床表现者。
- 头颅CT:
  - 适用于有颅脑外伤、局灶性神经学表现或无法排除有无颅内压升高者。

鉴别诊断

- 高热性谵妄。
- 高热寒战伴面色苍白及口唇发绀。
- 儿童高热伴屏气发作。
- 严重危及生命的事件。
- 其他导致癫痫发作的原因:
  - 伴有发热的非发热性癫痫。
  - 抗惊厥药物突然中断。
  - 感染:
    - 脑膜炎/脑炎。
    - 急性胃肠炎,常伴脱水。
  - 头部外伤。
  - 药物中毒:
    - 抗胆碱药。
    - 拟交感药。
    - 其他。
  - 组织缺氧。
  - 代谢性疾病。
  - 颅内占位。
  - 中枢血管病变。

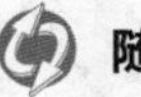

治疗

院前

- 气道保护。
- 给氧。
- 必要时呼吸支持。
- 提醒:
  - 注意防范发生惊厥时出现相关损害。
  - 避免过量使用苯二氮䓬类药物引起呼吸抑制和窒息。
  - 单纯的高热惊厥呈自限性,一般不需要应用抗惊厥药物或呼吸支持措施。

初步稳定/治疗

- 气道和呼吸支持措施。
- 苯二氮䓬类很少需要应用:
  - 持续的癫痫发作或药物耐受者。
  - 劳拉西泮、地西泮或咪达唑仑。
  - 应用地西泮纳肛,咪达唑仑喷或劳拉西泮喷鼻剂可能有较好疗效。

急诊治疗/程序

- 通常自限性,很少需要药物干预。
- 对苯二氮䓬类药物无法逆转的癫痫发作:
  - 左乙拉西坦。
  - 苯妥英或磷苯妥英。
  - 苯巴比妥。
  - 仔细检查排除其他病因。
- 若发现存在细菌感染,应酌情使用抗生素。
- 控制发热。
- 消除其父母的恐惧、焦虑并加强宣教非常重要。

药物治疗

- 对乙酰氨基酚:每次10~15 mg/kg,必要时口服;不超过5次/24 h或4 g/24 h。
- 地西泮:0.2 mg/kg,静脉注射(最大剂量8 mg);0.5 mg/kg,必要时(最大剂量20 mg)。
- 磷苯妥英:20 mg/kg,静脉注射,给药时间不少于20 min。
- 布洛芬:10 mg/kg,口服。
- 左乙拉西坦:20~60 mg/kg,静脉注射(最大剂量2.5 g),给药时间不少于15 min。
- 劳拉西泮:0.1 mg/kg,静脉注射(最大剂量4 mg)。
- 咪达唑仑:0.15 mg/kg,静脉注射;0.2 mg/kg,含服或肌内注射(最大剂量10 mg);0.3 mg/kg,椎管内注射(最大剂量10 mg)。
- 苯巴比妥:20 mg/kg,静脉注射(最大剂量1 g),给药时间15~30 min,监测呼吸,预防呼吸抑制。
- 苯妥英:20 mg/kg,静脉注射,给药时间30~45 min。

随访

进一步处理

入院指征

- 反复发作或长期发作。
- 来源不明的发热,不适合在门诊治疗者。

出院指征

- 单纯性发热惊厥:
  - 神经系统检查无异常。
  - 发热适合在门诊治疗。
- 消除父母的恐惧和疑虑。

随访建议

安排到基层内科医师处进行随访。

F

要点和误区

• 高热惊厥通常是自限性的，不需要特殊的抗惊厥治疗。

• 推荐使用退热药积极控制发热，但使用此类药物在减少癫痫的复发方面的获益目前尚存在争议。

• 治疗发热性疾病期间口服地西泮可降低惊厥复发风险；很少建议预防性使用或联用抗惊厥药，这类治疗方案存有争议，只有在与其父母进行充分沟通后方考虑采用。

反应性关节炎 Reactive Arthritis

Christopher M. Fischer 袁晓伟 童朝阳 译

基础知识

描述

• 典型症状包括三联征：结膜炎、尿道炎、关节炎。

• 也被称为"Reiter 综合征"，这个名字已经不受欢迎了：典型的被称为"看不见，不能尿，不能爬树"综合征。

病因

• 由于缺乏标准化的诊断标准，很难确定确切的发病率。

• 通常发生在胃肠道或泌尿生殖系统病原体感染后。

- 胃肠道：沙门菌、志贺杆菌、弯曲杆菌、耶尔森菌、艰难梭菌。
- 泌尿道：沙眼衣原体(最常见的原因)、淋病奈瑟菌。

• 好继发于上呼吸道感染后、尿路感染、卡介苗治疗膀胱癌。

• 好发年龄为 30 岁。

诊断

症状和体征

• 泌尿生殖系统：90%病例发生。

- 女性：宫颈炎，盆腔炎，膀胱炎(通常无菌尿)。
- 男性：尿道炎，附睾炎。

• 关节炎、肌腱炎和指炎。

- 典型的多关节，不对称性。
- 发病时间为最初感染数日至数周后。
- 膝和踝最常受影响。
- 也可能影响手指、背部、骶髂。
- 关节：40%的病例为跟腱炎。

• 眼科：30%～60%的病例发生。

- 结膜炎最常见：通常为双侧。
- 葡萄膜炎，角膜炎不太常见：通常是单侧的，通常在前 1～2 日眼睛不舒服。

• 黏膜与皮肤：在 HLA - B27 阳性患者中更为常见。

• 心脏：罕见，包括心传导阻滞、心包炎。

病史

• 症状一般在感染后 4 周内出现，可延迟至 1 年发病。

• 通常通过既往史及体格检查诊断。

• 只有 1/3 的患者有结膜炎、尿道炎、关节炎的三联征。

• 痢疾：通常出现在有症状的肠道感染之前，尤其是儿童。

• 最初的泌尿生殖道感染可能没有症状。

体格检查

• 一般情况：可能包括发热、疲劳、体重减轻、不适。

• 泌尿生殖：尿道炎、宫颈炎、前列腺炎。

• 四肢：肿胀，活动后疼痛，红斑。

• 腊肠指(全指弥漫性肿胀)：在 15%的病例中发生。

• 眼科：

- 结膜炎：常伴有黏液脓性分泌物。
- 症状从轻微的刺激到严重的炎症。
- 葡萄膜炎：眼痛、红肿、畏光、瞳孔缩小、眼睑痉挛。

• 皮肤/黏膜：

- 溢脓性皮肤角化病：开始于手掌和脚底的斑疹和水疱，发展为脓疱和暗色斑块。
- 外观与脓疱性牛皮癣相似。

• 环状阴道炎：见于 50%的男性：阴茎龟头上有斑块、水疱或丘疹。

• 溃疡性外阴炎：可能与阴道分泌物有关。

• 指甲变化：包括甲营养不良、甲周脓肿。

• 口腔病变：包括溃疡、地图样舌、腭部糜烂，通常无痛。

基本检查

• 临床诊断需基于体格检查，以及胃肠道病史、性传播疾病感染史及上呼吸道感染史。

• 必须排除其他需要及时治疗的严重的时间敏感性诊断。

诊断检查与说明

实验室检查

• 实验室检查不能确诊。

• 血常规可能表现为白细胞增多和轻度贫血。

• ESR 和 CRP 通常升高；尿液分析显示无菌性脓肿。

影像学检查

• 没有影像学检查能证实诊断。

• 可考虑肢体的 X 线平片，排除其他诊断，可能提示关节积液。

诊断步骤/外科

关节腔穿刺术：

• 如考虑感染性关节炎，应进行关节腔穿刺术。

• 滑膜液分析可能显示白细胞增多，中性粒细胞占优势：未见晶体，提示其他病理(痛风、假痛风)。

鉴别诊断

• 淋球菌的尿道炎。

• 类风湿关节炎。

• 梅毒。

• 痛风。

• 淋球菌的关节炎。

• 脓毒性关节炎。

• 脓疱性银屑病。

• 遗传病疾病。

• 接触性皮炎。

• 牛皮癣。

• 川崎病(儿童)。

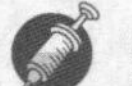

治疗

院前治疗

没有特殊的院前治疗。

■ 急诊治疗/程序

• 一旦排除其他严重感染，进行对症治疗。

• 对于初始胃肠道疾病，没有证据表明对轻中度疾病的抗生素治疗可以降低随后反应性关节炎的发病率。

• 不常规使用抗生素。

• 抗生素：由细菌感染引起的反应性关节炎，在滑膜(尤其是衣原体)中可能具有长期存在。

• 研究表明，多西环素、环丙沙星、阿奇霉素没有长期疗效。

• 短期的系统性皮质类固醇使用可能对于严重或长期的疾病有一定疗效。

• 关节炎：休息，冰敷，仰卧，非甾体抗炎药。

• 结膜炎：局部抗生素可缓解症状。

• 尿道炎：初次感染未被发现或治疗时应予以治疗。

■ 药物治疗

药物没有明确的作用。

 随访

■ 进一步处理

入院指征

一旦被确诊并且排除其他诊断，一般门诊治疗。

出院指征

大多数患者反应性关节炎可以出院，到初级保健医师处随访。

转诊问题

严重葡萄膜炎应转眼科密切随访。

■ 随访建议

初级保健医师随访。大多数病例病程较长(3～12个月)，大约25%可能有复发。

要点和误区

未诊断出严重的危及生命或肢体的病情。

• 脓毒性关节炎。

• 淋球菌的关节炎。

• 川崎病。

房室传导阻滞 Atrioventricular Blocks

Aaran B. Drake · James Scott 吴增斌 潘曙明 译

 基础知识

■ 描述

• 连接心房和心室之间的房室结或 His-purkinje 系统的传导破坏。

• 一度房室传导阻滞：

- 房室结传导延长。
- 室性冲动没有脱落。
- 多为良性的，可见于1.6%的健康成人。

• 二度房室传导阻滞：

- 心房冲动不能传导至心室。
- 莫氏Ⅰ型(Wenckebach)：
  - 通常继发于房室结的传导缺损。
  - PR间期逐渐延长直到出现非传导的P波和QRS波群脱落。
  - 通常是良性的，也可能是下壁心肌梗死的并发症。
- 莫氏Ⅱ型：
  - 传导缺损通常位于房室结下方。
  - PR间期固定直到单个或多个脉搏脱落。
  - 极易发展成完全性心脏阻滞。
  - 如伴有急性心肌梗死预后差。
  - 较Ⅰ型少见。

• 三度房室传导阻滞：

- 也称为完全性传导阻滞。
- 所有房性冲动不能到达室性传导系统，出现室性逸搏，导致房室分离。
- PP和RR间期固定，而PR间期不固定，因为PP和RR间期各自独立。
- 当阻滞点位于传导系统的位置越低症状越严重。
- 如果继发于药物的毒性作用，当停用药物后可缓解。

■ 病因

• 基本上是由于：心脏结构性病变；固有不应期增加；室上性周期明显缩短。

• 心肌梗死：下壁心肌梗死可伴有一度和二度Ⅰ型房室传导阻滞；这些阻滞是暂时性的，房室传导可恢复至正常而不增加死亡率和并发症；5%的前壁心肌梗死可伴有二度Ⅱ型房室传导阻滞，由于室性心律失常和左心力衰竭而增加死亡率。冠状动脉性心脏病：慢性心肌缺血可导致房室传导周围纤维化。

• 药物中毒：地高辛、β受体阻滞剂、钙通道阻滞剂、胺碘酮、普鲁卡因酰胺、1C类抗心律失常药(普罗帕酮、恩卡尼、氟卡尼)、可乐定。

• 先天性。

• 心脏瓣膜病。

• 外科创伤：冠状动脉搭桥术或瓣膜置换术后。

• 迷走张力增高。

• 感染：梅毒、白喉、锥虫病、结核、弓形虫病、莱姆病、心肌炎、心内膜炎、风湿热、室间隔脓肿形成。

• 胶原性血管病。

• 浸润性疾病：结节病、淀粉样变性、血色素沉着病。

• 心肌病。

• 电解质紊乱：高钾血症。

• 黏液性水肿。

• 低体温。

儿科注意事项

• 可见于儿童，但通常无症状。

• 新生儿的死亡率高。

• 通常伴有：先天获得来自母亲的抗体、先天性心脏病、风湿热或心肌炎。

• 对于新发作的房室传导阻滞要排除有无中毒。

诊断

■ 症状和体征

病史

• 一度：无症状。

• 二度Ⅰ型：脉搏不规则。

• 二度Ⅱ型和三度：运动不耐受、心悸、胸痛、晕厥、意识改变、气促、呼吸困难。

体格检查

• 一度：没有阳性体征。

• 二度Ⅰ型：不规则脉率。

• 二度Ⅱ型和三度：不规则脉率、低血压、意识改变、心力衰竭表现(啰音、发绀、颈静

F

脉怒张)。

诊断步骤/外科

• 12 导联心电图可诊断阻滞类型和明确心肌梗死。

• 一度：PR 间期＞0.20 s。

• 二度Ⅰ型：PR 间期逐渐延长直到出现非传导的 P 波和 QRS 波群脱落，可重复周期性出现，QRS 波群通常为窄波形。

• 二度Ⅱ型：PR 间期固定，房性冲动非间歇性传导，室性搏动偶发脱落，QRS 波群根据病变部位可以延长。

• 三度房室传导阻滞：P 波以固定间歇出现；QRS 波群与 P 波群互相独立；QRS 波群通常为窄波，除非房室结下传导紊乱或室性逸搏节律。

▪ 诊断检查与说明

实验室检查

• 电解质。

• 钙、镁。

• 心肌酶谱：特别是二度Ⅱ型和三度。

• 地高辛浓度。

影像学检查

• X 线胸片：可明确心肌病或心力衰竭。

• 心电图：可明确局部心室壁运动障碍或瓣膜病。

▪ 鉴别诊断

• 加速性结性心律。

• 室性自主心律。

• 窦性心动过缓。

• 窦房阻滞。

治疗

▪ 院前

• 不稳定的二度Ⅱ型和三度可经皮起搏。

• 阿托品：二度Ⅱ型避免使用，因为可加速完全性心脏阻滞；三度伴宽 QRS 波群禁用。

• 可尝试阻止迷走张力的增加。

▪ 初步稳定/治疗

• 经皮起搏：适合于有低灌注体征的不稳定患者：低血压、胸痛、呼吸困难、神志改变。

• 阿托品：可用于窄 QRS 波群的完全心脏传导阻滞，有症状的窦性心动过缓。

▪ 急诊治疗/程序

一度房室传导阻滞：无需治疗；避免可引起房室传导阻滞的药物；评估可能伴有的心肌梗死、电解质紊乱、药物过量。

二度Ⅰ型：通常无需治疗；如果有症状，阿托品可促进房室传导。

二度Ⅱ型：临时经皮或经静脉起搏；阿托品治疗无效且避免使用。

三度：一线治疗是紧急安装起搏器；窄 QRS 波群可能对阿托品短暂起效；如果是药物毒性引起的，特殊治疗包括：地高辛抗体(地高辛过量)、胰高血糖素和钙剂(β 受体阻滞剂和钙通道阻滞剂)。

▪ 药物治疗

• 阿托品：0.5～1.0 mg(儿童：0.01～0.03 mg/kg)，静脉推注，q5 min。

• 地高辛抗体：10 瓶(380 mg)是恰当的负荷剂量，血清浓度×体重(kg)＝所需瓶数。

• 胰高血糖素：5～10 mg(儿童 50 μg/kg)，静脉推注，5 min。

• 氯化钙：250～500 mg(儿童：20 mg/kg)，静脉推注。

随访

▪ 进一步处理

入院指征

• 二度Ⅱ型。

• 三度房室传导阻滞。

出院指征

• 无症状的一度和二度Ⅰ型。

▪ 随访建议

无症状的一度和二度Ⅰ型可在心脏科医师门诊随访。

要点和误区

• 对于有症状的患者快速心电图检查是至关重要的。

• 一旦诊断高度房室传导阻滞迅速启动经皮起搏。

• 获得完整的病史有助于明确中毒可能。

• 常见的缺陷：不能正确地解读心电图；不能正确地诊断房室传导阻滞；不能及时启动经皮起搏，不能及时咨询心脏科医师进行永久起搏。

F

非心源性肺水肿 Noncardiogenic Pulmonary Edema

Michael N. Cocchi · Christopher James Watson　朱妍 译

基础知识

▪ 描述

• 非心源性肺水肿(NCPE)是指与静水压力升高(肺毛细血管压正常)无关的因素使过量的液体和蛋白质聚集到肺泡内。

• 渗透率增加：

- 毛细血管-肺泡膜的功能破坏使得蛋白质和水分从血管内自由移动进入肺泡。

• 非心源性肺水肿和心源性肺水肿(CPE)之间的区别：

- 肺毛细血管楔压≤18 mmHg。

- 往往临床表现明显。

- 非心源性肺水肿患者，肺泡液中的蛋白质浓度与血管内空间的是相同的。

- 与 CPE 不同，NCPE 通常不会显示头部血流重新分布、肺积液或心脏增大。

• 通常情况下，水肿在有害损伤后 1～2 h 发生。

• 每年在美国约有 250 000 例，重症患者死亡率为 46%。

• 好坏参半：高达 20% 的急性呼吸窘迫综合征(ARDS)患者会伴有心力衰竭。

▪ 病因

• ARDS 是最常见的病因：

- 造成原因：

◦ 脓毒症。

◦ 肺炎。

◦ 创伤。

◦ 吸入有毒物质和送气。

◦ 弥散性血管内凝血(DIC)。

◦ 胰腺炎。

◦ 濒临溺水。

◦ S/p 体外循环。
◦ 输血相关急性肺损伤(TRALI)。
◦ 严重烧伤。
◦ 放射性肺炎。
• 高原肺水肿(HAPE)。
• 神经源性肺水肿。
• 阿片类药物过量。
• 肺栓塞。
• 子痫。
• 气胸再扩张或大量胸腔积液引流后复张性肺水肿。
• 水杨酸盐毒性。
• 吸入可卡因。
• 尿毒症。
• 病毒感染(即汉坦病毒心肺综合征)。

诊断

症状和体征

• 呼吸急促。
• 疲劳。
• 虚弱。
• 咳嗽。
• 萎靡不振。

体格检查

• 散在鼾音及水泡音。
• 缺氧。
• 呼吸困难。
• 呼吸急促。
• 辅助呼吸肌使用。
• 心动过速。
• 粉红色,泡沫痰。
• 除非同时出现心力衰竭,否则左侧和右侧心力衰竭的痕迹将会消失:
- 下肢肿胀。
- 颈静脉扩张。
- 心脏肥大。

基本检查

• 病史和体格检查通常已经足够来区分心源性肺水肿和非心源性肺水肿。
• 确定诊断和评估严重程度时 X 线胸片是必不可少的。

诊断检查与说明

实验室检查

一般的实验室异常对非心源性肺水肿无特异性,但有助于阐明潜在的病因。

影像学检查

X 线胸片:
• 早期可能是正常的。
• 肺水肿的经典蝴蝶征。
• 无心脏扩大。
• 发现出现后的几小时内,并将持续几日到几周。

诊断步骤/外科

肺动脉导管:
• 肺毛细血管楔压正常或接近正常,而心源性肺水肿压力升高。

急性呼吸窘迫综合征的柏林标准(2012年):
• 在已知的临床侮辱或新的或恶化的呼吸道症状后 7 日内发病。
• CXR 或 CT 上"与肺水肿一致"的双侧阴影。
• PaO_2 : $FiO_2 \leqslant 300$ mmHg。
- 轻度:PaO_2 : FiO_2 在 201~300 mmHg。
- 中度:PaO_2 : FiO_2 在 101~200 mmHg。
- 重度:PaO_2 : $FiO_2 \leqslant 100$ mmHg。

鉴别诊断

• 心源性肺水肿。
• 弥漫性肺泡出血。
• 肿瘤散在转移,如淋巴瘤或白血病、淋巴管扩散。
• 间质性肺病。
• 药物毒性(即博来霉素、胺碘酮)。
• 肺栓塞。
• 肺炎。

治疗

院前

• 保持气道通畅。
• 充分氧合。
• 注意事项:
- 治疗心力衰竭的常规措施无效。

初步稳定/治疗

• 补充氧气(鼻导管或非循环呼吸式)。
• 建立静脉通路。
• 持续心电监护。
• 连续血脉氧饱和度。

急诊治疗/程序

• NCPE 治疗的主要目标是识别和治疗潜在原因,并提供支持性护理。
• 推荐采用保守的液体疗法,但利尿剂不太可能有益。
• 可以考虑使用无创正压通气(NIV):
- 如果无创不能改善氧合或通气情况,则需要气管插管。
• 气管插管往往是必要的:
- 改善氧合和通气,并减少呼吸功。
- 使用低潮气量的 6~8 ml/kg 理想体重减少气压伤。
- 使用 5~10 cmH_2O 的呼气末正压通气(PEEP)减少肺不张和滴定。
- 最初使用 100%氧:
◦ 测量 PO_2,并相应的减少 FiO_2。
• 神经肌肉阻滞可以改善呼吸机的同步性和改善气体交换。
• 考虑俯卧位治疗顽固性低氧血症。
• 类固醇在降低死亡率方面还没有被证明是有效的。
• 尽管对呼吸机进行了优化,但如果无法充分通风或充氧,请考虑转到 ECMO 中心。
• 如果在高海拔地区和怀疑高原肺水肿,让患者转到低海拔的地方或使用高压氧舱。
- 硝苯地平是吸氧和降低海拔之外的辅助治疗。

F

随访

进一步处理

入院指征

所有有症状的患者应收入 ICU:

出院指征

无症状的患者(尤其是麻醉剂过量、高原肺水肿或吸入性):
• 急诊观察 6~12 h,如果没有肺水肿且氧合充足,则可出院并密切随访。

随访建议

患者出院后,应在 48 h 内进行随访。

要点和误区

• 快速识别和治疗诱因是改善预后的关键。
• 由于治疗方法不同,鉴别心源性和非心源性病因失败是一个误区。
• 周到的呼吸机管理可以改善预后。

非甾体抗炎药中毒 Nonsteroidal Anti-Inflammatory Poisoning

Michele Zell-Kanter 朱妍 译

基础知识

描述

• 抑制环氧合酶(COX),从而阻断花生四烯酸转化为前列腺素。

• 通常服用 NSAIDs 时发病率较低。

• 大多数关于非选择性 NSAIDs 毒性的文献提及布洛芬,可能是因为其非处方药的有效性。

• 死亡病例的报告与大剂量摄入有关。

• 更多潜在的毒性是关于充血性心力衰竭或肾衰竭:

- NSAIDs 导致钠水潴留,降低肾血流量。
- COX-2 抑制剂(塞来昔布)轻度过量的经验,治疗应该与传统 NSAIDs 相同。

病因

• 非甾体类药物均可通过处方和非处方获得。

• NSAIDs 包括:

- 双氯芬酸。
- 二氟尼柳。
- 依托度酸。
- 非诺洛芬。
- 布洛芬。
- 吲哚美辛。
- 酮洛芬。
- 酮咯酸。
- 甲氯芬那酸。
- 甲芬那酸。
- 美洛昔康。
- 萘丁美酮。
- 萘普生。
- 奥沙普秦。
- 吡罗昔康。
- 舒林酸。
- 托美汀。

诊断

症状和体征

• 胃肠道:

- 恶心。
- 呕吐。
- 上腹部疼痛。

• 中枢神经系统:

- 嗜睡。
- 头晕。
- 昏睡。
- 无菌性脑膜炎。
- 癫痫发作。

• 心血管系统:

- 低血压。
- 心动过速。

• 肺:

- 嗜酸细胞性肺炎。
- 窒息。
- 过度换气。

• 肾:

- 急性肾衰竭、高钾血症。
- 急性肾小管坏死。
- 急性间质性肾炎。

• 肝:

- 肝细胞损伤。
- 胆汁淤积性黄疸。

• 代谢:

- 轻度、短暂的代谢性酸中毒。

• 过敏症:

- 无菌性脑膜炎。
- 哮喘急性发作。
- 血管神经性水肿,荨麻疹。

基本检查

• 一般来说,摄入 NSAIDs 可导致轻微的毒副作用。

• 准确识别药物有帮助:

- 在 NSAIDs 之间微妙的毒理学差异。
- 无菌性脑膜炎多见于使用布洛芬。
- 肝毒性多见于使用双氯芬酸和舒林酸。

诊断检查与说明

实验室检查

• 电解质、尿素氮/肌酐、葡萄糖:

- 肾功能基础。
- 检查代谢性酸中毒。

• 血常规。

• 肝功能检查。

• 大剂量过量时查动脉血气。

• 凝血酶原时间(PT)和部分促凝血酶原激酶时间延长:

- 服用依托度酸时查胆红素/酮试纸呈假阳性。

• 对乙酰氨基酚和水杨酸水平:患者经常混淆水杨酸盐、对乙酰氨基酚和 NSAIDs 产品,认为它们都是相同的。

• NSAIDs 难以进行毒理学筛选且不利于管理。

鉴别诊断

其他药物引起代谢性酸中毒、精神状态改变和胃肠道刺激:

• 水杨酸。

• 异烟肼。

• 乙二醇。

• 甲醇。

• 异丙醇。

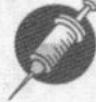

治疗

院前

在急诊室收集药瓶、药物做鉴定。

初步稳定/治疗

• 基础支持治疗。

• 意识状态改变患者使用纳洛酮、硫胺素、葡萄糖(或 Accu-Chek)。

急诊治疗/程序

• 支持治疗。

• 使用活性炭。

• 由于血浆蛋白结合率高,体外循环提高清除率的方法无益处。

药物治疗

• 活性炭浆:1~2 g/kg 至 90 g 口服。

• 葡萄糖:50% 葡萄糖 1 安瓿(50 ml 或 25 g;儿童:25% 葡萄糖 2~4 ml/kg),静脉注射。

• 纳洛酮(narcan):初始剂量 2 mg(儿童:0.1 mg/kg),静脉注射或肌内注射。

• 硫胺素(维生素 B_1):100 mg(儿童:50 mg),静脉注射或肌内注射。

儿科注意事项

吡罗昔康、萘普生、酮洛芬和甲芬那酸可引起小儿癫痫发作。

随访

进一步处理

入院指征

• 持续的呕吐、呕血。

• 中枢神经抑制、癫痫发作。

F

• 代谢性酸中毒。
• 心力衰竭、低血压、高血压。
• 肾衰竭。

转诊问题

患者服药后 6～8 h 无症状，即认为没有毒副反应。

随访建议

故意服药者予以精神病学随访/转诊。

要点和误区

• 调查所有非甾体抗炎药过量的摄入。
• 对所有表现出可能服用 NSAIDs 患者，检测其对乙酰氨基酚和水杨酸水平。
• NSAIDs 中毒一般是轻微的，除非有大剂量的过量；有潜在的心力衰竭，冠状动脉疾病的患者中毒的风险更高。

肥厚型心肌病 Cardiomyopathy, Hypertrophic

L. Kristan Arnold 彭沪 王毅鑫 译

基础知识

概述

• 影响肌小节的遗传性疾病：多种突变，多种表型变异。
- 肥厚的（局部或全心），不扩张的左心室或右心室很少在没有其他原因的情况下出现肥厚，如高血压或主动脉狭窄。
- 分型：
  ◦ 非梗阻性（HCM）：75％的患者。估计年死亡率约为 1％。
  ◦ 梗阻性（HOCM）：25％的患者。患者病情更严重，估计年死亡率约为 2％。
- 体现在所有年龄段，从新生儿到老年人。
  ◦ 最明显的表现在儿童和青少年，青春期的生长突增。
  ◦ 一般在年轻时被诊断出的更为严重。
  ◦ 小比例患者进展到左心室功能降低。
- 临床表现多见于中晚期：最初可能被误诊为哮喘、慢性阻塞性肺疾病、心律失常或睡眠呼吸暂停。
- 致命性心律失常在年轻患者中更为常见：年轻（35 岁以下）运动员非创伤性死亡的最常见原因。
- 室上性心律失常的发病率随年龄增加而增加：房颤常见，耐受性差。

• 患病率：每 500 个成人中就有 1 个是根据超声心动图诊断的。
• 病理结构：
- 心室壁不规则、明显增厚，增厚区肌原纤维排列紊乱，纤维蛋白沉积：
- 在梗阻状态下，高压对左心室的影响要高于右心室，但如果梗阻被清除，心肌肥厚就会减少。
- 某些表型的心肌肥厚随着年龄的增长而逐渐变薄，早期通常与较厚的壁相关。

• 增厚通常不对称，累及膈膜的程度要大于游离的心室壁；心房扩张继发于舒张期充盈不良；微血管扩张受损，伴有内膜增厚和血管周围胶原沉积。
• 门诊长期管理：
- 避免容量耗尽和心脏需求增加，取决于肥厚的程度和位置。
- 药理学：β受体阻滞剂或维拉帕米减慢和控制心率，从而延长舒张期充盈。
- 植入式心脏除颤器：有晕厥、心搏骤停、家族成员猝死、无症状性非持续性室性心动过速（VT）、运动血压异常反应、心肌大部肥厚等病史的患者。
- 无症状的非持续性室性心动过速（VT），运动时血压反应异常，大量肥大。
- 酒精消融治疗的导致流出道梗阻的间隔组织肥厚。
- 外科间隔肌切除术，通过更多中心提高统计数据。

风险因素

遗传学

• 遗传学基础确定的第一种心脏疾病（1989 年）。
• 常染色体显性遗传：
- 共发现大于 10 种相关基因，其中大多数编码肌小节的蛋白质，并识别出超过 700 个不同的突变。
- 高外显率。
- 可变表型表达。
- 某些基因型明显更具致命性：目前常规筛查不切实际；随着对原发性肌小节异常与其他遗传和非遗传因素之间相互作用的更多了解，其复杂性也在增加；某些突变影响直接细胞膜离子泵。因此，与心律失常也有一定相关性。

病因

见遗传学。

诊断

症状和体征

病史

• 梗阻症状与用力或突然采取直立姿势有关：减少静脉回流或心室充盈的活动；严重程度取决于室壁增厚的部位和程度。
• 气短。
• 劳力性呼吸困难。
• 劳力性或餐后心绞痛。
• 晕厥先兆。
• 晕厥。
• 充血性心力衰竭（CHF）。
• 心血管性虚脱。
• 心律失常：
- 阵发性心房颤动：当伴有充血性心力衰竭时，常常导致明显的、快速的临床病情恶化；血栓引起的 CVA 风险升高。
- 室上性心动过速。
- 非持续性室性心动过速。
- 缓慢性心律失常少见。
- 可能导致猝死的室性心动过速（VT）或心室颤动。

• 已知 HCM 的早期治疗可能包括手术或酒精注射以减少间隔体积：潜在传导阻滞；潜在间隔破裂。
• 已知的心律失常风险较高的病例可能植入了除颤器。
• 无明显诱因或已知 HCM 的猝死家族史。

儿科注意事项

由于青春期潜在的严重程度增加，任何没有明确病因的晕厥患儿，或与运动有关的患儿，应具有更广泛、更集中的家族性猝死史（标准为三代），并可能转诊进行评估。

体格检查

• 没有明显的体征表现。

- 大多数流出道梗阻患者的表现各不相同：
  - 左侧 S4 听诊响亮。
  - 胸骨中上部双心尖搏动。
- 杂音：左胸骨边缘渐进性-衰减性收缩中期杂音；向主动脉和二尖瓣区域放射，而不是向颈部或腋部；进行 Valsalva 动作或站立时强度增加；躺卧、蹲下或握手时杂音减少；二尖瓣反流频发。
- 梗阻越严重，放射到胸骨左缘的杂音越明显。
- 伴有二尖瓣关闭不全时杂音可向腋窝放射。

诊断检查与说明

心电图表现

- 超过 90% 的 HCM 患者心电图表现异常。
- T 波倒置 >1 mm^2 或+导联 V_2～V_6，Ⅱ和 AVF，或Ⅰ和 AVL 或>16 岁的非加勒比海血统运动员 V_4～V_6 中的深 TWI。
- 2 个或更多导联 ST 段压低>0.5 mm 则需要进一步检查。
- 除Ⅲ和 AVR 以外的至少 2 个导联中的 Q 波深度>3 mm 或持续时间>40 ms。
- P 波>120 ms，Ⅰ或Ⅱ导联的负部分>1 mm，V_1 导联>40 ms。
- 非特异性 IVCD>140 ms。

实验室检查

- 临床实验室检测没有帮助。
- 基因测试可能有助于门诊患者的检查，但在急诊中没有帮助。

影像学检查

- CXR：绝大多数正常，左心缘隆起代表左心室游离壁肥大；右心房或左心房增大；肺血管再分布。
- 经胸心脏回声/多普勒：左心室壁>15 mm，具有正常或较小的左心室腔(13～14 mm，具有其他特征；例如，成人的家族史)，在儿童中，年龄、性别、体型的标准差大于平均值的 2 倍；收缩期流出道梗阻，舒张期充盈异常。
- 心血管磁共振(CMR)：造影剂回声，允许更多的结构细节作为纤维化的证据。
- 应激铊和 PET 评估缺血。

诊断步骤/外科

基于急诊的程序没有诊断实用价值。

鉴别诊断

- 迷走神经和其他原因引起晕厥和晕厥前期。
- 中暑。
- 主动脉瓣狭窄。
- 肺动脉狭窄。
- 心室中隔缺损。
- 二尖瓣反流。
- 二尖瓣脱垂。
- 区分出现 CHF 或心绞痛的患者：在 HCM 的情况下更不可观。

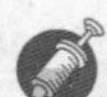

治疗

> **注意**
>
> 在标准治疗期间失代偿的 HCM 患者，考虑因 CHF、缺血或超 VT 及在运动期间或刚刚运动后的年轻运动员出现的虚脱(除外中暑)。由于舒张硬化，HCM 患者可能因静脉输液失代偿。

初步稳定/治疗

- ABC 管理。
- 静脉置管。
- 吸氧。
- 心电监测。
- 脉搏血氧饱和度测定。

急诊治疗/程序

- 取决于表现类型：心律失常、心力衰竭、胸痛或缺血。
- 了解对任何可能损害心脏充盈的情况的敏感性的基本原则。
- 患者可能需要保持仰卧。
- 标准的 CHF 或心绞痛血管扩张治疗可能导致心血管性虚脱；如果发生这种情况，用液体推注弹丸式治疗。
- 注意任何程度较小的低血容量都可能会显著损害心输出量。
- 控制心率和改善舒张期充盈(治疗 HCM 相关性心力衰竭和心绞痛的基本原则)：
  - β受体阻滞剂；维持治疗；减少节律紊乱和降低跨左心室流出道的压力梯度。
  - 钙通道阻滞药：维拉帕米通过降低收缩力和改善舒张期舒张和充盈来减少梗阻，硝苯地平因血管扩张而相对禁忌。
- 心律失常控制：
  - β受体阻滞剂和钙通道阻滞剂是治疗室上性心律失常的一线用药。
  - 胺碘酮：β受体阻滞剂和钙通道阻滞剂失效时室性心律失常的首选药物。
  - 电复律：HCM 合并心房颤动和心力衰竭时的早期应用。

药物治疗

面对可能的流出道限制，必须对所有药物的疗效进行评估：

- 胺碘酮：10 min 内 150 mg，6 h 后 360 mg，18 h 后 540 mg(儿童：5 mg/kg，静脉注射，快速静脉注射骨髓腔注射，参考制造商标示，但根据美国心脏协会指示，VT 具有脉冲的类别和 VF 和无脉性 VT 的类别不确定。不要在婴儿中使用)。
- 普萘洛尔：1～3 mg 缓慢静脉推注(儿童：0.01～0.1 mg/kg，缓慢静脉推注，超过 10 min；不超过 1 mg/剂)。
- 维拉帕米：2.5 mg[儿童：>1 岁：每次 0.1～0.2 mg/kg，超过 2 min；根据需要重复 q10～30 min；不超过 5 mg(第一剂量)或 10 mg(第二剂量)]，静脉推注超过 1～2 min，可在 15～30 min 内重复 5 mg。
- 苯肾上腺素：0.1～0.2 mg(儿童：1～20 μg/kg)缓慢静脉推注对液体推注无效的严重低血压(休克)。根据需要 10～15 min 重复，或开始静脉滴注以滴定 BP；或其他纯血管收缩剂(即无变力作用)，维持量：0.05 μg/(kg·min)[儿童：0.1～0.5 μg/(kg·min)]，静脉注射。

一线治疗

不适用。

二线治疗

地尔硫䓬：0.25 mg/kg(儿童：禁忌证<12 岁)静脉注射超过 2 min；可在 15 min 内以 0.35 mg/kg 重复给药。

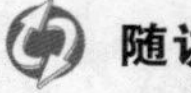

随访

进一步处理

入院指征

- 不明原因晕厥，尤其是年轻人。
- 晕厥发作、心力衰竭、心绞痛、血流动力学显著性快速性心律失常收入 ICU。

出院指征

- 当存在以下表现，且心室壁增厚是 ED 评估中的偶然发现时：无家族性猝死的病史(建议在怀疑时排除三代人)或个人晕厥病史。
- 需要心脏病专家的紧急随访。
- 咨询任何可能减少舒张期充盈的活动，等待随访：咨询身体运动专家，直到由心脏病专家评估。

转诊问题

见出院标准。

随访建议

见出院标准。

要点和误区

• 提高对“正常变异”定义中遗传和表型特征的认识：一些学者主张进行心脏超声筛查任何青少年参与体育运动；一些学者主张把 AICD 用于诊断。

• 如果考虑一个晕厥患者是 HCM，那就必须排除晕厥病因，因为它的重复发作很可能是致命的。

肺孢子虫病 Pneumocystis Pneumonia

Alan M. Kumar · Christine A. Babcock 瞿金龙 译

基础知识

描述

• 最初叫卡氏肺孢子虫肺炎，也叫卡氏肺囊虫肺炎。
• 一般机会性感染，如 HIV 患者。
• 可能通过呼吸传播：
- 孢囊吸入支气管内。
- 孢囊破裂后滋养体释放，并在肺泡内传播。
• 有很多可能与某些潜在的疾病再次发作有关。
• 确切的传播机制目前尚未清楚。

病因

• 卡氏肺孢子菌是真菌的一种。
• 一般发生于细胞免疫缺陷者：
- HIV 感染者。
- 肿瘤。
- 激素治疗。
- 器官移植。
- 营养不良。

儿科注意事项

患儿感染典型，更严重。

诊断

症状和体征

• 亚急性。
• 高达 7%的患者无症状。
• 吸入喷他脒的患者可能症状比较轻：
- 气胸的发生率高。
- 肺外疾病多。

病史

• 发热。
• 咳嗽，少量白痰。
• 呼吸困难在活动后或休息时。
- 数日进展快(非 HIV 感染患者)。
- 数周或者数月进展慢(HIV 感染患者)。
- 氧合下降。
• 畏寒。
• 劳累。
• 胸痛。
• 体重减轻。

体格检查

• 呼吸快。
• 心率快
• 肺部可及捻发音和干啰音。

基本检查

• 血常规。
• 电解质。
• 动脉血气。
• LDH。
• 血培养。
• 胸部 X 线。

诊断检查与说明

实验室检查

• ABG：
- 所有患者必查。
- 计算肺泡-动脉氧梯度。
- 泡-动脉氧梯度＞35 mmHg 或 PaO_2＜70 mmHg 患者给予激素治疗。
• LDH：
- 对于 HIV 感染患者进行评估。
- 高可能与预后差相关。

影像学检查

• X 线胸片：
- 鉴别双肺还是局部浸润。
- 25%的患者 X 线片正常。
- 早期和轻症患者敏感性差。
- 典型的表现：
◦ 肺叶浸润。
◦ 囊形成。
◦ 气胸。
◦ 胸膜浸润。
◦ 结节性浸润。
- 吸入喷他脒是发展为上肺叶的高危因素。
- 治疗后很长一段时间都会有影像学表现的不正常。
• 高敏感性 CT：
- HIV 感染患者敏感性高。
- 提示毛玻璃样高密度影。

诊断步骤/外科

• 深部痰：
- 最终确诊需要呼吸道内培养出肺孢子虫。
- 特异性 100%，但是敏感性可能因深部痰的质量和实验室技术有关。
- 对于吸入喷他脒和非 HIV 阳性的患者，敏感性较差。
• 支气管肺泡的灌洗：
- 痰培养阴性，仍怀疑 PCP 患者。
- 敏感性 80%～100%。

鉴别诊断

呼吸困难、发热、影像学提示浸润，少量或无痰的咳嗽，缓慢进展的非典型肺炎。
• 衣原体肺炎。
• 军团菌肺炎。
• 霉浆菌。
• 肺结核。
• 病毒性肺炎。

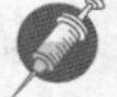

治疗

院前

为有症状患者提供充足的氧气。

初步稳定/治疗

• ABC 管理。
• 提供足够的氧气。
• 呼吸衰竭必要时行气管内插管。
• 对于低血压、严重脓毒症和脱水患者给予 500～1 000 ml 生理盐水扩容。

急诊治疗/程序

• 起始抗菌治疗：
- 复方新诺明是一线用药。
- 复方新诺明不耐受，可予以喷他脒静脉用药。

F

- 对于一般情况尚可的患者可予以口服药物治疗。
- 另一种治疗方法包括甲氧苄啶-氨苯砜、克林霉素-伯氨喹、阿托伐醌。
- 持续治疗 21 日。

• 皮质类甾醇类辅助治疗对于肺泡-动脉氧梯度>35 mmHg 或 PaO_2<70 mmHg：
- 必须首个 72 h 治疗。

• 必须对怀疑感染 PCP 患者进行隔离。

药物治疗

• 阿托伐醌：750 mg，口服，q12 h。

• 克林霉素-伯氨喹：克林霉素 900 mg，静脉注射，q8 h；或者 300～450 mg，口服，q6 h，伯氨喹 15～30 mg，qd，口服。

• 喷他脒：4 mg/(kg·24 h)，静脉注射，>1 h。

• 泼尼松：40 mg，口服，q12 h ×5 日；40 mg，口服，qd ×5 日；20 mg，口服，qd ×11 日。

• 甲氧苄啶-氨苯砜：甲氧苄啶 15～2 mg/(kg·24 h)，静脉注射，间隔 8 h＋氨苯砜 100 mg，口服，qd。

• 甲氧苄啶-磺胺甲噁唑(复方新诺明)：甲氧苄啶 15～2 mg/(kg·24 h)，静脉注射，q8 h 和磺胺甲噁唑 100 mg/(kg·24 h)，静脉注射，q6 h。

儿科注意事项

• 治疗选择：静脉给予甲氧苄啶-磺胺甲噁唑后，然后静脉给予喷他脒。

• 另外的药物选择没有设定。

随访

进一步处理

入院指征

• 中度到重度：肺泡-动脉氧梯度>35 mmHg 或者 PaO_2<70 mmHg。

• 不能耐受口服药物。

• 不能及时随访。

出院指征

• 无明显的临床症状。

• 轻度症状，无明显缺氧。

• 能够口服药物治疗。

• 可以及时至医院随访。

• 如果没有痰液，可以加用大环内酯类经验性治疗药物。

随访建议

对于门诊患者必须安排感染科医师会诊。

要点和误区

• 对于气短的免疫抑制患者，必须将 PCP 鉴别诊断。

• 对于诊断 PCP 患者，可能也有结核及非典型肺炎的高危因素。

• 对于有低氧血症患者可能有合并症的高危因素。

肺挫伤 Pulmonary Contusion

Kristen G. Moore 郑金浩 毛恩强 译

F

基础知识

描述

• 动能转移到肺，引起直接肺实质损伤，导致没有肺裂伤的肺出血和水肿。

• 死亡率为 10%～25%。

• 独立危险因素：
- 急性呼吸窘迫综合征。
- 肺炎。
- 长期呼吸衰竭。

病理生理

• 肺挫伤的发展过程。
- 可分为两个阶段：
  ◦ 第一阶段：与直接外伤有关，导致肺泡膜毛细血管破坏，血管内血液漏至间质和肺泡腔内。
  ◦ 第二阶段：在患者复苏阶段，静脉输液引起损伤加重。

• 导致：
- 肺内分流增加。
- 气道阻力增加。
- 肺顺应性降低。
- 呼吸做功增加。
- 低氧血症和酸中毒。
- 呼吸衰竭。

病因

• 钝性或穿透性胸部损伤。

• 突然减速或加压。

• 坠落。

• 交通事故。

• 殴打。

• 袭击。

诊断

症状和体征

病史

• 以任何方式引起的钝伤或穿透性胸部创伤。

• 受伤方式通过患者、家属或急救人员获得：
- 使用安全带。
- 方向盘损坏。
- 气囊展开。

• 胸痛。

• 呼吸困难。

• 咯血。

体格检查

• 听诊：
- 起始呼吸音正常或减弱。
- 发展到哮鸣音、啰音或呼吸音消失。

• 胸壁局限性瘀斑、水肿、红斑和胸壁疼痛。

• 肋骨骨折也引起骨畸形、捻发音、点压痛、反常性呼吸运动。

• 体表安全带位置的瘀斑又称为“安全带标志”。

• 方向盘冲击造成的瘀斑。

• 夹板呼吸。

• 发绀、心动过速、低血压。

• 呼吸困难、呼吸急促。

注意

• 外伤后 6～12 h 潜在的肺挫伤开始加重。

• 伤后 24～48 h 发生急性呼吸窘迫综合征和肺炎的高风险，尤其是老年患者。

基本检查

• X 线胸片。

• 肺挫伤的 X 线片可能在受伤后 6～12 h 开始成像。

• 斑片状肺泡浸润明显联合。

- 和胸内损伤有关：
  - 肋骨骨折。
  - 气胸、血胸。
  - 纵隔扩大。

诊断检查与说明

实验室检查

动脉血气可能提示低氧血症和肺泡动脉梯度升高。

影像学检查

- 胸部 X 线：
  - 挫伤的比例可以协助判断是否需要插管：
    - 挫伤比例<18%：往往不需要插管。
    - 挫伤比例>28%：往往需要插管治疗。
- 胸部 CT 对于发现肺损伤和不能在胸片显现的相关性胸内损伤很有临床意义：
  - 研究表示 CT 检查损伤大小有助于预后判断。
  - 肺挫伤面积大于肺容积 20%提示需要机械通气。
- 经研究超声是诊断肺挫伤最敏感迅速的检查方式。

鉴别诊断

- 成人呼吸窘迫综合征。
- 充血性心力衰竭。
- 血胸。
- 非心源性因素引起的肺水肿。
- 肺炎、脓肿或其他的感染。
- 气胸。
- 肺栓塞、肺梗死、肺血管内血栓形成。

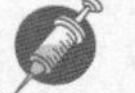

治疗

院前

有重要机制的胸部创伤或先前存在的肺部疾病应被送往最近的可用的创伤中心。

初步稳定/治疗

- 按挫伤情况进行气道管理和液体复苏。
  - 稳定相关的胸壁损伤(开放性气胸、连枷胸)。
- 建立静脉通路、吸氧、持续心电监护、指脉氧饱和度监测。
- 管理气道：
  - 气管插管的指征：
    - 严重低氧血症(PaO_2<60 mmHg，吸氧条件下 PaO_2<80 mmHg)。
    - 有明确的肺疾病。
    - 即将发展到呼吸衰竭。
  - 早期插管和常规给药呼气末正压：
    - 纠正低氧血症、高碳酸血症。
    - 减少呼吸做功。

急诊治疗/程序

- 保持呼吸道通畅和供氧。
- 监测血氧饱和度和呼吸频率。
- 在意识清楚的患者和严重患者，面罩吸氧是一线推荐。
- 如果使用高流量吸氧，患者氧饱和度仍然不能>80%：
  - 继续给予面罩正压吸氧。
  - 双水平正压通气(BiPAP)。
  - 早期气管插管和机械通气。
- 重度单侧损伤患者伴有大咯血和漏气，可以选择气管插管。

> **注意**
> - 避免过多的液体：
>   - 复苏所需的晶体液需要和增加肺间质水肿的风险要权衡。
> - 频繁的检查和重复行胸片以监测肺水肿情况。
> - 精神状态必须适合，患者必须对 BiPAP 配合保持警觉。
>   - 通常这只是一种姑息治疗，患者病情恶化应当立即插管。

药物治疗

- 充分的疼痛控制是最佳结果的关键。
- 激素没有效果的相关证据。
- 预防性抗生素没有提示有关证据。

儿科注意事项

胸壁的柔韧性提高肺挫伤的频率。

老年人注意事项

- 心肺功能储备不足和大容量液体复苏，增加了老年人肺挫伤病情恶化的可能。
- 肺挫伤已被确定为老年患者胸部挫伤预后不良的指标。

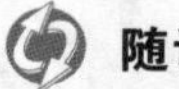

随访

进一步处理

入院指征

肺挫伤的患者需要住院观察，延缓发病的预期。

出院指征

- 患者胸部外伤轻微。
- 没有呼吸窘迫或低氧血症的依据。
  - 呼吸频率正常。
  - 指脉氧饱和度正常。
  - 胸片正常。
- 出院前应与患者进行严格的再入院标准：
  - 气短。
  - 咯血。
  - 疼痛难忍或加剧。
  - 咳嗽。

要点和误区

- 避免针对早期胸片低估了肺挫伤病情的严重性。
- 在住院治疗过程中未能意识到肺挫伤的严重性，可能导致严重后果。
- 联合基础疾病如慢性肺部疾病和肾衰竭增加需要机械通气的可能性。
- 严密监测和重新评估是重中之重。

肺栓塞 Pulmonary Embolism

Alan M. Kumar · Christine A. Babcock 郑金浩 毛恩强 译

基础

描述

- 肺栓塞大部分来自下肢和骨盆深静脉血栓。
- 血栓也起源于肾和上肢静脉。
- 肺栓塞后，血栓大小决定症状和体征。

病因

- 大多数患者肺栓塞有明确的危险因素：
  - 近期有手术。

- 妊娠。
- 先前有深静脉血栓形成(DVT)或肺栓塞。
- 脑卒中或近期瘫痪。
- 恶性肿瘤。
- 年龄大于 50 岁。
- 肥胖。
- 吸烟。
- 口服避孕药。
- 重大创伤。

• 血液学危险因素:
- 凝血因子 5。
- 蛋白 C 或缺乏 S。
- 抗凝血酶 3 缺乏。
- 抗磷脂抗体综合征。
- 狼疮抗凝物。

儿科注意事项

• 血栓栓子疾病鲜见。
• 小儿的危险因素:
- 中心静脉导管存在。
- 制动。
- 心脏病。
- 外伤。
- 恶性肿瘤。
- 手术。
- 感染。

F

诊断

▪ 症状和体征

• 体征和症状的变化多样使诊断困难。
• 共同特点:
- 呼吸困难。
- 胸膜炎性胸痛。
- 呼吸急促。

• 全身症状:
- 发热[很少高于 102 ℉(138.9 ℃)]。
- 出汗。

• 肺的症状:
- 咳嗽。
- 咯血(很少大量咯血)。
- 啰音。

• 心血管症状:
- 心动过速。
- 昏厥。
- 心脏杂音。

• 窘迫症状:
- 发绀。
- 血栓性静脉炎的表现。
- 下肢水肿。

• 腹痛。
• 如果患者年龄小于 40 岁,症状如老年人但通常更更轻。

▪ 基本检查

• 常规的实验室检查没有特异性。
• 胸片:
- 往往可以找出病因。
- 肺栓塞最常见的表现:
  ◦ 正常。
  ◦ 非特异性肺实质异常。
  ◦ 肺不张。
- 肺栓塞的其他表现:
  ◦ 胸腔积液。
  ◦ 肋膜的楔形(Hampton's hump 征)。
  ◦ 膈肌升高。
  ◦ 局部血流量减少(韦特马克征)。

• 心电图:
- 排除心脏病因。
- 肺栓塞患者心电图通常正常。
- 其他表现包括:
  ◦ 非特异性 ST-T 波改变(最常见的异常)。
  ◦ 窦性心动过速。
  ◦ 电轴左偏。
  ◦ 右束支传导阻滞。
  ◦ S1Q3T3 的图形罕见,对于诊断或排除肺栓塞无意义。

• 最新的威尔斯标准:
- 常用的标准,可以联合血浆 D-二聚体为危险因素分层。
- 每一条都有对应的量化评分,如果总分<4,D-二聚体阴性,肺栓塞的风险为<2%:
  ◦ 深静脉血栓的临床表现:3 pts。
  ◦ 肺栓塞为首要诊断:3 pts。
  ◦ 心率>100 次/分:1.5 pts。
  ◦ 4 周内有手术或制动 3 日的经历:1.4 pts。
  ◦ 有肺梗死或深静脉血栓形成的病史:1.5 pts。
  ◦ 咯血:1 pts。
  ◦ 6 个月内治疗过恶性肿瘤:1 pts。

• 肺栓塞排除标准(PEPC):
- 结合低临床可能性,低患病风险评定有临床价值。
  ◦ 年龄<50 岁。
  ◦ 心率<100 次/分。
  ◦ 氧饱和度≥95%。
  ◦ 没有咯血。
  ◦ 无雌激素应用史。
  ◦ 无深静脉血栓或肺栓塞病史。
  ◦ 无单侧下肢肿胀。
  ◦ 近 4 周无手术史、无需住院治疗的外伤史。
- 45 日内如果 PERC 评分为 0 分,肺栓塞或深静脉血栓的风险<1%。

▪ 诊断检查与说明

实验室检查

• 动脉血气分析:
- 可以提示低氧血压、低碳酸血症、呼吸性碱中毒或肺泡动脉氧浓度梯度。
- 肺栓塞时可能肺泡动脉氧浓度梯度正常。
- 不能辅助诊断肺栓塞。

• 血细胞计数:
- 贫血可能加重呼吸困难。
- 几乎所有的肺栓塞患者 D-二聚体水平都>500 mg/ml。
- 3 周内有手术史或恶性肿瘤治疗史的患者 D-二聚体水平同样会升高。
- 大量的研究证明,经酶联免疫试验测得 D-二聚体结合临床表现不符合肺栓塞可以排除肺栓塞的诊断。

影像学检查

• 胸部增强 CT:
- 可以明确其他肺病变。
- 可以准确识别肺栓塞部位的肺楔影:
  ◦ 检查前高度怀疑的患者,增强 CT 阳性的预测值为 96%。
  ◦ 检查前可能性不大的患者,增强 CT 的阴性预测值为 96%。

• 通气血流扫描(V/Q):
- 4%的肺栓塞患者通气血流比值正常或接近正常。
- 4%的肺栓塞患者通气血流比值降低,临床表现不典型。
- 16%~40%的肺栓塞患者通气血流比值降低,有典型的临床表现。
- 16%~66%的肺栓塞患者通气血流比例中等程度异常。
- 56%的肺栓塞患者通气血流比值升高,但临床症状不典型。
- 96%的肺栓塞患者通气血流比值升高,伴有典型的临床症状。

• 双下肢超声:
- 在需要另行肺动脉造影的患者应用。
- 如果存在深静脉血栓,需要和肺栓塞进行相同的抗凝。
- 下肢血管超声阴性不能排除肺栓塞。

• 超声心动图:
- 当有溶栓条件时,用于评估右有心功能,是否存在卵圆孔未闭。

诊断

- 肺血管造影。
- 诊断的金标准。
- 用于不能确诊的病例或用于排除诊断。
- 和其他方式相比，并发症发病率高。

鉴别诊断

- 焦虑性障碍。
- 主动脉夹层。
- 哮喘。
- 心律失常。
- 肋软骨炎。
- 心肌梗死。
- 心包炎。
- 肺炎。
- 气胸。
- 肋骨骨折。

治疗

院前

- 吸氧。
- 建立静脉通道。
- 心电监护。

初步稳定/治疗

- ABC 管理。
- 给予氧疗，确保氧饱和度正常。
- 如果氧饱和度低行气管插管术。
- 对于低血压患者，静脉输液需小心。
- 过多的液体负荷可能加重右心力衰竭。
- 静脉抗休克治疗可以确定低血压是否可以通过静脉补液纠正。

急诊治疗/程序

- 抗凝：
  - 防止血栓形成。
  - 稳定现有凝块，防止凝块脱落。
  - 治疗引起出血的风险。
- 普通肝素：
  - 剂量滴定法很困难，常引起治疗不充分。
  - 目标是保持部分凝血活酶时间在参考值（60～80 s）的 1.5～2.5 s。
- 低分子肝素：
  - 多中心随机对照试验证明，低分子肝素的效果不劣于普通肝素。
  - 治疗目标自动匹配基于体重给药剂量。
  - 和普通肝素相比更容易管理和监测，成本有优势。
- 华法林：
  - 长期抗凝的口服药物。
  - 治疗目标为把国际标准化比值（INR）的控制在 2～3。
- 拜瑞妥：
  - 口服凝血因子Ⅹ抑制剂。
  - 尽量推荐使用拜瑞妥治疗肺栓塞。
  - 使用剂量不需监测。
  - 在肾功能不全、肝功能不全及妊娠期妇女中不推荐使用。
  - 没有特效拮抗药，但半衰期短，以防出血。
- 溶栓：
  - 对于确诊肺栓塞血流动力学不稳定的患者进行溶栓。
  - 在血流动力学稳定的肺栓塞患者伴有严重的低氧血症、大面积肺栓塞或右心室功能不全的仍需考虑溶栓治疗。
- 下腔静脉过滤器：
  - 有抗凝禁忌证或抗凝治疗未能阻止肺栓塞的患者可植入下腔静脉过滤器。
- 手术或导管源性栓子清除术。
  - 对那些有溶栓禁忌或溶栓失败或确定治疗过程中不稳定的患者可以考虑。
  - 具体案例具体分析。

药物治疗

- 阿替普酶：100 mg（儿童不适用），静推持续 2 h。
- 依诺肝素：1 mg/kg（儿童：0.75 mg/kg），皮下注射，q12 h。
- 瑞替普酶：10 U（儿童不适用），静推 30 min 1 次，使用 2 次。
- 链激酶：250 000 U（儿童：3 500～4 000 U/kg），静推持续 30 min，然后 100 000 U（儿童：1 000～1 500 U/kg），静推维持 24 h 以上。
- 普通肝素：
  - 80 U/kg（儿童：75 U/kg），静推 10 min 以上。
  - 维持剂量：18 U/kg（儿童：20 U/kg），静滴。
  - 不用总体重估算肥胖患者的用药剂量。
- 华法林：5 mg[0.05～0.34 mg/(kg·d)] 口服每日 1 次，调整剂量至 INR 目标为 2～3。
- 拜瑞妥：15 mg 每日 2 次持续使用 3 周后，改为 20 mg 每日 1 次。

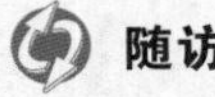

随访

进一步处理

入院指征

- 对于所有的肺栓塞患者均收入院进行抗凝和观察。
- 高度怀疑肺栓塞但病情稳定的患者，没有溶栓禁忌证，缺少通气血流比值或者未能行肺动脉造影，若医疗条件允许时间在情况可以考虑进行溶栓。

要点和误区

- 临床表现各种各样，并且无特异性，很多病例很难明确诊断。
- 患有恶性肿瘤的患者香豆素治疗失败的可能更大，即使国际标准化比值控制在目标范围内也有肺栓塞的风险。

肺水肿

Lee A. Replogle · Shamai A. Grossman　郑金浩　毛恩强 译

基础知识

描述

各种特殊非平衡的作用力引起肺毛细血管里的液体漏入肺泡和肺间质并积聚。

- 心源性的：
  - 心功能不全导致组织灌注不足。
  - 急性心力衰竭代偿期：在慢性心力衰竭的基础上急性水负荷过多。
  - 急性血管功能障碍：血管扩张或血管阻力增加。
- 非心源性的：
  - 肺泡膜通透性增加，非心源性肺泡积液。
  - 急性肺损伤：轻微。
  - 急性呼吸窘迫综合征（ARDS）：

• 氧合指数(PaO_2/FiO_2)≤200 mmHg。
• 纽约心脏协会分级(NYHA):
- 一级:日常活动没有症状。
- 二级:日常活动后出现乏力、呼吸困难或其他症状。
- 三级:日常活动受限。
- 四级:休息或任何活动后都会出现症状。

流行病学

• 美国 580 万患者。
• 发病风险随着年龄的增长而增长,75 岁的患者发病率为 10%。
• 每年有 30%~40%的心力衰竭患者住院治疗。
• 经过急性心力衰竭治疗后 1 个月内死亡率高达 11%。

病因

• 心源性:
- 心肌收缩力降低。
◦ 缺血性心脏病。
◦ 特发性心肌病。
◦ 心肌炎。
- 收缩压力过强:
◦ 主动脉狭窄。
◦ 二尖瓣反流。
- 限制性舒张功能障碍。
◦ 二尖瓣狭窄。
◦ 左心房黏液瘤。
◦ 肥厚型心肌病。
- 高心输出量状态:
◦ 甲状腺功能亢进症。
◦ 贫血。
◦ 动静脉瘘。
◦ 湿性脚气病(wet beriberi)。
- 先天性心脏病。
- 心内膜炎。
- 风湿性心脏病。
• 非心源性病因:
- 脓毒症。
- 急性肺炎。
- 吸入性肺损伤。
- 吸气。
- 溺水。
- 弥散性血管内凝血(DIC)。
- 胰腺炎。
- 肺挫伤。
- 严重外伤(不包括胸部)。
- 心肺旁路。
- 尿毒症。
- 高空性肺水肿。
- 神经性肺水肿。
- 麻醉用药过量。
- 水杨酸过量。
- 肺栓塞。
- 脂肪栓塞。
- 输血相关急性肺损伤。

诊断

症状和体征

病史

• 危险因素:
- 慢性心力衰竭的病史。
- 冠心病或心肌梗死的病史。
- 肥胖。
- 严重的全身性疾病。
• 症状:
- 迅速进展的呼吸困难,至静息时依然有呼吸困难。
- 端坐呼吸。
- 外周性水肿。
- 阵发性夜间呼吸困难。
- 体重迅速增加。
- 体弱、疲劳。
- 咳嗽。

体格检查

• 生命体征:
- 可能有高血压或低血压。
- 呼吸快。
- 低氧血症。
• 整体状况:
- 出汗。
- 畏寒、脸色苍白、皮肤青紫。
• 呼吸:
- 呼吸音。
- 气喘。
- 辅助呼吸肌参与呼吸运动。
• 心血管:
- 心动过速。
- 颈静脉充盈。
- 第二心音亢进,出现第三心音及第四心音。
- 肝颈反射阳性。
• 非心源性:
- 与呼吸体征相似,但是少有外周的症状。

基本检查

• 心电图:评估是否存在心肌梗死和心律失常。
• X 线胸片:评估疾病的严重性,可确诊本病。
• 实验室检查:BNP、心肌酶和肌酐。

诊断检查与说明

实验室检查

• BNP:
- 心力衰竭诊断和随访的实验室指标。
◦ <100 pg/ml:未必是慢性心力衰竭。
◦ 100~500 pg/ml:不确定。
◦ >500 pg/ml:可考虑为慢性心力衰竭。
- 可能在急性发作的慢性心力衰竭或者心室流入道梗阻并不升高。
- 在肾衰竭透析患者左心室肥厚可能会引起假阳性。
• BNP 前体:
- 和 BNP 意义相似。
• 肌钙蛋白:
- 心肌缺血引起肌钙蛋白升高进而导致急性心力衰竭或者急性心力衰竭影响心脏系统引起肌钙蛋白升高。
- 急性心力衰竭发作期可升高 20%。
- 预后不良的指标。
• 血生化:
- 肌酐升高:
◦ 无论什么病因引起的慢性心力衰竭患者中,血肌酐升高预示着预后不良。
◦ 提示急性末梢器官灌注不足。
◦ 提示需收入院或者留观。
- 低钠血症:提示严重心力衰竭。
- 心力衰竭的治疗过程常常引起电解质紊乱。
• 丙氨酸氨基转移酶、门冬氨酸氨基转移酶或胆红素升高提示慢性肝病。
• 如果有潜在病因合并血清脂肪酶升高,提示胰腺炎。
• 动脉血气:评估低氧血症、通气血流失衡、高碳酸血症和酸中毒。

影像学检查

• 胸部 X 线片:
- 肺重新分布:头端血管集中化。
- 心脏扩大:仅在 PA 检查中心影大于胸廓内径的 50%。
- 间质水肿:
◦ 胸腔积液。
◦ 克尔利(氏)B 线。
- 双侧肺门周围肺泡水肿引起的蝴蝶影。
- 非心源性:双侧间质或肺泡浸润均匀时通常没有心影扩大。
- 肺水肿常在出现 12 h 后才在影像学上有

F

所表现。

• 心电图：

- 评估潜在的心脏疾病。

◦ 急性心律失常。

◦ 急性冠状动脉综合征的表现。

◦ 电解质异常的表现。

◦ 30%～42%的房颤患者会出现急性心力衰竭。

◦ 心动过速和缓慢型心律失常均可降低心输出量。

• 超声心动图：

- 评估左心室功能。

- 评估急性心瓣膜病或心包疾病。

- 测量心输出量。

• 床边超声：

- 双侧B线：在左胸和右胸，彗星尾伪影从胸膜线开始延伸到很远的区域强度不减少。

▪ 鉴别诊断

• COPD急性发作。

• 肺炎。

• 哮喘。

• 肺栓塞。

• 心脏压塞。

• 气胸。

• 胸腔积液。

• 过敏反应。

• 酸中毒。

• 过度通气综合征。

治疗

▪ 院前

• 建立静脉通路。

• 吸氧。

• 确定用无重复吸气的面罩。

• 心电监护。

• 指脉氧监测。

• 硝酸酯舌下含服。

• 如果需要气门面罩，在允许的情况下使用PEEP。

• 重症患者行气管插管。

▪ 初步稳定/治疗

• 呼吸和循环的评估，保持气道通畅。

• 呼吸衰竭的患者行无创通气或气管插管。

• 静脉通路。

• 提供氧气。

• 指脉氧饱和度监测。

• 保持患者为直立体位。

• 低血压伴有器官功能障碍的患者进行强心治疗。

▪ 急诊治疗/程序

• 治疗取决于引起肺水肿的病因。

• 吸氧。

• 限制液体量。

• 无论有无导尿管均应注意尿量。

• BiPAP/CPAP。

- 改善氧饱和度，减少呼吸肌做功，减少左心室后负荷。

- 减少插管的概率，减少住院时间和死亡率。

• BIPAP的效果和CPAP无差别。

• 非心源性病因：常常需要正压通气。

- 推荐小潮气量机械通气(6 ml/kg)。

• 呼气末正压：提高供氧的有效措施。

• 低血压患者：

- 避免使用硝酸酯、血管紧张素转化酶抑制剂(ACEI)和吗啡类药物。

- 出现负性肌力：

◦ 多巴胺、多巴酚丁胺、去甲肾上腺素或米力农。

- 新发不稳定心房颤动患者直接心脏复律治疗。

• 血压正常或高血压患者：

- 硝酸酯(硝酸甘油或硝普钠)。

- 利尿剂(呋塞米或布美他尼)在初始稳定后可能最有效。

• 非心源性：治疗潜在的病因。

▪ 药物治疗

• 阿司匹林：抗血小板活性以降低ACS死亡率。

- 325 mg，口服；或650 mg经直肠给药。

• 呋塞米：可用于容量管理的利尿剂。

- 40～150 mg静脉注射。

• 托拉塞米：可用于容量管理的利尿剂。

- 20～40 mg静脉注射。

• 多巴酚丁胺：肌力调节剂和血管扩张剂β_1受体和β_2受体激动剂：

- 2～10 μg/(kg·min)，静推，滴定模式。

- 低血压可能由于血管舒张效应。

• 多巴胺：升压药和肌力调节剂a_1受体、a_2受体和β_1受体激动剂：

- 5～50 μg/(kg·min)，静推；滴定。

- 剂量>20 μg/(kg·min)可能导致心律失常。

• 去甲肾上腺素：升压药和肌力调节剂a_1受体和β_1受体激动剂：

- 0.05～0.5 μg/(kg·min)。

• 米力农：对高血压或血压正常的心力衰竭有用的血管扩张剂和肌力调节剂，负荷剂量50 μg/kg，静推滴定；而后10 min内输注0.375～0.75 μg/(kg·min)。

• 硝酸甘油：静脉扩张剂和血管扩张剂：

- 0.4 mg，舌下含服；重复口服至血压限制值。

- 贴于胸部：1～2 in。

- 5～20 μg/min静推滴定。

• 硝普钠：静脉扩张剂和血管扩张剂：

- 0.5～8 μg/(kg·min)滴注直至理想效果。

- 氰化物代谢物在慢性肾脏病中积聚。

• 地尔硫䓬：治疗室上性心动过速(SVT)的钙通道阻滞剂：

- 0.25 mg/kg，以0.35 mg/kg重复一次，如果成功则过渡到口服药物，如果不成功则滴注地尔硫䓬。

- 充血性心力衰竭禁忌证。

• 美托洛尔：B1特异性β受体阻滞剂(BB)，用于治疗室上性心动过速：

- 0.15 mg/kg静脉注射，最多重复3次，如果成功，随后过渡到口服药物或艾司洛尔滴注。

• 胺碘酮：用于室上性心动过速对BB或CCB无效或心律失常伴低血压的抗心律失常药物：

- 150 mg静脉滴注一次，维持1 mg/min滴注6 h，0.5 mg/min滴注18 h。

• 普鲁卡因胺：宽复合或窄复合室上性心动过速的抗心律失常。

- 17 mg/kg，20～50 mg/min，静脉滴注30 min。

随访

▪ 进一步处理

入院指征

• ICU：

- 正压通气。

- 呼吸肌需支持。

- 急性心肌缺血或心肌梗死。

- 急性呼吸窘迫综合征。

• 留观：

- 新发肺水肿。

- 心电图有所改变。

- 患者有死亡的危险因素，包括高龄、肾功能不全、低血压、使用地高辛、贫血。

出院指征

• 肺水肿大部分患者需要收入院或观察

24 h。

• 患者轻度基础疾病及轻度恶化已住院充分治疗，并且无院外死亡的风险或许可以考虑离院。

• 确保患者随访。

■ 随访建议

和患者的家庭医师联系，确保心内科医师参与随访。

• 继续利尿。

• 低盐饮食。

• 每日称重。

要点和误区

• 硝酸酯舌下含服、静推是降低前负荷的首选药物。

• BNP 对于鉴别急性左心力衰竭和其他疾病引起的肺水肿临床意义较高。

• 急性左心力衰竭早期在胸片上可能不能显像。

• 正常血压和高血压并对利尿剂和 ACEI 类药物抵抗可采用硝酸酯早期治疗改善临床症状。

• 正压机械通气对于非心源性肺水肿是必要的治疗方式，并且可以降低急性心力衰竭的插管率和死亡率。

肺炎(成人)

Jamie L. Adler · Jason C. Imperato　瞿金龙 译

基础知识

■ 描述

• 流行病学：

- 美国引起死亡的第 7 位原因，是感染的首要原因。

• 老年人及合并以下病情的患者死亡率高：

- 慢性心、肺、肝和肾脏疾病。
- 糖尿病。
- 酒精(乙醇)中毒。
- 恶性肿瘤。
- 脾切除术后。
- 免疫抑制。
- 近 3 个月使用抗生素。

• 分类：

- 病因：
  ◦ 社区获得性。
  ◦ 护理院获得性。
  ◦ 医院获得性。
  ◦ 呼吸机相关性。
- 症状：
  ◦ 典型。
  ◦ 非典型。

• 并发症：

- 菌血症。
- 脓毒症。
- 脓肿。
- 脓胸。
- 呼吸衰竭。

■ 病因

• 社区获得性 CAP(典型性)：

- 肺炎链球菌。
- 流感嗜血杆菌。
- 肺炎克雷伯菌肺炎。
- 黏膜炎莫拉菌。
- 化脓链球菌。
- 金黄色葡萄球菌。

• 社区获得性 CAP(非典型性)：

- 肺炎支原体。
- 肺炎衣原体。
- 军团菌。
- 病毒。

• HCAP、HAP 和 VAP：

- 革兰阴菌(假单胞菌、嗜麦芽假丝单胞菌)。
- 耐甲氧西林金黄色葡萄球菌(MRSA)。

• 免疫抑制。

- 肺炎分枝杆菌。
- 卡氏肺孢子菌。

• 吸入性。

- 化学品吸入，胃或口服误吸。

诊断

■ 症状和体征

病史

• 典型：

- 急性起病。
- 发热。
- 畏寒。
- 寒战。
- 咳嗽。
- 脓痰。
- 气短。
- 胸痛。

• 非典型：

- 亚急性起病。
- 病毒前驱症状。
- 咳嗽，少痰。
- 低热。
- 头痛。
- 肌肉酸痛。
- 全身乏力。
- 寒战和胸膜炎比较少见。

体格检查

• 生命体征：

- 呼吸急促。
- 心动过速。
- 低氧。
- 发热。

• 肺部体征：

- 叩诊浊音。
- 触诊震颤。
- 支气管咩音。
- 湿啰音。
- 干啰音。
- 呼吸音减弱。

• 注意，在没有上述症状及体征的情况下，也可能会出现肺炎。

老年人注意事项

• 老年人常常症状不典型。

• 老年人死亡率高。

■ 基本检查

临床和放射诊断。

实验室检查

• 一般检查：

- 血常规。
- 血生化。

• 其他：

- 血培养。
- 痰培养和痰涂片。

- 尿抗原检测(铜绿假单胞菌)。
- CRP(C反应蛋白)。
- 乳酸。
- 流感病毒检测。

影像学检查

X线胸片检查:

- 概述:
  - 影像学上变化对于感染的病原菌无特殊特点。
  - 可能在年轻患者或健康患者变现延迟。
  - 如果影像学结果阴性也不能排除使用抗菌药物。
- 阳性结果:
  - 侧位片:心脏的大小等。
  - 支气管造影片。
  - 节段或亚节段的实变改变。
  - 弥漫性改变。
  - 胸腔积液。
  - 脓胸。
  - 脓肿。
  - 空洞形成。

诊断步骤/外科

胸腔穿刺术:

- 大量胸腔积液、不明原因的肺炎或对标准治疗失败的。

鉴别诊断

- 哮喘发作。
- 支气管炎。
- 充血性心力衰竭(CHF)。
- 慢性阻塞性肺疾病(COPD)。
- 异物误吸。
- 气胸。
- 肺栓塞。
- 肿瘤。

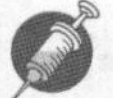

治疗

院前

- 建立静脉通路。
- 吸氧。
- 心电监护。
- 吸入支气管扩张药。
- 严重患者必要时气管内插管。

初步稳定/治疗

- 静脉通路,必要时液体复苏。
- 吸氧。
- 心电监护。
- 吸入支气管扩张药。
- 严重患者必要时气管内插管。

急诊治疗/程序

- 美国胸科协会经验性治疗指南:
- 门诊患者:
  - 既往健康,无合并其他疾病。
    - 大环内酯或多西环素。
  - 有合并症状(具体见上述)。
    - 联合β-内酰胺类药。
    - 呼吸喹诺酮类药物。
- 住院患者:
  - 轻症患者。
    - 联合β-内酰胺类药和大环内酯。
    - 单独呼吸喹诺酮类药物。
  - 严重患者。
    - 联合β-内酰胺类药和大环内酯或呼吸喹诺酮类药物。
    - 对假单胞菌:联合抗假单胞菌药物(哌拉西林三唑巴坦、亚胺培南、美罗培南)。
    - 对MRSA:万古霉素或利奈唑胺。
    - 吸入性肺炎:加克林霉素或甲硝唑。
    - 低于耐药的肺炎球菌:加万古霉素。

药物治疗

- 阿莫西林克拉维酸钾:500 mg,口服,q12 h。
- 氨苄西林-舒巴坦:1.5 g,静脉注射,q6 h。
- 阿奇霉素:0.5 g口服首日,0.25 g口服2~5日;或500 mg口服3日;或500 mg,每日1次。
- 氨曲南:1~2 g,静脉注射,q12 h。
- 头孢吡肟:2 g,静脉注射,q12 h。
- 头孢噻肟:1~2 g,静脉注射,q8 h。
- 头孢泊肟:200 mg,口服,q12 h。
- 头孢他啶:2 g,静脉注射,q12 h。
- 头孢曲松:1~2 g,静脉注射,qd。
- 头孢呋辛:0.75~1.5 g,静脉注射,q8 h。
- 多西定:100 mg,口服/静脉注射,q12 h。
- 厄他培南:1 g,静脉注射,qd。
- 左氧氟沙星:500~750 mg/d,口服/静脉注射。
- 利奈唑胺:600 mg/d,口服/静脉注射。
- 亚胺培南:500 mg,静脉注射,q6 h。
- 美罗培南:1 g,静脉注射,q8 h。
- 莫西沙星:400 mg/d,静脉注射。
- 哌拉西林-他唑巴坦:3.375~4.5 g,静脉注射,q6 h。
- 万古霉素:1 g,静脉注射,q12 h。

一线用药

- 门诊患者:
  - 健康患者。
    - 阿奇霉素:0.5 g口服首日,0.25 g口服2~5日;或者500 mg口服3日;或500 mg每日1次。
  - 合并症患者。
    - 左氧氟沙星:750 mg,口服,5日。
- 住院患者:
  - 非ICU:
    - 左氧氟沙星:750 mg,静脉注射,每日1次。
  - ICU:
    - 头孢曲松:1~2 g,静脉注射,每日1次,联合左氧氟沙星750 mg,静脉注射,每日1次±哌拉西林-他唑巴坦3.375~4.5 g,静脉注射,q6 h或±万古霉素1 g,静脉注射,q12 h。

二线用药

氨曲南替代β-内酰胺类药物作为ICU二线用药。

随访

进一步处理

入院指征

- 根据患者的严重程度、合并症、家庭的护理能力。
- 决定可以通过对患者进行分级评分,不能只看临床症状等。
- CURB-65评分:
  - 严重程度:
    - 神志情况。
    - Cr>7 mmol/L或BUN>19。
    - 呼吸频率≥30次/分。
    - 收缩压<9 mmHg,或平均动脉压<60 mmHg。
    - 年龄≥65岁。
  - 说明:
    - 0~1分:门诊治疗。
    - 2分:可以选择入院或门诊治疗。
    - 3~5分:ICU治疗。
- 肺严重程度评分:
  - 一般情况:
    - 男性:+年龄。
    - 女性:+年龄-10。
    - 家庭护理:+10。
  - 合并症:
    - 肿瘤:+30。
    - 肝脏:+20。
    - 慢性心功能不全:+10。
    - 脑血管病:+10。
    - 肾脏病:+10。

F

- 体格检查：
  - 生命体征变化：+20。
  - 脉搏≥125 次/分：+20。
  - 呼吸次数≥30 次/分：+20。
  - 舒张压＜90 mmHg：+15。
  - 体温＜35 ℃或≥40 ℃：+10。
- 实验室检查：
  - pH＜7.35：+30。
  - BUN≥30 mg/dl：+20。
  - Na^+＜130 mmol/L：+20。
  - 血糖≥250 mg/dl(13.8 mmol/L)：+10。
  - 血细胞比容：＜30%：+10。
  - $PaCO_2$＜60 mmHg：+10。
  - 胸腔积液：+10。
- 说明：
  - 0：Ⅰ级门诊治疗。
  - ＜70 分：Ⅱ级门诊，可以观察。
  - 70～90 分：Ⅲ级可家里静脉抗生素治疗和短暂的留院观察。
  - 90～130 分：Ⅳ级住院治疗。
  - ＞130 分：Ⅴ级住院治疗。
- 补充说明：
  - 前一年因肺炎住院。
  - 门诊治疗失败。
  - 条件有限，不适合门诊治疗。

出院指征

- 年龄＜65 岁。
- 无合并症。
- 无全身毒性反应。
- 无生命体征变化。
- 实验学检查正常。
- 随访 72 h 无特别。

随访建议

一般随访 72 h。

要点和误区

- 危重病患者延迟抗生素治疗。
- 被潜在的肺情况延误。
- 不能识别的肺结核(TB)和人类免疫缺陷病毒(HIV)。
- 免疫抑制或老年人可能症状不典型。

肺炎(儿童) Pneumonia, Pediatric

Gary D. Zimmer · Karen P. Zimmer 瞿金龙 译

基础知识

描述

- 机制不清。
- 口咽部吸入或血行感染。
- 分布主要是部位不同：间质性(支原体、病毒)、肺泡(肺炎球菌)、脓肿(葡萄球菌)、弥漫性(卡氏肺囊虫)。

病因

- ＜2 周：
  - 肺炎球菌 B 型。
  - 肠源性革兰阴性菌。
  - 呼吸道合胞病毒。
  - 单纯疱疹病毒。
  - 金黄色葡萄球菌。
- 2 周至 3 个月。
  - 衣原体。
  - 副流行性感冒。
  - 肺炎球菌。
  - 金黄色葡萄球菌。
  - 流行性感冒。
  - 百日咳博德特菌。
- 3 个月至 8 岁：
  - 病毒：
    - 呼吸道合胞病毒。
    - 副流行性感冒。
    - 流行性感冒。
    - 腺病毒。
  - 肺炎球菌。
  - 流行性感冒。
  - 肺炎球菌 A 型。
  - 金黄色葡萄球菌。
  - 百日咳。
- ＞8 岁：
  - 支原体。
  - 病毒。
  - 金黄色葡萄球菌。
- 近期发达国家的病原学变迁。
  - 支原体结核。
  - 流行性感冒病毒。
  - 百日咳。
- 免疫异常患者。
  - 卡氏肺囊虫。
  - 肺炎杆菌复合体。
  - 支原体结核。
  - 肺炎克雷伯菌。
  - 假单胞菌。
- 少见菌。
  - 真菌。
  - 立克次体(Q 热)。

诊断

症状和体征

- 一般(所有年龄)：
  - 咳嗽。
  - 啰音。
  - 发热。
  - 低氧。
  - 心率快。
  - 呼吸困难。
  - 呼噜音。
  - 皮疹、斑丘疹(超过 10%的患者)。
  - 非典型性中毒症状。
  - 肺部检查：
    - 呼吸音减低，机械通气。
    - 叩诊浊音。
    - 哮鸣音。
- ＜6 个月的婴儿：
  - 行为改变：没精打采，易发怒。
  - 呼吸困难。
  - 结膜炎。
  - 发绀。
  - 呼噜音。
  - 喂养差。
  - 体温不稳定。
  - 咳嗽时呕吐。
  - 咳嗽。
  - 鼻翼扇动。
  - 鼻充血。
  - 哮鸣。
  - 断断续续地咳嗽。
- ＞5 岁：
  - 胸痛。
  - 咳嗽、咳痰。
  - 畏寒、寒战。

病史

• 预防免疫史。
• 既往治疗史,包括免疫状态。
• 暴露史。
• 症状和体征。

体格检查

• 肺部检查有助,尤其 5 岁以上小孩。
• 外周或者中枢性发绀。
• 呼吸系统并发症。

■ 基本检查

• 指脉氧。
• X 线胸片:
- 诊断的金标准。
- 需要鉴别低位呼吸道感染,或者 36 个月内的白细胞明显升高(>15 000/mm^3)。
- 注意病毒和细菌的鉴别。
- 病毒和支原体主要间质改变。
- 细菌主要是肺叶、肺泡的改变。
- 肺炎球菌引起大叶性肺炎。
- 侧位片可以鉴别有无积液。

实验室检查

• 血常规检查:
- 白细胞增高。
- 敏感性和特异性差。
- WBC>20 000/mm^3 或者中性粒细胞(N)>9 000/mm^3 可能合并菌血症可能。
- 百日咳能引起淋巴细胞增多。
• 血培养:
- 培养阳性低。
- 推荐在小于 36 个月的儿童患者中应用。
- 一般在中毒症状很重的患者进行,需要住院处理。
• 动脉血气:用来观察有无呼吸衰竭。
• 电解质检查:排除抗利尿激素分泌异常综合征。
• 痰涂片和痰培养。
• 支原体 IgM 抗体和冷凝集试验。
- 怀疑这种病原菌时此检查有用。
- 危重病患者阳性的可能性更大。
• 鼻拭子或咽拭子直接抗体或者培养:
- 区分 RSV、百日咳等。

影像学检查

X 线胸片仍是影像学检查很好的选择。
• 有条件行后前位和侧位。
• CT 检查可以提供肺部细节情况和潜在的肺疾病。

■ 鉴别诊断

• 气道疾病急性发作(哮喘、气管炎等,年龄<2 岁)。
• 吸入性疾病:
- 胃食管反流。
- 血管环。
- H 型气管食管瘘。
- 异物。
- 碳氢化合物。
• 充血性心力衰竭。
• 先天性疾病:
- 囊性纤维化。
- 先天性肺叶缺损。
- 血管瘤。
• 肿瘤。
• 败血症。

治疗

■ 院前

• 指脉氧监测。
• 对于呼吸衰竭患者给予高流量吸氧。
• 补液(开始生理盐水 20 ml/kg)容量复苏,纠正低血压。
• 对于呼吸衰竭患者给予支持和插管治疗。

■ 初步稳定/治疗

• 如果病情较重:
- 保护气道,必要时气管插管机械通气治疗,如果合并严重脓毒症或感染性休克患者行气管插管治疗。
- 高流量吸氧。
- 扩容补液(开始生理盐水 20 ml/kg)容量复苏,治疗低血压。
• 心电监测。
• 指脉氧监测。
• 如果有机械通气,需动脉血气检查。
• 严重患者监测血糖变化:
- 对于血糖过低,需注射高糖 D_{25} 2 ml/kg(幼儿)、D_{10} 5 ml/kg(婴儿)。

■ 急诊治疗/程序

• 继续院前或初始稳定病情的处理和治疗。
• 早期广谱抗生素治疗以解决所在地区的局部耐药。
• 通常需要用支气管扩张剂治疗的特异性治疗的并发反应性气道疾病。临床试验可能有助于确定临床反应:
- 如果缺氧与 CXR 上的结果不成比例,则空气流动减少,或者存在特发反应性或哮喘/支气管炎的患者或家族史,这尤其重要。
• 如果胸腔积液损害呼吸功能或用于诊断测试,可在影像学引导下行胸腔穿刺。

■ 抗生素治疗

• 经验性给予抗生素治疗对于>6 个月的患者效果最佳。
- <2 个月:
◦ 无合并症或呼吸困难者可以继续门诊。
- 3 个月至 5 岁:
◦ 一线用药:
▫ 阿莫西林。
▫ 阿莫西林-克拉维酸。
◦ 二线用药:
▫ 甲氧苄啶-磺胺甲噁唑。
▫ 大环内酯类(阿奇霉素或克拉霉素等)。
- 5~18 岁:
◦ 一线用药:
▫ 大环内酯类(阿奇霉素或克拉霉素等)。
• 对于危重病患儿起始静脉治疗:
- 初生婴儿:
◦ 氨苄西林和头孢噻肟或庆大霉素。
◦ 对于敏感的衣原体或百日咳使用阿奇霉素。
- 1~2 个月:
◦ 氨苄西林和头孢噻肟。
◦ 对于敏感的衣原体或百日咳使用阿奇霉素或红霉素。
- >3 个月:
◦ 头孢噻肟、头孢呋辛或头孢曲松。
◦ MRSA 感染万古霉素。
◦ 大环内酯治疗支原体。
◦ 克林霉素 A 型链球菌。
• 对于不确定诊断可以请感染科会诊。
• 沙丁胺醇吸入治疗。
• 阿莫西林:80 mg/(kg·24 h),q6 h,静脉注射。
• 阿莫西林-克拉维酸盐:30 mg/(kg·24 h),q12 h,口服。
• 氨苄西林:100~150 mg/(kg·24 h),q6 h,静脉注射。
• 阿奇霉素:10 mg/(kg·24 h)第 1 日,然后 5 mg/(kg·24 h),持续 4 日。
• 头孢噻肟:50~75 mg/(kg·24 h),q8 h,静脉注射,最大剂量 2 g。
• 头孢曲松:100 mg/(kg·24 h),q12~24 h,静脉注射,最大剂量 2 g,q12 h。
• 头孢呋辛:100 mg/(kg·24 h),q8 h,静脉注射,最大剂量 2 g。
• 克拉霉素:15 mg/(kg·24 h),q12 h,口服,最大剂量 500 g。

F

• 克林霉素：30～40 mg/(kg·24 h)，q6～8 h，静脉注射。

• 庆大霉素：5～7.5 mg/(kg·24 h)，q6～12 h，静脉注射。

• 甲氧苄啶-磺胺甲噁唑：8～10 mg/(kg·24 h)，q12 h，口服。

• 万古霉素：10～15 mg/(kg·24 h)，q8～12 h，静脉注射，最大剂量 1 000 mg。

随访

进一步处理

入院指征

• 中毒反应严重。

• 呼吸衰竭

• 脱水或呕吐。

• 呼吸困难。

• 婴儿<2 个月。

• 婴儿<6 个月伴有肺炎。

• 低氧。

• 胸腔积液。

• 对门诊口服药物不耐受。

• 免疫抑制患儿。

• 对于不配合门诊治疗的父母。

出院指征

• 很多患者可以在家里治疗，如果没有明显的低氧和呼吸困难或呕吐等严重并发症。

• 可以随访 1～2 日。

转诊问题

呼吸衰竭、胸腔积液或中毒反应很重。

随访建议

治疗中必须要有定期随访。

要点和误区

• 对于严重脓毒症和感染性休克早期气道保护治疗。

• 避免抗菌药物的延迟。

• 出院患者必须要有明确的证据表明良好的支持、随访和无明显中毒症状。

• 本地的患者可能出现细菌耐药，必须及时使用敏感抗生素。

肺源性心脏病 Cor pulmonale

Ryan M. Kring · David T. Chiu　陈奇通 译

基础知识

描述

右心室肥大(RVH)或扩张导致肺动脉压力增高。全身性缺陷或先天性心脏病引起的 RVH 不被归入肺源性心脏病。

• 急性肺源性心脏病：
  - 右心室扩张伴心肌壁被拉伸变薄。
  - 因急性肺动脉高压(HTN)引起的过负荷。
  - 常因大的肺栓塞引起。

• 慢性肺源性心脏病：
  - RVH 最终发展至扩张伴右心衰竭。
  - 由慢性肺动脉高压的适应性反应造成。
  - 主要为肺泡低氧的结果引起的。

• 肺循环是一个低阻力低压力系统：
  - 肺动脉是薄壁且可扩张的。
  - 平均肺动脉压为 12～15 mmHg。
  - 正常左侧肺动脉压为 6～10 mmHg。
  - 驱动肺循环的实际压力差仅为 6～9 mmHg。

• 3 个因素影响肺动脉压力：
  - 心输出量。
  - 肺静脉压力。
  - 肺血管阻力。

• 肺动脉高压可因多种机制引起：
  - 心输出量明显增大。
  - 继发于先天性心脏病的左向右分流。
  - 低氧：
    ◦ 肺血管阻力增高的最常见病因。
    ◦ 低氧性肺血管收缩是对肺泡低氧的适应性血管舒缩反应。
    ◦ 肺动脉系统内可见代偿性压力增高，以维持通过肺血管床的血流。
  - 肺动脉栓子通过引起肺血流阻力导致相似的改变。
  - 明显提高血液黏度或胸内压同样阻碍血流。

• 肺动脉高压被分为 5 组。
  - 第一组：肺动脉性高压。
  - 第二组：左心疾病引起的肺动脉高压。
    ◦ 此分类中右心室功能不全不认为是肺源性心脏病。
  - 第三组：肺疾病和/或低氧引起的肺动脉高压。
  - 第四组：慢性血栓栓塞性肺动脉高压。
  - 第五组：未明确的多因素机制引起的肺动脉高压。

流行病学

发生率

• 每年约 86 000 位患者死于 COPD：
  - 相关的右心室衰竭在许多病例中为显著性因素，同时占美国心力衰竭入院的 10%～30%。

• 大于 50 岁的 COPD 的患者，50%发生肺动脉高压，并有发生肺源性心脏病的风险。

• 肺源性心脏病的病程通常与潜在疾病过程的进展有关。

• 一旦发展至肺源性心脏病，患者的 5 年生存率为 30%。

病因

• 慢性缺血。
  - COPD。
  - 高海拔居住者。
  - 睡眠呼吸暂停。
  - 胸部畸形。
    ◦ 脊柱后侧凸。

• 肺栓塞。

• 间质性肺疾病。
  - 硬皮病。
  - 系统性红斑狼疮。
  - 混合型结缔组织病。
  - 结节病。
  - 肺朗格汉斯细胞增多症。
  - 多发性神经纤维瘤。
  - 淋巴管平滑肌瘤病。

• 囊性纤维化。

• 重度贫血。

• 肥胖。

• 肺静脉阻塞疾病。

• 继发于肿瘤或腺瘤的肺血管阻塞。

• 血黏度增高。
  - 真性红细胞增多症。
  - 白血病。

• 胸内压增高。
  - 有呼气末正压的机械通气。

• 特发性肺动脉高压。

诊断

症状和体征

- 劳力性呼吸困难。
- 易疲劳。
- 虚弱。
- 劳力性晕厥。
- 咳嗽。
- 咯血。
- 无冠状动脉疾病出现劳力性心绞痛。
- 厌食。
- 右上腹不适。
- 喘鸣。
- 声嘶。
- 体重增加。
- 肝大。
- 腹水。
- 外周水肿。
- 终末期肺源性心脏病。
- 心源性休克。
- 少尿。
- 四肢发冷。
- 继发于左心室舒张功能受损的肺水肿。

病史

- 不耐受运动。
- 心悸。
- 胸痛。
- 头重脚轻。
- 晕厥。
- 下肢水肿。

体格检查

- 颈静脉扩张。
- 显著的A波和V波。
- 胸部直径增加。
- 水泡音和/或喘鸣音。
- 心脏触诊可及胸骨左缘起伏。
- 可能听到第二心音分裂或肺动脉瓣杂音。
- 肝颈回流征和肝脏搏动。
- 下肢凹陷性水肿。

诊断检查与说明

实验室检查

- 脉搏氧饱和度或动脉血气：
- 平静 PO_2 40～60 mmHg。
- 平静 PCO_2 常为 40～70 mmHg。
- 血细胞比容：
- 常增高。
- β-钠尿肽：
- 如增高，对中度到重度肺动脉高压敏感，且可能作为独立的死亡率预测工具。
- 单一的数值增高不足以建立肺源性心脏病的诊断。
- 其他实验室检查通常无帮助。

影像学检查

- X线胸片：
- 肺动脉高压的征象：
  - 大的肺动脉影（>16～18 mm）。
  - 增大的右心室轮廓。
  - 肺源性心脏病检查中可有大于90%者发现异常，但不能指示疾病严重程度。
  - 胸腔积液并非只在肺源性心脏病中出现。
- 心电图：
- 电轴右偏。
- 右束支传导阻滞。
- 右心室肥厚。
  - V_1 和 V_2 导联中R波为主波方向。
  - V_5 和 V_6 有大的S波。
  - 心前区导联为小的R波和深的S波。
- 右心房增大。
  - 高尖的P波（肺型P波）。
- S1Q3形式见于急性肺源性心脏病。
- 瞬时改变由低氧引起。
- 右侧心前区T波低平。
- 超声心动图：
- 优选的无创性诊断手段。
- 右心室扩张或右心室肥大。
- 评估三尖瓣反流。
- 多普勒定量测量肺动脉压力、右心室射血分数。
- 胸部CT、通气/灌注现象或肺动脉造影：
- 在急性肺源性心脏病时有作用。
- 磁共振：
- 评估右心室大小和功能较超声心动图更为优秀。
- 肺功能测试：
- 因肺动脉高压引起弥散能力受损。
- 右心导管：
- 最精准估计肺血管血流动力学。
- 准确测量肺动脉压力和肺毛细血管楔压。

鉴别诊断

- 左心原发病。
- 二尖瓣狭窄。
- 先天性心脏病。
- 艾森门格综合征。
  - 胎儿心脏的先天性缺损导致的左向右分流，导致肺血管血流增加，引起肺动脉高压。
- 甲状腺功能减退症。
- 肝硬化。

治疗

院前

- 支持治疗：
- 补充氧气。
  - 达到动脉氧饱和度90%的目标。
- 静脉通路。
- 心电监测。
- 脉搏氧饱和度监测。
- 治疗呼吸疾病相关的支气管痉挛：
- β受体激动剂雾化药物。
- 注意：
- 血管扩张剂和利尿剂不在此治疗内。
- 严重低氧的患者可能需要气管插管。

初步稳定/治疗

急诊治疗指向潜在的疾病过程和降低肺动脉高压。

急诊治疗/程序

- 补充氧气足以使动脉氧饱和度上升至90%：
- 提高氧合降低肺动脉血管收缩和右心室后负荷。
- 提高的心输出量增加对体内多余水分的利尿作用。
- 小心监测患者通气情况和 PCO_2，因高碳酸可能降低呼吸驱动和引起酸中毒。
- 可谨慎加用利尿剂，如呋塞米，因其可通过降低循环血容量来降低肺动脉压力：
- 当心容量不足和低钾血症。
- 患者应维持盐和液体限制。
- 治疗肺源性心脏病不需要使用地高辛。
- 支气管扩张剂：
- 支气管扩张剂治疗对于COPD患者特别有帮助。
- 选择性β肾上腺素能药物，如特布他林0.25 mg皮下注射可能有帮助。
- 支气管扩张剂影响和减低心室后负荷。
- 茶碱可能对提高膈肌收缩力和降低肌肉疲劳有作用。
- 血栓栓塞性疾病的高危患者可考虑抗凝。
- 急性失代偿性COPD患者：
- 早期激素治疗。
- 抗生素使用。
- 总的来说，潜在呼吸疾病的改善可使得右心室功能改善。

药物治疗

- 呋塞米：20～60 mg，静脉注射（儿童：

F

1 mg/kg,可提高到 1 mg/kg, q2 h,不超过 6 mg/kg)。

- 特布他林: 0.25 mg,皮下注射。

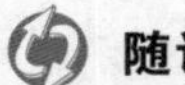

随访

进一步处理

入院指征

- 新发的低氧。
- 全身水肿。
- 严重呼吸衰竭。
- 潜在疾病过程的入院标准。

出院指征

无低氧或氧气需求平稳的患者。

转诊问题

- 潜在病因对紧急处理有反应者密切随访。
- 需要进行睡眠研究以评估睡眠呼吸暂停者,应与患者的负责医师协调。

随访建议

慢性缺氧的患者应确保家中吸氧。

要点和误区

- 体格检查对探查 COPD 患者是否存在肺心病是不可靠的,因为胸腔过度膨胀使得经典体征不清晰。
- 血管扩张剂治疗仅应在传统治疗和氧合失效时考虑使用。

分娩(无并发症) Delivery, Uncomplicated

Patricia De Melo Panakos · Ivette Motola 许磊 译

基础知识

病因

- 急诊分娩是罕见的:
  - 在美国急诊分娩的发生率是未知的。
  - 医疗保健系统中,患者有很少产前保健时往往急诊分娩的发生率更高。
- 急诊分娩通常发生以下 3 个场景:
  - 有过早产的多产孕妇。
  - 不能认清临产症状的未生育孕妇。
  - 患者缺乏产前保健,缺乏转运或早产。

诊断

症状和体征

- 临产时表现为宫缩发生至少每 5 min 一次,每次持续 30～60 s,并引起宫颈的变化。
- 有分娩史的重大阴道出血需要即刻评估前置胎盘或胎盘早剥。

病史

- 上次月经期及估计胎龄(EGA)。
- 近期感染。
- 妊娠史,并发症。
- 在此之前剖宫产。
- 产前检查。
- 腹部、盆腔痉挛。
- 接触性出血。
- 胎膜破裂(羊膜囊)。
- 可报告性尿失禁。
- 推动或有排便的冲动。
- 血性的黏液阻塞。
- 宫缩的发生和频率。

体格检查

- 即将分娩体征:
  - 完全消失和扩张子宫颈(足月婴儿 10 cm 左右)。
  - 胎儿可触及部分。
  - 会阴部胀。
  - 外阴阴道区域扩张。
- 经宫颈触诊或通过床旁超声尝试确定胎位和体位。

基本检查

- 无菌双合诊盆腔检查是最有用的工具用于评估分娩前兆和可能性存在的即刻分娩:
  - 评估扩张、位置和消失。
  - 不挤压,直到完全扩张。
  - 阴道流血时不应该行双合诊检查,直到超声(US)可以排除前置胎盘。
- 胎心音(FHT)应该进行多普勒检查。

诊断检查与说明

实验室检查

- 如果患者临产:
  - 全血细胞检查。
  - 血型。
  - Rh。
    - 胎儿血红蛋白酸洗脱试验应该在分娩后检查,如果 Rh 阴性的母亲生下 Rh 阳性的孩子。
    - Rh 免疫球蛋白可以用于 72 h 内分娩的母亲。
- 尿液检查,如果担心有尿路感染或先兆子痫。

影像学检查

- 并不需要的影像学检查: 无并发症的阴道分娩。
- 妊娠晚期阴道出血,急诊超声评估胎盘早剥或前置胎盘。
- 如果时间允许,B 超有助于找到位置胎盘的解剖。

鉴别诊断

- Braxton Hicks 收缩:
  - 不规则的子宫收缩不导致宫颈扩张或消失。
- 肌肉腰痛。
- 子宫圆韧带疼痛。
- 腹痛的其他原因,如扭转、卵巢、阑尾炎、肾结石。

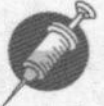

治疗

院前

- 患者取左侧侧卧位。
- 院前急救医疗服务(EMS)人员应有充分的培训,并有适当的设备可用于分娩。
- 分娩前对高危产科患者(OB)进行紧急医疗救治:
  - 降低新生儿发病率和死亡率。
  - 更快,更便于分娩后的新生儿转运。
- 使用航空运输产科患者已证明是安全和有效的:
  - 在飞行中,高度可导致胎儿缺氧,孕妇患者应放在补充氧气的地方。

初始治疗

- 对无阴道流血患者,立即行无菌妇科检查,以评估子宫颈扩张、消失、位置或呈现部分。

• 临产患者应立刻转移,除非分娩立马进行。

• 如果患者是完全扩张和胎儿部分在会阴边缘,准备急诊分娩。

■ 急诊治疗/程序

• 产科医师应通知分娩将在急诊发生。

• 儿科医师或新生儿和新生儿重症监护病房应通知。

• 准备新生儿复苏。

• 患者平卧位或半俯卧位。

• 开始静脉生理盐水或 D_5NS 和补充氧气,并把患者取截石位。

• 组装产科(OB)包装:

- Bulb 注射器。
- 2 无菌 Kelly 夹。
- Sterile Mayo 剪刀。
- Umbilical 夹。

• 新生儿复苏设备也应该是可用的。

• 如果时间允许,消毒阴道区使用聚维酮碘(Betadine)。

• 简单的阴道分娩应该发生:

- 当胎儿头先露发生时,分娩头部应该控制,通过阴道口引导它每一次收缩。
- 常规侧切是没有必要的,然而如果会阴撕裂,进行中线外阴切开术,通过将 2 个手指的背后会阴部,使直切口朝(但不包括)直肠用无菌 Mayo 剪刀。
- 后胎头娩出后,迅速吸鼻咽部,再感觉一下颈部颈背线:
  ◦ 如果存在,手动减少头动。
  ◦ 如果脐带绕颈过紧,双钳,切割,并迅速分娩婴儿。
- 取适量涂抹于胎头温和下行压力子宫收缩:
  ◦ 分娩前肩。
  ◦ 后肩和婴儿的其余部分将快速分娩。
- 分娩后,婴儿应与子宫口处在同一水平线并咽部再吸。
- 用无菌凯利双钳线,夹钳,并切断它们。
- 婴儿应刺激、加热、干燥处理:
  ◦ 如果发绀存在,婴幼儿应给予氧气和复苏。
  ◦ 按照新生儿复苏指南,如果必要。
- 将脐带钳夹。
- 胎盘会自发地提供在 20～30 min:
  ◦ 密切观察母亲产后出血。
- 子宫按摩可以帮助胎盘从子宫内分离和限制宫缩乏力:
  ◦ 避免将牵拉脐带,因为这可能导致子宫反转或者撕裂。
- 如果患者有严重出血和胎盘不能自发通过,应该立刻送到手术室。
- 胎盘分娩后,应检查任何不规则或破坏地区可以保留胎盘。

• 在简单的分娩中,使用的药物是不必要的:

- 胎盘分娩后,子宫按摩可以使子宫出血停止。

• 产后子宫出血是常见的:

- 子宫、阴道和会阴应检查对于裂伤。
- 如果没有发现裂伤,假设子宫收缩乏力。
- 如果子宫不能收缩对于子宫按摩,使用催产素静脉注射。
- 如果出血仍然存在子宫持续按摩可能会有所帮助,然后给甲基麦角马来酸(methergine)肌内注射。
- 如果以上措施不能控制出血,可使用卡前列素氨丁三醇(欣母沛)。
- 氨甲环酸(TXA)可减少产后出血的死亡。
  ◦ 一旦发生出血应尽快给药。

■ 药物治疗

• 卡前列素氨丁三醇(欣母沛):0.25 mg,肌内注射,q15～60 min(最多 2 剂)。

• 马来酸甲麦角(methergine):0.2 mg,肌内注射或静脉注射。

• 催产素:20～40 U,在 1 L 生理盐水注入,250～500 ml/h,静脉注射。

• 氨甲环酸:1 g(100 mg/ml),1 ml/min。

随访

■ 进一步处理

入院指征

• 所有妇女分娩并发症,无显著产后出血应被允许分娩或产后单位的关心和监控。

• 获得儿童或新生儿会诊,进入新生儿重症监护病房:

- 所有的婴儿呼吸窘迫。
- 胎龄<35 周。
- 重量<5 Ib(约 2.3 kg)。
- 低 Apgar 评分。

• 以无上述并发症的足月儿可被录取到幼儿园或母胎结合单元。

• 如果分娩后转运母亲和婴儿,考虑使用 2 辆救护车。

出院指征

• 分娩后充足的恢复,患者可以适当活动和分娩或产后单元。

• 患者不应该回家从急诊出来后。

要点和误区

• 要准备好处理并发症,如脐带脱垂、肩难产、臀位分娩。

• 准备好处理分娩后的患者——母亲和婴儿。

F

分娩(早产和胎膜早破)

Adam Z. Barkinr 何超 段立伟 译

基础知识

分娩包括婴儿经产道从子宫娩出过程中发生的所有一系列生理性事件。

■ 描述

• 分娩过程中子宫颈会发生改变,使婴儿能顺利地从产道娩出。

• 子宫产生协调同步的收缩。

• 子宫重要的、持续的、有节律的收缩过程会带来子宫颈的扩张和婴儿的娩出。

• 产程一般分为 3 个过程。

- 第一产程:从子宫开始收缩到宫颈完全打开。
- 第一产程可以进一步分为潜伏期和活跃期。
  ◦ 在潜伏期:子宫的轻度收缩,持续时间短(<45 s),节律不规则,子宫颈的变化不明显。
  ◦ 之后进入子宫收缩的活跃期,一般会在子宫颈扩张 3～4 cm 后开始,子宫收缩强有力,节律规则(每 2～3 min 一次),持续时间长(>45 s)。
- 第二产程:从子宫颈完全扩张到胎儿娩

出的过程。

- 第三产程：从胎儿娩出到胎盘娩出的过程。

• 分娩过程中的持续时间因每位妇女而差异明显。

• 对于初产妇，第一产程和第二产程的时间会比较长。

- 初产妇：第一产程一般平均 14.4 h，第二产程平均 1 h。

- 经产妇：第一产程平均 7.7 h，第二产程平均 0.2 h。

• 第二产程的时间受以下 3 个因素的影响较大，总结为 3P：

- passenger：胎儿的大小和胎位。

- passageway：骨盆的大小和软组织等因素。

- powers：子宫收缩的力量。

• 这三者中如何一项的异常都会造成分娩过程的异常。

- 如胎位不正、子宫收缩不良、头盆不称等。

• 假临产(Braxton Hicks 收缩)。

- 在真实临产前数日至数周发生的子宫不规则，无节律的收缩，通常不会引起子宫颈的扩张。

病因

• 8%～10%的孕妇会发生早产。

• 30%～40%的早产是由于子宫、宫颈和尿道的炎症引起的。

• 胎膜早破定义为孕妇妊娠 37 周前，产程开始至少 2 h 前出现的羊膜或绒毛膜的破裂。

- 约 3%的孕妇会发生胎膜早破，但 30%～40%的早产会发生胎膜早破。

诊断

症状和体征

• 分娩的症状：

- 间歇的下腹痛伴随或不伴随下腰痛。

- 至少每 5 min 发生一次规律性疼痛。

- 持续 30～60 s。

• 早产是发生在妊娠 37 周前出现的子宫收缩和宫颈扩张或消失。

• 分娩不伴随阴道流血：

- 患者出现 3 个月的腹痛或阴道流血应怀疑前置胎盘或胎盘早剥。

• 突发大量透明液体从阴道流出或感觉到会阴部潮湿应怀疑胎膜早破。

- 并不是分娩过程中的伴随症状，但是通常会导致分娩的到来。

病史

• 育龄期。

• 产前检查。

• 既往妊娠：

- 并发症。

- C 形切口。

• 近期感染。

体格检查

• 评估宫底高度：

- 从耻骨至子宫顶端的距离。

- 中期妊娠后与孕周平行。

- 帮助确定未知的孕周数。

• 进行无菌盆腔检查来评估宫颈扩张和成熟度。

> **注意**
> 如果阴道流血禁止行盆腔检查。

基本检查

• 对可能生产的孕妇立即行无菌盆腔检查，评估宫颈扩张和成熟度，以及即将来临的生产。

• 伴阴道流血的晚期妊娠患者禁止行双手盆腔检查，除非用超声先排除胎盘前置和胎盘早剥。

• 可疑羊膜破裂的患者应用无菌窥器在直视下检查宫颈，并收集阴道区域的液体。

• 提示羊膜破裂：

- 液体在玻片上干燥呈羊齿状结晶。

- 阴道内大量积水。

- 石蕊试纸颜色由黄色变绿色。

• 早产和宫颈改变的患者应行尿常规和培养、宫颈培养。

• 看见胎儿提示已经发动。

诊断检查与说明

实验室检查

• 如果患者正在生产，应送检血细胞计数、血型和筛查。

• 送尿常规检查是否有蛋白尿。

• 如果没有孕史，应行 Rh 因子和抗体筛查。

• 早产患者送宫颈和尿培养。

• 胎儿纤维连接蛋白。

- 用于评估早产。

- 是帮助羊膜囊"粘"在子宫内膜上的蛋白质。

- 如果阳性，意味着羊膜囊受到破坏，增加早产的风险。

- 只在 22～34 周，使用宫颈拭子送检。

- 通常由妇产科医师操作。

影像学检查

• 一般不需要。

• 妊娠晚期患者伴腹痛和阴道出血应急诊行超声来评估胎盘前置和早剥。

鉴别诊断

• Braxton Hicks 收缩(假产)是不伴宫颈改变的不规则的子宫收缩。

- 收缩可每 10～20 min 一次。

• 子宫圆韧带痛，肌肉骨骼性背痛。

• 其他导致腹痛的常见原因，如阑尾炎、卵巢囊肿、憩室炎、肾结石、泌尿道感染。

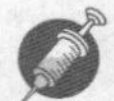

治疗

院前

• 急诊医疗服务人员应先给待产的患者吸氧，左侧斜位保证子宫最大氧供。

• 也可手动将子宫向左移位。

• 使用飞机运送待产孕妇时要保证孕妇充足的氧供以减少机舱的低气压对孕妇造成的伤害。

初步稳定/治疗

如果孕妇需要立刻进行分娩(可见胎先露部)，则需要准备在急诊室进行经阴道的分娩。

急诊治疗/程序

• 除外需要进行立刻分娩的孕妇，所有待产孕妇都要在产房里进行分娩。

• 在将孕妇转移至产房的过程中需要做到以下几步：

- 静脉使用抗生素预防一些未知的乙型链球菌感染。

- 在 30～60 min 静脉输注 1 L 生理盐水或葡萄糖。

- 孕妇进行必要的生命体征监测。

- 如果需要暂停分娩(胎儿早产)，给予宫缩抑制剂，包括特布他林或硫酸镁。

◦ 镁中毒表现为深部减反射减弱。

◦ 大剂量的镁会导致心律失常和呼吸抑制。

药物治疗

• 硫酸镁：前 30 min 内静脉使用 4～6 g，之后 2～6 g/h。

• 特布他林：0.25 mg 皮下注射，30 min 后相同剂量重复给药。

• 在出血的情况下，以 10～15 mg/kg 的剂量静脉注射氨甲环酸 10 min。

注意

既往有心脏损伤病史的患者要预防性给予抗生素治疗。

随访

进一步处理

入院指征

- 所有没有即刻分娩风险的患者都要收入产房进行分娩。
- 所有早产的患者都需要立刻进行产科监护并送入产房进一步治疗。

出院指征

- 假分娩的患者在进行充分的产科监护并确认胎儿健康后可以出院，但要进行密切的随访。
- 假分娩可能会进展为真正的分娩。

要点和误区

- 患者出现阴道流血时要注意排除胎盘早剥或前置胎盘。
- 当存在引导流血时避免进行指检。
- 对于正在分娩的患者进行骨盆检查时要确保无菌。
- 假分娩有可能会进展为真正的分娩。

风湿热 Rheumatic Fever

Christopher Gardner · Dalton Cox 何融冰 译

基础知识

描述

- 多种症状和体征(修订乔纳斯标准)。
- 继发于A组链球菌感染(GAS)，也称为酿脓链球菌，经常表现为咽炎。
- 在美国不常见，此种疾病在发达国家最常见，更常见于澳大利亚和新西兰的当地居民。
- 全世界范围内心脏方面致病和致死的主要原因，每年有超过230000人死亡。
- 在5～15岁儿童中最常见。

病因

- A组溶血性链球菌GAS咽炎(与GAS皮肤感染无关)。
- GAS感染致结缔组织炎性自身免疫反应。

诊断

乔纳斯标准中2个主要的或1个主要的和2个次要的条件加上新近GAS感染。

在有急性风湿热(ARF)病史的患者中，有3个次要的近期GAS感染标准也可诊断。

症状和体征

修订乔纳斯指标

- 低风险人群和中高风险人群的标准不同。
  - 低风险人群定义为：
    - ARF发病率<2/10万。
    - 儿童5～14岁。
    - 每年风湿性心脏病RHD发病率<1/1000。
    - 否则，被认为是中高风险。
  - 中高风险标准。
    - 儿童不确定来自低风险人群。
    - 这些标准在下面用斜体表示。
- 主要表现：
  - 35%～66%初次发作，以游走性多关节炎为表现。
    - 最早出现的症状。
    - 累及大关节：膝盖、髋部、踝、肘部和腕关节。
    - 下肢关节更易受累。
    - 一般对水杨酸盐和非甾体抗炎药反应迅速。
    - *在中高危人群中，单关节炎或多关节痛可达到"主要表现"标准。*
  - 心脏炎症发生于50%～70%的新病例中：
    - 心包、心肌和心内膜可能被累及(全心炎)。
    - 心肌炎可能导致心力衰竭，但通常无症状。
    - 风湿性心脏病(RHD)和心内膜炎是ARF最严重的后遗症。
    - 新的杂音、心动过速、奔马律、心包摩擦音或CHF提示心脏炎症。
    - 多普勒超声心动图可在没有听诊表现的情况下检测到瓣膜炎(亚临床性心炎)。
  - 舞蹈症发生在10%的病例中：
    - Sydenham舞蹈症主要发生于青少年女孩。
    - 四肢无目的，共济失调的动作，有时被称为St. Vitas舞蹈症。
    - 在焦虑期更明显。
    - 舞蹈症可以是ARF的唯一表现。
  - 边缘性红斑发生在<5%的病例中：
    - 为无瘙痒的淡红色丘疹，中心正常，边界清晰不规则。
    - 常分布于躯干和四肢。
  - SC结节见于<5%的病例：
    - 分批出现的小SC，无痛性结节大部分位于伸面。
- 次要表现：
  - 临床：
    - 发热(>38.5℃)(*38℃针对中高风险区域*)。
    - 多关节痛(*单关节痛针对中高风险区域*)。
  - 实验室表现：
    - ESR>60，CRP>3 mg/dl(*ESR≥30在中高风险区域*)。
    - PR间期延长。
- 新近GAS咽喉感染的证据：
  - 咽部细菌培养或快速抗体试验为阳性。
  - 抗体试验增加或上抬：抗链球菌溶血素O(ASO)滴度。

病史

- 发热(38.5℃，针对中高风险区域38℃)。
- 咽喉疼痛(通常在2～4周前)。
- 疹。
- 关节痛。
- 四肢异常运动。
- 呼吸困难。
- 下肢水肿。

体格检查

- 咽部红斑。
- 疹与边缘性红斑相关。
- SC结节。
- 与二尖瓣或主动脉疾病有关的心脏新杂音。
- 体液超负荷、CHF的证据。

基本检查

- 仔细检查皮肤病灶、关节肿胀。
- 仔细检查心脏和肺。
- 咽喉拭子快速检测链球菌或培养。

F

- 心电图。
- 胸部 X 线。
- 多普勒超声心动图。
- 见下实验室检查。

诊断检查与说明

实验室检查

- 快速链球菌抗原检测。
- 咽部细菌培养。
- ASO 滴度。
- CBC。
- ESR 或 C 反应蛋白。

影像学检查

- 多普勒超声心动图。
- X 线胸片。

鉴别诊断

- 青少年特发性关节炎。
- 感染性心内膜炎。
- 反应性关节病。
- 系统性红斑狼疮。
- 淋球菌感染后关节炎。
- 其他造成关节炎和心脏炎的感染性因素：
  - 柯萨奇 B 病毒和细小病毒属。

儿科注意事项

- 风湿热是一种常见的儿科疾病，但也可发生于年轻人。
- 在美国＜3 岁者不推荐行链球菌咽部测试，因为咽部链球菌的低发现率及罕见的 ARF。

妊娠注意事项

如果女性有风湿热的病史，推荐进行产前咨询，因为心脏疾病风险增加。

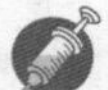

治疗

院前

- 需要时吸氧。
- 必要时给予监护。
- 谨慎建立静脉通道。

初步稳定/治疗

一些 CHF 患者需要进行气道管理。

急诊治疗/程序

- 心包积液可能需要引流。
- 在严重心脏炎时，可使用泼尼松。
- 在严重舞蹈症时，使用氟哌啶醇。
- 青霉素根除 GAS。
- 针对关节炎、关节痛、发热使用阿司匹林或萘普生。

药物治疗

- 阿司匹林：4～8 g/d[儿童：100 mg/(kg · d)]，口服，q4～6 h；不要超过 4 g/24 h。
- 阿奇霉素 500 mg 第 1 日，然后 250 mg，口服，再持续 4 日[儿童：10 mg/kg 第 1 日然后 5 mg/kg，每日 1 次，口服，再持续 4 日]。
- 地高辛：0.25～0.5 mg(儿童：0.04 mg/kg)，静脉注射。
- 呋塞米：20～80 mg(儿童：1 mg/kg)，静脉注射。
- 氟哌啶醇：2～10 mg[儿童：0.01～0.03 mg/(kg · d)；仅在＞2 岁和＞15 kg 使用]，q6 h，肌内注射或口服。
- 萘普生：10～20 mg/(kg · d)，每 12 h 分次给药，持续 1～2 周；不超过 1 g/d。
- 青霉素：120 万 U(儿童：600 000 U，对于＜27 kg)，肌内注射此后每月 1 次(预防)。
- 青霉素 VK：500 mg(儿童：250 mg)，口服，q8 h，持续 10 日(急性治疗)。
- 泼尼松：1～2 mg/(kg · d)，连续 14 日，接下来 2 周剂量逐渐减小。

一线用药

- 阿司匹林(心脏炎症患者)。
- 青霉素(根除 GAS)。
- 氟哌啶醇(治疗舞蹈症)。

二线用药

皮质类固醇类。

随访

进一步处理

新诊断的患者应入院稳定病情并进一步评估心脏疾病的严重性。

入院指征

- CHF。
- 新诊断。
- 未控制的舞蹈症。
- 未控制的疼痛。
- 心包积液。

出院指征

- 疼痛已受控制。
- 心血管状态稳定。
- 关于继续治疗和心内膜炎预防的教育。

转诊问题

- 所有患者需要其主治医师和心脏病学专家的密切随访。
- 考虑转诊到传染病专家和风湿学专家处。

随访建议

- 超声心动图检查，对亚急性细菌性心内膜炎给予预防建议。
- 传染病专家建议延长青霉素使用时间来预防复发。
- 慢性关节问题需要风湿病学专家来解决(不常用)。

要点和误区

- 风湿热在美国不常见，但必须谨慎治疗链球菌感染来预防疾病再发。
- 此种疾病在贫穷和人口众多的国家中更常见。
- 修订后的乔纳斯标准被修改为对中高风险人群更加敏感。
- 年龄小于 3 岁的儿童无需进行咽部细菌培养。
- 如果最初正常但怀疑 ARF，则在 2～4 周重复超声心动图。

风湿性关节炎 Arthritis, Rheumatoid

Stephen R. Hayden 汤璐佳 潘曙明 译

基础知识

描述

- 慢性系统性关节炎症疾病：
  - 非化脓性，增生性滑膜炎。
  - 关节软骨破坏。
  - 关节僵硬。
- 常常累及膝关节。
- 一些慢性病变可见 Baker 囊肿。
- 如累及脊柱可局限于部分脊椎区域：
  - 可引起寰枢椎半脱位。
  - 脊髓压迫少见。

儿科注意事项

幼年型风湿性关节炎(见"幼年型特发性关节炎")。

• 遗传学:

- 与 HLA - DR4 遗传有关。
- 女性与男性比例为 3∶1。
- 主要发病年龄为 30～50 岁。

病因

• 病因不明。

• 诱因可能为感染与自身免疫反应。

• 美国及全世界发病率约为 1%。

诊断

症状和体征

• 精神萎靡、乏力。

• 全身肌肉骨骼疼痛。

• 发病后数周至数月,患者关节开始出现肿胀、发热、疼痛。

• 早晨症状常较重。

• 常累及全身多系统及关节。

• 常以手足小关节起病:

- 后发展到腕关节、肘关节和膝关节。

• 远端指间关节少累及:

- 如累及远端指间关节应考虑其他类型关节炎。

• 可逐渐出现滑膜炎。

• 病程较长的患者可出现明显的关节改变:

- 掌指关节肿胀,尺侧偏移。
- 鹅颈畸形。

• 关节外并发症:

- 胶质结节。
- 血管炎。
- 心包炎或心内膜炎。
- 肺纤维化。
- 肺炎。
- 干燥综合征。
- 多发性神经炎。

• 近 1/3 的患者行心脏超声检查时可发现轻度心包炎。

• 这些患者应考虑进行心电图检查评估。

• 这些患者往往因疾病恶化或其他器官系统出现并发症而至急诊就诊:

- 环状软骨炎或喉结肿大可引起气道阻塞。
- 心脏传导阻滞、缩窄性心包炎、心脏压塞或心内膜炎。
- 肺纤维化、胸膜炎、肺内结节或肺炎。
- 肝炎。

• 神经系统改变多由于颈椎半脱位引起,部分患者眼部症状如巩膜炎及浅表巩膜炎。

- 可合并视网膜周围血管炎及反复发作的虹膜炎,如患者出现畏光、红眼、视力减退应考虑并发症,需由眼科医师进行评估。

• 长期使用类固醇的并发症:

- 感染。
- 骨质疏松和骨折。
- 胰岛素抵抗。
- 青光眼或眼内压升高,加速引起白内障。

• 患者还可能出现服用水杨酸盐或非甾体抗炎药引起的副作用,如消化道溃疡出血。

• 甲氨蝶呤、青霉素胺等药物也有毒副作用,大多数表现为消化道不适,也可表现为神经性副作用。

基本检查

• 急诊科通常无法确诊风湿性关节炎。

• 滑膜炎应持续至少 6 周,美国风湿病协会规定必须满足以下 7 条标准中的 4 条才可诊断:

- 晨僵至少 1 h。
- 3 个或 3 个以上关节肿。
- 腕、掌指关节或近端指间关节肿。
- 对称性关节炎。
- 骨突出部位,伸肌表面或关节周围类风湿结节。
- 类风湿因子显著升高。
- 放射学改变包括骨质侵蚀或骨质脱钙(非骨关节炎引起)。

• 其他相关病史:精神萎靡、乏力、体重下降、肌痛、滑囊炎、肌腱炎、不明原因的发热。

• 初步检查应重点排除其他原因引起的关节炎,特别是感染性关节炎、反应性关节炎、痛风。

• 可能需要进行关节穿刺抽液。

诊断检查与说明

心电图,胸部、颈椎或四肢摄片,当患者出现并发症时血红蛋白检测有意义。

实验室检查

• 全血细胞计数:轻度贫血、白细胞及血小板升高。

• 红细胞沉降率:常>30。参考值上限:男性年龄/2,女性(年龄+10)/2。如显著升高且视力突发明显下降需考虑合并巨细胞动脉炎。

• C 反应蛋白与侵袭性疾病相关。

• 30%～40%的患者抗核抗体阳性。

• 类风湿因子:约 70%的患者升高。

• 关节液分析:

- 白细胞 4 000～5 000/mm^3。
- 中性粒细胞明显增多。
- 显微镜下染色未见微生物及晶体。

• 心电图:可见传导阻滞,提示心包炎。

影像学检查

• 关节摄片。

- 渗出。
- 骨质侵蚀或骨质脱钙。
- 关节间隙狭窄。
- 软骨缺失。

• 磁共振检查可以比 X 线平片更早发现炎症。

• 胸片提示肺纤维化、胸膜改变、肺结节病或肺炎:

- 心内膜炎可引起心影改变。

• 颈椎摄片:

- 可出现寰枢关节半脱位。

鉴别诊断

• 骨关节炎。

• 感染性关节炎。

• 反应性关节炎。

• 淋球菌关节炎。

• 莱姆病。

• 痛风。

• 结缔组织疾病。

• 系统性红斑狼疮、皮肌炎、多肌炎、血管炎、Reiter 综合征和结节病。

• 风湿热。

• 肿瘤。

F

治疗

院前

必要时固定颈椎及开放气道。

初步稳定/治疗

• ABC 管理。

- 插管时注意固定颈椎。

• 治疗并发症。

急诊治疗/程序

• 水杨酸类及非甾体抗炎药为一线用药:

- 如果一种非甾体抗炎药失败,另一种不同类型的非甾体抗炎药可能会更有效。

• 发病 18 个月内的早期治疗对减少关节破坏可起重要作用。

药物治疗

• 糖皮质激素、甲氨蝶呤及其他二线用药需在风湿科专业医师指导下使用。

• 阿司匹林:成人:900 mg,口服,每日 4 次(2.6～5.4 g/d);儿童:60～90 mg/(kg · d),每日 4 次,最大剂量每日 3.6 g。

> **注意**
>
> 肠溶阿司匹林有延迟吸收性,其镇痛作用较普通阿司匹林有延迟。阿司匹林如需达到抗炎效果则需达到毒性剂量。患者在服用阿司匹林时应严密观察避免毒性反应。

• 金诺芬：3～9 mg/d[儿童：0.15 mg/(kg·d),最大剂量 9 mg],每日 2 次。

• 塞来昔布：100～200 mg,每日 2 次,口服;儿童：N/A。

• 羟氯喹：成人：200～600 mg/d,每日 2 次。

• 布洛芬：200～800 mg,每隔 6 h 口服(儿童：10 mg/kg)。

• 来氟米特：起始剂量为 100 mg,每日口服 1 次,共计 3 日;维持剂量为 10～20 mg,每日口服 1 次;儿童：N/A。

• 甲氨蝶呤：7.5 mg,每周 1 次。

• 泼尼松：维持剂量：5～10 mg,每日 1 次,口服;急性期：20～50 mg,每日 1 次,口服;儿童：维持剂量：0.1 mg/(kg·d),口服,急性期：2～5 mg/(kg·d),口服。

• 柳氮磺胺吡啶：成人：500～1 000 mg,每日 2 次,口服;儿童 30～60 mg/(kg·d),每日 2 次,最大剂量为 2 g。

- 不推荐 6 岁以下儿童使用。

• 可使用非甾体抗炎药和曲马多镇痛。

• 新型抗风湿病程改善药物和单克隆药物应在风湿科医师指导下使用,不建议在急诊科使用,这些药物包括：阿巴西普、阿达木单抗、阿那白滞素、依那西普、英夫利昔、利妥昔单抗、托珠单抗。

> **注意**
>
> 近期研究表明使用非甾体抗炎药尤其与 COX-2 类药物合用时可能增加心血管事件风险。

随访

进一步处理

入院指征

• 患者出现威胁生命的症状或并发症。

• 诊断不明的感染性关节炎或系统性血管炎。

• 一些需控制疼痛的病例。

• 患者无法保证日常生活。

• 伴有高热及关节炎症状的儿童。

出院指征

无明显并发症的患者可安排服用适当药物随访。

转诊

所有患者均应请相应科室如风湿科、心脏科、骨科会诊以明确治疗方案。

要点和误区

• 风湿性关节炎多为对称性。

• 风湿性关节炎患者也可出现感染性关节炎。

• 及时请风湿科会诊,不要在急诊室盲目使用类固醇或肿瘤坏死因子拮抗剂。

风疹 Rubella

Austen-Kum Chai 何融冰 译

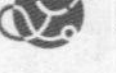

基础知识

描述

• 又称德国麻疹或 3 日麻疹。

• 通过呼吸道飞沫传播。

• 中度传染性。

- 在出疹期或患有先天性风疹综合征(CRS)的婴儿。
- 患有先天性风疹的婴儿会在数月到 1 岁之间释放大量病毒。

• 感染期：皮疹出现前 7 日至皮疹出现后 5 日。

• 潜伏期：14～21 日。

• 超过 50%的不明显或者亚临床型。

病因

• 风疹病毒(族：披膜病毒科;属：风疹病毒属)。

• 人类是唯一已知的储存宿主。

诊断

症状和体征

年龄较大的儿童和成人的前驱尿道炎、不适、低热和淋巴结病。

• 皮疹通常见于幼儿：

- 皮疹比麻疹更轻,不合并。
- 红色黄斑皮疹演变为粉红色黄斑丘疹,偶有瘙痒：
- 从面部开始,从头到脚。
- 第一日完成,3 日后消失。
- 可能有出血的表现。

• 淋巴结病：

- 耳后,枕下,颈后。
- 可能在出疹前 1 周开始,持续数周。

• 并发症：

- 不常见,多见于成人。

• CRS：感染主要发生在妊娠的前 3 个月。

- 关节炎：
  - 妇女中更常见(达 79%)。
  - 慢性关节炎少见。
  - 在起病 2～3 日后开始。
  - 膝盖、腕、手指受影响。
- 出血性表现。
  - 继发于血小板减少。
  - 儿童中更常见。
- 神经系统后遗症：
  - 脑炎在成人中更常见,预后通常较好。
  - 与孤独症无关。

儿科注意事项

• 麻疹、流行性腮腺炎和风疹±水痘(麻腮风三联疫苗 MMR 或水痘疫苗 MMRV)疫苗应在 12 个月或 12 个月后接种给儿童。第二剂是在 4～6 岁开始上学前服用的。

• 补种剂量与疫苗接种之间应间隔至少 4 周。

妊娠注意事项

• CRS：

- 预防 CRS 是疫苗接种的主要目标。
- 妊娠早期感染最严重。
- 可能影响所有器官造成各种先天性缺陷、胎儿死亡、自然流产、早产。
- 胎龄 20 周后所致感染导致胎儿缺陷罕见。

• 妇女妊娠期间不应接种 MMR 或 MMRV。

• 接种疫苗后至少 4 周内避免妊娠。

老年注意事项

1957 年以前出生的人通常被认为是免疫的。但是,如果血清学检测显示滴度为阴性,那些在卫生保健机构工作的人应该接种疫苗。

基本检查

基于临床发现进行诊断。

诊断检查与说明

实验室检查

• 全血细胞计数：
- 白细胞，血小板下降（儿童更常见）。
• 尿液分析：
- 血尿。
• 风疹的聚合酶链反应（PCR）。
• 风疹病毒 IgM。
• 风疹 IgG 抗体滴度：
- 与急性和恢复期血清标本相比，滴度显著上升。
- 对比婴儿和产妇血清检测 CRS。
- 细小病毒属，传染性单核细胞增多症，类风湿因子可造成假阳性。
- 可以用来检查有潜在暴露史的妊娠患者的免疫力。
• 病毒培养：
- 皮疹出现前 1 周至出现后 2 周期间，病毒可以从咽部分泌物中分离。
- 也可以从鼻腔分泌物、尿液、血液、脑脊液中分离出来。
• CSF：
- 脑炎时极少量白细胞（单核细胞）。

诊断步骤/外科

• 若怀疑脑炎行腰椎穿刺。
• 对无法解释的关节炎行关节穿刺术。

鉴别诊断

• 猩红热。
- "沙纸样"皮疹、帕氏线和草莓舌。
• 麻疹（风疹）：
- Koplik 斑、咳嗽、鼻炎、结膜炎和高热。
• 幼儿急疹：
- 春秋季。
• 落基山斑疹热：
- 皮疹开始于踝和腕部。
• 类风湿关节炎。

治疗

院前

使用防护措施，防止通过呼吸道分泌物的飞沫传播。

初步稳定/治疗

必要时行 ABC 管理。

急诊治疗/程序

• 对症治疗。
• 解热抗炎药物。
• 将风疹患者与易感人群隔离开（如孕妇）。
• 疫苗：
- 麻疹、流行性腮腺炎和风疹疫苗。
- 风疹疫苗是减活疫苗。
- 1 剂可能会使人终身免疫。
- 适应证：
  ◦ >12 个月到入学儿童。
  ◦ 易感的青春期后女性。
  ◦ 高风险人群（大学、部队、工作场所）。
  ◦ 非免疫性接触。
• 保健工作者和育龄妇女：
- 常见的主诉是发热、淋巴结病和关节痛。
• 免疫球蛋白：
- 不能防治病毒血症，但可以缓解症状。

药物治疗

• 对乙酰氨基酚：
• 布洛芬。
• 免疫球蛋白：0.5 ml 配制成小瓶装输注液皮下注射（0.25～0.50 ml/kg）。

随访

进一步处理

入院指征

• CRS。
• 脑炎。

出院指征

• 大多数患者可以回家。
• 询问家庭成员的疫苗接种状态。

转诊问题

• 可能接触病原体或患病的妊娠妇女。
• 并发症。
• 疑似 CRS 的儿童需要全面评估。

随访建议

疑似风疹或接触过病原体的妊娠妇女应进行病原体滴度随访，应请产科会诊进行咨询。

要点和误区

• 已感染个体应与易感人群隔开（孕妇、免疫力低下者）7 日。
• 针对未接种疫苗者，有发热皮疹、其他风疹症状和国际旅行史患者，应考虑风疹。
• 先天性风疹综合征与心脏、大脑、眼科和听觉有关。

蜂窝织炎 Cellulitis

John Mahoney · Dolores Gonthier 彭沪 王毅鑫 译

基础知识

描述

• 表浅皮肤组织和结缔组织的急性的播散性的红斑：
- 非化脓性皮肤和软组织感染（SSTI）：单纯性蜂窝织炎。
- 化脓性 SSTI："脓肿"中包括化脓性蜂窝织炎。
- 进展到深层组织能导致软组织感染坏死。
• 进展性的红斑，皮温增高，疼痛，触痛。
• 诱因：
- 淋巴水肿。
- 足癣。
- 之前存在的皮肤损伤（疖）。
- 之前存在的创伤和外科手术史。
- 体内残留异物。
- 血管或免疫功能不全。
- 滥用药物。
- 周期性 SSTI。

病因

• 单纯性蜂窝组织炎（非化脓性 SSTI）：
- A 型链球菌。
- 对甲氧西林敏感的金黄色葡萄球菌（MSSA）。
- 耐甲氧西林的金黄色葡萄球菌（MRSA）。

F

- 葡萄球菌感染的危险因素(MSSA 和 MRSA):
 ◦ 最近入院或长期护理。
 ◦ 最近的手术。
 ◦ 孩子。
 ◦ 军人。
 ◦ 被监禁者。
 ◦ 接触运动的运动员。
 ◦ 注射用药。
 ◦ 与男性发生性关系的男性。
 ◦ 透析治疗和导管。
 ◦ 穿透性创伤的历史。
- MRSA 感染的其他危险因素:
 ◦ 先前的 MRSA 感染。
 ◦ MRSA 定植。
 ◦ MRSA 高发地区。
 ◦ 与 MRSA 患者密切接触。
• 淋巴管破裂后的严重蜂窝织炎:
- 非 A 型溶血性链球菌(C、B、G 型)。
• 糖尿病患者蜂窝织炎:
- 病原体可以是金黄色葡萄球菌、链球菌、革兰阴性杆菌、厌氧菌,特别是合并皮肤溃疡时。
• 眶周蜂窝织炎:
- 金黄色葡萄球菌。
- 链球菌。
• 口腔蜂窝织炎:
- 具有厌氧性口腔菌群的微生物,与口腔内裂伤或牙齿脓肿有关。
• 不常见原因:
- 梭状芽孢杆菌。
- 炭疽。
- 巴斯德菌属亚种:通常在猫和犬咬伤后。
- 侵袭性艾肯菌:人咬伤口。
- 铜绿假单胞菌:
 ◦ Hot-Tub 毛囊炎:自限性。
 ◦ 足穿刺伤。
 ◦ 坏死性脓疮的中性粒细胞减少的患者。
- 丹毒丝菌属:生鱼片、家禽、肉及无症状携带者。
- 产气单胞菌:淡水中游泳。
- 弧菌属:海水及生海产品。

儿科注意事项

• 儿童面部蜂窝织炎:
- 链球菌属。
- B 型流感嗜血杆菌,由于流感嗜血杆菌疫苗的使用,发病率有了下降。
• 肛周蜂窝织炎:
- A 型链球菌。
- 与前期咽炎或脓疱病有关。
• 新生儿:
- B 型链球菌。

诊断

症状和体征

• 一般症状:
- 疼痛,触痛,皮温增高。
- 红斑。
- 水肿或硬化。
- 发热、畏寒。
- 局部淋巴结肿大。
- 淋巴管炎。
- 伴随腹腔脓肿可能。
- 初始抗生素治疗失败的应怀疑深部脓肿。
- 表面水疱。
• 口腔蜂窝织炎:
- 牙源性患者更加严重:
 ◦ 牙痛、喉痛或面部肿胀。
 ◦ 进展到颈部软组织伴发热、红斑、颈部肿胀和吞咽困难。

儿科注意事项

• 儿童严重的蜂窝织炎:
- 面部和眼睑部出现红斑肿胀。
- 进展迅速。
- 通常为单侧。
- 上呼吸道症状。
- 是海绵窦血栓和永久视神经损伤的危险因素。
• 肛周脓肿:
- 肛周数厘米至邻近的皮肤红斑和瘙痒。
- 排便疼痛。
- 大便带血丝。
- 化脓性分泌物

病史

• 葡萄球菌病因:创伤进展,创伤后。
• 链球菌病的病因:更急性,伴随恶心的毒素,已存在的淋巴水肿。

体格检查

• 葡萄球菌引起的:病灶脓肿常具有波动、黄色或白色中心,有中心点或"头",脓液流出,进展缓慢。
• 链球菌性:边界清楚,淋巴管炎,之前存在的淋巴水肿,毒素导致的恶心。
• 链球菌病的病因:边界清晰,淋巴管炎。
• 查找感染源。
• 识别足趾网异常
• 评估血管充盈。

基本检查

• 蜂窝织炎是临床诊断。

诊断检查与说明

实验室检查

• 白细胞通常不是必需的。
• 革兰染色和微生物培养明确抗生素的选择和揭示抗药性病原体(MRSA):
- 穿刺验证最重的点,如果没有伤口可以培养则进行穿刺活检。
- 治疗失败的患者施行此检查同时考虑收入院。
• 血培养:
- 简单的蜂窝织炎通常为阴性。
- 可用于明确以下患者致病微生物情况:
 ◦ 淋巴水肿。
 ◦ 面颊或眶周脓肿。
 ◦ 盐水或淡水来源。
 ◦ 发热或寒战。

影像学检查

X 线平片可以发现脓肿形成、腹腔气体或者异物:
• 进展到骨(骨髓炎)在早期平片无明显改变。
• 血管影像学检查(多普勒超声)能帮助排除深静脉血栓。
• 如果体检不确定或者有大面积的蜂窝织炎,超声对脓肿的诊断有益。
- 在蜂窝织炎中可看到特征性的"鹅卵石"改变和增厚的 SC 层,均由水肿导致。
• CT 或 MRI 能帮助排除坏死性的筋膜炎。

鉴别诊断

• 瘀滞性皮炎。
• 坏死性筋膜炎。
• 淋巴管炎或者淋巴腺炎。
• 血栓性静脉炎或深静脉血栓。
• 昆虫咬伤。
• 过敏反应。
• 急性痛风或假性痛风。
• 贝克囊肿破裂。
• 疱疹性指头炎。
• 肿瘤。
• 植物日光性皮炎。
• 莱姆病导致的慢性游走性红斑。
• 面部蜂窝织炎的鉴别诊断:
- 神经性水肿。
- 结膜炎。
- 挫伤。

儿科注意事项

肛周蜂窝织炎鉴别诊断:
• 念珠菌性间擦疹。
• 银屑病。

F

- 绦虫感染。
- 儿童虐待。
- 行为问题。
- 炎症性肠病。

治疗

初步稳定/治疗

- 纵深、范围广泛的面部或颈部蜂窝织炎可能会累及气道。
- 监测和支持败血症综合征的血压/通气。
- 评估全身症状的严重程度，包括 SIRS 标准（全身性炎症反应综合征）。
  - SIRS 标准：
    - 温度＞38℃或＜36℃。
    - HR＞90 次/分。
    - RR＞20 次/分。
    - 白细胞计数＞12 000/mm³ 或＜4 000/mm³。

急诊治疗/程序

- 一般原则：
  - 冷敷带来舒适感。
  - 镇痛药。
  - 肢体抬高。
  - 治疗足癣或其他足趾异常。
- 蜂窝织炎的护理原则：
  - 除常见原因外，还应考虑当地耐药菌的流行情况。
  - 通常的门诊治疗：
    - 5～10 日的抗生素。
    - 在 48～72 h 进行随访以评估改善情况。
  - 如果怀疑葡萄球菌可能是病原体，则抗生素应同时涵盖 MSSA 和 MRSA。
- 这种怀疑应基于临床检查，风险因素评估和全身症状的严重程度（SIRS 标准）。
  - 单纯性蜂窝组织炎＝非化脓性 SSTI。
  - 门诊：
    - 头孢氨苄。
    - 替代品：双氯西林，克林霉素。
  - 住院：
    - 静脉注射萘夫西林或头孢唑林。
    - 替代品：静脉用克林霉素。
    - MRSA 治疗：如果怀疑 MRSA 是病因，请添加以下内容。
  - 门诊：
    - 甲氧苄啶-磺胺甲噁唑。
    - 替代品：强力霉素。
  - 住院：
    - 静脉用万古霉素。
    - 替代品：静脉用利奈唑胺。
    - 具有严重全身症状的蜂窝织炎：
  - 定义为≥2SIRS 标准，加上低血压或免疫功能受损或疾病快速发展。
  - 静脉用万古霉素加静脉用哌拉西林-他唑巴坦。
- 淋巴受阻引起的末端蜂窝织炎：
  - 治疗同单纯性蜂窝织炎。
- 糖尿病患者蜂窝织炎：
  - 门诊患者：
    - 口服阿莫西林-克拉维酸＋甲氧苄啶-磺胺甲噁唑（覆盖社区获得性 MRSA）或克林霉素。
  - 住院患者：
    - 静脉用氨苄西林-舒巴坦或亚胺培南-西司他丁或等效药物；＋静脉用万古霉素（覆盖社区获得性 MRSA）。
- 成人眶周蜂窝织炎：
  - 门诊患者：口服阿莫西林-克拉维酸。
  - 住院患者：静脉用万古霉素。
- 成人口腔蜂窝织炎：
  - 门诊患者：口服双氯青霉素或阿奇霉素；＋甲氧苄啶-磺胺甲噁唑（覆盖社区获得性 MRSA）。
  - 住院患者：静脉用头孢曲松。
  - 牙源性感染：
    - 必要时引流。
    - 覆盖厌氧菌：克林霉素。
- 儿童面部蜂窝织炎：
  - 静脉用头孢曲松。
- 肛周蜂窝织炎：
  - 门诊患者：口服青霉素 V 钾。
  - 住院患者：静脉用青霉素（水化的）。
- 动物或人咬伤：
  - 门诊患者：口服阿莫西林-克拉维酸。
- 足穿刺伤：
  - 口服或静脉用环丙沙星或静脉用头孢他啶。

药物治疗

- 阿莫西林-克拉维酸：500～875 mg[儿童：45 mg/(kg·24 h)]，口服，每日 2 次；或 250～500 mg[儿童：40 mg/(kg·24 h)]，口服，每日 3 次。
- 氨苄西林-舒巴坦：1.5～3 g[儿童：40 kg 以下，100～300 mg/(kg·24 h)；超过 40 kg，给予成人剂量]，静脉使用，q6 h。
- 头孢他啶：500～1 000 mg[儿童：150 mg/(kg·24 h)；最大剂量 6 g/24 h；儿童患者使用耐盐形式]静脉使用，q8 h。
- 头孢曲松：1～2 g[儿童：50～75 mg/(kg·24 h)]，每日 1 次，静脉使用。
- 头孢氨苄：500 mg[儿童：50～100 mg/(kg·24 h)]，口服，每日 4 次。
- 环丙沙星：（仅用于成人）500～750 mg 口服，每日 2 次；或 400 mg，静脉滴注，q8～12 h。
- 克林霉素：450～900 mg[儿童：20～40 mg/(kg·24 h)]，口服或静脉滴注，q6 h。
- 双氯青霉素：125～500 mg[儿童：12.5～25 mg/(kg·24 h)]，口服，q6 h。
- 多西环素：成人 100 mg，口服，每日 2 次。
- 亚胺培南-西司他丁：500～1 000 mg(儿童：15～25 mg/kg)，静脉滴注，q6 h；最大量 4 g/24 h 或 50 mg/(kg·24 h)，以较少者为准。
- 利奈唑胺：600 mg，口服或静脉滴注，q12 h[儿童：30 mg/(kg·24 h)分开使用，q8 h]。
- 萘夫西林：1～2 g，静脉滴注，q4 h[儿童：50～100 mg/(kg·24 h)分开使用，q6 h]；最大量 12 g/24 h。
- 青霉素 V 钾：250～500 mg[儿童：25～50 mg/(kg·24 h)]，口服，q6 h。
- 青霉素(水成的)：400 万 U[儿童：10 万～40 万 U/(kg·24 h)]，静脉滴注，q4 h。
- 甲氧苄啶-磺胺甲噁唑：2 片，口服，q12 h[儿童：6～10 mg/(kg·24 h)磺胺甲噁唑分开口服，q12 h]。
- 万古霉素：1 g，静脉滴注，q12 h(儿童：10 mg/kg，静脉滴注，q6 h；年龄小于 5 岁剂量需做调整)；检查血肌酐水平。

随访

进一步处理

入院指征

- 中毒症状。
- 组织坏死。
- 有免疫抑制。
- 同时并存慢性内科疾病。
- 不能服用口服药物。
- 不稳定的患者。
- 门诊治疗失败。

出院指征

- 无中毒症状的轻微感染。
- 能服用口服抗生素。
- 没有免疫抑制病史和同时并存的内科疾病。
- 没有累及手或面部感染。
- 24～48 h 可完成充足的随访。

随访建议

- 随访 24～48 h。
- 尽快识别恶化的症状，包括新发的或恶化的淋巴管炎，红肿面积的增加，发热加重。

F

• 治疗前描记红斑的范围，帮助评估治疗反应性。

要点和误区

• 链球菌和葡萄球菌是常见病原菌。

• 如今 CA - MRSA 引起蜂窝织炎很常见，需保证足够的经验性治疗药物覆盖之。

• 临床医师在床旁不能准确识别 MRSA 感染。

• 深部脓肿可能错误地归类为蜂窝织炎。

• 使用临床怀疑论及超声避免遗漏脓肿。

辐射损伤

Robert J. Feldman 郑金浩 毛恩强 译

基础知识

描述

• 这一章所讲的辐射是指电离损伤。

• Alpha(α)：氦核，不穿透皮肤。

• Beta(β)：电子，可穿透皮肤数厘米。

• Gamma(γ)：光子，可穿透整身体。

• 中子：具有穿透性，虽然没有被盖革计数器探测到，但中子发射器也会发射 γ 射线。

• 放射性同位素/放射性核素：化学元素从原子核发出射线：

- 不能摧毁放射源，只能移除或采取防护措施。
- 放射源不能改变元素的理化功能，如重金属的毒性。

• 暴露/放射：患者处于电离辐射内：

- 全身或特定部位暴露。

• 污染：辐射性物质位于不应当出现的位置。

- 内部：体内(如肺)。
- 外部：体外(如皮肤、头发、衣服)。

• 剂量：组织吸收辐射能的量。

- 单位转换。
  - 1 Gy＝100 rad。
  - 1 Sv＝100 rem。
- 对于 β 和 γ 射线：
  - 1 Gy＝1 Sv＝100 rad＝100 rem。

> **注意**
>
> • 如果发生放射性事件，报告当地政府或中央部门指导工作。

儿科注意事项

• 儿童对于辐射损伤更敏感。

• 碘化钾对儿童有保护作用，如果怀疑儿童放射性物质(^{131}I)暴露，应给予适量碘化钾。

妊娠注意事项

• 发育过程中的胎儿对射线非常敏感。

• 妊娠期人员不应诊治体内含放射性物质的患者。

病因

• 电离辐射引起细胞损伤。

• 损伤血管，引起动脉内膜炎和组织缺血。

• 细胞增殖活跃的脏器对射线更敏感：

- 骨髓和胃肠道对射线非常敏感。
- 皮肤和神经对射线不敏感。

• 急性辐射综合征发生于以下全身暴露情况：

- 前驱期：急性辐射损伤引起急性炎性反应(0～48 h)。
- 潜伏期：如果急性损伤后得以存活，炎性反应和症状缓解(0～2 周)。
- 发病期：高辐射剂量，器官衰竭继而进展。
- 恢复期或死亡：往往继发感染。

• 辐射源包括医疗设备、核素治疗、核武器和含有放射源的工厂。

诊断

• 诊断辐射损害非常容易。

• 诊断和定量辐射暴露非常困难，可能需专家会诊。

症状和体征

• 基于不同暴露剂量，临床症状不同。

• 整体：

- 全身暴露：和高剂量化学毒物症状相似。
- 急性辐射综合征症状出现越迅速，暴露剂量越大。

• 局部暴露：

- 早期和烫伤或紫外线损伤相似。
- 晚期和缺血性溃疡相似。

病史

• 明确暴露：

- 职业、放疗、运输放射源泄露。

• 不知情的情况下发生暴露：

- 放射性分散设备，隐藏或未被识别的放射源。
- 工业医学放射源可能被做成颗粒，放射直径仅几毫米但放射量很强。
- 如果大量患者出现任何阶段的急性辐射综合征，无烫伤史出现烫伤表现或在非常发位置出现缺血性溃疡(如触碰不明物质的手或放射源放置口袋对应的臀部)应考虑辐射损伤。

体格检查

• 全身暴露：

- 恶心，呕吐：
  - 100 rad 以上的暴露，持续 3～6 h，辐射能量越大产生症状的时间越短。
  - 暴露 1 h 以内出现呕吐提示潜在致死性损伤(>600 rad)。
- 倦怠、乏力(>200 rad)。
- 发热：
  - 急性，由于炎性反应。
  - 发病期感染引起发热。
- 脱发，出血，腹泻可能随剂量>300 rad 加重。

• 皮肤暴露：

- 起初出现红斑。
- 继而出现水平或缺血性坏疽。

基本检查

• 使用盖格计数器测量辐射量，核医学单位或放疗单位都备有盖格计数器：

- 任何探测方式用于测量辐射量都被认可。
- 使用检查手套覆盖探头。
  - 防止探头污染。
  - 阻挡 α 射线，但是可以探测 β、γ 射线。
- 测量背景射线时需远离患者。
- 缓慢移动探头靠近患者皮肤。
  - 距离皮肤 1～2 cm。
  - 探头移动速度为 2～3 cm/s。
  - 辐射量为>2 倍以上的背景射线水平。
  - 记录所有强辐射区域。
  - 按照系统模式探测，避免遗漏。
  - 注意探测手掌、足底、头发。

F

• 淋巴细胞绝对计数是辐射损伤严重程度的最佳指标。
- <1 000/mm^3：中度暴露，200～600 rad。
- <500/mm^3：重度暴露，>600 rad。

诊断检查与说明

• 血细胞分类计数 q4～6 h(持续 24 h 或直至病情平稳)。
• 两侧鼻腔拭子，检测吸入的放射物质。
• 验血型和交叉配血。
• 如果怀疑体内含放射物质，留取 24 h 尿做放射性监测。

影像学检查

• 按临床提示相应的影像学检查辅助诊断。
• 如果高度怀疑体内有放射源，盖格计数器结果为阴性，排除体内放射源最好的检查方式为全身 γ 照相(无准直器)。

诊断步骤/外科

通过细胞学可以更精确地估测射线剂量：
• 抽取 10 ml 血压放入肝素-锂抗凝管中(乙二胺四乙酸也可以)。
• 暴露 24 h 后收集。
• 冷藏(4 ℃)然后送至射线紧急救援中心(REAC)或培训基地。
• 由于资源限制，只有极少数样本可以进行预处理。

鉴别诊断

• 全身性疾病：淋巴细胞减少，乏力，恶心：
- 在暴露和未暴露患者，心理影响因素常见，可能假装急性辐射综合征：
  ◦ 急性辐射综合征引起的呕吐等射线损伤应当伴有淋巴细胞计数降低，如果淋巴细胞计数正常并且稳定，考虑精神因素或其他疾病。
- 血液系统的恶性疾病。
- 化学武器(水疱/芥子气)。
- 获得性免疫缺陷综合征，免疫抑制。
• 皮肤损伤：
- 缺血性溃疡。
- 棕隐斜蛛咬伤。
- 坏疽性脓皮症。

治疗

个人防护设备(PPE)：
• 必须提供防护，远离放射粉尘(特别是吸入，如佩戴 N95 口罩、长袍、手套、头发、鞋套)。
• 射线防护围裙没有价值：射线防护围裙对于大部分 γ 射线均不能阻挡。

院前

危及生命(开放气道、人工呼吸、循环管理)。
• 对所有爆炸现场进行评估，判断有无放射性污染。
• 去除衣服可以消除约 80%的外部污染：
- 无放射污染：可以按救治常规处理患者。
- 如果放射源仍存在，评估医疗环境：
• 安全稳定：开始去除放射源。
• 有安全隐患：提供必要的处理和转移，使用床单等物控制放射源。

初步稳定/治疗

• 血细胞计数。
• 评估辐射损伤伤情。
• 如果患者病情尚平稳，清除辐射源后再转入救治场所。
• 营救人员辐射损伤最小化：
- 时间：在辐射污染区域时间最小化，常常通过移除放射源实现。
- 距离：使用长把手的工具处理放射源。
- 防护：把放射性物质放入铅容器(在核医学部常备)，X 线防护铅围裙效果不佳。

急诊治疗/程序

• 医院方面：
- 如有放射性污染的提示，启动医院灾难救护计划，调动相应医疗资源。
- 指定污染区域以及相对清洁区域。
- 发生突发放射泄露事件后，临时任命一名辐射安全指挥人员(RSO)指挥协调调动所有的患者、救援人员及医疗资源至相对安全的诊治区域。
  ◦ 如果需要，在急救起始阶段，经过专业培训使用盖氏测量仪和放射量测定器的任何参与救援人员都可被临时指定为辐射安全指挥员。
- 未经辐射的患者和无放射污染的物质不需要观察治疗及去污染。
- 寻求专家的帮助：医院的辐射安全指挥人员、当地核安全机构人员、健康机构或放射紧急救援中心。
• 救援人员方面：
- 如上所述，为救援人员提供个人防护设备(PPE)和心理疏导支持。
- 分派妊娠期救援人员至“无反射污染的区域”实施救援。
• 去除污染：
- 辐射物质去除的优先顺序：伤口>黏膜损伤>皮肤完整处。
- 使用洞巾防护邻近的皮肤。
- 使用肥皂和水并且确保不含其他化学物质。
- 皮肤完好的部位使用棉布擦拭；擦拭从一边开始，至中心区域，然后移开。
- 冲洗伤口：收集污水，防止污水溅出。
- 多重新评估去除放射物的效果。
- 避免擦伤皮肤。
- 如果放射物质不易被清除，覆盖污染区域，防止污染播散和移动，控制残余污染。
• 放射性布散装置(RDD)袭击：
- 急诊手术需尽快完成(36～48 h)，辐射暴露>200 rad 延迟 1～2 个月。
- 现场排除爆炸为放射性布散装置以前，任何爆炸受害者都应评估辐射剂量。
- 保护刑事案件现场证据。
• 治疗呕吐和脱水。
- 止吐药物(昂丹司琼)。
- 静脉补液。
• 不同的辐射源使用不同的药物，促进其在体内的排泄：
- 联络射线紧急救援中心 REAC 或培训基地(参考下述)。
- 普鲁士蓝(不溶性)可增强对体内放射性铊或铯的消除。
- 三胺五乙酸三钠钙和锌可增强对钚、镅和锔的消除。
• 辐射剂量>200 rad，可能需要输血和细胞因子支持治疗。
• 碘化钾：
- 仅用于预防放射性污染 4 h 内甲状腺摄入放射性碘(核反应堆中发现)，参考 www.remm.nlm.gov/potassiumiodide.htm。

药物治疗

• Ca DTPA(若可以获得，适用于首选 DTPA 的孕妇)：所有患者在初始剂量 Ca DTPA 后改用 Zn DTPA 进行后续螯合治疗。
- 成人：1 g 静推 3～4 min 以上。
- 儿童：14 mg/kg 缓慢静推，最大量至 1 g。
• 骨髓细胞因子(非格司亭，乙二醇化非格司亭)：剂量和治疗时间不同，见 https://www.remm.nlm.goy/cytokines。
• 昂丹司琼 8 mg 静推(或等价的 5-羟色胺受体阻滞剂)。
• 碘化钾：
- 成人：130 mg，口服，每日 1 次。
- 儿童：
  ◦ 3～18 岁：65 mg，口服，每日 1 次。
  ◦ 1 个月～3 岁：32 mg，口服，每日 1 次。
  ◦ <1 个月：16 mg，口服，每日 1 次。

F

- 普鲁士蓝(不溶性)：
  - 成人：3 g，口服，每日 3 次。
  - 儿童：2～12 年 1 g 口服，每日 3 次 2 岁以下剂量不确定。
- Zn DTPA：妊娠患者的初始剂量，以及在 Ca DTPA 初始剂量后的所有患者的第二次及以上剂量。
  - 成人：1 g 静推，持续 3～4 min。
  - 儿童：14 mg/kg 缓慢静推，最大量至 1 g。

随访

进一步处理

入院指征

- 暴露后 24～48 h，淋巴细胞计数<1 000。
- 暴露后 24～48 h，淋巴细胞减少 50% 以上。
- 怀疑急性放射量暴露>200 rad。
- 严重颅脑外伤或其他疾病。
- 无法控制的呕吐。
- 当对患者病情存在疑问时，复查血细胞计数，请相关科室会诊。

出院指征

- 无残余放射性污染物。
- 没有急性辐射量>100 rad 的证据。
- 可以口服流质。

随访建议

- 放射性物质内污染：联系射线紧急救援中心(REAC)或培训基地了解详情。
- 拨打急救电话。
- 不能移除的表面放射性污染。
- 所有的放射性物质暴露的患者需要剂量评估和风险咨询。

要点和误区

- 紧急医疗救护优先于洗消。
  - 目前还没有 1 例活的受污染患者的放射性会对急救人员造成直接危害。
- 不要低估任何涉及"辐射"的事件所造成的心理影响。
- 淋巴细胞计数可以帮助区分急性辐射综合征和心身疾病：如果呕吐是由于急性辐射综合征导致，淋巴细胞计数应该是低的，下降持续 4～8 h 及以上。

腐蚀性化学物中毒

Paul Kolecki　彭沪 译

基础知识

F

描述

- 碱：
  - 分解水产生 OH^-，从而导致液化坏死。
  - 咽下，主要损伤食管。
    - 也可以损伤胃(见"酸")。
  - 食管损伤(按损伤程度加重排序)包括：
    - 浅表面充血。
    - 黏膜水肿。
    - 浅表面水疱。
    - 渗出性溃疡。
    - 全层坏死。
    - 穿孔。
    - 纤维化食管狭窄。
  - 不会直接导致系统并发症。
- 酸：
  - 分解水产生氢离子(H^+，导致凝固性坏死和结痂)。
  - 咽下，通过食管快速进入可以损伤胃。
  - 胃损伤(按损伤程度加重排序)：
    - 水肿。
    - 炎症。
    - 即刻或继发出血。
    - 全层坏死。
    - 穿孔。
    - 纤维化导致胃排空功能障碍。
  - 大量吸收后可导致红细胞溶血和机体酸中毒。

病因

- 直接的化学损伤。
- 继发于酸和碱暴露后的损伤(皮肤、眼、呼吸道、胃肠道)。
- 很多腐蚀性的试剂(酸和碱)在生产生活中到处可见。
- 腐蚀性药物：
  - 氢氧化铵。
- 玻璃清洁剂：
  - 甲醛：
    - 防腐剂。
  - 盐酸：
    - 抽水马桶清洁剂。
  - 氢氟酸：
    - 玻璃雕刻制造业。
    - 微芯片制造业。
    - 除锈剂。
  - 碘酒：
    - 防腐剂。
  - 苯酚：
    - 防腐剂。
  - 氢氧化钠：
    - 下水道清洁剂。
    - 下水道去污剂。
    - 烤箱清洁剂。
  - 硼酸钠、碳酸盐、磷酸盐和硅酸盐：
    - 洗洁剂。
    - 洗碗机。
    - 次氯酸钠。
    - 漂白剂。
  - 硫酸：
    - 车用蓄电池。
    - 纽扣电池。

诊断

症状和体征

- 口咽部：
  - 疼痛。
  - 红斑。
  - 灼伤。
  - 腐蚀。
  - 溃疡。
  - 流涎。
  - 声嘶。
  - 喘鸣。
  - 失声。
  - 口咽部无可见伤口不能除外内脏损伤。
- 肺部：
  - 呼吸急促。
  - 咳嗽。
  - 吸入性肺炎。
- 胃肠道：
  - 疼痛。

- 呕吐或吐血。
- 黑便，吞咽困难。
- 吞咽疼痛。
- 食管或胃穿孔。
- 穿孔导致的腹膜炎。

• 心血管：
- 心动过速。
- 低血压。
- 直立性低血压。

• 血液系统：
- 酸摄入可导致红细胞溶血。

• 皮肤组织：
- 疼痛。
- 红斑。
- 1度、2度、3度烧伤。

• 眼睛：
- 疼痛。
- 红斑。
- 充血。
- 角膜灼伤。
- 全层角膜损伤。

• 代谢：
- 代谢性酸中毒。

■ 基本检查

• 暴露史或相关的症状体征。

• 无口咽部损伤不能除外内脏损伤。

■ 诊断检查与说明

实验室检查

• 血常规。

• 电解质、尿素氮、肌酐、葡萄糖。

• 动脉血气。

• 血培养：
- 在怀疑有纵隔炎症或腹膜炎症时。

• 测血型和交叉配血。

影像学检查

以下情况行X线胸片和腹部片：

• 食管穿孔或胃穿孔。

• CT检查可以发现重要消化道疾病。

■ 诊断步骤/外科

• 食管镜和胃镜。
- 对于有系统症状的患者明确有无其他损伤。
- 在摄入后第一个12～24 h施行。
- 建议在有呼吸窘迫时进行合适的气道管理。
- 在有严重的咽部损伤的情况下不建议施行。

• 钡餐造影不建议在急性期施行。
- 可以用于后续的狭窄评估。

■ 鉴别诊断

• 腐蚀性物品、酸、碱、干燥剂、起泡剂、氧化剂和还原剂。

• 异物吸入。

• 上气道感染或神经性水肿。

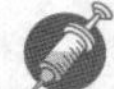

治疗

■ 院前

• 口部烧伤或相关症状：用大量清水或牛奶冲洗。

• 以下患者可用牛奶或清水冲洗：
- 能进水。
- 无腹痛主诉。
- 无气道狭窄和呕吐。

• 眼睛或皮肤的接触应该立即用大量清水冲洗。

■ 初步稳定/治疗

• ABC管理：
- 如果患者有呼吸道狭窄的证据，应该予以预防性插管。
- 禁止使用盲法鼻插管。
- 注意腐蚀性导致的气道水肿。
- 考虑使用地塞米松。
- 使用生理盐水静脉滴注进行液体复苏。

■ 急诊治疗/程序

• 去除残余接触：
- 真皮或口腔暴露：
  ◦ 用清水和生理盐水冲洗直到pH正常。
  ◦ 碱接触比酸接触需要更充分的冲洗。
- 催吐剂、活性炭、洗胃术(大口径的管或鼻胃管)，禁止使用酸或碱中和摄入的腐蚀性物品。

• 稀释：
- 在第一个30 min内使用清水或牛奶：
  ◦ 对于液体腐蚀性碱特别有用。
  ◦ 过多饮入可能诱发呕吐从而损伤食管。
- 如果怀疑有食管或胃穿孔则应禁止使用。

• 如果只有口服暴露保持患者NPD。

• 怀疑纵隔炎或腹膜炎的使用广谱抗生素。

• 对于恶心和呕吐使用止吐剂。

• 按标准烧伤指南治疗真皮的暴露损伤。

• 详细检查眼部暴露损伤情况。

• 静脉使用质子泵抑制剂或H_2受体阻滞剂缓解症状。

• 胃肠科和外科会诊。

• 使用激素治疗食管损伤目前存有争议：
- 可能阻止食管狭窄的形成。
- 可能导致细菌感染、免疫抑制及组织软化。
- 一旦决定使用激素要求整个团队来护理患者。
- 如果使用激素同时开始使用广谱抗生素。

• 穿孔和全层坏死者行腹腔镜检查或剖腹探查术。

• 局部的氢氟酸暴露(决定于损伤的严重性和部位)：
- 肌内注射5%葡萄糖酸钙(0.5 ml/cm^2皮肤，30G针头)。
- 10 ml 10%葡萄糖酸钙稀释于40 ml 5%葡萄糖溶液中。
- 颈动脉注射长于4 h。

■ 药物治疗

• 地塞米松：10 mg(儿童：6 mg/kg，总剂量为10 mg)，静脉注射。

• 甲泼尼龙：40 mg，q8 h[儿童：2 mg/(kg·d)]，静脉注射；治疗疗程为14～21日，之后逐渐递减。

• 昂丹司琼：4 mg(儿童：0.1～0.15 mg/kg)，静脉注射。

• 泮托拉唑：40 mg，静脉注射。

• 普鲁氯嗪(甲哌氯丙嗪)：5～10 mg，静脉注射(儿童：每次肌注量0.13 mg/kg)。

• 雷尼替丁(甲胺呋硫)：50 mg，静脉注射，q6～8 h。

随访

■ 进一步处理

入院指征

• 所有有症状的患者。

• 非意外的摄入。

出院指征

• 意外摄入且无吞咽困难的无症状患者。

• 轻微的口咽部疼痛，与可见的病变损伤一致；无流涎，无呼吸苦难；无喉部，胸部或腹部疼痛；吞咽无困难。

■ 随访建议

蓄意吞服的人建议精神科干预。

F

要点和误区

- 无论在家还是急诊室，在第一个 30 min 内用清水或牛奶冲洗。
- 眼睛或皮肤接触应该大量冲洗。
- 相比于酸，碱接触损伤应该更彻底的冲洗。

附睾炎和睾丸炎

Epididymitis/Orchitis

Matthew D. Cook · Kevin R. Weaver 单怡 译

基础知识

描述

附睾炎

- 定义：附睾的炎症或感染。
- 青春期前男性少见。
- 发病机制：
  - 起始期：
    - 细胞炎症开始于血管输送和下递至较低位的附睾区。
  - 急性期：
    - 附睾上下极水肿和变硬。
    - 精索增厚。
  - 睾丸由于被动充血或炎症而水肿。
  - 消退期：
    - 可完全恢复而无后遗症。
    - 附睾周围组织纤维化增生可使管腔阻塞。
- 并发症：
  - 2/3 的病例由于睾丸动脉部分血栓形成，导致附睾萎缩。
  - 脓肿和梗死少见(5%)。
  - 单侧附睾炎不孕症的发病率不明确。
    - 双侧附睾炎可有 50%的不孕症发病率。

睾丸炎

- 定义：睾丸的炎症或感染。
  - 通常是附睾炎病程的延续。
  - 单纯的睾丸感染少见：
    - 可通过细菌血行播散或流行性腮腺炎感染后发病。
- 分类：
  - 化脓性细菌性睾丸炎继发细菌性附睾炎。
  - 病毒性睾丸炎：
    - 最常见的是流行性腮腺炎病毒。
    - 青春前期男性少见，20%～30%青春期后男性可继发于流行性腮腺炎感染。
    - 发生在腮腺炎后 4～6 日，也可在无腮腺炎情况下发病。
    - 70%的患者是单侧发病。
    - 通常 6～10 日后恢复。
    - 30%～50%的睾丸有萎缩的残余效应，很少影响生育。
  - 肉芽肿性睾丸炎：
    - 梅毒。
    - 结核和真菌性疾病。
    - 通常发生于免疫力低下宿主。

病因

附睾炎

- 儿童：
  - 最常见于<1 岁儿童或 12～15 岁儿童。
  - 只有 25%的青春期前男性明确病因。
  - 大肠杆菌或假单胞菌感染。
  - 青春期前的性传播疾病少见。
  - 与下尿路畸形有关。
- 青年，<35 岁：
  - 通常通过性接触传播。
  - 沙眼衣原体感染(28%～88%)的炎症反应很强，但损害最小。
  - 淋病奈瑟菌感染(3%～28%)。
  - 大肠杆菌感染(7%～24%)。
    - 脓肿有高度破坏性倾向。
    - 大肠杆菌在男同性恋中更常见。
    - 解脲支原体(只有 6%案例中有此微生物的单纯感染)。
- 年龄较大人群，>35 岁：
  - 通常与泌尿系统病理性疾病相关(良性前列腺增生、前列腺癌、狭窄)。
  - 可能有急性或慢性细菌性前列腺炎。
  - 大肠杆菌感染更常见(23%～67%)，特别是经器械操作后。
  - 沙眼衣原体感染(8%～80%)。
  - 克雷伯菌属和假单胞菌属感染。
  - 淋病(15%)。
  - 革兰阳性球菌感染。
- 药物相关性：
  - 胺碘酮相关的附睾炎：
    - 通常胺碘酮水平大于治疗水平。
- 肉芽肿性：
  - 病因可能与分枝杆菌、梅毒或真菌感染有关：
    - 结核分枝杆菌是引起附睾炎肉芽肿性疾病最常见的原因。
    - 可能发生于 HIV 感染的患者。
    - 尿培养结核分枝杆菌常为阴性。
- 血管炎性：
  - 结节性多动脉炎。
  - 白塞病。
  - 过敏性紫癜。

睾丸炎

- 化脓性细菌性睾丸炎：
  - 大肠杆菌。
  - 肺炎克雷伯菌。
  - 铜绿假单胞菌。
  - 葡萄球菌。
  - 链球菌。
- 病毒性睾丸炎：
  - 流行性腮腺炎：
    - 20%可发展为附睾-睾丸炎。
    - 与腮腺炎病毒减活疫苗关系不大。
- 柯萨奇病毒 A 和淋巴细胞性脉络丛脑膜炎病毒。
- 肉芽肿性睾丸炎：梅毒、结核分枝杆菌和真菌性疾病：
  - 可能发生于获得性免疫缺陷综合征(艾滋病)患者。
- 真菌性睾丸炎：
  - 发生于芽生菌病流行地区。
  - 免疫抑制患者侵袭性念珠菌感染。
- 创伤性睾丸炎：炎症。

诊断

症状和体征

既往史

- 睾丸或阴囊轻至中度的进行性疼痛，通常为单侧。
- 进行性的阴囊肿胀。
- 排尿困难(30%)：
  - 近期尿路感染。
  - 膀胱功能紊乱病史。

- 尿道分泌物：
  - 淋菌性附睾炎患者，21%～30%无主诉尿道分泌物。
  - 50%无尿道分泌物。
- 发热(14%～28%)。
- 近期有过泌尿系统器械或导管操作。

体格检查

- 腹股沟、下腹部和阴囊压痛。
- 阴囊皮肤通常有红斑和发热。
- 早期：
  - 可能有肿胀，附睾硬结。
- 后期：
  - 可能无法区分睾丸和附睾。
  - 可能有脊髓水肿。
- 提睾反射正常。
- Prehn 征：
  - 抬高睾丸疼痛缓解。
  - 通常可见，但无特异性。
- 合并前列腺炎少见(8%)。
- 化脓性细菌性睾丸炎：
  - 患者通常急性发作。
  - 发热。
  - 强烈的不适感，睾丸肿胀。
  - 通常有反应性鞘膜积液。

基本检查

- 必须与睾丸扭转鉴别。
- 如果高度怀疑睾丸扭转，尽早请泌尿外科医师会诊。

诊断检查与说明

实验室检查

- 尿液分析和培养：
  - 在首段尿中白细胞酯酶阳性或首段尿沉积物中白细胞计数大于 10 个每高倍视野。
  - 15%～50%的附睾-睾丸炎患者有脓尿。
  - 24%的患者有尿细菌培养阳性。
- 淋病和衣原体病的核酸扩增试验(NAAT)。
  - 尿液是更好的样本。
  - 在检查前 2 h 内尽量保持膀胱充盈(以免降低敏感性)。
  - 尤其注意青春期后期青少年和性生活活跃者。
- 尿道分泌物革兰染色每个油浸视野≥2 个白细胞(确诊尿道炎)，白细胞内包含革兰阴性双球菌(确诊淋球菌感染)。
- 如有全身不适行血培养。

影像学检查

- 超声：彩色多普勒超声：
  - 对睾丸扭转或血流速低的敏感性为 82%～100%，特异性为 100%。
  - 附睾睾丸炎：
    - 充血。
    - 血管数目和血流量的增加。
  - 优点：
    - 能够评估附睾炎或其他造成阴囊疼痛的原因。
    - 诊断附睾炎敏感性为 70%，特异性为 88%。
  - 缺点：
    - 高度依赖于受检者。
    - 对婴儿或儿童难度大。
- 睾丸闪烁影像：
  - 放射性核素显像评估灌注情况。
  - 对于检测睾丸扭转的敏感性为 90%～100%，特异性为 89%～97%。
  - 炎症过程增加了造影剂的流动和吸收。
  - 许多机构不常规应用。

诊断检查与说明

手术探查指征：

- 阴囊脓肿。
- 不能排除扭转。
- 严重附睾炎引起的可疑或确诊的缺血。
- 单侧睾丸的患者。
- 阴囊固定：提示严重炎症和潜在脓肿。

鉴别诊断

- 睾丸扭转。
- 睾丸肿瘤。
- 睾丸附件扭转。
- 阴囊损伤。
- 急性疝。
- 急性鞘膜积液。

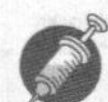

治疗

院前

- 建立静脉通路。
- 静脉输液，尤其是有全身系统疾病时。

初步稳定/治疗

- 建立静脉通路。
- 静脉输液，尤其是有全身系统疾病时。

急诊治疗/外科

- 抗生素治疗：
  - 怀疑性传播患者、抗衣原体及淋球菌治疗。
  - 抗大肠杆菌治疗：
    - 儿童或>35 岁成人。
    - 男同性恋者。
    - 非性接触传播者。
    - 近期性泌尿生殖系统操作(前列腺活检，输精管切除术)。
- 卧床休息，抬高，冰袋冰敷阴囊。
- 止痛和抗感染。

药物治疗

- 年龄在 35 岁以下或怀疑性传播淋病或衣原体病：
  - 头孢曲松钠 250 mg，肌内注射，每日 1 次+强力霉素 100 mg，口服，每日 2 次，连续 10 日。
- 年龄在 35 岁以上或近期泌尿生殖系植入史或沙眼衣原体、淋球菌培养、DNA 扩增阴性者：
  - 氧氟沙星 300 mg，口服，每日 2 次；或左氧氟沙星，500 mg/d，口服，连续 10 日。
- 细菌性附睾炎不常见于青春期前的男孩并且抗生素给药方案不推荐。
- 儿童患者避免使用喹诺酮类和四环素类。
- 对于肛交的男性同性恋者：
  - 头孢曲松钠 250 mg，肌内注射 1 次+氧氟沙星，300 mg，口服，每日 2 次；或左氧氟沙星 500 mg/d，口服，维持 10 日。

随访

进一步处理

入院指征

- 有手术指征。
- 老年患者需要住院明确检查者。
  - 许多可能有潜在的泌尿系统病理疾病。
- 全身性疾病、发热、恶心、呕吐。
- 阴囊脓肿。
- 难以控制的疼痛。

出院指征

- 未达到住院标准。
- 检查状态良好。
- 可口服抗生素治疗。

随访建议

- 初始抗生素治疗 3 日无效需要评估泌尿系统的情况。
- 经过充分的抗生素治疗，症状持续存在，寻找其他造成附睾炎的原因：
  - 结核或真菌性附睾炎、阴囊脓肿、肿瘤、梗死。
- 性伴侣怀疑或确诊沙眼衣原体、淋球菌感染，应该检查与治疗。
- 儿童需要泌尿外科医师评估是否有泌尿

系统解剖畸形。

要点和误区

• 所有初发的睾丸疼痛的患者需排除睾丸扭转。

• 35 岁以下男性发生附睾炎通常是由于性生活活跃导致性传播疾病。

• 35 岁以上男性发生附睾炎通常是由于大肠杆菌感染。

• 应一开始就使用抗生素治疗，可根据临床表现经验性使用抗生素。

复视 Diplopia

Jonathan A. Edlow · Kiersten L. Gurley 谭美春 译

 基础知识

描述

• 复视。

- 同时感知到两个图像。

- 可与另一图像成水平方向、垂直方向或对角线方向。

- 两种类型：单眼（眼科原因）和双眼（神经性原因）。

- 双眼和第Ⅵ对脑神经（CN Ⅵ）麻痹最常见。

• 复视通常由于眼外肌（EOM）异常运动造成，由Ⅲ对脑神经支配（CN）：

- 第Ⅲ对脑神经（CN Ⅲ）：上、下、内直肌和下斜肌。

- 第Ⅳ对脑神经（CN Ⅳ）：上斜肌。

- 第Ⅵ对脑神经（CN Ⅵ）：侧直肌。

• 脑干病变可损害脑神经核或其连接（内侧纵束，MLF），造成核间性眼肌麻痹（INO）。

• 脑神经紊乱。

- 穿过蛛网膜下腔和静脉窦受到压迫。

- 炎症。

- 脑脊液压力升高（或降低）可引起 CN Ⅵ麻痹。

• 影响眼眶和颅骨的疾病可以引起一个或两个眼睛或眼外肌运动受限。

病因

• 外伤性复视。

- 眼眶骨折。

- 挫伤。

- 血肿。

- 少见脑干挫伤或血肿。

• 单眼复视。

- 几乎总是由于眼睛自身的问题引起。

- 角膜表面圆锥形角膜。

- 晶状体半脱位。

- 眼睛内的结构缺陷。

- 功能性障碍，如转换障碍、人为障碍或躯体化。

• 非创伤性双眼复视。

- 脑与脑干功能障碍。

◦ 脑卒中。

◦ 多发性硬化。

◦ 大脑皮质问题（例如，偏头痛）是罕见的。

- 中枢神经系统功能紊乱。

◦ 后交通动脉瘤（CN Ⅲ麻痹）。

◦ 慢性淋巴细胞性脑膜炎（多发神经缺损）。

◦ 假脑瘤（CN Ⅵ麻痹）。

◦ 低压（自发性低颅压，CN Ⅵ麻痹）。

- 颅骨和眼眶：

◦ 肿瘤。

◦ 甲状腺疾病。

◦ 炎症（Tolosa-Hunt 综合征）。

- 眼外肌神经-肌肉接头（NMJ）：

◦ 重症肌无力（MG）。

诊断

症状和体征

病史

• 确定复视是否继发于头部损伤，是持续性或间歇性，以及持续时间。

• 确定复视是单眼还是双眼。

• 询问是否有绝对远视（HA）或其他神经或视觉症状。

• 两个图像是垂直、水平或对角线方向排列。

体格检查

• 单眼与双眼鉴别。

- 如果覆盖任一眼睛复视消失，它是双眼复视。

- 如果有一只眼睛存在复视，它是单眼复视（问题在于存在复视的眼睛上）。

• 鉴别外伤和非外伤性的复视。

• 单眼的复视。

- 仔细的眼科检查。

- 视敏度。

• 双眼复视：

- 完整检查眼睛（是否有上睑下垂、瞳孔不等大、眼外肌受限、眼球突出、突眼）矫正视力（VA）是否正常。

- CN Ⅲ：累及瞳孔，斜复视伴上睑下垂和瞳孔散大。

- CN Ⅲ：不累及瞳孔，斜复视伴正常眼睑和瞳孔。

- CN Ⅳ：垂直或斜复视，最不常见。

- CN Ⅵ：水平复视，当从受影响一侧侧面凝视结束时影像更加分离。

- 做一个完整的神经功能测试。

• 创伤性复视：

- 面部感觉缺失。

- 瞳孔大小不等。

- 眼球突出。

- 视敏度降低。

> **注意**
>
> • 患者可能在一般检查中表现良好，必须高度警惕并仔细进行神经或眼科检查。
>
> • 做一个系统性的体格检查，尽可能确定病灶位置。
>
> • 如果 CN Ⅲ麻痹，鉴别瞳孔未累及（通常是微血管梗死）和瞳孔累及的麻痹（通常为动脉瘤）。这通常由于未破裂的动脉瘤扩张引起。

• 如果面瘫（CN Ⅴ）伴复视，考虑海绵窦或眶上裂综合征。

• 如果视力减退，考虑眼眶或眶上裂综合征。

基本检查

精确的病史和体格检查是诊断的基础。建立创伤的病史是关键。在自发病例中，体格检查应该直接进行：

• 复视是否单独存在。

• 如果单独存在，哪对颅神经受累。

• 如果有其他神经缺损存在，努力定位病灶。

• 如果有 CN Ⅲ麻痹和瞳孔散大，进行某些

形式的脑动脉造影(CTA、MRA、DSA)。

■ 诊断检查与说明

实验室检查

• 急诊的实验室检查通常无用：

- 偶尔甲状腺功能检查有帮助。其他血清学试验(例如，重症肌无力不需要在急诊科做的)。

诊断步骤/外科

• 如果重症肌无力可能，考虑一个腾喜龙(依酚氯铵)测试或冰试验。

• 腰椎穿刺：如果考虑蛛网膜下腔出血、慢性淋巴细胞性脑膜炎、高或低脑脊液压力。

• 脑和脑血管成像：如果考虑肿瘤、动脉瘤、脑卒中、多发性硬化。具体的测试依赖于特定的鉴别诊断。

■ 鉴别诊断

• 创伤后的复视：

- 眼眶骨折、血肿伴脑神经直接损害或血肿限制眼外肌活动。

- 非常罕见，脑干挫伤影响脑神经核或MLF。

• 单眼复视：

- 几乎所有的眼部问题(角膜、晶状体、虹膜、视网膜问题和折射率)。

- 很罕见，皮质功能障碍导致双侧单眼复视。

• 双眼复视：

- 脑和脑干。

◦ 卒中或多发性硬化累及脑干，通常有单核脑神经麻痹或 INO。这一模式罕见于头外伤和挫伤后。

◦ 韦尼克脑病。

◦ 罕见："皮质"复视由于偏头痛或刺激性病灶和肉毒中毒。

- 脑神经损害。

◦ 脑神经麻痹由于拉伸、挫伤、缺血、脑脊液严重或异常压力。

◦ CN Ⅲ：关键是鉴别瞳孔累及(必须排除动脉瘤)和瞳孔未累及(糖尿病或高血压所导致的微血管梗死)。

◦ CN Ⅵ麻痹无定位结果。

◦ 当多个神经功能受累，可以考虑重症肌无力、淋巴细胞性脑膜炎、海绵窦病变。

◦ 当内核受累(降低内收)，但是没有明确的 CN Ⅲ麻痹，考虑核间性眼肌麻痹(INO)。

• 头骨和眼眶：

- 眼眶浸润性疾病(甲状腺、肿瘤、脓肿和 Tolosa-hunt 综合征)。

• 神经-肌肉接头：

- 重症肌无力和肉毒杆菌中毒。

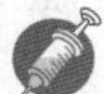

治疗

■ 初步稳定/治疗

绝大多数患者不要求稳定治疗。按照个体患者的病因开始治疗。

■ 急诊治疗/程序

• 腰椎穿刺：

- 如果是淋巴细胞学脑膜炎、假性脑瘤、自发性颅内高压，进行腰椎穿刺。总是测量开放压力。

• 依酚氯铵测试：

- 建议进行一次依酚氯铵或冰试验。

• 眼罩：

- 出院患者可以考虑眼罩控制症状。

儿科注意事项

相同的鉴别诊断。

妊娠注意事项

• 孕妇伴妊娠剧吐时可引发韦尼克脑病或眼眶出血，两者都可以表现为复视。

• 妇女产后可因为海绵窦血栓、硬膜穿刺后头痛或眼眶出血引发复视。

随访

■ 进一步处理

入院指征

• 入院是根据病因来判定。

• 很多患者收治入院是为了方便进行快速检查查找严重病因(包括高级脑部及血管影像学检查和专业咨询)。

出院指征

大部分单眼复视或外伤性复视，病因明确不需要急诊手术患者可安全出院。

■ 随访建议

所有伴有复视的出院患者都需要某些形式的随访，通常有神经科或眼科医师进行。

要点和误区

• 如果两个影像间距较近时复视可以表现为"视力模糊"。

• 永远不要把复视作为孤立的脑神经疾病，而不进行非常仔细的神经系统检查。

• 检查瞳孔避免遗漏颅内动脉瘤。动脉瘤性 CN Ⅲ麻痹通常由于未破裂的动脉瘤引起(CT 或腰椎穿刺正常)。除非有禁忌证，否则患有急性 CN Ⅲ麻痹的患者应该进行某种形式的无创血管造影。

• 重症肌无力可表现为间歇性复视，瞳孔总是正常。

• 监测面部感觉：感觉减退和复视定位病灶在海绵窦或眶上裂。

• 监测视力：纠正视力减退和复视通常是由于眼眶或眶上裂病变(可能是外科急诊)。

F

富尼埃坏疽

Gary M. Vilke · Peter H.D. Solomon　万健 译

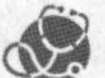

基础知识

■ 描述

• 局部卫生状况差导致皮肤浸渍及表皮剥脱：

- 使细菌进入组织。

• 一旦皮肤屏障遭到破坏，会阴部筋膜便可有细菌群生长。

• Colles 筋膜与泌尿生殖隔膜融合，延缓感染向两侧扩散。

• 前方的 Buck 筋膜与 Scarpa 筋膜相连续，可使感染向前方腹壁迅速蔓延，并延筋膜向两侧扩散。

• 睾丸和尿道通常不受累。

• 大部分患者存在以下 3 个解剖学上的病因：

- 下尿道原因(40%)：尿道狭窄，留置导尿管。

- 阴茎或阴囊原因(30%)：包茎、汗腺炎和龟头炎。

- 肛门直肠原因(30%)：瘘、直肠旁感染和痔。

• 罕见来源于腹腔的感染，如穿通性阑尾炎、憩室炎、胰腺炎等可通过侵入性感染引起本病。

■ 病因

• 多种菌株感染（需氧菌和厌氧菌混合感染）。
• 多种细菌产生相互协同的组织坏死效应。
• 皮下组织末端血栓形成，产生厌氧环境，加速感染扩散。
• 细菌毒素及组织坏死因子也可加重症状。
• 危险因素：
- 创伤。
- 糖尿病。
- 酒精中毒。
- 其他免疫抑制状态。
- 病态肥胖。
- 腹部手术。

诊断

■ 症状和体征

• 急性进行性会阴部皮下组织和筋膜坏死性感染，常累及肌层：
- 常见于糖尿病或免疫功能低下的患者。
• 感染往往来源于泌尿生殖道、直肠、阴茎及阴囊。

儿科注意事项

• 虽然儿童少见，但有约 50 例患者见诸报道。
• 多数是烧伤、包皮环切、龟头炎、严重尿布疹、昆虫叮咬。
• 致病微生物通常是葡萄球菌或链球菌。
• 儿童患者多以局部症状主，全身毒性症状较轻。

病史

• 持续性体征：
- 发热或寒战。
- 恶心和呕吐。
- 尿路感染症状。
• 典型的症状迅速发展。
• 如果患有糖尿病或免疫功能损害，可以提示本病。
• 患者常有嗜睡和表情淡漠等表现。

体格检查

• 患者常出现中毒症状，伴有恶心、呕吐、发热、寒战和疼痛表现。
• 疼痛在早期阶段和检查不相称，但最终死亡组织变得不敏感。
• 仔细检查生殖器及直肠周边区域。
• 认真评估皮肤。
- 皮肤呈现青铜色或紫色的异常颜色。
- 皮肤颜色异常处见浅棕色浆液渗出。
- 皮肤溃疡，水疱。
- 皮下捻发感染，皮下积气。
- 皮肤坏死和焦痂形成。

■ 基本检查

• 富尼埃坏疽（Fournier 坏疽）是一个临床诊断。
• 应特别重视病史与体格检查，尤其是会阴部。
• 评估感染表现。
• 尽早请外科会诊，急诊清创非常重要。
• 针对相关疾病进行检查，如糖尿病、免疫功能抑制等。

■ 诊断检查与说明

实验室检查

• 除对组织和引流物进行革兰染色外，尚无特异性实验室检查可以诊断 Fournier 坏疽。
• 所有患者均应做尿液分析。
• 白细胞增多、贫血、电解质紊乱、酸中毒、肾功能不全较为多见。
• 可出现弥散性血管内凝血（DIC），测定凝血酶原时间（PT）、活化部分凝血活酶时间（APTT）、纤维蛋白降解产物及纤维蛋白原水平有助于诊断。
• 若怀疑或已知患者患有糖尿病，应检测血糖、电解质及血清酮体，以评估糖尿病及糖尿病酮症酸中毒（DKA）。
• 尽可能进行血、尿和组织的培养。

影像学检查

• 影像学检查不应延迟手术评估，如果高度怀疑是 Fournier 坏疽。
• 拍摄骨盆 X 线平片以明确皮下气肿及肠梗阻。
• 如怀疑感染来源于腹腔或坐骨直肠，应行 CT 检查。
• 超声检查皮下气肿对区分阴囊的其他疾病很有帮助。

诊断步骤/外科

逆行尿路造影、肛门镜检、直肠乙状结肠镜检查、钡灌肠等可能有助于对感染源的定位。

■ 鉴别诊断

• 附睾炎或睾丸炎。
• 昆虫或人咬伤。
• 直肠周围炎。
• 阴囊脓肿或腹股沟脓肿。
• 阴囊蜂窝织炎。
• 睾丸扭转。
• 体股癣。

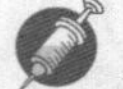

治疗

■ 院前

患者可能因脓毒症休克而发生低血压，需要液体复苏和血管活性药物。

■ 初步稳定/治疗

• 气道开放与复苏。
• 开放中心静脉通路，积极液体复苏，必要时应用血管升压药物：
- 避免从股静脉穿刺置管，避免从下肢外周静脉输液。
• 如发生脓毒症应给予早期目标导向治疗。
• 留置导尿管或耻骨上膀胱造瘘。

■ 急诊治疗/程序

• 经验性应用广谱抗菌药物。
• 早期急诊扩大清创。
• 尽早开始高压氧疗和外科重症监护。
• 纠正脱水和电解质紊乱。应给予血液制品，维持血细胞比容＞30%有利于减轻氧负债。
• 必要时注射破伤风疫苗。

儿科注意事项

• 采取更为保守的外科手段。
• 抗菌药物充分覆盖葡萄球菌。

■ 药物治疗

• 万古霉素（15～20 mg/kg）静脉注射（或其他抗 MRSA 药物）和克林霉素（600～900 mg）静脉注射[起抗毒素作用；儿童：40 mg/(kg·d)，q8 h]，以及碳青霉烯类或 β-内酰胺酶抑制剂。
• 如怀疑有真菌来源，可考虑静脉注射氟康唑（800 mg）或其他抗真菌药物。
• 必要时输入血液制品。
• 充分液体复苏后仍有低血压时，应用多巴胺或多巴酚丁胺静脉滴注，起始剂量为 5 μg/(kg·min)。
• 应用胰岛素调节血糖和酸中毒。

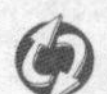

随访

■ 进一步处理

入院指征

• 所有 Fournier 坏疽患者均需要入院并收

入外科重症监护病房(ICU)治疗。

• 病死率为3%～38%，因此强调早期监护的重要性。

• 一旦病情允许应尽早转入能提供高压氧治疗的医疗机构。

出院指征

有Fournier坏疽症状的患者不可出院。

要点和误区

• 应对会阴外生殖器仔细检查，特别是儿童。

• 不应忽视过度的痛苦。

• 应当及时给予初始的抗菌药物治疗。

腹部穿透性创伤 Abdominal Trauma, Penetrating

Frances E. Rudolf · Allyson A. Kreshak 马林浩 林兆奋 译

基础知识

描述

• 实质脏器损伤通常会导致出血。

• 空腔脏器损伤可能会导致肠内容物溢出和腹膜炎。

• 相关的情况：

- 胸腹联合伤出现的概率为25%。

病因

腹部穿透伤常由枪击和刀刺导致明显的腹内损伤，最常见的损伤结构包括：

• 小肠。

• 肝。

• 结肠。

• 腹部血管结构。

诊断

症状和体征

• 刀、枪和其他异物均可导致穿透伤。

• 症状会从受伤的局部疼痛到腹膨隆甚至腹膜刺激征。

- 高速发射物会导致广泛的直接组织损伤。

- 出口部位损伤可能比入口部位更大，小的入口和出口损伤可能会掩盖巨大的内部损伤。

• 低血压、脉搏无力、心动过速可能反映出失血和明显的损伤。

• 记住腹部的边界：上至乳头(前面)或肩胛骨下缘(后面)下至臀褶。

基本检查

• 从前至后进行检查以评估损伤。

• 由枪击造成腹腔内损伤的诊断是由在手术室开腹后做出的。

• 探查局部前腹部的穿刺伤。

- 如果伤情穿透了前筋膜层，患者应该接受诊断性腹腔灌洗或床旁超声。

• 指肠检查可用来评估骨折或指肠和乙状结肠的损伤。

• 诊断性腹腔镜检查对于膈肌损伤和脾脏、肝脏的撕裂伤有帮助。

- 可以帮助避免不必要的手术。

• CT扫描对于怀疑后腹膜腔损伤患者的评估是有用的。

- 对于空腔脏器和膈肌损伤不可靠。

诊断检查与说明

实验室检查

• 血红蛋白或者血细胞比容。

- 多次检查来评估持续性出血的情况。

◦ 检查凝血标志物(血小板、凝血酶原时间和活化部分凝血活酶时间)。

• 尿液分析查找血液以评估可能的泌尿生殖道损伤。

• 动脉血气分析。

- 碱剩余缺乏可能有助于评估低容量和指导容量复苏。

• 为所有严重腹腔内损伤的患者行血型检测和交叉配血。

影像学检查

• X线平片。

- 能够获知异物、子弹、相关骨折及游离气体的位置信息。

• 床旁腹部超声(FAST：关注创伤后的腹腔超声)。

- 可能发现腹腔内的血液或者液体。

• 对于稳定的患者，有条件时行增强CT扫描。

- 评估可能的后腹膜腔和实质脏器损伤。

鉴别诊断

• 对于上腹部损伤患者，考虑胸腔内损伤的可能性。

• 对于下胸腔损伤的患者，考虑腹腔内损伤的可能性。

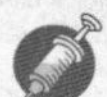

治疗

院前

• 注意：

- 使用消毒敷料打开创面并使用湿润的消毒敷料接触暴露的肠管。

- 固定钉入的异物，不要轻易去除它。

初步稳定/治疗

• 确保气道和呼吸稳定。

• 双腔深静脉导管输注晶体液。

• 如果输注1L晶体液仍无反应，输注2～4U红细胞悬液：

- 如果患者病情不稳定，最初可以使用Rh阴性的O型血。

- 可能时，进行血型检测和交叉配血。

• 面罩接100%氧气。

• 出血患者考虑TXA。

儿科注意事项

• 处于低血容量性休克的患儿应该接受20 ml/kg晶体液的冲击治疗。

• 处于严重低血容量性休克的患儿应该接受10 ml/kg的红细胞悬液。

急诊治疗/程序

• 放置鼻胃管。

- 会降低误吸风险。

- 可能减轻由于膈肌损伤腹腔内容物疝进胸腔而引起的呼吸窘迫。

- 胃管出血可能代表胃肠道出血。

• 放置导尿管。

- 排除尿路损伤后插入。

- 放置后快速评估泌尿生殖系统损伤。

- 帮助监测尿量。

F

药物治疗

• 破伤风类毒素：0.5 ml，肌内注射。

• 破伤风免疫球蛋白：没有接受完整破伤风类毒素治疗的患者，250 U，肌内注射。

• 可考虑使用镇痛药，避免非甾体抗炎药，可能引起出血。

• 静脉使用抗生素：使用覆盖革兰阴性菌和厌氧菌的抗生素。

• 视需要使用抗凝相关药物。

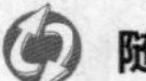

随访

进一步处理

入院指征

• 需要腹部手术的患者。

• 一些患者可能需要管理和持续 24 h 的腹部检查。

出院指征

穿刺伤没有造成筋膜穿透在急诊室观察后情况稳定者可以出院。

要点和误区

• 最好的暴露患者将最少地漏诊伤情。

• 为了进一步稳定病情，不要耽误不稳定患者进入手术室的时间。

• 脊柱固定并不需要，除非存在明显的脊髓损伤。

腹部创伤影像 Abdominal Trauma: Imaging

Richard Childers · Gary M. Vilke　马林浩　林兆奋 译

基础知识

描述

诊断步骤：在不稳定的创伤患者，及时超声探查可用于明确是否有开腹探查的必要。情况稳定的创伤患者怀疑腹内损伤时，可 CT 检查并静脉内造影增强，这也是诊断的一种思路。

诊断

症状和体征

• 单纯的腹部损伤到多系统损伤均会导致患者出现腹部创伤。

• 腹部创伤分为钝性创伤和贯穿伤。贯穿性腹部损伤可进一步分为穿刺伤和枪击伤。

• 血流动力学状态是初始最重要的评估重点。大多数不稳定的患者将需要早期外科干预，而稳定的腹部外伤患者可能不需要手术处置。

病史

• 病史应包括受伤的机制、是否使用约束及约束的方法、有无使用气囊或头盔、院前生命体征情况、最初的神志意识状态和神志状态的改变。

• AMPLE 病史（包括药物和造影剂过敏史、用药史、既往医疗和手术病史、最后一餐的时间和情况，以及与这次受伤有关的事件）。

体格检查

• 全面检查应从 ABCDE 评估开始，包括全面的暴露检视患者以及仔细的腹部触诊。

• 在喝醉（药物过量）、不配合及多系统损伤的患者中，腹部体格检查常常不准确或不满意。

基本检查

参见腹部钝性创伤和腹部穿透伤。

诊断检查与说明

腹部创伤患者影像学检查通常包括：

• 不稳定的创伤患者：

- 不稳定的患者需要立刻行床边超声（FAST）进行循环状态的评估。FAST 结果阳性提示腹腔内出血是低血压的原因。FAST 结果阴性提示可能存在腹膜后出血、血液丢失在腹膜后、不稳定骨盆骨折造成的出血或出血进入其他体腔内。

- 立刻请外科医师会诊准备对患者实施确定性手术。

• 稳定的创伤患者：以下 2 种主要的诊断手段适合腹部创伤后血流动力学稳定的患者，包括：

- 超声：也适用于血流动力学稳定患者的初始评估。稳定的创伤患者超声结果阳性提示存在循环状态恶化的可能性。CT 扫描及外科会诊需要在这些患者中快速实施。

- CT 扫描：是稳定的创伤患者的确定性检查手段。CT 扫描对于实质脏器损伤和腹膜后损伤均优于超声检查。CT 影像可以用于决定是否需要栓塞的措施来进行出血控制。在所有穿刺伤的患者中均有必要进行 CT 扫描。CT 扫描也适用于肉眼血尿的患者以寻找肾脏损伤。

实验室检查

• 血型检测与配型。

• 血常规。

• 电解质和肌酐。

• 尿常规。

影像学检查

• 超声：FAST 检查关注在腹腔内可能存在血液聚集的区域，包括肝肾间隙、脾肾间隙、耻骨上区域及心包。

- 优点：

◦ 快速，非侵入性，便携。

◦ 对腹内游离液体敏感性高（0～500 ml）。

- 缺点：

◦ 结果依赖于操作者水平。

◦ 实质性脏器损伤有时不可靠（如脾和肝脏撕裂伤），后腹膜损伤也不可靠。骨盆骨折严重出血的患者检查结果也可能是阴性的。对于肠管损伤也是不敏感的。

- 受限的情况：

◦ 肥胖，皮下气肿。

- 阳性检测：

◦ 检查区域包括右上腹肝肾间隙、左上腹脾肾间隙、耻骨上区域盆腔及心脏区域。

◦ 多次重复检查可提高敏感性。

• CT 扫描：

- 优点：

◦ 对于腹腔积血、实质脏器损伤、腹膜后损伤和邻近的脊髓损伤敏感性和特异性较好。

◦ 可以帮助实质脏器损伤处置，包括可能的观察及介入影像学操作。

- 缺点：

◦ 患者暴露于辐射和造影剂。

◦ 孤立的膈肌损伤、胰腺损伤、肠管损伤可能被遗漏，特别是刚受伤就实施 CT 检查的患者。

- 检查指征：
  ◦ 血流动力学稳定的患者。
- 禁忌证：
  ◦ 已经存在剖腹探查指征者；血流动力学不稳定；之前出现过造影剂反应。
- 建议：
  ◦ 许多机构对于多发创伤患者实施"pan-scan"的套餐检查，包括头、颈椎、胸部和腹部/骨盆的CT扫描套餐，这是有争议的，他们可能发现隐秘的损伤，而这些损伤可能是无关紧要的。
  ◦ 静脉注射造影剂对于腹部创伤患者已经足够。口服和直肠内造影剂并不需要。
  ◦ 血管造影：
    ▪ 不稳定的患者和骨盆骨折。
    ▪ 这种操作能够阻断来自骨盆、脾脏等部位的血管。

诊断步骤/外科

• 诊断性腹腔灌洗：很大程度上被FAST和CT取代，但在特定情形中还是有用的。
- 步骤：
  ◦ 首先，尝试吸取游离腹腔内血液。>10 ml的血液指示腹内损伤。
  ◦ 接着，若抽不出血液，通过向腹膜内打入液体的方法进行灌洗，然后回抽分析。
- 优点：
  ◦ 若在严重损伤的患者通过FAST评估后发现腹内创伤是低血压的原因，可以快速识别此类情况。
  ◦ 其他检查受限制时有时可以能够帮助检测肠系膜和空腔脏器损伤。
  ◦ 操作相关并发症概率低。
- 缺点：
  ◦ 有创1%～2%的并发症发生率。
  ◦ 不能识别具体的受损器官。
  ◦ 假阳性和假阴性可能因为技术失败而出现。
  ◦ 腹膜后出血敏感，在稳定患者可能导致不必要的开腹探查。
- 禁忌证：
  ◦ 绝对禁忌证：已经存在剖腹探查指征的患者。
  ◦ 相对禁忌证：既往腹部手术病史、严重腹部膨隆、妊娠中晚期患者。
- 建议：
  ◦ 开始这项操作前先插好导尿管和鼻胃管。
- 阳性检查：
  ◦ 吸引出超过10 ml的血液、胆汁、肠内容物或尿液。
  ◦ 诊断性腹腔穿刺的液体在尿液或者胸管中。
  ◦ 钝性创伤患者，诊断性腹腔灌洗液常规检测大于100 000红细胞/mm³。
  ◦ 贯穿性创伤患者，诊断性腹腔灌洗液常规检测大于1 000红细胞/mm³。

• 原位伤探查：可以决定刀刺伤探查深度，若伤口在腹腔表面，且患者其他条件适宜，可以安全回家。否则进一步诊断。

儿科注意事项

儿童腹部创伤诊断同成人。

妊娠注意事项

• 常规思路：
- 优先稳定母亲的情况，若母亲死亡会导致胎儿死亡。
- 孕周>20(触诊宫底位于脐上)，保持孕妇左侧30°卧位以改善灌注。
- 不孕症的患者要继续妊娠：不稳定患者行FAST评分决定是否急诊剖腹产，稳定患者是否需要CT检查。
- 评估创伤患者的所有必需的放射性检查射线剂量要低于婴儿致畸剂量。
- 当诊断的获益大于对胎儿的损伤时，推荐静脉造影检查。
- 因为MRI检查时间长，MRI很少用于创伤患者的紧急评估。
- 在首次评估母亲和胎儿情况均稳定后，可存活的胎儿(>24周)应该行持续4 h的心动图观察确保无胎盘剥离。
- 胎盘剥离发生于无弹性的胎盘从有弹性的子宫剥离时，超声和CT可帮助诊断但不够敏感，因此择机行胎儿监护。

鉴别诊断

参见腹部钝性创伤和腹部穿透性创伤。

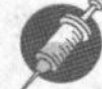

治疗

院前

所有存在严重受伤机制或怀疑存在严重创伤的患者应该被分诊到指定的创伤中心(最好是一级创伤中心)。

初步稳定/治疗

• 不稳定的患者，必须优先处置气道、呼吸、低血容量性休克液体复苏稳定循环及快速的控制大出血。

• 参见腹部钝性创伤和腹部贯穿伤。

急诊治疗/程序

• 参见腹部钝性创伤和腹部贯穿伤。

• 严重的腹部损伤通常都需要静脉输注晶体液。

• 双腔深静脉导管应该被留置好。

• 血流动力学不稳定的所有腹部创伤患者均有指征输血。Rh阴性的O型血或者Rh阳性的O型血可以被用于育龄期年龄之外的所有男女患者。

• 血流动力学不稳定存在神志意识状态改变及不能保护气道的创伤患者，在转运至手术室之前通常需要先行气管插管。

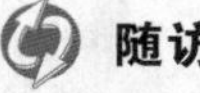

随访

进一步处理

入院指征

• 所有的不稳定创伤患者都需要住院治疗，而且其中大部分需要外科干预。

• 大多数的多系统创伤患者同时存在腹部创伤将需要住院治疗。

• 妊娠大于24周需要收住院进行胎儿-母亲监护。

• 稳定的患者分为以下3种类型。
- 腹部枪击伤：几乎所有患者都将需要住院。由于存在很大可能的器官损伤，这类患者进行外科探查的概率非常高。
- 腹部穿刺伤：筋膜穿透的患者需要住院治疗。超声、CT或者体格检查将有助于决定哪些患者需要手术处置。
- 腹部钝性创伤：超声、CT或检查决定哪些患者需要住院治疗。

出院指征

• 急诊室内血流动力学稳定的患者，各项检查均为阴性并且随访检查可靠的，可以考虑出院。

• 无法自行回到医院或者由于症状恶化联系120急救的患者必须考虑收住院治疗。

随访建议

少量出院的患者中可能存在未诊断的损伤(最常见的是肠道和胰腺损伤)。患者出院时必须被告知一旦恶化的腹痛、腹胀、呕吐或直肠出血，必须返回急诊室。

要点和误区

• 不稳定创伤患者，早期快速FAST试验有助于明确是否需要急诊开腹治疗。

• 稳定的创伤患者，CT是检查损伤并指导治疗的有效选择。

• CT结果阴性的患者，考虑膈膜、肠、胰腺和肠系膜损伤。

F

• 考虑行连续的超声检查。这对于存在血流动力学状态或者体格检查有异常的患者尤其重要。

• 许多稳定的成人和儿童创伤患者目前可以根据 CT 扫描的结果而通过非手术的方式处置。

• CT 套餐检查降低了漏诊的概率，但使患者暴露于射线、造影剂和增加的下游试验。

• 由于超声和 CT 的增加使用，诊断性腹腔灌洗和局部伤口探查在腹部创伤中应用减少。

• 误区：

- CT 阴性的患者仍可有临床重要的损伤。

- 让妊娠大于 24 周者回家而没有进行胎儿-母亲监护。

腹部钝性创伤

Abdominal Trauma, Blunt

Frances E. Rudolf · Allyson A. Kreshak 马林浩 林兆奋 译

基础知识

描述

• 受伤是由于腹部遭受突然增加的压力造成的。

• 实质脏器受损通常表现为出血。

• 空腔脏器受损导致出血和肠腔内容物污染可引起腹膜炎。

病因

• 机动车碰撞是最常见的受伤原因。

• 实质脏器较空腔脏器更容易受损伤。

• 脾脏是最常见的受损脏器（25%），其次为肝脏（15%）、肠道（15%）、腹膜后结构（13%）及肾脏（12%）。

• 不太常见的损伤包括肠系膜、胰腺、膈肌、膀胱、尿道和血管性结构。

儿科注意事项

• 小儿可能因为血容量少而快速丢失大量腹腔内血液。

• 由于胸廓容积较小脾脏和肝脏部分位于肋骨保护范围以外而更容易受伤。

• 若不能及时识别，小儿腹部创伤致死率很高。

诊断

症状和体征

• 症状与体征包括腹痛、腹膜刺激征及低血容量性休克。

• 恶心或呕吐。

• 膈肌受累或者上腹部损伤会使得呼吸费力。

• 左肩部吸气时疼痛（克尔征 Kehr 征）是由于出血刺激膈肌所致。

• 症状出现延迟可能与小肠损伤有关。

• 联合损伤（骨折，腹壁损伤）可能类似腹部损伤。

• 缺损或瘀斑可能预示着腹内损伤。

- 安全带样擦伤可能指示明显的腹内损伤。

- 胁和脐周瘀伤可能代表腹膜后出血（后期发现）。

• 腹膜后出血肠鸣音可能消失。

基本检查

• 评估并确保通畅气道、呼吸运动及循环状态。

• 初始评估应着眼于是否需要手术干预。

• 腹部检查来发现是否存在腹腔内出血或腹膜刺激征。

• 腹膜后和胸腔内的损伤很难通过触诊评估。

• 记住腹腔的概念包括靠上的膈肌（乳头与肩甲角连线）与髂前上棘围成的区域。

• 磨损和瘀斑可能是腹腔内损伤的征象：

- 把患者翻过来看看背后的情况。

- 安全腰带处的磨损可能是腹腔内损伤的重要指征。

• 由于腹膜刺激肠鸣音可能消失（晚期发现）。

•（如果尿道口没有血液、没有会阴部血肿、前列腺检查正常的话）留置导尿管获取尿液并记录尿量。

• 骨盆 X 线平片：

- 骨盆骨折和肉眼血尿可能提示泌尿生殖系统损伤。

- 通过逆行尿道膀胱造影、膀胱 X 线片及静脉肾盂造影来进一步检查这些结构。

• CT 对于是否需要手术干预的评估非常有必要并且可以评估腹膜后空间和实质脏器。

- 患者必须足够稳定可以接受 CT 检查。

- 对于怀疑的肾损伤也有帮助。

• 针对创伤的超声快速评估（FAST）检查是否存在腹腔积液。

- 超声快速无需造影剂并且无创。

- 对于操作者有一定要求。

诊断检查与说明

实验室检查

• 血红蛋白/血细胞比容：由于等容量性的血液丢失最初可能是正常的。

• 检查凝血标志物（血小板、凝血素和部分凝血酶原时间）。抗凝的效应在实验室检查可能无法准确评估。

• 血型检测与配型是必需的。对于不稳定的患者准备交叉配血红细胞悬液。

• 尿液分析。

- 存在休克的患者出现镜下血尿是进行泌尿生殖系统评估的指征。

• 孕龄期妇女要做妊娠试验。

• 动脉血气分析。

- 碱剩余缺乏可能提示低血容量性休克并且有助于指导液体复苏。

• 乙醇浓度。

影像学检查

参见基本检查。

诊断步骤/外科

参见基本检查。

鉴别诊断

• 下胸腔的损伤能够导致腹痛。

• 骨折（肋骨、骨盆）可能导致腹痛。

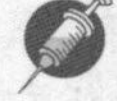

治疗

院前

• 滴定液体复苏至有临床反应。目标收缩期血压为 90～100 mmHg。

• 正常的生命体征并不能排除严重的腹腔内损伤病变。

初步稳定/治疗

• 确保气道通畅。

- 如果需要的话进行气管插管。

- 氧气面罩接100%氧气。
- 双腔深静脉通路进行晶体液输注。
- 输注2L晶体液后无反应则需要开始输注红细胞悬液。
- 如果患者处于严重休克状态可以考虑立即输注Rh阴性的O型血。
- 出血患者考虑TXA。
- 无法控制的休克，发现腹膜后出血，腹膜炎体征或观察期间临床症状加重建议经验丰富的外科医师剖腹探查行手术干预。

急诊治疗/程序

- 继续之前的稳定治疗措施。
- 鼻胃管排空胃部减少胃膨胀并降低误吸风险。
- 如果是膈疝导致的呼吸窘迫上述措施可以减轻症状。

药物治疗

- 破伤风类毒素增强剂：对于存在开放性损伤的患者0.5ml肌内注射。
- 破伤风免疫球蛋白：没有接受完整破伤风类毒素治疗的患者250U肌内注射。
- 临床指示明确时纠正凝血。
- 需要时使用镇痛药，因为出血风险，避免非甾体抗炎药。
- 静脉使用抗生素：使用类似于第二代头孢菌素覆盖广谱的需氧菌和厌氧菌。

儿科注意事项

- 患儿存在休克给予20ml/kg晶体液复苏。
- 红细胞悬液的剂量为1ml/kg。

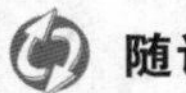

随访

进一步处理

入院指征

- 术后患者。
- 诊断性腹腔灌洗、超声检查及CT检查结果不明确的患者。

出院指征

- 患者有孤立的腹部钝伤并且临床情况稳定，腹部CT检查阴性(静脉造影增强)可以考虑安全出院。
- 怀疑腹部创伤的患者都不应该出院。

要点和误区

- 如果患者存在明显的休克即使血细胞比容正常也不要延迟使用血制品的时间。
- 所有育龄妇女都需要做妊娠试验。
- 不稳定的患者不要送去做CT影像学诊断检查。
- 考虑使用抗凝药物。

腹腔积液 Ascites

Paul J. Allegretti · Keri Robertson 祝青藤 王海嵘 潘曙明 译

F

基础知识

描述

- 腹膜腔病理性的浆液聚集。
- 门静脉高压(>12mmHg)液体潴留。
- 严重的钠水潴留。
- 潴留的水钠增加了血浆容量。
- 水排出受损。
- 抗利尿激素(ADH)的释放量增加。
- 尿钠潴留，体内钠总量增加，稀释性低钠血症。
- 低钠血症的程度是与疾病的严重度相关的预后因素。
- 低白蛋白血症导致血浆胶体渗透压下降。
- 感染、炎症、肿瘤可引起腹膜刺激征。

病因

- 肝实质疾病：
  - 肝硬化和酒精性肝炎：
    - 占到80%的成人患者。
  - 暴发性肝功能衰竭。
- 肝充血：
  - 充血性心力衰竭。
  - 缩窄性心包炎。
  - 静脉闭塞性疾病和布加综合征。
- 恶性肿瘤：
  - 腹膜转移癌。
  - 肝细胞癌或者癌细胞转移性疾病。
- 传染病：
  - 结核性、真菌性、细菌性腹膜炎。
- 低白蛋白血症：
  - 肾病综合征。
  - 营养不良，白蛋白<2.0g/dl。
- 其他情况：
  - 胰源性腹水。
  - 胆源性腹水。
  - 肾源性腹水。
  - 卵巢肿瘤。
  - 淋巴管渗漏所致的乳糜性腹水。
  - 结缔组织疾病。
  - 黏液性水肿。
  - 肉芽肿性腹膜炎。

儿科注意事项

很多儿科病例归因于：

- 恶性肿瘤(伯基特淋巴瘤、横纹肌肉瘤)。
- 肾病综合征。
- 营养不良。

诊断

症状和体征

- 腹胀不适。
- 体重增加；有时候体重减轻。
- 呼吸困难。
- 端坐呼吸。
- 水肿。
- 腹疝。
- 肌肉萎缩。
- 移动性浊音，侧腹饱满，液体波动，凹陷性水肿。
- 基础疾病的症状和体征。
- 慢性肝病的皮肤红斑。

病史

- 肝疾病的危险因素。
- 起始症状的描述。
  - 腹腔积液与肥胖症的鉴别。
  - 患者不能忍受的腹腔积液的迅速进展。
- 明确的肝硬化患者出现新发腹腔积液可能意味着下列情况之一：
  - 进展性肝脏疾病。
  - 叠加其他急性肝损伤(酒精性、病毒性

肝炎)。
- 肝细胞癌。

体格检查

• 肥胖患者检查困难。
• 侧腹饱满是一项典型的检查发现：
- 侧翻饱满约有 500 ml 腹腔积液。
- 液体波动。
- 移动性浊音。

基本检查

• 寻找肝疾病、充血性心力衰竭、结核病、恶性肿瘤及其他系统功能紊乱。
• 腹腔穿刺术：
- 对于下列情况是必需的：
◦ 新发的腹腔积液。
◦ 进展性脑病。
◦ 发热。
◦ 腹部疼痛/压痛。
• 确定是否有腹腔积液的感染及门静脉高压的存在。
• 腹腔积液的检测：
- 细胞计数及分类。
◦ 在快速诊断腹腔积液是否感染时很有帮助。
◦ 标本的顺序。
- 白蛋白。
- 总蛋白。
- 革兰染色。
- 10 ml 腹腔积液注入血培养瓶中，培养 2 次。
- 乳酸脱氢酶(LDH)。
- 葡萄糖。
- 结核培养。
- 淀粉酶。
- 甘油三酯(三酰甘油)。
- 细胞学检查。
- 胆红素。
- 癌胚抗原。
• 自发性细菌性腹膜炎(SBP)：
- 腹腔积液的感染无腹部手术治疗史。
- 发热，腹部疼痛/压痛，意识状态的变化。
- 多形核中性粒细胞>250/mm^3。
- 腹腔积液蛋白含量<1 g/dl。
- 低浓度的调理素。
• 继发性细菌性腹膜炎：
- 细菌性腹膜炎来源于腹部外科手术。
- 肠穿孔或腹腔脓肿(例如，肾周脓肿)。
- 继发性腹膜炎多形核中性粒细胞>250/mm^3，伴随革兰染色多种微生物感染。
◦ 总蛋白>1 g/dl。
◦ 葡萄糖<50 mg/dl。
◦ 血清乳酸脱氢酶>正常值上限。

诊断检查与说明

实验室检查

• 全血细胞计数。
• 基本生化检查。
• 肝功能检查。
• PT、APTT、INR。
• 动脉血气分析或氧饱和度检查。
• 尿液检测。
• 尿钠检测。
• 肝炎病毒检测。
• 淀粉酶/脂肪酶检测。
• 甲胎蛋白。
• 促甲状腺激素。

影像学检查

• 超声。
- 确诊腹腔积液，尤其是<500 ml。
- 评估肝、胰腺、脾，以及卵巢。
- 指导腹腔穿刺术。
• 多普勒超声检查：评估肝血流量。
• CT 扫描。
• 胸部 X 线检查：充血性心力衰竭、胸腔积液、空洞、肿块。
• 心电图。

诊断步骤/外科

• 腹腔镜检查：不明原因腹腔积液，尤其是结核。
• 腹腔穿刺。
- 无腹腔穿刺的自发性细菌性腹膜炎临床诊断是不充分的。
- 关于腹腔穿刺术的安全性：
◦ 70%的腹腔积液患者有凝血功能障碍。
◦ 诊断性的腹腔穿刺获益大于风险。
◦ 腹腔穿刺术仍然是可控制的，除非出现 DIC。
◦ 不推荐在腹腔穿刺术之前输注血浆或血小板。

鉴别诊断

• 常见的腹部膨胀原因(5F)：
- 腹腔积液(包括系统性的)。
- 肥胖。
- 胃肠胀气。
- 妊娠。
- 胃肠型。
- 其他：器官巨大症。
• 血清-腹水白蛋白梯度＝血清白蛋白—腹水白蛋白：
- 在腹水的鉴别诊断中取代了腹水总蛋白的检测。
- SAAG 的数值≥1.1 g/dl。
◦ 预测门静脉高压的精确性达 97%。
◦ 肝硬化。
◦ 酒精性肝炎。
◦ 心功能不全。
◦ 肝转移。
◦ 暴发性肝衰竭。
◦ 门静脉血栓。
◦ 静脉闭塞性疾病。
◦ 黏液性水肿。
◦ 布加综合征。
◦ 妊娠期脂肪肝。
◦ 自发性细菌性腹膜炎。
- SAAG 的数值<1.1 g/dl。
◦ 腹膜转移癌。
◦ 结核。
◦ 胰腺源性腹腔积液。
◦ 肾病综合征。
◦ 肠梗阻或梗死形成。
◦ 血管炎。
◦ 术后淋巴管渗漏。

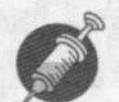

治疗

院前

有症状的血压过低：
• 开放气道，保持气道通畅，维持有效循环容量，生理盐水静脉滴注。

初步稳定/治疗

评估突然增加的腹围、疼痛，以及发热等需要紧急处理的并发因素，可能的并发因素如下。
• 感染。
• 肝癌。
• 胆道梗阻。
• 肝功能失代偿。

急诊治疗/程序

• 成功的治疗有赖于病因的准确诊断。
• 病因治疗。
• 在没有影响到有效血容量的情况下尽量减少腹腔积液和外周水肿。
• 并发症的早期发现是必要的。
- 自发性细菌性腹膜炎。
◦ 高度怀疑(的患者)。
◦ 降低腹腔穿刺的门槛。
◦ 及时治疗。
- 张力性腹腔积液和胸腔积液。

◦ 对症，吸氧。
◦ 呼吸困难的患者需要治疗性行胸腹腔积液穿刺术。
- 腹壁疝。
◦ 当心嵌顿、坏死及破裂。
◦ 治疗性穿刺术。
◦ 外科会诊。
- 穿刺点的持续性渗漏：
◦ 除去更多的液体。
◦ 小孔的屏障装置。
- 感觉异常性股痛。
◦ 由于压迫了侧面的股神经。
◦ 通过腹腔穿刺或利尿缓解压迫。
- 大量腹腔积液穿刺。
- 5～10 L(100 ml/kg)。
- 在保证循环稳定的前提下安全执行穿刺有效的腹腔积液量。
- 如果抽取液体量＞5 L，静脉滴注白蛋白(5～10 g/L液体移除)。
- 出院前监测患者8 h。
• 减少腹腔积液的非穿刺措施。
- 限盐。
◦ 小于2 g/d。
◦ 如果血钠小于120～125 mmol/L，限制水的摄入。
- 螺内酯。
◦ 尤其适用于肝硬化腹水。
◦ 替代选择：阿米洛利或氨苯蝶啶。
- 呋塞米。
◦ 尤其适用于其他原因所导致的腹水。
◦ 在肝硬化患者中与螺内酯联合用药，螺内酯/呋塞米比例为100 mg/40 mg。
◦ 对于反应差的患者增加甲苯喹唑磺胺。
- 利尿剂的使用原则：
◦ 执行利尿剂早晨单剂量法。
◦ 获取尿钠数值评估治疗效果。
◦ 当患者的尿钠数值＞10 mmol/L 时效果满意。
◦ 不存在水肿的患者利尿剂导致的体重下降不应超过2 lb/d(1 lb＝0.45 kg)，有水肿的患者不超过5 lb/d。
◦ 监测电解质和肾功能。
◦ 避免低血钾，因为低血钾会增加肾氨生成，血氨升高会诱发肝性脑病。
- 难治性腹腔积液：
◦ 比例约为腹水患者的10%。
◦ 确保患者对饮食及药物的依从性。
◦ 外科腹腔静脉分流术和门体静脉转流术治疗。
◦ 肝移植。
- 避免NSAID类药物的使用，因为该药可引起以下问题。
◦ 降低利尿剂的反应。
◦ 减少肾血浆流量和GFR。
◦ 引起钠潴留，减少尿钠排出。
- 治疗腹腔积液的根本病因，除肝硬化以外的情况。
◦ 结核、心力衰竭。

药物治疗

一线用药

• 白蛋白：腹水的排泄5～10 g/L，如果＞5 L使用。
• 头孢噻肟：2 g静脉滴注，q8 h。
• 螺内酯：100～400 mg/d(儿童：1～6 mg/kg)，口服，分为2次给药/日。
• 呋塞米：40～160 mg/d(儿童：1～3 mg/kg)，口服。

二线用药

• 阿米洛利：5～20 mg/d，口服。
• 甲苯喹唑磺胺：5 mg/d。
• 氨苯蝶啶：100～300 mg/d，口服，分为2次给药/日。

随访

进一步处理

入院指征

• 暴发性肝衰竭。
• 肝性脑病。
• 自发性细菌性腹膜炎。
• 肝肾综合征。
• 消化道出血。
• 对急诊处理无反应的张力性腹腔积液。

出院指征

对急诊处理有反应的患者。

随访建议

• 所有新增病例的专科检查。
• 社区医师或专科医师随访确诊病例。

要点和误区

• 新病例需要全面检查和专科咨询处理。
• 自发性细菌性腹膜炎的症状常不明显。
• 高度怀疑的自发性细菌性腹膜炎，必须降低腹腔穿刺术的门槛。
• 对于有凝血功能障碍的患者来说，为明确自发性细菌性腹膜炎而进行的腹腔穿刺术检查获益远大于出血风险。
• 在少量腹腔积液穿刺时，超声的指导是有帮助的。

腹痛 Abdominal Pain

Saleh Fares 马林浩 林兆奋 译

基础知识

描述

• 最常见的急诊就诊原因。
• 有很多病因，包括多种威胁生命的病因。
• 各种原因导致诊断困难，需要系统性考虑。
• 腹膜疼痛。
- 刺激性物质导致腹膜疼痛。
- 疼痛通过体神经传导。
- 腹膜张力的改变会加重疼痛。
- 疼痛是锐利感的，能够很好地被腹部的反跳痛和肌卫定位。
• 内脏痛。
- 疼痛的传入冲动是基于内脏胚胎学起源而不是真实器官的位置，从而导致疼痛定位的不准确。
◦ 前肠结构的疼痛位于上腹部。
◦ 从中肠结构来源的疼痛位于脐周部。
◦ 从后肠结构来源的疼痛位于耻骨上区域。
- 空腔或实质脏器包膜膨胀或肠肌纤维痉挛。
◦ 疼痛是持续性而剧烈的。
- 炎症。
◦ 一旦炎症累及腹膜会引起局灶性压痛。
- 血管急症引起的缺血。
◦ 疼痛是严重而弥漫性的。

• 牵扯痛。
- 病变脏器导致远隔部位的疼痛。
- 是由于被影响到的神经段重叠支配所致。
• 腹壁疼痛。
- 持续性的肌肉痉挛引起疼痛。
- 会影响到其他肌肉群。

■ **病因**

• 腹膜刺激物质。
- 胃液、粪便、异物、血液、胆汁、胰酶。
• 内脏梗阻。
- 小肠和大肠、胆囊、输尿管和肾脏、内脏缺血(小肠、肾脏和脾脏)。
• 内脏炎症。
- 阑尾炎、炎症性肠病、胆囊炎、肝炎、消化性溃疡、胰腺炎、盆腔炎性疾病、肾盂肾炎。
• 腹壁疼痛。
• 牵扯痛(如胸腔内疾病)。

诊断

■ **症状和体征**

病史

• 疼痛。
- 疼痛发作的性质。
- 疼痛发作的时间点与持续时间。
- 疼痛发作时的位置及目前的位置。
- 腹部以外的放射痛。
- 疼痛的剧烈程度(锐利痛、钝痛、痉挛痛)。
- 加重或者减轻的影响因素。
- 疼痛发作时的伴随症状。
- 之前的发作史。
• 厌食。
• 恶心。
• 呕吐(胆汁、咖啡色液体)。
• 全身乏力不适。
• 昏厥或者晕厥。
• 粪便性状改变(如黑便)。
• 血尿。
• 排便及排尿习惯改变。
• 创伤或内脏梗阻病史。
• 妇产科相关病史。
• 围手术期(如导致肠梗阻)。
• 家族史(如家族性主动脉动脉瘤)。
• 饮酒史与饮酒量。
• 用药史(如阿司匹林和非甾体抗炎药)。

体格检查

• 全身:
- 厌食。
- 心动过速。
- 呼吸急促。
- 低血压。
- 发热。
- 巩膜黄染(黄疸)。
- 远端脉搏和上下肢的脉压。
• 腹部:
- 瘢痕。
- 腹膨隆。
- 异常肠鸣音。
  ◦ 高调肠鸣音提示肠梗阻。
  ◦ 肠鸣音消失提示腹膜炎或麻痹性肠梗阻。
- 腹部波动性包块。
- 反跳痛、肌卫及咳嗽测试腹膜刺激征(如阑尾炎、腹膜炎)。
- 结肠充气试验,提示阑尾炎。
  ◦ 左下腹触诊导致右下腹疼痛。
- 腰大肌征提示阑尾炎(右侧)。
  ◦ 大腿伸展引发疼痛。
- 闭孔试验提示盆腔内阑尾炎(仅仅在右侧)。
  ◦ 大腿旋转,尤其内旋时引发疼痛。
- 麦氏点压痛与阑尾炎相关。
  ◦ 右侧髂前上棘与脐连线中外 2/3 交界处触诊导致疼痛。
- 墨菲征提示胆囊炎。
  ◦ 检查者胆囊点触诊时引发吸气时暂停。
- 腹壁触痛征(Carnett 征)提示腹壁疼痛。
  ◦ 患者仰卧位时抬头和肩膀收缩腹壁引起疼痛。
- 疝气部位触痛或者颜色改变。
- 直肠和盆腔检查。
  ◦ 盆腔腹膜刺激引起压痛。
  ◦ 宫颈抬举痛。
  ◦ 附件肿块。
  ◦ 直肠肿块或压痛。
  ◦ 大便隐血试验。
• 泌尿生殖系统。
- 胁腹痛。
- 排尿困难。
- 肋椎角压痛。
- 耻骨上压痛。
- 骨盆附件触痛。
- 睾丸痛。
  ◦ 可能是由于肾脏或阑尾疾病所致。
• 牵扯痛。
- 克尔征(Kehr 征)由于血液或其他刺激性物质引起膈肌刺激造成肩痛。
• 肢体。
- 脉搏缺失或者不对等的股动脉搏动。
• 皮肤。
- 黄疸。
- 肝病(脐周静脉曲张)。
- 出血。
  ◦ 格雷-特纳征(Grey-Turner 征)胁肋部位的出血征。
  ◦ 库伦征(Cullen 征)是脐周部位的出血。
- 带状疱疹。
- 蜂窝织炎。
- 皮疹[亨氏紫癜(HSP)]。

■ **基本检查**

• 妊娠期妇女腹痛就诊时必须要做妊娠试验。
• 超声可以诊断大多数的腹痛病因,超声检查阴性或者不确定者,需要做腹部 CT。

■ **诊断检查与说明**

实验室检查

• 全血细胞计数。
• 血电解质、肌酐和血糖。
• 红细胞沉降率。
• 肝功能检测。
• 乳酸。
• 血脂肪酶检测。
- 敏感性和特异性均优于血淀粉酶。
• 尿液分析。
• 粪便检测(隐血试验)和培养。
• 妊娠试验(育龄妇女)。

影像学检查

• 心电图。
- 存在冠心病危险因素的患者需要考虑。
• 腹部立卧位 X 线摄片。
- 怀疑内脏穿孔或肠梗阻者,CT 检查优于 X 线平片。
• 立位胸部 X 线检查。
- 气腹。
- 胸腔内疾病导致腹部疼痛。
• 超声。
- 胆道异常。
- 肾盂积水。
- 腹腔积液。
- 主动脉瘤。
- 肠套叠。
• US(多普勒超声)。
- 扭转和旋转不良。
- 睾丸和卵巢扭转。
- 肝炎、肝硬化和门静脉血栓形成。
• 腹部 CT 扫描。
- 螺旋 CT 平扫。
  ◦ 肾绞痛。

F

- ◦ 腹膜后出血。
- 仅经静脉造影剂增强 CT 扫描。
  - ◦ 稳定的患者怀疑血管破裂(如急性腹主动脉瘤、主动脉夹层)。
  - ◦ 缺血性肠病。
  - ◦ 胰腺炎。
- 静脉和口服造影 CT 扫描。
  - ◦ 炎症性肠病史。
  - ◦ 消瘦的患者(体质指数低)。
  - ◦ 憩室炎。
- CT 血管造影。
  - ◦ 肠系膜血栓。
  - ◦ 腹主动脉瘤。
- • 静脉尿路造影(IVP)。
  - 对于泌尿系结石,CT 检查已经取代静脉尿路造影。
- • 钡剂灌肠。
  - 肠套叠。
  - 治疗和确认肠套叠是由于空气灌肠所致。
- • 磁共振。
  - 考虑放射线暴露或者肾毒性(造影剂)。
  - 有金属植入物的患者存在磁共振的检查禁忌。

妊娠注意事项

超声和磁共振优先考虑以预防对于胎儿电离放射的暴露。

■ 鉴别诊断

- 急性腹主动脉瘤(AAA)。
- 腹型癫痫或者腹型偏头痛。
- 特发性食管破裂综合征。
- 肾上腺危象。
- 早期阑尾炎。
- 肠梗阻。
- 胆囊炎。
- 便秘±粪便嵌顿。
- 糖尿病酮症酸中毒。
- 憩室炎。
- 痛经。
- 异位妊娠。
- 食管炎。
- 子宫内膜异位症。
- 菲-休-柯三氏综合征。
- 胃肠炎。
- 肝炎。
- 嵌顿性疝。
- 感染性胃肠炎。
- 炎症性肠病。
- 肠易激综合征。
- 缺血性肠病。
- 梅克尔憩室。
- 肿瘤。
- 卵巢扭转。
- 卵巢囊肿(出血)。
- 胰腺炎。
- 盆腔炎性疾病。
- 消化性溃疡疾病。
- 泌尿系统结石。
- 肾梗死。
- 镰状红细胞危象。
- 蜘蛛(黑寡妇)咬伤。
- 脾梗死。
- 自然流产。
- 睾丸扭转。
- 输卵管卵巢脓肿。
- 泌尿道感染。
- 肠扭转。
- 牵扯痛。
  - 心肌梗死。
  - 肺炎。
- 腹壁痛。
  - 腹壁血肿或者感染。
  - 黑寡妇蜘蛛咬伤。
  - 带状疱疹。

儿科注意事项

- 2 岁以下患儿。
  - 先天性巨结肠。
  - 嵌顿性疝。
  - 肠套叠。
  - 肠扭转。
  - 吞食异物。
- 2～5 岁患儿。
  - 阑尾炎。
  - 嵌顿性疝。
  - 梅克尔憩室炎。
  - 镰状红细胞危象。
  - 亨氏紫癜(HSP)。
  - 便秘。

治疗

■ 急诊治疗/程序

- 鼻胃管减压和肠道休息。
- 静脉补液与纠正电解质异常。
- 止吐药膳是重要的舒适治疗。
- 麻醉药物与镇痛药不应被一律拒绝。
- 不稳定的患者送血型检测与交叉配血。
- 怀疑外科病因时及时请外科会诊。

■ 药物治疗

- 芬太尼：1～2 μg/kg,静脉注射,qh。
- 硫酸吗啡：0.1 mg/kg,静脉注射,q4 h,根据需要给药。
- 昂丹司琼：4 mg,静脉注射。
- 丙氯拉嗪：0.13 mg/kg,静脉注射、口服或肌内注射,q6 h,根据恶心症状的需要给药;成人剂量为 25 mg, q6 h。
- 异丙嗪：25～50 mg/kg,肌内注射、口服或灌肠。

随访

■ 进一步处理

入院指征

- 外科干预。
- 腹膜炎体征。
- 患者不稳定无法撤除液体。
- 疼痛控制不佳。
- 特殊病情(心肌梗死、糖尿病酮症酸中毒)需要住院治疗。
- 需要静脉使用抗生素。

出院指征

没有发现外科情况或者严重病因,患者病情稳定并能撤除液体,疼痛控制疗效好,并且能够遵从出院细节说明。

■ 随访建议

患者出现下列任一警示情况均需返回医院：

- 呕吐。
- 呕血、呕吐咖啡色液体,或者黑便。
- 皮肤或者巩膜黄染。
- 8～12 h 疼痛无改善,或者出现加重。
- 寒战,或者发热体温>38℃。

要点和误区

- 无法询问复杂病史及体格检查。
- 老年患者更容易出现不典型症状以及危及生命的病因而需要住院治疗。
- 如果直肠穹窿内没有粪便不要考虑便秘。
- 呕吐先于疼痛发作出现时,一般不存在需要外科干预的病因。
- 不要过度依赖实验室检查。

腹泻(成人)

Isam F. Nasr　谭美春 译

基础知识

描述

由于感染或中毒使排便表现为频繁(>3次/日)、松散和水样便。

病因

- 病毒：
- 占所有病例的 50%～70%。
- 侵袭性细菌：
- 空肠弯曲菌：
- 污染的食物或水、荒野水、鸟、动物。
- 最常见的细菌性腹泻。
- 60%～90%的患者可出现便血或粪隐血。
- 沙门菌：
- 污染的水、蛋、禽或奶制品。
- 伤寒(伤寒杆菌)，其特征为稽留热、腹痛、玫瑰疹、脾大和心动过缓。
- 志贺菌：
- 粪或口途径。
- 副溶血性弧菌：
- 生的和未熟透的海产品。
- 耶尔森菌：
- 受污染的食品(猪肉)、水和牛奶。
- 可表现为肠系膜淋巴结炎或拟阑尾炎。
- 细菌毒素：
- 大肠杆菌：
- 主要导致旅行者腹泻。
- 摄入被粪便污染过的食物和水。
- 金黄色葡萄球菌：
- 最常见的毒素相关疾病。
- 摄取食物后 1～6 h 出现症状。
- 蜡样芽孢杆菌：
- 经典传染源，留在蒸汽保温锅中的炒饭。
- 症状在 1～36 h 出现。
- 难辨梭状芽孢杆菌：
- 抗生素相关性肠炎与假膜性肠炎存在关联。
- 暴露后潜伏期在 10 日之内，或由使用抗生素引发。
- 嗜水气单胞菌：
- 水产品为主要来源。
- 影响 3 岁以下儿童。
- 粪便中无白细胞。
- 霍乱：
- 由霍乱弧菌产生的肠毒素引起。
- 大量水样便伴黏液(典型表现为淘米水样便)。
- 病原虫：
- 贾第鞭毛虫：
- 北美最常见的寄生虫胃肠炎病因。
- 高危人群：旅行者、托儿所中的儿童、收容所中的人、男性同性恋者、饮用未经处理山泉水的野外露营者。
- 小隐孢子虫：
- 通常在发生于艾滋病患者。
- 溶组织内阿米巴(内阿米巴病)：
- 5%～10%肠外表现(阿米巴性肝脓肿)。

儿科注意事项

- 大多数来源于病毒感染，有自限性。
- 轮状病毒占 50%。
- 志贺菌：感染伴有癫痫。
- 重点评估脱水情况。

诊断

症状和体征

病史

- 松散，水样大便。
- 血便带黏液。
- 腹痛和痉挛，里急后重，胀气。
- 发热，头痛，肌痛。
- 恶心，呕吐。
- 脱水，嗜睡，昏迷。

体格检查

- 黏膜干燥。
- 腹部压痛。
- 肛周炎，肛裂，肛瘘。

基本检查

- 直肠指检，以确定是否存在血便或潜血。
- 粪白细胞测定：
- 存在致病性细菌。
- 无法检测出原虫感染、病毒、毒素引起的食物中毒。

诊断检查与说明

实验室检查

- 全血细胞计数，适应证：
- 显著失血。
- 全身中毒。
- 电解质、血糖、尿素氮、肌酐，适应证：
- 嗜睡、显著脱水、中毒或精神状态改变。
- 使用利尿剂、持续性腹泻、慢性肝病或肾病。
- 粪便培养，适应证：
- 粪便中检出白细胞。
- 标志性病史：免疫力低下、旅游、同性恋。
- 公共卫生：食品处理、托儿所、保健工作者、收容所。
- 血培养，适应证：
- 怀疑菌血症或全身性感染。
- 需要住院的患者。
- 免疫力低下。
- 老年患者和婴幼儿。

影像学检查

腹部 X 线片：

- 没有价值，除非怀疑梗阻或中毒性巨结肠。

鉴别诊断

- 溃疡性结肠炎。
- 克罗恩病。
- 肠系膜缺血。
- 憩室炎、肛裂、痔。
- 肠易激综合征。
- 牛奶和食物过敏。
- 肠扭转不良。
- Meckel 憩室。
- 肠套叠。
- 阑尾炎。
- 药物和毒物：
- 甘露醇。
- 山梨醇。
- 酚酞。
- 含有镁的抗酸剂。
- 奎尼丁。
- 秋水仙碱。
- 蘑菇。
- 汞中毒。

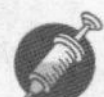

治疗

院前

- 严重脱水时静脉通道开放困难。
- 避免接触污染的衣服或排泄物。

初步稳定/治疗

- 基本支持治疗。
- 严重脱水时静脉输液用生理盐水(NS)液体复苏。

■ 急诊治疗/程序

• 轻度脱水时口服补液(佳得乐/电解质液体)。
• 静脉输液适用于：
- 低血压、恶心呕吐、反应迟钝、代谢性酸中毒、显著高钠血症或低钠血症。
- 生理盐水溶液：500 ml～1 L(儿童：20 ml/kg)复苏，生理盐水或 5% 葡萄糖(D_5W) 0.45%盐水(儿童：D_5W 0.25%盐水)维持足够的尿量。
• 次水杨酸铋(Pepto-Bismol)：
- 抑酸剂。
- 有效的临床缓解无不良反应。
• 白陶土-果胶制剂(kaopectate)：
- 减少大便流动性。
- 不影响病程。
• 抗动力药物：地芬诺酯(复方苯乙哌啶片)、洛哌丁胺(易蒙停)、镇痛剂、可待因：
- 适用于非感染性腹泻。
- 初始小剂量应用于感染性腹泻，以控制症状。
- 避免在感染性腹泻中长时间使用，可增加发热、腹泻和菌血症的持续时间，并且可以诱发毒性巨结肠。
• 抗生素治疗感染性病原体：
- 空肠弯曲菌：喹诺酮类或红霉素。
- 沙门菌：喹诺酮类药物或复方新诺明(TMP-SMX)。
- 伤寒：头孢曲松钠。
- 志贺菌：喹诺酮类、TMP-SMX 或氨苄西林。
- 副溶血性弧菌：四环素或强力霉素。
- 难辨梭状芽孢杆菌：甲硝唑或万古霉素。
- 大肠杆菌：喹诺酮类或 TMP-SMX。
- 贾第鞭毛虫：甲硝唑或奎纳克林。
- 溶组织内阿米巴(内阿米巴病)：双碘喹或甲硝唑。

■ 药物治疗

• 氨苄西林：500 mg[儿童：20 mg/(kg·24 h)]，口服或静脉注射，q6 h。
• TMP-SMX(复方新诺明)：1 片，口服 2/日[儿童：8～10 mg TMP/40～50 mg SMX/(kg·24 h)]；或 8～20 mg/(kg·24 h)TMP，静脉注射，每日 2～4 次给药。
• 头孢曲松钠：1 g[儿童：50～75 mg/(kg·12 h)]，肌内注射或静脉注射，q12 h。
• 环丙沙星(喹诺酮类)：500 mg，口服或 400 mg，静脉注射，q12 h(＞18 岁)。
• 强力霉素：100 mg，口服；或 100 mg，静脉注射，q12 h。
• 红霉素：500 mg[儿童：40～50 mg/(kg·24 h)]，口服，每日 4 次。
• 双碘喹：650 mg[儿童：30～40 mg/(kg·24 h)，每日不超过 2 g]，口服，每日 3 次。
• 甲硝唑：250 mg[儿童：35 mg/(kg·24 h)]，口服，每日 3 次(＞8 岁)。
• 四环素：500 mg，口服或静脉注射，q6 h。
• 万古霉素：125～500 mg[儿童：40 mg/(kg·24 h)]，口服，q6 h。

随访

■ 进一步处理

入院指征

• 低血压，静脉输液无反应者。
• 明显出血。
• 败血症或中毒征象。
• 顽固性呕吐或腹痛。
• 严重电解质紊乱或代谢性酸中毒。
• 精神状态改变。
• 儿童伴＞10%～15%脱水。

出院指征

• 轻症病例需要口服补水。
• 静脉补液有效的纠正脱水。

转诊问题

长期腹泻的病例可以为进一步检查咨询消化科医师。

■ 随访建议

由于腹泻是自限性，后续治疗是可以选择的。

要点和误区

• 避免感染性腹泻长时间使用抗动力药物。
• TMP-SMX(复方新诺明)、环丙沙星、强力霉素和四环素禁用于妊娠期。甲硝唑可以在妊娠晚期使用。
• 卫生服务提供者和食物处理人员有感染性腹泻记录的需要从当地卫生部门得到许可后才可恢复工作。
• 艰难梭菌导致的感染性腹泻发病率升高，尤其是住在疗养院里的患者。

F

腹泻(儿童) Diarrhea, Pediatric

Rajender Gattu · Richard Lichenstein 谭美春 译

基础知识

■ 描述

• 儿童常见病之一，在儿科急诊中发生率仅次于呼吸道感染，排第 2 位。
• 全世界范围内儿童疾病和死亡的主要原因。
• 急性感染性小肠炎(AIE)：
- 呕吐和腹泻。
- 在美国，＜5 岁的儿童几乎每年发病 2 次。
- 约占小儿科急诊和住院总就诊人数的 10%。
• 粪便性状的急性改变，导致排便次数和排便量增多，持续时间＜7 日。WHO 定义，每日粪便不成形或水样泻次数＞3 次。
- 慢性腹泻：腹泻持续时间＞2 周。
• 从病理生理学的角度来看，有两种基本机制参与其中，即渗透和分泌。除了这些机制之外，肠动力也会发生改变。

■ 病因

• 急性小肠炎：
- 感染性：
◦ 病毒：占病例的 70%～80%：
 ▪ 轮状病毒最常见。
 ▪ 肠道腺病毒。
 ▪ 诺如病毒(食源性疾病暴发)。
◦ 细菌：占 10%～20%：
 ▪ 大肠埃希菌、耶尔森菌、难辨梭状芽孢

杆菌。
- 沙门菌、志贺菌和弯曲菌。
- 霍乱弧菌。
- 嗜水气单胞菌。

◦ 寄生虫5%：
- 隐孢子虫病(水源性疾病暴发)。
- 贾第鞭毛虫。

- 非感染性：

◦ 感染后。
◦ 食物过敏和不耐受：
- 牛奶蛋白。
- 大豆蛋白。
- 甲基黄嘌呤。
- 乳糖不耐受症。

◦ 化疗/辐射引起。
◦ 药物引起：
- 抗生素、泻药、抗酸剂。

◦ 食入重金属——铜、锌。
◦ 摄入植物——风信子、水仙花、伞形毒菌类。
◦ 维生素缺乏：烟酸、叶酸。
◦ 维生素毒性：维生素C。

- 伴有其他感染。

◦ 中耳炎、尿路感染、肺炎、脑膜炎、阑尾炎。

• 慢性腹泻：

- 饮食因素：饮用大量果汁，过度摄入山梨醇或果糖。
- 免疫功能低下伴肠道感染。
- 营养不良。
- 内分泌：甲状腺功能亢进、嗜铬细胞瘤。
- 炎症性肠疾病：克罗恩病、溃疡性结肠炎。
- 吸收不良综合征(囊性纤维化、乳糜泻)。
- 肠易激综合征。

诊断

症状和体征

• 频繁，粪便稀溏。
• 大便性状：

- 水样泻。
- 血便。
- 黏液。

• 有时腹痛，发热，厌食、里急后重。
• 脱水的症状反映的机体脱水程度和脱水程度的变化：轻度<5%，中度5%～10%，重度>15%。
• 严重脱水：

- 精神状态变化：严重脱水时常见精神不振，与肌张力减弱相关。
- 黏膜：干。
- 皮肤弹性：减弱。
- 前囟：凹陷。
- 血压：降低。
- 脉搏：心动过速。
- 毛细血管充盈：时间延长(>2 s)。
- 尿量：减少。
- 眼睛：凹陷，无泪。
- 渴。

病史

• 发病及持续时间。
• 精神状态和外貌。
• 发热及相关症状(如腹痛、呕吐)。
• 粪便次数、粪便性状改变，可伴鲜血和黏液。
• 尿量。
• 喂养。
• 近期抗生素使用史。
• 近期旅行史。
• 可能吞食。
• 免疫缺陷。
• 潜在的肠道畸形(如先天性巨结肠症)。

体格检查

• 异常毛细血管充盈时间异常>2 s。
• 无泪。
• 黏膜干燥。
• 用于确定孩子脱水的3个典型体征：异常的呼吸模式、皮肤弹性异常和毛细血管充盈时间延长，也要观察黏膜。

- 在临床中综合多项查体的体征判断脱水病情比依据单一体征更准确。

基本检查

小儿急性腹泻多数不需要任何实验室检查。考虑检查，如果：

• 温度>103 ℉(39.4 ℃)。
• 全身性疾病。
• 血性腹泻。
• 病程迁延>2周。
• 里急后重。
• 轻度以上的脱水通常需要静脉给药治疗。
• 腹泻带血或黏液提示存在侵袭性炎症或细胞毒素介导的过程(沙门菌、侵袭性大肠杆菌)。

诊断检查与说明

实验室检查

• 全血细胞计数与白细胞分类、血培养、尿培养、尿酸，如果有全身感染的迹象。也要检测尿比重和尿酮体。
• 基础代谢包括电解质、尿素氮、肌酐、碳酸氢盐、严重脱水或出现异常体征的孩子均应当予以静脉输液治疗：

- 最近一项证据表明，血清碳酸氢盐对检测中度脱水特别有帮助。
- 粪便pH<5.5或粪便还原性物质阳性有助于诊断乳糖不耐受症。
- 粪便潜血。

• 粪便镜检：

- 粪便残渣每高倍视野>5个白细胞提示为侵袭性细菌感染：

◦ 志贺菌。
◦ 沙门菌。
◦ 弯曲杆菌。
◦ 耶尔森菌。
◦ 侵袭性大肠杆菌。

• 粪便培养：

- 在大多数情况下不需要，除非有极高可能性识别细菌病原体(隐血试验和/或粪便白细胞)，并且能够通过抗生素治疗改变临床病程和传染期。

• ≤12个月的发热患儿考虑尿培养。

影像学检查

影像通常不显示。如果临床高度怀疑其他诊断，如肠套叠、肠梗阻、阑尾炎，则行腹部X线或超声对诊断有帮助。

诊断步骤/外科

除非临床依据病史和体格检查高度怀疑其他诊断，否则通常不进行该项处理。

鉴别诊断

• 感染后：

- 急性、细菌性、病毒性肠胃炎，常与吸收不良相关，尤其是乳糖。

• 艰难梭菌感染中使用抗生素。
• 牛奶过敏。
• 肠旋转不良与肠扭转。
• 炎症性肠病。
• 肠套叠。
• 吸收不良综合征。
• 肠外感染。
• 药物改变肠道菌群，如抗生素(如阿莫西林-克拉维酸)。

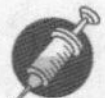

治疗

初步稳定/治疗

• 对于休克或接近休克的严重脱水的孩

子,静脉注射或骨内注射 20 ml/kg 生理盐水溶液,如果低血糖加用 1 g/kg 葡萄糖溶液。

- 或者,在严格的协议管理下皮下注射重组人透明质酸酶。
- 脉搏氧饱和度仪。
- 休克儿童必要时进行气管插管。

■ **急诊治疗/程序**

- 对于轻度脱水使用口服补液疗法(ORT),50 ml/kg 和 100 ml/kg,4 h 内中度脱水,分别予以下述处理:
  - 按照每次大便后 10 ml/kg ORT 的量补充持续失水量。
  - 理想的 ORT 溶液具有低渗透压摩尔浓度(210~250),葡萄糖约 2 g/L,钠含量 50~60 mmol/L。
- 对于中度至重度脱水,采用肠外补液维持量和缺损量。
- 如果腹泻不伴有脱水,按照每次大便后补充 10 ml/kg ORT 的量口服补液。
- 肠炎抗生素只用于诊断明确的急性肠炎:常规不推荐使用,仅用于任何严重的或感染性疾病、免疫功能低下的患者,或有严重的胃肠道基础疾病的患者。
  - 红霉素用于治疗空肠弯曲菌。
  - 甲氧苄啶-磺胺甲噁唑(复方新诺明):
    - 沙门菌——复杂(婴儿<6 月龄、传播、菌血症、免疫功能低下者、伤寒)。
    - 志贺菌。
    - 耶尔森菌。
    - 侵袭性大肠杆菌。
  - 甲硝唑或万古霉素:
    - 梭状芽孢杆菌肠炎(严重和/或持续性肠炎)。
  - 新霉素:用于侵袭性大肠杆菌。
  - 呋喃唑酮或甲硝唑:用于贾第鞭毛虫。
- 不推荐使用止泻剂。
- 益生菌:鼠李糖乳杆菌。
  - 益生菌降解和修饰食物性抗原并且平衡抗炎反应的细胞因子,可能会减少腹泻的持续时间。
- 急诊后饮食:
  - 尽可能补水,提供与儿童腹泻年龄相适应的饮食喂养。
  - 耐受性良好的食物:
    - 含复合糖类(米饭、土豆、面包)。
    - 瘦肉。
    - 酸奶。
    - 水果。
    - 蔬菜。
    - 全营养配方奶,高度怀疑存在乳糖不耐症的儿童除外。
  - 避免高脂肪食品和高单糖食品。

■ **药物治疗**

- 氨苄西林:50~200 mg/(kg · 24 h),静脉注射或口服,q6 h。
- 红霉素:40 mg/(kg · 24 h),口服,q6 h;10~20 mg/(kg · 24 h),静脉注射,q6 h。
- 甲硝唑:30 mg/(kg · 24 h),分成每日 4 次,口服,持续 7 日。
- 新霉素:50~100 mg/(kg · 24 h),口服,q6~8 h。
- 甲氧苄啶-磺胺甲噁唑:8~10 mg/(kg · 24 h),根据甲氧苄啶的用法分成每日 2 次,口服。
- 万古霉素:40~50 mg/(kg · 24 h),口服,q6 h。
- 洛哌丁胺(不适用于<6 岁儿童或粪便隐血阳性患儿):年龄 6~8 岁,2 mg,分成每日 2 次,口服;年龄 8~12 岁,2 mg,每日 3 次,口服。
- 头孢克肟:8 mg/(kg · d),口服,7~10 日。
- 头孢曲松钠:50 mg/(kg · d),静脉注射或肌内注射,7~10 日。
- 鼠李糖乳杆菌和鲍氏酵母菌:50 亿 U/d。
- 锌:10~20 mg/d,10~14 日(儿童<5 岁)。

一线用药

- 复方新诺明:用于沙门菌和志贺菌。
- 强力霉素:用于霍乱弧菌。
- 甲硝唑:用于艰难梭菌。

二线用药

- 头孢曲松和头孢噻肟:用于沙门菌和志贺菌。
- 红霉素:用于霍乱弧菌。
- 万古霉素:用于耐药的艰难梭菌。

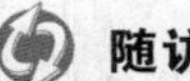

随访

■ **进一步处理**

入院指征

- 外科急腹症。
- 无法耐受口服补液。
- ≥10%的脱水。
- 疑似复杂沙门菌肠炎。
- 有中毒反应的儿童。
- 患有严重基础疾病的儿童。

出院指征

- 患者的病情缓解。
- 护理人员能够按照要求给予患儿适当的口服补液和饮食。
- 护理人员能够识别脱水的症状和体征。

转诊问题

- 免疫力低下的人群。
- 有肠道基础疾病。

■ **随访建议**

后续护理取决于腹泻的病程和严重程度、患儿的年龄,以及护理人员依从医嘱的能力:

- 单纯性腹泻通常不需要随访。
- 新生儿需要在短期内严格随访。

要点和误区

- 病史和体格检查有助于区分单纯腹泻与其他儿童严重疾病。
- 绝大多数小儿急性腹泻并不需要大量的实验室检查,这不会影响临床处置。
- 止泻药和抗生素对儿童腹泻的治疗作用非常有限。
- 需要考虑如下可能性诊断,如阑尾炎、肠套叠、尿路感染、败血症。

F

腹主动脉瘤 Abdominal Aortic Aneurysm

Adam S. Kaye · Carlo L. Rosen 马林浩 林兆奋 译

基础知识

描述

• 主动脉壁局部扩张膨大，直径增加超过50%(>3 cm)。
• 95%位于肾脏下方。
• 快速膨胀或破裂会导致临床症状。
• 可能破裂入腹膜内或者腹膜后空间。
• 腹膜内破裂通常迅速致死(20%的腹主动脉瘤)。
• 平均增大速度为每年 0.2～0.5 cm。
• 如果破裂：
- 总体死亡率为 90%。
- 抵达医院患者死亡率为 80%。
- 接受紧急修补患者死亡率为 50%。
• 有血管内主动脉瘤的患者行动脉瘤修补术(EVAR)，持续血流灌注可导致持续性动脉瘤增大和破裂。

老年注意事项

• 随着年龄增加，发病风险增大。
• 出现在：
- 4%～8%的 65 岁以上患者。
- 5%～10%的 65～79 岁男性患者。
- 12.5%的 75～84 岁男性患者。
- 5.2%的 75～84 岁女性患者。

病因

• 危险因素同其他血管疾病：
- 男性。
- 年龄大于 65 岁。
- 家族史。
- 吸烟史。
- 动脉粥样硬化。
- 高血压。
- 糖尿病。
- 结缔组织病。
◦ Ehlers-Danlos 综合征。
◦ 马方综合征。
• 少见的病因：
- 钝性腹部创伤。
- 先天性动脉瘤。
- 主动脉感染。
- 继发于心内膜炎的真菌性动脉瘤。
• 破裂的危险因素：
- 大小(年破裂率)。
◦ 动脉瘤 5～5.9 cm＝4%。
◦ 动脉瘤 6～6.9 cm＝7%。
◦ 动脉瘤 7.9～7 cm＝20%。
- 扩张：
◦ 小动脉瘤 6 个月内增大超过 5 cm 存在破裂高风险。
- 年龄：
◦ 对于相似大小的 4.0～5.5 cm 动脉瘤，女性发生破裂的概率是男性的 4 倍。

诊断

症状和体征

病史

• 腹部、后背或胁腹痛。
- 模糊的，钝性的。
- 持续性的，波动性的，疝气样痛。
- 急性、严重、持续存在的痛。
- 可放射到胸部、大腿、腹股沟区域或阴囊。
- 胁腹痛，见于 10%的患者。
• 下肢痛。
• 晕厥或近晕厥。
• 非破裂性的常常无症状。

体格检查

• 非破裂性的。
- 腹部肿块或者腹胀。
- 可触及的、无痛的、搏动性包块。
- 完整的股动脉搏动。
• 破裂性的。
- 经典三角(仅 1/3 病例)。
◦ 疼痛。
◦ 低血压。
◦ 搏动性腹部包块。
- 全身反应。
◦ 低血压。
◦ 心动过速。
◦ 系统性栓塞形成。
- 腹部。
◦ 搏动性、压痛的腹部包块。
◦ 肋腰部出血斑(Grey-Turner 斑)说明腹膜后出血。
◦ 动脉瘤直径>5 cm 的仅 75%可以触及。
◦ 腹部压痛。
◦ 腹部杂音。
◦ 胃肠道出血。
- 肢体。
• 肢体中的脉搏消失或不对称。
• 并发症：
- 大栓子：急性下肢疼痛。
- 微栓子：冰凉、疼痛、发绀的趾(“蓝趾综合征”)。
- 动脉瘤血栓形成：急性下肢缺血。
- 主动脉肠瘘：胃肠道出血。

基本检查

• 不稳定的患者：
- 床旁腹部超声。
- 无其他辅助设备检查的患者行剖腹探查。
• 稳定的、有症状的患者：
- 腹部 CT。

诊断检查与说明

实验室检查

• 血型检查及交叉配血试验。
• 全血细胞计数。
• 肌酐。
• 尿液分析。
• 凝血功能检查。

影像学检查

• 腹部超声。
- 检测破裂前腹主动脉瘤具有 100%敏感性和 92%～99%的特异性。
- 破裂后报道敏感性降低至 10%。急诊室内，对于测定腹主动脉瘤的存在很有帮助。
- 腹主动脉瘤的超声表现为增宽的主动脉直径大于 3 cm 或局部额主动脉扩张。
- 主动脉血栓发生而主动脉直径正常。主动脉壁外测量可以防止错估。
- 对于既往 EVAR 的患者，超声检查受限，推荐 CT 检查和专家评估。
• 腹部 CT 扫描。
- 诊断无需增强扫描，但制定外科手术方案是需要通过 CT 血管造影明确血管内结构。
- 会说明动脉瘤及破裂位置(腹膜内 *vs.* 腹膜后)。
- 能够更精确地测定主动脉的直径。

鉴别诊断

• 其他腹部动脉瘤(如髂动脉瘤或者肾动脉瘤)。
• 主动脉夹层。
• 肾绞痛。
• 胆绞痛。

F

• 肌肉骨骼的背痛。
• 胰腺炎。
• 胆囊炎。
• 阑尾炎。
• 肠梗阻。
• 肠穿孔。
• 肠系膜缺血。
• 憩室炎。
• 胃肠道出血。
• 主动脉血栓栓塞。
• 心肌梗死。
• 艾迪生病危象。
• 脓毒症。
• 脊髓压迫症。

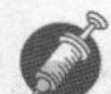

治疗

院前

• 建立2条快速静脉通道。
• 迅速转运至最近的能够实施备选手术的机构。
• 通知急诊室工作人员准备如下内容：
- 手术室。
- 万能供血者血液。
- 外科会诊。

初步稳定/治疗

• 2条快速静脉通路。
• 输注晶体液。
• 心电监护。
• 早期输血。

急诊治疗/程序

对于有症状的腹主动脉瘤患者：
• 紧急外科会诊和手术干预。
• 由血管外科医师行剖腹修补或主动脉血管内修补(EVAR)。
• 不能因诊断检查延误确定性治疗。

随访

进一步处理

入院指征

所有有症状的腹主动脉瘤患者都需要入院并接受紧急外科干预。

出院指征

仅无症状的患者。

随访建议

• 出院前一定要安排严密的血管外科医师随访。
• 有以下症状立即返回住院：
- 任何后背、腹部、肋腰部或下肢的疼痛。
- 任何头晕或晕厥。

要点和误区

• 任何出现腹痛、后背痛或肋腰部痛的患者都应鉴别是否为腹主动脉瘤。
• 有症状的腹主动脉瘤患者需要立即治疗。不要因为其他检查而耽误治疗。
• 血流动力学不稳定的患者(如低血压)不应去做CT扫描。

F

钙通道阻滞剂中毒 Calcium Channel Blocker Poisoning

Christopher S. Lim · Steven E. Aks 陈丽 译

基础知识

描述

- 3 类钙通道阻滞剂(CCB)：
  - 苯烷胺类(维拉帕米)：
    - 血管扩张导致血压下降。
    - 负性频率和肌力作用：降低血压时未出现反射性的心动过速。
  - 二氢吡啶类(硝苯地平)：
    - 降低血管阻力，导致血压下降。
    - 微弱的负性肌力作用：反射性心动过速。
  - 苯二氮䓬类(地尔硫䓬)：
    - 降低外周血管阻力，导致血压下降。
    - 心率(HR)和心输出量首先增加。
    - 直接负性肌力作用，导致心率下降。
- 钙通道阻滞作用：
  - 钙在心肌和平滑肌收缩中起着关键作用。
  - 钙通道阻滞剂可防止：
    - 钙内流，导致肌肉松弛。
    - 胰岛细胞释放胰岛素，导致高血糖。

诊断

症状和体征

- 心血管：
  - 低血压。
  - 心动过缓。
  - 反射性心动过速(二氢吡啶)。
  - 传导异常、心脏传导阻滞。
- 神经：
  - 中枢神经抑制。
  - 昏迷。
  - 癫痫发作。
  - 兴奋。
  - 精神错乱。
- 代谢：
  - 高血糖。

病史

- 询问是否错用药物。
- 询问是否有自杀意图。
- 询问儿科患者是否接触到此药物。

体格检查

- 低血压。
- 心动过缓。
- 皮肤温暖而不是湿冷。

基本检查

心电图：

- 心动过缓(硝苯地平的反射性心动过速)。
- 传导延迟：QRS 波群延长。
- 心脏传导阻滞。

诊断检查与说明

实验室检查

- 钙离子水平。
- 服用地高辛者地高辛浓度(钙用药安全性)。
- 全血细胞计数。
- 电解质、尿素氮、肌酐、血糖。
  - 在设定心动过缓、低血压和高血糖时建议考虑钙通道阻滞剂过量情况。
  - 非糖尿病患者高血糖的程度可能与钙通道阻滞剂中毒相关。
- 如果怀疑复合摄取药物应进行毒理学检测。

鉴别诊断

- β受体阻滞剂中毒。
- 可乐定中毒。
- 洋地黄中毒。
- 急性心肌梗死合并传导阻滞。

治疗

院前

- 运送药物、药瓶去急诊室。
- 用钙剂治疗确诊由钙通道阻滞剂过量引起的传导阻滞或不稳定患者。

初步稳定/治疗

- ABC 管理：
  - 按照指征保护气道。
  - 按需给予氧气。
  - 生理盐水静脉通道。
- 血流动力学监测。

急诊治疗/程序

目标

- 心率>60 次/分。
- 收缩压>90 mmHg。
- 充足的尿量。
- 提高意识水平。

清理胃肠道

- 吐根糖浆：院前或者急诊室是禁忌。
- 活性炭：
  - 可能有益，特别是在复合摄取药物时。

钙

- 通常只是暂时有效。
- 葡萄糖酸钙(10%)：
  - 每毫升包含 0.4 mg 钙离子。
  - 不会像氯化钙那样引起组织坏死。
  - 葡萄糖酸钙：酸血症时首选。
- 氯化钙(10%)：
  - 每升包含 1.36 mg 钙离子(比葡萄糖酸钙高 3 倍)。
  - 渗出可引起组织坏死和腐烂。
  - 静脉刺激作用强。
- 如果重复给予钙剂应监测血钙水平。
- 地高辛中毒是禁忌，因为在这种情况下钙可引起严重的不良反应。

心动过缓/低血压

- 静脉输液：
  - 在低血压患者中谨慎管理。
  - Swan-Ganz 导管或中心静脉压监测帮助追踪容量状态。
- 阿托品通常是无效的。
- 高剂量胰岛素：
  - 钙通道阻滞剂引起心肌胰岛素抵抗和抑制胰岛细胞释放胰岛素。
    - 低效脂肪酸代谢。
  - 高剂量胰岛更有效地促进心肌碳水化合物的代谢，并能改善血流动力学。
- 血管加压药：
  - 没有明确的证据表明，其中 1 种加压药比另外一种更有效。
  - 制订有创检测来帮助指导治疗。
  - 多巴胺：
    - 低剂量时为 $β_1$ 受体激动剂，对心肌有正性肌力作用。
    - 高剂量时为 α 受体激动剂，可以使血管收缩。
  - 肾上腺素：
    - 有效的 α 受体激动剂和 β 受体激动剂。
- 氨力农：
  - 选择性的磷酸二酯酶峰抑制剂。
  - 间接增加 cAMP 增加收缩力。
- 电起搏：当其他治疗方法失败时。
- 未来的潜在治疗方法：
  - 高渗碳酸氢钠。
  - 静脉脂肪乳剂(20%脂肪乳)。

药物治疗

- 氨力农：负荷剂量 0.75 mg/kg；维持量

2～20 μg/(kg·min)；据效果滴定。

• 阿托品：0.5 mg(儿童：0.02 mg/kg)静脉应用；重复给药 0.5～1 mg(儿童：0.04 mg/kg)。

• 氯化钙：10%氯化钙 5～10 ml 缓慢静脉泵入(儿童：0.2～0.25 ml/kg；如果需要，10 min 可重复给药)，然后 20～50 mg/(kg·h)滴注。

• 葡萄糖酸钙：10%葡萄糖酸钙 10～20 ml 缓慢静脉泵入(儿童：1 ml/kg；如果需要，10 min 可重复给药)。

• 葡萄糖：50%葡萄糖 50 ml(儿童：25%葡萄糖 0.25 g/kg)。

• 多巴胺：2～20 μg/(kg·min)；据效果滴定。

• 肾上腺素：1～2 μg/(kg·min)(儿童：0.01 mg/kg 或者 1∶10 000 肾上腺素 0.1 ml/kg)；据效果滴定。

• 去甲肾上腺素：开始 2～4 μg/min 静滴；静脉滴定至 1～2 μg/(kg·min)。

• 钾：40 mmol 口服或静脉给予。

高剂量胰岛素治疗方案

• 如果对液体复苏反应不佳，可以考虑应用。

• 胰岛素(常规胰岛素)：1 U/kg 静脉推注，然后 0.5～1 U/(kg·h)滴定到有临床效果。

• 管理葡萄糖，如果血糖<200 mg/dl。

• 管理钾，如果血钾<2.5 mmol/L。

• 在第一个 4 h 内，每 30 min 监测一次血糖和血钾浓度。

• 大约 24 h 的胰岛素需求量：成年患者需 1 500 U 的正规胰岛素。

一线用药

• 静脉输液。

• 钙。

• 高剂量胰岛素。

• 血管加压药。

二线用药

• 氨力农。

• 静脉脂肪乳剂。

• 试验性治疗：亚甲蓝，咨询当地毒物中心。

随访

进一步处理

入院指征

• 收治有症状的患者到监测床进行血流动力学监测。

• 收治所用摄入缓释型钙通道阻滞剂的患者进行 24 h 观察和检测，因为症状的延迟性。

出院指征

摄入速效制剂后 8 h 没有症状的患者可以出院。

随访建议

• 对所用自杀患者进行心理评估。

• 对有儿童误食的家长进行中毒预防指导。

要点和误区

• 低血压和心动过缓的患者考虑钙通道阻滞剂中毒。

• 在钙通道阻滞剂中毒的患者要考虑自杀行为。

• 如果液体复苏没有快速起效的话，要考虑高剂量胰岛素及葡萄糖和钾。

肝肾综合征

Hepatorenal Syndrome

Douglas W. Chesson · Matthew T. Keadey 陈奇通 译

G

基础知识

描述

• 肾衰竭患者合并有急慢性肝脏疾病，无其他明确的肾脏病理诱因。

• 肝肾综合征表现为由于严重肝脏疾病而导致的肾灌注显著下降。

- Ⅰ型肝肾综合征：
  - 肝脏疾病患者出现急性短暂性肾衰竭。
  - 快速进展。
  - 肌酐清除率降低 50%或 2 周内肌酐水平升高超过原来的 2.5 倍。
  - 3 个月内死亡率超过 90%。
  - 常见于急性肝衰竭或者酒精性肝病。
  - 少尿或无尿。
- Ⅱ型肝肾综合征：
  - 肾衰竭病程较长。
  - 见于难治性腹水的患者。
  - 比Ⅰ型肝肾综合征致死率低。

• 肝肾综合征的特征：

- 患者必须有肝硬化和腹水。
- 肾前性疾病。
- 急性肾损伤(AKI)的一种功能性形式，由于肾血管收缩。
- AKI 根据国际腹水协会(ICA)的标准。
- 可逆性肾血管收缩并且伴有轻微低血压。
- 肾脏组织结构正常。
- 血容量升高后，肾功能没有改善。
- 目前没有使用肾毒性药物。

• 肝脏疾病导致全身血管舒张和血容量减少：

- 交感神经反射性兴奋。
- 肾素-血管紧张素系统激活。
- 很多血管活性物质释放：一氧化氮、前列腺素、心房钠尿肽、血小板活动因子、内皮素、儿茶酚胺、血管紧张素Ⅱ、血栓素。

• 血管收缩的影响：

- 肾脏皮质血管扩张继而导致肾脏灌注增加。
- 肾血流量减少，肾小球滤过率减低。

• 尿钠降低。

• 肝肾综合征的发病率：第 1 年 18%，5 年内升高至 39%。

• 低钠血症和高肾素水平是危险因素。

病因

• 慢性肝疾病，尤其是酒精相关性肝病，如肝硬化和重症酒精性肝炎。

• 急性肝衰竭。

• 诱发因素：

- 血容量减少：失血、多尿腹腔穿刺大量引流。
- 使用肾毒性药物：非甾体抗炎药、氨基糖苷类抗生素。
- 败血症：自发性细菌性腹膜炎能够引起肾衰竭，有效预防后能够降低急性肾衰竭的发生率。

诊断

症状和体征

急慢性肝脏疾病的表现：

• 门静脉高压的征象。

• 腹水。

- 进行性少尿。
- 黄疸或干性脑病。
- 凝血功能障碍。
- 心动过速。
- 低血压。
- 腹水导致的呼吸困难或呼吸急促。

病史

- 急慢性肝病和门静脉高压：
- 肝功能恶化常先于急性肾衰竭发生。

体格检查

- 合并有严重肝脏疾病。
- 生命体征：
- 合并有败血症。
- 可有发热、低血压、内出血。

诊断检查与说明

实验室检查

- 血常规：
- 失血性贫血。
- 电解质
- 高钾血症
- 酸中毒。
- 血糖。
- 肌酐、尿素氮：
- 肌酐正常可伴有肾小球滤过率降低、肌肉萎缩、营养不良和腹水；
- 肌酐增高见于使用某些抑制肾小管分泌肌酐的药物，如西咪替丁(甲氰米胍)、甲氧苄啶及螺内酯(安体舒通)等。
- 凝血酶原时间和二聚体检查。
- 尿液检测
- 缺乏管型将 HRS 与急性肾小管坏死(ATN)区分开来。
- 检查 UT。
- 尿钠和尿肌酐和尿渗透压。
- 24 h 尿量：未使用利尿剂的情况下明显降低。
- 24 h 尿肌酐：
- 肾小球滤过率。
- 血、腹水及尿的细菌培养。
- 尿蛋白检测。

影像学检查

- 胸部 X 线片检测：充血性心力衰竭和体液潴留。
- 尿路造影：排除梗阻性尿路疾病。
- 超声：评估肾血管收缩情况。

诊断步骤/外科

- 心电图：心律失常或高钾血症征象。
- 尿管：评估尿量。
- 中心静脉：压评估血容量。

鉴别诊断

- 肝肾综合征是排除性诊断。
- 肾小球疾病：
- 乙型肝炎能够引起肾小球肾炎。
- 丙型肝炎由于冷球蛋白血症引起肾脏的实质性损伤。
- 急性肾小管坏死：
- 尿钠＞30 mmol/L。
- 等渗尿、管型尿。
- 细胞碎片。
- 肾前性氮质血症：
- 低血容量纠正后尿排量增加。
- 尿路梗阻。
- 感染或败血症。
- 药物相关性肾炎，如非甾体抗炎药。
- 间质性肾炎。
- 肝移植后肾功能不全：
- 移植肝功能衰竭导致肝肾综合征。
- 药物影响，如环孢素。
- 之前合并有肾脏疾病，血容量少。

治疗

院前

注重 ABC 管理：

- 严重脑病患者进行气道控制。
- 严重腹水患者出现的呼吸衰竭。
- 建立静脉通道，纠正低血容量。

初步稳定/治疗

- ABCs。
- 积极纠正血容量不足：
- 生理盐水。
- 胶体溶液：白蛋白 1 g/kg。
- 密切控制临床状态。
- 纠正肾前性氮质血症后，应当提高尿量。
- 处理威胁生病的急症：
- 高钾血症。
- 严重的酸中毒。
- 低氧血症。
- 尿毒症心包炎。

急诊治疗/程序

- 去除可逆性和可治性肝肾综合征的诱因。
- 支持疗法直到肝功能恢复。
- 禁用对肾脏有损伤的药物。
- 如非甾体抗炎药。
- 氨基糖苷类抗生素。
- 环孢素等。
- 积极治疗原发病。
- 治疗并存的肾脏疾病。
- 纠正电解质紊乱。
- 治疗相关的心肺功能异常和低氧血症。
- 怀疑败血症时尽早使用广谱抗生素。
- 治疗肝脏并发症：
- 梗阻性黄疸。
- 肝性脑病。
- 低血糖。
- 腹膜炎。
- 建立静脉通道，补充白蛋白。
- 提高渗透压以减轻腹水。
- 增加肾血流能够短暂的改善肝肾综合征。
- TIPS。
- 透析：纠正水电解质紊乱、酸碱平衡及肺水肿。
- 肝移植：
- 目前最有效的治疗方式。
- 在等待移植时是否考虑使用分子吸收剂循环系统(MARS)支持肝脏。

药物治疗

- 目前无一线药物，仅在排除其他原因引起的肾功受损情况下使用。
- 多巴胺：2～5 μg/(kg · min)。
- 可提高肾功能。
- 缓解症状。
- 甲氧胺福林(7.5～12.5 mg，口服，每日 3 次)和奥曲肽(100～200 μg，皮下注射，每日 3 次)：奥曲肽是生长抑素类似物，甲氧胺福林是拟交感神经药物。
- 去甲肾上腺素：
- 通过中心静脉通路在 ICU 环境中使用。
- 外周血管收缩作用于 α 受体。
- 米索前列醇 0.4 mg，口服，每日 4 次：人工合成的前列腺素 E 类似物。
- 鸟氨酸加压素：加压素类似物。
- 能够能加肾灌注压，改善肾功能。
- 在美国不能使用。
- 特利加压素 2 mg/d，用 2 日：
- 人工合成的血管加速素类似物。
- 具有内在血管收缩活性。
- 在美国不能使用。

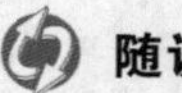

随访

进一步处理

入院指征

- 疑有肝肾综合征并伴有肾脏受损表现。
- 合并有心肺疾病、肝性脑病及严重的电解质紊乱应及时进入ICU。

出院指征

无

要点和误区

合并有肝脏疾病的患者出现任何程度的肾功受损的情况下要严密注意。

肝损伤 Hepatic Injury

Todd Baumbacher · Stephen R. Hayden 陈奇通 李文放 译

基础知识

描述

- 肝的大小和位置使其有很大的损伤风险：
  - 肝是穿透性损伤中最常见的实体器官。
  - 是腹部钝性损伤中第二常见的器官，仅次于脾。
  - 非常容易受到钝性伤害，直接打击或减速力。
- 损伤机制和力的描述是评估患者可能的肝损伤的重要因素：
  - 钝性损伤：
    - 获取任何减速或压缩力的力和方向（水平或垂直）的信息。
  - 穿透性损伤：
    - 武器的类型和口径。
    - 距离武器的距离。
    - 刀或刺入物的种类和长度。
- 肝损伤按严重程度分级，从包膜下血肿和破裂到严重肝碎裂。
- 相关情况包括肋骨骨折和脾、膈、肾、肺、胆囊、胰腺和血管的损伤。
- 据报道，肝损伤的总死亡率为8%～10%。
- 孤立性钝性肝损伤的非手术治疗越来越普遍。

儿科注意事项

肌肉组织发育不良，前后直径相对较小，使儿童肝抗压能力十分脆弱。

病因

- 创伤：
- 钝性创伤：
  - 减速。
  - 加速。
  - 压缩。
- 穿透性损伤：
  - 刺伤。
  - 枪伤。
  - 穿刺对象。

症状和体征

体格检查和病史多样。

病史

外伤史通常可从患者或院前医护人员处获得。

体格检查

- 肝损伤无敏感性与特异性检查。
- 与急性失血有关的全身症状：
  - 可能出现头晕和虚弱。
  - 休克症状包括心动过速和低血压。
- 局部体征：
  - 右上腹压痛。
  - 保护。
  - 腹胀。
  - 板状腹。
  - 反跳痛。
  - 压痛。
  - 挫伤/擦伤。
  - 右胸、侧腹或腹部的穿透性伤口。

基本检查

- 体格检查不可靠。
- 客观评估包括腹部影像学检查或手术探查。

诊断检查与说明

实验室检查

- 没有血液学检验针对肝损伤。
- 获取基线血红蛋白水平。
- 肝功能检查在急性期没有帮助。
- 如果怀疑活动性出血，考虑交叉配血。

影像学检查

- 基于受伤机制和体格检查考虑影像学检查。
- 腹部X线片：
  - 价值较小。
- 床旁超声：
  - 顿性和穿透性腹部损伤的筛查工具。
  - 不稳定患者的程序性检查。
  - 可能确定腹腔液在肝肾隐窝（Morison）或实质损伤。
  - 提示钝性多器官损伤患者腹腔出血。
- CT增强扫描：
  - 最好地描述了肝损伤的程度和对邻近器官的损伤。
  - 要求患者血流动力学稳定。
  - 动脉期CT显影剂外渗，提示血管或高度肝损伤需要手术干预。

诊断步骤/外科

- 诊断性腹腔灌洗（DPL）：
  - 少见，通常与创伤外科医师一起做。
  - 对腹腔积血敏感。
  - 对出血源无特异性。
  - 阳性者需手术和剖腹探查。
  - 对于病情不稳定和高度损伤的患者，必须手术治疗。
- 越来越多的轻度损伤在不做手术的情况下得到了成功的治疗。

鉴别诊断

- 导致腹腔内损伤的其他原因。
- 腹膜后损伤。
- 胸部受伤。
- 膈肌的伤害。
- 脾损伤。
- 血管损伤。

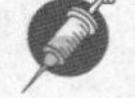

治疗

院前

- 获取损伤机制的详细信息。
- 开放大口径静脉通道：
  - 出血可能十分迅速，危及生命。
- 湿润盐水敷料覆盖穿透性伤口或内脏。
- 直接加压控制活动性出血。
- 除孤立性穿透性外伤外，全椎体固定。

初步稳定/治疗

- 初步治疗。

G

• 根据需要控制气道，可能有相关的损伤，包括头部损伤。

• 吸氧，心电监护，指脉氧监测。

• 足够的静脉通路，包括中心静脉、骨髓腔，并根据患者情况减少。

• 液体复苏，首先使用 2 L 晶体液(生理盐水或乳酸林格液)，然后是血液制品，如悬浮红细胞。

• 根据需要考虑新鲜冷冻血浆(FFP)。

▪ 急诊治疗/程序

• 对于有下列情况的急性损伤患者，立即剖腹手术：

- 血流动力学不稳定。
- 前腹部枪伤。
- 腹腔内出血的 Frank 征象。
- 根据诊断程序的适应证，如 DPL。
- 失败的非手术处理。

• 当腹腔内穿刺未被证实或不明确时，刺穿创面可以先进行局部创面探查，然后进行超声或 DPL 检查。

• 考虑以下患者非手术治疗：

- 血流动力学稳定，精神状态正常。
- 无其他腹腔内损伤的证据。
- 影像学检查证实的孤立性低度(1～3 级)肝损伤。
- 输血需求＜2 单位悬浮红细胞。
- 严重肝损伤(4、5 级)非手术治疗成功率低。

• 饮食：禁食。

• 活动：严格卧床。

• 特殊治疗：

- 血管造影加栓塞：选择性应用于持续性出血患者可能会减少手术治疗和输血的需要。
- 凝血因子Ⅶa、凝血酶原复合物被用于非手术治疗的辅助手段，控制大量出血。

▪ 药物治疗

• 晶体液：NS 或乳酸林格液。

• 红细胞。

• FFP。

• 重组因子Ⅶa：15～30 μg/kg，静脉注射，q4～6 h，直到止血。

• 凝血酶原复合物浓缩物(PCC)：50 U/kg，静脉注射。

• 创伤后 3 h 内给予氨甲环酸：初始标准剂量为 10 g，IVPB，10 min 以上，8 h 后给予 1 g。

 **随访**

▪ 进一步处理

入院指征

• 所有肝损伤的患者都需要住院接受明确的剖腹手术，或通过系列检查或 CT 扫描以及血细胞比容测量来密切观察血流动力学。

• ICU 通常在受伤后 48 h 内入院。

出院指征

确诊或疑似肝损伤的患者不应出院。

转诊问题

向当地有关部门报告所有枪伤和刀伤。

▪ 后续建议

随访超声、体格检查和血细胞比容水平不变对最初良性表现的患者至关重要。

要点和误区

• 对不稳定的患者尽早进行手术会诊。

• 未能进行适当的和充分的影像学检查是一个陷阱。

• 不依赖超声阴性结果排除肝损伤。

• 未能充分液体复苏和补充血液制品是一个陷阱。

• 如果肝损伤被证实，确保周围器官没有损伤。

• 检查女性是否妊娠。

G

肝性脑病 Hepatic Encephalopathy

Jeremy Graham · Matthew N. Graber 陈奇通 李文放 译

 **基础知识**

▪ 描述

肝性脑病(HE)的特征是行为、意识和运动障碍的改变，与肝功能不全和肝正常代谢物质的积累有关。其可能由以下原因导致：

• 氨(NH_3)的积聚：

- 肠道细菌分解蛋白质。
- 小肠、肾和肌肉中谷氨酰胺的脱氨作用。
- 积累的 NH_3 通过血脑屏障，星形胶质细胞摄取 NH_3 代谢成谷氨酰胺，引起细胞肿胀，最终导致脑水肿和大脑线粒体功能障碍。

• 其他神经毒素积聚：

- 短链脂肪酸。
- 锰中毒。
- 神经甾体。
- 酚类。
- 硫醇。
- 色氨酸等氨基酸。

• 抑制性神经递质水平升高：

- 苯二氮䓬类。
- γ 氨基丁酸(GABA)。
- 5-羟色胺。

• 兴奋性神经递质水平降低：

- 谷氨酸。
- 多巴胺。
- 天冬氨酸。
- 儿茶酚胺。

• 其他导致肝性脑病的因素：

- 脑血流和氧供降低。
- 葡萄糖消耗增加和低血糖可能。
- 缺锌。

• 遗传：

- 尿素循环的遗传性错误。

▪ 病因

• 基于第十一届世界胃肠病学大会的分类：

- A 型：合并急性肝损伤和暴发性肝功能衰竭(FHF)。
- B 型：与门静脉分流相关，无肝脏疾病。
- C 型：伴有肝硬化和门脉高压。

• 诱因：

- 胃肠道出血(老年人常见)。
- 低钾血症、低钠血症。
- 碱中毒可减少肾脏 NH_4^+ 的排泄。
- 脓毒症(如自发性细菌性腹膜炎 SBP)。
- 便秘。
- 慢性肝功能衰竭不服从治疗。
- 低血糖。
- 血容量不足(如穿刺大量排放腹水)。

- 氮质血症(如利尿剂或腹泻导致)。
- 麻醉剂或镇静剂,包括酒精。
- 锌缺乏,多种尿素循环酶需要锌。
- 肝细胞损伤。
- 病毒性或药物性肝炎。
- 门静脉分流术后。
- 复发性脑病可在无诱因的情况下发生。

诊断

症状和体征

• A型:迅速进展为癫痫发作、去大脑僵直、昏迷,常死于脑水肿。

• B型和C型是慢性疾病,可能表现为轻微或显性肝性脑病。显性肝性脑病可分为间歇性和持续性:

- 轻微肝性脑病:以精神运动速度、视觉感知、注意力和集中力受损,精神处理缓慢和记忆力丧失为特征。只有通过心理测试才能检测到。
- 显性肝性脑病:说话方式缓慢单调,精细运动能力丧失,反射亢进,阵挛,过度通气,锥体外系运动障碍,癫痫发作,神志不清,昏迷,去大脑/去皮质姿势。
- 显性肝性脑病发作:以数小时到数日的短时间意识变化为特征,通常通过治疗可以恢复到正常精神状态。在持续性肝性脑病中,患者不会恢复到正常的精神状态。

• 分级(West Haven标准):

- 0期:
  ◦ 无明显临床变化。
  ◦ 神经生理学和神经心理测试异常。
  ◦ 可能会出现跌倒和驾驶事故。
  ◦ 无扑翼样震颤。
- 1期:
  ◦ 性格变化、易怒、抑郁、欣喜。
  ◦ 睡眠倒错。
  ◦ 书写、绘画、加、减的障碍。
  ◦ 扑翼样震颤可能存在。
- 2期:显著的行为改变,通常是不恰当的。
  ◦ 嗜睡。
  ◦ 反应缓慢。
  ◦ 扑翼样震颤。
  ◦ 口齿不清。
  ◦ 共济失调。
- 3期:
  ◦ 定向力障碍。
  ◦ 健忘。
  ◦ 偏执。
  ◦ 眼球震颤。
  ◦ 反射减弱。
  ◦ 巴宾斯基征阳性。
  ◦ 半昏睡到昏睡。
- 4期:
  ◦ 瞳孔放大。
  ◦ 昏睡或昏迷。

基本检查

• 了解肝病病史和以前的肝性脑病发作情况。

• 寻找诱因(尤其是消化道出血和感染)。

• 检查电解质异常:即使轻微异常也可能表现为显著的临床变化。

诊断检查与说明

• 血氨水平:

- 血氨水平与肝性脑病分级或脑水肿的存在相关性不大。
- 在不明原因的精神状态改变(AMS)病例中有助于诊断肝性脑病。
- 可疑肝性脑病患者伴正常的 NH_3 水平需要寻找其他导致精神状态改变的原因。
- 必须保持冷藏并在30 min内化验检测。

• 考虑隐血试验和鼻胃管(NG)灌洗以排除消化道出血。

• 排除贫血。

• 电解质、尿素氮、肌酐、葡萄糖。

• PT/INR升高提示严重的肝功能衰竭。

• 肝功能/肝酶。

• 尿路感染。

• 尿、腹水培养,寻找感染病因。

• 对意识水平改变的原因进行毒理学筛查:

- 对乙酰氨基酚和酒精浓度检测是必要的。

• 根据临床情况的额外实验室检查:

- TSH。
- 血气。
- 镁。
- 病毒血清学。

影像学检查

• 胸部X线片:排除肺炎和充血性心力衰竭。

• 头颅CT:对于新发精神状态改变、局灶性神经功能缺损、疑似脑水肿或外伤。

• 头颅MRI对门体分流但无肝病的患者肝性脑病诊断特别有帮助。

诊断步骤/外科

• 心电图:心律失常和电解质紊乱。

• 脑脊液检查:

- 新发或不明原因的恶化的肝性脑病。
- 脑脊液谷氨酰胺水平与肝性脑病的严重程度有关。

• 腹穿及腹水培养:排除自发性腹膜炎。

• 脑电图通常是不正常的,最常见的表现为广义慢化和其他非特异性改变。

鉴别诊断

• 酒精戒断综合征,包括震颤、妄想。

• 脑血管意外。

• 充血性心力衰竭。

• 二氧化碳麻醉。

• 头部创伤合并脑震荡或颅内出血。

• 低钙血症或高钙血症。

• 低血糖症。

• 低钾血症。

• 脑膜炎或脑炎。

• 代谢性脑病。

• 神经精神疾病。

• 继发于毒性混乱状态:

- 镇静剂过量。
- 酒精中毒。
- 违禁药。
- 药物治疗。
- 尿毒症。

儿科注意事项

• 即使PT只是轻度延长,也要尽早考虑Reye综合征(儿童暴发性肝功能衰竭最常见的原因)。

• 考虑脂肪酸氧化障碍:

- 冷冻血清和尿液样本供后续检测。

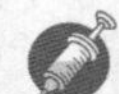

治疗

初步稳定/治疗

• 吸氧。

• 气道保护:

- 3期或4期患者可能需要插管以保护气道。丙泊酚是首选的镇静剂。

• 心电监测。

• 液体复苏。

• 精神状态改变初始治疗:

- 纳洛酮。
- 50%葡萄糖溶液(或床旁血糖测定)。
- 维生素 B_1。

急诊治疗/程序

识别和排除诱因是关键,可能会改善单独的临床印象。

> **注意**
>
> • 肝功能衰竭使患者易患低血糖和肝性脑病,这些都可能是临床表现的补充,因此频繁的血糖检查是绝对重要的。

• 早期脑水肿的识别很重要，因为必须保证脑灌注并防止脑疝(相关但不限于3、4期肝性脑病)。
• 并发症的治疗：
- 急性消化道出血。
- 脓毒症。
- 电解质酸碱紊乱。
- 凝血功能障碍。
- 肾脏和电解质紊乱。
• 尽量避免使用镇静剂/麻醉剂：
- 如必需，使用非肝脏代谢的药物。
• 促进 NH_3 的排除：
- 用不可吸收糖清洁肠道(乳果糖是主要的治疗药物)。3、4期肝性脑病首选保留灌肠。
• 减少产生 NH_3 的肠道菌群(联合乳果糖)：
- 新霉素(肾毒、耳毒)。
- 甲硝唑(口服)。
- 纠正锌缺乏。
• 预防对肝性脑病患者造成身体伤害。
• 肝移植可治疗严重的自发性或复发性肝性脑病。
• 可能有益：
- L-鸟氨酸-L-天冬氨酸(LOLA)-可能对抗乳果糖的HE有帮助。
- 支链氨基酸。
- 益生菌。
- 左卡尼汀。
- 白蛋白透析。
- 广谱抗生素覆盖范围。
- 防治作用。
- 代谢氨清除剂。
- 高渗盐水治疗脑水肿。
- 依地酸钙二钠与锰的螯合作用。

药物治疗

• 葡萄糖：50%葡萄糖，1～2安瓿(25 g)，(儿童：2 ml/kg 25%葡萄糖溶液)，静脉注射。
• 乳果糖：30 ml(儿童：0.3 ml/kg)，口服/鼻胃管 q6 h 滴定，每日2～3次软便，粪便 pH<5；或保留灌肠，300 ml 生理盐水或饮用水，q4～6 h。
• 甲硝唑：250 mg，口服/鼻胃管[儿童：10～30 mg/(kg · d)]，q8 h，2周。
• 纳洛酮：2 mg(儿童：0.1 mg/kg)，静脉注射或肌内注射，初始剂量。
• 新霉素：1～3 g[儿童：50～100 mg/(kg · d)]，口服，q6 h。
• 利福昔明：550 mg，口服或鼻胃管，q12 h(12岁以下儿童安全未知)。
• 甘露醇：0.5～1 g/kg，静脉注射。
• 硫胺素(维生素 B_1)：100 mg(儿童：50 mg)，静脉注射或肌内注射。
• 醋酸锌或硫酸锌：220 mg，口服或鼻胃管，q8 h。

入院指征

• 2、3、4期肝性脑病或社会保障不足者。
• A型肝性脑病(任何分期)和B、C型(2期或以上)应收进ICU并请消化科急会诊。
• 相关并发症(消化道出血和脓毒症)。
• 精神状态改变病因不明。

出院指征

• 已知慢性或间歇性肝性脑病。
• 0、1期，可逆性病因。
• 充分的监督和密切的跟踪。
• 适合出院的患者回家应继续：
- 低蛋白饮食。
- 乳果糖处方。

转诊问题

• 如果早期复发，请向主治医师或消化科咨询，考虑药物或饮食改变。
• 对于任何分期的A型肝性脑病，考虑转移到肝移植机构。

随访建议

• 饮食咨询。
• 酒精咨询。

要点和误区

• 考虑利福昔明治疗乳果糖抵抗性肝性脑病。
• 低血糖在肝性脑病患者中很常见。
• 尽可能避免使用镇静剂和麻醉剂。如有必要，使用非肝脏代谢的药物。

G

肝炎 Hepatitis

Duncan K. Wilson · Christopher T. Richards　陈奇通　李文放 译

基础知识

描述

• 由感染性、毒性和自身免疫性疾病引起的肝脏炎症。
- 从肝细胞损伤(肝炎)到瘢痕形成(肝硬化)的进展。

病因

• 5%～10%的急慢性肝炎病例和高达50%的暴发性肝衰竭(FHF)病因不明。
• 感染是急性肝炎最常见的病因。
• 甲型肝炎(HAV)：
- 传播：粪-口途经。
- 潜伏期：2～7周。
- 暴发性肝衰竭：0.1%。
- 无慢性期。
◦ 10%的患者会在几个月内复发。
• 乙型肝炎(HBV)：
- 传播：黏膜、经皮体液暴露、围生期。
- 潜伏期：30～180日。
- 70%为亚临床型。
- 暴发性肝衰竭：1%。
- 慢性肝炎的风险随着感染年龄和合并症的增加而增加：
◦ 新生儿：>90%。
◦ 婴儿：50%。
◦ 儿童：20%。
◦ 免疫功能正常成人：1%～5%。
◦ 免疫功能缺陷成人：50%。
- 肝硬化、肝细胞癌的风险。
• 丙型肝炎(HCV)：
- 传播：血液传播>>性传播和围生期传播。
- 潜伏期：15～160日。
- 暴发性肝衰竭少见。
- 80%慢性化。
- 有发生肝硬化、肝细胞癌的危险。
• D型肝炎(HDV)：
- 只有在HBV感染的情况下才能传播。
• 2种感染模式：同时感染HBV和HDV，或HDV重复感染一个慢性HBV患者。
- 传播：与HBV相同。
- 潜伏期：30～180日。
- 暴发性肝衰竭：3%。

- 5%慢性化。
- HDV 感染者患肝硬化的风险是单纯 HBV 感染者的 3 倍。
• E 型肝炎(HEV):
- 世界范围内最常见的急性肝炎和黄疸病因。
- 很少在发展中国家以外的地方发现。
- 通常为暴发。
- 传播:粪口,水源性,食源性。
- 潜伏期:14~60 日。
- 暴发性肝衰竭:健康成人 1%~2%,孕妇 10%~20%。
• 慢性感染几乎完全发生在免疫缺陷人群中。
• 酒精性肝炎:
- 与女性>14 杯/周和男性>21 杯/周有关。
- 长期使用的后遗症:
◦ 90%~100%的肝脂肪变性。
◦ 肝炎:10%~35%。
◦ 肝硬化:5%~15%。
- 与慢性病毒性肝炎的相关性增加。
- Maddrey 判别函数(MDF)≥32 只与 50%~65%的生存率有关。

MDF=4.6×(PT 延长)(s)+血清胆红素(mg/dl)。

• 脓肿性肝炎。
• 溶组织内阿米巴,化脓性。
• 继发性肝炎病毒。
• CMV、EBV、HSV、HIV。
• 药物和毒素诱导。
• 自身免疫性肝炎:
- 肝细胞的细胞介导的免疫攻击。
- 可能与自身免疫性疾病的个人或家族病史有关。
- 往往影响年轻到中年妇女。
• 非酒精性脂肪肝疾病:
- 是美国最常见的慢性肝病。
- 影响 25%的成人。
- 伴脂肪性肝炎,很少有肝硬化。
• 遗传性肝脏疾病:
- 威尔逊疾病。
- 血色沉着病。
- α-抗胰蛋白酶缺乏症。

儿科注意事项

• 绝大多数病例是由甲型肝炎引起的。
• 围生期 HBV 感染 90%发展为慢性疾病。

妊娠注意事项

• 妊娠期 HEV 的死亡率为 20%。
• 急性妊娠脂肪肝(AFLP):
- 可进展为 DIC。
• 溶血、肝酶升高和低血小板综合征(HELLP)。
• 妊娠期间免疫预防是安全的。

诊断

症状和体征

• 通常无症状。
• 黄疸前期:
- 发热,发冷。
- 乏力。
- 恶心,呕吐,厌食症。
- 关节痛。
- 厌恶吸烟。
• 黄疸期:
- 黄疸。
- 尿色深。
- 黏土色大便。
- 瘙痒。
- 皮疹。
- 右上象限疼痛。
• 急性肝衰竭:
- 出血。
- 精神改变。

病史

• 旅游史。
• 免疫接种史。
• 高危性行为,特别是男男性行为者(MSM)。
• 静脉吸毒史(IVDU)。
• 药物包括非处方药和草药补品。
• 使用酒精。
• 有肝脏疾病的家族史。

体格检查

• 黄疸前期:
- 发热。
- 关节炎。
- 脱水。
• 黄疸期:
- 发热。
- 皮肤、巩膜黏膜、鼓膜的黄疸。
- 非特异性斑丘疹或荨麻疹。
- 脱水
- 肝大可触及。
• FHF:
- 瘀血。
- 肝性脑病(HE)。
- 扑翼样震颤。

基本检查

• 肝炎危险因素的详细病史,包括毒物接触和药物使用。
• 病毒血清学是诊断病毒病因的主要方法。

诊断检查与说明

实验室检查

• 循环血液细胞 CBC 异常。
• 基础代谢检查:
- 暴发性肝衰竭中肝肾综合征伴氮质血症。
- 低血糖伴严重肝损伤。
- 低钠血症。
• LFT:
- 转氨酶升高反映肝细胞损伤。
- 升高的程度并不总是与严重程度相关。
- 如果碱性磷酸酶超过正常的 4 倍,应考虑原发性胆汁淤积,而不是病毒性肝炎。
- 由于排泄减少而导致的结合胆红素升高。
• 淀粉酶、脂肪酶可能提示胰腺或胆道的病因。
• PT、APTT、INR 和白蛋白:
- 测定肝脏综合功能。
- INR 延长反映了更严重的损伤。
• 氨水平:
- 精神状态改变者。
• 病毒血清学:
- HAV:
◦ 抗 HAV IgM:急性感染。
◦ 抗 HAV IgG:既往接触,免疫。
- HBV:
◦ HBsAG:急性感染(出现症状前),慢性感染。
◦ 抗-HBs:既往感染,带菌者状态,免疫后。
◦ 抗-HBc IgM:急性感染。
◦ 抗-HBc IgG:既往感染,慢性感染,带菌者状态。
◦ HBeAg:急性感染,一些慢性感染。
◦ 抗-HBe:既往感染,慢性感染,带菌者状态。
◦ 免疫者:只有抗-HBs 阳性。
- HCV:
◦ 抗-HCV:急性感染、慢性感染,首选检查项目。
◦ HCV RNA:急性感染、慢性感染,确诊。
- HDV:
◦ 抗-HDV 或病毒 RNA,非常规。
- HEV:
◦ 抗-HEV IgM:急性感染,仅 3~12 个月可检出。
◦ 抗-HCV IgG:持续数年。
• α 甲胎蛋白:
- 用于慢性乙肝或丙肝评估肝癌。
• Monospot:EBV。

G

· 尿胆红素分析。

影像学检查

· 头颅 CT 评估肝性脑病。

· 右上腹超声评估胆道梗阻。

· 肝超声多普勒评估血管闭塞情况。

鉴别诊断

· 病毒性肝炎。

· 中毒性肝炎。

· 非酒精性脂肪肝。

· 自身免疫性肝炎。

· 胆囊炎、胆管炎。

· 瑞氏综合征(Reye)。

· 肝脓肿。

· 肝豆状核变性(威尔逊病)。

· 中暑。

· Fitz-hugh-curtis 综合征。

· 缺血性肝炎("休克肝")。

· 充血性心力衰竭。

· 血色沉着病。

· Budd-Chiari 综合征。

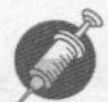

治疗

初步稳定/治疗

ABC 管理和静脉液体复苏治疗暴发性肝衰竭和重症肝性脑病。

急诊治疗/程序

· 等渗液体治疗低血容量症。

· 纠正电解质紊乱。

· 昂丹司琼、甲氧氯普胺治疗呕吐。

· 避免肝毒性药物：扑热息痛(对乙酰氯基酚)、酒精、吩噻嗪。

· 避免肝脏代谢药物：

- 镇静首选异丙酚(丙泊酚)。
- 止痛芬首选太尼。

· 活动性出血时纠正凝血功能障碍。

· N-乙酰胱氨酸(NAC)治疗对乙酰氨基酚诱导的肝炎和暴发性肝衰竭。

· 考虑类固醇治疗重症急性酒精性肝炎。

· 熊去氧胆酸或去氧胆碱治疗胆汁淤积性瘙痒。

· 腹腔穿刺术用于腹水导致的呼吸困难。

· 解毒剂和活性炭可选择性使用。

· 暴露后预防(PEP)：

- HAV：
  ○ HAV IG 0.02 ml/kg，肌内注射，接触 2 周内。
  ○ HAV 疫苗 1 ml(儿童：0.5 ml)，肌内注射。
- HBV：
  ○ HBV IG 0.06 ml/kg，肌内注射，接触 7 周内。
  ○ HBV 疫苗 1 ml(儿童：0.5 ml)，肌内注射。
- HCV 和 HDV 没有有效的免疫预防措施。
- 美国没有 HEV 疫苗。

药物治疗

· 胆碱胺：4 g，口服，每日 2～4 次，止痒。

· 甲氧氯普胺：10 mg，静脉注射或肌内注射，q6～8 h；10～30 mg，口服，每日 4 次。

· N-乙酰胱氨酸(NAC)：140 mg/kg，静脉注射，负荷剂量。

· 昂丹司琼：4 mg，静脉注射。

· 泼尼松：40 mg/d，口服。

· 维生素 B_1(硫胺素)：100 mg(儿童：50 mg)，静脉注射，肌内注射或口服。

- 如果营养不良，在葡萄糖摄入之前使用。

· 熊去氧胆酸：3 mg/kg，每日 3 次。

· 维生素 K：10 mg，静脉注射或口服。

随访

进一步处理

入院指征

· 顽固性呕吐、脱水或电解质失衡，急诊治疗无效。

· 有明显肝功能障碍的证据，收入 ICU，并考虑转移到 FHF 和急性肝炎的移植中心：

- PT＞正常值 50%或 INR＞1.5。
- 胆红素＞20 mg/dl。
- 低血糖。
- 白蛋白＜2.5 g/dl。

· 肝性脑病。

· 妊娠。

· 宿主免疫缺陷。

· 中毒性肝炎可能。

出院指征

· 电解质正常。

· 口服治疗耐受。

· 轻度肝损害。

转诊问题

· 肝病、胃肠病和传染病随访，以进一步进行血清学诊断和明确治疗。

· 酒精相关疾病的匿名戒酒互助社推荐和社会工作推荐。

随访建议

· 严格的个人卫生指导。

· 避免对乙酰氨基酚和酒精。

· 避免长时间体力活动。

要点和误区

· 急性肝炎常误诊为非特异性病毒综合征，通过血清肝功能和尿检筛查。

· 急诊治疗主要是支持性治疗。

· 详细的社会交往和旅游史。

· 暴发性肝衰竭患者早期转移到移植中心。

· 建议患者预防保健和个人卫生预防措施。

· 对症状相容的孕妇保持高度怀疑 AFLP 和 HELLP。

肝硬化 Cirrhosis

Paul J Allegretti · Rodney M. Fullmer 陈奇通 译

基础知识

描述

· 是炎症反应的发展过程，包括肝细胞损伤和坏死、弥漫性纤维化、再生结节形成。

· 小叶和血管结构缺失。

· 不可逆转的临床阶段。

· 由于肝血窦阻力增加，中央静脉受压，肝动脉和门脉系统之间出现交通吻合支，导致门静脉高压形成。

病因

· 慢性丙型肝炎(美国最常见的病因)。

· 慢性酗酒(美国第二常见原因)。

· 非酒精性脂肪肝(NAFLD)和非酒精性脂

肪性肝炎(NASH)。
• 其他：慢性乙型和/或丁型肝炎。
• 代谢障碍：
- 遗传性血色病(铁质沉着)。
- 肝豆状核变性。
- 卟啉症。
• 药物：
- 对乙酰氨基酚。
- 甲氨蝶呤。
- 胺碘酮。
- 甲基多巴。
• 肝淤血：
- 右心衰竭。
- 心包炎。
- 布-加综合征(肝静脉流出道受阻)。
• 浸润性/自身免疫性：
- 结节病。
- 淀粉样变性。
- 原发性胆管炎(PBC)或继发性(硬化性胆管炎)。
- 弥漫性浸润性肝细胞性肝癌。
• 感染：
- 布鲁菌病。
- 包虫病。
- 三期梅毒。
- 血吸虫病。

儿科注意事项

• 先天性：动肝发育不良，胆道闭锁。
• 囊性纤维化，α_1-抗胰蛋白酶缺乏。
• 代谢障碍。
• 果糖血症、酪氨酸血症、半乳糖血症、糖原累积症。
• 感染。
• 先天性乙型肝炎。

诊断

■ 症状和体征

病史

• 可能无症状。
• 起病隐匿而无特异性表现。
- 萎靡。
- 疲劳。
- 食欲不振。
- 恶心和呕吐。
- 体重减轻。
- 皮肤瘙痒。
- 皮肤色素沉着。
• 黄疸。
• 腹壁侧支循环形成，呈水母头状。
• 肝大。
• 脾大。
• 腹部不适或敏感。
• 发热。
• 肝臭。
• 扑翼样震颤。
• 低血压。
• 克-包氏杂音。
• 肾功能不全。
• 蜘蛛痣，毛细血管扩张。
• 肝掌。
• 掌腱膜挛缩。
• 腮腺和泪腺肿大。
• 特里指(趾)和白色横纹。
• 杵状指。
• 雌激素增多：
- 睾丸萎缩。
- 阳痿。
- 性欲减退。
- 男性乳房发育。
- 女性月经不调或闭经。
• 并发症：
- 并发症一旦出现，患者即考虑为失代偿期。
- 门静脉高压症。
- 腹水。
- 静脉曲张破裂出血：
◦ 1/3 的患者有静脉曲张破裂出血。
◦ 每一次出血事件有 33% 的死亡率。
◦ 肝静脉压力梯度>12 mmHg 增加出血发生率。
- 门静脉高压性胃病或消化性溃疡。
- 自发性细菌性腹膜炎。
- 肝性脑病(HE)，可能原因为：
◦ 上消化道出血。
◦ 感染。
◦ 摄入蛋白质增加。
◦ 低血钾。
◦ 镇静剂使用。
◦ 便秘。
◦ 氮质血症。
◦ 碱中毒。
- 肝性肾衰竭：
◦ 严重的肝硬化失代偿期肾血流灌注减少导致。
◦ 医源性：继发于利尿剂、非甾体抗炎药(NSAIDs)、静脉造影、氨基糖苷类抗生素、大量放腹水。
◦ 高死亡率。
- 肝肺综合征：
◦ 肺血管扩张和低氧血症。
◦ 肺泡动脉血流梯度增加的结果。

■ 基本检查

详细的病史和体格检查以发现肝病迹象。

■ 诊断检查与说明

实验室检查

• 全血细胞计数：
- 贫血。
- 巨红细胞。
- 白细胞减少症和中性粒细胞减少。
- 血小板减少。
• 肝功能损伤：
- 胆红素升高。
- 白蛋白降低。
- 球蛋白升高。
- PT 延长。
- 不同程度的 DIC。
- 低血糖症。
• 肝酶升高：
- 谷草转氨酶(AST、SGOT)、谷丙转氨酶(ALT、SGPT)——提示肝细胞损伤。
- 酒精性肝病 AST/ALT>2。
- 碱性磷酸酶和 5′核苷酸酶提示胆汁淤积。
- γ-谷氨酰转肽酶(γ-GT)。
- 在非活动期肝硬化可能正常。
• 电解质，尿素氮，肌酐。
• 低钠血症：
- 肾功能不全或肝肾综合征。
• 以下情况时查动脉血气或脉搏氧饱和度：
- 疑似肺炎。
- 充血性心力衰竭。
- 肝肺综合征。
• 寻找病因：
- 乙肝表面抗原。
- 丙肝抗体。
- 抗核抗体(ANA)和抗平滑肌抗体(自身免疫性肝炎)。
- 血清抗线粒体抗体(原发性胆汁性肝硬化，PBC)。
- 血清铁，转铁蛋白饱和度，铁蛋白(血沉着病)。
- 血浆铜蓝蛋白(肝豆状核变性，Wilson 病)。
- α_1-抗胰蛋白酶缺乏。
- 血清免疫电泳(PBC 时高 IgM)。
- 胆固醇(慢性胆汁淤积)。
- 甲胎蛋白(肝细胞癌)。

影像学检查

• 超声检查用于肝脏结构、胆道阻塞、腹水、

G

门静脉血栓、脾大。

• 腹部 CT 扫描来探索超声的异常发现。

• X 线平片用于检查胸腔积液、心脏肥大、充血性心力衰竭。

诊断步骤/外科

• 食管胃十二指肠镜（EGD）显示上消化道出血或静脉曲张检测。

• 静脉曲张套扎或内镜下硬化剂治疗。

• 大量腹水或自发性腹膜炎时行腹腔穿刺术。

■ 鉴别诊断

• 腹水：

- 右心压力增加。

- 肝门静脉血栓。

- 腹膜恶性肿瘤/感染。

- 胰腺疾病。

- 甲状腺疾病。

- 淋巴管阻塞。

• 上消化道出血：

- 消化性溃疡。

- 胃炎。

• 颅脑疾病：

- 代谢异常。

- 中毒。

- 颅内疾病过程。

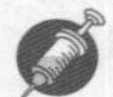

治疗

■ 院前

• 纳洛酮、右旋糖（或者 Accu-Chekk）、维生素 B_1 以改善精神状态。

• 静脉补液以纠正低血压防止急性缺血性肝损伤。

■ 初步稳定/治疗

• 处理并发症如上消化道出血或肝性脑病。

■ 急诊治疗/程序

• 若怀疑静脉曲张破裂出血：

- 静脉给予质子泵抑制剂。

- 静脉给予奥曲肽收缩内脏血管。

- 纠正凝血功能障碍。

◦ 输入新鲜冰冻血浆，1 U/h 直到出血控制。

◦ 去氨加压素（DDAVP），改善出血时间和 PT 延长。

- 三腔二囊管气囊压迫曲张静脉止血（很少使用，推荐预防性气管插管）。

- 紧急内镜下硬化剂治疗。

• 怀疑脓毒血症或自发性腹膜炎时立即开始使用广谱抗生素：

- 头孢噻肟。

- 替卡西林-克拉维酸。

- 哌拉西林-他唑巴坦。

- 氨苄西林-舒巴坦。

• 处理并发症，如腹水、肝性脑病、自发性腹膜炎。

• 治疗瘙痒症：

- 苯海拉明：25～50 mg，静脉注射或肌内注射，q4 h。

- 消胆胺、熊去氧胆酸或利福平。

- 纳洛酮：0.2 μg/(kg · min) 静脉输注以临时缓解危急情况。

• β受体阻滞剂（普萘洛尔）用于食管静脉曲张：

- 使脉搏下降至 60 次/分或者静息状态下脉搏减少 25%。

- 用或者不用硝酸异山梨酯。

- 减少再出血发生率。

- 可能延缓或阻止第一次出血发生。

• 用内镜、X 线或外科手术方法解除胆道梗阻（如狭窄）。

• 提供营养饮食，高热量和足够的蛋白质（1 g/kg），除非并发肝性脑病。

• 任何时候肝移植术后患者在急诊室出现肝功能异常，疑似脓毒血症或治疗相关并发症需及时咨询肝移植协调员。

■ 特殊治疗

• 血色病：静脉放血疗法或去铁胺（铁螯合剂）。

• 自身免疫性肝炎：泼尼松加或不加咪唑硫嘌呤。

• 慢性乙肝或丙肝：干扰素 α（肝硬化失代偿期避免使用）。

• 原发性胆汁性肝硬化：熊去氧胆酸。

• 肝豆状核变性：青霉胺。

• 肝移植是治疗肝硬化唯一的最先进的方法。

■ 药物治疗

• 咪唑硫嘌呤：1～2 mg/kg，每日口服。

• 头孢噻肟：1～2 g，q6～8 h[儿童：50～180 mg/(kg · d)，q6 h]，静脉注射。

• 消胆胺：4～6 g，口服，1～5 次/日。

• 去氨加压素（DDAVP）：0.3 mc/kg 加入 50 ml 生理盐水，输注时间超过 20～30 min。

• 右旋糖：$D_{50}W$ 1 安瓿（50 ml 或 25 g；儿童 $D_{25}W$ 2～4 ml/kg），静脉注射。

• 纳洛酮：初始剂量 0.2～2 mg（儿童：0.1 mg/kg），静脉注射或肌内注射。

• 乳果糖：15～30 ml，每日 3 次，目标是每日大便 2～3 次。

• 奥曲肽：静脉注射 25～50 μg，然后静脉滴注 50 μg/h。

• 哌拉西林-他唑巴坦：3.375 g，静脉注射，q6 h[儿童：100～400 mg/(kg · d)，静脉滴注，q6～8 h；肾功能计量给药]。

• 泼尼松：每日 40 mg（儿童：1～2 mg/kg），口服。

• 普萘洛尔：40 mg（初始剂量）～240 mg[儿童：1～5 mg/(kg · d)]，口服，每日 3 次。

• 利福平：每日 600 mg（儿童：10～20 mg/kg），口服。

• 维生素 B_1：100 mg（儿童：50 mg），静脉注射或肌内注射。

• 熊去氧胆酸：13～15 mg/(kg · d)，每日 3 次。

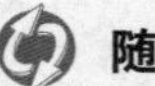

随访

■ 进一步处理

入院指征

• 有严重的失代偿或并发症情况。

• 在门诊不能进行病情检查的情况下，第一次临床表现为明显的肝硬化。

• 分级高的肝性脑病、脓毒血症、活动性上消化道出血、肝肾综合征和肝肺综合征需入住重症监护室。

• 晚期肝细胞癌。

出院指征

大多数代偿性肝硬化患者可以在门诊治疗。

■ 随访建议

所有新的胃肠道疾病病例。

要点和误区

• 预后是高度可变的。

• 患者出现各种各样的迹象和症状与晚期肝病有关。

• 新的情况需要全面检查和胃肠科会诊。

• 任何并发症可导致患者失代偿状态。

• 自发性腹膜炎症状经常是模糊的：

- 考虑为自发性腹膜炎时大多数是高度怀疑和低反应域而需腹腔穿刺术。

G

肛裂 Anal Fissure

Julia H. Sone　马林浩　林兆奋 译

基础知识

描述

- 坚硬粪便通过，割裂肛膜。
- 线性撕裂从齿状线延伸到肛膜：
  - 前中线 95%。
  - 前中线 5%。
  - 外部：形成皮赘或前哨痔。
  - 内部：形成肥厚的肛门乳头。
  - 慢性裂隙可能会发现前哨痔内侧括约肌纤维。

病因

- 压力或过度紧张的肛门括约肌导致后部外胚层的局部缺血。
- 腹泻或硬便会撕裂中胚层。
- 肛门性交或性虐待的局部创伤可能是原因。
- 侧裂指示潜在的全身性疾病：
  - 克罗恩病。
  - 肛门癌。
  - 白血病。
  - 梅毒。
  - 既往肛门手术。

诊断

症状和体征

- 通常在卫生纸上出现的来自直肠的红色血液。
- 排便时剧烈、切割、阵发性或灼痛：
  - 可能持续数小时。
- 便秘，由于疼痛无法通过粪便：
  - 硬而有棱角的粪便。

病史

- 硬便或便秘。
- 腹泻的表现。
- 在卫生纸有清楚的红色血液。

体格检查

肛门检查：

- 显露臀部并让患者忍耐以显示裂缝。
- 严重的疼痛通常会妨碍手动或指诊：
  - 在尝试直肠指诊之前使用利多卡因或外用利多卡因 ELA - Max5 软膏。
  - 需要排除脓肿或肿瘤。

儿科注意事项

可以使用透明试管作为肛门镜来观察肛管/裂隙。

基本检查

仔细的直肠检查。

诊断检查与说明

实验室检查

如果病史提示严重出血，查血细胞比容。

影像学检查

CT 骨盆：

如果直肠检查可触及肿块，排除肛门直肠脓肿、肿瘤。

鉴别诊断

- 克罗恩病。
- 慢性溃疡性结肠炎。
- 肛肠癌。
- 直肠周围脓肿。
- 血栓痔。
- 性虐待。
- 肺结核。
- 梅毒。
- 淋巴瘤。
- 白血病。
- 既往肛门手术。

治疗

院前

为直肠大出血患者建立静脉通道。

初步稳定/治疗

给有明显疼痛的患者服用止痛药。

急救治疗/程序

- 静脉、肌内注射或口服止痛药：非甾体抗炎药、对乙酰氨基酚、肌肉松弛剂缓解括约肌痉挛(环苯扎林、地西泮、2%地尔硫䓬软膏、0.3%硝苯地平软膏)。
- 表面麻醉药：5%利多卡因霜剂(ELA - Max5)、2%利多卡因凝胶剂。
- 坐浴(用温水)以缓解括约肌痉挛。

饮食

- 高纤维饮食指导：
  - 纤维/麸皮：20 g/d。
  - 车前草种子(metamucil 或 Konsyl)：1～2 茶匙(儿童：0.25～1 tsp/d)，口服，q24 h。
- 鼓励每日食用 10～12 oz 的水(1 oz 约 30 ml)。

药物治疗

- 环苯扎林(flexeril)：10 mg(儿童：未标明)，口服，每日 3 次。
- 地西泮(安定)：5 mg[儿童：0.12～0.8 mg/(kg · d)]，口服，每日 3 次，PRN 用于痉挛。
- 地尔硫䓬 2%软膏：适用于裂隙，每日 2 次。
- 多库酯钠(Colace)：50～200 mg(儿童：<3 岁，10～40 mg/d；3～6 岁，20～60 mg/d；6～12 岁，40～150 mg/d)，口服，q12 h。
- ELA - Max5(5%利多卡因肛肠膏)：适用于肛周区域 q4 h，PRN 疼痛(小儿剂量：不适合 12 岁以下者)。
- 布洛芬：400～600 mg[儿童：40 mg/(kg · d)]，口服，q6 h。
- 0.3%硝苯地平软膏：涂抹于裂隙，每日 3 次(儿童：未标明)。
- 0.2%硝酸甘油软膏：用棉签涂抹于裂隙，少量豌豆大小，每日 2～3 次(儿童：未标明)。

随访

进一步处理

入院指征

因粪便嵌塞引起的严重腹痛或腹胀。

出院指征

- 初始治疗是作为门诊患者的急性肛裂的保守疗法。
- 慢性肛裂的手术治疗。

随访建议

有症状的肛裂患者的结直肠或胃肠道随访。

要点和误区

- 对直肠区域进行仔细的检查，以描绘肛裂并排除其他病变。
- 为患有明显疼痛的患者提供缓解疼痛和肌肉松弛剂的组合治疗。
- 提供出院药物、指导以防止便秘。

高钙血症

Ryan A. Stroder · Ryan H. Wyatt 巩博 译

基础知识

描述

- 严重性与血清钙水平和上升情况有关。
- 0.1%～1%的患者常规筛查结果异常。
- 大部分情况为轻度高钙(<12 mg/dl),无症状。
- 高钙血危象,通常>14 mg/dl,引起严重的症状和体征。
- 血液中的钙存在 3 种形式:
  - 离子形式:45%。
  - 与蛋白质结合(主要是白蛋白):40%。
  - 与其他阴离子结合:15%。
- 离子钙:唯一有生理活性的形式。

病因

- 原发性甲状旁腺功能亢进症。
- 恶性肿瘤。
- 前两者占 80%。
- 其他多种原因。

诊断

症状和体征

病史

- 神经系统:
  - 头痛。
  - 疲乏与嗜睡。
  - 体弱。
  - 注意力不集中。
  - 意识混乱。
  - 抑郁与妄想。
  - 幻觉。
- 肾:
  - 多尿与多饮。
  - 少尿型肾衰竭相关疾病。
  - 慢性和以下相关的疾病:
    - 肾结石。
    - 肾钙质沉着症。
    - 间质性肾炎。
- 消化系统:
  - 厌食。
  - 恶心与呕吐。
  - 腹痛。
  - 便秘。
  - 慢性和以下相关的疾病:
    - 消化性溃疡。
    - 胰腺炎。
- 皮肤病:
  - 瘙痒。

儿科注意事项

- 发育不良。
- 发展迟缓。
- 可能出现精神发育迟缓。

体格检查

- 神经系统:
  - 易怒。
  - 嗜睡。
  - 昏睡。
  - 昏迷。
  - 反射减弱。
- 心血管系统:
  - 如果严重耗竭,出现低血压或高血压。
  - 窦性心动过缓。
  - 严重高钙血症出现心搏骤停(少见)。
- 肾:
  - 脱水的症状。
- 皮肤:
  - 带状角膜病变。
  - 异位钙化。

儿科注意事项

- 特征面相:狮子鼻、胖鼻梁、“丘比特之弓”样上唇。
- 张力减退。

基本检查

- 离子钙和总血清钙水平、白蛋白水平:
  - 正常总钙水平<10.5 mg/dl。
  - 必须校正蛋白结合钙,主要是白蛋白。
  - 校正总钙(mg/dl)=测得的总钙(mg/dl)+0.8×[4.0－白蛋白浓度(g/dl)]。
- 电解质、尿素氮/肌酐、葡萄糖。
  - 可能出现少尿型肾衰竭。
- 心电图:
  - QT 间期缩短。
  - PR 间期延长。
  - QRS 波群增宽。
  - 增强地高辛的副作用。
  - 窦性心动过缓、束支传导阻滞、房室阻滞、严重高钙血症出现心搏骤停(少见)。
  - 通常和低体温一起引起 Osborn J 波,出现在 QRS 波群的末端。
  - ST 段抬高。

诊断检查与说明

实验室检查

- 磷酸盐。
- 蛋白质。
- 尿液分析。
- 甲状旁腺激素(PTH)水平:
  - 如果升高或者正常高值,可能为原发性甲状旁腺功能亢进。
  - 如果<20 pg/ml,考虑检查 PTH 相关肽和维生素 D 代谢物。
- 维生素 D 代谢:
  - 25-羟基维生素 D(骨化二醇):
    - 如果升高,考虑外源性(如药物、维生素、补充剂)。
  - 1,25-二羟基维生素 D(骨化三醇):
    - 如果升高,考虑淋巴瘤或者肉瘤。
- 口服地高辛的话,监测地高辛水平。
- 甲状腺功能检查。

影像学检查

- 精神状态改变查头颅 CT。
- 如果没有其他引起高钙血症的原因,检查胸部 X 线,筛查潜在的恶性肿瘤。

诊断步骤/外科

甲状旁腺切除术:

- 原发性甲状旁腺功能亢进出现症状或者严重的高钙血症。
- 有些患者需要紧急甲状旁腺切除术。

鉴别诊断

- 原发性甲状旁腺功能亢进:
  - 门诊患者的常见病因。
  - 甲状旁腺腺瘤 80%;增生 15%;癌 5%。
  - 程度较轻,<11.2 mg/dl。
  - 患者可无症状或血钙缓慢上升。
  - 增强骨吸收,钙分泌相对减少,增强肠道钙吸收。
- 恶性肿瘤:
  - 住院患者的常见病因。
  - 通常血清钙快速上升。
  - 患者多数有症状。
  - 更高的血清钙浓度。
  - 常见于伴癌综合征。
  - 引起高钙血症的常见肿瘤:乳腺、肺、结肠、胃、宫颈、子宫、卵巢、肾、膀胱、头和颈部的肿瘤,以及多发骨髓瘤、淋巴瘤。

G

- 多数和 PTH 相关蛋白有类似作用。
- 可能与肿瘤产生的增强骨吸收的其他产物有关。
- 可能由局部溶骨性骨转移造成。

• 其他：
- 高钙血症相关的肉芽肿病。
- 过多的钙补充剂。
- 噻嗪类利尿药引起肾重吸收增加。
- 家族性低钙尿高钙血症。
- 急性维生素 A 中毒。
- 外源性维生素 D 摄入。
- 过多进食钙和不能吸收的抗酸药，如牛奶或者碳酸钙，会引起乳碱综合征。
- 长期锂治疗。
- 肾移植。
- 甲状腺功能亢进。
- 急性肾小管坏死。

儿科注意事项

鉴别诊断：与成人不同：

• 原发性甲状旁腺功能亢进：
- 比成人少见。

• 婴儿高钙血症：
- 原因不明。
- 可能高度敏感并且在宫内过度暴露于维生素 D。

• 制动性高钙血症：
- 常见于快速生长的青少年。
- 长期制动，尤其在牵引的患者，导致高钙尿，然后高钙血症。
- 大概因为骨吸收增强，同时骨矿化减少或者停滞。

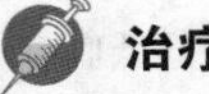

治疗

院前

常规稳定技术。

初步稳定/治疗

• ABC 管理，建立静脉通道，吸氧，心电监测。

• 低血压或者严重脱水患者生理盐水 1 L 快推(20 ml/kg)。

• 精神状态改变予纳洛酮、硫胺素、50%葡萄糖(或血清葡萄糖测量)。

急诊治疗/程序

• 整体治疗：
- 无论症状如何，严重高钙血症(校正总钙>14 mg/dl)都需要紧急治疗。症状性高钙血症也需要紧急治疗。
- 无症状或者轻度高钙血症不需要急诊治疗。

• 补液量：
- 生理盐水：
  ○ 200～300 ml/h，调整维持尿量 100～150 ml/h。
  ○ 一般每日需要 2～5 L。
  ○ 必须警惕超负荷补液。
  ○ 纠正其他电解质异常。
  ○ 有心血管疾病的患者需要检测中心静脉压来调整补液量。

• 肾排泄：
- 补液之后，如果需要避免液体超负荷，使用髓袢利尿剂(呋塞米)。
- 避免使用噻嗪类利尿剂。
- 在肾衰竭中，可能需要腹膜或者血液透析，使用低钙透析液。

• 抑制破骨活动：
- 减少骨钙动员。
- 当校正钙水平>14 mg/dl 或者出现症状体征时，使用药物治疗。
- 一线药物：
  ○ 二磷酸盐：帕米膦酸二钠(更有效，毒性可能更少)、依替膦酸钠。
  ○ 降钙素：起效快，适度速度下降。
- 其他潜在药物治疗：
  ○ 普卡霉素：有效但是有许多副作用。
  ○ 氢化可的松：伴有恶性肿瘤、肉芽肿疾病、维生素 D 中毒时，尤其有效。
  ○ 在合适的患者鼓励步行。

• 治疗潜在疾病：
- 对于有症状或者高钙血症的原发性甲状旁腺功能亢进，行甲状旁腺切除术。
- 如果药物引起高钙血症，终止药物治疗。

药物治疗

一线用药

• 唑来膦酸：4 mg，静脉注射 15 min。

• 帕米膦酸钠：60～90 mg，静脉注射单次 2～24 h 输液(儿童：咨询儿科医师)。

二线用药

• 降钙素：4 U/kg，肌内注射或皮下注射，q12 h。

• 氢化可的松：200～400 mg/d，静脉注射，持续 3～5 日(儿童：咨询儿科医师)。

• 泼尼松：40 mg/d，持续 2～4 日。

• 德尼单抗：向专家咨询剂量指导。

• 西那卡塞：向专家咨询用药指导。

儿科注意事项

• 婴儿很少需要髓袢利尿剂，因为它可能减少肾小球滤过率，加重高钙血症，对婴儿产生有害作用。

• 在儿童，二磷酸盐尚无大量研究资料，但是显示是安全的。

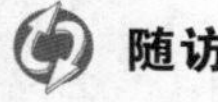

随访

进一步处理

入院指征

• 校正总钙水平>13 mg/dl。

• 高钙血症产生的症状和体征，尤其是心电图变化。

• 校正总钙水平>14 mg/dl 或者严重症状体征入住监控床或者 ICU。

出院指征

校正总钙水平<13 mg/dl，并且没有高钙血症的症状体征。

转诊问题

• 快速安排查找病因和长期治疗。

• 考虑内分泌科医师会诊。

随访建议

• 保持正常水合状态。

• 观察有无精神状态改变。

要点和误区

• 在症状和校正钙的基础上做决定。

• 不管症状如何，所有血清钙>14 mg/dl 的患者需要治疗。

• 足够重视心电图变化。

• 接受静脉补液的患者，需要密切监护：
- 他们一般需要大量液体，但是必须注意防止补液过多。

高钾血症 Hyperkalemia

Stella C. Wong 巩博 译

基础知识

描述

• 高钾血症：血清钾＞5.5 mmol/L。

- 轻度：5.5～6.4 mmol/L。
- 中度：6.5～7.5 mmol/L。
- 重度：＞7.5 mmol/L。

• 体内 98%的钾都在细胞内。

• 细胞钾离子梯度由 Na^+ - K^+ - ATP 酶维持。

• 细胞内和细胞外钾梯度的作用：

- 静息细胞膜电位。
- 心脏活动。
- 肌肉和神经活动。

病因

• 增加摄入量：

- 补充钾。
- 富含钾的食物。
- 红细胞输血。

• 排泄：受损。

- 急性肾损伤。
- 醛固酮减少症。
- 原发性肾小管缺损。

• 假性高钾血症：

- 溶血。
- 静脉注射钾液。
- 冷冻样本。

• 药物诱导：

- 血管紧张素转换酶抑制剂。
- 保留钾利尿剂。
- 青霉素钾。

诊断

症状和体征

• 虚弱。

• 心慌。

• 尿样改变。

• 呼吸急促。

病史

• 增加从食物中口服钾的摄入量。

• 服用含钾的药物。

体格检查

• 可以正常。

• 生命体征：血压正常、血压过高或低血压。

• 一般：虚弱。

• 心血管：心动过速、心动过缓、心音不规则。

• 腹部：腹部弥漫性压痛。

• 考虑自发性细菌性腹膜炎与腹膜透析患者的腹痛。需要送去腹膜透析液，与患者肾病医师商量，开始静脉注射抗生素。

• 神经：精神状态改变，反应迟钝。

• 检查透析导管、瘘管或移植物。

基本检查

• 电解质、BUN、肌酐、葡萄糖。

• 心电图。

诊断检查与说明

实验室检查

• 电解质，BUN，肌酐，葡萄糖。

• BUN 升高：肾衰竭。

• 静脉血气（VBG）：

- 酸碱状态。
- 快速评估钾。

• 尿钠：

- ＞25 mmol/L：计算肾小管钾梯度（TTKG）确定是否为盐皮质激素缺乏症。
- ＜25 mmol/L：急性肾损伤。

• TTKG＝［K（尿）/K（血）］×［渗透压（血）/渗透压（尿）］。

- TTKG＜6：肾元远端醛固酮生物活性受损。
- TTKG＞6：钾超载或细胞转移。

影像学检查

• 如果患者呼吸短促，请行胸部 X 线检查：

- 评估肺水肿、容量超负荷，尤其是透析患者。

• 心电图：

- 血钾＞5 mmol/L：T 波高尖。
- 血钾 6.5～7.5 mmol/L：P 波消失，QRS 延长，异位。
- 血钾＞7.5 mmol/L：正弦波。

鉴别诊断

不限于以下内容：

• 假高钾血症（实验室报道高钾血症为静脉切开溶血伪影）。

• 糖尿病的紧急情况。

• 病毒性疾病。

• 心肌梗死。

• 脑血管意外。

• 心律失常（由潜在心脏病引起）。

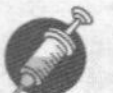

治疗

院前

• 监测。

• 生命体征。

• 如果可能的话，建立静脉通路。

• 心电图。

• 如果患者病情不稳定或心电图异常，呼叫医师指导。

• 送往最近的急救室。

初步稳定/治疗

• 基础生命支持。

• 心电监测。

• 心电图（即使用 EMS 也要重复）。

• 如果 EMS 没有做，建立静脉通路。

• 容量复苏，如果需要。

• 实验室（VBG 或 ABG 可以快速评估 pH 和钾值，特别是在紧急情况下）。

急诊治疗/程序

• 主要目的是稳定心肌细胞膜。

• 轻度至中度高钾血症（5.5～7.5 mmol/L）稳定且心电图无变化患者：

- 低血压患者静脉液体复苏（小心不要超载肾衰竭或 CHF 患者）。
- D_{50} 25 g，静脉注射。
- 胰岛素 5～10 mg，静脉注射（注意低血糖）。
- 葡萄糖酸钙 1 g，静脉注射，如果 $K^+ \geqslant$ 6 mmol/L。
- 沙丁胺醇（10～20 mg）雾化。
- 治疗潜在的原因。

• 生命体征异常、心电图改变、重度高钾血症（＞7.5 mmol/L）患者：

- 低血压患者静脉液体复苏（小心不要超载肾衰竭或 CHF 患者）。
- D_{50} 25 g，静脉注射。
- 胰岛素 5～10 mg，静脉注射（注意低血糖）。
- 氯化钙 1 g，静脉注射。
- 沙丁胺醇（10～20 mg）雾化。
- 如果酸中毒，考虑 50～100 mmol，静脉注射碳酸氢钠。
- 肾内科急会诊。
- 如果患者是透析患者：紧急透析。

• 心搏骤停：

G

- ACLS。
- 静脉输液复苏。
- D_{50} 25 g,静脉注射。
- 胰岛素 5～10 mg。
- 氯化钙 1 g,静脉注射。
- 碳酸氢钠 50～100 mmol。

■ 药物治疗

• 急性治疗:
- 葡萄糖酸钙:1 g,静脉注射。
- 氯化钙:1 g,静脉注射。
- D_{50}:25 g,静脉注射。
- 常规胰岛素:5～10 U。
- 沙丁胺醇:10～20 mg 雾化。
- 碳酸氢钠:50～100 mmol。

• 亚急性治疗:
- 聚苯乙烯磺酸钠(Kayexalate):15 g,口服,1～4 次/日;或灌肠 30～50 g, q6 h。

 随访

■ 进一步处理

入院指征

• 轻度高钾血症伴心电图改变、生命体征异常或治疗后持续高血钾。
• 中度血钾过高。
• 严重高钾血症。
• 伴有高钾血症的新急性肾损伤。

出院指征

• 轻度高钾血症,心电图无变化,生命体征正常,治疗后高钾血症消退后续建议。
• 肾脏和初级护理医师密切随访。

要点和误区

• 如果血钾>6 mmol/L 或有心电图改变,给予钙剂。
• 钙只是一种心脏膜稳定剂,其他高钾血症治疗也需要。
• 静脉注射胰岛素治疗高钾血症慎防低血糖。
• 静脉注射胰岛素前检查患者血糖。
• 透析(血液透析和腹膜透析)高钾血症患者需要透析。
• 腹膜透析患者的腹痛考虑自发性细菌性腹膜炎。

高钠血症 Hypernatremia

Linda Mueller 巩博 译

 基础知识

■ 描述

高钠血症的定义:血清钠>145 mmol/L。
• 轻度高钠血症:血清钠 146～155 mmol/L。
• 严重高钠血症:血清钠>155 mmol/L。

■ 病因

分为 3 种类别。

低容量性高钠血症

• 最常见。
• 水和钠丢失或不足,但是水丢失比钠丢失更多。
• 例如:
- 肾衰竭。
- 药物治疗(如利尿剂、乳果糖)。
- 渗透性利尿(甘露醇、糖尿、高蛋白质饮食)。
- 隐性水分丢失(烧伤、出汗)。
- 呼吸丢失。
- 缺陷性口渴机制。
- 腹泻与呕吐。
- 插管患者。

等容量性高钠血症

• 水不足不伴有钠丢失,自由水丢失。
• 例如:
- 发热。
- 下丘脑性尿崩症(DI):
◦ 头部创伤。
◦ 肿瘤。
◦ 先天性。
◦ 感染(结核、梅毒、真菌、弓形虫、脑炎)。
◦ 肉芽肿疾病(肉样瘤、Wegner 肉芽肿)。
◦ 脑血管意外。
◦ 动脉瘤。
- 肾性尿崩:
◦ 先天性。
◦ 药物(锂、两性霉素 B、膦甲酸、地美环素)。
◦ 梗阻性肾病。
◦ 慢性小管间质性疾病(镰状细胞性肾病、多发性骨髓瘤、淀粉样变性、肉状瘤病、系统性红斑狼疮、多囊肾)。
◦ 电解质紊乱(高钙血症、钾缺乏)。

高容量性高钠血症

• 摄入水和钠,获得的钠比水多。
• 例如:
- 医源性:最常见原因。
◦ 输注碳酸氢钠。
◦ NaCl 片。
◦ 肠外高渗性营养。
◦ 静脉注射高渗性液体。
◦ 高渗性透析。
◦ 高渗性药物治疗,如羟基噻吩西林和羧苄西林。
- 库欣病。
- 肾上腺增生。
- 海水淹溺。

儿科注意事项

• 更倾向于医源性原因。
• 更容易死亡或者有永久神经系统后遗症。
• 死亡率从 25%到 50%。
• 可能出现尖叫、昏睡、易怒、肌无力。
• 在新生儿,母乳喂养不良和不合适的配方奶粉是潜在原因。
• 如果高钠血症由酮症酸中毒引起,按照儿童酮症酸中毒方案进行液体复苏。
• 去氨加压素在 3 个月至 12 岁患儿可经鼻给药,5～30 μg/d。
- 考虑鼻胃管补液。

老年人注意事项

• 最常见的原因是肾浓缩功能受损和口渴机制下降。
• 如果根本原因是单纯脱水,考虑忽视它。

妊娠注意事项

• 可能遇到妊娠期短暂尿崩症。
• 去氨加压素和抗利尿激素是妊娠期 B 类别药物。
• 水合状态很难通过检查来精确评估。

诊断

■ 症状和体征

• 多数症状归因于根本病因(如脱水)。
• 多数有急性改变。
• 钠≥185 mmol/L,很有可能出现死亡。

G

- 通常钠≥160 mmol/L，可能出现下列症状：
  - 神经系统：
    - 头痛。
    - 震颤。
    - 烦躁。
    - 共济失调。
    - 精神错乱。
    - 谵妄。
    - 惊厥。
    - 昏迷。
    - 反射亢进。
    - 扑翼样震颤。
    - 舞蹈病。
    - 蛛网膜下腔、颅内、硬膜下出血。
    - 硬脑膜静脉窦血栓形成。
  - 骨骼肌系统：
    - 痉挛。
    - 肌无力。
    - 肌肉抽搐。
  - 其他：
    - 厌食。
    - 呼吸急促。
    - 皮肤弹性差。
    - 恶心与呕吐。

低容量性高钠血症

- 心动过速。
- 体位性低血压。
- 皮肤黏膜干燥。
- 尿少。
- 氮质血症。

高容量性高钠血症

- 肺水肿。
- 周围性水肿。

体格检查

- 评估水合状态。
- 观察黏膜、颈静脉及皮肤弹性。
- 进行完整的神经系统检查，在急救室期间，自始至终重复检查。
- 获取直立时生命体征。

基本检查

血清 Na^+ 水平。

诊断检查与说明

实验室检查

- 电解质、尿素氮/肌酐、血糖。
- 全血细胞计数。
- 尿液分析：
  - 尿比重。
  - 尿/血渗透压。
  - 尿 Na^+。

影像学检查

- X线胸片：
  - 检查感染/呼吸系统。
  - 高容量高钠血症伴有肺水肿。
- 脑CT：
  - 精神状态改变。
  - 硬脑膜静脉窦血栓形成。
  - 蛛网膜下腔出血。
  - 硬膜下血肿。

诊断步骤/外科

需要精确监测出入量时考虑尿管。

鉴别诊断

- 糖尿病酮酸中毒。
- 高渗性昏迷。
- 原发性中枢神经系统病变。

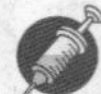

治疗

院前

如果低容量或者有血流动力学不稳的证据予以容量复苏。

初步稳定/治疗

- ABC管理。
- 严重低血压予以生理盐水快速静推。
- 精神状态改变予以纳洛酮、硫胺素、50%葡萄糖(或血糖检查)。

急诊治疗/程序

通用：

- 计算失水量：
  - 失水量＝0.6(体重 kg)×(1－需补钠/实际钠)。
- 不要快速纠正高渗至正常血渗透压：
  - 快速纠正可能引起惊厥。
  - 降低血清钠水平＜0.5～0.7 mmol/(L·h)。

低容量性高钠血症

- 使用生理盐水快速静推改善容量不足。
- 一旦容量补足或者血流动力学稳定改为5%葡萄糖注射液或低渗盐水。

等容量性高钠血症

- 计算失水量。
- 使用5%葡萄糖注射液或者低渗盐水纠正水不足：
  - 第一个24 h补充缺水量的一半，剩余部分通过1～2日补足。

高容量性高钠血症

- 使用利尿剂或透析去除多余的水。
- 补液时，使用5%葡萄糖补充水缺乏。
- 避免使用高渗性盐水溶液，因为患者已经有过多的钠。

尿崩症高钠血症

- 限制钠摄入。
- 去氨加压素：
  - 水剂加压素(DDAVP)。
  - 最佳治疗药物。
- 氯磺丙脲加强抗利尿激素在肾小管的作用。
- 卡马西平引起抗利尿激素释放。
- 氢氯噻嗪加强肾排泄。
- 停止使用引起尿崩的药物。

药物治疗

- 氯磺丙脲：100～500 mg/d。
- 抗利尿激素(DDAVP)：1～2 μg，静脉注射或皮下注射，q12 h，或者5～20 μg经鼻给药。

一线用药

纠正容量开始时使用盐水。

二线用药

治疗根本病因。

随访

进一步处理

入院指征

- 新诊断的血钠＞150 mmol/L，需要监测和治疗。
- 钠＞160 mmol/L或者有症状的患者入住ICU。

出院指征

- 钠＜150 mmol/L无症状的患者。
- 钠＞150 mmol/L有钠慢性升高病史的患者，而钠在他们的基线，且没有症状。

随访建议

1周内重复检测血钠水平。

要点和误区

- 高达30%的急性高钠血症患者将有神经系统后遗症，一份完整的证据充分的神经系统检查是必需的。
- 急性高钠血症的死亡率在28%～70%。
- 如果使用生理盐水监测高氯血症。
- 高龄患者伴有慢性疾病最容易出现神经系统并发症：
  - 进行性水丢失可能需要重新计算需要补充的水量。
  - 重复实验室检查以确认控制补钠量。

高黏滞综合征 Hyperviscosity Syndrome

Brooks L. Moore · Erika Phindile Chowa 巩博 译

 基础知识

■ 描述

- 高黏滞综合征(HVS)是血液黏稠度增加引起的临床症状。
- 经典临床症状三联征：黏膜出血、视力障碍和神经系统症状。
- 黏稠度是一种材料改变形状遇到的阻力。
- 血液黏稠度越高，血液流动的内部阻力越高。
- 需要提高心输出量使高黏稠血液维持足够的灌注。
- 经过微循环系统时流动缓慢，氧输送功能受损。微循环系统氧合障碍产生了该综合征的临床症状。

■ 病因

- 当血液中的细胞或非细胞成分增加，发生高黏滞综合征。
- 非细胞(蛋白质)性高黏血症：
  - 高黏血症最常见的病因(85%～90%)是γ球蛋白浓度增加：
    - 单克隆丙种球蛋白病：见于一些恶性疾病，如瓦氏巨球蛋白血症和多发性骨髓瘤。
    - 多细胞系丙种球蛋白病：常见于风湿性疾病(非常少见)。
- 细胞(血细胞)性高黏血症：
  - 少见(10%～15%)。
  - 在真性红细胞增多症中，红细胞数量增加。
  - 在急性和慢性白血病中，白细胞浓度增加(>100 000/mm^3)。
  - 血小板增多。

诊断

■ 症状和体征

- 经典三联征：
  - 黏膜出血。
  - 视力障碍。
  - 神经系统症状。
- 原发性：
  - 发热。
  - 消瘦。
  - 盗汗。
  - 疲劳。
- 血液：
  - 出血是最常见的表现。推测机制是血小板功能异常。
  - 鼻出血。
  - 牙龈、直肠、子宫出血。
  - 手术后长期出血。
  - 血液恶病质。
  - 红细胞破坏后产物引起皮肤瘙痒。
  - 脾脏增大。
  - 淋巴结病。
- 眼睛：
  - 视力改变：
  - 模糊。
  - 复视。
  - 视力下降。
  - 眼底检查血管呈"腊肠样"改变。
  - 视网膜血管呈交替性膨胀收缩。
  - 视网膜出血、脱落。
  - 微动脉瘤形成伴渗出。
  - 视乳头水肿。
- 肾：
  - 肾病综合征。
  - 血尿。
  - 无菌性脓尿。
- 神经系统：
  - 头痛。
  - 共济失调。
  - 精神状态改变，昏迷。
  - 头晕，眩晕。
  - 眼球震颤。
  - 耳鸣，听力下降。
  - 感觉异常，周围神经病变。
  - 癫痫。
  - 颅内出血。
- 心血管：
  - 心绞痛或心肌梗死。
  - 心律失常。
  - 充血性心力衰竭(CHF)。
- 皮肤：
  - 雷诺现象。
  - 网状青斑。
  - 可触及的紫癜。
  - 蜘蛛痣。
  - 手指梗死。
  - 周围性坏疽。
  - 舌头肿大。

病史

应在下列患者中考虑HVS：

- 任何患者出现经典三联征：黏膜出血、视力下降、神经系统症状。
- 任何患者已明确的免疫球蛋白引起的血液病，出现靶器官微循环损害或心脏代偿失调的症状和体征。
- 任何患者已明确的细胞过多引起血液病，出现靶器官微循环损害或心脏代偿失调的症状和体征。

体格检查

HVS没有特异性的异常体征，但是患者会出现和受累靶器官相关的异常症状。黏膜出血、瘀点或瘀斑、局部神经功能异常、失代偿性心力衰竭和眼底异常都被报道过。

■ 基本检查

- 评估靶器官缺血和出血。
- 测量血清或全血黏稠度。
- 如果因为血液淤积和高黏稠度引起分析仪堵塞，无法进行实验室检查，怀疑该诊断。

■ 诊断检查与说明

实验室检查

- 全血细胞计数：
  - 贫血或红细胞增多都可以出现。
  - 贫血常为正细胞性和正色素性。
  - 外周血涂片红细胞呈缗钱状是一条重要的诊断依据。
  - 白血病时检查白细胞。
- 电解质、尿素氮、肌酐和血糖：
  - 肾衰竭在HVS中很常见。
  - 多发性骨髓瘤出现高钙血症和伪低钠血症。
- 尿液分析：
  - 蛋白尿。
  - 血尿。
  - 无菌性脓尿。
- 凝血功能检查。
- 血清和尿蛋白电泳。
- 检查血清黏稠度(在急诊室常规没有此项检查)：
  - 奥氏黏度计。
  - 同水相比，血清黏稠度正常范围是1.4～1.8。
  - 出现症状的最小黏稠度是4 cP(1 cP=

G

10^{-3} Pa·s)。

- 白细胞碱性磷酸酶、乳酸脱氢酶、维生素 B_{12} 升高。

影像学检查

患者出现中枢神经系统功能障碍的症状或体征，应考虑检查头颅 CT，以排除颅内出血。

鉴别诊断

• 出血和凝血功能异常：
- 血小板异常（数量和质量）。
- 遗传性因子缺乏症。
- 获得性疾病（维生素 K 缺乏、肝脏疾病）。
- 弥散性血管内凝血。

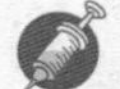

治疗

院前

出现出血进行静脉液体复苏。

初步稳定/治疗

• 补液：经静脉输注生理盐水。

• 出血或靶器官缺血可能不会对血浆置换外的任何治疗有效。

• 有贫血和白血病的患者，在血浆置换前不要输血，以免 HVS 恶化。

急诊治疗/程序

• 补液、支持治疗和及早血液科医师会诊是初期急诊室治疗方案。

• 静脉切开放血或紧急血浆置换：如果 HVS 患者出现严重的神经系统症状（如昏迷或癫痫），可以作为临时措施：
- 如果不能进行血浆置换，急重症患者在急诊室开展这些措施方便、有效。
- 放全血 100～200 ml，然后使用等渗盐水补充。
- 有条件的话，请血液科医师会诊。
- 真性红细胞增多症患者选择此治疗方法。

• 血浆置换/白细胞去除术：
- 稳定的患者：40 ml/kg。
- 危重患者：60 ml/kg。
- 副作用包括使用包含枸橼酸的抗凝剂引起的低钙血症和心律失常（少见）。
  ◦ 许多患者需要多次血浆置换。
  ◦ HVS 的确定性治疗方法：应当在血浆置换/血液科团队会诊后开展。
  ◦ 当患者有白细胞增多症（通常＞100 000/mm^3）时，进行白细胞去除术。

• 在危急情况，急诊科医师可以置入直径较大的透析管，同时注意避免操作过程中出血并发症。

随访

进一步处理

入院指征

• 有高黏血症的患者出现严重症状或者靶器官缺血或出血的证据，应当住院治疗血液疾病。

• 下列情况入住 ICU：
- 出血。
- 精神状态改变。
- 急性心肌梗死。

出院指征

针对根本病因进行确定性治疗后可以出院。

转诊问题

所有 HVS 患者都应转诊至血液科专科。

要点和误区

• HVS 患者避免使用利尿剂，因为利尿剂可以增加血液黏稠度。

• HVS 经典三联征包括黏膜出血、视力下降、神经系统症状。

高渗综合征 Hyperosmolar Syndrome

Matthew T. Robinson · Catherine D. Parker 巩博 译

基础知识

描述

• 由于未诊断或者未治疗的糖尿病胰岛素相对不足。

• 持续的高血糖造成渗透性利尿和脱水：
- 细胞内、外空间通过二者之间的渗透梯度差来维持。
- 细胞内液逐渐出现脱水。

• 人体丢失水、Na^+、Cl^-、K^+、PO_4^{3-}、Ca^{2+} 和 Mg^{2+}。

• 和糖尿病酮症酸中毒（DKA）不同，不出现严重的酮症酸中毒。
- 血循环中的胰岛素水平更高。
- 胰岛素的反调节激素很少上升。
- 高渗状态自身抑制脂肪分解和酮酸生成。

老年人注意事项

• 最常见于有 2 型糖尿病的老年人，严重的疾病促进高血糖状态进一步恶化，并且损伤肾功能。

• 在老年人，30%～40%的病例和糖尿病的初始症状相关。

儿科注意事项

高渗性高血糖状态很少出现在儿童。

病因

• 下列因素促进高血糖状态发生：
- 受损的外周胰岛素作用。
- 外源性或者内源性葡萄糖增加。
- 患者补充缺失液体的能力下降。

• 感染（尤指肺炎和尿路感染）是最常见的诱发因素。

• 其他诱因：
- 治疗/药物治疗缺陷。
- 脓毒症。
- 药物/毒品：
  ◦ 利尿剂。
  ◦ β 受体阻滞药。
  ◦ 钙通道阻滞剂。
  ◦ 非典型抗精神病药物。
  ◦ 糖皮质激素。
  ◦ 拟交感神经。
  ◦ 苯妥英。
  ◦ 西咪替丁。
  ◦ 苯丙胺。
  ◦ 乙醇。
- 心肌梗死。
- 脑血管意外。
- 肾衰竭。
- 中暑。
- 胰腺炎。
- 阑尾炎。
- 肠梗阻。
- 内分泌失调。

- 妊娠。
- 创伤。
- 烧伤。

诊断

症状和体征

病史

- 典型的症状体征进展时间可为数日到数周。
- 多尿,多饮,体重下降。
- 头昏,无力,疲劳。
- 视力模糊。
- 下肢痉挛。

体格检查

- 脱水。
- 心动过速。
- 眼眶凹陷。
- 低血压。
- 黏膜干燥。
- 皮肤弹性下降。
- 颈静脉塌陷。
- 昏迷,昏睡,睡眠过多。
- 在晚期前一直有小便排出。
- 癫痫或局部神经功能受损。
- 诱发其他疾病。

基本检查

诊断标准:

- 血糖≥600 mg/dl(常常>1 000 mg/dl)。
- 酮体很少。
- pH≥7.30, HCO_3^-≥15 mmol/L。
- 有效血浆渗透压>320 mOsm/kg:
  - =2×Na^++血糖/18。
  - 不包括尿素氮,因为它可以在不同体液间自由出入。

诊断检查和说明

实验室检查

- 检测相关检查以评估高渗透压综合征并查找诱因。
- 电解质:
  - K^+在液体不足的情况下也有可能上升,因为K^+从细胞内液迁移至细胞外液。
  - 高阴离子间隙代谢性酸中毒是因为乳酸、β羟丁酸升高或者肾功能减退。
  - 钠上升:高血糖时需要校正:校正$[Na^+]=[Na^+]+1.6\times[(血糖\ mg/dl)-100]/100$。
- 尿素氮、肌酐:
  - 氮质血症伴随上升的尿素氮/肌酐,是因为肾前性或肾性因素。
- 静脉血气或动脉血气,快速检测pH:
  - 评估混合性酸碱紊乱动脉血气是必需的。
- 血清酮体、β羟丁酸和乳酸水平:如果pH<7.3或阴离子间隙明显升高检查酮体、乳酸、β羟丁酸。
- 血渗透压。
- 全血细胞计数:
  - 白细胞增高是因为感染、应激或者血液浓缩。
  - 血红蛋白、血细胞比容上升是因为血液浓缩。
- 脂肪酶和淀粉酶:
  - 常见于胰腺炎。
  - 淀粉酶和脂肪酶上升而没有胰腺炎的证据。
  - 可能是因为唾液分泌、血液浓缩或肾清除率下降。
- 尿液分析:
  - 检查酮体/血糖。
  - 评估有无泌尿系统感染。
- 镁、钙、磷酸盐。
- 脓毒症查血培养。
- 横纹肌溶解查肌酸激酶:
  - 发生率高达17%。
- 生育期的妇女检查尿妊娠试验。
- 心肌梗死检查心肌酶和肌钙蛋白。

影像学检查

- 胸片查找可能潜在的肺炎。
- 头颅CT:查找局灶性神经功能缺损。

诊断步骤/外科

心电图:

- 评估电解质异常引起的传导异常。
- 评估缺血的症状作为触发事件。

鉴别诊断

同糖尿病酮症酸中毒鉴别:

- 如果出现酸中毒或者明显的阴离子间隙,必须查找原因(如酮症、糖尿病酮症酸中毒、低灌注、脓毒症或其他引起代谢性酸中毒的原因)。
- 高渗性高血糖状态和糖尿病酮症酸中毒混合出现于高达33%的患者。

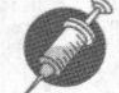

治疗

院前

静脉液体复苏,初步稳定病情。

初步稳定/治疗

ABC管理:

- 昏迷的患者保持气道通畅。
- 心电监测,使用18G针建立静脉通路。
- 不明原因的昏迷患者,使用纳洛酮、硫胺素,查血糖。
- 静脉补液,恢复血流动力学稳定。
- 第一个小时输注生理盐水1~2 L。
- 维持正常生命特征和尿量需要大量补液。

急诊治疗/程序

- 通用方案:
  - 频繁重复评估体液量和精神状态。
  - 电解质评估困难:
    - 血Na^+、K^+、PO_4^{3-}不能精确反映人体已丢失的溶质或者细胞内环境。
- 液体:
  - 在1~2 h予以生理盐水1~2 L进行复苏,以恢复血容量并且达到血流动力学稳定。
  - 初步复苏后使用0.45%盐水。
  - 计算人体总失水量(TBW)使用校正血钠公式:
    - TBW=0.6×体重(kg)×(1−140/校正Na^+)。
  - 平均失水量是8~10 L。
  - 在接下来的12 h补充失水量的一半。
  - 初次复苏后使用:
    - 生理盐水:如果血清钠低。
    - 0.45%盐水:如果血清钠升高/正常或患者高渗。
  - 当血糖<250 mg/dl,液体变为5%葡萄糖盐水。
- 钾:
  - 预期低血钾:
    - 人体总丢失5~10 mmol/kg(补充超过3日)。
  - 有小便后开始补钾。在无尿的患者或者起病时K^+>5 mmol/L,不要补钾。
  - 如果起病时K^+低(3~4 mmol/L),第一升液体补充40 mmol。
  - 如果血K^+<3 mmol/L,暂停胰岛素,补充10~20 mmol/h直到K^+>3.3 mmol/L,然后每升液体添加40 mmol。
  - 每1~2 h重复检测血钾,并且根据结果调整治疗方案。
- 胰岛素:
  - 不参与早期复苏。
  - 过早使用胰岛素可能导致高血糖快速纠正,伴随血管内容量下降、低血压、休克或者

G

低血钾、心律失常。
- 有些患者不需要使用胰岛素。
- 体液过多的患者（如急性肾衰竭），胰岛素可单独用药。
- 达到血流动力学稳定并且评估血钾情况后开始使用：
◦ 除非血 K^+＞3.3 mmol/L，不要使用。
- 由于吸收不稳定，不推荐皮下注射或者肌内注射。
- 血糖每小时下降 50～90 mg/dl 为最佳。如果出现进展性脑水肿，快速纠正血糖。
- 当血糖＜250 mg/dl，降低血糖，下降速度一半。
- 调整胰岛素维持血糖在 150～200 mg/dl。
• 磷酸盐：
- 不推荐常规补充。
- 如果血清水平＜1 mg/dl，24 h 补充 20～30 mmol 磷酸钾。
- 密切监测血钙水平。
• 镁：
- 第一个 3～4 h 在液体补充 0.35 mmol/kg 镁（70 kg 患者补充 2.5～3 g $MgSO_4$）。
- 在急性肾衰竭患者谨慎使用。
• 抗凝：
- 高渗状态可能并发动脉血栓：
◦ 考虑皮下注射肝素作为预防措施。
- 保持警惕栓塞并发症（如心肌梗死、肺栓塞、肠系膜缺血）。

■ 药物治疗

• 胰岛素：开始时每小时 0.05～0.1 U/kg，评估临床反应后调整用量。
• $MgSO_4$：50%（5 g/dl，静脉使用前至少稀释成 20%）。
• 纳洛酮：2 mg（儿童 0.1 mg/kg），静脉推注。
• 磷酸钾：血磷酸＜0.5 mg/dl，0.5 mmol/kg 静脉滴注，超过 4～6 h；血磷酸 0.5～1 mg/dl，0.25 mmol/kg 静脉滴注，超过 4～6 h。
• 磷酸钾：口服，每片含磷 250 mg、钾 1.1 mmol。
• 硫胺素：100 mg（儿童 10～25 mg），静脉推注。

随访

■ 进一步处理

入院指征

• 除了最轻的患者外，所有患者都应入住 ICU。
- 第一个 24 h 反复进行实验室检查。
- 快速补充液体和电解质，存在精神状态恶化和心律失常的可能性。需要密切监测。
• 轻症患者可在观察病房治疗超过 12～24 h。

出院指征

• 符合高渗透性综合征诊断标准的患者不应出院。
• 轻度高血糖患者伴随轻度液体不足和正常血渗透压，在补液纠正高血糖后可以出院。

转诊问题

患者应出院 1 周内转诊至内分泌医师，进行长期血糖监测和胰岛素治疗。

要点和误区

• 没有查出诱发事件或原因。
• 过快纠正血糖，可能导致低血压。
• 液体复苏后继续补充等渗液体可能导致高钠血症。
• 继续补充低渗液体不监测电解质可能引起细胞水肿或脑水肿。
• 未能阻止低血钾：呼吸抑制、心律失常。
• 在癫痫活动期间避免使用苯妥英：
- 抑制内源性胰岛素释放。

G

高铁血红蛋白血症 Methemoglobinemia

Natalie R. Neumann · Navneet Cheema 段立伟 译

基础知识

■ 描述

• 高铁血红蛋白是一种血红蛋白，含有氧化铁（Fe^{3+}），而不是亚铁（Fe^{2+}）状态。
• 高铁血红蛋白（MetHb）：
- 降低总携氧能力（功能性贫血）。
- 使血红蛋白氧解离曲线左移，影响 O_2 向组织中释放。
- 红细胞中的烟酰胺腺嘌呤二核苷酸（NADH）-高铁血红蛋白（细胞色素 B_5）还原酶系统使其保持在生理水平。
• 高铁血红蛋白血症是指存在超生理水平的高铁血红蛋白（即超过全身血红蛋白的 1%～2%），它可能是先天遗传性的或后天的。
• 高铁血红蛋白引起的症状：
- 通常发生在 MetHb 水平＞20%。
- 合并贫血时，病情更严重。
- 比同等程度的贫血更严重。
- 反映了 MeHb 合成速度和合成的量。
• 先天性高铁血红蛋白血症：
- NADH-高铁血红蛋白（细胞色素 B_5）还原酶缺乏（纯合或杂合）。
- 复杂高铁血红蛋白和其他异常血红蛋白类型。
• 红细胞氧化应激导致的获得性高铁血红蛋白血症：
- 一些高铁血红蛋白诱导剂是直接氧化剂（如亚硝酸盐）。
- 许多物质通过 N-羟基胺的代谢产物产生氧化损伤。
• 高铁血红蛋白血症的形成可能与接触的物质有关。
• 许多高铁血红蛋白诱导剂也可引起亨氏体溶血性贫血（HA）：
- 可由红细胞蛋白质的氧化损伤引起。
- 葡萄糖-6-磷酸脱氢酶（G-6-PD）缺乏的患者有较高的风险。
- 高铁血红蛋白血症患者应筛查 HA。
• 高铁血红蛋白血症可以作为基因异常的标志物指标：
- 杂合 NADH-高铁血红蛋白（细胞色素 B_5）还原酶缺乏。

■ 病因

• 氰化物（CN）的解毒剂：
- 通过仲戊基和亚硝酸钠诱导高铁血红蛋白血症。
- CN 优先与产生氰氧血红蛋白的高铁血红蛋白复合，该复合物随后被代谢成硫氰酸盐，硫氰酸盐被肾脏清除。
• 硝酸盐或亚硝酸盐（最常见）：
- 亚硝酸盐。

- 硝酸盐，如硝酸甘油，经代谢转化为亚硝酸盐。
- 一氧化氮(NO)。
- 染料：
- 苯胺染料。
- 亚甲基蓝（过量）。
- 抗寄生虫药（高铁血红蛋白形成可能性增加）：
- 氨苯砜。
- 伯氨喹。
- 氯喹。
- 局部麻醉药（高铁血红蛋白形成可能性增加）：
- 苯佐卡因。
- 利多卡因。
- 丙胺卡因。
- 止痛药：
- 非那吡啶。
- 非那西丁。
- 抗生素：
- 呋喃妥因。
- 砜。
- 磺胺类药物。
- 其他：
- 甲氧氯普胺（胃复安）。
- 萘（樟脑丸）。
- 百草枯（除草剂）。
- 砷气体（砷化氢）。
- 氯酸盐（高氯酸）。
- 酚（如二硝基酚、对苯二酚）。

诊断

症状和体征

- 中央型发绀，难治性缺氧：
- 对于非贫血患者来说，高铁血红蛋白占到总血红蛋白的10%～15%时，发绀症状明显（或高铁血红蛋白 1.5 g/dl 的血液）。
- 超过 20%，时常出现呼吸困难，气促。
- 胸痛，心律失常。
- 昏厥。
- 当其水平>50%，可出现精神状态改变。

病史

- 暴露于高铁血红蛋白诱导剂。
- 摄入的所有物质和摄入的时间(s)。
- G-6-PD 缺乏症。
- 自身状况对氧输送损伤敏感（如冠心病）。

体格检查

- 发绀。
- 重视精神状态和心血管系统结果。
- 黄疸或深色尿可伴随溶血性贫血。

基本检查

- 存在高铁血红蛋白血症时，脉搏血氧饱和度是不准确的。
- MetHb 干扰脉搏血氧饱和度的测量。
- 血氧饱和度降到 85%左右时，可能存在严重的高铁血红蛋白血症。
- 脉搏血氧饱和度测定不能用于指导治疗。
- 动脉血气(ABG)可检查以下指标：
- 动脉血氧分压。
- 动脉血二氧化碳分压。
- 碳氧血红蛋白监测：
- 高铁血红蛋白水平。
- 碳氧血红蛋白水平。
- 心电图。

诊断检查与说明

实验室检查

- 血液可呈典型的巧克力色。
- 包含人工分类计数的血常规检查、血液涂片检查以寻找溶血性贫血的证据。
- 在肺功能正常的情况下，尽管桡动脉处血氧饱和度较低（PaO_2 反映的是血浆，而不是血红蛋白饱和度），但预计血氧饱和度正常。

影像学检查

胸片排除其他肺部病变。

鉴别诊断

- 缺氧：
- 充血性心力衰竭(CHF)。
- 慢性阻塞性肺疾病(COPD)。
- 肺栓塞。
- 刺激性气体接触。
- 青变：
- 缺氧。
- 硫血红蛋白血症。
- 氰化物中毒。
- 硫化氢中毒。
- 过量的亚甲蓝管理。
- 碲毒性。
- 皮肤接触、沾染蓝色染料。

治疗

院前

- 把患者可能摄入的所有物质都带去医院。
- 询问目击者和观察现场以发现家用品及其他潜在的可摄入物：
- 记录和传达相关发现给急救医疗人员。
- 商业或工业场所：
- 获取相关材料安全数据表(MSDS)，以确定商业或化工产品。
- 避免皮肤暴露。

初步稳定/治疗

- 气道、呼吸和循环管理：
- 心电监测。
- 低血压时需给予等渗晶体溶液。
- 精神状态改变时可给予纳洛酮、硫胺素和葡萄糖($D_{50}W$)。
- 补充氧气。

急诊治疗/程序

- 去污：
- 如果急性摄入的时间在 1～2 h，呼吸道反射功能都完好无损，可给予 75 g 活性炭口服。
- 除去氧化应激源。
- 亚甲蓝：
- 指征：
  ◦ 无症状者，高铁血红蛋白水平>30%。
  ◦ 有症状的患者，高铁血红蛋白水平>10%～20%，特别是存在其他共患疾病。
- 剂量：
  ◦ 1～2 mg/kg，静脉注射超过 5 min。
  ◦ 几分钟内就可看到临床好转。
  ◦ 如果给药后 1 h 内没有改善，则重新给药。
- 亚甲蓝给药后，脉搏血氧饱和度的短暂恶化：
  ◦ 干扰脉搏血氧饱和度测定，无需特殊干预。
- 存在葡萄糖-6-丙酮酸脱羧酶缺乏症的患者应谨慎使用：
  ◦ 可能引起溶血。
- 如果用亚甲蓝无改善，应考虑氧化应激源未消除，或存在硫血红蛋白血症：
- 硫血红蛋白血症是由于硫分子结合血红蛋白导致的，表现类似于高铁血红蛋白血症，但为自限性。
- 红细胞输注：
- 可增加血液携氧能力。
- 特别是存在溶血性贫血时。
- 换血：
- 特别是新生儿或婴儿。
- 高压氧治疗：
- 增加氧气输送到组织的效率，不受血红蛋白影响。
- 如果可立即使用应在危及生命的高铁血红蛋白血症患者中使用。

G

儿科注意事项

• 儿童可因微量的摄入而导致严重的高铁血红蛋白血症。

• 症状可在摄入后几小时才发生，所以需要长时间的观察。

• 新生儿发生高铁血红蛋白血症的风险较高(由于 NADH 高铁血红蛋白还原酶的存储较少)。

药物治疗

• 低血糖患者应静脉给予 50%右旋糖：25 g (50 ml)(儿童：0.5 g/kg $D_{25}W$)。

• 亚甲蓝 1 mg/kg 的 1%溶液静脉注射，注射时间>5 min(成人和儿童)：

- 如果 1 h 内无改善可重复给予一次。
- 0.3～1 mg/kg 静脉注射对新生儿有效。

• 纳洛酮：0.4～2.0 mg(儿童：0.1 mg/kg)，静脉注射，当怀疑阿片类药物依赖时，可重复给药直达 10 mg。

• 硫胺素：100 mg(儿童：1 mg/kg)，肌内或静脉注射。

随访

进一步处理

入院指征

• 症状严重的患者。

• 需要大剂量亚甲蓝患者。

• 氨苯砜导致的长期的复发性高铁血红蛋白血症。

出院指征

高铁血红蛋白含量<20%，高铁血红蛋白含量逐渐下降其没有症状或合并症患者。

转诊问题

严重暴露应请毒理学专家会诊。

随访建议

职业相关暴露应转诊职业医疗中心。

要点和误区

• 高铁血红蛋白血症时，脉搏血氧饱和度是不准确的。

• 应进行血气分析检测。

• 对于严重病例应给予亚甲蓝治疗。

高血压急症 Hypertensive Emergencies

Hiren Patel · David F. M. Brown 巩博 译

基础知识

描述

• 高血压危象：

- 收缩压(SBP)显著上升>179 mmHg 或者舒张压(DBP)>109 mmHg。

• 高血压紧急状态：

- 血压显著上升，但没有靶器官损伤。

• 高血压急症：

- 显著上升的血压伴有急性靶器官损伤。

• 高血压急症时血压的自动调节机制失调：

- 小动脉收缩维持血压。
- 高血压使小动脉过度收缩并且出现内皮细胞损伤。
- 内皮损伤导致渗透性增加，凝血反应和血小板激活，纤维蛋白沉积。

• 激活肾素-血管紧张素系统和交感神经系统：

- 导致进一步的血管收缩，产生促炎因子。

• 靶器官缺血：

- 血管收缩剂重新释放。
- 压力排钠进一步加重。
- 触发一个恶性循环。

• 受累器官：

- 脑(脑病、脑血管意外、颅内出血)。
- 视网膜(出血、视乳头水肿)。
- 心脏(心肌梗死、主动脉夹层、急性心力衰竭)。
- 肾(急性肾衰竭)。
- 胎儿(子痫前期/子痫)。

病因

• 有高血压病史。

• 肾：

- 血管性疾病。
- 实质性疾病。

• 主动脉狭窄。

• 中枢神经系统疾病：

- 头部外伤。
- 脑血管意外或颅内出血。
- 脑瘤。
- 脊髓损伤。

• 内分泌：

- 嗜铬细胞瘤。
- 库欣综合征。
- 原发性醛固酮增多症。
- 肾素分泌瘤。

• 药物：

- 可卡因、苯环已哌啶、苯丙胺。
- 促红细胞生成素、他克莫司、环孢素、皮质类固醇、口服避孕药。
- 和单胺氧化酶抑制剂相互作用。
- 停用降压药物。
- 铅中毒。

• 自主神经高反应：

- 吉兰-巴雷综合征。
- 间歇性卟啉病。

• 术后疼痛或者麻醉并发症。

• 妊娠相关：

- 先兆子痫/子痫。

诊断

症状和体征

病史

• 询问下列问题：

- 使用的任何处方或者非处方药物。
- 已存在的高血压控制情况和持续时间。
  ◦ 已存在的靶器官损害。
- 降压治疗的细节。
- 合并疾病(肥胖、冠状动脉疾病、糖尿病)。
- 使用娱乐性药物。

• 按下列顺序评估靶器官损害：

- 呼吸困难。
- 胸痛。
- 头痛。
- 精神状态改变或意识混乱。
- 局灶性神经症状。

体格检查

• 测量双上肢血压。

- 使用合适的袖带。

• 评估靶器官损害：

- 神经：
  ◦ 意识水平。

○视野。
○局部运动或感觉缺陷。
-眼科：
○眼底镜检查(视网膜出血、视乳头水肿)。
-心血管：
○颈静脉怒张。
○肺部湿啰音。
○主动脉关闭不全杂音。
○第三心音。
○脉搏不对称。

基本检查

• 12 导联心电图：
-缺血改变，左心室肥大。
•评估肾功能：
-急性肾衰竭可能没有症状。

诊断检查与说明

实验室检查

•全血细胞计数。
-贫血和血小板减少可能在栓塞性微血管病中出现。
•胸痛时进行标准检查方案。
•尿素氮、肌酐。
•电解质。
-原发性盐皮质激素增多症可能出现低血钾。
•尿液分析：
-蛋白尿、血尿、管型尿。
•尿毒理学检查：
-如果怀疑使用娱乐性药物。
• HCG。

影像学检查

•胸部X线：
-如果出现心肺相关症状。
•头颅CT：
-如果出现头痛、意识模糊、神经学发现。
•胸腹部CTA检查：
-如果怀疑主动脉夹层。

诊断步骤/外科

•动脉管路。
•腰椎穿刺：
-排除蛛网膜下腔出血。

鉴别诊断

•急性冠状动脉综合征。
•急性心力衰竭。
•主动脉夹层。
•颅内出血。
•脑血管意外(缺血或者出血)。
•先兆子痫/子痫。
•戒断综合征：
-β受体阻滞剂。
-可卡因(中枢神经α_2受体激动剂)。
•儿茶酚胺过多：
-嗜铬细胞瘤。
-可卡因/拟交感神经药物中毒。
-使用单胺氧化酶抑制剂时口服酪胺。

治疗

院前

• ABC管理。
•考虑缓慢降压。

初步稳定/治疗

• ABC管理，心电监测，脉搏氧饱和度。
•吸氧。
•建立静脉通道。

急诊治疗/程序

•高血压紧急状态：
-不需要治疗，但是密切随访。
-只使用口服药物。
-延迟的家庭口服药。
-目标：在24～48 h缓慢降压。
•高血压急症：
-不要单纯降压，要治疗靶器官损害。
-在第1 h内平均动脉压(MAP)下降20%～25%。
-目标：2～6 h内收缩压降至160 mmHg，舒张压降至100 mmHg。
-通过静脉用药血压稳定后，在6～12 h转为口服药物治疗。
-推荐缓慢降压：
○中枢神经系统急性进行性损伤。
-推荐快速降压：
○主动脉夹层。
•高血压脑病：
-目标：在第1 h内MAP最多下降20%或者舒张压降至100～110 mmHg，然后在48～72 h将血压降至正常。
-药物选择：尼卡地平、氯维地平或拉贝洛尔。
•缺血性卒中：
-脑灌注压(CPP)=MAP-颅内压(ICP)。
-低血压(MAP低)CPP下降或脑水肿(高ICP)可能加重梗死。
-只有收缩压>220 mmHg或者舒张压>120 mmHg时治疗。
-溶栓患者血压应低于185/110 mmHg。
-目标：在第1个24 h内，MAP降低不超过15%～20%，舒张压不低于100～110 mmHg。
- t-PA溶栓后目标：血压<185/105 mmHg。
-药物选择：尼卡地平、氯维地平或拉贝洛尔。
•出血性卒中或者蛛网膜下腔出血：
-如果收缩压>180 mmHg/舒张压>100 mmHg，降压治疗。
-目标：在第1 h内MAP降低20%～25%或者收缩压降至140～160 mmHg。
-药物选择：尼卡地平、氯维地平或拉贝洛尔。
-避免使用扩张脑血管的药物硝酸甘油、硝普钠。
•急性冠状动脉综合征：
-目标：MAP降至60～100 mmHg。
-药物选择：拉贝洛尔或艾司洛尔与硝酸甘油联合使用。
-避免：肼屈嗪(反射性心动过速)和硝普钠(冠状动脉窃血)。
•急性心力衰竭：
-目标：MAP降至60～100 mmHg。
-药物选择硝酸甘油或者硝普钠与ACEI和/或袢利尿剂。
•急性肾衰竭、微血管病性贫血。
-在第1 h内MAP降低20%～25%。
-药物选择：尼卡地平、氯维地平或非诺多泮。硬皮病肾衰竭时选择ACEI。
•主动脉夹层：
-通过降低血压和心率来降低剪切力(dP/dT)。
-β受体阻滞剂优先于任何引起反射性心动过速的药物。
-目标：在第1个20 min内收缩压降至100～120 mmHg，心率<65次/分。
-药物选择：艾司洛尔联合二氢吡啶类钙通道阻滞剂或硝普钠。
-如果是A型夹层，请血管外科会诊。
•拟交感神经(嗜咯细胞瘤、可卡因、苯丙胺)：
-目标：在第1 h内MAP降低20%～25%。
-避免单独使用β受体阻滞剂(α受体未阻滞)。
-药物选择：酚妥拉明或者钙通道阻滞剂联合苯二氮䓬类药物。
-在可乐定戒断中使用可乐定。

妊娠注意事项

•先兆子痫：

- 定义：收缩压>140 mmHg 或者舒张压>90 mmHg 合并蛋白尿(24 h>300 mg 或者尿蛋白/肌酐>0.3 或者测量试纸 1+)。
- 妊娠>20 周，产后 4 周出现。
- 头痛、视力改变、周围性水肿、右上腹疼痛。
- 并发症：子痫，HELLP 综合征。
- 目标：收缩压降至 130～150 mmHg，舒张压降至 80～100 mmHg。
- 药物选择：拉贝洛尔、尼卡地平、肼屈嗪、镁。
- 产科会诊。

• 艾司洛尔：
- β_1 受体阻滞剂。
- 起效 60 s，持续 10～20 min。
- 急性心力衰竭、COPD、心脏传导阻滞等病避免使用。

• 拉贝洛尔：
- 有 α 和 β 受体阻滞作用。
- 起效 2～5 min，持续 2～6 h。
- 因为 β 受体阻滞作用没有反射性心动过速。
- COPD、急性心力衰竭、心动过缓时避免使用。

• 氯维地平：
- 第三代二氢吡啶类钙通道阻滞剂。
- 起效 2～4 min，持续 5～15 min。
- 排泄不依赖肝肾功能。
- 对豆制品和蛋制品过敏、脂质代谢缺陷和心房颤动人群避免使用。

• 尼卡地平：
- 第二代二氢吡啶类钙通道阻滞剂。
- 起效 5～15 min，持续 4～6 h。
- 急性心力衰竭、冠状动脉缺血避免使用。

• 硝酸甘油：
- 静脉舒张>动脉舒张。
- 起效 2～5 min，持续 10～20 min。
- 增加冠状动脉灌注，减少缺血。
- 引起反射性心动过速、快速耐药反应、高铁血红蛋白血症。

• 硝普钠：
- 短效动静脉扩张剂。
- 起效 3 s，持续 1～2 min。
- 并发症：
  ◦ 反射性心动过速、冠状动脉窃血，增加 ICP。
  ◦ 长期使用出现氰化物中毒。
- 孕妇、肾衰竭避免使用。

• 肼屈嗪：
- 小动脉扩张剂。
- 起效 5～15 min，持续 3～10 h。
- 较少出现低血压。
- 孕妇安全。

• 依那普利拉：
- ACEI。
- 起效 0.5～4 h 持续 6 h。
- 妊娠、急性心肌梗死避免使用。

• 非诺多泮：
- 选择性突触后多巴胺受体激动剂(DA1)。
- 起效 5～15 min，持续 1～4 h。
- 没有反射性心动过速。
- 维持肾灌注。
- 避免使用：青光眼。

• 酚妥拉明：
- α_1 受体阻滞剂，周围血管扩张药。
- 起效 1～2 min，持续 10～30 min。

■ **药物治疗**

• 氯维地平：1～16 mg/h，静脉滴注。
• 依那普利拉：每 6 h 1.25～5 mg，静脉推注。
• 艾司洛尔：80 mg，静脉推注，然后 150 μg/(kg·min)，静脉滴注。
• 非诺多泮：0.1～0.6 μg/(kg·min)，静脉滴注。
• 肼屈嗪：10～20 mg，静脉推注。
• 拉贝洛尔：每 10 min 20～80 mg，静脉推注(总量 300 mg)；然后 0.5～2 mg/min 静脉滴注。
• 尼卡地平：2～15 mg/h，静脉滴注。
• 硝酸甘油：5～100 μg/min，静脉滴注，使用非 PVC 的管路。
• 硝普钠：0.25～10 μg/(kg·min)，静脉滴注。
• 酚妥拉明：5～15 mg，q5～15 min，静脉推注。

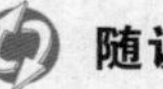

随访

■ **进一步处理**

入院指征

• 所有有靶器官损害的患者。
• 入住 ICU 进行心电、脉搏监测。

出院指征

• 没有靶器官损害。
• 很可能配合社区治疗。
• 已知高血压病史。
• 可逆转的病因(如药物、不配合)。
• 可以重新开始之前的药物治疗方案。
• 出现胸痛或者头痛复诊。

■ **随诊建议**

在家庭医师护理下开始一套合适的治疗方案。

要点和误区

• 高血压紧急状态时避免静脉用药。
• 高血压急症的目标是第 1 h 内 MAP 降低 20%～25%，除非出现缺血性卒中和主动脉夹层。
• 避免降压过快过多，可能引起靶器官损害。
• 主动脉夹层时避免反射性心动过速。
• 在儿茶酚胺过多时避免不阻滞 α 受体。

高压氧治疗 Hyperbaric Oxygen Therapy

Trevonne M. Thompson 巩博 译

基础知识

■ **描述**

• 在>1 atm 大气压(1 atm=1.013×10^5 Pa)的环境下(通常 2～3 atm)吸入纯氧。
• 作用机制：
- 在细胞水平，增加氧的可用性。
  ◦ 在 3 atm 下吸入纯氧，可以提供足够的溶解氧维持生命，不再需要血红蛋白参与。
  ◦ 压缩已形成的气泡(防止空气栓塞或减压病)。
• 2 种类型高压氧舱：
- 单人舱：
  ◦ 可以容纳一个仰卧的患者。

◦ 舱外有技术员监测。
◦ 纯氧舱。
- 多人舱：
◦ 容纳多个患者。
◦ 可容纳照顾患者的护理人员。

诊断

症状和体征

高压氧治疗的适应证：
- 动脉气体栓塞。
- 减压病。
- 一氧化碳中毒。
- 软组织感染：
◦ 气性坏疽。
◦ 坏死性筋膜炎。
◦ 难治性骨髓炎。
◦ 慢性不愈合伤口。
• 伤口护理：
- 辐射引起的组织损伤。
- 挤压伤。
- 烧伤。
- 受损的皮肤移植和皮瓣。

注意

急诊室内科医师应关注动脉栓塞、减压病、一氧化碳中毒，对这些疾病采取高压氧治疗。

基本检查

• 如上文描述，决定是否需要高压氧治疗。
• 开展全面的身体检查以筛除治疗的禁忌证，完善预处理基线检查。
• 治疗的禁忌证：
- 未处理的气胸是绝对禁忌证：
◦ 可能转变为张力性气胸。
- 心血管不稳定：
◦ 不稳定的患者不能在单人舱治疗。
◦ 如果收益超过风险，这样的患者可以在多人舱治疗。

诊断检查与说明

实验室检查

动脉血气分析：
• 在合适的情况下评估缺氧。

影像学检查

胸部X线：
• 评估隐匿性气胸。

治疗

初步稳定/治疗

• 基础生命支持。
• 建立静脉通道。
• 纯氧。
• 心电监测(恰当的时候)。

急诊治疗/程序

• 决定是否需要高压氧治疗。
• 将任何装置上的气囊(导尿管、气管内导管)充满液体，避免治疗期间破裂。
• 对使用减充血药引起任何鼻窦不适的患者进行预治疗。
• 在机械通气的患者或者有中耳疾病(如中耳炎)的患者，采取鼓膜切开置管术。

注意

高压氧治疗的并发症：
• 鼻窦疼痛。
• 气压伤：
- 鼓膜破裂。
- 张力性气胸。
• 癫痫：
- 可能是氧中毒的结果。
• 减压病：
- 当减压太快时。
◦ 当使用单人舱时，不能接受不稳定的患者。

随访

进一步处理

入院指征

• 动脉气体栓塞。
• 减压病。
• 严重一氧化碳中毒。

出院指征

患者稳定，症状已解决。

转诊问题

• 可能需要转运至有高压氧舱的医院。
• 当考虑转运一个不稳定的患者时，评估风险和受益。
• 潜水员报警：
- 为潜水相关伤害提供24 h救援电话咨询。

随访建议

随访进行重复高压氧治疗。

要点和误区

• 将任何装置上的气囊(导尿管、气管内导管)充满液体，避免治疗期间破裂。
• 检查隐匿性气胸。

G

高原病 High-Altitude Illness

Jeffrey J. Schaider　陈奇通 译

基础知识

描述

• 发生率依赖于：
- 上升率。
- 最终海拔。
- 睡眠时海拔。
- 海拔高度的持续时间。
• 急性高山病(AMS)的发生率：
- 最高67%的发生率：急速爬升(1～2日)>14 000 ft(4 267.2 m)。
- 在海拔7 000～9 000 ft(2 133.6～2 743.2 m)高度滑雪和睡眠的人中，发生率为22%。如果海拔高度为10 000 ft(3 048 m)，则发生率增高到40%。
• AMS的危险因素：
- 之前曾患高原病。
- 强体力活动。
- 年轻人(<50岁)。
- 未采取有效防护措施。
- 肥胖和肺部疾病增加风险。
• 高原性肺水肿(HAPE)的发生率：
- <1%～2%。
- 因上升率而异。
• 高原性脑水肿(HACE)的发生率<1%。
• HACE和HAPE多发生在海拔13 000 ft(4 000 m)。

妊娠注意事项

• 妊娠和高原病之间的联系并没有确定。

• 高海拔时常见妊娠高血压综合征、蛋白尿、外周性水肿，可能与孕妇血氧不足有关。

• 没有证据表明高海拔与自然性流产、胎盘早剥或前置胎盘的发生率有关。

• 旅行的孕妇和正常妊娠孕妇在中等海拔地区似乎是安全的，但当海拔＞13 000 ft 和复杂妊娠时仍需提高警惕。

老年人注意事项

老年人更易患有受海拔影响的潜在健康问题，如高血压（HTN）、慢性阻塞性肺疾病（COPD）和冠心病，但 AMS 的发生风险在 55 岁以上人较其他年龄组更低。

病因

• 在没有进行环境适应的情况下，急速上升＞8 000 ft（大约 2 500 m）是最常见的高原病原因。

• 急速上升、最后到达的海拔、睡眠时的海拔及个体差异等这些因素在高原病的发展中具有重要意义。

诊断

症状和体征

病史

• AMS：
- 头痛＋至少以下一项：
  ◦ 恶心或呕吐。
  ◦ 疲劳或精神不振。
  ◦ 头晕。
  ◦ 失眠。
- 在上升后 4～12 h 开始出现症状。
- 通常是良性和自限性的。
- 症状可能使人变得虚弱。

• HAPE：
- 在上升后 2～4 日开始出现，大部分出现在第二晚。
- 可以威胁生命。
- 咳嗽（一开始干咳，后来有痰）。
- 安静时呼吸困难。

• HACE：
- 威胁生命。
- 发生可在 HAPE 和/或 AMS 之前：
  ◦ 很少独立存在。
- 初始：
  ◦ 可以发生在 AMS 开始后的 12 h。
  ◦ 通常疾病进展需要 2～4 日。
- 精神状态改变。
- 严重或不断加重的头痛。
- 恶心及呕吐。

儿科注意事项

• AMS 在婴儿和小儿的表现：
- 变得更易激怒。
- 嬉闹减少。
- 食欲减退。
- 呕吐。
- 睡眠障碍。

• HAPE 更易发生在年轻个体（＜20 岁）。

• 暂时还没有＜4 岁的 HAPE 或 HACE 病例被报道。

体格检查

• AMS：
- 在出现 HAPE 或 HACE 前，体格检查一般均正常：
  ◦ 轻度 AMS 常被误诊为病毒综合征或酒醉后的不良反应。

• HAPE：
- 呼吸急促。
- 湿啰音。
- 发绀。
- 可能出现发热。
- 可能发生严重呼吸困难和死亡。

• HACE：
- 共济失调。
- 视神经乳头水肿，视网膜出血。
- 精神状态改变或脑病：
  ◦ 局部神经功能缺陷不常见。
  ◦ 癫痫（少见）。
  ◦ 昏迷。
  ◦ 被称为“晚期”AMS。

基本检查

• 临床诊断的确定依赖于所处海拔高度。

• AMS：
- 诊断确定依靠曾有头痛病史＋至少以下一项：
  ◦ 恶心或呕吐。
  ◦ 精神不振或疲倦。
  ◦ 头晕。
  ◦ 失眠。
- 没有实验室或影像学检查变化。

• HAPE：
- 劳力性呼吸困难：普遍出现在高海拔。
- 静止性呼吸困难：HAPE 的症状，尤以夜间严重。
- 湿啰音、发绀或咳嗽均支持诊断。
- 心动过速、呼吸急促常与疾病严重程度一致。

• HACE：
- 有小脑共济失调，伴随或不伴随其他症状的 AMS。
- 视神经乳头水肿、视网膜出血是相关表现。

诊断检查与说明

实验室检查

HAPE 的动脉血气分析：

• 提示血氧不足（氧分压在 30～50 mmHg）和呼吸性碱中毒。

影像学检查

• HAPE 行胸部 X 线检查：
- 显示斑片状肺泡浸润与斑块之间正常区域。
- 单侧或双侧浸润（右肺中叶受累最常见）。
- 心脏肥大，“蝙蝠”样浸润，Kerley B 线（尤其是心源性肺水肿）。HAPE 通常少见。

• CT 和 MRI 在 HACE 中的应用：
- 脑白质血管性水肿。

诊断步骤/外科

HAPE 中心电图的应用：

• 心动过速。

• 右心改变的证据。

鉴别诊断

• AMS：
- 喝酒后宿醉。
- 一氧化碳中毒。
- 脑炎。
- 疲惫。
- 脑膜炎。
- 病毒综合征。

• HAPE：
- 高原支气管肺炎和咽炎。
- 肺炎。
- 肺栓塞：
  ◦ 一开始进展迅速。
  ◦ 胸膜炎性胸痛。

• HACE：
- 脑血管意外或短暂脑缺血发作：
  ◦ 出现局灶性神经系统体征改变，提示血管病变。

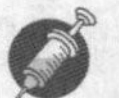

治疗

院前

• 重症患者需要立即转运至低海拔地区。

• 出现不适症状后不要继续向更高海拔前进。

• 氧输送或在高压氧舱模仿氧气下降的情

景(Gamow bag),是可以救命的临时措施。

■ 初始稳定/治疗

• HAPE 和 HACE:
- ABC 管理:
◦ 对于呼吸困难或行气道保护的患者可行气管插管术。
- 建立静脉通道。
- 辅助供氧和监测。
- 对 HAPE 行持续正压通气。

■ 急诊治疗/程序

• AMS:
- 轻度 AMS 通常为自限性:
◦ 对症治疗。
◦ 停止上升直到症状缓解。
- 为了缓解症状,对于严重患者可给予乙酰唑胺。
- 有头痛的患者可给予布洛芬或对乙酰氨基酚。
- 恶心、呕吐的患者可给予异丙嗪或昂丹司琼。
- 对于严重患者给予辅助供氧。
- 严重或持续症状的患者立即下降到低海拔。
- 乙酰唑胺可用于 AMS 的预防:
◦ 计划进行快速爬升的高危人群。
• HAPE:
- 对于中重度的患者应立即转运至低海拔地区。
- 轻度的患者在以下情况下可以不必转运至低海拔:
◦ 充足的氧气供应。
◦ 完备的医学检查。
◦ 临床状态出现恶化立即转运至低海拔地区。
- 卧床休息,避免剧烈运动诱导肺动脉高血压。
- 辅助供氧:
◦ 高流量吸氧(6～8 L/min)直到病情有所缓解,而后改为持续低流量吸氧。
- 当其他干预措施不能使用时,给予硝苯地平。
- β受体激动剂的吸入剂可能有所帮助。
- 高压氧治疗是可行的,而立即下降是不可能的。
• HACE:
- 立即转运至低海拔地区。
- 吸氧。
- 地塞米松。
- 头与床成 30°卧床休息,在严重病例颅内压增高需积极治疗。

■ 药物治疗

• 乙酰唑胺:
- AMS 疗法:250～500 mg(儿童:5 mg/kg),口服,2 次/日。
- AMS 预防:250 mg,口服,2 次/日(儿童:5 mg/kg),提前 24 h 服用。
• 地塞米松:8 mg,静脉注射;然后 4 mg,口服或静脉注射,3 次/日。
• 布洛芬:800 mg(儿童:5～10 mg/kg),口服,3 次/日。
• 硝苯地平:10 mg,口服;然后 30 mg 维持(SR 口服,1 次/日)。
• 异丙嗪:12.5～25 mg(儿童:0.25～1 mg/kg),口服、灌肠(经直肠)或肌内注射,q4～6 h。

一线用药

• 乙酰唑胺(AMS)。
• 硝苯地平(HAPE)。

二线用药

• 地塞米松。
• 目前文献中不支持多药治疗高海拔疾病的应用。

随访

■ 进一步处理

严重病例必须尽快转运至低海拔地区。

入院指征

• 在转运至低海拔地区后仍有持续症状者。
• HAPE。
• HACE。

出院指征

一旦临床症状改善,或者在海平面高度血氧饱和度＞95%,或更高海拔有正常氧饱和度。

转诊问题

• 提供预防性治疗,防止患者今后进入高海拔地区复发 AMS(乙酰唑胺)或高原性肺水肿(硝苯地平)。
• 高剂量的地塞米松(4 mg/6 h)可考虑用于高危情况,如军事或被空运到海拔超过 3 500 m 的地方的搜救人员,并可立即进行身体活动。

要点和误区

• 高原病的症状可以与轻度病毒感染症状相似。
• 缺乏对高原病的重视和认识程度不高。
• 当治疗高原病时,一旦出现病情加重,直到症状缓解前都不能向更高海拔移动。
• 共济失调和呼吸困难分别是 HACE 和 HAPE 早期可能出现的症状。
• HACE 与严重的 AMS 可通过神经学症状如意识混乱、共济失调或精神状态改变来区分。
• HACE 和 HAPE 可以同时发生。
• 当无法下降时,应考虑使用高压氧和辅助药物。

G

睾丸扭转 Testicular Torsion

Edward Newton・Taku Taira 范浩浩 李文放 译

基础知识

■ 描述

• 睾丸和血管蒂围绕精索旋转。
• 旋转经常发生在中间(2/3 的情况):
- 从不完全(90°～180°)到完全(360°～1 080°)的扭转。
- 根据扭转的程度:
◦ 发生血管闭塞。
◦ 超过 6 h 后的睾丸梗死热缺血。
• 睾丸补救:
- 73%～100%,缺血时间＜6 h。
- 50%～70%,缺血时间在 6～12 h。
- 缺血 12 h 后＜20%。
- 睾丸发病 24 h 后仍然值得尝试挽救。
• 睾丸梗死导致萎缩,可能会最终降低生育率。

■ 流行病学

扭曲的双峰分布：
- 婴儿和青春期发病率最高。
- 85%的病例发生在12～18岁，平均为13岁。
- 扭转在30岁后很少见，但仍然有可能。

■ 病因

- 先天性生殖器异常：
  - 鞘膜高位插入精索。
  - 多余的睾丸系膜。
  - 在其血管蒂上睾丸的活动性和扭曲性增加。
- 12%的人存在双侧解剖异常，所以两个睾丸都易受扭转。

诊断

■ 症状和体征

病史

- 突然发生单侧睾丸疼痛。
- 阴囊肿胀和红斑。
- 不太常见的是，扭转可能伴随着腹股沟或下腹部疼痛。
- 多达40%的患者主诉以前有类似情况。
  - 是因为自发性扭转。
- 50%的病例发生恶心和呕吐。
- 低热发生率为25%。
- 睾丸在疼痛发作之前通常有轻微的创伤史。
- 缺乏尿路感染的症状（排尿困难、尿频和尿急）。

体格检查

- 区分扭转和附睾炎，局部压痛对早期诊断有帮助；然而，一旦发生严重的阴囊肿胀，解剖结构变得模糊。
- 睾丸附件的扭转不那么疼痛，会威胁睾丸的生存能力。
- 以"蓝点"标志为特征。
- 受影响的扭转睾丸可能横向倾斜，与正常的垂直位置相反。
- 患侧睾丸扭转的提睾反射经常阴性。
- 灵敏度达96%，特异性达66%。
- Prehn征：
  - 附睾炎中睾丸升高时疼痛缓解。
  - 睾丸扭转时疼痛加剧或无变化。
  - 判断不准确。

■ 基本检查

- 在小孩或儿童中出现"急性阴囊症状"，青少年需要快速评估和立即咨询泌尿科医师。
- 这些患者需要无创血流研究或手术探查以确认扭转。
- 这些患者的3.3%（急诊）～30%（泌尿科检查）最终证明睾丸扭转。

■ 诊断检查与说明

实验室检查

- 50%的病例存在左移的白细胞计数升高。
- 尿液分析通常正常，但高达20%的病例有脓尿。
- 没有针对睾丸扭转的实验室测试。

影像学检查

> **注意**
> - 所有血流检查都存在局限性：
>   - 仅反映当前的灌注状态。
>   - 自发性睾丸扭转可能会显示正常甚至血流增加。
>   - 仍然处于反复扭转的高风险中。
> - 传统的标准一直是^{99m}Tc放射性核素扫描：
>   - 与未受影响的一侧比较，扭转睾丸的血流量减少。
>   - 获取扫描的时间通常滞后。
> - 多普勒超声：
>   - 直接可视化评估扭转精索的血流量。
>   - 取代了核扫描：
>   - 侵袭性较小。
>   - 更容易获得的检测。
>   - 结果可比较。
>   - 总体敏感度和特异度分别为76%～98%和100%，但区分睾丸扭转和附睾扭转的能力较低。
>   - 由于炎症反应，附睾炎会显示血流量增加。
>   - 扭转会显示血流减少或无血流。
>   - 彩色血流多普勒最常用。
>   - 使用多普勒造影材料可能会增强准确性。
>   - 高清晰度超声波（HDUS）正在兴起，可作为精索扭转的直接影像学的准确手段。

儿科注意事项

- 所有影像学技术在婴幼儿的应用中都有技术限制。
  - 睾丸血管很小。
  - 正常情况下睾丸的血流量最小。
- 可能需要进行阴囊探查。

诊断步骤/外科

- 可以在当地迅速完成麻醉阴囊探查，来诊断和治疗扭转。
- 两个睾丸的"铃铛"畸形应该通过睾丸股固定术来纠正。

■ 鉴别诊断

- 急性鞘膜积液。
- 附睾炎、睾丸炎。
- 过敏性紫癜。
- 嵌顿腹股沟疝。
- 睾丸肿瘤。
- 睾丸创伤或睾丸破裂。
- 睾丸附件扭转（31%～70%为急性阴囊病例）。
- 其他腹内情况：
  - 阑尾炎。
  - 胰腺炎。
  - 肾绞痛。

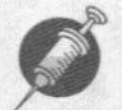

治疗

■ 院前

- 在该领域没有可以提供的确切治疗方法。
- 医院前工作人员必须认识到年轻患者的急性睾丸疼痛是紧急情况。
- 这些患者应该立即运送到急诊室。

■ 初步稳定/治疗

静脉输液，适当镇痛。

■ 急诊治疗/程序

- 快速分类和评估。
- 检查睾丸以排除原发性肿瘤。
- 确定诊断并进行适当进行泌尿外科护理。
- 在阴囊上敷冰袋可缓解疼痛：
  - 可延长缺血性睾丸的生存力。
- 如果明确有效的处理很可能从扭转开始延迟超过4～5 h，就可以尝试手动复位（26.5%～80%成功）。
  - 向外旋转受影响的睾丸与通常的向内侧方向扭转相反。
  - 继续，直到疼痛缓解、正常解剖位置恢复或超声多普勒显示流量回归。
  - 所有接受手动解旋的患者必须通过手术探查。

■ 药物治疗

镇痛。

随访

■ 进一步处理

入院指征

- 确认扭转的患者必须入院进行阴囊探查和双侧睾丸固定术。
- 血流动力学研究不确定和技术性限制要求通过手术进一步探查阴囊。

G

• 如果血流检查有任何被延迟获得的可能，急性阴囊急症患者必须入院接受手术探查：
- 出现明显自发性扭转的患者应进行选择性探查并行双侧睾丸固定术。

出院指征

• 阴囊探查阴性与血流检查正常的患者可以在适当的泌尿外科随访的情况下出院。
• 因为反复扭转的可能性，必须研究重返急诊室患者的数据。
• 明确诊断除外睾丸扭转的患者可以转院护理。

要点和误区

• 儿童睾丸扭转可以与急性阑尾炎形似。
• 请记住“时间就是睾丸的生命”，紧急处理并需要咨询。
• 所有年龄组患者均要维持高度怀疑睾丸的心态，睾丸扭转发病的高峰在青少年和新生儿中。
• 如果早期诊断出睾丸扭转，睾丸的挽救率可能接近100%。睾丸固定术不是未来不再扭转的保证，但是它确实减少了可能性。

膈肌外伤 Diaphragmatic Trauma

Sam L. Frenkel · Peter L. Steinwald · Karen B. Van Hoesen 谭美春 译

基础知识

描述

• 穿通伤：
- 尖锐物体损伤膈膜（刺伤和枪伤最常见）。
- 可能伤及膈膜的任何部分。
- 相比钝器损伤创面更小（更容易被漏诊）。
• 钝器伤：
- 增加的腹腔内压力或胸腔内压力被传递到膈肌，从而引起破裂。
- 通常伤及左侧：
◦ 左半膈有脆弱的胚胎发育点。
◦ 右侧膈肌有肝脏的保护。
◦ 损伤比穿透伤大（损伤范围在5～15 cm）。
• 膈肌缺损无法自行愈合是因为胸腹腔压力梯度：
- 最大呼吸运动之间压力梯度可能超过100 cmH_2O。
- 促进腹腔内容物通过膈膜撕裂形成膈疝。

流行病学

发病率

不常见，占所有创伤的比例＜1%。

病因

• 横向冲击躯干造成同侧膈肌破裂的可能性是正面碰撞的3倍。
• 可疑膈肌损伤：
- 胸腹区的穿透伤。
- 跨横膈平面损伤，可延伸至第4肋骨。

诊断

注意

在急性期，可能没有腹腔疝气的表现：

• 这种外伤很可能被最初的CT扫描、剖腹手术或腹腔镜检查遗漏。

症状和体征

• 取决于疾病的阶段，处于急性期、潜伏期或阻塞期：
- 急性期：
◦ 呼吸急促和低血压。
◦ 呼吸音消失或减弱。
◦ 腹胀。
◦ 胸部闻及肠鸣音。
- 潜伏期：
◦ 腹腔内容物进入胸腔导致间歇性腹部不适症状。
◦ 餐后腹部疼痛加剧。
◦ 仰卧位腹痛加剧。
◦ 疼痛放射到左肩。
◦ 恶心、呕吐、嗳气。
- 嵌顿：
◦ 剧烈腹痛。
◦ 顽固性便秘。
◦ 恶心、呕吐。
◦ 腹胀。
• 腹腔脏器嵌顿可能造成穿孔，腹腔内容可能扩散至胸腔。
• 呼吸受限、败血症、死亡。
• 可能有迟发型的嵌顿性损伤。

基本检查

胸片可以显示突入胸腔内的肠疝环或其他腹腔脏器：
• 病症表现为胃管出现在膈肌以上。
• 结果经常是非特异性的：
- 膈肌升高。
- 膈肌轮廓不规则。
- 纵隔偏向患侧。
- 单侧胸膜增厚或胸腔积液。
- 局限性肺不张或合并基础疾病。
- 小范围的血胸或气胸。
• 最初的胸片50%可能是正常的。
• 由于膈疝时现时消，导致潜伏期的诊断比较困难。
• 胃肠道的对比研究可能会有所帮助。

诊断检查与说明

实验室检查

• 没有相关的实验室检查能够证实或排除膈肌损伤。
• 检测胸腔积液淀粉酶可评估膈肌撕裂。

影像学检查

• 膈疝发生时胸片可以诊断90%的病例，但在非急性膈疝时诊断灵敏度受限。
• 胃肠对比度的研究是最有用的，穿过膈肌的腹腔内容物有助于诊断慢性膈疝。
• 可以使用超声，特别是在右侧伴随肝疝时。
• 常规CT很少用于诊断该病，其敏感性较差。
• 螺旋和多排CT(MDCT)已被成功应用于诊断微小的膈肌损伤。
• MRI可将膈膜作为独立结构进行可视化成像，但并不适用于急诊或急性梗阻检查。

诊断步骤/外科

• 诊断性气腹造影：
- 空气通过DPL导管注入。
- 气胸后胸片用于诊断膈肌损伤。
- 病情不稳定的患者耐受性较差，可能需要放置胸腔引流管。

• 需要进行胸腔镜和腹腔镜探查：

- 尤其当高度怀疑时应进行此项检查，即使结果阴性。

- 有利于微创修复。

• CT 胸膜造影：

- 造影剂通过胸腔导管注射。

- CT 显示腹部造影剂外渗与膈肌撕裂一致。

- 需要放置胸腔导管。

■ 鉴别诊断

• 肺不张。
• 血胸。
• 气胸。
• 肺挫伤。
• 胃扩张、腹腔内积液。
• 创伤性肺膨出。
• 膈下脓肿。
• 胸腔内囊肿。
• 脓胸。
• 先天性膈膜膨出。

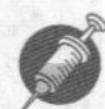

治疗

注意

• 膈疝的腹腔内容物进入胸壁，其症状可能类似于血胸或张力性气胸。

• 胸部闻及肠鸣音可以帮助鉴别。

• 怀疑胸部横向压缩导致膈肌损伤：

- 在胸廓造口术中放置针或导管时必须谨慎。

• 胸腔内有粪便提示肠破裂。

■ 初步稳定/治疗

• 遵循先进的创伤生命支持(ATLS)协议。

• 如果存在呼吸窘迫，立即留置胃管进行胃肠减压，可以解压并减少腹部疝内容物。

■ 急诊治疗/程序

• 插入胸管前需进行胸腔内脏器的触诊。

• 患者内脏穿孔化脓，需要超常规的液体复苏和抗生素治疗。

• 在内脏穿孔的情况下先进行经验性广谱抗生素治疗。

• 早期手术治疗是最重要的。

• 可在特定情况下进行微创修复。

■ 药物治疗

• 革兰阴性需氧菌：

- 庆大霉素：成人/儿童：初始剂量 2～5 mg/kg，静脉注射。

• 革兰阴性厌氧菌：

- 克林霉素：900 mg[儿童：20～40 mg/(kg・24 h)]，静脉注射，q8 h。

- 甲硝唑：1 g(儿童：15 mg/kg)静脉注射负荷，然后 500 mg(儿童：7.5 mg/kg)，静脉注射，每 6 h 一次。

• 需氧菌和厌氧菌：

- 氨苄西林-舒巴坦：1.5～3 g[儿童：100～400 mg/(kg・24 h)]，静脉注射，q6 h。

- 头孢替坦：2 g[儿童：40～80 mg/(kg・24 h)]，静脉注射，q12 h。

- 头孢西丁：2 g[儿童：80～160 mg/(kg・24 h)]，静脉注射，q12 h。

- 替卡西林-克拉维酸：3.1 g(儿童：50 mg/kg)，静脉注射，q12 h。

随访

■ 进一步处理

入院指征

• 怀疑存在膈肌损伤的患者必须收住入院进行外科手术。

• 窒息或呼吸窘迫的高风险患者应立即/监测或收入 ICU。

出院指征

确诊或高度怀疑其存在膈肌损伤的患者不能从急诊室出院。

■ 随访建议

膈肌损伤 S/P 修复患者必须创伤外科医师随访，以监测复发。

儿科注意事项

• 儿童的解剖差异使其受到较轻的外伤时更容易造成膈肌损伤：

- 更薄的腹壁。

- 多数膈膜呈水平方向。

- 肋骨多为软骨成分。

• 左右两侧膈肌外伤的发生率大致相等。

• 更容易造成单发伤。

要点和误区

• 依据有关机构报告，总死亡率为 18%～40%。

• 常伴发于严重的肝脾损伤、血胸、气胸、骨盆骨折外伤疾病。

• 如果存在左上腹和下胸部穿通伤，必须高度怀疑膈肌损伤。

• 延迟诊断将增加膈疝与腹腔脏器绞窄的风险。

• 要实时获取胸部影像学资料。

弓形虫病 Toxoplasmosis

Roger M. Barkin 张晟 林兆奋 译

基础知识

■ 描述

• 弓形虫：细胞内原生寄生虫。

- 3 种形式。

◦ 速殖子：无性侵袭形式。

◦ 组织囊肿：在慢性期持续感染宿主组织。

◦ 卵囊：含有孢子体，在猫肠寄居的性周期内产生。

• 传播：

- 摄取组织囊肿或卵囊：

◦ 摄入未煮熟的肉。

◦ 被卵囊污染的蔬菜。

◦ 通过猫或土壤接触猫粪。

- 胎盘。

- 血液制品。

- 器官移植。

■ 病因

• 70%的成人血清阳性。

• 大多数免疫功能正常的患者无症状。

• 全球范围已知猫是常见的宿主。

• 孵化期为 7 日，潜伏期为 4～21 日。

诊断

症状和体征

4种感染。

免疫力低下的宿主

- 中枢神经系统。
- 亚急性表现(90%)。
- 脑炎。
- 头痛。
- 精神状态改变。
- 发热。
- 癫痫。
- 颅神经麻痹。
- 脊髓病变。
- 小脑病变表现。
- 脑膜炎样症状。
- 运动障碍。
- 神经心理症状。
- ○精神病。
- ○偏执狂。
- ○痴呆症。
- ○焦虑。
- ○烦乱。
- 肺部。
- 肺炎。
- 干咳。
- 呼吸困难。
- 长期发热的疾病。

免疫活性宿主

- 90%无症状。
- 淋巴结肿大,通常是颈椎周围淋巴结。
- 发热。
- 心神不安。
- 伴有黄斑皮疹和肝脾大的单核细胞增多症样综合征。
- 头痛。
- 咽喉痛。
- 盗汗。
- 斑丘疹。
- 荨麻疹。
- 通常是自我限制的过程,在2～12个月消失。
- 很少出现肺炎或脑炎。

眼弓形虫病

- 视野模糊。
- 视野暗点。
- 疼痛。
- 畏光。
- 视网膜。
- 一小群黄白色的棉状斑块。
- 脉络膜视网膜炎,85%的未经治疗的先天性感染年轻成人受影响。

先天性弓形虫病

- 妊娠期间无症状急性感染的结果。
- 妊娠前期。
- 自然流产。
- 死胎。
- 在此期间发生严重疾病概率高达25%。
- 妊娠中期或妊娠后期。
- 有50%～60%的可能患获得先天性弓形虫病。
- 死亡率为2%。

弓形虫病

- 2%致命。
- 大多数出生时无症状。
- 延迟发病。出生时70%～90%无症状。
- 中枢神经系统疾病。
- 眼部疾病(数月至数年后失明)。
- 淋巴结肿大。
- 肝脾大。
- 出生时可能有斑丘疹、淋巴结肿大、肝大、脾大、黄疸、血小板减少症。

基本检查

- 通过以下方式诊断:
- 病原学培养。
- ○血液。
- ○脑炎时查脑脊液。
- ○肺炎时查支气管肺泡灌洗液。
- ○羊水。
- ○房水。
- 检测组织或体液中的速殖子。
- 淋巴结活检显示特征性病理。
- 彻底的眼科检查。
- 视网膜检查。
- 视敏度。

诊断检查与说明

实验室检查

- 与弓形虫病相关的LDH＞600 U/L。
- CBC。
- 异型淋巴细胞。
- 用于肺部症状的ABG/脉搏血氧仪。
- IgG抗体。
- 酶联免疫吸附试验(ELISA)终身存在。
- IgM后2周IgG阳性有助于确诊。
- IgG滴度高低与感染程度无关。
- 免疫球蛋白M(IgM)抗体。
- 在免疫功能正常的宿主缺少排他性诊断。可能需要重复。
- 诊断急性感染。
- 在5日内出现。
- 在数周至数月内消失。
- PCR具有较高的特异性和可变的敏感性。如果在第一周为阴性,可能需要重复。
- 新生儿检查结果与母体感染鉴别。
- 帕洛阿尔托医学基金会提供额外的测试。

影像学检查

胸部X线片显示肺部征象。

- 与网状结节状阴影相关的肺炎。
- 具有对比度的头颅CT。
- 多发性双侧低密度环强化病变。
- MRI脑部。
- T_2加权像上的高信号异常。
- 系列胎儿超声检查可用于探索先天性中枢神经系统或其他先天性感染症状。

诊断步骤/外科

脑活检用于脑炎确诊。

鉴别诊断

- 隐球菌性脑膜炎。
- 中枢神经系统淋巴瘤。
- 卡氏肺囊虫肺炎。
- 巨细胞病毒性视网膜炎。
- 分枝杆菌感染。

G

治疗

初步稳定/治疗

- 用地西泮和苯妥英钠按标准方式治疗癫痫发作。
- 如果由于肺炎引起的缺氧给予氧疗。

急诊治疗/程序

免疫功能正常的宿主

弓形虫淋巴结炎。

- 除非症状严重且无缓解,否则不用抗生素。
- 治疗有症状的患者,乙胺嘧啶和亚叶酸加磺胺嘧啶或克林霉素治疗3～4周。
- 克林霉素可能是一种有效的替代磺胺嘧啶的药物,因为后者的副作用以及人群对磺胺类药物易过敏。
- 乙胺嘧啶和磺胺嘧啶联合用药。
- 皮质类固醇可能对治疗眼部并发症和中枢神经系统症状有用。几乎没有证据支持。
- 重新评估以确定是否需要更长时间的治疗。

免疫力低下的宿主

- 通过血清学/症状确认急性感染。
  - 症状缓解后用乙胺嘧啶和亚叶酸＋磺胺嘧啶或克林霉素治疗 4～6 周。
  - 替代药物：
    - 甲氧苄氨嘧啶-新诺明。
    - 乙胺嘧啶和亚叶酸氨苯砜。
- CNS 症状＋CT 或 MRI 上的病变。
  - 用乙胺嘧啶和亚叶酸钙＋磺胺嘧啶或克林霉素进行经验性治疗。
  - 脑活检或脑脊液确认诊断。
  - 只有确认先兆癫痫才能使用抗癫痫药。
    - 服药抗癫痫药物患者的预后较差。
- 慢性无症状感染。
  - 不需要治疗。
  - 艾滋病和免疫抑制患者的弓形虫预防选择。
    - 甲氧苄氨嘧啶-磺胺甲噁唑（800 mg/160 mg）；咨询后 HIV 感染患者应考虑终身预防。
    - 乙胺嘧啶（75 mg/周）和氨苯砜（200 mg/周）和亚叶酸钙 10～25 mg，搭配单位剂量乙胺嘧啶。

眼科治疗

- 用乙胺嘧啶和磺胺嘧啶治疗 1 个月。
- 可加用克林霉素。
- 系统性类固醇用药治疗黄斑或视神经神经受累。没有确切的疗效证据。

妊娠急性感染

- 最初用螺旋霉素进行诊断性治疗并及时会诊。由于缺乏明确的有效性和毒性风险症状，起始治疗需要慎重且应在会诊后。
- 感染确认后，会诊后开始治疗。
  - 前 17 周用螺旋霉素。
  - 17 周后使用乙胺嘧啶和磺胺嘧啶。
- 螺旋霉素可能会降低先天性传播，但是如果胎盘感染，则胎儿无法受到治疗；母亲的治疗可能会降低先天性疾病的严重程度。
- 用磺胺嘧啶、乙胺嘧啶和亚叶酸，给药 12 个月治疗先天性感染。
- 未受弓形虫感染的妊娠期女性在接触猫或猫排泄物时防止暴露于弓形虫，这很重要。

药物治疗

- 克林霉素。
  - 600 mg[儿童：20～40 mg/(kg · 24 h)]，静脉，q6 h。
  - 300 mg[儿童：8～20 mg/(kg · 24 h)]，口服，q6 h。
  - 如果患者对磺胺过敏，则克林霉素很有用。
- 氨苯砜：每日 50 mg 口服或每周 200 mg 口服[儿童＞1 个月：2 mg/(kg · d)]。
- 亚叶酸钙：每日 10～25 mg 口服连同乙胺嘧啶和磺胺嘧啶治疗预防血液毒性。
- 乙胺嘧啶：首日负荷量 100 mg，每日 2 次，然后与磺胺嘧啶联合口服每日 25～50 mg，口服。
- 螺旋霉素：需要 FDA 授权。
- 磺胺嘧啶：500 mg～2 g[儿童：75～150 mg/(kg · 24 h)]，口服，q6 h。
- 甲氧苄啶-磺胺甲噁唑：5 mg/kg 甲氧苄啶组分，静脉或口服，q12 h。

随访

进一步处理

入院指征

- 伴严重全身症状的急性感染。
- 免疫功能低下的患者。
  - 弓形体病脑炎。
  - 肺炎。
  - 脓毒症。

出院指征

- 免疫功能正常的患者。
  - 症状轻微。
  - 眼睛症状消失。
- 轻微症状的先天性感染。

转诊问题

感染科会诊，探讨替代疗法及潜在并发症。

G

肱骨骨折 Humerus Fracture

Megan Tresenriter · Christanne H. Coffey　巩博 译

基础知识

描述

- 肱骨近端骨折：
  - 常为无移位、移位和/或骨折/脱位。
  - 占所有肱骨骨折的 5%。
  - 随着年龄增长，发病率增加。
  - 男女比例为 1∶4。
  - 大多数患者＞60 岁。
  - 是第三常见的骨质疏松性骨折，前 2 位是髋骨和桡骨远端骨折。
  - Neer 分类：一种识别骨折或骨折/脱位的位置、碎片数量、移位和角度的系统。
- 肱骨干骨折：
  - 占肱骨骨折的 3%。
  - 可能为螺旋形、斜形或横形。
  - 肱骨干骨折（AO 分型）：
  - 简单。
  - 楔形。
  - 粉碎性（复杂型）。

病因

- 肱骨近端骨折：
  - 通常有摔伤史（低能量）。
  - 常发生在摔倒时手臂撑开。
  - 由电击、癫痫或高能量损伤导致的强烈肌肉收缩少见。
- 肱骨干骨折：
  - 高能量直接创伤（穿透性或钝性）或扭曲力。
  - 由摔伤引起。
  - 投掷损伤引起的应力性骨折。

诊断

症状和体征

- 疼痛、肿胀，有压痛。
- 主动运动困难。
- 手臂常贴紧胸壁。
- 肢体短缩。
- 可能存在捻发音。
- 瘀斑。
- 神经血管损伤。

病史

- 左利手。
- 受伤机制。
- 共同危险因素（年龄、摔倒风险、恶性肿瘤）。
- 合并伤。

体格检查

• 完整检查患肢：
- 检查肩部和肱骨有无变形、短缩和开放性损伤。
- 评估肩部、肘部的活动度。
- 神经血管检查。

基本检查

• 评估单个神经：
- 桡神经(在肱骨干中段骨折中尤其注意)。最常见的损伤神经检测：三头肌力量，手腕伸展，掌指关节伸展和拇指伸展，感觉拇指指腹空间。
- 正中神经：拇指和示指对位做“O”手势。
- 尺神经。
- 腋神经(肩部侧面的感觉功能)。
- 肌皮神经(前臂伸肌的感觉功能)。
- 肩胛上神经——支配冈上肌和冈下肌，分别检查外展和外旋。

• 评估血供：
- 存在桡动脉、尺动脉、肱动脉搏动。
- 所有指端毛细血管再充盈良好。
- 放射学检查明确伤情。

儿科注意事项

• 发病年龄<3 岁或>12 岁。
• 分娩创伤导致的新生儿骨折：
- 常见于>4.5 kg 和臀位分娩。
- 可能出现假瘫。
- 关节固定术：通过吊带将前臂固定在胸腔 2 周。

• 较大的儿童：同成人一样的受伤机制。
• 儿童骨膜较厚，可限制肱骨干骨折移位。
• 肱骨近端骨折：
- 当近端肱骨影像学正常但是有明显疼痛时应考虑 SalterⅠ型骨折。
- SalterⅡ型骨折常见于年轻儿童。

• 尤其注意(特别是<3 岁)：
- 受伤类型：
  ◦ 横形(直接打击)。
  ◦ 斜形或螺旋形(牵拉或者肱骨旋转)。
  ◦ 干骺端骨折(桶柄式半月板破裂)。

诊断检查与说明

• X 线平片：
- 肱骨近端骨折(至少 3 个角度)：
  ◦ 前后位、侧位和腋位。
  ◦ 腋位评估结节移位、关节盂关节面、肱骨头和关节盂的关系。
- 肱骨干骨折：
  ◦ 必须行前后位和侧位检查。
  ◦ 包括肩关节和肘关节成像以排除并发关节受累。

• CT 扫描：
- 在肱骨近端骨折中有助于复杂/粉碎性骨折手术方式的确定。
- 在可疑骨折/脱位中有助于明确肱骨头和关节盂的关系。

诊断步骤/外科

不适用。

鉴别诊断

• 急性出血性黏液囊炎。
• 外伤性肩袖撕裂。
• 脱位。
• 肩锁关节脱位。
• 钙化性肌腱炎。
• 挫伤。
• 肌腱破裂。
• 神经失用症。
• 病理性骨折。

治疗

院前

注意：

• 避免手臂过度运动，可能导致进一步神经血管损伤。
• 使用肩悬吊带固定并转运。
• 出现神经或血管功能障碍时快速转运。

初步稳定/治疗

• 对相关损伤进行主要和次要检查。
• 固定：
- 舒适。
- 阻止骨折片移位。
- 阻止神经血管损伤。

• 可以使用腋垫使患者舒适。
• 控制疼痛。
• 使用冰块减轻肿胀。
• 开放性骨折：
- 使用无菌敷料覆盖。
- 预防破伤风。
- 注射抗生素。

急诊治疗/程序

• 患者在诊断和治疗伤情期间应接受合适的止痛治疗。
- 口服、肌内注射或静脉注射麻醉药品是首选治疗。

• 肱骨近端骨折：
- 使用 Neer 分类来描述基于移位部分/部件的数量：
  ◦ 根据 4 个部分的解剖关系：大结节、小结节、肱骨头(解剖性颈骨折)、骨干(外科颈骨折)。
  ◦ 考虑分开的断端与断端之间，如果>1 cm 分离或>45°成角。
- 单节段肱骨近端骨折：
  ◦ 无移位。
  ◦ >80%肱骨近端骨折。
  ◦ 可采取非手术治疗。
  ◦ 治疗采用肩悬吊带。
  ◦ 早期全范围关节运动(ROM 运动)。
- 移位、多节段肱骨近端骨折：
  ◦ 骨科复查和转诊适用于 2 节段或以上骨折。
  ◦ 可减少和非手术处理许多 2 节段骨折。
  ◦ 3～4 节段骨折可能需要 ORIF/半关节成形术。
  ◦ 手术选择不仅取决于骨折类型，而且还取决于患者的年龄、共病和患者对肢体功能的期望。
- 肱骨近端骨折会诊的适应证：
  ◦ 开放性骨折。
  ◦ 不能在急救室复位的骨折/移位。
  ◦ 血管损伤。

• 肱骨干骨折：
- 大多数肱骨干骨折可以采取非手术治疗的方式，不需要复位(90%)。
- 向前成角 20°或者内翻成角 30°可以被肱骨周围的肌肉组织耐受。
- 肱骨可以耐受 3 cm 的短缩，有较小的功能缺陷。

• 无移位的肱骨干骨折：
- 急救室可以使用夹板治疗。
- 除外横形骨折。
- 骨科医师可以使用功能支具。

• 横形骨折：
- 急救室应使用肩悬吊带。
- 骨折不愈合高发。

• 有移位的肱骨干骨折：
- 骨科医师可以使用悬吊石膏、复位移位或短缩。

• 肱骨干骨折骨科医师紧急会诊的适应证：
- 神经血管损伤。
- 多段骨折。
- 骨折延展至关节面。
- 开放性骨折。
- 浮肘(骨折并发同侧前臂骨折)。
- 严重软组织损伤。

G

- 筋膜室综合征。

儿科注意事项

接近骨成熟的儿童，判断移位程度或近端肱骨骨骺范围是精确复位的基础，这对于防止以后的生长障碍是重要的。

■ 药物治疗

• 止痛治疗：
- 麻醉药品（一线）。
- 非甾体抗炎药（二线）。
• 闭合性复位时给予镇静治疗（见操作时镇静）。

随访

■ 进一步处理

入院指征

• 开放性骨折准备行手术治疗和注射抗生素治疗。
• 骨折并发血管损伤。
• 移位的碎片不能通过闭合性复位手法复位。
• 并发严重损伤需要治疗和观察。

入院指征

• 无移位骨折。
• 闭合性复位治疗的骨折。
• 大多数闭合性肱骨干骨折不伴有其他伤情。
• 更多的复杂肱骨近端骨折（如肱骨近端骨折 Neer 3 型、4 型）可能需要非急诊手术。应当在骨科医师会诊后出院。

儿科注意事项

• 儿科患者表达能力差，对于制动的依从性差，他们可以在住院中受益。
• 评估环境安全，注意是否存在非意外创伤。

转诊问题

• 多数肱骨骨折应当转诊骨科门诊。
• 复杂肱骨近端骨折（Neer 2～4 型）应当和骨科医师一起评估，制订门诊就诊计划和可能的非紧急干预。
• 有些一部分移位的肱骨近端骨折可行经皮微创髋关节钢板螺钉系统治疗。
• 移位肱骨干骨折需要骨科医师进行确定性治疗（功能支具、悬吊石膏、切开复位内固定等）。

■ 随访建议

• 大多数患者需要密切随访，重复测试患肢，以确定合适的止痛治疗，到达急诊室后快速评估治疗方案。
• 稳定的肱骨近端骨折应该评估早期 ROM 治疗，以减少最小化粘连性关节囊炎的风险。

要点和误区

• 所有肱骨骨折患者应当接受神经血管测试：
- 复位后应当重复神经血管检查。
- 在肱骨干骨折中，桡神经损伤是最常见的功能缺陷。
- 大多数桡神经功能缺陷在一段时间（数月）后会自然消退。
• 在波及外科颈或关节面的肱骨近端骨折中，可能出现缺血性坏死。
• 多部分肱骨近端骨折（Neer 2 型或更高）的患者可能经常从急救室出院，但是需要和骨科医师制订下一步计划，患者可能需要外科干预和/或伴关节成形术。

汞中毒 Mercury Poisoning

Denise A. Whitfield · David A. Tanen 段立伟 译

G

基础知识

■ 描述

汞：

• 3 种存在形式：元素形式、无机盐形式和有机物形式。
• 与巯基反应，导致酶活性抑制和细胞膜改变。
• 可结合到酶的磷酰基基团、羰基基团、酰胺基基团和胺基基团。

■ 病因

• 通常由胃肠道和吸入途径进入体内导致暴露，也可经皮肤接触暴露。
• 制造氯气和氢氧化钠、利尿药、抗菌剂、防腐剂、温度计、电池、化石燃料、塑料、油漆、珠宝、灯具、炸药、焰火、氯乙烯和颜料时可导致暴露。
• 接触动物标本、摄影、口腔科、汞矿开采也可导致暴露。
• 食用受污染的海鲜。

诊断

■ 症状和体征

• 天然存在的汞会被转换成 3 种形式，每种形式的汞都有自己的毒理学效应：
• 元素汞：
- 通常为吸入性暴露，数小时内产生症状：
◦ 咳嗽和呼吸困难，可能发展成肺水肿。
◦ 金属味，流涎。
◦ 虚弱、恶心、腹泻、发热、头痛、视力障碍。
- 皮下沉积可表现为肉芽肿或脓肿。
- 静脉暴露症状与肺动脉栓塞症状一致。
- 尽管有发生阑尾炎的报道，但经口摄入元素汞相对无毒。
• 无机盐形式的汞摄入：
- 腐蚀性消化道损伤：
◦ 伴有恶心、呕吐、腹泻和腹痛。
◦ 金属味，咽喉肿痛。
◦ 伴有便血和呕血出血性胃肠炎。
- 急性肾小管坏死。
- 肢痛症（粉色病）：
◦ 特异反应性，主要发生于儿童。
◦ 四肢疼痛。
- 粉红色皮肤变色脱落。
• 有机汞：
- 子宫中的婴儿发生暴露时受影响最严重（如日本水俣湾）。
- 可以出现急性胃肠道症状。
- 延迟性中枢神经系统毒性症状占主导地位，可能需要几周到几个月才表现出来：
◦ 皮肤感觉异常。
◦ 共济失调。
◦ 麻痹。
◦ 视野受限。
◦ 构音障碍。
◦ 听力丧失。
◦ 智力减退。
◦ 死亡。

病史

- 询问汞产品工作地点、环境或意外暴露史。
- 记录患者最近几周的海鲜摄入情况。

体格检查

- 元素汞：
  - 如果吸入或静脉注射，可表现为咳嗽，并进展到呼吸困难。
  - 共济失调。
  - 如果注射摄入，可见皮下结节或肉芽肿。
- 无机汞：
  - 口腔烧伤。
  - 腹肌紧张。
  - 粪便隐血阳性。
- 有机汞：
  - 中枢神经系统异常：
    - 进展性认知恶化。

基本检查

- 工作场所和环境暴露病史。
- 体格检查要点：
  - 呼吸困难。
  - 腐蚀性胃肠道损伤。
  - 神经精神受损。
- 实验室检查：
  - 肾衰竭。
  - 血液和尿液汞水平。
    - 近期有食用海鲜史时，测量结果不可靠。

诊断检查与说明

实验室检查

- 无机汞暴露：
  - 血常规。
  - 电解质、BUN、肌酐、葡萄糖。
  - 24 h 尿液汞收集：
    - 正常尿液水平＜20 mg/dl。
  - 全血汞水平：
    - 正常血液水平＜10 mg/dl。
- 有机汞暴露：
  - 血常规，周围血涂片。
  - 电解质、BUN、肌酐、葡萄糖。
  - 全血汞水平：
    - 正常血液水平＜10 mg/dl。

影像学检查

- X线胸片：
  - 发现非心源性肺水肿。
  - 在肺血管发现静脉注射汞的证据。
- 腹部X线平片：
  - 故意口服患者，可有利于发现汞的存在。
- 头颅 CT：
  - 可能会检测出脑萎缩。

诊断步骤/外科

存在精神状态改变的患者要进行腰椎穿刺检查。

鉴别诊断

- 多系统受累时常与其他重金属中毒混淆。
- 脑血管意外。
- 老年性痴呆和阿尔茨海默病。
- 帕金森病。
- 消化性溃疡病。
- 消化道出血。
- 胰腺炎。
- 脓血症。
- 肺炎。
- 肺栓塞。

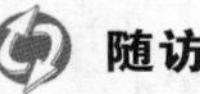

治疗

院前

- 脱离毒物暴露。
- 去污：
  - 清洗裸露的皮肤。

初步稳定/治疗

- ABC 管理和监测。
- 生理盐水。
- 低血压时给予静脉补液复苏：
  - 严重胃肠道出血者可给予输血治疗。

急诊治疗/程序

- 元素汞：
  - 对于吸入暴露患者，密切观察几小时以发现非心源性肺水肿。
  - 摄入的汞元素可通过肠道排泄，伴有少量的吸收。
  - 对于有症状的患者可考虑口服二巯基丁二酸(DMSA)进行螯合。
  - 对于皮下结节或脓肿，可切开引流。
- 无机汞：
  - 给予活性炭。
  - 大量生理盐水静脉补液/血制品以纠正低血容量性休克：
    - 水化和维持尿量[1 ml/(kg · h)]。
  - 有症状患者考虑螯合治疗。
    - 肌内注射二巯基丙醇。
    - 由于腐蚀性胃肠道损伤，口服 DMSA 效果有限。
- 有机汞：
  - 给予活性炭。
  - 口服 DMSA 进行螯合。

药物治疗

一线药物

- 二巯基丁二酸(DMSA)：10 mg/kg，口服，每日 3 次，共 5 日，然后每日 1 次，服用 2 周，轻度至中度中毒。
- 二巯基丙醇(BAL)：5 mg/kg，肌内注射，q4 h，用 48 h，然后 2.5 mg/kg，肌内注射，q6 h，用 48 h，然后 2.5 mg/kg，肌内注射，q12 h，用 7 日。

二线药物

- D-青霉胺：
  - 成人：250 mg，口服，每日 1 次，用 7～14 日。
  - 儿童：5～7 mg/kg，口服，每日 1 次，用 7～14 日。
  - N-乙酰-DL-青霉胺(NAP)是一种副作用较少的试验性药物。
- 二巯基丙磺酸钠：
  - 静脉或口服。如果有可能，请联系当地毒物中心。

随访

进一步处理

入院指征

急性有症状患者：

- 任何有呼吸功能减弱证据的患者。
- 口服摄入无机汞可能导致消化道损伤的患者。
- 肾脏损伤的患者。
- 需螯合治疗的患者。

出院指征

- 有摄入元素汞病史，消化道完整无症状的患者。
- 有吸入元素汞病史，观察 6 h 后仍无症状的患者。

转诊问题

- 有症状或需要螯合剂治疗的患者应转诊到毒理科。
- 转诊到胃肠科处理腐蚀性胃肠道损伤。
- 有吸入性损伤症状的患者应进入肺科 ICU 治疗。
- 进展性脑部功能恶化患者的评估要在神经科进行。
- 转诊毒物中心用以检测各种可疑暴露源。

随访建议

- 对于可能有工作场所或环境暴露的出院

G

患者，他们的初级保健医师要定期随访患者的 24 h 尿液和全血汞水平。
• 门诊疑似或确诊病例要转诊到毒理科。
• 对于无症状患者，限制患者食用海鲜 2 周后，复查 24 h 尿液汞水平。

要点和误区

• 当患者有胃肠道或神经精神方面的不适时，应仔细询问患者工作地点、环境和意外暴露病史。
• 吸入暴露的患者至少监测 6 h。
• 口服摄入无机汞可导致严重的腐蚀性胃肠道损伤。
• 实验室检查可出现假阳性结果，特别是对于食用海鲜的患者。

共济失调

Lara K. Kulchycki 王海嵘 潘曙明 译

 基础知识

描述

• 无法进行协调动作。
• 由小脑或小脑连接疾病导致的。
- 横向小脑损伤引起的身体同侧体征。
- 中线损伤引起的躯干共济失调。

病因

通常原发在小脑，但也可出现感觉、运动或前庭功能失调：
• 创伤。
• 重大损伤。
• 血管疾病。
• 感染或感染后进展。
• 毒物、药物。
• 代谢、内分泌性的精神紊乱。
• 脱髓鞘疾病。
• 先天畸形。
• 遗传疾病。
- 先天性代谢异常。
- 进行性共济失调退化。
• 营养缺陷。

诊断

症状和体征

• 失调步态。
- 共济失调通常伴有步态不稳。
- 行走初始的不安全感。
- 无法完成特殊技能(骑单车、滑雪、攀爬)。
- 不平衡感。
- 分腿站立姿势和蹒跚步态。
- 串联步态测试以检验细微的共济失调。
• 肢体共济失调。
- 不协调。
- 意向震颤。
- 书写，拾物，钉纽扣时动作笨拙。
- 辨距不良：指鼻试验和跟膝胫试验完成不佳。
- 轮替运动完成不佳：无法快速进行轮替运动。
• 躯干共济失调。
- 头部震颤。
- 躯体不稳。
- 蹒跚：静止时头、躯干摇摆。
• 构音障碍和延髓症状。
- 言语含糊。
- 说话断音。
- 吞咽不协调导致的哽咽。
• 视觉异常。
- 视力模糊。
- 眩晕：
◦ 鉴别中枢性眩晕和外周性眩晕。
◦ 外周性眩晕通常很严重，由运动触发，常伴随耳痛、听力丧失和耳鸣。
- 眼球震颤：
◦ 凝视引发的眼球震颤：快速反复由中点向侧边移动。
◦ 回弹的眼球震颤。
• 肌肉、骨骼和力量的异常。
- 等距试验：双手使用中很难维持恒定力量：
◦ 让患者使用轻微，稳定的力度握检查者的手指(检查者会感到不规则的压力)。
- 小脑疾病导致的肌力减退或不寻常的肌张力减退。
• 感觉失调：
- 感觉异常。
- 麻木。
- 小心翼翼的跨域步态。
- 标志性的闭眼协调性减退：
◦ Romberg 征阳性是典型的感觉失调表现。
- 位置感、震动感丧失。
- 精细动作困难。

病史

• 如果出现由疼痛、衰弱、头晕、眩晕或共济失调导致的步态改变，详细的病史是必需的。
• 起病：
- 数小时至数日：急性。
- 数周至数月：亚急性。
- 数月至数年：慢性。
• 对称或病灶的症状。
• 发热、精神改变、衰弱、感觉缺失或尿失禁的表现。
• 新近的病毒感染或免疫接种。
• 创伤史或中毒史。
• 运动疾病家族史。

体格检查

• 彻底的检查，包括神经系统及步态测试。
• 评估急性、危及生命的疾病的症状和体征，如出血、脑卒中或中枢感染：
- 精神状态的改变。
- 头痛。
- 神经系统局部病灶。
- 颅内压升高：
◦ 心动过缓、高血压、呼吸节律异常。
◦ 视神经乳头水肿。
◦ 囟门突出。
- 发热。
- 假性脑膜炎。
- 眼球震颤。
- 恶心、呕吐。
- 耳检查和眼球震颤的刺激性试验(Dix-Hallpike)。
• 怀疑中毒者应记录中毒表现。

基本检查

详细的病史和体格检查能帮助确定需要的必要检查。

诊断检查与说明

实验室检查

• 血糖水平。

G

• 血清电解质。
• 毒物筛查：
- 运动失调患者不包括在标准组。
• 甲状腺功能检测。
• 可能的额外检测，比如抗惊厥物质。

影像学检查

• CT：
- 头颅 CT 能鉴别大量的出血、亚急性的脑梗死或脑积水。
- 如果怀疑大量，不论有无静脉对照，考虑 CT。
- CT 血管造影可以用于评估血管性疾病。
• MRI：
- 用于评估急性缺血、大面积、脱髓鞘损伤和血管畸形是极好的。
- 颅后窝的影像较明确。
- 如果高度怀疑血管畸形，推荐头颈的 MRI 血管造影。
• 心电图：
- 不推荐用于共济失调的病情检查中，但对于评估非特异性头晕是有用的。

诊断步骤/外科

• 腰椎穿刺：
- 怀疑颅内感染或吉兰-巴雷综合征时推荐。

鉴别诊断

• 急性对称性共济失调：
- 头颅外伤。
- 药物、中毒：
◦ 酒精。
◦ 锂。
◦ 苯妥英。
◦ 巴比妥类。
◦ 酰胺咪嗪。
◦ 镇静安眠剂。
◦ 丙戊酸。
◦ 苯二氮。
◦ 苯海拉明。
◦ 右美沙芬。
- 急性病毒性小脑炎。
- 脑膜炎/脑炎。
- 脑积水。
- 感染后综合征。
- 低血糖。
- 低钠血症。
- 严重中暑。
• 急性局灶性共济失调。
- 后循环梗死。
- 大脑前动脉综合征。
- 基底动脉供血不足(VBI)。
- 脑出血。
- 硬膜下血肿。
- 脑脓肿。
- 脑脊髓炎的急性播散。
- 复杂的偏头痛。
- 非典型癫痫。
• 亚急性对称性共济失调：
- 药物/中毒：
◦ 汞。
◦ 铅。
◦ 碳氢化合物。
◦ 吸胶毒(嗅胶)。
◦ 细胞毒性化疗。
◦ 有机磷酸酯类。
- 维生素 B_1 或维生素 B_{12} 缺失。
- 癌旁综合征：
◦ 乳腺癌/卵巢癌。
◦ 霍奇金淋巴瘤。
◦ 成神经细胞瘤。
- 莱姆病。
- 弓形虫病。
- Creutzfeldt-Jakob 病。
• 亚急性局灶共济失调。
- 小脑胶质瘤。
- 转移肿瘤。
- 淋巴瘤。
- 多发性硬化。
- 吉兰-巴雷综合征。
- 艾滋病相关进行性多发病灶的脑白质病。
- 脊髓空洞症。
- 颈椎病。
• 慢性共济失调：
- 酒精相关性的小脑退变。
- 神经胶质过多征。
- 遗传疾病：
◦ 脊髓小脑共济失调。
◦ Friedreich 共济失调。
◦ 共济失调毛细管扩张。
◦ Niemann-Pick 病。
- 甲状腺功能减退。
- 维生素 E 缺失。
- 背部脊髓结核。
- 先天畸形。
◦ Arnold-Chiari。
◦ Dandy-Walker。
• 导致外周性眩晕的疾病可以出现共济失调步态：
- 良性阵发性的位置性眩晕。
- 急性内耳炎。
- 梅尼埃病。

儿科注意事项

• 会出现拒绝行走。
• 儿童急性共济失调通常是良性的、自限性的过程：
- 60%的病例由急性小脑共济失调或药物导致。
• 急性小脑共济失调：
- 感染后小脑脱髓鞘。
- 通常出现于 2～5 岁的小儿。
- 在诱发疾病发生后 1～3 周出现。
- 约 1/4 的病例出现于水痘后，但与许多病毒感染和免疫接种相关。
- 精神状态正常。
- 没有发热，没有病灶或癫痫。
- 轻症可在家治疗，但须接受伤害预防咨询。
- 大多数儿童可在 3 个月内完全康复。
• 药物/中毒：
- 预期中的精神改变。
- 评估用药途径和制定合适的毒物学测试。
• 吉兰-巴雷综合征：
- 15%的病例以感觉共济失调为表现。
- Miller-Fisher 变体：共济失调，反射消失，眼肌麻痹三联征。
• 肿瘤：
- 超过 50%的儿童脑瘤发生于脑干和小脑。
- 斜视眼阵挛-肌阵挛-共济失调综合征：
◦ 癌旁自身免疫综合征影响小脑。
◦ 超过 50%病例由成神经细胞瘤引起。
• 脑卒中：
- 儿童罕见，但也可发生于镰红细胞病或血液高凝状态。

老年人注意事项

• 老年人的步态疾病常是多因素的。
• 潜在的认知缺失使疾病很难同晕厥前期、衰弱、眩晕和不协调鉴别。
• 脑血管后循环综合征，比如 VBI 和脑卒中，在老年人中更常见，常表现为不明确的症状，如头晕。
• 评估静止平衡位或锥体外系疾病，如帕金森病。

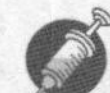

治疗

院前

注意：

• 急性共济失调发作可能预示着脑卒中或出血。

G

• 意识状态减退可能预示着气管插管。

■ 初步稳定/治疗

• 心肺复苏。
• 建立静脉通道。
• 给氧。
• 心电监测。
• 指尖针刺测血糖。
- 低血糖者给予葡萄糖。
- 酗酒者和营养不良者考虑硫胺素。

■ 急诊治疗/程序

• 制定预防措施。
• 治疗必须根据患者的表现和潜在病因制定。
• 小脑梗死会导致严重的脑水肿和脑疝：
- 需要神经外科会诊决定是否需要行颅骨切除减压术。

■ 药物治疗

• 葡萄糖：D_{50} W(50 ml 或 25 g)(D_{25} W 2～4 ml/kg)静脉使用。
• 硫胺素(维生素 B_1)：100 mg 静脉使用。

随访

■ 进一步处理

入院指征

• 急性和亚急性共济失调，特别是良性病因不能确定的话。
• 无法安全步行的患者。
• 因小脑出血或严重并发症入住 ICU。

出院指征

• 可逆或轻症。
• 正常的精神状态。
• 能够安全步行。

■ 随访建议

遵循初级护理或在症状基础上的神经病学。

要点和误区

• 未能将真实的共济失调与其他不稳步态疾病鉴别。
• 醉酒患者未能记录创伤。
• 在评估颅后窝时未能认识到 CT 扫描的局限。
• 在小脑损伤，包括脑卒中的病例中未能认清脑疝的风险。

股骨干滑脱 Slipped Capital Femoral Epiphysis

Stephen R. Hayden 周健 潘曙明 译

基础知识

■ 描述

• 股骨骨骺相对于股骨头/颈向后和向下移位(滑脱)。
• 分类系统：
- 股骨头滑脱度占股骨颈直径的百分比：
◦ 轻度，1 级：<33.3%。
◦ 中度，2 级：33.3%～50%。
◦ 严重，3 级：>50%。
• 时间：
- 急性期：<3 周。
- 慢性：>3 周的症状。
- 慢加急性：>3 周的症状，现在伴有急性疼痛。
• 稳定性：
- 稳定：能承受没有拐杖的重量。
- 不稳定：不能承受重量。

■ 流行病学

• 最高年龄：12～14 岁(男孩)，11～12 岁(女孩)。
- 男性>女性(1.5：1)。
• 双侧滑脱：20%；双侧进展 20%～40%。
- 非典型股骨头骨骺滑脱症(SCFE)：内分泌病相关：
- 患者年龄可小于 10 岁，>可小于 16 岁，体重可小于 50%。
- 双侧鳞状细胞癌的高风险(高达 100%)。

■ 病因

• 青春期髋部近端位置由水平向斜位改变，髋力由"压迫"向"剪切"转变。
• 股骨干剪切力>肌无力最弱点＝肥厚区。
• 风险因素：
- 肥胖：可能有助于剪切力。
- 甲状腺功能减退、生长激素缺乏、肾性骨营养不良(2°)、甲状旁腺功能亢进等内分泌病：可能导致生长板功能减弱。

诊断

■ 症状和体征

病史

经常性表现为跛行，体力活动可增加疼痛。
• 确定慢性症状和患者是否能承受体重。
• 膝盖、大腿、腹股沟或臀部的疼痛(指闭孔神经引起的疼痛)：
- 慢性 SCFE 数周内感觉模糊和迟钝。
- 急性鳞状细胞增生症(SCFE)的严重和突然发作，通常发生在创伤环境中。

体格检查

• 如稳定，则表现为跛行或劳力跛行。
• 如果不稳定(患者不能走动)，避免进一步的走动尝试。
• 通常表现为腿外翻。
• 内旋、外展、屈曲受限(不能触及大腿至腹部)。
• 前髋关节压痛。
• 试验：轻柔被动屈髋→髋外旋＋外展→高度提示 SCFE。
• 步态：
- Antalgic(患者在"站立"阶段步态时在受影响一侧采取短步以减少负重)。
- Trendelenburg 征(躯干移至患髋)。
◦ 轻微/严重滑倒迹象。
- 摇摆(双边 SCFE 的标志)。

■ 基本检查

• X 线平片：
- 在会诊医师的帮助下进一步成像。
• 整形咨询。

■ 诊断检查和说明

实验室检查

• 如果没有诊断性的 X 线异常，医师可以考虑以下方法来帮助风险分层可能的替代诊断：
- CBC 具有差异性、红细胞沉降速率、C 反应蛋白。

• 如怀疑内分泌失调，可考虑甲状腺功能检查。

影像学检查

• 为了比较，应该对两边的臀部进行成像。

• 在急性 SCFE 中，一些临床医师更倾向于采用交叉表侧位视图，而不是蛙式位（理论上的移位恶化风险）。

• 前后的 X 线摄片：

- 肿瘤变宽或不规则。
- 鸟喙外观的骨骺。
- 从股骨头上滑下来。
- Klein 线：从股骨颈上缘画出的平行线，与正常人骨骺相交侧放（蛙式位或跨桌）。

• 侧位 X 线片（蛙腿或横卧位）。

• CT 通常不需要，也不优于 X 线平片。

• MRI 能更好地发现 X 线平片未见的早期、有症状的预测。

诊断步骤/外科

如果怀疑化脓性髋关节，可能需要抽吸和穿刺液检查排除。

鉴别诊断

• Legg-Calve-Perthes 病：

- 典型见于 4～9 岁年龄段。

• 髋关节感染性关节炎。

• 骨髓炎。

• 中毒性滑膜炎。

• 股骨或骨盆骨折。

• 腹股沟疝或股疝。

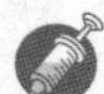

治疗

院前

如怀疑有髋部骨折或脱臼，应将患者固定以方便转运。

初步稳定/治疗

• 固定髋部，保持非承重。

• 不要试图减少。

急诊治疗/程序

• SCFE 是一种紧迫的骨科疾病；延误诊断可导致慢性不可逆髋关节功能障碍。

• 立即咨询矫形外科以确定制动或手术干预。

药物治疗

疼痛管理；如果计划手术干预，避免口服药物。

随访

入院指征

• 急性、慢性和双侧 SCFE 需要骨科住院进行紧急手术固定（通常为原位单空心螺钉固定）。

• 慢性 SCFE 可采用延迟手术固定治疗。

出院指征

无（由于并发症风险，包括骨坏死和/或软骨溶解，观察或闭合复位尝试无作用）。

随访建议

应该由骨科专家安排。

要点和误区

• 克莱恩线可以是一个有用的工具，发现 X 线平片的异常。

• 当孩子出现膝盖或大腿部疼痛时，记得检查臀部。

股骨骨折 Femur Fractures

Alexander D. Miller　万健 译

基础知识

描述

骨折的分类根据：

• 骨折的部位：

- 近端 1/3 段（粗隆以上区域）。
- 中段 1/3。
- 远端 1/3（远侧干骺端骨干连接处）。

• 骨折的几何形状：

- 螺旋形。
- 横形。
- 斜形。
- 节段性。

• 软组织损伤的程度：

- 开放性。
- 闭合性。

• 股骨骨折有两种常用的分类系统：AO/OTA 和 Winquist、Hansen 分类。

• 粉碎的程度：Winquist 和 Hansen 分类：

- Ⅰ级：骨折碎骨片小于股骨干宽度的 25%；股骨长轴方向受力和旋转都是稳定的。
- Ⅱ级：骨折为股骨干宽度的 25%～50%；股骨长轴方向受力稳定，旋转力可稳定或不稳定。
- Ⅲ级：骨折大于股骨干宽度的 50%；股骨长轴方向受力和旋转都是不稳定的。
- Ⅳ级：两断端没有皮质相连；股骨长轴方向受力和旋转都是不稳定的。

病因

• 通常由严重的高能量的创伤所致。

• 患者通常为年轻成人，由高能量造成损伤（车祸、枪伤、坠落伤）。

- 高处坠落伤伴有脊柱骨折。

• 如损伤机制轻微需考虑病理性骨折。

• 偶可由反复运动造成压力性骨折。

• 合并伤包括骨筋膜室综合征、脂肪栓塞、成人呼吸窘迫综合征（ARDS）和出血。

老年人注意事项

• 不典型的股骨骨折与使用二磷酸盐药物有关。

儿科注意事项

• 70%大于 3 岁的儿童股骨骨折是非意外伤所致。

• 股骨旋转性骨折提示非意外伤。

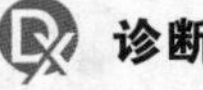

诊断

症状和体征

病史

• 股骨疼痛、畸形、肿胀及股骨缩短。

• 髋关节或膝关节运动障碍。

• 通常合并多处损伤。

- 胸部、腹部、骨盆、臀部、膝盖损伤，包括脱位。

体格检查

• 除贯通伤外，少有开放性骨折。

• 患者可因股骨出血造成低血压。

• 患者可因股骨远端供血不足和骨筋膜室综合征使足部血液循环造成损害。

■ 基本检查

• X线检查。

• 评估末端脉搏、触摸筋膜间隙，评估感觉和运动功能。

• 如脉律不齐或无法触及，需行床旁多普勒或血管造影检查。

• 探查合并伤。

• 怀疑非意外损伤，需行骨骼检查及骨扫描。

■ 诊断检查与说明

实验室检查

全血细胞计数、血型及交叉配血。

影像学检查

• 骨盆前后位、髋关节正侧位、股骨正侧位和全膝关节片。

• 基础胸部X线及外伤所提示的其他部位X线检查。

■ 鉴别诊断

• 髋关节骨折或脱位。

• 膝关节骨折或脱位。

• 大腿挫伤或血肿。

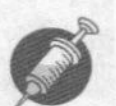

治疗

■ 院前

• 肢体固定和夹板牵引很重要，可以进一步防止大腿内出血。

- 肢体后部的固定、稳定的夹板牵引可以使肢体远端处于舒适的位置。

• 牵引的禁忌证：

- 靠近膝关节的骨折。

- 同侧髋关节的骨折或脱位。

- 骨盆骨折。

- 小腿下部的骨折。

• 不要在野外对开放性骨折进行复位，用无菌敷料包扎伤口。

• 密切监测失血性休克的进展，因为大腿能容纳4～6 U的血量。

■ 初步稳定/治疗

• 依次处理气道、胸部和腹部损伤。

• 持续监测血压，注意失血性休克的体征。

■ 急诊治疗/程序

• 维持远端肢体的稳定。

• 去除夹板和敷料。

• 镇痛：

- 单纯的股骨损伤：口服镇痛药物。

- 多处损伤或儿童患者：股骨神经阻滞。

• 所有的股骨骨折均需整形科医师会诊：

- 如神经血管受累时紧急处理。

- 开放性骨折需直接进入手术室冲洗和清创。

• 应用抗生素：

- 需要手术的骨折：开放性骨折伴撕裂，应用头孢唑林(头孢菌素过敏时应用克林霉素)。如远处软组织损伤或污染：考虑庆大霉素、妥布霉素及破伤风抗毒素。

- 如伤口严重污染：应用能覆盖梭状杆菌的青霉素。

• 股骨骨折伴远端脉搏触摸不清或消失、逐渐扩大的血肿或可触及的搏动性肿块时，需要立即行血管造影或股骨动脉探查。

• 如患者不能立即行手术治疗应给予骨骼牵引。

■ 药物治疗

• 抗生素：

- 一线：

◦ 头孢唑林：2 g肌内注射或静脉注射(儿童：50～100 mg/kg，肌内注射或静脉注射，q6～8 h，最大量1 g)。

- 二线：

◦ 克林霉素：450～900 mg，肌内注射或静脉注射，q6～8 h；最大剂量4.8 g/d[儿童：20～40 mg/(kg·d)，肌内注射或静脉注射，分3～4次给药]。

• 适当镇静：

- 依托咪酯：0.1～0.3 mg/kg，静脉注射1次(小于12岁患儿不建议使用)。

- 芬太尼：50～100 μg静脉注射，每次注射时间超过1～2 min(儿童：大于6个月，1～2 μg/kg静脉注射1次)。

- 氯胺酮：0.07 mg/kg，肌内注射；或1 mg缓慢静脉注射，每次2～3 min，最大量5 mg(儿童：0.25～0.5 mg/kg，口服，最大口服剂量20 mg；6个月到5岁，0.05～0.1 mg/kg静脉滴定，最大量0.6 mg/kg；6～12岁，0.025～0.05 mg/kg静脉滴定，最大剂量0.4 mg/kg)。

- 异丙酚：2～10 mg，静脉注射，q4 h；滴定镇痛(儿童：0.1 mg/kg，静脉注射，q4 h；滴定镇痛最大剂量每次15 mg)。

儿科注意事项

• 非意外伤的评估：

- 伤情延迟出现。

- 病史与发病机制同损伤不一致。

- 单独的股部损伤，如烧伤、钝器伤或线性擦伤。

• 评估股骨上段干骺端脱位。

• 考虑到患者的年龄和骨折类型，儿科骨折不全需要手术治疗。

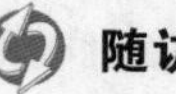

随访

■ 进一步处理

入院指征

• 除不符合出院指征者外，所有股骨骨折患者必须住院。

• 任何怀疑非意外伤的儿童。

出院指征

对于相当罕见环境下出现的病理性骨折，或不能下地活动的股骨骨折患者和不能耐受手术固定的患者，只有适当控制了疼痛并确保随访的条件下，经整形科医师会诊后，可考虑出院。

■ 随访建议

由手术医师根据临床病程确定随访。

要点和误区

• 由于高能量机制引起股骨骨折，必须排除其他相关的创伤。

• 初始评估即需要治疗神经血管功能，并且反复评估。

• 考虑到患者的年龄和骨折类型，儿科骨折不全需要手术治疗。

G

股骨头骨骺炎 -Perthes Disease

Brenna Derksen · Charlotte A. Sadler 何超 段立伟 译

基础知识

描述

- 儿童(4～12 岁)股骨头原发性无血管性坏死。
- 基因：
  - Ⅴ因子变异和抗心磷脂抗体频率增高。
  - 与 2 型胶原 *COL2A1* 基因突变相关，比例很小。

儿科注意事项

儿科专有疾病。

病因

- 因血管闭塞导致股骨头血液供应中断所致的特发性缺血性坏死，随后出现再骨化、畸形和骨的机械性损害。
- 可能是多因素的。
- 危险因素包括吸烟、二手烟、出生低体重、出生体长＜50 cm，骨骼发育迟缓、创伤、凝血功能障碍。
- 疾病的进展包括 4 个阶段。
  - 起始阶段：厚重的股骨头导致间歇性滑膜炎。
  - 碎裂：股骨头变软、变形，运动能力下降。
  - 恢复：股骨头新骨形成。
  - 残余：恢复的股骨头伴有畸形。
- 常于 3～7 岁发病。男孩中常见：男性＞女性，约为 4∶1。
- 高加索人种常见。
- 10%～15%病例为双侧性。
- 与身材矮小、人口贫困、延迟和不成比例生长相关。

诊断

症状和体征

病史

- 多隐匿起病。
- 主诉多为跛行。
- 无发热表现。
- 疼痛：
  - 髋部、腹股沟区、股前内侧区或膝前内侧疼痛。
  - 可能较轻。
  - 活动后加重，休息后缓解。
  - 病程早期常诉有肌痉挛。

体格检查

- 间歇性跛行。
- 髋关节前面有压痛。
- 髋部关节僵硬：
  - 早期能发现内旋受限或疼痛。
  - 外展受限。
  - 后期发现患侧肌萎缩、腿缩短。
- 健侧表现正常，无发热。
- 可能无症状。

基本检查

- 在急诊内，髋部 X 线最重要。
- 考虑并排除化脓性关节炎(通常是一种急性发热性疾病)和一过性滑膜炎。

诊断检查与说明

实验室检查

- 没有对儿童股骨头缺血性坏死有特异性诊断价值的实验室检查。
- 若考虑化脓性关节炎需检查全血细胞计数、C 反应蛋白(CRP)或红细胞沉降率。

影像学检查

- 特征性影像学表现结合一致的病史和体格检查可确诊。
- X 线平片、MRI、核闪烁扫描(骨扫描)是应用的主要检查手段。
- 髋关节 X 线：
  - 患侧前后位和蛙式侧位片。
  - 拍摄双侧髋关节检查对侧。
  - 评估分期、程度和严重性。
  - 第一个 3～6 个月可表现正常。
  - 就诊时通常表现为异常。
  - 可观察到连续的 5 期：
  - 股骨头骺部停止生长：患侧股骨头骺部缩小，关节腔增大。
  - 软骨下骨折。
  - 骨吸收。
  - 新骨再骨化。
  - 恢复期。
- CT：
  - 显示股骨头和髋臼准确的解剖关系。
  - 在计划手术和分期中有一定作用。
- MRI：
  - 诊断 LCP 敏感，提供良好的解剖信息。
  - 能比 X 线平片更早检测出异常。
  - 用于评估股骨头梗死的程度。
  - 应用的影像学方法不同，发现也不同。
- 骨扫描：
  - 比 X 线的改变平均提前 3 个月。
  - 评估再血管化和再通的模式。
- 超声：
  - 显示髋部渗出，但对 LCP 非特异。
  - 评估滑膜增厚。
  - 评估股骨头畸形和大小。
- 关节成像：
  - 用于评估治疗手段。

诊断步骤/外科

髋关节穿刺术是排除化脓性关节炎的确定性检查，可能需要矫形外科会诊。

鉴别诊断

- 涉及单侧：
  - 一过性(又称中毒性)滑膜炎。
  - 化脓性关节炎。
  - 骨化性肌炎。
  - 镰刀细胞性贫血。
  - 青少年类风湿性关节炎。
  - 风湿热。
  - 创伤：
    - 股骨颈骨折。
    - 髋关节脱位。
    - 股骨头骨骺移位。
  - 结核。
  - 肿瘤。
- 涉及双侧：
  - 甲状腺功能减退。
  - 骨骺发育不良。
  - Gaucher 病。

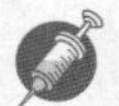

治疗

院前

临床表现为亚急性，较少通过急救车就诊。

初步稳定/治疗

不是威胁生命的状况，临床不稳定的需鉴别其他疾病。

急诊治疗/程序

- 急诊室主要治疗是止痛。
- 限制负重。

药物治疗

一线用药

- 布洛芬：10 mg/kg 每剂，口服，q6～8 h，疼痛必要时。

G

• 对乙酰氨基酚：每次 10～15 mg/kg，24 h 内不要超过 4 g。

二线用药

地西泮：0.1～0.2 mg/kg 每剂(最大 5 mg)，口服，q6～8 h，肌痉挛必要时。

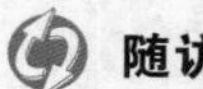

随访

进一步处理

入院指征

需要收治的较少，指征为：

• 经口药物治疗不能控制的严重疼痛和肌痉挛。

• 社会考虑，在家卧床/照顾不可行。

出院指征

• 经口药物治疗疼痛完全控制。

• 安排 1～2 周矫形外科随访。

注意事项

• 发病年龄影响预后，6 岁前发病预后较好，8 岁后预后较差。

• 对更严重的疾病，要使用一系列治疗措施，包括保守治疗、矫正、牵引和截骨术，取决于矫形外科医师会诊结果。

• 退变性关节炎和需要关节置换是主要的远期并发症。

随访建议

矫形外科会诊决定未来治疗计划，可以门诊随访。

要点和误区

突然起病，表现为发热、状况不稳定的患者或有毒性表现，考虑诊断不是 LCP。

骨骺骨折 Epiphyseal Injuries

Erica Lash · Neha Raukar 单怡 译

基础知识

描述

儿童骨有四部分组成：骨干或骨体，干骨后端(骨中最宽部分，是骨发育起始部)，生长部位、骨骺(生长面末端，第二成骨部位)。

骨骺骨折占儿童长骨骨折的 21%～30%，其中 30%可导致成长畸形：

• 多见于桡骨、尺骨远端和胫骨、腓骨远端和趾骨。

• 在儿童，比韧带损伤多见。

- 儿童骨骼的抗拉能力较邻近韧带差。
- 骨骺是儿童骨骼最薄弱的部位。
- 成人同样的损伤易导致扭伤。

• 成长高峰时较常见：

- 女性：9～12 岁。
- 男性：12～15 岁。
- 婴幼儿少见，因为婴幼儿骨骺未骨化，因此起到减震作用。

• 女性骨骼发育成熟早，故发病率为男性的 2 倍。

• Salter-Harris(SH)分类，最简单和最常用的分类系统：

- 骨折 SH 分级可能与随后的成长障碍有关，较高的 GH 分级往往伴随较差的预后。
- SALTER 有助于帮助记忆分类：
  ◦ 垂直型：Ⅰ型。
  ◦ 上型：Ⅱ型。
  ◦ 下型：Ⅲ型。
  ◦ 穿通型：Ⅳ型。
  ◦ 消除型：Ⅴ型。
- Ⅰ型：
  ◦ 横向骨折线局限于骨骺。
  ◦ 骨骺和干骺端完全分离。
  ◦ 若骨膜完整，骨骺不会移位。
  ◦ 根据骨骺的强度做出临床诊断。
  ◦ 最常见例子是 SCFE(骨股头骨骺滑脱)。
  ◦ 成长滞缓少见。
- Ⅱ型：
  ◦ 最常见，占骨骺骨折的 80%。
  ◦ 骨折沿长骨体生长横向延伸并波及干骺端(Thurston-Holland 征)。
  ◦ 骨折的对侧骨膜破裂。
  ◦ 生长滞缓少见。
- Ⅲ型：
  ◦ 少见。
  ◦ 骨骺骨折延伸并贯穿长骨体生长部。
  ◦ 胫骨远端受累多见。
  ◦ 若移位，需行解剖复位。
  ◦ 即使解剖复位也难以避免生长障碍。
- Ⅳ型：
  ◦ 骨折起于关节面。
  ◦ 贯穿长骨生长部并延伸到干骺端和骨骺。
  ◦ 肱骨远端受累多见。
  ◦ 有 Thurston-Holland 碎片。
  ◦ 必须解剖复位，移位片段需行切开复位内固定术。
  ◦ 即使治疗得当，生长滞缓多见。
- Ⅴ型：
  ◦ 由骨骺严重的挤压暴力导致。
  ◦ 无直接可视的 X 线表现改变，故早期诊断困难。
  ◦ 压缩损伤导致骨骺损伤和生长障碍。
  ◦ 多在回顾病史时发现。

• Ogden 修订 SH 系统以包括周围解剖组织——骨膜、软骨膜和骺生长板周围环的损伤：

- Ogden Ⅰ～Ⅴ型与 SH Ⅰ～Ⅴ型相似。
- Ogden Ⅵ型：累及软骨膜和骺生长板周围环。
- Ogden Ⅶ型：仅累及骨骺。
- Ogden Ⅷ型：累及干骺端且导致骺板缺血。
- Ogden Ⅸ型：累及骨干和干骺端骨膜，可能造成骨膜生长和成骨障碍。

• Peterson 分类系统，1994：

- 10 年回顾性研究的成果显示 16%骨骺损伤不能用 SH 系统分类。
- 分类包括 6 种骨折类型，包含了 2 种没有被 SH 分类和 Ogden 分类系统描述的类型：
  ◦ Peterson Ⅰ型：骨折沿长骨体生长横向延伸并波及干骺端，是最常见的骨折方式。
  ◦ Peterson Ⅵ型：开放性外伤导致骨骺、长骨体的部分丢失，伴严重的生长障碍。

病因

• 娱乐竞技损伤。

• 外伤。

• 虐待儿童。

• 严寒。

• 辐射损伤。

• 遗传、神经病变和代谢性疾病。

诊断

症状和体征

现病史

• 多发生于坠落后。

• 严寒和辐射可损伤骨骺板。

体格检查

• 局部触痛。
• 肿胀。
• 活动受限。
• 若下肢受累，患者不能负重。
• 关节松弛：
- 可能因骨干损伤，而无韧带损伤。

■ 基本检查

• X线检查评估损伤程度。
• 评估损伤部位远端肢体的脉搏、运动感觉功能。
• 评估远端的运动和感觉功能。
• 评估伤域皮肤的完整性。
• 定位和处理合并损伤。

■ 诊断检查与说明

影像学检查

• 损伤部位X线平片：
- Ⅰ型骨折：
◦ 常见。
◦ 轻微的骺骨分离或相应的关节积液征象。
◦ 与对侧关节对比发现小损伤。
◦ 随访可见硬化征。
- Ⅱ～Ⅳ型：X线平片诊断骨折。
- Ⅴ型：
◦ 伤后首次摄片正常。
◦ 后续摄片示：损伤处骨过早形成，生长停滞。
• 婴幼儿软骨未骨化，超声有助于诊断。
• CT检查：有助于评估定位粉碎性骨折，通常不会改变治疗方案。
• MRI：
- 损伤急性期最精确的检查。
- 可发现生长停滞线。
- 诊断模棱两可时推荐应用，确认某一特殊骨折时可改变治疗策略。

■ 鉴别诊断

• 拉伤。
• 扭伤。
• 挫伤。

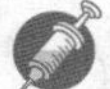

治疗

■ 院前

• 评估患肢远端的神经血管功能。
• 不影响血管状态时患肢制动于受伤体位。
• 冰敷损伤处。
• 检查其他合并损伤。

■ 初步稳定/治疗

• 止痛。
• 止血并用无菌敷料覆盖开放伤口。

■ 急诊治疗/程序

• 复位/矫正错位的骨折。
- 需要达到解剖复位。
• 远处血管或神经的损伤需要立即处理。
• 制动所有可疑的或X线证实的生长板损伤：
- 夹板固定伤部相邻的远近关节至解剖复位和神经复位。
- 限制伤肢的活动。
• 开放性骨折：
- 根据发病机制和获得的培养结果，针对金黄色葡萄球菌、A组溶血链球菌和潜在的厌氧菌静脉注射抗生素。
- 生理盐水充分冲洗。
- 无菌纱布覆盖。
- 骨科医师会诊。
• 会诊：
- 开放性骨折。
- 错位的Ⅱ型骨折和Ⅲ型及以上骨折。

■ 药物治疗

疼痛控制：

• 苏太尼：2～3 μg/kg，静脉注射；透皮糖丸5～15 μg/kg最大剂量；体重<10 kg禁用。
• 吗啡：0.1 mg/kg，静脉注射或肌内注射。

若开放性骨折：

• 头孢唑林：25～50 mg/(kg·d)，静脉注射或肌内注射，q6～8 h。
• 青霉素：10万～30万U/(kg·24 h)，肌内注射或静脉注射，分4～6次。对于在农场受伤的患者更好地覆盖链球菌和棒状杆菌感染。
• 庆大霉素：5～7.5 mg/(kg·d)，用于明显污染的损伤。

随访

■ 进一步处理

入院指征

• 开放性骨折。
• 需要开放性手术复位。
• 考虑为Ⅲ型和Ⅳ型骨折。

出院指征

• 低分级的骨折和确定随访的高分级的骨折。
• 夹板固定良好。
• 止痛。
• 冰敷。
• 抬高患肢。
• 1周内骨科医师随访。

转诊问题

所有累及骨骺的损伤需要肌肉骨骼专家的随访。

■ 随访建议

通常需要监测患肢长度，尤其是高级别损伤。

• 包括阶段性的体格检查和影像学评估。

要点和误区

• 远期并发症：
- 若整个骨骺板受损，肢体长短不一。
- 若仅部分骨骺受损，肢体成角。
• 怀疑SH骨折而影像学检查正常者，制动且于几日后随访。

G

骨盆骨折 Pelvic Fracture

Andrew T. LaFree · Theodore C. Chan 王虑 译

基础知识

■ 描述

• 占全身骨折发生率的3%。
• 骨盆是由骶骨和2块髋骨组成。
- 髋骨由坐骨、髂骨和耻骨组成。
• 骨盆结构的稳定是通过骨盆区域的韧带、肌肉和其他软组织协同实现的。
• 骨盆前稳定是通过耻骨联合和耻骨支的作用实现的。
• 骨盆后稳定是通过骶骨关节和骨盆底的作用实现的。

- 骨盆能起到保护该区域下尿路、胃肠道、生殖系统、血管和神经的作用：
  - 骨盆骨折有较高的发病率和致死率，需要尽快诊断和治疗。
- 不稳定骨盆骨折有发生以下伤的高风险：
  - 骨盆出血和出血性休克。
  - 腹腔和胃肠道损伤。
  - 泌尿生殖器和尿路损伤。
  - 子宫和阴道损伤。
  - 神经损伤。
  - 动脉静脉淋巴系统损伤。

病因

- 65%的骨盆骨折是因为车祸伤，包括行人被机动车撞伤。
- 10%因为摔倒。
- 10%因为挤压伤。
- 其他的原因包括运动、穿刺伤或非创伤性损伤。
- 骨盆骨折的病死率为 6%～19%：
  - 开放性骨折或出血性休克的死亡率增加。
- 严重的出血会致体征不稳、高能骨盆骨折（B 型和 C 型骨折）：
  - 出血常见于骨盆后骨折累及血管和淋巴结。
  - 腹膜后出血会占据封闭的骨盆空间。

Tile 分类系统

- 包括稳定的单一骨骨折及撕裂性骨折和骨盆环骨折。
- 需要手术修复。
- A 型：稳定的骨盆环骨折。
  - A1：髋骨撕裂性骨折（坐骨结节、髂骨）。
  - A2 - 1：髂嵴骨折。
  - A2 - 2：孤立的支骨骨折，最常见的骨盆骨折。
  - A2 - 3：4 柱前环骨折。
  - A3：骶骨和尾骨横断骨折。
- B 型：部分稳定型骨盆环骨折（旋转不稳定，但垂直稳定）：
  - B1：单侧翻书型骨盆骨折。
  - B2：单侧压缩性骨折。
    - B2 - 1：同侧双支骨折和后侧骨折。
    - B2 - 2：对侧双支骨折和后侧骨折（桶柄型骨折）。
    - B2 - 3：双侧 B 型骨折。
- C 型：不稳定的骨盆环骨折、旋转和垂直不稳定，马尔盖涅骨盆骨折：
  - 耻骨联合前分离或 2～4 耻骨支骨折伴移位和通过骶骨、骶髂关节或回肠的不稳定骨折。
    - C1：单侧垂直剪骨折。
    - C2：单侧垂直剪骨折和对侧 B 型骨折。
    - C3：双侧垂直剪骨折。
- 髋臼骨折（后唇骨折、中央/横向骨折、前柱骨折或后柱骨折）。

Young 分类系统

- 根据受伤机制分类。
- 仅包括骨折致骨盆环破坏的情况；不是单一骨，撕裂或髋臼骨折。
- 预测受伤的发生率和死亡风险：
  - LC：侧面压缩。
  - APC：前后压缩。
  - VS：垂直剪切。
  - CM：复合性受伤模式。

儿科注意事项

- 儿童可能出血更严重。
- 注意非事故性创伤。

妊娠注意事项

妊娠子宫有受伤的风险，包括子宫破裂。

诊断

症状和体征

- 疼痛，肿胀，瘀斑，臀区、腹股沟、会阴部和下背部触痛。
- 常同时伴随着其他创伤，包括神经系统、腹腔、泌尿生殖系统、会阴、直肠和阴道损伤。
- 失血性休克表现。
- 骨盆整体稳定性缺失。

病史

- 创伤史（摔倒、车祸、挤压伤、运动伤）。
- 髋关节运动、行走、坐、站立、排便均会疼痛。

体格检查

- 瘀斑，肿胀，骨隆突会阴部、耻骨、骨盆区和下背部触痛。
- 下肢缩短或旋转。
- 髋关节活动受限。
- 不能主动或被动地执行受累髋关节的活动范围。
- 骨盆耻骨支、耻骨联合和骶髂关节触痛。
- 直肠、阴道或泌尿道出血提示可能有开放性骨折。
- 出血性休克：
  - 心动过速，低血压，脉压变小。
  - 精神状态改变。
  - 四肢冰凉苍白。

基本检查

- 骨盆放射影像学检查是开始最常做的检查。
- 当怀疑骨折时骨盆前后位 X 线平片应尽快完成以协助诊断。
  - 大部分不稳定骨盆骨折都能通过骨盆前后位 X 线平片发现。
- 其他拍摄位包括：
  - 进口位：30°坐位，有后弓视角。
  - 出口位：30°头测角，有骶骨视角。
  - Judet 斜视角：评估髋臼情况。

诊断检查与说明

实验室检查

- 血型鉴定和匹配。
- 血细胞比容测定、血小板计数、凝血机制（凝血时间、部分凝血时间）。

影像学检查

- CT 检查能进一步显示骨盆骨折情况、腹膜后出血情况及内脏损伤情况：
  - 增强 CT 能发现出血位置，但患者血流动力学需稳定。
- 严重的创伤需要行腹腔超声检查，但要区分骨盆骨折是腹膜内出血还是腹膜后出血还是很困难的。
- 磁共振检查能发现神经系统损伤。

诊断步骤/外科

- 尽管诊断很大程度上依靠超声和 CT 检查，但诊断性腹腔灌洗仍然是快速诊断腹腔出血的方法。
- 血管造影和选择性静脉栓塞用于骨盆出血：
  - 尤其用于小动脉静脉出血。
- 手术：
  - 在临床发现和骨科/普外科医师的意见。
  - 通过骨盆填塞使其稳定。
  - 手术直接控制出血。

鉴别诊断

- 韧带损伤。
- 脊髓损伤。
- 腹腔损伤和出血。

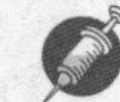

治疗

院前

- 静脉补液复苏。
- 骨盆制动和固定等处理。

初步稳定/治疗

- 创伤治疗基础支持治疗。
- 阴性或少见的血型患者血流动力学不稳

定的，可静脉补充血制品或晶体液：

- 避免使用下肢静脉通路。

• 适当制动和固定骨盆去避免进一步损伤和减轻出血：

- 加压装置：像钳子似的折叠装置将粗隆边包裹以固定骨盆。

- 充气抗休克服：在急诊使用还有争议，但能迅速制动并压缩骨盆以减缓出血。

- 外部固定器：比抗休克服需要更长时间去放置，但固定骨盆的原理相似。但对于粉碎性骨盆骨折是禁忌。

- 放置固定装置不能影响后续的治疗工作(如超声、诊断性腹腔灌洗)。

急诊治疗/程序

• 先判断骨盆骨折是稳定型还是不稳定型的。

• A 型骨折常是稳定型骨折。

• B 型和 C 型骨折是不稳定型骨折。

• A 型骨折：

- 传统治疗方法包括卧床休息、镇痛和安抚措施；治疗措施需有骨科医师会诊意见。

- 对于四柱前环损伤，需做 CT 检查以评估后骨盆伤情。

- 确保骨盆环没有其他的损伤。

• B 型和 C 型骨折：

- 骨科医师会诊意见。

- 需急诊骨盆制动措施。

- 评估骨盆出血情况。

• 马尔盖涅骨折：

- 注意可能严重的出血和伴发的损伤。

• 髋臼骨折：

- 立即骨科会诊。

• 骨盆出血：

- 不稳定骨折的机械固定(常使用外置骨盆固定装置)。

- 血管造影术和选择性静脉栓塞。

- 直接手术控制骨盆出血。

• 检查的优先次序：CT、血管造影或手术：

- 血流动力学不稳定患者：

◦ 开放性 B 型和 C 型骨折：手术探查。

◦ 封闭性骨折：诊断性腹腔灌洗或超声能协助决定是紧急手术探查还是选择性血管造影或栓塞。

• 对于血流动力学稳定的患者，可以在适当外固定条件下行 CT 检查以评估腹腔、骨盆和腹膜后情况。

药物治疗

• 晶体液：2 L 静脉快速输注生理盐水或林格液(20 ml/kg)。

• 血液制品：交叉配血，血型鉴定(10 ml/kg)。

随访

进一步处理

入院指征

• 血流动力学不稳定和骨盆出血患者。

• B 型和 C 型骨盆骨折。

• 髋臼骨折。

• 其他合并损伤(如泌尿系统损伤、腹腔损伤、神经损伤)。

• 难控制的疼痛。

出院指征

A 型骨盆骨折；血流动力学稳定并且没有其他伤情的证据。

出院的患者需密切随访。

随访建议

出院患者需接受骨科医师的随访和建议。

要点和误区

• 骨盆骨折是典型的高能量消耗的创伤：

- 分析潜在的腹部/骨盆损伤包括：消化系统、泌尿生殖系统、血管和神经系统损伤。

• 早期的复苏，骨盆的制动固定，需在充分考虑骨折稳定性或开放性骨折情况或出血部位的前提下。

• 明确诊断/治疗的手段包括 CT 平扫或增强，选择性血管造影，手术取决于患者的血流动力学状态，潜在的伤情和骨折的类型。

• 所有的马尔盖涅骨折患者需在骨科医师会诊后收入院。

G

骨髓炎 Osteomyelitis

Stephen R. Hayden 朱妍 译

基础知识

描述

• 骨髓炎(OM)：伴随持续性炎症性损害的骨骼感染。

• 细菌性常见，但真菌性骨髓炎也存在。

• 急性或慢性、血源性的或非血源性的。

病因

• 血源性骨髓炎：

- 主要见于儿童、老年人或滥用静脉药物滥用者(IVDA)。

- 细菌通过血液循环从远隔感染部位播散到骨骼。

- 儿童通常患急性骨髓炎，成人更常患亚急性或慢性骨髓炎。

- 成人长骨的血源性骨髓炎罕见。

- 大部分急性血源性骨髓炎的儿童没有前驱症状。

- 1/3 的患者受累部位有陈旧性创伤史。

- 在不同年龄骨髓炎中金黄色葡萄球菌是最常见的致病菌。

- 新生儿：金黄色葡萄球菌、肠杆菌、A 组和 B 组链球菌和大肠埃希菌。

- 儿童：金黄色葡萄球菌、A 组链球菌、流感嗜血杆菌和大肠埃希菌。

- 沙门菌：常见于镰状细胞病。

- 成人：金黄色葡萄球菌、肠杆菌、假单胞菌属、革兰阴性杆菌、表皮葡萄球菌、革兰阳性厌氧菌，尤其是消化链球菌属。

- 使用药物不当：念珠菌、假单胞菌属、黏质沙雷菌。

- 持续中性粒细胞减少：念珠菌、曲霉菌、根霉菌、芽生菌、球孢子菌。

• 血源性脊柱骨髓炎：

- 不常见。

- 常见于>45 岁成人。

- 涉及上下两个椎体及椎间盘的。

- 通常发生在长期留置导尿管、静脉药物滥用者、癌症、血液透析或糖尿病患者。

- 静脉药物滥用者：发生于耻骨联合、胸锁关节、骶髂关节(SI)的骨髓炎。

- 腰椎最常见，然后是胸椎，再是颈椎。
- 向后扩散导致硬膜外或硬膜下脓肿或脑膜炎。
- 向前扩散可能导致椎旁、咽后、纵隔、膈下、腹膜后或腰大肌脓肿。
- 直接或邻近的骨髓炎：
- 通过创伤病原菌直接播散至骨骼，尤其是开放性骨折：
  - 从邻近感染部位或愈合不良的软组织伤口播散。
- 在成人和青少年中更常见。
- 金黄色葡萄球菌、肠杆菌、假单胞菌属。
- 正常的血管：
  - 金黄色葡萄球菌、表皮葡萄球菌、革兰阴性杆菌和厌氧菌。
- 脉管炎和糖尿病：
  - 足部小骨是好发部位。
  - 感染造成轻微创伤、感染指甲床、蜂窝织炎或皮肤溃疡。
  - 多种微生物，包括厌氧菌。
- 针刺伤通过网球鞋：金黄色葡萄球菌、厌氧菌。
- 锁骨骨髓炎多为锁骨下静脉导管置入术的并发症。
- 慢性骨髓炎：
- 持续或复发性骨髓炎。
- 突出的特征是必须清除的坏死骨（死骨片）。
- 表皮葡萄球菌、金黄色葡萄球菌、铜绿假单胞菌、黏质沙雷菌、大肠埃希菌。

G

诊断

症状和体征

病程的多样化。

病史

- 主要为非特异症状。
- 通常在几日内逐渐出现症状。
- 疼痛：在运动或不运动时都可发生的局限的、深部的、迟钝的和搏动性疼痛。
- 急性骨髓炎受累部位的隐匿性疼痛。
- 慢性骨髓炎可能在受影响部位出现疼痛、红斑或肿胀。
- 发热和寒战：在慢性骨髓炎比较少见。
- 萎靡、恶心、呕吐。
- 四肢不愿意活动。
- 适当治疗难以治愈的溃疡。
- 把骨髓炎作为骨折不愈合的一个病因。
- 诱因：糖尿病、血管病变、静脉滥用药物、侵入性操作、肿瘤。

体格检查

- 触诊骨时轻柔、温暖，红斑，水肿，活动受限。
- 窦道流脓。
- 深部溃疡和骨擦感（+"probe to bone"试验有很高的积极预测价值）。
- 如果溃疡面积 $>2\ cm^2$ 且深度 >3 mm，很可能涉及骨骼。

基本检查

- 血常规。
- 红细胞沉降率和C反应蛋白。
- X线片。
- 血和伤口分泌物培养和药物敏感试验。

诊断检查与说明

实验室检查

- 血常规：白细胞可以升高但通常都正常。
- 红细胞沉降率，在>90%的患者中都升高。
- C反应蛋白（通常升高）。
- 血培养（在大概50%的患者中阳性）。
- 骨髓炎的明确诊断需要从受累骨骼的活检中获得培养，这可能与伤口培养不同。

影像学检查

- 在诊断时有决定性意义。
- 开始时做X线平片，其他检查也需要。
- X线片：
- 在症状开始的2～3周可能是正常的。
- 最早改变是骨膜增厚，伴随着骨皮质侵蚀，然后新骨形成。
- 40%～50%的病灶骨丢失需要检测其在X线片上的透光度，少于1/3的病例在10日时有诊断性发现。
- 如果怀疑肺结核应拍摄胸片。
- MRI：
- 是最好的获得详细解剖、软组织分布和骨髓累及范围的方法。
- 敏感度和特异度在90%左右。
- 先于X线片发现骨髓水肿、骨皮质破坏、骨膜反应、关节表面破坏和软组织累及。
- 有效的早期检查（感染发生的开始3～5日）。
- 选择MRI来确定椎体骨髓炎和继发于糖尿病足部溃疡的骨髓炎。
- 创伤患者偶有假阳性结果，尤其外科手术或神经接头疾病。
- 症状出现1周后如MRI检查阴性则排除急性骨髓炎。
- CT：
- 不能做MRI时可选择。
- CT可显示X线平片不能发现的骨髓水肿、皮质破坏、骨膜反应、小点状气体或破坏、关节表面破坏和软组织累及。
- 对椎体、胸骨、跟骨、骨盆的骨髓炎诊断有帮助。
- 对指导外科医师清创和活检有帮助。
- 骨扫描：
- ^{99m}Tc亚甲基二磷酸盐（^{99m}Tc-MDP）。
- 骨代谢活动度的测量方法增加。
- 大约95%的敏感度，但是特异性比MRI差。
- 在症状出现2～3日后骨扫描可异常。
- 在创伤、手术、慢性软组织感染，肿瘤可能会发生假阳性。
- 高辐射负担，在疑有多部位疾患时有用。
- 如果金属硬件无法进行MRI或CT，核扫描是首选检查。
- 白细胞闪烁扫描法：
- ^{111}In标记的白细胞。
- 比骨扫描特异性更高，但敏感性更低。
- 很难区别是骨骼还是软组织的炎症（如蜂窝织炎、肿瘤、反应性关节炎）。
- 超声：
- 特别在儿童骨髓炎患者选用的一种紧急方法。
- 骨膜变高或增厚，骨周积液常见。
- 骨髓炎患者超声比X线平片可能更早发现异常。
- 对指导活检有作用。

诊断步骤/外科

- 诊断的金标准是有组织学和组织革兰染色的骨活检，包括培养和药物敏感试验。
- 细针穿刺比开放性活检敏感度低。
- 伤口窦道和引流液培养会误诊，与金黄色葡萄球菌有很好的相关性，但没有其他微生物可靠。

儿科注意事项

- 70%～85%的儿童有38.5℃以上发热。
- 新生儿一般无发热。
- 仅1/3的儿童可能有白细胞升高。
- 血培养阳性率约为50%。
- 超声。

鉴别诊断

- 蜂窝织炎。
- 甲沟炎、化脓性指头炎。
- 滑囊炎、中毒性滑膜炎、化脓性关节炎。
- 肢体骨折。
- 镰状细胞患者的骨梗死。
- 急性白血病、恶性骨肿瘤。

- 机械的背部疼痛。
- 硬脊膜外脓肿。
- 布鲁菌病，尤其是在髂关节。
- 结核，胸椎最多见(Pott 病)。

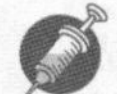

治疗

初步稳定/治疗

如果存在脓毒症或由于脊髓受累引起神经功能缺陷需紧急治疗。

急诊治疗/程序

- 在可能的情况下，抗生素治疗应该推迟到可以进行骨培养的时候。
- 无并发症的非血源性骨髓炎(无硬件，患者不是脓毒症)的最佳治疗方法是在使用抗生素之前清除坏死骨并培养受累组织。
- 培养应该指导随后的抗生素方案。
- 抗生素：依赖于患者的年龄和微生物(见药物治疗)。
- 骨科及传染病科会诊。
- 外科干预可能需要优化治疗(如骨折或内固定感染、骨坏死)。
- 对于血源性骨髓炎(如脊椎)，急诊的经验性抗生素治疗应该对 MRSA 和革兰阴性菌有活性。
- 肠外抗生素治疗 4～6 周。

药物治疗

- 新生儿至 4 个月：耐青霉素酶的合成青霉素(如萘夫西林：37 mg/kg，静脉推注，q6 h)加第三代头孢菌素[如头孢曲松钠：50～75 mg/(kg · d)，静脉注射]；如果怀疑耐甲氧西林金黄色葡萄球菌(MRSA)选择万古霉素(40～60 mg/kg，静脉注射，q6 h)加第三代头孢菌素(注：剂量是基于年龄>28 日)。
- 儿童(>4 个月)：耐青霉素酶的合成青霉素(如萘夫西林：32 mg/kg，静脉推注，q6 h，每日最大剂量 8～12 g)。如怀疑 MRSA，选用万古霉素(40～60 mg/kg，静脉注射，q6 h 至最大剂量 2～4 g/d)。如果怀疑革兰阴性杆菌或存在革兰染色阳性，加用第三代头孢菌素[如头孢曲松 50～75 mg/(kg · d)，静脉注射至最大剂量 2～4 g/d]。
- 成人：耐青霉素酶的合成青霉素(如萘夫西林 2 g，静脉注射，q4 h)；如怀疑 MRSA，万古霉素(15 mg/kg，静脉注射，q12 h)。
- 革兰阴性菌(包括铜绿假单胞菌)所致慢性骨髓炎：环丙沙星 750 mg，口服，每日 2 次；或左氧氟沙星 750 mg，口服，每日 1 次。
- 镰状细胞贫血合并骨髓炎：环丙沙星 400 mg，静脉注射，q12 h；或左氧氟沙星 750 mg，静脉注射，q24 h(儿童禁用)；替代药：第三代头孢菌素。
- 钉子扎透网球鞋后的骨髓炎：环丙沙星 750 mg，口服，每日 2 次；或左氧氟沙星 750 mg，口服，q24 h；备选药品：头孢他啶 2 g，静脉注射，q8 h。
- 涉及骨科假体或器具：针对金黄色葡萄球菌的给药方案需添加利福平[10 mg/(kg · d)，口服或静脉注射至最大剂量 600 mg/d]。通常需要取出假体。
- 创伤后的骨髓炎：万古霉素和头孢他啶。
- 如存在耐万古霉素肠球菌：利奈唑胺 600 mg，静脉注射，q12 h×6 周。

儿科注意事项

血源性骨髓炎的儿童患者可能经历短疗程静脉注射抗生素，然后换成口服补充 1～2 个月。

随访

进一步处理

入院指征

- 急性骨髓炎的患者需收入院。
- 慢性骨髓炎患者如需外科干预、清创术和获得骨培养和组织学标本通常需收入院。

出院指征

可以在家使用抗生素、骨标本已获取及坏死骨已清除或不需要的情况下，亚急性或慢性骨髓炎患者可以门诊治疗。

- 通过清创和抗生素治疗难以治愈的病例可以把高压氧作为标准治疗方案的辅助手段并从中获益。
- 大约 2/3 的患者将获益。

要点和误区

- 很多患者白细胞可能正常，尤其是慢性骨髓炎。
- 在症状出现的第一个 2～3 周，X 线表现可能都正常。
- 在抗生素治疗时进行伤口培养具有很低的阳性率。

骨折(儿童) Fractures, Pediatric

Adam Z. Barkin 万健 译

基础知识

描述

- 发生急性损伤的患儿中有 20% 会伴有骨折。
- 男童较女童更常见。
- 解剖：
  - 骨干：长骨生长部，管状长骨。
  - 骨骺：接近骨末端的软骨中心，是骨生长的部位。
  - 骺板：放射线下在长骨干骺端与骨骺之间有一盘状软骨结构。
  - 干骺端：长骨末端软骨迅速生长为骨小梁的部位，位于骨干和骨骺之间。
  - 大多数长骨在骨化在青春期后期结束。
- 儿童骨有很强的韧性、弹性和抗折性。
- 以下几种骨折在成人中难以见到：
  - 青枝骨折。
    - 对侧骨皮质不完全断裂的骨折。
  - 螺旋(扣带)骨折。
    - 通常在干骺端和骨干连接处。
    - 一侧骨皮质有压缩。
  - 塑形畸形。
    - 骨有弯曲，但没有骨皮质的断裂。
  - 骨折包含了长骨生长部。
- 软骨生长部是潜在的损伤部位。
- 韧带较骨骺板更能耐受损伤。
- Slater-Harris 分型：按对生长发育影响的危险度的增加可分Ⅰ～Ⅴ型。
  - Ⅰ型：
    - 骨骺的分离从干骺端开始，没有骺板的损伤或移位。
    - 疼痛和压痛局限于骺板处。
    - X 线检查通常正常。
    - 对生长发育影响罕见。
  - Ⅱ型：

◦ 干骺端骨折延伸到骨干。
◦ 最常见。
◦ 对生长发育影响罕见。
- Ⅲ型：
◦ 关节内骨折通过骨骺延伸到骨干。
◦ 最常见于胫骨远端骨骺。
◦ 对生长发育可能有影响。
- Ⅳ型：
◦ 骺、骨骺和干骺端的骨折。
◦ 肱骨外髁是最常见的部位。
◦ 很有可能影响生长发育。
- Ⅴ型：
◦ 骺板挤压伤导致生长停滞。
◦ 通常发生于只有一个平面的关节，如膝关节。
• 骨折通常伴有脱位。
• 如果病史与体格检查不一致，多为非意外创伤。

■ 病因

• 致伤机制有助于确定损伤类型和潜在危险性前臂直接受到打击。
• 肥胖和生长过快是危险因素。
• 非意外损伤：
- 任何<1 岁的小儿的骨折的病史与损伤不完全一致。
- 干骺端"成角"断裂是病理性的。
- 后肋骨折。
- 股骨螺旋骨折。
- 骨折愈合阶段不同。
- 颅骨骨折跨越了骨缝线，尤其是在<1 岁的小儿。
- 小儿或家长非寻常的习惯。

G

诊断

■ 症状和体征

• 肢体活动减少，拒动。
• 肿胀。
• 压痛。
• 畸形。
• 出血斑。
• 捻发音。
• 跛行。
• 手足末梢神经血管异常状态。
• 骨筋膜室综合征。
- 严重的疼痛，尤其在前臂、小腿和足部。
- 被动伸展手指、足趾时疼痛。
- 手足末梢感觉下降。
- 末梢低温。
- 末梢脉搏减弱。
• 开放性骨折可以很明显，也可能很隐秘(收集皮下积血时发现脂肪微粒)。

病史

• 致伤机制：
- 车速(小车、自行车等)。
- 坠落高度。
• 神经损伤。
• 受伤环境。
• 其他损伤。

体格检查

• 全面的反复检查，寻找畸形、青紫和其他损伤体征。
• 评估神经血管状况。
- 运动或感觉神经。
- 末梢脉搏。
- 毛细血管充盈。
• 包含所有关节的运动范围检查。
• 排除伴发的损伤。
• 确保病史和损伤的一致性。

■ 基本检查

• 及时固定。
• 影像学检查。

■ 诊断检查与说明

实验室检查

• 仅在有伴随损伤、有预期手术或有多部位/重要骨折时需要。
• 怀疑感染时需要查 CBC、ESR。

影像学检查

• 后前位、侧位、斜位 X 线检查是必要的，摄片需涵盖骨折的上下关节。
• 对比摄片对骺板骨折检查有益。
• 7～10 日后复查 X 线有助于排除股骨头缺血性坏死或 Salter Ⅰ型骨折。
• 骨扫描、CT 或 MRI 对有助于排除 X 线平片不能发现的骨折或评估感染。

诊断步骤/外科

• 如怀疑感染，可考虑关节穿刺术。

■ 鉴别诊断

• 关节扭伤或肌肉劳损。
• 擦伤(挫伤)。
• 感染。
• 肿瘤。
• 神经缺损。
• 小关节错位，如桡骨头半脱位。
• NAT。

治疗

■ 院前

固定。

■ 初步稳定/治疗

• 伴发伤的急救处理。
• 固定。

■ 急诊治疗/程序

• 处理好威胁生命的伴发伤。
• 控制疼痛。
• 错位需要及时评估，并注意神经血管损伤。
- 致伤机制有助于减少复位方向上的用力。
• 复位非常重要，尤其是骨折包含关节面时。
• 关于 NAT 的适当报告。

Salter-Harris 骨折

• Ⅰ型和Ⅱ型骨折需要固定，并进行骨科随访。
• Ⅱ型股骨远端骨折需紧急骨科会诊。
• Ⅲ型和Ⅳ型骨折需要紧急的骨科会诊进行解剖复位。
• Ⅴ型骨折需要固定和会诊。
• 解剖复位并不能消除对生长发育影响的可能性。

锁骨骨折

• 保持舒适的夹板固定或悬吊(如 8 字形)。
• 第三型锁骨远端骨折需考虑到第一时间悬吊和包扎，或者行肩关节的固定。

肘部骨折

• 所有儿童骨折的 10%。
• >50%为髁上骨折。
- 10%～15%有神经损伤。
• 可能仅在侧位 X 线上显示肘后方积液。
• 因有潜在的血管神经并发症故需骨科会诊。
• 肱动脉损伤发生在 6%～20%的髁上骨折。
• 髁上骨折发生正中神经损伤占 10%～20%。
• 髁上骨折后可出现前臂掌侧室综合征：
- 在受伤后 12～24 h 进展。
- 会导致 Volkmann 缺血性挛缩。
◦ 肘关节固定屈曲，前臂旋前，腕关节屈曲，掌指关节伸直。
• 骺损伤伴长期的生长发育异常。

桡尺骨远端骨折

• 儿科骨折最常见的部位：桡骨远端。
• 复位成角>15°的骨折。

• 沿桡骨掌侧的旋前肌脂肪垫暗示隐匿的骨折。
• Colles 骨折。
- 通过对畸形线的牵引来减弱碎片的致畸作用，减轻对远端碎片背侧的压力和近端碎片掌侧的压力。
- 矫正影像偏差。
- 腕、肘关节固定(Sugar-tong 夹板)。
- 骨科会诊。
- 螺旋骨折(不完全骨折，屈曲或成角仅在骨压缩侧)。
- 最常见于前臂远端。
- 青枝骨折(长骨骨干张力侧的不完全性骨折)。
- 固定。
- 复位(婴儿，成角畸形>30°；儿童，成角畸形>15°)。

胫腓骨骨折

• 单纯的腓骨骨折：跛行。
• 未错位的胫骨骨折：长夹板后方固定，避免承重。
• 错位的胫骨骨折和复合骨折需要会诊。
• 幼儿骨折：
- 无移位的、斜形骨折，远端胫骨骨折。
- 可能需要正侧位片或骨扫描帮助诊断。
- 可疑骨折时应夹板固定，并在 7～10 日后 X 线摄片复查。
• 可将渥太华的足踝规则应用到儿童身上。

股骨头骨骺撕脱

• 股骨头骨骺撕裂伤。
• 需要 AP 或蛙形腿 X 线检查。
• 青年男孩过度负重。
• 疼痛可向膝、大腿或腹股沟放射。
• 相伴的非负重所致的骨病。
• 常常为双侧性的。

股骨骨折

最常见的长骨骨折。

应力性骨折

• 越来越常见。
• 起病隐匿。
• 定位不清的疼痛。
• 常与激烈的活动相关。
• 治疗：
- 选择性支架支持。
- 运动矫正。

开放性骨折

• 盐水纱布包扎。
• 制动。
• 轻度撕裂或轻微污染时应用头孢唑林。
• 轻度污染、高能损伤或有明显的软组织损伤时应用庆大霉素。
• 怀疑与梭状芽胞杆菌(农田、粪便或土壤污染)时应用青霉素。
• 小的伤口伴有软组织损伤时可能需要口服抗菌药物，并在骨科医师指导下制动处理。
• 预后好于成人。

儿童跛行

• 仔细检查和询问风湿病、感染或恶性肿瘤病史。
- 白血病患儿起始症状可能是跛行。
• CBC、SER、CRP 和关节穿刺检查可能有所发现。
• 一过性滑膜炎与臀部感染。
- 需高度怀疑感染感染：
◦ 发热。
◦ ESR/CRP 上升。
◦ WBC 升高。
◦ 拒绝承重。

药物治疗

• 对乙酰氨基酚：10～15 mg/kg(口服，q4～6 h；或纳肛，24 h 不超过 5 次)。
• 头孢唑林：25～100 mg/kg，每日 1 次，肌内注射或静脉注射，分 3 次，q8 h。
• 庆大霉素：2.5 mg/kg，肌内注射或静脉注射，q8 h；或 6.5～7.5 mg/kg，肌内注射或静脉注射，q24 h。
• 治疗血肿：1% 利多卡因不加肾上腺素(最大剂量：3～5 mg/kg)。
• 布洛芬：10 mg/kg，口服，q6～8 h(一线治疗)。
• 吗啡：0.05～0.2 mg/kg，皮下、肌内或静脉注射，q2～4 h。

随访

进一步处理

入院指征

• 不做特殊处理(或只接受社工服务)。
• 开放性骨折。
• 潜在神经血管损伤和骨筋膜室综合征：
- 髁或髁上骨折。
- 股骨干骨折。

出院指征

• 无并发症的骨折：无合并伤或神经血管损伤和骨筋膜室综合征。
- 随访已安排好且父母了解如何应对损伤情况。

转诊问题

所有的 Salter-Harris 骨折均应有骨科医师访视。

要点和误区

• 评估 NAT 时病史非常重要。
• 必须让父母完全理解 NAT。
• 不必顾忌上夹板或请骨关节医师会诊。
• 镇痛常被低估，应予以重视。
• 远端桡骨骨折常与其他骨折密切相关：尺骨骨折、肘部骨折、腕骨骨折等。
• 髁上骨折可能导致神经或血管损伤。

骨质疏松症

Stephen R. Hayden　王虑 译

基础知识

描述

• 逐步扩散的骨骼质量整体下降。
• 骨骼脆性和增加骨折风险。
• 骨小梁(尤其是椎骨和股骨)更早受累也最为常见。
• 从青春期就发病，但 50 岁以后才容易发生骨折。
• 女性患者多于男性，尤其是绝经后；与雌激素缺乏或年龄有关。

病因

• 骨骼的再吸收增加超过了新骨的合成。
• 年龄的增加是最大的危险因素。
• 年轻时钙摄入不足也是重要原因。
• 缺少运动的生活方式也是危险因素(体重

会影响新骨的合成）。

• 绝经后雌激素分泌减少是女性患骨质疏松的关键因素。

• 其他危险因素包括：长时间类固醇激素的使用、酗酒、服用甲氨蝶呤、吸烟、低体重。

• 家族性或遗传因素。

儿童注意事项

骨质疏松可于青少年期起病，儿童时期也可无症状。

诊断

症状和体征

• 平时无症状，直到出现病理性骨折。

• 无明显病因的骨折和反复的骨折是其特点。

• 脊柱最常受累。

• 多个脊柱压缩性骨折常导致驼背和脊柱侧弯。

• 臀部骨折（股骨颈股骨粗隆骨折）也十分常见。

病史

• 无明显原因的疑似骨折或有骨折病史均提示骨质疏松。

• 骨质疏松家族史是重要的危险因素。

体格检查

主要是发现骨质疏松所致的急性骨折的相关体征。

基本检查

• 无原因的骨折和患病危险因素：这两点最为重要。

• 仔细地对股骨或足部骨折的神经血管进行检查。

• 排便排尿困难提示有脊柱骨折。

• 放射检查发现可以，骨折可能提示存在骨质疏松。

• CT 检查能对脊柱骨折的病情做出更好的评估。

– 椎管损害常常 X 线平片无法发现。

– 确保 CT 检查能对损伤的脊髓上下层面做全面扫描。

诊断检查与说明

实验室检查

一些生化指标比如钙、甲状旁腺素和碱性磷酸酶等对于鉴别诊断有意义。

影像学检查

• X 线平片能够诊断是否骨折，但陈旧性骨折靠 X 线平片难以发现。

• 骨扫描或 CT 能帮助发现陈旧性骨折，尤其是脊柱的骨折。

诊断步骤/外科

骨密度扫描有助于判断预后并指导治疗。用双能 X 线骨密度仪测定骨密度 T，分数≤2.5：可诊断为骨质疏松。

鉴别诊断

• 多发性骨髓瘤或其他转移性肿瘤。

• 成骨不全（常见于儿童）。

• 甲状旁腺功能亢进症。

• 佩吉特病。

• 其他脱骨质疾病。

• 非意外创伤/虐待老人。

治疗

院前

注意：

• 院前多获得些患病信息对诊断病理性骨折有较大帮助。

• 不要额外搬动患者，这有可能使骨折加重。

初步稳定/治疗

固定骨折。

急诊治疗/程序

• 骨折没及时得到的治疗延迟或不完全愈合。

• 预防比治疗更有效。

• 长期治疗更为有益（见药物治疗），通常由专科医师或会诊医师发起。

• 矫正支架和背心的使用应当参考脊柱科医师的建议。

• 适度运动对治疗也很有帮助。

• 必须在使用类固醇或甲氨蝶呤治疗和导致骨质疏松症的风险这两者之间寻求平衡。

药物治疗

• 阿仑膦酸钠：10 mg/d 或每周 70 mg，另外可选的是利塞膦酸钠：5 mg/d，每周 35 mg 或每月 150 mg。

• 唑来膦酸：5 mg 静推，每年 1 次。

• 雷洛昔芬（选择性雌激素受体调节剂）：60 mg，口服，每日 1 次。

• 钙：1 200 mg，每日 1 次（日常膳食加另外补充）。

• 维生素 D：800 U/d。

• 降钙素：喷鼻 200 U/d。

• 狄诺塞麦（单克隆抗体）：60 mg，皮下注射，每 6 个月 1 次。

• 甲状旁腺素（1 - 34）：20 μg，皮下注射，每日 1 次。

• 雌激素：0.625 mg/d（可同时服用或不用醋酸甲羟孕酮）。

儿科注意事项

确保日常膳食，摄入充足的钙质。

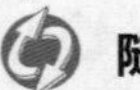

随访

进一步处理

入院指征

• 按照正常骨科入院原则，兼顾考虑患者年龄和社会环境。

• 压缩性骨折通常比较稳定，但必须排除爆裂性骨折可能导致的脊髓压迫。

• 颈部骨折或伴有神经症状的患者，在听取神经外科和骨科医师建议后应急诊入院并接受紧急外科干预。

• 收治入院后因为减少了走动，有利于减轻疼痛。

出院指征

• 按照正常骨科出院原则，兼顾考虑患者年龄和社会环境。

• 若患者伤情较轻，能在适当帮助下在家照顾自己，并且移动造成的疼痛可控，可以在骨科医师的随访下予以出院。

• 在急诊室进行物理治疗评估可能会有所帮助。

转诊问题

急性损伤需转诊到骨科。

随访建议

• 急性损伤患者要正常随访。

• 随访主治医师应确保鼓励患者继续治疗，并预防骨折再发。

要点和误区

• 无明显诱因的复发性骨折往往提示骨质疏松症。

• 若 X 线平片上显示骨密度下降则高度提示可能有骨质疏松，应立即行进一步检查和治疗。

• 双膦酸盐类药物是治疗骨质疏松症的一线用药，通常不在急诊使用。

鼓膜穿孔 Tympanic Membrane Perforation

Andrew K. Chang · Kirsten L. Morrissey 张晟 林兆奋 译

基础知识

描述

穿孔有几种不同的分类方式。
- 持续时间。
- 急性(<3个月)。
- 慢性(>3个月)。
- 部位。
- 紧张部。
- 松弛部。
- 范围。
- 限于1个象限(<25%)。
- 2个或更多象限。
- 全部穿孔。

病因

- 感染(急性中耳炎)。
- 造成急性穿孔最常见的病因。
- 钝性创伤(扇耳光)。
- 家暴、街斗。
- 侵入性创伤(棉签)。
- 鼓室造口术管的挤压。
- 快速压力变化(潜水、飞行)。
- 常在100～400 mmHg范围内发生破裂(深度变化2.6 ft,压力变化达60 mmHg)。
- 极度噪声(爆炸)。
- 闪电。
- 急性坏死性鼓膜炎(β溶血性链球菌)。
- 炉渣烧伤(焊接或金属工艺)。
- 外科手术的并发症。
- 鼓膜切开术、鼓室成形术、鼓膜切开置管术。

诊断

症状和体征

病史
- 耳痛(轻度)。
- 患耳严重疼痛或完全听力丧失提示存在额外的损伤。
- 耳鸣。
- 眩晕(尤其当穿孔在水下发生时)。

体格检查
- 听力丧失(部分的)。
- 外耳道脓性或血性分泌物。
- 气动耳镜的喷射。
- 仅在鼓膜静止时,小的穿孔可能会明显。
- 如果压力可经瘘传导至中耳并进入迷路瘘道,保持压力15 s(瘘试验)可能导致眼球震颤或眩晕。
- 韦伯试验(音叉位于中线骨)。
- 双侧声音应一致或患侧声音略大,声音持续性衰减传播。
- 声音局限于一侧提示可能有听神经损伤。
- Rinne试验(音叉位于乳突部)。
- 常正常(空气传播在骨传导衰减后才被感觉到)或者显示轻微的传导损失。

基本检查

临床检验。
- 直接可视的耳镜鼓膜检查。
- 双耳听力测试。
- 耳屏阻塞外耳道(瘘的标志)位置或压力变化时记录任一侧眼球震颤。

诊断检查与说明

实验室检查

如果出现耳道引流液,进行引流物培养是有必要的。

影像学检查
- 颅脑CT。
- 如果临床怀疑颞骨骨折,拍摄CT会有用。

鉴别诊断

- 颞骨骨折。
- 浆液性中耳炎。
- 感染性中耳炎。
- 外耳炎。
- 耳垢影响。
- 气压伤。
- 声音相关的创伤。
- 异物。
- 虐待儿童。

治疗

初步稳定/治疗

- 创伤治疗及护理。
- 颈椎制动,根据情形查看颅内损伤。

急诊治疗/程序

- 小心清除外耳道异物。
- 不可灌洗,因为这样会导致更多污染物进入中耳。
- 如果耳垢嵌塞看不见鼓膜,但高度怀疑鼓膜穿孔时,人工清除耳垢或者吸引清除。
- 如果临床证据怀疑颞骨骨折,做CT扫描以排除。
- 不建议预防性使用抗生素。
- 如果有感染的证据、水或污染物进入外耳道则使用抗生素。
- 阿莫西林。
- 奥格门汀。
- 头孢克肟、头孢曲松。
- 头孢地尼。
- 头孢呋辛。
- 阿奇霉素。
- 克林霉素。
- 如果疼痛需要,用止痛药。
- 除氟喹诺酮类的例外,针对耳的用药因其耳毒性的风险还有争议。
- 当有分泌物流出时,大多数人支持抗生素,因其可治疗或预防外耳道感染并减少中耳感染的扩散。
- 针对耳的抗生素在中耳内形成高浓度,药物浓度可能超过机体可耐受的最小药物浓度。
- 耳用氟喹诺酮类是慢性化脓性中耳炎的一线用药,在创伤性鼓膜怀疑有水进入中耳时也作为一线用药。
- 有以下情形时紧急咨询耳鼻喉科专家:
- 眩晕、眼球震颤或共济失调。
- 感觉性听力丧失。
- 严重耳鸣。
- 活动性出血或严重出血。
- 面肌麻痹。

药物治疗

- 阿莫西林:500 mg口服,每日3次[儿童:80～90 mg/(kg·24 h),口服,每日2次],连用7～10日。
- 奥格门汀:875 mg[儿童:90 mg/(kg·24 h)],口服,每日2次,连用7～10日。
- 头孢克肟:400 mg[儿童:8 mg/(kg·24 h)],口服,每日1次,连用7～10日。
- 头孢地尼:300 mg口服避孕药;或600 mg,q24 h(儿童:14 mg/kg口服避孕药,q24 h)。
- 头孢呋辛250 mg,口服,每日2次,连用7～10日[儿童:30 mg/(kg·24 h),口服,每日2次]。
- 头孢曲松:1～2 g静脉注射或肌内注射

G

（儿童：50 mg/kg，肌内注射，最大剂量 1 g）1 剂。

• 阿奇霉素：2 g（儿童：30 mg/kg，最大剂量 1 500 mg），口服 1 剂。

• 克林霉素：150～450 mg［儿童：30 mg/(kg · 24 h)］，口服，每日 4 次，连用 7～10 日。

• 环丙沙星-地塞米松：滴耳用每日 2 次，每次 4 滴，连用 7～10 日。

• 新霉素-多黏菌素 B-氢化可的松：滴耳用悬浮液：1 只耳 4 滴，每日 3～4 次（儿童：3 滴每日 3～4 次），最大剂量用 10 日，患耳朝上侧躺 5 min。

一线用药

• 阿莫西林和奥格门汀是急性中耳炎伴鼓膜穿孔主要用药。

- 奥格门汀应用于有复发性感染的患者或应用抗生素不足 1 个月的患者。

- 环丙沙星和地塞米松滴剂用于慢性化脓性中耳炎和创伤性鼓膜穿孔怀疑水或污染物进入中耳。

二线用药

• 青霉素过敏的患者可用头孢菌素。

- 有呕吐或其他并发问题的患者更适合头孢曲松肌内注射。

• 对青霉素呈高敏感Ⅰ型超敏反应的患者可能适合用阿奇霉素或克林霉素。阿奇霉素对流感嗜血杆菌和肺炎链球菌的疗效有限，只能在必要/有限的情况下使用。

随访

进一步处理

入院指征

• 相关的外伤需要处理。

• 严重的眩晕影响行动。

出院指征

几乎所有患者都能出院。

转诊问题

• 1 周内安排门诊耳鼻喉科随访。

- 在详细检查和正规听力测试后，大多数耳鼻喉科医师进行观察等待，因为大多数鼓膜穿孔可自发愈合。

- 穿孔大小扩大并且穿孔位置明显变化时听力损失增加。

- 手术修复（修补或鼓膜成形术）适用于 10%～20% 无法自我恢复的患者。

随访建议

• 提供详细的出院指导。

- 洗澡时用浸润石油或抗生素软膏的棉花塞住外耳道防止水进入中耳，否则会痛且会加重感染。

- 仅在有合适的耳塞时游泳。

- 避免用力擤鼻涕。

• 预期结果。

- 大多数穿孔在数日至数月可自发愈合，一个关于儿童的研究指出，儿童鼓膜穿孔 70% 在 1 周内愈合，94% 在 1 个月内愈合。

- 自发性愈合和穿孔大小、感染类型和耳道干性还是浆液性环境相关。

- 湿性穿孔倾向于更快愈合。

- 由融化的金属或电烧伤造成的穿孔很少自发性愈合；并发症包括：

◦ 感染。

◦ 听小骨移位。

◦ 外淋巴液漏。

◦ 胆脂瘤。

要点和误区

• 急性中耳炎是造成鼓膜穿孔最常见的病因。

- 小的穿孔可能只能经气动耳镜喷射才能诊断。

- 异物、耳垢或分泌物应被吸引清除或人工清除，怀疑鼓膜穿孔时禁忌耳道灌洗。

- 耳用氟喹诺酮类用于慢性化脓性中耳炎的抗生素治疗，创伤性鼓膜穿孔怀疑伴异物、水或污染物进入时也可应用。

- 大多数穿孔可自愈，然而必须要进行护理防止感染载体进入中耳。

• 有鼓膜穿孔时，慢性中耳炎可造成中耳或乳突气室复发性感染。

• 当鼓膜穿孔处有持续性脓性引流物 >6 周，可诊断为慢性化脓性中耳炎。

• 使用新霉素-多黏菌素 B-氢化可的松耳用悬浮液治疗外耳炎症伴鼓膜穿孔。

关节损伤

Ilona A. Barash　何超　段立伟 译

基础知识

描述

• 交叉韧带损伤：

- 前交叉韧带：

◦ 能够防止胫骨的过度前移、内旋和膝关节的过伸。

- 后交叉韧带：

◦ 是前交叉韧带的 2 倍强韧和 2 倍厚，因此不常发生。

◦ 从胫骨中间区域的前外侧骨节至胫骨的后侧。

• 半月板撕裂：

- 中段半月板的损伤最常发生。

◦ 与关节囊的连接最紧密，因此活动性比外侧半月板差。

- 撕脱来自股骨和胫骨骨节之间的牵拉和压力。

- 半月板的撕裂造成的游离组织会存在于关节内部，引起真性的闭锁关节。

• 内侧副韧带：

- 从中间腓骨的后侧骨节至胫骨，关节远端。

- 通常伴随其他的损伤。

◦ 关节外旋产生的压力。

流行病学

发病率和患病率预测

• 前交叉韧带：

- 在膝关节韧带损伤中最常见。

- 每年美国有 200 000 例的前交叉韧带损伤的发生。

- 约 2/3 的前交叉韧带损伤是非接触性的。

- 女性：3 倍的风险。

• 伴随的损伤：

- 50% 的前交叉韧带损伤伴有半月板的撕裂。

- 通常伴有软骨和软骨下的损伤。

• 半月板：

- 内侧半月板损伤的发生率是外侧半月板损伤的 10 倍。

- 真性关节闭锁的发生占 30%。

■ 病因

• 交叉韧带损伤：
- 前交叉韧带：屈伸或旋转运动过程中减速产生的应力损伤或过伸损伤。
◦ 通常会是运动相关性的，如滑雪或足球运动带来的损伤。
- 后交叉韧带：
◦ "汽车仪表盘损伤"：屈曲的膝受到来自近端胫骨前方的直接力量的打击(交通撞击或直接创伤)。
◦ 屈曲的膝关节坠落伤。
• 半月板撕裂：
- 突然的膝关节的蹲膝、旋转、翻转、弯曲和旋转运动。
- 伴随蹲着或跪着姿势的体育活动。
• 内侧副韧带的损伤：
- 屈曲的膝关节外翻产生的外翻应力。

儿科注意事项

• 前交叉韧带是儿童膝关节韧带损伤最常见的部位。
• 生长板闭合前单纯性内侧副韧带损伤少见(<14 岁)。

诊断

■ 症状和体征

病史

• 交叉韧带损伤：
- 膝关节的失去控制感或撕裂感。
- 多数的患者反映会立刻出现膝关节的功能障碍，但是有一些患者即使发生完全的前交叉韧带撕裂仍能步行，这是因为一些支撑性结构保持了关节的稳定性。
- 会即刻出现大量的渗出，患者诉关节肿胀严重。
• 内侧副韧带：
- 在膝关节的内侧立刻出现失去控制感和剧烈的疼痛。
- 相比于完全撕脱，韧带的不完全的撕脱的疼痛和压痛更明显。
• 内侧半月板损伤：
- 患者自述关节失去控制感。
- 关节伸直体位下的不稳定性。
- 约 50％的患者会出现关节内渗出，一般在受伤后的 6～12 h 出现。
- 不同于韧带的损伤，患者一般会在活动之后自诉疼痛。
- 退行性半月板损伤的发生具有隐匿性，表现为一些非创伤性的症状、肿胀不严重、关节疼痛模糊，有时会出现机械力学方面的症状，通常伴发骨关节炎。

体格检查

• 避免受伤关节的承重。
• 触诊寻找疼痛的位置：
- 骨折处的骨突起。
- 儿童患者的骨骺板。
- 内外侧的关节线(半月板和侧副韧带的损伤)。
• 关节的活动范围：
- 闭锁：前交叉韧带、半月板损伤或游离体出现。
- 在疼痛、渗出和痉挛的情况下会出现假性闭锁。
• 渗出：
- 即刻发生的渗出(2～3 h)通常提示包括前交叉韧带损伤在内的关节内的严重损伤。
- 约有 70％的急性关节内血肿是由于前交叉韧带的损伤引起，但是如果没有渗出时不能排除前交叉韧带的损伤。
- 内侧副韧带、半月板、后交叉韧带的损伤所引起的渗出比较迟发(12～24 h 发生)。
- 如果出现皮温高，皮肤红斑考虑感染。
• 神经血管检查：
- 远端动脉搏动。
- 踝关节或足趾的背曲。
• 压力测试：将损伤侧的关节与未损伤侧进行比较。
- 在损伤的急性期疼痛和痉挛会限制压力测试的检查。
- 对于前交叉韧带损伤，Lachman 测试更加可靠。
◦ 膝关节屈曲 20°，患者平卧，大腿部进行支撑，臀部轻度外旋，一只手固定近端胫骨，另一只手在髌骨上端固定股骨，迅速将胫骨向股骨前侧复位。
◦ 疼痛但尚有运动功能：韧带的部分撕脱或损伤。
- 轴移测试：
◦ 患者仰卧位，膝关节完全伸展，内旋。临床医生的远端一只手保持踝关节内旋，另一只手放在胫骨平台外侧，有轻微外翻应力。临床医生慢慢屈膝。如果在前 30°屈曲期间胫骨平台半脱位与对侧不同，则为阳性。
◦ 对前交叉韧带损伤更为特异，但在非麻醉情况下不可靠，疼痛剧烈。不建议在急诊室做常规检查。
- 前后抽屉试验：
◦ 膝关节屈曲呈 90°，患者仰卧位，臀部屈曲 45°，足部呈中立性稳定位。
◦ 后纵韧带损伤时出现胫骨的前方松弛。
◦ 后抽屉试验(后纵韧带)：向后施压出现胫骨向后移动。
◦ 前抽屉试验(前纵韧带)：向前施压出现胫骨向前移动。
- 股四头肌收缩试验(后纵韧带)：
◦ 患者仰卧位，膝关节屈曲成 90°，臀部屈曲呈 45°。
◦ 嘱患者抵抗检查者的施压将膝关节向前伸直。
◦ 若股四头肌活动时出现胫骨的向前移位则该试验阳性。
- 内翻、外翻应力试验：膝关节伸直并 20°屈曲检查内侧副韧带和外侧副韧带的松弛度。
- 同时伴有支点损伤、渗出和 Lachman 阳性，在交叉韧带撕裂中 LR>17。
• 半月板：在急性疼痛得到缓解后进行检查。
- McMurray 试验：触摸关节线，伸膝，而后自内向外旋转膝关节。疼痛和弹响表示阳性。
- Apley 试验：患者俯卧位，屈膝 90°，施加轴向压力，并分别向内/外侧旋转小腿。疼痛为阳性。

儿科注意事项

• 儿童和青少年检查的表现比成人更松弛。
• 如果考虑髋部病变，检查髋并获取放射图像(特别是股骨头骺脱位)。
• 要高度怀疑骨骺生长板损伤。

G

■ 诊断检查与说明

实验室检查

• 如果膝关节渗出原因不是创伤，将滑液抽取物送细胞计数、革兰染色、培养、结晶。
• 创伤后一般不进行关节穿刺术，除非为了缓解张力性渗出导致的症状。

影像学检查

• Ottawa 膝关节规则(成人)：有以下 5 个表现的需要拍 X 线平片。
- 年龄≥55 岁。
- 单侧膝关节压痛。
- 腓骨头压痛。
- 不能屈至 90°。
- 不论即刻还是在急诊室中都不能承受重量。
• 标准 X 线。
- 对可疑高风险骨折的 ACL 损伤均应拍摄。
- 对评估儿童胫骨脊和生长板骨折很重要。
- 体位：前后位、侧位、斜位、切迹。

- 特别注意正中/侧胫骨脊和侧胫骨平台的撕脱性骨折，这种 ACL/PCL 损伤更易通过手术修复。
- 骨折的液性脂肪水平。

• MRI 对 ACL 撕裂和其他关节内异常(半月板、PCL、骨坏死、骨软骨损伤、隐性骨折)有约 95%的敏感性和更高的特异性，但紧急情况下较少应用。

• 对可疑脱位需用动脉超声评估血管完整性。

• 超声对检查囊肿和腘动脉瘤很有帮助。对前交叉韧带和半月板损伤的诊断很有帮助。今后可能会看到超声使用的越来越多。

儿科注意事项

Ottawa 规则对儿童不适用。

基本检查

• 神经血管评估。
• 排除骨折和感染。
• 评估多向不稳。
• 屈曲 20°加压外翻/内翻。
• 伸肌机制功能。
• 对 ACL 损伤进行 Lachman 检查。

鉴别诊断

• 生长板损伤。
• 胫骨平台骨性损伤，其他骨折。
• 暂时性的髌骨脱位。
• 髋关节损伤产生的疼痛。
• 非创伤性因素引起的膝关节肿胀和疼痛包括化脓性膝关节炎、痛风、化脓性骨关节炎、风湿性关节炎。

G

治疗

院前和初步稳定/治疗

• 进行心肺复苏的抢救和后续的高级生命支持。
• 膝关节制动。
• 记录是否存在神经和血管的损伤。
• 进行冰敷、悬吊和止痛治疗。

急诊治疗/程序

• 在第一个 24 h 内，减轻对于由于半月板损伤带来的膝关节交锁。
- 让患者坐下，并且利用检查桌将患肢进行悬吊，结合止痛药物能够有效地缓解关节交锁。
- 协助患者轻柔的牵引并旋转胫骨。

• 关节穿刺术能够缓解严重的关节肿胀并且避免关节交锁的发生。

• 治疗(不合并骨折)：
- 休息，冰敷，压迫，置高。
- 适当的承重，必要时使用拐杖。
- 进行膝关节的保护性制动，但是在充分支撑的条件下可以鼓励患者进行一定的活动。
- 如果使用膝关节固定器，需要每日从膝关节固定器中取出进行 20～30 次屈曲/伸展运动，外加每日 2～4 次 10～20 次直腿抬高，除非有禁忌证。

药物治疗

• 疼痛控制：NSAIDs 类止痛药优于阿片类止痛药。
• 布洛芬：400～600 mg(儿童：5～10 mg/kg)，每日 3 次，口服。

随访

进一步处理

入院指征

• 单发的前交叉韧带、后交叉韧带、半月板或副韧带的损伤一般不需要急诊收治入院。
• 膝关节的脱位损伤一般不太需要心电监护。
• 一旦发生骨折则需要进行切开复位内固定来减少创伤后关节炎的发生。

出院指征

大部分患者经过恰当的治疗后可以出院。

随访建议

• 对于急诊检查不能明确诊断或患者的病史提示存在更加严重的损伤时，推荐在 48 h 后复查。
• 如果损伤 1～2 周后存在韧带的损伤，需要进行整形外科随访。
• 对于希望今后拥有运动等活动性较大的生活方式的患者推荐进行手术的损伤修复。

要点和误区

• 损伤后要进行仔细的血管神经检查，同时检查范围一般包括疼痛关节相关的上下各一关节。
• 对于多个方向关节不稳或多个韧带损伤的患者高度怀疑存在全膝关节脱位。
• 不要遗忘：膝关节脱位、骨折、化脓性关节炎、髋关节损伤的牵涉痛、血管神经损伤。

管饲并发症

Colleen N. Hickey 万健 译

基础知识

描述

• 导管脱落：
- 无意或有意的。
- 鼻饲养管比经皮内镜下胃造瘘管、胃管或空肠造瘘管更常见。

• 导管阻塞：
- 导管管径过小：
  ◦ 多见于鼻饲管。
- 药丸碎片导致阻塞。
- 冲管不充分。
- 管饲物和药物间生理学不相容。
  ◦ 管饲物残渣黏附于导管内壁。
- 必须排除导管位置不当、结构问题和移位等。

• 外口感染：
- 危险因素：
  ◦ 营养不良。
  ◦ 造口渗漏。
  ◦ 局部刺激。
  ◦ 外口护理不当。
  ◦ 免疫功能低下。
  ◦ 糖尿病。
  ◦ 外口愈合不良。
  ◦ 肥胖。
  ◦ 恶性肿瘤。
- 导管过度牵拉：
  ◦ 导致胃与皮肤间的导管通路延迟形成。
  ◦ 造口渗漏增加。

• 造口渗漏：
- 远端阻塞问题(机械性或肌张力障碍性)，多见于胃大量残留时。

- 导管移动过度。
- 更容易发生在营养不良和糖尿病患者。

• 吸入性肺炎：
- 高危因素：
◦ 咳嗽/咽反射异常。
◦ 肠梗阻胃排空延迟。
◦ 梗阻。
◦ 胃轻瘫。
◦ 胃食管反流(常见于较粗的鼻饲管)。

• 腹泻：
- 医源性：
◦ 抗生素。
◦ 促胃肠动力药。
- 难辨梭状杆菌、其他细菌或念珠菌过度生长。
- 高渗的管饲物。
- 低蛋白血症。

• 喂养不耐受：
- 大量残渣提示胃肠动力障碍。
- 喂养速度过快。
- 高渗管饲物。
- 乳糖或脂肪不耐受。
- 低白蛋白血症。

• 少见并发症：
- 腹壁血肿。
- 瘘管：
◦ 肝胃部。
◦ 胃结肠部。
◦ 结肠与皮肤。
- 穿孔(通常由置管引起)。
- 压疮和溃疡。
- 消化道出血。
◦ 食管炎、胃应激性溃疡、消化道溃疡。
- 消化道出口梗阻。
◦ 临时置管时胃幽门部或十二指肠被导管或球囊部分或完全阻塞。
- 内固定器植入综合征。
◦ 少见但较严重。
◦ 由于压力过大引起消化道溃疡，使内固定器嵌入胃壁和皮肤之间。
- 经皮内镜下胃造瘘管周围肠扭转。

儿科注意事项

误吸风险增加。

• 延迟胃排空。
• 食管下括约肌发育不良。

诊断

症状和体征

• 导管脱落：
- 导管从固定部位脱出。

• 阻塞：
- 液体不能通过导管。

• 导管移动：
- 经皮内镜下胃造瘘管远端放置不当。
- 远端或幽门部的梗阻。
- 倾倒综合征。
- 局部缺血。
- 套叠。
- 管外发现远端脱落征象(如有标记)。

• 外口感染：
- 蜂窝织炎。
- 脓肿形成。
- 坏死性筋膜炎。

• 小口渗漏：
- 小口周围鼻饲物、胃内容物的渗漏。

• 吸入性肺炎：
- 咳嗽。
- 呼吸困难。
- 缺氧。
- 肺分泌物中可见食物颗粒。
- 发热。

• 鼻导管误插入肺支气管：
- 气胸。
- 胸腔积液。
- 渗出性胸膜炎。
- 气管胸膜瘘。
- 肺炎。

• 腹泻：
- 常见稀便。
- 脱水。

• 肠内营养不耐受：
- 胃残留增加。
- 误吸风险增加。

基本检查

• 仔细检查置管部位和鼻饲管放置情况。

• 可疑导管移位时，应用水溶性造影剂做影像学检查来确定导管在腹部、胃、小肠内的位置。

诊断检查与说明

实验室检查

• 造口周围的感染：
- 严重感染时行全血细胞计数检查。
- 全身感染时行血培养检查。

• 吸入性肺炎：
- 脉氧测定或血气分析。
- 全血细胞计数。
- 电解质、尿素氮/肌酐、血糖。
- 血培养和痰培养。

• 腹泻：
- 粪便查白细胞、粪培养、难辨梭状杆菌毒素。

• 消化道出血：
- 连续监测全血细胞计数。

影像学检查

• 胸部 X 线检查：
- 鼻导管位置。
- 吸入性肺炎。

• 怀疑导管移位时水溶性影像学造影检查。

诊断步骤/外科

内镜下评估是否有导管移位。

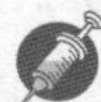

治疗

院前

> **注意**
> 如发生导管脱落，将患者和导管一起转运便于再次置管。

初步稳定/治疗

• ABC 管理。
• 脱水、脓毒症时给予静脉液体复苏。

急诊治疗/程序

导管脱落

• 鼻饲管：
- 在急诊室重新置管。
- 使用前行 X 线检查确定位置。

• 经皮内镜下胃造瘘管和胃空肠管：
- 胃皮通道、瘘管成形需 4～6 周。
- 不恰当或粗暴地放置导管会破坏胃皮通道，引起腹膜炎。
- 经皮内镜下胃造瘘管放置＞4 周：
◦ 在急诊室重新放置(选择尺寸匹配的导管)。
◦ 行水溶性造影剂检查确定位置。
◦ 将导管固定于腹壁上以避免移位。
- 经皮内镜下胃造瘘管放置＜4 周：
◦ 不需要在急诊室重新放置。
◦ 有腹腔内移位的风险。
- 外科胃造瘘管或空肠造瘘管：
◦ 与经皮内镜下胃造瘘管处理相似。
◦ 3 日内早期松脱需急诊外科会诊并给予抗生素控制腹膜炎。
◦ 如放置时间＜4 周可能需要内镜下重新放置导管。

G

导管阻塞

• 可试着先用生理盐水、蒸馏水、苏打水和含胰酶液体轻轻冲洗。

• 如冲洗失败则重新放置导管。

• 不要使用蛋白类软化剂。

导管移位

• 如能撤出导管并且耐受良好。

- 固定导管外部。

- 行初步饲管试验后即可出院回家。

• 如管饲不耐受，或出现持续梗阻及腹膜炎体征：

- 转至合适的胃肠外科机构会诊。

• 如体外导管被切断(无意或有意)而体内导管仍在腹腔内：

- 体内置入部分常滑入胃肠道(1 周内完成 XR 确认)。

- 有过梗阻、穿孔、腹膜炎的报道，尤其是儿童患者。

置管周围感染

• 局部创口处理。

• 使用抗生素：

- 第一代头孢菌素(头孢唑林或头孢氨苄)。

- 氨苄西林-舒巴坦。

- 阿莫西林-克拉维酸。

- 克林霉素(适用于青霉素过敏者)。

• 较轻病例门诊处理。

• 较重病例需请外科会诊决定是否行引流/清创及住院治疗。

• 严重感染(腹膜炎、坏死性筋膜炎)需要拔管。

• 放置导管前预防性应用抗生素(头孢唑林)可减少创口感染(3%*vs*18%感染率)。

导管周围渗漏

• 从间断输注改为连续性输注。

• 输注速度减慢。

• 营养状态的优化。

• 解除导管过大的张力。

• 给予促胃动力剂(如甲氧氯普胺)。

• 不要放置过粗的导管。

• 局部护理：

- 置管部位保护清洁干燥。

- 黏附剂。

吸入性肺炎

• 停止肠内营养。

• 给予氧疗和广谱抗生素治疗。

• 呼吸衰竭时气管插管机械通气，保证气道通畅。

• 预防吸入性肺炎的措施：

- 床头抬高。

- 监测胃残留量。

- 采用分级的持续输注。

- 采用促胃动力药。

腹泻

• 病因处理。

• 纠正水电解质紊乱。

• 试用等渗、低渗、无脂肪或无乳糖配方。

• 如上述配方失效，试用高纤维素配方。

• 抗动力药：

- 洛哌丁胺。

- 果胶。

- 消胆胺。

配方制剂不耐受

• 促胃动力药促进胃排空。

■ 药物治疗

• 阿莫西林-克拉维酸(奥格门汀)：500～875 mg[儿童：25～45 mg/(kg·24 h)]，口服，q12 h。

• 氨苄西林-舒巴坦：1.5～3 g[儿童：100～200 mg/(kg·24 h)]，静脉注射，q6 h。

• 头孢唑林：500 mg～1 g[儿童：25～100 mg/(kg·24 h)]，静脉注射，q6 h。

• 头孢氨苄：250～500 mg[儿童：25～50 mg/(kg·24 h)]，口服，q6 h。

• 消胆胺：2～4 g(儿童：大于 6 岁，80 mg/kg，q8 h)，口服，q6～12 h。

• 克林霉素：150～300 mg(儿童：5～10 mg/kg)，静脉注射，q6 h。

• 果胶：30 ml(儿童：3～6 岁，7.5 ml；6～12 岁，15 ml)，每次稀水便后口服，每日不超过 7 次。

• 洛哌丁胺(易蒙停)：首剂 4 mg，2 mg(儿童：13～20 kg，1 mg，q8 h；20～30 kg，2 mg，q12 h；30 kg 以上，每日总量不超过 9 mg)，口服，每日总量不超过 16 mg。

• 甲氧氯普胺：5～10 mg[儿童：0.1～0.2 mg/kg，最大剂量 0.8 mg/(kg·d)]口服/静脉注射/肌内注射，q6 h(餐前 30 min 和睡前)。

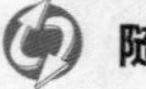

随访

■ 进一步处理

入院指征

• 经皮内镜下胃造瘘管在置入 1 周内脱落者。

• 胃造瘘管或空肠造瘘管在置入 3 日内脱落者。

• 置管周围严重感染。

• 吸入性肺炎。

• 与脱水相关的腹泻。

• 活动性消化道出血。

• 腹膜炎。

出院指征

• 喂养管脱落后再次成功置入后。

转诊问题

在急诊室喂养管重置不成功时应请消化科或外科会诊。

■ 随访建议

反复出现喂养管并发症时应加强基础护理或消化科随访。

要点和误区

• 应行 X 线检查来确认喂养管置管在位。

• 不要在急诊室尝试重置新近放入的经皮内镜下胃造瘘管、胃管或空肠管。

过度通气综合征 Hyperventilation Syndrome

Robert F. McCormack 巩博 译

基础知识

■ 描述

• 过度通气综合征描述了一系列症状：

- 最常见：呼吸急促、胸痛、头晕和感觉异常。

• 每分通气量由非生理性增加产生：

- 增加每分通气量可以通过增加呼吸频率或者潮气量来实现。

• 在诊断过度通气综合征前必须排除病理性或生理性原因导致的过度通气。

• 流行病学：

- 10%~15%的普通人群发病。
- 女性更常见。
- 25%~83%的焦虑症患者。

■ **病因**

• 病因不清楚：
- 通常是对心理性压力因素的反应。
• 对于某些疾病引起过度通气存在争议：
- 低碳酸血症。
- 低磷酸血症。
- 低钙血症。

诊断

■ **症状和体征**

病史

• 既往史：
- 持续时间。
- 触发因素。
- 过去治疗情况。
- 常常发作的时间点。
• 心脏：
- 胸痛。
- 呼吸急促。
- "氧饥饿"。
- 心慌。
• 神经系统：
- 眩晕。
- 头昏眼花。
- 晕厥。
- 感觉异常。
- 头痛。
- 手足痉挛。
- 手足僵直。
• 精神状态：
- 十分害怕、焦虑。
- 濒死感。
- 眼花。
- 不真实感。
• 一般情况：
- 疲乏。
- 虚弱。
- 心神不安。

体格检查

• 临床症状少见：
- 呼吸急促最常见。
- 但是呼吸急促不一定出现。患者增加的可能是潮气量而不是呼吸频率。
- 心动过速。
- 手足痉挛：
◦ 可能出现眩晕。
◦ 可能出现沃斯特克征。

■ **基本检查**

• 排除性诊断：
- 必须查找和排除过度通气原发性病理性或生理性病因。
• 临床诊断以病史和体格检查为依据。
• 生命体征包括脉搏氧饱和度。
• 过度通气综合征不会引起低氧。

■ **诊断检查与说明**

实验室检查

• 只需要排除病理/生理原因。
• 妊娠试验。
• 考虑低氧患者的 ABG 来评估 a-a 梯度，在过度通气综合征中是正常的。
• 怀疑酸中毒/糖尿病酮症酸中毒要考虑电解质、尿素氮、肌酐和葡萄糖水平。
• 考虑检查是否摄入有毒酒精。
• 如果出现胸痛，考虑心电图和肌钙蛋白。

影像学检查

任何缺氧患者或肺部检查异常的患者检查胸部 X 线。

■ **鉴别诊断**

• 病理性。
• 缺氧：
- 哮喘。
- 充血性心力衰竭(CHF)。
- 肺栓塞。
- 肺炎。
• 严重胸痛。
• 中枢神经系统功能障碍。
• 酸中毒(糖尿病酮症酸中毒)。
• 肺动脉高压。
• 肺栓塞。
• 低血糖。
• 轻度哮喘。
• 药物：
- 阿司匹林中毒。
- 戒断综合征(如酒精、苯二氮䓬类)。
• 低血糖症。
• 甲状腺毒症。
• 妊娠。
• 发热。
• 高原反应。
• 撤药反应。

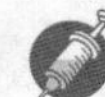

治疗

■ **院前**

• 生命体征异常的患者需要建立静脉通道，监测脉搏氧饱和度。
• 如果患者缺氧，给予吸氧。

■ **初步稳定/治疗**

• 生命体征异常的患者需要建立静脉通道，监测脉搏氧饱和度。
• 病理性或生理性原因引起的过度通气立即开始治疗。

■ **急诊治疗/程序**

• 如果检查不支持病理性或生理性病因，而病史及体格检查支持过度通气综合征，按过度通气综合征治疗方案开始治疗。
• 安慰患者，使患者平静，向患者解释症状中的自主原因，经常立刻取得良好效果。
• 不要使用纸袋呼吸增加 PCO_2。文献上不支持这种方法。
- 这可能会使缺氧患者或由生理性、病理性原因引起过度通气的患者陷入危险。
• 阐明心理压力因素的作用有助于患者避免将来再次发作。
• 评估患者是否需要精神病评估(如自杀观念)。
• 抗焦虑药：
- 如果症状持续，使用苯二氮䓬类打破焦虑和过度通气的循环。
- 短期使用抗焦虑药可能有助于患者应对临时压力因素。

■ **药物治疗**

• 急诊治疗：
- 阿普唑仑：0.25~0.5 mg，口服。
- 劳拉西泮：1~2 mg，口服或静脉注射。
- 地西泮：2~5 mg，口服或静脉注射。
• 门诊患者治疗：
- 丁螺环酮：5 mg，口服，3 次/日。
- 地西泮：2~5 mg，口服，2~3 次/日。
- 阿普唑仑：0.25~0.5 mg，口服。

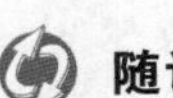

随访

■ **进一步处理**

入院指征

过度通气综合征不需要住院。

出院指征

• 排除或已治愈引起过度通气综合征的原

发生理性或病理性原因。

• 不存在急性精神性问题。

• 初级保健医师提供恰当的随访。

■ 随访建议

• 初级保健医师随访。

• 评估是否需要精神科随访。

要点和误区

• 排除引起过度通气的生理性或病理性原因。

• 过度通气综合征不会引起缺氧。

• 轻度哮喘可能与过度通气综合征相似。

• 就潜在的心理压力源作为病因向患者提供咨询。

过敏 Anaphylaxis

Sean-Xavier Neath 马林浩 林兆奋 译

基础知识

■ 描述

• 过敏是个体在接触抗原的几分钟之内发生的一种急性的分布性休克。

• 总体过敏反应似乎正在增加，特别是在儿童中。

• 根据当前数据估计，总发病率约为 50/(10万人 · 年)：

- 幸运的是，进入急诊室的患者的病死率很低(0.1%～0.3%)。

• 涉及从炎症细胞释放生物活性分子，如组胺、白三烯和前列腺素：

- 介质释放导致血管通透性增加，血管舒张，平滑肌收缩和上皮分泌增加。

- 在生理上，这表现为总外周阻力，静脉回流，心输出量及血管内容积减小。

■ 病因

• IgE 介导的：

- 抗生素，特别是青霉素类。

- 毒液，特别是蜜蜂和黄蜂。

- 胶乳。

- 疫苗。

- 食品(贝类、大豆、花生、坚果、小麦、牛奶、鸡蛋、硝酸盐/亚硝酸盐)。

- 单克隆抗体疗法。

• 非特异性 IgE 介导的：

- 碘造影剂。

- 阿片类药物。

- 万古霉素。

◦ 通常可以通过降低输液速度来预防。

- 精液。

- 锻炼。

儿科注意事项

对于儿童，食品是 IgE 介导的过敏性反应的一个重要触发来源：

• 牛奶、鸡蛋、小麦和大豆(MEWS)是最常见的食物过敏原。但任何食物都会产生反应。

诊断

■ 症状和体征

• 症状出现在接触抗原后的几秒到几分钟内。

• 过敏反应几乎总是涉及皮肤或黏膜。90%以上的患者有荨麻疹、红斑、瘙痒或血管性水肿。

• 部分患者在最初症状发生后可有濒死的感觉。

- 呼吸系统：打喷嚏、鼻塞、支气管痉挛和喉头水肿。

- 心血管系统：低血压、心律失常、心肌缺血。

- 胃肠道反应：恶心、呕吐、腹泻。

- 眼部：眼痒和流泪，结膜充血。

- 血液：激活的内源性凝血途径有时会导致弥散性血管内凝血，血小板减少。

- 神经系统：癫痫发作。

病史

• 过敏反应的诊断是临床诊断。

• 一个简短的病史应该包括以前的过敏史或过敏反应，以及暴露于潜在的新的触发物质。

体格检查

• 一般将包括 2 个或多个以下的系统改变：皮肤、呼吸道、胃肠道或心血管系统。

• 低血压或呼吸衰竭并不常见。

■ 基本检查

• 诊断是依据临床症状做出的。

• 在早期阶重要的是不要低估过敏反应潜在的严重性。

• 患者有心脏病史或心肌缺血症状应进行心电图检查，老年人应常规进行。

■ 诊断检查与说明

实验室检查

过敏反应的诊断通常是基于临床表现；在急性情况下实验室检查通常对诊断帮助有限。类胰蛋白酶水平持续升高，对一个疑似过敏后确诊是有帮助的。

影像学检查

胸片上可见过度通气表现。

■ 鉴别诊断

• 肺栓塞。

• 急性心肌梗死。

• 气道阻塞。

• 哮喘。

• 张力性气胸。

• NSAID 反应。

• 迷走血管性虚脱。

• 遗传性血管性水肿。

• 血清病。

• 系统性肥大细胞增多症。

• 嗜铬细胞瘤。

• 类癌综合征。

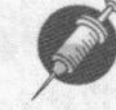

治疗

■ 院前

• 静脉通路，吸氧，心脏和脉搏血氧饱和度监测。

• 早期气管插管主要依据疾病的进程和对治疗的反应决定：

- 喉水肿和痉挛可迅速进展。

- 喉头水肿可以在插管之前使用去氧肾上腺素。

• 皮下肾上腺素注射可早于静脉注射在途中应用。

注意

目前的指南主张使用肌内或皮下注射肾上腺素。

■ 初步稳定/治疗

• 基础生命支持。
• 保证通气量。
• 气道管理：
- 经口气管插管是基本的气道技术。
- 如果喉头水肿、痉挛或软组织肿胀存在，考虑使用更高级的气道辅助工具。
- 如果软组织肿胀不能经口插管，考虑经鼻盲插气管插管。
- 经皮气管切开或环甲膜切开可能是必要的气道控制。
• 肾上腺素静脉注射或皮下注射或气管内给药：
- 直接注射到舌根静脉丛是一种选择。
• 用晶体液和胶体进行容量复苏。

■ 急诊治疗/程序

• 连续的心脏和生命体征监测，直到稳定。
• 持续性支气管痉挛可以用 β_2 受体激动剂治疗。
• 低血压应补充容量，升压药可以提供帮助。
• 抗组胺药(包括 H_1 和 H_2 受体阻滞剂)已经被证明在防止靶组织与组胺相互作用时很有帮助。
• 糖皮质激素有助于防止过敏症的进展或复发。
• 胰高血糖素可用于肾上腺素耐药的过敏症。

■ 药物治疗

注意

患者使用β受体阻滞剂可拮抗肾上腺素的作用。对于这些患者考虑使用胰高血糖素，因为它增加细胞内环磷腺苷水平，并不依赖β受体。

一线用药

• 苯海拉明：成人 50 mg(儿童：1～2 mg/kg)，缓慢静脉注射。
• 肾上腺素：0.3～0.5 mg，用 1∶1000 稀释皮下注射和 1∶10 000 静脉注射(儿童：肾上腺素 0.01 mg/kg，皮下注射或静脉注射)。
• 氢化可的松：成人 500 mg，静脉注射(儿童：每次 4～8 mg/kg)。
• 甲泼尼龙：成人 125 mg，静脉注射(儿童：1～2 mg/kg)。
• 泼尼松：成人 60 mg，口服(儿童：1 mg/kg)。
• 沙丁胺醇：0.5 ml 的 0.5%溶液溶解在 2.5 ml 等渗盐水中进行喷雾器治疗。

二线用药

• 去氧肾上腺素：2.25%溶液(0.5 ml 置于 2.5 ml 的生理盐水中)。
• 胰高血糖素：成人 1～2 mg，静脉注射、肌内注射或皮下注射。
• 雷尼替丁：成人 50 mg，静脉注射；或西咪替丁，300 mg，静脉注射。

随访

■ 进一步处理

• 过敏性疾病的治疗方法和持续时间应根据急诊内治疗过程中持续监测的结果进行个性化：
- 对于具有严重过敏反应风险因素(如哮喘，先前的双相反应或先前的长期过敏反应)有病史的患者，应进行更长时间的观察。
- 具有这些危险因素且对治疗无反应的患者应在临床解决方案后至少观察 4～8 h。

入院指征

• 呼吸困难或气管插管的患者应该入重症监护室。
• 对初始治疗没有反应的患者应该密切监护。
• 患者显著全身反应和症状持续存在，已知会发生双相或迟发反应，应留院观察 24 h。

出院指征

• 经过急诊留观，患者的症状完全消失几小时后可以出院。
• 请注意可能会导致第二次延迟的未经授权的过敏反应峰值(“双相反应”)：
- 没有强有力的证据表明给予皮质类固醇激素可以防止反应延迟。
• 任何重大过敏反应后从急诊出院的患者在出院时应使用肾上腺素自动注射器。

转诊问题

• 在进行脱敏治疗及应用抗生素治疗感染的时候咨询过敏症/免疫学家是正确的。
• 在进行造影检查时如果患者有造影剂过敏反应风险的情况，关于预处理和选择造影剂需要放射科医师会诊。

■ 随访建议

• 患者发生过敏反应后应随访 48 h，从而评估门诊治疗的有效性。
• 将发生过敏性休克、血管神经性水肿或荨麻疹的患者从急诊转诊给过敏症专家，进行后续的皮肤测试和脱敏治疗。
• 应建议患者进行某种准备，可以用在未来发生过敏反应的情况下，如预充式注射器。
• 患者对已知的过敏原应严格避免接触。

要点和误区

• 如果不能早期识别过敏性休克后果可能是灾难性的，如血流动力学不稳定和气道塌陷。
• 早期给予肾上腺素是最重要的干预措施。
• 有过敏史者应接受避免接触过敏原的教育并指导其正确使用肾上腺素自动注射笔。

过敏性紫癜 Henoch-Schonlein Purpura

Michele R. McKee 陈奇通 李文放 译

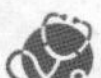

基础知识

■ 描述

血管炎。

■ 病因

• 机制：血清 IgA 复合物增加，血管沉积，补体途径的激活。
- 肾小球系膜沉积可引起系膜增生，形成新月形肾小球肾炎。
• 尽管原因未明，但是有许多相关因素：
- 感染(A 族链球菌、支原体、水痘、EB

病毒）。
- 药物：青霉素、四环素、阿司匹林、磺胺类、红霉素。
- 过敏原：昆虫叮咬、巧克力、牛奶、小麦。
• 高危人群：学龄儿童和青年人，4～6 岁是高发人群。
• 白种人更常见。
• 男性＞女性。
• 冬春季易发。
• 多系统受累时可危及生命或导致长期并发症：
- 肠套叠。
- 增生性肾小球肾炎。
- 慢性肾衰竭：更常见于年龄较大的儿童和成人（13%～14%），在血尿和肾病范围蛋白尿患者中风险较高。
- 颅内出血（罕见）。

诊断

症状和体征

• 一般：
- 儿童可仅表现为皮疹。
- 近期或当期有上呼吸道感染。
- 不适。
- 低热。
- 高血压，合并肾衰竭。
• 3 个月以下的婴儿可能只有皮肤表现。
• 2 岁以下儿童可只表现为面部水肿。
• 皮肤：
- 紫癜性皮疹：
◦ 发生于 50% 的患者。
◦ 所有患者均出现紫癜。
◦ 最初表现为粉红色圆形丘疹，并逐渐变白。
◦ 24 h 内进展为 2～3 cm 的圆形紫癜，可分散或融合。
◦ 皮疹始于腿部和臀部的重力依赖性区域，可能扩展至上肢和躯干。
◦ 对称性分布。
◦ 可能累及下背部、会阴部。
◦ 很少累及面部。
◦ 皮疹复发率达 40%（6 周）。
• 腹部：
- 腹部疼痛：
◦ 发生于 70%～80% 的患者。
◦ 严重绞痛。
◦ 腹部症状可早于皮疹四周出现。
- 胃肠道出血：
◦ 发生于 75% 的患者。
◦ 程度从隐血至严重出血均有。
◦ 肠套叠（回肠或回结肠）。
• 泌尿生殖系统：
- 无症状性血尿：
◦ 发生于 80% 的患者。
- 阴囊疼痛。
- 睾丸肿胀。
- 肾衰竭。
• 四肢：
- 关节炎：
◦ 发生于 70%～80% 的患者。
- 游走性关节疼痛。
- 最常见于膝关节和踝关节。
- 血管性水肿。
• 神经系统：
- 头痛。
- 癫痫。
- 精神状态改变。
- 焦点缺陷±视觉异常和语言障碍。

病史

• 体征：
- 发热。
• 皮疹：
- 皮疹的位置、时间、持续时间和进展。
• 相关症状：
- 腹痛，呕吐，少见有面部水肿。
- 症状的时间、持续时间和进展。

体格检查

• 一般情况：
- 反应水平，生命体征（高血压）。
• 心血管系统：
心音。
- 末梢灌注情况（脉搏、毛细血管再灌注情况）。
• 胃肠道：
- 腹胀，压痛，肿块，血便。
• 泌尿生殖系统：
- 睾丸肿胀，压痛。
• 皮肤：
- 皮疹部位。
- 苍白或非苍白。
- 红斑或紫色隆起病变（丘疹、紫癜）或黄斑病变（瘀斑）。
- 儿童很少出现进行性出血性大疱。
• 神经系统：
- 意识水平。
- 存在局灶性病变。

基本检查

如果条件允许，需排除导致瘀斑、紫癜、严重腹痛、血尿和中枢神经系统症状的致命性病因。

诊断检查与说明

实验室检查

• CBC：
- 血小板计数正常。
- WBC 通常升高。
• PT、APTT（出血或休克时；或诊断不确定，担心凝血功能异常时）。
• ASO。
• 电解质（高血压或尿检异常时）。
• BUN、肌酐（高血压或尿检异常时）。
- 合并严重肾脏并发症时可能升高。
• 尿液分析可能是唯一最重要的实验室：
- 血尿常见。
- 蛋白尿提示肾小球肾炎。
• 培养：排除常见感染。

影像学检查

• 腹部影像学检查：
- 有腹痛或消化道出血的表现。
- 限制使用直立位腹部 X 线片。
- 可能需要腹部超声、钡灌肠或 CT 扫描排除肠套叠。
• 睾丸超声：
- 睾丸疼痛和肿胀的患者。
• 头部 CT：
- 有神经系统病变需排除出血的患者。

诊断步骤/外科

腰椎穿刺，按临床要求。

鉴别诊断

• 腹痛：
- 肠胃炎。
- 阑尾炎。
- 炎症性肠病。
- 肠套叠。
- 梅克尔憩室。
• 关节痛：
- 急性风湿热。
- 结节性多发性关节炎。
- 幼年类风湿关节炎。
- 系统性红斑狼疮。
• 皮疹：
- 感染：
◦ 脑膜炎球菌血症。
◦ 细菌性脓毒症：链球菌或葡萄球菌。
◦ 落基山斑疹热。
◦ 传染性单核细胞增多症。
◦ 细菌心内膜炎。

◦ 病毒性皮疹。
- 创伤/儿童虐待。
- 功能性血小板疾病。
- 血小板减少症。
- 血管炎。
- 结节性红斑。
- 药物/毒素。
• 肾脏疾病：
- 急性肾小球肾炎。
• 睾丸肿胀：
- 嵌顿疝。
- 睾丸炎。
- 睾丸扭转。

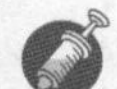

治疗

■ 院前

按临床要求稳定症状。

■ 初步稳定/治疗

• 静脉补液抗休克。
• 大量消化道出血患者输注红细胞。

■ 急诊治疗/程序

• 对预危及生命的情况紧急干预。
• 非甾体抗炎药(布洛芬)：
- 关节疼痛。
• 泼尼松：
- 排除危及生命病因的严重腹痛。
- 可考虑用作镇痛的辅助治疗。
- 肾脏疾病(需要大剂量甲泼尼龙冲击治疗)。
- 累及中枢神经系统。
• 免疫抑制剂：
- 严重危及生命的疾病合并过敏性紫癜肾炎。
• 免疫抑制剂、多克隆 Ig 治疗、抗血小板和抗凝药物存在争议，建议肾病会诊。

■ 药物治疗

一线用药

• 布洛芬：每剂 10 mg/kg，q6 h，最大剂量 600 mg。
• 泼尼松：每日口服 1～2 mg/(kg·d)，连续 5～7 日，每日最大剂量 60 mg。

随访

■ 进一步处理

入院指征

• 剧烈腹痛。
• 中枢症状。
• 消化道出血。
• 肠套叠。
• 肾衰竭表现。

出院指征

• 血小板计数正常。
• 肾功能正常。
• 无或轻度腹痛。
• 如果开始使用类固醇，请在 24 h 内进行随访。

转诊问题

• 胃肠道：
- 严重腹痛。
• 肾：
- 肾功能不全或肾衰竭的证据。

■ 随访建议

• 初级保健医师：
- 密切监测血压，根据临床复查 CBC，尿液检查(儿童建议至少 6 个月)。

要点和误区

• 排除危及生命的病因。
• 通常给予足量的非甾体抗炎药。
• 大多数患者不需要全身性应用皮质类固醇，因为没有证据表明其会影响过敏性紫癜肾炎的预后。

G

海绵窦血栓 Cavernous Sinus Thrombosis

Joanna W. Davidson 彭沪 译

基础知识

描述

• 颅内主要静脉回流系统分支血栓。
• 大部分为感染性。
• 感染源多为面部、牙齿或者鼻窦。
• 少部分为高凝状态导致。

解剖

3 个主要的血栓来源：
• 海绵窦——最常见：
- 表浅静脉的回流系统。
• 上外侧蝶窦和鞍区周围：
- 脑神经Ⅲ、Ⅳ、V1 和 V2 穿过鼻窦的侧壁。
- 脑神经Ⅵ和颈内动脉占据了鼻窦的中间部分。
• 横窦和表浅的矢状窦。

病理生理学

• 脸、耳或颈部感染通过血行通路进入静脉回流系统。
• 直接从鼻窦腔的感染(蝶骨、筛骨>额骨)。
• 细菌过度生长导致的感染和高凝状态，从而导致血栓。
• 海绵窦静脉充血能引起邻近部位的感染：
- 脑神经Ⅲ、Ⅳ或者Ⅵ感染导致眼肌麻痹。
- 脑神经Ⅲ感染导致瞳孔固定。
- 脑神经Ⅴ1 和Ⅴ2 感染导致额面部感觉异常或缺失。

病原学

• 感染性来源：
- 70%为金黄色葡萄球菌。
- 部分为链球菌肺炎、革兰阴性杆菌和厌氧菌。
- 真菌少见；包括曲霉菌属和根霉菌属。
• 非感染性来源：
- 少见。
- 肉芽肿(结核)。
- 其他综合作用(颅骨肿瘤、动脉瘤)。
• 高凝状态：

儿科注意事项

• 小儿可表现为肺感染的症状如精力下降、呕吐、发热。
• 小儿一旦具有耳炎或咽炎以及更糟糕的一些症状，精神疲软，或以下颅内压(ICP)增高的症状均应高度怀疑：
- 高血压、心动过缓、嗜睡、呕吐、行走不稳。
• 新生儿更常见，而诊断却非常困难。

诊断

症状和体征

• 症状：
- 90%的患者存在头痛。
- 发热。
- 眼睛或眼球后头痛。
- 面部肿胀。
- 视力缺陷。
- 嗜睡或精神状态改变。
• 体征：
- 眼眶水肿是最早的征象。
- 球结膜水肿伴视网膜静脉充血。
- 眼睑下垂，眼球突出。
- 脑神经麻痹：
○ 外侧凝视(脑神经Ⅵ)。
○ Ⅴ1 和Ⅴ2 神经过敏/迟钝(脑神经Ⅴ)。
- 假性脑膜炎。
- 意识改变或昏迷。
- 癫痫。
- 脓毒症伴循环系统不稳定或衰竭。

病史

高风险既往史包括：
• 外伤史。
• 耳鼻喉或神经外科植入史。
• 面部疖肿挤压史。
• 糖尿病或免疫缺陷状态(HIV、使用激素、肿瘤)可能增加风险。

基本检查

• 临床诊断：静脉充血，视觉系统，单侧症状变成双侧，进展迅速。
• 非特异的实验室检查。
• 细致的影像学检查。

诊断检查与说明

实验室检查

• 缺乏特异性和敏感性。
• 血常规：
- 白细胞增多。
- 杆状核细胞增多。
• 凝血酶原时间/部分凝血酶原时间/国际凝血指数。
• 红细胞沉降率和 D-二聚体通畅增高。
• 腰椎穿刺/脑脊液：脑膜外感染或直接脑膜炎。

影像学检查

• CT 扫描：
- 在疾病的早期作为标准检查。
- 非增强 CT 能显示增加的密度。
- 增强 CT 能显示充盈缺损。
○ 可鉴别感染的原发部位(如鼻窦炎)。
○ 眼上静脉扩张。
○ 颅内压增高的信号：脑室变小，脑缝消失。
• 磁共振血管造影(MRA)/磁共振静脉造影(MRV)：
- 可选择的诊断方法。
- 可直接显示颅内血管和鼻窦。
- 能看到各阶段的血栓。

鉴别诊断

• 脑膜炎、脑炎。
• 颅内脓肿。
• 眶周和眼窝蜂窝织炎。
• 颈内动脉动脉瘤或瘘管形成。
• 假性脑瘤。
• 急性闭角型青光眼。
• 颅内出血。
• 托洛萨-亨特综合征：海绵窦罕见的肉芽肿炎症。

注意
• 诊断及极困难。
• 患者出现中毒症状合并最近的耳鼻喉感染或者难以忍受的头痛和高凝状态或者有颅内感染，均应高度怀疑。

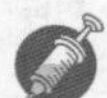

治疗

院前

注意
• 患者病情容易很不稳定。
• 需要迅速评估和稳定气道、呼吸以及循环。

初步稳定/治疗

• 仔细评估意识状态，必要的时候行气管插管保护气道通畅。
• 一旦出现循环系统不稳定进行积极的液

体复苏。

■ 急诊治疗/程序

• 广谱抗生素联用：
- 覆盖革兰阳性菌、阴性菌及厌氧菌。
- 萘夫西林或万古霉素[用于耐甲氧西林的金葡球菌(MRSA)]＋头孢曲松：
◦ 严重感染时增加甲硝唑或克林霉素。
◦ 一项研究表明，用利奈唑胺比万古霉素治疗效果更好。
• 肝素：
- 减少血凝块的播散和降低发病率/死亡率。
- 横窦和矢状窦由于容易导致继发出血应用存在争议。
- 在CT扫描排除了出血后再安排入院。
- 低分子肝素是否由于普通肝素仍存疑问。
- 严重的顽固型病例使用组织型纤维蛋白溶酶原激活物。
• 全身激素：
- 合并脑垂体功能不足和感染或炎症时应用确定获益。
- 外科会诊主要感染中心的引流情况(如牙脓肿或鼻窦炎)。

■ 药物治疗

• 头孢曲松钠：2 g/d，静脉注射[儿童：80～100 mg/(kg・d)，q12 h]。
• 克林霉素：300～900 mg，静脉注射，q6～12 h[新生儿：10～20 mg/(kg・24 h)，静脉注射，q6～12 h；儿童：25～40 mg/(kg・24 h)，q6～8 h]。
• 利奈唑胺：600 mg，静脉注射，q12 h(儿童：10 mg/kg，静脉注射，q8～12 h)。
• 甲硝唑：500 mg，静脉注射，q6 h[新生儿：7.5～30 mg/(kg・24 h)，q12～24 h；儿童：30 mg/(kg・24 h)，静脉注射，q6 h]。
• 萘夫西林：1～2 g，静脉注射，q4 h[儿童：50～75 mg/(kg・24 h)，静脉注射，q8～12 h，依年龄而变]。
• 万古霉素：1 g，静脉注射，q12 h[儿童：10～20 mg/kg，静脉注射，q8～12 h，依据年龄而变]。

一线治疗
• 广谱抗生素。
• 抗凝治疗。

二线治疗
• 静脉注射地塞米松或氢化可的松。
• 具有适应证的病例使用溶栓治疗。

随访

■ 进一步处理

入院指征
• 所以窦血栓形成患者应该住院并进行监护。
• 考虑收入ICU。

出院指征
无。

■ 随访建议

神经科和神经外科会诊。

■ 并发症

• 失明。
- 1/6的患者遗留视力障碍。
• 中枢神经麻痹。
• 脑膜炎或颅内脓肿。
• 癫痫，特别是上矢状窦血栓。
• 由于局部侵犯导致的脑垂体坏疽和功能降低。
• 细菌性栓子。
• 脓毒症和休克。
• 30%死亡率。

要点和误区

• 诊断依赖于临床评估和确切的实验室诊断临床需要高度警惕。
• 非增强头部CT常为阴性或非特异。MRI/MRV是具有诊断价值的影像学方法，对于高度怀疑病例应予以检查。
• 早期静脉使用抗生素，特别在疾病面容合并有耳鼻喉或神经学主诉的患者。
• 高凝状态导致中心和外周静脉血栓。检查和处理时必须考虑全身性血栓可能。

海洋生物蜇伤 Marine Envenomation

Armando Marquez Jr・Timothy B. Erickson 王胜云 译

H

基础知识

■ 描述

指的是由脊椎动物或无脊椎海洋物种刺痛或咬伤而引起的中毒。

■ 病因

• 海绵动物：
- 包括锋利带有刺激物的针骨，会引起皮肤瘙痒。
• 腔肠动物(刺胞动物水母)：
- 包括它们触须上的刺细胞。
- 含流体的囊肿通过接触喷出刺激性的空的螺纹状管。
- 螺纹管出渗入皮肤，并将毒针注入受害者体内。
- 箱形水母能在几分钟内把人杀死。
• 海星：
- 锐利且坚硬的体刺上附有黏滑的毒液。
• 海胆：
- 中空且锋利的体刺上充满了各种毒素。
• 海参：
- 中空的触须分泌出海参素，一种液体毒素。
• 锥形薄壳：
- 通过飞镖状可拆分的牙齿将毒液注入。
- 活性多肽干扰神经肌肉传导。
- 体现为刺伤感，类似于黄蜂蜇痛。
• 黄貂鱼：
- 人类海洋毒液最常见的原因。
- 锥形体刺将毒液注入受害者体内。
• 蝎子鱼：
- 狮子鱼通常很温和，石鱼则会威胁生命。
- 鱼的背部及骨盆处有锋利的体刺。
- 经常会不注意踩到。
- 毒害神经的毒液。
• 鲇鱼：
- 背部及胸部体刺含有毒腺。
• 海蛇：
- 中空的毒牙有毒腺。
- 高度毒害神经的毒液会阻滞神经肌肉传导。

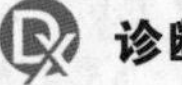

诊断

■ 症状和体征

• 海绵动物：

- 接触后数小时内出现发痒及灼烧感。
- 局部肿胀及软组织水肿。
- 发热。
- 心神不安。
- 头晕。
- 恶心。
- 肌肉痉挛。
- 严重情况下，10 日到 2 个月内出现脱皮现象。

• 腔肠动物(刺胞动物水母)：
- 轻微毒液蜇入疼痛：
  ◦ 即刻刺痛感。
  ◦ 瘙痒。
  ◦ 感觉异常，灼烧感。
  ◦ 搏动痛。
  ◦ 起疱，局部水肿，形成水疱。
- 适度/严重：
  ◦ 神经系统：共济失调、瘫痪、谵妄、癫痫。
  ◦ 心血管：过敏、溶血反应、低血压、节律障碍。
  ◦ 呼吸系统：支气管痉挛、喉水肿、肺水肿、呼吸衰竭。
  ◦ 骨骼肌系统：肌肉痉挛或抽搐、关节痛。
  ◦ 胃肠：恶心、呕吐、腹泻、吞咽困难、唾液分泌过多/口渴。
  ◦ 眼科：结膜炎、角膜溃疡、眼内压增大。

• 棘皮动物：
- 海星：
  ◦ 即刻疼痛。
  ◦ 出血。
  ◦ 轻微水肿。
  ◦ 严重的话，会感觉异常、恶心、呕吐。
- 海胆：
  ◦ 剧烈疼痛，严重的局部肌肉酸痛。
  ◦ 恶心，呕吐。
  ◦ 感觉异常，低血压，或者呼吸困难，伴有蜜蜂蜇伤的疼痛感。
- 海参：
  ◦ 轻微接触性皮炎。
  ◦ 角膜及结膜感染：反应严重会导致失明。

• 软体动物：
- 锥形薄壳：
  ◦ 刺伤，类似于黄蜂蜇伤。
  ◦ 剧烈烧痛及刺痛。
  ◦ 感觉异常表明严重的蜇刺毒作用。
  ◦ 会演化成肌肉麻痹、呼吸衰竭、吞咽困难、晕厥、弥散性血管内凝血。

• 黄貂鱼：
- 刺伤或锯齿状撕裂伤。
- 局部剧烈疼痛、水肿、出血；严重的话出现细胞坏死。
- 恶心、呕吐、腹泻。
- 出汗。
- 头痛。
- 心跳过速。
- 痉挛。
- 发热。
- 高血压。

• 蝎子鱼：
- 剧烈疼痛持续 6～12 h。
- 红疹，并演变为蜂窝织炎。
- 头痛。
- 恶心、呕吐、腹泻。
- 面色苍白。
- 精神错乱。
- 痉挛。
- 发热。
- 高血压。

• 鲇鱼：
- 局部疼痛，局部缺血性症状，产生红疹。
- 肿胀，出血并水肿。
- 局部肌肉痉挛。
- 出汗。
- 神经病变、肌束震颤、虚弱、晕厥。

• 海蛇：
- 咬伤后，开始会引起轻微疼痛感。
- 对针形的牙齿印。
- 发病时间 5 min 到 6 h。
- 肌肉痛、下肢瘫痪、关节痛。
- 牙关紧闭、视力模糊、吞咽困难。
- 严重迹象包括：
  ◦ 上行性麻痹。
  ◦ 误吸。
  ◦ 昏迷。
  ◦ 肾衰竭和肝衰竭。
- 如果得不到治疗，25%的死亡率。

病史

• 毒液蜇入时间。
• 被毒液蜇入的身体部位。
• 被毒液蜇入时进行的活动(斯库巴潜水、游泳、冲浪、钓鱼、划船、照顾宠物)。
• 水的类型(咸水、淡水、养鱼池)。
• 地理位置(度假区、国际范围、偏远处、当地、水族馆、动物园、宠物店)。
• 发病症状，疼痛。
• 精神状态变化。
• 几乎淹溺。

体格检查

• 关键迹象。
• 呼吸道。
• 精神状态。
• 心肺检查。
• 皮肤检查，异物，蜂窝织炎，起疱。

基本检查

• 仔细留意病史，反复评估受伤部位。
• 呼吸道、呼吸和循环流转的评估。

诊断检查与说明

实验室检查

• 全血细胞计数。
• 电解质、血尿素氮、肌酸酐和葡萄糖水平。
• 肝功能检查。
• 尿液分析。
• 症状严重，进行动脉血气分析。

影像学检查

软组织拍 X 线片以检测异物。

鉴别诊断

• 过敏反应。
• 蜂窝织炎。
• 肠胃炎。
• 吸入性肺炎。
• 几乎淹溺。

治疗

院前

• 使患者离开水源。
• 控制呼吸道和呼吸。
• 控制出血。
• 按下述方法，以创口冲洗器解毒。

初步稳定/治疗

• ABC 管理。
• 以生理盐水进行静脉注射。

急诊治疗/程序

• 一般情况：
- 以抗准备过敏反应(肾上腺素、类固醇)。
- 如需要，准备插管。
- 苯海拉明治疗发痒、灼伤、荨麻疹。
- 破伤风预防。
- 以皮质类固醇治疗严重局部反应。
- 严重疼痛，以麻醉镇痛。
- 以抗生素预防：
  ◦ 大面积撕裂或灼伤。
  ◦ 较深刺伤。
  ◦ 严重污染伤口。
  ◦ 老年或慢性病患者。

H

- 抗生素选择：
  ◦ TMP-SMX。
  ◦ 四环素。
  ◦ 环丙沙星。
  ◦ 第三代头孢菌素。
• 海绵动物：
- 轻轻使皮肤干燥，去除骨刺。
  ◦ 胶布有助于骨刺去除。
- 5%乙酸(醋)(或40%～70%异丙醇)浸泡10～30 min，每日4次。
• 腔肠动物(刺胞动物水母)：
- 以盐水或海水清洗伤口：
  ◦ 低渗的(淡水或自来水)，刺激刺细胞。
- 不要摩擦皮肤，避免刺细胞释放出来。
- 5%乙酸(醋)浸泡30 min灭活毒素。
- 用剃刀和蛤壳去除剩余刺细胞。
- 一旦去除刺细胞，使用表面麻醉药。
- 可使用海里安全的水母防晒产品。
- 箱水母毒液蜇入(澳大利亚)紧急病例：
  ◦ 使用箱水母抗毒素：1氨苄西林(20000 U)与1∶5晶体稀释。
- 以皮质类固醇治疗严重反应。
• 海星：
- 以非滚烫的水浸泡减轻疼痛。
- 冲洗和寻找所有刺伤。
- 严重伤口使用预防性抗生素。
• 海胆：
- 以非滚烫的水浸泡减轻疼痛。
- 去除所有剩余脊椎。
- 严重伤口使用预防性抗生素。
• 海参：
- 以非滚烫的水浸泡减轻疼痛。
- 5%乙酸浸泡。
- 眼部病变：
  ◦ 丙美卡因为了缓解疼痛。
  ◦ 用生理论盐水充分冲洗。
  ◦ 仔细的裂隙灯检查。
• 锥壳：
- 浸入热水缓解疼痛。
- 准备好心脏或呼吸支持。
• 黄貂鱼：
- 去除可见的刺后充分冲洗。
- 局部抽吸是具有争议的。
- 热水浸泡缓解疼痛。
- 毒品缓解疼痛。
- 高发病率的细菌感染：
  ◦ 管理预防重大的创伤。
• 蝎子鱼：
- 热水浸泡缓解疼痛和毒液失活。
- 去除可见的刺后充分冲洗。
- 局部利多卡因或局部阻塞为了缓解剧烈疼痛。
- 手术探查为了深层渗透/异物。
- 石鱼抗蛇毒血清为了缓解严重的表面变质：
  ◦ 1支2 ml氨苄西林用50 ml生理盐水稀释缓慢注射。
  ◦ 可能会导致血清病。
• 鲇鱼：
- 热水浸泡缓解疼痛和毒液失活。
- 去除可见的刺后充分冲洗。
- 局部利多卡因或局部阻塞或麻醉：为了缓解剧烈疼痛。
- 手术探查：为了深层渗透/异物。
- 让穿刺伤口打开愈合。
- 考虑对手、足或深层伤口使用预防性抗生素。
• 海蛇：
- 固定伤口末端。
- 使用压力绷带使静脉闭塞(就医前)。
- 保持伤员温度和静止。
- 多价海蛇抗蛇毒素降低死亡率至3%：
• 可能需要3～10支氨苄西林(每支1000 U)。
• 早期准备辅助通风。

■ 药物治疗

• 头孢克肟：400 mg[儿童：8 mg/(kg·24 h)]，每日1次，口服。
• 环丙沙星：500 mg，每日2次，口服。
• 肾上腺素：0.3～0.5 ml比例1∶1000(儿童：0.01 ml/kg)。
• 四环素：500 mg，每日4次，口服(小心光敏性)。
• TMP-SMX：1贴[儿童：5 mg液体(40/200/5 ml)/10 kg每剂]，每日2次，口服(小心光敏性)。

随访

■ 进一步处理

入院指征

系统性参与的重要迹象或有抗蛇毒管理的需求。

出院指征

在8 h的观察后没有系统性疾病的迹象。

转诊问题

动物园、水族馆有抗蛇毒素供应。

要点和误区

• 随着近期海洋气候变化、沿海人口转移和全球旅行，人类与有毒海洋生物的接触越来越多。
• 大部分毒素通过温度变化(热水)或通过pH变化(酸性更强)可解毒。
• 特定的抗箱型水母、石头鱼和海蛇表面变质的抗蛇毒素有供应但有限，在疗程早期获得。

横纹肌溶解

Vishnu Parthasarathy · Gabriel Wardi 袁晓伟 童朝阳 译

基础知识

■ 描述

系统性肌肉内容物异常释放：字面意思是"骨骼内容物的溶解"。定义为肌肉内容物的病理性释放——肌酸激酶(CPK)、肌红蛋白、钾、磷酸盐、尿酸盐——伴有全身并发症。由创伤、肌肉直接压迫、中毒、感染、原发性肌肉疾病和许多其他疾病状态引起。并发症包括：

• 肌红蛋白导致的肾衰竭，成人中有15%～50%，儿童中只有5%。
• 高钾血症导致的猝死。
• 低钙血症和酸中毒。
• 血管内低血容量：体液滞留在受损肌肉内或导致其他基础疾病。
• 25%发生肝衰竭。
• 弥散性血管内凝血(DIC)。

■ 流行病学

发病率

• 美国每年有26000例发病。
• 严重事故导致成百的肾衰竭病例。

危险因素

- 外伤，尤其是挤压伤。
- 脓毒症。
- 长时间固定。
- 遗传性肌病。
- 酒精或药物滥用。
- 使用某些药物治疗。
- 伴或不伴危险因素的用力过度。

病理生理

- 肌膜中的离子泵通常通过 ATP 依赖的过程使细胞内钙、钠、钾保持低水平。
- 心肌细胞损伤降低了 ATP 的利用率，破坏了离子通道的活性。
- 长时间的细胞内高钙引起持续的肌原纤维收缩和进一步的 ATP 耗竭导致缺血。
- 钙依赖性蛋白酶引起细胞膜溶解。
- 细胞内容物逸出：肌红蛋白、钾、磷酸盐、CPK、乳酸盐等。
- 肌红蛋白可引起肾脏直接毒性，并与其他蛋白质沉淀，阻碍肾小管血流。
- 容量减少也会导致肾血管收缩和衰竭。
- 高钾血症导致心律失常。
- 钙与磷酸盐沉淀，导致全身性低钙血症。

病因

- 病因一般较明显，但不总是这样：
- 成人：外伤、中毒、感染。
- 儿童：病毒性肌炎、外伤。
- 由于外伤、挤压、烧伤、电击性休克导致的肌肉损伤：最常见病因。
- 肌肉用力过度：剧烈运动、马拉松、在湿热环境中锻炼、遗传性疾病或缺乏锻炼的人运动、癫痫持续状态震颤性谵妄、僵直性痉挛、精神躁动。
- 肌肉缺血：广泛血栓形成、多处栓塞、休克、镰状细胞危象。
- 手术：固定、低血压、血管钳夹引起的缺血。
- 大量血液输注。
- 体温过高，体温过低(NMS，MH)。
- 无外伤的过长时间制动。
- 药物及中毒：酒精、可卡因、苯丙胺类及其类似物(甲基苯丙胺、摇头丸)、甲苯、阿片类、LSD、苯环利定(PCP)、咖啡因、一氧化碳、蛇毒、蜜蜂/胡蜂毒液、铁杉、水牛鱼、破伤风毒素、蘑菇中毒(口蘑属)。
- 药物：最常见。
  - 氟哌啶醇、吩噻嗪类、HMG－CoA 还原酶抑制剂(他汀类)尤其是与贝特类药物(吉非罗齐)联合使用。
- 运动补充剂：包括麻黄、咖啡因、雄激素类固醇、肌酸、利尿剂。
- 神经阻滞剂恶性综合征(特异性的且与剂量无关)。
- 代谢障碍：低钾血症、低磷酸盐血症、低钙血症、高钠和低钠血症、糖尿病酮症酸中毒、高渗状态、甲亢状态(少见)、嗜铬细胞瘤(少见)。
- 感染：
  - 病毒性：柯萨奇病毒、疱疹病毒、HIV、流感病毒 B、巨细胞病毒、EB 病毒、埃可病毒、腺病毒。
  - 细菌性：军团菌、化脓性肌炎、脓毒症。
  - 寄生虫(恶性疟原虫)、原虫(钩端螺旋体病)、立克次体。
  - 遗传性肌病性失调：McArdle 病、Tarui 病、CPT 缺乏。
- 免疫缺陷：皮肌炎、多肌炎。
- 特发性疾病。

普遍相关疾病

- 挤压综合征。
- 骨筋膜间室综合征。
- 酒精及药物滥用。
- 年老长期不动(在地板上发现)。

诊断

症状和体征

病史

- 变化剧烈，反映基本疾病过程。
- 创伤、挤压和劳累后通常很明显。
- 考虑非意外病史不明的损伤。
- 如果无损伤，考虑药物中毒、心脏疾病、制动、用力过度。
- 询问有无酱油色尿液和尿量减少。
- ＜9 岁儿童最常见的非创伤原因是合并肌炎的病毒性疾病。

体格检查

- 低体温或高体温。
- 反应灵敏或迟钝。
- 肌痛(只有 40％～50％)。
- 如果怀疑筋膜间室综合征，则累及的肌肉群有神经血管症状。
- 血容量不足、黏膜干燥、皮肤肿胀、心动过速、低血压。
- 尿量下降。
- 茶色尿是早期症状(少数病例有)。
- 儿童通常无体征。

诊断检查与说明

实验室检查

初始实验室检查。

- 血清 CPK 水平＞1000 U/L 或 5 倍实验室限值是最常见的诊断临界值，尽管没有绝对临界值，CPK 水平应根据适当的临床情况进行解释。
- 血清和尿肌红蛋白水平由于快速代谢和排泄通常正常。
- 发展为急性肾小管坏死的危险因素包括 CPK 水平、电解质异常、酸中毒、治疗延迟。
- 血红素尿试纸检测阳性，但无红细胞，提示横纹肌溶解。
- 显微镜下尿分析查找色素沉着管型。
- 儿童血红素尿试纸检测＜2＋，与急性肾衰竭(ARF)危险降低相关。
- 血清电解质(钾、钙、镁、磷、BUN、肌酸、尿酸、碳酸氢盐)。
- 附加考虑：
  - 动静脉血气(ABGA、BG)。
  - 尿/血清肌红蛋白。
  - 血糖。
  - 肝功能检查(LFT)包括 GGTP、LDH、白蛋白。
  - 无身体损伤则行毒物筛查。
  - 如果怀疑 DIC，则行 PT、APTT、血小板计数、纤维蛋白原、纤维蛋白裂解产物检查。

影像学检查

- 肾超声检查排除长期肾衰竭(肾小、萎缩)或肾梗阻(肾积水)。其他影像学检查可用于评估外伤、感染评估。

诊断步骤/外科

- 早期心电图：在血清检查进行之前可发现高钾血症或低钙血症。
- 在严重横纹肌溶解症患者中放置导尿管以监测尿量。
- 如果怀疑骨筋膜室综合征，则测量筋膜室压。

鉴别诊断

可能呈现血清 CPK 升高表现，但非横纹肌溶解：

- 非创伤性肌病：包括肌肉营养障碍和遗传性肌病。
- 慢性肾衰竭。
- 肌内注射。
- 心肌损伤。
- 卒中。

H

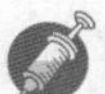

治疗

院前

- 挤压损伤的快速脱离。
- 早期给药，甚至在完成拔出之前，以防止受伤肢体恢复血流的并发症（低血容量、高钾血症等）。
- 儿童推荐：首先0～15 ml/(kg·h)生理盐水，然后换成(0.45%)低张盐水直至到达医院。增加50 mEq碳酸氢盐到第2日或3 L中，使尿液碱化。

初步稳定/治疗

- 进行ABC管理。
- 固定创伤/挤压伤。
- 成人挤压伤的治疗方案可由儿童治疗方案推断。
- 管理的基础是积极的液体复苏晶体以逆转低血容量和防止肌红蛋白肾功能衰竭。

急诊治疗/程序

- 目标是确保尿量至少为200～300 ml/h，2.5 ml/(kg·h)的晶体液体量适合大多数没有明显液体过载的患者。
- 近年来，由于缺乏有意义的人类数据，用碳酸氢钠进行尿碱化（防止肌红蛋白分解成血红素和血红蛋白，这两种都是肾毒性药物）近年来已失去了人们的青睐。它改善了结果，但可以在个别案情况下考虑（例如，严重酸中毒伴高钾血症）。
- 甘露醇20%：50 ml（每升添加10 g），最多120～200 g/d[1～2 g/(kg·d)]：利尿剂，自由基清除剂。可能有助于室间隔综合征（有争议的是，与单纯晶体治疗相比，这种疗法从未被证明能改善预后）。
- 呋塞米和其他利尿剂二线治疗积极晶体液复苏后少尿（<500 ml/d）肾衰竭；有争议。
- 通过血清水平和心电图来监测高钾血症。高钾血症与较严重的损伤相关。
- 一般治疗高钾血症不使用钙剂，除非病情严重。
- 低钙血症：仅在有症状（手足抽搐或癫痫发作）或心律失常时治疗。磷酸钙结晶可能发生并恶化肾衰竭。
- 停止服用违禁药物。
- 肾替代疗法适用于危及生命的电解质异常（如高钾血症）、严重酸中毒或严重的容量超负荷。

手术治疗

- 血液透析治疗难治性高钾血症、液体过载、无尿、酸中毒。
- 考虑中心静脉容量监测。
- 筋膜切开术治疗筋膜室综合征。

随访

进一步处理

入院指征

- 尽管有液体复苏，但CPK升高或最小程度降低（入院时没有CPK值）。
- 经过液体复苏后或者血液透析，急性肾衰竭改善甚微。
- 严重的电解质紊乱（高钾血症、低钙血症）。
- 血流动力学不稳定。
- 骨筋膜室综合征。
- 潜在的严重疾病/共病或严重的诱发事件（如大面积挤压伤、感染性休克、DIC）。

出院指征

在肾功能正常的情况下降低CPK水平，引起横纹肌溶解症的病因确定、逆转，无其他入院指征。

并发症

- 肌红蛋白性肾衰竭。
- 高钾血症。
- 骨筋膜室综合征。
- 低钙血症。
- 酸中毒。
- 死亡。

要点和误区

- AST(95%)和ALT(73%)的升高在横纹肌溶解症中经常被忽视，这些酶都存在于骨骼肌中，高水平的表达预示着骨骼肌的破坏。
- 早期和积极复苏失败会导致肾衰竭和需要透析。

H

红细胞增多症

Walla A. Alfaraj · Michelle D. Lall　瞿金龙 译

基础知识

描述

- 血红蛋白比正常增加：
  - 男：血红蛋白>165 g/L，血细胞比容>49%。
  - 女：血红蛋白>160 g/L，血细胞比容>48%。
- 症状一般与血黏度升高有关，如血细胞比容>60%。

病因

- 继发性红细胞增多：
  - 继发于血容量减少。
  - 急性：脱水。
  - 慢性Gaisbock综合征：肥胖、高血压、中年吸烟者。
- 原发性红细胞增多：
  - 真性红细胞增多：骨髓异常增生引起红细胞、白细胞、血小板增加，以红细胞增加为特征：
    - JAK2酶突变，在EPO受体信号通路上起作用。
    - 中位年龄为60岁，5%<40岁，最高在70岁以上。
    - 在北欧犹太教徒发病率最高，亚洲和非裔美国人较少。
    - 中位生存期约14年。
    - 可能发展为骨髓纤维化或急性白血病。
- 继发性红细胞增多：
  - 缺氧引起红细胞增多：
    - 慢性肺疾病。
    - 睡眠呼吸障碍(5%～10%)。
    - 肥胖通气不足综合征（Pickwickian综合征）。
    - 先天性心脏疾病（右向左分流）。
    - 高海拔。
    - 吸烟者的红细胞增多。
    - 一氧化碳中毒（慢性）。

◦ 慢性高铁血红蛋白血症。
- 肾脏原因引起红细胞增多症：
◦ 肾细胞癌。
◦ 肾动脉粥样硬化狭窄。
◦ 局灶性肾小球肾炎。
◦ 肾移植后。
◦ 慢性肾积水。
◦ 多囊肾疾病。
- 自发性红细胞增多。
◦ 肝细胞瘤。
◦ 小脑血管母细胞瘤。
◦ Wilms 肿瘤。
◦ 甲状旁腺肿瘤。
◦ 卵巢肿瘤。
◦ 肾上腺腺瘤和癌。
◦ 子宫肌瘤。
- 人为干预：
◦ 促红细胞生长素的滥用。
◦ 自体输血。
- 药物滥用。
◦ 慢性可卡因滥用。
◦ 雄激素的使用。
• 遗传性红细胞增多：
- 高亲和力的血红蛋白变种。
- 生理性磷酸甘油酸盐缺陷。
- Von Hippel-Lindau 综合征。
- Chuvash 红细胞增多症。
- 红细胞生成素受体变异。
- 先天性高铁血红蛋白血症。
• 感染：
- 病毒性肝炎、获得性免疫缺陷综合征(AIDS)。

诊断要点

• 主要因素：
- 血红蛋白＞165 g/L(男性)或 160 g/L(女性)。
- 通过 PCR 技术发现 *JAK2* 缺陷明确诊断。
- 氧饱和度＞92%，没有继发性红细胞增多的因素。
• 次要因素：
- 促红素减少。
- 骨髓穿刺提示骨髓异常增生。
• 其他：
- 血小板＞400 000/mm^3。
- ANC＞10 000(WBC＞12 000/mm^3)。
- 脾大。
- 白细胞碱性磷酸酶升高。
- 维生素 B_{12}＞900 pg/ml，未结合维生素 B_{12}＞2 200 pg/ml。

诊断

体征和症状

病史

• 一般情况：
- 呼吸困难。
- 体弱、疲乏。
- 容易出汗。
- 鼻出血、牙龈出血。
- 瘙痒(40%)：
◦ 全身。
◦ 热水澡后加重。
◦ 抓痕症。
- 痛风或痛风石出现。
• 神经病学：
- 头痛。
- 头晕、眩晕。
- 昏睡、意识错乱。
- 感觉错乱。
- 脑血管意外或 TIA 发作。
• 视力变化。
- 黑矇。
- 暗点或视物模糊。
- 眼科性偏头痛。
• 心血管系统。
- 慢性心力衰竭。
- 心绞痛或心肌梗死。
- 深静脉血栓形成。
- 高血压。
• 四肢。
- 红斑性肢痛病：
◦ 继发于毛细血管沉积。
◦ 四肢烧灼样疼痛。
◦ 四肢温暖、红斑、水肿。
◦ 肢体末端感觉异常。
◦ 晚上加重。
◦ 冷敷或阿司匹林明显改善。
◦ 脉搏正常。
- 指(趾)溃疡形成。
• 肝损伤。
- 肝大、脾大。
- 突发脾大。
- 上腹部不适或饱胀感。
- 消化性溃疡和出血。
- Budd-Chiari 综合征(肝静脉血栓形成)。

体格检查

• 高血压。
• 结膜充血。
• 胃底：静脉曲张。
• 面色红润、多血症。
• 四肢、甲床发红。
• 抓痕症。
• 脾大(75%)。
• 肝大(30%)。
• 血栓并发症：
- 2/3 动脉，1/3 静脉。
- 发生率每年 2%～5%。
- TIA、心肌梗死、脑梗死。
- 不寻常的静脉血栓：
◦ 脾、肠系膜静脉。
◦ 肝静脉、下腔静脉血栓。
◦ 静脉窦血栓。
- 深静脉血栓、肺栓塞。
• 血黏度增加的并发症：
- 嗜睡、意识障碍。
- 头痛，头晕，视觉改变。
- 慢性心力衰竭、捻发音。
• 出血并发症：
- 出血斑。
- 鼻出血。
- 牙龈出血。

基本检查

全血细胞检查和血小板检查。

诊断检查与说明

实验室检查

• 首先：区分继发性红细胞增多：
- 容量恢复后复查全血细胞。
• 其次：其他激发因素评估：
- 指脉氧＜92%。
- 碳氧血红蛋白水平。
- 红细胞生成素水平(正常或继发升高)。
- 胸部 X 线、CT 检查，肺功能检测。
- 睡眠质量。
- 血红蛋白电泳。
• 红细胞质量。
- ^{51}Cr 标记红细胞。
- ^{131}I 标记白蛋白。
- 血红蛋白＞185 g/L(男)或 165 g/L(女)。
- 红细胞质量＞35 mg/kg(男)或 31 mg/kg(女)。
- 降低的血容量伴正常的红细胞质量与红细胞增多相关。
- 增高的红细胞质量提示原发或继发红细胞增多。
- 铁缺乏假性降低。
• 高度怀疑红细胞增多，以下情况：
- Hgb＞185 g/L(男)，165 g/L(女)。

- 中性粒细胞计数>10 000/mm³。
- 血小板>400 000/mm³。
- 指脉氧>92%。
- 红细胞生成素水平降低。
- 维生素 B_{12} 水平增高 30%。
- 尿酸增高 40%。
- 白细胞碱性磷酸酶增加 70%。
- *JAK2* 基因检测可以诊断(97%)。

影像学检查

腹部的超声或 CT 可以检查是否合并脾大。

鉴别诊断

见病因学。

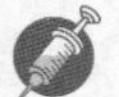

治疗

初步稳定/治疗

如果无慢性心力衰竭,重点放在容量复苏。

急诊处理

血黏度高或血细胞比容>60%的急诊处理

• 液体复苏来稀释血液。
- 除非有慢性心力衰竭的证据。
• 紧急放血同时输注相同量的生理盐水 250～500 ml, 1～2 h 完成。
• 24 h 以上放血 1 000～1 500 ml,并通过补液来实现血细胞比容<60%,或者症状缓解。
- 保持血细胞比容>45%。
- 通过等量盐水稀释。
• 在静脉放血治疗时,对于年龄大的和心血管疾病的患者要慢:
- 隔日放血治疗。
• 静脉放血治疗:
- 静脉放血防止血栓形成。
• 血小板增多治疗:
- 阿司匹林口服,如果血小板在 500 000～1 500 000/mm³,无出血并发症。
• 苯海拉明治疗瘙痒症。

长期处理

• 静脉切开放血治疗:主要对于血细胞比容>45%(男),42%(女)。
• 如果有血栓形成,阿司匹林 81 mg/d。
• α 干扰素:
- 尤其对顽固性瘙痒和脾大。
- 建议用于<60 岁的有症状患者。
• 阿那格雷。
- 血栓形成。
- 无白细胞增多的高危因素,主要用于治疗放血治疗后的预防血栓形成的治疗。
- 可以单独起作用,或者降低化疗的次数。
• 羟基脲。
- 对于>60 岁,需要多次放血治疗、血栓形成风险大的患者。
• 白消安类药物。
- 老年人顽固发作。
- 有白细胞增多的高危因素。

妊娠注意事项

暂时不予处理。

儿科注意事项

• 初生婴儿定义:静脉血细胞比容>65%,血红蛋白>220 g/L:
- 标本必须妊娠后 6 h 取。
- 毛细血管的血细胞比容和血红蛋白比静脉高 10%(以静脉为依据)。
- 1%～5%的婴儿。
- 50%的患儿发生子宫内发育延迟。
• 病因:
- 胎儿缺氧继发于母亲的心肺疾病、糖尿病、先兆子痫、高血压或吸烟等。
- 延迟的脐带结扎,导致增加的脐带血回输。
• 症状和体征:
- 肢端发绀症。
- 呼吸困难、呼吸窘迫。
- 过敏、嗜睡、神经过敏、喂养差。
• 低血糖和高胆红素血症。
• 治疗:
- 观察和检测全血细胞。
- 每日 100 ml/kg 静脉滴注(有症状的患儿)。
- 部分血交换:同等量的生理盐水替换 20 ml/kg 的血(对于严重和持续发作的患儿)。
- 如果低血糖应补充葡萄糖。

老年人注意事项

注意放血治疗的速度和液体复苏的速度。

随访

进一步处理

入院指征

• 新诊断的红细胞增多症患者。
• 无症状但是血细胞比容>60%的患者。
• 生命体征不稳定,或者合并其他疾病。

出院指征

• 诊断红细胞增多症,无症状并且血细胞比容<60%。
• 生命体征平稳。

转诊问题

所有患者必须经血液科医师或相关科室医师会诊。

要点和误区

• 低氧后的红细胞增多症的静脉切开放血治疗的标准不明确。
• 如果红细胞增多症有血栓形成的高危因素,必须明确原发性红细胞增多还是继发性的因素。
• 接触水后的瘙痒和红斑性肢痛病是红细胞增多症特征性的表现。

H

红眼 Red Eye

Franklin D. Friedman 何融冰 译

基础知识

描述

• 几乎所有的眼部疾病都可引起。
• 通常是良性的,但也可能是系统性疾病的表现。
• 由结膜血管充血引起。
• 主要病因包括炎症、过敏、感染和创伤。
• 结膜炎是最常见的病因。

病因

• 炎症:
- 葡萄膜炎:
◦ 前部和后部。
- 虹膜炎(下边缘充血)。
- 巩膜外层炎(常见,但一般良性)。
- 巩膜炎(50%与系统性疾病有关)。
- 全身性炎症反应。

- 过敏：
  - 由于组胺释放和血管通透性增加导致结膜水肿(球结膜水肿)、水样分泌物及瘙痒，通常是双侧的。
- 感染：
  - 角膜炎。
  - 传染性结膜炎。
  - 眼眶蜂窝织炎
    - 一般由鼻窦、皮肤或血液传播。
  - 泪囊炎。
    - 因为泪管堵塞。
  - 泪小管炎。
  - 眼内炎。
    - 眼内感染，可能是手术后所致。
- 创伤性：
  - 角膜擦伤。
  - 结膜下出血(SCH)。
  - 异物。
  - 隐性穿孔。
- 其他。
  - 睑裂斑、翼状胬肉、出血、睑炎、干眼综合征、急性闭角型青光眼、新生儿眼炎、结膜肿瘤。

诊断

症状和体征

病史

- 年龄(通常为新生儿或年龄>50 岁)。
- 发作时间，症状持续时间。
- 暴露(如化学制品、过敏原)。
- 患者职业(如金属品制造工人)。
- 相关症状和体征(头痛、全身性症状、其他感染)。
- 眼部症状：
  - 疼痛。
  - 畏光。
  - 异物感。
  - 视力改变。
  - 分泌物。
  - 瘙痒。
- 使用隐形眼镜。
- 其他合并症。

体格检查

- 彻底的体格检查。
  - 耳前或下颌下腺病。
  - 酒渣鼻(可以引起眼睑炎)。
  - 面部或皮肤损害(疱疹)。
- 眼科学。
  - 视敏度。
  - 一般状况：
    - 广泛或局部眼睛变红。
    - 结膜充血。
    - 眼睑累及。
    - 脓性或清澈分泌物。
    - 明显异物。
    - 眼球突出。
    - 畏光。
    - 倒睫毛(倒睫症)。
  - 瞳孔检查。
  - 对抗性视野检查。
  - 眼外肌功能。
  - 荧光素裂隙灯检查：
    - 前房细胞或闪光。
    - HSV 针眼或树突状损伤。
    - 角膜擦伤。
    - 异物。
  - 睑外翻。
  - 眼底检查和眼压测量。

基本检查

- 考虑红眼的系统性疾病。
- 进行如上所述的体格检查。

诊断检查与说明

针对红眼可疑病因进行检查。

- 泪囊炎：培养分泌物。
- 角膜溃疡：刮角膜进行培养(经常由眼科医师执行)。
- 细菌性结膜炎：
  - 轻度分泌物：获得结膜拭子进行常规细菌培养和敏感测定(未接种的儿童通常为金黄色葡萄球菌、链球菌和流感嗜血杆菌)；然而，不一定需要，因结膜炎通常进行诊断性治疗。
  - 严重分泌物：淋病奈瑟菌。
  - 根据可疑病因标记特殊培养基和方法(如 GC 用 Thayer-Martin 培养基)。

儿科注意事项

- 沙眼衣原体是最常见的新生儿结膜炎感染原因(单眼或双眼、脓性或黏脓性分泌物)。
- 淋病奈瑟菌是另一种新生儿感染病原，典型者发生在出生后 2～4 日内，以脓性分泌物、球结膜水肿、眼睑水肿为标志。
- 可能有严重并发症。

实验室检查

- 经常是不明确的。
- 如果病因是系统性疾病则是有用的。
- 如果是双侧，再发的，怀疑是肉芽肿性葡萄膜炎，做全血细胞计数、红细胞沉降率、抗核抗体、梅毒血清学试验、荧光密螺旋体抗体吸附、纯化蛋白衍生物、ACE 水平、胸部 X 线片(肉瘤样病和结核病)、莱姆病滴度、HLA-B27、弓形虫和巨细胞病毒(CMV)滴度。

影像学检查

如果怀疑异物，眼眶疾病或外伤，做眼眶的 X 线平片和/或 CT 平扫。

诊断步骤/外科

- 如果考虑青光眼则测量眼压。
- 钴蓝光荧光素裂隙灯检查：
  - 儿童采用荧光紫外线照射灯检查。
- 移除简单的角膜异物。
- 评估化学接触的 pH。

鉴别诊断

- 局部：感染、过敏、外伤(也要考虑病因)。
- 急性闭角型青光眼。
- 系统性(一般为炎症反应)：
  - 关节炎。
  - 强直性脊柱炎。
  - 溃疡性结肠炎。
  - Reiter 综合征。
  - 肺结核。
  - 疱疹。
  - 梅毒。
  - 肉瘤样病。
  - 弓形虫病。
  - 巨细胞病毒。

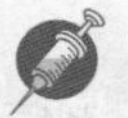

治疗

院前

- 止痛和安抚措施。
- 化学物质接触的初步冲洗。
- 如果眼球穿透则给予保护眼罩。

初步稳定/治疗

- 如果可以，移除隐形眼镜。
- 及时冲洗化学品引起的创伤。
- 如果可以，进行系统性疾病的治疗。

急诊治疗/程序

- 针对特殊病原的直接治疗。
- 按指示用药。
- 特别提醒：
  - 区分角膜擦伤和角膜溃疡。
  - 眼部修补不再被推荐，通常为擦伤禁忌。
  - 受伤后重新进行破伤风免疫。
  - 禁止使用隐形眼镜。

- 不要传染到未感染的眼睛或尚未感染的人。
- 淋球菌或沙眼衣原体导致的结膜炎的诊断需要对患者或传染源的系统性感染进行治疗。
- 如果怀疑系统性疾病必须进行检查和治疗。

特殊类型

角膜擦伤

- 非隐形眼镜佩戴者：
- 药膏或滴剂：
  - 红霉素软膏：q4 h。
  - 硫酸多黏菌素 B 和甲氧苄啶滴眼液：4 次/日。
- 隐形眼镜佩戴者需覆盖假单胞菌属：
- 妥布霉素、氧氟沙星或环丙沙星滴剂：4 次/日。
- 用 1%～2%环喷托酯，2～4 滴每日来扩瞳缓解虹膜炎疼痛。
- 不经修补的擦伤会愈合。
- 系统性镇痛药、阿片类或非阿片类。
- 局部麻醉剂可用于 72 h 而不损害角膜上皮愈合。
- 如果 48 h 仍有症状，重新评估。

角膜溃疡

- 非隐形眼镜佩戴者：
- 硫酸多黏菌素 B 和甲氧苄啶滴眼液：4 次/日。
- 氧氟沙星、环丙沙星滴剂：q2～4 h。
- 隐形眼镜佩戴者需覆盖假单胞菌属（如上文所述）。

严重或影响视力的角膜溃疡

- 中心＞1.5 mm 或伴有严重的前房反应。
- 依上述治疗并增加抗生素滴剂使用频率，如前 6 h 每 15 min 1～2 滴，然后持续每 30 min 一次。
- 眼科会诊进一步治疗，可能包括环丙沙星 500 mg，口服，每日 2 次；或由药剂师配制的强化抗生素滴剂。
- 眼科医师会诊后通常建议住院。

急性闭角型青光眼

- 典型症状包括迅速起病、剧烈眼部疼痛、发红、视力下降、瞳孔中度扩大及无反应性。
- 其他症状包括：
- 恶心和呕吐。
- 头痛。
- 视力模糊和/或看到光周围有色圈。
- 流泪增加。
- 当眼压测量发现眼压升高（＞21 mmHg），诊断进一步明确。

结膜下出血

- 如果量大且在排除眼球穿刺伤情况下。
- 对于少量 SCH，安抚措施和润滑滴剂可加速愈合。

单纯或带状疱疹

- 1%曲氟尿苷（三氟甲基脱氧尿苷），2 滴，9 次/日；或 3%阿糖腺苷软膏 5 次/日（儿童首选软膏）。
- 请眼科会诊。

儿童注意事项

疱疹感染：

- 通常与 HSV-2 感染相关。
- 可能与脑炎相关，也可为单独的损伤。
- 新生儿出生后 1～2 周发病。
- 表现：通常单眼，严重分泌物，轻微结膜感染。

> **注意**
>
> 眼睛 HSV 感染有引起视觉丧失的严重风险。

创伤或葡萄膜炎

排除异物。

药物治疗

- 抗生素滴剂：
- 0.3%环丙沙星：1～2 滴，q1～6 h。
- 0.3%庆大霉素：1～2 滴，q4 h。
- 0.3%氧氟沙星：1～2 滴，q1～6 h。
- 硫酸多黏菌素 B 和甲氧苄啶滴眼液：1 滴，q3～6 h。
- 10%磺胺醋酰：0.3% 1～2 滴，q2～6 h。
- 0.3%妥布霉素：1～2 滴，q1～4 h。
- 0.1%曲氟尿苷：1 滴，q2～4 h。
- 抗生素软膏（眼科）：
- 杆菌肽：500 U/g ½条状，q3～6 h。
- 0.3%环丙沙星：½条状，q6～8 h。
- 0.5%红霉素：½条状，q3～6 h。
- 0.3%庆大霉素：½条状，q3～4 h。
- 新孢霉素：½条状软膏，q3～4 h。
- 多链丝霉素：½条状软膏，q3～4 h。
- 10%磺胺醋酰：½条状软膏，q3～8 h。
- 0.3%妥布霉素：½条状，q3～4 h。
- 阿糖腺苷：½条状，5 次/日。
- 散瞳药和睫状肌麻痹剂：
- 1%或 2%阿托品：1～2 滴，每日 1～4 次。
- 0.5%、1%或 2%环喷托酯：1～2 滴，必要时。
- 2%后马托平：1～2 滴。
- 0.12%、2.5%或 10%苯肾上腺素：1～2 滴，每日 2～3 次。
- 0.5%、1%托吡卡胺：1～2 滴 PRN。
- 皮质醇抗生素联合滴剂（仅用于眼科会诊）：
- 磺胺醋酰泼尼松龙滴眼液 1～2 滴，q1～8 h。
- cortisporin：1～2 滴，q3～4 h。
- maxitrol：1～2 滴，q1～8 h。
- Pred G：1～2 滴，q1～8 h。
- 妥布霉素地塞米松滴眼液：1～2 滴，q2～6 h。
- 青光眼类药物（往往用于眼科会诊）：
- 乙酰唑胺：250～500 mg，口服，每日 1～4 次。
- 0.25%或 0.5%倍他洛尔：1～2 滴，每日 2 次。
- 1%卡替洛尔：1 滴，每日 2 次。
- 0.25%或 0.5%左布诺洛尔：1 滴，每日 1～2 次。
- 1%地匹福林：1 滴，每日 2 次。
- 甘露醇：1～2 g/kg，静脉滴注，超过 45 min。
- 毛果芸香碱（0.25%、0.5%、1%、2%、3%、4%、6%、8%或 10%）：1～2 滴，每日 3～4 次（仅用于机械性闭合已排除时）。
- 0.25%或 0.5%噻吗洛尔：1 滴，每日 2 次。
- 局部麻醉。
- 0.5%盐酸丁卡因滴眼液：1 滴，必要时，而不超过 72 h。

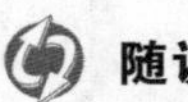

随访

进一步处理

入院指征

- 眼内炎。
- 穿孔性角膜溃疡。
- 眼眶蜂窝织炎。
- 并发伤（如外伤）。
- 如有系统性疾病指征。

儿科注意事项

怀疑有淋病奈瑟菌感染的新生儿结膜炎应住院，使用静脉抗生素（头孢噻肟）并考虑进行化脓性检查。

出院指征

能够遵循门诊指示。

转诊问题

- 泪囊炎。
- 角膜溃疡。

• 巩膜炎。
• 闭角型青光眼。
• 葡萄膜炎。
• 眼球突出。
• 眼眶蜂窝织炎。
• 视力丧失。
• 诊断不明确。
• 淋病或衣原体性结膜炎。

■ 随访建议

• 如果超过预期时间症状未缓解需重新评估。
• 避免使用隐形眼镜直至眼科医师同意。

要点和误区

• 未能辨别和治疗溃疡、疱疹性感染、新生儿细菌性感染、闭角型青光眼和穿透性创伤。
• 甾类药物经眼科医师会诊后方可应用。

虹膜炎 Iritis

Rene Mack · Yasuharu Okuda 倪沁赟 译

基础知识

■ 描述

• 前葡萄膜炎症。
• 虹膜炎、前葡萄膜炎和虹膜睫状体炎是同义词。
• 继发于外伤的虹膜炎又称外伤性虹膜炎。
• 急慢性表现。

■ 病因

• 大部分病例是特发性，但也有可能是创伤性或与感染性/非感染性全身性疾病相关。
• 最常见于 30～50 岁的患者。
• 男女比例是相等的。
• 可以是急性或慢性。
• HLA - B27 单倍型导致高达 50％的病例。
- 强直性脊柱炎。
- 炎症性肠病。
- 反应性关节炎/Reiter 综合征。
- 银屑病性关节炎。
• 非感染性全身性疾病包括：
- 类风湿性关节炎。
- 多发性硬化症。
- 结节病。
- 白塞病。
- 幼年型类风湿关节炎。
- 川崎病。
- 间质性肾病。
- Ig A 肾病。
- 药物反应。
- 干燥综合征。
• 感染性疾病包括：
- 病毒感染：
◦ 单纯疱疹病毒，1 型（最常见）。
◦ EB 病毒。
◦ 基孔肯亚病毒。
◦ 登革热病毒。
◦ 寨卡病毒。
◦ 风疹病毒。
◦ 麻疹病毒。
◦ 腺病毒。
◦ 单纯疱疹病毒。
◦ HIV。
◦ 流行性腮腺炎。
◦ 水痘。
◦ 巨细胞病毒。
◦ 西尼罗病毒。
- 细菌：
◦ 结核。
◦ 梅毒。
◦ 百日咳。
◦ 布鲁菌病。
◦ 莱姆病。
◦ 衣原体。
◦ 立克次体。
◦ 淋病。
◦ 麻风。
◦ 钩端螺旋体病。
◦ 猫抓病。
- 真菌：
• 恶性肿瘤包括：
- 白血病。
- 淋巴瘤。
- 多发性硬化。
- 多发性骨髓瘤。
- 视网膜母细胞瘤。
• 其他原因包括：
- 使用可卡因。
- 农药暴露。
- 角膜异物。
- 钝性创伤。
- 术后并发症。

诊断

■ 症状和体征

病史

• 可能是由于外伤或自发性发作。
• 急性表现：
- 单侧眼痛。
- 红眼（结膜炎）。
- 畏光。
- 通常在发病数小时至数日内进行评估。
- 流泪，但通常没有出院。
- 视力模糊/视力下降。
• 慢性表现：
- 反复发作。
- 很少或没有急性表现。
- 双眼受累。

体格检查

• 弥漫性结膜注射伴周围血管突出（睫状体冲洗）。
• 瞳孔不规则，反应迟钝。
• 自发性畏光。
• 前房细胞和光斑。
• 表面麻醉对缓解疼痛可能无效。
• 虹膜粘连（虹膜与晶状体或角膜粘连）可见于慢性病。
• 虹膜和睫状肌痉挛引起的瞳孔缩小。
• 由于睫状体功能不全和产水量减少而导致的低眼压（偶尔可能很高）。

■ 基本检查

• 病史和系统回顾：
- 高达 50％的患者发病可能与全身性疾病相关。
• 裂隙灯检查：
- 在前房见炎症细胞（白细胞）或发红（像“耀斑”一样）即可诊断。

H

-"耀斑"是蛋白漏出至眼房水中形成的均匀的雾状改变。
-使用短、宽光束可最佳观察细胞和"耀斑"。
-细胞沉积常伴随更严重的炎症。
• 眼内压测定。
• 视力。
• 瞳孔反射检查。
• 荧光素染色可能导致角膜损伤或感染。

诊断检查与说明

• 通常无特别征象，特别是：
-首次出现。
-单方面的。
-健康个体。
-无临床意义的病史和体格检查。
• 如果患者的病史、症状和体征强烈指向某个原因，需要给予患者特别的检查（转诊至眼科、风湿科或内科）。

实验室检查

• 任何培养物的 PCR 和 ELISA 检测。
• 结核：
-纯化蛋白衍生物(PPD)。
• 强直性脊柱炎：
- ESR。
- HLA-B27。
• 炎症性肠病：
- HLA-B27。
• Reiter 综合征：
- HLA-B27。
-结膜和尿道的培养。
• 银屑病关节炎：
- HLA-B27。
• 莱姆病：
-免疫测定法。
• 幼年型类风湿关节炎：
-抗核抗体。
-类风湿因子。
• 结节病：
- ACE(血管紧张素转换酶)。
-血清溶菌酶水平。
• 性传播疾病：
-快速血浆反应素或性病研究试验室试验。
-荧光密螺旋体抗体吸收试验。
-合适的培养。

影像学检查

• 强直性脊柱炎：
-骶髂关节脊柱 X 线片。
• 结节病：
-胸部 X 线片。
• 结核：
-胸部 X 线片。

诊断步骤/外科

• 生物显微镜可用于病理诊断。
• 前房穿刺术。

鉴别诊断

• 急性闭角型青光眼。
• 结膜炎。
• 角膜擦伤。
• 角膜异物。
• 巩膜炎。
• 眼内异物。
• 角膜炎。
• 眼后段肿瘤。

治疗

院前

• 目标：
-降低炎症反应。
-减轻痛苦。
-预防并发症。

急诊治疗/程序

• 如果有指征使用外用类固醇激素：
-小心使用，随时与眼科专家保持联系。
-可能导致明显的并发症（如单纯疱疹病毒性角膜炎发展）。
• 睫状肌麻痹症：
-通过缓解睫状体痉挛来控制疼痛。
-防止后粘连的发展。
-治疗继发性青光眼。
• 支持措施：
-戴墨镜。
-口服镇痛。
• 确定原因并处理：
-非感染性全身性疾病。
-传染性。
-恶性。
-创伤性。

药物治疗

一线用药

• 局部皮质类固醇（应在咨询眼科医师后使用）：
-醋酸泼尼松龙 1%：2 滴，每 15～30 min×4 滴，然后 q6 h，持续 23 日。

二线用药

• 睫状肌麻痹/散瞳：
-霍马托品 5%：1 滴，q6 h，最多 4 日。
-环孢素 1%：1 滴，q8 h，最多 4 日。
• 止痛：
-口服非甾体抗炎药。
-泰诺。
-麻醉止痛药。

儿科注意事项

• 散瞳不建议 6 岁以下儿童使用：
-可能导致全身抗胆碱能毒性伴随视力模糊、面部潮红、心动过速、低血压和幻觉。
• 可待因不建议 12 岁以下儿童使用。

妊娠注意事项

妊娠和哺乳期间不建议使用可待因。

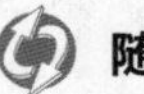

随访

进一步处理

入院指征

除非有全身症状，否则无入院指征。

转诊问题

• 虹膜炎：
- 24 h 内联系眼科医师做后续护理和可能的类固醇治疗。
• 如果不太可能是特发性原因，请咨询相关专业人员。

要点和误区

• 如果局部麻醉可减轻疼痛，可能不是虹膜炎。
• 必须区别于其他，危害视力的眼痛形式：
-角膜炎。
-单纯疱疹性结膜炎。
-细菌性结膜炎。
-急性闭角型青光眼。
-外伤性眼球破裂。
• 如果担心前房浅，避免睫状肌麻痹：
-可能进展为急性角型青光眼。
• 未经适当治疗的并发症。
-白内障。
-视力丧失。
-青光眼。
-黄斑水肿。

喉骨折 Larynx Fracture

Katja Goldflam · David Della-Giustina 何超 段立伟 译

基础知识

描述

• 强大的外力导致的喉部的直接离断。
• 从单纯的黏膜撕裂到喉软骨断裂和粉碎，再到喉与气管分离：
- 不成对：甲状腺、环状软骨和会厌软骨。
- 成对：杓状软骨、角质软骨和楔形软骨。
• 发生率：急诊患者患病率为 1/5 000～1/42 000。
• 占钝性损伤的不足 1%。
• 最近的数据显示这种情况可能更为常见：CT 可以诊断几乎 1%的颈部外伤患者。
• 院前死亡率可能高达 80%，但在确保气道安全后，死亡率降低到＜5%。

病因

• 交通车祸或暴力损伤对于颈前部的暴力或贯穿性打击。
• 最常见的病因是对于颈前部暴露区域的直接高压打击。
• "晾衣绳"损伤也是一种常见损伤原因(患者由于绳索、条带等物质缠绕于颈部所带来的损伤)。
• 近些年来在老年患者中医源性病因比较常见。

儿科注意事项

自行车手把：
• 儿童将颈部置于自行车手把，一旦出现外力的冲撞会造成颈椎的骨折和喉部的损伤。

H

诊断

症状和体征

• 症状可能会持续数小时。
• 高达 10%的患者入院时无症状。
• 症状和外部症状并不与实际伤害的严重程度相关。
• 对于钝性损伤造成的喉部骨折的诊断比较困难。
• 出血、衣领或多发伤会提供一些隐匿的发现。
• 颈部压痛。
• 颈前部的挫伤或擦伤。
• 声音沙哑等音色的改变。
• 咯血。
• 呼吸困难。
• 喘息。
• 纵隔气肿。
• 发声困难。
• 气胸。
• 颈部正常软骨标志物的消失。

基本检查

• 内镜检查优于影像学检查，因为黏膜的水肿造成气道受压情况比骨折损伤更常见。
• 颈椎 X 线成像：
- 当 X 线平片不能获得清晰的判断时可以选择颈部 CT。
• X 线胸片：
- 检查是否存在气胸、胸腔积液和纵隔气肿。
• 颈部 CT：
- 应进行软组织和骨窗的二维和三维重建，因为平扫可能会造成漏诊。
- 使用对比剂可以发现是否存在血管损伤。
- 对于不是立刻进行外科手术治疗的患者都推荐使用 CT 检查。
- 即使对于症状不严重并且直接喉镜检查未发现明显异常的患者，使用 CT 检查是有帮助的。
• 血氧饱和度监测。

> **注意**
>
> 不推荐 MRI。
> • 时间耗费长。
> • 对气道受伤的患者难以进行密切气道监测。
> • 对于颈部骨折的患者诊断作用不大：
> - 在无骨化患者中可能有用，CT 无法显示高度怀疑骨折的儿童软骨。

诊断检查与说明

实验室检查

对于呼吸困难的患者行动脉血气检查。

诊断步骤/外科

• 纤维喉镜
- 选择经鼻喉镜检查，能够直视下观察气道、声带的损伤情况。
• 血管造影：
- 锐器损伤时。
- 当考虑可能存在血管损伤时选择进行。
• CT 血管成像技术比传统的血管造影更具有优势：
- 创伤性更小，患者接受度更好。
- 能够快速地进行。
- 检查术后的并发症较少。
- 能够较好地评估颈部软组织、消化道、椎管和脊髓的损伤。
• 纤维支气管镜和喉镜检查。
• 手术。
- 严重的损伤时。
- 条件紧急时可以选择急诊手术。
- 目前已经证明，早期的手术可以减少 40%的声音和气道并发症。

鉴别诊断

相关损伤：
• 颅内损伤(13%)。
• 开放的颈部损伤(9%)。
• 颈髓损伤(8%)。
• 食管损伤(3%)。
• 颈动脉损伤。
• 膈神经损伤。
• 脑缺氧性损伤。
• 气道水肿。
• 气胸。
• 气体栓塞。

儿科注意事项

• 儿童的喉部在颈部的位置较高，同时软骨含量和移动性较成人都更好，所以容易发生喉部骨折。
• 由于喉部黏膜下组织疏松，因此容易发生软组织的损伤、严重水肿及血肿。
- 由于气道本身直径不大，所以很快便会出现呼吸困难和气道受压。
• 症状包括颈部压痛、声音嘶哑、呼吸困难和喘鸣。
• 在儿童患者中 CT 检查并无内镜或体格检查常用，因为在 CT 中不能清晰地辨别儿童喉部的微小骨折。

治疗

院前

• 注意：
- 可以选择进行侵入性的气道管理：吸氧，吸痰。
- 颈椎制动。
- 院前时可能会因为其他损伤或缺乏系统

的检查，颈部的损伤可能会被忽视。

- 争议：
  - 不推荐选择性插管，尤其是缺乏经验的操作者。

初步稳定/治疗

最重要的是对气道的管理：

- 早期进行气管插管有利于之后避免更多的气道并发症。
- 环状软骨压迫是禁忌。
- 避免进行反复的经口气管插管尝试。
  - 应该请经验丰富的操作者。
  - 降低呼吸阈值。
- 对于严重的颌面部损伤或环状软骨损伤的患者推荐环甲膜切开气管插管。
- 当存在环甲膜下出血或环状气管环的破坏时不采取环甲膜切开术。
- 如果时间允许，在手术室进行正式气管切开术可能比气管插管或环甲膜切开术更好。
  - 可防止气管内操作对受伤部位的进一步损害。
- 气道损伤严重时可行紧急气管切开术。

儿科注意事项

- 不推荐选择性插管。
- 气管插管应尽可能在纤维喉镜直接观察下进行。
- 对诊断和治疗过程有困难，可行 CT 扫描。

急诊治疗/程序

- 开通静脉通道。
- 气道湿化给予吸氧。
- 头部抬高以减轻头颈部的软组织水肿。
- 禁食。
- 避免发声。
- 耳鼻喉科医师会诊，评估是否需要进行手术。
- 对于严重肺损伤合并气胸、急性呼吸窘迫的患者进行呼气末正压和容量控制模式的机械通气。

药物治疗

- 对于喉部损伤合并纵隔气肿的患者：
  - 考虑到上呼吸道的黏膜与颈部的深部组织相通：
    - 氨苄西林：1.5～3 g，静脉给药（儿童 50 mg/kg，静脉给药），q6 h。
    - 克林霉素：600～900 mg，静脉给药，q8 h 重复给药[儿童：25～40 mg/(kg·24 h)，静脉给药]。
    - H_2 受体拮抗剂：抑制损伤黏膜的渗出[雷尼替丁 150～300 mg，静脉给药，儿童 2～4 mg/(kg·d)]，或质子泵抑制剂（如泮托拉唑 40 mg，静脉给药）。
- 对于喉部水肿患者可以使用一定的类固醇激素。
  - 对于严重的水肿有一定疗效，但是不推荐长期使用。
  - 甲泼尼龙：250 mg，静脉给药，q4 h（起效快）。
  - 地塞米松：8～10 mg，静脉给药，q8 h。

随访

进一步处理

入院指征

- 对于确切的喉部损伤的患者都应该收治入院进行气道的管理和监测，必要时进行外科手术修复。
- 对于怀疑存在喉部损伤的患者也应收治入院，视情况选择纤维喉镜的检查。

出院指征

- 在急诊室进行 6 h 的观察后，如果患者没有出现严重喉部损伤伴有气道水肿和受压的症状后可以出院。
- 患者在损伤后的数小时内可以表现正常，没有相应的症状，这时候如果有任何怀疑都应该收治入院后进行相应的监测。

喉头炎 Croup

Dale W. Steele 陈奇通 译

基础知识

描述

- 上呼吸道的病毒感染。
- 最常见于 6 个月至 3 岁婴幼儿：
  - 喉气管炎、喉气管支气管炎。
  - 由于胸外气道梗阻导致的吸气性喘鸣。
  - 呼气性喘鸣音提示累及下呼吸道。
  - 声门下区炎性水肿。
  - 小儿气道最狭窄的部分。
  - 也称为喉气管支气管炎。
- 可能病情进展为呼吸衰竭。

病因

- 副流感病毒 1 型、2 型和 3 型。
- 人类冠状病毒 NL63。
- 甲型流感。
- 腺病毒。
- 人类冠状病毒。
- 呼吸道合胞病毒。
- 麻疹。
- 肺炎支原体。
- 单纯疱疹。

诊断

症状和体征

病史

- 非特异性呼吸道前驱症状，有或没有发热。
- 咳嗽：常“海豹状”。
- 疾病病程。
- 有震颤：进行性，静息或活动时有震颤。
- 气管插管史或人工气道。
- 可疑的异物吸入史。
- 以前的发作情况。
- 喘息的病史。
- 疫苗接种情况[B 型流感嗜血杆菌（HIB）、白喉、百日咳、破伤风（DPT）]，流感。

体格检查

- 通常无中毒。
- 发绀（在大多数患者不存在。如果存在，表明非常严重的疾病）。
- 喜欢保持直立姿势。
- 类似啼哭声。
- 流口水、口齿不清、颈部后伸受限建议其他科室协助诊断。
- 精神状态。
- 喘息，呼吸频率增加。
- 水化状态。
- 韦斯特利的喉炎评分（最高分：17）：
  - 喘鸣（吸气，双相）：

◦ 0＝没有。
◦ 1＝在休息状态，使用听诊器可闻及。
◦ 2＝在休息状态，不使用听诊器可闻及。
- （辅助肌群的）收缩：
◦ 0＝没有。
◦ 1＝轻微。
◦ 2＝中等。
◦ 3＝严重哮吼评分。
- 吸气入口：
◦ 0＝正常。
◦ 1＝减少。
◦ 2＝严重下降。
- 发绀：
◦ 0＝无。
◦ 4＝伴焦虑不安。
◦ 5＝静息状态。
- 意识水平：
◦ 0＝正常。
◦ 5＝意识障碍。

诊断检查与说明

实验室检查

• 持续的脉搏血氧饱和度的监测，缺氧意味着严重的疾病。
• 其他的检查不常使用。

影像学检查

颈椎的正侧X线位片：
• 尖塔征显示声门下气管狭窄。
• 除了不典型的临床表现和疾病过程，否则不需要常规检查。
• 因容易被误诊，不应该作为排除会厌炎的唯一手段。
• 在儿童中因对于会厌炎和细菌性气管炎的怀疑，手术室中确定性的可视化气管插管不应被延迟。
• 如果做影像学检查，因对婴幼儿进行监护。

鉴别诊断

• 感染：
- 细菌性气管炎。
- 咽后或咽旁脓肿。
- 会厌炎。
- 扁桃体周围脓肿。
- 白喉。
• 异物（气道或食管）。
• 血管性水肿。
• 先天性气道异常：
- 喉软化，气管软化，喉裂。
• 获得性声门下狭窄。
• 声带麻痹。
• 热或化学损伤上气道。
• 血管瘤。
• 喉乳头状瘤。
• 声带功能障碍（VCD）（青少年）。

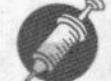

治疗

院前

• 允许患儿保持舒适的体位。
• 延迟以下可能使患儿痛苦的干预措施：
- 静脉注射。
- 肌内注射。
• 如果呼吸窘迫：
- 立即雾化吸入肾上腺素。

初步稳定/治疗

• 如果静息时存在呼吸窘迫或喘鸣，雾化吸入外消旋肾上腺素或肾上腺素：
- 左旋肾上腺素仅包含活性异构体已被证明是与外消旋肾上腺素疗效相当。
- 可以进行背靠背治疗，一般20 min一次。
- 如果反应良好，在出院前，必须观察治疗后至少2～3 h，不得出现喘鸣或疼痛。
• 氧疗（通过吹气、插管或面罩，如果可以忍受的话）用于怀疑或记录的缺氧。缺氧与严重疾病有关。
• 雾化疗法有时使用，但无循证依据。
• 地塞米松：
- 减少插管的需求，缩短医院的停留时间，减少住院和复诊，可能在30 min内起效。
- 轻症喉头炎患者中依然有效（韦斯特利的喉炎评分≤2）。
• 如果对雾化吸入外消旋肾上腺素或左旋肾上腺素反应很差：
- 考虑试验氦：
• 氦氧混合气，在能够使用时，已被用于减少对肾上腺素反应不佳的患者的呼吸功。
• 尽管已经使用了上述的治疗，但即将发生或已经存在呼吸衰竭：
- 请能够找得到的最有经验的人行气管插管。
- 使用比通常的小0.5～1 mm的不充气囊的气管插管（ETT）。
• 如果怀疑会厌炎或异物：
- 入手术室，行吸入麻醉，直接喉镜，插管。
- 外科医师随时准备紧急气管切开术。

急诊治疗/程序

见初步稳定/治疗。

药物治疗

• 2.25%消旋肾上腺素：0.25～0.5 ml加入到生理盐水2.5 ml雾化吸入。
• 1∶1000左旋肾上腺素：5 ml（5 mg）雾化吸入。
• 地塞米松：单剂量0.6 mg/kg（最大剂量10 mg），口服（使用压碎片）或静脉注射。
• 准备（4 mg/ml）调味糖浆口服。口服、静脉注射或肌内注射是等效的。低剂量也许是有效的。
• 氦氧混合气（氦70%∶30%氧通过面罩或氧帐混合来使用）。
• 抗生素：无指征。

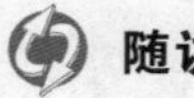

随访

进一步处理

入院指征

• 婴幼儿，已经存在上气道梗阻。
• 静息状态持续或复发喘鸣对肾上腺雾化无反应，或在肾上腺素雾化后2～3 h观察期复发。
• 病因不明。
• 儿科ICU：
- 持续重度梗阻。
- 需要频繁使用肾上腺素或氦氧混合气治疗。
- 气管插管辅助通气。

出院指征

• 呼吸室内空气时氧合正常。
• 休息时无喘鸣在短暂的观察后（可出院）。
• 最初服用肾上腺素的儿童，如果在治疗后没有喘息或任何痛苦，应观察至少2～3 h。
• 可靠的看护，通信，转运。

转诊问题

• 关注潜在的解剖异常（年龄小、气管插管史、频繁复发）。
• 反复的喉头炎。

随访建议

• 绝大部分哮吼的患儿不需要特殊的随访。
• 已经有持续很长时间的喘鸣和喘鸣急性加重的患者应去初级保健医师处就诊或返回急诊室。

要点和误区

• 谨防婴幼儿喘鸣（考虑先天性异常的高发率）。
• 轻度和早期会厌炎或细菌性气管炎可能和哮吼相仿。
• 流口水，口齿不清，颈部伸展受限，提示其他诊断。

H

喉炎 Laryngitis

Yi-Mei Chng 何超 段立伟 译

基础知识

描述

- 喉黏膜的炎症。
- 通常是由上呼吸道病毒感染引起。
- 也可能是由声带损伤引起的：
  - 咳嗽或清喉过度。
  - 在上呼吸道感染时，讲话过度。
  - 尖叫或大声叫喊。
  - 过度讲话。
  - 在嘈杂的环境中讲话。
  - 吸烟。
- 流行病发病的高峰与呼吸道病毒的流行病学特点呈平行关系。
- 在秋末、冬季及早春多发。

病因

- 急性喉炎最常见的病因是病毒性上呼吸道感染：
  - A型和B型流感病毒。
  - 1型和2型副流感病毒。
  - 腺病毒。
  - 鼻病毒。
  - 不常见(或见于免疫功能低下者)：柯萨奇病毒、呼吸道合胞病毒、疱疹病毒、HIV等。
- 细菌感染相对少见：
  - β溶血性链球菌。
  - 肺炎链球菌。
  - 嗜血杆菌。
  - 卡他莫拉菌。
  - 百日咳杆菌。
  - 白喉。
  - 结核。
  - 梅毒。
  - 麻风。
- 由于胃食管反流症造成的食管咽喉反流病(成人多见)。
- 真菌感染(多见于长期使用吸入性糖皮质激素或使用免疫抑制剂患者)。
- 过敏。
- 用嗓过度。
- 吸入或食入具有腐蚀性的物质或其他刺激性物质。
- 自身免疫性(合并类风湿关节炎、复发性多发慢性炎症、魏格纳肉芽肿或结节病)。
- 创伤。

儿科注意事项

- 急性痉挛性喉炎。
- 感染的发生较多：
  - 如果排除自身免疫性因素首先考虑嗜血杆菌、白喉等。
- 异物。

诊断

症状和体征

病史

- 声音嘶哑。
- 声调异常。
- 喉头水肿。
- 喉部瘙痒。
- 喉部生硬感。
- 有持续性清嗓的强迫感。
- 咳嗽。
- 发热。
- 精神萎靡。
- 食欲不振。

体格检查

- 区域性淋巴结肿大。
- 婴儿尖锐的哭声。
- 声音嘶哑。
- 咽部红斑，渗出，肿大。
- 当存在异物时表现为不对称的呼吸音。

基本检查

- 急性喉炎：
  - 在大部分病例中，通过仔细询问病史和喉部检查能够区分感染性和肺感染性喉炎。
    - 感染性喉炎一般会持续7～10日。
  - 对于非流感嗜血杆菌感染的患者需要排除是否存在会厌炎。
- 慢性喉炎(>3周)。
  - 试验检查要进一步明确慢性感染的病因，是否存在胃食管反流症、神经功能的异常和肿瘤。
  - 一般情况下需要直视下对喉部进行检查。
  - 患者需要经过耳鼻喉专科医师的进一步检查。

诊断检查与说明

实验室检查

颈部软组织成像：

- 一般不选择做颈部软组织成像，因为喉镜检查能够提供更加合适的病情评估。
- 当怀疑存在会厌炎或喉部异物的患者可以采用。

影像学检查

纤维喉镜：

- 声带炎症，红肿，声带边缘增厚。
- 偶尔会出现出血或渗出。
- 细菌性喉炎的患者会出现喉内部的化脓性改变。
- 咽部出现假膜是白喉的特征性表现。

鉴别诊断

- 哮喘。
- 会厌炎。
- 食管反流病。
- 局部结节。
- 咽部或甲状腺恶性肿瘤。
- 格鲁布性喉头炎。
- 异物嵌塞或创伤。

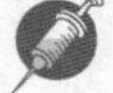

治疗

院前

必要的支持治疗，但是不推荐使用救护车进行运送。

> **注意**
> - 儿童出现喘鸣提示咽部或支气管呼吸道的阻塞。
> - 颈部创伤后的喉炎需要耳鼻喉科专科医师进行疾病评估。
> - 注意伴随喉炎发生的食管损伤。
> - 当存在呼吸窘迫情况时提示伴发会厌炎，注意：
>   - 运送过程中保持直立。
>   - 吸氧。
>   - 这时候进行插管是困难的，只有对于情况紧急的患者才尝试插管。

初步稳定/治疗

当患者出现呼吸窘迫时需要进行稳定性治疗：

- 以无创呼吸机进行氧疗。
- 在时间允许的情况下在手术室进行经口气管插管治疗。
- 同时颈部消毒，准备好相关器械以备气管

H

切开。

■ 急诊治疗/程序

• 对于急性喉炎的成年患者不考虑将抗生素治疗作为一线方案。

- 在一项随机对照试验的回顾性研究中，比较使用抗生素和安慰剂发现，抗生素治疗并不能明显改善症状。

• 使声带休息（避免耳语，因为这样会使喉部功能亢进）。

- 如果患者一定要说话，可以使用较轻柔的声音。

• 呼吸湿润的空气。

• 增加饮水。

• 使用止痛药物。

• 避免吸烟。

• 病毒引起的喉炎一般会在 7～10 日后症状消失。

• 如果症状超过 14 日，需要转诊。

• 传统治疗方案是使用吸入性糖皮质激素，但并不是目前最好的临床选择。

■ 药物治疗

根据喉炎的病因而定：

• 上呼吸道感染或过敏时使用一些化痰剂，如愈创甘油醚。

• 病毒感染时可使用对乙酰氨基酚或 NSAIDs 类药物缓解症状。

• 胃食管反流症相关的喉炎使用质子泵抑制剂：

- 埃索美拉唑：20～40 mg（1～11 岁的儿童使用 10 mg），口服，每日给药。

- 奥美拉唑：20 mg，口服，每日给要 2 次。

• 对于念珠菌性喉炎使用大扶康治疗。

• 格鲁布性喉头炎：地塞米松 0.6 mg/kg，口服或肌内注射。

• 抗组胺类药物能够使声带变得干燥，不利于黏液和渗出液的排出。

• 全身使用糖皮质激素有时可在紧急时使用，但目前证据不足。

- 最好由耳鼻喉科专家来会诊。

• Cochrane 回顾性研究发现使用抗生素治疗急性喉炎对患者并无益处。

- 但抗生素可用于治疗一些高危患者或经细菌性培养证实革兰阳性菌感染的患者。

 随访

■ 进一步处理

入院指征

• 结核性喉炎。

- 具有传染性，所以必须进行隔离。

• 出现会厌炎的症状，或呼吸窘迫、颈部创伤或过敏性症状。

出院指征

大多数患者如果没有出现合并的会厌炎并且没有呼吸困难的症状则可以出院，注意充分湿化。

■ 随访建议

• 慢性喉炎的患者需要进行耳鼻喉随访。会厌炎＞3 周但找不到明显病因的患者需要排除肿瘤等恶性情况。

• 有以下症状立即返回住院：

- 2～3 周症状尚未好转需要进行耳鼻喉科随访。

- 有胃食管反流症症状的患者需要进行消化方面的特别护理。

要点和误区

• 大部分的急性喉炎是由于病毒感染，因此抗生素治疗不一定有效。

• 考虑到发声改变的一些威胁生命的病因，如会厌炎。

• 不合并上呼吸道感染的喉炎一般与胃食管反流症相关。

• 存在慢性或久治不愈的喉炎需要进行耳鼻喉科的随访。

呼吸机管理 Ventilator Management

Kristen G. Moore　周秋香　毛恩强 译

 基础知识

■ 描述

• 机械通气是机器产生的气体流入和流出肺部，代替正常的呼吸功能。

• 成功的呼吸机管理需要了解呼吸衰竭的原因和影响肺力学的病理生理学。

■ 生理学和肺动力学

• 自然呼吸模式包括负压通气：

在肺的功能残气量（FRC，静息状态）下，肺泡的表面张力由胸壁的弹性回缩平衡；肺泡压力等于大气压力。

- 吸气时，肺泡压变为负值，空气进入肺部。

- 呼气通常是被动的，但可以通过使用辅助肌肉来主动呼气。

- 呼吸功（WOB）等于克服气流阻力（阻力 WOB）和肺静息状态下（弹性 WOB）所需的力乘以呼吸频率。

• 机械通气是正压通气，因为强制气体输送在吸气时产生正压力。

• 通气指的是从血液中功能性地清除二氧化碳；这会影响 $PaCO_2$、pH 和 $ETCO_2$：

- 分钟通气量（MV）＝呼吸频率（RR，次/分）×潮气量（TV，标准呼吸）。

- 无效腔（DS）＝不参与气体交换的呼吸量；DS 随着气道受损或肺泡供血减少而增加（如肺栓塞）。

- $ETCO_2$ 通常为 2～5 mmHg＜$PaCO_2$；其值受 DS、通气/灌注（V/Q）不匹配、代谢性 CO_2 生成和静脉回流的变化影响。

• 氧分压（PaO_2）受吸入氧（FiO_2）和呼气末正压（PEEP）的影响：

- PEEP 有助于维持肺泡扩张，减少 V/Q 比例失调。

- PEEP 可以改善氧合，但高水平时存在肺泡损伤风险。

• 顺应性是指肺膨胀性（容积随压力变化而变化）：

- 随着软组织受损（如肺炎、ARDS）或胸壁/胸膜问题（如肥胖、腹胀）而顺应性降低。

• 顺应性决定平台压力，这是在正压通气过程中分配到小气道和肺泡的稳态压力；使用吸气保持动作测量；目标值≤30 mmHg。

• 气道阻力是指压力随气流的变化；这主要由气道半径决定：

- 由于呼吸道问题（如支气管痉挛）、气管插管（如分泌物）或呼吸机导管问题，阻力增加。

- 阻力决定了气道峰压（大气道中的压力）；目标值≤40 mmHg。

■ **基本通气方式**

• 无创正压通气(NIPPV,见"无创通气管理"):
- 持续气道正压(CPAP):在整个呼吸循环中设定压力支持。
- 双水平正压(BiPAP):吸气压力高于呼气压力以支持呼吸功和增加通气。

• 持续强制通气(CMV):
- 呼吸只能以固定的速率进行。
- 时间是每次呼吸的触发因素:
  ◦ 容量控制(或容量循环)CMV:每次呼吸时提供设定的容量,并保证一定的分钟通气量。
  ◦ 压力控制(或压力循环)CMV:提供恒定气流,直到设置吸气压力以限制峰值压力。
  ◦ 放松呼吸肌肉,但通常需要大量镇静剂,不常用。

• 容量控制/辅助控制(VC/AC):
- 病人或时间触发呼吸,但同样是机器控制的呼吸(设定容量或流量)。
- 降低呼吸功和保证潮气量,但可能导致过度换气或吸气压力过大。

• 同步间歇指令通气(SIMV):
- 患者或时间触发呼吸在一个设定的 RR。
- 患者呼吸由压力控制,机器呼吸由气流或压力控制。
- 减少对心血管功能的干扰,但增加患者对两种呼吸方式的适应能力。

• 压力支持通气(PSV):
- 呼吸机以设定的压力增加患者的自发呼吸。
- 改善患者的舒适度并降低呼吸功,但存在换气不足或呼吸暂停的风险。

诊断

■ **症状和体征**

• 机械通气指征:
- 缺氧(PaO_2<60 mmHg)。
  ◦ V/Q 异常(如肺炎、PE、ARDS、肺水肿)。
  ◦ 分流(如 AVM、心脏缺陷、严重 ARDS)。
  ◦ 弥散性障碍(如间质性肺病)。
  ◦ 通气不足(如过量服用阿片类药物、慢性阻塞性肺病、神经肌肉疾病、胸壁僵硬、气道阻塞)。
  ◦ 严重休克(供氧不能满足组织供氧)。
- 通气障碍($PaCO_2$>50 mmHg,低 pH)。
  ◦ 麻醉/镇静。
  ◦ 神经肌肉无力(如高位脊髓损伤、吉兰-巴雷综合征、重症肌无力)。
  ◦ 胸壁功能不全(如胸部水肿、腹部压力增加、肥胖、大量胸腔积液)。
  ◦ 增加死腔(如肺气肿、急性呼吸窘迫综合征、大出血)。
  ◦ 代谢性酸中毒(需要更高的 MV 来补偿)。
- 患者安全/评估需求。
- 预测临床预后恶化。

病史和体格检查

• 体征、症状、病史和检查有助于确定呼吸衰竭的病因。

• 检查内容应包括血氧饱和度、血流动力学状态、听诊肺音/空气流动、观察胸壁上升和触诊腹胀。

• $ETCO_2$ 波形(电容图)的评估可能非常有用:
- 对支气管扩张剂治疗的反应,气道阻塞的波形有更陡的上坡(延长的呼气相)而不是平台。
- 评估心肺复苏的充分性(将看到具有良好按压的波形恢复)。

• 通气策略应具体针对机械通气的适应证:
- 哮喘与慢性阻塞性肺病。
  ◦ NIPPV 可作为慢性阻塞性肺疾病患者和选择性哮喘患者的治疗对象。
    ▪ 吸气压力支持可能增加 5 cmH_2O 到 20/5。
    ▪ 密切监测插管需要情况(疲劳、持续低氧血症、高碳酸血症)。
  ◦ 如果插管:
    ▪ 限制气道压力和分钟通气量以防止空气滞留。
    ▪ 设置低 RR(10~12)和高 I∶E(1∶4、1∶5)。
    ▪ 允许性高碳酸血症(pH 保持>7.2)。
    ▪ 考虑神经肌肉阻滞。
- 心源性肺水肿:
  ◦ 考虑一下 NIPPV 的试验:
    ▪ 降低呼吸功,降低死亡率和插管需要。
    ▪ PEEP 改善左心室功能(吸气压力 12~15,呼气压力 8~10)。
- ARDS:
  ◦ 肺保护策略:低潮气量(6 ml/kg PBW),限制平台压(<30 mmHg),避免氧中毒(FiO_2<0.6)。
  ◦ 允许性高碳酸血症。
  ◦ 如果是顽固性低氧血症,考虑神经肌肉阻滞、俯卧位、吸入一氧化氮、气道压力释放通气(高级模式)或 ECMO。
- 感染性休克。
  ◦ 包括高通气需求和呼吸肌灌注减少,导致高呼吸功、耗氧量和肌肉疲劳;机械通气减少呼吸功和氧气需求。
  ◦ 建议对脓毒症肺损伤患者采取保护性措施。
- 心肺骤停。
  ◦ 需要立即使 O_2(PaO_2 70~100 mmHg)和 CO_2($PaCO_2$ 40~50 mmHg)正常化。
  ◦ 低潮气量、肺保护措施与 ARDS 相似。
  ◦ 感染的早期诊断和治疗。

■ **诊断检查与说明**

实验室检查

• 动脉血气(ABG):
- 动脉血气(ABG)用于评估氧合(PaO_2);静脉血气(VBG)足以评估通气(pH 和 PCO_2)。
- 应在机械通气开始后 15~30 min 检查,并在临床状态发生任何变化时重复检查。
- 使用 SaO_2 和 $ETCO_2$ 可以减少对频繁 ABG 或 VBG 的需要。

• 血清生化检查可以帮助评估酸碱状态,这将影响通气策略。

• 血红蛋白含量将有助于描述携氧的能力。

影像学检查

影像学检查可能包括超声、胸部 X 线检查和胸部 CT 检查,以评估内镜乳头管放置和肺和胸壁的病理生理学。

■ **鉴别诊断**

见上面机械通气的指征。

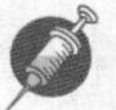

治疗

■ **院前**

每个当地急救团队的呼吸支持。

■ **初步稳定/治疗**

• 建立静脉通路。
• 心电监护。
• 血压监测。
• 脉搏血氧仪。
• 若有条件呼气末二氧化碳监测。

■ **急诊治疗/程序**

• 急性呼吸衰竭管理目标。
- 减少呼吸功。
- 选择性使用 NIPPV(见要点和误区)。
- 针对即将发生的呼吸衰竭早期插管治疗。

- 标准管后护理：
  - 镇静和/或镇痛(见药物治疗)。
  - 抬高床头。
  - 确认管路位置(CXR)。
  - 放置 NG/OG 管和折叠管。
- 病因治疗。

• 呼吸机管理的关键措施。
- 选择适当的初始呼吸机设置。
- 重新评估患者并调整设置。
  - 优化气体交换。
  - 确保患者-呼吸机同步。
  - 限制呼吸机相关性肺损伤(VILI)风险。
  - 以 ABG、VBG、$ETCO_2$ 和生命体征为指导。

• 初始呼吸机设置。
- 模式：如上所述，通常使用容量控制模式。
- 潮气量：通常 8～10 ml/kg 预测体重(PBW)，ARDS 使用较低的潮气量(6 ml/kg)。
- 呼吸频率：通常为 12～20 bpm 但可能低于(10～12)COPD 或哮喘或更高，以弥补严重代谢性酸中毒(DKA，水杨酸中毒)。
- FiO_2：通常从 100%开始；如果在 ABG 或指脉氧上的氧合稳定(对于 ARDS，sat 92%～94%或>88%)，应迅速下降(目标<60%)。
- PEEP：通常从 PEEP 5～10 cmH_2O；如果胸壁顺应性较差，考虑 10～15 cmH_2O。
- 吸呼比例(I∶E)：确定流速；通常为 1∶2，但在阻塞性气道疾病中增加呼吸分数以防止呼吸堆积(1∶4 或 1∶5)。

• 机械通风风险：
- 呼吸机相关性肺损伤：肺高压引起的过度膨胀会导致肺水肿和肺泡损伤。
- 减少损伤：以用适当的 PEEP 来降低因为肺泡反复开放和塌陷引起的炎症和损伤。
- 由于周期性再充气(即气胸、气腹、皮下气肿)导致的肺外气压伤。
- 氧中毒。
- 由于胸内压升高，静脉回流下降和随后心输出量/血压下降。
- 由于气体输送模式改变导致的通气血流比例不匹配增加(在自然呼吸中通常不会显著输送气体的肺泡将导致更多的气体交换，而没有任何增加的供血，并且肺泡的过度膨胀可能导致肺泡血液供应的压缩)。
- 上呼吸道感染。
- 相关的镇静风险(谵妄、长期卧床、疾病转为慢性)。
- 制动的相关风险(严重肌病、血栓形成、长期疾病等)。
- 应激性溃疡形成。
- 与气管导管或气管切开术有关的问题，如气管瘤性声带麻痹。

• 呼吸机故障排除：
- 保持足够的镇静和镇痛。
- 通过调整潮气量和呼吸频率来控制通气。
- 通过调节 PEEP 和 FiO_2 来控制氧合。
- 调整 FiO_2(目标<60%)。
- 使用 pH 来确定适当的通气量。
- 气道阻力高(支气管痉挛、分泌物或管扭结)可导致峰值压力升高；评估是否存在空气潴留，增加呼吸时间，根据需要降低呼吸频率。
- 平台压力(用吸气暂停评估)由肺和胸壁顺应性决定，并可能因 ARDS、肺纤维化、肥胖或水肿而升高；如果高，使用超声或 X 线进行气胸 r/o 检查，并评估合适 PEEP：
  - 当压力波形没有返回到设置 PEEP 时，就会出现自动 PEEP(需要呼气保持动作)。
  - 如果是自动 PEEP，则降低呼吸频率，增加吸气流量或增大 PEEP 设置。
- 如果明显低血压(胸腔内高压限制静脉回流)，断开患者与通气口的连接，手动减压胸廓，手动气囊，IVF，闭合性/开放性气胸。

药物治疗

• 镇静和镇痛策略应优先考虑控制疼痛，确定可能的最低镇静水平，并在采用输液之前采用间歇性推注治疗。

• 过量和苯二氮䓬类药物都伴有重症谵妄的风险。

• 异丙酚：0.3～1 mg/kg 静脉输注负荷剂量，维持 5～50 μg/(kg·min)静脉输注维持。引起血管舒张和相关的低血压。尤其是用药丸剂量，输注异丙酚有延长输液时间的风险。

• 右美托咪定：0.2～1.4 μg/(kg·h)，可用于负荷 1 μg/kg 的推注。不会导致呼吸抑制，可以与显著的心动过缓相关。

• 氯胺酮：负荷 1～3 mg/kg，维持 1～2 mg/kg。潜在的好处是可以避免血流动力学障碍。苯二氮䓬剂量可以帮助预防出现噩梦。关于使用氯胺酮增加颅内压的患者存在争议，但它可能实际上有助于维持机械通气患者的脑灌注压。

• 芬太尼：推注 0.5～1.5 μg/kg 肌内注射或缓慢静脉注射。输注速率从 1 μg/(kg·h)开始。给药时应考虑是否服用过阿片类药物。

• 沙丁胺醇：通过在线气管内输送，q4 h，2.5～5 mg/5 ml 盐水。

• 溴化异丙托溴铵：0.5 mg/2.5 ml 盐水，q4 h，小瓶经气管内输送。

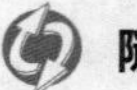

随访

进一步处理

入院指征

所有插管患者都需要 ICU 入院。

要点和误区

• 了解机械通气的适应证是选择通气和排气装置设置中最适用和危害最小的模式的关键。

• 用理想或 PBW 计算潮气量。

• 通过将 FiO_2 调整至 60%以防止氧气中毒。

• 哮喘和慢性阻塞性肺病患者需要限制性的气道压力和延长的呼气时间。

• 成功的 NIPPV 可能阻止插管，但是失败的 NIPPV 需要插管与死亡率增加相关。
- NIPPV 禁忌证：无法保护气道、呕吐、血流动力学不稳定、分泌物过多或不能容忍 NIPPV 口罩而意外脱落。
- NIPPV 对 COPD 和失代偿 CHF 最有益，但与低氧性呼吸衰竭、肺炎和 ARDS 患者预后不良有关。
- 在气管插管前，针对患有生理性分流患者进行预充氧有益。
- 在选择患者时必须谨慎，反复评估，并在需要时尽早插管。

H

呼吸窘迫 Respiratory Distress

Christopher James Watson · Michael N. Cocchi　袁晓伟　童朝阳 译

基础知识

描述

呼吸窘迫是病人呼吸困难的生理表现，是急症患者的常见主诉。

病因

- 上呼吸道梗阻：
- 过敏性反应。
- 会厌炎。
- 喉气管支气管炎（哮吼）。
- 异物。
- 血管性水肿。
- 脓液/积液。
- 咽后脓肿。
- 脓性颌下炎。
- 扁桃体周围脓肿。
- 心血管性：
- 肺水肿、充血性心力衰竭。
- 心律失常。
- 心肌缺血。
- 肺栓塞。
- 心包炎。
- 心脏压塞。
- 心肌病。
- 瓣膜病。
- 空气栓塞。
- 肺部：
- 哮喘。
- 慢性阻塞性肺疾病（COPD）、肺气肿。
- 肺炎。
- 流感。
- 恶性肿瘤/上腔静脉综合征。
- 病毒性感染（流感、呼吸道合胞病毒等）。
- 成人呼吸窘迫综合征（ARDS）。
- 胸腔积液。
- 胸腔积液、乳糜胸。
- 误吸。
- 毛细支气管炎。
- 生物武器（炭疽、鼠疫、兔热症、出血性病毒）。
- 外伤：
- 气胸。
- 张力性气胸。
- 血胸。
- 肋骨骨折。
- 肺挫伤。
- 高位颈椎损伤。
- 长骨骨折脂肪栓塞。
- 神经肌肉性：
- 吉兰-巴雷综合征。
- 重症肌无力。
- 代谢性、系统性和中毒性：
- 贫血。
- 碱中毒。
- 甲状腺功能亢进症。
- 脓毒症。
- 来自静脉药物的脓毒性栓子或留置导管感染。
- 药物过量（阿片类药物、镇静剂、乙醇、水杨酸盐）。
- 拟交感神经药物（可卡因、苯丙胺、嗜铬细胞瘤）。
- 肥胖（退化、限制性肺疾病）。
- 吸入性伤害（烟雾、一氧化碳）。
- 精神性：
- 焦虑障碍。
- 换气过度综合征。

儿科注意事项

- 呼吸衰竭是婴儿心脏停搏的最常见原因。
- 细支气管炎。
- <2 岁。
- 呼吸窘迫，轻微啰音，充血。
- 鼻导管吸氧和高流量氧气。
- 哮喘。
- ≥2 岁。
- 呼吸困难，喘息。
- 沙丁胺醇-异丙托品喷雾剂，类固醇，氧气。
- Croup 综合征包括：
- 6 个月至 6 岁。
- 呼吸窘迫，狂吠样咳嗽，喘鸣。
- 全身使用类固醇激素。
- 如果静息状态下喘鸣，予以去氧肾上腺素。
- 异物。
- 儿童，通常小于 3 岁。
- 可能呼吸窘迫，喘鸣。
- 直立和侧卧位 X 线片。
- 考虑到阻塞恶化的风险，请专家取出物体。
- 会厌炎：
- 2～4 岁发病率最高。
- 突然发作的呼吸窘迫及喘鸣。
- 气道分泌物过多，烦躁不安。
- 紧急送往急诊室进行起到管理并静脉给予抗生素。

妊娠注意事项

- 肺栓塞：包括血栓栓塞、羊膜栓塞和脓毒性流产或子宫感染的脓毒栓塞。
- 围生期扩张型心肌病。

诊断

症状和体征

- 低氧血症型呼吸衰竭。
- 呼吸过速，心动过速，躁动，低 SpO_2/PaO_2，低 $PaCO_2$，发绀，辅助肌肉使用。
- 最终导致呼吸肌疲劳及的高碳酸血症，如下所示。
- 高碳酸血症型呼吸衰竭。
- 呼吸迟缓，心动过缓，嗜睡，迟钝，高 $PaCO_2$。
- 上呼吸道损伤的体征：
- 喘鸣、喘息、声音嘶哑、分泌物控制不良、呼吸功增加/辅助肌肉使用。
- 下呼吸道损伤的体征：
- 气喘、啰音、多产性咳嗽（化脓、泡沫、血液）、呼吸音丧失、气管偏移、呼吸功增加、辅助肌肉使用。

病史

- 已知的心肺、肿瘤、肾脏、神经、肝脏、自身免疫、精神病、毒理学疾病。
- 近期发热或上呼吸道感染、咳嗽、咳痰、咽喉痛、全身性疾病、外伤。
- 最近旅游或病患接触史。
- 感染的危险因素。
- 免疫状态。
- 全身症状。

体格检查

- 视诊：呼吸频率、精神状态、痛苦程度、呼吸功/辅助肌肉的使用、颈静脉扩张、皮肤颜色。
- 触诊：远端肢体脉搏、胸壁、外周器官水肿。
- 叩诊：肺部浊音或共振、腹部膨胀或肝大。
- 听诊：气流运动、啰音或喘息、上呼吸道喘鸣音、心脏杂音、摩擦音、奔马律。

儿科注意事项

- 观察凹陷、行为、呼吸频率、呼吸音和

H

肤色。

• 新生儿窘迫的症状：新生儿哭声微弱、呼吸性呻吟、鼻翼扇动、气促、心悸及发绀。

基本检查

• 脉氧测定。
• 监护心脏及血压。
• X线胸片。
• 如怀疑心源性可行心电图。

诊断检查与说明

实验室检查

• 动脉血气分析反映疾病严重程度和酸碱比例。
• CBC。
• 基本代谢指标。
• 根据病情，考虑：
- 痰培养、涂片和革兰染色。
- B型利钠肽（BNP）：用于尚未区分的气短或慢性心力衰竭严重程度。
- D-二聚体。
- 肌钙蛋白。
- 病毒测试，包括流感。
- 毒理学检测。
- 记录尿排出量监测肺水肿。

影像学检查

• CXR：
- 肺炎。
- 气胸。
- 通气过度。
- 肺不张。
- 肺水肿。
- 脓肿、空洞性病变或其他浸润性疾病。
- 结核。
• 超声：
- 气胸。
- 胸腔积液。
- 肺水肿。
- 肋骨骨折。
• 超声心动图：
- 心脏压塞。
- 全心收缩力和左右心室扩大。
- 心室壁异常运动。
- 瓣膜运动异常。
• 用颈部CT或X线片评估会厌，软组织间隙，有无异物。
• 肺栓塞行CT血管造影或通气/灌注扫描。

儿童注意事项

• 胸、颈部X线可显示异物或Croup综合征的"尖顶征"。
• 有异物可行胸部X线透视评估呼吸运动。

诊断步骤/外科

• 纤维喉镜检查评估会厌、声带和咽腔。
• 支气管镜检查气管或支气管中异物。
• 严重CHF、ARDS、肺水肿行肺动脉（Swan-Ganz）置管。

鉴别诊断

见病因。

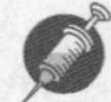

治疗

院前

• 患者处于舒适体位。
• 高流量氧气：
- 鼻插管，面罩，面罩吸入器。
- 辅助性囊-瓣面罩（BMV）通气。
• 气道辅助装置（经口或鼻）来维持气道通畅。
• 严重呼吸系统疾病行插管。
• 有可疑张力性气胸行针穿刺抽吸。

初步稳定/治疗

• ABC管理。
• 保证呼吸道通畅，严重呼吸窘迫或呼吸停止应行BVM辅助或插管。
• 低血压静脉补液。
• 面罩100％给氧：
- 严重COPD或慢性CO_2潴留患者应谨慎使用。
• 监测血压、心率、呼吸、脉氧。
• 心律失常或停搏的高级心脏生命支持。

急诊治疗/程序

• 适当处理潜在病因。
• 呼吸隔离预防措施。
• CHF或心源性肺水肿：
- 利尿剂。
- 硝酸甘油。
- 高血压使用硝普钠。
- 病情严重进行肺动脉置管。
- 严重时可插管。
• 哮喘、支气管炎、COPD：
- 沙丁胺醇-异丙托铵喷雾器。
- 激素。
- 镁治疗严重哮喘。
- 感染应用抗生素。
- 流感应用抗病毒药物。
- 严重时插管。
• ARDS。
- 机械通气与肺保护通气策略（低潮时气量为6 ml/kg，目标平台压力＜30 cmH_2O）。
- 激素使用有争议。
• 肺炎：
- 抗生素。
- 考虑耐药微生物的风险因素。
• 气胸：
- 可疑张力性气胸应立刻减压。
- 胸腔闭式引流术（见气胸）。
• 胸腔积液：
- 明确病因。
- 诊断性和治疗性胸腔穿刺。
• Croup综合征：
- 冷的、湿润的空气或氧气。
- 激素。
- 去氧肾上腺素。
- 抗生素治疗细菌性感染。
• 会厌炎：
- 尽量在手术室行插管或气管造口术立即稳定呼吸道。
- 针对流感嗜血杆菌使用抗生素。
• 过敏反应，血管性水肿：
- 静脉给予激素。
- H_1/H_2受体阻滞剂。
- 皮下注射或静脉给予肾上腺素。
- 早期插管。
- 考虑C1酯酶抑制剂或新鲜冷冻血浆遗传性血管性水肿。
• 脓肿：
- 引流。
- 静脉给予抗生素。
- 耳鼻喉科会诊。
• 心脏：
- 治疗心律失常或缺血。
- PE抗凝或溶栓。
- 心脏压塞行心包穿刺术。
- 心包炎使用非甾体抗炎药或阿司匹林。
• 神经肌肉：
- 必要时给予无创通气（NIV）或插管。
- 重症肌无力使用溴吡斯的明或新斯的明。
- 吉兰-巴雷综合征的血浆置换或IVIG治疗。
• 代谢性和中毒性：
- 治疗病因。
• 精神性的：
- 抗焦虑剂。

儿科注意事项

• 如果无法插管行经气管喷射通气（＜10岁儿童不推荐环甲膜切开术）。

• 毛细支气管炎：
- 支气管扩张剂。
- 呼吸道合胞病毒用抗病毒药物。
- 感染使用抗生素。
• 痉挛性哮吼：
- 对湿润空气非常敏感。
• 细菌性哮吼（假膜性喉气管支气管炎）：
- 覆盖金黄色葡萄球菌。

妊娠注意事项

• 对羊水栓塞及肺栓塞（PE）行支持性供氧和肝素治疗。
• PE 运用肝素。
• 脓毒性栓塞静脉输注抗生素。

■ 药物治疗

根据不同病因。

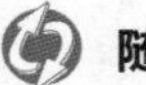 随访

■ 进一步处理

入院指征

• 需持续供氧。
• 心脏或血流动力学不稳定：
- 需输液。
- 需密切监测呼吸道或重复治疗。
- 呼吸道隔离。
• 基本病因或明显合并疾病的需要。

出院指征

• 根本病因纠正。
• 呼吸道情况稳定。
• 不需要紧急供氧。

转诊问题

根据具体病因。

要点和误区

• 注意免疫缺陷状态。
• 认为呼吸窘迫是心脏和毒性/代谢病理的继发性表现。
• 对脓毒症患者尽快开始抗生素治疗。

呼吸困难 Dyspnea

Matthew M. Hall · Christopher James Watson 姜颢 张连东 译

基础知识

■ 描述

不能舒适地呼吸。

• 许多可能的潜在疾病的一个症状。
• 是否与呼吸功增加相关。
• 通常是一种无意识的活动，呼吸困难是主观感觉，从轻微的不适到感觉到窒息。
• 是 3.5%急诊患者就诊的原因。
• 由于难以维持气体交换和酸碱平衡状态而引起。
• 可以反映通气、灌注、代谢功能或中枢神经系统驱动功能的损伤。
• 控制呼吸的机制：
- 控制中枢：
◦ 脑干和大脑皮质影响呼吸的自动和自主控制。
- 化学、牵张和刺激性感受器：
◦ CO_2 受体位于中枢和 O_2 受体位于外周。
◦ 机械感受器存在呼吸肌和牵张反应。
◦ 肺内机械对感受器化学刺激、充血反应、伸展做出反应。
- 呼吸中枢输出的效应器位于呼吸肌上，对中枢性刺激做出反应，使气体进出。
- 膈肌和呼吸肌的运动感觉的控制都是通过 $C_3 \sim C_8$ 神经和 $T_1 \sim T_{12}$ 神经控制。
• 任何神经感受器通路紊乱都导致产生呼吸困难：
- 呼吸困难感觉的多种病因都归因于控制呼吸的复杂机制。

■ 病因

• 上呼吸道：
- 会厌炎。
- 喉梗阻。
- 气管炎或支气管炎。
- 血管性水肿。
• 肺部：
- 气道肿块。
- 哮喘。
- 支气管炎。
- 胸壁创伤。
- 充血性心力衰竭。
- 药物引起的情况（例如，快克肺、阿司匹林过量）。
- 积液。
- 肺气肿。
- 肺癌。
- 转移性疾病。
- 肺炎。
- 气胸。
- 肺栓塞（PE）。
- 肺动脉高血压。
- 限制性肺疾病。
• 心血管：
- 心律失常。
- 冠状动脉疾病。
- 心内分流。
- 左心室衰竭。
- 黏液瘤。
- 心包疾病。
- 心脏瓣膜病。
• 神经肌肉：
- 中枢神经系统疾病。
- 肌病和神经病变。
- 膈神经和膈肌疾病。
- 脊髓疾病。
- 系统性神经肌肉疾病。
• 代谢性酸中毒：
- 脓毒症。
- 酮症酸中毒（糖尿病、酒精、饥饿）。
- 肾衰竭（容量过负荷、尿毒症）。
- 深硫胺素缺乏。
• 中毒：
- 高铁血红蛋白血症。
- 水杨酸中毒。
- 细胞窒息。
◦ 一氧化碳。
◦ 氰化物。
◦ 硫化氢。
◦ 叠氮化钠。
- 酒精中毒。
• 腹部压迫：
- 腹水。
- 妊娠。
- 重度肥胖。
• 心音性：
- 换气过度综合征。
- 焦虑。
• 其他：

- 高海拔。
- 过敏。
- 贫血。

老年注意事项

• 急诊就诊老年患者中最常见的诊断伴有呼吸困难。
- 失代偿性心力衰竭。
- 感染(肺炎、泌尿系统感染)。
- 慢性阻塞性肺病/哮喘。
- 肺栓塞。

儿科注意事项

• 在年龄<2 岁患者中,常见的鉴别诊断:
- 哮喘。
- 假膜性喉炎。
- 先天性气管畸形。
- 先天性心脏病。
- 异物误吸。
- 鼻咽部梗阻。
- 休克。

妊娠注意事项

• 孕妇肺活量下降,且有贫血倾向。

• 当仰卧位时,妊娠子宫压迫下腔静脉,导致呼吸困难和低血压。

• 妊娠期和产后不久发生 PE 的风险增加,同时围生期和产后发生羊水栓塞的风险增加。

诊断

症状和体征

• 困难、吃力或不舒服的呼吸。
• 上呼吸道:
- 喘鸣。
- 上呼吸道梗阻。
• 肺:
- 呼吸急促。
- 使用辅助呼吸肌。
- 气喘。
- 啰音。
- 呼吸音不对称。
- 呼吸运动减弱。
- 呼气相延长。
• 心血管:
- 第三心音奔马律。
- 舒张期杂音。
- 颈静脉怒张。
• 中枢神经系统:
- 意识水平改变。
- 肌力下降。
• 一般情况:
- 皮肤湿、冷与热、干。
- 面色苍白。
- 直立性体位。
- 杵状指。
- 发绀。
- 水肿。
- 酮症气味。

病史

• 有呼吸困难病史。
• 病程,发病急缓度,诱因和严重程度。
• 喘鸣或呼吸困难史。
• 运动(活动)耐力。
• 药物和近期依从性。
• 接触过敏原。
• 既往史。
• 伴随症状:
- 胸痛。
- 发热。
- 咳嗽。
- 咯血。
- 出血。

体格检查

• 急性呼吸窘迫综合征:
- 精神状态改变。
- 发绀。
- 呼吸频率。
- 吸气凹陷征表明严重疾病。
• 听诊肺部异常呼吸音:
- 哮鸣音。
- 啰音。
- 喘息音。
- 呼吸音减弱。

基本检查

• 脉搏血氧计:
- 可能会由于通气量增加或一氧化碳而假性升高。
- 给氧后仍 SPO_2 低的患者提示生理性分流或高铁血红蛋白血症。
- 在判断前确保波形良好。
- 可能需要清除指甲油或夹在耳上。
• 呼气末 CO_2:
- 快速提示 CO_2 分压。
- 波形能为病因提供线索。
• 胸部 X 线平片:
- 对大部分稳定的患者进行胸部正位和侧位片检查。
- 诊断肺部情况。
- 评估心脏大小和充血性心力衰竭的证据。
• 静脉血气分析:
- 用于评估 pH、PO_2 和 HCO_3^-。
- 和动脉血气(ABG)相比,静脉血气分析通常就够了,且更简单、更少痛苦、能更安全的获得。
- 静脉 pH 大约比动脉 pH 低 0.03。
- 静脉 PO_2 和动脉 PO_2 无相关性。
- 静脉 HCO_3^- 大约比动脉高 1.41 mEq。
• 动脉血气分析:
- 通常不是必须做的,由于有静脉血气分析,但是在高碳酸血症≥45 mmHg 或严重休克时,仍然有必要测定 $PaCO_2$。
- 计算动脉-肺泡梯度:
  ◦ a(在海平面)$=150-(PO_2-PCO_2)/0.8$,正常为 5~20。

诊断检查与说明

实验室检查

• 全血细胞计数:
- 评估贫血。
- 中性粒细胞计数帮助感评估染进程。
• 电解质、尿素氮、肌酸激酶、血糖:
- 怀疑有特定的代谢紊乱时应考虑。
- 充血性心力衰竭可能有 B 型利尿钠肽(BNP)升高。
• 毒理学检查。
• 高铁血红蛋白、一氧化碳血红蛋白水平。
• 甲状腺功能测试。
• D-二聚体(ELISA):
- 如正常可排除肺栓塞,但特异性相对较差。
- 减少为了肺栓塞而过度检测的策略包括:
  ◦ 对于>50 岁的患者,使用年龄调整的 D-二聚体(年龄×10)。
  ◦ 低风险的<50 岁的患者使用 PERC 判定原则。

影像学检查

• 渗出、浸润、气胸或者血管融合者查胸部 X 线平片。

• 怀疑肺栓塞者行 CT 肺血管造影(在稳定患者中,如果造影剂使用禁忌,通气-肺灌注扫描可能更有效)。

• 怀疑上呼吸道阻塞者行颈部软组织摄片、颈部 CT 或可视纤维镜。

诊断步骤/外科

• 怀疑心肌缺血、充血性心力衰竭、心包积液/压塞者行心电图。

• 床旁超声心动图评估右心劳损、心壁运动异常、心肌病、大体瓣膜病理。

• 评估气道反应性疾病者行最大呼气量/肺活量测定。

• 重症肌无力者行腾喜龙试验。

H

■ 鉴别诊断

- 抗胆碱能或肾上腺素能中毒综合征。
- 甲状腺危象。
- 孟乔森综合病征。

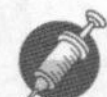

治疗

■ 院前

- 给所有患者补充供氧、脉搏血氧计、呼气末 CO_2，以及心脏监护仪。
- 当提示以下引起呼吸困难的可疑病因时，开始针对病因治疗：
  - 哮喘。
  - 慢性阻塞性肺疾病。
  - 充血性心力衰竭。
- 对即将发生的呼吸衰竭者应用高级气道。
- 许多呼吸困难可以用无创正压通气改善。

■ 初步稳定/治疗

- 常规治疗。
- 对即将发生呼吸停止者立即行气管插管：
  - 意识状态改变。
  - 生命体征不稳定。
- 危重患者应用 BiPAP：
  - 禁忌证：
    - 心脏不稳定。
    - 怀疑上呼吸道阻塞。
    - 精神状态萎靡。
    - 上消化道出血。

■ 急诊治疗/程序

- 基于潜在的病因：
  - 早期使用抗生素和液体治疗感染/脓毒症。
  - 针对慢性充血性心力衰竭的患者使用无创正压通气和利尿剂。
  - 针对哮喘的支气管扩张剂和皮质激素。
  - 针对心肌梗死的阿司匹林、肝素及 lyrics 导管试验。
  - 针对其他病因的必要治疗措施。
- 阿片类药物姑息治疗用于缓解终末期患者的呼吸困难。

随访

■ 进一步处理

入院指征

- 辅助通气。
- 在休息或运动时缺氧。
- 动脉-肺泡梯度>40。
- 身体状况需住院治疗。

出院指征

- 足够的氧合。
- 可以门诊处理的稳定疾病。
- 足够下地行走的脉氧和呼吸功。

转诊问题

基于可疑的潜在病因。

■ 随访建议

- 应当告知患者戒烟的短期和长期获益。
- 患者出现以下问题时应当返院：
  - 24 h 内无好转或加重。
  - 新发胸痛、压迫、压榨或紧缩样。
  - 寒战，或发热>102 ℉。
  - 新发或加重的咳嗽或喘息。
  - 腹痛、呕吐、剧烈头痛。
  - 头晕、惊慌或行为改变。
  - 任何症状出现重大变化，或任何相关的新发症状。

要点和误区

- 意识状态改变是严重呼吸困难患者需立即气道管理的指征。
- 呼吸困难可以并且应当被量化。
- 呼吸困难和呼吸急促的发生可能不伴有呼吸道疾病，而是由于代谢紊乱或严重中枢神经系统疾病。

呼吸暂停(儿童)

Sarah M. Halstead 李岩 王瑞兰 译

H

基础知识

■ 描述

- 呼吸性气流暂停 20 s，伴或不伴心率降低。
  - 中枢性呼吸暂停。
    - 呼吸信号在脑干和下行神经肌肉通路中的传播中断。
  - 阻塞性呼吸暂停。
    - 用力呼吸但没有气流。
    - 结构性气道阻塞，常伴有反常的胸壁运动。
    - 气道塌陷引起的功能性阻塞。
  - 混合性呼吸暂停。
- 简要解决的无法解释的事件(BRUE)：
  - 小于 1 岁的婴儿突然发作，短暂发作，现已消退并与以下一项或多项有关：
    - 青紫或苍白。
    - 缺乏、减少或不规则的呼吸。
    - 音调明显变化。
    - 响应度改变。
    - 经过适当的病史和体格检查后的临床表现和排除诊断。

■ 病因

- 感染：
  - 脓毒症。
  - 脑膜炎或脑炎。
  - 肺炎。
  - 百日咳和衣原体。
  - 呼吸道合胞病毒和其他呼吸道病毒感染。
- 呼吸系统：
  - 阻塞性气道病变：
    - 扁桃体和腺样体肿大。
    - 声带功能障碍。
    - 喉气管畸形。
    - 血管环。
    - 异物。
    - 颅面异常。
    - 胆道闭锁或狭窄。
  - 气道塌陷的功能性阻塞。
  - 感染。
  - 对缺氧、高碳酸血症的通气反应异常。
- 神经系统：
  - 癫痫发作。
  - 颅内出血。
  - 颅内压增高。
  - 肿瘤。
  - Arnold-Chiari 畸形或其他中枢神经系统畸形。
  - 摄入。
  - 毒素。
  - 缺氧性损伤。

- 神经肌肉疾病。
- 中心性肺换气不足综合征。
- 心脏：
- 节律紊乱。
- 先天性心脏病。
- 充血性心力衰竭。
- 心肌炎。
- 心肌病。
- 胃肠道：
- 胃食管反流病。
- 扭转。
- 肠套叠。
- 虐待儿童。
- 内分泌/代谢：
- 低血糖。
- 电解质紊乱。
- 先天性代谢异常。
- 其他：
- 短暂的窒息发作。
- 喉痉挛。
- 周期性呼吸。
- 屏气。

诊断

> **注意**
>
> 如果患者无呼吸，必须立即开始治疗。

症状和体征

呼吸暂停可能是目前存在的，之前发生的，或即将发生的。可以伴或不伴有心率或呼吸音改变。

病史

- 呼吸暂停持续时间。
- 状态：
- 睡着，醒着，哭着，与饮食、仰卧有关，容易发生。
- 用力呼吸：
- 没有呼吸，浅的呼吸，呼吸加深，挣扎着呼吸，窒息。
- 体表及部位颜色的变化。
- 眼睛的位置。
- 运动和肌肉张力的描述。
- 照顾者的干预措施。
- 前期症状，如发热或咳嗽。
- 之前的创伤。
- 过去的病史，包括早产、心肺、胃肠道、神经系统状况。
- 该患者有任何过往的 BRUE 病史或家庭成员猝死史。

体格检查

- 生命体征与温度。
- 生长参数：
- 体重。
- OFC。
- 动脉血氧饱和度。
- 气道和肺检查：
- 评估即将发生的呼吸暂停。
- 喘鸣或上气道阻塞的其他证据。
- 快或慢的呼吸。
- 辅助呼吸肌的使用。
- 外膜的肺鸣音。
- 心脏检查：
- 心律不齐、心动过速或心动过缓。
- 杂音。
- 慢性心力衰竭的证据。
- 神经系统检查：
- 评估精神状态。
- 评估外伤、癫痫发作或中毒综合征。
- 肌肉张力和反射。
- 眼底镜检查。

基本检查

- 完整的病史和体格检查。
- 病史因素和检查将直接影响诊断性评估和治疗。
- 酌情检查，清理上呼吸道。
- 酌情移除或抽吸气道分泌物。
- 对于考虑隐匿性创伤的要确保正确的头部定位。

诊断检查与说明

实验室检查

根据检查结果进行适当的检查：

- 血糖检查。
- CBC。
- 尿液分析。
- 集落刺激因子。
- 血液、尿液和脑脊液培养。
- 电解质(包括钙)。
- 尿素氮、肌酐。
- 血气分析。
- 呼吸道合胞病毒和呼吸道病毒的研究。
- 百日咳和衣原体试验。
- 考虑毒理学筛查(包括有毒的醇和对乙酰氨基酚)。
- 肝功能和氨检查。

影像学检查

根据报告进行适当的检查：

- 胸部 X 线片。
- 头颅 CT 或 MRI。
- 心电图。
- 上消化道检查。
- 怀疑中枢或阻塞性睡眠呼吸暂停的患者随访做多导睡眠图。
- 脑电图随访。

鉴别诊断

- 如前所述的多种病因。
- 特别注意事项：
- 屏气发作。
- 用力呼气导致反射性呼吸停止。
- 发绀和苍白。
- 发生在 0.1%～5%的健康儿童 6 个月至 6 岁龄时的突发事件。
- 新生儿周期性呼吸。
- 3 次或以上的呼吸暂停持续>3 s 且<20 s。
- 可能是正常的事件。

> **注意**
>
> 在新生儿中，需考虑隐匿性脓毒症。

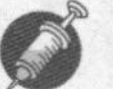

治疗

院前

- 呼吸支持。
- 如果呼吸恢复给予高流量氧气。
- 检查/清理上气道。
- 压迫环状软骨并给予面罩通气。
- 如果持续性呼吸暂停给予气管内插管。
- 静脉输液，吸氧，心电监护。
- 寻找潜在原因：
- 药物。
- 记录基本的神经系统检查：
- GCS 评分。
- 瞳孔。
- 肢体动作。
- 外伤的所有征象。
- 与家人或院前工作人员谈话，获得信息。

初步稳定/治疗

- 稳定病情。
- 检查/清除口咽部分泌物。
- 移除或吸除气道分泌物。
- 确保正确的头部定位。

急诊治疗/程序

- 如果目前处于窒息状态，给予呼吸面罩通气和高流量吸氧。
- 如果持续呼吸暂停，需要气管内插管。
- 给予适当复苏药物和抗生素。
- 如果怀疑屏气或呼吸衰竭，请提供支持和咨询。

药物治疗

- 急救抗生素剂量：
  - 头孢曲松：50 mg/kg，静脉注射。
  - 万可霉素：15 mg/kg，静脉注射。
  - 新生儿：氨苄西林：50 mg/kg，静脉注射；庆大毒素：2.5 mg/kg，静脉注射。
- 葡萄糖：2～4 ml/kg D_{25} W，静脉注射；或5～10 ml/kg D_{10} W，静脉注射。
  - 新生儿：1 个月，2～4 ml/kg D_{10} W，静脉注射。
- 纳洛酮：0.01～0.1 mg/kg，静脉注射、肌内注射、皮下注射或气管内给药。
  - 注意：长期使用阿片类药物的患者可能会出现戒断综合征。

随访

进一步处理

- 已有或即将发生窒息的患者应收入院适当的监测。那些持续生命体征异常的患者需要加强监护。

推荐参考儿童评估和随访转诊说明。干预措施可能包括进一步的观察、抗反流药物或咖啡因治疗，以及居家观察。

要点和误区

- 尤其是在新生儿中应考虑隐匿性脓毒症。
- 考虑隐性损伤。

华法林的并发症 Warfarin Complications

Joanne C. Routsolias　吴昊　李文放 译

基础知识

描述

- 最常见的口服抗凝血剂。
- 抑制维生素 K 的新陈代谢，以抑制Ⅱ、Ⅶ和Ⅹ因子。
- 抑制的外源性凝血途径和共同途径。
- 通常用于静脉血栓栓塞和人工心脏瓣膜或心房纤维性颤动后预防血栓形成。
- 基于国际标准化比值（INR）进行药物调整。
- 典型的控制范围在 2～3。
- 对于机械瓣膜和抗磷脂综合征控制在 2.5～3.5。
- 任何情况下出血或不良反应的风险超过临床效益的禁忌证。
  - 过敏史。
  - 皮肤反应。
  - 近期手术。
  - 活跃的或潜在的胃肠道、颅内的或者泌尿生殖器的出血。
  - 跌倒风险。

病因

- 出血并发症：
  - 每年 15%的患者。
    - 4.9%大出血事件。
    - 高达 0.8%的致命，最常见的颅内出血。
  - 出血风险与 INR 直接相关。
    - 当高于 4 时出血风险显著增加。
- 非治疗性疾病的危险因素：
  - 年龄>75 岁。
  - 高血压、脑血管疾病、严重心脏病。
  - 糖尿病、肾功能不全。
  - 酒精中毒或肝病。
  - 代谢过盛、发热。
  - 甲状腺功能亢进。
  - 癌症。
  - 胶原血管疾病。
  - 遗传华法林抵抗。
  - 细胞色素 P450 多态性。

常见药物反应

表 1

INR 增高	INR 下降
多种抗生素	卡马西平
NSAIDs	巴比妥酸盐
胺碘酮	利福平
普萘洛尔	氟哌啶醇
泼尼松	圣约翰麦芽汁
西咪替丁	高维生素 K 的食物
葡萄柚、大蒜	
银杏	

妊娠注意事项

- 妊娠等级 X。
- 穿过胎盘导致自发性流产和出生缺陷。

诊断

症状和体征

- 表现可能是隐匿性或剧烈性的。
- 需要高度怀疑潜在威胁生命的并发症。
- 开始使用或低 INR：血栓形成。
- 治疗性和超过有效浓度范围的：消化道、中枢神经系统、腹膜后出血。
- 皮肤坏死和肢体坏疽：
  - 华法林皮肤坏死和肢体坏疽的典型病变开始于第 3～8 日。
  - 皮下脂肪（皮肤坏死）的毛细血管性血栓形成和下肢静脉循环阻塞（肢体坏疽）。
  - 通常与蛋白质 C 缺乏有关。
  - 需鉴别焦痂与瘀斑。
- 药物过量。
  - 可能无症状。
  - 超级华法林（鼠药）会导致较长时间的出血风险（数月）。
  - 连续随访 INR。
  - 不要以经验的方法开始补充维生素 K，可能会掩盖 INR 升高的后期发展。
  - 考虑活性炭治疗。

基本检查

- 完整病史。
  - 许多主诉都因抗凝而变得复杂。
    - 抗凝治疗的原因、最近的剂量变化、依从性、最近的 INR 测试、其他处方、非处方和替代药物。
    - 精神状态的微妙变化，最近的“轻微跌倒”或流血。
- 检查生命体征异常：
  - 早期出血性休克。

H

- 高血压和心动过缓继发于颅内出血的库欣反应。
- 心脏药物往往掩盖了生命体征的重要变化。
• 细致检查：
- 苍白、挫伤、擦伤、瘀伤，在受影响的肢体和皮肤损伤中明显的脉搏。
- 检查粪便。

■ 诊断检查与说明

实验室检查

• PT、APTT、INR：
- 即使在 INR 治疗范围内也可能发生严重的出血。
- 在中毒时 APTT 也可升高。
- 在剂量过高时，升高可以延迟。
• 血常规：
- 早期的血细胞比容不准确测量急性快速出血。
- 血小板：阿司匹林和 ADP 抑制剂（氯吡格雷）导致了正常的血小板水平，但有功能上的缺陷。
• 电解质、BUN、肌酐、肝功能、葡萄糖：
- 升高的 BUN 可能提示胃肠道出血。
- 如果有服用药物的话，这些指标需要检测。
• 血型及交叉配血。

影像学检查

• 低阈值 CT 成像检测隐性出血而不是威胁生命的出血。
• 头部 CT：
- 无丧失意识情况下，头部创伤的较小病因。
- 在颅脑出血症状出现之前检测。
• 腹部 CT：
- 腹部钝挫伤，无压痛。
- 腹膜后出血。
- 实体器官或内脏损伤。

■ 鉴别诊断

• 所有出血的原因：
- 胃肠道、腹膜后、中枢神经系统，以及创伤性创伤。
• 皮肤出血性病变：
- 血小板障碍等止血功能障碍。
- 血管性紫癜包括糖皮质激素的使用、维生素 C 缺乏、紫癜风、弥散性血管内凝血、紫癜性肾炎、蛋白质 C 缺乏。

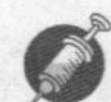

治疗

■ 院前

• ABC 管理。
• 建立两路大剂量静脉输液通路和生理盐水输液治疗低血压。
• 心脏和脉搏血氧测定。

■ 初步稳定/治疗

• 对于早期液体复苏效果不佳患者，建立中心静脉通路。
- 仅对于浓缩情况。
• 尽早补充补充丢失血液。
- 早期给予 O 型阴性血液直至可以输注特定血型血液。
- 对于儿童 10 ml/kg 快速补液。

■ 急诊治疗/程序

• 根据 INR、出血、抗凝的原因，以及患者的依从性，进行性针对性治疗。
- INR<5 并且没有出血：
◦ 降低服用剂量或暂停下一次服用。
◦ 在 24 h 内重新检查 INR。
- INR 5～9 并且没有出血：
◦ 停用下 1 剂或 2 剂，或停用 1 剂，并给予 1～2.5 mg，口服维生素 K。
◦ 如果增加出血或术前的风险，则服用维生素 K 1～5 mg，口服，INR 将在 24 h 内降低。
◦ 在 24 h 内重新检查 INR。
- INR>9 并且没有明显出血：
◦ 停用华法林并提供维生素 K 2.5～5 mg，口服。
◦ INR 将在 24～48 h 大幅降低。
- INR>20，有轻微出血或危及生命的出血，不考虑 INR：
• 停用华法林，慢静脉输液 10 mg，维生素 K。
◦ 新鲜冷冻血浆（FFP）或凝血酶原复合物（PCC），视剂型和适用性而定。
◦ PCC 能快速纠正 INR 以及止血；然而，在患者预后上中没有明显的益处。
◦ 在脑出血、大出血及容量过载中，优先考虑 PCC。
• 在控制出血的背景下，保持 INR 在较低的水平上：
- 1.5～2 的心房纤维颤动。
- 2～2.5 和机械心脏瓣膜。
• 在转移患者之前使用拮抗药物以获得更好的预后。

■ 药物治疗

• 维生素 K_1。
- 副作用：
◦ 静脉或口服过敏反应。
◦ 皮下注射吸收不可预测。
◦ 肌内注射可能会导致血肿的形成。
◦ 血栓栓塞纠正后，高剂量维生素可增加风险。
- 10 mg 静脉输液 10～30 min（建议用于危及生命的活动出血），1～2 h 后开始起效。
• FFP：
- 通常，3～4 U 的 FFP（1 L）可以在短期内控制持续的出血，而不会有过多的血栓栓塞风险。
- 必要时可能需要增加用量。
- 密切复查 INR。
- 患者的反应是无法预测，可能与 INR 的纠正不相关。
- 副作用：
◦ 液体负荷量增加。
◦ 罕见输注病毒导致感染。
◦ 输注相关的急性肺损伤：罕见。
• PCC：
- 保存期长和易于重组成高度浓缩的体积（20 ml 等效于 1 L 的 FFP/剂）。
- 快速输注不加重液体负荷。
- 副作用：
◦ 血栓形成。
◦ 比 FFP 更少发生病毒传播。
- 多项研究显示，与 FFP 相比，INR 的快速拮抗华法林作用，减少出血量。
- 与患者预后的关系还没有被证明。
- 4 因子 PCC（Kcentra）同时含 FFP 的分馏后的 4 种凝血因子，包含等量的 Ⅱ、Ⅶ、Ⅸ 和 Ⅹ 因子：
◦ FDA 在 2013 年批准了，但没有得到广泛的应用。
◦ 对于 INR2～3.9 的患者，给予 25 U/kg；INR4～5.9，35 U/kg；INR>6，50 U/kg。
- 3 因子 PCC（bebulin - VH，profilnide - SD）包含非常少量的 Ⅶa 因子。
◦ 根据可用性，单独使用 Ⅶa 或联合使用 Ⅶa。
◦ 50 U/kg 的 PCC 以及 1～2 mg FⅦa。
◦ 考虑 FFP 补充 FⅦa 不可用。
◦ 在美国更广泛地应用。
◦ 拮抗华法林是超说明书使用。

随访

进一步处理

入院指征

- 胃肠道活动性出血、腹膜后出血或中枢神经系统出血。
- 具有出血的证据的抗凝血创伤患者：
  - 抗凝血和血液置换。
  - 手术干预，早期外科咨询。
  - 在最初的稳定之后，需转运至 LEVEL Ⅰ水平的创伤中心进行进一步的治疗的情况。
- 皮肤坏死和肢体坏疽出现后，需要在与血液科医师协商后，予以替代抗凝治疗。
- 可能需要适当的抗凝治疗肝素或低分子肝素，以防止出现血栓栓塞患者：
  - 对于门诊依诺肝素治疗的患者，调整华法林使用和密切的随访，以减少不必要的住院治疗。

出院指征

- 无症状的稳定 INR 患者，经过以下评估：
  - 抗凝的适应证、超过有效治疗范围的原因、潜在的共病、出血的总体风险、跌倒的风险、社会状况、可靠性和随访的可用性。
- 具备以下条件的无症状抗凝患者：有轻微的创伤、治疗性的 INR、稳定的血红蛋白、正常的影像学和可靠的护理人员，可以通过密切的随访来出院。

转诊问题

- 患者应在 24～48 h 对初级护理医师或专科医师进行随访，复查 INR 并进行进一步的华法林调整。
- 对于故意用药过量者，建议精神科随访。

随访建议

- 对患者进行宣教，密切监大量出血和/或新的血栓事件的体征和症状。

要点和误区

- 对于创伤患者，华法林需保持低阈值。
- 对于 INR<5 不出血，不使用维生素 K。
- 维生素 K 静脉给药可能导致致命的过敏反应：
  - 此类患者仅在 INR>20 合并少量出血的患者中使用，或有危及生命的出血患者。
  - 其他患者予以口服。
- 为了快速拮抗华法林作用，FFP 仍然被认为是一线治疗。
- 4-因子 PCC 或 3-因子/FⅦa 应该用于治疗颅内出血、限制液体量或大量出血患者。

滑囊炎 Bursitis

Patrick H. Sweet · Uziel Sauceda　沈黎蔚 译

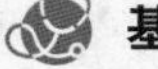

基础知识

描述

- 滑囊是充满滑液的囊。
  - 约有 150 个滑囊分布于骨骼、韧带、肌腱、肌肉和皮肤。
- 它们在行动时提供润滑以减轻摩擦。
- 滑囊炎是由于创伤、过度使用、感染、结晶沉积或全身系统性疾病引起的滑囊的炎症。
- 慢性滑囊炎会引起滑囊的增生性改变。
- 常受累的部位。
  - 肩部(肩峰下)。
  - 肘部(鹰嘴)：通常继发于创伤。
  - 髋关节(大转子、坐骨、髂腰肌)：常发生于老年人。值得注意的是，转子滑囊炎并不像此前认为的那么常见，更常见的疼痛是由外展肌附着点病变引起的。
  - 膝关节(髌前和鹅掌)：继发于创伤或关节炎。
  - 足(跟骨)：最常继发于穿不合适的鞋/鞋跟。

病因

- 创伤(最常见的原因)。
  - 关联关节的特殊创伤或反复使用。邻近肌腱撕裂(如急性肩袖撕裂)。
- 感染：二次直接渗透，可能是明显的或微观的。
  - 糖尿病、慢性酒精过量、尿毒症、痛风、免疫抑制患者患病的风险更高。
  - 90%的患者由葡萄球菌引起。
- 结晶沉积：磷酸钙、尿酸。
- 全身系统性疾病：类风湿性关节炎、痛风、强直性脊柱炎、银屑病关节炎、狼疮、风湿热。

诊断

症状和体征

病史

- 急性或慢性。
- 有创伤、过度使用或长时间受压史。
- 随着轴关节的活动增加或受压而出现疼痛。
- 功能性主诉(如跛行)。
- 有局部肿胀病史。
- 全身系统性疾病的局部症状。
- 有痛风、假性痛风或风湿性疾病史。
- 滑囊有近期损伤史(如穿刺抽吸术、感染等)。

体格检查

- 无菌性滑囊炎有轻微的触痛。
- 活动时会有局部的疼痛。
- 由于调整被动的关节活动度通常会降低主动的关节活动度(ROM)。
- 局部肿胀，特别是浅表滑囊。
- 滑囊表面有皮肤创伤。
- 皮温升高且有红斑。
- 脓毒性滑囊炎可能会发热。
- 脓毒性滑囊炎通常会有红斑、发热、肿胀、轻微触痛的综合征。

基本检查

- 全面评估邻近的骨骼肌肉组织。
- 任何怀疑感染的滑囊的穿刺抽吸术(特别是鹰嘴和髌前的滑囊)。
- 避免针道直接穿过关节紧张处的横向方法。
- 在超声引导下或依据相关意见行髋关节或其他深部关节的穿刺抽吸术。

诊断检查与说明

实验室检查

- 血清学检查：
  - 怀疑感染：CBC。
  - 相关的系统性疾病的评估(如痛风患者的

尿酸水平)，风湿性疾病患者的 ESR 和 CRP 水平。

- 行滑囊液体抽吸术的患者的血糖。

• 滑囊液体分析：

- 滑囊液的全细胞数、葡萄糖、总蛋白、晶体测定、革兰染色及微生物培养。

- 微生物培养通常是需要的。

- 正常的滑囊液：滑囊液通常是黄色的，有 0～200 个白细胞，0 个红细胞，低蛋白、葡萄糖和血清中相同。

- 创伤性滑囊炎：滑囊液是血性/黄色的，有＜1 200 个白细胞，大量红细胞，低蛋白，葡萄糖正常。

- 脓毒性滑囊炎：液体是浑浊的黄色，有＞50 000 个白细胞，少量红细胞，蛋白质升高，葡萄糖降低，细菌革兰染色。

- 风湿以及警惕性炎症(无菌性滑囊炎)：液体是黄色的，偶尔是浑浊的，有 1000～40000 个白细胞，少量红细胞，蛋白少量增加，葡萄糖水平是可变的，晶体的显微镜检查。

影像学检查

• X 线检查显示软组织肿胀或邻近的慢性关节改变或钙沉积。

- 特别推荐用于排除骨折性创伤或异物，也推荐用于评估老年患者的肿瘤转移和病理性骨折。

• MRI 和超声可以用于诊断深部滑囊炎及确定脓毒性滑囊炎的范围。

• CT 检查也有助于从非特殊性滑囊炎中区分特殊性滑囊炎。

鉴别诊断

• 关节炎：感染性、炎症性、风湿性及退行性关节炎(骨关节炎)。

• 痛风及假性痛风。

• 肌腱炎、筋膜炎、外上髁炎。

• 骨折、肌腱/韧带撕裂、挫伤、扭伤。

• 骨髓炎。

• 神经卡压。

• 也发生在髋关节：神经炎、腰椎病、骶髂关节炎。

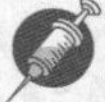

治疗

院前

从该病中区分出骨折可能有些困难；可疑的关节应该被固定，特别是在创伤患者中。

初步稳定/治疗

• 疼痛严重时应该固定关节。

• 肩部应该固定＞2～3 日，因为有粘连性关节囊炎的风险。

急诊治疗/程序

• 非脓毒性滑囊炎。

- 注意休息并去除使疾病加重的因素(如避免直接的压力及过度使用关节，必要时使用保护垫)。

- 冰敷患处 10 min，每日 4 次直到症状好转，后改为热敷。

- 使用 NSAIDs 药物至少 7 日，最好在症状好转后继续使用 5 日以避免复发。

- 如果有波动感，将液体抽出并使用敷料压紧。

- 如果 5～7 日后症状好转且已排除感染(通过微生物培养)，需考虑使用利多卡因和皮质类固醇注射。

• 用 2 ml 利多卡因与适量的 depo-糖皮质激素混合，使用消毒注射器将 1～3 ml 混合液注入滑囊腔内。

• 4 周内只能行 1 次类固醇注射，未经专业意见的情况下每个滑囊腔注射不能＞2 次。

- 炎症消退后通常需要行物理治疗。

• 脓毒性滑囊炎。

- 浅表滑囊：在严密监测的情况下可以使用滑液抽吸术及抗生素。

- 其他的大部分滑囊：使用抗生素及关节引流术(放置引流管可以减少治疗周期并避免最后行滑囊切除术)。

- 发热的患者需静脉注射抗生素。

- 结合革兰染色结果或者依据当地细菌感染经验选择抗生素。

• 找到革兰阳性球菌选用耐青霉素酶青霉素，如果球菌成簇出现时抗生素需覆盖到 MRSA。

• 如找到革兰阴性菌，需行血培养并寻找其他的主要的感染源。

• 抗生素需使用 5～7 日直到感染症状消失(并且仍需要随访)。

• 需治疗相关疾病(如痛风)。

治疗药物

• NSAIDs(很多选择，这里列举一小部分)。

- 萘普生：500 mg，口服，q12 h。

- 布洛芬：600 mg，口服，q6 h(儿童：5～10 mg/kg，口服，q6 h)。

- 酮咯酸：30 mg，静脉注射或肌内注射，q6 h；或 10 mg，口服，q4～6 h。

- 美洛昔康：7.5 mg，口服，q12 h；或 15 mg，口服，每日 1 次。

• 滑囊内感染的皮质类固醇治疗。

- 曲安奈德：20～40 mg(一次)。

- 醋酸甲基氢化泼尼松：20～40 mg。

- 醋酸地塞米松/钠：8 mg。

- 倍他米松磷酸钠/醋酸酯：3 mg。

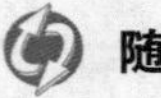

随访

进一步处理

• 大部分患者可以院外治疗。

• 大部分患者 3～4 日对治疗就有反应，并需每周或需要时随访。

• 脓毒性滑囊炎需每 3～5 日反复行滑囊抽吸术直到无液体产生。

入院指征

• 有系统性炎症反应综合征(SIRS)，广泛蜂窝织炎，不能口服抗生素，院外治疗失败或免疫抑制的患者。

• 机体异常，原发部位在滑囊外或深部滑囊受累的患者。

出院指征

• 可以耐受疼痛。

• 脓毒性滑囊炎在接受了适合的治疗以及严密随访下可以安全出院。

转诊问题

风湿科或骨科推荐给对于关节内注射类固醇无反应或复发性滑囊炎或需要手术治疗的患者。

随访建议

• 脓毒性滑囊炎患者密切随访。

• 症状加重的患者必要时可去急诊室，除此之外推荐于初级保健医师处随访。

要点和误区

• 单项检测以区分创伤和脓毒性滑囊炎是不可靠的。

- 抽吸术和滑液分析可能是区分的唯一方法。

• 当心口服 NSAIDs 药物相关的消化道出血及酮咯酸相关肾损伤。

• 如果出现 4 个感染症状(肿、痛、红、热)，那么很可能是脓毒症，但是仍然需要抽吸术和培养。

• 晶体沉积病、黏液囊炎因酷似感染而“声名狼藉”。

• 抽吸感染囊时要注意相邻关节间形成赘生物的可能。

H

化学武器中毒 Chemical Weapons Poisoning

Patrick M. Whiteley 庄育刚 张中琳 译

基础知识

描述

当受害者暴露于化学制剂后导致的中枢神经系统、呼吸系统、心血管系统、皮肤、眼睛或胃肠道系统的损伤。

病因

- 全身中毒制剂：氰化物。
  - 通过抑制细胞呼吸结合铁离子在细胞色素氧化酶 a-a3 和解偶联氧化磷酸化。
- 起泡剂：硫芥子气、氮芥、糜烂性毒气、光气肟。
  - 烷基化和交联的嘌呤碱基的 DNA 和氨基酸导致核酸结构的变化导致核酸、蛋白质和细胞膜结构的变化。
- 催泪剂和防暴剂：1-氯苯乙酮(CN，Mace)、邻氯苯亚甲基丙二腈(CS)、脂溶性的辣椒喷雾(OC)、三氯硝基甲烷、亚当式毒气(DM)。
  - 黏膜刺激剂。
- 肺刺激物(窒息物)：
  - 高水溶性毒物：氨。
    - 眼睛和上气道的黏膜刺激物。
  - 中水溶性毒物：氯。
    - 以盐酸、次氯酸的形式，形成游离小分子刺激上气道和肺组织。
  - 低水溶性毒物：光气。
    - 最初只是轻微的刺激反应，之后 24 h 后出现延迟的肺水肿。
    - 当吸入的毒物水解为盐酸可以直接导致肺损伤。
- 神经毒物：
  - 抗胆碱酯酶抑制剂-胆碱能过度刺激导致毒蕈碱样、烟碱样和中枢神经反应。
- 失能剂：二苯羟乙酸-3-喹咛环酯(BZ)：
  - 抗胆碱能(抗毒蕈碱)。

诊断

症状和体征

病史

有多名受害者、火灾、明确的暴露病史。

体格检查

- 血液毒物(氰化物和氰化物)：
  - 主要体征：
    - 呼吸急促和呼吸过度(早期)，呼吸衰竭(晚)。
    - 高血压和心动过速(早期)，低血压和心动过缓(晚)。
    - 几秒至几分钟死亡。
  - 神经系统：
    - 头痛。
    - 精神状态。
    - 癫痫。
  - 肺水肿：
    - 呼吸困难。
    - 非心源性肺水肿。
    - 发绀。
  - 消化系统：
    - 苦杏仁的味道(有时)。
    - 口腔和咽喉的烧灼感。
    - 恶心、呕吐。
- 水溶性毒物(芥气、路易斯毒气)：
  - 一般情况：
    - 死亡率为 2%～4%。
  - 皮肤损伤：
    - 皮肤接触毒物后 2～24 h 出现的皮肤红斑、水肿、瘙痒。
    - 皮肤接触毒物后 2～18 h 出现皮肤坏死和水疱形成。
  - 头、眼、耳、鼻和喉(HEENT)：
    - 由于气道分泌物、气道塌陷引起的气道阻塞。
    - 喉头痉挛、咽喉疼痛、鼻窦炎。
    - 眼睛疼痛、畏光、流泪、视物模糊。
    - 眼睑痉挛、眼周围水肿。
    - 结膜水肿、角膜溃疡。
  - 呼吸道症状：
    - 支气管痉挛、支气管炎。
    - 呼吸衰竭。
    - 频繁咳嗽。
  - 消化道症状：
    - 恶心、呕吐。
  - 血液系统：
    - 白细胞减少。
- 催泪剂和防爆剂(催泪性毒气)：
  - 头、眼、耳、鼻和喉(HEENT)：
    - 眼睛疼痛。
    - 流泪。
    - 眼睑痉挛。
    - 一过性失明。
  - 皮肤疾病：
    - 皮肤刺激。
    - 丘疹、水疱(催泪性毒气较多见)。
    - 浅度烧伤。
  - 呼吸系统：
    - 咳嗽。
    - 胸部紧迫感。
    - 咽喉干涩。
    - 窒息感。
    - 当在密闭环境吸入高浓度毒气后出现的肺水肿。
- 肺部刺激剂(窒息剂)：
  - HEENT。
    - 咽痛、流泪、眼睑痉挛。
  - 肺部症状：
    - 呼吸急促、咳嗽、支气管痉挛。
    - 胸痛。
    - 接触毒物后最迟 24 h 发生的肺水肿(光气中毒)。
- 神经毒素[沙林、二甲氨基氰磷酸乙酯、甲氟膦酸频那酯、维艾克斯(VX)]：
  - SLUDGEBAM 综合征：
    - 流涎(S)。
    - 流泪(L)。
    - 尿失禁(U)。
    - 腹泻(D)。
    - 消化道痉挛(G)。
    - 呕吐(E)。
    - 支气管炎、支气管收缩、心动过缓(多数危及生命)(B)。
    - 胃肠道紊乱(A)。
    - 瞳孔缩小(M)。
  - HEENT。
    - 瞳孔缩小。
    - 唾液分泌过多、多汗、流泪、支气管淋巴结增大。
  - 神经系统：
    - 易激惹、神经质。
    - 眩晕。
    - 乏力、倦怠、抑郁。
    - 共济失调、惊厥、昏迷。
  - 肺部症状：
    - 支气管痉挛。
    - 支气管炎。
  - 消化系统：
    - 恶心、呕吐、腹泻。
    - 腹部疼痛、痉挛。

H

◦ 大小便失禁。
• 失能剂(BZ):
- 抗胆碱能(抗毒蕈碱的)中毒综合征:
◦ 发热。
◦ 口干。
◦ 皮肤潮红。
◦ 失明。
◦ 精神失常。
◦ 高血压。
◦ 心动过速。
◦ 尿潴留。
◦ 肠鸣音减弱。

基本检查

• 毒物接触的病史和症状是关键。
• 体格检查:
- 氰化物(苦杏仁味、昏睡、降血压药、代谢性酸中毒)。
- 芥末(虚弱、甜芥末味、大蒜味、水疱、脱落的皮肤、呼吸困难)。
- 检查 SLUDGEBAM 综合征。
- 催泪剂(眼睛刺激、流泪、睑痉挛)。
- 令人窒息的毒物(支气管痉挛引起的呼吸困难)。

诊断检查与说明

实验室检查

• 动脉血气分析:
- 氰化物:
◦ 动静脉血氧饱和度差值减小。
◦ 乳酸酸血症与高阴离子间隙代谢性酸中毒。
◦ 静脉血的动脉血化。
◦ 氰化物水平无法在临床相关的时间内进行检测。
• 全血细胞计数(CBC):
- 白血球减少症、接触芥子导致的血小板减少贫血。
• 电解质、尿素氮、肌酐、血糖。
• 尿常规。
• 肌酸磷酸激酶。
• 神经毒气的红细胞胆碱酯酶活性。

影像学检查

X线片。

鉴别诊断

• 哮喘、COPD。
• 史蒂文斯-约翰逊综合征。
• 中毒性表皮坏死松解症。
• 慢性天疱疮。
• 烫伤样皮肤综合征。
• 有机磷和氨基甲酸酯农药中毒。
• 肉毒中毒。
• 辐射中毒。
• 充血性心力衰竭。
• 过敏反应。

治疗

院前

• 应避免环境污染和医源性污染。
- 使用 A 级或 B 级的个人防护装备。
- 去除污染:
◦ 皮肤湿性去污主要用于神经和起泡剂。
◦ 干去污(去除衣服和首饰)适用于其他毒物。
• 使用阿托品,即使患者心动过速,因为环境可能导致患者缺氧。

初步稳定/治疗

• ABC 管理。
• 患者去污:
- 刷去化学粉尘。
- 用大量清水或生理盐水冲洗皮肤和眼睛。
- 转移和处置的衣物要使用双层的包装。
• 对医护人员的防护:
- A 级或者 B 级的个人防护套装。
- 化学防护套装。
- 厚重的橡胶手套和靴子,氯丁橡胶手套。
• 给予吸氧,心电监测,氧饱和度测定。
• 建立静脉通路补充生理盐水。

急诊治疗/程序

• 去除污染:避免二次污染。
• 血液毒物:
- 高流量 100% NRB 氧气。
- 苯二氮䓬类药物治疗癫痫发作。
- 羟钴胺素(一线用药)。
- 氰化物解毒剂(二线用药),可能会重复使用。
• 发泡剂:
- 支持性护理。
- 基础代谢管理。
- 阿托品,缓解眼睛疼痛。
- 监测容量、电解质平衡,完整的血液生化指标。
- 监测全血细胞计数。
- 脓毒症、贫血、出血的支持性护理。
- 粒细胞集落刺激因子(G-CSF)对症治疗中性粒细胞减少症。
• 窒息剂、催泪剂和防爆剂:
- 支持性护理,给予支气管扩张剂治疗。
- 冲洗眼睛。
- 拍摄胸部 X 线片和密切监测呼吸道并发症。
- 若是光气中毒,要求 24 h 内严密监测防止延迟肺水肿的发生。
• 神经毒气:
- 支持性护理:
◦ 吸入 100%氧气。
◦ 增加吸痰次数。
- 阿托品 2 mg,静脉注射,q5 min 直到支气管的黏液分泌减少、支气管狭窄、支气管狭窄和血氧不足情况改善。
◦ 患者可以出现毒蕈碱样反应和一些中枢神经系统反应,但是没有导致肌肉骨骼的乏力或呼吸衰竭。
◦ 瞳孔散大和心率增快不是判断阿托品化的指标。
- 患者恢复意识和自主呼吸后停止阿托品(可能会周期性复发),尽可能多地去扭转呼吸抑制。
- 氯解磷定(2-PAM 或氯磷定制剂)。
◦ 胆碱酯酶复活剂通过逆转磷酸化起作用(除非已经发生了老化)。
◦ 减少异常的骨骼肌运动,改善肌无力,同时扭转松弛性瘫痪。
◦ 可以重复首次剂量或开始持续滴注。
◦ 如果首次剂量后患者情况改善,在 60~90 min 可以再次给予重复。
- 地西泮:控制癫痫发作。
• 失能剂(BZ):
- 支持治疗。
- 积极的静脉补液。
- 苯二氮䓬类用于亢奋和肌肉活动增强的患者。
- 毒扁豆碱中毒的患者应该考虑与中毒中心联系。

药物治疗

• 沙丁胺醇喷雾:2.5 mg 融入 2.5 ml 生理盐水中(儿童:每次 0.1~0.15 mg/kg)。
• 阿托品:2 mg 肌内注射或静脉注射(严重中毒的成人患者使用 5~6 mg;儿童:0.02~0.08 mg/kg),然后每 5~10 min 根据临床效应给予滴定式治疗。连续输注 2 mg/min 或更高的剂量已用于有机磷酸盐中毒。
• 氰化物解毒剂:
- 吸入亚硝酸异戊酯 30 s qmin 直至亚硝酸钠药物的使用。
- 亚硝酸钠:10 ml 3%浓度的溶液或 300 mg 3~5 min 静脉注射(儿童:0.15~0.33 ml/kg)。

◦ 监测血红蛋白水平使其变化小于30%。
- 硫代硫酸钠：25%浓度的溶液50 ml，静脉注射或12.5 g(儿童：1.65 ml/kg)。
• 地西泮：5～10 mg，超过3～5 min，静脉注射(儿童：0.2～0.4 mg/kg，最大剂量为10 mg大于2～3 min，静脉注射)。
• 维生素 B_{12}：5 g，静脉注射。
• 氯解磷定(2-PAM，氯解磷定制剂)：1～2 g，超过20～30 min 静脉注射或600 mg 肌内注射(溶解为300 mg/ml 的浓度)，阿托品剂量(儿童：每次25～50 mg/kg，静脉注射)，如果肌无力无明显改善的情况下2 h内可再追加一次，根据病情需要，在4～6 h可再次给予治疗有机磷中毒患者给予500 mg/h持续静滴。

随访

进一步处理

入院指征

• 有显著临床症状的患者收入ICU。
• 有起水疱、窒息、催泪剂，失能剂中毒的患者需要进一步观察的患者收入院。
• 至少12 h的神经毒剂暴露观察(低水平暴露最初可能主要表现为胃肠道症状)。

出院指征

• 控制风险。
• 如果症状消失进一步在急诊观察6 h可出院。

要点和误区

必须进行足够的去污处理。

踝关节骨折/脱位 Ankle Fracture/Dislocation

Samantha E. M. McGlone · Leslie C. Oyama 马林浩 林兆奋 译

基础知识

描述

踝关节的常见机制及损伤模式：
• 损伤机制：
- 反转损伤：
◦ 外踝撕脱性骨折。
◦ 内踝斜形骨折。
- 外翻损伤：
◦ 内踝撕脱性骨折。
◦ 腓骨斜形骨折。
- 外旋损伤：
◦ 胫腓联合的中断，或远端腓骨骨折。
◦ 伴有远端胫腓骨分离的胫骨前方或后方骨折(不稳定骨折)。
- 反转和外旋骨折(Maisonneuve 骨折)：
◦ 内踝撕脱性骨折或三角韧带撕裂。
◦ 胫腓联合的破坏。
◦ 腓骨近端的斜形骨折。
- 反转和背屈(滑雪者骨折)：
◦ 距骨外侧突骨折。
- 后脱位最常见。足底屈脚向后力的结果，常伴有胫腓韧带破裂或外踝骨折。
• 流行病学：
- 大多数踝部骨折是踝。
- 常见于年轻男性和50～70岁女性。
- 与吸烟和高BMI相关。

儿科注意事项

• 儿童踝关节骨折常累及骺板(生长板)：
- 可能会导致因生长板损伤所引起的慢性畸形。
- 小于10岁的儿童，生长板弱于骨骺。
• Tillaux骨折：由外翻及侧旋引起的胫骨侧方骨骺的Salter-Harris Ⅲ型损伤。
• 三平面骨折：骨折线在3个不同平面(冠状面、横断面和矢状面)的胫骨远端异常骨折。

诊断

症状和体征

• 外伤史。
• 局部踝关节疼痛、肿胀、畸形。
• 无法负重。
• 软组织损伤、肿胀、瘀斑、皮肤隆起、皮肤苍白。
• 神经血管损害。
- 毛细血管再充盈减慢。
- 胫后(PT)或足背(DP)脉搏减弱。
• 关节活动度受限。

病史

• 弄清受伤时踝关节位置。
• 确定患者伤后是否能够立即行走或者后来行走是否需要帮助。
• 询问患者是否听到有响声，因为这可能表明肌腱部分或全部断裂。

体格检查

• 渥太华踝关节规则，100%敏感，对疑似损伤到踝和足中部的患者开放射学检查的决策规则。
- 踝部(如果存在以下任一发现，而后足踝X线片证实)：
◦ 踝后缘或远端6 cm(A点和B点)有骨压痛。
◦ 在受伤后和急诊室，不能连续走4步。
- 足弓区(如果存在以下任一发现，而后足部X线片证实)：
◦ 在第5跖骨基底(C点)有骨压痛。
◦ 舟骨中部(D点)有骨压痛。
◦ 在受伤后和急诊室，不能连续走4步。
- 被认为是5岁以上儿童的可靠评估工具。
• 评估皮肤是否肿胀、瘀斑、破裂或缺血。
• 仔细评估末梢血管状况。
- 毛细血管再灌注。
- 足背和胫骨后部脉搏触诊或超声多普勒。
• 触诊腓骨近端压痛，尤其当内踝或三角韧带出现压痛：
- 当伴有Maisonneuve骨折时，腓总神经有损伤的风险。
◦ 环绕腓骨头。
◦ 测试胫骨前肌和踇长伸肌。
◦ 评估空间感觉。

诊断检查与说明

影像学检查

• X线：
- 如果踝部有压痛，从前后(AP)、横向、复合(腿内旋20°)的角度观察踝关节。
- 评估复合的角度，使内侧空间增宽至大于4 mm和胫腓间隙大于6 mm。
- 以下特殊情况下考虑X线检查：
◦ 感觉改变或肢体远端的感觉减退。
◦ 多处疼痛及损伤。
◦ 评估10日前发生的损伤。
• 不稳定踝关节骨折或脱位要求夹板治疗后的3个平面的复位X线片。

• 如果临床上怀疑有 Maisonneuve 骨折，需要做前后和横向的胫、腓骨 X 线片。

• 如果患者将在 3～7 日复查，不必在急诊室对疼痛膝关节进行韧带的压力测试。

• 踝关节的应力 X 线片通常是不必要的。

• CT 扫描或 MRI。

- 评估胫骨远端的损伤程度。

诊断步骤/外科

N/A。

鉴别诊断

• 踝关节扭伤。

• 跟腱损伤。

• 三角骨骨折。

• 第 5 跖骨骨折(琼斯骨折)。

• 腓骨肌腱脱位或损伤。

• 距骨骨折。

• 距骨穹窿骨折/损伤。

• 距下关节脱位。

• 跟骨骨折。

• 足部骨折。

• 踝关节分离。

• 响尾蛇咬伤。

儿科注意事项

• 生长板损伤可能在 X 线平扫上不明显。

• 如果临床怀疑是有依据的，即使 X 线片不支持，也要考虑固定、非负重状态和骨科转诊。

• 可以进行 CT 扫描或 MRI 检查来观察损伤的程度。

• 对于伤到骨骺的患者，要告知父母有生长发育异常的可能性。

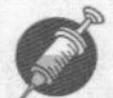

治疗

院前

• 软夹板固定以减少疼痛、出血和进一步损伤。

• 注意事项：

- 牵引装置通常是不必要的。

◦ 开放性损伤禁忌。

- 不应复位突出的骨，伤口应使用干净的敷料覆盖。

初步稳定/治疗

• 避免负重。

• 冷敷。

• 加压。

• 抬高。

急诊治疗/程序

• 踝关节骨折：

- 所有的踝关节骨折或脱位均需骨科会诊或转诊。

- 开放性踝关节骨折：

◦ 清理污染物。

◦ 应用湿润无菌敷料。

◦ 评估破伤风免疫。

◦ 抗生素。

◦ 急诊骨科会诊。

- 闭合性踝关节骨折：

◦ 必要时进行闭合复位。

◦ 后夹板固定。

◦ 后夹板用大量的敷料将足部固定在 90°位置，并由足底的(后方的)和接骨(U 型板)夹板材料覆盖。

- 稳定性损伤(只有踝部一个面受到损伤)：

◦ 不累及中间部的外踝独立性损伤几乎都是稳定的。

◦ 使用后夹板。

- 不稳定性损伤(足踝的两个面受到损伤)：

◦ 紧急骨科会诊。

◦ 与稳定性损伤相同的后夹板固定。

◦ 可能需要在出现明显肿胀之前进行紧急切开复位内固定(ORIF)。

- 神经血管损伤需要紧急骨科会诊。

• 踝关节脱位：

- 应尽快进行闭合复位以降低皮肤缺血和距骨缺血性坏死的风险。

- 皮肤皱褶和神经血管受累的证据是立即复位的指征，甚至优于 X 线片。

- 大多数踝关节脱位需切开复位内固定治疗。

- 复位后，放置后夹板。

药物治疗

• 闭合性骨折：

- 主要是镇痛药(阿片类药物)。

• 需要闭合复位的脱位或移位骨折：

- 短效苯二氮䓬类(咪达唑仑 0.05～0.1 mg/kg，静脉注射)或巴比妥类(美索比妥 1～1.5 mg/kg，静脉注射)与阿片类镇痛剂。

• 开放性骨折：

- 头孢唑林：2 g 负荷剂量(儿童：50 mg/kg)，静脉注射。

- 万古霉素：如果青霉素过敏，1 g 负荷剂量(儿童：10 mg/kg)，静脉注射。

- 破伤风类毒素(如果有需要)。

- 如果受到严重污染，则添加破伤风免疫球蛋白和氨基糖苷类[庆大霉素：q24 h，5～7 mg/kg(儿童：2.5 mg/kg，q8 h)，静脉注射]。

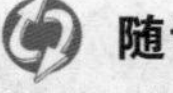

随访

进一步处理

入院指征

• 不稳定的踝关节骨折需要紧急骨科会诊，并且可能需要入院治疗。

• 应该进行清创、灌洗、静脉注射抗生素的开放性踝关节骨折和脱位。

• 开放或闭合复位治疗的踝关节脱位。

• 涉及骨筋膜室综合征、神经血管损伤。

出院指征

单纯无移位且无神经血管损伤的稳定性踝关节骨折可给予夹板治疗，患者可出院。

随访建议

• 夹板。

• 抬高受影响的下肢。

• 配备拐杖，并展示如何使用。

• 受影响的关节放置在非负重状态，直到骨科医师复查。

要点和误区

• 为了减少关节移位，患肢膝关节部分屈曲将减少对跟腱和踝关节的张力。

• 通过体格检查鉴别踝关节骨折和距下关节骨折：后者是罕见的，而且很难复位。

• 切记要寻找其他损伤，包括腰椎、臀部、胫骨、腓骨，尤其是腓骨近端颈部和足部(胫骨干骨折合并踝关节损伤合并症的 25%)。

H

踝关节扭伤 Ankle Sprain

Joseph R. Brown · Christopher J. Coyne 李岩 王瑞兰 译

基础知识

描述

• 踝关节的韧带损伤。
• 踝关节是由胫骨、腓骨、距骨组成的铰链关节。
• 损伤范围从轻微损伤的拉伤(Ⅰ级)到部分中断(Ⅱ级)再到完全中断(Ⅲ级)。

病因

• 足踝受内翻和外翻暴力。
• 强力碰撞。
• 85%~90%踝关节扭伤会有侧韧带损伤:
- 前距腓韧带(ATFL)。
- 后距腓韧带(PTFL)。
- 跟腓韧带(CFL)。
- 通常由内翻损伤所致。
- 前距腓韧带最易受伤。
- 如果踝关节在中立位受伤,CFL 经常受损。
- 后距腓韧带很少单独受损。
• 三角韧带(连接到内踝到距骨和舟骨)损伤通常是由外翻损伤所致:
- 常伴有内踝撕脱或距骨插入。
- 很少作为独立的损伤被发现。
- 怀疑相关的外踝骨折或腓骨近端骨折(Maisonneuve 骨折)。
• 韧带扭伤(胫腓韧带或小腿骨间韧带损伤):
- 最常见于碰撞与运动。
- 下胫腓韧带损伤("高踝关节扭伤")有较高的发病率和潜在的长期并发症。

儿科注意事项

• 小于 10 岁,有创伤性踝关节疼痛而无骨折的影像学证据的儿童最易发生 Salter Harris 骨折。
• 韧带实际上比开放的骨骺更强韧。

诊断

体征和症状

病史

病史可以预测损伤的类型,应包括:
• 受伤时间。
• 机制。
• 是否产生碎裂声。
• 既往创伤史。
• 相关的医疗状况(如骨或关节疾病)。
• 入院前处理。
• 在现场和急诊室的伤后负重能力。

体格检查

• 旨在检测关节不稳定和任何相关的损害。
- 注意内外踝后缘及第 5 跖骨基底部是否存在骨压痛。
• 记录远端神经血管的损伤状态。
• 评估活动范围并与健侧比较。
• 在急诊室的压力测试往往受疼痛限制,并可能不利于韧带损伤的检测。
• 挤压测试有助于确定韧带联合损伤:
- 在小腿中部挤压胫骨和腓骨,感到足踝疼痛表明测试结果阳性。
• 评估受伤上方和下方的关节的运动范围、强度和关节稳定性。
- 具体来说,评估腓骨近端对触诊的压痛。

基本检查

• 渥太华踝关节规则是对成人做 X 线片的一个选择策略,它认为足部或踝部 X 线检查是不必要的,除了以下任何一种情况:
- 在任一踝关节远端 6 cm 的后缘或尖端有骨压痛。
- 在第 5 跖骨或舟骨的基底部有骨压痛。
- 受伤时和急诊室中不能独立行走 4 步。
• 该规则已被原作者前瞻性地验证,并被美国、英国、法国和其他国家的团体独立地验证。

诊断检查与说明

影像学检查

• 考虑有骨折的踝关节损伤应拍摄 X 线片。
• 在急诊拍摄应力 X 线片几乎没有用,除非会诊医师要求,否则不应作为常规要求。

鉴别诊断

• 踝关节骨折(外侧、内侧或后踝)或脱位。
• 跟腱损伤。
• Maisonneuve 骨折。
• 三角骨骨折。
• 第 5 跖骨骨折(琼斯骨折)。
• 距骨穹窿软骨骨折。
• 腓骨肌腱脱位或损伤。

治疗

院前

固定踝关节是必要的。

初步稳定/治疗

• 防止进一步的损伤;如果有疼痛感,避免负重。
• RICE(休息,冷敷,加压,抬高)。

急诊治疗/程序

• 治疗的目标是减少疼痛和恢复正常活动而无长期疼痛或关节松弛。
• 现有的证据支持早期运动和功能治疗:
- 不稳定的踝关节(如Ⅲ级)或有严重疼痛的人可能会受益于短暂的固定后早期恢复功能治疗。
• Ⅰ级或Ⅱ级扭伤可以采用功能支持治疗(弹性绷带、空气夹板、凝胶夹板等):
- 最近的研究表明,弹性绷带与空气箍夹板一起穿戴优于其他形式的固定。
• Ⅲ级扭伤可采取固定(U 型夹板或后路夹板或弹性绷带加上空气箍夹板)和早期骨科会诊或转诊。
• 早期为了缓和痛苦可能需要拐杖,但鼓励Ⅰ级和Ⅱ级患者忍受负重。
• 一旦急性疼痛和肿胀已经缓解,加强锻炼和本体感觉训练(如平衡板、绕小圈行走)可以提高踝关节的强度和功能,以及防止再次损伤。
• 只有当跑步和转动已无痛苦的时候,才可以恢复完整的体育活动。
• 踝关节夹板、空气或凝胶夹板都能减少在高危运动(如篮球、排球、足球和跑步)中再次受伤的风险。
• 最新证据表明,损伤严重程度并不一定与功能预后相关。

药物治疗

• NSAIDs 对治疗急性疼痛有效:
- 布洛芬:800 mg(儿童:5~10 mg/kg),口服,每日 3 次。
• 局部 NSAIDs 已显示可控制疼痛并缩短急性脚踝扭伤的愈合时间:
- 双氯芬酸钠 1%凝胶:将 4 g 涂于患处,每日 4 次。

• 严重的疼痛可能需要麻醉性镇痛药。

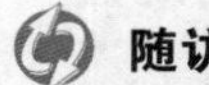

随访

进一步处理

入院指征

单纯踝关节扭伤不需入院治疗。

出院指征

单纯性踝关节扭伤通过合适的治疗、用药、治疗后指导和转诊可以安全地从急诊出院。

转诊问题

患者的任何影像学资料副本都可能促进早期随访。

随访建议

• 应通知Ⅰ级和Ⅱ级扭伤的患者在 1～2 周联系初级保健医师。

• Ⅲ级扭伤和韧带联合损伤的患者应该在 7～10 日转交给骨科医师或运动医学专家。

要点和误区

• 记住要在体格检查中充分评估皮下腺损伤。

• 渥太华踝关节规则可能会减少影像学的需要。

• 用弹性绷带加上空气箍夹板固定后早期功能治疗可缩短愈合时间。

坏疽 Gangrene

Karen B. Van Hoesen · Stephen R. Hayden 祝各亮 译

基础知识

描述

• 气性坏疽或梭菌性肌坏死。

• 一种急性的，快速进展的，形成气体的肌肉和皮下组织的坏死性感染。

• 从邻近区域连续发展或血液繁殖。

• 常见于创伤后及手术后。

• 会不断入侵和破坏正常的肌组织。

病因

• 梭状芽孢杆菌：

- 兼性厌氧、可形成芽孢、革兰阳性杆菌。
- 能产生许多毒素，最普遍和最致命的是 α 毒素。

• 产气荚膜梭菌是最为常见的菌种，80%～90%的伤口上都能找到它。

• α 毒素是组织破坏的主要原因。

• 其他的菌种包括诺维梭菌、腐败梭菌、溶组织梭菌、双酶梭菌和谲诈梭菌。

• 2 种产生梭状芽孢杆菌的机制：

- 创伤和术后。
- 孢子进入深层组织，在厌氧环境中繁殖。
- 与糖尿病、周围血管病变、酒精中毒、静脉吸毒、恶性肿瘤相关的病变。

诊断

症状和体征

• 肢体及受累部位突然出现的剧烈疼痛。

• 低热。

• 心率增快且高于体温所对应的范围。

• 受累部位的皮肤呈褐色，进一步发展可呈紫色或红色。

• 捻发音。

• 形成疱疹或水疱。

• 稀薄的有甜味的浆液性渗出物。

• 病变范围迅速扩展。

• 感觉减退。

• 全身毒性反应。

体格检查

• 触诊软组织中的乳突是最敏感的物理发现。

• 远端神经血管检查。

基本检查

• 病史和查体，特别注意软组织捻发音等体征。

• 软组织 X 线片可以探测到筋膜平面的气体：

- 没有探测出气体，也不能排除坏疽可能。

• 伤口渗出物革兰染色可见革兰阳性菌及少量白细胞。

诊断检查与说明

实验室检查

• 血常规、电解质、血尿素氮和肌酐。

• 炎性标志物、CPR、ESR。

• 凝血功能。

• 血型鉴定。

• 伤口渗出物做革兰染色。

• 伤口或组织的厌氧菌培养。

• 血培养。

影像学检查

• X 线片可以看见软组织内的气体。

• 气体位置特殊，难以发现时可行 CT 以进一步检查。

诊断步骤/外科

所有气性坏疽患者必须行外科清创处理。

鉴别诊断

• 蜂窝织炎。

• 坏死性筋膜炎。

• 非梭状芽孢杆菌性肌炎和肌坏死。

• 其他原因致外界、呼吸道或胃肠道气体进入组织内。

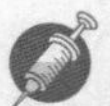

治疗

院前

建立静脉通道，注入等渗液体。

初始稳定/治疗

气道管理及复苏：

• 如果需要及时行气管插管。

• 供氧：

- 必须行心电及氧饱和度监测。

• 深静脉置管：监测中心静脉压对于脓毒症患者是必要的。

• 快速扩容：如果出现感染性休克需大量补充晶体、血浆、红细胞、白蛋白。

急诊治疗/程序

• 抗生素治疗：

- 初始的经验性治疗必须覆盖梭状芽孢杆菌和 A 型链球菌，覆盖需氧菌和厌氧菌。
- 哌拉西林他唑巴坦联合克林霉素。
- 初步明确诊断后的治疗以青霉素＋克林

霉素为主。
- 替代药物：头孢曲松＋红霉素。
- 如果存在混合感染：青霉素＋克林霉素、甲硝唑、万古霉素及覆盖革兰阴性菌的庆大霉素。
- 根据当地脓毒症治疗方案。
• 外科会诊：
- 清创、截肢或筋膜切开术。
• 辅助高压氧治疗：
- 早期高压氧治疗可以起到挽救生命的作用。
- 缺乏随机对照试验的证据，但非随机研究表明其有效。
• 破伤风预防。
• 防止主要并发症包括急性呼吸窘迫综合征、肾衰竭、心肌过激和 DIC。
• 多价抗毒素不是在美国研制出来的，研究尚未证明其疗效：
- 因为会出现严重的过敏反应，所以这不是常规推荐的治疗方法。

药物治疗

• 头孢曲松：2g[儿童：100mg/(kg・24h)，最多不超过 4g]，q12h，静脉注射。
• 克林霉素：900mg[儿童：40mg/(kg・d)，q6h]，q8h，静脉注射。
• 红霉素：1g[儿童：50mg/(kg・d)]，q6h，静脉注射。
• 庆大霉素：2mg/kg(儿童：2mg/kg)，q8h，静脉注射。
• 甲硝唑：500mg(儿童：安全标准未建立)，q8h，静脉注射。
• 青霉素：2400万 U/24h[儿童：25万 U/(kg・24h)]，q4～6h，静脉注射。
• 哌拉西林-他唑巴坦：4.5g，静脉注射，q8h[儿童：2～9个月，240mg/(kg・d)静脉注射，q8h；9个月，<40kg：300mg/(kg・d)，静脉注射，q8h；>40kg：3.375～4.5g，静脉注射，q8h]。
• 破伤风免疫球蛋白：500U，肌内注射。
• 破伤风类毒素：0.5mg，肌内注射。

随访

进一步处理

入院指征

• 所有气性坏疽以及有肌坏死证据的患者都需要外科清创及静脉输注抗生素。
• 高压氧治疗是非常重要的辅助手段。

出院指征

所有坏疽患者都需住院治疗。

转诊问题

清创及应用抗生素稳定病情后可以考虑转移进行高压氧治疗。

要点和误区

• 菌血症的出现概率为 15%并且可以快速进展为血管内溶血。
• 高压氧治疗作为清创及早期应用抗生素的辅助治疗的前提是患者血流动力学稳定。

坏死溃疡性龈炎 Necrotizing Ulcerative Gingivitis

Stephen K. Epstein・Laura B. Glicksman 伍力学 译

基础知识

描述

• 该病是一种牙周疾病。
• 以龈乳头呈"火山口状"为特征。
• 症状：
- 急性坏死溃疡性龈炎。
- 牙周炎。
- 黏膜溃疡性口炎(vincent disease)。
- 梭菌螺旋体性龈炎。
• 无传染性。
• 在发展中国家的儿童和青年人中高发。
• 主要发生在撒哈拉沙漠以南地区。
• 较罕见，最常发生在免疫缺陷的患者。
• 男性发病率高于女性。
• 可进展成更严重的疾病。
- 坏死性口炎：
◦ 与坏死溃疡性龈炎相似，但可扩展到舌部和颊黏膜。
- 坏死性溃疡性牙周炎：
◦ 与坏死溃疡性龈炎类似，伴有牙周组织松动和牙槽骨受累。
- 颜面部的坏疽(坏疽)。

病因学

• 由口腔菌过度繁殖而引起。
• 中间普雷沃菌。
• 螺旋体。
• 诱因(非诊断必要条件)：
- 口腔卫生不良、牙龈炎。
- 免疫缺陷(如 HIV)。
- 免疫抑制。
- 营养不良。
- 吸烟。
- 精神与生理压力。
- 某些化学药物接触史(如二亚甲基双氧苯丙胺或者迷幻药等)有关。

诊断

症状和体征

• 主要临床特征：疼痛性的龈炎。
- "火山口状"龈乳头溃疡灶。
- 溃疡灶易出血或自发出血。
• 次要临床特征：
- 坏死碎屑"假膜"包裹住溃烂部位。
- 口臭。
- 发热、精神萎靡。
- 通常发病迅速。

病史

• 急性的弥漫性口腔疼痛。
• 牙龈出血：
- 自发的或轻微触碰即出血。
• 口臭。
• 萎靡不振。
• 低热。

体格检查

• 牙间乳头缺失(重要的临床特征)。
• "火山口状"龈乳头溃疡灶。
• 坏死性碎屑常出现在溃疡面。
• 炎性细胞和坏死细胞形成"假膜"。
• 覆盖在溃疡病灶上。
• 去除后表面出血。
• 淋巴结肿大，尤其是下颌下部位。
• 口臭。
• 低热。

基本检查

• 考虑全身性疾病：

- 中性白血球减少症。
- HIV。

• 其他原因导致的免疫抑制或免疫损害。

• 排查有无并发症：
- 进展为坏死性口炎或溃疡性牙周病。
- 损害蔓延至牙周韧带和牙槽骨。

• 牙槽骨毁坏。
- 进展为面部坏疽(坏疽性口炎)。

诊断检查与说明

实验室检查

实验室检查对临床意义不大。

影像学检查

多无提示意义。

鉴别诊断

• 其他疾病很少表现为龈乳头"火山口状"溃疡改变。

• 急性疱疹性龈口炎。
- 影响整个牙龈，而不只是龈乳头。
- 常伴低热。
- 有传染性。

• 病毒：
- 病毒感染：EB 病毒、水痘-带状疱疹病毒。

• 鹅口疮。

• 放射菌病。

• 链球菌性、淋球菌性龈炎、口腔炎。

• 梅毒二期。

• 白喉。

• 囊泡性疾病。

• 天疱疮。

• 类天疱疮。

• 口腔扁平苔藓。

• 系统性红斑狼疮。

• 创伤：
- 牙签。
- 用力刷牙或用牙线洁牙。

• 免疫系统受损：
- 白血病。
- 粒细胞缺乏(恶性粒细胞缺乏)。
- HIV。

治疗

初步稳定/治疗

针对脱水进行液体复苏。

急诊治疗/程序

• 处理全身性和局部的疼痛。
- 很少需要使用麻醉药物。
- 利多卡因。

• 清除假膜。
- 以浸湿双氧水的纱布或棉签局部清理。

• 有以下情形者需使用抗生素(青霉素、甲硝唑或克林霉素)：
- 发热。
- 淋巴结肿大。
- 考虑存在免疫抑制的患者应用广谱抗生素、抗真菌及抗病毒药物。

• 门诊治疗：
- 消除诱因。
- 用稀释后的双氧水冲洗。
- 葡萄糖酸氯己定(洗必泰)。
- 必要时应用抗生素。
- 避免刺激物(辛辣食物、热饮)。
- 止痛剂用于控制疼痛。
- 每日通过刷牙及牙线清洁，促进口腔卫生。

药物治疗

一线药物

• 口腔冲洗：
- 葡萄糖酸氯己定 0.12%(洗必泰)：15 ml 漱口，每日 2 次。
- 双氧水(3%双氧水稀释至 1 倍)：最多冲洗每日 12 次，适用于儿童局部使用。

• 利多卡因。

• 疼痛控制：
- 非甾体抗炎药(如布洛芬)，对乙酰氨基酚。

二线药物

• 甲硝唑：250～750 mg[儿童：30 mg/(kg·24 h)]，口服，每日 4 次，共 7 日。

• 青霉素：500 mg[儿童：<12 岁，25～50 mg/(kg·24 h)]，口服，每日 4 次，共 10 日。

• 克林霉素：300 mg[儿童：6～8 mg/(kg·24 h)]，口服，每日 3 次。

• 抗生素治疗的免疫抑制患者应考虑使用抗真菌药物。

• 镇静、镇痛治疗。

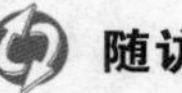

随访

进一步处理

入院指征

• 疾病蔓延出现全身症状者。

• 严重脱水、无法接受口服补液者。

• 颜面部坏疽征象：口、面部感染。
- 不治疗者死亡率达 70%。

出院指征

可保证正常液体补充者。

随访建议

紧急转诊到口腔科或牙周病专科医师进行刮牙、清创术。

要点和误区

• 应考虑有无 HIV 或者免疫抑制情况存在。

• 若不治疗，病情进展恶化极快。

坏死性软组织感染 Necrotizing Soft Tissue Infections

Jamie L. Linker 伍力学 译

基础知识

描述

• 坏死性软组织感染(NSTI)是指有坏死性改变的任一皮肤或软组织层面所发生的感染。
- 包括蜂窝组织炎、筋膜炎和肌炎。
- 通常沿着组织层面快速蔓延。

• 作为群体有以下特征：
- 保留皮肤的广泛的筋膜及肌肉出现广泛坏死而皮肤受累相对较轻。
- 死亡率高。
- 有全身中毒症状。

• 坏死性蜂窝组织炎：
- 皮肤的龟裂和气体。
- 保留较深的结构。
- 可能缺乏全身毒性。

• 坏死性筋膜炎：
- 大多数 NSTI 的经典名称(通常描述不准确)。

- 进行性、快速蔓延的感染，筋膜和皮下脂肪广泛剥离和坏死。
- 最初经常保留皮肤和肌肉。

• 富尼耶(Fournier)坏疽。
- 会阴有氧-厌氧混合感染所致的坏死性软组织感染。

• 据美国疾控中心报道，美国每年有 500～1 500 例病例。
• 通常难以被识别。
• 危险因素包括：
- 高龄。
- 慢性全身性疾病：
◦ 糖尿病。
◦ 肥胖。
◦ 外周血管病。
◦ 肾衰竭。
- 抽烟。
- 酗酒。
- 静脉药物滥用。
- 免疫抑制。
- 近期手术。
- 创伤性伤口。

• 病死率达 14%～40%。
• 有下列疾病的患者发病率较高：
- 经常需要截肢。
- 肾衰竭、心肌病、多系统器官功能障碍。

病因

• 导致 NSTI 的常见原因有：
- 大多数来自局部组织创伤并有细菌入侵。
- 较少是由于局部缺血或非穿透性创伤，以及如上所述的宿主防御能力降低。

• Ⅰ型 NSTI：
- 多种微生物的混合感染，包括至少 1 个厌氧菌。
- 需氧和厌氧菌。
- 包含富尼耶坏疽。
- 更多见于老年人、有潜在疾病的人或最近的手术后。
- 占 NSTI 的大多数。
- 链球菌属是最为常见的需氧菌。
◦ 金黄色葡萄球菌、肠球菌和大肠杆菌、克雷伯菌也很常见。
- 拟杆菌是最为常见的厌氧菌。

• Ⅱ型 NSTI：
- 单一微生物。
- 最常见的 A 组链球菌。
- 金黄色葡萄球菌，包括耐甲氧西林金黄色葡萄球菌(MRSA)，第二常见。
- 通常为年轻健康的患者。
- 几乎一半没有皮肤破溃。
- 通常在成像上看不到气体。
- A 组链球菌与 A 组链球菌的大约一半在全身中有多个地方，其余的是与链球菌中毒性休克综合征相关的小病例。
- 易感因素包括皮肤损伤、静脉用药、手术、分娩。

• Ⅲ型 NSTI：
- NSTI(<5%)。
- 进展迅速。
- 包括梭状芽孢杆菌、弧菌、产气单胞菌和革兰阴性细菌的感染。
- 通常发生在穿透性伤口或挤压伤或暴露于水之后。

• Ⅳ型 NSTI(罕见)：
- 包括念珠菌和接合菌在内的真菌病原学。
- 发生在免疫受损的。

• 所涉及的微生物包括：
- A 组 β_2 溶血性链球菌(GABHS)。
- B 组链球菌。
- 葡萄球菌。
- 肠球菌。
- 杆菌。
- 铜绿假单胞菌(绿脓杆菌)。
- 大肠埃希菌。
- 变形杆菌。
- 克雷伯杆菌
- 肠杆菌。
- 拟杆菌。
- 巴氏德杆菌。
- 梭状芽孢杆菌。
- 霍乱弧菌。
- 产气单胞菌。
- 假丝酵母菌。
- 接合菌。

儿科注意事项

• 新生儿的危险因素：
- 脐炎。
- 小手术：包皮环切、疝气。

• 儿童的危险因素还包括：
- 慢性疾病。
- 手术。
- 近期水痘感染。
- 先天性和获得性免疫缺陷。

诊断

症状和体征

病史

• 有无发热(可能没有或被药物抑制)。
• 有无神志改变。
• 有无慢性疾病。
• 有无静脉药物依赖。
• 恶心、呕吐、腹泻(伴有 GABHS)。
• 皮肤(可能早期没有皮肤发现，只是剧烈疼痛)：
- 疼痛进行性加重及受累部位的肿胀。
- 在第一个 24 h 内出现局部红、肿、热、痛并进行性加重。
- 1～5 日，局部呈蓝紫色，伴水疱和大疱形成(通常为出血性)，区域麻醉。
- 恶臭味的稀薄液体(从坏死的脂肪和筋膜中流出的“洗碗机”样脓液)。

• 尽管使用抗生素，但仍有进行性感染。

> **注意**
> 非甾体抗炎药的使用与更糟糕的结果相关，不清楚这是因为它掩盖了体征和症状，还是因为它抑制了中性粒细胞功能。

体格检查

• 全身毒症状：
- 发热。
- 心动过速。
- 呼吸急促。
- 血压降低。
- 神志改变。

• 剧烈疼痛与体检结果不成比例。
• 皮肤：
- 发红。
- 肿胀。
- 浅灰色或深色创面引流物。
- 水疱或大疱形成。
- 坏死。
- 溃疡。
- 有捻发音(为特征性体征，但只见于 10%～37%的病例)。
- 疼痛部位可超越可见的感染或可触摸到的硬结区域。
- 皮肤麻醉(局部破坏)。

• 四肢比躯干或会阴更容易受累。

儿科注意事项

• 最常见的症状。
• 局部疼痛(97%)。
• 皮疹(73%)。
• 血压过低、神志改变及休克表现相对较少。

基本检查

• 诊断较困难。
• 高危患者：对上述症状和体征进行仔细

检查。

• 感染部位之外的区域有疼痛的患者：须怀疑是否存在 NSTI。

• 诊断可能需要切开或穿刺活检：

如果手指很容易从切口穿过筋膜或"洗碗水"样脓液剥离，则"手指测试"呈阳性。

诊断检查与说明

实验室检查

• 全血细胞计数：

- 核左移的白细胞升高。
- 血细胞比容下降。

• 代谢水平：

- 血清钠下降。
- 肾功能肌酐升高。
- 血清钙下降(由于广泛的脂肪坏死)。
- 白蛋白下降。
- 谷草转氨酶升高。

• DIC 相关检测(凝血病)。

- 肌酸磷酸激酶升高。

• C 反应蛋白升高大于 150。

• 乳酸升高。

• 对病灶行革兰染色和需氧/厌氧菌培养或组织活检。

• 血培养(Ⅰ型 20%的阳性率，Ⅱ型 60%的阳性率，可能不包括所有的致病微生物)。

影像学检查

• X 线排查有无软组织气肿：为特征性表现，但不到一半的病例出现。

• CT 扫描：

- 在排查皮下气肿方面优于 X 线片。
- 坏死性软组织感染缺乏特异性筋膜强化的 CT 增强扫描。
- 还可识别深部脓肿或其他原因所致的感染。

• MRI：

- 能够显示感染扩散的范围。
- 非特异性筋膜增厚看起来类似于其他原因引起的全身性炎症。
- 可能过于敏感和耗时。

• 超声：

- 筋膜增厚和筋膜间隙的积液。
- 皮下软组织水肿、空气或脓肿。

> **注意**
>
> 影像检查不应延误疾病或快速进展性感染的清创手术，越早手术效果越好。

诊断步骤/外科

- 所有疑似 NSTI 患者均需行外科清创术。
- 深部组织活检和培养是诊断的金标准。
- LRINEC 分数不敏感或不特异。

鉴别诊断

• 蜂窝织炎。

• 气性坏疽。

• 坏疽脓皮病。

• 脓性肌炎。

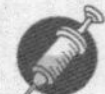

治疗

院前

• 静脉液体复苏。

• 必要时开放气道。

初步稳定/治疗

• 依病情给予开放气道和液体复苏治疗。

• 根据需要行快速诱导麻醉插管。

• 监测生命体征与心电监护。

• 建立静脉通路和积极的液体复苏。

• 根据当前脓毒症指南进行护理：

- 注意：使用升压药患者的 MAP 远远大于 65 可能会降低外周灌注。

急诊治疗/程序

• 抗生素：早期应用可覆盖需氧革兰阳性菌、需氧革兰阴性菌及厌氧菌的广谱抗生素。

• 治疗耐甲氧西林金黄色葡萄球菌直到清除为止：

- 万古霉素或利奈唑胺或达托霉素。

• 克林霉素抑制链球菌感染/中毒性休克外毒素和细胞因子的产生。

• 外科会诊：

- 及早清创，切开受累筋膜并彻底引流筋膜间的积液从而清除所有坏死组织至关重要。

• 高压氧辅助治疗。

- 研究冲突，不应推迟手术。
- 可能会导致更大的组织挽救和存活率。

• 静脉注射免疫球蛋白(IVIG)：

- 有争议，不是 IDSA 推荐的。
- 可能对 A 组链球菌导致的 NSTI 有作用。

• 观察有无严重并发症，包括急性呼吸窘迫综合征、急性肾衰竭、心肌应激、心肌病变和 DIC。

> **注意**
>
> 怀疑 A 组链球菌或梭状芽孢杆菌感染时应尽快开始克林霉素治疗。

药物治疗

儿科每日剂量不应超过成人每日剂量。

• 头孢曲松：2 g[儿童：100 mg/(kg · 24 h)]，静脉注射，q24 h。

• 环丙沙星：400 mg，静脉注射，q12 h。

• 克林霉素：900 mg(儿童：10 mg/kg，q6 h)，静脉注射，q8 h。

• 达托霉素：4 mg/kg，静脉注射，q24 h。

• 庆大霉素：2 mg/kg，静脉注射，q8 h。

• 亚胺培南-西司他汀：1 000 mg，静脉注射，q6 h(儿童：25 mg/kg，q6 h)。

• 多西环素：100 mg，静脉注射，q12 h。

• 左氧氟沙星：750 mg，静脉注射，q24 h。

• 利奈唑胺：600 mg，口服或静脉注射，q12 h(儿童：20 mg/kg，口服或静脉注射，q8 h)。

• 美罗培南：1 g[儿童：20 mg/(kg · d)，q8 h]，静脉注射，q8 h。

• 甲硝唑：500 mg[儿童：13.3 mg/kg，q8 h，40 mg/(kg · d)]，静脉注射，q8 h。

• 青霉素：200 万～400 万 U，q24 h(儿童：60 000～100 000 U/kg，q6 h)，静脉注射，q4～6 h。

• 哌拉西林-他唑巴坦：3.375～4.5 g(儿童：75 mg/kg 哌拉西林，静脉注射，q6 h)，静脉注射，q6 h。

• 替加环素：首次 100 mg，静脉注射；续以 50 mg，静脉注射，q12 h(儿童限量：1.2 mg/kg，q12 h)。

• 万古霉素：15～20 mg/kg，静脉注射，q8～12 h(儿童：15 mg/kg，静脉注射，q6 h)。

一线药物

推荐的初始急诊联合疗法：

• 哌拉西林-他唑巴坦＋万古霉素＋克林霉素。

只有在类型确定的情况下才能使用狭义抗生素：

• Ⅰ型感染：

- 哌拉西林-他唑巴坦＋克林霉素＋万古霉素。
- 亚胺培南-西司他丁、美罗培南或厄他培南。
- 重度青霉素超敏反应：克林霉素＋氨基糖苷类或氟喹诺酮。

• Ⅱ型感染(链球菌)：

- 克林霉素＋青霉素。
- 重度青霉素过敏：万古霉素、利奈唑胺或达托霉素。

• Ⅲ型感染(水生生物)：

- 多西环素＋头孢曲松。

H

随访

进一步处理

入院指征

• 所有 NSTI 患者必须接受外科清创术和静脉抗生素治疗和支持性护理。

• 大多数患者将需要 ICU 级别的护理。

出院指征

存在 NSTI 的患者均不应从急诊出院。

随访建议

在接受抗生素治疗和外科清创术后，病情稳定者，可以考虑转复杂的伤口护理和高压氧辅助治疗。

要点和误区

• 临床医师必须对 NSTI 有高度警惕性，因为早期的皮肤症状并不十分显著。

• 疼痛范围明显大于体检所见的病灶区域是一个重要表现。

• 如果仅使用抗生素治疗而不清创，死亡率接近 100%。

• 对于 NSTI 的评分体系(比如 LRINEC)作用有限。

• 治疗 NSTI 的 4 条原则：

- 液体复苏和纠正代谢紊乱。
- 早期抗生素治疗。
- 早期外科清创。
- 脏器功能衰竭的治疗。

环/束带移除损伤 Ring/Constricting Band Removal

Carl K. Hsu · Bradley Peckler 何融冰 译

基础知识

描述

• 原发性束带：带子紧扣末端肢体造成肿胀和疼痛(如 1 根头发缠绕在幼儿足趾端)。

• 继发性束带：带子过紧引起的损伤或疾病导致肿胀和水肿(如压紧的戒指合并下方手指骨折)。

• 如果不经治疗，束带会嵌入并破坏皮肤完整性。

• 任何原因引起的缩窄都会导致止血带综合征，给远端组织带来影响。

儿科注意事项

对于还未学会说话的儿童来说，束带可能是受虐待或忽视的表现；也可能是造成无法安抚的哭泣的原因。

老年人注意事项

认知力受损的疗养院居住者或阿茨海默病患者可能无法表达受伤或疼痛。

病因

止血带综合征可能由过敏性、皮肤、医源性、内分泌、感染性、肿瘤性、代谢性、生理性或创伤性疾病引起，也可能与妊娠相关。

诊断

症状和体征

• 束带引起组织或肢体末端皮肤的肿胀，通常涉及 1 根手指。

• 水肿组织和皮肤周围形成收缩带，这可以由任何材料(垫圈、螺母、金属丝、头发、绳子、橡皮筋、扎带、避孕套)导致。

• 部位如腕、踝、足趾、脐、耳垂、乳头、鼻间隔或鼻翼、阴茎、阴囊、阴道、唇、悬雍垂、或舌。

• 活动肢体末端或束带时有疼痛。

病史

• 通常很清楚，但对无法言语的患者来讲，可能是造成不明确疼痛的原因。一个无法安抚的哭泣的新生儿可能是由于 1 根头发缠绕而引起疼痛。

体格检查

• 评估涉及范围。

• 对于无法安慰的哭泣婴儿或不安的无法言语的成人，检查手指、足趾和生殖器。

基本检查

• 原发性束带：可通过特别注意神经血管症状的病史和体格检查而做出诊断。

• 继发性束带：通过影像学和实验室检查结果来诊断基础病因。

诊断检查与说明

实验室检查

• 紧急治疗不需要。

• 检测电解质、BUN、肌酐、甲状腺功能检查，水疱状损害的 Tzanck 检查有助于明确诊断。

影像学检查

X 线平片评估潜在骨折或束带移除后有无残留异物。

鉴别诊断

造成明显肿胀和水肿诱发止血带综合征的疾病。

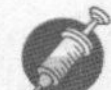

治疗

院前

在发展为止血带综合征前移除环或其他可能存在的束带。

• 尤其在肢体创伤区域。

初步稳定/治疗

控制疼痛或镇静。

急诊治疗/程序

• 通过抬高带远侧或分离带来移除束带。

• 以下辅助措施可以单独或联合使用：

- 抬高患肢可减轻血管充血。
- 用冰水或冷水降低四肢温度，可减轻水肿和红斑。
- 用肥皂或矿物油润滑可使其从发炎或水肿部位滑脱。用 1%～2% 利多卡因不使用肾上腺素进行指端阻滞可降低移除或处理基础损伤时的不适感。
- 指(趾)端阻滞可能；增加局部肿胀。考虑局部阻滞。
- 处理带时可能用到纱布或持针器。

• 远侧肿胀的手指，特别是近端指间关节，是束带移除很重要的障碍。

• 从远端到近端序贯挤压可减轻水肿：

- 胶带从远端到近端包扎在带上方，形成一光滑的减压区域。
- 在试图移除之前，用 Penrose 外科引流管或从小号手套切下的一个手指套拉伸越过远端肿胀组织。
- 经过润滑后引流管远端拉伸穿过环下端，

H

在环上形成一个套，通过远端牵拉环套可以将束带从减压部位抬高。

- 缝合材料(0号线、牙线或脐带胶布)从远端至近端方向拉紧经过水肿上方；缝合材料的近侧尾端或牙线挤进环内；通过润滑、拉紧的尾端向远处拉伸并无损伤地，迫使环脱离分层的缝合材料和减压区域。

• 分离法移除缩窄环：

- 可用剪刀先提起再剪掉压缩幼儿足趾或阴茎的纤维性条带。
- 切缘朝上的11号手术刀片可有效切断由头发、纤维或塑料条带形成的束带。
- 一种商业使用的脱毛发剂可以用来分离因局部水肿而无法辨别清楚的可疑头发。
- 一种手提式金属丝切割剥离器可以在对潜在的损伤造成最小程度不适的情况下分离小型金属环。然而这种移除方式会对环造成彻底破坏，修复困难。
- 一种在大多数手术室或医院器械部门都有的长柄切割器可以用来分离大型或较宽的环：
  ◦ 长柄有利于切割大型环。
  ◦ 加强的刀片切缘可能不太容易穿过伴随毗邻组织及皮肤肿胀的缩窄环。
  ◦ 一种手动的医用环形切器(Steinmann针状剪和1个MacDonald抬高器)可用来分离小型软金属(金/银)束带。
  ◦ 使用这种方式进行的整齐切割有利于后续环修补。
  ◦ 缺点是手动环切割器劳动强度大，可加重潜在损伤的疼痛。
  ◦ 一种机动的高RPM切割装置无论环的大小和形状都可进行快速分割，它可以在手术间由DC或AC驱动或空气驱动。

• 切割程序：

- 先割开肢体掌侧的环面。
- 可以用持钩撕开软金属质地的条带。
- 第二次切割时条带应在肢体上旋转180°，使对条带的第二次切割在肢体的掌面进行。

• 机动切割：

- 移走工作区域的易燃液体。
- 每位在场人员，包括患者，应佩戴护目镜。
- 在患者皮肤和环之间放置铝夹板(按环的弯曲度塑形)作为保护下面组织的屏障。
- 在切割前和切割过程中用冰水冲洗法冷却夹板和切缘。
- 限制机械装置切割的最长时间为5 s。中间间隔60～90 s来使用冰水冲洗防止局部过热。

• 脱毛霜：

- 怀疑在"无法解开或切除"部位存在由头发引起的缩窄时使用。
- 肿胀的组织堆积在头发周围，可看不到头发，只看到可能在下面埋有头发的褶皱。
- 应用于褶皱的脱毛膏可以在10 min内解除头发缩窄。

• 分离后治疗：

- 下方的损伤需要彻底冲洗来移除金属颗粒，防止异物反应和肉芽肿形成。
- 如果需要可进行破伤风预防。

▪ 药物治疗

• 破伤风预防接种：破伤风菌疫苗0.5 ml肌内注射。

• 无需特殊用药，除非有感染的证据或风险。

• 少数病人可能需要程序镇静取决于位置和预期的疼痛；详见镇静篇。

一线用药

• 头孢唑林：1 g，静脉注射或肌内注射(儿童：20～40 mg/kg，静脉注射或肌内注射在急诊室单剂量)。

• 头孢氨苄：500 mg，口服[儿童：25～50 mg/(kg·d)]，每日4次，持续7日。

• 阿莫西林/davulanate：875/125 mg，口服[儿童：25 mg/(kg·d)]，每日2次，持续7日。

二线用药

如果患者青霉素过敏：

• EES：800 mg，口服，然后400 mg，口服，q6 h，持续7日。

• 克林霉素：300 mg，口服，q6 h，持续7日。

 随访

▪ 进一步处理

入院指征

• 神经血管损伤或伤口需要外科修补。
• 伴发感染或坏死。
• 虐待或忽视的调查。

出院指征

成功移除条带并恢复血供。

转诊问题

有感染高风险的伤口需密切随访1～2日。

▪ 随访建议

疼痛加重，感觉减退，发麻，发红，肿胀引流，发热或其他临床症状改变。

要点和误区

• 未能彻底检查易激惹婴儿的手指；足趾和生殖器。

• 头发导致的缠绕缩窄可能被水肿和堆起的组织皮肤遮盖。

• 肢体远端创伤时戒指必须早期移除。

缓慢性心律失常 Bradyarrhythmias

Benjamin S. Heavrin　李兰玉 译

 基础知识

▪ 描述

• 心室率<60次/分。

- 窦性心动过缓可能为生理性变异。
- 其他心动过缓均为病理性。

• 可无症状，或有低血压、意识状态改变、疲劳、恶心、晕厥等表现。

• 治疗方法因心电图及临床表现不同而异。

▪ 病因

• 生理性：

- 见于健康的运动员。

• 心源性疾病：

- 窦房结功能异常，如病态窦房结综合征(缓慢性心律失常可与心动过速相交替)。
- 房室传导阻滞。
- 交界性或室性逸搏心律。
- 浸润性疾病：
  ◦ 淀粉样变性、肉状瘤病、血色素沉着病。

- 胶原血管病：
  ◦ 系统性红斑狼疮(SLE)、硬皮病、类风湿关节炎。
- 解剖学异常：
  ◦ 先天性、手术后、移植后、放射后。
- 肌肉疾病：
  ◦ 强直性肌营养不良。
- 心脏传导组织损伤。
• 非心源性疾病：
- 低氧。
- 心肌损伤和心肌坏死：
  ◦ 右冠状动脉(RCA)坏死可引起窦性心动过缓。
  ◦ 左前降支动脉(LAD)梗死引起高度阻滞。
- 酸中毒。
- 药物和中毒：
  ◦ β受体阻滞剂(BB)、钙通道阻滞剂(CCB)、地高辛、可乐定、抗心律失常药、锂、有机磷等。
- 电解质紊乱：
  ◦ 低钾血症、高钾血症、低血糖症、低钙血症、高钙血症、高镁血症。
- 生命体征异常：
  ◦ 低氧、低体温、低血压、高血压等。
- 内分泌紊乱：
  ◦ 甲状腺功能减退。
- 感染性疾病：
  ◦ 莱姆病、美洲锥虫病(原虫感染性心肌炎)、白喉、心内膜炎、心肌炎等。
- 神经性疾病：
  ◦ 出血性脑血管意外、头部损伤、颅内压增高、迷走神经张力增高、颈动脉窦高敏、脊柱损伤等。
  ◦ 可被排尿、排便、咳嗽、呕吐、压迫眼球或其他瓦氏动作诱发。

儿科注意事项

低氧血症是儿童缓慢性心律失常最常见的病因。对婴儿，如 HR<60 次/分且有症状者，立即开始胸外按压。

妊娠注意事项

母亲的 SLE 可导致孩子先天性完全性心脏传导阻滞。

诊断

症状和体征

• 通常没有症状，也可有以下表现。
• 脚步轻浮，迷糊，疲劳，意识水平下降。
• 呼吸困难，发绀，苍白。
• 胸痛、胸闷，出汗。
• 低血压。
• 晕厥。
• 低体温。
• 心脏停搏。

病史

• 用药改变，尤其是心脏药物。
• 尿量：
- 利尿剂引起的低钾血症。
- 肾衰竭引起的高钾血症。
• 外伤史：
- 颅内损伤。
- 心肌挫伤。
• 症状发生时正在进行的活动：
- 迷走神经张力增高。

体格检查

• 呼吸状态。
• 灌注状态，脉搏。
• 心律是否规则。
• 意识状态，进行神经系统检查。
• 身体一般情况，观察皮肤、毛发、指甲等。
• 体温。

基本检查

• 心电图和持续心电监测。
• 指脉氧。
• 血压监测。
• 血糖和电解质。
• 毒物鉴定。

诊断检查与说明

实验室检查

• 血糖。
• 血电解质。
• 血尿素氮和肌酐。
• 心肌酶谱。
• 地高辛浓度。
• 甲状腺功能检查。
• 抗核抗体、类风湿因子及其他免疫学指标。
• 莱姆病毒滴度。
• 血清铁。
• 毒物的检测。

影像学检查

• X线胸片。
• 头颅 CT(如果患者出现意识水平改变)。

诊断步骤/外科

心电图：

• 窦性心动过缓：
- 每个 QRS 波群前都有 P 波，每个 P 波后都有 QRS 波群，通常都是窄 QRS 波群。
• 窦房传导阻滞：窦房结和心房间传导异常。
• 窦性停搏：
- 没有窦房结活动，没有 P 波。
• 房室传导阻滞：心房及心室间传导异常。
- 一度房室传导阻滞：PR 间期>0.2 s，每个 P 波经传导产生一个 QRS 波群群。
- 二度Ⅰ型房室传导阻滞，又称莫氏Ⅰ型或文氏房室传导阻滞：PR 间期逐渐延长，直至脱落一个 QRS 波群，此现象周而复始。
- 二度Ⅱ型房室传导阻滞，又称莫氏Ⅱ型房室传导阻滞：PR 间期固定不变，间断性脱落 QRS 波群，发展成为三度房室传导阻滞的风险较高。
- 三度房室传导阻滞，又称为完全性房室传导阻滞：心房活动和心室活动完全分离，有恒定的 PP 间期及恒定的 RR 间期，但两者之间毫无关联，节律通常不稳定。
• 房室交界性节律：
- 失去心房传导，房室交界区起搏点逸搏节律为 40～60 次/分。
- 逆行性 P 波可位于 QRS 波群之前、之中或之后，且 QRS 间期可长可短。
• 宽 QRS 群。
- 可能提示药物过量。
• 室性逸搏心律：
- 既没有窦房活动，又没有房室活动，希氏束或浦肯野纤维以 30～40 次/分的节律逸搏。
- QRS 间期多>0.12 s。
- 多为临终节律。

鉴别诊断

• 正常生理变异。
• 心肌缺血。
• 药物中毒。
• 起搏器功能障碍。
• 缺氧。
• 低体温。
• 电解质紊乱。
• 肾衰竭。
• 甲状腺功能减退。
• 感染。
• 风湿性疾病。
• 神经肌肉病变。
• 颅内压增高。
• 心肌挫伤。

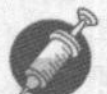

治疗

院前

- 救治患者，而不是单纯提高心率。
- 吸氧：
- 适用于所有患者，尤其是儿童。
- 如果阿片类药物过量可使用纳洛酮。
- 如果体温低，为患者保暖，并予以补镁治疗。
- 速度不要过快：轻移患者，粗暴操作可能会诱发室颤。
- 阿托品或去甲肾上腺素：
- 仅用于低血压或意识状态改变的患者。
- 对于三度房室传导阻滞患者通常是无效甚至是有害的。
- 经皮起搏：
- 其他治疗措施无效时。

初步稳定/治疗

- 基础支持治疗。
- 氧气治疗。
- 应用起搏器并持续心电监测。
- 建立静脉通路。

急诊治疗/程序

- 无症状性心动过缓。
- 监测病情变化。
- 症状性或不稳定性心动过缓。
- 吸氧。
- 阿托品。
- 窦性心动过缓、一度和二度Ⅰ型房室传导阻滞。
- 通常高度房室传导阻滞无效。
- 肾上腺素。
- 经皮起搏。
- 如经皮起搏无效则经静脉起搏。
- 寻找病因并治疗。
- 阿片类药物过量：
- 纳洛酮。
- 低血糖：
- 高糖溶液。
- 低钙血症：
- 葡萄糖酸钙。
- 高钙血症：
- 生理盐水±呋塞米。
- β受体阻滞剂（BB）或钙通道阻滞剂（CCB）过量：
- 钙通道阻滞剂过量：
- 一线：静脉使用钙剂，高剂量胰岛素疗法，去甲肾上腺素或肾上腺素。
- 二线：增加剂量的高剂量胰岛素治疗，如果心肌功能障碍，静脉脂乳疗法，安装心脏起搏器。
- 高钾血症：
- 静脉注射钙剂、加胰岛素的高糖溶液、沙丁胺醇，存在酸中毒应用碳酸氢钠、呋喃苯胺酸、磺苯聚乙烯酸钠及透析。
- 低钾血症：
- 补钾。
- 地高辛中毒：
- 地高辛抗体（地高辛免疫抗原结合片段）。
- 心肌梗死：
- PCI、抗血小板、起搏器。
- 甲状腺功能减退：
- 左旋甲状腺素。
- 低体温：
- 积极给予保暖复温。
- 温氧、温液体输注、加温器、毛毯、加热灯，考虑温暖的膀胱和胃灌注，体外循环。
- 感染：
- 针对性的抗生素治疗、抗病毒或抗真菌治疗。
- 心肌挫伤：
- 支持治疗。
- 颅内压增高：
- 应用甘露醇，神经外科会诊。
- 起搏器故障：
- 检查起搏器，心脏内科会诊。
- 特发性：
- 心内科评估入住ICU和起搏器安置情况。

药物治疗

- 阿托品：0.5～1 mg（儿童：0.02 mg/kg，最小剂量：0.1 mg），静脉注射，q3～5 min；最大剂量3 mg或0.04 mg/kg。
- 葡萄糖酸钙：1 000 mg（儿童：60 mg/kg），静脉注射，q3～5 min，最大剂量，3 g。
- 高糖溶液：1～2安瓿（儿童：D_{10}或者D_{25} 2～4 ml/kg），静脉注射。
- 氯化钙含有3倍氯离子，而葡萄糖酸钙对静脉的腐蚀性较小。对于接近于心跳停止的患者，应使用氯化钙。
- 地高辛免疫抗原结合片段：剂量因地高辛的摄入量变化，一般6瓶（儿童：平均剂量，1瓶）一次性静脉注射；看说明书。
- 肾上腺素：0.1～0.5 mg[儿童：0.01～0.03 μg/(kg·min)]，静脉注射，q3～5 min；静脉泵注2～10 μg/min[儿童：0.1～1 μg/(kg·min)]。
- 胰高血糖素：BB或CCB过量时应用，3～5 mg（儿童：0.05 mg/kg），静脉注射，可重复一次；静脉泵入1～5 mg/h[儿童：0.07 mg/(kg·h)]，静脉注射。
- 常规胰岛素：BB或CCB过量10 U（儿童：0.1 U/kg）一次，联合胰高血糖素静脉推注。毒物测定后应用更大的剂量。

一线用药

阿托品、肾上腺素、起搏器。

二线用药

特定疾病的治疗。

随访

进一步处理

入院指征

- ICU：
- 血流动力学不稳定的心动过缓。
- 二度Ⅱ型房室传导阻滞或三度房室传导阻滞。
- 经皮或经静脉起搏器置入。
- 需要升压治疗。
- 急性心肌梗死或缺血。
- 远程监测：
- 血流动力学稳定的心动过缓。

出院指征

无症状的窦性心动过缓。

转诊问题

- 所有没有初级保健医师的患者都应由全科医师随访。
- 一度和二度Ⅰ型房室传导阻滞需要心脏科转诊。
- 严重内分泌疾病、风湿性疾病、感染、肾脏或者神经疾病需要相关专科转诊。

随访建议

- 轻微的实验室异常不需要住院治疗的需要PCP随访。
- 除了无症状的窦性心动过缓外其他患者均需要心脏科随访。
- 特定的疾病需要相关的专科随访。

要点和误区

- 无症状的窦性心动过缓是唯一可能正常的缓慢性心律失常。其他心动过缓均需治疗或随访。
- 血糖水平有助于区分β受体阻滞剂过量（低）和钙通道阻断剂过量（高）。

• 所有患者均需吸氧、指脉氧测定、开通静脉通道、心电图检查。

• 儿童心动过缓可能是继发于缺氧。

• 所有有症状的患者均应备起搏垫。

• 针对病因的治疗最重要。

幻觉 Hallucinations

Michael Ganetsky 朱雨锋 李文放 译

基础知识

描述

幻觉是一种症状或特征，而不是诊断。它们可能是听觉的、视觉的、触觉的、味觉的或嗅觉的。幻觉和类似的现象通常被定义为如下。

• 幻觉：

- 感官知觉：在没有外部刺激相关感觉器官的基础上出现的真实的知觉，并通过该器官形成一种感觉的经历。
- 患者可能不会认为他们有幻觉。

• 错觉：

- 对于真正外部刺激的误解或曲解。

• 闪回：

- 复发的记忆、感觉或过去经历中的真实感知。

• 假性幻觉：

- 不通过感觉器官产生的幻觉（如头部的声音或身体内在是声音而不是听到的声音）。

流行病学

发病率和患病率估计

• 一般人群幻听终身发病率为4.8%（由于定义模糊或假性幻觉，估计值可能略高）。

• 超过50%的老年痴呆症患者会出现妄想或幻觉。

病因

引起幻觉的原因有很多，下列是常见的病因：

• 精神病：

- 精神分裂症。
- 双相情感障碍，躁狂。
- 重度抑郁症。

• 急性中毒：

- 乙醇。
- 大麻：
- 合成大麻类（如K2香料）。
- 拟交感神经药：
  ◦ 苯丙胺。
  ◦ 冰毒。
  ◦ 可卡因。
  ◦ 合成性卡西酮（如MDPV、“浴盐”）。
- NMDA受体拮抗剂：
  ◦ 氯胺酮。
  ◦ 普斯普剂。
  ◦ 右美沙芬。
- 血清素：
  ◦ 亚甲二氧基甲基苯丙胺（摇头丸）。
  ◦ D-麦角酸二乙胺。
  ◦ 皮约特仙人掌（麦司卡林）。
  ◦ 蘑菇（裸头草碱）。
  ◦ 2C系列（如2CB、2CT-7）。
  ◦ 5-MeO系列（如5-MeO-DMT）。
- κ阿片受体激动剂：
  ◦ 鼠尾草（引起痛感，如听到颜色或闻到声音）。
- 阿片类药物。
- 吸入剂：
  ◦ 甲苯。
  ◦ 一氧化二氮。

• 药物：

- 抗胆碱能药物。
- 类固醇。
- 哌醋甲酯。

• 停药反应：

- 乙醇。
- 苯二氮䓬类。
- 巴比妥类药物。
- γ-羟基丁酸盐。

• 药物诱导的精神失调：

- 甲基苯丙胺相关性精神病：
  ◦ 精神病时间延长，听觉幻觉和复发。
- 大麻诱导的精神病。

• 感染：

- 脑膜炎。
- 脑炎。
- 在老年痴呆症患者，任何感染（如泌尿系统、肺部感染）均可引起幻觉。

• 代谢：

- 低血糖。
- 电解质紊乱。
- 甲状腺疾病。
- 肾上腺疾病。
- 威尔逊病。
- 硫胺素缺乏。

• 神经系统：

- 癫痫发作：
  ◦ 部分单纯或复杂的癫痫发作会导致视觉、听觉、嗅觉和味觉幻觉。
- 偏头痛。
- 中枢神经系统出血或肿瘤。
- 咳嗽变异性哮喘。
- 抽动秽语综合征。
- 神经退行性疾病：
  ◦ 帕金森病。
  ◦ （路易体痴呆、老年痴呆症）。
  ◦ 艾滋病。

• 眼：

- 青光眼。
- 黄斑变性。
- Charles Bonnet综合征。

• 其他：

- 食物，感觉，睡眠剥夺。
- 疲劳，极限应激。
- 热相关疾病。
- 宗教或仪式活动。
- 入睡和觉醒。

儿科注意事项

幻觉在儿童和青少年中是比较常见的，通常发育正常。大多数儿童的幻觉并不是因为精神病。幻觉可以作为精神错乱的一部分，发热亦可引起幻觉。与成年患者一样，需仔细地进行一次医疗或神经系统的病因检查。

老年人注意事项

在老年患者中，幻觉最常因器官性病变引起，通常伴随着痴呆、抑郁、药物反应和药物滥用，而且经常伴随着躁动的发生。非典型抗精神病药是治疗老年人幻觉的有效药物。

H

诊断

症状和体征

病史

- 往往难以准确和全面地获取病史：
  - 应该从旁观者、快递员、警察、家人、家庭医师了解病史。
- 评估行为的变化。
- 探查妄想或被害观念。
- 幻觉以前的情节。
- 药物变化。
- 物质滥用史。
- 时间进程：认知改变迅速，在短时间内情绪快速变化提示谵妄。
- 头痛可能会提示中枢神经系统病变或偏头痛。

体格检查

- 急性精神病：
  - 杂乱无章的思维。
  - 对内部刺激产生应答。
- 躁狂症：
  - 说话过多或压迫式的讲话。
- 谵妄：
  - 意识水平的改变。
  - 无目的性。
  - 异常的生命体征。
- 中枢神经系统损伤：
  - 脑神经缺损。
  - 失语。
  - 任何局灶性神经系统发现。
  - 步态异常。
  - 创伤的外部体征。
- 全身性或感染性疾病：
  - 扑翼样震颤。
  - 发热。
  - 颈强直。
  - 肌阵挛。
  - 黄疸。
  - 腹水。
- 中毒或停药反应：
  - 拟交感神经毒素、乙醇类、苯二氮䓬类药物停药。
    - 激动，兴奋性谵妄。
    - 瞳孔散大。
    - 心动过速和高血压。
    - 体温上升。
    - 出汗。
  - 合成大麻类。
    - 躁动，兴奋谵妄。
    - 嗜睡。
    - 局灶性神经功能障碍。
    - 心动过速。
    - 呕吐。
  - 阿片类药物：
    - 瞳孔缩小。
    - 呼吸过缓。
    - 针尖样瞳孔。
  - 血清素：
    - 心动过速和高血压。
    - 反射亢进。
    - 阵挛。
    - 震颤。
  - NMDA 受体拮抗剂：
    - 眼球震颤。

诊断检查与说明

- 常规检验：
  - 血常规和生化指标。
  - 乙醇、对乙酰氨基酚、水杨酸浓度。
  - 尿常规。
- 检查重点应根据患者的基础疾病或临床状况而定：
  - 毒品尿检：
    - 结果的信服度可能不够，因为这是一个对于是否使用而不是中毒与否的测试。此外，它不适合用来检测新型毒品，虽然其中的一部分会产生反应。
  - 心电图。
  - 甲状腺功能。
  - 肝功能试验。
  - RPR、叶酸、维生素 B_{12} 和硫胺素。
  - 特定药物浓度。

影像学检查

- 脑部影像学(CT、MRI)。
- 胸部 X 线平片。

诊断步骤/外科

- 如果怀疑存在药物原因，应当考虑如下操作：
  - 腰椎穿刺。
  - 脑电图。
- 如果幻觉是急性精神疾病或慢性精神病失代偿引起的：
  - 精神科急会诊。

基本检查

有明确的精神病史和特征性症状患者仅需基本检查(血常规、生化)。然而，难以区分的幻觉，特别是那些高危人群患者需要积极的检查。

鉴别诊断

急诊室评估的主要目的是区分精神性或非精神性疾病产生的幻觉：

- 更可能是精神性疾病：
  - 听觉幻觉和指令性幻觉。
  - 将幻觉和幻想并入妄想系统。
  - 发病年龄在 13～40 岁。
  - 情感平淡。
  - 行为目的性正常。
  - 注意力混乱。
  - 生命体征正常。
- 下列人群高度考虑非精神性疾病：
  - 老年人。
  - 物质滥用史。
  - 没有预先存在的精神病史。
  - 存在前驱疾病。
  - 社会经济水平较低。
  - 症状迅速发作。
  - 生命体征异常，发热。
- 下列情况视觉幻觉较常见：
  - 谵妄。
  - 老年痴呆症。
  - 偏头痛。
  - 促多巴胺治疗(如卡比多巴)。
  - 脑梗死后。
  - 发作性睡病。

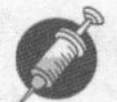

治疗

院前

需仔细患者周围环境中的细节，以便获取更多有用的信息：

- 杂乱无章的生活环境。
- 吸毒用具。

初步稳定/治疗

- 如果患者呈现出任何生命体征不稳定，需进行心肺复苏(如缺氧时需供氧)。
- 测血糖。
- 硫胺素 100 mg 静脉注射或口服。
- 治疗急性躁动(见躁动)。
  - 消减技术。
  - 身体约束。
  - 化学镇静。

急诊治疗/程序

- 如果基础疾病原因确定：
  - 治疗病因。
  - 这些患者通常不需要抗精神病药物。

• 对于急性精神病和慢性精神病失代偿患者：

- 使用抗精神病药物和苯二氮草类药物。

• 因中毒产生兴奋性精神错乱的幻觉患者：

- 一般支持治疗。
- 避免高热。
- 在没有化学限制的情况下避免使用物理限制。
- 苯二氮草类药物。

• 如果痴呆伴幻觉：

- 如果有，进行基础疾病的病因治疗。
- 典型抗精神病药物有利也有害（脑血管意外、锥体外系症状）。

> **注意**
>
> 处理因急性中毒导致的伴有兴奋性谵妄的幻觉时（除乙醇中毒），应当用苯二氮草类药物。

随访

进一步处理

入院指征

根据医疗条件或精神科评估来处置。一些毒品如冰毒或大麻所致的幻觉，可以在药物代谢后依然发挥作用。

• 医疗条件决定的入院指征。

• 急性精神病或慢性精神疾病失代偿需要精神科住院治疗。

• 一些中毒的幻觉，如甲基苯丙胺或大麻，甚至在药物代谢后仍可能持续存在。

出院指征

• 症状已经缓解或药物原因已解除（如中毒、尿道感染）。

• 慢性精神病失代偿已得到纠正，家庭环境适宜与心理健康随访可行。

转诊问题

酌情进行酒精、药物的治疗。

随访建议

适当的医疗或慢性精神状态随访。

要点和误区

• 不要认为听觉幻觉总是由精神性疾病引起的，而视觉、触觉、嗅觉和味觉的幻觉是由非精神性疾病引起的，需进行全面评估。

• 虽然10%的精神分裂症发生在45岁以上的患者，但是不要认定老年幻觉患者是精神性原因引起的而不进行积极的检查。

• 不要用抗精神病药物处理因急性中毒导致的伴有兴奋性谵妄的幻觉（除酒精中毒）。

黄疸 Jaundice

Andrew K. Chang · Sean P. Geary 何超 段立伟 译

基础知识

描述

• 血清胆红素＞2.5 mg/dl 时，机体出现高胆红素血症，表现为组织或体液的黄染。

- 血红素的降解产物。
- 不溶于水，与白蛋白结合。
- 溶血性：
  ◦ 产生大量的非结合胆红素。
- 肝性：
  ◦ 肝脏对胆红素的降解、分泌功能降低：
    ▪ 摄入障碍：药物的影响、Crigle-Najjar 综合征。
    ▪ 结合障碍：Gilbert 综合征。
    ▪ 干细胞分泌胆红素障碍：药物、Dubin-Johnson 综合征。

• 结合性高胆红素血症：

- 结合性胆红素具有水溶性。
- 在结合性高胆红素血症中，胆红素在肝脏形成结合胆红素后返回血流，而不是流入胆管。
- 肝细胞功能障碍：
  ◦ 肝炎。
  ◦ 肝硬化。
  ◦ 肿瘤侵袭。
  ◦ 重度损伤。
- 肝内胆汁淤积。
- 肝外胆汁淤积。

病因

• 肝前性：

- 溶血性（病态细胞、其他血红蛋白性疾病）。
- 红细胞生成障碍。
- 药物性因素。
- Gilbert 综合征：初始症状以遗传性非结合胆红素血症为主。
- 长时间的禁食。

• 肝细胞性：

- 肝炎（感染、酒精性、自身免疫性、毒性、药物性）。
- 肝硬化。
- 缺血引起的损伤。
- 血色素沉着病。

• 肝内胆汁淤积：

- 先天性胆汁淤积。
- 药物。
- Dubin-Johnson 综合征。
- Rotor 综合征。
- 良性反流性胆汁淤积。
- Familial 综合征。
- 脓毒症。
- 手术后黄疸。
- 淋巴瘤。

• 肝外阻塞：

- 胆总管结石。
- 胆管狭窄。
- 细菌性胆道炎。
- 硬化性胆道炎。
- 肿瘤。
- 胰腺炎、胰腺假性囊肿。
- 胆道出血。
- 十二指肠息肉。
- 蛔虫病。
- 胆囊切除术后综合征。
- 先天性胆道闭锁。
- 先天性胆总管囊肿。

儿科注意事项

肝内胆汁淤积症：

• 心血管疾病（先天性心脏病、充血性心力衰竭、休克、窒息）。

• 代谢性或遗传性（α_1-抗胰蛋白酶缺乏症、18和21三体综合征、囊性纤维化、戈谢病、尼曼-皮克病、糖原贮积病Ⅳ型）。

• 传染性疾病（细菌性败血症、巨细胞病毒、肠道病毒、单纯疱疹病毒、风疹、梅毒、结核

H

病、水痘、病毒性肝炎)。

• 血液系统疾病(严重免疫性溶血病)。

诊断

症状和体征

• 皮肤巩膜黄染:
- 长时间黄绿色。
- 在面部、躯干和巩膜处最明显。
- 在白天光照是比在非自然光下更明显。

• 瘙痒:
- 与胆红素水平和黄疸持续时间成正比。

• 合并高胆红素血症时,尿呈深黄色或棕色。

• 无胆汁粪便:
- 白色、灰色或黏土色。
- 完全性胆道梗阻。

病史

• 胆汁淤积:
- 大便颜色变浅。
- 尿液颜色加深。

• 恶性:
- 厌食。
- 体重降低。
- 精神不振。

• 腹痛。

体格检查

• 巩膜和舌部黄染。

• 右上腹压痛。
- Courvoisier 定律:
  ◦ 胆囊可触、无痛伴有无痛性黄疸提示恶性的胆总管阻塞。

• 结节性肝硬化:
- 腹部侧支循环的建立包括脐周静脉扩张形成海蛇头征、肝脾大、肝脏萎缩。
- 腹水。
- 蜘蛛痣。
- 肝掌。
- Dupuytren 挛缩。
- 扑翼样震颤。
- 肝性脑病。
- 男性乳房发育。

• 胆囊可触及。

• 肝大。

• 脾大。

• 腹部包块。

• 恶病质。

• 皮肤抓痕(胆总管硬化、阻塞)。

• Kayser-Fleicher 环:
- Wilson 病。

基本检查

• 病史、体格检查、常规的实验室检查能够对 80%的病例进行诊断。

• 胆汁酸水平:能够提示病因。
- 恶性疾病会伴有胆汁酸的严重升高(10~30 mg/dl)。
- 胆汁淤积性疾病很少超过 15 mg/dl。

实验室检查

• 尿试纸检查对于胆红素的检查有 74%的敏感性。

• 碱性磷酸盐:
- 在没有骨性疾病和妊娠的情况下,碱性磷酸盐升高提示胆管功能的损伤。
- 2 倍正常值:肝炎、肝硬化。
- 3 倍正常值:肝外胆管阻塞和肝内胆汁淤积。

• 转氨酶:提示肝细胞损伤。
- 丙氨酸转氨酶(ALT, SGPT):主要存在于肝脏。
- 天冬氨酸转氨酶(AST, SGOT):存在于肝脏、心脏、肾脏、肌肉和脑。

• γ-谷氨酰胺转氨酶:存在于肝脏胆道系统、胰腺、肾脏、心脏、肺脏:
- 提示胆道系统疾病的最敏感指标。

• 5′-核苷酸酶:组织发布广泛。

• 白蛋白:在严重肝脏疾病中会降低。

• 凝血时间:急性肝炎患者中延长具有重要的诊断意义。

诊断检查与说明

影像学检查

• 腹部超声:
- 对于 90%患者能够诊断胆石症。
- 肝脏和胰头的肿瘤通常能很好地被发现。
- 区分肝脏实体瘤和囊性结构。
- 胆管扩张是提示肝外阻塞的有效征象。
  ◦ 胆囊和胆总管扩张提示远端阻塞,肝内胆管扩张但不合并胆总管扩张提示近端阻塞。

• 肝脏肿瘤和胰头癌能够在影像学检查中发现。

• 注意区分实体肝脏肿瘤和囊性病变。

• X 线平片。
- 能够显示肝脏、脾脏的扩大或胆汁性钙化。

• 肝脏核扫描(肝胆的亚氨基二乙酸扫描):
- 能够准确地诊断急性胆囊炎和胆囊管阻塞。
- 比较费时(耗时几小时)。

• CT 扫描:
- 相比于超声,对于胰腺的疾病和腹部肿瘤的诊断更优越。
- 能够区分液性结构。
  ◦ 诊断性操作或手术。
  ◦ 内镜下逆行胰胆管造影(ERCP)。

• MRCP:
- 优点:可以确定 80%~100%导管扩张的原因,并消除内镜检查和导管插管导致穿孔和胰腺炎的风险。
- 缺点:诊断性的而非治疗性的。

诊断和外科治疗

经内镜逆行胰胆管造影(ERCP):

• 诊断:
- 有结石存在时会在胆管内腔形成充盈缺损。
- 当存在恶性病变时胆管内腔会异常狭窄。

• 治疗:
- 去除胆总管结石,并能够扩张旁路通道缓解恶性狭窄。
- 能够在直视下留取组织活检。

鉴别诊断

治疗

初步稳定/治疗

• 脱水时补充等渗液体。

• 存在中毒症状的患者:
- 供氧,心电监护。
- 经鼻饲管吸出,插好导尿管。

急诊治疗/程序

• 细菌性胆管炎或脓毒症患者,进行血培养和抗生素治疗:
- 氨苄西林-舒巴坦、哌拉西林-他唑巴坦。
- 碳青霉烯类抗生素。
- 替代用药环丙沙星、甲硝唑或第三代头孢菌素。

• 阻塞性肝外黄疸:
- 考虑手术治疗。
- 经内镜逆行胰胆管造影/支架置入术。

• 胆总管结石:
- ERCP 乳头状切开术、球囊或吊篮取出术、开放性胆囊切除术伴胆管探查术、经皮肝穿刺胆管造影术(PTC)或经皮胆囊造瘘管放置术。

• 梗阻性肝内黄疸或非梗阻性黄疸:
- 解除酒精性或药物性诱因。

H

- 应用干扰素治疗乙型、丙型肝炎。
- 应用青霉胺和静脉切开治疗 Wilson 病和血色沉着病。
- 应用糖皮质激素治疗自身免疫性疾病引起的慢性肝炎。

儿科注意事项

• 需要治疗：
- 根据早产和并发症，分为低、中、高 3 个风险阶段。
- 使用新生儿胆红素计算器或 AAP 绘制新生儿胆红素列线图。

• 治疗措施：
- 照光疗法可在 4～6 h 降低总胆红素 2～3 mg/dl，并在最初 24 h 内降低 30%～40%。
- 血浆置换：
  ◦ 存在胆红素引起神经功能障碍或改善照光疗法失败的患者。
  ◦ 胆红素/白蛋白>6.8(高危儿)；>7.2(中度风险婴儿)；>8.0(低风险婴儿)。
- 使用免疫球蛋白：如果总胆红素水平在光疗后仍在上升，或者血浆置换在 2～3 mg/dl 的范围内时，可以考虑使用免疫球蛋白治疗。

• 苯巴比妥钠：针对脓毒症或药物引起的黄疸，主要降低结核性胆红素。

• 金属卟啉：实验性的血红素氧化酶抑制剂。

药物治疗

• 雷帕西林：儿童 25 mg/kg，静脉滴注，q6～8 h。

• 头孢西丁：2 g，静脉滴注，q6 h[儿童：40～160 mg/(kg · d)，q6～12 h]。

• 庆大霉素：1.5～2 mg/kg，静脉滴注，8 h。

• 甲硝唑：7.5 mg/kg，静脉滴注，q6 h(儿童：同前)。

• 哌拉西林-他唑巴坦：3.375 g，静脉注射，q6 h[儿童：300 mg/(kg · d)div，q6 h]。

• 美罗培南：1 g，静脉滴注，q8 h(儿童：20 mg/kg，q8 h)。

• 厄他培南：1 g，q24 h(无儿童剂量)。

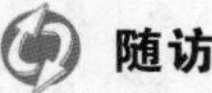

随访

进一步处理

入院指征

• 细菌性胆管炎。
• 难治性疼痛。
• 难治性呕吐。
• 与病情相关的胰腺炎发作。
• 凝血酶原时间延长。

出院指征

• 感染被治愈，不再有感染的证据。

会厌炎(成人) Epiglottitis, Adult

Jonathan Fisher · Aubri S. Carman 单怡 译

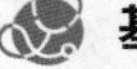

基础知识

描述

• 进行性加重的会厌部及周围组织炎症导致气道受压。

• 成人疼痛表现不及儿童明显，成人可快速进展至完全气道阻塞。

• 儿童会厌炎发病率在降低，而成人发病率在升高。

• 声门上炎症：
- 会厌炎：
  ◦ 水肿是最初的气道表现。
  ◦ 可原发或及继发于邻近结构。
- 会厌谷炎。
- 杓状软骨炎。

• 感染来源常来自咽后壁。

• 成人每年发病率为(1～4)/10 万且仍在增长。

• 男性更多见，男女比例为 3∶1。

• 成人死亡率为 7%(儿童死亡率<1%)。

• 合并下列因素患者往往病情较重：
- 糖尿病。
- BMI>25 kg/m^2。
- 合并肺炎。
- 会厌脓肿。

• 抽烟和滥用药物者更易伴发并发症。

• 免疫力低下患者尤其严重，临床表现不典型，常为少见病原体感染(念珠菌和铜绿假单胞菌)。

• 并发症：
- 完全气道阻塞。
- 咽后壁脓肿。
- 急性呼吸窘迫综合征。
- 肺炎。

病因

• 感染因素：
- A 型、B 型及不可分型流感嗜血杆菌。
- 副流感嗜血杆菌。
- 肺炎链球菌。
- 金黄色葡萄球菌。
- β溶血性链球菌：A、B、C、F、G 亚型。
- 奈瑟菌脑膜炎。
- 单纯疱疹。
- 铜绿假单胞菌。
- 其他少见病原菌。

• 物理因素：
- 化学和热力损伤。
- 毒品或非法药物吸入。

• 创伤、器械操作。

诊断

症状和体征

病史

• 全身症状：
- 发热。

• 上呼吸道感染症状。

• 大多病例无前驱症状。

• 头、眼、耳、鼻、咽喉：
- 咽痛。
- 吞咽困难。
- 声音低沉。
- 声音改变。
  ◦ 发音含糊不清。
  ◦ 声音嘶哑。
- 咽喉异物感。
- 流涎。
- 扁桃体、扁桃体周围、悬雍垂相关表现。

• 呼吸系统：
- 气道阻塞的主观感觉。
- 气短。

体格检查

• 全身症状：
- 发热。

H

- 心动过速。
- 呈“三角架式”坐姿。
• 头、眼、耳、鼻、喉:
- 典型表现为会厌樱桃红色,50%可表现为苍白色或水肿。
- 留取口咽部分泌物。
- 淋巴结炎。
• 呼吸系统:
- 吸入性喘鸣。
- 突发气道阻塞。
- 呼吸困难需要用辅助呼吸肌呼吸。

> 注意
> 呼吸困难患者易迅速进展至完全气道阻塞,需紧急行气道处理。

基本检查

如果有明显的呼吸困难:
• 避免侵入性诊断检查。
• 经验应用抗生素,保持气道通畅以利于进一步的诊断性检查。

诊断检查与说明

实验室检查

• 全血细胞计数。
• 血培养。
• 咽部细菌培养。
- 仅在无呼吸困难症状时或成功建立气道管理。

影像学检查

• 有中重度呼吸困难患者,在影像学检查前行气管插管。
• 便携式颈部侧位 X 线:
- 会厌“拇指纹征”:
◦ 会厌增厚,见于 77%~88%的患者。
- 会厌谷征。
- 杓状会厌皱襞和杓状软骨水肿。
- 椎前软组织水肿。
- 明显假阴性结果。
- 怀疑阴性结果的真实性。
• CT 检查:
- 无法行喉镜检查或怀疑合并软组织并发症时。
- 同时也用于提示疾病复发时排除是否存在潜在组织畸形或其他发现。

诊断步骤/外科

• 有呼吸困难时,首先行气管插管。
• 鼻咽镜(迷你光导纤维视野)。
• 间接喉镜。

鉴别诊断

• 格鲁布性喉头炎。
• 气道异物。
• 过敏反应。
• 声带功能紊乱。
• 咽炎/扁桃体炎。
• 口咽部脓肿(扁桃体周或咽后)。
• 细菌性气管炎。
• 先天性异常。
• 悬雍垂炎症。
• 白喉。
• 上呼吸道肿瘤。

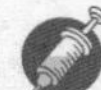

治疗

院前

• 转移患者至舒适区域。
• 吸氧,避免焦虑。
• 一度呼吸困难时气管插管。
• 吸入剂、消旋肾上腺素和β受体阻滞剂无效。

初步稳定/治疗

• ABC 管理。
• 手边准备确定性气道管理的所有设备,包括手术建立气道,直到排除此诊断或转运至 ICU。
• 气道检查可引起气道梗阻。
• 通过紧扣面罩的高流量环路给予氦氧混合气能够通过增加氧气层流充当临时计量仪。
• 有气道梗阻或严重呼吸困难的患者要经口气管插管:
- 呼吸困难、呼吸衰竭的发生可以是毫无预料的。
- 如果患者可能是困难气道/需要手术建立气道,请五官科/外科会诊。
• 如果气管插管失败,又无法立即手术建立气道,环甲膜穿刺可能是暂时性的抢救措施。

急诊治疗/程序

• 湿化氧气支持。
• 脉氧饱和度和心肺功能监测。
• 建立静脉通道,并应当水化治疗。
• 开始经验性使用有效抗生素治疗。
• 激素的使用意见不一但现在较推荐。

药物治疗

一线用药

• 头孢噻肟:2 g,静脉注射,q8 h+万古霉素:15 mg/kg,静脉注射,q12 h。
• 头孢曲松:2 g,静脉注射,q24 h+额外覆盖葡萄球菌抗生素。
• 平均疗程 7~10 日。

二线用药

• 氨苄西林-舒巴坦:初始 3 g,静脉注射,续贯 200~300 mg/(kg · d)分 4 次+万古霉素 1 g 静脉注射,q12 h。
• 甲氧苄氨嘧啶-磺胺甲噁唑:初始 320 mg 甲氧苄氨嘧啶,静脉注射及 1 600 mg 磺胺甲噁唑静脉滴注;续贯 4~5 mg/kg,静脉注射,q12 h。
• 呼吸道喹诺酮类。
• 如培养得 MRSA、中重度脓毒症和/或脑膜炎并不影响,考虑使用以下方案替代万古霉素治疗:
- 萘夫西林:2 g,静脉输注,q4 h。
- 克林霉素:600~900 mg,静脉输注,q8 h。
• 预防性的使用利福平:
- 成人:600 mg/d,连续口服 4 日。
- >1 个月的儿童:20 mg/(kg · d),连续口服 4 日。
- <1 个月的儿童:10 mg/(kg · d),连续口服 4 日。

随访

进一步处理

入院指征

疑似或确诊会厌炎的患者都应收住 ICU 给予静脉抗生素治疗和气道管理。

出院指征

• 只有经验丰富的医师通过检视声门上结构排除会厌炎才可出院。
• 与患者密切接触者应接受利福平预防性治疗。

转诊问题

应当请五官科医师会诊。

要点和误区

• 未能及时处理气道问题。
• 气道通畅前避免不必要的操作。
• 成人会厌炎病死率为 7%。

H

会厌炎(儿童) Epiglottitis, Pediatric

Roger M. Barkin 单怡 译

基础知识

描述

• 会厌及周围组织的炎症,当进行性的气道阻塞时可危及生命。
• 儿童发生上气道阻塞的风险更大:
- 小儿上呼吸道管径小(阻力与半径的 4 次方成反比)。
- 黏膜表面疏松及黏膜血管丰富易产生黏膜水肿。
- 气道的动力性塌陷。
• 流感嗜血杆菌疫苗的接种使小儿会厌炎的发生率大为降低,但是接受免疫的儿童中由于疫苗接种失败偶有发生小儿会厌炎。
• 由于接种 B 型流感嗜血杆菌疫苗,会厌炎的平均发病年龄在增加,与学龄前和学龄期儿童相比,青少年和成人的发病率更高。
• 全年均可发病。

> **注意**
> 怀疑会厌炎的患者需重症监护和处理。有可能快速进展为气道阻塞。

病因

• 感染:
- B 型流感嗜血杆菌。
- 肺炎链球菌。
- A 组 β 溶血性链球菌。
- 链球菌。
- 金黄色葡萄球菌。
- 病毒。
- 少见病原如克雷白杆菌、假单胞菌、念珠菌。
• 腐蚀。
• 烫伤。
• 创伤。
• 移植后淋巴组织增生障碍。
• 先天性血管性水肿。

诊断

症状和体征

现病史

• 常突然发病而没有前驱症状。
• 全身症状:
- 烦躁不安,咽喉痛(主诉非常难受的咽喉疼痛),发热,呼吸音粗。
- 进行性中毒反应和呼吸困难。
- 成人常在诊断前就诊过 1 次以上。成人会主诉"这辈子咽喉从没这么痛过"。

体格检查

• 全身检查:
- 中毒性面容。
- 典型的高热。
- 急性发病并快速进展。
• 咽喉:
- 流涎。
- 吞咽困难。
- 言语含糊不清。
- 老年人咽喉痛明显。
• 呼吸系统:
- 快速进展的呼吸困难(成人仅 1/3 出现呼吸困难)。
- 小儿常表现为上身挺直、向前倾斜着张口呼吸("三脚架体位")以尽可能多吸气。
- 喘鸣呈进行性加重(成人仅 10%出现喘鸣)。
• 并发症:
- 气道阻塞是最严重的并发症。
- 会厌脓肿。
- 并发肺炎和肺不张。

基本检查

• 会厌炎是临床诊断。
• 小儿怀疑有会厌炎时应避免间接喉镜或其他可直视会厌的检查,除非一切急救措施准备就绪(青少年或成年人,无气道阻塞的患者应做纤维鼻咽镜检查)。
• 若怀疑感染,在气道保护的前提下,在喉镜检查时留取会厌部培养标本。

诊断检查与说明

实验室检查

• 气道保护前避免实验室检查。
• 气道保护后行喉部病原学培养。
• 气道保护后行血培养:
- 当嗜血杆菌感染时血培养常为阳性。

影像学检查

• 颈侧软组织 X 线检查:
- 非诊断必需。
- 可增加延迟保护气道的风险,刺激患儿发生气道阻塞,并且常把患儿从急诊室转运至未知的环境。患儿绝对不能在无人陪伴下行 X 线检查。必须配备控制气道所需要的设备和医护人员。
• X 线的各种表现:
- 正常。
- 会厌及声门上组织肿胀(拇指指纹征)。
- 下咽部鼓起。
- 会厌谷闭塞。
- EW/C3W(即会厌宽度与第 3 颈椎体宽度)比例>0.5。

诊断步骤/外科

喉镜:
• 在急救措施完善的环境随时可进行喉镜检查。
• 气道保护后在喉镜检查的同时行会厌病原学培养,有助于确定致病菌并指导治疗。
• 会厌可表现为肿胀、炎症、发红。

鉴别诊断

• 其他感染性疾病:
- 细菌性气管炎。
- 咽后脓肿。
- 扁桃体周围脓肿。
- 格鲁布综合征(即哮吼),主要发生于幼儿,但在发病年龄上与会厌炎有重叠。
- 百日咳。
- 单核细胞增多症。
- 路德维希咽峡炎。
- 白喉。
• 血管性水肿的过敏反应。
• 遗传性血管水肿。
• 上呼吸道异物。
• 喉部创伤。
• 喉部痉挛。
• 吸入毒物(如碳氢化合物)。
• 气道灼伤(与可卡因相关)。
• 过度通气。
• 中枢神经系统功能障碍。

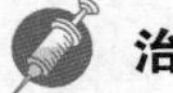

治疗

院前

干预程度和方式必须取决于阻塞程度、转运的时间和方式、护理者的能力等。咨询并通知接收的医院。

初步稳定/治疗

• 对病情严重的患儿实行气道管理。

H

• 纯氧面罩通气及环状软骨加压能够提供足够的通气，争取时间将患儿送至安全的环境，如手术室。
• 经口气管插管：
- 选择比患儿年龄或气道长度所应使用的气管插管小 1 号或 2 号的导管。
- 直接压迫颈前部声门位置有助于暴露肿胀的声门时看到气泡。
- 辅助应用困难气道所需的设备。
• 若口气管插管失败：
- 患儿年龄＞10 岁，紧急行环甲膜切开或穿刺术。
- 患儿年龄＜10 岁，则行环甲膜穿刺术。

■ 急诊治疗/程序

• 患者可耐受纯氧。
• 允许患者保持舒服的体位，迫使患者平躺可能会加重气道阻塞。
• 尽管未经证实，在等待建立确定性气道时，雾化吸入右旋/左旋肾上腺素可以暂时稳定症状。但必须小心操作以免引起刺激。
• 避免引起患儿刺激的操作。

■ 药物治疗

一线用药

• 头孢噻肟：2 g，静脉注射，q8 h。
• 头孢曲松：2 g，静脉注射，q24 h。

二线用药

• 氨苄西林-舒巴坦：初始 3 g，静脉注射，续贯 200～300 mg/(kg · d)，分 4 次＋万古霉素 1 g，静脉注射，q12 h。
• 甲氧苄氨嘧啶-磺胺甲嘧啶：初始 320 mg，静脉注射；续贯 4～5 mg/kg，静脉注射，q12 h。
• 考虑增加用药覆盖金黄色葡萄球菌感染：
- 萘夫西林：每日 150～200 mg/kg，静脉注射，分 4 次。
- 克林霉素：600～800 mg，静脉注射，q8 h。
• 预防性使用利福平：
- 成人：600 mg/d，连续口服 4 日。
- ＞1 个月的儿童：20 mg/(kg · d)，连续口服 4 日。
- ＜1 个月的儿童：10 mg/(kg · d)，连续口服 4 日。

随访

■ 进一步处理

入院指征

疑似或确诊会厌炎的患者都应收住 ICU，给予静脉抗生素治疗和气道管理。

出院指征

• 只有经验丰富的医师通过检视声门上结构，排除会厌炎才可出院。
• 与患者密切接触者应接受利福平预防性治疗。

转诊问题

应当请五官科医师会诊。

要点和误区

紧急气道管理。患者需要随时监测，并有能建立确认性气道的医师陪同。

昏迷 Coma

Gregory D. Jay · Linda C. Cowell　陈奇通 译

基础知识

■ 描述

• 轻度昏迷：
- 对疼痛有反应。
• 深度昏迷：
- 对疼痛无反应。
• 无反应性：
- 觉醒和认知的丧失。
◦ 觉醒丧失。
◦ 觉醒主要为脑干功能。
◦ 网状激活系统受损。
◦ 认知丧失。
◦ 双侧大脑半球功能异常。
- 木僵。
◦ 深度睡眠，并非无意识。
◦ 表现出少量或者无自主活动。
◦ 刺激能觉醒。
◦ 觉醒后无运动或言语。
• 缓和：
- 意识迟钝伴轻度或中度警觉下降。
• 谵妄：
- 浮夸的异常意识状态。
- 易激惹。
- 无休止活动。
- 短暂幻觉。
- 定向异常。
- 错觉。
• 意识模糊：
- 意识障碍。
- 对当前刺激的清楚思考或感知，反应和记忆能力受损。

■ 病因

• 弥漫性脑功能不全(69%)：
- 营养缺乏：
◦ 低血糖。
◦ 低氧。
- 中毒：
◦ 乙醇。
◦ 异丙醇。
◦ 乙烯甘醇。
◦ 甲醇。
◦ 水杨酸。
◦ 镇静催眠药。
◦ 麻醉剂。
◦ 抗惊厥药物。
◦ 异烟肼。
◦ 重金属。
◦ 阿片类。
◦ 苯二氮䓬类。
◦ 抗胆碱能药物。
◦ 锂。
◦ 苯环己哌啶。
◦ 氰化物。
◦ 一氧化碳。
- 感染：
◦ 细菌性、结核性、梅毒性脑膜炎。
◦ 脑炎。
◦ 疟原虫性脑膜炎。
◦ 伤寒发热。
◦ 狂犬病。
- 内分泌紊乱：
◦ 黏液性水肿昏迷。
◦ 甲状腺素毒性。
◦ Addison 病。

H

◦ Cushing 病。
◦ 嗜铬细胞瘤。
- 代谢紊乱：
◦ 肝性脑病。
◦ 尿毒症。
◦ 卟啉病。
◦ Weinicke 脑病。
◦ 氨基酸血症。
◦ Reye 综合征。
◦ 高碳酸。
- 电解质紊乱：
◦ 高钠血症、低钠血症。
◦ 高钙血症、低钙血症。
◦ 高镁血症、低镁血症。
◦ 低磷血症。
◦ 酸中毒、碱中毒。
- 体温调节：
◦ 低体温。
◦ 中暑。
◦ 安定药恶性综合征。
◦ 恶性高体温。
- 尿毒症。
- 发作后状态，癫痫持续状态。
- 精神疾病。
- 休克。
- 脂肪栓塞。
- 高血压脑病。
• 幕上病灶(19%)：
- 出血(15%)：
◦ 实质细胞内出血。
◦ 硬膜外血肿。
◦ 硬膜下血肿。
◦ 蛛网膜下腔出血。
- 梗死(2%)：
◦ 血栓性动脉闭塞。
◦ 栓塞性动脉闭塞。
◦ 静脉闭塞。
- 肿瘤或脓肿(2%)：
◦ 脑积水。
◦ 脑疝。
◦ 邻近血管侵蚀引起的出血。
• 幕下损伤(12%)：
- 梗死。
- 出血。
- 肿瘤。
- 基底部偏头痛。
- 脑干脱髓鞘。

妊娠注意事项

子痫。

诊断

症状和体征

病史

持续的意识损害。

体格检查

• 无自主睁眼。
• 对疼痛刺激反应缺失。
• 无肢体活动。
• 规律的心血管呼吸功能。
• Glasgow 昏迷量表(GCS)评分：
- 睁眼(E)：
◦ 自主睁眼：4。
◦ 语言命令睁眼：3。
◦ 疼痛睁眼：2。
◦ 无反应：1。
- 最好的运动反应为遵言语命令：
◦ 遵指令：6。
- 对疼痛刺激的运动反应：
◦ 疼痛定位：5。
◦ 疼痛躲避：4。
◦ 异常肢体屈曲：3。
◦ 异常肢体伸张：2。
◦ 无反应：1。
- 言语反应(V)：
◦ 表达正确且可对答：5。
◦ 表达混乱且可对答：4。
◦ 有简单重复的言语：3。
◦ 只能发音：2。
◦ 无反应：1。
- GCS＝E＋M＋V。
• 低体温：
- 感染、低血糖、黏液水肿性昏迷、酒精和镇静催眠药物中毒。
• 发热：
- 感染、甲状腺毒症、抗胆碱能药物、拟交感药物、安定药恶性综合征、下丘脑出血。
• 高血压。
• 结构性损害，高血压脑病。
• 低血压。
• 瞳孔放大。
- 有机磷酸酯类。
• 瞳孔缩小：
- 麻醉剂。
- 抗胆碱能药物。
- 脑桥损害。
• 瞳孔反射消失或双侧瞳孔不对等：
- 结构性损害。
• 头颅创伤的证据。
• 颈项强直：
- 脑膜炎。
- 蛛网膜下腔出血。
• 去皮质姿势：
- 肘和腕关节屈曲。
- 双侧肩关节内收内旋。
- 前臂后旋。
- 提示中脑以上水平严重损伤。
• 去大脑姿势：
- 肘和腕关节伸张。
- 双侧肩关节内收内旋。
- 前臂外旋。
- 提示中脑水平或间脑水平损伤。
• 不对称运动：
- 结构性损害。
- 单个肢体持续抽动：
◦ 癫痫持续状态。

基本检查

• 寻找和治疗可逆转的病因。
• 立即排除类昏迷状态：
- 关注被动翻开眼睑时的阻力，脑卒中(中风)时有眼睑扑动，有迅速关闭眼睑，眼球有扫视样运动(而不是徘徊不定)，或发现眼球后翻。
- 冰水热量试验可触发眼球震颤。
- 在给一个患者麻醉插管前，应尝试寻找是否存在闭锁综合征。
- 患者能够在口头命令下眨眼，可诊断闭锁综合征。
- 气管插管可预防误吸。

诊断检查与说明

实验室检验

• 测末梢血糖。
• 全血细胞检查。
• 电解质。
• 血和尿液毒物筛查。

影像学检查

头颅 CT：
• 出血和中线移位的诊断。
• 怀疑脑血管意外可行 CT 血管造影。

诊断步骤/外科

• 腰椎穿刺：
- 所有病因未知的昏迷患者，特别是有发热者。
- 腰椎穿刺前抗生素可使用长达 48 h。
- 如有颅内压增高、肿物、外伤史或局部表现的证据，应在腰椎穿刺前行 CT 检查。
• 有颅内肿物的患者行腰椎穿刺出现小脑

扁桃体疝的风险非常小。

• 脑电图：
- 排除可疑的癫痫发作。
- 在急诊评估时作用小。
- 与在实验室进行的脑电图不同，灯光会造成伪差。

■ 鉴别诊断

• 闭锁综合征。
• 精神性无反应性。
• 木僵。
• 紧张症。
• 运动不能性缄默。

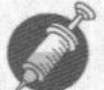

治疗

■ 院前

• 如果气道开放受影响行气道管理。
• 对昏迷鸡尾酒治疗无反应则行气管插管。
• 静脉通路。
• 葡萄糖或血糖试纸检查。
• 纳洛酮。
• 寻找潜在病因的体征：
- 医疗警示手环。
- GCS 评分。
- 瞳孔。
- 四肢运动。

■ 初步稳定/治疗

• 气道管理。
• 经验性纳洛酮使用。
• 经验性使用葡萄糖注射液：
- 如果无法在床边测量血清血糖浓度，则使用葡萄糖。
- 在硫胺素前可安全使用。
- 对脑卒中(中风)患者不会恶化预后。

■ 急诊治疗/程序

• 一旦明确病因，相应的特异性治疗即开始。
• 病因未明确的昏迷患者可以考虑经验性使用抗生素。
- 选用抗菌谱广且有好的脑脊液渗透性的抗生素，如头孢曲松。
• 使用苯二氮䓬类、苯妥英、苯巴比妥药物停止癫痫发作。
• 毒物摄取的经验性治疗：
- 活性炭。
• 纠正体温：
- 体核温在 32～35℃的患者应给予主动复温，小于 32℃者行有创性复温。
- 严重高热者在浸湿的暴露皮肤上放置冰毯和风吹。

药物

• 头孢曲松：100 mg/kg，静脉注射。
• 葡萄糖：1～2 ml/kg D_{50} W，静脉注射；新生儿 10 ml/kg D_{10} W，静脉使用；儿童 4 ml/kg D_{25} W，静脉使用。
• 地西泮(安定)：0.1～0.3 mg/kg，缓慢静脉注射(单次最大剂量 10 mg)，q10～15 min×3 次。
• 氟马西尼：0.20 mg，静脉使用，qmin×(1～5)次。
• 甲吡唑：15 mg/kg，静脉使用。
• 劳拉西泮：0.05～0.1 mg/kg，静脉使用(单次最大剂量 4 mg)，q10～15 min。
• 甘露醇：0.25～1 g/kg，静脉使用超过 20 min。
• 纳洛酮：0.01～0.1 mg/kg。
• 苯巴比妥：10～20 mg/kg，静脉注射，监测呼吸抑制情况。
• 苯妥英钠：输注小于 50 mg/min；18～20 mg/kg，静脉/骨髓腔输注；或磷苯妥因 15～20 mg/kg，静脉/骨髓腔输注。
• 毒扁豆碱：0.5～2 mg，静脉注射。
• 硫胺素：100 mg，肌内注射；或 100 mg 硫胺素溶于 1 000 ml 静脉液体中畅滴。
• 维生素 B_6：70 mg/kg，静脉注射(最高剂量 5 g，与 INH 过量呈 1∶1 比例)。

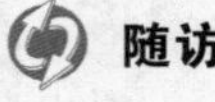

随访

■ 进一步处理

入院指征

无法轻易识别，且病因无完全逆转的昏迷患者应收治入院。

出院指征

可纠正的低血糖和对积极急诊处理有反应的阿片类中毒的昏迷患者，可予以出院。

转诊问题

进一步描述或者防止可能的药物不良反应。

■ 随访建议

• 如果出院需要紧急初级保健医师随访。
• 药物不良反应的考虑。
• 出院后观察 24 h。
• 在阿片类药物中毒的情况下，讨论药物辅助治疗的选择和纳洛酮的使用。

要点和误区

• 快速药物稳定。
• 神经影像学检查寻找结构性病灶。
• 代谢性和中毒性因素评估。
• 明确不常见的昏迷原因。
• 可出院患者血药急诊观察时间。
• 推荐药物滥用。

霍纳综合征

Richard S. Krause 巩博 译

基础知识

■ 描述

眼睛单侧交感神经受损产生霍纳综合征的病症：

• 上眼睑和下眼睑收缩的肌肉松弛。
- 上睑下垂(眼睑下垂)。
• 支配瞳孔扩大的神经消失。
- 瞳孔缩小(无对抗的瞳孔收缩)。
• 汗腺的交感神经刺激消失。
- 无汗症。

■ 病因

• 40%病因不明。
• 肺癌或转移至颈部淋巴结：
- 可能干扰节前交感神经纤维(在胸交感神经干和颈上神经节之间)。
• 创伤：穿透性颈部伤直接损伤交感神经纤维。
• 气胸：
- 张力性气胸可引起纵隔移位，导致交感神经纤维受到牵拉。
• 颈部淋巴结感染或浸润：
- 类肉状瘤病、结核病。
• 血管疾病：
- 偏头痛或丛集性头痛。
- 颈动脉夹层。
• 单侧延髓梗塞产生霍纳综合征，是延髓背外侧综合征的一部分。
- 出现眩晕和共济失调，这些可能掩盖霍纳综合征。
• 海绵窦血栓形成可能出现霍纳综合征的部分症状。
- 常引起头痛和/或眼痛。
- 眼部体征包括眼麻痹、疼痛、球结膜水肿及眼球突出。

儿科注意事项

• 遗传性霍纳综合征：
- 患侧蓝虹膜（或不规则颜色）。
- 健侧棕色（虹膜异色）。
• 分娩损伤：
- 可能对交感神经链产生损伤。
• 儿童新发霍纳综合征应快速检查肿瘤（神经母细胞瘤）。

诊断

症状和体征

• 霍纳综合征的特点：
- 上睑下垂：患侧眼睑下垂，通常为轻度。
- 瞳孔缩小：患侧瞳孔直径变小（瞳孔不对称≥1 mm）。
- 无汗症（患侧面部出汗少）。
- 常为单发，很少多发。
• 霍纳综合征的要点是并发某些特定疾病。

病史

预先处理在霍纳综合征之前存在的疾病或这些疾病的危险因素：
• 肿瘤、血管疾病和创伤：
- 颈动脉夹层前常出现小的创伤。
• 心血管风险。
• 暴露：
- 假性霍纳综合征。
• 疼痛：
- 提示颈动脉夹层。

> **注意**
> • 急性霍纳综合征伴颈部或面部疼痛：
> - 假定颈动脉夹层直到排除：
> ◦ 许多颈内动脉解剖都表现为疼痛性霍纳综合征。

体格检查

关注神经系统检查以确定霍纳综合征并排除其他神经系统疾病：
• 一般体格检查应注意识别其他可疑疾病的病征，如肿瘤。

基本检查

• 病史和体格检查应当关注神经系统症状。
• 胸部 X 线筛查肿瘤或气胸。

诊断检查与说明

激发试验：
• 药物（可卡因）试验可明确交感神经眼损伤的诊断。
- 一滴 5%眼用可卡因液体滴双眼。
- 在 1 h 内，同健侧相比，患侧瞳孔扩张失败（阳性结果）。

实验室检查

对霍纳综合征本身无用。
• 经常用来检查病因或并发症。

影像学检查

• 霍纳综合征伴有胸部疾病，常行胸部 X 线检查。
• 在某些指征或综合征，可行头部、颈部、胸部 CT 或 MRI。
• 对于可疑颈动脉夹层：
- 头部和颈部 MRA 或 CTA：
◦ 其他合适的检查。
◦ 病变和霍纳综合征位于同侧。
• 可疑脑卒中患者选择神经影像检查严重依赖本地资源。
- 如果怀疑脑卒中，至少行脑部 CT 检查排除出血性脑卒中。
- 如果怀疑急性脑卒中（<3 h），且患者准备溶栓治疗，在技术团队的支持下进行影像学检查。

诊断步骤/外科

如果怀疑急性青光眼，进行眼压测定。

鉴别诊断

• 颅内压增高。
- 总是与意识水平的改变、头痛相关。
• 单纯瞳孔不等（假性霍纳综合征）：
- 15%～20%的人瞳孔不等大，3%～4%有瞳孔缩小和上睑下垂。
- 可可因试验阴性（双侧瞳孔同等扩张）。
- 检查身份证照片是否有预先存在的瞳孔不等大。
- 局部用药或暴露是瞳孔缩小的常见原因。
• 偏头痛或丛集性头痛。
• 青光眼、炎性眼部疾病或眼外伤。

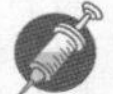

治疗

院前

注意：
• 霍纳综合征并发一些严重的潜在性疾病。
• 应尽快识别伴有颅内压增高的或张力性气胸的患者，并且尽快治疗。
• 如果怀疑脑卒中，可能的话应尽快送至指定脑卒中中心。

初步稳定/治疗

• 如果怀疑颅内压增高，启动控制颅内压的措施：
- 插管，渗透性利尿。
• 张力性气胸：
- 胸腔穿刺并引流。

急诊治疗/程序

霍纳综合征本身不需要急诊治疗。
• 原发疾病或并发疾病可能需要急诊治疗。

药物治疗

可卡因：5%（成人），2.5%（儿童）滴眼液：每只眼 1 滴，作为诊断性治疗使用。

随访

进一步处理

入院指征

单纯霍纳综合征没有必要住院治疗：
• 原发疾病可能需要住院治疗。

出院指征

• 单纯霍纳综合征且病情稳定的患者可以出院，并安排合适的门诊随诊以继续检查：
- 当怀疑霍纳综合征时，在出院前应排除脑卒中或颈动脉夹层等紧急情况。

随访建议

神经科医师和眼科医师应经常参与霍纳综合征的诊治和复查。

要点和误区

必须考虑有无潜在的病因。

机会性感染 Opportunistic Infections

Karen J. Bowers · Michelle D. Lall 朱妍 译

基础知识

描述

当宿主对正常非致病微生物抵抗力下降时发生的不常见的感染。

病因

• 在 $CD4^{+}$ T 淋巴细胞计数降到 200/mm^3 或淋巴细胞计数中占比＜14％的 HIV 患者中发生：
- 肺孢子菌肺炎(PCP)。
- 播散性结核。
- 隐孢子虫病。
- 微孢子虫病。
- 等孢子球虫病。
- 弓形虫病。
- 组织胞浆菌病。
- 隐球菌病。
- 鸟分枝杆菌复合体。
- 结核性心包炎或脑膜炎。
- 巨细胞病毒。
- 人类疱疹病毒 8 型(Kaposi 肉瘤)。
- JC 病毒(进行性多灶性脑白质病)。
- 乙型肝炎病毒。
- 马尔尼菲青霉病。
- 各种细菌。

• 细胞介导的缺陷：
- 恶性血液病。
- 淋巴瘤。
- 高剂量糖皮质激素治疗。
- 自身免疫失调。
- 病毒感染。
- 细胞毒性药物、化疗。
- 放射治疗。
- 伴随：
  ◦ 军团菌病。
  ◦ 诺卡菌病。
  ◦ 沙门菌。
  ◦ 分枝杆菌。

• 粒细胞减少或缺乏：
- 细胞毒性药物。
- 再生障碍性贫血。
- 药物反应：
  ◦ 氨苯砜。
- 肿瘤侵犯骨髓。
- 砷。
- 青霉素。
- 氯霉素。
- 普鲁卡因胺。
- 维生素缺乏。
- 伴有：
  ◦ 葡萄球菌和 A 型溶血性链球菌。
  ◦ 肠道微生物和厌氧菌。
  ◦ 侵袭性曲霉病。

• 免疫调节药物：
- TNF－α 抑制剂。
  ◦ 英夫利昔单抗＞依那西普。
  ◦ 利妥昔单抗。
  ◦ 阿达木单抗。
- 硫唑嘌呤。

• 考虑肝炎、带状疱疹和结核分枝杆菌的再激活。

诊断

症状和体征

• 新发或加重的乏力症状。
• 呼吸急促。
• 发热。
• 寒战。
• 盗汗。
• 肺源性感染：
- 咳嗽。
- 充血。
- 啰音。

• 泌尿系统来源感染：
- 排尿困难。
- 尿频。
- 尿潴留。

• 胃肠来源感染：
- 腹痛。
- 呕吐。
- 腹泻。
- 出血。
- 黏液或脓性大便。
- 黄疸。

• 中枢神经系统来源感染：
- 精神混乱。
- 局灶性神经功能缺损。
- 头痛。
- 癫痫。

病史

• HIV/AIDS 病史。
• 恶性肿瘤放化史。
• 器官移植史。
• 自身免疫紊乱史。
• 炎症性肠病病史。
• 使用细胞毒药物。
• 使用高剂量糖皮质激素。
• 免疫调节药物的使用：
- 使用一种以上药物时的叠加效应。

体格检查

• 完整详细的体格检查表明在免疫功能低下的患者中感染征象可能更轻微。
• 系统性炎症反应综合征的征象：
- 体温＞38 ℃或＜36 ℃。
- 心率＞90 次/分。
- 呼吸频率＞20 次/分或 PCO_2＜32 mmHg。

• 感染性休克。
• 局灶性神经功能缺失。
• 新发震颤。
• 肺孢子菌肺炎患者活动后缺氧。
• 肺炎导致的湿啰音和/或干啰音。
• 腹胀或腹膜炎
• 皮肤/黏膜缺损是感染的入口。
• 口咽念珠菌病是免疫抑制的征象。

基本检查

免疫功能不全的患者需进行完整的检查：

• 感染体征在免疫功能低下的患者中可能不表现。
• 可能会表现出轻微的体征并迅速恶化。
• 发热等体征提示患者需完整的评估。
• 彻底的检查对寻找感染源至关重要。

诊断检查与说明

实验室检查

• 血常规可以鉴别中性粒细胞减少和白细胞增多症：
- WBC＞12 000/μl 或＜4 000/μl 是系统性炎症反应综合征的标准。
- 中性粒细胞减少：
- 中性粒细胞计数绝对值(ANC)＜1 500/μl。
- ANC ＝ WBC(细胞数/μl)× 百分比(PMNS＋杆状核细胞)/100。

• 培养(需氧菌、厌氧菌、真菌、病毒)：
- 尿。
- 血。

J

- 伤口。
- 粪。
- 痰或微型 BAL(在插管患者中)。
- CD4 细胞计数：
- 如果 CD4 细胞未知，淋巴细胞计数绝对值(ALC)<1000/μl 提示 CD4<200。
- ALC=WBC(细胞数/μl)×百分比(淋巴细胞)/100。
• 尿常规出现 WBC、亚硝酸盐、白细胞酯酶。
• 电解质、尿素氮/肌酐、葡萄糖，阴离子间隙升高型酸中毒提示严重感染。
• 酸中毒时的静脉血葡萄糖。
• 乳酸水平：升高提示严重感染。
• PT、APTT 是弥散性血管内凝血(DIC)的证据。
• 乳酸脱氢酶(LDH)：PCP 患者升高。

影像学检查

• 胸部 X 线检查：
- 预测特殊感染病因的非特异性检查。
◦ 肺炎：
◦ 节段性或亚节段的浸润。
◦ 支气管充气征。
◦ 脓肿。
◦ 空泡。
◦ 积脓。
◦ 胸膜渗出。
- PCP：
◦ 典型表现是双侧间质性或中央性肺泡浸润。
◦ 高达 25%的患者放射影像是正常的。
• 心脏超声：
- 对肺状态、心功能、液体状态的床边评估。
- 疑似肝脏病理的 RUQ。
• 高分辨率胸部 CT：
- 早期研究提示在 HIV 阳性患者中诊断 PCP 敏感性高。
- 表现为斑片状毛玻璃影。
• 头颅 CT：
- 弓形虫脑炎病灶可被对比剂增强，通常在基底节区。
• 腹部和盆腔增强 CT：
- 如果临床体检怀疑为胃肠道来源的感染推荐该检查。

诊断步骤/检查

腰椎穿刺：
• 如果怀疑中枢神经系统感染行脑脊液常规检查。
• 诊断性穿刺。
• 免疫抑制肝病患者检查自发性细菌性腹膜炎(SBP)。

治疗

初步稳定/治疗

• ABC 管理。
• 低血压快速静脉补液：给予生理盐水与平衡盐溶液。
• 吸氧。
• 生命体征不稳者行心电监护。
• 早期开始抗生素治疗。

急诊治疗/程序

• 严格隔离。
• 抗生素：结合超广谱青霉素(美洛西林、羟基噻吩青霉素、哌拉西林)和氨基糖苷类(阿米卡星、妥布霉素)。
- 如果使用氨基糖苷类药物有禁忌，单药疗法可使用第三代头孢菌素(头孢他啶、头孢吡肟)、氟喹诺酮(左氧氟沙星、加替沙星)或其他广谱抗生素(亚胺培南-西司他丁)单药治疗。
- 如果区域内有高发耐甲氧西林的病原菌，可使用万古霉素。
- 如果患者使用充分的抗生素治疗 1 周，可考虑使用抗真菌药(两性霉素 B、氟康唑)。
- 甲氧苄啶-磺胺甲噁唑可以用于 PCP 感染(次选：戊烷脒、克林霉素+伯氨喹)。
• 类固醇激素：泼尼松用于伴低氧血症的 PCP 患者。

药物治疗

• 两性霉素 B：0.25 mg/(kg·d)，静脉注射。
• 头孢吡肟：1～2 g，q12 h，静脉注射。
• 头孢他啶：
- 成人：1～2 g，静脉注射，q8～12 h。
- 儿童：100～150 mg/(kg·24 h)，静脉注射，q8～12 h。
• 氟康唑：400 mg 首剂，之后 200～400 mg/d 静脉注射[儿童：6～12 mg/(kg·24 h)，静脉注射，q12 h]。
• 加替沙星：400 mg/d，静脉注射。
• 亚胺培南-西司他丁：500～1000 mg，静脉注射，q6～8 h，极量 50 mg/(kg·d)或 4000 mg/d。
• 左氧氟沙星：500 mg/d，静脉注射。
• 万古霉素：1～2 g，静脉注射，q12 h[儿童：10～50 mg/(kg·24 h)，静脉注射，q6 h]。
• 甲氧苄啶 15～20 mg/kg+磺胺甲噁唑 75 mg/kg，口服或静脉滴注，q8 h。
• 泼尼松：40 mg，口服，2 次/日×5 日；之后 40 mg 口服，1 次/日×5 日；之后 20 mg，口服，1 次/日×11 日。
  * 肺孢子菌肺炎应在 72 h 内使用抗生素。

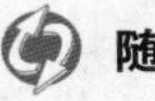

随访

进一步处理

入院指征

疑诊或确诊系统性感染。

出院指征

排除系统性感染。

转诊问题

考虑感染科会诊。

随访建议

系统性机会感染的患者应被收入院。

要点和误区

• 免疫抑制的患者可能并不表现出感染的征象。
• 可能会表现出细微的征象并迅速恶化。

J

肌腱撕裂伤

NichoJIe D. Bromley　范浩浩　李文放 译

基础知识

注意

撕裂伤附近肌腱必须通过完整的运动范围来探查以排除损伤。

描述

• 取决于受伤机制
• 外部创伤：
- 贯穿伤：
◦ 枪击。
◦ 玻璃。
◦ 刀。
◦ 异物。
- 闭合性损伤：
◦ 过伸造成挤压或撕脱。
• 内部创伤：
- 骨折导致的夹闭、撕裂伤(罕见)。

病因

肌腱损伤大致分为影响上下肢的因素。

• 与工作场所、家庭、袭击或企图自杀相关的上肢损伤。
• 下肢损伤最常见的是工作或机动车事故相关性损伤。

诊断

症状和体征

• 疼痛是主要症状。
• 功能缺陷。
• 软组织损伤：
- 肿胀。
- 瘀斑。
- 伤口。
- 出血。
• 四肢处于异常的静止位置或大关节不稳，应重点怀疑肌腱损伤的可能。

基本检查

• 细致的病史回顾：
- 机制、受伤时间。
- 受伤时手的位置。
- 手的主导地位。
- 药物过敏。
- 药物。
- 既往史。
- 破伤风疫苗的接种状态。
• 体格检查：
- 检查手的休息位置(休息时有手指的自然弯曲角度由正常的径向向尺侧增加)。
- 检查初始损伤位置的伤口。
- 在当地医院进行麻醉，在麻醉状态下行神经血管检查。
- 分别检查每个手指。
- 测试对抗阻力的能力。
- 直视下检查肌腱全方位的运动能力。
• 趾深屈肌受伤：
- 目前无法弯曲远端指间(IP)关节。
- 检查包括当患者试图屈曲远端指间关节时固定的近端指间关节在充分伸展的位置。
• 指浅屈肌损伤：
- 存在无法弯曲近端指间关节的手指。
- 通常通过标准的浅表肌腱试验来建立诊断：
◦ 将未受伤的手指全部保持伸直位置，患者试图弯曲受影响的手指的近端指间关节。
◦ 如果深度功能正常，则为假阴性。
- 远端指间关节伸直测试：
◦ 可以使这个诊断更加明显。
◦ 要求患者进行拇指和受伤手指之间精确捏合。
◦ 然后要求将近端指间关节弯曲以便于远端指间关节过度伸展。
◦ 确认指浅屈肌的完整性。
• 前臂和腕部屈肌受伤：
- 表现为无法弯曲尺侧或桡侧。
◦ 手腕或在阻碍拇指到小指运动的同时弯曲手腕。
• 伸肌腱损伤：
- 可通过远端指骨对抗阻力时无力或不能伸直而发现该损伤。
- 表示部分或完全中断。
- 最好由患者将手掌放在平面上并要求患者尝试单独伸直手指来确定。
- 检查每根肌腱。
- 正常张力丧失表示受伤。
• 局部麻醉(1%利多卡因或0.5%布比卡因)后在出血少光线充足的手术领域进一步探索附近的肌腱和伤口：
- 必须探查伤口附近完整范围内的肌腱。
- 最好探明远端或近端的肌腱损伤到的皮肤伤口。

儿科注意

• 更难以获得足够的检查。
• 愈合过程通常更快，相关功能往往可完全恢复到受伤前状态。

诊断检查与说明

实验室检查

创伤后12 h以上才进行第一次检查或伤口明显的感染应该进行培养。

影像学检查

• 经常需要X线片识别不透射线的异物或骨折。
• 高频超声可用于完整的识别肌腱撕裂：
- 部分肌腱撕裂难以影像学显示。
- 当试图对一个极度疼痛的肢体进行影像学检查时，水浴可能会有帮助。
• 超声可能有助于指导清除异物。

鉴别诊断

• 排除相关的异物或骨折。
• 近端指间关节涉及伸肌的侧带或中央索机制：
- 由于不适当的处理成的胸花畸形。
• 破坏远端的伸肌腱中央索导致槌指畸形。
• “泽西手指”是一个封闭的创伤性指深肌腱撕裂的损害，常见于一名员抓住另一名球员的手指卡住了。
• 远端屈曲趾浅部皮肤撕裂可能有或没有关联撕脱性骨折：
- 怀疑手指被快速移动的物体撞击时。

治疗

院前

• 请勿在现场移除患者身上的异物。
• 固定和运输患者。
• 加压止血。
• 评估远端神经血管状态。
• 在尝试采取任何控制损伤的措施之前联系医疗机构。

初步稳定/治疗

• 评估肢体并控制出血。
• 去除所有首饰或束缚性穿戴。

急诊治疗/程序

• 按需要给予镇痛。

• 根据需要施用破伤风类毒素。

• 用1L生理盐水进行大量冲洗。

• 广谱抗生素，如第一代头孢菌素（头孢唑林）。

• 与人咬伤有关的肌腱断裂：

- 必须大量灌洗。

- 联合应用抗生素，包括口腔厌氧菌（氨苄西林-舒巴坦）。

- 固定和抬高手部。

• 去除所有异物并进行无血运组织清创术。

• 累及肌腱横截面积的20%以上的撕裂必须修复。

• 在急诊室中可以修复简单的伸肌腱撕裂：

- 1区：通常为锤状指，远侧指间关节延伸部分用夹板固定。

- 1～4区和6区：可在急诊室修复。

- 5区：可疑的"打斗咬伤"，需要立即请手外科会诊进行冲洗和手术修复。

- 7区、8区：拇指受累、开放性骨折或严重污染应转诊手外科进行修复。

- 使用3-0或4-0非可吸收缝线行8字形缝合或改良凯斯勒缝合术。

• 所有可疑的屈肌腱、手腕和远端前臂肌腱撕裂需要请外科医师会诊，最好在12h内。

• 近端指间关节的肌腱撕裂可能导致胸花样畸形：

- 咨询手外科医师。

• 手腕掌侧面的多种肌腱、神经血管容易受到穿透性创伤的伤害：

• "意大利面手腕"或"满屋"：

- 至少10个结构参与手腕掌侧的裂伤。

- 需要及时与手外科医师协商。

• 与骨折相关的肌腱撕裂推荐进行手术修复。

• 如果外科医师没有及时处理：

- 大量灌洗。

- 关闭肌腱而不修复肌腱。

- 用足够的敷料和手掌夹板固定受伤的手。

- 手腕屈曲20°～30°。

- 掌骨关节屈曲60°～70°。

- 指端关节屈曲10°～15°。

药物治疗

• 氨苄西林-舒巴坦：3g，静脉滴注，q6h［儿童：200mg/(kg·d)，肌内注射或静脉滴注，q6h］。

• 头孢唑林：1g，静脉滴注［儿童：100mg/(kg·d)，肌内注射或静滴，q6h，其次是40mg/(kg·d)口服每日1次用5～7日］。

• 破伤风类毒素：0.5ml肌内注射（儿童：<7岁，百白破疫苗是首选；>7岁，成人剂量破伤风类毒素，如果免疫系列没有完全完成）。根据需要注射破伤风免疫球蛋白，肌内注射，250U。

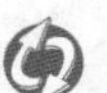

随访

进一步处理

入院指征

• 感染性肌腱撕裂的患者必须接受手术清创。

• 任何继发于人咬伤的肌腱损伤患者必须承认咬伤史才能进行手术清创和静脉滴注抗生素。

• 任何有明显屈肌腱撕裂伤的患者应及时手术修复或转移到最近的手外科医师处。

出院指征

• 伸肌腱裂伤患者没有感染，也没有其他显著相关损伤或基底骨折，通过急诊医师的处理，适当的固定，及时手术随访可以出院。

• 伸肌腱裂伤患者要求外科医师转诊进行修复（手腕、前臂、近端指间关节），已经被正确治疗并使用抗生素，可出院并进行及时的手术随访。

要点和误区

• 局部撕裂是常见的，但比完全中断更难以诊断，因为他们可以表现出完整的功能：

- 正常休息手位置的改变可能提示存在部分裂伤。

• 掌指关节出现裂伤应考虑是人咬伤的可能，除非证明是其他情况：

- 掌指关节弯曲时寻找相关的伸肌腱损伤。

• 力量测试非常重要，因为肌腱发生高达90%的全层裂伤仍可以有正常的运动范围。因此，需要测试抗抗力量。

• 横截面积>20%的肌腱裂伤需要修复。

肌腱炎 Tendonitis

James Killeen · Christian Dameff 范浩浩 李文放 译

J

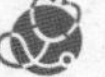

基础知识

描述

• "肌腱炎"一词在了解病理基础之前已被用来描述慢性疼痛性肌腱损伤。这一术语导致了对潜在障碍的病因、慢性和治疗的混淆。术语"肌腱病"或"肌腱病变"应用于描述慢性肌腱疾病。

• 过度使用综合征：

- 慢性疼痛与肌腱增厚的临床综合征。

- 滑膜细胞的厚度增加。

- 关节滑膜积液过多。

- 持续刺激。

• 如果没有进一步的损伤发生，急性过程可能持续48h至2周。

• 肌腱变性被描述为存在无炎症细胞的纤维化，并且症状持续时间超过3个月。

病因

• 机械超负荷或肌腱单位的重复性微创伤：

- 内在因素：

◦ 不灵活。

◦ 肌肉无力或不平衡。

- 外在因素：

◦ 过度偏差、频率或活动。

- 在肌腱疾病中，胶原是一种破损的状态，在肌腱及其衬里中有神经血管组织的修复增殖和慢性刺激。

• 血管活性化学介质释放：

- 血管扩张和细胞水肿增加PMN的数量和活性。

诊断

症状和体征

病史

• 患者的病史可提示什么运动导致了损伤。

• 反复的压力和机械过载：典型的炎性征象包括红、肿、热、痛症状。

• 最初疼痛在运动后会迅速消失，只遗留运动后的阵痛。

体格检查

• 仅定义为肌腱的炎症。

• 肌腱炎与腱鞘炎（炎症程度）的区别很小。这些现在被称为肌腱病。

• 临床发现：

- 发热。
- 存在积液。
- 运动范围受限。
- 不稳定。
- 运动时疼痛。
- 肌腱部位变软。

冈上肌特殊状态

肌腱病变

冈上肌和其他肩袖肌腱：

• 肱骨和肩峰之间受压。

• 过度使用可能导致肌腱和纤维的微创伤。

• 内尔分类法：

- 第一阶段：
  ◦ 年龄＜25 岁。
  ◦ 常见于需要重复高举上肢的运动（如游泳或投手）。
  ◦ 肌腱的水肿和出血。
  ◦ 屈曲-外展运动会引发疼痛。
  ◦ "钝痛"。
- 第二阶段：
  ◦ 25～40 岁。
  ◦ 疼痛持续不断，夜间更明显。
  ◦ 主动运动受到疼痛的限制。被动运动范围被限制。
  ◦ 弥漫性，剧烈的疼痛。
  ◦ 肌腱增厚和纤维化。
- 第三阶段：
  ◦ 部分或全部肌腱撕裂。
  ◦ 在保留肩胛骨旋转的情况下，强迫向前屈曲抬高肱骨头有冲击感。

钙化性肌腱炎

• 年龄＞40 岁，病因未知。

• 肩袖的任何肌腱都可能受到影响，但是倾向于冈上肌。

• 大多数病例无症状，常规 X 线片可以找到钙化灶。

• 随着时间的推移，钙会沉积在肌腱内，经历自发性吸收，引起疼痛。

• 晶体释放可能导致急性发作。

肱二头肌肌腱病

• 前肩部疼痛，沿桡骨向下放射。

• 当在肩上滚动或触探臀部口袋或背部拉链时不适。

• 局灶性压痛位于肱骨大结节和小结节之间。

• 亚格森试验：

- 屈肘 90°和手臂对着身体。
- 疼痛随着腕关节反旋而增加。

• 速度测试：

- 疼痛沿肱二头肌沟蔓延，前屈和前臂后旋受阻。

外侧上髁炎（网球肘）

• 重复旋转运动引起疼痛。

• 肘部外侧的隐痛感随着肱骨外上髁的插入而增加。

• 肱骨外上髁上伸肌腱附着点的炎症反应。

• 抵抗腕关节的主动背屈和中指对阻力的伸展可以增加肘关节的疼痛。

• 桡侧腕屈肌在内侧上髁上的炎症反应：

- 保龄球、高尔夫球手、投手。
- 主动抵抗手腕的弯曲导致疼痛。

手腕/手

• 肌腱与支持带滑膜衬里的炎症变化。

• De Quervain 腱鞘炎：

- 拇长伸肌和拇短伸肌的炎症反应。
- 芬克尔斯坦测试：
  ◦ 患者用拇指蜷缩在手掌握拳。
  ◦ 腕部在尺骨方向偏离。
  ◦ 第一伸肌发生疼痛。
- 腕掌关节骨关节炎或 GC 腱鞘炎引起相同的疼痛。

扳机指

• 手掌屈肌腱鞘的近端部分由于手指移动而变得狭窄而卡顿。

• 从疼痛到屈曲锁定的症状各不相同。

踝

• 跟腱病：

- 男性常见的过度使用损伤。
- 引起炎症的创伤或全身性疾病。
- 反复的压力、瘢痕组织形成和肌腱变性。
- 患者会有疼痛，运动范围缩小或晨僵。

• 跟腱断裂。

- 在 30～40 岁的运动员中更常见。
- "爆裂感觉"。
- 急性力量减退，无法继续活动。
- 感觉像是踢腿或在腿后部打。
- 最初可能触诊阴性，其次是瘀斑和隐隐作痛。
- 足底无法弯曲足跟。
- 汤普森测试：
  ◦ 患者趴在床边上，下肢搭在床边。
  ◦ 医生挤压小腿肌肉并寻找跖屈。
  ◦ 20%～30%的跟腱断裂在初次就诊时漏诊，因为临床医师因患者有屈曲或步行能力而失去警觉。
  ◦ Matles 试验：患者俯卧，膝关节屈曲至 90°。与未受伤侧相比，观察受影响的足是否背屈或中立（均为异常），其中足应该出现跖屈。

儿科注意事项

• 骨骺中心的儿童发生骨关节炎：

- 内上髁的小关节。
- 胫骨结节 Osgood Schlatter 综合征。

• 缺血性坏死（AVN）：

- 关节周围出现疼痛和肿胀。
- 可发生在各个部位。
- 广为认可的部位：
  ◦ 肱骨小头。
  ◦ 跗骨舟骨。
  ◦ 跖骨头。
  ◦ 股骨头。
  ◦ 常需矢状面 X 线平片诊断，排除骨折、AVN、剥脱性骨软骨炎或骨肿瘤。

基本检查

体格检查。

诊断检查与说明

实验室检查

血常规、C 反应蛋白（CRP），怀疑有严重感染检查 ESR。

影像学检查

• 放射检查：

- 关节病因的关节外。
- "SECONDS"：
  ◦ 软组织肿胀。
  ◦ 腐蚀。
  ◦ 钙化。
  ◦ 骨质疏松症。
  ◦ 缩小。
  ◦ 畸形。
  ◦ 分离。

• 超声检查。

- 评估关节积液。
- 比 MRI 更敏感。
- 在紧急情况下被频繁使用。
- 局灶肌腱增厚。
- 局灶性低回声区。
- 不规则和界限不明的边界。
- 瘙痒性水肿。

• MRI：

- 肌腱和肌腱的内部形态及周围的结构。
- 有助于诊断跟骨滑囊炎和插入性腱鞘炎。

- 肌腱变厚和信号增加伴有慢性肌腱异常。
• 闪烁照相术：
- ^{99m}Tc 酸盐磷酸盐(结合与血浆蛋白质)并且集中在关节空间中(滑囊炎)。

■ 鉴别诊断

• 化脓性关节炎。
• 骨折。
• 骨关节炎。
• 类风湿关节炎。

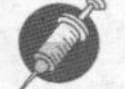

治疗

■ 院前

按照指南固定受伤的肢体。

■ 初步稳定/治疗

冰敷，固定，等待后续处理。

■ 急诊治疗/程序

• 一般：
- 休息。
- NSAIDs。
- 冰敷(10～20 min 间隔)。
- 练习运动的范围。
- 离心运动是指在延长的肌肉中增加负荷的运动方式(及肌肉劳力)。
- 局部注射用于控制疼痛。
- 门诊管理。
- 只有手术或严重残疾可收入院。
- 6～12 周治愈。
- 最近的研究已经报道了成功研究性治疗。
- 增生疗法、超声引导下注射葡萄糖和利多卡因刺激修复。
- 硬化剂注射聚己醇降低新生血管的硬化治疗。
- 抑肽酶是一种广谱蛋白酶和基质金属蛋白酶(MMP)抑制剂，被注射于病灶周围。
• 钙化性肌腱炎。
- 最近低能量无线电冲击波疗法能够显著缓解疼痛。
◦ 可能是因为增加钙的吸收。
◦ 西咪替丁已被用于减轻疼痛。
• 扳机指：
- 保守疗法，如休息、夹板(拇指角)和应用 NSAIDs。
- 一些医师建议可的松注射(治愈率 84%～91%)。
- 可能需要手术释放 A-1 滑轮。
• De Quervain 腱鞘炎。
- 休息，冰敷，NSAIDs。
- 拇指角夹板 3～5 日经常有帮助缓解病情。
• 跟腱炎：
- 休息，冰敷，应用 NSAIDs。
- 矫形器或跟楔。
- 冷冻疗法已被证明有利于控制炎症。
- 跟腱断裂应该轻微跖屈：
◦ 根据患者的需要，考虑骨科手术。

■ 药物治疗

• 布洛芬：400～800 mg，口服，q6～8 h(最大剂量 2 400 mg/d)；儿童：5～10 mg/kg，口服，q4～6 h[最大剂量 50 mg/(kg·d)]。
• 对乙酰氨基酚：10～15 mg/kg，q4～6 h；不要超过对乙酰氨基酚 4 g/24 h(儿童：24 h 内不要超过 10～15 mg/kg 5 次剂量)。

随访

■ 进一步处理

入院指征

需要手术或其他更严重的疾病/伤害的患者收入院。

出院指征

大多数患者可以作为门诊患者进行治疗，可适当转诊。

转诊问题

• 所有完全性肌腱断裂都值得转诊以进行手术咨询。
• 部分肌腱撕裂和慢性肌腱疾病，3～6 个月保守治疗未能改善，可向以下机构或专业人员求助：诊所、物理医学和康复专家、物理治疗师或整形外科医师。

■ 随访建议

预防再次受伤是后续护理的关键。

要点和误区

• 氟喹诺酮类。
• 在氟喹诺酮类药物中，成人肌腱断裂的报道很少见，但已有的报道多数选用氟喹诺酮类药物。

肌萎缩侧索硬化症 Amyotrophic Lateral Sclerosis

Richard S. Krause 马林浩 林兆奋 译

J

基础知识

■ 描述

• 发生于成人的进行性、无法治愈的疾病。
• 各级运动系统的神经退行性疾病。
• 一些患者有痴呆症。
• 表现：
- 肌肉无力。
- 消瘦。
- 肌束震颤。
- Babinski 征阳性。
- 反射亢进。
• 主要包括上运动神经元和下运动神经元受累。
• 多发于运动系统，其他神经元无影响。
• 可能从吞咽困难和发音障碍的延髓症状开始。
• 著名的棒球运动员受到该病影响，因此也被称为"Lou Gehrig 病"。
• 最终导致呼吸道功能受损，继发膈肌和其他呼吸肌肉的肌无力。
• 80%的病例年龄在 40～70 岁。
• 死亡(通常来自呼吸麻痹)通常发生在诊断后的 3～5 年。
• 50%在 3 年内死亡。
• 约 10%的 ALS 患者存活 10 年或更长时间。
• 男性发病多于女性。

■ 病因

• 肌萎缩侧索硬化症(ALS)的病因尚不清楚。
• 10%的患者有另一个家庭成员患病。
• 吸烟和重金属暴露可能是危险因素。
• 西太平洋有一个疾病群。
• 病理学上，上、下运动神经元细胞均有损失。

诊断

症状和体征

- 不对称肢体无力是 ALS 最常见的表现(80%)。
- 可以从手臂(颈髓起病)或腿部(腰髓发作)开始:
  - 后半肢体受到影响。
- 延髓的 ALS:
  - 通常表现为构音障碍或吞咽困难。
  - 第二常见的表现。
- 下运动神经元(无力和肌肉萎缩)和上运动神经元征(Babinski 征阳性和反射亢进)出现。
- 呼吸肌和声带受影响较晚。
- 肌肉震颤很常见,但患者表现可能并不明显。
- 眼外肌、括约肌、认知和感觉都得以保留。

病史

- 大多数患有 ALS 的急诊患者都可以确诊。
- 病史采集应该关注急性临床表现和功能衰退的线索。
- 基于"虚弱"的主诉而怀疑肌萎缩侧索硬化时,考虑到这种情况会发生在许多疾病中,包括:
  - 肺病。
  - 心脏病。
  - 贫血。
  - 内分泌失调。
  - 中毒综合征。
  - 肌肉或关节的疾病。
  - 脊髓异常。
  - 抑郁症。
- 区分真正的虚弱:呼吸短促、胸痛、关节疼痛、疲劳、运动耐量差等。
- 真正的虚弱往往无法完成遵嘱动作:
  - Bulbar 麻痹:
    - 面部无力。
    - 舌头无力和僵硬。
    - 构音障碍。
  - 颈髓 ALS:
    - 洗头发、用梳子很困难。
    - 夹持运动能力受损。
  - 腰椎发作 ALS:
    - 频繁继发于足后坠。
    - 难以走上楼梯。

体格检查

- 详细而彻底的神经系统检查是诊断的关键,但通常不在急诊室中进行。
- 上运动神经元疾病引起缓慢的不协调运动和僵硬。
- 下运动神经元疾病导致伴有萎缩和肌肉痉挛的无力很常见。
- 常见征象:
  - 快速反应。
  - 肌肉萎缩。
  - 肌肉消瘦。
- 检查应侧重于排除或确认其他条件。

基本检查

- 以前未确诊的 ALS:
  - ALS 依靠临床诊断,很少在急诊室中进行:
    - 认识到这种疾病的可能性就够了,并要求转诊进行检查。
  - 如果怀疑是 ALS,应该进行用力肺活量(FVC)测定。
- 已知的 ALS 患者:
  - 患有已知疾病和进行性症状的患者:
    - 根据实验室和影像学检查评估潜在的可治疗并发症。
  - FVC 是呼吸肌无力的敏感指标:
    - FVC<预计的 50%被认为是疾病进展。
    - FVC<50%通常需要通气支持。
    - 条件允许应尽快开始非侵入性正压通气。
    - 与患者之前的基线值比较。
  - 胸部 X 线检查可能显示吸入或肺炎或合并症,如 CHF。
  - 脉搏血氧饱和度和血气分析有助于诊断呼吸衰竭。
  - 电解质和其他血液生化检查可能发现某些进行性的肌无力的可逆病因。

诊断检查与说明

实验室检查

- 在肌无力无变化的情况下,考虑 CPK 测量以及血液化学检查:
  - 升高的 CPK 与肌病有关。
- 电解质异常如低钾血症、高钙血症等可能导致全身无力,但这通常与其他体征和症状相关。
- 可能需要 CBC、UA 寻找感染源。

影像学检查

跌倒(ALS 常见)或排除其他情况时可能需要影像学检查,其他骨骼 X 线检查或头部 CT。

诊断步骤/外科

- 检查 FVC。
- 肌电图(EMG)可能有助于确诊(通常不是急诊检查)。

鉴别诊断

- 颈椎按压:
  - 类似症状,但通常伴有疼痛和感觉改变的急性发作。
  - 脊柱 MRI 或脊髓造影诊断。
- 甲状腺毒症可能类似 ALS:
  - 通常有明显的全身症状。
- 重金属中毒(铅、汞、砷)。
- 梅毒和莱姆病。
- 淋巴瘤可能具有相关的下运动神经元综合征,其类似 ALS。
- 延髓起病型 ALS(Bulbar-onset ALS)。
  - 食管癌。
  - 重症肌无力。

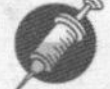

治疗

- 药物利鲁唑是一种谷氨酸释放抑制剂,已被证明能延长 ALS 患者的生存期平均数月。
- 依达拉奉是一种自由基清除剂,可减缓功能恶化:
  - 在 ALS 诊断后 2 年内对 137 例患者进行的安慰剂对照研究。
  - 依达拉奉组 24 周的功能下降较小。
  - 差异具有临床意义。
- 急诊处理主要围绕对症治疗和并发症的鉴别和治疗。

院前

争议:

- 许多患者将接受积极的干预措施:
  - 立即干预至关重要,在确定指令之前,应避免插管。
  - 可以首先尝试无创通气支持手段。

初步稳定/治疗

- 呼吸功能不全或衰竭:
  - 确定任何高级干预。
  - 无创通气支持。
  - 气管插管。
- 脱离呼吸机非常困难:
  - 机械通气后的平均生存时间为 19 个月。

急诊治疗/程序

- 镇静和镇痛:
  - 关节疼痛可能对 NSAIDs 有反应。
- 挤压疼痛引起的失眠(由于不能动)使用苯海拉明或阿米替林可能有效。
  - 失眠也可用苯二氮䓬类药物治疗。

•分泌物误吸或流涎可用阿米替林、阿托品或莨菪碱(干性分泌物)治疗。

•肌肉痉挛可能对巴氯芬或替扎尼定有反应。

•便秘与不能动和饮食有关:

-用泻药、大便软化剂和调整饮食来治疗。

■ 药物治疗

•阿米替林:25~100 mg,口服,每晚睡前。

•阿托品:0.4 mg,口服,q4~6 h。

•巴氯芬:10~25 mg,口服,每日3次。

•苯海拉明:每晚睡前25~50 mg,口服。

•替扎尼定:2~4 mg,口服,每日2次。

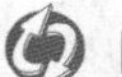

随访

■ 进一步处理

入院指征

•需要呼吸支持。

•脱水。

•由于疾病的进展,无法在家照顾。

•并发症(如感染)或需要入院的其他诊断。

出院指征

•疑似肌萎缩侧索硬化症:如果一般情况允许,则考虑门诊评估,并排除其他需要入院的严重情况。

•已知ALS的并发症:如果门诊治疗可用并且呼吸状态稳定,则出院。

■ 随访建议

如果考虑诊断为肌萎缩侧索硬化症,应及时联系神经科医师进行随访。

要点和误区

•ALS是一种进行性神经退行性疾病,影响运动系统的所有组成部分。

•许多ALS患者都有高级生命支持的条件-优先或积极干预。

•FVC<50%通常需要机械通气支持。

肌张力障碍反应

Kenneth C. Jackimczyk 姜颢 译

基础知识

■ 描述

•中枢神经系统神经传递的正常模式由多巴胺能受体和胆碱能受体的平衡来维持:

-某些药物在基底核拮抗多巴胺受体可引起多巴胺能和胆碱能兴奋失衡。

-这种失衡导致面部或颈部(躯干、骨盆或四肢也可被涉及)不自觉的肌痉挛。

•这种痉挛会令人不适和恐惧,但除了在极罕见病例中涉及喉部肌肉时外,它不会引起生命危险。

•通常发生在摄入后数小时内:

-几乎总是在应用引发问题的药物后1周内。

•危险因素:

-儿童和青壮年风险更高。

-很少发生在45岁以上的患者。

-男性更容易受影响。

-肌张力障碍提前发作会显著增加风险。

-近期使用可卡因会增加风险。

■ 病因

•经常发生在患者服用抗精神病药、止吐药、抗抑郁药之后。

•肌张力障碍反应的发生率依据药效变化较大(2%~25%)。

•强效药物的发生率较高(氟哌啶醇、氟非那嗪)。

•弱效药物的发生率较低(氯丙嗪、甲硫达嗪)。

•不典型的抗精神病药的发生率最低(喹硫平、奥氮平、利培酮)。

•止吐药:

-甲氧氯普胺(灭吐灵)。

-普鲁氯嗪(甲哌氯丙嗪)。

-异丙嗪(非那根)。

-氟哌利多(达哌啶醇)。

•其他药物:

-环类抗抑郁药。

-H_2受体阻滞剂。

-一些抗疟药。

-抗组胺药。

-一些抗痉挛药。

-多虑平。

-锂盐。

-苯环己哌啶。

儿科注意事项

儿童在脱水或发热时特别容易出现肌张力障碍反应。

诊断

■ 症状和体征

病史

•在症状开始的数周内摄入抗精神病药、止吐药或其他药物:

-可以发生在服用抗精神病药中增加抗精神病药剂量或减少治疗锥体外系症状药物(抗胆碱能药)用量的患者。

•发声困难。

•完全警觉并且能够回答问题,涉及面部肌肉,可引起言语困难。

•不自主肌肉收缩或痉挛常累及面部或颈部(参看体格检查):

-躯干、骨盆或四肢肌肉也可受累。

体格检查

•典型的不自主肌肉痉挛发生。

•动眼神经危象:

-涉及眼和眶周肌肉。

-进展成眼球向上或侧向运动困难。

•眼睑痉挛:

-不自主的眼睑闭合。

•颊舌危象:

-累及面部肌肉和舌。

-可能有言语困难。

-扮鬼脸。

-牙关紧闭。

-伸舌。

-吞咽困难。

•痉挛性斜颈:

-颈部扭曲。

•骨盆歪斜危象:

-腹壁肌肉痉挛。

•角弓反张:

-累及躯干和背部肌肉。

-脊柱扭曲成弓形。

•喉部肌张力障碍:

-非常罕见但可能危及生命。

-由于喉痉挛可能发展成气道阻塞。

- 表现为言语障碍或喘鸣。

基本检查

- 临床诊断基于典型的症状与体征，以及可能的药物暴露史。
- 确诊依靠对治疗的反应：
- 对治疗缺乏反应时应当考虑另外的诊断。

诊断检查与说明

实验室检查

- 不需常规行实验室检测。
- 如果对治疗无反应，应当考虑低钙血症并检测钙水平。

影像学检查

不需要影像学检查。

鉴别诊断

- 迟发性运动障碍：
- 长期抗精神病药治疗的并发症。
- 经常出现舞蹈样动作。
- 使用抗胆碱能药不能快速改善。
- 静坐不能：
- 不自主的运动不宁。
- 可出现焦虑。
- 惊厥：
- 有痉挛发作史。
- 对口头刺激无反应。
- 强直阵挛性肌肉运动而非痉挛。
- 癔症或假性发作：
- 剧烈情绪事件史。
- 强直阵挛性肌肉活动而非持续痉挛。
- 强直。
- 士的宁中毒。
- 慢性肌张力障碍：
- 大脑瘫痪，家族性舞蹈病。
- 肌张力障碍史经常与慢性神经疾病进展有关。
- 蝎毒蜇入：
- 动眼神经危象和角弓反张是蝎毒蜇入的常见临床表现。
- 患者缺乏药物暴露史。
- 脑膜炎和脑炎可能表现为类肌张力障碍发作的不典型癫痫。
- 下颌脱臼。
- 低钙血症。

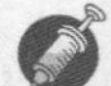

治疗

院前

- 极少危及生命。
- 首先注意喉舌痉挛，确保肌张力障碍反应不会引起呼吸损害。
- 询问家属或朋友是否服用抗精神病药、止吐药以及消遣性毒品。
- 提交药瓶。

初步稳定/治疗

稳定气道以防止喉或舌痉挛引起呼吸损害。

急诊治疗/程序

- 给予苯海拉明（苯那君）或甲磺酸苯托品（苯甲托品）：
- 通过恢复中枢神经系统的胆碱能-多巴胺能平衡快速解除肌肉痉挛。
- 优先应用静脉注射给药。
- 2～5 min 后开始减轻。
- 30 min 后症状完全缓解。
- 肌内注射给药可作为备用的治疗路径。
- 15～30 min 后开始起效。
- 继续口服给药 3 日以防症状复发。
- 地西泮（安定）：
- 在肌张力障碍对足量的抗胆碱能药物无反应的情况下给药。
- 对标准治疗无反应时医师应当考虑其他诊断。

药物治疗

- 甲磺酸苯托品（苯甲托品）：1～2 mg 静脉推注（超过 2 min）或肌内注射，继之以 1～2 mg 口服，每日 2 次，持续 2～3 日：
- 不得用于 3 岁以下儿童。
- 对于 3 岁以上儿童：0.02 mg/kg 静脉推注（超过 2 min）或肌内注射，继之以 0.02 mg/kg 口服，每日 2 次，持续 2～3 日。
- 苯海拉明（苯那君）：1～2 mg/kg 至 100 mg 静脉推注（超过 2 min）或肌内注射，继之以 25～50 mg（儿童：1～2 mg/kg）口服，q6～8 h，持续 2～3 日。
- 地西泮（安定）：5～10 mg 静脉推注，继之以 5 mg，口服，q4～6 h，必要时持续 2～3 日。

一线用药

苯海拉明（苯那君）。

二线用药

甲磺酸苯托品（苯甲托品）：
- 不得用于 3 岁以下儿童。
- 地西泮。

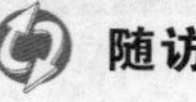

随访

进一步处理

入院指征

- 症状经治后没有消除，需要维护气道，或诊断不明确时。
- 如肌张力障碍反应引起喉痉挛，应当在症状解除后观察患者 12～24 h。

出院指征

- 症状解除后出院。
- 应当终止致病因素。
- 患者在服用镇静剂时不应驾驶或进行需高度注意力的工作。

随访建议

- 服用高危药物患者需至处方医师处随访。

要点和误区

- 有相关服药史、经适当治疗后症状完全解除，可诊断急性肌张力障碍。
- 一线药物是苯海拉明。
- 对治疗无应答应当考虑其他诊断。

J

吉兰-巴雷综合征 Guillain-Barr´e Syndrome

Paul A. Leccese · Jeffrey Druck 祝各亮 译

基础知识

描述

- 一组以自身免疫性脱髓鞘为特征的周围神经障碍和周围神经轴索变性导致急性上行性麻痹的疾病（GBS）。
- 体液和细胞免疫介导的。
- 全球引起软瘫的首要原因（自急性脊髓灰质炎疫苗接种后）。
- 可由细菌、病毒感染引起。
- 发病率随着年龄的增长而增加，男性好发：

- 平均为1.1/(10万人·年)。
• 肌肉无力会在2～4周恶化。
• 数周至数月后会出现自行恢复：
- 80%的患者在1年左右会完全恢复。
- 20%的患者在6个月左右无法行走。
- 5%的患者死于并发症。
◦ 肺栓塞。
◦ 感染。
◦ 心血管事件。
• 急性炎症性脱髓鞘多发性神经病(AIDP)：
- 吉兰-巴雷综合征最常见的形式(约占90%)。
- 脱髓鞘有时会伴有轴突丧失。
• 其他形式的GBS：
- 急性炎性脱髓鞘型多神经病(AMAN)：
◦ 纯运动轴索受累。
◦ 67%空肠弯曲杆菌阳性。
◦ 往往恢复迅速。
◦ 常是儿童患者。
- 急性运动感觉性轴索神经病(AMSAN)：
◦ 没有明显的炎症或脱髓鞘的运动，以及感觉神经变性。
◦ 与AMAN相似，但也累及感觉神经。
- 急性自主神经病：
◦ 很少见。
◦ 包括交感神经和副交感神经。
◦ 体位性低血压、心律失常、心动过速和高血压。
◦ 视力模糊，眼干，无汗。
◦ 逐渐恢复，但往往是不完全的。
- 米勒-费雪综合征：
◦ 少见。
◦ 迅速发展的不伴有肌无力的共济失调、腱反射消失和眼肌麻痹。
◦ 第Ⅱ和Ⅵ脑神经、脊神经节和周围神经出现脱髓鞘和炎症。
◦ 在1～3个月可恢复。

病因

• 感染后：
- 2/3的患者有前驱感染，常为呼吸道或消化道。
- 不同自身抗体与不同亚型相关。
- 前驱疾病和神经症状之间间隔1～3周。
- 空肠弯曲菌是最常见的前驱感染菌。
- 巨细胞病毒是最常见的前驱感染病毒。
- EB病毒、水痘-带状疱疹病毒、HIV病毒、支原体也与之相关。
- 出现与寨卡病毒相关的病例，尚不清楚寨卡病毒感染后是否需要其他病毒促发GBS。
- 也与免疫调节剂(如阿达木单抗)相关。
- 与疫苗的关系值得怀疑。
- 流感疫苗导致的风险略有增加。
◦ 发病率每百万疫苗接种2例。
◦ 低于与病情进展相关的风险。
- 有青少年脑膜炎球菌疫苗接种后GBS病例报告。
◦ 在更大的研究中没有明确的联系。

诊断

症状和体征

病史

• 快速进展(数天到数周)的对称性上行麻痹。
• 无或轻度的感觉症状(如手指或足趾的感觉异常)，通常是轻微的。
• 疼痛常见于：
- 骨盆。
- 肩带。
- 大腿后侧。
• 脑神经受累可影响吞咽、面部肌肉和眼球运动。
• 前驱细菌或病毒感染。
• 症状进展超过8周不称为GBS，而是慢性炎症性脱髓鞘多发性神经病(CIDP)。

体格检查

• 上升性对称性肌无力，下肢比上肢更明显。
• 深反射丧失。
• 寻找脑神经受累证据。
• 呼吸功能不全(25%的患者需要气管插管)。
• 感觉功能检查正常或轻微异常。
• 其他亚型：
- 自主神经功能障碍：
◦ 高血压。
◦ 体位性低血压。
◦ 梗阻。
◦ 心律失常。
◦ 尿潴留。
- 米勒-费雪综合征：
◦ 共济失调。
◦ 反射消失。
◦ 肌麻痹。
◦ 轻度肢体无力。
◦ 延髓介导的肌无力。
◦ 气道损害。
• 出现以下症状时考虑其他诊断：
- 发热。
- 反射正常。
- 上运动神经元体征。
- 非对称性神经功能缺损。
- 感觉平面分界清楚。

诊断检查与说明

• 一般根据临床证据可以做出诊断。
• 实验室和影像学检查可以帮助诊断和排除其他引起症状的原因。

实验室检查

• 电解质(一部分患者有抗利尿激素分泌失调综合征)。
• 腰椎穿刺：
- 蛋白质细胞分离：蛋白质增加伴无或少量的白细胞。
- 蛋白质通常为55～350，只有当发病后7～10日，进展为血脑屏障功能障碍时才会出现蛋白升高。
◦ 症状出现后早于7日可假性正常，白细胞正常不能排除GBS。
- 白细胞大于10～50提示其他病因。
- 开放压力正常。

影像学检查

CT或MRI以排除脊髓压迫。

诊断步骤/外科

电生理学检查会出现异常(神经传导试验)。

鉴别诊断

• 多发性神经病：
- 急性间歇性卟啉病。
- 慢性重金属中毒。
- 白喉。
- 莱姆病。
- 副肿瘤疾病。
- 脊髓灰质炎。
- 结节病。
- 蜱麻痹。
- 血管炎。
• 脊髓疾病：
- 脊髓压迫。
- 横贯性脊髓炎。
• 神经-肌肉接头疾病：
- 肉毒杆菌中毒。
- 兰伯特-伊顿综合征。
- 重症肌无力。
• 肌肉疾病：
- 急性多发性肌炎。
- 危重症肌病。

J

• 其他：
- 低钾血症。
- 精神性，诈病。

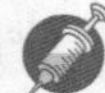

治疗

院前

注意气道管理。

初步稳定/治疗

气道评估与管理：

• 呼吸衰竭进展可以相当迅速。

急诊治疗/程序

• 气道管理：
- 25%需要呼吸机支持治疗。
- 在发病的 24～28 h 需要插管。
- 避免琥珀酰胆碱，因为有可能导致高钾血症。
- 密切监测呼吸参数：
◦ 用力肺活量(FVC)或最大吸气负压(NIF)。
◦ 如果 FVC<20 ml/kg 或 NIF<30 cmH_2O，则有进入 ICU 的指征。
◦ 如果 FVC<15 ml/kg，则推荐气管插管。

• 检查是否存在自主神经功能紊乱。

• 头部、肘部无力，咳嗽或站立不稳，或急性呼吸衰竭(从症状出现到入院的时间<7 日)。

• 支持疗法(分泌物、血流动力学支持、血栓栓塞预防)。

• 早期神经科会诊。

药物治疗

• 血浆或静脉注射免疫球蛋白(IVIG)，需咨询神经科：
- 使用这两种方法都未显示明显受益，使用任何一种临床上均得到相同的结果。
- 对米勒-费雪综合征或轻度 GBS 是否有益尚不清楚。

• IVIG：400 mg/(kg·d)，5 日。

• 疼痛控制：
- 对乙酰氨基酚：500 mg，口服，q6 h，不超过 4 g/24 h。
- 布洛芬：400～800 mg，口服，q8 h。
- 加巴喷丁：初始剂量 300 mg，口服，1 次/日。

• 皮质激素对于改善疼痛或神经功能缺损没有帮助：
- 口服激素会延迟恢复。
- 静脉激素亦无益处。

随访

进一步处理

入院指征

• 所有 GBS 患者或疑似 GBS 患者都应入院进行密切观察。

• 呼吸功能障碍、自主神经功能紊乱或需要经常监测病情进展的患者需进入监护病房。

出院指征

神经科会诊后认为可以不入院治疗的患者。

随访建议

• 由神经科专家决定随访细节。

• 不良预后大多源于：
- 高龄。
- 持续时间长。
- 需要呼吸机支持治疗。
- 前驱腹泻及空肠弯曲菌感染。

要点和误区

• 要点：
- 检查 FVC 和/或 NIF 以决定气道管理方案。
- 如果脑脊液白细胞计数在 10～50 及以上，考虑其他病因。

• 误区：
- 未能进行适当的大脑和脊髓影像学检查以排除其他潜在原因。
- 对于怀疑 GBS 的患者不进行神经科会诊或入院观察。

急性冠脉综合征：冠状动脉血管痉挛

Acute Coronary Syndrome: Coronary Vasospasm

Jamie L. Adler · Shamai A. Grossman 马林浩 林兆奋 译

J

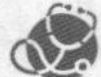

基础知识

描述

• 冠状动脉血管痉挛导致的胸痛自发性发作，正常或病变的冠状血管所支配的心肌需氧量增加。

• 也称为变异型心绞痛，最初描述于 1959 年。

• 最常见于年轻患者和男性。

• 通常发生于无心脏危险因素或冠状动脉疾病的患者，但可能同时发生于阻塞性冠状动脉疾病。

• 持续 12 个月以上的冠状动脉痉挛继发心肌梗死事件等同于急性心肌梗死伴单支或双支血管疾病。

• 危险因素：
- 吸烟(高达 75%的病例)。
- 高血压。
- 高胆固醇血症。
- 糖尿病。
- 使用可卡因。

病因

• 冠状动脉血管扩张功能异常，通常来自内皮细胞。

• 微血管和心外膜血管受累的患病率高。

• 分为三类：
- 病灶：局部的，通常在单个动脉狭窄处或附近。
- 多部位：同一动脉的 2 段或 2 段以上。
- 多血管：涉及不同冠状动脉。

• 氧需求增加的情况消失之后可能出现。

• 无拮抗的 α 交感神经刺激。

• 内源性激素的交感神经高反应性刺激可能导致血管收缩。

• 与此相反，也与迷走神经张力增加或迷走神经张力减退有关，乙酰胆碱激发试验证实了这一点。

• 由血管收缩介质引起的冠状动脉超敏反应。

• 内皮功能障碍可能来自一氧化氮合酶的基因突变。

• 最新研究表明平滑肌细胞中 p 激酶活性

可能增加。

诊断

症状和体征

• 胸痛或胸口不适：
- 胸骨后。
- 放射至颈部、下颌、左肩或手臂。
- 休息时出现。
- 在晚上或早上更频繁地出现。
- 与体位无关。
- 可能与出汗、恶心、呕吐、头晕有关。

• 心悸。
• 晕厥或晕厥。
• 少数患者伴有偏头痛和雷诺病。
• 可能在寒冷天气或压力下发生。
• 与典型心绞痛相比，可能持续时间延长。
• 过度通气可引起。
• 可通过运动引起。
• 昼夜节律模式，通常在迷走神经张力高的夜间或清晨。
• 冠状动脉痉挛疾病国际学术组(COVADIS)诊断标准：
- 硝酸盐反应性心绞痛。
- 短暂缺血性 ECG 改变。
- 血管造影术可发现高级别的短暂冠状动脉痉挛证据。

病史

可能与心绞痛类似，在清晨发生的血管痉挛症状应高度怀疑与本病相关，但也要询问与压力、锻炼和寒冷天气的关系。

体格检查

体格检查对诊断帮助小。

基本检查

• 必须包括心电图。
• 利用基于病史的其他检测。

诊断检查与说明

• 心电图。
- 短暂 ST 段抬高是典型特征，是很明显的表现。
- 经常发生双向的变化。
- 伴 ST 段压低或 T 波倒置。
- 冠状动脉痉挛期间伴有心律失常。
- 心脏阻滞伴右冠状动脉痉挛。
- 室性心动过速伴左主干痉挛。
- 在长期血管痉挛期间可出现猝死(罕见)。

实验室检查

• 肌钙蛋白。
• CK/CK-MB。

毒理学检查

如果怀疑可卡因是胸痛的病因。

影像学检查

• 胸部 X 线检查：
- 可以帮助排除其他病因，如肺炎、气胸或主动脉夹层。

• 无创冠状动脉成像(核灌注、冠状动脉 CTA、冠状动脉 MR)：
- 通常只有在与兴奋测试相结合时才有用。

诊断步骤/外科

• 运动压力测试：
- 通常没有帮助，但可以帮助确定哪些真正的缺血性疾病。

• 无创性兴奋过度通气。
- 高度特异性，中度敏感，往往有利于那些疾病活动增加的人。
- 配合心电图或心电图加＋灌注成像。

• 动态心电图监护仪：
- 有助于沉默病例或心律失常。

• 心脏磁共振造影。
- 可以识别多至 87%患者的潜在病因。

• 冠状动脉造影：
- 轻度动脉粥样硬化通常是常态。
- 乙酰胆碱激发试验是金标准。

鉴别诊断

• 心绞痛。
• 焦虑和恐惧症。
• 主动脉夹层。
• 可卡因胸痛。
• 食管破裂。
• 食管痉挛。
• 食管炎。
• 胃食管反流。
• 二尖瓣脱垂。
• 肌肉骨骼胸痛。
• 心肌梗死。
• 消化性溃疡病。
• 心包炎。
• 气胸。
• 肺栓塞。
• Takotsubo 心肌病。

治疗

院前

治疗任何其他急性冠状动脉综合征。

初步稳定/治疗

• 静脉通路。
• 氧。
• 心脏监测。
• 生命体征和氧饱和度。

急诊治疗/程序

• 所有胸心痛患者都应考虑心肌缺血，应该在抵达急诊室时接受阿司匹林治疗：
- 可能会增加变异型心绞痛的严重程度，因为抑制了使冠状动脉血管扩张的前列环素的生物合成。

• 仍应给予硝酸甘油，通常有助于缓解缺血性和血管痉挛性胸痛。
• 如果临床病史与冠状动脉痉挛一致，则需要进行钙通道阻滞剂试验。
• 肝素和 β 受体阻滞剂对真正的冠状动脉血管痉挛没有帮助：β 受体阻滞剂可能由于无法拮抗的 α 受体介导的血管收缩而有害，胸痛应避免使用可卡因。

药物治疗

• 阿司匹林：325 mg，口服。
• 地尔硫䓬：240～360 mg，口服(速释型)。
• 硝酸甘油。
- 0.4 mg，舌下含服。
- 10～20 μg/min 静脉注射非 PVC 管，滴定更有效。
- 应用 1～2 次经皮硝酸甘油涂剂。

• 维拉帕米：40～80 mg 口服(速释型)。

一线用药

• 地尔硫䓬/维拉帕米。
- 尽管采用了钙通道阻滞剂治疗，仍有 40%的患者会复发血管痉挛型心绞痛。

• 长效硝酸盐。

二线用药

• α 受体阻滞剂。
• 他汀类药物治疗。
• 针对血管痉挛区内病灶的支架植入治疗目前仍有争议，可导致冠状动脉树其他区域的痉挛。
• 心脏起搏器置入：有复发性晕厥或 AV 节阻滞的血管痉挛性心绞痛。

随访

进一步处理

入院指征

• 新发胸痛。
• 使用阳性生化指标进行治疗或进行激发试验。
• 使用阳性生化指标或压力测试进行治疗。

J

• 以往许多住院的患者现在可以在胸痛观察单元或临床决策单元进行有效评估。

出院指征

• 病情稳定(慢性胸痛)。

• 心肌缺血相关检查结果阴性。

随访建议

• 7 日内心脏科随访急诊评估。

• 戒烟教育。

要点和误区

• 5 年生存率为 95%。

• 除吸烟外，典型患者不会有传统的冠心病危险因素。

• 钙通道阻滞剂是一线用药。

• 30%～40%的患者难以治疗，并且会重复发作。

• 可能以 ST 段抬高型心肌梗死的形式发病，但是真正的梗死几乎患有先前存在的冠状动脉粥样硬化疾病的患者。

• 由于无法拮抗的 α 受体血管收缩，β 受体阻滞剂可导致血管痉挛恶化。

• 血管痉挛性心绞痛和偏头痛的患者，避免使用曲普坦。

• 长期血管痉挛的患者可出现 ST 段抬高型心肌梗死、室性心律失常和猝死。

急性冠脉综合征：无 Q 波(非 ST 段抬高)心肌梗死

Acute Coronary Syndrome: Non-Q-Wave (Non-ST-Elevation) MI

Nathaniel Mann · David F. M. Brown　马林浩　林兆奋 译

基础知识

描述

• 非 ST 段抬高心肌梗死(NSTEMI)是临床综合征的一部分，其他急性冠脉综合征的类型还包括不稳定型心绞痛和 ST 段抬高 MI (STEMI)。

• 由冠状动脉血流的闭塞引起：

- 常为不完全缺血事件。

• 冠状动脉斑块破裂。

- 内皮细胞被破坏暴露内皮下胶原和其他血小板黏附体，血管性血友病因子(vWF)和纤维连接蛋白。

- 组织因子激活因子Ⅶ和外部途径。

• 血栓生成：

- 通过糖蛋白(GP)Ⅰa/Ⅱa 与胶原蛋白黏合；GP Ⅰb 到 vWF。

◦ 血小板激活：释放 ADPf 血栓素 A2 和 5-羟色胺改变 GP Ⅱb/Ⅲa 受体，同时引起局部血管收缩

◦ 血小板聚集：GP Ⅱb/Ⅲa 受体结合纤维蛋白原，交联血小板，形成局部血小板栓塞。

- 血小板稳定：凝血酶将纤维蛋白原转化为纤维蛋白，提供纤维蛋白网，稳定血小板聚集。

• 可能发生下游冠状动脉微栓塞。

• NSTEMI 患者多为高龄且比 STEMI 患者有更多合并症。

病因

• 冠状动脉血栓形成。

• 冠状动脉痉挛、特发性或可卡因诱发。

• 原位血栓形成、高凝状态。

• 栓塞事件(如心内膜炎、PFO 反常栓塞)。

• 动脉炎。

诊断

症状和体征

病史

• 疼痛。

- 压力或紧张或沉重。

- 胸骨下、上腹部。

- 辐射至手臂、下颚、背部。

- 更可能是无体位性、无胸膜性、触诊无明显改变。

• 恶心、呕吐。

• 出汗。

• 咳嗽。

• 呼吸困难。

• 焦虑。

• 头晕目眩。

• 晕厥。

• 服用可卡因或苯丙胺。

• 冠状动脉疾病家族史。

• 非典型表现常见，尤其是女性、糖尿病患者和老年人。

老年人注意事项

患者可能出现非典型症状或无症状缺血。

体格检查

• 苍白或发汗。

• 高血压或低血压。

• 心律失常。

• 第四心音奔马律。

• 体格检查通常是正常的。

基本检查

心电图、心肌标志物，CXR。

诊断检查与说明

实验室检查

• 心肌标志物。

- 肌钙蛋白：心肌梗死的特异性指标，在 MI 后 2～4 h 上升，1～2 日达到峰值，10 日回降。

- 肌酸激酶(CK)：在 3～4 h 上升，在 18～24 h 达到峰值，在 3～4 日下降；CK-MB 对心源性更具特异性。

- 肌红蛋白：在 1～6 h 上升，在 24 h 内恢复到基线，高度敏感但非特异性。

- LDH：24 h 内上升，3～6 日达到峰值，在 8～12 日下降。

• CBC。

• 电解质，包括镁离子。

• 接受华法林治疗患者 PT、APTT、INR。

• NT-proBNP：较高水平与 NSTEMI 患者的死亡率增加相关。

影像学检查

• 心电图。

- ST 段压低或瞬时升高表明风险增加。

- T 波倒置不增加风险，有助于区分心脏疼痛和非心脏疼痛。

- 深(>2 mm)心前区 T 波倒置表明心肌缺血。

• CXR：

- 评估心脏大小，肺水肿、充血或确定胸痛的其他原因。

• 超声(通常不是急诊评估的一部分)：

- 识别室壁运动异常并评估心室功能。

• 放射性核素(如果是保守治疗，一般不是急诊评估的一部分)：

- Sestamibi 扫描：识别存活心肌。
- ^{99}Tc：识别新发梗死的心肌。

诊断步骤/外科

冠状动脉造影（±PCI），通常是住院患者，取决于患者的风险状况和并发症。

鉴别诊断

- STEMI。
- 肺栓塞。
- 主动脉夹层。
- 急性心包炎、心肌炎。
- 气胸。
- 胰腺炎。
- 肺炎。
- 食管痉挛、胃食管反流。
- 食管破裂。
- 肌肉骨骼疼痛、肋软骨炎。

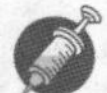

治疗

院前

- 静脉通道。
- 吸氧管理。
- 12 导联，心电监护，治疗心律失常。
- 阿司匹林，镇痛，抗焦虑。

初步稳定/治疗

- 吸氧管理（如果 SpO_2＜95%）。
- 静脉通道。
- 12 导联，心电监护，治疗心律失常。

急诊治疗/程序

- 抗缺血治疗减少心肌的需求，增加心肌的供氧：
  - β受体阻滞剂：持续疼痛的高血压给予静脉注射，否则在 24 h 内口服，心力衰竭者忌用。
  - 硝酸盐：禁用于严重 AS，怀疑 RV 梗死或最近使用磷酸二酯酶抑制剂（如西地那非）。
  - 吸氧。
  - 吗啡。
  - 钙通道阻滞剂（非二氢吡啶类，如地尔硫䓬、维拉帕米）可用于持续缺血和β受体阻滞剂禁忌的患者。

  心力衰竭禁忌。
- 双重抗血小板治疗，以减少血小板聚集：
  - 阿司匹林：只有在有过敏反应的情况下才停止使用。
  - ADP 抑制剂：氯吡格雷（超敏反应时可替代 ASA），替格拉或普拉格雷（如果出血风险低，不太可能出现 CABG，无 CVA 病史，年龄＜75 岁）。
- GP Ⅱb/Ⅲa 抑制剂（替非罗班）：
  - 只有持续缺血，心脏标志物阳性和 PCI；可以按照住院治疗。
  - 如果在 PCI 至少 6 h 前给予氯吡格雷负荷剂量或用于抗凝治疗比伐卢定，可省略。
- 抗凝治疗预防血栓：
  - 普通肝素或依诺肝素是一种治疗方法。
  - 磺达肝癸钠（Ⅹa 因子抑制剂）是一种合理的替代方案，尤其适用于医学管理的患者；可能会降低出血风险。
  - 对已知的肝素诱导的血小板减少症患者保留比伐卢定（凝血酶抑制剂）。
- 抗焦虑药抑制拟交感神经释放。

药物治疗

一线用药

- 阿司匹林 162～325 mg，口服，每日 1 次。
- β受体阻滞剂：
  - 阿替洛尔：起始剂量 5 mg，静脉注射，5 min，之后 5 mg，静脉注射，10 min，之后 50～100 mg 口服每日（静脉注射后 1～2 h）。
  - 艾司洛尔：100 μg/(kg · min)，静脉注射[50 μg/(kg · min)，q15 min 增加，直到最大剂量 300 μg/(kg · min)]。
  - 美托洛尔：5 mg 静脉注射 q5 min，之后 25～50 mg，口服，每日 2 次。
  - 普萘洛尔：0.5～1 mg 静脉注射，之后 40～80 mg，口服，q6～8 h。
- 氯吡格雷：300～600 mg，口服之后 75 mg/d。
- 肝素：
  - 低分子肝素：1 mg/kg，皮下注射，q12 h，可在给药前给予 30 mg（注意肾功能不全患者）。
  - 肝素：60 U/kg 静脉滴注，12 U/(kg · h) 输注（最大值）。最多 4 000 U，注射速率 1 000 U/h（目标是 APTT 50～75 s）。
- 吗啡：1～5 mg，静脉注射，q5～30 min。
- 硝酸甘油：0.3～0.6 mg 舌下含服或 0.4 mg，q5 min 后静脉滴注 10～20 μg/min，如果疼痛持续（最大值），剂量 200 μg/min。
- GP Ⅱb/Ⅲa 抑制剂：
  - 依替巴肽：180 μg/kg 静脉注射之后 2 μg/(kg · min) 滴注 72～96 h。
  - 替罗非班：0.4 μg/(kg · min) 静脉注射超过 30 min；之后 0.1 μg/(kg · min) 滴注 12～24 h。

二线用药

- 钙通道阻滞剂：
  - 地尔硫䓬：起始 0.25 mg/kg，15 min 后 0.35 mg/kg 30 mg，口服，q6 h：速释片。
  - 维拉帕米：起始 5～10 mg 静脉注射 30 min 后如果有必要的时候重复给药，然后 80～160 mg，口服，q8 h：速释片。
- ADP 阻滞剂：
  - 替格瑞洛：PCI 时 180 mg，口服×1；或 PCI 后 1 h，90 mg，每日 2 次。
  - 普拉格雷：PCI 时 60 mg，口服×1；或 PCI 后 1 h，10 mg/d。
- 劳拉西泮：1～2 mg，静脉注射，PRN。
- 抗凝（不是普通肝素）：
  - 磺达肝葵钠：2.5 mg，皮下注射，每日 1 次。
  - 比伐卢定（仅在 PCI 之前）：0.75 mg/kg 静脉注射，之后 1.75 mg/(kg · h) 静脉注射持续 4 h，之后 0.2 mg/(kg · h) 静脉注射持续 20 h。

随访

进一步处理

入院指征

- 患者的所有心脏生物标志物均为阳性，根据临床预测（TIMI、GRACE、PURSUIT）有较高的不良结局风险，或急性冠状动脉综合征的临床概率显著，在出现症状后 12～24 h 进行紧急或早期侵入性治疗。
- ICU 监测不稳定的患者。

出院指征

只有在排除了在急性冠状动脉综合征/非 Q 波梗死之后的患者才能安全地离院。

随访建议

只有排除急性冠状动脉综合征的患者才能安全出院：

- 出院的患者应在 1～2 日与其初级保健医师或心脏病专家一起随访。
- 门诊压力测试应在 72 h 内完成。

要点和误区

- 在抵达急诊后，所有的胸痛患者均应在 10 min 内做心电图。
- 早期药物干预可以降低 NSTEMI 患者死亡率。
- 注意：
  - 不排除基于初始或单组心脏标志物的梗死，特别是症状发作的时间＜4～6 h。
  - 注意询问苯丙胺或可卡因的使用情况。
  - 在给予硝酸甘油之前，不要忘记询问西地那非、伐地那非或他达拉非的使用情况。

J

急性冠脉综合征：心肌梗死 Acute Coronary Syndrome：Myocardial Infarction

Joshua W. Joseph · Shamai A. Grossman 马林浩 林兆奋 译

基础知识

描述

- 心肌供血和耗氧量失衡。
- 急性冠状动脉综合征(ACS)包含一系列疾病。
  - 不稳定型心绞痛。
  - 急性心肌梗死(AMI)。
  - ST 段抬高心肌梗死(STEMI)。
  - 非 STEMI。

病因

- 冠状动脉狭窄的动脉粥样硬化。
- 血管痉挛(变异型心绞痛)。
- 微血管性心绞痛或弥漫性血管，疾病血管异常松弛。
- 斑块破裂。
- 血栓形成。
- 动脉炎：
  - 狼疮。
  - 大动脉炎。
  - 川崎病。
  - 类风湿关节炎。
- 持续性低血压。
- 贫血/缺血：
  - 血红蛋白<8 g/dl(80 g/L)。
- 一氧化碳/碳氧血红蛋白升高。
- 冠状动脉气栓。
- 甲状腺危象。
- 冠状动脉结构异常：
  - 放射性纤维化。
  - 动脉瘤。
  - 扩张。
- 可卡因或苯丙胺引起的血管痉挛。
- 心脏危险因素包括：
  - 高胆固醇血症。
  - DM。
  - HTN。
  - 吸烟。
  - 一级相关家族史<55 岁。
  - 男性，年龄>55 岁。
  - 绝经后女性。

诊断

症状和体征

病史

- 胸痛。
  - MI 最常见的症状。
  - 胸骨后。
  - 疼痛。
  - 挤压。
  - 燃烧感。
  - 紧缩感。
- 没有胸痛的 MI 症状：
  - 腹痛。
  - 晕厥。
  - 出血。
  - 恶心或呕吐。
  - 虚弱。
- 疼痛或放射到手臂、肩膀、背部、颈部或下颌。
- 相关症状：
  - 呼吸困难。
  - 晕厥。
  - 疲劳。
  - 出血。
  - 恶心。
  - 呕吐。
- 症状通常由劳累、进食、暴露于寒冷或情绪压力引起。
- 症状通常持续 30 min 或更长时间。
- 休息或劳累时可能会出现症状。
- 通常在递增型心绞痛之前。
- 可以通过休息或硝酸甘油来改善或缓解。
- 症状通常与位置或吸气无关。
- 胸部正面或胸部紧缩感提示心绞痛。
- 症状期间血压通常会升高。

体格检查

- 体检通常不会发现。
- 偶尔的体格检查发现包括：
  - S3 或 S4 收缩或舒张杂音。
  - 由乳头肌功能障碍引起的中度反流。
  - 外周脉搏减弱。
  - 失代偿 CHF 的体格发现。

基本检查

在鉴别 MI 与非心脏病因方面，病史至关重要。

诊断检查与说明

实验室检查

- 电解质。
- 钙、镁。
- 心脏酶。
- 地高辛水平。

影像学检查

- 胸部 X 线检查。
  - 鉴别心肌病或 CHF。
  - 主动脉夹层。

诊断步骤/外科

- 心电图。
  - 区分 ST 段抬高的非缺血性原因。
    - 心包炎。
    - 良性早期复极。
    - 左心室肥厚。
    - 既往 MI 合并左心室动脉瘤。
    - 高钾血症。
- STEMI 的心电图标准。
  - 新发 ST 段从 J 点抬高，出现在至少 2 个相邻导联，男 0.2 mV，女 0.15 mV 在 V_2～V_3 或 0.1 mV 在其他的胸导联或肢体导联。
  - V_1～V_2 ST 段压低可能是损伤的先兆。
  - 新发或推测左束支阻滞被认为等价于 STEMI。多数情况下 LBBB 表现为非陈旧性但之前的心电图不可靠。
  - 修改后的 Sgarbossa 标准对于 LBBB 中的心肌梗死或同步节律诊断为：
    - QRS 综合征阳性伴导联协调的 ST 段抬高>1 mm。
    - V_1～V_3 导联协调的 ST 段压低>1 mm 伴 QRS 综合征阴性。
    - ST 段(从 J 点测量)和 R 或 S 波不协调(无论哪个更大，从 PR 测量)比值<−0.25。
- 超声：
  - 可以识别局部室壁运动异常或瓣膜功能障碍。

J

■ 鉴别诊断

- 主动脉夹层。
- 焦虑。
- 胆绞痛。
- 肋软骨炎。
- 食管痉挛。
- 食管反流。
- 带状疱疹。
- 食管裂孔疝。
- 二尖瓣脱垂。
- 消化性溃疡病。
- 心理症状。
- 恐惧症。
- 心包炎。
- 肺炎。
- 肺栓塞。

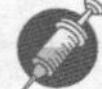

治疗

■ 院前

- 静脉通道。
- 阿司匹林。
- 吸氧。
- 心电监护。
- 舌下含服硝酸甘油。
- 如果可以，将12导联心电图传至接收医院。

■ 初步稳定/治疗

- 建立静脉通路。
- 吸氧。
- 心电监测。
- 血氧饱和度。
- 持续血压监测和血氧饱和度监测。

■ 急诊治疗/程序

- STEMI需要尽快进行再灌注治疗：
- 如果可行的话，经皮冠状动脉介入治疗(PCI)是首选的诊断和治疗方式。
- 目标是在首诊90 min内进行初级PCI。
- 如果在首诊后120 min内无法使用PCI，应使用溶栓药物(参见“心脏再灌注治疗”)。
- 患者抵达无PCI能力的医院应在30 min内立即转至有相应能力的医院。
- 患者院外心脏事件接受复苏后心电图显示STEMI应立即接受PCI。
- 除非已知过敏，否则应首先给所有疑似MI患者服用阿司匹林。
- 糖尿病蛋白Ⅱb/Ⅲa抑制剂(如阿昔单抗)可在PCI开始时使用。
- 普拉格雷或氯吡格雷应在PCI开始时使用。
- 普拉格雷不应给予有既往卒中史或TIA史的患者。
- 对于给予纤维蛋白溶解剂的患者，氯吡格雷是推荐的ADP受体抑制剂。
- 剂量减少(＜75岁，300 mg；＞75岁，75 mg)。
- 如果血压＞90～100 mmHg，则给予舌下含服硝酸甘油，或静脉注射，若没有心电图或右心室梗死的临床证据。
- 舌下含服硝酸甘油片后持续存在的症状强烈提示AMI或非心脏病因。
- 如果没有禁忌证(如心脏传导阻滞、心率＜60次/分、心力衰竭、低血压或阻塞性肺病的迹象)存在，则应在第一个24 h内开始β受体阻滞剂。
- 在PCI或ED治疗前给药无益。
- 可以给予吗啡来缓解疼痛、焦虑和增加携氧能力。
- 肝素(UFH)或比伐卢定应用于接受直接PCI的患者，比伐卢定适用于出血风险高的患者。
- 在接受溶栓治疗的患者中，肝素(UFH)、依诺肝素或磺达肝素是合适的。
- 如果患者出现心源性休克，应尽快将患者送至心导管实验室进行血管成形术和主动脉内球囊反搏(参见“充血性心力衰竭”)。
- 室性心律失常(参见“室性心动过速”)。
- 心动过缓伴低血压应使用阿托品或外置起搏治疗。
- 传导干扰：
- 一度房室传导阻滞和莫氏Ⅰ(Wenckebach)通常是自限性的，不需要治疗。
- 莫氏Ⅱ，完全心脏传导阻滞，新的右束支传导阻滞(RBBB)，RBBB加左前支阻滞或左后束支阻滞，左束支阻滞加一度房室传导阻滞可能需要临时起搏器。
- 再灌注后可出现室性心律加快(AIVR)，表现为室性心律，心率低于120次/分。
- 只有持续治疗电复律或碳酸氢钠。
- 利多卡因和其他抗心律失常可能导致心搏停止。

■ 药物治疗

- 阿司匹林：162～325 mg，口服。
- ADP受体抑制剂。
- 氯吡格雷：600 mg，口服。
- 普拉格雷：60 mg，口服。
- 替格瑞洛：180 mg，口服。
- 比伐卢定：0.75 mg/kg，静脉注射，之后1.75 mg/(kg·h)维持。
- 低分子肝素：1 mg/kg，皮下注射，q12 h。磺达肝素：2.5 mg，静脉注射。
- 糖蛋白Ⅱb/Ⅲa抑制剂：
- 阿昔单抗：仅在PCI使用之前，0.25 mg/kg，静脉注射。
- 依替非巴肽：180 μg/kg静脉注射1～2 min，之后2 μg/(kg·min)维持72 h。
- 替罗非班：0.4 μg/(kg·min)维持30 min，之后0.1 μg/(kg·min)维持48～108 h。
- 肝素：60 U/kg静脉注射(最大4 000 U)，之后12 U/(kg·h)(最大1 000 U/h)。
- 美托洛尔：5 mg静脉注射q5～15 min后接受25～50 mg口服起始剂量耐受(注意：禁用于可卡因胸痛)。
- 吗啡：2 mg静脉注射，若没有呼吸系统恶化且SBP＞90 mmHg可以2 mg递增，以缓解疼痛。
- 硝酸甘油：最高0.4 mg舌下含服q5 min，3剂。
- 硝酸甘油：静脉注射5～10 μg/min，使用非PVD管。
- 硝酸盐：1～2 in透皮给药。
- 溶栓：参见“心脏再灌注治疗”。

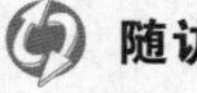

随访

■ 进一步处理

入院指征

- AMI患者需要入院治疗。
- 如果诊断不清楚，进入医院或急诊观察，可能连续心肌酶、心电图及运动压力测试和/或心脏导管插入(如果需要)有用。

出院指征

如果没有AMI即可离院。

转诊问题

- 如果治疗机构无法获得PCI，特别是患者出现心源性休克，则应将其送往另一家医院在120 min内启动PCI。
- 再灌注失败的患者应该被紧急运送到支持PCI的设施。
- 作为侵入性策略的一部分，接受再灌注治疗的患者在3～24 h被转移到具有PCI功能的机构实施治疗将使其获益。

要点和误区

- 如果PCI不可行，溶栓治疗的目标是30 min内。
- 新的或可能是新的LBBB很少发生，不应被视为单独诊断AMI。

急性冠脉综合征：心绞痛 Acute Coronary Syndrome: Angina

Margaret J. Lin · Shamai A. Grossman 马林浩 林兆奋 译

基础知识

描述

- 由于心肌血液供应和氧气需求不平衡导致的胸部不适。
- 加拿大心血管学会心绞痛分类：
  - 第一类：普通体力活动没有心绞痛。
  - 第二类：正常活动受轻微限制，在步行、爬楼梯或情绪紧张时发生心绞痛。
  - 第三类：普通活动严重受限制，在水平面上行走1～2个街区或爬上一段楼梯时即发作的心绞痛。
  - 第四类：在休息时无法进行任何身体活动而不会出现不适或心绞痛症状。
- 通常分为稳定型或不稳定型。
- 稳定型心绞痛：可预测，随着劳累发作，并随着休息而改善。
- 不稳定型心绞痛(UA)：新发，发作的频率，持续时间或下限阈值增加；休息时也发作或>20 min。
- UA与透壁性心肌梗死和心脏病死亡风险增加有关。
- 高敏感心脏标志物使得UA和NSTEMI分界模糊。

病因

- 心脏危险因素：
  - 年龄：
    - 男性>35岁。
    - 女性绝经。
  - 高胆固醇血症。
  - 糖尿病(DM)。
  - 高血压(HTN)。
  - 吸烟。
- 冠状动脉粥样硬化：
  - 稳定型心绞痛：慢性、运动时导致血流动力学不稳定。
  - UA：运动或休息时斑块急性破坏，可导致症状恶化。
- 血管痉挛：心绞痛、毒品相关(可卡因、苯丙胺)。
- 微血管心绞痛或血管异常松弛，如果弥漫性血管疾病。
- 动脉炎：狼疮、高山病、川崎病、类风湿关节炎。
- 贫血。
- 高压氧、一氧化碳血红蛋白(HbCO)升高。
- 冠状动脉结构异常：放射、动脉瘤、扩张。

诊断

症状和体征

病史

- 胸痛：
  - 胸骨后疼痛、沉重、紧绷、灼烧或挤压。
  - 放射痛至颈部、下颌、左肩或手臂。
- 局部疼痛，内脏疼痛。
- 心绞痛包括：
  - 呼吸困难。
  - 上腹部不适。
  - 虚弱。
  - 发汗。
  - 恶心、呕吐。
  - 腹部疼痛。
  - 晕厥。
- 症状通常由劳累、进食、冷暴露、情绪压力引起。
- 症状通常不是体位性的或胸膜炎性的。
- 通常休息或硝酸甘油可缓解。
- 对于稳定型心绞痛常持续数秒但<20 min且症状的模式和频率没有改变。

老年人注意事项

- 女性、糖尿病患者、少数民族以及>65岁或经常出现非典型症状的患者。
- 非典型症状患者预后更差。

体格检查

- 莱文征：拳头紧握放于胸口，最典型的表现。
- 在出现症状时，血压通常会升高。
- 体检可获得的信息有限。
- 可及第三心音(S3)/第四心音(S4)。乳头肌无功能伴二尖瓣反流或新的杂音，外周动脉搏动减弱。

基本检查

心电图：

- 标准12导联：
  - 对于急性胸痛患者，应在10 min内获得并阅读。
  - 在检测急性MI方面非常有帮助，尤其是UA。
  - 与先前的心电图比较(如果有)很重要。
  - UA患者新出现ST改变或可疑TWI。
    - T波低平或双向T波。
    - ST压低≤1 mm持续80 ms，是UA的典型特征。
    - 可见陈旧性缺血，高张或梗死的证据，如陈旧性的TWI、Q波、ST段压低。
    - 连续ECG有助于区分稳定型和不稳定型心绞痛。
    - 急性MI单次心电图约60%的敏感性，90%的特异性。
- 心电图还有助于诊断胸痛的其他原因心包炎：
  - 弥漫性ST段抬高，T波倒置和脉速降低。
  - 肺栓塞S1Q3T3型，不明原因心动过速，右心劳损征象。

> **注意**
>
> 患有正常或非特异性心电图的患者AMI发生率为1%～5%，UA发生率为4%～23%。

诊断检查与说明

实验室检查

- 对于稳定型心绞痛，心肌酶未显示异常，但如果病史可疑为急性MI，应进行检查。
- CK-MB和肌钙蛋白I或T：
  - 高敏肌钙蛋白转阳性且随时间相应变化可以排除
  - CK-MB 12～24 h达到峰值，回到基线在2～3日。
  - 肌钙蛋白12 h达到峰值，回到基线7～10日。
- 血细胞量(贫血增加缺血风险)。
- 凝血情况。
- 电解质，特别是Cr和K^+。

影像学检查

- 胸部X线检查：
  - 通常没有发现。
  - 可以显示心肌肥大或者肺气肿，CHF可能提示UA。
  - 可能在识别其他的病因，如肺炎、气胸或者主动脉夹层方面具有一定作用。
- 冠状动脉CTA：
  - 适用于低风险的没有冠状动脉疾病

(CAD)图像的患者去排除心肌缺血症，以及评估冠状动脉狭窄所引起疼痛的病因的可能性。

- “三重排除原则”适用急性冠状动脉坏死综合征、心包积液和主动脉夹层。

• 床旁超声：检查室壁运动异常及其他休克、心包积液、气胸的病因。

• 心肌^{99}Tc静息成像：心肌对于放射性核素的灌注摄取。

诊断步骤/外科

• 运动压力测试：

- 如果剧烈胸痛并有中度至高度缺血的可能，则不适用。

• 若基线ECG异常，行影像学压力测试(铥显影、砣或超声)。

• 其他影像学形式包括MRI、PET也被使用。

• 冠状动脉造影：

- CAD诊断金标准。

鉴别诊断

• 焦虑和恐惧症。
• 主动脉夹层。
• 胆绞痛。
• 肋软骨炎。
• 食管反流。
• 食管痉挛
• 食管炎。
• GERD。
• 带状疱疹。
• 食管裂孔疝。
• 二尖瓣脱垂。
• 肌肉骨骼胸痛。
• MI。
• 心肌炎。
• 心肌缺血的非动脉粥样硬化原因：
- 冠状动脉痉挛。
- 冠状动脉栓塞。
- 先天性冠状动脉疾病。
- 冠状动脉剥脱。
- 瓣膜病：AS、AI、肺动脉狭窄、二尖瓣狭窄。
- 先天性心脏病。
• 消化性溃疡病。
• 心包炎。
• 肺炎。
• 心理因素。
• 气胸。
• 肺栓塞。

治疗

院前

• 静脉通道。
• 阿司匹林。
• 氧气。
• 生命体征和氧饱和度。
• 心脏监测。
• 12导联心电图，如果可能的话。
• 舌下含服硝酸甘油。

初步稳定/治疗

• 静脉通道。
• 氧气。
• 心电监测。
• 生命体征和连续氧饱和度。

急诊治疗/程序

• 所有胸心痛患者应考虑心肌缺血，应在抵达急诊室后接受阿司匹林。

• 舌下含服硝酸甘油：如果3次舌下给药后症状持续存在，提示UA、AMI或非心脏病因。

• 疼痛控制。

• 抗凝治疗。

药物治疗

一线用药

• 阿司匹林：325 mg口服或81 mg×4嚼服。

• 阿司匹林过敏患者：氯吡格雷300～600 mg，口服；或普拉格雷60 mg，口服；或替卡格雷180 mg，口服。

• 对于中度至高度风险的UA患者，应给予双抗血小板治疗，选择有侵入性策略的患者，如导管插入术或手术。

• 硝酸甘油：
- 0.4 mg舌下含服。
- 静滴5～10 μg/min。
- 1～2粒硝酸甘油片。
- 注意维持血压稳定(RV梗死：Q波出现在Ⅱ、Ⅲ、aVF；STE在右侧V_3、V_4)。
- 注意若患者有无勃起功能障碍史并且在最近的48 h内使用磷酸二酯酶抑制剂如西地那非(伟哥)或他达拉非(西力士)。

• 吗啡：
- 无呼吸抑制，收缩压>90 mmHg时，4 mg静脉推注，缓解疼痛。

• β受体阻滞药：
- 美托洛尔：25～50 mg口服或5 mg静脉推注q5～15 min治疗难治性HTN和心动过速。
- 禁忌：反应性呼吸道疾病、充血性心力衰竭、心动过缓、低血压、心肌梗死、可卡因使用者。
- 当患者到达急诊室，该药不是必需的药品，但建议在AMI 24 h内服用。

二线用药

• 可根据机构不同而变化，推荐给予住院患者专业的抗凝方案。
- 肝素：60 U/kg静脉推注，之后12 U/(kg·h)(目标APTT 50～70)。
- 依诺肝素：如果Cr清除率<30 ml/min，1 mg/kg，皮下注射，q12 h或q24 h。

• 糖蛋白Ⅱb/Ⅲa抑制剂：
- 依替巴肽(整合素)：在1～2 min 180 μg/kg静脉推注，之后2 g/(kg·min)至72 h。
- 罗替非班：0.4 μg/(kg·min)持续30 min，然后0.1 μg/(kg·min)持续48～108 h。
- 阿西单抗：0.25 mg/kg静脉推注，然后0.125 μg/(kg·min)。
- 比伐卢定、磺达肝癸钠。

• 出血风险高的患者包括老年人、女性、贫血症患者、慢性肾衰竭患者。

• 对稳定型心绞痛患者，持续性的管理预防治疗包括肝素，血压控制(β受体阻滞剂、钙通道阻滞剂、长效硝酸盐)及生活方式改变(减重，减少脂肪/糖摄入，戒烟)。
- 新型抗心绞痛药物包括雷诺嗪可能也是健康管理的一部分。

随访

进一步处理

入院指征

• UA患者需要进医院。

• 心脏导管插入术的早期干预可能会降低心肌酶升高、持续性心绞痛或血流动力学不稳定的患者的死亡率。

• 诊断不明确的患者可能会因到急诊观察心肌酶谱、心电图和压力测试/导管插入术而受益。

出院指征

稳定型心绞痛患者。

随访建议

稳定型心绞痛或检查阴性胸痛的患者应在急诊后几日内与他们的PCP或心脏病专家进行随访。

J

要点和误区

• 病史是区分不稳定型心绞痛和非心脏性疼痛的最重要因素。

• 所有患有胸痛或心脏病症状的患者应立即进行心电图检查，且连续心电图对 ACS 很有必要。

• 一次心肌酶学阴性不能排除胸痛患者存在 ACS。

• 女性、糖尿病患者、少数民族和 65 岁以上的患者需要降低 ACS 检查门槛，因为他们经常有不典型的表现。

• 与住院部心脏病专家/介入专家讨论因医院不同而调整抗凝方案是非常重要的。

急性精神病 Psychosis, Acute

Timothy M. Scarella 郑金浩 毛恩强 译

基础知识

描述

大脑功能紊乱，其特征是不合逻辑的、怪异的或妄想的信念、不正常的感知，以及情绪、思想和行为的混乱。

病因

精神病学

• 原发性神经病：

- 精神分裂症：6 个月以上有超过以下 2 种症状：幻觉、妄想、阴性症状、思维混乱、行为紊乱。
- 如果症状＜1 个月，则为简单精神障碍；如果症状为 1～6 个月，则为分裂样障碍。
- 分裂情感障碍：伴有精神病失代偿的显著情绪症状。
- 妄想性障碍：没有其他精神病症状的僵硬妄想的存在。

• 情绪障碍：

- 精神病性躁狂。
- 精神病性抑郁症。

• 精神病学上对精神病的模仿(不是真正的精神病，但可能很像)：

- 创伤后应激障碍：可能涉及强烈的参考性思维和对与客观现实脱节的危险恐惧。
- 边缘性人格障碍：可能涉及强烈的指涉思维和相关的情感不稳定。
- 强迫症：强迫症的本质可能是如此不合逻辑和僵化，以至于看起来像是精神病。
- 神经发育障碍：自闭症或智力残疾的人可能有奇怪的或不切实际的信念，或者将内心的想法体验为“声音”。

精神科

• 神经系统疾病：

- 妄想症(明显的混乱、注意力不集中、意识消退；可能包括知觉障碍和不合逻辑或妄想)。
- 头部损伤。
- 痴呆症(任何痴呆症都可能出现幻觉和妄想，包括阿尔茨海默症、路易体痴呆症、额颞叶痴呆症)。
- 脑血管意外(急性或慢性)。
- 癫痫发作(发作间或发作后)。
- 占位性病变(肿瘤、脓肿、囊肿)。
- 脑积水。
- 脱髓鞘疾病(多发性硬化症)。
- 神经精神障碍(帕金森病、亨廷顿病、威尔逊病)。
- 朊病毒病。

• 感染性疾病。

- 脑膜炎/脑炎(细菌、病毒或真菌)。
- HIV 感染。
- 三期梅毒。
- 三期莱姆病。

• 代谢性疾病：

- 中毒(精神兴奋剂、致幻剂、氯胺酮、苯环利定、大麻素、摇头丸、右美沙芬)。
- 药物副作用(环孢菌素、环丝氨酸、皮质类固醇、氟喹诺酮、金刚烷胺、左旋多巴、普拉克索、左乙拉西坦)。
- 高钙血症。
- 维生素 B_{12} 缺乏症。
- 重金属中毒(砷、汞)。
- 卟啉症。

• 内分泌系统疾病：

- 甲状腺疾病。
- 库欣综合征。
- 肾上腺功能不全。

• 自身免疫性疾病：

- 狼疮脑炎(通常伴随癫痫发作的神经系统症状)。
- 自身免疫性脑炎(即抗 NMDA)。
- 副肿瘤综合征。

• 毒素：

- 重金属。
- 有机磷酸酯类。
- 一氧化碳。

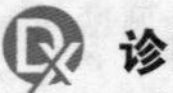

诊断

症状和体征

• 顽定的错觉，错误的信念：

- 不受外部逻辑的影响。
- 往往涉及持久的，与宗教或躯体相关的内容。

• 幻觉：

- 在没有外部刺激的情况下的感官体验。
- 可以涉及任何感官形态，听觉和视觉是最常见的。
- 与幻形想不同，幻想是对真实刺激(即被认为是人的衣帽架)的感觉加工和改变，常见于谵妄，但也发生在精神病中。

• 杂乱无章的想法：

- 独特的逻辑、松散的联系、不切实际的讲话。
- 语言异常：新词、新奇联想、词语混乱。

• 无组织的行为：

- 不可预测或不适当的行为。
- 冲动。
- 奇怪或无目的的行为。
- 无法执行普通任务。

• 阴性症状：

- 情绪低落。
- 冷漠。
- 快感缺乏。
- 社交隔绝。
- 思想内容贫乏。

• 紧张症：

- 更常见于医疗状况和情绪障碍。
- 可能发生在精神病中。
- 运动表现：僵硬、缺乏运动或运动过度、姿势、蜡样屈曲、奇怪/无目的的运动。
- 模仿动作(模仿测试者的动作)。
- 模仿语言(模仿测试者的语言)。
- 自动服从、消极(对指令的抗拒)、抓握

J

反射。

- 生命体征异常。
- 提示非精神病因的特征：
- 突然发作。
- 新发病＞30 岁。
- 过程波动。
- 局灶性神经症状。
- 异常生命体征。
- 视觉、嗅觉、味觉或触觉幻觉。
- 定向、注意力或认知功能受损。

病史

- 筛选所有精神病症状，包括发作、持续时间、触发因素和内容。
- 妄想：
- "你有危险吗？你觉得有人想伤害你，还是有人在监视你？"
- "有人试图给你发信息，解读你的想法，或者阻止你的思考吗？"
- "你有什么特殊能力吗？"
- 幻觉：
- "你曾经看到或听到过别人看不见或听不见的东西吗？"
- "你有没有听到过有人告诉你做一些伤害自己或伤害他人的事情？"
- 自杀或杀人行为或威胁。
- 既往病史和精神病史。
- 社会地位和照顾自己的能力。
- 最近药物或酒精的使用、增加或停止。
- 尽可能从朋友、家人和治疗者那里获取病史。

体格检查

寻找医学病因的迹象：

- 生命的迹象。
- 一般测试特别注意毒素的迹象和症状。
- 神经学检查，包括认知评估。
- 秘密评估谵妄迹象。

基本检查

工作是具体的，主要基于相关病因。

诊断检查与说明

实验室检查

- 电解质、尿素氮、肌酐、葡萄糖、钙。
- 毒理学检测。
- 全血细胞计数变化。
- 促甲状腺激素。
- 尿分析。
- 进一步的具体研究应该被怀疑的潜在的病因。

影像学检查

- 头颅 CT：
- 考虑新的精神病症状，具有表明非血清学病因的特征。
- 排除颅内出血。
- MRI：
- 如果怀疑颅内病变而不是出血。

诊断检查/外科

当临床需要时，考虑：

- 腰椎穿刺术。
- 心电图：
- 评估 QT 间期延长。
- 脑电图：
- 考虑以非典型精神病排除复杂的部分性癫痫发作。
- 即使在活跃的癫痫发作期间，这些发现也可能显得非特异或不显著。

鉴别诊断

参考病因学。

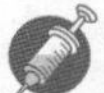 治疗

初步稳定/治疗

- 患者和工作人员的安全至关重要，可能需要安保人员在场。
- 首先应该使用行为干预。
- 提供一个平静、包容的环境。
- 移除所有潜在危险物品。
- 用令人安心的声音和平静的举止来设定界限和口头重定向。
- 如果安全是一个问题，患者需要不断接受观察。
- 在决定进行约束之前，先口服药物。
- 只有在维护患者和工作人员安全的情况下，才需要物理或化学约束。

急诊治疗/程序

- 如果怀疑有非精神病因，识别并治疗潜在的疾病。
- 抗精神病药物可减少急性激动：
- 鼓励在注射前自愿服用口服药物。
- 避免多药。
- 快速镇静可以通过添加苯二氮䓬来实现。
- 监测和治疗抗精神病药物的不良反应：
- 锥体外系症状（肌张力障碍、静坐不能、假性帕金森综合征和迟发性运动障碍）。
- 神经安定恶性综合征是一种危及生命的并发症，其特征是高热、肌肉僵硬、自主神经不稳定和意识改变。

药物治疗

- 导致对患者或其他人造成伤害的急性激动（如果反应不充分，给药并在 20～30 min 后重复）。
- 氟哌啶醇：2～10 mg，口服、静脉注射或肌内注射，重复 q20～60 min，必要时，最大剂量 100 mg/d；老年人 0.5～2 mg/剂。
- 羟哌氟丙嗪：2.5～10 mg，口服或肌内注射。
- 阿立哌唑：2～15 mg，口服或肌内注射，最大剂量 30 mg/d。
- 齐拉西酮：10～20 mg，肌内注射，最大剂量 40 mg/d，注意监测 QT 间期。
- 上述药物通常用 1～2 mg 劳拉西泮静脉注射进行镇静，用 0.5～1 mg 苯妥英或 25～50 mg 苯海拉明静脉注射进行预防急性肌张力障碍或静坐不能。
- 氯丙嗪：25 mg，口服或肌内注射，重复 25～50 mg q60 min 必要时，最大剂量 1 000 mg/d。注意：体位性低血压，避免在老年人中使用。
- 奥氮平：2.5～20 mg，口服或肌内注射，可重复剂量 q2～4 h，必要时，最大剂量 30 mg/d；老年人 2.5～5 mg/剂。注意：同时使用肌内注射奥氮平和静脉苯二氮䓬类药物可能会增加心肺衰竭的风险。
- 如果怀疑没有急性激动和原发性精神障碍，可以在精神处置未决期间开始口服抗精神病药物治疗。
- 紧张症状需要用苯二氮䓬类药物治疗。

老年人注意事项

抗精神病药物带有一个黑匣子警告，指出老年痴呆相关精神病患者接受抗精神病药物治疗会增加死亡风险。

妊娠注意事项

所有抗精神病药物都是丙类，除了氯氮平是乙类。没有致畸作用是已知的。新生儿适应综合征的风险。可能会增加早产风险，但对出生体重、神经发育结果或新生儿死亡率没有已知影响。

- 急性抗精神病药物给药：注意急性肌张力障碍（包括喉部肌张力障碍）、急性静坐不能、直立性。
- 慢性给药：迟发性运动障碍（肌张力障碍、运动障碍、帕金森综合征）、体重增加、糖尿病、高脂血症。

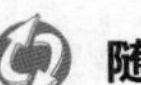 随访

进一步处理

入院指征

- 如果是非精神病因，接受适当的医疗

服务。

• 如果精神病病因和患者在医学上是稳定的，如果由于精神病，患者是：

- 有伤害自己的危险。
- 有可能对他人造成伤害。
- 严重残疾，因精神病不能自理。
- 非自愿承诺的标准因地域而异。

出院指征

• 患者没有伤害自己或伤害他人的表现，日常生活自理。

• 躯体疾病好转，精神症状缓解，患者病情允许时可离院。

■ 随访建议

如果担心患者对自己或他人有危险，无法照顾自己，或担心精神病影响医疗决策，建议进行精神病学咨询后续建议。

• 如果出院，与医疗和精神病学提供者一起计划适当的门诊随访。对于不符合住院标准的急性症状，考虑转诊到强化门诊或部分医院项目。

• 考虑转诊与物质使用相关的精神病患者戒毒。

要点和误区

• 精神症状需评估是否由躯体疾病引起，不要直接否认躯体疾病的病因，即使知道患者存在精神疾病。

• 出现视觉、嗅觉、味觉或触觉的幻觉应当及时进行医疗检查。

• 避免使用肌内注射奥氮平静脉苯二氮䓬类药物，它们可以增加心肺衰竭的风险。

• 最近开始或增加抗精神病药物的患者出现发热、强直、自主神经不稳定和精神状态改变时，应进行评估。

急性肾损伤 Kidney Injury, Acute

Michael D. Burg · Matthew N. Graber 段立伟 译

基础知识

■ 描述

• "肾衰竭"是一个过时的术语。

• 急性肾损伤(AKI)由肾脏疾病改善全球预后(KDIGO)新定义为：

- 48 h 内血清肌酐≥0.3 mg/dl。
- 7 日内血清肌酐增加至平时水平的 1.5 倍以上。
- 尿量 0.5 ml/(kg·h)，持续 6 h。

• 血清肌酐或尿量的变化决定 AKI 分期。

• KDIGO 分期：

- 第 1 期：Cr≥0.3 mg/dl 或 1.5～1.9 倍基线或尿量<0.5 mg/(kg·h)×6 h。
- 第 2 期：Cr 超过平时水平 2～2.9 倍或尿量 0.5 mg/(kg·h)×12 h。
- 第 3 期：Cr≥平时水平 3 倍或≥4 mg/dl；或 UO<0.3 mg/(kg·h)×24 h 或无尿≥12 h 或开始肾脏替代治疗。

• AKI 导致的后果包括：

- 体内废物堆积。
- 电解质紊乱。
- 液体潴留。
- 免疫力下降。
- 其他器官功能障碍。

• AKI 导致发病率和死亡率增加。

• AKI 生物标志物对于早期诊断、鉴别诊断和预后将变得越来越重要。

■ 病因

• 肾前性 AKI：

- 肾脏低灌注。
- 肾组织保持正常，除非存在严重/长期低灌注。

• 肾性 AKI：

- 由肾实质疾病引起的。

• 医源性 AKI，原因包括：

- 氨基糖苷类抗生素。
- 非甾体类药物。
- 血管紧张素转换酶抑制剂。
- 血管紧张素受体阻滞剂。
- 静脉造影对既往有重大疾病的患者也是一个危险因素。

• 肾后性 AKI：

- 由于尿路梗阻（如前列腺肥大、前列腺炎）。

诊断

■ 症状和体征

• 通常无症状，通常根据常规实验室指标来进行诊断。

• 少尿(<400 ml/d)。

• 液体潴留表现为：

- 呼吸困难。
- 高血压。
- 颈静脉怒张。
- 肺水肿和外周水肿。
- 腹水。
- 心包积液和胸腔积液。

• 呕吐。

• 皮肤变化或皮肤瘙痒。

• 精神变化。

肾前性 AKI

• 血管内液体相对或绝对不足。
• 黏膜干燥。
• 低血压。
• 心动过速。
• 心排量低。
• 充血性心力衰竭。
• 全身性血管扩张（如败血症、过敏反应）。

肾性 AKI

• 过敏性间质性肾炎：

- 发热。
- 呼吸困难。
- 关节痛。
- 近期发生心肌梗死。

• 肾静脉血栓：

- 肾病综合征。
- 与肺栓塞相关。
- 腰痛或腹痛。

• 肾小球肾炎，血管炎。

• 溶血性尿毒综合征。

• 血栓性血小板减少性紫癜(TTP)：

- 轻度 BUN 或 Cr 升高。
- 发热。
- 精神状态改变。
- 贫血和血小板减少症。
- 昏迷、癫痫、头痛、神志改变。

肾后性 AKI

• 腹痛或腰痛。
• 膀胱扩张。
• 少尿或无尿。

J

AKI 并发症

- 尿毒症:
- 精神状态改变。
- 扑翼样震颤。
- 反射异常。
- 局部神经异常。
- 癫痫。
- 不宁腿综合征。
- 心包炎。
- 心包积液或心脏压塞。
- 肠梗阻。
- 血小板功能障碍。
- 瘙痒。
- 血液病:
- 贫血。
- 出血时间延长和血小板功能不全。
- 白细胞增多。

病史

- 既往有 AKI 病史。
- AKI 危险因素:CHF、DM、HTN、其他疾病。
- 肾毒性药物史。
- 体重变化。

体格检查

- 生命体征:低血压、高血压、发热、心动过速。
- 精神状态改变。
- 眼:眼底镜检查。
- CV 检查:颈静脉怒张。
- 肺部:啰音。
- 腹部:腹部压痛,肾脏可触及。
- 水肿。
- 皮肤:表皮脱落、"尿毒症霜"、皮肤干燥。

老年人注意事项

- 易患肾前性 AKI。
- 肌酐会随肌肉质量变化,因此"正常"的 Cr 可能对于老年病人代表 Cr 升高。
- 药物会增加发生 AKI 风险。

儿科注意事项

- 新生儿肾前性 AKI 要被考虑到。
- 先天性解剖结构异常。

妊娠注意事项

- 肾源性氮质血症。
- 子痫。
- 局部缺血:产后出血、胎盘早剥、羊水栓塞。
- 非法人工流产药物的毒性作用。
- 产后血栓性血小板减少症,微血管病。

基本检查

- 电解质包括 Ca^{2+}、Mg^{2+}、PO_4^{3-}。
- BUN/Cr。
- 尿液检查
- 离心标本有助于鉴别 AKI 的病因。
- 管型、血液、白细胞和晶体。
- 钠和/或尿素的排泄分数(FE)。
- 全血细胞计数:常见由慢性病引起的贫血。
- 排空后残余容积(>100 ml 表示梗阻)。
- 尿路梗阻,尤其是老年男性(如前列腺肥大、前列腺炎)。
- 心电图,但是需要注意的是,心电图对于致命性的高钾血症并不敏感。
- 生物标志物(在未来临床上可用的):NGAL、KIM-1、IL-18、L-FABP、cystatin-C。

诊断检查和说明

实验室检查

肾前性

尿液:

- 尿比重>1.018。
- 渗透压>500 mmol/kg。
- 钠<10 mmol/L。
- 透明管型。
- BUN/Cr>20。
- 钠分次排泄率<1%。
- 肾脏灌注正常后肾功能可迅速恢复。

肾性

- BUN/Cr<10~15。
- 钠分次排泄率>2%。
- 肾小球肾炎,血管炎:
- 尿液检查中发现红细胞或颗粒状管型。
- 补体和自身抗体。
- 溶血性尿毒综合征或血栓性血小板减少性紫癜:
- 尿液检查正常。
- 贫血。
- 血小板减少。
- 碎裂的红细胞。
- 肾毒性急性肾小管坏死(ATN):
- 尿液:
  - 褐色颗粒或上皮细胞管型。
  - 比重=1.010。
  - 尿渗透压<350 mmol/kg。
  - 尿钠>20 mmol/L。
- 乙二醇摄入:
- 尿液:草酸钙结晶。
- 阴离子间隙性代谢性酸中毒。
- 渗透压低。
- 横纹肌溶解:
- 血清 K^+、PO_4^{3-}、肌红蛋白、肌酸激酶、尿酸升高。
- 血清钙离子降低。
- 肾小管间质性疾病。
- 过敏性间质性肾炎。
- 尿液内有白细胞管型、白细胞、红细胞和蛋白尿。
- 嗜酸性粒细胞增多。

肾后性

尿液:

- 通常是正常的。
- 可能存在血尿,但是没有管型和蛋白尿。
- 钠分次排泄率通常>4%。
- 尿渗透压<350 mmol/kg。

影像学检查

- 超声:
- 可以排除 98%的梗阻性病因。
- CT:
- 对梗阻不敏感。
- 可发现肾内的问题。
- 双功能彩色超声:
- 肾动脉或静脉血栓。
- 肾动脉造影:
- 可明确诊断肾动脉血栓,肾梗阻。
- 下腔静脉和肾血管造影诊断肾静脉血栓形成。
- 静脉肾盂造影(很少)。

诊断步骤/外科

心电图:

- 继发于容量超负荷的高血压可能导致缺血性表现。
- 可检测到急性电解质变化,但对危及生命的高钾血症敏感性较差。

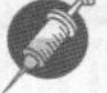

治疗

院前

- ABC 管理。
- 缺氧时,及时给氧。
- 容量不足时,及时静脉补液。

初步稳定/治疗

- ABC 管理。
- 缺氧时及时给氧。
- 容量不足时,及时静脉补液。
- 纠正电解质紊乱。
- 紧急透析指征(与肾脏科医生商议)。
- 顽固性高血压。
- 容量过多、充血性心力衰竭。
- 尿毒症脑病、出血或心包炎。

J

- 难以纠正的代谢性酸中毒。
• 避免使用肾毒性药物。
• 监测病人状态。
• 心电监护。

急诊治疗/程序

肾前性 AKI：
• 静脉补充晶体液纠正容量不足。
• 出血或 2 次补液后效果不佳，使用红细胞悬液。
• 如无法评估心力衰竭或低容量时，使用有创监护。
• 对补充晶体液后反应良好是反映低血容量情况的一个很好的指标。

> **注意**
> 在肝衰竭伴有腹水时，谨慎补充晶体液。

肾性 AKI
• 肾小球肾炎：
- 糖皮质激素或血浆置换。
• 急性肾小管坏死
- 容量治疗。
• 低钠血症：限制饮水。
• 高钾血症：
- 当血钾>6.5 mmol/L 或心电图符合高钾表现时：
◦ 沙丁胺醇雾化吸入。
◦ 高糖和胰岛素。
◦ 如果患者不是无尿状态，使用呋塞米。
◦ 钙高钾血症时心肌细胞有稳定作用。
◦ 葡萄糖酸钙对病情稳定患者有治疗作用。
◦ 无脉患者使用氯化钙。
◦ 难以纠正的高钾血症，可透析治疗。
• 代谢性酸中毒：
- 慢性病程的患者在 pH<7.2 或 HCO_3^-<15 mmol/L 才可使用碳酸氢钠。
- 高磷血症：
◦ 碳酸钙。
◦ 氢氧化铝。
- 肌红蛋白尿时，积极进行液体复苏。

> **注意**
> • 心电图仅在 PR、QT 或 QRS 间期增宽会受到钙离子影响。T 波峰值本身并不是一种指标。
> • 碳酸氢钠对于无尿/少尿患者造成的负担过重，需谨慎使用。

药物治疗

• 沙丁胺醇：10～20 mg，雾化吸入。
• 氢氧化铝：0.5～1.5 g，口服。
• 碳酸钙：0.25～3 g，口服。
• 葡萄糖酸钙：10%溶液 10 ml，大于 5 min 静脉注射(5 min 后可重复给药一次)。
• 氯化钙：10%溶液 10 ml。
• 葡萄糖：25 g。
• 呋塞米：20～400 mg，静脉注射。
• 胰岛素：0.1 U/kg 常规静脉注射葡萄糖(严重肾脏和/或肝脏疾病的剂量减少 50%)，并静脉注射右旋糖酐。
• 碳酸氢钠：1～2 mEg/kg，静脉注射。

> **注意**
> • AKI 是不建议使用利尿剂和多巴胺(在没有容量超负荷时)。
> • SPS(聚磺苯乙烯)不再推荐使用。

随访

进一步处理

入院指征
• 新发的 AKI。
• 高钾血症、严重的电解质异常。
• 缺氧、充血性心力衰竭导致的液体过多。
• 尿毒症。
• 精神状态改变。

出院标准
• 病情稳定。
• 电解质正常。

随访建议

要点和误区

• 对于严重的肝脏或肾脏疾病，应减少高钾血症的胰岛素剂量，以避免低血糖。
• 任何程度的 AKI 都应避免使用非甾体抗炎药。

脊髓灰质炎 Polio

Waleed Mohammed Hussein · Philip Shayne 瞿金龙 译

J

基础知识

描述

• 脊髓灰质被感染引起。
• 潜伏期 7～14 日。
• 持续时间<1 周。
• 临床表现如下：
- 亚临床病变(不明显的)90%～95%。
- 无症状的脊髓灰质炎 4%～8%：
◦ 临床表现和其他病毒感染的区别不明显(发热、肌痛、不舒服)。
◦ 在疾病流行期常怀疑为脊髓灰质感染。
- 非瘫痪的小儿麻痹症 1%～2%：
◦ 和无症状的脊髓灰质炎的区别是有脑膜刺激表现。
◦ 和无菌性脑膜炎的病程相似。
- 脊髓灰质炎瘫痪 0.1%，进一步细分为：
◦ 脊髓型脊髓灰质炎。
◦ 延髓型脊髓灰质炎(占脊髓灰质炎患者的 10%)：受脑神经支配的肌群瘫痪；延髓的呼吸和循环中枢常受累死亡率高。
◦ 混合型脊髓灰质炎。
- 脊髓灰质炎后综合征：
◦ 新出现的进行性肌肉无力、疼痛，局部或普遍肌肉萎缩。
◦ 在疾病活动期后发生在 8～70 岁，常发生于先前受累的肢体。
◦ 风险因素包括感染脊髓灰质炎的年龄、恢复的程度和性别。
◦ 逐步进展。

病因

• 脊髓灰质炎病毒。
- 小核糖核酸病毒。
- 小的，未封装 RNA 肠病毒属。
- 3 个亚型：1、2、3。
• 粪口传播途径。
- 从口腔进入体内。
- 病毒在咽部、消化系统和淋巴系统复制。

• 人类是唯一的天然宿主。

• 脊髓灰质炎病毒选择性摧毁运动系统和自主神经系统。

• 天然(野生)病毒株在美国 1979 年后已经完全消灭了。

• 口服脊髓灰质炎疫苗(OPV):

- 仅统计了美国的脊髓灰质炎患者。
  - 每年 8～10 例疫苗相关小儿麻痹症:源于疫苗病毒出现神经毒转变,后来随着灭活脊髓灰质炎病毒的广泛使发病率大大下降。
  - 疫苗相关小儿麻痹症发生在免疫接种落后地区,接受了野生病毒株。
  - 在一些第三世界国家发病率有所上升。

诊断

■ 症状和体征

• 主要表现是没有症状。

• 病毒感染症状:发热,头痛,全身不适。呼吸系统综合征:咽痛;消化系统:恶心,呕吐。

• 非瘫痪性无菌性脑膜炎:颈强直,有时还有背部强直。

• 肌肉痛和无力。

• 进行性衰弱,时间在 1 周以内。

• 若有吞咽困难和发音困难则有延髓受累。

病史

• 接种疫苗史。

• 脊髓灰质炎感染。

• 最近有口服脊髓灰质炎疫苗史。

• 最近有到疫区国家旅游史(尼日利亚、巴基斯坦、印度、阿富汗)。

• 有免疫系统缺陷特别是 B 淋巴细胞系统紊乱(如低丙球蛋白血症)。

体格检查

• 发热(37～39 ℃)。

• 头痛、畏光。

• 颈背部僵硬。

• 神经病学改变:

- 肌肉疼痛变为严重的肌肉痉挛,后迅速进展为肌肉无力和瘫痪。
- 瘫痪不对称四肢远端多于近端。
- 尿潴留(50%的瘫痪患者)。
- 起初神经反射极度活跃,随后缺失。
- 不安和易怒,偶尔表现为嗜睡。
- 无与运动缺陷相关的感觉丧失。

儿科注意事项

大多可能有双相急性病程。

• 病毒性症状持续 1～2 日。

• 症状缓解期 1～2 日。

• 主要症状突然出现。

■ 基本检查

• 临床诊断。

• 和其他急性瘫痪原因的鉴别。

• 当怀疑该诊断时通知公共卫生管理人员。

■ 诊断检查与说明

实验室检查

• 血细胞计数:

- 白细胞正常或轻度升高。

• 诊断确诊需:

- 比较恢复期和急性期血清抗原滴度。
- 从血液、脑脊液、排泄物、咽喉分泌物分离病毒(1 周内的感染)。

诊断步骤/外科

• 腰椎穿刺/脑脊液分析:

- 无菌性脑膜炎的典型异常情况(淋巴细胞和蛋白质升高)。
- 脊髓灰质炎病毒很少能从脑脊液分离。

• 电反应诊断:

- 运动功能由正常变慢。
- 感觉功能完好。

■ 鉴别诊断

• 无症状的脊髓灰质炎和其他病毒感染表现类似。

• 非麻痹性脊髓灰质炎和其他病毒性,无菌性脑膜炎不易鉴别。

• 麻痹性脊髓灰质炎:

- 肌萎缩性脊髓侧索硬化症。
- 吉兰-巴雷综合征。
- 急性横断性脊髓炎。
- 脊髓压迫/梗死。
- 多重硬化症。
- 横纹肌溶解。
- 急性间歇性卟啉病。
- 西尼罗病毒感染。
- 白喉。
- 肉毒中毒。
- 蜱瘫痪。
- 脑炎。

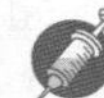

治疗

注意

极少有病例有呼吸困难的,如有需要迅速予以通气支持。

■ 初步稳定/治疗

对于呼吸困难的患者,积极的肺灌洗和早期气管插管很有必要。

■ 急诊治疗/程序

• 支持和对症处理。

• 对于肌肉痛和痉挛用止痛药。

• 卧床休息,防止麻痹加重。

• 脊髓灰质炎麻痹患者建议将肢体固定,肌内注射或受伤常先于感染 2～4 周发生。

- 应避免任何不必要的组织损伤。
- 没有抗病毒药物可用。

• 预防。

• 灭活脊髓灰质炎疫苗:

- 费用高。
- 疼痛。
- 不能产生免疫力。
- 不会发生疫苗相关小儿麻痹症。

• 口服脊髓灰质炎疫苗:

- 仅统计了美国的脊髓灰质炎患者(8～10 例/年)。
- 疫苗相关小儿麻痹症发生率:1/900 000(免疫功能不全:1/1 000)。
  - 最主要的风险在免疫功能低下的年轻人群。
- 对于未注射疫苗可能经粪口途径感染的人群可考虑服用。
- 不昂贵。
- 美国已没有。
- 仍被世界卫生组织推荐推广使用的疫苗。

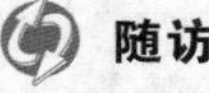

随访

■ 进一步处理

入院指征

所有脊髓灰质炎麻痹急性期需严格卧床以观察呼吸系统症状的患者。

• 隔离未接受疫苗的人群。

出院指征

没有神经系统受累证据和对未接受疫苗人群没有危险性者。

• 肌力减退症状在 3～5 日后好转。

■ 随访建议

物理治疗:

• 仅 1/3 急性麻痹症患者能完全恢复肌肉力量。

• 拉莫三嗪能减轻疼痛,缓解症状改善生活质量。

• 静脉注射免疫球蛋白能改善肌肉力量，但还没有证据表明能减轻疼痛和改善生活质量。

要点和误区

• 大多数病例是无症状的，症状多是病毒感染和急性的肌肉麻痹无力。

• 灭活脊髓灰质炎疫苗是美国唯一可用的疫苗，然而口服脊髓灰质炎疫苗仍为全球使用。

• 诊断多是临床诊断，确诊需根据从血液、脑脊液、排泄物或咽喉分泌物分离出的病毒。

• 如果诊断明确，所有急性期的脊髓灰质炎麻痹患者需收入院，密切监测呼吸系统功能。

• 如果患者从急性期存活，麻痹的呼吸系统和吞咽困难的症状能完全恢复。

• 脊髓灰质炎麻痹能在病毒感染后数十年后发病。

脊髓综合征 Spinal Cord Syndromes

Stephe n R. Hayden 江伟伟 李文放 译

基础知识

描述

• 全脊髓综合征：
- 脊髓远端的感觉、自主运动和神经支配完全丧失。
- 通常由外伤引起，但其他原因包括梗死、出血和外源性压迫。
- 持续>24 h 的症状通常是永久性的。

• 脊髓未完全损伤：
- 3 种主要类型：中央脊髓综合征、Brown-Sequard 综合征和前脊髓综合征。
- 以保留某些脊髓功能为特征。

• 中央脊髓综合征：
- 最常见的不完全性脊髓综合征。
- 通常发生在有颈椎狭窄的老年患者。
- 他们在跌倒时发生过伸性损伤。
- 强迫过度伸展使黄韧带屈曲，造成脊髓中央部分的剪切损伤。

• 脊髓前综合征：
- 最常见的是脊髓前动脉闭塞。
- 可发生在主动脉手术或创伤后。
- 其他原因包括低血压和感染。

• Brown-Sequard 综合征：
- 传统上由于穿透性伤口造成脊髓的分段。
- 很少单侧脊髓受压。

• 脊髓圆锥综合征：
- L_1 或 L_2 水平的损伤。
- 原因包括中央椎间盘突出、肿瘤和直接创伤。

• 马尾部综合征：
- 马尾部神经根损伤，而不是脊髓本身。
- 原因包括中央椎间盘突出和直接创伤。
- 临床上可类似于脊髓圆锥综合征。

病因

• 脊髓综合征是由神经传递的局部破坏引起的，并表现出混合运动和感觉缺陷。最常见的机制是创伤。

• 患有关节炎、骨质疏松症、转移性疾病或其他慢性脊柱疾病的患者轻微创伤也有发生脊髓损伤的风险。

诊断

症状和体征

急性运动和/或感觉功能丧失在创伤之后。

体格检查

• 脊髓完全综合征：
- 低于损伤水平的弛缓性轻瘫。
- 继发于交感神经张力丧失的自主神经症状：心动过缓、低血压（神经性休克）和阴茎勃起。
- 脊髓休克：损伤急性期肌肉张力和反射的丧失。通常小于 24 h，以完成球海绵体反射的恢复为标志。

• 中央脊髓综合征：
- 运动功能丧失对上肢的影响比下肢更严重。
- 最严重的缺陷发生在远端上肢。
- 感官损失更加多变。

• 前索综合征：
- 损伤水平以下双侧痉挛性瘫痪和痛温觉丧失。
- 保留背柱功能（本体感觉和位置觉）。

• Brown-Sequard 综合征（侧索综合征）：
- 同侧痉挛性麻痹和背柱功能丧失（本体感觉和位置觉）。
- 疼痛和温度感觉的对侧丧失。
- 缺陷通常在损伤下 2 个平面。

• 脊髓圆锥综合征。
- 可出现鞍区麻木。
- 典型的双侧，轻微的运动症状。
- 膀胱和直肠括约肌控制受损。

• 马尾综合征：
- 可出现鞍区麻木。
- 典型的单侧，明显的运动症状。
- 膀胱和直肠括约肌控制障碍。

• 感官缺陷水平：
- L_2：枕骨。
- C_4：锁骨区。
- L_6：拇指。
- C_8：小指。
- T_4：乳头线。
- T_{10}：脐。
- L_1：腹股沟区域。
- L_5：足背。
- S_5：肛周区域。

• 感官缺陷水平：
- C_5：屈肘。
- C_7：肘关节伸展。
- C_8：手指屈曲。
- T_1：手指外展。
- L_2：髋关节屈曲。
- L_3：膝盖延伸。
- L_4：踝关节背屈。
- S_1：踝关节跖屈。

基本检查

• 详细的神经系统查体，着重于确定是否存在任何缺陷，试图确定受伤程度。

• 如果考虑到脊髓圆锥或马尾综合征，检查尿潴留。

• 在大多数情况下，建议神经外科会诊。

诊断测查与说明

实验室检查

检查后指示的命令；通常对脊髓综合征的检查没有帮助。

影像学检查

临床怀疑的所有区域都应使用普通 X 线

片进行成像。

当X线平片正常或模棱两可时，行脊柱CT：

• CT允许评估椎管和任何骨碎片撞击。

• MRI是检测脊髓损伤的首选成像方式，在急性情况下，MRI的适应证为：

- 神经学上的缺陷不能用CT或X线平片解释。

- 脊髓损伤的临床表现有加重趋势。

- 明确有无急诊手术指征。

- MRI的缺点包括：

◦ 在进行研究时充分监测患者的不适性。

◦ 与某些金属设备不兼容。

◦ 检查耗时较长。

老年人注意事项

由于严重的DJD，普通放射线拍摄难以解释的病例，使用CT可能更合适。

诊断步骤/外科

• 当MRI不可用或无法执行时，脊髓造影可与CT一起使用。

• 如果考虑吉兰-巴雷综合征、多发性硬化症或横贯性脊髓炎，可能需要腰椎穿刺。

鉴别诊断

背根伤：

• 周围神经损伤。

• 吉兰-巴雷综合征。

• 多发性硬化症。

• 横向性脊髓炎。

• 硬膜外脓肿。

• 脑血管意外。

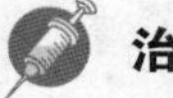

治疗

院前

• 全脊柱固定。

• 应建立静脉通路，以进行神经源性休克时的液体复苏。

• 应该将患者运送到最近的创伤中心：

- 及时评估和神经外科干预可能会导致更好的结果。

儿科注意事项

颈托必须是合适的尺寸；用毛巾和胶布夹住头部和身体是一个合理的选择。

初步稳定/治疗

• 脊椎固定必须始终保持。

• 气管插管操作时应保持脊柱固定，但插管需要颈部活动方可完成，可适度调整位置。

• 静脉输液应维持常规速度，除非出现休克：

- 脊髓创伤可导致低血压，因失去交感神经张力，液体复苏是首要治疗。

- 低血压的其他原因（如出血）应该在脊髓损伤（SCI）之前考虑。

- 一般而言，低血容量性休克导致心动过速，而神经性休克导致心动过缓。

- 如果在液体复苏后血压没有改善，并且排除其他原因引起低血压，可能需要使用血管活性药物；α受体激动剂是优选的。

• 减少低氧和低血压，预防继发性脊髓损伤。

急诊治疗/程序

• 其他伤害必须按照指示处理。

• 脊髓损伤的水平应该被确定作为改善或恶化的基线。

• 高位颈髓损伤，膈神经损伤时密切监测呼吸状态（C_3～C_4水平）。

• 一旦怀疑脊髓损伤，即使X线平片正常，也必须咨询神经外科医师；早期手术减压或固定可能会降低发病率。

• 脊髓损伤患者选择适合的局部创伤或脊柱中心进行治疗：

- 如有必要，其他伤害允许的情况下应尽快进行转移。

• 对穿透性损伤的患者给予抗生素和破伤风预防。

• 神经源性休克的治疗需要静脉升压药物。

药物治疗

• 肾上腺素：静推0.5～2 μg/kg，然后滴注50～100 μg/min。

• 头孢唑林：1 000 mg，q8 h。

注意

在20世纪90年代早期，在第二次和第三次国家急性脊髓损伤研究报告（NASCIS Ⅱ，NASCIS Ⅲ）中指出，广泛采用高剂量甲泼尼龙输液作为标准治疗，然而这种疗法的广泛的系统回顾和支持它的证据证明，这种疗法不建议作为脊髓损伤的常规治疗。

随访

进一步处理

入院指征

所有脊髓综合征患者必须入住ICU。

出院指征

没有脊髓损伤症状的患者应该出院。

要点和误区

• 详细的神经系统检查和记录神经症状的脊柱水平是至关重要的。

• 早期神经外科会诊，因为在许多情况下，预后与时间相关。

• 急诊医师不应为急性脊髓损伤进行泼尼松龙治疗。

J

脊椎滑脱和脊椎前移 Spondylolysis/Spondylolisthesis

Lisa G. Lowe Hiller 江伟伟 李文放 译

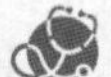

基础知识

描述

• 滑脱：

- 骨缺损在峡部（上下骨之间的峡部）。

- 可以是单侧或双侧的。

- 双侧型滑脱或松动的可能性高于单侧型。

- 85%～95%发生在L_5，5%～15%发生在L_4，很少发生与L_1以上节段。

- 4%多节段受累。

- 比脊柱移位更常见。

• 前移：

- 一个椎体向前滑动到另一个椎体。

- 脊椎关节退行性变可导致脊柱前移，在5%的人群中有所体现，男性发病率是女性2～4倍。

- 脊椎关节炎患者中，50%在其一生中会出现一定程度的脊柱前移，其中50%会出现症状：

- 文献未将运动与滑动发病率联系起来。

- 脊柱前移诱发神经根受累和坐骨神经痛。

- 分类：
- 1 型发育不良型：神经弓或关节方面的先天性缺陷与隐性脊柱裂相关。
- 2 型峡部型：峡部应力性骨折。
- 3 型退变型：椎间长期不稳定。
- 4 型创伤型。
- 5 型病理型：全身或局部骨病。
- 1 型有最高的进展风险约 32%，与运动相关；而峡部裂则只有 4%的进展风险。
- 根据滑脱程度将脊椎滑脱分为 4 级（Meyerding 分级系统）：
  - Ⅰ级：高达椎体宽度的 25%。
  - Ⅱ级：高达椎体宽度的 26%～50%。
  - Ⅲ级：高达椎体宽度的 51%～75%。
  - Ⅳ级：高达椎体宽度的 76%～100%。
- 脊柱滑脱最常见的位置是 L_5 在骶骨上移位（85%～95%），其次是 L_4 在 L_5 上移位。

儿科注意事项

- 脊椎关节松解症是儿童严重腰痛的最常见原因，但最常见的是无症状。
- 多见于 10～15 岁青春期生长儿童。
- 常见于运动青少年，特别是在背部过度伸展的运动中（如体操、潜水、足球）。
- 急性症状与创伤有关。

病因

未知。理论包括先天性肢体畸形、骨密度改变及复发性亚临床应激损伤。

诊断

症状和体征

病史

- 发病通常是渐进的，除非是创伤性的。
- 常伴有椎旁肌肉僵硬或痉挛。
- 站立和行走加重了背部和近侧腿部的疼痛。
- 坐下和向前弯曲可缓解疼痛。
- 不同程度的运动后，站立或咳嗽会出现疼痛：
- 加重因素可能包括重复过度伸展运动。
- 缓解因素可以包括休息，尽管过程是不同和缓慢的，但通常是坐下或弯腰。
- 全身性/神经症状：极少，除非有明显的创伤或“滑倒”。

体格检查

- 过度前凸姿势：
- 躯干可能缩短。
- 肋骨接近髂嵴。
- 腘筋紧张：
- 膝盖弯曲让患者直立。
- 只有“典型”是单腿过伸：
- 1 条腿站立，向后倾斜，使同侧疼痛。
- 触诊可及显著滑脱的 L_5 突出棘突。
- 神经系统检查通常是正常的：
- 如果异常疼痛和感觉失调是在皮肤分布。
- 考虑疝或腰椎滑脱。
- 如果怀疑撞击/神经根病，运动检查应包括踝关节背屈（主要是 L_4）、踇趾伸展（主要是 L_5）和踝足底外翻和外翻（S_1）的测试。
- 对于影像学上有神经根病或高度脊椎滑脱症状的患者需行马尾综合征的相关检查。

儿科注意事项

- 少于 10 岁的儿童脊椎松解是罕见的，这些患者应该注意以下几点：
- 数周的持续疼痛。
- 晚上自发疼痛。
- 疼痛与学校、游戏或运动有关。
- 疼痛伴有明显的僵硬、运动受限、发热或神经症状。
- 在骶骶连接处疼痛。

诊断检查与说明

实验室检测

没有必要行实验室检查。

影像学检查

- 对于没有明显征象（如发热、夜间疼痛、神经或胃肠道不适或免疫抑制剂/平时应用类固醇激素等）的患者，可能不需要行影像学检查。
- 腰骶椎 X 线片：
- 脊柱侧位和斜位片最有用。
- 峡部裂会表现为在峡部透亮缺损，斜视图可见“白领”或“断颈”症。
- 次级影像学征象可能包括峡部裂水平的隐性脊柱裂和对侧椎弓跟硬化。
- 多数（80%～95%）在 L_5～S_1 水平，15%在 L_4～L_5。
- 脊椎滑脱将表现为一个椎体向前滑动（在侧视图上看到）。
- 单光子发射型计算机断层扫描（SPECT）更适合于腰背部疼痛和脊椎溶解，尤其是在怀疑其他病理性改变时，优于普通 CT。
- CT 扫描：
- 病理上比 X 线平片表现更清楚。
- 可以区分急性和慢性病变。
- 局限性包括高辐射暴露。全腰椎 CT 为约 6 mSv。
- 局部 CT 聚焦可低至 1.5 mSv，但对治疗计划的制订帮助较小。
- MRI：
- 是最有用的检查，推荐用于需要进一步检查的儿童患者：
- 好处包括缺乏电离辐射。
- 磁共振可发现软组织异常，如椎间盘病理、骨骺炎和椎间盘炎。
- 用于定义神经根撞击、中央管和神经根狭窄。
- 可能有助于异常评估的敏感性。
- 可以替代病理诊断。
- 局限性包括骨折分期困难，可能会夸大某些损伤的程度。
- 有利于恢复运动期和康复治疗时的评估。
- Tesla 磁共振成像在未来的诊断中更有潜力。

儿科注意事项

- 影像学检查的指征更低。
- 比成人更容易发生渐进性滑倒。

鉴别诊断

- 结核病（Pott 病）。
- 椎间盘炎。
- 骨或脊髓肿瘤。
- 肾盂肾炎。
- 腹膜后感染。
- 背部肌肉或关节受伤。
- 先天性髋关节脱位。
- 佝偻病。
- 椎间盘破裂。
- 血管跛行。
- 骨髓炎。
- 骨样骨瘤。
- 主动脉瘤。

治疗

院前

除非近期有创伤史，否则不需要脊柱预防措施。

初步稳定/治疗

不应该进行牵引力试验。

急诊治疗/程序

- 临床需要控制疼痛和松弛肌肉。
- 如果症状轻微，支持疗法。
- 限制活动 3～6 周，因为重复性创伤可能会加重疾病（如运动），然后在无症状时开放运动。

J

• 防止脊柱前凸(有争议的)或物理疗法。
• 骨科急会诊适用于神经系统疾病,例如马尾神经症状或感染性病变者。
• 如果中度至重度或支持治疗无效,则转往骨科治疗。
• 外科手术通常是在弯曲位置行脊柱融合:
- 有 50%的腰椎滑脱症状患者需要手术。
• 所有Ⅲ级或Ⅳ级滑脱的有症状的患者都应该行外科手术。
• 锻炼没有被证实有好处。

儿科注意事项

• 如果没有症状,活动限制是不必要的。
• 文献指出保守治疗对年轻运动员有好处。

药物治疗

• 肌肉松弛剂:
- 美索巴莫:1 000～1 500 mg,口服,每日 4 次(对<12 岁儿童的安全性和有效性不确定)。
- 地西泮:2～10 mg,口服,每日 3～4 次。
- 环苯扎林:5～10 mg,口服,每日 3 次(年龄>15 岁安全)。
• 非甾体抗炎药:
- 布洛芬:200～800 mg,口服,每日 3～4 次(5～10 mg/kg,口服,q6 h)。
• 阿片类药物(剂量因口服药物而异):
- 硫酸吗啡:0.1 mg/kg,最多 2～4 mg 静脉。
- 对乙酰氨基酚/氢可酮:5/500 mg 1～2 片,口服,每日 4 次;对乙酰氨基酚不要超过 4 g/24 h(24 h 分 5 次使用,不要超过 10～15 mg/kg)。
- 对乙酰氨基酚/羟考酮:5/32 mg 1～2 片,口服,每日 4 次;对乙酰氨基酚不要超过 4 g/24 h(24 h 分 5 次使用,不要超过 10～15 mg/kg)。
- 对乙酰氨基酚/可待因:300/30 mg 1～2 片,口服,每日 4 次[片剂:0.5～1 mg/kg 可待因,口服,q4～6 h;最大 60 mg/d;>3 岁患者 75 mg/(kg·d),～4 g/d];对乙酰氨基酚不要超过 4 g/24 h(24 h 分 5 次使用,不要超过 10～15 mg/kg)。

随访

进一步处理

入院指征

• 不能行走。
• 由于疼痛或社会状况而无法在家处理。
• 新的或进行性神经功能缺陷。

出院指征

• 骨科随访安排。
• 社会支持。
• 疼痛控制。
• 患者教育。

儿科注意事项

强制性密切随访。

脊椎损伤(成人,颈部) Spine Injury: Cervical, Adult

Gary M. Vilke 张溢燛 伍力学 译

基础知识

描述

• 颈部损伤导致脊髓、颈椎或支撑颈椎的韧带受伤。
• 可能同时存在一个以上的致伤机制。
• 屈曲性损伤:
- 简单的楔形骨折:通常是稳定性骨折。
- 前半脱位:后骨韧带复合体破坏但无骨性损伤,属于潜在的不稳定性损伤。
- Clay shoveler 骨折:C_7、C_6 或 T_1 棘突的撕脱性骨折,属于稳定性骨折。
- 屈曲型撕裂骨折:极度不稳定性骨折;可能与急性前颈髓综合征有关。
- 寰枕关节脱位:不稳定性损伤。
- 双侧小关节脱位:可发生于 C_2～C_7;该损伤不稳定。
• 屈曲/扭转性损伤:
- 单侧小关节脱位:稳定型损伤。
- 扭转性寰枢椎脱位:不稳定性损伤。
• 伸展性损伤:
- 伸展型撕裂骨折:涉及椎体前下角的撕脱骨折;伸展时不稳定,屈曲时稳定。
- C_1 后弓的骨折:在过度伸展中,后弓在枕骨和棘突之间被压缩;属不稳定性骨折。
- 寰椎前弓撕脱骨折:C_1 椎体横向骨折伴周围软组织肿胀。
- Hangman 骨折:涉及 C_2 椎弓根的椎间盘外伤性滑脱;属不稳定性骨折。
- 过度伸展脱位:这是一类颈椎影像学正常的瘫痪综合征。
• 伸展-扭转性损伤:
- 柱骨折:一般属于稳定性骨折。
• 垂直压缩(轴向受力)损伤:
- 杰斐逊骨折:C_1 前后弓的爆裂性骨折;极度不稳定性骨折。
- 爆裂性骨折:椎体粉碎性骨折,椎体后部碎片突入椎管。

病因

• 钝性创伤是颈部受伤的主要原因:
- 交通事故:占 50%以上。
- 高处坠落:占 20%。
- 运动性损伤:占 15%。
- 严重关节炎患者的轻微创伤可导致颈部损伤。
• 穿通性损伤。

诊断

症状和体征

• 颈部疼痛,触诊压痛。
• 上肢或下肢麻木、乏力、感觉异常。
• 以下情况考虑颈椎损伤:
- 创伤后或发生了存在创伤可能的不明事件后,出现意识改变(意识丧失、醉酒、药物或缺氧)。
- 创伤后或发生了可能存在创伤的不明事件后,无法沟通者(智力障碍、语言障碍或气管插管)。
- 弥漫性损伤。
- 涉及头部或颈部的钝性外伤。
• 不完全性颈髓综合征(参见单独章节):
- Brown-Sequard 综合征:穿透伤损伤导致的半切综合征(同侧运动性麻痹/对侧感觉减退)。
- 前索综合征:颈椎屈曲损伤导致脊髓挫伤(瘫痪/位置觉、触觉、振动觉减退)。
- 中央脊髓综合征:颈椎退行性关节炎伴被动过度屈曲体位(上肢相较下肢缺陷更明显)。

J

病史

• 获取头部或颈部创伤的病史。

• 明确有无强直性脊柱炎或其他骨病的病史。

• 特异性症状:

- 颈部疼痛。
- 乏力。
- 麻木。
- 刺痛。

体格检查

• 直接观察颈部是否有挫伤或畸形。

• 触诊棘突。

• 运动、感觉和上下肢反射检查。

■ 基本检查

依据临床征象,完善体格检查和影像学检查。

■ 诊断测查与说明

影像学检查

• 标准 X 线片包括 3 个方位的图像:保持固定不动,行齿状突的侧位,前后位和开口位摄片。

• 侧位 X 线片必须包括 $C_1 \sim T_1$;以覆盖较低平面的损伤。

• 仰卧斜位片可能有助于识别细微的扭转性损伤。

• 当 X 线平片提示颈椎骨折、脱位、软组织肿胀或 X 线平片正常,但有原因不明的颈部疼痛/神经功能缺损时,应行 CT 检查。

• 相较 X 线平片,CT 是更好的选择。

• 当神志清楚,可配合检查的患者主诉疼痛明显,但静态影像学无阳性发现时,可能需要屈-伸位影像(或 MRI)来评估动态韧带损伤情况。

• MRI 已成为评估患者神经功能缺损的很有价值的工具,包括 X 线平片上无异常的脊髓损伤的患者。

J

■ 鉴别诊断

• 颈部肌肉拉伤(甩鞭样损伤)。

• 颈椎脱位。

• 颈椎骨折脱位。

• 复杂或单纯的颈椎骨折。

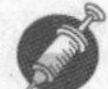

治疗

■ 院前处理

• 如果怀疑颈椎损伤、用硬领、颈托和木板固定。

• 行颈椎制动的患者在呕吐的情况下需要密切观察。

• 只在存在神经功能缺损的情况下,颈部穿透伤患者才需要固定颈椎。

• 如果致伤物扔在损伤部位,固定颈部以避免进一步的伤害,并且不要移除致伤物,除非它妨碍呼吸。

■ 初步稳定/治疗

• 使用硬领固定颈椎,并在侧面用胶带、毛巾或轻质泡沫衬垫。

• 开放气道,建立静脉通道,维持循环稳定:

- 最好的方式是颈椎固定后经口气管插管。
- 纤支镜引导下的插管设备应备在床旁,确保需要时能用。

■ 急诊治疗/程序

• 评估患者的其他伤害,仅靠关注颈椎受伤患者的腹部体格检查是不可靠的,需要进一步的客观检查结果来明确。

• 具有强直性脊柱炎或其他脆性骨疾病的患者,即使是较弱的损伤,也有发生骨折和脊髓损伤的风险。

• 如果有以下情况的患者可临床排除,不需要行颈椎影像学检查(基于 NEXUS)。

- 感觉平面没有改变。
- 意识没有异常兴奋和改变。
- 后颈正中线没有压痛。
- 没有弥漫性疼痛和损伤。
- 没有局灶性神经缺陷。

• 加拿大的颈椎治疗原则:对于处于觉醒状态,GCS 15 分,病情平稳的患者,暂不需要行颈椎影像学检查,但需要进一步评估下列危险因素:

- 评估所有骨折的高危因素,如年龄大于 65 岁,存在致伤机制或感觉异常等,如果存在这些因素则需影像学检查。
- 高危致伤因素包括从大于 3 或 5 级台阶上摔下,头部纵向受力,高速的机动车交通事故。
- 存在某些低危因素,但适度活动颈部来进行评估仍是安全的。
- 这些低危因素包括:常规的机动车后排交通事故,患者在急诊可保持坐位或随意走动,迟发性颈部疼痛或无脊柱中线压痛者。
- 如果仅有低危因素,则患者可以自行使颈部向左侧和右侧旋转至少 45°。
- 如果可以安全的转动颈部,则无需影像学检查。

如果存在神经缺陷,请咨询神经外科。

• 如果 X 线平片或 CT 存在异常,请咨询神经外科或脊柱矫形医师。

- 如果 X 线片正常,但有明显颈部疼痛的患者,若意识清楚,能配合检查的,可考虑屈伸平片、CT 或 MRI,如果结果不正常,请咨询神经外科。

• 如果考虑合并颈部血管损伤,可行 CTA 检查。

• 对于颈部穿通伤患者,应给予静脉抗生素和预防性破伤风注射。

• 神经源性休克患者可能需要静脉血管活性药物支持。

治疗药物

• 苯肾上腺素:0.5~2 μg/kg 快速推注,续以 50~100 μg/min 静滴维持。

• 头孢唑林:1 000 mg,q8 h。

> **注意**
>
> 在 20 世纪 90 年代,依据第二版和第三版《急性脊髓损伤研究报告》(NASCIS II, NASCIS III)的建议,大剂量甲泼尼龙作为标准治疗被广泛使用;但是,随着针对这一疗法大量的文献回顾和证据结果的出现,目前不推荐将大剂量甲泼尼龙用作急性脊髓损伤的常规治疗。

随访

■ 进一步处理

入院指征

• 对于颈椎骨折或脱位伴有神经功能缺损的,或任何不稳定性骨折或脱位的患者应入 ICU 或进行心电监测。

• 稳定的颈椎骨折或脱位。

• 在 X 线平片上与任何神经缺陷或不稳定性无关的孤立的棘突骨折。

• 单纯无神经功能缺损的颈椎楔形骨折。

出院指征

• 急性颈椎劳损。

• 与轻度至中度疼痛相关的肌肉损伤,无神经损伤,影像学正常。

转诊问题

• 患者颈椎影像学正常,但持续疼痛者,出院需颈托固定,到骨创伤科做必要的随访。

• 对于持续性刺激症状的患者,应该在 3~4 周对肌电图进行随访。

■ 随访建议

如果疼痛增加,并出现麻木、乏力、刺痛或

其他临床变化,需到急诊进行评估。

要点和误区

• 强直性脊柱炎或其他脆性骨病患者发生轻微颈部损伤即可能导致严重伤害。

• 在没有影像学检查的情况下,需要系统的应用 NEXUS 标准来安全评估和排除临床上显著的脊柱骨折。

• 急诊科医师不应独自开始使用甲泼尼龙治疗急性脊髓损伤。

脊椎损伤(儿童,颈部) Spine Injury: Cervical, Pediatric

Roxanna A. Sadri 江伟伟 李文放 译

基础知识

描述

• 严重钝性创伤患者相对少,占1%~2%。

• <8 岁的儿童更容易上颈椎损伤(C_1~C_3),并且有生长板损伤的风险:

- 脊柱支点较高(出生时 C_2~C_3)。
- 头相对于身体较大。
- 较弱的宫颈肌肉组织。
- 韧带松弛。
- 未成熟的椎关节。

• >8 岁的儿童:

- 宫颈损伤的发生率增加。
- 椎体和椎弓骨折。
- 下颈椎脊柱损伤更常见。

• 重点关注:

- 唐氏综合征。
- Klippel-Feil 综合征。
- Morquio 综合征。
- 拉森综合征。

• 无放射学异常的脊髓损伤(SCIWORA):

- 根据研究结果,4.5%~35%的脊髓损伤发生在儿童患者中。
- 在<8 岁的儿童中更常见。
- 可能存在明确的脊髓损伤:
  ◦ 脊髓休克。
  ◦ 神经功能缺陷。
- 症状可能是暂时的,在评估时已经缓解:
  ◦ 感觉异常。
  ◦ 手烧灼感。
  ◦ 乏力。
- 症状通常在损伤后立即发生,但可能延迟发作(几分钟至几日不等)。

病因

• 出生:臀部阴道分娩。

• <8 年:机动车碰撞(MVC)和坠落伤。

• >8 年:MVC 和运动受损。

诊断

症状和体征

• 局部颈椎疼痛。

• 运动范围受限。

• 神经功能缺陷(可能是短暂的)。

• 可能被意识状态改变或分布性伤害所掩盖。

• 生命体征异常:

- 低血压。
- 心动过缓。
- 通气不足或呼吸骤停。

• 颈部标志:

- 颈椎的触诊。
- 运动范围受限。
- 肌肉痉挛。

• 神经系统体征:

- 感觉异常或感觉缺陷。
- 肌张力下降。
- 肠鸣音减弱。
- 麻痹。

• 麻痹:

- 前索综合征:
  ◦ 过屈性损伤。
  ◦ 麻痹。
  ◦ 疼痛感、触觉和本体感觉丧失。
- 中央脊髓综合征:
  ◦ 过伸伤。
  ◦ 上肢损伤较下肢重。
  ◦ 手及手指灼烧感。
- Brown-Sequard 综合征:
  ◦ 脊髓半横断损伤。
  ◦ 患侧瘫痪。
  ◦ 对侧痛觉丧失。
- 霍纳综合征:
  ◦ 交感神经系统受损。
  ◦ 同侧上睑下垂,瞳孔缩小,无汗。
  ◦ 也要考虑颈动脉解剖结构。
- 四肢瘫痪。
- 无反应。

• 儿童可能无法表达症状,或可能无法配合检查。

基本检查

• 需行颈椎影像学检查:

- 颈椎压痛。
- 意识状态改变。
- 神经系统缺陷(即使是短暂的)。
- 分散性损伤。
- 有损伤机制。

• 如果普通 X 线片不确定或临床检查提示有损伤,可以行其他影像学检查(CT、MRI)。

• Nexus 标准可以安全地应用于>8 岁儿童,但更小的不行。

诊断检查与说明

影像学检查

• 颈椎 X 线片:

- 标准初始视图:正位、仰卧位和齿状突开口位。
- 仰卧水平摄片能识别 80%的骨折、脱位和半脱位。
- AP 和齿状突的加入提高了敏感性。
- 需要包括所有 7 个颈椎和 C_7~T_1 连接处。
- C_1 前弓与齿状突前之间的距离:
  ◦ 小孩 5 mm 或更小,成人 3 mm。
- 椎前软组织增厚:
  ◦ 提示潜在的骨折或韧带损伤。
  ◦ 颈部屈曲、呼气、吞咽也会发生。
  ◦ 对于高度敏感的测量来说存在太多的可变性。
  ◦ 声门下方的软组织应比声门上方厚约 2 倍。
- C_2 的假脱位:
  ◦ 正常变异。

◦ 这是韧带松弛的结果,并且通常在 8 岁时就可以解决。
◦ C_2 在 C_3 前面位移。
◦ 颈椎后路线正常关系。
◦ C_1 和 C_3 的棘突的前方的连线应该在 C_2 的棘突的前方 2 mm。
◦ >2 mm 的空间表明潜在的枢椎椎弓骨折。
◦ 只能在 $C_1 \sim C_3$ 应用。
- C_3 和 C_4 的前椎体楔入:
◦ 可能被误认为是压缩性骨折。
- 骨骺生长板可能类似于骨折:
◦ C_1 的后弓在 4 岁融合。
◦ C_1 的前弓在 6 岁时融合。
◦ 齿状突的基部与 C_2 的椎体在 7 岁时融合。
- 伸屈视图:
◦ 属限制性操作。
◦ 如果怀疑隐匿性韧带损伤,可能会有用。
◦ 颈椎片阴性。
◦ 没有神经功能异常。
• CT 扫描:
- X 线平片阴性,怀疑骨折。
- 进一步证实平片的骨折。
- X 线片上可疑骨折。
- 影像学资料不足。
• MRI:
- 无论在 X 线平片或 CT 上有无异常,疑似脊髓损伤。

■ **鉴别诊断**

• 颈肌劳损。
• 斜颈。
• 子宫颈腺炎。
• 咽后脓肿。
• 脑膜炎。

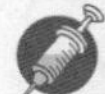

治疗

■ **院前**

• 固定所有有潜在颈椎损伤的婴儿和儿童。
• 大小适合的颈托。
• 如果颈托不适用,则使用胶带、毛巾、垫子与木板固定。
• 将垫子放置在颈部、肩膀和背部下面,因为较大的头盖骨会引起弯曲。
• 如果正在体育运动,头盔不用取下。

■ **初步稳定/治疗**

• 颈椎固定术。
• 轴线翻身。
• 如果需要气管插管,需固定颈椎。

■ **急诊治疗/程序**

• 任何具有与脊髓损伤一致的神经功能缺损的创伤患者都应该考虑使用甲泼尼龙。
• 神经外科会诊:
- 真正的半脱位。
- 骨折。
- 暂时或持续性神经功能缺损。

■ **药物治疗**

存在争议:
• 甲泼尼龙:1 h 内静脉负荷剂量 30 mg/kg;在接下来的 23 h 内维持输注 5.4 mg/(kg · h);在受伤后 8 h 内开始。
• 可能导致免疫抑制并增加感染风险。
• 在使用之前与神经外科进行讨论。

随访

■ **进一步处理**

入院指征
• 意识状态改变。
• 脊髓损伤的症状和体征。
• 骨折。
• 会诊:
- 神经外科。
- 整形脊柱外科。

出院指征
• 完全正常的意识状态。
• 影像学正常。
• 无暂时或持续性神经功能缺陷。
• 交代家长:
- SCIWORA 可能出现延迟症状。
- 如果出现感觉异常、虚弱或瘫痪,患者应该返回医院。

■ **随访建议**

• 听外科医师或神经外科医师的建议。
• 如果怀疑脑震荡,随访。
• 有重大创伤的儿童应心理科随访。

要点和误区

• 检查期间保持固定状态。
• 在大多数情况下,行普通 X 线片初始筛查。
• 了解小儿颈椎的独特特征。
• SCIWORA 的症状可以是暂时的或延迟的。

脊椎损伤(尾骨) Spine Injury: Coccyx

Gary Schwartz 江伟伟 李文放 译

基础知识

■ **描述**

• 患者通常是坐位落下。
• 通常从高处坠落。
• 可发生在分娩过程中,大多数情况发生在需要使用器械的分娩过程中。
• 女性更常见。

■ **病因**

请参阅“描述”。

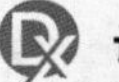

诊断

■ **症状和体征**

• 压痛局限于尾骨。
• 臀沟瘀斑。
• 坐着时感到疼痛,特别是向前倾和排便时。

病史

患者或目击者提供完整的经过,包括任何可能影响摔倒或损害机制的早期事件。

体格检查

全面的:
• 包括直肠检查,评估尾骨的触痛或活动性。
• 在单纯尾骨骨折中应该没有神经功能

缺陷。

■ 基本检查

最常见的单纯尾骨骨折，但如果出现其他脊柱损伤问题，应该固定脊柱。

■ 诊断检查与说明

影像学检查

常规影像学检查不必要：

- 临床上可以诊断时，影像学检查可能对生殖腺产生不必要的影响。
- 如果考虑到其他脊柱损伤，则需行影像学检查。
- X线片可能很难解释，因为尾骨具有正常的变异位置，可能与骨折混淆。
- 侧位X线片是骨折和脱位的最佳视角。

■ 鉴别诊断

- 尾骨痛。
- 提肛肌综合征。
- 潜毛性囊肿。
- 肛周脓肿。
- 蛛网膜囊肿。
- 尾骨刺。

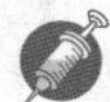

治疗

■ 院前

- 疼痛管理。
- 评估其他伤害。

■ 初步稳定/治疗

- 通常不需要；如果患者不稳定，请考虑其他诊断。
- 用药治疗疼痛。

■ 急诊治疗/程序

- 止痛药。
- 复位移位的尾骨骨折，但通常是不必要的。

■ 治疗一般措施

建议使用甜甜圈形坐垫，以获得舒适感。

■ 用药

- 根据需要，服疼痛药。
- 大便软化剂。

■ 手术/其他过程

如果尾骨骨折明显，可考虑行复位术，但很少需要和成功。

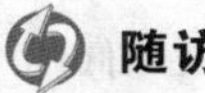

随访

■ 进一步处理

入院指征

通常不需要入院。

出院指征

尾骨骨折可以在门诊处理，除非合并有其他损伤考虑住院。

门诊随访

明确慢性疼痛的病因诊断为运动过度和脱位非常重要。

脊椎损伤(胸部) Spine Injury: Thoracic

Gary M. Vilke　江伟伟　李文放 译

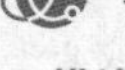

基础知识

■ 描述

- 以下损伤占胸部大部分骨折和脱位：
  - 轴向压缩。
  - 弯曲旋转。
  - 剪断。
  - 屈曲牵张。
  - 过伸。
- 3个解剖学上不同的支撑；如果3个支撑中的2个被破坏，则脊柱不稳定：
  - 后部分：后骨弓和相互连接的韧带结构。
  - 中间部：椎体的后方、后环空纤维化和后纵骨。
  - 前部分：前纵韧带、前环纤维化和前椎体。
- 主要与次要骨折：
  - 次要骨折。
    - 单纯关节骨折。
    - 横突骨折。
    - 棘突间骨折。
    - 峡部骨折。
  - 主要骨折：
    - 压缩性骨折。
    - 爆裂性骨折。
    - 安全带损伤。
    - 骨折脱位。
- 压缩性骨折(前方或外侧屈曲)：
  - 具有完整的中柱的椎体前部的骨折。
  - 可能是后列中断。
  - A型：通过两端板断裂。
  - B型：通过上端板断裂。
  - C型：通过下端板骨折。
  - D型：两个端板完好无损。
- 爆裂性骨折(轴向负荷)：
  - 通过脊柱中柱破裂。
  - 可能后部和椎板骨折进入椎管内，导致神经损害。
  - A型：通过两个端板断裂。
  - B型：通过上端板断裂。
  - C型：通过下端板骨折。
  - D型：中柱爆裂，旋转受伤导致半脱位。
  - E型：前柱不对称压缩，中柱爆裂。
- 安全带损伤(屈曲分离)：
  - 后柱和中柱与前柱完好分离。
  - 通常由没有肩带的安全带引起。
  - A型：通过骨。
  - B型：主要为韧带。
  - C型：骨穿透中柱。
  - D型：通过韧带和椎间盘，没有中柱破裂。
- 骨折脱位：
  - 压缩，拉伸，旋转或剪切后，所有3个支撑损伤。
  - A型：屈曲旋转，高处坠落。
  - B型：躯干长轴的剪切暴力。
  - C型：屈曲分离，双侧小关节脱位。

■ 病因

- 由于需支撑肋骨和肋椎关节，胸椎是硬的：
  - 胸椎椎管最窄。
- 创伤性胸椎骨折需要巨大的力量。大多数骨折是由于汽车和摩托车碰撞、汽车撞击行人和高处坠落(尤其是从>10 ft 高处)：
  - 一小部分是由穿透性损伤引起的(参见

J

"脊髓综合征")。

- 50%的脊柱骨折和40%的脊髓损伤发生在胸腰段(T_1～H_2)。

儿科注意事项

• 如果没有明确的机动车造成胸椎损伤的病史,可怀疑虐待儿童。

• 后肋骨骨折需考虑虐待儿童,并需要仔细检查胸椎和全身隐匿性损伤。

老年人注意事项

由于老年人(>65岁)的骨密度降低,所以老年人更容易造成损伤,很小的高度就可能造成损伤。

诊断

症状和体征

• 产生胸椎骨折需要很大的力量。

• 骨折部位或骨碎片对附近结构引起疼痛。

• 由于肋骨的原因,需要更大的力量才能引起胸椎脱臼:

- 应怀疑伴有内部损伤。

- 胸椎骨折脱位较胸腰椎骨折脱位较少,但神经功能障碍的发生率较高。

- 脊柱损伤应高度怀疑胸部损伤,反之亦然。

• 常见体征和症状:

- 局部软组织缺损。

- 瘀瘢或血肿:

◦ 肩胛挫伤。

- 椎间盘间隙的缩短、畸形或扩大(更具体)。

- 疼痛或压痛(更敏感):

◦ 定位:局部疼痛和棘突压痛。

◦ 提示:椎旁、前胸、腹部。

- 椎旁肌肉痉挛。

- 感觉迟钝或感觉异常。

- 虚弱(局部或全身)。

- 远端反射消失、弛缓性瘫痪。

- 大小便失禁。

- 阴茎异常勃起。

- 体温不能调节。

- 脊柱休克,伴有心动过缓的低血压。

病史

• 损伤机制。

• 合并症。

基本检查

• 快速评估ABC。

• 初级和次级创伤调查。

• 详细的神经检查,包括肠鸣音和肛周感觉。

• 彻底的脊椎检查,以确定畸形或压痛。

• 体格检查中任何压痛、分散性损伤、意识状态改变或有关机制的损伤都需要行影像学检查。

• 如果存在断裂,则确定其是否稳定。

• 评估脊髓休克中球海绵体反射。

诊断检查与说明

影像学检查

• 胸椎疼痛或压痛,重大机动车事故或高处跌倒需行脊柱前后侧X线平片。

• 对于在X线平片上有脊柱骨折和平片正常,但患者有明显的脊柱疼痛,并有严重损伤机制的患者,均应显示薄层CT扫描。平片纵隔扩大的患者也应对胸椎损伤或主动脉损伤进行评估。

• 任何有胸椎骨折处的患者都需要使用普通X线片对整个脊柱进行成像,至少10%的患者将会有附加骨折。

• 越来越多的胸、腹部、骨盆CT数据被重新明确创伤性胸腰椎:

- 比普通照相更敏感,无辐射,成本更少。

• MRI用于进一步评估可疑的脊髓损伤、压迫或韧带撕裂。

鉴别诊断

• 关节炎(退行性和类风湿关节炎)。

• 强直性脊椎炎。

• 脊柱裂。

• 先天性畸形。

• 退行性椎间盘疾病。

• 肿瘤。

• 病理性骨折:

- 骨质疏松。

- 良性或恶性骨肿瘤。

治疗

院前

• 如果患者最初可以放置固定板,则应该放置,直到患者完全排除该病。

• 神经功能缺陷患者应该输送到创伤中心。

初步稳定/治疗

• 按指示管理呼吸道和复苏:

- 气道干预固定颈椎。

- 确定有无继发于出血和神经源性的低血压。

- 伴有创伤的低血压患者,应该被视为由于出血导致的血容量减少,直到明确诊断为其他原因。

- 先使用血液制品,后使用晶体进行液体复苏。

• 稳定脊柱,保护残余的脊髓功能,并防止进一步的损伤。

急诊治疗/程序

• 在患者全脊柱固定的情况下进行所有需要的复苏和诊断测试。初次检查期间不应取下脊柱固定板。

• 躁动的患者可能需要镇静、肌松剂和气管插管。

• 请脊柱骨科或神经外科会诊。

• 适当镇痛。

• 如果CT证实稳定性损伤且患者的神经功能完整,以下情况可保守治疗:

- 孤立棘突、横突骨折。

- 机会性骨折。

- 楔前压缩性骨折(<50%)。

- 稳定型的爆裂性骨折。

• 如果怀疑脊髓损伤,考虑给予大剂量激素,请脊柱外科医师会诊。

• 如果怀疑有脊椎骨折或韧带损伤而没有神经损伤,应请神经外科或整形脊柱外科会诊,同时行CT或MRI扫描。

• 应尽快控制疼痛,非甾体抗炎药、阿片类药物和苯二氮䓬类药物是治疗的主要药物。

• 神经源性低血压表现为心动过缓或心率正常,患者会因周围血管舒张而变得温暖。这与低血容量性休克时发生的心动过速和四肢冷却相反:

- 神经源性低血压应该用晶体进行复苏,但仍可能需要血管升压药。

注意

20世纪90年代初,根据第二次和第三次全国急性脊髓损伤研究报告(NASCIS Ⅱ,NASCIS Ⅲ)报告的推荐,大剂量甲泼尼龙一度作为标准治疗方案而被广泛采用;然而,对这种疗法的系统回顾和相关支持证据表明,这一疗法并不推荐用于脊髓损伤的常规治疗。

药物治疗

排除禁忌证后可应用麻醉类药物镇痛。

• 由于缺乏支持使用激素的证据和激素使用不良反应的风险,不建议使用大剂量激素。

• 如果予以激素的话,必须在受伤后8h内,并在医院内按规定使用。

• 甲泼尼龙：30 mg/kg，静推 15 min 以上，45 min 后维持输液，如果在伤后 3 h 内开始，则在接下来的 23 h 内为 5.4 mg/(kg·h)；如果伤后 3～8 h，考虑继续 48 h。

• 受伤后 8 h 以上不建议使用大剂量激素治疗。

随访

进一步处理

入院指征

• 有明显脊髓损伤或脊柱损伤的患者应该在区域创伤中心接受治疗。

• 不稳定的脊柱损伤。

• 脊髓或根部损伤。

• 肠梗阻。

• 控制疼痛。

• 合并其他创伤性损伤。

• 受伤严重，需 ICU 级护理。

出院指征

骨科或神经外科评估稳定的轻微骨折。

随访建议

急诊或住院患者评估和治疗后，门诊骨科随访。

要点和误区

• 如何创伤患者需怀疑并评估腰椎损伤。

• 有创伤机制、压痛、全身性损伤、意识状态改变都需要行 CT 评估。

• 保持脊柱固定不动，直到影像学和体格检查排除。

• 尽早请脊柱外科医师会诊，确定是否存在骨折、神经功能缺损或不稳定。

• 在院前急救医疗服务(EMS)中的不恰当制动并不能使患者受益。

• 急诊科医师不应自行开始应用大剂量甲泼尼龙治疗急性脊髓损伤。

脊椎损伤(腰部) Spine Injury: Lumbar

Dunya Nasrallah Alfaraj · Gary M. Vilke　江伟伟　李文放 译

基础知识

描述

• 屈曲压缩骨折：

- 楔形压缩：
  - 如果＜50%椎体前方受压，认为损伤稳定。
  - 没有韧带损伤。
  - 没有神经缺陷。
- 爆裂性骨折：
  - 椎体骨折伴骨神经管骨化。
  - 侧位 X 线片可见明显脊柱后弯。
  - 后方韧带损伤。
  - 前部压缩，下肢、跟骨骨折。
  - 可能存在神经功能缺陷。

• 屈曲扭伤(腰带损伤)：

- 可能有腹部受伤。
- 可能有断裂：
  - 纯粹的骨伤；骨折线穿过棘突、椎弓根和椎体。
  - 侧位片无明显脊柱后凸。
  - 通常没有神经功能缺陷。
- 小关节脱位：
  - 主要是软组织损伤，没有骨折。
  - 完全破坏后部韧带和椎间盘。
  - 神经功能缺陷可能存在。

• 屈曲旋转：

- 不稳定的伤害。
- 经常出现神经功能缺陷。

• 伸展：

- 不稳定，不常见。
- 前纵隔和椎间盘破坏。
- 很少有神经系统后遗症，但可能有。

• 剪切伤(平移伤)：

- 上椎体在下一椎体的前、后或侧向平移。
- 韧带断裂。
- 存在神经功能缺陷。

• 简单骨折：

- 孤立性棘突骨折：
  - 韧带撕裂。
  - 没有神经缺陷。
- 孤立的横突骨折：
  - 韧带破裂。
  - 根部损伤可能出现神经功能缺陷，罕见。

病因

• 腰部轴向牵拉、轴向压缩或水平方向的钝挫伤。

• 高处跌落、足(相关的跟骨骨折)或臀部着地。

• 机动车事故(MVA)。

儿科注意事项

• 罕见的虐待儿童表现为腰椎骨折导致下肢弛缓性麻痹。

• 脊髓在新生儿中终止于 L_3，成人终止于 T_{12}，腰椎高位骨折患儿可能直接损伤脊髓。

• 终板撕脱骨折：青春期损伤通常在 L_4～L_5 或 L_5～S_1 水平，韧带剥离椎体终板，有相关的神经系统表现。

• 穿透伤：原发性枪伤。

诊断

症状和体征

• 腰部中线疼痛或局部压痛。

• 腰部有瘀斑或畸形，可触及的畸形，椎旁肌痉挛。

• 触诊棘突间距增宽。

• 触诊触及脱位(前方或后方移位棘突)。

• 腰脊神经引起的神经功能缺损：

- 失去膀胱控制。
- 运动：髋屈曲(L_1～L_4)、腿伸展(L_3、L_4)、踝背屈(L_4、L_5)、足趾伸展(L_5)。
- 感觉：肠弯曲(L_1)、大腿内侧(L_2～L_3)、膝外侧(L_4)、外侧小腿(L_5)。
- 反射：膝部猛拉(L_2～L_4)。

• 疼痛可能被相关的损伤(如骨盆、跟骨骨折)所掩盖。

• 多发性损伤和精神状态改变的患者临床检查不可靠，需要进行影像学检查。

• 马尾综合征：L_2 以下的损伤，以会阴或双侧腿痛、肠或膀胱功能障碍、肛管周围麻痹、直肠括约肌张力减弱和下肢无力为特征。

病史

可能对腰部损伤的机制：

• 机动车事故。

• 高处坠落。

• 直接作用于腰部区域。

体格检查

- 腰椎中线压痛或畸形。
- 与腰椎神经相关的神经功能。

老年人注意事项

- 不确定机制情况下考虑虐待。
- 服用香豆素或其他抗凝剂的患者，需考虑出血的可能，如脊柱血肿。

基本检查

遵循高风险胸腰椎(TL)脊柱损伤的标准，并完善影像学检查：

- 胸腰椎疼痛或触痛。
- 意识水平降低(格拉斯哥评分＜14 分)。
- 药物过量，疼痛感有变化。
- 神经功能缺陷(如上所述)。
- 痛苦，分布性损伤。
- 严重的伤害机制(如机动车事故、汽车撞击行人、从＞10 ft 高处坠落)。
- 腰椎 X 线片(详见影像学检查)。
- 神经系统检查包括：
  - 评估肠鸣音。
  - 提睾反射。
  - 会阴部感觉。

诊断检查与说明

实验室检查

- 标准多发伤实验室(如果有指定的话)：
- 血常规。
- 生化。
- 凝血功能。
- 尿常规。

影像学检查

- 腰椎 X 线，前后位和侧位片。不稳定骨折的特征包括：
  - 棘突间或椎弓根间距增宽。
  - 脊柱后凸＞20°。
  - 平移＞2 mm。
  - 椎体高度减少＞50%。
  - 关节骨折。
- X 线可能无法识别 25%的爆裂性骨折。
- 如果发现骨折，应对整个脊柱进行影像学检查以评估相关损伤。
- 棘突间骨折、横突骨折或单纯横骶骨骨折，如果患者神经功能完好，并且没有不稳定损伤的证据，则需要行屈伸动态检查。
- 应进行 CT 或 MRI 以进一步评估 X 线平片上可疑骨折，以评估脊髓完整性。
- CT 只能评估骨骼状况。MRI 对于评估无影像学异常(SCIWORA)、软组织损伤、韧带、爆裂性骨折分类和手术适应证是必不可少的。

诊断步骤/外科

导尿或超声检查评估残余尿，以确定尿潴留。

鉴别诊断

- 挫伤。
- 病理性骨折(转移性癌)。
- 骨质疏松。
- 骨盆骨折。
- 外伤性椎间盘突出。
- 低位肋骨骨折。
- 结核性脊椎炎(Pott 病)。
- 强直性脊柱炎。
- 成骨不全(儿科)。
- 先天性脊柱侧凸伴半椎体畸形(误认为是外侧楔形骨折)。
- 虐待儿童。
- 脊髓血肿。
- 硬膜外脓肿。

治疗

院前

院前很难确定伤情是否稳定，任何疑似脊髓损伤的患者应该被固定以防止进一步的损伤。

- 脊柱固定术仍然是 EMS 方案的一个组成部分，尽管这一措施目前缺乏有效性的证据和而且存在引起相关并发症的担忧，尤其是在穿透性创伤患者中。

初步稳定/治疗

- 如果在危及生命的条件下需制动。
- 开放气道、人工呼吸和维持循环。

急诊治疗/程序

- 保持脊柱固定。
- 对于运动过度的患者可能需要镇静、肌松和气管插管。
- 任何神经功能缺陷的可给予大剂量甲泼尼龙治疗(最好咨询专家)。
- 咨询骨脊柱科或神经外科。
- 适当的镇痛。
- 以下的稳定性损伤患者，如果 CT 提示损伤稳定，且患者的神经功能无缺陷，则可以保守治疗：
  - 单纯棘突、横突骨折。
  - Chance 骨折。
  - 前部楔形压缩(＜50%)骨折。
  - 稳定的爆裂性骨折。
- 矫正装置长期使用可能是有用的，限制性活动、俯睡、避免枕头和软床垫，可能会加重畸形。

> **注意**
>
> 20 世纪 90 年代初，根据第二次和第三次全国急性脊髓损伤研究(NASCIS Ⅱ，NASCIS Ⅲ)报告的推荐，大剂量甲泼尼龙一度作为标准治疗方案而被广泛采用；然而，对这种疗法的系统回顾和相关支持证据表明，这一疗法并不推荐用于脊髓损伤的常规治疗。

药物治疗

- 无禁忌证情况下可予以止痛药。
- 大剂量激素方案：甲泼尼龙：第一个小时静脉注射 30 mg/kg，然后在接下来的 23 h 内接受 5.4 mg/(kg · h)；在受伤后 8 h 内开始使用。

一线用药

- 泰诺：1 g(15 mg/kg)，口服，q4 h。
- 布洛芬：400～800 mg(10 mg/kg)，口服，q6 h。
- 盐酸二氢吗啡酮：1～2 mg(0.015 mg/kg)，静推或肌内注射，q3 h。
- 吗啡：2～10 mg(0.1～0.2 mg/kg)，静推或肌内注射，q3 h。
- 酮咯酸：30 mg 静推或 60 mg 肌内注射(0.5 mg/kg 静推或 1 mg/kg 肌内注射)q6 h。
  - 对于＞65 岁的患者使用酮咯酸时剂量减半。

二线用药

- 盐酸环苯扎林：5～10 mg，口服，q8 h。
- 肌安宁：350 mg，口服，q8 h。
- 枢复宁：4～8 mg，静推或口服(＞4 岁，4 mg，静推或口服)，q8 h。
- 甲哌氯丙嗪：5～10 mg，静推、肌内注射或口服(2.5 mg 口服)，q8 h。
- 异丙嗪：12.5～25 mg，肌内注射、口服或静推(0.5～1 mg/kg 肌内注射)，q8 h。
  - 异丙嗪静推有组织坏死的报道，而不推荐使用。

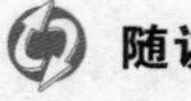

随访

进一步处理

入院指征

- 创伤性腰椎骨折患者应行稳定性手术，静脉止痛，可能的肠梗阻处理以及相关损伤评估。
- 所有脊髓综合征患者必须收入重症监护病房。

出院指征

• 与脊柱外科医师一起评估稳定损伤的神经功能正常的患者。

• 单纯压缩(楔形)骨折的患者,且无神经功能缺陷,如果可以控制疼痛和定期随访,那么可以考虑门诊治疗。

• 单纯性骶骨骨折、棘突骨折和横突骨折也可用于门诊治疗。

• 患者必须神经功能正常,生活状况稳定;CT和屈伸位检查确认稳定性骨折。

老年人注意事项

患有脊椎骨折且仅有轻微相关损伤的老年人可能需要入院,以便于评估跌倒风险并加快康复。

转诊问题

出院时患有稳定损伤的患者应在1周内接受初级保健或矫形外科手术,以监测康复情况并评估潜在并发症。

随访建议

• 如果有新的神经系统症状或出院所带药物控制不了的疼痛,立即返回急诊治疗。

• 按上所述进行随访。

要点和误区

• 腰椎骨折在儿科很少见。如果机制不明确,积极查找病因。

• 老年人可能有腰椎病的潜在病因。寻找疼痛的其他原因,如血肿和感染。对于服用抗凝剂的患者提高警惕。

• CT应根据X线平片上的压缩性骨折来评估稳定性和潜在的椎管受累。

• 如果检查结果令人放心,那么机动车事故后仅背痛的健康的可活动的患者可以在没有影像学检查的情况下安全出院。

家庭暴力 Domestic Violence

Leslie A. Bilello 姜颢 张连东 译

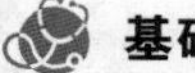

基础知识

描述

• 亲密伴侣暴力(IPV)是被现任或前任伴侣在其身体、性或心理上进行虐待。

• 发生在成人和青少年之间通过社会经济形成亲密的关系中。

病因

• 大多数受害者是被男性行凶者伤害的妇女。

• 在同性关系中,成人包括男性也可能成为受害者。

• 亲密伴侣暴力的危险因素包括女性、青少年(20～24岁)和被分离的伴侣/配偶。

诊断

症状和体征

• 外伤:

- 各种各样的陈述。
- 通常有难以觉察到的头、颈、面部损伤。
- 生殖器或乳房受伤。
- 前臂的擦伤或骨折说明一个防御性的姿势。
- 在不同阶段的外伤。

• 精神病学:

- 慢性疼痛综合征。
- 抑郁。
- 心理问题躯体化。
- 焦虑。
- 自杀。
- 药物滥用。

> **注意**
>
> 临床线索:
>
> • 病史和体格检查结果之间的差异。
>
> • 伴侣拒绝让患者和服务提供者单独相处。
>
> • 寻求照顾拖延。
>
> • 在妊娠期间受到的伤害。
>
> • 患者和伴侣之间的互动表明人际关系问题。
>
> • 没有明显的体格检查结果的多个症状。

病史

• 针对IPV的筛选问题,对发现家庭暴力的受害者是有用的。

• 争议在于是否有可行的证据说明筛选提高健康结果。

• IPV筛选由联合委员会的要求一些专业的医疗组织支持。

• 筛选应该是直接的、无偏见的、支持性和私密性的。

• 计算机筛选急诊患者为IPV提供一些有效证据。

• 考虑药物滥用/中毒的IPV患者,因为他们可能会有更大的风险和不太可能被确定。

体格检查

• 仔细检查外伤。

• 精神状态检查。

基本检查

• 鉴定为IPV后,立即检查外伤和急性药物或行为健康疾病。

• 评估患者将来的伤害/受害风险。

鉴别诊断

患者有外伤、行为健康问题。医疗投诉(例如,生殖、泌尿、多种心理躯体化疾病)时高度怀疑IPV是非常重要的。

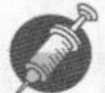

治疗

院前

• 一般创伤评估和治疗。

• 急性医疗服务对事件的准确描述应该纳入医疗记录。

初步稳定/治疗

• 提供及时和适当的医疗照顾。

• 在检查和治疗中提供适当的情感支持。

急诊治疗/程序

• 在一个没有任何家庭成员在场的、私人的、安全的情况下与患者会面。

• 当有语言障碍时,使用医学翻译(不是家庭成员)进行交谈。

• 提供完整、仔细的文件,包括使用患者的原则话,作为法庭证据。

• 详细描述受伤部位和范围。图表或照片非常有帮助。

• 如果病情稳定予以出院,评估危险情况。

- 危险因素包括:频率和严重程度增加的暴力,来自伴侣杀人或自杀的威胁,致命武器的使用能力。
- 与患者一起合作制订符合他(她)意愿的最佳出院计划。
• 安排转诊和随访:
- 门诊受害人服务。
- 紧急避难信息。
- 热线。
- 法院禁止令信息。
- 法律服务。
• 美国各州的强制性报告要求多样:
- 美国各州对于 IPV 报告要求多样化。
- 当受害者不愿警方或社会服务机构报告的情况下,强制性报告可能使受害者更加危险,给医师创造伦理困境。
- 告诉受害者官方报告的所有要求,报告可能产生的后果。

用药

• 对乙酰氨基酚:650～975 mg,口服(对乙酰氨基酚含量 24 h 不超过 4 g)。
• 硫酸吗啡:0.1 mg/kg,静脉或肌内注射。

随访

进一步处理

入院指征

• 根据创伤持续的程度,使用适当的入院指南。
• 当患者病情稳定可以出院,但其安全风险性在迫在眉睫时需要先制定安全出院计划然后住院。

出院指征

受害者的安全可以得到保证并且其所受伤害可以让门诊处理时,可以考虑出院。

转诊问题

宣传服务能力相当多样化。

随访建议

提供关于门诊服务和紧急保护的信息。

要点和误区

• 无法根据患者的主诉鉴别诊断时可以考虑为 IPV。
• 无法提供充分的、客观的关于攻击细节和体检结果的文件。
• 无法充分评估患者出院时的安全,并提供适当的报告。
• 强制报告法律仍存在争议可能引发对患者导致意想不到的后果。

甲苯中毒 Toluene Poisoning

Michael E. Nelson　范浩浩　李文放 译

基础知识

描述

• 典型挥发性碳氢化合物。
• 透明无色液体,有甜味。

病因

• 滥用其欣快作用。
• 职业暴露。
• 用作以下有机溶剂:
- 油画颜料和污渍。
- 油漆稀释剂。
- 胶水、油墨、染料、修正液。
- 冷却剂。
- 石油产品。
- 雾化家用产品。
- 脱脂剂。
• 生产和使用汽油是最大的暴露源。

儿科注意事项

• 青春期年龄组多见:
- 廉价且来源广泛。
- 许多滥用者有心理问题。
• 可能发展为慢性神经功能障碍。
• 机制:
- 吸入迅速吸收。
- 迅速穿越血脑屏障,脑中的浓度升高。
- 可能使心肌对儿茶酚胺的致心律失常作用更加敏感。
- 抑制心肌电压门控钠通道和内向整流钾通道。
- 肺泡排泄和肝脏代谢。
• 中毒的途径:
- 嗅闻:直接从容器中吸入物质。
- 呼吸:通过饱和蒸气吸入。
- 袋装:从含该气体的包装袋中吸入蒸气。
• 毒性范围:
- 100 ppm:精神运动和知觉障碍表现。
- 500～800 ppm:头痛、嗜睡、恶心、虚弱和混乱、潜在的致命性。
- >800 ppm:惊厥、共济失调、步态蹒跚。
- 10 000～30 000 ppm:1 min 内麻醉。

诊断

症状和体征

• 急性:
- 神经系统:
◦ 抑郁症。
◦ 欣快。
◦ 共济失调。
◦ 头晕。
◦ 癫痫发作。
- 心脏:
◦ 致命性心律失常。
- 肺部:
◦ 化学性肺炎。
◦ 肺水肿。
- 电解质:
◦ 低钾血症。
◦ 低钙血症。
◦ 高氯代谢性酸中毒,可能来自马尿酸代谢物。
- 胃肠道:
◦ 腹部疼痛。
◦ 恶心、呕吐。
◦ 呕血。
- 肾:
◦ 远端肾小管性酸中毒。
◦ 血尿。
◦ 蛋白尿。
- 肌肉骨骼:
◦ 全身乏力。
• 慢性:
- 神经系统:
◦ 周围神经病变(弥漫性脱髓鞘)。
◦ 白质脑病。
◦ 脑/小脑萎缩。
◦ 视神经萎缩。
◦ 痴呆。
◦ 认知/神经行为异常。
- 心脏:

◦ 节律失常。
◦ 扩张型心肌病。
- 肾：
◦ 远端肾小管酸中毒。
◦ 肾衰竭。
◦ 范科尼综合征。
- 肌肉骨骼：
◦ 横纹肌溶解症。
- 精神科：
◦ 成瘾/戒断。

妊娠注意事项

• 报告来自妊娠时长期滥用甲苯的母亲，有胎儿溶剂综合征，它类似于胎儿酒精综合征。
• 婴儿更可能是早产、低出生体重、小头畸形和发育迟缓。

病史

• 详细地询问嗅闻、呼吸、装袋或其他滥用涂料/溶剂病史。
• 职业暴露。

体格检查

• 口唇、鼻或衣服上有毒剂(金属油漆中浓度最高)。
• 慢性吸入或从装袋吸入引起的口周湿疹性皮炎。
• 溶剂的气味。

基本检查

• 详细的体格检查。
• 怀疑肺炎查 CXR。

诊断检查与说明

实验室检查

• 电解质、BUN、肌酸酐、葡萄糖：
- 低钾血症。
- 正常或高阴离子间隙代谢性酸中毒。
- 高氯血症。
- 肾功能受损。
- 严重低钙血症/低磷血症。
• 尿液分析：
- 检查肌红蛋白(横纹肌溶解症)。
- 血尿和蛋白质经常出现。
• 肌酸激酶，如果怀疑横纹肌溶解。
• 酒精水平，通常产生促成剂。
• 肝酶、PT、APTT、INR，可能会导致肝毒性。
• 马尿酸(甲苯代谢物)的尿液：
- 确认暴露但与全身的影响不相关。
• 血清水平只能在暴露后短时间检测到。

影像学检查

• 心电图：
- 心房和心室节律失常。
• CXR：
- 指示呼吸困难或低氧饱和度。
- 化学性肺炎。
• 头部 CT：
- 精神状态改变、慢性暴露。
- 脑/小脑萎缩，白质低密度。

诊断步骤/外科

CSF 常常无明显改变但可能需要注意精神状态的改变，以排除其他病因。

鉴别诊断

• 酒精中毒。
• 其他碳氢化合物滥用。
• 其他吸入剂(一氧化二氮、二氟乙烷、丁烷等)。
• 甲醇。
• 乙二醇。
• 水杨酸盐。
• 重金属暴露。
• 吉兰-巴雷综合征。
• 代谢异常。

治疗

院前

• 中毒迅速发生。
• 突然心脏节律失常可能导致死亡(突然嗅到死亡)，通常来自儿茶酚胺激增(如逃避警方)。
• 根据需要进行局部去污。
• 未指明强制呕吐：
- 意识水平的降低可能导致误吸。

初步稳定/治疗

• 检查气道、呼吸、循环。
• 补充氧气。
• 心电监测。
• 生理盐水静脉输入。
• 纳洛酮、硫胺素，如精神状态改变，检查葡萄糖。

急诊治疗/程序

• 以标准方式治疗心脏节律障碍：
- 考虑用于快速心律失常的＞β受体阻滞剂。
• 如果有明显吸入毒剂的表现，使用脉搏血氧仪 CXR 和 ABG 监测呼吸状态。
• 不建议使用类固醇治疗肺炎。
• 纠正代谢异常：
- 钾。
- 钙。
- 磷酸盐。
• 酸中毒时给静脉输液。
• 如果横纹肌溶解，保持高尿量。
• 口服中毒时洗胃很少有用且可能造成伤害。
- 木炭不能很好地结合碳氢化合物，胃扩张可能易于呕吐并致误吸。

药物治疗

• 葡萄糖：$D_{50}W$，1 瓶：50 ml 或 25 g(或者：$D_{25}W$，2～4 ml/kg)，静脉注射。
• 纳洛酮(narcan)：2 mg(儿童：0.1 mg/kg)，静脉注射或肌内注射，初始剂量。
• 硫胺素(维生素 B_1)：100 mg(口服：50 mg)，静脉注射。

随访

进一步处理

入院指征

• 精神状态改变。
• 心律失常。
• 肝功能障碍。
• 肾衰竭。
• 横纹肌溶解症。
• 严重的代谢紊乱。
• 难治性低钾血症。

出院指征

观察 4～6 h 后：
• 稳定的精神状态。
• 没有心脏、代谢或神经系统紊乱的证据。

随访建议

• 请精神科会诊并评估故意或一再的摄入毒剂是不是上瘾所致。
• 停止使用毒剂是最重要的介入措施。

要点和误区

• 对儿茶酚胺过敏的心肌：
- 突发心律失常、死亡的可能性。
- 心脏节律失常预后不良。
• 监测调整充电解质异常。

J

甲醇中毒 Methanol Poisoning

Kirk L. Cumpston 段立伟 译

基础知识

描述

• 无色挥发性液体。
• 30～60 min 吸收。
• 由肝脏代谢。
• 半衰期：4～8 h。
• 病理生理：
- 代谢物甲醛和甲酸产生毒性作用。
- 抑制细胞色素氧化酶。
• 甲酸：
- 决定酸中毒、症状和死亡率。
- 直接作用于视网膜和视神经。
• 甲醇：
- 第一步：甲醇在乙醇脱氢酶作用下产生甲醛。
- 第二步：甲醛在醛脱氢酶作用下产生甲酸。
- 第三步：甲酸在叶酸依赖性作用下形成二氧化碳和水。
- 第一步和第三步是非限制性步骤。

病因

甲醇常见的来源：
• 木醇。
• 挡风玻璃清洗液(>60%的患者)。
• 吸入的滥用化油器清洁剂。
• 燃料防冻液。
• 福尔马林。
• 汽油。
• 油漆溶剂。
• 家用清洁剂。
• 固体酒精罐。
• 假酒。
• 飞机燃料。
• 影印液。
• 香水。

诊断

症状和体征

胃肠道：
- 厌食。
- 恶心、呕吐。
- 腹痛。
• 中枢神经系统：
- 头痛。
- 头晕。
- 谵妄。
- 醉酒。
- 昏迷。
- 痉挛。
• 眼科：
- 视物模糊。
- 畏光。
- "雪地视野"。
- 失明。
- 中心暗斑。

病史

• 有意或无意的甲醇摄入。
• 没有病史，但患者出现不明原因的高阴离子间隙、代谢性酸中毒。
• 原因不明的血清渗透压增大。

体格检查

• 视神经盘：
- 充血或苍白。
- 视神经乳头水肿。
• 瞳孔传入障碍。
• 呼吸急促。
• 精神状态改变。

基本检查

• 摄入史。
• 询问视觉症状。
• 眼底镜检查。
• 同时记录：
- 动脉血气分析。
- 血清甲醇、乙二醇、异丙醇、乙醇的水平。
- 电解质、BUN、肌酐和葡萄糖。
- 测量血浆渗透压(通过凝固点方法)。

诊断检查与说明

实验室检查

• 计算阴离子间隙 = (Na^+) − (Cl^- + HCO_3^-)。
- 正常值：8～12。
• 决定渗透压间隙的因素：
- 渗透压间隙 = 血浆渗透压测量值 − 血渗透压计算值。
- 血渗透压计算值 = 2(Na^+) + 血糖/18 + 尿素氮/2.8 + 乙醇/4.69(单位 mg/dl)。
• 渗透压间隙：
- 甲醇的显示器(甲醇渗透活性高，但毒性代谢产物低)。
- 甲醇摄入或合并乙醇摄入，在甲醇代谢为有毒物质早期渗透压间隙就能敏感地反映出来。
- 习惯上，渗透压间隙>10 表明排除甲醇摄入。然而甲醇中毒可以出现渗透压间隙<10。
- 渗透压间隙正常并不能排除甲醇暴露。
- 乙醇对乙醇脱氢酶具有比甲醇更高的亲和力。同时摄入乙醇渗透压间隙减小、酸中毒较轻，因为只有少量的甲醇转化为酸性代谢物。
• 血清甲醇浓度确定甲醇中毒：
- 摄入甲醇后可能表现为高阴离子间隙，严重代谢性酸中毒。
• 在相关的实验室检查中乙醇浓度具有临床意义。
• 凝血功能检查。

影像学检查

头颅 CT。

鉴别诊断

• 高渗透压间隙。
• ME DIE A：
- 甲醇。
- 乙醇。
- 利尿剂或稀释剂(甘露醇、甘油、山梨糖醇、丙二醇)。
- 异丙醇。
- 乙烯。
- 乙二醇。
- 丙酮、氨。
• 提高阴离子间隙代谢性酸中毒：*A CAT MUDPILES*：
- 酒精性酮症酸中毒。
- 氰化物、一氧化碳、硫化氢等。
- 对乙酰氨基酚。
- 抗反转录病毒药物(NRTI)。
- 甲苯。
- 二甲双胍。
- 尿毒症。
- 糖尿病酮症酸中毒。
- 三聚乙醛、苯乙双胍、丙二醇。
- 铁剂、异烟肼。
- 乳酸酸中毒。
- 乙烯醇水杨酸、乙酰水杨酸(ASA、阿司匹林）。

- 饥饿酮症。

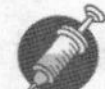

治疗

院前

• 移除所有可能摄入的物质。

• 去除衣物清理皮肤上残留的甲醇并用肥皂水清洗。

• 检测气道和中枢神经系统改变。

初步稳定/治疗

• ABC管理。

• 葡萄糖、纳洛酮和硫胺素改善精神状态。

• 防止进一步的甲醇吸收：

- 留置胃管洗胃：

◦ 甲醇吸收迅速，>1 h可能不会有帮助。

- 活性炭：

◦ 可能有效。

◦ 不吸附甲醇。

◦ 存在精神症状的患者风险大。

急诊治疗/程序

• 使用甲吡唑防止甲醇转化为有毒物质或乙醇静脉滴注。

• 甲吡唑。

- 竞争性抑制乙醇脱氢酶。

- 适应证：

◦ 有意摄入。

◦ 少量无意超过一小口。

◦ 不明原因的精神状态或视觉症状改变和/或高渗透压间隙，高阴离子间隙代谢性酸中毒。

◦ 如果故意摄入或无意超过一小口在血清甲醇水平回报前即开始使用。

◦ 维持给药至血清甲醇水平<20 mg/dl。

- 优点：

◦ 不需要连续灌注。

◦ 不造成醉酒及中枢神经系统抑制。

◦ 方便给药。

◦ 不造成低血糖、低钠血症、高渗。

◦ 无需检测血药浓度。

◦ 减少护理和监控。

◦ 隐匿性甲醇暴露第2日使用也是必要的。

- 缺点：

◦ 视物模糊。

◦ 一过性肝功能受损。

• 乙醇疗法：

- FDA未批准用于治疗甲醇中毒。

- 乙醇对乙醇脱氢酶的亲和力大于甲醇。

◦ 通过竞争性抑制减缓甲醛和甲酸的新陈代谢。

- 若不能使用甲吡唑，乙醇为第二治疗方案。

- 血清甲醇水平回报前即开始使用。

◦ 治疗剂量100 mg/dl。

- 维持给药至血清甲醇水平<20 mg/dl。

- 适应证：

◦ 有意摄入。

◦ 少量无意超过一小口。

◦ 不明原因的精神状态或视觉症状改变和/或高渗透压间隙，高阴离子间隙代谢性酸中毒。

◦ 血清甲醇浓度>20 mg/dl。

- 优点：

◦ 容易获取。

◦ 口服和静脉途径。

- 缺点：

◦ 中枢神经系统抑制，特别是儿童。

◦ 呼吸抑制。

◦ 低钠血症或高钠血症。

◦ 低血糖。

◦ 高渗血症。

◦ 连续注入。

◦ 血药浓度监测。

◦ 孕妇禁用。

◦ 胰腺炎。

◦ 胃炎。

• 血液透析加强消除甲醇与和有毒代谢产物。

- 降低甲醇的消除半衰期。

- 去除甲醛和甲酸。

- 适应证：

◦ 摄入>1 ml/kg 100%甲醇。

◦ 严重的眼科症状。

◦ 退碳酸氢钠治疗效果欠佳的严重代谢性酸中毒。

◦ 持续性电解质紊乱或代谢性酸中毒。

◦ 肾功能不全。

◦ 血清甲醇水平>20 mg/dl。

- 维持治疗至血清甲醇水平<20 mg/dl且酸中毒得到纠正。

• 叶酸和亚叶酸(甲酰四氢叶酸)：

- 叶酸：甲酸转换成二氧化碳和水必须因子。

- 营养不良的个人(酗酒者)需补充叶酸。

• 纠正酸碱平衡失调。

- 碳酸氢钠纠正酸碱平衡失调(pH<7.1)。

- 碳酸氢钠滴的目标是保持正常血清的pH。

药物治疗

• 活性炭：1 g/kg，口服。

• 葡萄糖：50%葡萄糖50 ml或25 g[25%葡萄糖2～4 ml/kg]，静脉滴注。

• 甲吡唑：

- 负荷剂量：15 mg/kg 缓慢静注 30 min以上。

- 维持剂量：10 mg/kg，q12 h，共4剂；然后15 mg/kg，q12 h，直至血清甲醇水平<20 mg/dl。

- 血液透析相关剂量：

◦ 如果最后一次给药时间<6 h，请不要在透析开始时给药。

◦ 如果上一次给药时间>6 h，则再一次给药。

◦ 透析期间剂量q4 h。

◦ 如果上一剂量与透析结束之间的时间距离上一次剂量<1 h，则不能使用新剂量。

◦ 如果从上一次剂量到透析结束的时间是从上一次剂量开始的1～3 h，则给予下一次预定剂量的1/2。

◦ 如果上一剂量与透析结束之间的时间距上一剂量超过3 h，则给予下一次预定剂量。

• 乙醇：

- 口服：50%乙醇溶液(100°白酒)经胃管：

◦ 负荷量2 ml/kg。

◦ 维持量0.5 ml/(kg·h)。

◦ 血液透析维持量1 ml/(kg·h)。

- 静脉注射：在D_5W中加入10%乙醇：

◦ 负荷量8 ml/kg，30～60 min。

◦ 维持性输液2 ml/(kg·h)。

◦ 血液透析期间维持性输液4 ml/(kg·h)。

• 叶酸：50 mg，静脉注射，q4 h，24 h。

• 碳酸氢钠：1～2 mEq/kg加入1 L D_5W和40 mEq KCl，250 ml/h。

J

随访

进一步处理

入院指征

• 即使最初没有症状，也有大量的历史甲醇摄入。

• 对于生命体征或精神状态不稳定，或需要血液透析的患者，收住ICU。

• 如果需要血液透析或解毒剂，但无法满足，则转移到其他医院。

出院指征

如果血清甲醇水平<20 mg/dl；酸碱状态和电解质正常。

■ 随访建议

自杀/抑郁患者的精神病随访。

要点和误区

• 渗透压间隙<10 mmol/L 不可排除甲醇暴露。

• 如果你有一个阴离子间隙升高的患者，并且在鉴别诊断中考虑存在接触甲醇，应立即给药福美哌唑，开始血液透析，并用血清浓度确认中毒情况。

• 如果您无法确认患者是否接触甲醇，或没有全天候血液透析功能，或没有解毒剂，请将患者转移到具备所有这些功能的医院。

• 并非所有的患者都会有一个升高的渗透压和阴离子间隙。早期的患者只会有一个渗透压间隙，因为甲醇具有渗透活性，而且还没有毒性代谢物。晚期出现者可能只有阴离子间隙，因为渗透活性化合物已经代谢成有毒的酸中毒代谢物。介于两者之间的患者会有一个阴离子间隙和一个渗透压间隙的组合。

甲沟炎 Paronychia

Gene Ma　王恵 译

基础知识

■ 描述

• 甲板和甲襞之间的密闭空间被破坏，细菌得以进入。

• 甲襞在甲板周围的炎症反应。

■ 病因

• 急性甲沟炎：主要致病菌是金黄色葡萄球菌，还可见链球菌、假单孢菌和厌氧菌感染。

• 慢性甲沟炎：多重致病因素包括真菌的过敏刺激反应，主要是白色念珠菌，该菌常与葡萄球菌共生。

诊断

■ 症状和体征

• 在甲襞的近端和侧面出现红、肿、热、痛的表现，一般在创伤后 2～5 日出现。

• 症状持续 6 周以上的才符合慢性甲沟炎的标准。

病史

• 急性甲沟炎：甲癖，吮吸指甲，过度修剪或使用指甲，指甲创伤后感染。

• 慢性甲沟炎：因职业原因手长期潮湿的；洗盘工、调酒师、外周血管病和糖尿病患者中发病人数也有所增加。

儿科注意事项

患有咬甲癖儿童常有口腔厌氧菌滋生。

体格检查

• 表现为肿、痛，红斑出现在甲襞的背外侧角并从甲板处鼓出。

• 表皮下和角质层下出现脓肿。

• 指甲颜色变绿提示假单胞菌感染。

• 甲床过度增生提示可能真菌感染。

■ 基本检查

• 仔细询问病史和体格检查，尤其对伴随的感染如指头脓肿或蜂窝织炎做特别的关注和评估。

• 破伤风的评估。

■ 诊断检查与说明

实验室检查

• 没有特异性的检查指标。

• 微生物培养不是常规检测。

• 当怀疑化脓性指头炎时需做涂片或微生物培养。

影像学检查

如果怀疑有异物可行软组织 X 线片检查，怀疑骨髓炎也可行常规影像学检查。

诊断步骤/外科

数字压力测试(将拇指和受累指头相对)能帮助判定早期指甲下脓肿的范围。

■ 鉴别诊断

• 疽。

• 化脓性指头炎。

• 创伤或异物。

• 原发性鳞状细胞癌。

• 转移性癌。

• 骨髓炎。

• 银屑病。

• 莱特尔综合征。

• 坏疽性脓皮病。

• 甲真菌病。

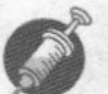

治疗

■ 急诊治疗/程序

急性甲沟炎

• 甲沟炎早期没化脓时可以用热水泡每日 4 次，口服抗生素，也可以不服用；也可以考虑局部用抗生素和糖皮质激素。

• 早期皮下脓肿：

- 用 11 号刀片(18 号针或小钳子)在甲板和甲襞之间最柔软部位中间将其划开。

- 可以行手指神经阻滞。

• 部分甲受累：

- 如果病灶扩大到指甲以下，可对指甲行纵行切开。

- 凡士林和碘伏纱布包裹伤口 24 h。

• 周边脓肿：

- 如果病灶超过指甲表面到另一边，则通过在甲襞背外侧边缘做 2 个小切口以切除 1/4～1/3 近端指甲，并用凡士林或碘伏纱布包裹甲襞，防止伤口粘连。

• 大范围甲下脓肿：

- 去除整个指甲。

• 早期无脓肿的甲沟炎可以仅用热水浸泡；其他甲沟炎如果伴有蜂窝织炎、脓肿或全身炎症反应等推荐使用抗生素。

• 甲氧苄啶-磺胺甲噁唑、双氯西林、阿莫西林-克拉维酸作为一线抗生素，根据病情严重程度使用 5～10 日。

• 如果有咬甲癖或口腔接触应使用克林霉素或阿莫西林-克拉维酸钾。

慢性甲沟炎

• 避免暴露和化学物刺激。

• 局部使用类固醇药物作为一线药物，局部抗真菌药可使用或不用。

J

• 抗金黄色葡萄球菌治疗。
• 难治病例。
- 切开引流术，包括去除甲襞近端处新月形皮肤，还有就是去除增生的增厚组织但不包括生发层基质。
- 口服抗真菌药治疗。

■ 药物治疗

一线用药

• 阿莫西林-克拉维酸：875 mg，口服，每日 2 次，持续 7 日[25 mg/(kg·d)，口服，q12 h]。
• 甲氧苄啶-磺胺甲噁唑（复方新诺明）口服，每日 2 次，持续 7 日。
• 双氯西林：500 mg 口服，每日 3 次，持续 7 日[12.5～50 mg/(kg·d)，口服，q6 h]。

二线用药

• 克林霉素：300 mg 口服，每日 3 次，持续 7 日[20～40 mg/(kg·d)，q6 h，口服，静脉注射，肌内注射]。
• 局部用抗生素：多黏菌素 B/杆菌肽，新霉素有极高的超敏反应发生率，百多邦、庆大霉素药膏每日 3 次，持续 5～10 日（0.1% 药膏）。
• 局部抗真菌药和类固醇混合制剂：制霉菌素-曲安奈德，每日 2～3 次，直至痊愈，但使用不超 1 个月。
• 所有的局部用抗生素都是少量用于患处每日 2～3 次。

随访

■ 进一步处理

入院指征

甲沟炎患者还患有其他疾病。

出院指征

• 患者甲沟炎程度轻病情简单，可予以出院随访指导治疗。
• 患者有切开填塞治疗的需 24 h 后再评估。

转诊问题

治疗难治的慢性甲沟炎。

要点和误区

• 急性甲沟炎采取减压治疗效果好，无论有无合并使用抗生素。
• 慢性甲沟炎大多是由于慢性暴露于过敏或刺激物引起。
• 莱特综合征和银屑病会有甲沟炎似的表现。
• 复发的甲沟炎应怀疑有化脓性指头炎可能。
• 对化脓性指头炎病情的评估。

甲状旁腺功能减退症 Hypoparathyroidism

Rami A. Ahmed · Patrick G. Hughes 倪沁赟 译

基础知识

■ 描述

• 甲状旁腺功能减退症继发于甲状旁腺激素缺乏。
• 假性甲状旁腺功能减退症继发于终末器官对甲状旁腺激素无反应。
• 甲状旁腺激素（PTH）：
- 尿路 Ca^{2+} 丢失减少。
- 尿路 PO_4^{3-} 丢失增加。
- 在肾脏刺激维生素 D 由 25-OH-D_3 转换成 1,25-$(OH)_2$-D_3。
- 从骨质释放 Ca^{2+} 和 PO_4^{3-}。
• 低钙血症是主要的代谢紊乱表现。
• 降钙素：
- 改善骨质 Ca^{2+} 和 PO_4^{3-} 的沉积（主要由甲状腺 C 细胞分泌产生）。
• 镁：
- 生成甲状旁腺激素（PTH）的辅因子。
- 在目标脏器使甲状旁腺激素（PTH）活化的主要因子。
• 甲状旁腺功能减退症：
- 原发性甲状旁腺功能衰竭（可能与 Addison 病有关）。
• 假性甲状旁腺功能减退症：
- 组织对升高的甲状旁腺激素（PTH）无反应性。
- 与甲状旁腺功能减退症和性腺功能减退症有关。
• 遗传因素：
- 先天性缺陷。
- 巴特综合征：
◦ 可能伴随低钾血症和代谢性碱中毒。
- 迪格奥尔格(DiGeorge)综合征：
◦ 甲状旁腺功能减退症。
◦ 胸腺发育不良。
◦ 严重免疫缺陷。
- 威尔逊(Wilson)病：
◦ 因铜沉积导致的腺体的破坏。
- Ⅰ型自身免疫性多内分泌腺综合征。
◦ 甲状旁腺功能减退症。
◦ 肾上腺功能不全。
◦ 黏膜皮肤念珠菌病。
- 奥尔布赖特（Albright）综合征（遗传性骨病）：
◦ 身材矮小。
◦ 肥胖。
◦ 圆脸。
◦ 短颈
◦ 第 4 和第 5 掌骨和跖骨短小（Ⅰ型假性甲状旁腺功能减退症）。

■ 病因

• 甲状旁腺功能衰竭：
- 自身免疫功能低下。
- 外科因素导致的血供中断或腺体切除。
- 放射性损伤。
- 低镁血症（PTH 辅助因子）。
• 终末器官对 PTH 无反应。

诊断

■ 症状和体征

> **注意**
> 最常见的症状常常出现在甲状旁腺手术术后。

儿科注意事项

新生儿/婴儿：
• 出生第 1 年发生短暂的甲状旁腺功能减退症。
• 低智商与低钙血症持续时间成比例。
• 牙齿发育不全。

病史

• 绝大部分症状常常出现在甲状旁腺切除术或甲状腺切除术术后的患者。
• 其次会出现在长期严重低镁血症、饮酒或

J

大剂量使用利尿剂的患者，且症状出现较慢；常缺乏临床症状。

体格检查

- 症状发生的严重程度和速度，低钙血症的持续时间。
- 一般检查：
  - 乏力。
  - 萎靡。
- 神经肌肉系统：
  - 感觉异常（尤其在口周和四肢末端）。
  - 手足痉挛。
  - 触发潜在的痉挛发作：
    - 面神经叩击试验即 Chvostek 征（轻叩外耳道前面神经引起面肌非随意收缩）。
    - 束臂加压试验即 Trousseau 征（血压计包绕于前臂充气至收缩压以上 20 mmHg 持续 3 min）。
  - 喉痉挛与支气管痉挛。
  - 睑痉挛。
  - 肌肉痉挛。
  - 手足搐搦。
  - 癫痫发作（1/3 的甲状旁腺功能减退症患者出现该症状）。
  - 颅内压升高伴有视乳头水肿表现。
  - 帕金森样症状和其他锥体束外神经症状。
  - 脊髓病变。
- 心血管系统：
  - QT 间期延长（与 ST 段延长有关）。
  - 心脏传导阻滞。
  - 充血性心力衰竭。
  - 心室颤动。
  - 血管收缩。
- 精神系统：
  - 记忆力下降。
  - 混乱。
  - 幻觉。
  - 痴呆。
- 皮肤：
  - 头发和指甲脆性增加。
  - 甲床的真菌感染。
  - 银屑病。
  - 白癜风/黏膜与皮肤的念珠菌病。
- 色素沉着：
  - 晶状体浑浊。

基本检查

- 患者有低钙血症但是无低钙血症的临床表现，应检查白蛋白水平：
  - 低蛋白血症纠正后，若低钙血症仍未纠正，应检查离子钙水平。
- 患者总钙水平正常但是有低钙血症的临床表现，应检查有无碱中毒：
  - 如果没有碱中毒，应检查离子钙水平。
  - 代谢性或呼吸性碱中毒会导致离子钙和白蛋白结合增加，从而降低离子钙水平。
- 患者离子钙水平低且有低钙血症的临床表现，应检查甲状旁腺激素水平：
  - 原发性甲状旁腺功能减退症及维生素 D 缺乏患者，PTH 水平低。
  - 假性甲状旁腺功能减退症及肾衰竭低钙血症患者，PTH 水平高。

诊断检查与说明

实验室检查

- 钙离子：根据白蛋白水平用下面的公式校正钙离子浓度：
  - 校正后 Ca^{2+} (mg/dl) = 所测得的 Ca^{2+} (mg/dl) + 0.8[4.0 − 白蛋白(g/dl)]。
- 总钙水平低且患者有临床症状，需监测离子钙水平。
- 电解质、尿素氮、肌酐和血糖。
- 血镁。
- 总钙水平正常但患者有临床症状，需监测动脉血气分析。
  - pH 每升高 0.1，离子钙水平下降 3%～8%。
- 血磷：
  - 若因缺乏维生素 D 而导致低钙血症发生时，血磷水平亦下降。
  - 当钙/磷乘积 > 60 时，因组织钙沉积而出现钙代谢增加，最终导致低钙血症。

诊断步骤/外科

心电图：

- QT 间期延长：
  - 因低钙血症导致 ST 段延长。

鉴别诊断

- 必须与各种原因导致的低钙血症进行区别。
- 实验室检查鉴别：
  - 无症状的低钙血症（白蛋白校正后），总钙水平降低是比较常见的。
- 碱中毒：
  - 有症状的低钙血症，但是总钙水平正常。
- 低镁血症（甲状旁腺激素分泌时所需）。
- 甲状旁腺激素抵抗。
- 维生素 D 缺乏（低 Ca^{2+} + 低 PO_4^{3-}）：
  - 抗惊厥药物的使用（可以降低维生素 D 的吸收）。
  - 肝脏疾病。
  - 维生素 D 抵抗。
  - 营养不良或饮食缺乏。
- 脓毒症（革兰阴性菌感染）。
- 肾衰竭或肾病综合征。
- 螯合作用：
  - 胰腺炎（脂肪酸与钙离子螯合）。
  - 氟化氢铵（轮胎清洁剂）。
  - 氢氟酸。
  - 柠檬酸。
  - 急性高磷血症：
    - 快速灌肠剂。
    - 横纹肌溶解。
    - 急性肾衰竭。

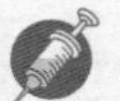

治疗

院前

- 如果知道患者存在甲状旁腺功能减退症或可疑存在低钙血症，在发生心室颤动或癫痫持续状态时，除了给予常规的药物，立即给予补钙治疗。
- 喉痉挛患者会出现喉鸣音。

初步稳定/治疗

- ABC 管理：
  - 针对喉痉挛患者及时进行气道的管理。
- 针对心律失常或手足搐搦的患者，静脉给予钙剂负荷量（盐水或糖水溶解均可）：
  - 除非患者临床正常明显，一般情况下缓慢静脉补充钙剂更安全。
- 室性心律失常包括心室颤动，需时刻做好准备。
- 预防癫痫。

急诊治疗/程序

- 纠正血钙水平：
  - 10%氯化钙（27.2 mg Ca^{2+}/ml）：
    - 在危及患者生命的情况下：静脉推注 10 ml(1 g)，持续时间不少于 5 min。
  - 10%葡萄糖酸钙（9 mg Ca^{2+}/ml）：
    - 在危及患者生命的情况下：静脉推注 20～30 ml(2～3 g)，持续时间不少于 3～5 min。
  - 在非危及患者生命的情况下，在 6～24 h 缓慢静脉补充 Ca^{2+} 500～1 000 mg[儿童：Ca^{2+} 100 mg/(kg · 24 h)]。
  - 持续心电监护。

J

－当出现心动过缓时停止输注。
－反复监测血钙水平。
－补钙过程中可能会加速洋地黄中毒的发生。
－尽可能将血钙水平纠正至患者无临床症状时的最低水平，然后改为口服治疗：
◦当钙/磷乘积60时，可能发生软组织钙化。
• 纠正低镁血症。
• 结合磷：
－当肌酐＜2时，使用氢氧化铝。
－当合并肾衰竭(肌酐＞2)时，使用乙酸钙或碳酸钙。
－磷酸盐结合剂或碳酸盐(磷结合剂)。
• 补充维生素D。
• 避免饮用碳酸饮料(含磷量高)。
• 评估相关的内分泌疾病。

■ 药物治疗

一线用药

• 葡萄糖酸钙：10%(9 mg Ca^{2+}/ml)：在危及生命的情况下20～30 ml静脉推注，至少持续3～5 min；否则缓慢静脉滴注(儿科患者：10%葡萄糖酸钙20 mg/kg或者Ca^{2+} 2 mg/kg)。
－缓慢静脉滴注：成人1～3 mg/(kg·h)(葡萄糖酸钙10 g溶于5%葡萄糖注射液)。
－相对于氯化钙来说，葡萄糖酸钙对静脉刺激或对外周静脉的损伤更小。
• 硫酸镁：静脉输注2 g(儿科患者：25～50 mg/kg至2 g)，持续时间至少2 h。严重患者可静脉输注6 g，持续时间至少6 h。
• 10%氯化钙(27.2 mg Ca^{2+}/ml)：在危及生命的情况下，静脉推注10 ml(1 g)，持续时间至少5 min；否则缓慢静脉滴注。

二线用药

• 醋酸钙：667 mg(167 mg Ca^{2+})，1或2片，每日3次，随餐服用。
• 碳酸钙：1 250 mg(500 mg Ca^{2+})，1或2片，每日4次(2～4 g/d)[儿童：45～65 mg Ca^{2+} mg/(kg·d)，每日4次]。
• 司拉维姆(磷酸盐结合剂)：800 mg，1或2片，每日3次，随餐服用。
• 氧化镁：400 mg，1片，每日1次或2次。
• 维生素D：400 U，口服，每日1次，若按常规剂量无效，则考虑骨化三醇[1,25-$(OH)_2$-D_3]0.25 μg，每日1次；滴定至0.5～2 μg/d。
－推荐其他长效维生素D类似物，对患者更有效，且费用低，起效快。
• 噻嗪类利尿剂：氢氯噻嗪25～100 mg，每日1次。

随访

■ 进一步处理

入院指征

• 有症状的低钙血症。
• 异常心电图。
• 无法口服维生素D或钙剂。
• 校正后的血钙水平＜5 mg/dl。

出院指征

• 无症状的低钙血症。
• 未达到入院指征。

■ 随访建议

• 任何需要治疗或需要复查实验室检查的患者。
• 1～2日复查电解质(钙、磷、镁)。

要点和误区

• 甲状旁腺切除术后临床症状出现快。
• 临床症状常与过度通气或者焦虑患者混淆。
• 在没有手术或严重低镁血症的情况下，需要明确低钙血症不是由脓毒症或则横纹肌溶解引起。
• 在非危及生命的情况下，避免静脉快速使用钙盐。

甲状旁腺功能亢进症 Hyperparathyroidism

Rami A. Ahmed · Jennifer Yee 巩博 译

基础知识

■ 描述

• 甲状旁腺激素(PTH)过多，由于PTH作用产生的症状：
－尿Ca^{2+}减少。
－尿PO_4^{3-}增加。
－刺激维生素D在肾脏从25-OH-D_3转变为1,25-$(OH)_2$-D_3。
－从骨骼中释放Ca^{2+}和PO_4^{3-}。
－高钙血症是主要的代谢性表现。
• 高钙血症引起的高钙尿(尽管尿排出减少)导致尿镁排出增加。
• 镁(负反馈阻止高钙血症导致低镁血症)：
－产生PTH的辅因子。
－PTH在靶组织作用的基础。
• 遗传因素：
－和1型多发性内分泌腺瘤相关：
◦甲状旁腺功能亢进(2A型，2B少见)。
◦甲状腺髓样癌(2A和2B型，2A型恶性程度较低)。
◦嗜铬细胞瘤(2A和2B型)。
◦黏液性神经瘤(2B型)。

■ 病因

• PTH释放过多的因素：
－原发性甲状旁腺功能亢进(腺瘤85%，增生14%，癌＜1%)。
－继发性甲状旁腺功能亢进(对维生素D缺乏的反应或者慢性肾衰竭伴随高磷酸血症)：
◦钙正常或低，但是PTH水平上升。

诊断

■ 症状和体征

结石、骨痛、消化道不适、精神改变。

> **注意**
> • 高钙危象(通常由原发性甲状旁腺功能亢进引起)：
> －少尿、无尿。
> －思维迟钝。
> －厌食、恶心、呕吐。

病史

决定于高钙血症的严重程度和上升速度。

儿科注意事项

• 婴儿：

J

- 肌无力，肌张力减退，精神萎靡。
- 由甲状旁腺功能减退的母亲喂养。

• 婴儿高钙血症：
- 额头宽大。
- 内眦赘皮。
- 鼻梁宽平。
- 上唇突出。

体格检查

• 脱水。

• 心血管：
- 高血压(即使处于脱水状态)。
- 心脏传导异常(和高钙血症程度不成比例)。
- 心动过缓型心律失常。
- 束支传导阻滞。
- 完全性心脏传导阻滞。
- 心搏骤停。
- QT 间期缩短(ST 段变短)。
- 增强洋地黄作用(高钙血症＋洋地黄＝洋地黄中毒)。

• 神经：
- 头痛。
- 反射下降。
- 近端肌肉无力。
- 痴呆。
- 嗜睡。
- 昏迷。

• 精神：
- 人格改变。
- 抑郁。
- 注意力不集中。
- 焦虑。
- 精神错乱。

• 消化道：
- 厌食、恶心与呕吐。
- 便秘。
- 消化性溃疡。
- 胰腺炎。

• 一般状态：
- 疲劳。
- 体重减轻。
- 多饮与多尿。

• 肌肉骨骼：
- 痛风/假性痛风。
- 骨痛与骨囊肿(骨炎性囊肿)。
- 关节痛。
- 软骨钙质沉着。

• 肾：
- 肾结石。
- 肾钙质沉着。
- 肾脏浓缩功能下降。
- 尿量减少。

基本检查

• 血钙。

• 白蛋白：
- 白蛋白上升：造成钙上升的假象。
- 白蛋白下降：造成钙更低的假象。

• 评估高钙血症的症状，尤其是即将发生的甲状旁腺危象(高血钙危象：厌食、恶心、呕吐、精神恍惚进展至昏迷)。

• 评估服用药物史(见鉴别诊断)。

• 在下列情况不需要进一步急诊检查：
- 无症状。
- 心电图正常。
- 纠正白蛋白干扰后，钙＜14 mg/dl。

• 有症状的，血钙＜14 mg/dl 或者任何患者钙＞14 mg/dl，应完善以下检查：
- 离子钙。
- 胸部 X 线(充血性心力衰竭或肿瘤)。
- 磷。
- 电解质、肌酐及尿素氮。
- 红细胞沉降率。
- 碱性磷酸酶。
- 镁。
- 促甲状腺素(TSH)。
- 全血细胞计数。

诊断检查与说明

实验室检查

• 校正白蛋白干扰：
- 校正 Ca^{2+} (mg/dl)＝测得的 Ca^{2+} (mg/dl)＋0.8[4－白蛋白(g/dl)]。
- 酸中毒：
  ◦ 降低白蛋白的亲和力，增加离子化(有代谢活性)Ca^{2+}。
  ◦ PH 每下降 0.1 U 增加离子化 Ca^{2+} 3%～8%。

• 磷：
- 在原发性甲状旁腺功能亢进时降低。
- 在继发性甲状旁腺功能亢进时常常升高。
- 在恶性肿瘤相关的高钙血症中正常或升高。

• Cl^-/PO_4^{3-} 比例：
- ＞33：甲状旁腺功能亢进。
- ＜30：恶性肿瘤。

• 碱性磷酸酶：
- 甲状旁腺功能亢进的患者增加 50%。
- 维生素 D 过多的患者正常。

• 红细胞沉降率(ESR)：
- 甲状旁腺功能亢进的患者正常。
- 在恶性肿瘤或肉芽肿性疾病中升高。

• 贫血：
- 出现在恶性肿瘤或肉芽肿性疾病。
- 不出现在甲状旁腺功能亢进。

• 镁：
- 降低或者正常低限。

• PTH：
- 原发性或者继发性甲状旁腺功能亢进都升高。

• PTH 相关肽：
- 见于肺癌、头颈部鳞状细胞癌、肾癌、膀胱癌、腺癌和淋巴瘤。

影像学检查

• 胸部 X 线：
- 评估静脉补液期间充血性心力衰竭的风险。
- 如果高钙血症病因不清楚，筛查恶性肿瘤和肉芽肿性疾病。
- 评估双侧肺门腺病的结节病，当高钙血症病因不明时。

诊断步骤/外科

根治性治疗手段是甲状旁腺切除术和查找甲状旁腺功能亢进的病因。

鉴别诊断

• PTH 相关：
- 原发性或继发性甲状旁腺功能亢进。
- 家族性低尿钙性高血钙。

• 恶性肿瘤相关：
- 溶骨性肿瘤分泌 PTH 相关肽或者 Ca^{2+}。

• 维生素 D 相关：
- 肉芽肿疾病患者服用过多维生素 D 或者维生素 D 产品。

• 固定：
- 和 Paget 病有关。

• 药物诱发：
- 噻嗪类利尿剂。
- 锂。
- 含铝制酸药。
- 三苯氧胺。
- 雌激素。
- 雄激素。
- 维生素 A。

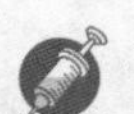

治疗

院前

可能以精神错乱为首发症状。

■ 初步稳定/治疗

• 如果有下列情况心电监测：
- 有症状的高钙血症。
- Ca^{2+} >14 mg/dl。
• 使用生理盐水静脉补液。
• 纠正酸中毒。

■ 急诊治疗/程序

• 治疗高钙血症：
- 予以最小 250 ml/h 的速度补充生理盐水，除非出现充血性心力衰竭：
◦ 24 h 内降低钙 1.5～2 mg/dl。
◦ 达到尿量 100 ml/h。
- 在充分补液或者出现充血性心力衰竭时予以呋塞米（速尿）或者其他襻利尿剂：
◦ 常见错误：充分补液前使用呋塞米。
◦ 如果尿钠超过补充的钠，肾会妨碍钙排泄。
- 避免使用噻嗪类利尿剂（阻碍钙排泄）。
- 考虑使用糖皮质激素（降低消化道吸收，增加 Ca^{2+} 从肾脏排泄）；在维生素 D 中毒或者肉芽肿疾病中最有效。
- 和主治医师商量使用二膦酸盐（帕米膦酸二钠或依替膦酸钠，抑制骨钙动员）。
• 使用标准方式治疗心脏心律失常。
- 纠正酸中毒。
• 查找高钙血症的病因。
• 停用所有可能引起高钙血症的药物。
• 极度谨慎使用地高辛。
• 可能出现充血性心力衰竭或电解质紊乱时，反复查看患者，监测血电解质和镁水平。
• 如果不能补液可使用降钙素。
• 肾衰竭紧急透析。

■ 药物治疗

一线用药

• 生理盐水补液：根据患者发生充血性心力衰竭的倾向，开始时 250～300 ml/h。
• 呋塞米：在合适补液后，40 mg 静脉注射，q2～4 h。
• 泼尼松：40～60 mg 口服或氢化可的松 100 mg（儿童 1～2 mg/kg），静脉滴注。

二线用药

• 请内分泌科医师会诊。
• 如果存在补液禁忌证，予以鲑鱼降钙素 4 U/kg 皮下注射。
- 试验剂量：推荐 10 U/ml 溶液 0.1 ml，皮内注射。
- 初始剂量：4 U/kg，皮下注射，q12 h。
- 二膦酸盐：最适合用于癌症相关高钙血症。
• 帕米膦酸二钠：
- 如果白蛋白校正后的 Ca^{2+} 12～13.5 mg/dl：60 mg，静脉滴注，时间超过 2 h。
- 如果白蛋白校正后的 Ca^{2+} >13.5 mg/dl：90 mg，静脉滴注，时间超过 4 h。
- 在肾功能受损的患者不应调整剂量，可延长滴注时间，减少潜在的肾毒性，但是没有正式的建议（妊娠类别 D——母亲受益可能超过胎儿风险）。
• 唑来膦酸：4 mg，静脉滴注，时间超过 15～30 min（由于使用方便有效本应为一线药物，但是因为缺少一般使用经验而很少选择）。
• 拟钙素（西那卡塞）：30 mg，口服，每日 1 次或 2 次（拟钙素用于继发性甲状旁腺功能亢进或甲状旁腺癌）。

 随访

■ 进一步处理

入院指征

• 校正 Ca^{2+} >14 mg/dl。
• 有症状的高钙血症。
• 有心脏节律异常或者传导异常的证据。

出院指征

• 不符合入院指征。
• 可以维持正常补液。

转诊问题

如果怀疑此诊断，转诊检查 PTH，检查治疗效果。

■ 随访建议

• 如果怀疑甲状旁腺功能亢进，安排随访并且检查 PTH 水平。
• 应指导患者维持正常水合状态，并且停止使用引起高钙血症的药物（见鉴别诊断）。

要点和误区

• 甲状旁腺功能亢进引起的高钙血症很少有症状出现，很少出现 Ca^{2+} >14 mg/dl（更高的血钙大部分是因为肿瘤性疾病）。
• 诊断的目的在于防范远期并发症。
• 血钙水平应计算离子 Ca^{2+} 或校正白蛋白后 Ca^{2+}。
• 充分补液前使用襻利尿剂将会加重高钙血症，有些专家建议将襻利尿剂不再用于此种情况。

甲状腺功能减退症 Hypothyroidism

Bradley A. Wallace · Terry Singhapricha 倪沁赟 译

 基础知识

■ 描述

• 有效血液循环中的甲状腺素水平下降，导致代谢率下降和对儿茶酚胺的敏感性下降。
• 女性和老年患者多见。
• 黏液性水肿性昏迷是少见但十分严重的甲状腺功能减退症的一种临床表现，以精神状态改变和体温调节异常为主要临床特征。

■ 病因

• 原发性：
- 特发性。
- 先天性。
- 自身免疫性：
◦ 甲状腺炎。
◦ 桥本病。
- 医源性：
◦ 术后。
◦ 外部放射。
◦ 放射治疗。
◦ 药物（碘化物、锂、胺碘酮、舒尼替尼、贝沙罗汀、干扰素、麻醉药物、镇静药物）。苯妥英和卡马西平增加甲状腺功能减退患者 T_4 清除率。
- 肿瘤：原发性（癌症）或继发性（浸润）。
- 感染：病毒（需氧或厌氧菌少见）。

J

- 碘缺乏(世界范围内最常见的原因)。
- 中心性(非常少见):
- 因药物或其他严重疾病导致垂体或者下丘脑功能障碍。
- 可能会导致其他激素的缺乏。
- 黏液性水肿性昏迷:
- 甲状腺功能减退症患者因为应激、长期在寒冷的环境下会导致失代偿表现。应激因素包括:
  - 感染。
  - 体温。
  - 中毒。
  - 药物。
  - 脑血管意外。
  - 心功能衰竭。
  - 创伤。

妊娠注意事项

- 甲状腺功能减退与早产、胎盘早剥、先兆子痫、低出生体重和剖宫产率增加有关。
- 患有甲状腺功能减退症的妊娠患者需要增加外源性甲状腺素补充。
- 产后甲状腺炎发生在超过10%的女性患者:
- 经常发生在产后3～6个月。
- 通常不经治疗炎症可自行消退。

诊断

症状和体征

病史

- 疲乏。
- 寒冷耐受不良。
- 头痛。
- 听力下降。
- 肌痛和肌无力。
- 月经量多。
- 不孕不育。
- 腕管综合征。
- 便秘。
- 体重增加。
- 抑郁、幻觉或偏执。
- 认知功能障碍。

体格检查

- 眶周水肿。
- 头发粗糙、稀疏、脆甲症。
- 眉毛1/3缺如。
- 声音沙哑或嘶哑。
- 皮肤发黄、干燥、苍白、发凉和粗糙。
- 黏液性水肿(皮肤干燥、淀粉样肿胀)。
- 四肢非凹陷性水肿。
- 黏液性水肿性昏迷:
- 精神状态改变。
- 低血压。
- 体温。
- 呼吸衰竭。
- 心动过缓。

儿科注意事项

- 未确诊的甲状腺功能减退症的婴儿,大部分在出生时可通过常规筛查排除。
- 儿童时期的甲状腺功能减退症通常考虑为桥本病。
- 儿童可表现为身材矮小,智力低下,性发育延迟。

老年人注意事项

甲状腺功能减退症的典型症状常被误认为由于衰老而引起。

基本检查

评估诱发的病因。初始的实验应包括:TSH和游离T_4。甲状腺功能减退症或黏液性水肿性昏迷无法在急诊室进行实验室确诊,治疗则基于临床疑诊。

诊断检查与说明

寻找黏液性水肿性昏迷的基本病因。

实验室检查

- 甲状腺功能:
- 总甲状腺素(TT_4)和游离甲状腺素(FT_4)水平低下。
- 总三碘甲状腺氨酸(TT_3)和游离三碘甲状腺氨酸(FT_3)水平低下。
- 促甲状腺激素(TSH):
  - 原发性甲状腺功能减退症患者TSH水平升高,但是因中枢病变导致的甲状腺功能减退症患者TSH水平正常或降低。
- 贫血。
- 低钠血症。
- 低血糖。
- 低氧血症。
- 高碳酸血症。
- 呼吸性酸中毒。
- 乳酸脱氢酶、肌酸激酶、胆固醇及肌酐水平升高。
- 高脂血症。

影像学检查

X线胸片:因心包积液可见心影增大。

诊断步骤/外科

心电图:

- 窦性心动过缓、低电压、PR间期延长、束支传导阻滞、QT间期延长及非特异性ST-T改变。
- 严重低温过低患者可能看见Osborn波。

鉴别诊断

- 慢性肾炎。
- 慢性肾病。
- 心力衰竭。
- 抑郁症。
- 低蛋白血症。
- 恶性贫血。
- 肾病综合征。
- 脓毒症。

> **注意**
> - 甲状腺功能正常的病态综合征:
> - 疾病、手术、空腹可能会导致甲状腺功能检查结果异常。
> - 在急性甲状腺疾病期间检查甲状腺功能可能会出现异常结果,解读该结果时需要引起注意。

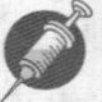

治疗

初步稳定/治疗

- ABC管理:
- 必要时行气管插管和机械通气。
- 心电监护。
- 维持血压。
- 维持氧和以保证代谢需要。
- 纠正低体温:
- 首先被动复温。
- 积极的复温可能出现因血管扩张导致血压的突然下降。

急诊治疗/程序

- 轻度甲状腺功能减退症:
- 同门诊患者一样,通过口服甲状腺激素进行替代治疗。
- 黏液性水肿性昏迷:
- 危及生命。
- 如果高度怀疑,立即开始甲状腺激素替代治疗:
  - 立即通过静脉替代治疗改善生存率。
  - 现存的方案仍存在争议。
  - 甲状腺素(T_4)和三碘甲腺原氨酸(T_3)。
  - 初始剂量治疗后4h重新评估。
  - 老年患者或有心脏疾病的患者可使用小剂量T_4、避免使用T_3,防止发生急性缺血。
- 使用氢化可的松预防肾上腺皮质危象。
- 使用葡萄糖治疗低血糖。

  - 静脉补液治疗低血压：
    - 如果可能应尽量避免使用血管活性药物，可能会导致心律失常。
    - 甲状腺素替代治疗开始之前，患者对血管活性药物反应差。
    - 甲状腺素治疗后会增加血管活性药物的反应性。
  - 严重低钠血症患者给予高渗盐水治疗。
  - 纠正潜在的急性情况。

■ 药物治疗

一线用药

在黏液水肿昏迷，给予 T_4、T_3 或组合：

- 初始联合治疗：
  - T_4：200～400 μg。
- 该剂量范围的下限应用于老年患者或有冠状动脉疾病或心律失常病史的患者。
- 如果在 6～12 h 没有明显的临床反应，可给予重复剂量，使总剂量在前 24 h 达到 400 μg。
- 补充治疗：
  - T_3：5～20 μg，静脉注射。
- 随后的治疗：
  - T_4：每日 1.6 μg/kg（静脉注射可达 75%）。
  - T_3：2.5～10 μg，静脉注射，q8 h，此范围内低剂量，仅限老年患者或有冠心病或心律失常病史的患者使用。

二线用药

- 氢化可的松：100 mg[儿童：4 mg/(kg · 24 h)]静脉，q6～8 h，治疗未确诊伴肾上腺功能不全，直至排除。
- 葡萄糖：50～100 ml D_{50}（儿童：5 ml/kg D_{10}），静脉注射，治疗低血糖。
- 在传染病病因被排除之前，考虑使用经验性抗生素。

随访

■ 进一步处理

入院指征

所有有黏液性水肿性昏迷的患者均需要 ICU 治疗。

出院指征

可以按照门诊甲状腺功能减退症患者治疗。

转诊问题

- 初级保健单位一般普遍可以治疗甲状腺功能减退症。
- 当甲状腺激素替代治疗之前，妊娠患者、老年患者和存在心肌缺血的患者需要特殊考虑。

■ 随访建议

- 患者应该至初级保健单位开始口服甲状腺激素替代治疗。
- 一些没有治疗的有甲状腺功能减退症的妊娠患者，可能会影响胎儿的大脑发育，导致产科相关的并发症。

要点和误区

- 甲状腺功能减退症的临床表现及体征没有特异性，可能会与其他精神或身体疾病混淆。
- 治疗甲状腺功能减退症起效可能需要数周的时间，最好在初级保健医师的指导下开始治疗。
- 黏液性水肿性昏迷的患者有精神状态的改变，基础合并有甲状腺功能减退症。
- 黏液性水肿性昏迷的患者病死率高，需要更积极治疗。但是老年患者和有心脏疾病的患者避免使用肠外 T_3 治疗。

甲状腺功能亢进症 Hyperthyroidism

Todd A. Taylor · Bradley A. Wallace 巩博 译

基础知识

■ 描述

- 甲状腺功能亢进是由于甲状腺分泌不适当的甲状腺激素。
- 发生在美国约 1.2%的人中。
- 甲状腺素激素过多，通过甲状腺激素的直接生理效应和提高儿茶酚胺敏感性导致一系列疾病：
  - 亚临床或轻度甲状腺功能亢进。
  - 甲状腺毒症。
  - 甲状腺危象伴有威胁生命的表现：
    - 1%～2%的甲状腺功能亢进症患者出现。
- 甲状腺素的调控：
  - 来自下丘脑的促甲状腺素释放激素(TRH)作用于垂体前叶。
  - 垂体前叶释放促甲状腺素(TSH)，导致甲状腺释放三碘甲腺原氨酸(T_3)、四碘甲腺原氨酸(T_4)增加：
    - 血液中大部分甲状腺素是 T_4，在外周转变为 T_3。
    - 和 T_4 相比，T_3 半衰期短，具有更强的生物活性。
- 遗传：
  - 基因和环境相互影响。
  - Graves 病和 HLA - B8、HLA - DR3 有关。
  - 在有些家族，可以看到非毒性甲状腺肿常染色体显性遗传。
- 甲状腺功能亢进的病因可分为 4 类：
  - 过度的甲状腺刺激。
  - 甲状腺激素合成不当。
  - 释放大量的激素。
  - 激素过多(内源性或外源性)。

■ 病因

- 原发性甲状腺功能亢进症：
  - 毒性弥漫性甲状腺肿(Graves 病)。
  - 毒性多结节性(Plummer 病)或单结节性甲状腺肿。
  - 摄入过多的碘(Jod-Basedow 病)。
- 甲状腺炎：
  - 产后甲状腺炎。
  - 放射性甲状腺炎。
  - 亚急性甲状腺炎(de Quervain 病)。
  - 胺碘酮相关甲状腺炎。
  - 慢性甲状腺炎(桥本病或淋巴结细胞性甲状腺炎)。
- 转移性甲状腺癌。
- 甲状腺异位(卵巢甲状腺瘤)。
- 垂体瘤。
- 药物诱发：
  - 胺碘酮。
  - 锂。
  - 干扰素 α。
  - 白细胞介素-2。
  - 碘(影像学造影剂)。

J

- 甲状腺素过多(人为的甲状腺毒症)。
- 阿司匹林过量。

诊断

注意

甲状腺危象是一种威胁生命的情况，可以由下列因素诱发：

- 感染。
- 创伤。
- 糖尿病酮症酸中毒。
- 有机磷中毒。
- 细胞毒药物化疗。
- 心肌梗死。
- 脑血管意外。
- 手术。
- 抗甲状腺药物突然停药或者急性摄入甲状腺药物。

症状和体征

- 症状和体征反映靶器官对甲状腺素的反应性：
  - 症状：
    - 发热。
    - 心动过速，脉压增大。
    - 出汗。
    - 充血性心力衰竭。
    - 休克。
    - 震颤。
    - 定向障碍及精神症状。
    - 甲状腺肿。
    - 甲状腺凝视、眼球突出及下睑迟滞。
    - 反射亢进。
    - 胫前黏液性水肿。
  - 体征：
    - 尽管饮食增加，但体重减轻。
    - 继发于甲状腺肿大的吞咽困难或呼吸困难。
    - 皮疹、瘙痒和多汗。
    - 心悸和胸痛。
    - 腹泻和呕吐。
    - 肌肉疼痛与无力。
    - 精神紧张或焦虑。
    - 月经不规则。
    - 热耐受不良。
    - 失眠、疲乏。
- 甲状腺危象出现更严重的甲状腺毒性症状和体征：
  - 严重心动过速及心律失常。
  - 充血性心力衰竭。
  - 休克。
  - 定向障碍，精神状态改变，包括昏迷和癫痫。
  - 血栓栓塞事件。

老年人注意事项

淡漠型甲状腺功能亢进症：

- 由于多结节甲状腺肿，常常有非毒性甲状腺肿病史。
- 常常表现出单一系统脏器功能失调：
  - 充血性心力衰竭(CHF)。
  - 难治性心房颤动。
  - 体重减轻。
  - 抑郁、情绪不稳定、情感匮乏。
  - 震颤。
  - 好动。

病史

逐步出现前面提到的症状和体征。

体格检查

- 生命体征：
  - 发热。
  - 心动过速。
  - 收缩压上升。
  - 脉压增大。
  - 呼吸急促/低氧。
- 脱发。
- 眼球突出或下睑迟滞。
- 甲状腺肿大，甲状腺杂音。
- 皮肤薄、多汗。
- 心跳不规则。
- 肺部啰音(CHF)。
- 右上腹压痛或黄疸。
- 肌肉萎缩或无力。
- 震颤。
- 精神状态改变或昏迷。

基本检查

- 发现根本病因及诱发因素。
- 血浆 TSH 是急诊室首选检查：
  - 正常水平可排除甲状腺功能亢进症：
    - TSH 水平可能下降，T_4 正常。检查 T_3 以排除 T_3 甲状腺毒症。
  - 如果无法检查 TSH，临床怀疑应积极开始治疗。

诊断检查与说明

实验室检查

- 下列情况检查甲状腺功能：
  - 甲状腺功能亢进症状。
  - 老年患者新发 CHF。
  - 新发心房颤动/室上性心动过速(SVT)。
  - 无明显病因的发热。
- TSH(常常下降)。
- 游离 T_4(常常升高)：
  - 如果不能获取游离 T_4，检查总 T_4 和 T_3 树脂摄取试验。
  - 5%的患者有 T_3 甲状腺毒性症状，如果 TSH 下降而 T_4 正常，检查 T_3 排除 T_3 甲状腺毒症。
- 实验室检查通常没有帮助/非特异性，进行需要的检查以查找潜在诱发因素：
  - 全血细胞计数排除贫血。
  - 生化检查：
    - 脱水时尿素氮、肌酐可能上升。
    - 低血钾、高血糖。
- 肝功能检查(转氨酶升高)。
- 动脉血气分析检查缺氧和酸中毒。
- 心脏标志物。
- 感染引起。
- 甲状腺危象的诊断尚无公认的标准。Burch-Wartofsky 评分系统可用于预测甲状腺危象的存在。所有有甲状腺功能亢进症状的病人疑似甲状腺危象。

影像学检查

胸部 X 线(在 CHF 或脓毒症患者)。

诊断步骤/外科

心电图：

- 最常见窦性心动过速。
- 排除心肌梗死诱发甲状腺危象。
- 新发心房颤动。

鉴别诊断

- 嗜铬细胞瘤。
- 脓毒症。
- 摄入拟交感神经药物。
- 精神病。
- 震颤性谵妄。
- 恶性高热。
- 抗精神病药恶性综合征。
- 下丘脑卒中。
- 人为甲状腺毒症。

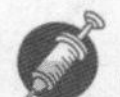

治疗

院前

稳定病情，给予支持治疗。

初步稳定/治疗

- ABC 管理。
- 管理气道、呼吸和循环。
- 心电监测。

• 吸氧。
• 静脉补液。
• 开始采用降温措施。
• 发热时使用对乙酰氨基酚。
◦ 避免阿司匹林(从甲状腺球蛋白替换出甲状腺素,游离 T_4 升高)。
• 冰毯。

■ 急诊治疗/程序

• 确认和治疗诱发因素。
• 对于甲状腺危象,临床怀疑时依次进行下面列出的治疗方案。
• 抑制激素合成使用硫代酰胺类:
• 丙基硫氧嘧啶(PTU):
◦ 首选药物。
◦ 降低激素合成,同时可减少外周 T_4 转变。
• 甲硫咪唑(MMI)。
• 只有在使用上述方法阻断激素合成后,才可以使用碘阻止激素释放。
• 口服卢戈尔溶液(碘化钾饱和溶液)。
• 碘番酸。
• 使用硫代酰胺 1 h 后使用碘组织激素释放。
• 对碘过敏的患者考虑使用锂。
• 阻断甲状腺素的外周效应:
- β受体阻滞剂:
◦ 普萘洛尔(心得安)是一线药物,因为它也可以抑制 T_4 转变 T_3。
◦ 艾司洛尔,选择性 β_1 受体阻滞剂,可以用在伴有活动性 CHF、哮喘等。
- 利血平、胍乙啶。
- 白蛋白溶液。
- 消胆胺减少肠道甲状腺素重吸收。
• 地塞米松或氢化可的松:
- 阻止外周 T_4 转变 T_3。
• 治疗继发于甲状腺炎的甲状腺毒症:
- β受体阻滞剂。
- 抗感染药物。
• 通用甲状腺毒症治疗:
- 高热时使用对乙酰氨基酚。
- 使用常规方法治疗 CHF。
- 使用10%葡萄糖溶液治疗脱水,同时补充消耗的肝糖原。
• 发现并治疗相关和潜在疾病(感染、酮症酸中毒、肺栓塞、脑卒中等)。

■ 药物治疗

• 消胆胺:4 g,口服,1 次/日。
• 艾司洛尔:500 μg/kg,静脉注射,时间超过 1 min;接下来 50 μg/(kg·min),静脉注射,持续滴定维持效果。
• 氢化可的松:开始 100 mg,静脉注射;在接下来 24~36 h,100 mg,静脉注射,q8 h。
• 碘番酸:1 g,静脉注射,第 1 个 24 h 中每 8 h1 次;然后 500 mg,静脉注射,2 次/日。
• 碳酸锂:300 mg,口服,1 次/日[儿童:15~60 mg/(kg·d),分次服用,1~3 次/日]。
• 卢戈尔溶液:5 滴(250 mg),口服,q6 h。
• MMI:60~80 mg/d,分 3 次口服[儿童:0.2 mg/(kg·d)]。
• 普萘洛尔:0.5~1 mg 静脉注射+随后 2~3 mg 静脉注射,注射时间 10~15 min,每几小时重复 1 次;或者 60~80 mg 口服,q4 h。
• PTU:开始时 100~150 mg,口服,q8 h;随后 200~250 mg 口服,q4 h[儿童:5~7 mg/(kg·d)分 3 次]。

一线用药

• PTU。
• 普萘洛尔。
• 碘治疗(卢戈尔溶液),口服 PTU 1 h 后。

二线用药

• MMI。
• 艾司洛尔。
• 锂(只在碘过敏时使用)。
• 胍乙啶(有支气管痉挛的患者)与利血平。

妊娠注意事项

• 和妊娠有关的生理变化可能与甲状腺功能亢进的许多症状类似。
• 甲状腺功能检查的参考范围在怀孕的不同阶段有所变化。
• 妊娠期控制不佳的甲状腺功能亢进可能导致:
- 妊娠剧吐。
- 早产。
- 先兆子痫。
- 低体重儿。
- 自发性流产。
- 死产。
• 甲状腺危象常常由应激因素诱发,包括感染、临产及分娩。
• 治疗:
- 在未妊娠时开始治疗稳定病情(ABC 管理,支持治疗)。
- 目前认为 PTU 比 MMI 安全。两者都可通过胎盘。PTU 应≤200 mg/d。
- 普萘洛尔可安全使用。
- 当妊娠或哺乳时,放射性碘是绝对禁忌证。
- 妊娠时如果不能耐受 PTU,甲状腺切除术是唯一选择。
• 产后甲状腺炎:
- 在 6 个月内生产的妇女中有 5%~10%出现产后甲状腺炎。
- 可能需要抗感染药物。
- 50%的患者在 1 年内甲状腺功能恢复正常。
- 随后可能出现短暂性甲状腺功能减退。

随访

■ 进一步处理

入院指征

• 甲状腺危象。
• 需要静脉用药控制心率。
• 症状严重或者不稳定的患者。

出院指征

症状缓解,口服治疗反应良好。

■ 随访建议

• 根据症状,在数周内应当有私人医师随访。
• 可能从转诊内分泌科中受益。

要点和误区

• 甲状腺危象可以是致命的。诊断需要高度怀疑,怀疑本病时就需要开始治疗。
• 孕妇伴甲状腺功能亢进,放射性碘绝不是一个可选择的治疗。
• 所有怀孕的甲状腺功能亢进/甲状腺危象患者都应该由专家处理。
• 甲状腺危象时,在使用 PTU 或 MMI 阻断激素合成前,绝对不要使用碘。

J

贾第虫病 Giardiasis

Roger M. Barkin · Benjamin Mattingly 祝各亮 译

基础知识

▪ 描述

• 非侵袭性腹泻。
• 全世界均有发病：
- 发达国家患病率为 2%～15%。
- 发展中国家患病率为 20%～40%。
• 占所有旅行者腹泻的 5%。
• 美国最常见的肠道寄生虫病：
- 夏秋季节发病率最高。
- 1～9 岁的儿童和 30～39 岁的成人中发病率最高。
- 在 2010 年有 19 888 个案例在美国被报道(大部分来自北部地区)。
• 粪-口传播：
- 人是主要传染源。
- 水源性及食源性传播。
- 动物传染源是畜养和野生的哺乳动物。
- 污染的地表水是传播媒介。
• 高危人群：
- 到特定地方(发展中国家、美国的荒野)的旅行者。
- 日间护理中心的儿童以及与他们密切接触的人。
- 收容在社会福利机构中的人。
- 肛门性生活者。

▪ 病因

• 蓝氏贾第鞭毛虫：
- 一种原生动物鞭毛虫。
• 也叫肠贾第虫或十二指肠贾第鞭毛虫。
• 贾第虫附着于小肠绒毛吸收营养。
• 改变肠道刷状缘酶，阻碍乳糖和其他糖类的消化。
• 不产生毒素。

诊断

▪ 症状和体征

病史

• 接触后的 1～2 周开始发病。
• 感染可能是无症状的(最常见的)。
• 腹泻作为急性发病症状(90%的症状性患者)：
- 恶臭的粪便。
- 脂肪泻。
- 非血性。
- 2～4 周具有自限性。
- 在免疫功能低下患者和存在患肠道疾病患者中会更严重。
• 胀气和腹胀(70%～75%)。
• 腹痛(70%)。
• 恶心(70%)。
• Roger 病。
• 不适(86%)。
• 厌食症(66%)。
• 体重下降(60%～70%)。
• 发热较少见(15%)。
• 30%～50%急性病例发展为慢性贾第虫病(>4 周)：
- 脂肪吸收不良。
- 继发于叶酸缺乏的严重的巨幼细胞贫血。
- 继发性乳糖酶缺乏(20%～40%的患者)。
• 在免疫抑制的患者中，感染会更严重并难以根除。

儿科注意事项

• 急性感染：
- 严重脱水。
• 慢性感染：
- 发育不良。
- 生长迟缓与认知功能障碍。
- 由于营养吸收不良。

体格检查

• 腹部检查是良性的。
• 肠外表现(10%的患者)：
- 多发性关节炎。
- 荨麻疹。
- 阿弗他溃疡。
- 斑丘疹。
- 胆道疾病。

▪ 基本检查

• 病史：
- 可能接触传染源。
- 高危人群成员。
• 体格检查：
- 如果直肠指检时发现便血或隐血，则贾第虫病的可能性较低。

▪ 诊断检查与说明

实验室检查

• 粪便样本显微镜(虫卵和寄生虫)：
- 1 个样本具有 50%～70%的敏感性。
- 2 日的时间间隔(理想)取 3 个样品具有 85%～90%的敏感性。
- 100%特异性。
- 有能力检测其他寄生虫。
• 粪便 ELISA 或免疫荧光抗体(IFA)检测：
- 95%的敏感性，95%～100%的特异性。
- 不能检测其他寄生虫。
• 直接免疫荧光法(DFA)。
• 一般不需要粪便白细胞检测和粪便培养，除非出现肠道侵袭症状(发热、血便)。
• 抗贾第虫的抗体血清对于急诊发病患者并没有作用。
• 电解质、尿素氮/肌酐、葡萄糖：
- 如果长期腹泻或有脱水表现。
• 血常规：
- 慢性贾第虫病常有巨幼细胞性贫血。
- 在急性贾第虫病中无诊断价值。

影像学检查

腹部 CT 或超声可显示肠壁增厚和十二指肠皱襞扁平(非特异性)。

诊断步骤/外科

• 十二指肠取样：
- 肠试验(患者吞下一根负重的线，之后会被取回并在显微镜下检查贾第虫)。
• 内镜：
- 十二指肠穿刺。
- 内镜下十二指肠活检。

▪ 鉴别诊断

• 病毒性胃肠炎：
- 诺沃克病毒。
- 轮状病毒。
- 甲型肝炎。
• 细菌感染：
- 金黄色葡萄球菌。
- 大肠埃希菌。
- 志贺菌。
- 沙门菌。
- 耶尔森菌。
- 空肠弯曲菌。
- 艰难梭状芽孢杆菌。
- 霍乱弧菌。
• 其他原生生物：
- 隐孢子虫。
- 微孢子虫。

J

- 等孢球虫。
- 内阿米巴。
• 炎症性肠病。
• 肠易激综合征。
• 乳糖酶缺乏。
• 热带口炎性腹泻。
• 药物和毒素：
- 抗生素。
- 钙通道阻滞剂。
- 镁的抗酸剂。
- 咖啡因。
- 酒。
- 山梨醇。
- 泻药滥用。
- 奎尼丁。
- 秋水仙碱。
- 汞中毒。
• 内分泌：
- 艾迪生病。
- 甲状腺疾病。
• 恶性肿瘤：
- 结直肠癌。
- 甲状腺髓样癌。

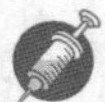

治疗

初步稳定/治疗

• ABC 管理。
• 如果存在明显脱水体征，静脉补充生理盐水。

儿科注意事项

• 严重脱水(>10%)：
- 静脉补充生理盐水 20 ml/kg。
- 心电监护。
- 血糖测定。

急诊治疗/程序

• 轻度脱水时口服补液盐。
• 纠正血电解质紊乱。
• 粪便取样送检。
• 如果粪便检验结果为阳性：按下文药物治疗。
• 如果粪便检验结果为阴性：
- 向胃肠病专家寻求进一步专业的检查。
- 如果高度怀疑贾第虫病，考虑使用甲硝唑进行经验性治疗。

药物治疗

一线用药

• 甲硝唑或替硝唑是首选用药：
- 任何一个具有 90% 的治愈率。
• 甲硝唑：250～500 mg[儿童：15 mg/(kg·24 h)]，口服，q8 h，持续 5～10 日。
• 替硝唑：2 g[儿童(>3 岁)：50 mg/kg]，口服，1 次。

二线用药

• 阿苯达唑(78%～90%有效率)、奎纳克林(90%有效)、硝唑尼特(75%有效)，如果一线治疗失败。
• 阿苯达唑：400 mg[儿童：10～15 mg/(kg·24 h)]，口服，每日 1 次，持续 5～7 日。
• 呋喃唑酮：100 mg[儿童：6～8 mg/(kg·24 h)]，口服，q6 h，持续 5～7 日。
• 硝唑尼特：500 mg(儿童：2～3 岁，100 mg；4～11 岁，200 mg)，口服，每日 2 次，持续 3 日。
• 巴龙霉素：500 mg[儿童：25～30 mg/(kg·24 h)]，口服，q8 h，持续 5～10 日。

儿科注意事项

• 甲硝唑是一线用药(80%～95%有效)。
• 替代药物：
- 呋喃唑酮(80%～85%有效)。
- 硝唑尼特(60%～95%有效)。
- 巴龙霉素(55%～90%有效)。

妊娠注意事项

• 甲硝唑在妊娠早期禁忌。
• 阿苯达唑、替硝唑、奎纳克林在妊娠期禁忌。
• 使用硝唑尼特替代。
• 如果只有轻微症状，考虑推迟到妊娠晚期或产后进行治疗。

免疫功能低下

• 对于免疫功能低下的患者，严格按照药物标准治疗方案进行治疗存在风险：
- 尝试不同类/不同机制药物或甲硝唑＋奎纳克林治疗至少 2 周。

注意

• 只能年龄较大的儿童中使用呋喃唑酮，因为它会：
- 引起婴儿溶血性贫血。
- 引起 G－6－PD 缺乏者溶血性贫血。
• 避免肾衰竭患者使用巴龙霉素。

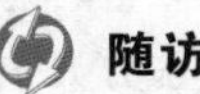

随访

进一步处理

入院指征

• 低血压或心动过速，静脉补液无改善。
• 严重电解质紊乱。
• 儿童出现>10%的脱水。
• 出现脓毒症或中毒症状(在单独贾第虫病中很少出现)。
• 患者不能维持足够的口服补液：
- 极端的年龄，认知功能障碍，明显的伴发疾病。

出院指征

• 能够维持足够的口服补液。
• 静脉补液后脱水症状改善。

随访建议

• 如果在药物治疗情况下，症状持续>4 周，需寻求胃肠病学专家进行诊断性内镜检查。
• 可能会进展为获得性乳糖不耐受症，可持续数周至数月。
• 与感染后疲劳综合征相关。

要点和误区

诊断是该病的最大挑战：
• 所有腹泻患者都应与贾第虫病鉴别：
- 家庭用水中偶尔也会被查出贾第鞭毛虫。
- 患者往往不会自行说明经典病史和危险因素。
- 根据 1 个粪便样品结果往往无法做出诊断。
• 预防至关重要。

J

间室综合征 Compartment Syndrome

Chester D. Shermer 陈奇通 译

基础知识

描述

• 密闭空间内的组织压力增高会阻断毛细血管内血流。
• 正常组织压力小于 10 mmHg。
• 间室内毛细血管血流的阻断压力大于 20 mmHg。
• 压力大于 30 mmHg 时肌肉和神经可发生缺血性坏死。
• 体检发现远端搏动消失，可能存在肌肉坏死。
• 腿部 4 个间室是最常受累及的，但是间室综合征可以在上臂、前臂、手、脚、肩部、臀部和大腿发生。

病因

• 间室体积减小：圆环状手镯、烧伤痂皮或军事抗休克外裤(MAST)。
• 间室内容物增加：直接外伤、骨折、肌肉过度活动、造影剂外漏、欢愉药品注射、缺血后、长时间侧卧挤压肢体导致的水肿或血肿挤压间室。

诊断

注意
• 保持肢体在心脏水平以增加动脉血流，但又不减少静脉回流。
• 怀疑间室综合征时不要使用冰袋，它会减少微循环。

症状和体征

• 间室部位持续严重的疼痛与损伤范围不成比例。
• 主动肌肉收缩和被动拉伸会增加疼痛。
• 肌肉无力。
• 感觉减退。
• 6P 征：疼痛、压力、瘫痪、感觉异常和脉搏存在。

病史

• 在合适的临床环境下引出上述症状。
• 6P 征。

体格检查

• 肌肉间室的触痛。
• 评估运动和神经功能。

诊断检查与说明

影像学检查

如果怀疑骨折应行放射学检查。

诊断步骤/外科

• 利用如 Stryker IC 压力监测系统测量间室压力，持续压力监测连接 18G 针头或内在导管。
• 技术如下：
- 局部皮肤用消毒药水消毒。
- 局部麻醉仅可穿透至皮下组织，注意不要注射到肌肉内。
- 用于测压的针头穿过皮肤直至有突破感时提示已穿透筋膜。
- 0.2 ml 生理盐水注射用以清理针管腔，随后即可读取间室内压力。
- 为了保证间室内针头正确放置，外部压力作用于肌肉间室，否则肌肉会被动牵拉而瞬时增加间室内压力；一旦该操作停止，压力应降至基线并保持稳定。

鉴别诊断

• 慢性间室综合征。
• 筋膜疝出。
• 应力性骨折。
• 动脉闭塞。
• 神经失用症。
• 蜂窝织炎。
• 骨髓炎。
• 腱鞘炎。
• 滑膜炎。

治疗

初步稳定/治疗

• 急性肢体损伤。
• 保持肢体在心脏水平。

急诊治疗/程序

• 急性间室综合征是外科急症。
• 治疗的重点在于筋膜切开，特别是间室压力大于 30～40 mmHg。

药物治疗

• 在间室综合征中，包括激素和血管扩张剂等药物均无帮助。
• 确定诊断和会诊评估后，止痛药物是重点。

一线药物

虽然多数时候疼痛非常剧烈，且仅能依靠手术室中减压缓解疼痛，静脉使用麻醉镇痛药物仍可部分减轻疼痛。

二线药物

口服麻醉镇痛药物和非甾体药物无法在短时间里提供益处。

随访

进一步处理

入院指征

• 间室压力大于 30 mmHg 应请急诊整形外科或外科医师会诊。
• 对于间室压力大于 20 mmHg 而小于 30 mmHg 者，应请求外科会诊并收治入院。
• 对于间室压力在 15～20 mmHg 者，反复测量间室压力；如果患者无法可靠地返回行重复间室压力测量者，应收治入院。

出院指征

间室压力 10～15 mmHg 或以下：患者应给予控制症状的治疗，并告知如疼痛增加、水肿、出现感觉异常应返回医院。

转诊问题

如医师怀疑为慢性间室综合征，需迅速转诊至整形外科医师。直接交流能最好地表达你的考虑。

要点和误区

• 必须测量间室压力，如无相应能力应转运至更高级医疗单位。
• 测量间室压力时应小心，避免损伤肌腱、神经和血管。
• 在挤压类损伤中必须考虑合并的横纹肌溶解。

J

肩关节脱位

Stephen R. Hayden 周健 潘曙明 译

基础知识

描述

• 肩关节是经常活动的关节，容易受伤。
• 前脱位(90%～96%)：
- 损伤源自外展和外旋臂施加的直接或间接力量。
- 损伤也可能源自对肩部后外侧的直接打击。
• 后脱位：
- 经常被忽视。
- 对内收和内旋臂施加的力量导致肱骨头相对于肩胛窝后脱位。
- 常见机制是癫痫发作和后肌群突然收缩。
- 其他机制包括电击和对前肩部的直接打击。
• 下脱位(罕见)：
- 肩关节直立脱位。
- 肩臂过度外展，旋转被困在喙突和肩胛窝下；肱骨头常见于头顶 180°旋转。
- 经常在从高处摔落后出现：
◦ 胳膊在下降时撞到物体并向上推。
- 通常伴有神经血管损伤和骨折。

儿科注意事项

在儿童中，肩关节脱位很少见；应怀疑骨骺骨折。

老年人注意事项

脱位经常伴随有骨折。

病因

• 从高处跌落。
• 冲击伤。
• 上臂牵拉伤。
• 癫痫发作。
• 触电。

诊断

症状和体征

• 受影响的肩部剧烈疼痛。
• 前脱位：
- 肩部呈方形。
- 突出的肩峰和可触及的前部凸起；肱骨头应在肩峰下方存在缺损。
- 手臂稍微外展和外旋。
• 后脱位：
- 树突突出，可触及后部突起。
- 手臂稍微内收和内旋。
• 下脱位(直立脱位)：
- 罕见但易于识别。
- 手臂缩短且固定在头顶上方，好像在举手提问。
• 肱骨头可能可于侧胸壁上被触及。

基本检查

• 评估下肢神经血管情况。
• 测试肩部顶端(腋神经情况)。
• 在任何干预后重新检测神经血管状况。
• 脱位需要及时治疗：
- 如果不及时处理，创伤后关节炎的发生率会随时间推移而增加。
- 应立即进行肩部 X 线检查。
- 即使在临床上明显的病例中，也应在干预之前进行摄片检查，除非摄片会导致显著的诊疗延迟。
- 如果进行干预，受压的肱骨头骨折可能会变成移位的肱骨头骨折。

诊断检查与说明

影像学检查

• 至少应获取 2 个视图。
- 前后位(AP)：
◦ 用于观察脱位和骨折。
- 经肩胛 Y 形或腋下视图：
◦ 用于观察前方或后方。
• 前脱位：
- 肱骨头后外压缩性骨折(Hill-Sachs 畸形)。
- 前侧关节盂边对应病变为 Bankart 病变：
◦ 这些不需要治疗。
- 肱骨头大结节骨折在 15%～35%病例中可见：
◦ 如果复位后位移超过 1 cm，则可能需要手术干预。
• 后脱位：
- 在前后位片上常被忽略。
• X 线片上重叠程度较小且向上位移，产生“半月板征”。
• 旋转的肱骨在前后位视图上呈现“灯泡在杆上”的表现：
- 可能还会看到由前内侧肱骨头的压缩性骨折引起的反向 Hill-Sachs 畸形。

鉴别诊断

• 肱骨头骨折。
• 肱骨干骨折。
• 肩锁关节损伤。
• 肩关节感染。
• 肩关节血肿。
• 肩胛骨骨折。
• 颈椎损伤。

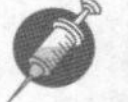

治疗

院前

应识别出神经血管损伤，手臂应该固定在最舒适的位置。

初始稳定/治疗

• 根据需要进行气道管理和复苏。
• 排除更严重的伤情，尤其是在多发伤患者中。
• 确保腋神经或血管没有受伤。

急诊治疗/程序

• 充分的镇痛和肌松对于成功复位至关重要。
- 使用短效阿片类药物和苯二氮䓬类药物进行程序性镇静。
- 或者单独使用氯胺酮、美托咪醇或依托咪酯。
- 在配合的患者中，仅进行关节内阻滞(在肩关节注入 20 ml 1%利多卡因或 0.5%布比卡因)。
• 前脱位复位技术。
- 肩胛骨操作：
◦ 患者取坐位，水平平面上牵引手臂，另一只手在锁骨上施加对抗牵引。
◦ 另一个人使肩胛尖端内收，移动肩窝。
- Stimson 法：
◦ 患者取俯卧位，手臂悬挂在侧边，手腕挂上 10～15 磅的重物；肌肉疲劳持续 20～30 min。
◦ 可同时使用肩胛骨操作。
◦ 仅需 1 人操作。
- 牵引/对抗牵引：
◦ 患者取仰卧位，对患侧手臂进行持续纵向牵引。
◦ 胸部包裹着的布料提供对抗牵引。
◦ 如果数分钟后仍不成功，手臂内外旋转。
- 外旋转：
◦ 患者取仰卧位；肘部呈 90°；轻柔、缓慢地外旋和外展手臂。

J

◦ 应该与患者配合着缓慢地进行。

• 后置脱位复位技术：

- 可使用 Stimson 法或牵引/对抗牵引技术，同时前置肱骨头进行操作。

• 下脱位复位技术：

- 患者取仰卧位；轻轻向头部牵拉以使肱骨头分离。

- 用覆盖在斜方肌和胸部上的布单进行轻柔的对牵拉。

- 将手臂缓慢从 180°旋转至 0°。

• 文献中描述了多种替代的复位方法。

• 复位后诊疗护理：

- 复位后摄片。

- 复位后立即放置托带和绑带或肩关节固定器。

- 年轻患者应该保持肩部固定 2～3 周。

- 年长患者的固定时间应该较短，以避免发生冻结肩关节。

■ 药物治疗

• 0.5%布比卡因：20 ml，肩关节内注射。

• 地西泮：5～10 mg，静脉注射（儿童：0.2 mg/kg）。

• 艾托咪酯：0.2 mg/kg，静脉注射（成人和儿童）。

• 芬太尼：50～100 μg，静脉注射（儿童：2～4 μg/kg）。

• 氯胺酮：1～2 mg/kg，静脉注射；2～4 mg/kg 肌内注射（成人/儿童）。

• 利多卡因 1%：20 ml，肩关节内注射。

• 甲巴比妥：1～1.5 mg/kg，静脉注射（儿童：不常规使用）。

• 米达唑仑：2～5 mg，静脉注射（儿童：0.035～0.1 mg/kg）。

• 吗啡：2～8 mg，静脉注射（儿童：0.1 mg/kg）；使用无防腐剂配方。

• 丙泊酚：1～2 mg/kg，静脉注射。

• 程序性镇静。

随访

■ 进一步处理

入院指征

• 如果未能复位肩膀，可能需要进行全麻下的复位或开放性复位手术。

• 有神经血管损伤的患者。

出院指征

• 通过 X 线确认成功复位的患者可以带着适当的固定器出院，并进行骨科随访。

• 复发性脱位可能需要选择性手术。

• 因受伤或操作而残留神经症状的患者可以安全出院，但应遵循医嘱，大多数症状会缓解，但应进行神经学随访。

■ 随访建议

• 残留神经症状的患者应建议去看神经科医生。

• 所有成功复位的患者都应建议进行常规骨科会诊。

要点和误区

在复位前一定要记录腋神经感觉检查。

肩锁关节损伤 Acromioclavicular Joint Injury

Gina T. Waight · Aleksandr M. Tichter 马林浩 林兆奋 译

基础知识

■ 描述

• 肩锁关节（AC）是由锁骨远端和肩胛肩峰连接而形成的。

• 由 AC 韧带、喙锁（CC）韧带、三角肌和斜方肌附着而稳定。

- AC 韧带负责水平稳定性。

- CC 韧带负责垂直稳定性。

• Rockwood 分类（序贯损伤模式）：

- Ⅰ型：

◦ 无可见畸形。

◦ AC 韧带扭伤（AC 关节韧带）。

◦ 完整的关节囊。

◦ 无 CC 韧带损伤。

◦ 无三角肌或斜方肌损伤。

◦ 无放射学异常（临床诊断）。

- Ⅱ型：

◦ 交趾韧带断裂（AC 关节代偿）（锁骨远端水平不稳）。

◦ 关节囊破裂。

◦ 扭伤的 CC 韧带（CC 韧带代偿）。

◦ 最小的三角肌和斜方肌损伤。

◦ 射线照片显示 AC 关节略微扩大（正常<5 mm）。

◦ 正常 CC 空间（11～13 mm）。

- Ⅲ型：

◦ 交趾韧带断裂（AC 关节屈服）（锁骨远端水平不稳）。

◦ 关节囊破裂。

◦ CC 韧带断裂（CC 韧带触痛）（锁骨远端垂直不稳）。

◦ 分离三角肌和斜方肌。

◦ 完全的 AC 分离。

◦ 射线照片显示 AC 关节变宽。

◦ 增加 CC 空间，远端锁骨位于肩峰上方（100%位移）。

- Ⅳ、Ⅴ、Ⅵ型：

◦ 比Ⅰ型、Ⅱ型和Ⅲ型引起更大的疼痛。

◦ 横向、腋下 X 线片最佳可视化。

◦ 全部需要手术治疗。

◦ 长期残疾的风险更大。

- Ⅳ型：

◦ 与Ⅲ型相同的韧带、肌肉损伤模式。

◦ 锁骨向斜方肌后移位。

◦ 检查时可能会触及后方移位的锁骨。

◦ 可能导致皮肤后隆起。

- Ⅴ型：

◦ 很少见。

◦ 与Ⅲ型相同的韧带/肌肉损伤模式。

◦ 锁骨位移超过斜方肌（CC 空间增加 100%～300%）。

◦ 肩膀严重下垂。

◦ 锁骨可以皮下触诊。

◦ 可能导致皮肤出现隆起、缺血或中断。

- Ⅵ型：

◦ 通常与严重创伤有关。

◦ 与Ⅲ型相同的韧带、肌肉损伤模式。

◦ 锁骨下位移到肩峰下或腋下位置。

◦ 肩部呈扁平状。

◦ 伴有神经血管损伤很常见。

■ 病因

• 在接触性运动中最常见于年轻活跃的男性。

• 最常见的机制是手臂内收时直接伤及上肩或侧肩，通常是在摔倒时。

- 肩峰自下而上移位。
- 锁骨通过胸锁韧带保持稳定。

• 也可以通过伸直的手或肘部的坠落间接发生，并将力传递到AC关节。

诊断

■ 症状和体征

病史

• 外伤后肩部前部或上部疼痛。
• 手臂在胸部、背部或头顶移动会加重疼痛。
• 机制/力量将决定对伤害的怀疑和模式。
• 相关的神经血管症状。
• 颈椎症状。

体格检查

• 在站立或坐姿时进行检查，仰卧位会抵消重力，从而掩盖关节的不稳定性。

• 检查：瘀斑、擦伤、肿胀、对称、交感关节畸形、皮肤拉伤或撕裂。

- 锁骨突出，肩峰下垂表明AC关节破裂(Rockwood Ⅱ型或以上损伤)。

• 触诊：胸锁骨关节、锁骨长度、AC关节、CC韧带、喙突、肩胛骨和肱骨近端的序贯检查。

- AC关节上的压痛提示AC韧带损伤(Rockwood Ⅰ型损伤或更严重)。
- 锁骨远端水平不稳提示AC韧带断裂(Rockwood Ⅱ型损伤或更严重)。
- CC韧带压痛提示CC韧带损伤(Rockwood Ⅱ型或以上损伤)。
- 锁骨远端垂直不稳提示CC韧带断裂(Rockwood Ⅲ型损伤或更严重)。

• 特殊检查：

- 跨身内收试验：
  ◦ 手臂抬高90°，肘关节屈曲90°，向内收越过胸口。
  ◦ 肩膀上方疼痛提示AC损伤。
  ◦ 敏感度77%，特异性79%。
- O'Brien测试：
  ◦ 手臂抬高90°，肘关节伸直，内收10°～15°，前臂最大内旋。
  ◦ 检查者对抵抗力施加向下的力。
  ◦ 肩膀上方的疼痛提示AC损伤。
  ◦ 敏感性16%～93%，特异性90%～95%。

• 完整的末梢神经血管检查，包括臂丛。

• 谨慎的颈髓检查。

■ 基本检查

• 寻找导致AC关节损伤和相关暴力的机制。

• 身体检查以评估损伤类型、神经血管损害和排除其他疼痛原因。

• 放射学评估，如下所述。

■ 诊断检查与说明

影像学检查

• 特定的AC关节X线片。

- 如果怀疑AC损伤，则建议使用。
- 应包括双侧AC关节(以作比较)。
- 标准的肩部视野会穿透AC关节，可能会掩盖细微的损伤。
- 不推荐应力视图。

• Zanca视图(10°～15°头倾斜)用于有限的初始视图。

• 观察Ⅲ～Ⅳ型损伤的腋窝，以确定锁骨远端的位置。

• CT或MRI用于进一步评估手术病例(Rockwood Ⅳ～Ⅵ型)。

- 血管造影可用于评估相关的神经血管损伤。
- 如果CT、MRI不可用。

■ 鉴别诊断

• 肩膀脱臼。
• 肩峰或锁骨骨折。
• 肩袖损伤。
• 肌腱炎。
• 囊炎。
• 颈神经根病。
• 骨关节炎。
• 骨髓炎。

儿科注意事项

• 包裹在骨膜管中的小儿锁骨。

- CC管内韧带。
- AC管外韧带(更易受到伤害)。

• AC关节损伤很少单独发生在儿科人群中。

• 当确实发生伤害时，通常是Ⅰ型或Ⅱ型。

• 通过植骨形成的锁骨远端骨折比Ⅲ型AC关节脱位更常见。

治疗

■ 院前

• 冰袋。
• 悬吊固定。
• 如果需要，颈椎固定。

■ 初步稳定/治疗

• 冰敷。
• 吊带固定。
• 如果需要，颈椎固定。
• 镇痛(NSAIDs，其他镇痛药)。

■ 急诊治疗/程序

• Ⅰ型和Ⅱ型：

- 放置，冰敷，镇痛药。
- 吊带固定(通常3～7日)。
- 运动范围(ROM)和加强运动需要被限制。
- 运动范围和力量恢复正常活动(2～4周)。

• Ⅲ型：

- 休息，冰敷，镇痛药。
- 固定和早期(72 h内)骨科转诊。

• 治疗计划存在争议缺乏有效的证据表明一种管理策略优于另一种管理策略(保守与手术)。

- 选择何种方法可能取决于患者的总体健康状况、活动水平、职业、手部优势和再次受伤的风险。
- 现下的趋势是尽可能不手术，但是若6～12周后仍有持续的症状及功能受限，需要手术治疗。

• Ⅳ型、Ⅴ型、Ⅵ型：

- 休息，冰敷，镇痛药。
- 固定和立即骨科转诊。
- 需要早期手术治疗。

• 特殊情况：AC关节损伤的潜在并发症是关节炎。

儿科注意事项

• Ⅰ型和Ⅱ型：

- 保守管理(休息，冰敷，镇痛药，吊带)。
- 应该在没有重大后遗症的情况下治愈。

• Ⅲ型：

- 年龄<15岁，保守管理。
- 年龄>15岁可能需要更积极的治疗。

• Ⅳ型、Ⅴ型和Ⅵ型：

- 手术修复。

■ 药物治疗

• 布洛芬：600 mg(儿童：4～10 mg/kg)，口服，每日4次。

• 酮咯酸：30 mg(儿童：0.5 mg/kg，最大剂量30 mg，如果>6个月)，肌内注射或静脉注射，q6 h(15 mg，肌内注射或静脉注射，q6 h，如果>65岁或<50 kg)。

随访

进一步处理

入院指征

- 开放伤。
- 需要手术的Ⅳ型、Ⅴ型和Ⅵ型。

出院指征

- Ⅰ型和Ⅱ型可以通过骨科转诊进行出院。
- Ⅲ型应该有紧急的骨科转诊。

建议

- Ⅰ型和Ⅱ型：2～4 周内进行骨科随访。
- Ⅲ型：早期(72 h 内)骨科随访。
- Ⅳ～Ⅵ型：即刻骨科转诊。
- 所有儿科损伤都应及时进行骨科随访，Ⅳ～Ⅵ型损伤需要立即转诊。

要点和误区

- Ⅰ型和Ⅱ型 AC 伤害：
  - 不增加 CC 空间。
  - 保守管理，休息，冰敷，吊索和 ROM/力量练习。
- Ⅲ型伤害：锁骨远端位移 100%。
  - 管理有点争议。
  - 需要早期骨科随访。
- Ⅳ～Ⅵ型伤害：
  - Ⅲ型的韧带和肌肉损伤。
  - 根据锁骨远端位置的差异。
  - 手术管理是标准的护理。

减压病 Decompression Sickness

Nicole L. Lunceford 许磊 译

基础知识

描述

由于惰性气体气泡(氮气)从溶液中逸出进入体液和组织而引起的多系统疾病过程。

病因

- 机制：
  - 增加环境压力导致氮分压增加(根据亨利定律)。
  - 在组织氮气积累，浓度增加的时间越长，环境压力越高。
  - 减压病的结果是，当环境压力保持在溶液中氮减少的过快时，防止氮气逐渐去除体内多余的负担。
  - 随着除氮梯度的增加，组织变得过分饱和，并有气泡产生。
- 亨利定律：
  - 在给定的温度下溶解的气体的量与气体的分压成正比。
  - 增加分压导致大量的气体溶解在组织里。
  - 减小分压导致气体从溶液中流出。
- 气体被看作是有身体的炎症反应和溶血反应的异物：
  - 导致血管通透性增加，血容量和血液浓度减少。
- 气泡位置决定临床效果：
  - 血液和淋巴阻塞导致缺血、梗死或者淋巴水肿。
  - 组织机械扩张导致疼痛。
- 减压病的风险因素：
  - 潜水因素：
    - 深度。
    - 长时间潜水。
    - 一日内多次潜水。
    - 快速上升。
    - 冷水。
  - 人为因素：
    - 肥胖。
    - 并发疾病。
    - 肺部疾病。
    - 脱水。
  - 正确使用潜水表和计算机不能消除减压病的风险。
  - 潜水前积极运动可能减少风险。
- 50%的患者在 1 h 内出现症状，90%的人在 6 h 内出现症状。
- 下降飞行的飞机可以引起减压病是由于较低的机舱压力。

诊断

症状和体征

- 皮肤：
  - 猩红热、丹毒、斑点、红疹：
    - 斑点(表皮鳗鲡)经常预示更严重的疾病。
  - 皮肤出现橙色是由于淋巴阻塞。
- 肌肉骨骼(减压病)：
  - 疼痛：
    - 迟钝，深肌肉痛。
    - 经常在一个关节(肘和肩最常见)。
    - 通常运动不会加剧或者减少触诊。
- 胃肠：
  - 恶心和呕吐。
  - 腹痛。
- 肺(窒息)：
  - 肺部血管阻塞，由于大量气泡(静脉气体栓塞)所致。
  - 急性呼吸窘迫。
    - 胸骨痛、挤压。
    - 咳嗽。
    - 呼吸困难。
    - 缺氧。
- 中枢神经系统：
  - 虚弱和疲劳。
  - 麻木及感觉异常。
  - 激动。
  - 头痛。
  - 头晕。
  - 眩晕。
  - 抽搐。
  - 膀胱和/或直肠失禁。
  - 昏睡。
  - 视觉障碍。
  - 最常见影响脊髓(下胸椎和腰椎区域)。
- 内耳(眩晕症)：
  - 前庭损伤。
  - 头晕、眩晕、耳鸣和恶心。
  - 类似症状内耳气压伤，但是预后更差。

病史

有过潜水史，包括时间、深度、上升史且发病症状。

体格检查

全面体格检查，包括详细的神经检查。

基本检查

- 临床诊断：识别危险因素和各种临床表现。

J

- 全面神经系统检查，记录可能减弱的症状。
- 压力试验：
  - 在高压舱内再压缩迅速缓解症状可能是诊断减压病的唯一途径。

诊断检查与说明

实验室检查

- 全血细胞计数：
  - 血细胞比容增高继发于血液浓缩。
- 电解质、血尿素氮、肌酐、葡萄糖。
- 尿检：
  - 尿比重增加可能表明血管内血容量不足。
- 动脉血气分析、脉搏、血氧饱和度：
  - 检测氧合。

影像学检查

- 胸部X线：
  - 伴随肺部气压伤。
  - 非心源性肺水肿来源于减压病。
- 末端X线：
  - 排除外伤疼痛的原因。
- 头部CT，当神经状态改变或者精神功能障碍。

鉴别诊断

- 无关气泡形成的肌肉损伤。
- 内耳或中耳气压伤。
- 动脉气体栓塞。
- 脑血管意外(CVA)。
- 创伤。

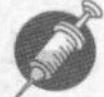

治疗

院前

- 慎重：
  - 识别减压病。
    - 潜水后下肢疼痛经常归因于肌肉损伤。
    - 严重的神经症状经常很小，因为潜水员没有考虑到减压病。
  - 如果需要：
    - 极限海拔高度低于1 000 ft或使用增压机。
- 争议：
  - 水内再压缩：
    - 回到受伤的潜水员(患者)的潜水深度，在那里症状可改善。
    - 非常困难。
    - 需要大量的表面的支持。

初步稳定/治疗

- ABC管理。
- 通过面罩或者气管插管(ETT)提供常压氧(100%)：
  - 增加惰性气体(氮气)从组织中消除，减少气泡的量。
  - 增加氧气向损伤组织运输。
- 保持患者仰卧位以防止进一步的脑损伤。
- 尽早在加压高压舱内治疗。

急诊治疗/程序

- 静脉补液生理盐水(NS)以保持尿量在1～2 ml/(kg·h)。
  - 潜水员经常脱水，归因于利尿剂、运动、呼吸干燥压缩空气和血管通透性的增加。
  - 增加血流有助于气体输出和氮气的溶解。
- 高压氧加压治疗(看高压氧治疗)：
  - 安排运送到最近的高压氧舱。
  - 预防胸部内简单的气胸，防止转化为张力性气胸。
  - 在气管内或者导管内添加水或者盐水，以避免在整个压缩过程中出现压缩、损伤。
  - 参考美国《海军潜水手册》的加压治疗方案。
- 潜水员警报网(DAN)：
  - 24 h紧急热线为治疗潜水损伤提供医疗咨询并转到高压氧舱。
- 止痛药和止吐药。
- 地西泮(安定)治疗严重的眩晕。
- 辅助治疗的非甾体抗炎药和/或丹阳混合气体可能减少再压缩治疗的次数。

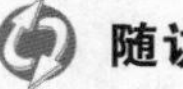

随访

进一步处理

入院指征

- 所有疑似或者减压病的患者需要高压治疗。

出院指征

- 症状较轻、稳定的患者可以出院后在行高压氧治疗。
- 航空旅行可能加重症状，由于环境压力减小。

随访建议

高压转诊。

要点和误区

- 很难区别肌肉骨骼减压病与肌肉骨骼疼痛。
- 显著疲劳可能是减压病的唯一症状。
- 即使轻微的症状或者症状分析怀疑减压病，应该在高压氧治疗。
- 在减压病很可能诊断时，不要拖延加压治疗的实验室检查和影像学检查。
- 避免水加压治疗。

J

睑腺炎和睑板腺囊肿 Hordeolum and Chalazion

Shari Schabowski · Kevin J. McGurk 巩博 译

基础知识

描述

- 由于炎症沿睫毛波及眼睑的腺体。
  - 睑腺炎：急性腺体堵塞导致炎症和脓肿形成。
  - 睑板腺囊肿：以腺体内容物滞留和慢性肉芽肿性炎为最终结果。
- 睑腺炎：
  - 由于一个或多个眼睑腺的流出道梗阻。
  - 梗阻的腺体可能导致继发感染。
  - 可能导致局部脓肿形成或并发眶周蜂窝织炎。
- 睑板腺囊肿：
  - 位于睑板腺的慢性肉芽肿性炎：
    - 源于滞留的分泌物。
    - 睑缘的腺导管堵塞可导致腺体内容物释放到眼睑周围软组织。
    - 继发脂性肉芽肿性炎。
    - 睑板腺囊肿可发生继发性感染。
    - 可能由内睑腺炎未完全排出发展而来。

病因

睑腺炎：

- 可发生继发性感染：
  - 葡萄球菌最常见。
- 诱发条件：
  - 睑板腺功能障碍。
  - 睑缘炎。
  - 红斑痤疮。
  - 有睑腺炎病史。

诊断

症状和体征

- 睑腺炎：
  - 当腺体流出道梗阻时病情进展迅速。
  - 睑缘红、肿、疼痛。
  - 常为单发，很少多发。
  - 局部炎症。
  - 可复发。
  - 不同腺体感染的表现：
    - 外睑腺炎：
    - 导管位于睫毛间的表面皮脂腺或者汗腺堵塞。
    - 有触痛的小肿块常朝向表面。
    - 内睑腺炎：
    - 导管位于睑缘内侧的皮脂腺堵塞。
    - 通过眼睑可触摸到有痛感的小肿块。
    - 可导致眼睛异物感和视觉障碍。
    - 通常更红，更大，更疼痛。
    - 可指向内部或穿透表皮。
  - 非全身性进程。
  - 可能并发：
    - 结膜炎。
    - 眶周蜂窝织炎。
- 睑板腺囊肿：
  - 坚硬、局限、无痛或微痛小结节。
    - 通常长期存在。
  - 非炎症性。
  - 症状常决定于物理性质：
    - 破坏眼睛的自然闭合。
    - 妨碍视野及周围视觉。
    - 对眼球造成压力。
    - 因为角膜暴露导致角膜干燥或者损伤。
  - 非急性、非紧急进程，不需要紧急干预，除非出现继发角膜或明显眼球压力。

病史

- 睑腺炎：位于眼睑边缘的突发、局限、疼痛肿块。
- 无全身性症状。

体格检查

- 发生于眼睑外部或者内部腺体伴有疼痛的局部炎症。
- 可见很小的周围性水肿。
- 脓肿可局限在睫毛线，从睑结膜或向外穿透眼睑皮肤。

基本检查

- 完整的眼科学检查包括裂隙灯检查和角膜评估。
- 评估相关蜂窝织炎和/或全身性检查。
- 睑腺炎：
  - 识别脓肿的起源。
- 睑板腺囊肿：
  - 检查睑板腺囊肿的特性是否导致角膜暴露和损伤。

诊断检查与说明

培养引流物对帮助治疗作用有限。

鉴别诊断

- 睑缘炎。
- 泪囊炎。
- 泪腺炎。
- 化脓性肉芽肿。
- 皮脂细胞癌。
- 基底细胞癌。
- 鳞状细胞癌。

治疗

急诊治疗

- 睑腺炎：减轻梗阻并阻止脓肿形成。
  - 热敷 15 min，每日 4～6 次。
  - 轻柔按摩结节以排出阻塞物质。
  - 严重内睑腺炎需要切开引流：
    - 常由眼科医师完成。
    - 如果指向结膜，行垂直切口，避免瘢痕导致睑板腺损伤并减少角膜损伤。
    - 很少需要外部皮肤切口。
    - 如果需要，可行横行切口。
    - 切除单个病灶包括睫毛可能对某些少见的严重外睑腺炎有益。
    - 肉毒杆菌。
- 睑板腺囊肿：通常抱怨影响美容和难处理的肿块。
  - 可能自发解决。
  - 通常对保守疗法有反应，每日敷几次，持续 4～6 周。
  - 推荐眼科学切开及切除或类固醇注射。
  - 润滑滴眼剂可减缓症状。

药物治疗

保持眼睛舒适，眼部保湿剂是必需的。

随访

进一步处理

出院指征

没有迹象表明需要住院，除非出现继发性并发症（如明显的眶周蜂窝织炎伴全身性症状）。

转诊问题

- 如果认为有切开和引流内睑腺炎的指征，应当考虑眼科医师紧急会诊。
- 睑板腺囊肿应交付眼科医师行根治性治疗。

随访建议

- 眼科随访 1～2 日来评估保守治疗的反应。
- 症状应在 1～2 周完全消失。
- 在>2 个月出现的睑板腺囊肿更有可能需要眼科的明确治疗。

要点和误区

- 睑腺炎采取热敷和轻柔按摩的保守治疗手段是标准治疗：
  - 大多数病例不需要进一步干预。
  - 紧急切开和引流的指征很少见，只适用在极端病例。
  - 切开和引流可能导致长期并发症，包括角膜损伤、瘘管形成和美容并发症。
- 睑板腺囊肿不需要紧急干预：
  - 可以自行解决还是保守处理。
  - 必要时转介眼科进行彻底治疗。

J

碱中毒 Alkalosis

Matthew T. Robinson · Catherine D. Parker 马林浩 林兆奋 译

基础知识

描述

- 呼吸性碱中毒：
- 血清 pH 升高继发于肺泡过度通气和 $PaCO_2$ 减少。
- 通过 2 型受体的刺激发生高通气：
  - 中枢受体：位于脑干和对降低的 CSF pH 有反应。
  - 胸部受体：位于主动脉弓且对低氧血症有反应。
- 增加的肺泡通气继发于：
  - 引起酸中毒的疾病。
  - 低氧血症。
  - 通过中枢神经系统或胸部疾病引起对这些受体的非生理性刺激。
- 通常 pH 低于 7.50 很少有生命危险。
- 代谢性碱中毒：
- 血清 HCO_3^- 的原发性增加，继发于失去 H^+ 或获得 HCO_3^-。
- 发病机制需要一个初始过程，产生代谢性碱中毒伴有继发性或重叠过程维持碱中毒。
- 通过以下机制中的一项生成：
- 通过摄入或输注获得碱。
- 通过胃肠道或肾脏的 H^+ 损失。
- 氢离子进入细胞内。
- 细胞外液（ECF）体积的减小伴 HCO_3^- 损失。
- 液体不足。
- 需要肾脏维持继发于肾脏排出 HCO_3^- 的巨大能力的代谢性碱中毒，通过以下内容发生：
- 降低 GFR（肾衰竭、ECF 耗竭）。
- HCO_3^- 的高效管状重吸收。

继发于低氯血症、醛固酮增多症、低钾血症、ECF 耗竭。

- 如果 pH＞7.55，死亡率为 45%；如果 pH＞7.65，死亡率为 80%。

病因

- 呼吸性碱中毒：
- 中枢神经系统：
  - 过度通气综合征。
  - 疼痛。
  - 焦虑、精神病。
  - 发热。
  - 脑血管意外（CVA）。
  - 中枢神经系统感染（脑膜炎、脑炎）。
  - 中枢神经系统肿块（肿瘤、创伤）。
- 低氧血症：
  - 海拔高度。
  - 贫血。
  - 分流。
- 药物：
  - 黄体酮。
  - 甲基黄嘌呤。
  - 水杨酸盐。
  - 儿茶酚胺。
  - 尼古丁。
- 内分泌：
  - 甲状腺功能亢进症。
  - 妊娠。
- 胸部刺激：
  - 肺栓塞。
  - 肺炎。
  - 气胸。
- 其他：
  - 败血症。
  - 肝功能衰竭。
  - 中暑。
- 代谢性碱中毒：
- 氯离子缺乏：
  - 消化道丢失：
    - 呕吐。
    - 鼻胃管（NG）吸引。
    - 高输出回肠造口丢失。
    - 氯丢失性腹泻（绒毛状腺瘤）。
  - 肾脏损失：
    - 利尿剂（襻利尿剂和噻嗪类利尿剂）。
    - 术后（慢性）高碳酸血症。
    - 药物（羧苄西林）。
    - Gitelman 综合征（氯丢失）。
    - 氯摄入少。
    - Batter 综合征（氯丢失）。
- HCO_3^- 潴留：
  - $NaHCO_3$ 输液。
  - 输血。
  - 盐皮质激素过量。
    - 醛固酮增多症。
- 其他：
  - 乳碱综合征。
  - 严重钾缺乏。

诊断

症状和体征

- 继发于以下情况的体征和症状：
- 小动脉血管收缩。
- 钙与白蛋白结合增加继发电离钙减少的低钙血症。
- 相关的低钾血症。
- 原因不明。
- 虚弱。
- 癫痫发作。
- 心理状态改变。
- 强直。
- Chvostek 标志。
- Trousseau 标志。
- 心律失常。
- 肌痛。
- 腕骨痉挛。
- 口周刺痛、麻木。
- 低氧血症。
- 脱水。

基本检查

- 电解质：
- HCO_3^- 升高与代谢性碱中毒。
- 评估低钾血症和低钙血症。
- BUN、肌酐：
- 评估肾衰竭或脱水。
- 血气（动脉、静脉）：
- pH。
- 呼吸性碱中毒 PCO_2 减少。
- 低氧血症 PO_2 减少。
- 静脉血气与动脉血气相比。
  - pH：良好相关性在 0.03～0.04 单位内。
  - pCO_2：良好的相关性，虽然 VBG 可能与严重休克无关。
  - HCO_3^-：良好的相关性。
  - 基础过剩：良好的相关性。
- 计算补偿以识别混合酸碱障碍：
- 急性呼吸性碱中毒：
  - HCO_3^- 降低继发于细胞内转移和缓冲对在 10～20 min 内的效应。
  - PCO_2 每降低 10 mmHg 预计 HCO_3^- 减少 2 mEq/dl。
- 慢性呼吸性碱中毒：

J

◦ HCO_3^- 降低继发于肾脏分泌继发 HCO_3^- 变化。
◦ 最大代偿需要48～72 h。
◦ 预计 PCO_2 每下降10 mmHg，HCO_3^- 下降5 mEq/dl。
◦ 如果 HCO_3^- 大于预测值，则伴随代谢性碱中毒。
◦ 如果 HCO_3 低于预测值，则伴随代谢性酸中毒。
- 代谢性碱中毒：
◦ 预计 $PCO_2=0.9[HCO_3^-]+9$。
◦ 如果 PCO_2 大于预测值，则伴随呼吸性酸中毒。
◦ 如果 PCO_2 低于预测值，则伴随呼吸性碱中毒。
• 尿氯化物：
- 比尿 Na^+ 更准确地显示患者的容量状态：
◦ UCl<20 mEq/L，提示血容量不足。
◦ UCl>40 mEq/L 提示血容量过多或水肿状态。
• 有助于确定盐水反应与耐盐水的代谢性碱中毒的原因。

诊断检查与说明

实验室检查

• 葡萄糖。
• 离子钙。
• 镁水平。
• 尿妊娠。
• 评估潜在病因的其他实验室检查：
- CBC 败血症的血培养。
- LFT 评估肝功能衰竭。
- 阿司匹林水平。
- 尿液毒理学筛选。
- 尿液利尿剂筛查(暴食症)。
- 尿液利尿剂筛查(私自滥用利尿剂)。
- Renin 级别。
- 皮质醇水平。
- 醛固酮水平。
- TSH、T_4。
- D-二聚体。

影像学检查

CXR：
• 可以识别心肌病或 CHF。
• 潜在的肺炎。

诊断步骤/外科

心电图：
• 可以识别局部室壁运动异常或瓣膜功能障碍。
• 评估传导干扰。

鉴别诊断

• 呼吸性碱中毒：
- 在诊断过度通气综合征或焦虑症状态之前排除器质性疾病至关重要。
• 代谢性碱中毒：
- 盐敏感(尿液 Cl^- - 20 mEq/dl)：
◦ 胃分泌物丢失。
◦ 失氯性腹泻。
◦ 利尿剂。
◦ 术后(慢性)高碳酸血症。
◦ CF。
- 耐盐：
◦ 醛固酮增多症。
◦ 库欣综合征。
◦ 巴特综合征。
◦ 外源性盐皮质激素或糖皮质激素。
◦ 吉特曼综合征。
◦ 低钾血症。
◦ 低镁血症。
◦ MIJK-碱综合征。
◦ 外源性碱输注/摄入。
◦ 输血。

治疗

初步稳定/治疗

呼吸道，呼吸，循环(ABC)：
• 精神状态改变者早期插管和气道控制。
• 静脉注射，氧气和心脏监测。
• 精神状态改变用纳洛酮、$D_{50}W$(或 Accu-Chek)和硫胺素。

急诊治疗/程序

• 呼吸性碱中毒：
- 潜在疾病治疗。
- 极少危及生命。
- 镇静/抗焦虑药物治疗焦虑，精神病或药物滥用。
- 过度通气综合征用呼吸循环的面罩(谨慎使用)。
• 代谢性碱中毒：检查尿液氯化物可以将病因分为氯化物耗竭或非氯化物耗竭性碱中毒：
- 氯化物<10 mEq/L 表示氯化物耗竭：
◦ 评估水合状况以确定治疗方法。
◦ 用氯化钾输注血容量/容量过大状态。
◦ 用生理盐水治疗血容量不足可通过增加肾脏 HCO_3^- 排泄降低血清 HCO_3^-。
- 尿氯化物>30 mEq/L 表示无氯消耗的病因。
- 治疗潜在疾病：
◦ 低钾状态的钾补充。
◦ 醛固酮与螺内酯的拮抗作用。
◦ 乙酰唑胺可增强水肿状态的肾脏 HCO_3^- 排泄。
- 其他：
◦ 呕吐止吐药。
◦ 质子泵抑制剂用于 NG 抽吸患者。
◦ 密切关注通气状态。
◦ 纠正电解质异常。
◦ 考虑血液透析治疗严重的电解质异常。

药物治疗

• 葡萄糖：$D_{50}W$ 1 安瓿(50 ml 或 25 g；儿童：25%葡萄糖和水 2～4 ml/kg)，静脉注射。
• 氯化钾(K-Dur、Gen-K、Klor-Con)：每日20～120 mEq 口服。
• 纳洛酮：2 mg(儿童：0.1 mg/kg)静脉注射或肌内注射初始剂量。
• 硫胺素(维生素 B_1)：100 mg(儿童：50 mg)静脉注射或肌内注射。
• 0.1～0.2 mol HCl(100～200 mEq/L)：以不超过0.2 mmol/(kg·h)的速率并通过中心静脉注入24～48 h以防止静脉硬化。

随访

进一步处理

入院指征

• 以下情况可入住 ICU：
- pH>7.55 或精神状态改变。
- 心律失常。
- 严重的电解质异常。
- 血流动力学不稳定。
• 合并需要入院治疗的疾病。

出院指征

碱中毒好转。

要点和误区

• 分钟通气量增加是呼吸性碱中毒的主要原因，其特征在于 $PaCO_2$ 降低和 pH 升高：
- 代谢性碱中毒通常是由于 HCO_3^- 的增加，继发于容量，钾或 Cl^- 损失的重吸收所致。
- 传统思想将碱中毒分为收缩性和非收缩性碱中毒；然而，新的文献表明，这实际上是一种氯化物耗竭或非氯化物耗竭性碱中毒，

J

导致血浆 HCO_3^- 浓度增加。

- 可能存在混合酸碱紊乱的线索是正常 pH、PCO_2 或 HCO_3^- 异常，当 HCO_3^- 和 PCO_2 沿相反方向移动时，或者当 pH 沿与预期相反的方向变化时。已知的原发性疾病。

腱鞘炎 Tenosynovitis

James Killeen · Brenna Dersen 范浩浩 李文放 译

基础知识

描述

- 定义：
  - 肌腱和肌腱鞘的炎症和疼痛。
  - 由急慢性炎症、过度使用或感染引起。
  - 导致疼痛、活动度下降、坏死和肌腱断裂。
- 解剖：
  - 滑膜鞘在肌腱穿过骨纤维隧道时覆盖肌腱：
  - 滑膜的脏层和壁层润滑和滋养肌腱。
- 病理生理学：
  - 炎症：纤维组织增生引起疼痛的摩擦，冲击/收缩肌腱。与糖尿病类和类风湿性关节炎高度相关。
  - 过度使用：重复性微创伤导致炎症和纤维化。
  - 感染：最常见的急性情况如下：
    - 进入腱鞘通过：
      - 皮肤损伤/穿刺最常见。
      - 血行播散。
- 手屈肌腱鞘炎(FTS)：屈肌肌腱闭合性感染，见于骨科急诊。
  - 最常见的机制是手指屈折处的穿透伤。
  - 原因包括：
    - 穿透性创伤。
    - 咬伤。
    - 高压注射(喷漆机、油枪)。
    - 气动工具。
    - 液压设备：表面看起来很轻微，但与 FTS 的高发病率有关。
    - 血源性或从深处或关节感染直接传播。

病因

- de Querrain 腱鞘炎：
  - 过度使用导致。
  - 炎症。
  - 2 种拇指肌腱：拇长展肌(APL)和拇短伸肌(EPB)。
  - 在拇指根部附近，APL 和 FPB 穿过一层厚的纤维鞘，在桡骨茎突处形成隧道。
  - 过度使用会导致伸肌支持带增厚和管腔狭窄。
- 非淋球菌感染性腱鞘炎：
  - 金黄色葡萄球菌和链球菌常见于穿透性损伤，但常见多种微生物感染。
  - 多杀巴斯德菌常见于猫咬伤。
  - 啮蚀艾肯菌在人类叮咬中很常见。
  - 糖尿病或海洋相关伤害的患者中可见假单胞菌。
  - 免疫力低下的患者可能出现分枝杆菌：怀疑是慢性惰性疾病。
- 淋球菌性腱鞘炎：
  - 传播性淋病奈瑟菌。
- 真菌性腱鞘炎可由荆棘或木本植物造成的刺伤引起。

诊断

症状和体征

- Kanavel 针对 FTS 的主要标志包括：
  - 沿着屈肌腱鞘压痛。
  - 梭形肿胀(香肠指)。
- 手指屈曲位。
- 手指被动伸展引起疼痛。

手

- De Quervain 腱鞘炎：
  - 拇指和其他手指的反复捏合动作。
- 装配线工人。
- 木匠。
- 园林绿化或除草人员。
  - 沿手腕桡侧疼痛。
  - 活动时疼痛加剧，休息时疼痛改善。
  - 拇指被动活动范围疼痛。
  - 抓伤或折断伤。
  - 芬克尔斯坦测试：
    - 拇指握于拳内时手腕部尺侧疼痛。
- 扳机指：掌侧屈肌腱鞘炎。
  - 常影响拇指和无名指。
  - 手指屈曲时锁定，突然松开后手指疼痛。
  - 近端腱鞘压痛，增厚，结节状。
- FTS：
  - 手部穿透伤。
  - 卡内韦尔征阳性。
- GC 腱鞘炎：
  - 最常见的影响：
    - 青少年。
    - 女性。
    - 踝、手和手腕。
  - 发热，发冷，多关节疼痛很常见。
  - 红斑，触诊压痛，疼痛涉及肌腱的运动范围。
  - 通常无阴道或阴茎分泌物。
  - 远端肢体或躯干可能出现皮炎或出血性斑疹或丘疹。

前臂

创伤性腱鞘炎可能是在前臂下部受到直接打击后出现的。

踝

- 狭窄性腱鞘炎：
  - 腓骨肌腱下支持带常见。
  - 患者通常年龄>40 岁，有一些易感创伤。
  - 运动增加疼痛。
- 类风湿性腱鞘炎：
  - 内侧，常累及胫后肌腱和拇长屈肌腱。
  - 侧方累及腓骨肌总腱鞘。
  - 前方累及胫骨前肌腱。
  - 活动增加了疼痛。
  - 可能会发生自发断裂。

病史

- 评估传染性病因：
  - 性传播疾病暴露史；然而往往无阴茎或阴道分泌物。
- 获取机制的病史：
  - 高压注射。
  - 刺伤，咬伤。
  - 环境暴露。
- 评估破伤风状况和共病因素(如糖尿病和免疫功能低下)。

体格检查

- 检查卡内韦尔征。
- 记录神经血管状态。
- 如果存在急性腱鞘炎，肌腱鞘则会肿胀。

• 识别系统性疾病的体征和症状，以及其他潜在的感染部位。

■ 基本检查

详细的病史和体格检查通常会引导出正确的诊断。

■ 诊断检查与说明

实验室检查

• 如果关注感染性病因：

- CBC、ESR。
- 考虑 GC 培养（尿道、宫颈、直肠或咽下肌），如果是 GC 的危险因素还有 LFT。

影像学检查

• 射线意义小，除非保留不透射线的软组织异物的怀疑。

• MRI 已被证明可以协助诊断腱鞘炎：

- 急诊治疗通常不需要。

诊断步骤/外科

• 握拳尺偏试验。

• 怀疑化脓性关节炎则进行关节穿刺。

■ 鉴别诊断

• 脓肿。
• 踝关节、软组织损伤。
• 滑囊炎。
• 腕管综合征。
• 蜂窝织炎。
• 间隔综合征。
• 指关节炎
• 心内膜炎。
• 瘭疽（化脓性指头炎）。
• 淋病。
• 痛风和假性痛风。
• 手部感染。
• 高压手部受伤。
• 骨关节炎。
• 软组织损伤。
• 赖特综合征。
• 风湿热。
• 类风湿关节炎。

治疗

■ 院前

• 延迟确诊治疗导致发病率明显增加和功能丧失。

• 应进行患肢的抬高和制动。

■ 初步稳定/治疗

• 按照指南管理呼吸道和复苏：

- 感染性休克。

• 抬高，受影响的肢体制动。

• 建立静脉通路。

• 破伤风免疫。

• 程序：

- 如果关节积液伴腱鞘炎，建议行诊断性关节穿刺：
  ◦ 大多数播散性 GC 感染的患者往往合并化脓性关节炎。
  ◦ 50%的患者的培养是阴性的。
  ◦ 25%的 GC 关节炎是多关节的。

■ 急诊治疗/程序

手

• 手部高压注射伤害：

- 外科急诊。
- 立即手外科医师会诊。
- 疼痛管理。

• 手感染性 FTS：

- 立即进行手外科医师会诊。
- 广谱抗生素覆盖。

• De Quervain 腱鞘炎：

- 休息，NSAIDs 治疗和拇指角状夹板。
- 如果情况没有好转，使用利多卡因/皮质类固醇注射剂。
- 超声药物透入疗法（每日在桡骨茎突区应用氢化可的松凝胶）。
- 如果疼痛或肿胀持续 2～6 周，则将糖皮质激素注射到第一伸肌室的皮损部位。

• 掌侧屈肌腱鞘炎（扳机指）：

- 休息，非甾体抗炎药，夹板固定。
- 腱膜周围利多卡因-皮质类固醇注射。
- 可能需要最终的手术肌腱松解。

• GC 腱鞘炎：

- 静脉抗生素治疗。
- 作为替代方案。
- 如果使用抗生素不能改善病情，可能需要手术引流。
- 疼痛管理。

• 非淋球菌感染性腱鞘炎：

- 如果诊断不明确，患者应该接受静脉抗生素治疗并请手外科医师会诊。
- 治疗覆盖葡萄球菌、链球菌，以及厌氧菌。
- 糖尿病或免疫功能低下的患者抗感染方案覆盖假单胞菌。
- 可添加氨基糖苷类药物以实现双重覆盖。
- 疼痛管理。

前臂

• 创伤性腱鞘炎：

- 休息，冰敷，抬高，制动，NSAIDs。

踝

• 狭窄性腱鞘炎：

- 休息，冰敷，抬高，制动，NSAIDs。

• 类风湿性腱鞘炎：

- 休息，冰敷，抬高，制动，NSAIDs。
- 羟基氯喹，甲氨蝶呤，口服类固醇，类固醇注射。

■ 药物治疗

• 阿奇霉素：1 g，口服，一次。

• 头孢唑林：1～2 g，静脉滴注，q8 h[儿童：50～100 mg/(kg・d)，静脉滴注，div，q8 h]。

• 头孢噻肟：1 g，静脉滴注，8 h[儿童：50～200 mg/(kg・d)静脉滴注/肌注，div，q6～8 h]。

• 头孢替坦：1～2 g，静脉滴注，q12 h[儿童：50～100 mg/(kg・d)静脉滴注，div，q12 h]。

• 头孢西丁：1～2 g，静脉滴注，q8 h[儿童：80～160 mg/(kg・d)静脉滴注，div，q6～8 h]。

• 头孢唑肟：1 g，静脉滴注，q8 h[儿童：100～200 mg/(kg・d)静脉滴注，div，q6～8 h]。

• 头孢曲松：1～2 g，静脉滴注，q12 h[儿童：50～100 mg/(kg・d)静脉滴注，div，q12 h]。

• 克林霉素：600～900 mg，静脉滴注，q8 h[儿童：20～40 mg/(kg・d)，静脉滴注，div，q8 h]。

• 青霉素：1 200 万～2 400 万 U，静脉滴注，div q4～6 h[儿童：100 000～40 000 U/(kg・d)，静脉滴注，div，q4～6 h]。

• 替门汀：3.1 g，静脉滴注，q6 h[儿童：200～300 mg/(kg・d)，静脉滴注，div，q4～6 h]。

• 妥布霉素：1 mg/kg，静脉滴注，q8 h；或者 5 mg/(kg・d)，静脉滴注，q24 h[儿童：2～2.5 mg/kg，静脉滴注，div，q8 h]。

• 哌拉西林钠：3.375 g，静脉滴注，q6 h[儿童：200～400 mg/(kg・d)，静脉滴注，div，q6～8 h]。

一线用药

• FTS：

- 头孢唑林：1～2 g，静脉滴注，q6～8 h。
- PCN 过敏：克林霉素，600 mg，静脉滴注，q8 h。

• GC 腱鞘炎：

- 头孢曲松：1 g，静脉滴注/肌内注射，q24 h，PLUS。
- 阿奇霉素：1 g，口服。

• 德奎尔万和炎症情况：

- NSAIDs：400～800 mg，口服，q6～8 h(儿童：5～10 mg/kg)。

二线用药

• FTS：见上文"用药"部分。

• GC 腱鞘炎：

- 头孢噻肟 1 g，静脉滴注，q8 h；或头孢唑肟 1 g，静脉滴注，q8 h，PLUS。

- 阿奇霉素 1 g，口服，顿服。

妊娠注意事项

妊娠 30 周后注意 NSAIDs 禁忌证。

儿科注意事项

非甾体抗炎药在 6 个月前禁用。

随访

进一步处理

• FTS 患者需要立即请手外科专家会诊并收入院。

• 症状持续 24～48 h 的患者可能需要更多保守治疗，包括制动、抬高、静脉滴注抗生素，并密切观察。

• 如果患者在第一个 24 h 内没有改善，或在 48 h 内阳性体征没有缓解则推荐外科清创术。

• 超过 48 h 的患者需要在手术室进行手术清创。

• 手外科医师可能会尝试持续导管冲洗肌腱鞘。

入院指征

• 病因为感染性或高压性腱鞘炎的患者应该被收入院。

• 疑似淋菌性腱鞘炎。

出院指征

炎症病因可以在适当转诊的状况下门诊治疗。

随访建议

• de Quervain 腱鞘炎和掌侧屈肌腱鞘炎：

- 初级保健医师或手病专家门诊转诊。

• 类风湿相关 FTS：

- 风湿病转诊。

要点和误区

• 类固醇注射应该慎用。

- 如果直接注射到肌腱中有害。

- 多次注射会削弱肌腱并有破裂的风险。

• 急诊就诊不推荐口服类固醇。

降糖药中毒 Hypoglycemic Agent Poisoning

Timothy J. Meehan 倪沁赟 译

基础知识

描述

• 口服或肠外药物可能导致低血糖或其他代谢紊乱。

• 降糖药中毒可能是有意或无意的事件。

病因

• 胰岛素：

- 促进葡萄糖向细胞内转移。

- 限制大脑的葡萄糖供应(大脑对低血糖非常敏感)。

- 影响钾离子的转移(低钾血症)。

• 磺酰脲类和格列奈类药物：

- 作用于胰岛 β 细胞促进胰岛素的释放，降低肝脏葡萄糖的产生，增加外周胰岛素的敏感性。

- 降血糖作用增强通过：

◦ 多种药物(药物的相互作用)。

◦ 饮酒和肝功能衰竭(营养不良)。

◦ 肾功能不全(清除下降)。

• 胰高血糖素样肽 1(GLP1)调节剂：

- 艾塞那肽是一种胰高血糖素样肽-1 类药物。

- 列汀类药物是一种二肽基肽酶Ⅳ抑制剂类药物(DPP4 抑制剂)，通常抑制 GLP1。

- 净效应：增强胰岛素分泌，延迟胃排空，增加饱腹感。

- 药物过量后对血糖的代谢效应尚不明确(目前缺乏数据)。

• 双胍类药物(二甲双胍)：

- 降糖药：

◦ 降低升高的血糖水平。

◦ 单独使用一般不引起低血糖。

- 在胰岛素存在的情况下，双胍类药物的作用：

◦ 促进葡萄糖向细胞内转移。

◦ 限制大脑的葡萄糖供应(大脑对低血糖非常敏感)。

◦ 影响钾离子的转移(低钾血症)。

◦ 降低胃肠道对葡萄糖的吸收。

◦ 降低肝脏的糖异生。

◦ 在肠道细胞的将葡萄糖代谢成乳酸，乳酸积累后可能导致酸中毒。

• 葡萄糖钠协同转运体 2 抑制剂：

- 依帕列净和卡格列净。

- 干扰过滤后葡萄糖的肾脏再摄取。

- 导致渗透性利尿，但通常用于单一治疗时降血糖：

◦ 可以增强胰岛素/磺脲类药物的效果。

◦ 可导致明显的低血糖组合。

◦ 报告导致血糖正常的 DKA。

• 噻唑烷二酮类：

- 在胰岛素存在的情况下，噻唑烷二酮类药物增加血糖的吸收和利用，降低糖异生。

• α-葡萄糖苷酶抑制剂：

- 通过降低胃肠道对碳水化合物的吸收，降低血糖水平。

诊断

症状和体征

• 胰岛素或磺脲类药物：

- 过量使用导致低血糖。

- 当血糖＜40～60 mg/dl 时常有症状发生(糖尿病患者在更高水平即出现症状)。

- 使用 β 受体阻滞剂症状减弱。

- 面部潮红、出汗、面色苍白、立毛。

- 饥饿、恶心、腹部绞痛。

- 呼吸困难、呼吸暂停。

- 头痛、视力模糊。

- 感觉异常、虚弱、共济失调、震颤。

- 焦虑、易怒、行为怪异、混乱、恍惚、昏迷、癫痫发作。

- 心悸、心动过速、心动过缓(发生较晚)。

- 低血压。

- 低体温。

• 双胍类药物：

- 中毒主要源于乳酸积累。
- 恶心、呕吐、腹痛。
- 兴奋、混乱、嗜睡、昏迷。
- Kussmaul 式呼吸。
- 低血压、心动过速。

儿科注意事项

• 通常在母体使用磺脲类药物后出现新生儿低血糖。

• 摄入 1 片磺脲类药物即可导致儿童低血糖：
- 曾有报道在使用 1 片磺脲类药物后死亡的病例。

• 出现低血糖症状可能会延迟 8 h。

病史

• 诊断糖尿病的患者。

• 糖尿病药物：
- 如果发生在医疗环境下（如医院、养老院），需考虑以下原因：
  ◦ 药物剂量错误。
  ◦ 人为因素（恶意）。

体格检查

• 生命体征：
- 心动过速（可能需要使用β受体阻滞剂）。

• 神经系统：
- 混乱、反应迟钝、昏迷。
- 共济失调、其他小脑体征。

▪ 基本检查

• 基于临床表现和准确的既往史诊断。

• 监测血糖。

• 监测生命体征和神经系统表现。

• 双胍类药物使用后监测电解质和乳酸值。

• 噻唑烷二酮药物使用监测肝功能指标。

▪ 诊断检查与说明

实验室检查

• 治疗前后监测血糖。

• 电解质：
- 明确是否存在低钾血症。
- 酸中毒情况下的 AG 值（阴离子间隙）。

• 尿素氮、肌酐：
- 肾功能不全可能会导致药物累积。

• 全血细胞计数

• 酒精水平。

• 乳酸水平（特别是使用双胍类药物的患者）。

• 肝功能指标。

• 动脉血气分析。

• 免疫反应性胰岛素和 C 肽水平的分析：
- 在低血糖的情况下，如果胰岛素水平高而 C 肽水平低，确定有无外源性胰岛素的使用。
- 与临床症状的敏感性并不相同。

影像学检查

• 心电图：窦性心动过速、室性期前收缩、房性心律失常。

• 脑电图：弥漫性改变而不是局灶性异常。

• CT 扫描：如果低血糖时间长，会有脑水肿表现。

• X 线胸片：肺炎或者肺水肿。

▪ 鉴别诊断

• 艾迪生病（肾上腺皮质功能不全）。

• 垂体功能减退症。

• 脓毒血症。

• 胰岛素瘤。

• 神经内分泌肿瘤。

• 肝硬化。

• 慢性酒精中毒。

• 酒精摄入。

• 水杨酸摄入。

• β受体阻滞剂摄入。

• Ackee 果实中毒。

治疗

▪ 院前

携带所有的药物包括药瓶，在急诊室明确是否药物过量。

▪ 初步稳定/治疗

• 基础支持治疗：
- 保持气道通畅。
- 吸氧。
- 静脉通道建立。
- 心电监护和指脉氧监测。

• 如果精神状态改变，给予纳洛酮、维生素 B_1、D_{50}（或 Accu-Chek）。

▪ 急诊治疗/程序

• 低血糖：
- D_{50} 药丸，然后：
  ◦ 静脉注射 5% 或 10% 葡萄糖注射液维持正常血糖或轻度低血糖。
  ◦ 饮食疗法（在患者心理状态改善或正常的情况下）。

• 神经低血糖：
- 血糖纠正后症状持续时间短。
- 症状持续存在则需要更多的葡萄糖继续治疗。

• 清除过量口服药物：
- 可选择活性炭（磺脲类药物或双胍类药物）。

• 支持治疗。

• 低血压：
- 生理盐水输注。
- 使用血管活性药物多巴胺或去甲肾上腺素：
  ◦ 可能会导致乳酸产生增加。
  ◦ 双胍类药物导致乳酸酸中毒，血管活性药物需要谨慎使用。

• 双胍类药物导致乳酸酸中毒，pH<7，则使用碳酸氢钠。

• 癫痫发作的患者使用苯二氮䓬类药物。

• 磺脲类药物过量导致的低血糖，需要抑制胰岛素的分泌：
- 奥曲肽。
- 氯甲苯噻嗪（避免低血压的发生）。

• 针对双胍类药物导致乳酸酸中毒，早期行血液透析可能有益：
- 纠正酸碱平衡失调。
- 增强药物的清除。

▪ 药物治疗

• 活性炭：1 g/kg，口服。

• 葡萄糖：50% 葡萄糖 50～100 ml，静脉注射（儿童患者：20% 葡萄糖 2 ml/kg，至少 1 min），必要时可重复。

• 地西泮：5～10 mg，静脉注射，q10～15 min（儿童患者：0.2～0.5 mg/kg）。

• 氯甲苯噻嗪：200 mg，口服；或 1～3 mg/kg，静脉推注[婴儿：8～15 mg/(kg · 24 h)，q8～12 h，口服或静脉推注；儿童：3～8 mg/(kg · 24 h)，q8 h，口服或静脉推注]。

• 胰高血糖素：1～2 mg（儿童患者：0.03～0.1 mg/kg），肌内注射、皮下注射或静脉推注。

• 劳拉西泮：2～4 mg（儿童患者：0.03～0.05 mg/kg），静脉推注，q10～15 min。

• 奥曲肽：50～100 μg，q8～12 h，皮下注射或静脉推注。

• 维生素 B_1：100 mg（儿童患者：50 mg），静脉推注或肌内注射。

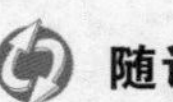

随访

▪ 进一步处理

入院指征

• 因磺脲类药物（可能需要监测数日）或长效胰岛素使用所导致的低血糖。

• 需要持续静脉输注葡萄糖来维持正常血糖。
• 故意过量使用药物或胰岛素的患者需要住院行 24 h 的血糖监测。
• 所有意外吞食磺脲类药物的儿童患者。
• 因双胍类药物摄入或积累所导致的代谢改变。

出院指征

• 糖尿病患者使用短效胰岛素所导致的一过性低血糖：
- 必须耐受口服治疗。
- 确保恢复基础的心理状态。
• 在观察的 4 h 内，血糖正常。

转诊问题

• 意外摄入毒物，需要行毒物咨询的患者。
• 故意中毒（如自杀），需要行精神评估的患者。

随访建议

密切随访以帮助监测血糖和调整合适的药物剂量。

要点和误区

• 磺脲类药物半衰期长，清除时间长：
- 低血糖发生延迟和低血糖恢复慢比较常见。
- 最小剂量使用时即需要观察。
• 血糖正常的 DKA。
- 与 SGLT－2 抑制剂报道。
- 通过脂肪分解和脂肪酸/酮释放增加胰高血糖素的产量。
• 使用静脉造影剂以后，二甲双胍会在体内至少保持 48 h：
- 静脉造影可延长双胍类药物的肾脏清除。
- 可导致二甲双胍相关性乳酸酸中毒。

焦虑症 Agitation

Lee A. Replogle · Maura Kennedy　马林浩　林兆奋 译

基础知识

描述

焦躁不安，极度不安的状态。
• 以语言和运动活动增加为特征。
• 可能包含各种医学（器质性）和精神（功能）疾病的症状。
• 严重程度。
- 从过度健谈到威胁或暴力行为。
- 包括兴奋性谵妄综合征。
◦ 以躁动、酸中毒、过度放射性神经功能紊乱为特征。
◦ 伴有心源性猝死，特别是暴力斗争后。

流行病学

发病率和患病率

• 6%的急诊是针对行为障碍的。
• 每年约有 170 万次急诊涉及患有激动的患者。

病因

药物（有机）因素。
• 传染性：
- 中枢神经系统感染。
◦ 神经性。
◦ 梅毒。
◦ 脑炎脑膜炎。
◦ 脓肿。
- 继发于败血症的活动过度或混合性谵妄。
• 代谢紊乱：
- 电解质紊乱。
◦ 低钠血症。
◦ 低钙血症。
◦ 低血糖。
- 肾衰竭。
- 酸性或碱性紊乱。
- 肝性脑病。
- Wernicke 脑病。
- Wilsons 病。
• 内分泌疾病：
- 甲状腺风暴。
- 甲状旁腺功能亢进。
• 肺部病因：
- 低氧血症。
- 高碳酸血症。
• 毒理学原因：
- 氧化酶。
◦ 拟交感神经。
◦ 抗胆碱能。
◦ 胆碱能。
◦ 酒精中毒。
◦ 酒精戒断。
- 抗精神病药物恶性综合征（NMS）。
- 血清素综合征（SS）。
• 神经学原因：
- 肿瘤。
- 中枢神经系统感染（见上文）。
- Huntington 病。
- 缺血性脑血管意外。
- 外伤性颅内出血。
- 蛛网膜下腔出血。
- 癫痫发作后。
• 精神病（功能性）病因。
• 躁狂/躁郁症。
• 精神分裂症等精神疾病。
• 焦虑障碍。

诊断

症状和体征

详细的病史和体格检查是区分躁动的医学和精神病因的关键。

病史

• HPI 在检测精神病患者的医疗疾病方面有 94%的敏感性。
- 如果患者无法获得详细的 HPI，可向家人、朋友和院前护理人员寻求相关信息。
• 需要：
- 创伤。
- 最近的疾病和发热。
- 头痛、意识丧失、神经功能障碍或视觉幻觉。
- 目前的药物。
- 病史：
◦ 精神疾病。
◦ 药物滥用。
◦ 癌症。
◦ 艾滋病病毒/免疫抑制状态。
◦ 神经系统疾病，包括癫痫。

体格检查

彻底的检查对于区分器质性病因和功能性病因至关重要。
• 生命体征异常应促使对器质性病因进行

全面评估。

- 发热可能提示感染性病因、NMS、SS 或兴奋性谵妄综合征。

• 进行以毒素为导向的检查，包括：

- 瞳孔评估。
- 皮肤评估。
- 尿潴留评估。

• 必须进行详细的神经系统检查。

- 任何神经系统缺陷都需要对潜在的医学疾病进行全面的评估。
- 有躁动的患者应保持完整的定位、记忆和注意力。
  ◦ 改变方向和记忆中谵妄和痴呆。
  ◦ 注意力不集中，如无法描述 1 周内的事，应该提高对谵妄的怀疑。
- 应评估肌肉张力和反射。
  ◦ 肌肉硬度可能表明 NMS。
  ◦ 反射亢进和阵挛可能表明 SS。

▪ 诊断检查和说明

诊断工作由病史、体格检查和对躁动的医学病因的潜在怀疑指导。

▪ 基本检查

至少所有患者都应该具备：

• 完整的生命体征。

• 完整的体格检查，包括详细的神经系统检查、认知和注意力测试。

• 血糖。

▪ 诊断检查与说明

诊断检查应以怀疑患者躁动的器质性病因、病史和体格检查作为依据。

影像学检查

创伤患者或有神经缺陷的患者应考虑头颅 CT。

诊断步骤/外科

• 患者应考虑腰椎穿刺：

- 脑膜征。
- 怀疑感染是躁动的病因，但没有发现病因。

▪ 鉴别诊断

躁动可能是潜在疾病、药物滥用、戒断或精神疾病的表现症状。

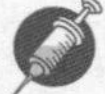

治疗

▪ 院前

院前工作人员经常遇到焦虑或暴力的患者，应该：

• 遵守关于物理和化学限制的区域协议。

• 在运送焦虑或暴力患者时提供预先通知，以便接收医院可以调动必要的资源。

• 在可行的情况下获得指间血糖。

▪ 初始稳定/治疗

• ABC 管理。

• 酌情治疗危及生命的医疗/创伤性疾病。

• 严重烦躁的患者可能会变得暴力，对工作人员和其他患者造成伤害。

- 患者应换上病号服，并搜查是否携带武器。
- 必要时应使用物理和化学约束装置，以确保患者和工作人员的安全。

▪ 急诊治疗/程序

• 怀疑或诊断出器质性病因时。

• 治疗应针对潜在病因。

• 怀疑或诊断出功能性病因时。

• 指示紧急精神科转诊。

• 焦虑管理。

• 言语减压技术是轻度或中度焦虑的第一道防线。

- 考虑言语降级的“十个步骤”：
  ◦ 尊重个人空间。
  ◦ 不要挑衅。
  ◦ 建立语言联系。
  ◦ 简明扼要。
  ◦ 识别需求和感受。
  ◦ 仔细聆听患者的讲话。
  ◦ 同意或不同意。
  ◦ 放下法律并设定明确的界限。
  ◦ 提供选择和乐观。
  ◦ 向患者和工作人员汇报。

• 药物控制包括：

- 苯二氮䓬类。
  ◦ 一线疗法，用于无法区别的躁动，要戒酒。
  ◦ 劳拉西泮或咪达唑仑（半衰期较短）。
  ◦ 副作用：呼吸抑制，过多的嗜睡，反常的抑制作用（罕见）；老年医学考虑：可能出现谵妄或谵妄恶化。
- 抗精神病药：
  ◦ 躁动/精神病的精神病学患者的第一线。
  ◦ 第一代：氟哌啶醇或氟哌利多（半衰期较短）。
  ◦ 第二代：奥氮平、利培酮或齐拉西酮（镇静作用少，锥体外系症状少）。
    ▪ 副作用：QTC 延长和锥体束外症状：
    ▪ 当言语降级不成功时，低剂量可用于精神错乱的老年患者。
- 氯胺酮：
  ◦ 在以下情况下可考虑用于严重躁动患者：抗精神病药和苯二氮䓬类药物失败，疑似兴奋谵妄综合征。
  ◦ 副作用：口腔分泌物增多、呕吐、喉痉挛（罕见）、高血压、心动过速、呼吸抑制，出现现象：
    ▪ 应密切监测生命体征、精神状态和呼吸状态。
    ▪ 劳拉西泮可同时服用以防止氯胺酮出现现象。
    ▪ 在院前环境中进行剧烈躁动可能会与高比例的急诊插管有关。
- 联合疗法：
  ◦ 可能比单药治疗产生更快的镇静作用。
  ◦ 高度激动/暴力患者应考虑。

• 咪达唑仑、氟哌利多、劳拉西泮和氟哌啶醇身体约束的使用：

• 应使用化学镇静剂以尽早停止身体约束。

• 医师和护士必须记录使用情况和使用理由。

• 长时间使用会导致：

- 热疗。
- 横纹肌溶解。
- 如果四肢长时间保持在同一位置，则会造成神经损伤。
- 兴奋谵妄综合征。

▪ 用药治疗

• 氟哌利多 2.5～5 mg，静脉注射或肌内注射，q3 h。

• 氟哌啶醇 2～10 mg，静脉注射或肌内注射，q3 h。

• 氯胺酮：

- 肌内注射：2～4 mg/kg（最大剂量 400 mg）。考虑起始剂量为 2 mg/kg（最大剂量 200 mg），在 5 min 内重复 prn×1，最大剂量为 4 mg/kg。
- 静脉注射：0.5～1 mg/kg。考虑起始剂量为 0.5 mg/kg，5 min 后重复 prn×1，最大剂量为 1 mg/kg。

• 劳拉西泮 0.5～2 mg，静脉注射或肌内注射。

• 咪达唑仑：

- 0.07 mg/kg，肌内注射；或 1 mg，静脉注射缓慢 q3 min，至 5 mg。

随访

▪ 进一步处理

入院指征

• 进一步处理最终取决于躁动的潜在原因，

以及该情况是否得到解决。

• 如果有潜在的医学或精神疾病需要住院治疗，住院是必要的。

出院指征

出院应限于那些根本原因解决的个人（如物质使用、滥用）和/或可以安全地作为门诊患者对待。

转诊问题

• 适当的精神病学推荐。

• 适当的酒精/药物治疗。

随访建议

随访由病因、医疗或精神状况决定。

要点和误区

寻找可能引起躁动的病因。

• 提示病因的因素包括：
- 新发病时年龄＞45 岁。
- 生命体征异常。
- 局部神经系统异常。
- 急性起病。
- 视觉幻觉。
- 记忆异常或认知测试注意力不集中。
- 注意头部创伤的证据。

• 未评估躁动的潜在原因。

• 不脱衣服和排查武器。

• 镇静剂/抗精神病药物剂量不足。

• 未能调整肢体位置以防止神经并发症。

• 无法记录需要克制的情况。

• 过度用药的患者需要插管或逆转。

角膜擦伤 Corneal Abrasion

Tracy MacIntosh · Yasuharu Okuda 陈奇通 译

基础知识

描述

• 角膜上皮的任何撕裂或缺损。

• 可能是外伤性的，自发性的，由于异物或佩戴隐形眼镜引起。

病因

• 创伤性。
- 人的指甲。
- 隐形眼镜操作。
- 环境要素：树枝、沙子或石头。
- 化学灼伤。
- 气囊调配。
- 胡椒粉喷雾。
- 化妆敷抹器。

• 相关异物：
- 木头。
- 玻璃。
- 金属。
- 铁锈。
- 塑料。
- 纤维玻璃。
- 植物物质。
- 眼睑异物。

• 接触镜片相关：
- 过度佩戴。
- 不适当安装或清洗。

• 自发性：
- 常为先前创伤性角膜擦伤或角膜上皮潜在缺损。

诊断

症状和体征

• 严重眼球疼痛。

• 异物感。

• 流泪。

• 眼睑痉挛。

• 畏光（特别是如果继发性创伤性虹膜炎存在时）。

• 结膜充血。

• 视物减退或模糊。

病史

• 对眼球的直接伤害。

• 已知或潜在的异物。

• 接触镜片使用。

• 既往角膜擦伤的病史。

• 眼睛、眼旁手术。

• 先前存在的视力损害。

• 发作时间。

• 相关症状和合并损伤。

• 就诊前处理。

• 职业风险：使用安全眼镜（敲击、钻孔、研磨金属）或眼镜。

• 全身性疾病（糖尿病、自身免疫性疾病）。

• 破伤风状态。

儿科注意事项

• 症状和体征可能不同：
- 极度哭泣。

• 小于 12 个月：
- 常无眼外伤史。
- 可能表现为哭泣且无法安慰的婴儿。
- 在 1～12 周婴儿中可能是偶然的发现，而不是烦躁不安或哭泣。

• 大于 12 个月：
- 更常有小的眼部外伤病史。
- 阳性眼部体征。

体格检查

• 如可以，注意在首次检查时评估其他危及生命的损伤。

• 完整眼科检查：
- 重点评估是否存在穿透损伤和/或感染的证据。
- 全面视力检查。
- 视觉敏锐度。
- 手电筒检查以评估结膜充血、瞳孔形状/反应性和角膜浸润或斑块的证据。
- 翻起上眼睑以检查残留异物。
- 裂隙灯检查评估异物、前房反应、浸润、角膜裂伤和穿透伤。
- 荧光染料以分辨角膜上皮缺陷的大小和位置。
- 局部麻醉药的应用通常可以改善症状。

基本检查

完成眼部检查，排除眼球破裂，包括视力、大体检查和荧光素。

诊断检查与说明

儿科注意事项

手持裂隙灯和 Wood 灯：儿童眼镜检查中有作用。

鉴别诊断

• 结膜炎，病毒或细菌。

• 角膜溃疡。
• 青光眼。
• 带状疱疹。
• 角膜炎，病毒或细菌或紫外线引起。
• 复发性角膜腐蚀综合征。
• 葡萄膜炎。
• 较角膜擦伤更广泛病变：
- 角膜裂伤。
- 角膜穿孔。
- 前房积血。
- 前房积脓。
- 虹膜下垂。
- 晶状体破裂。
- 眼球破裂。

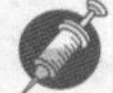

治疗

初步稳定/治疗

灌注局部麻醉(丙美卡因、丁卡因)。

急诊治疗/程序

• 浅表异物的去除：
- 残余的锈环不需要急诊去除。它可以在24～48 h去除。
• 口服止痛：
- 口服对乙酰氨基酚、非甾体抗炎药或麻醉剂：大多数小擦伤(≤4 mm)可在一夜之间愈合。
• 局部麻醉剂：
- 目前的证据是有争议的，目前不推荐；短期并发症可能包括视力下降、畏光、疼痛、撕裂、角膜浸润和水肿。
• 局部止痛药：
- 研究证明有效，然而有零星不良反应的报道。
- 另一只眼睛表面疾病和手术后的患者应避免使用。
- 局部双氯芬酸或酮咯酸。
• 睫状肌麻痹(可选，考虑作用时间 24～36 h与副作用)：抑制瞳孔收缩，从而防止对光的反应疼痛和畏光：
- 环孢素。
- 霍马托品。
• 局部抗生素：
- 软膏较滴眼液更好，因其亦为一种湿润剂。
- 症状消失 24 h 即停用抗生素。
- 接触镜佩戴者必须有抗假单胞菌覆盖：
• 眼修补：
- 不能改善疼痛或愈合，不推荐。
- 需要更多研究以评估超过 10 min 的擦伤进行修补的效益。
• 接触镜片。
- 不佩戴接触镜直至擦伤预后且停用药物 1 周眼部感觉正常。
• 破伤风预防：
- 擦伤不需要常规破伤风疫苗。
- 如果擦伤由有机物或泥土导致或污染，则注射破伤风疫苗。
• 眼内异物残留、眼球穿透伤(或其他更严重的损伤)、角膜浸润、白斑或混浊，提示溃疡、下睑，需紧急眼科会诊。

药物治疗

• 外用抗生素：
- 红霉素：药膏质量分数为 0.5%。
- 环丙沙星：0.35%溶液，1 滴，每日 4 次。
- 磺乙酰胺：每日 4 次和 qhs 为 10%软膏，或每 3 h 滴加 1～2 滴溶液。
- 隐形眼镜配戴者必须具备。
- 覆盖假单胞菌：
◦ 环丙沙星：0.3%软膏剂或溶液 1 滴剂。
◦ 氧氟沙星：0.3%溶液，2 滴，每日 4 次。
◦ 庆大霉素：0.3%软膏或溶液，2 滴，q6 h。
◦ 妥布霉素：每 6 h 含 0.3%软膏；或每 6 h 2 滴溶液。
• 独眼症：
- 荷马碱：2.5%～5%溶液，每日 1 滴。
- 环戊酸酯：0.5%或 1%，1 滴，每日 2 次。
• 止痛药：
- 双氯芬酸：0.1%溶液，1 滴，每日 4 次。
- 酮咯酸：0.5%溶液，1 滴，每日 4 次。
- 普鲁卡因：0.5%溶液，1 滴，单次给药。
- 丁卡因：1%溶液，1 滴，单次给药。

随访

进一步处理

入院指征

相关损伤需要住院者。

出院指征

所有简单角膜擦伤。

转诊问题

理想随访无研究。操作推荐表明所有角膜擦伤需要随访以确保无感染或瘢痕的愈合，特别是有严重外伤史，治疗后症状恶化，周围有擦伤浸润，反复出现糜烂综合征。

随访建议

• 24 h 内与眼科医生进行随访，以发现大缺陷，脓性分泌物，视力明显下降，小儿擦伤并持续引流，以及不愿睁开眼睛。
• 可以在 48～72 h 重新评估简单的磨损。

要点和误区

• 始终排除对地球的穿透性创伤。
• 认真评估感染证据。
• 避免给出院患者用任何表面麻醉剂。
• 不要给有青光眼病史的患者使用瞳孔放大剂。
• 建议不要使用接触镜，直到通过眼科检查。

角膜异物 Corneal Foreign Body

Carl G. Skinner 陈奇通 译

基础知识

描述

• 异物处于角膜上皮以上或者以内。
• 角膜上皮断裂：
- 如仅有上皮断裂则为擦伤。
- 角膜深层受损则有瘢痕。

病因

• 异物引起炎症反应：
- 可能引发结膜炎、角膜水肿、虹膜炎和坏死。
• 耐受性差：
- 有机材料(植物物质、昆虫碎片)。
- 有氧化性的无机材料(铁、铜)。

- 耐受性好：
- 惰性物质（油漆、玻璃、塑料、纤维玻璃、非氧化性金属）。

诊断

症状和体征

- 异物感。
- 眼痛。
- 结膜和巩膜充血。
- 流泪。
- 视物模糊或视力下降。
- 畏光。
- 可见异物或锈环。
- 虹膜炎。

病史

常见主诉：有物体降落、飞过或停留在眼睛上。

- 热的高速射流在起始时可能不引起疼痛。

体格检查

- 全面眼部检查：
  - 视力敏锐度。
  - 视野。
  - 眼外肌运动。
  - 眼睑和睫毛。
  - 瞳孔。
  - 巩膜。
  - 结膜。
  - 前房。
  - 眼底。
  - 缝隙灯和荧光素检查。
    - 执行赛德尔测试（荧光素缝隙灯检查时可见房水穿过角膜穿孔处）。
  - 如果无穿孔证据则测量眼内压。

基本检查

- 损伤史判断异物类型和穿孔可能。
- 排除眼内异物：
  - 高速机制需怀疑眼内异物，如机器操作或金属锤击、阳性侧壁试验或前房积血。

诊断检查与说明

影像学检查

- 怀疑眼内异物时行眼球 CT 或 B 超。
- 眼球 X 线平片用于筛查眼内金属异物。

注意

可能为金属异物时避免行 MRI。

鉴别诊断

- 结膜异物。
- 角膜损伤。
- 角膜穿孔伴有或不伴有眼内异物。
- 角膜溃疡。
- 角膜炎。

治疗

院前

放置 Fox 护具并使患者竖直位。

初步稳定/治疗

局部麻醉以减少眼睛不适并协助检查。

急诊治疗/程序

- 深部异物：
  - 穿透包曼氏膜的患者（上皮下一层）应联系眼科医师，因为可能出现永久性瘢痕。
- 浅表异物：
  - 冲洗清除异物技术。
- 局部麻醉。
- 直接用生理盐水以倾斜于角膜的角度尝试将异物冲离角膜。
  - 25G 针头或异物铲移除技术：
    - 使用缝隙灯固定患者头部并获得好的视线。
    - 以拇指和示指夹住针头（斜面向上），其他手指固定于患者面颊。
    - 将异物挑离角膜，保持针头与角膜表面平行。
- 锈环移除：
  - 含铁异物在 3 h 内氧化角膜，并在相邻上皮遗留锈斑。
  - 因锈环延迟愈合并成为刺激源，故建议移除。
  - 可随异物或其后 24 h，用针头和环形钩移除。
- 移除后治疗：
  - 再次行赛德尔检查以排除角膜穿孔。
  - 以抗生素或软膏治疗角膜擦伤。
  - 角膜炎可疑时使用抗生素眼药水或睫状肌麻醉剂药物。
  - 预防破伤风。
  - 开始口服镇痛。

儿科注意事项

可能需要镇静以方便检查和异物移除。

药物治疗

- 睫状肌麻醉剂：
  - 1%～2%环戊通：1 滴，每日 3 次（持续 2 日以上）。
  - 2%或 5%后马托品：1 滴，每日（持续 3 日以上）。
- 局部抗生素使用 3～5 日：常被使用，单未证实存在益处。
  - 红霉素软膏：细条，q6 h。
  - 环丙沙星：1 滴，q6 h。
  - 氧氟沙星：1 滴，q6 h。
  - 多黏菌素、甲氧苄氨嘧啶：1 滴，q6 h。
- 局部 NSAIDs：
  - 酮咯酸：1 滴，q6 h。
  - 双氯芬酸：1 滴，q6 h。

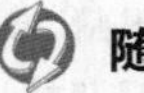

随访

进一步处理

入院指征

眼球贯穿。

出院指征

所有角膜异物。

转诊问题

- 眼科医师会诊：
  - 存在溃疡风险的植物性物质移除。
  - 任何感染或溃疡的证据。
  - 多个异物。
  - 异物移除不完全。
- 眼科医师随访 24 h：
  - 视野区域擦伤。
  - 大的擦伤。
  - 症状持续或第 2 日恶化的擦伤。
  - 锈环移除。

随访建议

如果症状持续或在 1～2 日恶化的患者需回访或联系医师。

要点和误区

- 需考虑眼内异物，特别是存在高喷射物或工业工具的病史者。
- 临床证据不支持眼睛斑片后有疼痛或愈合。
- 移除以后，大部分角膜异物能够按擦伤治疗，常可获得较好疗效而不需进一步处理。
- 局部麻醉药物不得作为家用处方。

角膜灼伤

Ryan A. Stroder · Ryan H. Wyatt 陈奇通 译

基础知识

描述

- 角膜被不适宜地暴露于化学制剂、高热、寒冷、电或放射性能量导致角膜损伤，常累及附近结构。
- 损伤的严重程度与液体暴露时长、物质类型、阴离子浓度和 pH 水平有关。
- 碱性物质：
  - 立即导致 pH 增高。
  - 溶液中高度可溶，故能快速渗透眼睛，导致严重的角膜损伤，如果未经干预将随时间持续渗透。
  - 渗透可在 1 min 内发生。
  - 例外：钙盐碱性洗涤液的渗透稍弱于肥皂成分；其可引起角膜斑块形成，故外在表现较差；但实际上较其他碱性物质烧伤其有更好的预后。
- 酸性物质：
  - 角膜上皮的蛋白立即凝聚。
  - 导致斑块形成。
  - 凝聚灶成为进一步渗透的阻碍。
  - 例外：氢氟酸(HF)的亲油性使它的化学行为更接近于有更快渗透率的碱。
- 温度烧伤：
  - 对眼睑较眼球影响更大，因为反射性眨眼和 Bell 现象(眼球向上外方旋转)。
  - 对角膜直接损伤。
  - 损伤首要取决于高热接触时长和程度。
- 电损伤：
  - 出现于电流通过头部，且输入端处于或靠近眼睛。
- 放射性损伤：
  - 因角膜暴露于超紫光。
  - 经常是双侧的。
  - 症状通常在暴露后 6～12 h 增加。

病因

- 碱性物：
  - 氨：
    - 肥料、冷却剂、家用氨水、清洁剂。
  - 氢氧化钾：
    - 腐蚀性钾盐。
  - 氢氧化镁：
    - 烟火、照明弹、爆竹。
  - 碱性液：NaOH：
    - 腐蚀性苏打、吸水剂。
  - 石灰：$Ca(OH)_2$ 或 $Mg(OH)_2$：
    - 新鲜石灰、生石灰、水合钙、熟石灰、水合石灰、石膏、石灰浆、水泥、石灰水。
  - 非特异性碱：
    - 汽车气囊膨胀时释放碱性物质。
    - 洗涤剂豆荚。
- 酸性物：
  - 硫酸：H_2SO_4。
    - 汽车电池中的酸、厕所清洁剂。
  - 亚硫酸：H_2SO_3。
    - 保鲜剂(水果和蔬菜)。
  - 乙酸：CH_3CO_2H。
    - 醋。
- 漂白粉。
- 冷冻剂：
  - HF 酸：
    - 蚀刻硅/玻璃。
    - 清晰砖头。
    - 电子打磨金属。
    - 酒窖中控制发酵。
    - 商业/住家去除铁锈。
- 温度：
  - 热的溶液、熔化的金属。
  - 火焰。
  - 热的烟雾/气体。
  - 电弧灼伤。
  - 蒸汽。
  - 香烟灼伤。
- 放射：
  - 太阳灯。
  - 日光浴。
  - 较高海拔的阳光。
  - 雪、水的反射。
  - 电弧焊接。

儿科注意事项

考虑虐待或忽略儿童。

诊断

症状和体征

- 严重的眼球疼痛。
- 畏光。
- 流泪。
- 异物感。
- 结膜充血。
- 角膜水肿。
- 角膜斑块。
- 视觉分辨力下降。
- 边缘黄化。
- 晶状体斑块形成。
- 清凉液体的小疱(低温损伤)。
- 血性液体的小疱。
- 虹膜、睫状体坏死。

病史

- 暴露类型：
  - 检查与患者携带瓶内的活性或非活性成分。
- 暴露物的载体：
  - 气溶胶：常见。
  - 挥发剂：可能导致眼球内异物、穿孔。
- 暴露时长。
- 发作时间。
- 灌洗起始时间。
- 之前的视力受损情况。
- 防护眼镜。
- 接触镜片。
- 抵达前的处理情况。

体格检查

完整的眼部检查(灌洗以后)。
- 视觉敏锐度。
- 白色亮光用于肉眼检查角膜、结膜、缘。
- 缝隙灯用于评估前部炎症。
- 荧光素染色：
  - 角膜上皮损伤：
    - 紫外线放射性灼伤患者，从下缝隙可见点状角膜病灶，其下缘不连续。
  - 穿孔(赛德尔试验)。
- 检查晶状体清晰度。
- 基底部检查。
- 测量眼内压(特别是延迟表现的患者)。
- 眼睑、睫毛严查。
- 检测酸性、碱性灼伤的 pH，可使用石蕊试纸或尿检测片上的 pH 指示剂。

诊断检查与说明

诊断步骤/外科

- 荧光素染色。
- 测量 pH。

鉴别诊断

- 感染：

J

- 病毒性角膜炎。
- 角膜溃疡。
- 角膜腐蚀综合征：
- 角膜异物。
- 角膜擦伤。
- 低温损伤。

儿科注意事项

手持缝隙灯和 Wood 灯在儿童眼镜检查中有帮助。

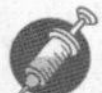

治疗

院前

- 除非有其他并存的危及生命的情况需要立即转运，否则应在现场灌洗 15～30 min。
- 把装有物质的瓶子或容器带到医院以帮助诊断。
- 在通往医院途中持续使用生理盐水或清水灌洗。

初步稳定/治疗

- 化学药物暴露：
  - 暴露于未知物质的患者应怀疑酸或者碱。
  - 使用任何可以稀释液体进行灌洗，但优选清水或生理盐水。
- 温度暴露：
  - 湿冷敷料并加盖冰袋。

急诊治疗/程序

- 化学制剂暴露：碱/酸/氯乙酰苯：
  - 持续灌洗使 pH 7.3～7.5（1～2 L 通过 Morgan 透镜>30～60 min）：
    - 每 30 min 测量 pH。
    - 将 pH 试纸蘸入结膜下穹窿。
  - 局部麻醉（丙美卡因或丁卡因）可能在灌流期间是必要的。
  - pH 需要在灌流后 5 min 和 30 min 时评估以保证 pH 正常。
  - 停止灌溉后等待 5～10 min，让稀释剂被吸收。
  - 仔细评估穹窿和眼睛最大运动范围，以保证所有微小的化学物质被去除。
  - 抗生素预防葡萄球菌、假单胞菌直至上皮化已完成：
    - 庆大霉素软膏＋红霉素或者杆菌肽。
    - 甲氧苄啶/多黏菌素 B 或氟喹诺酮滴剂。
  - 睫状肌麻痹剂以虹膜后粘连形成：
    - 1%环戊通。
    - 1%阿托品。
  - 口服止痛药。
  - 如眼内压增高：
    - 立即眼科医师会诊。
    - 给予乙酰唑胺 125 mg，口服，每日 4 次和 0.5%噻吗洛尔数滴，每日 2 次。
- 局部激素以控制前葡萄膜炎（眼科会诊）。
- 眼补片（眼科会诊）。
- 完全角膜穿透可能需要外科干预。
- 轻度损伤可电话会诊眼科医师。
- 所有中度到重度损伤立即请眼科医师会诊；如果医院内无眼科医师，安排转运至最近的眼科中心。
- HF 酸：
  - 如上治疗，＋1%葡萄糖酸钙滴眼液。
  - 24 h 全身性镇痛。
- 温度暴露：
  - 经常更换湿敷料。
  - 抗生素滴眼液每日 3 次。
  - 多使用湿润剂。
  - 眼睑严重损伤时进入保湿室。
  - 激素（眼科医师会诊；>1 周者不使用）。
  - 眼睑 2 度或 3 度烧伤时请眼科医师会诊。
  - 烟灰盒热的液体飞溅常导致角膜上皮损伤。
  - 治疗如角膜擦伤。
- 电击损伤：
  - 灌流。
  - 创伤护理。
  - 抗生素软膏。
  - 睫状肌麻醉剂（如前葡萄膜炎）。
  - 镇痛剂。
- 放射性损伤：
  - 局部麻醉。
  - 短效睫状肌麻醉剂。
  - 抗生素软膏。
  - 考虑口服阿片类药物以控制疼痛。

儿科注意事项

- 修补耐受差。
- 可能需要全身性止痛药物以完整检查。

药物治疗

- 人工眼泪。
- 阿托品：0.5%、1%、2%滴眼液（睫状肌麻醉 5～10 日，瞳孔扩大 7～14 日）1 滴，每日 3 次。
- 杆菌肽软膏：每日 4 次。
- 环丙沙星：0.35% 1 滴，每日 4 次。
- 环戊通：0.5%、1%、2%滴眼液（睫状肌麻痹 1～2 日，瞳孔放大 1～2 日）1 滴，每日 3 次。
- 红霉素：0.5%软膏，每日 4 次。
- 庆大霉素：0.3%软膏或 0.3%滴剂。
- 霍马托品：5%滴 1～2 滴，每日 2～3 次。
- 普罗帕卡因：q5～10 min 滴 1 滴，每次 5～7 次。
- 磺胺乙酰胺：1～2 滴。
- 丁卡因：q5～10 min 滴 1～2 滴，最多 5 剂。
- 妥布霉素：1～2 滴。
- 甲氧苄啶/polymix B：1 滴眼，q4 h。

随访

进一步处理

入院指征

- 顽固性疼痛。
- 眼内压增高。
- 角膜穿透需要理解手术干预。
- HF 酸灼烧；需 24 h 全身性镇痛者收治入院。
- 怀疑儿童虐待。

出院指征

所有轻度角膜灼伤。

随访建议

眼科医师强制性随访 12～24 h，在患者出院前安排事宜。

要点和误区

- 化学暴露是，延迟检查直至眼镜已经灌洗结束。
- 所有上皮缺损的患者需要眼科医师 12～24 h 随访。
- 不给出院患者开具局部麻醉药物的处方。

接触性皮炎 Contact Dermatitis

Christian D. Magallanes · Jeffey Druck 陈奇通 译

基础知识

描述

- 刺激物：
- 立即出现湿疹（主要在表皮的浅表炎症过程）。
- 最常见的皮炎。
- 刺激物直接损害皮肤导致非免疫性炎症反应，出现红肿、干燥、破裂或裂隙。
- 通常是由于反复暴露于轻度刺激物（如水、肥皂、热、摩擦、金属）。
- 病灶瘙痒或灼烧感：
- 常逐渐出现，边界不清晰。
- 最常见于手。
- 可能出现小疱或裂隙。
- 干燥、发红和粗糙的皮肤。
- 常见刺激物包括：
  - 水泥。
  - 染发剂。
  - 湿纸尿裤。
  - 橡胶手套。
  - 洗发水。
  - 经常洗手。
- 过敏：
- 延迟型（Ⅳ型）超敏反应（需要之前致敏）。
- 过敏原导致的免疫反应。
- 局部水肿、小疱、红肿、瘙痒或灼烧感。
- 常对应于非常明确的接触史（如手表带）。
- 常在 12～48 h 发作，伴有先前的致敏；可能经过 14～21 日的前期暴露。
- 常见来源：
  - 镍。
  - 金。
  - 新霉素。
  - 杆菌肽。
  - 防腐剂。
  - 香料。
  - 染色剂。
- 毒藤。
- 光接触：
- 皮肤上其他无害物质和紫外线相互反应。
- 常见来源：
  - 剃须洗液。
  - 遮光剂。
  - 磺胺类软膏。
  - 香水。

儿科注意事项

- 过敏性接触性皮炎在儿童尤其是婴儿中较少见。
- 儿童接触性过敏的主要来源：
- 金属、鞋、防腐剂、化妆品的香料、局部药物和植物。
- 尿片皮炎：典型的儿童刺激物接触性皮炎。
- 口周皮炎：见于婴儿和小儿，可能由某些事物引起（刺激或过敏反应）。

病因

- 刺激源（80%接触性皮炎），如：
- 肥皂、溶剂。
- 化学制剂（雾化农药）。
- 某些食物。
- 尿液、排泄物。
- 尿片。
- 持续或反复暴露于潮湿（洗手）。
- 纸、玻璃和羊毛纤维。
- 鞋相关的皮炎：常见；判别病灶局限于足远端背面，常不累及足趾间皮肤。
- 水泥（长时间暴露可能会导致严重的碱烧伤）。
- 环氧溶剂。
- 橡胶（如弹性腰带）或皮革中的化学品。
- 过敏性：
- 植物、毒藤、橡树、漆树（漆树皮炎）。
  - 北美最常见的过敏性接触性皮炎。
  - 直接：对植物的油性树脂漆酚有反应。
  - 间接：接触表面或皮毛上沾有油性树脂的宠物或衣物，或焚烧树叶的烟雾。
  - 病灶可在前期致敏（首次暴露后 12～21 日）后的暴露 3 日出现，可持续长达 3 周。
  - 小疱内液体无感染性，不引起新的病灶。
- 宠物或衣物上的油性树脂仍有接触传染性，直至被清除。
- 豚草花粉。
- 金属（特别是镍、金）。
- 乳液、化妆品。
- 局部药物（如新霉素、氢化可的松、苯佐卡因、尼泊金）。
- 某些食物。
- 对某些抗原起反应可能是基因决定的。
- 光照性皮炎：
- 暴露于刺激物（常为植物树液）和阳光而出现的炎症反应。
- 典型案例在无阳光时无反应。

诊断

症状和体征

病史

- 发病时间。
- 病灶的模式。
- 与工作的相关性。
- 是否有瘙痒。
- 黏膜是否累及。
- 暴露于新产品（如洗剂、肥皂和化妆品）、食物、药物和珠宝。

体格检查

- 特别注意皮疹的特征和分布。
- 急性病灶：皮肤红肿和瘙痒：
- 可见水肿、丘疹、小疱、大疱、浆液流出或硬痂。
- 亚急性：更少的水疱。
- 慢性病灶：可见鳞皮、苔藓样硬化、色素沉着或裂隙伴少量或无水疱；可能有特征性分布模式。

诊断检查与说明

实验室检查

暂无特异性急诊检查是有帮助的。

影像学检查

暂无特异性急诊检查是有帮助的。

诊断步骤/外科

- 修补检查：
- 一般不在急诊进行；通知过敏/免疫学医师。
- 淋巴细胞转化测试（基于血液的测试）在使用中存在争议。

鉴别诊断

- 异位性皮炎：与异位性家族史有关。
- 脂溢性皮炎：鳞状或硬痂“油脂”病灶。
- 钱币状湿疹性皮痒：钱币样病灶。
- 擦烂：同位结构皮肤处的皮炎（腋窝、腹股沟）。
- 感染性湿疹性皮炎：继发于细菌感染的皮炎，常为金黄色葡萄球菌。
- 蜂窝织炎：温暖、发白、疼痛的病灶。

J

• 脓疱病：黄色硬痂。
• 疥疮：极度瘙痒，常有指间痕迹。
• 牛皮癣：银白相邻的、鳞片状、清楚的病灶，影响伸肌表面、头皮和生殖器部位。
• 单纯疱疹：成组小疱、疼痛、灼烧感。
• 带状疱疹：疼痛，有皮节模式。
• 大疱性类天疱疮：分散的大疱病灶。
• 癣：最大累及边缘、Wood 灯下发出荧光。
• 白糠疹：独立的、无症状的、色素减退的病灶。
• 荨麻疹：突起的发痒病灶（风疹块），常伴有在周围红疹（底部散开）。
• 湿疹（汗疱疹性皮炎）：
• 药疹。
• Stevens-Johnson 综合征（SJS）。
• 中毒性表皮坏死松解症（TEN）。
• 结节性红疹（EN）。

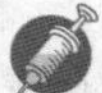

治疗

初步稳定/治疗

无合并病变是很少需要处理。

急诊治疗/程序

主要

• 首要对症、支持治疗。
• 以软肥皂和清水冲洗病变区域。
• 去除或避免刺激性物质（包括清洗衣物）。
• 清凉潮湿地挤压：在急性水疱期非常有效。
• 止痒药物：
- 局部：
◦ 炉甘石洗剂、皮质激素（不透过水疱）；避免使用含苯佐卡因的产品，这些产品可能进一步使皮肤过敏。
- 全身性：抗组胺药物、皮质激素。
• 醋酸铝（Burrows）溶液：涂抹表面。
• 局部激素（倾向于软膏）每日 2 次，2～3 周：
- 面部：低效能。
- 手臂、腿和躯干：中效能。
- 双手和双脚：高效能。
• 严重病例可口服激素。

漆树皮炎（常春藤/橡树/漆树）

• 主要方法加上：
- 清洗与植物有接触的所有衣物和宠物；油脂可持续存在且有接触致病性。
- 胶体燕麦浴或小苏打可以缓解疲劳。
- 大疱的无菌性吸入可缓解不适。
- 严重反应（>10% TBSA）：全身皮质激素治疗 2～3 周并逐步减量：
◦ 过早停止皮质激素治疗可能导致症状的快速反弹。

鞋相关的皮炎

• 主要方法加上：
- 穿戴露脚趾、帆布或者乙烯树脂的鞋。
- 控制流汗：更换袜子、使用吸收粉。

尿片相关性皮炎（可以接触或过敏）

• 主要方法加上：
- 局部氧化锌、凡士林软膏或阿夸福尔。
- 每次大便后更换尿片。

药物治疗

全身性：

• 抗组胺药物（H_1 受体拮抗剂，第一代和第二代）：
- 西替利嗪：成人和儿童>6 岁，5～10 mg，口服，每日 1 次（儿童：年龄 2～6 岁，2.5 mg，口服，每日 2 次）。
- 盐酸苯海拉明：25～50 mg，静脉注射、肌内注射、口服，q6 h，必要时[儿童：5 mg/(kg·24 h)分次 q6 h PRN]。
- 非索非那定：60 mg，口服，每日 2 次；或者 180 mg，口服，每日（儿童：年龄 6～12 岁，30 mg，口服，每日 2 次）。
- 盐酸羟嗪：25～50 mg，口服或肌内注射至每日 4 次 PRN[儿童：2 mg/(kg·24 h)，口服，分次 q6 h；或 0.5 mg/kg，肌内注射，q4～6 h，必要时]。
- 氯雷他定：10 mg，口服，每日 2 次。
- 顽固性瘙痒：多虑平，75 mg，口服，每日可能有效。
• 皮质激素：
- 泼尼松：40～60 mg，口服，[儿童：1～2 mg/(kg·24 h)，最大 80 mg/24 h]分次，每日 2 次。
• 顽固性瘙痒：多虑平，75 mg，口服，每日可能有效。

局部：

• 醋酸铝（Burrows）溶液：局部使用 20 min，每日 3 次，直至皮肤干燥。
• 炉甘石洗剂：q6 h，必要时。
• 局部皮质激素：
- 氢化可的松 1%或 2.5%（最低效力）。
- 丁酸氢化可的松 0.1%（低效）。
- 丙酸氟替卡松 0.05%（中等效力）。
- 氟嘧啶 0.05%（高效）。
- 每日给药 1～3 次。
◦ 注意：不可用于面部或眼睑。

一线用药

• 局部激素。
• 口服抗组胺药物。

二线用药

口服激素。

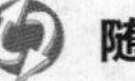

随访

进一步处理

入院指征

很少需要，除非有严重全身性反应或严重的继发感染（SJS、TEN、EB、坏死性筋膜炎）。

出院指征

• 症状缓解。
• 负责医师或皮肤科医师充分随访。

随访建议

• 负责医师随访，并 2～3 日复诊。
• 返回急诊：面部肿胀、呼吸困难、黏膜受累导致口服摄入下降。

要点和误区

• 去除刺激物。
• 预防过敏反应（如乳汁过敏）。
• 注意伴发的细菌感染。
• 局部类固醇是治疗的主要手段。
• 用肥皂和水（衣服、动物）清洗后，引起皮肤炎的漆树油不再有效。

结肠损伤 Colon Injury

Richard Childers · Gary M. Vilke 陈奇通 译

基础知识

描述

- 创伤导致结肠穿孔可引起其所处腔体的炎症。
- 由空腔脏器穿孔引起的腹膜炎常需要数小时进展。
- 由钝性损伤所致的肠系膜撕裂可引起出血和肠缺血。
- 延迟性穿孔可发生在缺血或坏死的肠段。
- 腹膜炎和脓毒症可由肠腔内菌群外渗发展而来。
- 升结肠和降结肠处于腹膜后。
- 结肠损伤的延迟诊断会提高发病率和病死率。

病因

- 穿透性腹腔创伤：
  - 结肠在穿透性创伤中为第二常见的受损器官。
  - 大约 1/3 的因枪伤而剖腹手术的创伤病例中，结肠损伤是最常见的损伤部位。
- 钝性腹部创伤：
  - 结肠钝性损伤是一种少见且难以诊断的损伤。
  - 钝挫伤的内脏空心损伤通常发生在高能量转移的环境中，并伴有其他损伤。
  - 闭襻性肠段受压可出现暴发性损伤。
  - 在钝性物体(安全带)和椎体或者骨盆之间的肠道可能受到挤压。
  - 突然减速可能引起肠管-肠系膜断裂，继而导致血流阻断。
  - 在减速时，乙状结肠和横结肠最易受损。
- 经肛门损伤：
  - 医源性内镜或钡剂灌肠损伤。
  - 在性行为时使用的外来物可能到达并损伤结肠。
  - 如在汽车修理厂的高压压缩气体可导致结肠穿孔，即使压缩喷头未完全插入肛门。
  - 吞下的尖锐物品(牙签)可能穿透结肠，特别是盲肠、阑尾和乙状结肠：
    - 大部分外来物能顺利通过，无并发症。

儿科注意事项

与成人不同，儿童发生的钝性和穿透性结肠损伤有相同概率。

诊断

症状和体征

- 结肠损伤常联合其他腹腔内和腹腔外的损伤，常累及小肠。
- 显著危重的损伤在可能仅有小的早期发现。
- 一般无法通过体格检查来确定特定脏器的损伤。
- 体检时评估：
  - 腹膜刺激征。
  - 安全带挤压后下腹的瘀斑或血肿。
  - 方向盘挤压后上腹部区域的瘀斑。
  - 腹膜后出血引起的 Grey Turner 征(侧腹血肿)。
  - 肛指发现异物或带血(如怀疑为尖锐物体，检查时需小心)。
  - 注意：即使存在损伤，腹壁瘀斑或血肿并非总是存在。
  - 注意：肠鸣音无帮助。

基本检查

- 因炎症需要一定时间进展，故应做多次腹部检查。
- 稳定患者最佳的诊断性检查为腹部增强 CT。
- 超声和诊断性腹腔抽液对于潜在不稳定患者有帮助。

诊断检查与说明

- 目前不存在单一或组合性诊断工具能够排除钝性结肠损伤。
- 肠道损伤后出现腹膜刺激征一般需要数小时。

实验室检查

很少有助于结肠损伤的诊断。

影像学检查

- 腹部 X 线平片可显示腹膜内和腹膜后游离气体等间接征象。
- 快速超声检查对结肠损伤没有特异性或敏感性。
- 在穿透性腹部创伤中，常规的 CT 扫描通常是保留在背部和侧面的有计划的非手术治疗的患者。
- 在稳定的外伤患者中，CT 是评估腹部创伤的首选方法。
- 一般来说，在钝性腹部创伤中，口服造影剂不是必需的，但在选择临床稳定的患者中可能是合适的。
- 空腔脏器损伤相关的 CT 表现包括肠壁缺损、腔外气体或造影剂、肠系膜脂肪条带、肠系膜血管突然终止、游离液体无实体器官损伤。
- CT 对诊断内脏凹陷损伤的敏感性中等，但异常表现较为典型。
- 水溶性荧光灌肠剂在其他检查无法确诊时有帮助。
- 直肠异物的评估，影像学检查不是强制性的，但可以用来识别异物的形状和位置，并排除穿孔。
- 见“腹部创伤，钝性”；“腹部创伤，影像”。

诊断步骤/外科

- DPL 很少做，但可以增加结肠损伤诊断的敏感性。
- 在钝性创伤中，DPL 常探测不到腹膜后损伤和肠道损伤，因为这些损伤中腹腔内出血是有限的。
- DPL 分析中发现 Fecal 或蔬菜物质提示空腔脏器损伤。
- 迟发性腹膜炎的腹水样本的白细胞反应可能为阴性。
- 空腔脏器损伤中的腹水样本白细胞计数与红细胞比值较实质脏器损伤时增高。

鉴别诊断

- 其他腹腔内损伤。
- 对于儿童，骨盆骨折的临床表现可与腹腔内损伤相近。

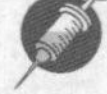

治疗

院前

- 注意：
  - 根据创伤标准院前处理指南进行处理(ABC 管理)。
  - 不去除穿透性异物。
  - 不尝试移除断裂的肠管；用湿盐水敷料覆盖。
  - 获取损伤机制相关的病史、车祸和安全带使用。

初步稳定/治疗

- 告知腹部创伤事项。
- ABC 管理应在腹部评估之前进行。

■ 急诊治疗/程序

• 早期外科会诊；外科手术是关键治疗手段。外科医生将确定结肠切除或一期吻合术是否合适。通常是指一期吻合。
• 将断裂肠管用湿盐水纱布覆盖，并置于非重力依赖的位置。
• 确保破伤风预防。
• 对直肠异物患者保持专业和无偏见的态度，考虑攻击或潜在的精神病诊断。

■ 药物治疗

• 所有腹部穿透伤患者术前应用广谱需氧和厌氧的单剂量预防性抗生素。以下各项均可接受：
• 氨苄西林-舒巴坦 3 g(儿童：50 mg/kg)，静脉注射，q6 h。
• 哌拉西林-他唑巴坦 3.375 g，静脉注射，q6 h(儿童：100 mg/kg，静脉注射，q8 h)。
• 头孢曲松 1 g(儿童：100 mg/kg)，q24 h＋甲硝唑 500 mg(儿童：10 mg/kg)，静脉滴注，q8 h。
• 替代方案包括联合氟喹诺酮＋甲硝唑，或单用碳青霉烯类药物。
• 对于急性损伤患者，预防性抗生素的持续使用时间不必超过 24 h。

随访

■ 进一步处理

入院指征

• 结肠损伤需要入院性外科手术修补或监测。
• 所有的穿透性异物必须去除，防止脓毒症。
• 有腹部瘀斑的患者需要住院并观察，因其有未诊断的空腔脏器损伤的可能。

出院指征

• 无严重腹部损伤，腹部检查完全正常，正常血流动力学状态，且无其他损伤的患者可考虑给予适当的警示并出院。
• 如有结肠损伤可能的怀疑，患者应住院并观察。

要点和误区

患者初始缺乏症状：
• 如果损伤机制提示严重钝性腹部损伤，需观察和反复体格检查。

结核 Tuberculosis

Martine Lory Camille · Michelle D. Lall 张晟 林兆奋 译

基础知识

■ 描述

结核是表现千变万化的传染性疾病，全球范围内引起显著的流行率和死亡率。

机制

• 呼吸道吸入传染性的飞沫。
• 细菌经咳嗽、打喷嚏、说话、唱歌四处弥散。
• 原发性结核/潜在的结核感染。
- 当细菌进入肺泡被巨噬细胞吞噬并经由区域淋巴结入血，初次感染就发生了并通过区域淋巴结扩散到血液。
- 患者通常无症状。
- 在免疫受抑制个体，病原体会进展甚至致死。
- PPD 试验阳性说明既往暴露史或感染史。
- PPD 试验阴性不能排除结核活动期。
- 可进展为活动性肺结核(5%～10%)。
• 活动性肺结核。
- 潜在的结核感染进展为活动性肺结核。
- 全身(15%)和肺部(85%)症状。
• 美国结核病发病率为 2.9/10 万。
• 2016 年报告的新病例数最低。
• 在报告的约 9 200 例新病例中，67% 为外国出生，86% 为 HIV 阳性。
• 结核病是全球 HIV 感染者的首要死亡原因。
• 估计单在美国仍有 1000 万～1500 万被感染。

■ 病因

• 结核分枝杆菌是一种生长缓慢，需氧的抗酸杆菌，此菌感染后致病。
• 人类是唯一所知的宿主。
• 最近结核病流行病学：
- HIV 感染者好发。
- 多药耐药结核分枝杆菌感染。
- 广泛耐药结核分枝杆菌感染(死亡率高，有效药物少)。

诊断

■ 症状和体征

• 取决于感染部位，人类所有组织都有被感染的风险。
• 肺结核。
- 咳嗽。
- 发热、盗汗。
- 全身乏力、体重降低。
- 咯血。
- 胸膜炎式的胸痛。
- 呼吸急促。
• 肺外结核。
- 中枢神经系统感染。
◦ 脑膜炎。
◦ 脑神经感染、复视。
◦ 头痛、发热、全身乏力。
◦ 意识模糊。
◦ 急性缺血性脑卒中。
- 心包炎。
◦ 斜卧位胸膜痛加重。
- 肾脏感染。
◦ 发热。
◦ 腰痛。
- 脊柱结核。
◦ 后背痛、僵硬、定点压痛。
◦ 发热。
◦ 活动范围减小。
- 颈部淋巴结炎。
◦ 单侧，无疼痛。
◦ 可能形成窦道。
- 粟粒性结核。
◦ 多器官系统病变。
◦ 弥漫性腺病。
◦ 肝大。
◦ 脾大。
◦ 体重减轻、发热。

病史

结核的易感因素和发病条件。
• HIV 感染和其他免疫功能不全状态(器官移植、肾衰竭、糖尿病)。
• 酗酒和药物滥用。
• 贫穷，无家可归(生活在棚户区)。

J

- 制度原因(护理院、监狱)。
- 来自结核流行区的移民。
- PPD试验阳性/有感染史。

体格检查

- 发热。
- 心动过速。
- 缺氧。
- 恶病质。
- 异常呼吸音。
- 颈部淋巴结肿大。

■ 基本检查

- 由于临床表现多样导致诊断困难。
- 胸片：活动性肺结核最有意义的检查。
- 皮肤试验：PPD。
- 干扰素γ释放试验：T-斑点试验或QuantiFERON-TB Gold检测。

■ 诊断检查与说明

实验室检查

- 全血细胞计数。
- 电解质、尿素氮、肌酐、血糖、肝功能。
- 低钠血症(由于不适当应用利尿剂所致综合征)。
- 用来评估氧合情况和通气状况的动态脑电图。
- 痰抗酸染色寻找结核杆菌。
  - 可快速推定诊断。
- 痰、脑脊液、血液、尿液、腹水培养。
  - 诊断结核的金标准。
  - 培养阳性的平均耗时3～6周。
  - DNA PCR更快出结果。
- 腰椎穿刺行脑脊液检查。
  - 适用于疑似结核性脑膜炎者。
  - 以淋巴细胞为主的白细胞升高。
  - 蛋白升高。
  - 葡萄糖正常或偏低。

影像学检查

- 胸片。
  - 可能正常。
  - 在原发性肺结核，肺实质浸润伴单侧肺门淋巴结肿大是最经典的影像学表现。
  - 继发性肺结核典型表现是空洞侵蚀伴或不伴钙化，常发生于肺上叶。
  - 粟粒性结核常表现为单侧肺部弥漫2mm结核结节。
  - AIDS或免疫缺陷患者胸片结果不能确诊结核。
  - 在原发或继发性肺结核均为单侧胸膜腔积液。
  - 气管移位伴瘢痕或肺不张。
  - Ghon点：瘢痕钙化/已愈合的原发性感染。
  - Ghon综合征：原发性结核浸润伴相连单侧肺门淋巴结结节。
- 脊柱X线片(Potts disease)。
  - 可表现正常。
  - 椎体前路受侵袭，椎间盘受破坏。
- 胸部CT。
  - 对病变范围定位清楚。

诊断步骤/外科

皮肤试验

- 前臂皮内注射0.1 ml PPD。
- 阳性表示以前或现在感染结核分枝杆菌。
- 在注射后48～72 h读取结果。
- 结果阳性的解读：＞5 mm硬结。
  - 与结核患者密切接触。
  - 结核的典型胸片结果。
  - HIV阳性。
  - 器官移植或其他免疫抑制状态。
- ＞10 mm硬结。
  - 静脉注射毒品者。
  - 从发病率高的国家移民而来(5年内)。
  - 伴随疾病(糖尿病、肾衰竭、恶性肿瘤)。
  - 医务工作者。
  - 监狱服刑人员。
  - 制度因素(护理之家，无家可归者)。
- ＞15 mm硬结。
  - 低感染风险个体。

血清监测

- 干扰素-γ释放分析：
  - T-Spot试验或Quantiferon-TB Gold Test。
  - 可用于诊断结核病感染，但不能区分活动性和潜伏性结核病。
  - 两者都测量血液中针对特定Mtb抗原的T细胞应答(IFN-Y)。
  - 在接受卡介苗接种的人中，对结核病的特异性比TST更强。
  - 更适合那些可能不会回来复诊的人。
  - 结果可以是阳性的、阴性的或不确定的。
  - TST是小于5岁儿童最适合的检验。
- TB-LAMP检测：
  - 世界卫生组织推荐的新开发的结核病检测。
  - 手动检测，可在＜1 h内完成。
  - 可以取代痰涂片镜检，仅在有与结核病有关的体征和症状的成人患者中诊断结核病。
  - 也可以作为痰涂片阴性后需要进一步检测的人的二次检测。
- 纳米盘：
  - 2017年开发的这一检测方法能够使用血清快速诊断活动性结核病。
  - 这是一种基于血清的定量检测方法，可以在健康和免疫受损人群中以更高的灵敏度和特异性检测特定的结核分枝杆菌肽片段。
  - 尚未商业化。

■ 鉴别诊断

- 细菌性肺炎。
- 支气管扩张。
- 球孢子菌病。
- 组织胞浆菌病。
- 肺脓肿。
- 肺癌。
- 淋巴瘤。
- 肺孢子菌肺炎。
- 肺栓塞。
- 结节病。

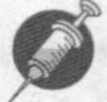

治疗

■ 院前

- 将患者进行呼吸隔离(负压房)。
- 给患者戴上口罩防止呼吸道传播。
- 开始治疗，静脉用药，吸氧，测脉搏及血氧饱和度。
- 严重咯血或呼吸困难的患者可能需要气管插管。
- 患者应佩戴亚微米滤过的口罩(N95口罩)。
- 通知亲密接触者。

■ 初步稳定/治疗

- ABC管理。
  - 按需要管理气道。
  - 按需要给氧。
  - 进行心电监测，脉搏、血氧饱和度监测。
  - 建立静脉通路，输入生理盐水。
- 隔离患者于负压房，每小时换气6次。
- 保护工作人员(N95口罩)。

■ 急诊治疗/程序

- 隔离和严密的预防呼吸道传播。
- 由于多重耐药病例增加，治疗要加强。
- 任何方案必须包含2种结核分枝杆菌敏感的药。
- CDC最近推荐初期治疗应包括4种一线用药。
- 潜在感染者而胸片正常给异烟肼9个月或者12周异烟肼加利福喷丁。
- 当用抗反转录疗法治疗HIV感染者时，咨询传染病专家的意见。
- 结核性脑膜炎加用地塞米松治疗。

J

• 结核脓胸可能需要手术引流，咨询胸椎外科专家。

• 为确保特定人群依从性，直接观察治疗(DOT)可能是有必要的。

• 间断治疗（双周）可能显示出更好的患者依从性。

药物治疗

药物敏感性测试

• 异烟肼和利福平的治疗应在以下患者群体中进行：

- 所有 HIV 患者。
- 那些在美国境外出生或在中度结核病流行国家>1 年的人。
- 那些与耐多药结核病患者有过接触的人。
- 那些以前治疗过结核病的人。

一线用药

• 异烟肼：5 mg/kg，最大剂量 300 mg（儿童：10～15 mg/kg，最大剂量 300 mg），口服或肌内注射，每日 1 次。

- 超剂量可能发生难治性癫痫，可用吡哆醇 5 g 静脉注射，时间>5 min，或者口服。
- 注意不可与酒精同服；肝炎患者慎用。

• 利福平：10 mg/kg，最大剂量 600 mg（儿童：10～20 mg/kg，最大剂量 600 mg）口服或静脉注射，每日 1 次。

• 吡嗪酰胺：20～25 mg/(kg·d)，最大剂量 2 g[儿童：15～30 mg/(kg·d)]或：

- 体重<55 kg：1 g，口服，每日 1 次。
- 体重 56～75 kg：1.5 g，口服，每日 1 次。
- 体重>75 kg：2 g，口服，每日 1 次。
- 不建议孕妇服用。

• 乙胺丁醇：15～20 mg/kg，最大剂量 1600 mg（儿童：15～30 mg/kg，最大剂量 1 g）口服，每日 1～3 次；<13 岁不建议服用，非用不可要查视力。

• 利福喷丁：10 mg/kg 最大剂量 900 mg（儿童：<13 岁不建议服用）1 周口服 1 次，或者：

- 体重 10～14 kg，每周口服 300 mg。
- 体重 14.1～25 kg，每周口服 450 mg。
- 体重 25.1～32 kg，每周口服 600 mg。
- 体重 32.1～49.9 kg，每周口服 750 mg。
- 体重>50 kg，每周口服 900 mg。

• 利福布丁：5 mg/kg，最大剂量 300 mg（儿童：不详），口服，每日 1 次。

二线药物

• 链霉素：15 mg/(kg·d)，最大剂量 1 g[儿童：20～40 mg/(kg·d)]，肌内注射或静脉注射，每日 1 次。

- 致畸：孕妇禁忌。

• 乙硫酰胺：0.5～1 g[儿童：10～20 mg/(kg·d)]，口服或静脉滴注，每日 4 次。

• 左氧氟沙星：750 mg（儿童禁用），口服或静脉注射，每日 1 次。

多重耐药 TB 的治疗

• 贝达奎林：每天 400 mg，连用 2 周，然后每周 3 次，共 200 mg，共 22 周。

- FDA 批准用于成人泛耐药结核病的治疗。
- 自 1971 年以来批准的第一种直接治疗结核分枝杆菌的药物。
- 应作为治疗多重耐药结核病的联合疗法的一部分。

随访

进一步处理

入院指征

• 呼吸困难。

• 怀疑诊断。

• 不能在门诊完成治疗。

• 门诊不具备治疗条件（无 PCP）。

• 不符合规定的门诊患者非自愿入院。

- 了解有关非自愿入院的各自州法律（咨询传染病专家的意见）。

出院指征

• 无呼吸困难。

• 有家庭隔离的条件。

• 有能力和意愿进行长期治疗。

• 可获得适当的门诊随访和治疗。

• 必须通知公共卫生部门。

转诊问题

转去公共卫生机构做 DOT。

随访建议

• 定期查痰以记录病菌清除状况。

• 药物毒性监测。

- 异烟肼、利福平、吡嗪酰胺：监测肝功能预防肝损伤。
- 吡嗪酰胺：检测尿酸水平。
- 乙胺丁醇：视力测试防止色盲。

要点和误区

• 早隔离和预防呼吸道传播。

• 详细询问既往史以明确风险因素。

• 胸片和 PPD 试验是诊断的辅助手段。

• 活动期疾病开始需 4 药合用。

• 未坚持的活动性肺结核患者被认为妨害公共卫生；在数个地区有相应的法律来规范这样的问题。

结节病 Sarcoidosis

Jesse B. Cannon 何融冰 伍力学 译

基础知识

描述

• 这是一种以 T 淋巴细胞和单核巨噬细胞局部堆积形成的非干酪性上皮样肉芽肿为特征的慢性多系统功能障碍性疾病。

• 其症状主要由于局部组织结构破坏导致的器官功能障碍所引起：

- 以肺部症状为主。

• 由于肉芽肿组织的分泌作用，血管紧张素转化酶和维生素 D 水平可能增加。

• 在美国和欧洲发病率为(10～20)/10 万。

• 可见于几乎所有种族和地域的人群。

- 非洲裔人群较为高发。
- 在美国，黑种人的发病风险为 2.4%，而白种人为 0.85%。

• 典型症状一般首发于 10～40 岁。

病因

尚不明确，表现为一种针对不明自身或非自身抗原的细胞介导的过度的免疫反应。其发病呈家族群集性，这提示该病可能与遗传相关。

诊断

■ 症状和体征

病史

- 全身性：
- 疲劳，全身无力。
- 体重减少。
- 发热。
- 皮肤(25%)：
- 皮疹，皮损。
- 心脏/呼吸(可见于90%患者)：
- 呼吸困难。
- 胸痛。
- 心悸。
- 咳嗽。
- 咯血。
- 神经系统：
- 颅神经麻痹。
- 癫痫。
- 精神异常。
- 眼部(可见于20%患者)：
- 眼痛。
- 视力模糊或失明。
- 肾脏：
- 腰肋部疼痛。
- 骨骼肌肉：
- 关节痛。

体格检查

- 全身性：
- 发热。
- 昏睡。
- 皮肤：
- 结节性红斑。
- 皮下结节。
- 斑丘疹。
- 斑块。
- 浸润性瘢痕。
- 冻疮样狼疮。
- 眼耳鼻喉：
- 角膜结膜炎，葡萄膜炎。
- 腮腺肿大。
- 神经系统：
- 神经麻痹(通常累及面神经)。
- 呼吸：
- 啰音。
- 气促少见。
- 心脏(约5%患者可见)：
- 心律失常、传导异常、房室传导阻滞。
- 慢性心衰(由于限制性心肌病)。
- 杂音(由于乳头肌功能障碍)。
- 肾脏：
- 肾结石。
- 肌肉骨骼的：
- 多发关节痛。
- Lofgren 综合征：
- 双侧肺门淋巴结肿大。
- 结节性红斑。
- 伴或不伴多发性关节痛。
- Heerfordt-Waldenstrom 综合征：
- 发热。
- 葡萄膜炎。
- 腮腺肿大。
- 伴或不伴面神经麻痹。

儿科注意事项

- <4 岁的儿童典型表现为合并皮疹、葡萄膜炎和关节炎“三联征”。
- >4 岁的儿童临床表现与成人相似。

■ 基本检查

- 体格检查重点在肺、皮肤、眼睛、心脏和肌肉骨骼系统。
- 脉氧饱和度/动脉血气分析。
- 心电图(心律失常、传导阻滞)。
- 眼部裂隙灯检查。

■ 诊断检查与说明

实验室检查

- 75%的病例血清 ACE 升高。
- 白细胞减少，可能伴有嗜酸性粒细胞增多。
- 肝功能检查：轻微，通常无症状，主要是碱性磷酸酶或转氨酶可能轻微升高。
- 血清钙：由于维生素 D 水平升高而引起的高钙血症。
- 尿液：高尿钙。
- 高丙种球蛋白血症。
- 脑脊液检查：淋巴细胞为主型，血管紧张素转化酶水平抬高。

影像学检查

胸部 X 线片：90%以上的类肉瘤病患者存在异常，因此很多患者是在检查中偶然发现该病：

- 1 型：双侧肺门淋巴结病变。
- 2 型：淋巴结病变和肺实质改变(网格样阴影)。
- 3 型：肺实质性改变，主要在上肺，伴有肺门淋巴结退行性改变。
- 4 型：网格样阴影，肺纤维化，尤其在上叶。
- 放射性核素扫描可辨别肉芽肿性疾病，但不具特异性。
- CT 扫描的结果与 X 线片相似。

诊断步骤/外科

- 活检：
- 支气管镜和支气管肺泡灌洗。
- 如有条件，可取皮损处活检。
- Kveim-Siltzbach 试验：
- 皮下注射抗原，与 PPD 试验相似。
- 很少用。

■ 鉴别诊断

- HIV、CVID。
- 其他肉芽肿性疾病。
- 血管炎，如 Wegener、Churg-Strauss。
- 因组织异物引起的肉芽肿。
- 淋巴瘤。
- 真菌感染(如组织胞浆菌病)。
- 尘肺。
- 分歧杆菌感染。
- 甲状旁腺疾病。

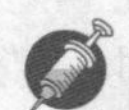

治疗

■ 院前

给氧。

■ 初步稳定/治疗

- 给氧。
- 监测心律失常。

■ 急诊治疗/程序

- 鉴于50%的患者可自发缓解，可先观察暂不治疗。
- 有一个以上上述表现的，应开始激素治疗：
- 有症状或Ⅱ期进展型肺疾病。
- Ⅲ期肺疾病。
- 恶性高钙血症。
- 严重眼部疾病。
- 神经系统后遗症。
- 鼻咽部、喉部受累。
- 考虑局部使用皮质类固醇和睫状肌麻痹剂治疗前葡萄膜炎或皮肤症状。

■ 药物治疗

- 泼尼松：10～80 mg(儿童：0.5～2 mg/kg)，口服，每日 1 次。
- 低剂量治疗高钙血症肾病和轻到中度病变。

- 高剂量治疗神经类肉瘤病。

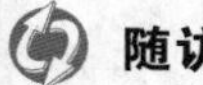

随访

进一步处理

入院指征

- 低氧血症。
- 有中度到重度呼吸系统症状的患者。
- 出现明显的心脏传导延迟。
- 重度血小板减少症。

出院指征

后续能确保有效随访者。

转诊问题

- 心脏疾病：
  - 任何传导障碍或慢性心衰。
- 风湿性疾病：
  - 常规治疗和随访：
    - 处于疾病活动期患者每2个月使用一次激素，无症状患者每3～4个月一次激素。
- 肺部疾病：
  - 进行规范的肺功能检查（来监测限制性肺疾病的进展）和肺活量测定及肺一氧化碳弥散量（DLCO）。
- 眼科疾病：
  - 发病48 h内的急性葡萄膜炎。

随访建议

- 限制饮食中的钙过量摄入。
- 监测与长期激素治疗相关的并发症。

要点和误区

- 通过胸片检查评估患者的疾病分期和进展情况。
- 泼尼松是疾病进展时可选择的治疗药物。
- 监测高钙血症征象和相关并发症。
- 关注急性神经系统和眼部后遗症。

结节性红斑 Erythema Nodosum

Kate E. Hughes 单怡 译

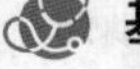

基础知识

描述

结节性红斑（EN）特征为下肢伸肌表面多个对称非溃疡疼痛结节。

- 年轻人常见。
- 高发年龄在30岁后。
- 女性更常见（4∶1）。
- 结节边缘不清楚，大小由1～10 cm不等。
- 皮损最初是红色的，经3～6周逐渐消退呈瘀斑。
- 脂肪小叶间隔炎症引起皮肤损害（间隔性脂膜炎）。
- 3～6周病变自然消退。
- 主要病变包括：
  - 游走性结节性红斑（通常是轻度单侧病变，很少或无全身症状）。
  - 慢性结节性红斑（病程较长，相关的全身症状往往较轻）。

病因

- 免疫介导反应。
- 30%～50%为特异性病因。
- 常常是一种潜在疾病的标志，特殊病因包括：
  - 药物反应：
    - 口服避孕药。
    - 磺胺类药物。
    - 青霉素。
  - 感染包括：
    - 链球菌性咽炎。
    - 结核杆菌（TB）。
    - 非典型分枝杆菌。
    - 球孢子菌病。
    - 肝炎。
    - 单纯疱疹病毒。
    - 传染性单核细胞增多症。
    - 梅毒。
    - 衣原体。
    - 立克次体。
    - 沙门菌。
    - 弯曲菌。
    - 鼠疫。
    - 寄生虫。
    - 麻风。
  - 全身性疾病：
    - 结节病。
    - 炎症性肠病。
    - 白塞病。
    - 结缔组织疾病。
  - 恶性肿瘤如淋巴瘤和白血病。
  - 猫抓病。
  - HIV感染。
  - 很少由肝炎疫苗和结核病卡介苗引起。
  - 妊娠。

儿科注意事项

结节性红斑通常在咽炎2～3周后发病。

诊断

症状和体征

- 分布于双小腿伸侧皮下结节。
- 病变偶尔发生于手指、手、手臂、小腿和大腿上。
- 长期卧床患者可能累及受压部位。
- 发热、乏力、关节痛、关节炎、白细胞增多、单侧或双侧肺门淋巴结肿大等此病的表现。

病史

- 一般症状可先于或伴随皮疹出现：
  - 发热。
  - 全身不适。
  - 多发性关节炎。
- 结节性红斑的一般症状可能是以下疾病的标志：
  - 炎症性肠病。
  - 细菌性肠炎。
  - 胰腺炎。
  - 白塞病。
  - 旅行史很重要，因为病因有地区差异。

体格检查

- 仔细的检查很重要，因为潜在的病因各不相同。
- 胫前区病变最常见，但也可能出现在大腿、上肢和颈部，面部较少。
- 下肢非典型病变。
- 可有下肢水肿。
- 应评估淋巴结肿大。

基本检查

详细的病史和体格检查旨在找出病因。

诊断检查与说明

实验室检查

- 全血细胞计数。

- 咽拭子、抗链球菌溶血素O滴度。
- 红细胞沉降率(血沉)。
- 合理的化学检查。
- 肝功能试验。
- 流行地区的球孢子菌病血清学试验。
- 流行地区结核皮肤测试。

影像学检查

X线胸片：肺门淋巴结肿大可能是结节病、球孢子菌病、肺结核或其他真菌感染。

诊断步骤/外科

- 深部活检和组织病理学可明确诊断(穿刺活检可能并不足够)：
- 当考虑为结核病时，通常不典型。

鉴别诊断

- 结节性筋膜炎。
- 各种类型的脂膜炎与结节性红斑类似。
- 可通过组织病理学鉴别。
- 其他疾病包括：
  - 结节性动脉周围炎。
  - 游走性血栓性静脉炎。
  - 浅表性血栓闭塞性脉管炎。
  - 硬皮病。
  - 系统性红斑狼疮。
  - α-抗胰蛋白酶缺乏症。
  - 白塞综合征。
  - 脂肪代谢障碍。
  - 白血病脂肪浸润。
  - 与使用类固醇相关的脂膜炎、寒战和感染。

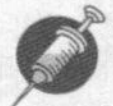

治疗

儿科注意事项

- 儿童罕见，咽炎是最可能的病因。
- 应考虑猫抓病。

院前

坚持常规预防措施。

初步稳定/治疗

气道、呼吸和循环(ABC管理)，建立静脉通路，供氧，监测。

急诊治疗/程序

- 应针对潜在的疾病治疗。
- 支持疗法包括休息，抬高肢体和应用止痛剂。
- 糖皮质激素和碘化钾可能有助于缓解症状。
- 某些潜在的感染(如结核或球孢子菌病)，全身应用糖皮质激素可能加快播散，故应禁用。
- 甲状腺功能亢进症(甲亢)和孕妇禁忌使用碘化钾。

药物治疗

- 阿司匹林650 mg，口服，必要时4～6 h给1次(儿童：禁忌使用)。总量不超过4 g/24 h。
- 布洛芬：400～800 mg，口服，q8 h(儿童：5～10 mg/kg，口服，q6 h)。
- 萘普生：250～500 mg，口服，q12 h(儿童：5～7 mg/kg，口服，q12 h)。
- 吲哚美辛：25～50 mg，口服，q8 h。
- 碘化钾/碘化钾饱和溶液(用于顽固性疾病，甲亢禁忌使用)：360～900 mg，口服，q8 h，持续3～4周。
- 全身性糖皮质激素治疗：40 mg/d，口服，由主治医师确定用药时间。

一线药物

- 休息或支持治疗。
- 抬高患肢。
- 非甾体抗炎药。
- 治疗基础疾病。

二线药物

- 碘化钾。
- 类固醇。

随访

进一步处理

入院指征

根据症状的严重程度和病因。

出院指征

- 无中毒表现，能够口服药物的患者。
- 应安排随访日程。

转诊问题

- 结节性红斑通常具有自限性，在3～6周好转。
- 不典型的病例可能需要活检。
- 类固醇和钾的治疗需要主治医师监测。
- 难治或反复发作患者需转诊皮肤科。
- 妊娠患者可能需要妇产科会诊协助用药方案。

随访建议

- 随访评估初诊医师或皮肤科医师治疗方案。
- 可能需要转诊至专科评估潜在的病因。

要点和误区

- 结节性红斑是通常是特发性的，但也可能是全身性疾病的首发征兆。
- 如果潜在的病因未得到治疗，病变可以复发。
- 非典型性和慢性病变可提示其他诊断并需要活检。
- 服用钾或类固醇的患者需要密切随访。

J

结膜炎 Conjunctivitis

Kendra Amico · Yasuharu Okuda 陈奇通 译

基础知识

描述

结膜的感染性和非感染性炎症，大多数情况是自我限制的。

病因

传染性

通常称为“红眼睛”：

- 细菌：
  - 金黄色葡萄球菌(大多数成人感染)。
  - 肺炎链球菌。
  - 卡他莫拉菌。
  - 流感嗜血杆菌(流行率下降)。
  - 铜绿假单胞菌。
  - 淋病奈瑟球菌(GC)：
    - 新生儿或成人。

◦ 眼科急症。
- 沙眼衣原体：
◦ 新生儿或亚急性感染(青少年/成人)。
• 病毒：
- 腺病毒最常见。
◦ 一些血清型引起暴发性形式：流行性角结膜炎(EKC)和眼科急症。
- 单纯疱疹病毒(HSV)和水痘-带状疱疹病毒(VZV)：
◦ 眼科急症。

非感染性

• 过敏：
- 花粉，动物皮屑，环境抗原。
• 接触/毒性/化学物质：
- 可能是由于化学刺激、防腐剂、药物、洗发水、氯、灰尘、烟气引起的超敏反应。
- 假单胞菌通常与隐形眼镜配戴者有关。

诊断

排他性诊断。

症状和体征

• 主要：
- 红眼(整个角膜充血刺激)。
- 沙粒感，异物感。
- 灼热、发痒的眼睛。
- 流泪增加。
- 晨起眼睑结痂或粘连，分泌物增多。
- 结膜水肿(球结膜水肿)和眼睑水肿。
- 24 h 内出现溃疡、瘢痕和穿孔，导致失明。
• 淋球菌性：
- 超急性多量脓性分泌物，通常在接触后 12 h 发作。
- 严重的球结膜水肿。
- 常无耳前淋巴结肿大。
- 24 h 内侵犯完整结膜和角膜，并引起溃疡、瘢痕和穿孔导致失明。
• 衣原体：
- 黏脓性分泌物。
- 伴有或不伴有畏光。
- 合并生殖器感染(>50%)。
• 病毒：
- 泪液、黏液或少量黏液脓性分泌物。
- 24～48 h 扩散至另一只眼睛。
- 眼睑结膜可能有凹凸不平的表现。
- 与上呼吸道疾病相关。
• EKC：
- 结膜充血。
- 球结膜水肿。
- 角膜浸润。
- 视力下降。
• HSV 和 VZV：
- 与附近皮肤的疼痛或感觉异常有关。
- 眼缘或眼球旁皮肤处有皮肤病灶或小疱。
- 角膜受累及树突状病灶。
- 结膜上很少形成囊泡或溃疡。
• 过敏：
- 特征：发痒。
- 水样分泌物。
- 乳头肥大。
- 经常有过敏、特应性、鼻漏的病史。
• 化学品：
- 急性症状导致角膜穿孔。
- 正常视力敏锐度和眼内压。

基本检查

• 病史：
- 炎症起始时间。
- 环境或工作相关暴露。
- 不洁接触史。
- 性行为、分泌物、皮疹。
- OTC 或者化妆品使用。
- 全身性疾病。
• 视力测试。
• 荧光素染色和裂隙灯检查(如有需要)。

诊断检查与说明

实验室检查

• 腺病毒快速抗原检测。
• 革兰染色和培养(常规情况下未显示)：
- 适应证：
◦ 新生儿结膜炎。
◦ 疑似淋球菌性结膜炎。
◦ 免疫功能低下的宿主。
◦ 全身疾病的体征和症状。
◦ 由于 MRSA 结膜炎增加，48～72 h 后抗生素治疗无效(依从性良好)。

鉴别诊断

“红眼”体征和症状包括畏光，视力下降，头痛和恶心，脊柱侧弯，瞳孔固定，睫毛潮红，应迅速考虑其他诊断。
• 急性后角闭角性青光眼(最严重病因)。
• 前葡萄膜炎。
• 角膜擦伤。
• 干眼。
• 异物。
• 虹膜炎。
• 角膜炎。
• 鼻泪管梗阻。
• 巩膜炎或巩膜外层炎。
• 结膜下出血。

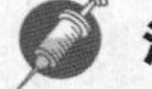

治疗

初步稳定/治疗

• 经验性使用广谱抗生素局部药物(如果担心细菌原因)。
• 添加针对淋球菌、衣原体和脑膜炎球菌结膜炎，新生儿结膜炎及所有严重感染的全身疗法，无论其原因如何。
• 咨询眼科医师，处理疱疹性眼部感染和 EKC。

急诊治疗/程序

• 总体管理与咨询：
- 经常用湿的一次性湿布擦去眼睛的分泌物。
- 隐形眼镜佩戴者应扔掉受影响的隐形眼镜并停止使用，直到：
◦ 症状已解决——24 h 无发红，无分泌物。
◦ 抗生素治疗完成。
- 经常洗手。
- 不合用毛巾、纸巾、化妆品、亚麻衣物。
• 细菌性结膜炎：
- 外用抗生素(小儿科首选药膏)。
- 症状缓解后继续治疗 48 h。
- 如果 48～72 h 无改善则停止治疗并留取培养(依从性良好)。
• 抗生素—全身性：
- 淋球菌感染需强制肠道外治疗。
- 衣原体患者的性伴侣和新生儿父母需接受全身性治疗。
• 病毒性结膜炎：
- 无特异性抗病毒治疗。
- 局部抗组胺药或解充血药物的作用有限。
- 非抗生素润滑剂。
• EKC：
- 可能需要局部使用类固醇，咨询眼科后决定。
• 过敏性结膜炎(预期可改善 2 周)：
- 抗组胺药或减充血药。
- 肥大细胞稳定剂、抗组胺药或 NSAIDs 滴眼液作为二线药物。
- 人工眼泪。
• 非感染性：
- 非抗生素眼药水或药膏。

药物治疗

• 主要：

- 全部接触镜佩戴者需假单胞菌覆盖。
- 在结膜炎的一般治疗中不使用糖皮质激素。
• 细菌治疗 5～7 日：
- 杆菌肽：500 U/g 眼膏 0.5 in，每日 1 次。
- 杆菌肽多黏菌素 B：0.5 in，每日 1 次。
- 0.3%环丙沙星：1 滴，每日 4 次（抗假单胞菌）。
- 0.5%红霉素：0.5 in，每日 4 次（便宜）。
- 0.3%氧氟沙星：1～2 滴，每日 4 次（抗假单胞菌）。
- 甲氧苄氨嘧啶-多黏菌素 B：1～2 滴，每日 4 次。
• 衣原体（局部无效）：
- 新生儿/儿科：
◦ 一线：阿奇霉素每天 20 mg/kg，口服×3 日。
◦ 二线：红霉素 12.5 mg/kg，口服，每日 4 次×14 日。
- 成人：
◦ 一线：阿奇霉素 1 g，口服一次（包括衣原体覆盖）。
◦ 二线：强力霉素：100 mg，口服，每日 4 次×7 日。
• 淋球菌：
- 新生儿/儿童：
◦ 一线：头孢噻肟 100 mg/kg，静脉注射。
◦ 二线：头孢曲松钠 50 mg/kg，静脉注射或肌内注射（新生儿高胆红素血症的风险）。
- 成人：
◦ 头孢曲松：250 mg，静脉注射一次（包括衣原体覆盖）。
• 病毒性：
- 眼药水或药膏：人造眼泪或 Lacri-Lube。
- Naphcon-A 或 Visine AC：1 滴或 2 滴，每日 4 次 PRN，持续不少于 1 周。
• HSV（局部和口服治疗具有相似的功效）：
- 一线：更昔洛韦 0.15%乳油凝胶，每日 5 次；或阿昔洛韦口服 400 mg，每日 5 次，持续 7～14 日。
- 二线：三氟胸苷 1% 1 滴，q2 h，持续 14 日（角膜上皮毒性风险）。
- 无糖皮质激素。
• VZV：
- 一线：伐昔洛韦，口服，1 g，每日 3 次，7～14 日。
- 二线：阿昔洛韦，口服，400 mg，每日 5 次；或泛昔洛韦，口服，500 mg，每日剂量×7 日（具有免疫能力）。
- 阿昔洛韦：口服，10 mg/kg，每日 3 次（免疫抑制）。
- 补充治疗：泼尼松龙 1%：1～2 滴，q2 h。
• 过敏性：
- 一线：萘甲唑啉（Naphcon-A）：1 滴，每日 2～4 次，或 Opcon-A 或 Visine-A。
- 二线：色苷酸钠 4%，1 滴，每日 4 次。
- 仅短期使用（<2 周），否则会出现反弹性充血。
• 非感染性和非过敏性：
- 眼湿润剂滴眼液或软膏：人工眼泪或 Lacri-Lube。
• 经验性治疗：
- 0.5%红霉素软膏，0.5 in，每日 4 次。

儿童注意事项

• 婴儿中常为全身性疾病的表现。
• 新生儿眼炎定义为生命的前 4 周内的结膜炎。
• 硝酸银不能根除沙眼衣原体。
• 一些用红霉素治疗的新生儿仍会发展成淋球菌性结膜炎。
• 出生第一个 36 h 出现的结膜炎常是化学药剂性的，其由出生时使用的硝酸银导致。
• 新生儿在通过产道期间通过垂直传播受到感染-淋球菌、疱疹、衣原体生物最常见。
• 软膏较滴眼液更合适，因滴眼液使用时存在困难。

随访

进一步处理

入院指征

已知或者可疑的淋球菌感染（任何年龄组）。

出院指征

所有病例密切随访。

转诊问题

EKC 和细菌性结膜炎的诊断需眼科医师会诊。

随访建议

所有有细菌性结膜炎或其他与单纯性结膜炎不一致的非典型检查结果的患者需要立即进行眼科随访。

要点和误区

• 结膜炎（和 EKC）极易传染；病毒病因具有长达 2 周的传染性。
• 确保给患者使用的裂隙灯和坐椅不被感染，以避免污染。
• 使用皮质激素时需非常小心，因为它们可能使潜在的 HSV 感染恶化或威胁健康视力。
• 如果出现“红眼”症状，请考虑其他诊断方法，并征询专家的意见。

疥疮 Scabies

Charles S. Graffeo 周健 潘曙明 译

基础知识

描述

• 疥螨属于节肢动物类，蛛形纲，螨亚纲，疥螨科。
• 疥螨可以繁殖，但不能在人类宿主身上繁殖。
• 严重时雌性疥螨形成洞穴，每日将 2～3 个卵沉积角质层，还有粪便、皮肤真菌和唾液存入角质层。
• 可发生继发感染，通常是由金黄色葡萄球菌或溶血链球菌引起的，可导致肾脏和心脏后遗症。
• 在拥挤、资源贫乏的社区和难民人口中，结核病是一个重大的全球卫生问题。

儿科注意事项

• 疥疮在儿童中以各种形式出现，与成人不同。
- 炎症性更强（水疱性或大疱性）。
- 包括面部、头皮、手掌或足底。
• 2 岁以下儿童患病率最高。

病因

• 流行病学：
- 流行报告涉及面很广。

- WHO 报道可能有 1.3 亿人感染。
- 疾病负担在热带气候国家最高，尤其是在拥挤和贫困地区。

• 通过(15～20 min)直接与皮肤接触，或不常通过感染的床上用品或衣物传播。
- 这是一种过度拥挤和贫穷情况下的常见疾病，而不是反映出卫生不佳。
- 家庭成员、性接触和机构环境都容易导致传播。

• 症状是由于对螨、卵、唾液和粪便的Ⅳ型超敏反应延迟(在初次暴露中为 2～4 周)。
- 炎症反应会导致强烈的夜间瘙痒，这是一个超敏反应症状。
- 疥疮(挪威语)的特点是感染高达数百万螨，具有高传染性在免疫功能低下患者中常见。

• 螨虫食用溶解的人体组织(不以血液为食)，在宿主体外可以活 3 日。

• 平均而言，宿主上的螨虫数量为 5～15，除非这表明有巨大的虫害。

诊断

症状和体征

全身和强烈的瘙痒，晚间更严重，通常头部和面部没有瘙痒。

病史

• 指间和皱褶皮肤病变最常见。

• 初期可能无症状。

• 可影响腋窝、乳晕、脐、生殖器、膝盖和脚踝。

• 皮疹史应包括生活条件、家庭成员和密切接触者作为潜在的皮疹源。

• 全身、强烈的瘙痒性疹：
- 瘙痒在夜间增强。

• 暴露和感染后 10～30 日发病，立即(1～3日)引起瘙痒。
- 挪威疥疮患者通常免疫功能受损，炎症反应减弱，瘙痒较少。

体格检查

常见的误诊包括湿疹、脓疱病、体癣(癣)和牛皮癣。

• 皮肤上的发现通常很少。

• 原发病灶：线形、高、白灰色洞穴(身长 1 cm，头发丝宽度)、最初无症状，末端有黑点(肉眼几乎看不到螨虫)：
- 手指、手腕和肘部屈肌表面、腰围、脐周皮肤、腋窝皱褶、臀部、阴茎、阴囊、外阴和乳晕周围的网隙对称分布。
- 成人很少受影响，但婴儿和儿童更常见。

• 继发性病变：炎症性丘疹、结节、脱皮，或继发性脓疱炎或毛囊炎：
- 继发性病变通常比洞穴多且突出，但如果使用局部类固醇也可能较少。

• 长时间的感染导致慢性的皮疹、湿疹、色素过多和脂化皮肤。

• 结痂的挪威疥疮在手部、足部、头皮和承压区域产生大面积的角质斑块：
- 鳞片会变疣状。
- 裂隙可能出现。
- 指甲受累是常见的。

• 所有疑似疥疮的病例都应检查生殖器。

儿科注意事项

• 皮疹通常是弥漫性的，有更多的小疱、脓疱，与脓疱类似。

• 新生儿疥疮与营养不良、体重增加和严重感染有关。

基本检查

• 仔细检查病史和皮肤特征。

• 患者可能会说他们的皮肤“像爬行一样”瘙痒。

• 诊断很容易被忽略，在任何持续性全身瘙痒患者中都应该考虑。

诊断检查与说明

实验室检查

• 没有诊断的“金标准”的实验室检查。

• 存在的结块或传播感染，需要积极检查是否存在全身感染。

• 筛查其他性传播疾病。

影像学检查

荧光显微镜和皮肤镜检查可用于在体内检查洞穴、粪便、螨虫。

诊断步骤/外科

使用皮肤镜或显微镜结合皮肤刮擦或表皮活检等设备进行直接可视化可能有助于诊断，特别是在多个部位取样时。

• 由于典型疥疮中螨虫数量少，负面刮除并不排除感染。

• 灵敏度＜50%，受采样点数量和采样者经验的影响。

• 使用新的程序，如荧光素和 Wood 灯或洞穴墨水测试可能有助于诊断，虽然都不是高灵敏度或特异性。

鉴别诊断

在最初的表现上，误诊很常见。

• 特应性皮炎。

• 湿疹。

• 疱疹样皮炎。

• 丘疹性荨麻疹。

• 毛囊炎。

• 扁平苔藓。

• 妊娠瘙痒性荨麻疹丘疹和斑块。

• 成人线性 IgA 大疱性皮肤病。

• 梅毒。

• 虱病。

• 玫瑰糠疹。

• 脓疱病。

• 脂溢性皮炎。

• 跳蚤叮咬和臭虫。

• 药物作用暴发。

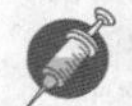

治疗

院前

保持常规预防措施。

初步稳定/治疗

• 不需要特定的稳定性。

• 前期筛查是入院的重要途径，通过对高危患者的筛查，可以及早发现感染患者。

治疗

• 治疗不应该是广泛性瘙痒患者的经验性治疗，而应该是有暴露史、典型的特征性疹分布或两者兼而有之的患者。

• 治疗患者和所有接触过局部杀菌剂的人：
- 同时治疗所有接触者，不论有无症状。

• 渗透率 5%时 89%～92%有效，耐受性良好(B类妊娠)：
- ＜2%氯菊酯被皮肤吸收，潜在毒性低：
  ◦ 儿童＞2 个月。
  ◦ 从头到足涂抹(避开眼睛和嘴)8～14 h 后淋浴。
  ◦ 1～2 周重复 1 次 10%的杀菌剂是 50%～60%有效的，当其他的杀菌剂不能耐受时使用。

• 伊维除虫菌素口服 2 次，间隔 7～14 日，其疗效与氯菊酯类似(但不适用于孕妇或哺乳期妇女或＜15 kg 的儿童)：
- 对不能耐受局部疥疮的患者或耐药或结痂的挪威疥疮患者有效。
- 可能对生命周期的所有阶段都无效(可能无法对疥疮卵进行消毒)。
- 在地方病人群中，大规模给药已被证明优于其他药物。

• 1%林丹疗效可能略低，对中枢神经系统有潜在毒性：
- 林丹吸收(通过皮肤、肺或肠黏膜或黏膜)

J

约为 10%。

◦ 副作用包括恶心、头痛、眩晕、弱视、易怒和癫痫。

- 不用于儿科患者或广泛的擦伤或皮炎患者。

• 10%克罗米通的疗效为 50%～60%，在其他 scabicide 不能耐受时使用(妊娠C类)。

- 连续使用两晚，第二次使用 48 h 后移除。

- 对婴儿安全。

• 挪威疥疮需要用角化液去除角化过度的鳞屑，以促进杀伤剂的进入。

• 治疗建议：

- 以患者为中心的关于预防治疗密切接触者的决定是必要的，因为证据是不确定的。

- 热循环(60 ℃)或干燥清洁处理后 2 日内穿的所有的衣服和床上用品，或将物品放在塑料袋中。

- 用真空吸尘器清扫家用地板、地毯、床垫和家具。

- 不建议进行高压灭菌、漂白或熏蒸。

- 皮肤炎症反应杀死螨虫后，瘙痒可持续 1～4 周。

- 局部类固醇和口服抗组胺剂可以减少瘙痒症状。

- 复发可以发生在未经处理的区域，如头皮和舌下区域。

- 治疗失败往往是由于患者认识不清和患者教育不到位造成的。

药物治疗

• scabicides：

- 克罗米通 10%乳液或乳霜：在儿童和成人的整个皮肤表面局部涂抹 2 个晚上，然后在最后一次使用后冲洗 48 h。

- 伊维菌素 3 mg 片剂：第一次口服剂量为 200 μg/kg，第二次口服剂量为 200 μg/kg 7～14 日(妊娠类 C)。

- 1%林丹乳液或乳霜：在 8～12 h 后从颈部向下涂抹，然后冲洗干净；在婴儿、妊娠、哺乳期、过度脱皮或癫痫发作时禁忌。

- 5%氯菊酯面霜：适用于成人颈部以下，儿童全皮肤；8～14 h 后冲洗(B级妊娠，母乳喂养安全性未知)。

- 5%～10%硫沉淀在凡士林油中：连续 3 个晚上在夜间使用，然后在 24 h 后清洗。

• 止痒剂：

- 低抗/选择性抗组胺药：

◦ 西替利嗪(仙特明)：成人和婴幼儿＞6 岁：5～10 mg/d；6～12 个月：2.5 mg/d，口服；12～24 个月：2.5 mg/d，口服；2～6 岁：2.5～5 mg/d。

◦ 盐酸非索非那定：成人和儿童＞12 岁：180 mg/d 或 60 mg；2～5 岁：15～30 mg；6～11 岁：30 mg，口服。

◦ 氯雷他定：成人和儿童＞6 岁：10 mg/d 婴幼儿；2～5 岁：5 mg/d。

- 镇静/非选择性抗组胺药：

◦ 苯海拉明：成人和儿童＞12 岁：25～50 mg 口服，q4～6 h；2～6 岁：6.25 mg 口服，q4～6 h；6～12 岁：12.5～25 mg，q4～6 h。

◦ 多虑平：25～50 mg，口服，剂量目前不可用。

◦ 羟嗪(Atarax)：成人和儿童＞12 岁：25～100 mg 口服 q6～8 h；＜6 岁：2 mg/(kg·d)口服，q6～8 h；6～12 岁：12.5～25 mg 口服，q6～8 h。

一线用药

氯菊酯 5%乳液。

二线用药

依维菌素或克罗米通 10%洗液或乳液。

随访

进一步处理

入院指征

• 严重局部或全身超级感染的患者。

• 耐药性或复发病例。

出院指征

出现常规症状的无毒患者。

随访建议

1～4 周后重新评估复发。

• 正确应用治疗后瘙痒可持续 4 周。

• 治疗失败往往是由于不正确的局部用药，或如果发现活螨虫后没有治疗所有的接触。

要点和误区

• 疥疮是一种常见的寄生虫感染，通过长时间的皮肤和皮肤直接接触传播。

• 儿童的疥疮与成人不同。

• 硬痂的挪威疥疮具有大量螨虫的特征，在免疫缺陷或生活不能自理患者中可见。

• 治疗失败很常见：

- 适当的患者教育可以减少治疗失败。

J

紧急剖宫产 Cesarean Section, Emergency

John A. Guisto · Gregory L. Gaskin 庄育刚 译

基础知识

• 产妇心搏骤停时的紧急分娩。

• 需要立即识别并开始复苏。

• 必须快速评估病因以进行直接治疗。

• 快速分娩为孕产妇和胎儿的生存提供了最佳机会。

• 同义词：复苏性子宫切开术。

注意

• 无论何种原因导致的妊娠 20 周以上的孕妇发生心跳呼吸停止，并且初期的心肺复苏无效果，急诊内科医师可紧急行死亡过程的急诊剖宫产，也是急诊内科医师唯一的手术适应证。

• 胎儿能否存活的重要预测因素是孕妇发生心跳停止和剖宫产之间的时间差。

- 剖宫产应在心跳停止 4 min 内进行。

- 目标是 1 min 内娩出胎儿。

• 产科医师、儿科医师和外科医师(创伤相关)急会诊。

- 相关医师到来前不要耽误启动流程。

• 20 周以内不要剖宫产。

病因

• 产前产妇心搏骤停罕见：

- 1/12 500 产妇。

• 孕产妇生存率为 17%～59%。

• 胎儿存活率为 61%～80%：

- 88%～100%的存活婴儿神经系统完整。

• 产妇心搏骤停的最常见原因：

- 出血：45%。
 ◦ 可能与创伤有关。
- 羊水栓塞：13%。
- 败血症：11%。
- 麻醉并发症：8%。
- 创伤：3%。

诊断

■ 症状和体征

病史

• 妊娠 20 周(通过宫底高度测定)以上女性发生心跳呼吸停止。

体格检查

妊娠 20 周，宫底高度在脐部或脐部以上。

■ 基本检查

• 对明显妊娠女性的内科检查确认呼吸停止和无脉搏。
- 迅速评估可逆转的心跳呼吸停止原因：
 ◦ 低氧。
 ◦ 血容量过低。
 ◦ 酸中毒。
 ◦ 低血钾/高血钾。
 ◦ 低体温。
 ◦ 创伤。
 ◦ 血栓形成。
 ◦ 中毒。
 ◦ 张力性气胸。
 ◦ 心脏压塞。
- 仰卧位低血压综合征(增大的子宫压迫下腔静脉)。

• 通过宫底高低评估妊娠时间。
• 耻骨到高低高度的厘米值大致与孕周一致。例如：20 cm＝20 周。
• 若能进行急诊超声对胎儿的评估则更有益，但不要延迟美国确认胎龄的程序。

■ 诊断检查与说明

影像学检查

• 无必要。
• 不需要把宝贵的时间应用于胎心监测。

■ 鉴别诊断

心跳呼吸停止是最终途径。

• 评估可能的原因。

治疗

■ 院前

• 时间最短。
• 手动将子宫移至左侧(建议)或将患者置于左侧卧位，避免压迫下腔静脉(仰卧位低血压综合征)。
• 创伤患者需要脊髓保护：
- 子宫可移到左侧。
- 右髋抬高 45°。

■ 初步稳定/治疗

• 标准心肺复苏。
- 急诊插管。
 ◦ 使用比未妊娠女性略小 0.5～1 mm 的气管导管。
- 高流量给氧。
- 心电、血压监测。
- 两条外周血管通路：
 ◦ 液体复苏。
 ◦ 可考虑输注 O 型血。

• 胎儿存活和母体存活与合适与初始孕妇复苏有关。
• 若妊娠不足 24 周，使用高级生命支持和高级创伤生命支持方案进行孕妇心肺复苏。
- 不要进行急诊剖宫产。

• 不建议将患者从现场转移到手术室，因为这可能会延迟剖宫产，并且在行进过程中会导致较低质量的压迫。
• 妊娠 20 周以上，使用 4 min 定律：
- 进行 4 min 高级生命支持和高级创伤生命支持。
- 若无反应，则行紧急剖宫产。
- 目标是 1 min 内娩出胎儿。
- 若孕妇无明显存活希望，立即进行死亡过程的紧急剖宫产。

■ 急诊治疗/程序

• 产科、外科、小儿科急会诊：
- 等待会诊过程中不要延误抢救。

• 不影响启动程序的情况下插入导尿管，并保证导尿管在位。
• 剖宫产：
- 使用腹部黑线作为正中垂直切口。
- 从阴毛线到脐上 5 cm 切开腹壁。
- 切口经过筋膜和腹膜。
- 回拉膀胱，使其处于耻骨联合下。
- 从膀胱头侧位置的下段子宫做一纵切口。
- 向头侧用剪刀延长切口。
 ◦ 手进入子宫。
 ◦ 向上推挤子宫壁避免损伤胎儿。
- 胎儿娩出。
- 两把止血钳夹住脐带，中间切断脐带。
- 手工取出胎盘。
- 此时迅速评估孕妇生命体征，因为可能有孕妇恢复自主循环。
- 合适方法持续孕妇心肺复苏。
- 0 号线锁边缝合子宫。
- 0 号线缝合腹膜和筋膜关腹。
- 缝合皮肤。
- 使用广谱抗生素。

• 若孕妇自主循环恢复，亚低温治疗。

■ 药物治疗

一线药物

• 使用高级生命支持指导药物对孕妇进行复苏。
• 治疗可能的病因。
• 分娩后考虑使用子宫收缩剂控制出血。

二线药物

• 可能需要新生儿心肺复苏。
• 经口气管插管。

随访

■ 进一步处理

入院指征

• 新生儿需要进入 NICU。
• 若孕妇心肺复苏成功，应进入 ICU。

出院指征

新生儿和孕妇没有急诊出院指征。

要点和误区

• 仅 20 周以上孕妇发生心跳呼吸停止才适用以上程序。
• 需在 4 min 内决定是否需要行围死亡期紧急剖宫产。
• 手术要在 1 min 内完成。

J

进食障碍 Eating Disorders

Rohn S. Friedman 姜颢 译

基础知识

描述

神经性厌食症(AN)

- 限制摄入,导致体重、身高和/或发育过程明显低于同龄。
- 对体重增加或变得肥胖的强烈恐惧,或阻止体重增加的行为。
- 严重的体像障碍,对体重和体型自我评价的不当影响,或否认低体重的严重性。
- 在美国女性终身发病率为0.9%,男性为0.3%。
- 好发于青春期至青年期。

神经性暴食症(BN)

- 暴饮暴食反复发作的特点:
 - 在一段不连续的时间里吃超乎寻常的大量食物。
 - 发作期间的一种对过食的失控感。
- 反复出现阻止体重增加的不适当补偿行为:
 - 自我诱导的呕吐。
 - 泻药或灌肠的滥用。
 - 利尿药。
 - 减肥药。
 - 禁食。
 - 过度锻炼。
- 暴饮暴食和补偿3个月内平均至少1周发生1次。
- 被体重或体型过度影响的自我评价。
- 终身患病率:在美国女性中为1.5%,男性中为0.5%。
- 通常在青春晚期或成年早期发病。

暴食症(BED)

- 暴饮暴食反复发作的特点:
 - 在一段不连续的时间里吃多于平常的食物。
 - 在发作期间的一种对过食的失控感。
- 暴食症与下列3项或更多有关:
 - 比平常吃得快得多。
 - 吃到因过饱而感到不适。
 - 当生理上没有感觉饥饿时吃大量食物。
 - 因对个人的食量感到尴尬而独自进食。
 - 在过食后对自己感到厌恶、沮丧或非常愧疚。
- 对暴食的显著窘迫。
- 3个月内平均至少1周发生1次暴食。
- 无补偿行为。
- 终身患病率:在美国女性为3.5%,男性为2%。
- 在青春晚期或成年早期发病。

病因

- 对孪生的研究强烈支持遗传学因素。
- 从文化角度上,瘦被暗示为一个重要特质。
- 被描述有气质或人格属性的完美主义、焦虑及行为刚性。
- 家庭矛盾或压力是常见因素。
- 曾被报道有神经化学性(血清素)和神经内分泌性(瘦素、肾上腺轴)失调。
- 节食是一种常见的即时沉淀剂。

诊断

症状与体征

病史

- 快速或持续的体重减轻。
- 典型的每日详细饮食模式表明限制和/或暴食行为。
- 清除(呕吐、泻药、利尿药、灌肠)。
- 过度锻炼。
- 眩晕、晕厥。
- 腹胀(胃轻瘫)、便秘、腹痛。
- 疲劳、嗜睡。
- 心悸。
- 不耐寒。
- 闭经、无性欲。
- 饮食失调和肥胖家族史。
- 共患精神失调(如情绪障碍、药物滥用、人格障碍)。

体格检查

- 神经性厌食症者体重<85%理想体重,或体质指数$<17.5\ kg/m^2$。
- 低体温症。
- 低血压,体位性低血压。
- 心动过缓,心律失常。
- 皮肤:干燥的皮肤、胎毛(胸部和手臂上柔软的体毛)、胡萝卜素黄皮病。
- 乳房萎缩。
- 腮腺肿胀,颌下腺肿胀。
- 异常齿列。
- 手背擦伤(Russell征)。
- 皮肤破裂,伤口愈合不良。
- 周围性水肿。
- 肌无力。

基本检查

- 病史。
- 体格检查。
- 实验室检查。
- 营养评估。
- 精神检查:
 - 并发的精神疾病。
 - 自杀风险评估。
 - 探查社会心理环境。
- 当患者同家人居住时进行家庭评估。

诊断检查与说明

实验室检查

- 全血细胞计数(贫血、白细胞减少症、血小板减少症)。
- 电解质、尿素氮、肌酐、血糖(低钠血症、低钾血症、低血糖、脱水、代谢性碱中毒)。
- 钙、镁、磷、白蛋白(低钙血症、低镁血症、低磷血症、低蛋白血症)。
- 肝功能试验(肝功能异常)。
- 尿酸,包括比重。
- 毒性筛查。
- β人绒毛膜促性腺激素(β-HCG)。
- 淀粉酶(如果呕吐测定唾液淀粉酶,胰腺炎)。
- 脂肪酶(比淀粉酶在预测胰腺炎时更准确)。
- 考虑检查促甲状腺激素。

影像学检查

特异性检查可能有助于鉴别诊断,如MRI(排除脑肿瘤)、腹部CT(排除梗阻)。

诊断步骤/外科

- 心电图(QTc间期延长、心律失常)。
- 如果大量减重,考虑心脏超声[神经性厌食症(AN)或吐根引起的心肌病]。
- 骨密度(骨质疏松症)。

鉴别诊断

- 身体状况:
 - 胃肠道疾病(如克罗恩病、炎症性肠病、乳糜泻)。
 - 内分泌失调(如糖尿病、甲状腺功能紊乱、肾上腺皮质功能不全)。

J

- 癌症。
• 精神状况：
- 边缘型人格障碍。
- 情绪障碍。
- 强迫性障碍。
- 药物滥用。

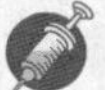

治疗

初步稳定/治疗

• 常规治疗。
• 明确低血压是由于心功能不全还是容量不足导致；慎重的液体复苏避免出现外周组织水肿或肺水肿。
• 注意脱水时的液体复苏，以避免突发外周或肺水肿。
• 充足的磷酸盐和维生素 B_1，由于再进食时两者都可能下降。
• 纠正低钾血症、低镁血症、低钙血症。
• 纠正低血糖。
• 为严重低体温症者提供暖毯。

急诊治疗/程序

• 初步检查。
• 药物稳定。
• 精神科会诊（包括评估自杀风险和精神疾病）。

药物治疗

一线用药

• 还没有药物被证明对 AN 本身是有益的：
- 小型试验表明，非典型抗精神病药物可能从中受益，特别是奥氮平 2.5～10 mg 口服，每日 1 次。
- 这可能有助于治疗精神疾病。
• 其他 SSRIs 很常用，但只有 20～60 mg 氟西汀口服，每日 1 次经 FDA 说明可用于 BN。有证据显示三环类抗抑郁药与托吡酯一样可用。
• 苯丙胺是目前 FDA 第一个批准的用于治疗暴食症的药物。有证据表明丙米嗪、舍曲林、艾司西酞普兰/依他普仑和托吡酯可治疗 BED。

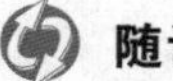

随访

进一步处理

入院指征

• 身体风险：
- 极低体重（<75%理想体重或 BMI<14）。
- 快速失重。
- 血清电解质紊乱（钾<3，血糖<60）。
- 心动过缓<40 次/分。
- 血压<90/60 mmHg。
- 体位性低血压（>20 次/分或>20 mmHg/10 mmHg）。
- 低温<97 ℉（36.1 ℃）。
- 心律失常或心力衰竭。
- 肝或肾功能不全。
• 精神风险：
- 严重抑郁、精神病或其他精神疾病诊断。
- 自杀。
- 缺乏治疗的动机或合作。
- 门诊治疗失败。
- 严重功能受损。
- 不良的家庭环境。

出院指征

• 身体和心理上安全到可以在门诊处理。
• 多模式、多学科小组来处理身体、营养和心理问题。

转诊问题

• 门诊治疗需要一个由下列组成的团队方法：
- 精神科医师和/或心理医师。
- 营养师，最好是专门从事饮食失调者。
- 儿科医师或内科医师。
- 家庭治疗师。
- 团体治疗师。
- 口腔医师。
• 预后：
- AN 和 BN：
◦ 20%慢性病程。
◦ 30%改善。
◦ 50%恢复。
- AN 每 10 年的死亡率为 5.6%。
- 早期诊断和治疗可改善结局。

随访建议

• 对于门诊治疗：团队必须建立适度的目标和明确的指标，包括厌食症患者的预期体重增加和随访的依从性。
• 内科医师/儿科医师：监测生命体征、体重、体质指数、电解质和心电图。
• 营养师：控制饮食、热量的摄入，运动。
• 精神疗法：
- 认知行为疗法和人际心理治疗是 BN 心理治疗的最有效方式。
- 认知行为疗法、家庭治疗和心理治疗都对 AN 有益。
- 基于家庭的治疗是青少年 AN 者的首选治疗方式，对于青少年 BN 者也是有前景的。
• 药物治疗：
- 只在有心理治疗的情况下适用，尤其是伴发精神疾病。
- 对 AN 来讲，没有可接受的药物治疗：
◦ 个案研究表明第二代抗精神病药对 AN 可能有益。
◦ 除了体重恢复和营养钙补充之外，没有针对骨质疏松症的特殊疗法的明确证据。
- 抗抑郁药物显著减少暴食与清除行为：
◦ 氟西汀是研究最好的药物。
◦ 苯丙胺被推荐用于进食障碍的治疗。

要点和误区

• 饮食失调与高身体风险和自杀风险相关，优先考虑安全性评估。
• 快速恢复营养、容量复苏和/或未能补足维生素和电解质，可引发致命的再进食综合征。
• 避免试图“搞定”妄想症患者。
• 与初级保健医师（PCP）和多学科小组的其他成员协作。

惊恐发作 Panic Attack

Juliana H. Chen · Bernardino Vaccaro 王虑 译

基础知识

描述

• 急性发作的特征性体征，极度的恐惧在 10 min 到达顶峰并在 20 min 后缓解。
• 患者也有没有恐惧的变异表现。

恐惧症

• 复发的、意外的惊恐发作持续>1 个月：
- 担心受到另外攻击。
- 担心攻击的暗示和结果。
- 行为的改变，如回避恐惧和相关的进攻。
- 有或没有广场恐惧症：恐惧相关的焦虑逃跑。
• 片段性、复发或慢性攻击。
• 长期伴有抑郁表现、滥用药物、残疾、自杀倾向。

遗传学

• 可能和遗传有关。
• 有恐慌和焦虑家族史。
• 羟色胺和苯二氮䓬受体功能功能改变。

病因

机制

边缘系统，去甲肾上腺释放，神经传导物质(如羟色胺)功能紊乱，导致“打架或迁徙”反应。

风险因素

• 发病前 1 年内生活的一些重大事件。
• 有恐慌和焦虑家族史。
• 身体疾病和滥用可卡因的病程。
- 在疾病和滥用药物控制后，症状还持续。
• 在女性中常见，患病人数是男性的 2 倍。

诊断

症状和体征

• 自主神经系统症状。
• 心脏：
- 心悸。
- 心律失常。
- 胸痛或不舒服。
• 呼吸系统：
- 气促。
- 窒息。
- 窒息感。
• 神经系统：
- 震颤。
- 头昏。
- 头晕。
- 感到头昏无力。
- 麻木。
- 刺痛。
- 出汗。
- 寒战。
- 脸红。
- 不真实感和超然感。
• 消化系统：
- 恶心。
- 腹部肌肉抽筋。
- 腹痛。
• 强烈恐惧感：
- 自动的，刻板的。
- 濒死感。
- 心脏打击感。
- 羞辱感。
- 失去控制，“发疯”。

病史

• 已知的医疗条件。
• 所有的药物。
• 中草药治疗。
• 娱乐性药物、饮酒。
• 咖啡因摄入。
• 发病年龄。
• 初始生活事件或压力因素。
• 儿童经历。
• 回避结果。
• 对先前药物治疗的反应。
• 有恐慌和焦虑家族史。
• 家庭药物和酒精服用史。

体格检查

• 彻底的体格检查和神经系统检查。
• 特征性的体征指导。

基本检查

详细的病史，适当的体格检查：
• 根据表现和最初临床发现提示病情。
• 可能症状和轻微。

诊断检查与说明

实验室检查

• 毒物检测。
• 三环抗抑郁药水平。
• 全血细胞计数。
• 电解质、尿素氮/肌酐、血糖。
• 促甲状腺激素。
• 血氧饱和仪和动脉血气。

诊断步骤/外科

• 怀疑二尖瓣脱垂行心电图检查，排除潜在的心脏病，服用三环类药物需监测 QRS 波形。
- 年龄>40 岁。
- 心脏症状。
• 24 h 动态心电图：
- 如果有心悸表现时采用此检查。
• 禁睡脑电图。

鉴别诊断

• 考虑器官因素：
- 年龄大出现了恐慌的表现(年龄>50 岁)。
- 没有儿童病史或家族史。
- 没有最初或生活的一些重大事件。
- 没有严重的恐慌和逃避感。
- 服用抗焦虑或抗抑郁药反应不佳病史。
• 药物：
- 精神安定剂(静坐不能)。
- 支气管扩张药。
- 洋地黄。
- 抗胆碱能类药物。
- 中枢兴奋剂。
- 减肥药。
- 中药支持治疗。
• 呼吸系统：
- 哮喘。
- 换气过度。
- 慢性阻塞性肺疾病。
- 肺栓塞。
- 细菌性肺炎。
- 肋软骨炎。
• 心血管系统：
- 心绞痛。
- 心肌梗死。
- 心律失常。
- 贫血。
- 二尖瓣脱垂。
• 药物性：
- 刺激性药物滥用。
- 回撤反应(酒精、镇静催眠药)。
- 抗镇静剂中断综合征(中断、减量、抗抑郁

J

或抗 5-羟色胺药物中断)。
- 咖啡因摄取过多。
• 内分泌:
- 甲状腺功能亢进。
- 低血糖。
- 甲状旁腺功能减退。
- 嗜铬细胞瘤。
• 其他代谢紊乱:
- 低钾血症。
- 低镁血症。
- 低磷血症。
• 神经系统:
- 复杂的局部痉挛发作(恐惧、认知扭曲、身体症状)。
- 短暂缺血表现。
- 内耳迷路炎。
- 良性位置性眩晕。
• 精神病学:
- 强迫症。
- 创伤后压力心理障碍症。
- 特定对象恐惧症或社会恐惧症。
- 躯体形式障碍。
- 佯病症。
- 急性悲痛。
• 家庭暴力。

儿科注意事项

心律失常。

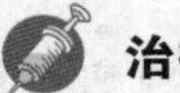

治疗

院前

• 如果诊断是基于以前的发生的事件和病史的:
- 使其放心并转移。
- 不需要紧急看护。
• 如果是首次发病,根据患者的具体表现治疗和转送。

初步稳定/治疗

• 使平静和放心。
• 大多惊恐发作不处理在 20～30 min 会自行缓解。
• 恐惧会触发又一次惊恐发作。

急诊治疗/程序

• 患者教育,新的认知能力:
- 对异常的警报能有正常的反应。
- 对于症状合适的心理解释。
• 长效苯二氮䓬类药物(药物的选择):
- 氯硝西泮:
◦ 不作为急诊紧急使用药物。
◦ 起效慢作用时间长。
◦ 最适合维持治疗防止惊恐再发作的治疗。
- 阿普唑仑:
◦ 起效快。
◦ 会出现焦虑的反跳,因为药物作用时间短和消耗快。
◦ 持续使用会致用量增大。
- 劳拉西泮(氯羟去甲安定):
◦ 快速起效。
◦ 优势在于能舌下给药。
◦ 比阿普唑仑作用时间长。
• 避免服用短效的苯二氮䓬类药物:
- 地西泮(安定)。
- 利眠宁。
• 5-羟色胺再摄取抑制剂能治疗惊恐复发,可以也可不联合使用氯硝西泮:
- 不是立即起效。
- 不需要紧急服用该药,特别在没有合适的随访计划建立起来时。
• 关于非典型抗精神病药(奥氮平、利培酮)治疗难治性恐慌症的研究很少。
• 出院后治疗:
- 几片氯硝西泮药片,以防惊恐复发。

> **注意**
> 阿普唑仑的快速消耗(回撤)可能会触发惊恐发作加剧。

药物治疗

一线用药

• 氯硝西泮:在急诊 0.5 mg,口服;最初在门诊治疗患者 0.25～0.5 mg,口服,每日 2 次。
• 5-羟色胺再摄取抑制剂:
- 门诊患者一开始就使用。
- 惊恐症患者可能需要比抑郁表现的患者更大的剂量和用药时间。

二线用药

• 劳拉西泮:1 mg,口服。
• 三环类药物:
- 门诊患者一开始就使用。

妊娠注意事项

• 控制苯二氮䓬类药物使用。
• 5-羟色胺再摄取抑制剂相对安全,少用三环类药物(如去甲替林、地昔帕明)。
• 对于有发病倾向的妇女,妊娠期和产后的生理和自发反应会触发惊恐发作。

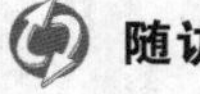

随访

进一步处理

入院指征

• 医学排除器质性疾病。
• 符合精神病学入院标准(自杀、杀人)。

出院指征

大多惊恐发作患者不需要入院治疗。

转诊问题

• 对于心理健康状态的管理。
• 从精神病学和认知能力治疗的角度评估恐慌的再发。
• 耻辱。
• 随访关注心理健康和精神状态的话题。

随访建议

• 安排主要的看护医师或心理健康的特别治疗。
• 避免刺激性,如咖啡因、兴奋剂、酒精。

要点和误区

• 恐慌有“传染性”,别被患者紧迫的感觉影响去处理发作症状;症状都能自行的缓解。
• 冷静不增加患者的警觉感,但要积极使患者感觉受到注意并放松警惕。
• 认知行为治疗可以在急诊开始,对症状的生理因素做简洁的解释。
• 注意对于儿童和年轻人,苯二氮䓬类药物别使用终身;认知行为治疗(5-羟色胺再摄取抑制剂治疗)效果好副作用少。
• 尽量避免使用阿普唑仑,尤其对于持续治疗。

J

精神分裂症

Sarah E. Herold 周健 潘曙明 译

基础知识

描述

- 以妄想、幻觉、行为与情绪障碍和认知缺陷为特征的慢性精神障碍：
  - 发病前的阶段：
    - 出现阴性症状：冷漠、快感缺乏、贪婪、健忘，反应迟钝。
    - 个人、社会和智力功能恶化。
  - 活跃的阶段：
    - 发展积极错觉、幻觉和怪异的行为。
    - 可能因压力事件加剧。
    - 残余型和未分化型阶段。
    - 患者留下社会和认知能力受损。
  - 精神病症状可能会持续存在。
- 通常在成年早期发病。
  - 男性：18～25 岁，女性：25～35 岁。
  - 很少发生在儿童时期或>45 岁。
- 共同滥用药物（酒精、大麻、烟草和兴奋剂）很常见。
- 暴力可能是由于判断力受损、偏执狂和产生幻觉。
- 平均预期寿命比一般人口低 28.5 岁：
  - 心血管疾病是最常见的死亡原因。
  - 41%的患者患有代谢综合征，死于心血管疾病的风险增加。
- 思维紊乱、行为异常和妄想可能会影响对疾病的诊断。
- 药物治疗的不依从性是导致精神疾病失代偿和急诊报道的一个关键原因。

病因

- 病理生理学不清楚，但多巴胺通路与此密切相关。
- 遗传成分（同卵双生双胞胎中 50%的一致率）。
  - 可能的多基因紊乱：具有小的、加性效应的多基因的影响。
  - 补体成分 C4：在神经发育过程中与突触修剪增加相关的表达增加。
  - DiGeorge 综合征的高危人群（22q11.2 缺失）。
- 围生期危险因素：
  - 妊娠中期的流感。
  - 母亲和产后感染。
  - 高龄。
- 使用大麻可以解除潜在患者的精神病。

诊断

症状和体征

《精神障碍诊断和统计手册》(DSM－5)的标准要求在 1 个月以上出现至少 2 种以下症状：

- 错觉（固定的、错误的信念）：
  - 奇异的、偏执的或浮夸的。
  - 通常是迫害的、宗教或身体的内容。
- 幻觉：
  - 通常是听觉的或视觉的，但可能涉及任何感觉方式。
- 思维障碍：
  - 语无伦次，从奇怪的、特殊的逻辑到语无伦次。
- 严重的无组织或紧张症行为。
- 阴性症状：
  - 冷漠和失去动力。
  - 注意力不集中。
  - 社会孤立。
  - 快感缺乏症。
  - 言语和情感表达能力降低。
- 至少一个主要的功能领域：学习、工作、人际关系、自我照顾。
- 持续至少 6 个月。

基本检查

- 完成一般和神经系统检查，包括生命体征和精神状态检查。
- 精神病的表现：
  - 错觉：
    - 你觉得有人想伤害你，或者你被跟踪吗？
    - 幻想任何人试图给你发送消息，偷窃，控制，或者阻止你在想什么？
  - 幻觉：
    - 你有没有看到或听到的东西，别人不能看到或听到？
    - 你曾经听到的声音告诉你做事，如伤害自己或他人？
- 评估自己或他人潜在的危险：
  - 筛选过去的暴力或自我伤害。
  - 探讨精神病症状的内容，以评估安全性。
    - 你需要保护自己或他人吗？如果是这样，如何？
- 患者病史和服药依从性可能不可靠。从其他来源获取附属历史：
  - 朋友和家人、医生、精神病学家。
- 评估情感性精神病（躁郁症、重度抑郁症或精神分裂症）。
- 评估是否患有谵妄或痴呆。
  - 精神分裂症不影响定向。
- 评估药物诱导的精神病（见精神病，急性）。
- 应排除因医学病因引起的精神病。

诊断检查与说明

实验室检查

- 毒理学。
- 电解质、BUN、肌酐、葡萄糖、钙。
- CBC 的差异性。
- TSH。
- 尿液分析。

考虑对未确定病因的新发精神病或新发神经症状的患者进行头部成像。

影像学检查

心电图监测 QT。

鉴别诊断

- 精神错乱。
- 药物引起的精神病。
- 继发于一般医疗条件的精神病，如 MSf LBD。
- 双相情感障碍。
  - 有精神病特征的重度抑郁症。
- 分裂情感障碍：
  - 精神分裂症，有明显的抑郁和/或躁狂症状。
- 妄想障碍。
- 分裂型人格。
- 短暂精神病发作：
  - 症状相似，持续时间<1 个月。
- 精神分裂症样的障碍：
  - 症状相似，持续时间 1～6 个月。

治疗

院前

- 患者会表现出不可预知的暴力行为。
  - 对自己和他人的行为。
- 患者可能需要警察在场和/或限制以保持安全。
  - 与一般人群相比，需要法律干预的患者的死亡风险高 3 倍。

• 美国各州法律因适用于非自愿急诊评估而有所不同。准则可包括下列任何一项：
- 对自己造成即时伤害的风险。
- 对他人造成即时伤害的风险。
- 在社区中无法照顾自己。

■ 初步稳定/治疗

• 医护人员和患者的安全至关重要；可能需要安全存在。

• 行为干预应该是首要的：
- 提供一个平静、包容的环境。
- 有潜在危险的物品应该从患者的房间里取出。
- 使用可靠的声音和冷静的态度来设定界限，并对患者进行直接口头指导患者方向。
- 如果考虑到安全问题，患者需要持续观察。

• 急性躁动可用抗精神病药物或苯二氮䓬类药物或两者联合。
- 鼓励患者自愿服用药物。
- 抗精神病药物包括氟哌啶醇、奥氮平、氯丙嗪（监测矫形术）、齐拉西酮（监测 QT）和阿立哌唑。
- 奥氮平，不应与静脉苯二氮䓬类联合使用，因为这会增加心肺衰竭的风险。

■ 急诊治疗/程序

• 精神分裂症失代偿患者进行心理咨询。

• 抗精神病药物是治疗的主要手段。

• 高效典型抗精神病药物：
- 与较少的 QT 延长有关。
- 更容易出现锥体外系症状：
  ◦ 肌张力障碍。
  ◦ 震颤麻痹。
  ◦ 静坐不能。
  ◦ 迟发性运动障碍四氟哌啶醇与锥体外系症状少于口服或肌内注射。

• 低效力典型的抗精神病药物：
- QT 延长的风险较高。
- 更少的锥体外症状。
- 更镇静。
- 直立性低血压（必须监控）。
- 抗胆碱能副作用。
- 降低发作阈值。

• 非典型抗精神病药物：
- 用更少的 EPS 更好的耐受性。
- 与代谢综合征和体重增加有关。
- 可引起直立性低血压。
- 几乎所有抗精神病药物均增加 QT 间期：
  ◦ 更有可能（齐拉西酮）。
  ◦ 不太可能（阿立哌唑）。
- 氯氮平是唯一一种对降低精神症状和自杀风险更有效的抗精神病药物：
  ◦ 需要密切监测白细胞粒细胞缺乏症。
  ◦ 高度镇静剂、降血压药、降低癫痫发作阈值。
  ◦ 可以引起 QT 间期延长。

• 长效抗精神病药物（2 周至 3 个月给 1 次）包括：
- 氟非那嗪癸酸。
- 氟哌啶醇癸酸。
- 奥氮平库（Relprew）。
- 帕潘立酮（抗抑郁药）棕榈酸酯（Sustenna）。
- 利培酮微球（Consta）。
- 阿立哌唑（Maintena）。

• 如果开始使用高效的常规抗精神病药物，40 岁以下的患者可以开始服用苄托平（Cogentin）2 mg，减少 10 日的肌张力障碍反应。

■ 药物治疗

• 典型抗精神病药物（第一代）：
- 高效力：
  ◦ 氟哌啶醇：0.5～100 mg/d。急性期 2.5～10 mg，口服、静脉注射或肌内注射。根据需要重复，q20～60 min。
  ◦ 氟奋乃静：10 mg/d。
  ◦ 氨砜噻吨：1～30 mg/d。
- 中等效力：
  ◦ 奋乃静：2～24 mg/d。
  ◦ 三氟拉嗪：1～20 mg/d
- 低效力：
  ◦ 氯丙嗪：50～200 mg/d，分 3 次。
  ◦ 洛沙平：5～100 mg/d。
  ◦ 甲硫哒嗪：50～800 mg/d，分 2～3 次。

• 非典型抗精神病药物（第二代）：
- 阿立哌唑：5～30 mg/d。
- 阿西那平类药物：5～20 mg/d(SL)。
- 氯氮平：12.5～900 mg/d。
- 伊洛哌酮：1～24 mg/d。
- 鲁阿西酮：20～160 mg/d。
- 奥氮平：5～20 mg/d。
- 帕利哌酮：6～12 mg/d。
- 喹硫平：25～800 mg/d。
- 利培酮：1～16 mg/d。
- 齐拉西酮：20～160 mg/d。

• 苯二氮䓬类。
- 氯拉西泮（Ativan）0.5～2 mg 每剂急性期增加抗精神病药老年的考虑。

黑盒警告

接受抗精神病药物治疗的老年痴呆症患者的死亡风险增加。

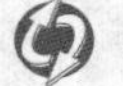 随访

■ 进一步处理

入院指征

• 如果患者病情稳定且新发的精神病和医学病因已经被排除。

• 在转移到精神病院之前，患者必须解决急性医疗和外科问题。

• 非自愿精神病院的标准因州而异。

出院指征

• 患者不会对自己或他人造成危险，能够进行日常生活活动。

• 安排精神病学随访。

• 精神病症状可能在出院时持续存在。

■ 随访建议

• 门诊精神药理学随访应在出院后 1 周内进行。

• 服用抗精神病药物（尤其是非典型药物）的患者应监测 QT 延长和肥胖及相关的代谢综合征。

• 辅助认知行为疗法和其他心理社会疗法可以帮助患者管理精神病症状，提高药物依从性。

• 讨论戒烟和转诊：
- 50%～80%的精神分裂症患者吸烟。

要点和误区

• 视觉上、嗅觉上、味觉上或触觉上的幻觉应能促使对精神疾病的次要原因进行医学检查，非典型发病年龄（>35 岁）也应如此。

• 抗精神病药物和社会干预的早期治疗一直与更好的精神分裂症预后相关。

• 避免在Ⅳ类苯二氮䓬类药物中使用奥氮平，因为这会增加心肺衰竭的风险。

• 最近开始服用抗精神病药物的患者，其发热、僵硬、自主神经不稳定，以及精神状态的变化，都应被评估为神经毒性恶性综合征。

精神症状的躯体因素和精神因素 Psychosis, Medical vs. Psychiatric

Eric C. Hyder · Laura J. Macnow 郑金浩 毛恩强 译

基础知识

描述

精神错乱包括幻觉、错觉导致与现实严重不符的很荒唐的行为：

• 复杂很难理解的病理生理。

• 多巴胺通路过度激活可能是引起此病的一个原因。

• 精神错乱范围从相对平和的错乱到紧张症。

• 可能由于以下损伤中枢神经系统导致精神表现：

- 神经系统病变。
- 代谢状态。
- 毒物和药物不良反应。
- 感染。

• 遭受精神疾病的高危因素：

- 幻觉和错觉形成妄想系统。
- 青春晚期/成年早期。
- 定位正常。

• 遭受躯体疾病的高危因素：

- 中老年人出现。
- 急性起病。
- 有药物滥用的病史。
- 没有出现精神症状的病史。
- 没有精神疾病的家族史。
- 呈现出之前存在的躯体疾病。
- 社会经济水平较低。
- 近期记忆遗忘。
- 方向障碍或注意力分散。
- 生命体征异常。
- 视觉幻觉。
  ◦ 谵妄。
  ◦ 痴呆。
  ◦ 偏头痛。
  ◦ 经多巴胺激动剂治疗(如甲基多巴)。
  ◦ 脑梗死后。
  ◦ 发作性睡病。

病因

• 神经病：

- 颅脑外伤。
- 占位性病变。
- 脑血管事件。
- 癫痫。
- 脑水肿。

• 神经精神疾病：(帕金森病、舞蹈症、阿尔茨海默病、PICK、肝豆状核变形)。

• 感染：

- 老年人局灶性感染(尿路感染、肺炎)。
- HIV。
- 神经梅毒。
- 脑炎。
- 莱姆病：螺旋体。
- 寄生虫病。
  ◦ 脑疟疾。
  ◦ 中枢神经系统感染猪肉绦虫幼虫。
  ◦ 血吸虫病。
  ◦ 钩形虫。
  ◦ 锥虫病。

• 代谢疾病：

- 电解质紊乱。
- 低血糖。
- 低氧血症。
- 卟啉症。
- 撤药反应综合征。

• 内分泌系统：

- 甲状腺疾病。
- 甲状旁腺疾病。
- 糖尿病。
- 垂体异常。
- 肾上腺异常。

• 终末器官衰竭。

- 心力衰竭、呼吸衰竭。
- 肾衰竭。
- 肝衰竭。

• 营养缺乏：

- 恶性贫血。
- 韦尼克-科尔萨科夫综合征。
- 糙皮病。
- 维生素 B_6 缺乏。

• 自身免疫疾病：

- 系统性红斑狼疮。
- 结节病。
- 重症肌无力。
- 副肿瘤综合征。

• 退髓鞘病。

- 多发性硬化。
- 脑白质营养不良。

• 术后状态：

- 谵妄。

• 中毒疾病：

- 酒精。
- 苯二氮䓬类。
- 巴比妥酸盐。
- 兴奋剂(可卡因、苯丙胺)。
- 迷幻剂。
- 阿片制剂。
- 抗胆碱化合物。
- 吸入剂。
- 大麻。

• 毒素：

- 溴化物。
- 一氧化碳。
- 重金属。
- 有机磷酸盐。

• 药物不良反应：

- 糖皮质激素。
- 抗胆碱能类。
- 镇静催眠药。

• 精神病学：

- 抗抑郁药。
- 抗精神病药。
- 碳酸锂。

• 抗帕金森病药物。

• 抗痉挛药物。

• 抗生素(喹诺酮类、异烟肼)。

• 抗高血压药。

• 治疗心脏疾病药物(洋地黄、利多卡因、普萘洛尔、普鲁卡因)。

• 干扰素。

• 肌松药。

• 非处方用药：

- 伪麻黄碱。
- 抗组胺药。

• 精神类药物：

- 精神分裂症。
- 情感分裂样精神病。
- 妄想症。
- 双相情感障碍。
- 抑郁症与精神病性特征。
- 应激反应包括创伤后应激障碍。
- 发作性睡病(在睡眠和觉醒的交界处出现幻觉)。
- 产后精神病。

J

诊断

症状和体征

• 精神病特点：
- 真实性体验受损。
- 不适当情感。
- 冲动的控制性差。

• 局部或分散的中枢神经系统损害可能导致以下情况紊乱：
- 知觉。
- 思考内容。
- 思考方式。

• 幻觉：
- 感受器没有外界刺激的情况下能感觉到真实的感觉，描述的感觉真实性很强。

• 妄想：
- 不合实际的信念顽固、无法纠正。
- 通过类型和主题归类如下：
  ◦ 奇特或非奇特。
  ◦ 情绪一致或中立。
  ◦ 被害或夸大妄想。
  ◦ 初级或中级。

• 思维障碍。
• 情感症状可能包括狂躁、抑郁或紧张症。

病史

• 时间过程：急性、慢性、片段性。
• 来自家庭或门诊医师的替代药物。
• 使用药物。
• 药物依赖。
• 家族史。
• 相关症状：发热、体重减轻、食欲缺乏、近期外伤或手术。

体格检查

• 生命体征。
• 神经系统查体：
- 认知检查：注意力和认知能力。
- 监控下测试：语气、不正常动作。

基本检查

详细的病史和体格检查包括神经系统查体。

诊断检查与说明

实验室检查

• 如果有患者有精神病既往史，无躯体疾病病史，体格检查均正常，临床意义不大。

• 一线试验：
- 血细胞计数。
- 电解质包括血钙、尿素氮、肌酐、葡萄糖。
- 尿和血的毒物筛查。
- 尿常规。
- 肝功能。
- 甲状腺功能。
- 维生素 B_{12} 和叶酸。

• 参考病史和体格检查情况的二线检查：
- 血氨。
- HIV 抗体。
- 梅毒螺旋体抗体全套(血清反应素不足以排除神经梅毒)。
- 血浆铜蓝蛋白。
- 尿重金属。
- 红细胞沉降率、C 反应蛋白、抗核抗体。

影像学检查

• 常规行 CT 或 MRI 临床意义不大。
• 指示：
- 病史或体格检查提示神经性疾病。
- 首次精神异常在 50 岁以上。
• 没有证据说明 MRI 优于 CT。

诊断步骤/外科

• 心电图注意 QT 间期是否正常。
• 不推荐以下筛查项目：
- 腰椎穿刺。
- 脑电图。

鉴别诊断

• 米切尔玛莎效应。
- 一个临床医师错误地判断患者感知的真实事件为妄想的过程。
• 闭锁综合征。
• 周期性瘫痪。
• 转换障碍。

治疗

院前

• 确保患者、旁观者、医护人员的安全。
• 监测生命体征、末梢血糖。

初始稳定/治疗

• 安全。
• 评估。
• 监测血氧饱和度和血糖。
• 如果患者不合作，有危险行为，控制患者的行为。

急诊稳定/治疗

• 治疗现有的躯体疾病，以及药物滥用障碍。
• 使用神经抑制剂前行心电图，监测有无 QT 间期延长。
• 氟哌啶醇联合劳拉西泮：
- 安全，速效，对检查项目影响较小。
• 非典型抗精神病药。
- 很少有锥体束以外的不良反应。
- 奥氮平和齐拉西酮可以肌内注射。
- 奥氮平(zydis)和维思通片可以溶于水，便于准备。
- 肌内注射劳拉西泮和奥氮平有呼吸衰竭的风险，避免同时使用。

药物治疗

一线用药

• 氟哌啶醇 2～10 mg，肌内注射或静脉推注；劳拉西泮 0.5～2 mg，肌内注射或静脉推注。

二线用药

• 神经松弛剂：
- 奥氮平：5～10 mg，口服、直肠给药或肌内注射。
- 利培酮：1～2 mg，口服或直肠给药。
- 喹硫平：25～100 mg，口服。
• 苯二氮䓬类：
- 地西泮 5～10 mg，静脉推注。

老年人注意事项

• 经典和非经典的抗精神药物均会增大大于 65 岁患者的致死风险。
• 以低剂量开始用药(氟哌啶醇 2 mg 静脉推注，奥氮平 2.5～5 mg 口服、直肠或肌内给药注射)。
• 注意兴奋的患者避免使用苯二氮䓬类，苯二氮䓬类有抑制解除的风险。

妊娠注意事项

抗精神药物中第一代抗精神药物，如氟哌啶醇，有在妊娠期使用安全的最佳证据。

随访

进一步处理

入院指征

• 如果基础疾病为躯体疾病并且有入院治疗的指征，是否收入院取决于具体的医疗条件。
• 如果基础疾病为精神病因素(如精神分裂症)收入精神卫生中心：
- 对自己及他人构成危害。
- 不能照顾自己。
- 疯狂的想法模式可能伤害到自己或者他人。
- 首次：评估和巩固。
- 各州法律对于强制住院治疗的要求各不

J

相同。

出院指征

• 稳定的医疗条件。
• 没有自伤或伤人想法。
• 可以照看自己。
• 可以做医疗方面的决定。

转诊问题

• 医疗保险范围确定住院和门诊精神病的治疗方案。
• 精神卫生中心需要个案管理和社会服务。

随访建议

• 如果精神症状首次发病，确定 1～2 周内随访以提供心理健康指导。
• 评估继续使用抗精神病药物的后续收益和风险。

要点和误区

• 对于有精神症状的患者，通常方式也许不能解释他们的症状。获取周围信息并对患者提供的信息保持怀疑态度。
• 对于精神病患者，疾病归咎于精神病最重要的前提是排除器质性病变。

精神状态改变 Altered Mental Status

David W. Schoenfeld · Christopher J. Shestak 马林浩 林兆奋 译

基础知识

描述

• 上脑干中的网状激活系统或 1 个或 2 个大脑半球的大面积的功能障碍。
• 定义：
- 精神混乱：一种意识清楚度，连贯性，理解力和推理能力降低的行为状态。
- 嗜睡：患者不易被触摸或噪声轻易唤醒，并且在一段时间内无法保持警觉性。
- 昏睡：精神状态受抑制，患者可能会觉得清醒，但对自我的和周围环境意识不强，无法唤起全部功能。
- 昏迷：患者只能通过剧烈的刺激来唤醒，并且努力避免不舒服或累积刺激。
- 深度昏迷：患者不能被刺激唤醒，也没有有目的的活动来避免疼痛的刺激。
- 谵妄：由于注意力和意识障碍而导致认知波动的急性发作，从精神混乱到昏迷都可出现。

病因

• 缺氧：
- 严重的肺部疾病。
- 贫血。
- 休克。
- 心脏分流(尤其是小儿科)。
• 新陈代谢：
- 低血糖或高血糖。
- 糖尿病酮症酸中毒。
- 非酮症高渗性昏迷。
- 低钠血症或高钠血症。
- 低钙血症或高钙血症。
- 低镁血症或高镁血症。
- 低磷血症。
- 酸中毒或碱中毒。
- 脱水。
- 缺乏症：硫胺素、叶酸、烟酸。
- 高血氨症(肝性脑病)。
- 尿毒症(肾衰竭)。
- CO_2 麻醉。
• 毒理学：
- 毒性醇。
- 水杨酸。
- 镇静和麻醉品。
- γ-羟基丁酸(GHB)。
- 抗痉挛药。
- 精神药品。
- 异烟肼。
- 重金属。
- 一氧化碳。
- 氰化物。
- 毒性植物(曼陀罗、蘑菇等)。
- 拟交感神经药。
- 抗胆碱能、胆碱能。
- 止吐药。
- 抗帕金森病药物。
- 戒断反应(特别是酒精、镇静剂)。
• 传染性：
- 泌尿道感染(尤其是老年人)。
- 肺炎。
- 脓毒症、菌血症。
- 脑膜炎、脑炎、脑脓肿。
• 内分泌：
- 黏液水肿性昏迷。
- 甲状腺功能亢进症。
- 甲状腺功能减退症。
- 艾迪生病。
- 库欣病。
- 嗜铬细胞瘤。
- 甲状旁腺功能亢进。
• 环境：
- 低温。
- 高热、心脏病。
- 高海拔脑水肿。
- 恶性精神抑制综合征。
• 血管：
- 高血压脑病。
- 脑血管炎。
- TTP、DIC、高黏度。
- 多发性血管炎。
• 原发性神经系统：
- 癫痫发作、非惊厥性癫痫持续状态和发作后状态。
- 头部创伤、脑震荡。
- 弥漫性轴索损伤。
- 结构性脑损伤：
◦ 出血(硬膜下、硬膜外、蛛网膜下腔、实质内)。
◦ 梗死。
◦ 肿瘤。
◦ 脱髓鞘疾病。
- 颅内高压(假瘤)。
- HIV 相关性脑病。
- 自身免疫、炎症性脑炎。
- 类脑膜炎。
- 原发性神经元或神经胶质疾病：
◦ 克罗伊茨费尔特-雅各布病。
◦ Marchiafava-Bignami 病。
◦ 肾上腺脑白质营养不良。
◦ 脑胶质瘤病。
◦ 进行性多灶性白质脑病。
• 外伤、烧伤。
• 卟啉症。
• 精神病。

J

- 多因素(尤其是老年人)。

诊断

▪ 症状和体征

精神错乱

- 难以保持连贯的思维和心理表现：
  - 考虑教育水平、语言和可能的学习障碍。
- 注意力不集中。
- 记忆缺陷：
  - 无法跟踪任务，有选择地专注于重要信息。
  - 无法回忆以下任何内容：
    - 日期，包括周、月、日、年。
    - 确切的地方。
    - 众所周知的信息。
    - 为什么患者在医院。
    - 地址、电话号码或社会安全号码。
- 精神表现受损：
  - 难以保持向前7位和向后4位。
  - 难以命名普通对象。
  - 标准计算：3到30减法测试。
- 杂乱无章的语言：
  - 可能会被误认为是失语症。
- 发热：
  - 传染性病因、药物毒性、内分泌失调、中暑。
- 严重的高血压和心动过缓：
  - 存在库欣反射时建议颅内病变。
- 低血压：
  - 传染性、毒理学病因、心输出量减少。
- 眼球运动：
  - 圆形摆动：
    - 缓慢周期性联合向下的眼球运动，快速回到中间位置。
    - 双侧脑桥受损，代谢紊乱和脑干受压。
- 眼部浸渍：
  - 眼睛慢、周期性、共轭、向下运动，然后迅速恢复到中间位置。
  - 见于弥漫性皮质缺氧损伤。
- 瞳孔测试：
  - 几乎所有致昏迷的毒性和代谢原因都使瞳孔反射迟钝，但双侧反射完整。
- 焦点发现(指示中枢神经系统过程)：
  - 偏瘫。
  - 偏盲。
  - 失语症。
  - 肌阵挛。
  - 抽搐。
  - 颈项强直。
- 扑翼样震颤：
  - 无节奏的扑动震颤(几乎总是双侧)。
  - 见于肝功能衰竭或严重肾衰竭。

病史

- 询问目击人、家人、院前人员。
- 基础心理状态。
- 病史(免疫抑制、肝功能衰竭、抑郁症或慢性病)。
- 近期事件：创伤、发热、疾病。
- 详细的药物清单。
- 药物滥用史。

体格检查

- 生命体征。
- 头部：创伤的迹象、瞳孔。
- 眼底镜检查：出血、视乳头水肿。
- 颈部：僵硬、瘀伤、甲状腺肿大。
- 心肺功能。
- 腹部：器官肿大、腹水。
- 四肢：发绀。
- 皮肤：发汗/干燥、皮疹、瘀点、瘀斑、碎片出血、针迹。
- 神经系统检查。
- 心理状态检测。

▪ 诊断检查与说明

实验室检查

- 血糖检查试纸和葡萄糖。
- CBC。
- 电解质(包括钙、镁、磷)。
- BUN、肌酐。
- 毒理筛选(包括有毒醇类)。
- 心电图。
- 尿液分析。
- 血液和尿液培养(疑似感染)。
- PT、PTT(抗凝、肝衰竭患者)。
- 考虑LFT、甲状腺功能测试、氨、血清渗透压、动脉血气。
- 考虑维生素 B_{12}、叶酸、RPR、尿中胆色素原、重金属筛查。

影像学检查

- 头部CT扫描：
  - 非增强CT只是为了排除出血和肿块效应。
- 胸片：诊断肺炎。
- MRI(如果有)：
  - 当怀疑缺血性脑卒中或其他中枢神经系统异常时。
  - 在接纳患者时可以推迟部分住院患者的检查。

诊断步骤/外科

- 腰椎穿刺(LP)：
  - 在实验室和CT扫描后病因仍不清楚时进行。
  - 疑似脑膜炎的患者，在LP之前应给予强效抗生素。
- 脑电图(住院患者)：对于疑似癫痫发作、非惊厥性癫痫持续状态。
- 前庭器官行热量刺激，以评估无反应的患者。

▪ 鉴别诊断

- 锁定综合征：
  - 由皮质脊髓束、皮质脑桥束损伤引起，导致四肢瘫痪和缄默症，伴意识保留。
  - 可以通过眼球运动建立沟通(保持垂直眼球运动)。
- 神志反应缺乏：
  - 转换反应。
  - 紧张症。
  - 伪装。
  - 动态缄默症。
- 痴呆：
  - 多种进行性认知缺陷。
  - 注意力在早期阶段得到保留。

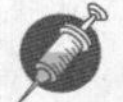

治疗

▪ 院前

- 如果呼吸道不通畅进行气道管理。
- 静脉接入，补充氧气，心电监测。
- 如果合并潜在创伤，固定脊柱。
- "昏迷鸡尾酒"：
  - 葡萄糖。
  - 纳洛酮。
  - 硫胺素。
- 寻找潜在原因的体征：
  - 药物，药物警戒手链。
  - 记录基本的神经系统检查、GCS评分、瞳孔、肢体运动。
  - 创伤的总体体征。
- 争议。
  - 如果Dextrostix不可用，经验性使用葡萄糖。
    - 葡萄糖可在硫胺素前安全给药。

▪ 初步稳定/治疗

- 静脉输入 D_{50}。
- 纳洛酮。
- 硫胺素。

▪ 急诊治疗/程序

- 考虑经验性地使用抗生素改变未确定病

因的精神状态：

- 具有良好 CSF 液体渗透性的广谱抗生素，如头孢曲松和万古霉素。
• 如果怀疑有毒摄入，则进行经验性治疗。
• 维持体温正常。
• 针对潜在病因的特异性治疗。

■ **药物治疗**

• 阿昔洛韦：10 mg/kg，q8 h。
• 头孢曲松钠：2 g[儿童：50～75 mg/(kg·d)，q12～24 h]，静脉注射，q12～24 h。
• 葡萄糖：1～2 ml/kg D_{50}W(儿童：2～4 ml/kg D_{25}W)，静脉注射。
• 地西泮：0.1～0.3 mg/kg，缓慢静脉注射(最大剂量 10 mg)，q10～15 min×3 剂量。
• 劳拉西泮：0.05～0.1 mg/kg，静脉注射(最大剂量 4 mg，q10～15 min)。
• 甘露醇：0.5～1 g/kg，静脉注射。
• 纳洛酮：0.01～0.1 mg/kg，静脉注射、肌内注射、皮下注射或经气管通路给药(ET)。
• 硫胺素：100 mg 肌内注射或 100 mg 硫胺素在 1 000 ml 静脉注射液体中开放。
• 万古霉素：1 g(儿童：10 mg/kg，q8～12 h)，静脉注射，q12 h。

随访

■ **进一步处理**

入院指征

所有精神状态急性和持续变化的患者都需要入院。

出院指征

• 与胰岛素治疗有关的低血糖，症状消失。
• 精神状态慢性改变(如痴呆)没有基本状况变化。
• 通过观察和药物将急性药物中毒与患者精神状态恢复到正常，且没有潜在的延迟毒性。

■ **随访建议**

初级保健随访，以管理导致精神状态改变的病因(即调整药物剂量，药物滥用治疗转诊)。

要点和误区

• 考虑可逆的原因。
- 低血糖(检查葡萄糖，给予右旋糖)。
- 过量服用(纳洛酮试验)。
- 噻嗪缺乏症(硫胺素试验)。
• 对于任何病因不明或神经异常的患者，请考虑头部 CT。
• 在发热或病因不明的患者中考虑经验性抗生素。

颈部绞窄伤和悬吊伤 Injury by Strangulation/Hanging

David Della-Giustina · Karen Della-Giustina 伍力学 译

 基础知识

■ **描述**

• 颈部绞窄伤：
- 绳索：用绳索等材料勒压颈部结构。
- 手掐：以手用力掐压颈部结构。
- 体位性挤压：以身体重量压迫而致气道梗阻(压在某一物体上)或体位不当压迫气道(多见于婴儿)。
• 上吊是另一勒颈窒息方式：
- 完全性：受害人整个身体离地悬吊。
- 不完全性：受害人身体部分接触地面，呈不完全悬吊。
- 典型：悬吊着力点位于枕部中心。
- 非典型：悬吊着力点不在枕部中心。
- 主观故意型：如自杀、他杀、自慰、窒息游戏等。
- 意外事故型：如儿童或衣物被绞入机器中。
- 悬吊未遂：见于非司法性质的绞刑中的获救者。

■ **病因**

• 绞刑(司法性)：
- 受刑者从至少与其身高相当的高处突然跌落。
- 巨大的力量将其头部与躯干分离而产生类似于斩首型损伤(颈椎骨折并颈髓离断)。
• 绞刑(非法性)：
- 跌落高度相对较低。
- 损伤与普通绞窄伤类似。
• 颈部绞窄伤：
- 由于颈部受到外部压力而导致的颈部血管和/或气道关闭造成的窒息。
- 三个原因：上吊，结扎勒死、手动勒死。
- 除了司法性质的绞刑外，颈髓损伤并不常见。
• 死亡：
- 继发于血管或气道受外力压迫。
- 发生在颈动脉窦受压后引发迷走反射，出现严重心动过缓而心搏骤停。
- 继发于直接的脊髓损伤。
- 继发于悬吊未遂者的肺部并发症。
- 继发于脑部缺氧。

■ **常见的并发损伤**

• 颈髓损伤。
• 脑部缺氧损伤。
• 动静脉破裂、血栓形成。
• 舌骨骨折：
- 通常见于非司法性质的颈部绞窄伤。
• 环状软骨损伤(罕见)。
• 甲状软骨损伤：
- 多见于非司法性质的颈部绞窄致死案例。
• 膈神经损伤。
• 气道水肿。
• 急性呼吸窘迫综合征(ARDS)。
• 吸入性肺炎(可能发生较晚)。
• 神经源性肺水肿(可能为发生较晚)。
- 由于交感兴奋使肺间质渗出增加所致。
• 梗阻后肺水肿(迅速起病)：
- 大气道梗阻时，吸气相胸膜腔负压增加所致。
• 气体栓塞：
- 当气肿和血管损伤同时存在时应考虑该病。

诊断

■ **症状和体征**

• 气道破坏：
- 肺气肿。
- 呼吸困难。
- 发音困难或喘鸣。
- 正常软骨标记缺失。
• 颈髓损伤：

J

- 呼吸骤停。
- 瘫痪。
• 神经损伤：
- 声嘶。
- 吞咽困难。
- 情志改变。
- 神经功能缺陷。
• 呼吸系统后遗症。
- 呼吸窘迫。
- 肺水肿、急性呼吸窘迫综合征（ARDS）、肺炎。
• 软组织损伤：
- 擦伤、挫伤、瘀斑、绳印或手印。
• 血管损伤：
- 血肿扩大。
- 脉搏无法触及或闻及杂音。
- 脑梗死征象。
- 塔帝厄斑（Tardieu spots）：颈部勒痕以上部位的皮肤、黏膜和结膜出血。

儿科注意事项

• 颈部结构较成人更软，更易移位。
• 对挤压损伤和骨折耐受性较好。
• 由于气道口径小，轻度软组织水肿后可能很快出现气道梗阻。

病史

• 颈部绞窄发生的方式：
- 患者体位：
◦ 通过体位判断绞窄发生的机制。
◦ 推测其他潜在损伤。
- 跌落位置越高则受力越大：
◦ 常见于斩首式损伤。
- 绳结的位置：
◦ 在典型的悬吊中动脉更易被压闭。
- 绳索材料：
◦ 绳索的弹性可减低受力程度。
◦ 仅静脉被压闭也可能导致意识丧失和死亡。
• 出事的环境：
- 是否意外事故、自杀或他杀、NAT、性窒息或窒息游戏等。

体格检查

• ABC 管理：
- 气道梗阻或呼吸窘迫。
- 颈椎预防性保护措施。
• 功能障碍：
- 昏迷，AMS，神经功能障碍，瘫痪。
• 进一步检查：
- 评估颈部损伤情况：
◦ 有无软组织损伤、皮下气肿及血管损伤。
- 其他因跌落所致的创伤、自伤（自杀）、冲突性损伤（他杀/NAT）。

基本检查

• 颈椎 CT 检查。
• 头部 CT 检查：
- 了解有无颅脑出血、蛛网膜下腔出血、血肿、水肿和缺氧损伤的征象。
• 颈部血管 CT：
- 了解有无血栓及血管内膜破裂。
• X 线片：
- 评估有无肺气肿、吸入性肺炎和肺水肿。
• 指脉氧监测。
• 心电监护。

诊断检查与说明

实验室检查

• 检测动脉血气分析：
- 评估低氧血症或呼吸功能障碍状况。
• 检测血细胞比容了解失血状况。
• 血管损伤者应完善输血前血型检测及交叉配血试验。
• 如果发现血管血栓或内膜瓣并且患者接受了抗凝治疗，则可将凝血曲线作为显著失血或作为基线。
• 毒物检测（ASA、APAP、ETOH）：
- 排除是否有服毒自杀可能。

影像学检查

• 颈部 MRI 检查：
- 高分辨率 MRI 排查软组织、骨骼及软骨损伤。
- 对软组织损伤的诊断价值优于 CT。
• 血管造影：
- 可确切评估有无隐匿的血管损伤。

诊断步骤/外科

• 纤维内镜：
- 直视下评估有无气管-食管损伤。
- 可协助插管。
• 外科探查。

鉴别诊断

颈部绞窄伤的病因鉴别：
• 意外事故、他杀、自杀、NAT、自慰、窒息游戏等。

治疗

院前

• ABC 管理。
• 早期积极行开放气道：给氧，吸痰，插管：
- 及时解开绳索。
• 心电监护。
• 颈椎固定：
- 依据患者体位、颈部绞窄方式、是否有跌落过程、绳结位置、有无窒息游戏等征象等实际情况而定。

初步稳定/治疗

• ABC 管理。
• 及时给予有创气管插管并行颈椎预防性保护措施至关重要：
- 有气道梗阻者及早插管。
- 加强给氧。
- 有严重的颌面部损伤者可能需要行环甲膜切开术或气管切开术。
◦ 如有血肿覆盖环甲膜或环状软骨破坏征象，应避免行环甲膜切开。
◦ 上述情形需安排紧急气管切开术（详见喉部骨折）。
• 通过直接压迫方式控制出血：
- 切勿在急诊室行伤口探查。

急诊治疗/程序

• 静脉通路。
• 请耳鼻喉科或创伤外科医师会诊颈部软组织损伤。
• 请血管外科医师会诊血管损伤。
• 请神经科医师会诊可疑的脑缺血性损伤（血栓、栓塞等）。
• 针对可疑的颅内压升高、脑水肿给予支持治疗：
- 抬高床头。
- 保证充足的氧供和脑灌注。
- 预防继发的神经损伤。
- 依病情请神经外科协助监测颅内压或行外科引流。
• 颈部损伤伴气肿：
- 假定上呼吸道黏膜与颈深部组织相贯通。
- 使用抗生素。
• 喉头水肿：
- 应用激素。
• 评估相关的损害：
- 对自杀病例应考虑有无服毒。
- 对于可疑的儿童患者非意外损伤应向相关机构报告。

药物治疗

• 缺氧性脑损伤：
- 甘露醇：0.25～1 g/kg 静脉注射（对考虑存在颅内压增高者应用，但儿童不常规应用）。

J

- 高渗盐水：剂量依病情而定(对考虑存在颅内压增高者应用)。
- 苯妥英钠：癫痫发作时，根据需要可给予15～20 mg/kg，静脉注射(负荷量)。
• 颈部损伤伴气肿(皮下气肿)：
- 氨苄西林-舒巴坦：1.5～3 g[儿童：100～400 mg/(kg·d)]，静脉注射，q6 h。
- 克林霉素：600 mg[儿童：25～40 mg/(kg·d)]，静脉注射，q8 h。
• 气道水肿：
- 地塞米松：0.5～2 mg/(kg·d)(儿童：0.25～0.5 mg/kg)，静脉注射，q6 h。

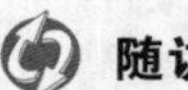

随访

进一步处理

入院指征

• 将颈部绞窄伤或悬吊伤的患者收入监护病房以观察有无气道塌陷或神经系统症状(可能为迟发表现)。
• 咽喉、食管或颈部血管损伤需要外科手术治疗者。
• 有神志状态改变、新发神经功能障碍或昏迷者。
• 呼吸窘迫：
- 因肺水肿、ARDS、肺炎而需要支持治疗者。
• 所有怀疑自杀或他杀所致的颈部绞窄伤患者均应请精神科会诊或联系社会服务机构。
• 对儿童患者：
- 怀疑是非意外损伤者，应考虑其居家安全。

出院指征

无颈部绞窄或悬吊伤者可在急诊室行适当的观察后方可出院，以确保无气道塌陷、血管损伤、神经功能障碍、自杀或他杀等情况存在。

随访建议

• 神经精神评估。
- 评估有无缺氧性脑病。
• 精神病学、心理学干预：
- 针对自杀或他杀患者。
- 自慰或窒息游戏患者给予药物、认知、行为方面的干预治疗。
• 外科随访：
- 损伤迁移未愈者。

要点和误区

• 颈椎损伤在非司法性悬吊伤受害者中并不常见：
- 脑部缺氧是最可能的死亡原因。
• 及时行有创气管插管至关重要。
• 透彻评估有无附带损伤。
• 所有绞窄或悬吊伤患者均应收入院观察。
• 预后：
- 入院时的 GCS 评分无法预测预后情况。
- 以下情形提示预后不良：
◦ 头颅 CT 提示脑部缺氧表现。
◦ 悬吊神经较长。
◦ 在事发现场或抵达急诊后出现过心搏骤停。

颈部腺炎 Cervical Adenitis

Julie A. Zeller 庄育刚 译

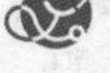

基础知识

描述

• 颈部淋巴结急性细菌感染。
- 经常继发于头部或颈部的细菌感染。
• 儿科常见。
- 近年来合并有免疫抑制(HIV、肿瘤、移植患者)成人也常见。
• 任何颈部结节均可感染。
- 超过 50%的病例涉及下颌下结。
- 临床表现为直径 3～6 cm 的温暖，柔软，肿胀，红斑。
- 结节通常是移动的。

病因

• 40%～89%的病例是由金黄色葡萄球菌(越来越多的 CA-MRSA)或 A 组 β 溶血性链球菌(GAS)感染引起的。
• B组链球菌(GBS)可表现为婴儿蜂窝织炎/腺炎。
• 厌氧菌：
- 考虑与牙齿或牙龈感染有关。
• 土拉菌(*Francisella tularensis*)。
- 接触被感染的动物(兔子、仓鼠、啮齿动物)后发生的高热疾病。
- 在美国，大多数病例都发生在中南部地区。
- 小脑上腺综合征(发炎的淋巴结引流区的丘疹病变)。
• 猫抓病(*Bartonella henselae*)。
- 从咬伤或刮伤接种后，症状在 1～4 周开始。
- 30%的患者出现发烧和轻度全身症状。
- 腋窝淋巴结最常受影响，但 1/4 的儿童可能患有孤立的宫颈淋巴结。
- 病态缓慢，但通常在 4～6 周后自发消退。
• 非结核分枝杆菌(NTM)。
- 鸟分枝杆菌复合物(MAC)最常见的原因。

儿科注意事项

• 儿童颈部包块常见原因。
• 总体上 A 群链球菌和金黄色葡萄球菌感染最常见。
• 新生儿由 B 群链球菌引起的蜂窝织炎和腺炎常见。
- 通常见于 3～7 周的男童，表现为发热、下颌下腺或者面部蜂窝织炎，同侧中耳炎。
- 94%合并菌血症。
• 金黄色葡萄球菌感染过程缓慢，出现化脓概率增高。
• 病毒感染会导致后继细菌感染。

老年注意事项

• 此类人群要考虑恶性肿瘤可能性，尤其没有发热和白细胞增高患者。
• 无痛固定硬结节可能不是颈部腺炎。

诊断

症状和体征

• 增大、压痛的颈部淋巴结。
• 单侧多见、质硬。
• 局部皮温高，红斑样。
• 早期坚硬，后期有波动感。
• 有或无发热。
• 萎靡。
• 新生儿或者儿童常见烦躁不安。

J

• 通常合并头部或者颈部感染。
- 咽炎、扁桃体炎、扁桃体周围脓肿。
- 中耳炎、内耳炎。
- 牙齿感染。
- 头皮感染。

病史

• 发病时间。
• 伴随症状：发热、体重下降、皮疹。
• 接触、旅行史。
• 新生儿出生史、合并症。

体格检查

出现头颈临床症状尤其要注意气道的评估。

■ 基本检查

• 颈部腺炎是一个临床诊断。
• 寻找头颈部感染源（中耳炎或者扁桃体炎）。
• 未发现头颈部感染源需要。
• PPD试验寻找可能的结核感染。
• 病毒感染可能。

■ 诊断检查与说明

实验室诊断

• 若能明确感染源可不需要。
• 病因不明，以下实验室诊断可能有帮助：
- 白细胞计数。
- 传染性单核细胞增多症检测试剂盒。
- 咽拭子培养。
- 抗体检测（EB病毒、CMV病毒、弓形体）。

影像学检查

• 胸片、颈部侧位片或曲面X线成像。
- 有助于寻找感染源和深部感染。
- 胸片有助于发现结核感染。
• 颈部CT/MRI。
- 有助于排除或者描绘发育异常。
• 超声。
- 能区分实质组织中的囊性结构，但是其他发现无特异性。
- 体格检查不能完全确定的深部脓肿。
• 活检。
• 细针抽吸。
- 所有波动性肿块须行细针抽吸。
- 标本送革兰染色，抗酸染色，需氧/厌氧培养，分枝杆菌培养和真菌培养。
- 若怀疑结核性淋巴结炎，不做抽吸穿刺以免慢性窦道形成和结核播散。
• 皮试。
- 分枝杆菌和猫抓综合征。

■ 鉴别诊断

• 淋巴结病（淋巴结非细菌性感染性炎症）是全身性疾病的征象，通常累及多发和双侧淋巴结。
• 病毒感染通常由于以下病毒引起：
- 呼吸道病毒（腺病毒、鼻病毒和肠道病毒）。
- EB病毒、单纯疱疹病毒、水痘病毒、CMV。
- 腮腺炎病毒、风疹病毒和麻疹病毒。
• 小儿特殊疾病：
- 川崎病。
- 组织细胞性坏死性淋巴结炎。
- 周期性发热、手足口病、PFARA。
• 弓形虫病。
• 先天异常：
- 腮裂囊肿、甲状舌管囊肿、水囊瘤。
• 恶性肿瘤：
- 白血病、淋巴瘤、横纹肌肉瘤、甲状腺肿瘤。
- 2%以下儿童有罕见的非特异性肿块。
• 其他全身疾病：
- 狼疮、结节病。

治疗

■ 初步稳定/治疗

• 吸氧，监测气道。
• 注意生命体征。

■ 急诊治疗/程序

• 治疗头和颈部感染。
- 若诊断不明，治疗A群链球菌和金黄色葡萄球菌。
- 若治疗效果不佳，考虑MRSA。
• 波动性肿块细针抽吸。
• 给予口服抗生素。
- 头孢氨苄。
- 头孢羟氨。
- 阿莫西林-克拉维酸。
• 怀疑牙齿、牙周或者厌氧菌感染：
- 克林霉素。
- 阿莫西林-克拉维酸。
• CA-MRSA：
- 克林霉素。
- 复方新诺明。
- 万古霉素或者利奈唑胺。
• 疗程至少10日，即使症状消失。
• 局部温热湿敷。
• 必要时给予镇痛。

■ 药物治疗

一线药物

• 头孢羟氨：500 mg，口服，q12 h；儿童30 mg/(kg·24 h)。
• 头孢氨苄：250～500 mg，口服，q6 h；儿童25～50 mg/(kg·24 h)。
• 阿莫西林-克拉维酸：250～500 mg，口服，q8 h；儿童20～40 mg/(kg·24 h)。
• 克林霉素：300 mg，口服，q8 h；儿童8～25 mg/(kg·24 h)。
• 复方新诺明：2片，每日2次。

二线药物

• 头孢唑林：1～2 g，静脉滴注，q8 h；儿童25～50 mg/(kg·24 h)。
• 新青霉素：1～2 g，静脉滴注，q4～6 h；儿童50～200 mg/(kg·24 h)。
• 克林霉素：600～900 mg，静脉滴注，q8 h；儿童20～40 mg/(kg·24 h)。
• 阿莫西林-舒巴坦：1.5～3 g，静脉滴注，q6 h；儿童200 mg/(kg·d)。
• 万古霉素注射液：10～15 mg/kg，静脉滴注，q12 h；儿童40～60 mg/(kg·d)，分q8 h用。
• 利奈唑胺注射液：600 mg，静脉滴注，每日2次；12岁以上儿童，30 mg/(kg·8 h)，12岁以下不超过1 200 mg。

随访

■ 进一步处理

入院指征

• 新生儿。
• 气道梗阻。
• 表现为病重。
• 免疫抑制。
• 不能口服药物。
• 口服抗生素无明显改善。

出院指征

• 大部分患者可带口服药出院。
• 2～3日密切随诊。
• 可以经口进流质、服药。
• 以下情况需回急诊：
- 症状加重。
- 脓肿进展。
- 声音改变。
- 呼吸困难加重。
- 全身症状加重。

转诊问题

临床检查要涉及恶性肿瘤和先天性异常

J

(腮裂囊肿、甲状舌管囊肿、水囊瘤)。

■ **随访建议**

- 48 h 强制回访以明确症状改善。
- 有需要口腔科或口腔内科随诊。

要点和误区

- 颈部腺炎是临床诊断。
- 单侧红、肿、热、有压痛的淋巴结。
- A 群链球菌和金黄色葡萄球菌是常见病原学。
- 儿童考虑 B 群链球菌,标准药物治疗效果不佳需考虑 MRSA。
- 临床特点决定治疗策略。

颈前部穿透伤 Penetrating, Anterior

Thien H. Nguyen · Anthony J. Medak　伍力学 译

基础知识

■ **描述**

- 创伤的严重程度可由颈阔肌所受暴力的程度来衡量。
- 颈部由 3 部分区域组成:
  - 区域一:在锁骨与环状软骨之间。
    - 涉及血管、肺、气管、食管和甲状腺。
    - 在这个部位的穿通伤死亡率最高,由于伤及胸部解剖结构。
  - 区域二:在环状软骨和下颌角之间。
    - 涉及血管、气管、食管、颈椎和脊髓。
    - 此区域为暴露部位,发生在此处的伤害最为常见。
  - 区域三:位于下颌角之上直到颅底。
    - 部位较深,外科处理困难。
- 较新的文献支持另一种"禁区"方法:
  - 外伤通常与内伤不符。

儿科注意事项

儿童的喉头在颈部较高位置,因此受到下颌骨和舌骨较好的保护。

■ **病因**

- 枪伤。
- 刺伤。
- 其他(如玻璃碎片、金属片、动物咬伤等)。

诊断

■ **症状和体征**

- 血管损伤"强指征":
  - 活动性、持续性出血或血肿。
  - 动脉搏动消失。
  - 霍纳综合征(颈动脉损伤)。
  - 颈部血管震颤或杂音。
  - 静脉气体栓塞。
- 气管食管损伤"强指征":
  - 呼吸窘迫。
  - 喘鸣。
  - 咳血。
  - 气管移位。
  - 肺气肿。
  - 气胸。
  - 负压吸引所致的损伤。
  - 声嘶、失声、发声困难。
  - 吞咽困难、吞咽痛。
- 神经系统损伤"强指征":
  - 中枢或周围神经系统功能缺陷。

病史

- 损伤跨越中线提示损伤较重。
- 利器戳伤。
  - 利器的大小。
  - 大多是低能量的穿通伤。
- 枪伤。
  - 枪的类型。
  - 长距离还是短距离。

体格检查

- 仔细检查伤口,明确损伤范围及是否穿透颈阔肌。
- 避免盲目探查伤口:
  - 可能会导致不可控的出血。

■ **基本检查**

- 颈阔肌损伤:
  - 无:处理伤口后予以出院。
  - 有:
    - 如病情不稳定,或存在任何"强指征":考虑建立紧急气道,然后进行或探查。
    - 如病情稳定:两个可接受的选项:
      - 区域方法:检查取决于损伤的区域。
      - "无区域"方法:CT 血管造影(CTA)。

■ **诊断检查与说明**

实验室检查

- 血型与交叉配血试验。
- 血细胞计数、常规化验、凝血功能检查。

影像学检查

- 行颈部 X 线侧位片评估软组织损伤程度并查看异物。
- 用行胸片检查有无血气胸及纵隔气肿。
- 区域一:
  - 血管造影:评估血管创伤的金标准,属有创检查。
    - 随着 CTA 的不断改进,使用频率降低。
  - CT 血管造影:速度快,无创。
    - 肩部有条纹状伪影,且锁骨下血管显影欠佳。
    - 可能会漏掉咽食管损伤。
  - 以水溶性造影剂或稀钡行食管 X 线片:
    - 敏感性低。
    - 需联合食管镜检查来排除是否存在损伤。
    - 指征:伤口接近、穿越中线,有皮下气肿。
- 区域二:
  - 无症状:观察。
  - 有症状:收入观察室。
- 区域三:
  - 有症状:血管造影法或 CT 血管成像。
- 使用"禁区"方法规定,任何有颈阔肌侵犯的稳定患者都要进行 CTA。

诊断步骤/外科

- 支气管镜检查法有助于评估气管损伤。
- 所有穿透颈阔肌的损伤均应请外科会诊。
  - 手术探查:
    - 血肿扩大或搏动性血肿。
    - 活动性出血。
    - 减小或不相等的外围脉冲。
    - 咳血。
    - 霍纳综合征。
    - 杂音。
    - 皮下气肿。
    - 呼吸窘迫。
    - 伤口有气体冒出。

■ 鉴别诊断

- 外周或中枢损伤。
- 颈髓损伤。
- 头部或胸部创伤。

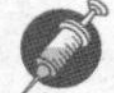

治疗

■ 院前

- 反复吸引清除气道中的血液、分泌物及呕吐物。
- 建立 2 个大孔径静脉通路。
- 高流量给氧。
- 避免使用球囊面罩通气，防止可能的颈部损伤或气体通过气管及喉部伤口进入皮下组织内导致气道受压。
- 密切观察气道，水肿或血肿扩大可导致气道受压。
- 早期插管的指征：
  - 有呼吸窘迫的临床表现。
  - 喘鸣。
  - 缺氧。
  - 呼吸疲劳。
  - 颈部血肿扩大。
- 经鼻气管插管可加重穿透伤。

注意

- 大的静脉损伤应予以密闭包扎以预防气体栓塞。
- 无局部神经功能障碍或颈椎损伤的常规颈椎固定无需行颈部制动。
  - 颈部制动可能限制对颈部的直接视诊和触诊，从而遗漏致命性征象。

■ 初步稳定/治疗

- 紧急气管插管指征：
  - 患者有出现呼吸窘迫或昏迷症状。
  - 注意有无声音改变或吞咽疼痛。
  - 对情况尚稳定，无明显呼吸窘迫者也可行预防性有创气管插管或利用床边气道监测设备密切观察病情。
  - 快速麻醉诱导后经口气管插管是颈部穿透伤患者确定型人工气道的构建方式。
  - 窒息、严重面部损伤或气道变形的患者禁忌使用经鼻盲插置管。
  - 在纤维支气管镜引导下行气管插管，患者处于清醒状态，可直视声门和损伤病灶，很有优势。
  - 当经口或经鼻气管插管失败时，需要经皮气管通气：
    - 上部气道梗阻者禁忌使用。
    - 可能导致气压伤。
  - 如环甲膜上有明显的血肿形成则禁忌行环甲膜切开术。
    - 在这种情况下，行气管切开术更为保险。
  - 呼吸：
  - 区域一损伤可引发气胸或锁骨下静脉损伤和血胸：
    - 可能需要穿刺减压或胸腔置管引流。
- 循环：
  - 外部出血：
    - 直接压迫止血。
    - 如压迫止血失败，可将 Foley 导尿管置入伤口内并充起球囊局部压迫止血。
    - 禁忌盲目钳夹血管，以免进一步加重神经血管损伤。
  - 出血难以控制或血流动力学不稳定者：直接送观察室。
  - 行气管插管后，颈部可以重物压迫包扎止血。
  - 血胸：胸腔置管引流。

■ 急诊治疗/程序

- 鼻胃管可能增加鼻咽部血肿破裂的风险，不宜留置。
- 考虑预防性抗生素：
  - 污秽/污染的伤口。
  - 疑似咽食管损伤。
  - 免疫功能受损的患者。
- 合理的抗生素选择包括：头孢西丁、克林霉素、青霉素＋甲硝唑。
- 预防破伤风。

■ 药物治疗

- 头孢西丁：1～2 g[儿童：80～160 mg/(kg·d)，静脉滴注，q6 h]，静脉注射，q6～8 h。
- 克林霉素：600～900 mg[儿童 25～40 mg/(kg·d)，静脉滴注，q6～8 h]，静脉注射，q8 h。
- 青霉素：400 万 U/d[儿童：100 000～400 000 U/(kg·d)，静脉注射，q4～6 h]，静脉注射，q4 h，联合甲硝唑。
- 甲硝唑：1 g 负荷量，续以 500 mg[儿童：30 mg/(kg·d)，静脉滴注，q6 h]，静脉注射，q6 h。

随访

■ 进一步处理

入院指征

- 所有颈部穿透伤患者均应入院观察。
- 应将患者留置在便于提供有效的手术治疗的区域进行观察。
- 提示有气道或血管损伤者应收入 ICU。

出院指征

- 无症状且检查结果为阴性者可在观察期后以予出院。
  - 应与外科一起进行最终处置。
- 对于仅发生未及颈阔肌的表浅损伤患者可直接从急诊室出院。

要点和误区

- 未能识别颈阔肌侵犯。
- 对困难气道插管预估不足。
- 未能识别即将发生的气道受压状况。

J

颈前部钝性创伤 Neck Trauma, Blunt, Anterior

Thien H. Nguyen · Anthony J. Medak 伍力学 译

基础知识

■ 描述

- 颈前部钝性创伤可由各种颈部结构损伤而导致。
  - 血管损伤：
    - 颈动脉损伤（包括颈内动脉、颈外动脉和颈总动脉）。
    - 椎动脉损伤。
    - 血肿、血管内膜撕裂、血栓形成和假性动脉瘤。
    - 出血或颈部血肿。

- 喉部和气管损伤：
  - 喉部损伤：舌骨骨折，甲状软骨、环状软骨骨折或环状软骨与气管断裂。
  - 声带损伤。
  - 杓状软骨移位。
  - 气管损伤：出血或断裂。
- 咽部和食管损伤：
  - 咽部：血肿、穿孔。
  - 食管：血肿、穿孔。
- 神经系统：
  - 颈交感走行于颈动脉周围：损伤后可出现霍纳综合征。
  - 迷走神经和喉返神经。
  - 颈神经根和脊髓。
- 颈椎：
  - 椎体、横突、棘突骨折等。
  - 移位。

病因

- 机动车交通事故（最常见原因）：
  - 在正面碰撞中由于惯性作用颈部与仪表盘或方向盘发生撞击而发生损伤。
  - 安全带也可能导致颈前部剪切样损伤。
- 颈前部受到拳打、脚踢或其他物品击打。
- “晾衣绳损伤”：
  - 发生在驾驶摩托车、雪地车、滑雪橇或全地形车过程中。
  - 驾驶者颈部与悬挂在两个物体之间的绳索或电缆等发生撞击。
- 绞窄伤。

儿科注意事项

- 儿童身体的头占比较大，使发生在颈部的加速-减速损伤的风险增加。
- 发生在口腔内的软腭时可能导致颈动脉血栓（如儿童含在口内的棒冰等，可能戳伤软腭）。

J

诊断

症状和体征

- 临床表现因致伤机制和受伤部位而异：
  - 血管损伤：
    - 出血、瘀斑、水肿。
    - 颈动脉杂音或震颤（血管损伤的特征性表现）。
    - 神经系统功能障碍（常为迟发性）。
  - 喉部和气管损伤：
    - 声音改变、嘶哑或失声。
    - 呼吸困难、吸气性喘鸣、劳力性呼吸困难、缺氧症状。
    - 皮下气肿，有触痛。
  - 咽部和食管损伤（少见）：
    - 吞咽困难、吞咽疼痛、咯血、血性唾液。
    - 局部有触痛。
    - 感染、脓毒症（迟发表现）。
  - 神经损伤：
    - 中枢或外周神经系统功能缺陷。

病史

- 结合症状和体征向患者详细了解病史（如患者尚能提供的话）：
  - 包括颈部所有结构及颈外生理结构的情况（颈部创伤常牵涉胸部、头部等处）。

体格检查

- 确保气道处于通畅状态。
- 请患者发声以评估他们的嗓音质量：
  - 评估发音困难、声音嘶哑。
- 详查颈部有无出血、血肿、瘀斑、水肿或解剖畸形：
  - 评估侧颈是否有安全带标志。
- 听诊颈动脉杂音、震颤。
- 触诊了解有无压痛及气肿。
- 行神经系统检查，了解有无缺血性损伤、脊髓损伤或外周神经损伤。
- 完善体格检查排除胸腹等部位的损伤。

基本检查

依据病史及体格检查所发现的情况而定。

诊断检查与说明

实验室检查

- 血型和交叉配血试验。
- 全血细胞计数。
- 应在行影像学检查前完善尿素氮、血肌酐（增强 CT 或 MRI）。

影像学检查

- 颈椎和颈部 X 线侧位片。
- X 线平片诊断价值有限，但仍可发现声门下狭窄、椎前软组织水肿、皮下气肿及喉部钙化骨的骨折等。
- X 线平片可发现胸部相关损伤（气胸、纵隔气肿等）。
- 颈动脉多普勒超声是一种无创快速诊查血管损伤的方法。
  - 相关回顾性研究显示其敏感率可达 92%，但效果取决于操作者水平，且血管分叉以上的可视程度较差。
- CT 可用于病情稳定的患者的喉部及气管的损伤、软骨破裂或颈髓损伤等的评估。
- CT 血管造影（CTA）：
  - 考虑在有血管损伤的明确迹象的钝性颈部创伤后进行 CTA。
  - 然而，最近的一项研究发现，孤立的安全带征象和异常的 CTA 之间的相关性很弱（r=0.007）。
- 磁共振血管成像（MRA）：
  - 与血管造影相比，MRA 对颈动脉和椎动脉损伤的初步研究的敏感性（49%）和特异性（99%）较低。
- 下列情形提示需行血管造影（考虑硬信号和软信号）：
  - 存在颈动脉杂音或颤动。
  - 搏动性出血。
  - 颈部血肿扩大。
  - 神经功能发生障碍，但 CT 未见颅内病理性改变。
  - 霍纳综合征。
  - 意识状况恶化。

诊断步骤/外科

- 不稳定的患者应及早进行手术评估和干预，以识别和治疗危重脑血管损伤。
- 喉部和食管损伤：
  - 纤维喉镜可直视声门下气道情况，判断气管插管有无困难并评估气道的通畅性及损伤程度。
- 食管损伤：
  - 首选检查：泛影葡胺吞咽试验（对胸膜的刺激较小）或吞钡试验。
- 内镜检查的适应证：
  - 吞咽痛。
  - 呕血或唾液中带血。
  - 皮下气肿。

鉴别诊断

- 外周或中枢神经损伤。
- 颈髓损伤。
- 头部或胸腔的相关损伤。

治疗

院前

- 应及早确保气道通畅，并密切监测：
  - 水肿或血肿扩大可加重气道受阻。
- 经口气管插管为开放气道的一线措施。
- 呼吸窘迫的临床表现：
  - 喘鸣。
  - 气短。
  - 劳力性呼吸困难。
  - 颈部血肿扩大。
- 避免经鼻盲插方式行气管插管：
  - 可能存在解剖结构异常和血肿破裂风险

增加。

• 在评估和气道干预期间必须保持颈椎稳定。

▪ 初步稳定/治疗

在颈椎固定的同时加强气道管理：

• 对于已经出现气道梗阻症状或随时可能发生此情况者，立即行气管插管。

• 若经口气管插管失败可能需要行环甲膜切开或紧急气管切开术。

– 甲状腺/环状软骨周围存在挫伤或血肿者为气管切开术的禁忌证。

• 在有气管插管作为气道保障后可通过用厚纱布压迫的方式控制咽部出血。

• 病情不稳定者需直接送入手术室。

▪ 急诊治疗/程序

• 对怀疑有血管、气管或食管损伤患者，应请外科会诊。

• 对有症状的血管、气管、咽喉或食管损伤患者，应立即行外科手术。

• 喉部损伤不一定需要立即行外科修复手术。

• 继发于管腔狭窄和血栓的血管损伤，推荐使用抗凝治疗：

– 有利于改善神经系统疗效。

– 在初始治疗前请外科会诊。

▪ 药物治疗

• 抗凝治疗(见上)。

– 开始使用普通肝素 15 U/(kg·h)(不推注)并监测 APTT。

• 有食管损伤者推荐预防性使用抗生素以预防脓肿形成(应覆盖厌氧菌)：

– 头孢西丁：2 g，静脉滴注，q8 h[儿童：80～160 mg/(kg·d)，q6 h]。

– 或者克林霉素：600～900 mg，静脉滴注，q8 h[儿童：25～40 mg/(kg·d)，q6～8 h]。

– 或者青霉素：240 万 U/d，静脉滴注，q4～6 h[儿童：15～25 U/(kg·d)]，联合甲硝唑。

– 甲硝唑：1 g 负荷量，续以 500 mg，静脉滴注，q6 h[儿童：30 mg/(kg·d)，q12 h]。

随访

▪ 进一步处理

入院指征

• 有症状、有异常检查结果或有明确的钝性创伤史的患者，须收入院接受创伤诊疗，并观察至少 24 h。

• 怀疑有气道或血管损伤证据者须收入 ICU。

> **注意**
>
> 接受抗凝药物治疗的患者应在损伤后 6 h 内在急诊室进行观察，并重新评估是否有延迟后遗症的迹象。

出院指征

只有那些损伤轻微且检查结果为阴性的患者可在仔细评估和观察后允许从急诊出院。在个案的基础上，注意病案追踪与回访。

▪ 随访建议

应明确告知患者如有迟发性血管、气管及神经系统损伤表现，须及时来急诊就诊。

要点和误区

• 钝性颈部血管和空气消化损伤可能有轻微或延迟的表现。

• 颅脑 CT 正常的闭合性颈部外伤患者要高度怀疑隐匿性血管损伤。

• 预测气道困难时，考虑早期麻醉或耳鼻喉科会诊(如果可行)。

胫骨粗隆骨软骨病 Osgood-Schlatter Disease

Stephen R. Hayden　朱妍 译

基础知识

▪ 描述

• 髌腱附着处的胫骨结节骨软骨炎。

• 是 10～15 岁儿童膝关节疼痛最常见的原因。

• 疼痛和胫骨结节的水肿：

– 压痛位于髌韧带连接点，因为髌韧带位于膝关节正下方。

• 关节外疾病：

– 疼痛活动后加重，休息后缓解。

– 是由于重复的压力所致，常见于参加运动的儿童。

• 良性、自限性的膝关节疾病。

▪ 病因

• 病因有争议。

• 主要学说：牵拉造成的粗隆处的微裂纹。

• 活动时髌韧带连接胫骨结节处反复受压会导致疼痛发生。

诊断

▪ 症状和体征

• 胫骨结节上方疼痛及肿胀。

• 跑步或跳跃后疼痛加剧。

• 休息后疼痛减轻。

病史

• 危险因素：

– 年龄：10～15 岁，与青春期快速生长有关。

– 多见于男孩。

– 运动：跑步、跳跃、快速改变方向的运动(如足球、篮球、花样滑冰)。

• 膝关节疼痛活动后加重，休息后缓解。

• 一般为单侧，约 20%的患者为双侧。

体格检查

• 胫骨结节上方突起及软组织肿胀。

• 膝关节抗阻力拉伸时疼痛复发。

• 胫骨结节上方髌韧带连接处压痛。

• 相对于健侧来说，患侧的股四头肌和股后肌群更紧绷。

• 胫骨结节处可能存在红斑。

• 膝关节检查正常。

▪ 基本检查

诊断主要依靠体格检查：

• 疼痛、肿胀和局限于胫骨结节的压痛。

▪ 诊断检查与说明

影像学检查

膝关节 X 线平片：

• 可以做出临床诊断。

• 考虑对非典型症状进行 X 线检查。

• 可以看到胫骨结节不规则骨化和断裂。

• 超声在观察周围软组织影像时有优势。

■ 鉴别诊断

• 髌骨应力性骨折。
• 髌骨或股四头肌肌腱炎。
• 髌前或髌下滑囊炎。
• 剥脱性骨软骨炎。
• 骨髓炎。
• 髌股关节疼痛综合征。
• 脓毒症性关节炎。
• 髌骨下极牵拉性骨突炎(Sinding-Larsen-Johansson 病)。
• 创伤性脂肪增生(Hoffa 病)。
• 复发性疼痛,尤其是臀部。

 治疗

■ 初步稳定/治疗

• 将下肢固定在舒适的位置。
• 膝关节冰敷。

■ 急诊治疗/程序

• 休息避免活动引起疼痛。
- 限制活动 6～8 周。
- 避免切割和跳跃运动,如篮球、足球、排球等。
• 冰敷患区。
• 镇痛药物。
• 伸展股四头肌和股后肌群。
• 加强股四头肌力量的练习。
• 在活动时膝关节前使用保护性敷料。
• 戴护膝 6～8 周。
• 避免注射皮质激素。
• 本病是个良性、自限性的疾病。

■ 药物治疗

一线用药

止痛药物:
• 布洛芬:10 mg/kg,口服,q6 h。
• 对乙酰氨基酚:15 mg/kg,口服,q4 h;请勿超过 4 g/24 h。

 随访

■ 进一步处理

入院指征

没必要住院。

出院指征

在家治疗。

转诊问题

• 如果保守治疗失败,那么倾向于儿科骨科手术。
• 极少情况下,需要外科手术切除,但是通常推迟到骨骼发育成熟后进行。

■ 随访建议

避免令人疼痛的活动并在 2～3 周至儿科医师处随访并复查。

要点和误区

• 诊断是临床诊断。
- 疼痛、肿胀和局限于胫骨结节的压痛。
◦ 锻炼时和锻炼后压痛和疼痛加重。
- 风险因素:
◦ 10～15 岁。
◦ 有跑步和跳跃的体育活动。
• 采取保守治疗:
- 治疗主要是休息、冰敷和 NSAIDs 药物。
- 避免体育运动直到疼痛缓解。

胫骨和腓骨骨折 Tibial/Fibular Shaft Fracture

Colleen J. Campbell 范浩浩 李文放 译

 基础知识

■ 描述

骨折描述

胫骨
• 80%有相关的腓骨骨折。
• 开放性损伤(24%)与闭合性损伤。
• 软组织损伤的程度。
• 开放性骨折的 Gustilo-Anderson 分类。
- Ⅰ型:
◦ 伤口<1 cm。
◦ 软组织损伤小。
◦ 无挤压伤害。
- Ⅱ型:
◦ 创伤>1 cm。
◦ 适度的软组织损伤。
◦ 很少或没有失活的软组织。
- Ⅲ型:严重软组织损伤。
◦ A:适当的骨软组织覆盖。
◦ B:组织丢失/骨膜剥离。
◦ C:神经血管损伤需要手术。
• 解剖位置:
- 近端、中间或远端 3 部分。
- 关节接合延长。
• 移位。
• 缩短程度。
• 角度。
• 形状:
- 螺旋状、横向或斜向。
- 粉碎、蝴蝶形碎片或多个片段。

腓骨
• 近端:
- 伴有腓神经损伤。
- 踝关节韧带的破坏(Maisonneuve 断裂)。
• 中间。
• 远端。

儿科注意事项

• 儿童第三常见的长骨骨折。
• 第二常见的非意外创伤的长骨骨折(通常是骨突或干骺角)。
• 非骺板骨折模式:
- 压缩(圆环):远端干骺端。
- 不完全拉伸压缩(松枝骨折)。
- 塑料/弓形畸形可能发生。
- 完整的骨折。
• 生长的骨折模式:
- 胫骨干骨折可能扩展到腓骨中 Salter-Harris Ⅱ模式。

■ 病因

• 高能量与低能量伤害。
• 软组织损伤由所涉及的能量程度决定,软组织损伤决定预后。
• 间接力量:经常低能量创伤。
- 经常由旋转和压缩力导致斜形和螺旋形骨折。
• 滑雪、摔倒、虐待儿童。
• 直接暴力:高能量创伤。
- 直接打击腿往往导致横向和纵向粉碎性骨折。

- 行人与汽车、机动车碰撞(MVC)：
  - 支点弯曲力产生楔形蝴蝶形粉碎分段。
- 滑雪者的靴子、足球铲球、MVC。

儿科注意事项

- 自行车辐条伤害：
  - 脚和小腿夹在框架和辐条之间。
  - 挤压伤是主要问题。
  - 软组织的良性外观常有欺骗性：
    - 可以在几日内发生全层皮肤损失。
  - 所有辐条相关骨折应请骨科会诊。
- 幼儿骨折：
  - 扭转力导致胫骨远端3度的螺旋骨折，腓骨无骨折。
  - 年龄范围是9个月至6岁，最常见的是学习行走的时候。
  - 中线或更多横向骨折暗示着无意外的创伤。

诊断

症状和体征

病史

- 创伤史。
- 疼痛通常是即刻的，严重的，并且很好地局部化到骨折部位。

体格检查

- 在骨折部位可见或可触及的畸形。
- 高能量创伤导致显著的软组织损伤。
- 如果涉及胫骨，则无法负重：
  - 如果单纯腓骨骨折，可能会行走。
- 因腓神经围绕非骨头、腓神经易受损导致伤脚下垂。
- 室间隔综合征。

儿科注意事项

- 依靠父母提供的病史信息。
- 孩子可能会出现跛行而无明显畸形。

基本检查

- 仔细评估软组织。
- 小心神经血管检查(与对侧)。
- 检查相关伤害。
- 完全暴露患者损伤部位，注意保温及隐私保护。
- 评估室间隔综合征。

注意

- 室间隔综合征。
- 见于8%的骨干骨折，更常见于年轻患者。
- 胫骨骨折相对常见的并发症并且可能在受伤后24 h才出现。
- 疼痛与预期不成比例。
- 患者可能有肿胀、室间隔张力增高，但是并不总是有室间隔触诊疼痛。
- 被动伸展时疼痛，足趾疼痛。
- 感觉障碍。
- 运动减弱是一个晚期表现。
- 无脉搏不是室间隔综合征的标志症状：
  - 除非有动脉损伤，否则室间隔综合征总是可以触及脉搏。
- 4个腿部隔间：前部、侧面、深处后部和浅表后部。
- 前部室间隔综合征：
  - 腓深神经。
  - 感知第1趾间皮肤。
  - 踝关节和趾背屈。
  - 胫前动脉供应足背动脉。
- 侧隔间：
  - 腓浅神经。
  - 感觉足背。
  - 足外翻。
- 后部深层：
  - 胫神经。
  - 感觉到足底。
  - 踝和趾跖屈。
  - 胫后动脉和腓动脉。
- 浅表后房：
  - 腓肠神经分支。
  - 足侧边感觉。

诊断检查与说明

实验室检查

如果考虑室间隔综合征，要查肌酸磷酸激酶水平。

影像学检查

- 正面和侧面的腿、膝盖和踝。
- 如果X线片未显示，1～4日再查，怀疑幼儿骨折或应力性骨折。
- 对复杂骨折模式甚至螺旋骨折排列不齐进行CT扫描评估。
- CT或MRI用于病理性骨折。
- 应力性骨折的MRI可能是必要的。

诊断步骤/外科

室间隔压力：

- 压力大于30 mmHg表示需要骨科会诊和筋膜切开术。
- 五P症状或舒张血压与隔室压力差值<20表示室间隔综合征。
- 随着时间的推移在距离骨折部位5 cm处重复进行压力测量，是必要的。

儿科注意事项

斜位X线片检查无移位骨折。

鉴别诊断

- 应力性骨折。
- 病理性骨折。
- 骨髓炎。

儿科注意事项

- 肉瘤。
- 病理性骨折。
- 骨髓炎。
- 非事故的创伤。

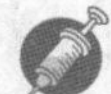

治疗

院前

- 寻找高能量的相关伤害机制。
- 评估神经或血管危害。
- 适当的固定对预防进一步受伤至关重要。

初步稳定/治疗

- 按照指示管理呼吸道和复苏。
- 威胁生命的伤害优先。
- 固定肢体。
- 使用冰块。
- 严格的NPO。
- 疼痛控制。

急诊治疗/程序

- 闭合性骨折：
  - 如果骨折异位，轻柔复位(不要多次尝试复位，可能会增加室间综合征的风险)。
  - 固定：
    - 肢体夹板固定，填充空隙。
    - 10°～20°屈曲膝盖。
  - 避免管形石膏固定。
  - 如果固定后疼痛持续存在，则怀疑：
    - 室间隔综合征。
    - 避免在怀疑室间隔综合征时抬高腿部，它降低了对肢体的灌注。
    - 神经受压。
  - 拐杖。
- 开放性骨折：
  - 去除污染物并覆盖伤口，用湿润、无菌敷料。
  - 抗生素。
  - 预防破伤风。
  - 固定好长腿后夹板。
  - 即时骨科手术会诊。
  - 清创和骨折固定。

J

• 单纯腓骨骨折：
- 通常对症处理：
◦ 加垫夹板。
◦ 抬高。
◦ 冰敷。
◦ 在肿胀消退之前不承重。
- 拐杖，如果不承重。

■ 药物治疗

• 开放性骨折的革兰阳性球菌覆盖：头孢唑林 2 g 负荷剂量，然后 1 g[儿童：50 mg/(kg · d)]，静脉滴注/肌内注射，q8 h。
• Gustilo-Anderson Ⅲ型，增加革兰阴性杆菌的覆盖：庆大霉素 3～5 mg/kg(儿童：2.5 mg/kg)，静脉滴注，q8 h。
• 农业事故，增加梭菌的覆盖范围：青霉素 1 000 万 U[儿童：250 000～400 000 U/(kg · d)]，静脉滴注，q6 h。
• 破伤风 0.5 ml 肌内注射和破伤风免疫球蛋白 250 U 肌内注射，根据伤口的类型和初次免疫次数来定。
• 如果青霉素过敏：万古霉素 1 g(儿童：10 mg/kg)，静脉滴注，q12 h。

随访

■ 进一步处理

入院指征
• 多发伤。
• 高能机制。
• 软组织受累。
• 室间隔综合征的风险。
• 所有开放性骨折。
• 偏移、有角度、横向、缩短、粉碎的和其他不稳定的骨折。
• 关节内损伤。
• 神经血管危害。
• 疼痛控制不足。
• 病理性骨折。
• 儿童非意外的创伤。

出院指征
• 低能量损伤最小限度地移位骨折机制。
• 闭合性骨折随访。
• 依从性好的骨筋膜室综合征患者反馈数据。
• 如果骨折>48 h，则骨筋膜室综合征是不太可能发展；如果没有发生，则出院。
• 标准可能更加宽松。

■ 随访建议

• 大多数儿科骨折均采用长腿石膏进行治疗 4～6 周。
• 未发生位移和最小移位骨折，成年人可以长腿石膏处理并关闭减少。
• 开放性骨折合并污染宜选择外固定和清创。
• 髓内钉治疗可以提早进行运动和允许范围内的承重。
• 克氏针有时用于治疗。

要点和误区

• 高能创伤相关的高损伤发生率：
- 相关的伤病通常包括：
◦ 股骨骨折(“浮膝伤”)。
◦ 头部创伤。
◦ 脊柱骨折。
- 胫骨骨折后的患者，深静脉血栓形成发生在 10%～25%。

胫骨平台骨折 Tibial Plateau Fracture

Kelly K. DiLorenzo · Leslie C. Oyama　范浩浩　李文放 译

基础知识

■ 描述

• 同义词：胫骨髁骨折。
• 邻近胫骨的关节表面骨折或受压。
• 外翻或内翻力轴向加载到胫骨平台上。

胫骨平台骨折的 Schatzker 分类

骨折
• 1 型：
- 胫骨平台侧边分离骨折而无平台受压。
• 2 型：
- 平台侧边分裂骨折和受压。
- 伴有外侧半月板损伤。
• 3 型：
- 一侧平台中央受压。
- 伤情可能不稳定。
• 4 型：
- 胫骨平台中间的分裂。
- 可能导致其他结构损坏：
◦ 膝后窝血管。
◦ 腓神经。
◦ 内侧副韧带。
◦ 外侧半月板。
◦ 侧副韧带。
◦ 十字韧带。
◦ 胫骨棘。
◦ 骨筋膜室间隔综合征。
• 5 型：
- 胫骨平台双髁骨折。
- 与 4 型相同的伤害。
• 6 型：
- 平台双髁严重粉碎性骨折。
- 骨干干骺分离。
- 与 4 型和 5 型相同的伤害。

■ 病因

• 约 66% 发生在外侧，25% 在内侧，11% 在双髁。
• 受伤机制：
- 1 型和 2 型来自有轴向负荷的外翻力，一般是低能量损伤。
◦ 与接触运动相关，扭动运动(如滑雪)或经典的行人受到汽车保险杠袭击。
- 3 型是骨质疏松合并低能量损伤。
- 4～6 型通常是高能量伤害，常来自机动车辆、自行车碰撞和高处坠落，引起中间平台骨折。
◦ 伴有神经血管损伤。
• 年龄相关。
- 1 型：年轻的松质骨患者，胫骨平台持续受压。
- 2 型和 3 型：压力性骨折见于骨质疏松的老年人的骨。

儿科注意事项

胫骨平台骨折在儿童少见，因其胫骨平台是密集的疏松质骨。

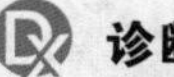

诊断

■ 症状和体征

• 膝盖疼痛肿胀。

• 无法承受重量。
• 膝关节积液(关节积血)。
• 主动和被动动作范围有限。
• 沿着胫骨近端和关节线变形。
• 膝盖可能出现内翻或外翻畸形。
• 由于关联韧带损伤可能导致联合关节不稳定。

病史

• 侧膝受伤。
• 从轴向负荷的高度跌落。
• 扭伤。

体格检查

• 使用放射摄影的决策工具:
- 渥太华膝盖规则(高度敏感):膝盖如果出现以下任何情况,建议拍X线片:
  ◦ 年龄>55岁。
  ◦ 腓骨头变软。
  ◦ 无法弯曲到90°。
  ◦ 孤立的髌骨压痛。
  ◦ 无论在伤后即刻还是在急诊,无法向4个方向转移负重。
  ◦ 可以跛行。
- 匹兹堡膝盖规则(高度敏感性和特异性):
• 在跌伤或钝性创伤出现以下情况时,拍膝关节X线片:
  ◦ 年龄<12岁或>55岁。
  ◦ 在急诊室中无法承受4个步骤的全部负重。
  ◦ 跛行是不允许的。
• 匹兹堡膝关节规则应谨慎适用于<18岁的患者。
• 神经血管检查:
- 高能机制带来神经血管损伤和骨筋膜室间隔综合征风险。
- 注意持续的疼痛、肌肉无力、紧张的肌肉肿胀、感觉过度或麻醉、被动伸展肌肉的疼痛。
- 检查腘窝、胫骨后部和足背脉搏。
- 检查腓神经的完整性:
  ◦ 踝和蹈趾背屈。
  ◦ 在蹈趾和第二趾间感觉是否正常。

诊断检查与说明

影像学检查

• 普通X线摄影:
- 胫骨平台视图:
  ◦ 屈曲位置前后(AP)视角在10°~15°以评估胫骨棘,骨折延伸到关节的线和压迫。
- 髌骨的斜上视图:
  ◦ 在识别髌骨骨折时非常有用,而它在AP或侧面视图上不可视。
- 十字桌侧视图:
  ◦ 评估平台中央并显示积脂积液情况(脂肪液面)。
- 斜视图:
  ◦ 识别在其他图像中不明显的裂缝,并提供更多关于骨折的信息。
- 注意韧带附着区域,这是可能发生撕脱骨折的地方:
  ◦ 内侧和外侧股骨髁。
  ◦ 胫骨脊柱(髁间隆起)。
  ◦ 腓骨头。
• CT用于揭示在X线平片上未见的隐匿性骨折并详细显示已知的骨折。
• MRI用于识别软组织损伤(韧带和半月板损伤)。
• 动脉造影有助于对受伤部位进行定位,但不应该延迟血运重建,并在以下情况时进行:
- 高能损伤机制。
- Schatzker 4型、5型或6型骨折。
- 远端脉搏的改变。
- 血肿扩大。
- 异常的声音。
- 损伤解剖相关的神经。

诊断步骤/外科

• 关节穿刺术寻找脂肪球和代表关节内骨折的骨髓质:
- 进行此操作的指征:有液体流出但X线平片上骨折不可见。
• 若出现以下情况,进行室间隔压力测量:
- 疼痛不在骨折部位。
- 被动拉伸疼痛。
- 感觉异常。
- 远端脉搏减少。
- 室内压力>30 mmHg时紧急骨科会诊。

鉴别诊断

• 膝关节脱位。
• 近端腓骨骨折。
• 股骨髁骨折。
• 髌骨骨折。
• 胫骨髁下骨折。
• 胫骨粗隆骨折。
• 胫骨脊柱骨折。
• 十字韧带撕裂。
• 侧副韧带撕裂。
• 半月板的撕裂。

儿科注意事项

包括斜视图作为常规X线摄影的一部分。

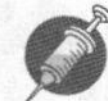

治疗

院前

注意事项:
• 高能损伤机制,相关主要损伤优先考虑。
• 固定以防止进一步的神经或血管损伤。

初步稳定/治疗

• 多重创伤患者的稳定。
• 长腿夹板全长。
• 冰敷。
• 患肢抬高。
• 弗兰克错位伴血管受损,需要立即在急诊室减压。

急诊治疗/程序

• 解除负重状态。
• 疼痛控制。
• 未移位的骨折或最小程度的移位(<8 mm)一侧平台骨折不伴韧带损伤。
- 关节积血吸引和注射局部麻醉剂麻药。
- 检查韧带不稳定性。
- 如果膝关节稳定:
  ◦ 加压包扎。
  ◦ 冰敷和抬高48 h。
  ◦ 避免负重、拐杖辅助。
- 膝关节不稳定,如果骨折导致血管损伤或室间隔综合征。
  ◦ 不稳定的膝盖骨折需要紧急骨科会诊。
• 开放性骨折:
- 去除污染物。
- 使用湿润的无菌敷料。
- 评估破伤风免疫力。
- 抗生素。
- 在2~3 h及早用抗生素。
- 骨科参与早期手术清创。

药物治疗

开放性骨折:氨基糖苷类+头孢菌素。
• 头孢唑林:2 g,静脉注射(儿童:50 mg/kg)。
• 庆大霉素:2~5 mg/kg,静脉注射(儿童:2.5 mg/kg)。
• 若需要,给予破伤风抗毒素。
• 万古霉素:如青霉素过敏,1 g,静脉注射负荷剂量(儿童10 mg/kg)。

J

随访

进一步处理

入院指征

- 开放性骨折，需要清创、冲洗和静脉输液抗生素。
- 粉碎性双髁骨折需要牵引。
- 高能量损伤机制，观察神经血管状态与骨筋膜室综合征的发展；损伤 24 h 后可能发生。
- 疼痛控制。

出院指征

没有移位或移位最小，一侧平台的稳定骨折。

随访建议

整形外科随访：

- 长腿夹板，冰敷，抬高和受影响关节的非负重状态。

要点和误区

- 考虑高能量腘后动脉损伤伤害机制。
- 关节穿刺术可见脂肪性关节积血（血液和脂肪球），特别见于膝关节内骨折。
- 胫骨平台骨折、Segond 骨折和 Salter-Harris 1 型骨折在膝关节 X 线片上很容易漏掉。

静脉功能不全

Bo E. Madsen 周秋香 毛恩强 译

基础知识

描述

- 静脉瓣功能不全导致静脉回流受阻，导致下肢水肿。
- 下肢血管功能不全的慢性病。
- 静脉系统中的正常血流是从浅静脉到深静脉单向运行。
- 腿部肌肉组织收缩和静脉瓣膜功能维持这种单向流动。
- 瓣膜损坏，如 DVT 后，导致瓣膜僵硬，失去适当的逆行血流的能力。
- 从下肢静脉回流减少导致静脉压力增加和扩张，这反过来导致瓣叶分离。
- 下肢静脉瓣膜功能不全导致慢性静脉功能不全和静脉曲张。
- 静脉瓣膜功能不全导致静脉引流受损，导致轻度水肿。
- 慢性静脉功能不全和由此导致的增加的静脉压传入皮肤微循环，导致大分子和红细胞外渗，造成损伤，导致皮肤完整性改变、溃疡形成和愈合不良。

病因

- 主要的瓣膜功能不全（最常见）。
- 深静脉血栓形成（DVT）。
- 风险因素：
  - 高龄（估计患病率为 5%～30%的成人）。
  - 性别（女：男为 3：1）。
  - 静脉曲张家族史。
  - 深静脉血栓形成或者静脉炎。
  - 腿部水肿。
  - 肥胖。
  - 妊娠。
  - 下肢创伤。

诊断

症状和体征

病史

- 无症状阶段：
  - 静脉扩张从静脉扩张发展到小静脉曲张。
- 症状阶段：
  - 踝关节和小腿肿胀。
  - 平静的疼痛、腿部疼痛：
    - 由于长期站立而变得更严重。
    - 腿抬高后缓解。
  - 烧灼感。
  - 瘙痒症。
  - 夜间抽筋。
  - 静脉曲张。
  - 皮肤变色、色素沉着。
  - 溃疡形成。
  - 脂性硬皮病。

体格检查

- 静脉曲张。
- 踝和小腿水肿。
- 小腿和踝的依赖性水肿。
- 毛细血管扩张。
- 网状静脉。
- 褐色至红紫色色素沉着。
- 瘀血性皮炎。
- 硬化、固结和皮肤萎缩。
- 脂肪性皮肤硬化。
- 静脉曲张出血。
- 静脉性溃疡：
  - 通常位于踝关节或小腿内侧。
  - 远端脉搏微弱或缺失时需考虑动脉功能不全。
- 细菌感染。
  - 溃疡迅速增长。
  - 四肢溃疡伴周围蜂窝织炎或化脓性引流。
  - 发热。
  - 淋巴管炎。
- 下列情况应怀疑除下肢近端静脉功能不全外的其他病因：
  - 心力衰竭或缺血性心脏病。
  - 肝病史。
  - 伴有腹水的周围水肿和溃疡。
  - 眶周水肿。
  - 端坐呼吸。
  - 肝颈静脉回流症。
  - 颈静脉扩张。

基本检查

体格检查对诊断至关重要。

诊断检查与说明

实验室检查

- 实验室检查对体检诊断没有帮助，除非是排除一些其他疾病。
- 如果考虑到其他引起腿部水肿的原因，可以行心脏标志物、脑钠肽、白蛋白和肾功能检查。

影像学检查

- 多普勒听诊（DopA）：
  - 可评估下肢动脉多普勒信号，以便在存在问题时(脉搏微弱或无法触及、外周动脉疾病病史、踝臂指数降低、四肢溃疡)区分静脉功能不全和动脉功能不全。

• 多普勒超声(DUS):
- 诊断慢性静脉功能不全的最常见的方法。
- 可使用B型灰度和脉冲多普勒评估来确定超深静脉分布中静脉血流的存在、通畅性和流向。
- 可以评估深静脉血栓形成(DVT)、瓣膜功能不全、功能不全和逆行性血流。

• 侵入性检查:
- 静脉造影检查。
- 血管内超声造影。
- CT/MR静脉造影。
- 动态静脉压监测。

诊断步骤/外科

臂-踝指数:

• 如果怀疑动脉供血不足,应该测量。

鉴别诊断

• 静脉瓣膜功能。
• 深静脉血栓形成(DVT)。
• 动脉功能不全。
• 淋巴障碍或阻塞。
• 软组织感染(糖尿病足溃疡)。
• 创伤:
- 室间综合征。
- 血管或淋巴管破坏。
- 炎症反应。
• 破裂的贝克囊肿。
• 坏疽性脓皮病。
• 充血性心力衰竭。
• 肺动脉高压。
• 肾病:
- 肾病综合征。
- 肾衰竭。
• 肝病伴腹水。
• 血管炎或自身免疫性疾病:
- 多动脉炎。
- 甲状腺功能减退伴黏液水肿。
- 系统性红斑狼疮。
• 妊娠合并或不伴子痫前期。
• 药物(非甾体抗炎药、钙通道阻滞剂)。

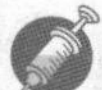

治疗

初步稳定/治疗

• 腿部抬高到心脏水平之上。
• 用直接加压控制肿胀。
• 可能需要应用有限的硝酸银或缝线放置,以有效控制持续肿胀。

急诊治疗/程序

• 腿部抬高,高于心脏的水平。
• 弹力袜或者针对ABI>0.8的患者进行辅料加压。
• 用于溃疡的保湿伤口敷料。
• 如果确诊DVT,使用抗凝剂。
• 如果有感染迹象,特别是蜂窝织炎或感染的溃疡,需使用抗生素。
• 阿司匹林(改善溃疡愈合率)。
• 表面活性物质用于瘀血性皮炎、瘙痒症、皮肤干燥。
• 抗组胺药治疗瘙痒症。

药物治疗

• 阿司匹林:325 mg,每日1次,口服。
• 力百汀:875 mg,每日2次,口服。
• 头孢氨苄:500 mg,每日4次,口服。
• 双氯青霉素:500 mg,每日4次,口服。
• 苯海拉明:12.5~25 mg,每日4次,口服。
• 依诺肝素:1 mg/kg,每日2次,皮下注射。

随访

进一步处理

入院指征

• 急性或严重慢性动脉功能不全。
• 蜂窝织炎、淋巴管炎或骨髓炎的证据可能需要入院,特别是门诊治疗失败或免疫功能低下的病例。
• DVT且存在以下情况:
- 广泛血栓形成或怀疑盆腔血栓形成。
- 并发肺栓塞需要住院治疗。
- 患者因抗凝而出血的风险很高。
- 使用低分子量肝素(伊诺肝素)的门诊患者需密切随访。
• 除主要静脉功能不全外,下肢病变的治疗与患者的其他合并症状。

出院指征

• 下肢脉搏存在。
• 没有出血或室间隔综合征的证据。
• DUS检查已排除DVT或患者风险低。
• 没有细菌感染。
• 适当的随访。
• 已经给患者提供了伤口护理、换药和弹力袜的使用说明。

转诊问题

应该将患者转诊给他们的初级保健医师。如果患有外周血管疾病,应将其转诊给血管外科医师。

随访建议

• 家庭医疗保健或密切跟踪,门诊提供患者的溃疡护理。
• 运用弹力袜。
• 静脉曲张不需要立即手术。
• 静脉剥离,静脉结扎,硬化疗法和静脉热消融治疗难治性病例的选择:
- 这些不会改善溃疡的严重程度,但可减少溃疡复发。
- 所有这些方法都会引起不可逆的静脉血管改变,从而导致水肿复发,并增加未来DVT的风险。

要点和误区

• 在确定静脉功能不全的病因之前,要确保动脉功能不全不是根本原因:
- ABI<0.9(在ABI>0.8的情况下,可以使用未经修改的压力治疗)。
- 无可触及的脉搏。
- 四肢剧痛。
- 四肢溃疡。
- 外周动脉疾病的危险因素。
• 对于患有周围血管疾病且ABI<0.8的患者,禁止使用非改良压迫疗法。
• 蜂窝织炎的患者应禁用压力治疗。
• 对孤立性慢性静脉功能不全的初步建议应包括压缩袜试验、运动和减肥(如适用)。
• 注意CVI并发蜂窝织炎和慢性皮肤变化。

静脉曲张 Varices

GaLeta C. Clayton 周秋香 毛恩强 译

基础知识

描述

- 门静脉压力增加导致门静脉系统分流。
- 胃食管结扎分流导致黏膜下食管静脉曲张。

病因

- 占所有出血性胃肠道病例的 10%～30%。
- 占肝硬化合并上消化道出血病例的 90%。
- 30%的肝硬化患者出现静脉曲张出血：
  - 50%会自发止血。
  - 30%的死亡率。
  - 70%患者会再次出血。
- 在成人中：
  - 肝硬化的原因是酗酒或慢性肝炎。
  - 胆汁淤积：Wilson 或血色素沉着症。
  - 中东部地区：血吸虫病。
  - 门静脉高压。
- 在儿童中：
  - 肝内胆管硬化阻塞。
  - 胆道闭锁。
  - 囊性纤维化。
  - β抗胰蛋白酶缺乏。
  - 肝炎。

诊断

症状和体征

- 一般情况：
  - 虚弱和疲劳。
  - 心动过速。
  - 呼吸急促。
  - 低血压。
  - 湿凉的皮肤，毛细管再填充延迟。
- 腹部：
  - 急性的上消化道出血：
    - 呕血。
    - 便血。
    - 黑便。
    - 可能的总血量损失的 20%～40%。
  - 腹痛。
- 严重肝功能不全致皮肤红斑：
  - 黄疸。
  - 蜘蛛痣。
  - 手掌红斑。
  - 足踝水肿。
  - 肝脾大。
  - 腹水。
- 门静脉高压病史：
  - 最常见的是酒精性肝硬化。
  - 其他，包括：
    - 原发性胆汁性肝硬化。
    - 血吸虫病。
    - Budd-Chiair 综合征。
    - 严重慢性心功能不全。
    - 结节病。
- 心血管系统：
  - 胸部疼痛、呼吸短促。
- 中枢神经系统。
  - 昏厥。
  - 起初为躁动。
  - 后为嗜睡和倦怠。

儿科注意事项

- 大量的呕血：典型的初始表现。
  - 低血压可能是一个后期的表现。

病史

- 50%的肝硬化患者存在胃底及食管静脉曲张，并与疾病密切相关。
- 最重要的出血预测指标是静脉曲张的大小。其他因素包括静脉曲张的数量、肝脏疾病的严重程度和内镜检查结果。
- PBC 患者在疾病早期即出现静脉曲张和静脉曲张出血，甚至是肝硬化的主要发展。

体格检查

- 生命体征可能是正常的，也可能表现为心动过速(早期)和低血压(晚期)。
- 神志意识状态改变或脑灌注不良。
- 活动性出血。
- 酒精性肝病的特点：
  - 腹水。
  - 一般水肿。
  - 黄疸。

基本检查

- 胃管放置：
  - 确定该患者是否正在积极出血。
  - 减压可能有助于减少胃出血。可能会降低误吸风险。
  - 便于内镜检查。
  - 不会增加或引起食管静脉曲张出血。
- 紧急内镜检查。

诊断检查与说明

实验室检查

- 血型和交叉配血 6～8 U：
  - 输血需要。
- 动脉血气分析：
  - 酸中毒。
  - 低氧血症。
- 血细胞计数：
  - 快速失血早期血细胞比容是不可靠指标。
  - 进行连续 CBC 以跟踪血液丢失。
- 电解质、BUN、肌酐、葡萄糖：
  - 评估肾功能。
  - BUN/肌酐＞30 表明胃肠道以及上消化道来源有明显的积血。
- PT、APTT、INR 和血小板：
  - 凝血功能障碍。
  - 延长出血时间。
  - 血小板减少。

影像学检查

- 胸部 X 线片排除穿孔。
- 心电图排除心肌缺血。

鉴别诊断

- 出血、消化道溃疡穿孔。
- 糜烂性胃炎。
- 马洛里-韦斯综合征。
- Boerhaave 综合征。
- 主动脉瘘。
- 胃静脉曲张。
- 胃血管扩张症。

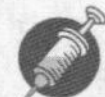

治疗

院前

- 气道稳定。
- 低血压，生理盐水通过 2 个 16G 大口径针头或深静脉输注。
- 心脏和脉搏血氧监测。

初步稳定/治疗

- 早期气管插管生命支持：
  - 容易插管就早期插管。
  - 对于 AMS 或大量咯血。
  - 紧急内镜检查。
- 对初始液体推注血压无反应的需建立中

心静脉通路行血管内监测。
• 尽快补充失血：
- 开始可用 O 型血直到有合适的血液可用。
- 对于儿童按照 10 ml/kg 输注。
- 可能需要输注新鲜冰冻血浆和血小板。
- 根据需要纠正凝血功能障碍。
• 经鼻胃管(清醒)或口服(插管)。
• 争议：
- 过度积极的补液增可能导致门静脉高压反弹、再出血和肺水肿。
- 绝大多数患者输血目标是血红蛋白 70 g/L。
- 老年患者或严重合并症患者的输血目标是血红蛋白 80 g/L。

儿科注意事项

• 如果外周血管通路不易建立的患者，可考虑骨内通路。
• 在儿童，大多数出血会自发停止。
• 在儿童生命体征改变出现的可能比较晚：
- 精神状态、毛细血管再充盈、轻微的心动过速或立位变化的细微变化可能意味着显著的失血。
- 婴儿的过度输液可以很快导致显著的电解质异常。

急诊治疗/程序

• 急性出血需急诊胃镜：
- 使用药物和压塞装置作为暂时性止血措施。
• 内镜：
- 鼻胃管处置急性活动性出血，12 h 内进行。
- 急性食管出血。
- 食管结扎相当于硬化疗法，并发症少：
◦ 在大量出血的情况下可能难视野不佳。
- 大量出血的硬化疗法。
- 由于再出血率高，胃静脉曲张不适于内镜修复：
- 在手术时间使用抗生素以降低自发性细菌性腹膜炎的风险：
◦ 氟喹诺酮或头孢曲松。
• 药物疗法：
- 特利加压素是一线治疗(在美国没有广泛应用)，因为它具有更高的疗效和更少的副作用。
- 当生长抑素无法使用时，奥曲肽是治疗的一线药物：并发症包括高血糖症和腹部痉挛。
- 血管加压素由于容易继发血管缺血，被奥曲肽、生长抑素所替代。
- PPIs 不适用于静脉曲张出血的治疗。
• 气囊填塞。
- 应用于大规模无法控制的流血。
- 三腔二囊管。
- 接加压，但存在食管穿孔和溃疡、气管压迫窒息和误吸的风险。
- 只有有经验的临床医师在遇到大量无法止住出血时才使用。
- 只有暂时的好处，在内镜检查之前用作稳定的手段。
• 外科疗法
- 门腔静脉分流术。
- 食管横断。
- 胃食管交界处断流术。

药物治疗

• 头孢曲松：2 g(儿童：50～75 mg/kg)，静脉滴注，q24 h。在 Child 评级 B/C 或喹诺酮耐药区。
• 头孢噻肟：2 g[儿童：50～180 mg/(kg · 24 h)]，静脉滴注，q8 h。
• 红霉素：250 mg，静脉注射。
- 有助于胃部清洁，以便在内镜检查时更好地显示。
• 诺氟沙星 400 mg，口服或环丙沙星 400 mg，静脉滴注；如果不能耐受口服(儿童禁用)。
• 奥曲肽：50 μg/kg 初始剂量，然后 50 μg/h 输注 5 日。儿童剂量：1～2 μg/kg 推注(最多 50 μg)，然后 1～2 μg/(kg · h)输注。老年人：25 μg 剂量，然后 25 μg/h 输注 5 日。
• 特利加压素：2 mg，静脉注射，q4 h。
• 生长抑素(如果奥曲肽不可用)：250 μg，静脉推注，然后静脉滴注 250 μg/h，持续 5 日。
• 血管加压素(如果奥曲肽不可用)：儿童剂量：0.002～0.005 U/(kg · min)[滴定至最大值 0.01 U/(kg · min)]。

一线用药

• 生长抑素(当生长抑素不可用时使用奥曲肽)。
• 诺氟沙星口服或环丙沙星静滴。

二线用药

• 依托红霉素。
• 头孢曲松钠。

随访

进一步处理

入院指征

• 严重静脉曲张出血，血流动力学不稳定，需要气道管理。
• 近期静脉曲张出血史。
• 早期再出血高风险：
- 年龄＞60 岁、肾衰竭、初始血红蛋白计数＜80 g/L。

出院指征

无静脉曲张出血。

转诊问题

• 持续出血需要手术或更高级别的护理。
• 肝移植。

随访建议

• 及时胃肠道门诊随访：
- 需要每年进行一次内镜检查。
• 药物和生活方式改变。

要点和误区

• 早期气管插管，尤其对于肝性脑病或血流动力学不稳定的患者。
• 在胃镜检查前开始预防性使用抗生素。
• 在美国，由于副作用，奥曲肽已经取代了加压素。如果需要加压素，可以使用静脉注射硝酸甘油来缓解末端器官局部缺血。
• 在放置球囊止血装置之前处理好气道，此方法优先于手术和 TIPS。
• 便血是血流动力学不稳定的患者的证明。
• 尽早咨询您的胃肠专家，因为内镜检查是第一道诊断和治疗程序，目标是出血后 12 h 内进行内镜检查。

酒精戒断 Withdrawal, Alcohol

Trevonne M. Thompson 吴昊 李文放 译

基础知识

描述

• 酒精戒断是急诊最常见的戒断症状。
• 神经兴奋是酒精戒断的标志。
• 酒精戒断症状可能危及生命。
• 更严重的症状和体征出现在之前的戒断症状中，这一过程被称为"点燃"。
• 酗酒在老年人中并不少见。
• 与年龄相关的酒精敏感性增加。
• 与酒精相关的问题可能被误诊为衰老的正常结果。

病因

• 慢性酒精的使用降低了 GABA（抑制）受体兴奋性，上调了 NMDA（兴奋）受体兴奋性。
• 由于这些受体的适应性，戒断或者减少酒精的使用会增加肾上腺素能活性。
• 酒精戒断的 4 个组成部分：
– 早期戒断症状。
– 戒断癫痫。
– 酒精幻觉症。
– 震颤性谵妄（DTs）。
• 有 5%的患者出现酒精戒断症状。
• DTs 有 5%～15%的死亡率。

诊断

症状和体征

• 早期戒断反应：
– 发生：最后一次饮酒后 6～8 h。
– 持续时间：1～2 日。
◦ 抖动。
◦ 焦虑。
◦ 心悸。
◦ 恶心。
◦ 厌食症。
• 戒断性癫痫发作。
– 发生：在最后一次饮酒之后 6～48 h。
– 持续时间：2～3 日。
• 全身性癫痫，一般短暂。
• 酒精性幻觉症：
– 发生：在最后一次饮酒之后 12～48 h。
– 持续时间：1～2 日。
◦ 视觉幻觉（最常见）。
◦ 触觉幻觉。
◦ 听觉幻觉。
◦ 通常其他感官是清楚的。
• 震颤性谵妄：
– 发生在最后一次饮酒后 48～96 h。
– 最多可以持续 5 日。
– 不一定是在出现幻觉或癫痫之前。
◦ 心动过速。
◦ 高血压。
◦ 发汗。
◦ 精神错乱。
◦ 焦虑。
◦ 感觉器官通常不清楚。

病史

• 酒精滥用历史：
– 最后使用物质的时间。
– 以前的戒酒史和严重程度。

体格检查

彻底的身体检查是必要的。

基本检查

通过彻底的病史和身体检查评估生命体征。

诊断检查与说明

实验室检查

• 电解质、BUN、肌酐、葡萄糖、镁。
• 血常规。
• 酒精含量。
• 尿液药物筛选很少改变管理。
• 尿液检查。
• 血/尿培养：
– 疑似感染。

影像学检查

• 如果早期戒断反应是明确的，那就没有必要了。
• 头部 CT：
– 精神状态改变或者与临床情况不对等的情况。
• 胸片。
– 如果怀疑是继发性感染（如吸入性肺炎）。

诊断步骤/外科

必要时做临床心电图。

鉴别诊断

• 苯二氮䓬类戒断。
• 巴比妥酸盐戒断。
• 脑内出血。
• 中枢神经系统感染。
• 癫痫。
• 低血糖症。
• 甲状腺功能亢进。
• 脓毒症。
• 药物中毒。
• 精神病。
• 电解质紊乱。

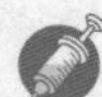

治疗

院前

• 评估生命体征。
• 评估末梢血糖。

初步稳定/治疗

• 气道/呼吸/循环管理。
• 建立静脉通路。
• 静脉液体管理。
• 心肺监测。

急诊治疗/程序

• 积极的支持性护理。
• 苯二氮䓬类。
– 苯二氮䓬类药物药效基本一致。
– 通常需要高剂量来控制症状和体征。
• 巴比妥酸盐。
– 可代替苯二氮䓬类药物使用或作为苯二氮䓬类药物的辅料。
• 在严重的情况下也可以使用丙泊酚，作为苯二氮䓬类或巴比妥类药物的辅助用药。

药物治疗

• 对于轻度症状和体征：地西泮：5～20 mg 口服。对于严重症状和体征：5～10 mg 静脉推注，可重复。
• 劳拉西泮：2 mg 口服，q2～4 h 重复，用于轻度症状和体征。在必要时重复服用 2 mg 静脉推注，以应对严重的症状和体征。
• 苯巴比妥：30～60 mg 的轻度症状和体征；15～20 mg/kg 缓慢静脉注射治疗严重症状或癫痫状态。
• 丙泊酚：以 25～75 g/(kg/min)开始，然后在必要时滴定。

随访

进一步处理

入院指征

- 中-重度的症状。
- 尽管治疗但症状持续存在。
- 震颤性谵妄或即将震颤性谵妄。
- 具有其他伴随疾病。

出院指征

轻度症状和治疗有效。

随访建议

转诊至戒毒项目或中心。

要点和误区

- 误诊为戒断综合征的医学疾病。
- 误解戒断综合征与共患病之间的关系。
- 给予足够数量的苯二氮䓬类药物来控制症状。

酒精性酮症酸中毒 Alcoholic Ketoacidosis

Nicholas M. V. Schulack · Ketan Patel · Ross P. Berkeley　马林浩　林兆奋 译

基础知识

描述

- 由于以下原因导致酮体产量增加：
  - 脱水(恶心、呕吐、ADH 抑制)导致压力荷尔蒙产生增加进一步增加酮形成。
  - 肝脏中的糖原储备消耗殆尽(营养不良、减少碳水化合物摄入量)。
  - 由乙醇代谢引起的 NADH/NAD 增加。
  - 增加游离脂肪酸的产生。
- NADH/NAD 升高导致 β-羟基丁酸酯(BHB)产生占主导地位并超过乙酰乙酸(AcAc)的生成量。

病因

- 营养不良、慢性酒精滥用者近期的重度酒精消费：
  - 产生恶心、呕吐或腹痛。
  - 导致酒精摄入停止。
  - 症状通常在 12～72 h 出现。

诊断

症状和体征

- 恶心、呕吐和腹痛：最常见的症状。
  - 通常以非特异性压痛扩散。
  - 上腹痛很常见。
  - 罕见：反弹压痛、腹胀、肠鸣音弱。
    - 这些发现要求寻找另一种并存的疾病。
- 心动过速(常见)归因于：
  - 脱水及相关体位变化。
  - 同时戒酒。
- 呼吸急促：
  - 常见。
  - 深快 Kussmaul 呼吸，并伴有严重酸中毒。
- 血容量不足导致尿量减少。
- 除非有潜在的感染，否则不会发热。
- 精神状态：
  - 由于血容量不足和可能酒精中毒导致的轻微改变。
  - 精神状态改变要求考虑其他联合存在的情况：
    - 头部受伤、脑血管意外(CVA)或颅内出血。
    - 低血糖。
    - 酒精戒断。
    - 脑病。
    - 毒素。
- 视觉障碍：
  - 用通用 AKA 评估孤立的视觉障碍。

病史

慢性酒精使用：
- 最近滥用。
- 突然停止。

体格检查

- 脱水最常见。
- 可能有酮症气味。
- Kussmaul 呼吸。
- 手掌红斑(肝硬化)。
- 腹部压痛，无反跳痛和肌紧张。

基本检查

- 存在继发于酮的阴离子间隙增加的代谢性酸中毒。
- 区别于酒精摄入性中毒和其他导致阴离子间隙代谢性酸中毒的原因。

诊断检查与说明

实验室检查

- 酸碱失调：
  - 阴离子间隙增宽型代谢性酸中毒的标志。
  - 混合酸碱干扰常见：
    - 呼吸性碱中毒。
    - 继发于呕吐和脱水的代谢性碱中毒。
    - 高氯性酸中毒。
  - 轻度乳酸性酸中毒常见。
    - 由于脱水和直接乙醇代谢的影响。
    - 严重的乳酸性酸中毒应该考虑其他疾病，如癫痫发作、缺氧和休克。
  - 尿液酮酸测试和血清硝普钠反应阳性。
    - 可能无法反映潜在酮症酸中毒的严重程度，因为 BHB 占主导地位，且不能通过该测试测量。
    - 因为更多的 AcAc 产生，可能产生假阳性结果。
  - β-羟基丁酸酯测定法(如果可用)在检测酮酸中更准确：
    - 在 AKA 中，BHB↑↑↑，在 DKA 电解质中，只有↑。
- 电解质：
  - 降低血清碳酸氢盐。
  - 由于呕吐引起的低钾血症。
  - 低钙血症。
  - 低磷酸盐血症可能会加剧中毒。
  - 低镁血症：
    - 血清镁水平可能无法准确反映出全身镁消耗情况。
  - 最初可能会出现高钾血症和/或高磷血症(尽管整体缺钾)：
    - 将纠正酸中毒的治疗。
- 葡萄糖：
  - 可能减少、正常或轻度升高。
  - 应经常监测，如 DKA。
- 酒精度可能为负。
- BUN 和肌酐因脱水而轻度升高，除非潜在的肾脏疾病。
- 尿液分析：
  - 无糖尿症的酮尿症。

J

• 脂肪酶(更特异性)/淀粉酶:
- 可能伴有急性胰腺炎。
• 渗透压间隙:
- 可能会升高。
- 升高>20 mOsm/kg 时应迅速评估其他摄入(甲醇和乙二醇)。
- 通过将乙醇含量除以 4.6 来校正渗透压间隙中的乙醇含量。
• LFT:
- 可能轻度升高了 LFT。
• 血红蛋白 A1C:可能有助于区分 AKA 与 DKA:
- 高血糖>250 mg/dl 在 AKA 中较少见:
◦ 正常 A1C 使 AKA 发生的可能性更高。
- A1C 升高的正常血糖增加了正常血糖 DKA 的可能性[例如,由于使用了 SGLT2(钠-葡萄糖共转运蛋白 2)抑制剂]。
• CBC:
- 轻度白细胞增多:既不敏感也不特异性。
- 慢性酒精中毒引起的血小板减少症和贫血。

心电图

• 可能表明继电解质异常和酸碱紊乱之后 QT 间隔和/或 QRS 持续时间的变化。
• 根据电解质和潜在的心脏状况,可能会出现心律不齐,包括心房颤动和可能的室性心动过速。

影像学检查

• 如果怀疑合并肺炎,行 CXR 检查。
• 出现急性腹痛,拍腹部 X 线平片查看腹腔游离气体。
• 如果合并头部创伤或无法解释的精神状态改变进行头部 CT 扫描。

鉴别诊断

• 阴离子间隙升高的代谢性酸中毒(ACCA MUDPILES):
- 酒精酮症酸中毒。
- 氰化物、CO、H_2S 等。
- 对乙酰氨基酚:
◦ 急性摄入罕见。
◦ 慢性摄入很少见。
◦ 暴发性肝功能衰竭。
- 抗反转录病毒药物(NRTI)。
- 甲苯。
- 甲醇、二甲双胍。
- 尿毒症。
- 糖尿病酮症酸中毒。
◦ 考虑使用 SGLT2 抑制剂进行正常血糖 DKA。
- 三聚乙醛、苯乙双胍、丙二醇。
- 铁、INH。
- 酸中毒。
- 乙二醇。
- 水杨酸盐、乙酰水杨酸(ASA,阿司匹林)、饥饿酮症。
• 低血容量:
- 胃肠道出血。
- 脓毒症。
• 腹痛,恶心,呕吐:
- 胰腺炎。
- 胃肠道出血。
- 胃炎、食管炎。
- 肝炎。
- 穿孔性溃疡。
- 酒精戒断。
- DKA。
- 梗阻/肠梗阻。
- 自发性细菌性腹膜炎。
- 病毒性疾病。

治疗

院前

• 支持性措施,包括静脉补充生理盐水,吸氧气和心电监护。
• 询问可能的其他病因的病史,如摄入毒性物质或糖尿病史,考虑可能的情况。
• 考虑其他可能的共存疾病,如消化道出血。

初步稳定/治疗

• 心脏监护和供应氧气。
• 如果神志状态改变,给纳洛酮、硫胺素和葡萄糖。
• 启动生理盐水静脉滴注。
- 500 ml~1 L 推注。
- 必要时进行液体复苏。
- 促进酮体经肾排泄。

急诊治疗/方法

• 止吐剂:昂丹司琼、异丙嗪或丙氯拉嗪。
• 苯二氮䓬类药物用于酒精戒断反应。
• 使用含右旋糖的溶液(D5NS):
- 比单独使用生理盐水更快速地解决代谢异常问题。
- 速率比维持耐受高,直到酸中毒解除。
- 避免出现明显的高血糖。
- 帮助充满糖原储备。
- 通过刺激内源性胰岛素的产生,减少酮体的产生。
• 葡萄糖给药前的硫胺素补充(IV),以避免沉淀 Wernicke 脑病。
• 碳酸氢钠很少使用:
- 没有经过同行评审的证据支持使用。
- 考虑严重的酸血症(pH<7.0)并伴有心血管功能障碍或激动的情况。
- 必须考虑严重酸血症的替代/伴随病因。
• 电解质替换:
- 低钾血症随治疗而发生,应该预判。
- 治疗可能发生低磷血症。
- 低镁血症和低钾血症都要补充钾。
• 胰岛素使用与否不确定,可能会导致低血糖。

治疗药物

• $D_{50}W$:1 安瓿 50% 右旋糖(25 g),静脉推注。
• 劳拉西泮(苯二氮䓬类):静脉注射 2 mg,滴定至起效。
• 纳洛酮:2 mg,静脉推注。
• 昂丹司琼:4~8 mg,静脉推注。
• 丙氯拉嗪:缓慢加入 5~10 mg,静脉推注(不是>5 mg/min)。
• 异丙嗪:12.5~25 mg,静脉推注。
• 硫胺素:100 mg,静脉推注。

随访

进一步处理

入院指征

• 持续代谢性酸中毒。
• 持续出现血容量不足的迹象。
• 持续恶心和呕吐。
• 病因不明的腹痛。
• 合并症需要入院治疗。
• 由于电解质异常需要继续治疗,需要床旁监测。

出院指征

• 许多患者可以在观察单位进行管理超过 12~24 h。
• 口服液体耐受良好。
• 解决代谢异常问题。
• 没有其他相关疾病需要额外的治疗。
• 大多数人观察后可出院。

随访建议

酒精戒断咨询。

要点和误区

• 含有葡萄糖液体的积极补液是关键。

• 容易漏诊,可与 DKA(血糖正常的 DKA/血糖正常的 AKA)混淆。
• 必要时补充生理盐水,补充硫胺素。
• 监测治疗前后的电解质无法识别的渗透压间隙增加。
• 避免胰岛素。
• 葡萄糖水平监测不足。
• 无法识别由治疗引起的初始电解质异常和电解质移位。
• 必须放在心脏监护仪上:
- AKA 突然死亡的案例:
◦ 可能的酒精性心肌病。
◦ 心律失常。
◦ 电解质紊乱。

酒精中毒 Alcohol Poisoning

Timothy J. Meehan 马林浩 林兆奋 译

基础知识

描述

• 酒精是急诊科患者中最常见的被滥用的娱乐性饮料。
• 经常与创伤有关。

病因

• 酒精中毒:
- 直接抑制中枢神经系统功能。
- 血液酒精水平下降 15～40 mg/(dl·h)取决于个体变量和长期性酒精饮用情况。
• 酒精戒断反应:
- 在慢性酒精滥用者身上部分或完全戒酒出现。
- 血清酒精水平＞100 mg/dl(如"中毒")时也可能出现。
- 主要是由于慢性中枢神经系统抑制的丧失:
◦ 中枢神经系统极度兴奋。
◦ 增加儿茶酚胺释放和肾上腺素能紧张性。

诊断

症状和体征

急性酒精中毒

• 中枢神经系统效应范围:
- 松弛。
- 欣快。
- 镇静。
- 记忆丧失。
- 定向障碍。
- 共济失调。
- 言语不清。
- 缓和或昏迷。
• 也可能导致胃肠道功能障碍。

酒精戒断综合征

• 早期或轻微戒断:
- 最后一次饮酒后＜8 h:
◦ 宿醉的症状。
◦ 头痛。
◦ 恶心或呕吐。
- 最后一次饮用后 12 h:
◦ 轻度震颤、焦虑。
◦ 厌食、恶心、呕吐。
◦ 虚弱。
◦ 肌痛。
◦ 多梦、噩梦。
- 最后一次饮用后 12～36 h:
◦ 烦躁、激动。
◦ 心动过速、高血压。
◦ 手和舌的震颤。
- 最后一次饮酒后 24～48 h:酒精性幻觉症:
◦ 视觉幻觉最常见(小虫爬行)。
◦ 幻听(嗡嗡声、咔哒声)。
◦ 存在于小规模和高强度戒断。
- 酒精戒断性癫痫发作:
◦ 末次饮后 8～12 h。
◦ 简短,自发地减轻强直-阵挛性活动。
◦ 前驱震颤性谵妄(DT)。
• 延迟戒酒或重大戒断:
- 最后一次饮用后 48 h。
- DTs:
◦ 意识模糊和谵妄。
◦ 困惑、定向障碍。
◦ 激动、好斗。
◦ 心动过速、高血压。
◦ 高热。
◦ 发汗。

病史

• 通常由 EMS 提供(家人或朋友)。
• 注意急诊室中的"常客":
- 有时还有其他原因导致 AMS:
◦ 肝病、脑病。
◦ 癫痫发作(发作后)。
◦ 低血糖。
◦ 头部受伤或颅内出血。

体格检查

• 生命体征:
- 急性中毒:正常或受抑制。
- 戒断:通常是升高的。
• 精神状态:
- 急性中毒:嗜睡、迟钝或昏睡的。
- 戒断:敏感性高,易激动。
• 肝损伤的迹象:
- 黄疸。
- 蜘蛛样血管。
- 扑翼样震颤。
- 肝大。
• 营养不良的迹象:
- 秃头征。
- 牙齿松动。
- 肌肉质量差。
- 腹部消瘦。
- 暂时的消瘦。

基本检查

• 获得准确的酒精摄入和戒酒史。
• 调查危及生命的癫痫发作原因:
- 低血糖(获得快速床边葡萄糖)。
- 颅内出血。
- 中枢神经系统感染。
- 电解质异常。
• 评估隐匿性创伤。
• 经常监测所有生命体征:
- 超高热代表预后不良。

诊断检查与说明

实验室检查

• 精神状态异常时的酒精含量。
• 尿液毒理学检查。
• 电解质、BUN、肌酐和葡萄糖。
• CBC。
• 镁、钙和磷酸盐。
• 如果怀疑患有凝血病,查 APTT、PT、INR。

- 疑似肝脏疾病查 LFT。
- 怀疑肝性脑病要测氨水平。
- 如果是怀疑酒精酮症酸中毒，查尿酮或血清丙酮。

影像学检查

- 以下情况可行头部 CT：
  - 精神状态的改变超过预期基于血清酒精浓度的 AMS 程度。
  - 预计头部创伤。
  - 颅内压升高或神经检查的局灶性发现。
  - 新发作的癫痫发作。
  - 未改善或恶化的意识。
- EEG 区分酒精戒断癫痫发作和特发性癫痫。
- 疑似误吸或肺炎行胸部 X 线检查。

鉴别诊断

- 急性酒精中毒：
  - 低血糖。
  - 二氧化碳麻醉。
  - 混合药物过量。
  - 乙烯、乙二醇、甲醇或异丙醇中毒。
  - 肝性脑病。
  - 精神病。
  - 严重的眩晕。
  - 精神运动性癫痫发作。
- 酒精戒断和癫痫发作：
  - 催眠-镇静药戒断。
  - 急性中毒：
    - 一氧化碳。
    - 异烟肼(特别是如果长时间癫痫发作没有进行标准治疗)。
    - 苯丙胺。
    - 抗胆碱能药。
    - 可卡因。
  - 继发癫痫发作：
    - 感染。
    - 脑膜炎。
    - 脑炎。
    - 脑脓肿。
  - 外伤。
  - 颅内出血。
  - CVA。
  - 肿瘤。
  - 抗惊厥药物抵抗。
  - 甲状腺疾病。

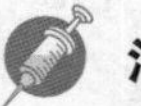

治疗

院前

- 给苯二氮䓬类药物用于治疗癫痫发作。
- 给予纳洛酮、氧气和右旋糖治疗昏迷患者。
- 根据气道保护需要进行气管插管防止误吸。
- 如果怀疑是创伤，可以进行 C 形脊柱固定。

初步稳定/治疗

- ABC 管理。
- 如果怀疑创伤，评估 C 形脊柱固定。
- 初始静脉补液，生理盐水，然后 D_5 0.45% 盐水。
- 若意识状态改变给纳洛酮、硫胺素和葡萄糖(或 Accu-Chek)。
- 癫痫者给苯二氮䓬类药物(可能需要大剂量)。

儿科注意事项

- 幼儿肝糖原储量减少。
- 无法对增加的葡萄糖需求进行适当的反应。
- 快速床边葡萄糖(Accu-Chek)是必需的：
  - 如果病情需要，则给予葡萄糖 D_5 (10 ml/kg)、D_{10} (5 ml/kg)或 D_{25} (2 ml/kg)，取决于年龄和大小。

急诊治疗/程序

- 酒精中毒：
  - 静脉输液体补充水分。
  - 纠正电解质异常：
    - 镁。
    - 钾。
    - 叶酸。
    - 硫胺素。
    - 多种维生素。
- 酒精酮症酸中毒：
  - 使用 D_5 生理盐水进行充分补液。
  - 排除阴离子间隙增宽的其他原因酸中毒。
- 酒精戒断综合征：
  - 酒精戒断临床评估量表更新。
    - 评估戒断严重程度的经验证的量表。
    - 指导初始药物治疗。
    - 测量对治疗的反应和需要重复给药("症状触发"治疗)。
  - 苯二氮䓬类是首选药物：
    - 酒精交叉耐受。
    - 增加 GABAA 介导的传播。
    - 抗惊厥作用。
    - 明显的戒断需要大剂量频繁给药。
    - 可以停止进入 DT。
  - 巴比妥类药物(苯巴比妥)：
    - 严重戒断或用大剂量的苯二氮䓬类药物效果不佳的 DT 有用。
  - 丙泊酚：
    - 插管患者的首选药剂。
    - 完全抑制癫痫发作。
    - 需要插管或通气。
    - 如果低血压，小心使用。
  - β 受体阻滞剂(拉贝洛尔、艾司洛尔或美托洛尔)：
    - 使异常的生命体征正常化。
    - 不治疗中枢神经系统的酒精并发症或戒断反应。
  - α 受体激动剂：
    - 集中作用 α_2 受体激动剂。
    - 使异常的生命体征正常化。
    - 不要治疗中枢神经系统的酒精并发症或戒断反应。
  - 苯妥英：
    - 不能判断酒精戒断引起的癫痫。
    - 表示癫痫发作由特发性癫痫引起，或创伤后癫痫或持续状态。

治疗药物

- 右旋糖：D_{50} W 1 安瓿(50 ml 或 25 g；儿童：D_{25} W 2～4 ml/kg)，静脉注射。
- 右美托咪定(precedex)：0.2～1.4 μg/(kg · h)，静脉连续输注。
- 地西泮(安定)：5～10 mg，静脉注射，5～10 min，直到患者冷静。
- 劳拉西泮(ativan)：0.5～4 mg，静脉注射或肌内注射，q5～10 min，直到患者平静。
- 纳洛酮(narcan)：0.4～2 mg(儿童：0.1 mg/kg)，静脉注射或肌内注射，初始剂量。
- 苯巴比妥：10～20 mg/kg，静脉注射(负荷剂量)，监测呼吸抑制。
- 苯妥英钠：15～18 mg/kg，不超过 25 mg/min。
  - 给予 fosphenytoin 15～20 mgPE/kg，最高速率为 150 mgPE/min。
- 异丙酚：25～75 μg/(kg · min)，静脉注射(负荷剂量)；5～50 μg/(kg · min)(维持剂量)。
- 硫胺素(维生素 B_1)：100 mg(儿童：50 mg)，静脉注射或肌内注射。

随访

进一步处理

入院指征

- 无法控制癫痫发作或口服药物无法控制

戒断症状。

• 肝功能衰竭、感染、脱水、营养不良、心血管衰竭、心律失常或外伤。

• 幻觉、生命体征异常、剧烈震颤或极度激动。

• 韦尼克脑病。

• 意识不清或谵妄。

出院指征

• 临床清醒。

• 无癫痫发作 6 h(如果是第 1 次,则进行阴性排除检查)。

转诊问题

与社会工作者和/或警察讨论,儿科患者和儿科患者家庭服务部门讨论。

随访建议

药物滥用参照周期性酒精中毒患者治疗。

要点和误区

• 慢性酗酒者由于非酒精性因素而无法参考淀粉酶的原因:

- 血清水平应下降 15～40 mg/(dl·h)。

- 如果精神状态没有改善(或恶化)需要进一步调查。

• 未能充分使用苯二氮䓬类药物治疗:

- 可能需要大剂量(如 200～300 mg 地西泮)来控制。

- 如果无法控制,请考虑其他 GABAergic 药物(苯巴比妥、异丙酚)。

• 未能将低血糖作为常见现象来考虑:

- 可能类似于酒精中毒的症状。

- 导致不良后果。

- 经常发生在慢性酗酒者和孩子。

巨细胞动脉炎 Giant Cell Arteritis

Donald J. Lefkowits 祝各亮 译

基础知识

描述

• 巨细胞动脉炎(GCA)是大中血管的慢性炎症,常发生于 50 岁以上患者。

• 常见的是颞动脉炎(TA)。

• 发病年龄的中位数是 72 岁。

• 最常见的动脉炎症来源是主动脉弓。

• 虽然大部分无临床症状,但胸主动脉的炎症仍会涉及少数一部分患者,且可能会导致主动脉瘤或主动脉夹层。

• 胸主动脉瘤是其晚期表现,发病率是无 TA 人群的 17 倍。

• 巨细胞动脉炎(GCA)患者中腹主动脉瘤的发病率增加 1 倍。

• 病理特点为单核肉芽肿性炎症导致明显的内膜增厚,血管腔闭塞。

• 闭塞性动脉炎可能会造成眼动脉栓塞,导致前部缺血性视神经病变(AIQN)和急性视力丧失。

• 动脉炎症涉及咀嚼肌,导致下颌运动障碍和舌部不适。

• 年龄是最大的危险因素:

- 50 岁以下人群少有发病。

- 90%以上患者年龄>60 岁。

- 50 岁以上患者的患病率约为 1/500。

• 在北纬地区发病率增加,斯堪的纳维亚后裔发病率最高。

• 女性发病率是男性的 2～4 倍。

• 在黑种人中少有发病,白种人中较常见。

• 与风湿性多肌痛(PMR)呈强相关(50%)。

基因

60%的患者在 *HLA-DR*4 上可以找到相关的易感位点。

病因

• 不明。

• 与遗传、环境和自身免疫因素有关。

诊断

• 满足下列 3 个或以上条件的需考虑动脉炎:

- 红细胞沉降率>50。

- 年龄>50 岁。

- 新出现的局部头痛。

- 颞动脉搏动减弱。

- 新出现的视力症状,尤其是暂时性单眼失明。

- 颞动脉病理活检提示坏死性动脉炎。

症状和体征

• 可以表现为急性、亚急性或慢性症状:

- 头痛是最常见的症状(70%)。

- 常为局部的钻痛或撕裂样痛。

- 位置常被描述为单侧太阳穴上方。

• 咀嚼时舌或下颌运动障碍是常见症状(50%)。

• 全身症状:

- 疲劳。

- 不适。

- 厌食。

- 体重下降。

- 虚弱。

- 关节痛。

- 低热。

• 视力症状:

- 通常表现为单侧。

- 出现其他症状后可进展至数周、数月。

- 可以波动,但视力障碍通常不随着时间的推移而改善,即使是在治疗中。

- 一过性黑矇。

- 失明。

- 复视。

- 上睑下垂。

- 眼外肌无力。

- 视野盲区。

- 视力模糊。

• 头皮触痛,尤其是在颞动脉上方。

• 颞动脉搏动:

- 早期病变时搏动增强。

- 晚期病变时搏动减弱。

• 头皮动脉上方出现红斑、发热、肿胀或结节。

• 大动脉血管杂音或搏动减弱,肢体跛行。

• 咽痛、咳嗽和吞咽困难。

• 罕见症状:

- 呼吸系统症状。

- 缺血性胸痛。

- 充血性心力衰竭。

• 神经系统问题:

- 发生于多达 1/3 的患者:

◦ 周围神经病变。

◦ 短暂性脑缺血发作。

◦ 脑血管意外。

J

• 隐匿表现包括：
- 舌炎。
- 舌梗死。
- 雷诺现象。

• 多达 30%的可能不出现头痛、头皮触痛、视力变化或下颌运动障碍的经典表现。

• 与 PMR 密切相关(高达 50%)：
- 肌肉僵硬。
- 近端肌肉酸痛。
- 早晨症状加重，运动后症状减轻。

• 常伴有滑膜炎，特别是在膝盖处。

基本检查

• 体格检查的重点内容：
- 颞动脉与头皮异常。
- 完整的神经系统检查。
- 眼科检查，包括视力和视野检查。

• 眼底检查：
- 初始通常正常。
- 虹膜炎和细玻璃体混浊可早期发现。
- 视神经水肿。
- 视盘肿胀、光滑和边缘模糊。
- 苍白。
- 出血。
- 散在棉织物样点。
- 之后出现血管充血和分泌物渗出。

• 注意四肢血管的搏动改变或大血管的杂音。

诊断检查与说明

实验室检查

• 红细胞沉降率上升，常＞100 mm/h：
- 红细胞沉降率＜40 很少见。

• C 反应蛋白超过 2.45 mg/dl。

• 血常规(CBC)：
- 典型表现为轻度正色素性贫血。
- 血小板增多(通常是略高)。
- 白细胞计数可以是正常或轻微的升高，分类通常是正常的。

• 肝功能、凝血酶原时间可能升高；肌酸激酶、肾功能检验、尿检验一般正常。

• 白细胞介素-6(IL-6)升高。

影像学检查

• 多普勒超声：
- 在颞动脉、面动脉和眼动脉血流减少。
- 出现晕征高度提示活动性颞动脉炎。

• MRI：
- 大动脉确诊性检查。

• 血管造影：
- 光滑，锥形闭塞或狭窄。

诊断步骤/外科

• 颞动脉活检：
- 用糖皮质激素进行初始治疗后即可进行，应在多部位取活检标本。
- 诊断的金标准。
- 如果初次结果为阴性，但又高度怀疑是动脉炎，建议在对侧进行活检。

鉴别诊断

• 血管炎：
- 结节性多动脉炎。
- 过敏性血管炎。
- 系统性红斑狼疮。
- 多发性大动脉炎。
- 韦格纳肉芽肿病。

• 视网膜、眼及颞动脉栓塞。

• 莱姆病。

• 非动脉炎性前部缺血性视神经病变(NAAION)。

治疗

院前

• 急性症状可与脑卒中混淆。

• 启动适当的监测和氧气装置。

• 患者可因为以下罕见后遗症中的一种出现低血压(主动脉夹层动脉瘤、腹主动脉瘤或心肌梗死)。

初步稳定/治疗

• 虽然罕见，但患者仍可能出现血管病变，如主动脉夹层动脉瘤、心肌梗死，需要适当、积极、早期处理。

• 肢体跛行、血压不对称和血管杂音可能是大血管受累的表现。

急诊治疗/程序

• 糖皮质激素：
- 当临床怀疑较高时，安排 TA 活检不应延误类固醇治疗。
- 开始类固醇治疗后 46 周出现组织病理学证据。
- 在颞动脉活检前开始使用需要强烈的临床指征。
- 早期、积极的治疗能显著降低失明的发生率。
- 糖皮质激素可以在几日到几周内有效地控制全身和局部症状。
- 泼尼松治疗可能会持续数年，一般疾病的病程是 3～4 年。

• 有指征时用非甾体抗炎药、水杨酸盐和/或麻醉药进行止痛处理。

药物治疗

• 泼尼松：60～100 mg，每日 1 次，症状减弱前至少 2 周。

• 急性视觉症状发作，考虑 1 000 mg 甲泼尼松在症状出现后前 1～3 日进行静脉注射。

• 低剂量阿司匹林治疗以减少血栓形成的风险。

• 非甾体抗炎药或麻醉药进行疼痛管理。

随访

进一步处理

入院指征

• 即将出现血管并发症或有急性局灶性神经系统表现的患者。

• 急性视力丧失或视力下降的患者。

出院指征

• 症状较少，没有终末器官受累证据的患者。

• 随访安排在后续 1～2 日。

转诊问题

• 风湿科。

• 有视觉症状时咨询眼科。

• 出现急性局灶性神经系统表现时咨询神经科。

随访建议

• 风湿科随访进行类激素管理和相关结缔组织病咨询。

• 神经科和眼科进行视觉障碍和神经系统表现的随访。

要点和误区

• 永久性视觉丧失是 GCA 最令人畏惧的并发症。

• 如果临床高度怀疑 GCA 或已存在视觉改变，不要因为等待活检而延迟糖皮质激素的治疗。

• 下颌活动障碍和一过性黑矇，是容易注意到的症状，但患者常常忘记向医师说明。如果考虑是 TA/GCA 的患者，可以直接向他们询问。

• 25%～50%的患有单眼急性视力下降的患者不治疗会进展为双眼失明。

卡马西平中毒 Carbamazepine Poisoning

James W. Rhee 高婷 译

基础知识

描述

- 卡马西平的治疗用途：
  - 抗惊厥。
  - 治疗慢性疼痛。
  - 预防偏头痛。
  - 稳定情绪。
- 作用机制：
  - 抗胆碱能。
  - 与苯妥英钠及三环类抗抑郁药类似。
  - 钠通道阻滞剂。
  - 抑制突触传递。

病因

卡马西平中毒可能由于以下原因引起：

- 自杀。
- 误食。
- 超治疗剂量服用。
- 药物间相互作用。

诊断

症状和体征

- 神经系统表现常见。
- 心脏毒性较罕见，除非在超大药物过量中。
- 中枢神经系统：
  - 共济失调。
  - 头晕。
  - 嗜睡。
  - 眼球震颤。
  - 幻觉。
  - 烦躁。
  - 昏迷。
  - 癫痫发作。
- 呼吸系统：
  - 呼吸抑制。
  - 吸入性肺炎。
- 心血管系统：
  - 低血压。
  - 传导阻滞(多发生在老年患者)。
  - 室上性心动过速。
  - 窦性心动过速或心动过缓。
  - 心电图改变：
    - PR、QRS及QTc间期延长。
    - T波改变。

儿童注意事项

神经系统表现发生率更高。

病史

- 卡马西平或缓释剂摄入剂量。
- 摄入时间。
- 药瓶是否还在。
- 有意或无意摄入。
- 是否同时摄入其他毒性物质。

体格检查

- 可出现癫痫发作或意识状态改变。
- 可出现烦躁或嗜睡。
- 窦性心动过速(大剂量卡马西平过量)。
- Brady 心律失常(通常发生在轻度卡马西平过量的老年患者中)。
- 抗胆碱能表现：
  - 肠鸣音减弱。
  - 瞳孔散大。
  - 潮红。
  - 尿潴留。
- 神经肌肉表现：
  - 震颤。
  - 口齿不清。
  - 肌阵挛。
  - 舞蹈样动作及手足徐动症。

基本检查

- 持续心电监测。
- 血清卡马西平浓度：
  - 治疗剂量为6～12 μg/L。
  - 血清浓度＞25～40 μg/ml与严重毒性反应相关：
    - 昏迷。
    - 癫痫发作。
    - 呼吸衰竭。
    - 传导阻滞。
  - 血清卡马西平水平无法明确地预测临床毒性反应，主要原因为：
    - 无法检测其活性代谢产物10,11-环氧化卡马西平水平。
    - 神经系统表现有赖于中枢神经系统中卡马西平的水平而非其血清含量。
  - 由于卡马西平吸收的不稳定性，需连续监测卡马西平浓度。
- 心电图：
  - 传导阻滞。
    - QRS间期延长。
    - PR间期延长。
    - QTc延长。
  - 心律失常。
- 血清对乙酰氨基酚水平。

诊断检查与说明

实验室检查

- 血常规：
  - 白细胞减少或白细胞增多。
- 电解质、尿素氮/肌酐及血糖：
  - 低血糖。
  - 低钾血症。
  - 低钠血症。
- 动脉血气分析。
- 尿检：
  - 尿糖阳性。
  - 尿酮体阳性。
- 妊娠检测。
- 谷丙转氨酶、谷草转氨酶、胆红素及碱性磷酸酶：
  - 可轻度升高。
  - 通常无临床症状。

影像学检查

X线胸片：

- 吸入性肺炎。
- 肺水肿。

鉴别诊断

- 引发意识状态下降的药物：
  - 酒精。
  - 抗胆碱能药物。
  - 巴比妥类药物。
  - 苯二氮䓬类药物。
  - 锂。
  - 阿片类药物。
  - 吩噻嗪类药物。
- 引发癫痫的药物：
  - 酒精截断。
  - 抗胆碱能药物。
  - 樟。
  - 异烟肼。
  - 锂。
  - 吩噻嗪类药物。
  - 拟交感神经药物：
    - 苯丙胺。
    - 可卡因。

K

- 三环类抗抑郁药。
• 引起运动异常药物：
- 抗组胺药。
- 丁酰苯类。
- 咖啡因。
- 可卡因。
- 左旋多巴。
- 杜冷丁。
- 苯环利定类。
- 吩噻嗪类。
- 苯妥英钠。
- 三环类抗抑郁药。

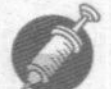

治疗

院前

• 不要催吐。
• 如果出现明显的呼吸抑制或气道损伤需气管插管。
• 开放静脉通路。
• 采集所有潜在摄入物品的信息。

初步稳定/治疗

• 基础支持(ABC 管理)。
• 开放静脉通路，如出现低血压则行液体复苏。
• 氧气吸入。
• 心电监测。
• 如出现精神症状可给予纳洛酮、硫胺素、50%葡萄糖或罗康全。

急诊治疗/程序

• 基础治疗：
- 活性炭治疗：
◦ 口服山梨糖醇及单剂量活性炭。
◦ 胃肠道活动减少患者慎用。
◦ 肠鸣音消失患者禁用。
- 多剂量活性炭：
◦ 降低卡马西平平均半衰期。
◦ 在消化道与未吸收的卡马西平结合。
◦ 阻断肝肠循环。
◦ 不与山梨糖醇同时服用。
- 体外治疗：
◦ 卡马西平可适度透析。
◦ 患者通常在无需血透或碳罐吸附情况下支持治疗效果好。
◦ 在严重卡马西平中毒(如多次发作，危及生命的心律失常)难以支持治疗和多剂量活性炭的情况下，建议进行体外治疗。
◦ 间歇性血液透析是体外治疗的首选形式。
◦ 间歇性血液灌流或连续性肾脏替代治疗是体外治疗的替代方法。
• 呼吸抑制：
- 气管插管。
- 通气支持。
• 低血压：
- 静脉输注等渗晶体溶液。
- 对液体复苏无反应患者可予以去甲肾上腺素。
• 癫痫发作：
- 地西泮(首选药物)。
- 苯巴比妥(在地西泮无效时)。
- 在大多数药物毒性引起的癫痫发作中，苯妥英钠治疗无效。
• 心脏传导延迟：
- QRS 波群增宽(>100 ms)：
- 碳酸氢钠(对抗钠离子阻滞剂)。
• 严重中毒的体外治疗行肾内科会诊。
• 如果有自杀倾向需精神科会诊。

药物治疗

一线药物

• 活性炭(初始剂量)：口服 1～2 g/kg 泥浆，最大剂量为 100 g。
• 多剂量活性炭：初始治疗后每 2 h 口服 25 g(儿童：0.25 g/kg)；或每 6 h 口服 50 g。

二线药物

• 葡萄糖：静脉注射 50%葡萄糖 50 ml 或 25 g(儿童：25%葡萄糖 2～4 ml/kg)。
• 地西泮：静脉注射 5～10 mg(儿童：0.2～0.5 mg/kg)。
• 纳洛酮：初始剂量为静脉注射或肌内注射 2 mg(儿童：0.1 mg/kg)。
• 去甲肾上腺素：起始剂量为 2～4 μg/min [儿童：0.05～0.1 μg/(kg · min)]逐渐加量滴定至有效剂量。
• 碳酸氢钠。

随访

进一步处理

入院指征

• 任何时间出现的意识状态恶化(血药浓度的波动易导致复发患者)。
- 复发后观察至少 24 h。
• 癫痫发作。
• 心律失常。
• 精神状态尚未恢复的自杀患者。

离院指征

• 观察 6 h 无症状。
• 精神状态正常。
• 初始心电图正常。
• 有胃肠道动力。
• 意图自杀患者恢复精神状态。

转诊建议

推荐给予意图自杀患者精神类疾病评估。

随访建议

对于需服用超治疗剂量药物治疗基础疾病的患者，需由内科医师指导监测用药。

要点和误区

• 在治疗过程中卡马西平血药浓度经常反跳至高水平。因此，在大剂量摄入的患者中需连续监测其血药浓度。
• 需密切监测心律失常。
• 大剂量摄入卡马西平患者需多剂量活性炭治疗。
• 在严重中毒反应中常常需要体外循环治疗。
• 出现反常癫痫发作，可用苯二氮䓬类药物治疗(地西泮为首选药物)。

咯血 Hemoptysis

Jason A. Kopec · Navneet Cheema 陈奇通 译

基础知识

描述

• 痰中带血来源于气管支气管树。
• 出血的来源：
- 支气管动脉(90%)，通常出血量较大。
- 肺动脉(5%)，通常出血量较少。
- 肺外动脉(5%)，包括肋间动脉、冠状动脉、胸椎和膈下动脉。
• 大咯血的阈值：
- 24 h 从 100 ml 到 1 000 ml。
- 100 ml/h。

- >8 ml/(kg·d)。
- 儿童 200 ml/24 h。
• 死亡率：
- 大咯血(>500 ml/24 h)：38%。
- 轻度到中度出血(<500 ml/24 h)：4.5%。
- 恶性肿瘤和凝血功能障碍会增加死亡的风险。

病因

• 感染(最常见的原因)：
- 急性或慢性支气管炎。
- 肺炎。
- 坏死性肺炎或肺脓肿(克雷伯杆菌、肺炎链球菌、铜绿假单胞菌、金黄色葡萄球菌、肺炎双球菌)。
- 肺结核。
- 病毒(流行性感冒、水痘)。
- 真菌(曲霉、球孢子菌、组织胞浆菌、芽酵母菌)。
- 寄生虫(蛔虫、阿米巴、肺吸虫、棘球绦虫)。
• 肿瘤：
- 鳞状细胞,小细胞,类癌。
- 支气管癌。
- 转移性癌。
• 肺部：
- 支气管扩张。
- 肺动脉栓塞、肺梗死。
- 囊性纤维化变性。
- 支气管胸膜瘘。
- 结节病。
• 心脏：
- 二尖瓣狭窄。
- 感染性心内膜炎。
- 心力衰竭。
• 全身性疾病：
- 肺出血肾炎综合征。
- 全身性红斑狼疮。
- 血管炎(韦格纳肉芽肿病、过敏性紫癜、白塞病)。
• 血液系统：
- 凝血功能障碍。
- 血小板减少症。
- 血小板功能异常。
- 弥散性血管内凝血(DIC)。
• 血管：
- 肺动脉高压。
- 动静脉畸形。
- 主动脉瘤。
- 肺动脉瘤(膜斯默森动脉瘤、霉菌性：动脉炎)。
- 主动脉支气管动脉瘘。
• 药物或毒素：
- 阿司匹林、抗血小板治疗。
- 抗凝血药物。
- 青霉胺、胺碘酮、丙基硫氧嘧啶、贝伐单抗。
- 可卡因肺。
- 有机溶剂。
• 创伤：
- 气管破裂。
- 肺挫伤。
• 医源性：
- 支气管镜及肺活检。
- 肺动脉或中心静脉导管插入术。
- 经气管抽取。
• 其他：
- 异物吸入。
- 月经期咯血(子宫内膜异位症)。
- 淀粉样变性病。
- 特发性或原因不明(根据患者人群有5%~30%)。

诊断

症状和体征

• 胸痛。
• 呼吸困难。
• 发热。
• 虚弱。
• 疲倦。
• 盗汗。
• 体重减轻。

病史

• 询问之前是否患有肺、肾脏或心脏瓣膜病。
• 吸烟史。
• 化学品(石棉)或者传染性职业病暴露。
• 旅游史(考虑寄生虫或真菌感染)。
• 阿司匹林、NSAIDs 或抗凝药的使用。
• 如果病史中之前出现血尿,应考虑肺出血肾炎综合征。
• 反复发生的或慢性咯血,应高度怀疑动静脉畸形、支气管扩张症或囊性纤维化。

体格检查

• 杵状指(慢性炎性肺疾病)。
• 皮肤瘀斑(血液病或抗凝血药物)。
• 口疮性溃疡(白塞病)。
• 鼻中隔穿孔(韦格纳肉芽肿病)。
• 血尿(肺出血肾炎综合征)。
• 单侧下肢水肿考虑深静脉血栓形成(DVT)。
• 假性咯血：
- 鼻窦炎、鼻出血、鼻漏、咽炎、上呼吸道感染及误吸。

儿科注意事项

• 全面的头部、眼、耳、鼻及咽喉检查,以排除非肺源性的出血。
• 肺部检查多正常。
• 喘息可能提示梗阻(如异物)。
• 湿啰音多提示潜在的肺疾病(如肺炎、血胸、心力衰竭)。
• 毛细血管扩张或血管瘤应考虑存在动静脉畸形。

基本检查

• 区分咯血与假咯血：
- 注意诱发因素、症状持续时间、出血的量与性状。
- 肺源性：
  ◦ 出血颜色为鲜红色。
  ◦ 表面呈泡沫状。
  ◦ 痰与血混合可能来源于肺。
  ◦ pH>7。
• 胃肠道来源：
  ◦ 出血为暗红色或棕色。
  ◦ 多连同胃内容物一起咯出。
  ◦ 有明显的恶心及呕吐。
  ◦ pH<7。
  ◦ 洗胃可以用来排除胃肠道来源的出血,但是鼻腔或其他外伤可引起进一步出血。

诊断检查与说明

实验室检查

• 全血细胞计数。
• 基础代谢功能检查试验组合。
• PT、INR、APTT。
• 尿液分析。
• 发热患者或疑似传染性疾病：
- 血培养。
- 痰培养和革兰染色。
- 细胞学检查。
- KOH 真菌培养。
- AFB 结核菌染色。
• 低血压患者(大咯血患者)：
- 血型与交叉配血。
- 全面的代谢功能检查(肝、肾功能)。
- 凝血病组合检查：
  ◦ 纤维蛋白和纤维蛋白原降解产物(FDP)或抗凝血酶Ⅲ。
• 儿童患者：

K

- 如果怀疑囊性纤维化病应考虑行汗氯试验。

影像学检查

• 胸部X线片检查：
- 病理特征(如肿瘤、空洞、渗出、气胸)。
- 早期的肺出血可能出现渗出。
- 20%的患者胸片正常。

• CT：
- 高分辨率CT已经成为诊断支气管扩张的金标准。
- 理想研究对于病情稳定和胸部X线检查正常的咯血患者。
- 根据空洞的存在以及腺泡结节发现活动性肺结核。
- 高灵敏度的外围肿瘤可能在支气管镜检查中并不明显。

• CTA：
- 可以发现变异性支气管动脉供血。
- 可以识别支气管动脉的起源和存在变异。
- 确定肺栓塞。

• V/Q：
- 体格检查可疑，同时患者不能行CTA检查。
- X线检查异常的患者使用意义不大。

诊断步骤/外科

支气管镜检查：

• 对肿瘤、异物、肉芽肿、炎性渗出可直接可视化。

• 收集支气管分泌物从而行细胞学和组织学检查。

• 对于支气管壁外的病灶、支气管远端狭窄或阻塞，以及周边病变诊断的阳性率有限。

鉴别诊断

假咯血：

• 鼻出血。

• 咽部出血。

• 胃肠道出血。

治疗

院前

• 呼吸系统和接触预防措施。

• 气道管理：
- 吸氧。
- 必要时吸痰。
- 如果呼吸道破坏、严重的呼吸窘迫或血氧不足可行气管插管。

• 建立2条快速静脉通道。

• 容量复苏。

• 连续脉搏血氧仪、血流动力学和心脏监测。

初步稳定/治疗

• 气道和呼吸：
- 呼吸衰竭的患者行气管插管术。
- ＞8F的气管插管便于吸引和支气管镜检查。
- 肺部未出血的患者选择气管插管，可根据情况选择单管或双管插管。
- 必要时可予以辅助供氧。
- 连续脉冲血氧定量法和心脏监测。

• 大咯血：
- 对生命的最大威胁不是出血而是窒息。
- 建立2条快速静脉通道。
- 必要时可给予大量晶体液或血液制品进行复苏。

急诊治疗/程序

• 如果考虑或诊断为感染所致的大咯血，应行抗菌治疗。

• 纠正低氧血症和/或凝血功能障碍。

• 如果大咯血：
- 通过静脉通路给予大量晶体液或血液制品进行复苏。
- 患者应采取直立位或侧卧位(受影响的肺处于下方)。
- 气管插管可以保护呼吸道，改善呼吸衰竭，方便支气管镜检查。
- Foley导管或Fogarty导管支气管填塞(＜4F)，或双腔气管导管(临时措施)。
- 支气管镜检查可同时实施包括血管收缩剂局部治疗、支架或球囊填塞、电灼、促凝物质等治疗。
- 支气管动脉栓塞(成功率高达98%)，有20%的病例出现再出血。
- 手术：
  ○ 如果栓塞未成功，有胸动脉瘤、肿瘤或者动静脉畸形的患者，可行肺叶或全肺切除术。
  ○ 手术切除对于病灶局限和有足够心肺储备的患者最有效。

药物治疗

参照特定病因。

随访

进一步处理

入院指征

• ICU：
- 气管插管。
- 大咯血。
- 血流动力学不稳定。
- 低血容量性休克。
- 呼吸衰竭。
- 气道狭窄。

• 普通病房：
- 轻度咯血。
- 肺结核(隔离)。
- 稳定的异物。
- 肺脓肿。
- 空洞性肺疾病。

出院指征

• 血流动力学稳定。

• 轻度咯血。

• 凝血功能正常。

• 不需要吸氧。

• 慢性稳定的咯血病史。

• 密切随访。

转诊问题

• 7～10日的PCP。

• 专家通过病因学认定需要转诊的患者。

随访建议

• 建议患者戒烟。

• 避免药物可能会增加出血的风险，包括草药补充剂，如大蒜、银杏、人参。

• 有以下症状患者应立即返回医院：
- 呼吸急促。
- 胸痛。
- 严重的眩晕。
- 晕厥。
- 持续或恶化的咯血。

要点和误区

• 考虑早期气道管理与临床表现相符。

• 如果因严重的单侧出血导致低氧血症，请将患者“受损的肺”处于下方。

• 支气管动脉栓塞很有效，应尽早与IR讨论病例。

K

开放性骨折

Christy Rosa Mohler 万健 译

基础知识

描述

- 皮肤连续性中断，骨折伤及部位包括伤口至骨外露。
- 属外科急症，延误处理会增加感染和并发症的发生率。
- 患者易发生并发症的相关因素：
  - 大面积软组织损伤。
  - 伤口严重污染。
  - 血管损伤。
  - 不稳定性骨折。
  - 患者有某些基础疾病（如糖尿病、血管病等）。

病因

开放性骨折通常是由严重钝性或锐性创伤所引起。

诊断

症状和体征

- 患部畸形及附近皮肤受损。
- 可能伴有神经血管损伤。
- 常有与创伤相关的其他表现。

病史

明确的创伤史。

体格检查

- 认真检查神经血管情况。
- 全面检查创伤引起的其他损伤。

基本检查

- 包含损伤部位与其相邻的上下关节的 X 线摄片。
- 应根据损伤机制和创伤相关损伤的证据来指导检查。

诊断检查与说明

实验室检查

- 对于大的骨折（股骨、骨盆）或多发伤患者应进行全血细胞计数、生化检查、凝血功能等检查。
- 大量失血或潜在失血者应予以定血型和交叉配血。
- 清创前后细菌培养价值不大，不予推荐。

影像学检查

怀疑血管损伤者应予以多普勒或血管造影检查：

- 膝关节后部脱位。
- 严重缺血。
- 高危区域大面积软组织损伤。

诊断步骤/外科

- 考虑筋膜室间隔综合征时应测量筋膜室内的压力。
- 可疑关节损伤者应予以动脉注射盐水或亚甲蓝关节造影。
- 若非侵入性手段不足以明确血管损伤时应予以血管造影。
- 水温冷却很快，立即加入温水或替换原有的水来保持温度在合适的范围。
- 过热的水温可致热损伤，过冷的水温使解冻减慢，都使得组织存活减少。

鉴别诊断

非连续性划伤或擦伤。

治疗

院前

- 无菌敷料覆盖开放伤口。
- 患处相近上下关节制动。
- 局部压迫控制出血。
- 当肢体离断或难以控制性出血时可考虑使用止血带。
- 如果肢体损伤严重远端脉搏消失应予以纵向牵引。

初步稳定/治疗

- 基本生命支持。
- 脱掉衣服和任何接触到的污染物、异物。

急诊治疗/程序

- 建立静脉通路。
- 禁食。
- 必要时注射破伤风疫苗。
- 开放性骨折者应尽早在急诊处理时就给予抗菌药物治疗以降低早期感染发生率。
- 最大限度地减少更换敷料的次数，以避免继发性感染。
- 常规检查肢体伤情，有无筋膜室间隔综合征和神经血管损伤。
- 某些大关节（踝、肘、膝）开放性骨折/畸形应减少在急诊室内的诊查。
- 骨科急会诊，予以正规伤口冲洗、清创或行骨折固定。
- 潜在血管损伤者应请血管外科医师会诊。

药物治疗

一线用药

- 头孢唑林：1～2 g，静脉注射（儿童：20 mg/kg，肌内注射或静脉注射）。
- 加用庆大霉素：1.5～2 mg/kg，静脉注射。它适用于损伤严重、大面积挤压和高度污染的伤口（儿童：2～2.5 mg/kg，静脉注射）。
- 加用青霉素：400 万～500 万 U，静脉注射。它适用于田园劳作时受伤、血管损伤、伤口受梭菌污染风险高等（儿童：5 万 U/kg，静脉注射）。
- 硫酸吗啡：2～10 mg（儿童：0.05～0.1 mg/kg），每剂量静脉注射或其他等效镇痛药物。

二线用药

- 克林霉素：900 mg，静脉注射（严重 β-内酰胺过敏）。
- 氨曲南：1 g，静脉注射（严重 β-内酰胺过敏/污染/大面积伤口）。

儿科注意事项

- 白喉-百日咳-破伤风疫苗用于 7 岁以下儿童。

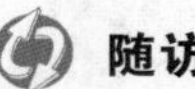

随访

进一步处理

入院指征

多数患者需要入院治疗，包括冲洗伤口、清创、静脉注射抗菌药物、手术固定等处理。

出院指征

单一轻微的开放性骨折可能只需要骨科会诊后在急诊室彻底冲洗，制动处置。患者可带口服抗菌药物出院。

转诊问题

多数开放性骨折患者需请骨科急会诊，还需要创伤救治团队评估其他合并创伤。

随访建议

患者经急诊室处置后应在 1～2 日到骨科随访。

要点和误区

• 开放性骨折是外科急症，应有骨科专科会诊。

• 40%～70%的开放性骨折患者合并其他创伤性损害。

• 快速彻底的急诊评估与处置可以显著降低开放性骨折患者的伤残率。

抗胆碱能药中毒 Anticholinergic Poisoning

Patrick M. Whiteley　李岩　王瑞兰 译

基础知识

描述

• 中枢和外周胆碱能阻断。

• 取决于所涉及的药物，拮抗作用发生在 M 受体(最常见)、R 受体或两种受体同时发生。

• 反应的发生：摄入 15～30 min 后。

• 影响持续时间：2～24 h。

病因

• 许多药物都含有抗胆碱能性质：

- 治疗剂量反应轻微。
- 过量会危及生命。

• 抗胆碱能药：

- 抗组胺药。
- 颠茄生物碱及其合成物。
- 抗帕金森药。
- 循环抗抑郁药。
- 抗精神病药物(抗精神病药)。
- 散瞳药。
- 骨骼肌松弛药(苯海拉明、环苯扎林)。
- 解痉药。
- 蘑菇——毒蝇鹅膏。
- 植物——致命的茄属植物、曼德拉草、天仙子。
- 曼陀罗——烟熏或摄入。

诊断

体征和症状

病史

• 症状的发生和持续时间。

• 摄入/暴露的类型和程度。

体格检查

• 经典的中毒综合征：

- “疯了”——精神状态改变。
- “热的像野兔一样”——高热。
- “红的像甜菜”——皮肤发红。
- “干的像骨头”——皮肤和黏膜干燥。
- “瞎的像蝙蝠”——瞳孔散大，继发视力模糊。

• 一般状况：

- 体温过高。
- 精神状态改变。

• 眼：

- 非反应性瞳孔散大。
- 不能调节。

• 心血管系统：

- 窦性心动过速。
- 心律失常(除非大量摄入，否则罕见)。
- 低血压/HTN。
- 心源性肺水肿。

• 肺：

- 呼吸急促。
- 呼吸衰竭。

• 消化道：

- 肠鸣音增强/减弱。
- 吞咽困难。
- 胃肠运动降低。
- 唾液分泌减少。

• 泌尿生殖系统(GU)：

- 尿潴留。

• 体表：

- 出汗减少。
- 皮肤发红。
- 干燥的皮肤和黏膜。

• 中枢神经系统：

- 精神状态改变。
- 幻听或幻视。
- 昏迷。
- 癫痫发作。

基本检查

诊断基于临床表现和准确的病史。

诊断检查与说明

实验室检查

• 尿液毒理学筛查来排除其他中毒。

• 电解质、血肌酐、尿素氮和葡萄糖。

• CBC。

• 如果怀疑横纹肌溶解，需测肌酸磷酸激酶(CPK)。

• 尿液分析。

• 对乙酰氨基酚水平：

- 检测隐匿性摄入(例如，对乙酰氨基酚 PM)。

影像学检查

心电图：

• 窦性心动过速最常见。

• QRS 间期延长。

• 房室传导阻滞。

• 束支传导阻滞。

• 心律失常。

鉴别诊断

• 拟交感神经中毒。

• 戒断综合征。

• 急性精神障碍。

• 脓毒症。

• 甲状腺疾病。

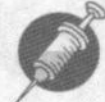

治疗

院前

在急诊中为了鉴别要提供所有涉及过量的药片及药瓶。

初步稳定/治疗

• ABC 管理：

- 气道控制至关重要。
- 补充氧气。
- 建立静脉通路。
- 心电监护和动脉血氧饱和度。

• 纳洛酮、硫胺素，如果精神状态改变使用 D_{50}(或罗康全)。

急诊治疗/程序

• 支持治疗：

- 静脉注射补生理盐水。
- 高热采用标准化积极降温措施。
- 使用地西泮治疗焦虑：

K

◦ 吩噻嗪类具有抗胆碱能作用，要避免使用。
- 用地西泮和巴比妥类治疗癫痫发作。
- 心律失常：
◦ 使用标准抗心律失常药。
◦ 避免使用Ⅰa类抗心律失常药，因为许多抗胆碱能药物具有奎尼丁样作用。
◦ 碳酸氢钠可逆转奎尼丁样作用。
• 净化：
- 口服药物中毒使用活性炭。
- 眼药水接触中毒要眼睛灌洗。
• 毒扁豆碱（水杨酸毒扁豆碱制剂）：
- 可透过血脑屏障的可逆性乙酰胆碱酯酶抑制剂。
- 逆转中枢和外周的抗胆碱能作用。
- 出现外周抗胆碱能症状和以下情况可证实：
◦ 对常规治疗无效的癫痫发作。
◦ 不可控制的兴奋。
- 由于存在心律失常（特别是心脏停搏）、癫痫发作和胆碱能危机的风险，所以要谨慎使用：
◦ 重视心脏监测。
◦ 观察胆碱能症状。
- 禁忌证：
◦ 循环抗抑郁药物过量（增强毒性）。
◦ 心血管疾病。
◦ 哮喘和支气管痉挛。
◦ 肠梗阻。
◦ 心传导阻滞。
◦ 周围性血管疾病。
◦ 膀胱梗阻。

■ 药物治疗

• 活性炭：1 mg/kg，口服。
• 葡萄糖：50～100 ml D_{50}（儿童：2 ml/kg D_{25}，超过 1 min），静脉给药；必要时重复给药。
• 地西泮（安定）：5～10 mg（儿童：0.2～0.5 mg/kg）每 10～15 min，静脉给药。
• 多巴胺：2～2 μg/(kg·min)，滴定至产生效果。
• 劳拉西泮：2～4 mg（儿童：0.03～0.05 mg/kg）每 10～15 min，静脉给药。
• 毒扁豆碱：0.5～2 mg（儿童：0.02 mg/kg），静脉给药超过 5 min，必要时在 30～60 min 内重复给药。
• 苯巴比妥：10～20 mg/kg，静脉给药（负荷剂量）。
• 硫胺素（维生素 B_1）：100 mg（儿童：50 mg），静脉给药或肌内注射。

一线用药

劳拉西泮或地西泮。

二线用药

毒扁豆碱（谨慎使用，考虑咨询医药毒理学家）。

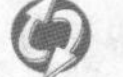

随访

■ 进一步处理

入院指征

• 中度至严重的抗胆碱能症状准许收入ICU（控制兴奋，控制温度，并观察癫痫发作或心律失常）。
• 任何接受毒扁豆碱的患者。

出院指标

• 轻度及急诊观察 6～8 h 后抗胆碱能中毒症状改善的患者。

转诊问题

• 成瘾性抗胆碱能药物滥用的患者需药物滥用转诊。
• 无意（意外）中毒的患者需要中毒预防咨询。
• 故意中毒（例如，自杀）的中毒患者需要精神科评估。

■ 随访建议

故意中毒的患者需要适当的精神科转诊。

要点和误区

• 积极治疗高热。
• 退热药对中毒性高热无效。
• 谨慎使用毒扁豆碱，条件允许时咨询医学毒理学家。

抗利尿素分泌异常症 Syndrome of Inappropriate Antidiuretic Hormone Secretion (SIADH)

Matthew D. Bitner · Andrew Connor 范浩浩 李文放 译

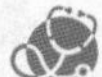

基础知识

■ 描述

• 住院患者低钠血症的最常见原因（在一些研究发现使住院患者死亡率增加 1 倍）。
• 是水平衡问题，不是钠平衡问题。
• 水平衡的正常调节：
- 抗利尿激素（ADH）：
◦ 水平衡的整体控制器。
◦ 增加集水管的透水性，导致游离水重吸收。
◦ 由下丘脑合成，但由垂体后叶分泌。
- 水分丢失（增加血浆渗透压）刺激分泌，如下所述：
◦ 渗透压感受器、心房牵张力感受器。
◦ 颈动脉压力感受器。
◦ 主动脉弓、肺静脉。
• 低钠血症：
- 轻度：血清钠<135 mmol/L。
- 中度：血清钠<130 mmol/L。
- 严重：血清钠<125 mmol/L。
- 相对于钠来说，细胞外有过量的水。
- 消耗性低钠血症：
◦ 钠消耗可能由饮食、胃肠道损失、利尿剂及肾或肾上腺疾病引起。
◦ 通常伴随着细胞外液的消耗。
◦ 低钠血症与低血容量临床症状相关。
◦ HCT、BUN、Cr 升高。
◦ 尿钠排泄<20 mmol/L。
- 稀释性低钠血症。
◦ 体内钠在正常情况下，细胞外液量增多。
◦ 可能是由于药物或医疗条件导致液体摄入量增加（口服或静脉补充）。
◦ 水肿。
◦ HCT、BUN、Cr 正常或降低。
◦ 尿钠排泄>20 mmol/L。
◦ 不合适的 ADH 分泌是稀释性低钠血症的一种形式。
• SIADH 的定义：
- 没有高渗或低血容量时 ADH 分泌。引起抗利尿激素水平的异常升高，作用于水孔蛋白从而使肾小管增强对水的重吸收。
• 定义标准：

K

- 必要特征：
  ◦ 低钠血症：但是纠正了高血糖症、高蛋白血症或高脂血症。
  ◦ 容量平衡：没有低容量症状（低血压、心动过速）或高容量症状（水肿、腹水）。
  ◦ 血浆渗透压：<275 mOsm/kg H_2O。
  ◦ 正常的肾、肾上腺和甲状腺功能。
  ◦ 没有最近的利尿剂使用。
  ◦ 尿液量>100 mOsm/kg H_2O。
- 补充特征：
  ◦ 血浆尿酸<4 mg/dl。
  ◦ BUN<10 mg/dl。
  ◦ FEN_a>1%。
  ◦ 输注生理盐水（NS）后未能纠正低钠血症。
  ◦ 异常水负荷试验（不能在 4 h 内排出 20 ml/kg 水的>90%）。

病因

- 恶性疾病：
  - 产生 ADH 的肿瘤。
  - 癌症（小细胞、胰腺、前列腺）。
  - 垂体肿瘤。
  - 胸腺瘤。
  - 淋巴瘤。
- 肺部疾病：
  - 肺炎。
  - 肺结核。
  - 肺脓肿。
  - 慢性阻塞性肺疾病。
- 神经系统障碍：
  - 肿块（肿瘤/脓肿/硬膜下血肿）。
  - 脑膜炎。
  - 脱髓鞘病变（多发性硬化/吉兰-巴雷综合征）。
  - 蛛网膜下腔出血。
  - CVA。
  - 急性精神障碍。
  - 头部受伤。
- 药物：
  - 促进 AVP 释放的药物（尼古丁、三环类、吩噻嗪类）。
  - 改变肾脏功能的药物（去氨加压素、缩宫素、血管加压素、前列腺素合成抑制剂，非甾体类解热镇痛抗炎药）。
  - 血管紧张素转化酶抑制剂（ACEI）和噻嗪类利尿剂，尤其是联合使用时。
  - 噻嗪类利尿剂。
  - 氯磺丙脲。
  - 长春新碱。
  - 抗惊厥药（卡马西平）。
  - 抗抑郁药（三环类、SSRs）。
  - 抗精神病药。
  - NSAIDs。
  - 摇头丸（MDMA）。
  - 加压素类似物（DDAVP、催产素、加压素）。
- 短暂的：
  - 耐力运动。
  - 全身麻醉。
  - 疼痛。
  - 压力。
- 其他：
  - 遗传。
  - 正压通气。
  - HIV。
  - 特发性。

注意

在精神病患者中较难诊断，由于：

- 症状与基础的精神疾病相似。
- 许多精神疾病（如精神分裂症、烦渴症、强迫性饮酒行为、厌食症相关的水过载等）和药物可引起抗利尿激素分泌异常综合征（详见病因学中的药物相关内容）。

注意

脑耗盐综合征（CSWS）与 SIADH 类似。

- 见于脑肿瘤或蛛网膜下腔出血和神经外科患者。
- 病因不详。
- 大量消耗钠时，水适量重吸收（尿 Na>30～40 mmol/L）。
- 限制液体可区分两者：
  - 在 SIADH：低尿酸血症将改正。
  - 在 CSWS 中：低尿酸血症将持续存在。
- CSWS 的治疗可能与 SIADH 不同：
  - 输注生理盐水。
  - 激素治疗。

诊断

体征和症状

- 血清钠<135 mmol/L：
  - 可能无症状。
- 血清钠<130 mmol/L：
  - 乏力、嗜睡。
  - 体重增加。
  - 头痛。
  - 厌食。
- 钠血清<120 mmol/L：
  - 意识状态改变。
  - 癫痫/昏迷。
- 慢性低钠血症：50%无症状。
- 急性低钠血症的死亡率高。

病史

- 既往用药史。
- 病程（急性、亚急性或慢性）。

体格检查

- 容量状态。
- 精神状态。
- 恶性肿瘤的恶病质。

基本检查

- 诊断是排除性的，需要评估其他原因：
  - 消耗性或稀释性低钠血症。
- 电解质、BUN、Cr、葡萄糖、蛋白质、血脂：
  - 低钠血症（血清钠<135 mmol/L）。
  - 血浆渗透压（血清渗透压<275 mOsm/kg）。
- 尿渗透压：
  - 无法排泄稀释的尿液。
  - 尿渗透压>100 mOsm/kg。
- 尿钠：
  - 继续尿钠排泄。
  - 尿钠>20 mmol/L。

诊断检查与说明

实验室检查

- 血清蛋白水平。
- 血脂水平。
- 葡萄糖水平。
- 血清渗透压。
- LFT 和甲状腺功能测试。
- 早晨皮质醇水平。

影像学检查

行影像学检查（胸片、头部 CT）来筛选 SIADH（肿瘤）引起的病症。

鉴别诊断

低钠血症的原因

- 见上面的病因。
- 细胞外液增多（稀释性低钠血症）：
  - 肾衰竭/不足。
  - CHF。
  - 终末期肝病。
- 正常细胞外液（稀释性低钠血症）：
  - SIADH。
  - 黏液性水肿。
  - 席汉综合征（产后垂体功能减退症）。
  - 渗透压重置综合征（在低于正常钠水平的情况下稀释尿液）。
- 细胞外液减少（耗竭性低钠血症）：

K

- 消耗增加：
  ◦ 过度出汗(耐力运动)。
  ◦ 消化道流失(呕吐、腹泻)。
- 至第三间隙。
- 利尿剂使用。
- 醛固酮缺乏症：
  ◦ 艾迪生病。
- 失盐肾病：
  ◦ 肾小管酸中毒。

• 假性低钠血症(见高血糖、高蛋白血症、高脂血症)。

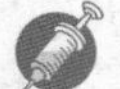

治疗

院前

• 在精神状态改变的患者中，气道的维持和保护至关重要。

• 怀疑有低血容量时，应开始适当的液体复苏。

• 快速的患者评估和转运是很重要的。

初步稳定/治疗

• 伴有中枢神经系统表现的严重症状性低钠血症。

• 对需要气道保护的患者进行气管插管。

• 识别/处理其他原因引起的意识改变。

• 用苯二氮䓬类药物治疗癫痫发作。

• 继续进行低钠血症治疗。

急诊治疗/程序

• SIADH 最有效的治疗方法是成功的消除根本原因。

• SIADH 引起的低钠血症与各种原因导致低血容量性低钠血症的治疗是相同的。

轻度症状性低钠血症、伴有轻微症状的慢性低钠血症和无症状性低钠血症

• 血清钠通常>125 mmol/L。

• 液体限制 500 ml/d，单独或与以下配合使用：
- 生理盐水输注和/或静脉推注呋塞米。

• 正确地升高血清钠不超过 0.5 mmol/(L·h)(5～6 mmol/d)：
- 血清钠水平过快校正可诱发中脑桥髓样髓鞘化，伴随延髓麻痹、四肢瘫痪、癫痫发作、昏迷和死亡。

严重低钠血症

• 有症状患者血清钠<125 mmol/L。

• 在第 1 个 24 h 内以 1 mmol/(L·h)的速率增加血清钠水平，不超过 12 mmol/L(当血清钠低于 125 mmol/L 时为 8～12 mmol/d，当血清钠水平升高至 125 mmol/L 时，调至 5～6 mmol/d)。

• 目标水平：125 mmol/L。

• 用 3%盐水溶液治疗具有显著神经学症状的患者。

• 血清钠实验室每 1～2 h 测一次。

急性危及生命的低钠血症

• 血清钠通常<120 mmol/L。

• 与癫痫发作或昏迷相关。

• 临床目标：癫痫停止发作，改善意识状态。

• 治疗目标：与严重低钠血症相同。

• 用高渗盐水溶液(3%)。

• 当症状(即癫痫发作)解决时停止高渗盐水，并换为生理盐水。

• 静脉呋塞米可促进利尿并诱导负向液体平衡。

• 一旦血清钠=125 mmol/L，进一步静脉输液应为生理盐水溶液。

• 血清钠恢复至正常水平应在 48 h 后。

• 抑制 ADH 分泌/作用的药物：
- 当 SIADH 不能自我调控和病因无法纠正时。
- 考尼伐坦-托伐普坦(通过竞争性结合 V_2 受体，拮抗血中 AVP 水平的升高效应)。
- 地美环素(阻断 ADH 的作用)。

药物治疗

• 盐酸考尼伐坦：20 mg，静脉注射，超过 30 min(严重低钠血症，入院后使用)。

• 去甲四环素：300 mg，口服，每日 2～4 次。

• 高渗盐水溶液(3% NaCl)：250～500 ml(最大初始剂量 5 ml/kg)：
- 25～100 ml/h。
- 血钠限制在 0.5～1 mmol/(L·h)。
- 癫痫停止发作或血清钠达到 125 mmol/L 时停止使用。
- 血清钠升高 4～6 mmol/L 通常足以阻止癫痫发作。

• 生理盐水：维持液体。

• 利尿剂：1 mg/kg 至 20～40 mg。

随访

进一步处理

入院指征

• 严重的危及生命的低钠血症。

• 有症状低钠血症。

• 无论症状如何，血清钠<125 mmol/L。

• 新发作的 SIADH，必须诊断并治疗潜在的原因或并发症。

• 患者的依从性是一个问题。

出院指征

• 无症状性慢性低钠血症。

• 血清钠>125 mmol/L。

• 没有不稳定的其他因素。

• 明确诊断 SIADH。

随访建议

所有符合出院标准的低钠血症患者仍需要随访以检查是否解决疾病，同时监测和/或诊断 SIADH/低钠血症的潜在原因。

要点和误区

• SIADH 是排除性的诊断。

• 必须评估其他原因以及肾脏、甲状腺、肾上腺、心脏和肝功能。

• 了解彻底的药物治疗史。

• 仔细筛查恶性肿瘤的危险因素。

K

抗抑郁药中毒 Antidepressant Poisoning

Patrick M. Lank 李岩 王瑞兰 译

基础知识

描述

• 抗抑郁药是美国最常用的精神科药物。

• 过量服用抗抑郁药的患者可能会服用各种抗抑郁药，分为 SSRI、SNRI 和非典型抗抑郁药。并用非典型抗精神病药和稳定情绪的药物是很常见的，其中一些药物已获得 FDA 批准用于治疗抑郁症。

• 可以为多种其他适应证开具抗抑郁药，包括慢性疼痛综合征、焦虑症、进食障碍、药物滥用和睡眠障碍。

• 三环抗抑郁药(TCA)在单独的章节中介绍。

病因

机制

• 选择性5-羟色胺(5-HT)再摄取抑制剂(SSRI):
- 通过阻止突触前神经元重新摄取5-羟色胺来增加突触处的5-羟色胺。
- SSRI包括帕罗西汀、氟西汀、舍曲林、西酞普兰和艾司西酞普兰。

• 5-羟色胺-去甲肾上腺素再摄取抑制剂(SNRI):
- 类似于SSRI,但也抑制去甲肾上腺素的再摄取。
- 研制是因为据说在治疗剂量下比SSRI副作用更少,尽管毒性并非如此。
- SNRI包括文拉法辛、地文拉法辛和度洛西汀。

• 非典型抗抑郁药:
- 对5-羟色胺、去甲肾上腺素和多巴胺有不同的影响。
- 包括米氮平、曲唑酮和安非他酮。

• 非典型抗精神病药:
- 大多数抗精神病药物在多巴胺受体上都有活性,尽管不同的药物和多巴胺受体有不同的激动性/拮抗性。
- 增加在5-羟色胺或肾上腺素能、组胺和毒扁豆碱受体的活性。

• 精神科药物也有不同的钾和钠通道阻滞,导致心脏毒性(QT和QRS分别延长)。

诊断

症状和体征

• SSRI类药物:
- 传统的SSRI(氟西汀、帕罗西汀):
  ◦ 镇静。
  ◦ 5-羟色胺综合征。
  ◦ 在单药过量中,很少会引起严重的医疗影响。
- 西酞普兰和依他普仑:
  ◦ 嗜睡,呕吐,心动过速。
  ◦ QTc延长。
  ◦ 癫痫发作(西酞普兰中较常见)。
  ◦ 表现出延迟毒性(摄入后长达24 h)。

• SNRI:
- 度洛西汀:
  ◦ 嗜睡,呕吐,心动过速。
  ◦ 癫痫发作罕见。
- 文拉法辛和去甲文拉法辛:
  ◦ 癫痫发作。
  ◦ QTc延长。

• 非典型抗抑郁药:
- 安非他酮。
  ◦ 镇静。
  ◦ 癫痫发作。
  ◦ QRS和QTc延长。
- 曲唑酮:
  ◦ 镇静。
  ◦ QTc延长。
  ◦ 低血压。
  ◦ 阴茎异常勃起。
- 米氮平:
  ◦ 镇静。
  ◦ QTc延长。
  ◦ 长期用药可能引起中性粒细胞减少症。

• 非典型抗精神病药:
- 与典型的抗精神病药相比,开发用于减少锥体束外症状(EPS),特别是迟发性运动障碍。
- 服用过量的最常见症状包括镇静、心动过速和瞳孔缩小。
- 氯氮平:
  ◦ 粒细胞缺乏症(长期服用者占1%)。
  ◦ 流口水。
  ◦ 心肌病。
  ◦ 抗胆碱能谵妄。
- 奥氮平:
  ◦ 抗胆碱能谵妄。
  ◦ QTc延长。
- 喹硫平:
  ◦ 明显的α_1拮抗作用引起的低血压。
  ◦ QTc延长。
  ◦ 抗胆碱能谵妄。
- 齐普拉西酮:
  ◦ 镇静。
  ◦ QTc延长→扭转风险增加。
- 阿立哌唑:
  ◦ 无QTc延长。
  ◦ 低血压。
  ◦ 中枢神经系统功能障碍。

基本检查

• 确定摄入的药物、剂量和摄入的时间:
- 调查同时服用的药物。

• 如果精神状态改变,需测床边快速血糖(Accu-Chek)。

诊断测查与说明

实验室检查

• 特定的药物水平很少,通常不指导临床管理。
• 心电图:
- 评估QT间期和QRS波群宽度。
• 尿妊娠试验:
- 育龄期妇女。
• 电解质、尿素氮、肌酐、葡萄糖。
• 血浆渗透压:
- 不能依靠血清渗透压排除其他药物的摄入,如有毒性的酒精。
• 常规毒理学筛查:
- 很少改变临床管理。
• 水杨酸和对乙酰氨基酚的水平。
• 血浆乙醇:
- 排除酒精中毒是精神状态改变的原因。
- 如果测量渗透压摩尔需要。
• 动脉/静脉血气(ABG/VBG)。
- 检测pH。

影像学检查

• 脑部CT用于评估精神状态改变的其他原因。
• 如果气管插管或缺氧需做CXR。

鉴别诊断

• 三环类抗抑郁药物过量。
• 酒精过量。
• 异烟肼过量。
• 低血糖。
• 低氧血症。
• 低钠血症。
• 低钙血症。
• 戒断综合征。
• 5-羟色胺综合征。
• 头部外伤。
• 阿片类药物中毒。
• 镇静催眠药中毒。
• 情绪稳定剂、抗癫痫药过量。
• 糖尿病酮症酸中毒。

治疗

院前

• 在疑似服药过量的情况下,将所有的药物和患者都带到医院去。
• ABC管理。
• 为了维持血压稳定,静脉注射生理盐水。
• 苯二氮䓬类药物用于癫痫发作。

▪ 初步稳定/治疗

• ABC 管理：
- 吸氧。
- 重视心电监护和监测动脉血氧饱和度。
- 用生理盐水建立静脉通路。
- 气管插管来保护气道或维持呼吸状态。
• 快速床边血糖测定。
• 表明有精神状态改变需给予纳洛酮，硫胺素和 $D_{50}W$：
- 氟马西尼不推荐用于混合性药物过量的患者、患者有潜在的癫痫发作或者患者长期使用苯二氮䓬类药物。
• 可以给予苯海拉明 25～50 mg，肌内注射或静脉注射；或苄托品 1 mg，口服，EPS。

▪ 急诊治疗/程序

• 胃肠道净化：
- 不要尝试在一个没有稳定气道的患者身上进行清洗。
- 尽管气管插管可单独用于净化的目的，但不常用。
- 50～75 g 活性炭口服或经鼻胃管（NGT）打入，如果患者气管插管早期过量服用可能会获益。
- 单独使用本章列出的药物过量的患者，一般不需要洗胃。
• 对于 QRS 波群增宽的患者，采用碳酸氢钠静脉推注。
• 治疗性对静脉输液反应迟钝的低血压，由于 α_1 受体的拮抗作用，采用去甲肾上腺素而非多巴胺。
• 治疗癫痫：
- 初始治疗：苯二氮䓬。
- 难治性癫痫发作：苯巴比妥。
• 治疗 5-羟色胺综合征的症状（发热、AMS、心动过速、死板、反射亢进）用苯二氮䓬类。

▪ 药物治疗

• 活性炭：口服初始剂量 50～75 g；最好允许每 1 g 摄入的异生物素含 10 g 木炭，最高可耐受 100 g 口服。
• 苯革平：1 mg，口服或静脉注射。
• 地西泮：静脉推注 5～10 mg（儿童：0.1 mg/kg，静脉注射；或 0.5 mg/kg 直肠）。
• 苯海拉明：25～50 mg，肌内注射或静脉注射（儿童：1 mg/kg）。
• 劳拉西泮：静脉推注 2～4 mg（儿童：0.03～0.05 mg/kg）。
• 纳洛酮：初次推注 0.4～2 mg（儿童：0.1 mg/kg），最多可以重复 10 mg。
• 去甲肾上腺素：0.5～2 μg/kg，静脉注射。
• 苯巴比妥：15～20 mg/kg，静脉注射，最大剂量为 2 g；注意：静脉内负荷剂量可能发展为呼吸抑制。
• 碳酸氢钠：静脉推注 1 mmol/kg（成人：8.4%；儿童：<50 kg，4.2%）。

随访

▪ 进一步处理

入院指征

• 摄入以下物质可进行 24 h 遥测：西酞普兰、依西酞普兰、文拉法辛、去甲文拉法辛、安非他酮。
- 服用其他抗抑郁药 6 h 后无症状的患者无需入院。
• 昏迷。
• 精神状态改变。
• NMS 的症状。
• 血流动力学紊乱。
• 心电图改变。
• 自杀的患者应给予一对一的观察。

出院指征

• 摄入后 6 h 内毒性较小的抗抑郁药的无症状患者可通过医学检查以接受精神科入院。
• 仅无自杀倾向的无症状患者(即意外接触)。

▪ 随访建议

故意过量的患者需精神科转诊。

要点和误区

• 对于 QRS 波群增宽，给予碳酸氢钠静脉推注。
• 治疗性对静脉输液反应迟钝的低血压，由于 α_1 受体的拮抗作用，采用去甲肾上腺素而非多巴胺。

咳嗽 Cough

Alison Sisitsiky Curcio　陈奇通 译

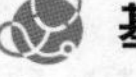

基础知识

▪ 描述

• 一种气道强烈的收缩导致气体从肺部释放，经常伴有独特的声音：
- 深吸气。
- 声门关闭。
- 呼气肌的收缩。
- 肺内压力的增加。
- 声门的开放。
- 高压气体的呼出。
- 分泌物和异物排出。
- 声带、支气管管壁、肺实质的共振。
• 清除气道异物与分泌物的防御机制：
- 自主或非自主的咳嗽。
• 非自主的咳嗽由迷走神经的传入神经调节：
- 自主咳嗽由皮质中枢控制。
- 因为大脑皮质的控制，安慰剂可以对咳嗽产生显著的影响。
- 咳嗽反射包括呼吸道受体的激活，通过传入神经元传到咳嗽中枢，随后输出到呼吸肌。
- 在喉、气管、隆突的机械受体，以及触觉和位移觉感受器。
- 在喉、气管及支气管的化学受体对气体和烟雾敏感。
- 被刺激物、黏液、水肿、脓液和热刺激所激活。
• 严重咳嗽的并发症：
- 鼻出血。
- 结膜下出血。
- 晕厥。
- 气胸。
- 纵隔气肿。
- 呕吐。
- 疝。
- 直肠脱垂。
- 尿失禁。
- 癫痫发作。
- 脑炎。
- 颅内出血。

- 脊髓硬膜外出血。
- 杵状指。
- 发痒的皮疹。

病因

- 急性(<3 周)。
- 肺炎。
- 急性支气管炎。
- 鼻窦炎。
- 百日咳。
- 肺结核。
- 上呼吸道感染。
- 咳嗽变异性哮喘。
- COPD 加重。
- 支气管扩张症。
- 肺栓塞。
- 左心室衰竭。
- 气道阻塞(食品、药丸)。
- 胃食管反流病。
- 过敏。
- 支气管痉挛。
- 亚急性(3～8 周)。
- 感染后咳嗽。
- 百日咳。
- 支气管炎。
- 细菌性鼻窦炎。
- 哮喘。
- 胃食管反流。
- 肺栓塞。
- 慢性(>8 周)。
- 鼻后滴漏。
- 哮喘。
- 胃食管反流病。
- 慢性支气管炎。
- 肺结核。
- 支气管扩张症。
- 嗜酸粒细胞性支气管炎。
- 血管紧张素转换酶抑制剂。
- 支气管癌。
- 癌病。
- 结节病。
- 左心室衰竭。
- 吸入综合征。
- 心理因素/习惯。

儿科注意事项

- 最常见的原因:
  - 哮喘。
  - 病毒性疾病。
  - 急性支气管炎。
  - 肺炎。
  - 鼻窦炎。
  - 胃食管反流。
- 不太常见的原因:
  - 气管支气管软化症。
  - 纵隔肿瘤。
  - 非紫绀型先天性心脏病。
  - 室间隔缺损。
  - 动脉导管未闭。
  - 肺动脉狭窄。
  - 法洛四联症。
  - 卡入的异物。
  - 慢性吸入的牛奶。
  - 环境暴露。
- 需要考虑的问题:
  - 新生儿的病史。
  - 喂养史。
  - 生长发育史。
  - 过敏。
  - 湿疹。
  - 睡眠障碍。
  - X 线胸片的适应证:
  - 怀疑误食异物。
  - 怀疑误吸。

诊断

症状和体征

- 痰的性状:
  - 泡沫(肺水肿)。
  - 黏液脓性。
  - 提示细菌性肺炎或支气管炎,但也可见于病毒感染。
  - 铁锈色(肺炎球菌肺炎)。
  - "葡萄干果冻样"(肺炎克雷伯菌)。
  - 咯血。
  - 咳嗽后晕厥或呕吐(表明百日咳)。
  - 呼吸急促。
  - 胸部疼痛。
  - 冷或热。
  - 夜间盗汗。
  - 气喘。
- 胃食管反流:
  - 烧心(上腹部烧灼感)。
  - 吞咽困难。
  - 反流。
  - 嗳气。
  - 早饱。
- 恶性疾病的表现:
  - 体重下降。
  - 食欲不振。
  - 疲劳。

病史

- 根据咳嗽的持续时间分为急性、亚急性和慢性。
- 如果存在痰液、咯血应描述其性状。
- 咳嗽后呕吐、晕厥、阵发性咳嗽表明百日咳。
- 有胃肠道症状的病史提示胃食管反流。
- 在慢性咳嗽中,体重减轻和盗汗提示肺结核。

体格检查

- 生命体征。
- 呼吸音异常:
  - 缺失或减少。
  - 气流减少与过度充气。
  - 啰音:打开闭合的肺泡爆裂音:
    - 湿啰音、干啰音、细啰音、粗啰音。
  - 鼾音:当大气道阻塞时会发出打呼噜的声音。
  - 哮鸣音:狭窄气道所产生的高调、尖锐的声音。
  - 喘鸣:上气道梗阻。
- 呼吸窘迫的证据:
  - 使用辅助肌。
  - 腹式呼吸。

基本检查

- 完整医学史:
  - 时间。
  - 相关症状。
  - 患者的接触史。
  - 吸烟暴露史。
  - ACE 抑制剂(ACEI)的使用。
  - 获得性免疫缺陷综合征(艾滋病)或免疫功能低下的状态。
  - 潜在暴露于结核。
- 心电图:
  - 心脏疾病史。
  - 相关的胸痛或异常的体征。
  - 缺乏感染症状。

诊断检查与说明

实验室检查

- 根据症状和体征:
  - 血白细胞计数。
  - 痰革兰染色、痰培养和药物敏感性。
  - 抗酸杆菌培养。
  - CD4 细胞计数。
  - 百日咳的抗体滴度。
  - D-二聚体。
  - 流感咽拭子检查(具有高危因素和有接触

K

史的患者）。

影像学检查

• 胸部 X 线片：
- 免疫功能低下的患者。
- 在急性咳嗽和咳痰的健康患者中有以下至少一项：
  ◦ 心率＞100 次/分。
  ◦ 呼吸率＞24 次/分。
  ◦ 口腔体温＞38℃。
  ◦ 胸部的检查发现有局部的实变、羊鸣音及震颤。
- 病态衰弱的出现。
- 慢性咳嗽性状的变化。
- 停用 ACEI 后仍持续的咳嗽。
- 抑制剂。

• 胸部 CT。
- 胸片异常。
- 评估肺栓塞。

诊断步骤/外科

• 峰流速。
• 纤维支气管镜检查：
- 胸部 X 线发现的不明性质的肿块。
- 咯血。
- 疑似癌症。

鉴别诊断

见病因。

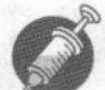

治疗

初步稳定/治疗

评估气道、呼吸和循环。

急诊治疗/程序

病因治疗：

• 呼吸道感染：考虑抗生素、抗病毒药物（流感）、减充血剂和止咳药。
• 哮喘：吸入 β_2 受体激动剂和类固醇。
• 胃食管反流：H_2 受体阻滞剂、质子泵抑制剂和抗酸剂。
• 怀疑百日咳：大环内酯类和 5 日隔离。
• 慢性支气管炎急性发作：吸入 β_2 受体激动剂和类固醇。
• 恶性肿瘤：支持治疗。

药物治疗

• 抗生素：
- 挑选合适的抗菌药物覆盖疑似细菌。

• 抗病毒药物：
- 达菲：75 mg（儿童：30～75 mg），口服，每日 2 次×5 日。

• 镇咳药：
- 可待因：10～20 mg[儿童：1～1.5 mg/(kg·d)]，q4～6 h，口服。
- 右美沙芬：10～20[儿童：1 mg/(kg·d)]，q6～8 h，口服。
- 氢可酮：5～10 mg[儿童：0.6 mg/(kg·d)]，q6～8 h，口服。

• 支气管扩张剂：
- 沙丁胺醇：2.5 mg 加入 2.5 ml 生理盐水中（儿童：每次 0.1～0.15 mg/kg）q20 min 吸入。
- 异丙托溴铵：0.5 mg 加入 3 ml 生理盐水中（儿童：喷雾器每次 250～500 μg，q6 h），q3 h。

• 减充血剂：
- 扑尔敏：4～12 mg（儿童：2 mg，口服，q4～6 h），口服，q4～12 h。
- 苯丙醇胺：25～50 mg（儿童：6.25～12.5 mg，口服，q4 h），口服，q4～8 h。

• 黏液溶解剂：
- 愈创木酚甘油醚：200～400 mg（儿童：2～5 岁，50～100 mg，口服；6～11 岁，100～200 mg，口服，q4 h），必要时。

• 类固醇：
- 地塞米松：2 喷/鼻吸入，每日 2 次。
- 甲泼尼龙：60～125 mg，静脉[儿童用药：1～2 mg/kg]，静脉/口服，q6 h]。
- 泼尼松：40～60 mg[儿童用药：1～2 mg/(kg·d)，q12 h]，口服。

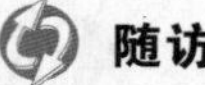

随访

进一步处理

入院指征

• 低氧血症或危重状态。
• 胸部 X 线检查结果阳性的疑似肺结核。
• 免疫功能低下合并发热。
• 有菌血症或脓毒症的风险。

出院指征

• 患者的氧合达标。
• 口服药物。
• 家里环境安全。

转诊问题

密切随访至初级保健医师进行门诊管理。

随访建议

• 戒烟，避免被动吸烟或吸入其他如石棉等有害物质。
• 改变饮食：
- 避免咖啡、茶、苏打水。
- 睡觉前至少 4 h 避免进食。
- 用枕头保持头在夜间抬高。
• 有以下情况应立即就医：
- 胸痛。
- 咯血。
- 气短。
- 晕倒。

要点和误区

• 对于临床上符合因胃食管反流而引起咳嗽的患者来说，推荐在最初的诊断做出后即启动治疗。
• 对于假设诊断为急性支气管炎的患者，没有理由证明常规抗生素治疗是有效的，同时也不应提供给患者。

可卡因中毒 Cocaine Poisoning

Steven E. Aks 陈奇通 译

基础知识

描述

• 拟交感。
• 抑制神经末梢对神经递质的重吸收。
• 代谢：
- 肝脏降解。
- 非酶催化的水解。
- 胆碱酯酶代谢。

病因

• 静脉、经鼻或口服摄入可卡因。
• 口服吸收。
- 人体填塞毒品者：

- 为逃避警察而吞入装有可卡因的袋子。
- 人体包裹毒品者：
  - 将装有可卡因的袋子藏在运输者的口腔、直肠或阴道内以走私。
  - 大量的可卡因被隐蔽地包在口袋中。

诊断

症状与体征

- 拟交感中毒症状。
- 心血管系统：
  - 高血压。
  - 心动过速。
  - 胸痛(心绞痛)。
- 呼吸系统：
  - 呼吸过快。
  - 胸膜性胸痛。
    - 纵隔气肿。
    - 气胸。
    - 支气管炎。
    - 肺栓塞。
  - 咳嗽。
- 中枢神经系统：
  - 躁动。
  - 震颤。
  - 昏迷。
  - 癫痫发作。
  - 脑卒中(中风)。
- 其他：
  - 体温增高(预后差)。
  - 肢体缺血(无意的动脉内注射)。
  - 角膜溃疡(中毒吸食可卡因烟者)：
    - 因局部化学和温度刺激而破坏了角膜上皮的完整性。
  - 横纹肌溶解。

病史

对于身体包裹和填塞者：

- 摄取的时长。
- 摄取的途径(经口、直肠或者阴道)。
- 摄取的袋数。
- 包装的物质和方式。

体格检查

拟交感中毒症状：

- 高血压。
- 心动过速。
- 呼吸增快。
- 流汗。
- 瞳孔放大。
- 神经肌肉高反应性。

基本检查

- 识别由可卡因导致的拟交感性中毒症状。
  - 与抗胆碱能中毒症状鉴别。
- 中毒症状的识别：
  - 拟交感性：
    - 心率(心动过速)。
    - 血压(增高)。
    - 皮肤潮湿。
    - 肠鸣音存在。
    - 体温(增高)。
    - 无尿潴留。
  - 抗胆碱能：
    - 心率(心动过速)。
    - 血压(增高)。
    - 皮肤干燥。
    - 肠鸣音消失。
    - 体温(增高)。
    - 尿潴留存在。

诊断检查与说明

实验室检查

- 全血计数。
- 电解质、尿素氮、血肌酐和血糖。
- 尿肌红蛋白检查。
- 心肌酶谱[肌钙蛋白、磷酸肌酸(CPK)]用于存在有：
  - 心绞痛性胸痛。
  - 异常心电图。
- 存在肌红蛋白尿者需行 CPK 检查。
- 毒物筛查。

影像学检查

- 心电图：
  - 存在心绞痛性胸痛者。
  - 可卡因相关胸痛考虑存在心肌梗死可能者。
- 胸片：
  - 存在胸痛或气短者。
  - 寻找纵隔气肿、气胸或主动脉破裂。
- 腹部摄片：
  - 为身体藏毒、填塞走私者。
  - 填塞走私者常检查为阴性结果，因毒品常被玻璃纸松散包裹。
  - 身体藏毒者常检查为阳性，因毒品包裹紧密，摄片常表现为斑块影。
- 腹部增强 CT：
  - 当身体藏毒、填塞走私者的采集病史不可靠，腹部摄片无发现时使用。
- 头颅 CT 扫描：
  - 存在意识改变或有严重头痛者。
  - 寻找脑缺血或出血。

鉴别诊断

- 其他具有拟交感作用的药物。
- 茶碱。
- 咖啡因。
- 苯丙胺。
- 沙丁胺醇。
- 三环类抗抑郁药。
- 抗组胺药。
- 苯环利定(PCP)。
- 甲状腺毒症。
- 安定药恶性综合征。
- 致幻药。

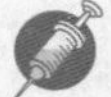

治疗

院前

- 开放静脉通路。
- 心电监护：
  - 胸痛可能为缺血性的。
  - 苯二氮䓬用于控制烦躁。
- 如果毒品为“快球”(海洛因和可卡因混合物)，应使用纳洛酮加速逆转昏迷。

初步稳定/治疗

- ABC 管理。
- 建立静脉通路。
- 进行心电监护。
- 使用纳洛酮(narcan)、硫胺素、葡萄糖(或 Accu-Check)改善意识情况。

急诊治疗/程序

- 对于症状轻微的患者进行支持治疗。
- 苯二氮䓬类药物：
  - 用于烦躁和震颤。
  - 用于高血压和心动过速的起始药物。
- 体温增高的降温方法：
  - 蒸发-对流方式。
- 横纹肌溶解的治疗：
  - 使用生理盐水水化。
  - 对于严重的患者静脉使用碳酸氢钠进行碱化。
- 心源性胸痛：
  - 阿司匹林。
  - 硝酸盐药物。
  - 氧气。
  - 阿片类药物。
  - 避免使用 β 受体阻滞剂，因 α 受体刺激无法被拮抗。
  - 急性心肌梗死需进行血管造影、血管成形术、溶栓。

• 高血压、心动过速。
- 苯二氮䓬类药物为起始药物。
- 如对苯二氮䓬类药物无反应，则单用 α 受体阻滞剂（酚妥拉明）或与 β 受体阻滞剂（普萘洛尔、艾司洛尔）合用。
- 谨慎使用拉贝洛尔（含有的 α 受体和 β 受体阻滞剂成分不等量）。
- 严重无反应性高血压者，静脉使用硝酸甘油、硝普钠。
• 身体藏毒者、身体填塞走私者。
- 不典型或轻微症状的身体藏毒者和身体填塞走私者的治疗：
◦ 单次剂量的活性炭适用于不典型或轻微症状的身体填塞者。
◦ 聚乙烯乙二醇电解质灌洗液全肠道灌洗（效用未知）。
- 有症状的身体藏毒和填塞者应请外科医师会诊。
◦ 如果使用之前所述药物治疗未能轻易控制药物毒性者，需手术取出毒品包。

药物治疗

一线药物

• 地西泮（安定）：每次增加 5 mg，静脉注射。
• 劳拉西泮：每次增加 2 mg，静脉注射。

二线药物

• 活性炭悬浊液：1～2 g/kg 至 90 g，口服。
• 葡萄糖：$D_{50}W$ 1 安瓿（50 ml 或者 25 g）（儿童：$D_{25}W$ 2～4 ml/kg），静脉使用。
• 艾司洛尔：50～200 μg/（kg · min），静脉输注，滴定至药效。
• 纳洛酮（narcan）：2 mg（儿童：0.1 mg/kg 至 2 mg），静脉或初次肌内注射。
• 硝酸甘油：10～100 μg/min，静脉输注。
• 硝普钠：0.3 μg/（kg · min），静脉使用[滴定至药效可达到 10 μg/（kg · min）]。
• 酚妥拉明：每 15～24 min，静脉使用 5 mg（滴定至临床效果）。
• 聚乙烯乙二醇（Golytely）：1～2 L，口服/h 直至毒品包排出（效用存在争议）。

 随访

进一步处理

入院指征

• 意识状态改变。
• 生命体征异常：心率大于 100 次/分，舒张压大于 120 mmHg，或低血压。
• 体温增高。
• 可卡因所致的心肌缺血。
• 身体藏毒和身体填塞走私者。
• 中至重度中毒者收治 ICU。

出院指征

• 观察 6 h 后意识状态和生命体征正常。
• 毒品包确认排出且无中毒临床表现的身体藏毒或填塞走私者。
• 携带非复杂性毒品包且无症状 12～24 h 的身体填塞者可出院。

要点和误区

• 苯二氮䓬类药物为可卡因拟交感中毒的一线治疗。
• 高动力性可卡因中毒的患者应避免使用 β 受体阻滞剂。
• 可卡因相关的胸痛有较广的鉴别诊断需考虑。
• 腹部平片对身体藏毒者有一定用处，但对身体填塞者的毒品包成像无价值。

口腔溃疡 Aphthous Ulcers

Matthew R. Berkman　李岩　王瑞兰 译

 基础知识

描述

口腔或生殖器黏膜发生的疼痛性圆形或卵圆形溃疡：
• 通常被称为“口腔溃疡”。

病因

• 单一病因：未知。
• 可能与多种因素有一定的相关性：
- 免疫功能紊乱，细胞介导的免疫系统激活。
- 感染。
- 食物过敏（即麸质）。
- 维生素缺乏。
- 妊娠。
- 月经。
- 创伤。
- 应激。
- 免疫缺陷。
- 药物：β 受体阻滞剂、抗感染药物。
• 流行病学：通常发生在儿童和年轻的成人（10～30 岁），占总人口的 20%～30%。
- 更常见于女性。
- 不太常见于吸烟者。
- 可能是家族性遗传。

诊断

症状和体征

• 少见的口腔溃疡。
- 占所有口腔溃疡的 70%～90%。
- <直径为 8 mm，一次可同时出现 5 个。
- 疼痛，浅溃疡伴中心坏死。
- 边缘隆起和红色晕。
- 灰白色假膜。
- 影响前口腔非角化黏膜。
◦ 唇、颊黏膜。
◦ 口底。
◦ 舌腹侧表面。
- 很少发现在舌背、硬腭或牙龈。
- 持续 10～14 日，不留瘢痕。
- 发热或全身症状很少出现。
• 主要的口腔溃疡或 Sutton 病。
- 占所有口腔溃疡的 10%～15%。
- 外观直径>1 cm，一次 1～10 个溃疡。
- 较深。
- 涉及包括咽、软/硬腭在内的所有口咽。
- 持续数周至数月，可以瘢痕愈合。
- 常伴有基础疾病。
- 很少发热。
• 疱疹样口腔溃疡：
- 占所有口腔溃疡的 7%～10%。
- 多个小簇。
- 直径 1～3 mm，任意时间可存在 10～100 个，可融合成斑块。
- 疱疹样性质，但病变部位培养不会出现单纯疱疹病毒。

K

- 持续 7～30 日，可能会产生瘢痕。

病史

• 燃烧或刺伤口腔黏膜 1～2 日感觉出现溃疡的前驱症状。
• 询问 SLE、炎症性肠病(IBD)、Behçet 病、Reiter 病 HIV、癌症家族史。
• 询问有性生活史的患者梅毒或疱疹病毒史。
• 询问目前使用的药物：
- 非甾体抗炎药。
- β受体阻滞剂。

体格检查

• 见症状和体征。
• 寻找脱水的迹象：
- 生命体征应在正常范围内。
- 评估黏膜状况。
• 评估继发感染的症状。
• 评估溃疡的系统性原因的症状(见病史)。

基本检查

• 由病史和临床表现获得诊断。
• 排除系统性疾病的口腔表现：
- 如果持续大于 3 周或与体质的症状相关。
• 关注眼、口、生殖器、皮肤、胃肠道、过敏的症状和饮食情况，以及身体状况。

诊断检查与说明

实验室检查

常规实验室检查不能确诊：
• 只有当怀疑系统病因导致溃疡时。
• 应以病史和体格检查为指导：
- CBC 系列。
- 快速血浆反应素试验。
- 荧光螺旋体抗体吸收试验。
- 抗核抗体试验。
- Tzanck 涂片：包涵体巨细胞(疱疹病毒)。
- 活检：多核巨细胞(巨细胞病毒)。
- 真菌培养。

诊断步骤/外科

任何溃疡>3 周应考虑门诊活检。

鉴别诊断

• 创伤：
- 咬伤。
- 补牙。
- 支架。
• 药物暴露：
- 非甾体抗炎药。
- 尼可地尔。
- β受体阻滞剂。
• 感染：
- 疱疹病毒属：
◦ 水疱。
◦ 附着黏膜溃疡。
- 巨细胞病毒：
◦ 免疫功能低下的患者。
- 水痘病毒：
◦ 典型的皮肤病变。
- 柯萨基病毒：
◦ 囊泡前溃疡。
◦ 手、足、臀部病变。
- 梅毒：
◦ 其他皮肤或生殖器病变。
- 多形性红斑：
◦ 唇部结痂。
◦ 独立的或与之连接的皮肤黏膜损害。
- 隐孢子虫感染毛霉、组织胞浆菌病。
- 坏死性牙龈炎。
• 潜在的疾病：
- Behçet 综合征：
◦ 生殖器溃疡。
◦ 葡萄膜炎。
◦ 视网膜炎。
- 反应性关节炎(Reiter 综合征)：
◦ 葡萄膜炎。
◦ 尿道炎。
◦ HLA-B27 相关性关节炎。
- Sweet 综合征：
◦ 发热。
◦ 皮肤红斑或结节。
◦ 与肿瘤有关。
- IBD：
◦ 血性或黏液性腹泻。
◦ 消化道溃疡。
◦ 体重降低。
- 红斑狼疮：
◦ 颧部红斑。
◦ ANA 阳性。
- 大疱性类天疱疮和寻常类天疱疮：
◦ 连接性和独立的黏膜水疱性病变。
◦ 弥漫性皮肤受累。
- 周期性中性粒细胞减少症：
◦ 周期性发热。
- 鳞状细胞癌：
◦ 慢性。
◦ 头/颈部淋巴结肿大。
• 免疫功能低下的患者：
◦ 艾滋病。
◦ 粒细胞缺乏症。
◦ 恶性肿瘤。

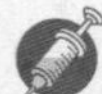

治疗

院前

• 以症状严重程度和持续时间为导向的治疗。
• 目标是缓解疼痛和减少炎症。

药物治疗

• 轻度至中度疾病：
- 避免口腔创伤/酸性食物。
- 保持良好的口腔卫生。
◦ 使用软牙刷、牙线、不含酒精的漱口水。
- 表面麻醉剂：
◦ 氢氧化镁/盐酸苯海拉明 5 mg/5 ml，1/1 混合，吐出。
◦ 2%～5%黏性利多卡因：饭后用于溃疡每日 4 次，直至痊愈。
- 保护性生物黏合剂：
◦ 曲克芦丁悬浮液。
◦ 外用非处方药制剂(Orabase，Anbesol)：饭后用于溃疡，每日 4 次，直至痊愈。
- 外用抗炎：
◦ 5%氨来昔洛糊剂(阿帕索尔)：饭后用于溃疡，每日 4 次，直至痊愈。
- 抗菌漱口水：
◦ 0.12%葡萄糖酸氯己定含漱液(培立思)：饭后漱口，每日 4 次，直至痊愈。
• 严重的疾病：
- 全身性用药。
◦ 泼尼松片：口服泼尼松 30～60 mg/d，持续 4～7 日。
◦ 秋水仙碱：0.6～1.2 mg/d 直至症状改善。
◦ 沙利度胺：每日 50～200 mg 口服×4 周。

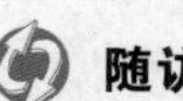

随访

进一步处理

入院指征

• 适当的镇痛后不能饮食或饮水。
• 异常生命体征或脱水的证据。

出院指征

• 可以进行流体饮食。
• 足够的镇痛。
• 生命体征正常。

转诊问题

如果病变没有在 2 周内得到解决，需要后续的基本医疗服务。

K

■ 随访建议

• 避免口腔创伤(硬食物)或酸性食物。

• 如果怀疑有潜在的疾病要转诊至相关专家。

要点和误区

• 口腔溃疡绝大多数是良性的、自限性的,需对症处理。

• 急诊医师必须考虑潜在的全身性溃疡的原因。

口腔念珠菌病 Candidiasis, Oral

Adam Z. Barkin 陈丽 译

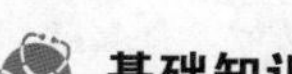

基础知识

■ 描述

• 念珠菌是一种真菌。

• 念珠菌是机会性感染。

• 口腔黏膜可以感染任何类型的念珠菌。

• 80%的分离株为白色念珠菌(最常见)、光滑念珠菌和热带念珠菌。

• 念珠菌通常作为口腔菌群存在于60%的健康人群中。

• 携带率随年龄增长递增。

• 变种包括:

- 假膜(鹅口疮)。
- 慢性和急性念珠菌萎缩。
- 口角炎。
- 增生性念珠菌病。

• 新生儿、老年人和口服免疫抑制剂的患者更常见。

• 在健康患者中通常是良性过程。

• 在免疫力低下的患者更可能是复发或是非白色念珠菌种。

• 在艾滋病病毒感染的患者中可能是早期表现。

• 典型的局限性。

• 系统感染的危险因素:

- 艾滋病-口腔表现最常见。
- 糖尿病。
- 住院患者。
- 免疫抑制治疗。
- 恶性肿瘤。
- 中性粒细胞减少。
- 器官移植。
- 早产。

■ 病因

• 当口腔环境改变时通常有白色念珠菌的过度生长。

• 可能是药物引起,常用的有抗生素、吸入或全身用类固醇、化疗药物、免疫抑制剂。

• 唾液流量的改变或减少:

- 抗胆碱能或精神药物。
- 干燥病。
- 头或颈部放射。

• 义齿(假牙)或其他正畸存在:

- 发生在50%~65%的牙颌。
- 慢性萎缩性念珠菌病病因。

• 上皮屏障中断(咬颊症)。

• 内分泌疾病(糖尿病,甲状腺功能减退)。

儿科注意事项

• 急性假膜性念珠菌病(鹅口疮)常见于婴儿期,因为他们的免疫系统不成熟,缺乏成熟的口腔菌群。

• 起始的症状可能是喂养困难,它继发于吞咽困难。

• 可能有念珠菌合并尿布疹。

• 如果母乳喂养,考虑母体治疗:

- 念珠菌在产妇乳房定植可引起持续性鹅口疮。询问产妇有无乳房疼痛、灼热、瘙痒或皮肤破裂。

老年人注意事项

• 念珠菌生物体常作为口腔菌群存在于65%~88%的老年人或那些长期护理设施里。

• 义齿可导致念珠菌增生。

• 口角炎多见于中老年人,它继发于面部皱纹。

诊断

■ 症状和体征

• 假膜性念珠菌病(鹅口疮):

- 无痛白色黏膜斑。
- 贴壁但可移除斑。
- 红斑基底。
- 可融合成大片或凝聚。
- 厌食,吞咽困难。

• 念珠菌性红斑病:

- 也称为红斑念珠菌病。
- 口腔或舌有烧灼感。
- 红斑很少,如有白色斑块,通常在上腭或舌背。
- 舌可能是鲜红色,类似于营养缺乏。
- 很少有白斑。

• 义齿性口炎:

- 也称为慢性萎缩性念珠菌病。
- 刺激义齿周围黏膜。
- 光滑或颗粒状红斑常局限于硬腭。
- 常与角性唇炎相关。
- 65%的义齿佩戴者常发生。

• 口角炎:

- 在口角有开裂或红斑。
- 病变可无症状、瘙痒或疼痛。
- 与葡萄球菌或链球菌二重感染是常见的。

• 增生性念珠菌病:

- 慢性,侵袭性溃疡。
- 白色、牢固黏附的斑点或板块。
- 通常为双侧。
- 通常在舌或颊黏膜横向边界。
- 在吸烟者中癌变率较高。

• 症状可能有所不同:

- 可能无痛。
- 灼痛。
- 言语障碍。
- 味觉受损。
- 无法进食。

■ 基本检查

• 在其他方面正常的婴儿简单的检查就可以做出临床诊断。

• 确定是否有破坏宿主因素的原因。

• 如有没有找到原因,评估HIV感染或糖尿病的可能性。

• 排除全身性感染。

■ 诊断检查与说明

• 临床诊断通常就足够了。

• 如果怀疑严重感染行CBC检查。

K

· 血糖测试。

· PAS 染色法、KOH、真菌培养：

- 分枝、线状菌丝、孢子或假菌丝可能被找到。

- 如果一线治疗失败或者高危人群（HIV/AIDS、中性粒细胞减少症、移植等），需行培养和药敏试验。

鉴别诊断

· 毛状白斑。

· 扁平苔藓。

· 鳞状细胞癌。

· 食物或牛奶黏附。

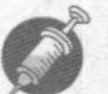

治疗

急诊治疗/程序

· 如果脱水和/或不能忍受口服流体的要静脉输液。

· 外用镇痛："神奇漱口水"。

- 2%黏性利多卡因、抗酸药和苯海拉明等分混合。

- 漱口 1～2 min，然后吐出。

· 外用抗真菌药物：

- 悬浮液，含片，锭剂。

- 软膏（口角炎）。

· 全身用药用于那些严重过感染或者耐药患者的治疗。

· 提供口腔卫生教育：

- 指导那些用类固醇吸入器的患者，用后应立即漱口。

- 义齿和正畸护理。

药物治疗

儿科注意事项

· 含片溶解在奶瓶里。

· 悬浮液患者果汁并冻成冰棒。

· 用棉签蘸取悬浮液处理基底面。

· 指导家长对牙刷、奶嘴、奶瓶进行消毒和更换。

老年人注意事项

· 口角炎：用外用制霉菌素药膏治疗。

· 义齿（假牙）：夜间去除，刷，浸泡。考虑隔夜用 2%洗必泰（氯己定）冲洗。

一线用药

· 制霉菌素：口服混悬液；新生儿 10 万 U；较大婴儿：20 万 U；儿童/成人：40 万～60 万 U。

· 每日 3 次漱口并咽下，维持 7～14 日。

· 制霉菌素锭剂：20 万 U 口服，每日 4 次，共 7～14 日。

· 克霉唑锭剂：10 mg 溶解后口服，每日 5 次，共 7～14 日（儿童>3 岁）。

二线用药

· 口服氟康唑：第 1 日负荷剂量 200 mg（儿童：6 mg/kg），然后 100 mg（儿童：3 mg/kg）每日口服，共 7～14 日。

· 伊曲康唑溶液：200 mg（儿童：>5 岁，2.5 mg/kg，每日 2 次，未经 FDA 批准）每日口服，共 7～14 日。

· 泊沙康唑：第 1 日 100 mg（儿童：>13 岁参照成人剂量），每日 2 次口服，然后每日 100 mg 口服，持续 13 日。

· 两性霉素 B（0.3 mg/kg）：每日口服，为治疗孕妇念珠菌的首选。

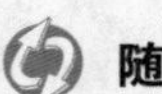

随访

进一步处理

入院指征

· 不能耐受口服摄入。

· 新诊断的免疫功能低下状态。

· 全身性感染。

出院指征

如果念珠菌感染不能威胁患者的水合状态，出院。

随访建议

在大龄儿童和成人不明原因的念珠菌感染中，关于免疫缺陷的额外检查是必需的。

要点和误区

· 没有识别的免疫缺陷。

· 没有识别的其他口腔病变，如鳞状细胞癌。

库欣综合征 Cushing Syndrome

Rami A. Ahmed · Brad D. Gable 陈奇通 译

基础知识

描述

· 库欣病：垂体腺瘤产生过量的促肾上腺皮质激素（ACTH）。

· 库欣综合征：过度的糖皮质激素效应。

危险因素

遗传因素

· 1 型多发内分泌肿瘤（男性）。

· Carney 综合征（色素痣、心房黏液瘤与库欣病生殖细胞肿瘤）。

病因

· 治疗性或私自使用是最常见的外源性糖皮质激素获得的途径。

· 垂体腺瘤分泌促肾上腺皮质激素。

· 肾上腺腺瘤、癌或结节性疾病均可分泌肾上腺皮质激素。

· 肿瘤产生的异位促肾上腺皮质激素：

- 肺小细胞癌：

◦ 最常见的。

- 子宫颈癌。

- 胰腺胰岛细胞瘤：

◦ Ⅰ型多发性内分泌腺瘤（MEN）综合征。

- 甲状腺髓样癌。

- 嗜铬细胞瘤。

- 神经节细胞瘤。

- 前列腺癌和黑色素瘤。

- 类癌：

◦ 肺。

◦ 胰腺。

◦ 消化道。

◦ 胸腺。

◦ 卵巢。

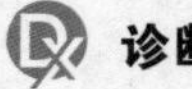

诊断

症状和体征

> **注意**
>
> · 在急诊室库欣综合征最重要的方面是：应意识到在应激期间有潜在 Addison 病（肾上腺危象）的可能。
>
> · 尽管非急症，但早期识别库欣综合征可以预防和降低发病率与死亡率。

K

儿科注意事项

怀疑肥胖增加而未能在生长图上保持身高，或发现与年龄不符（如骨质疏松症、高血压）。

妊娠注意事项

库欣综合征很少使妊娠过程复杂化，但与重度子痫前期和 HELLP 综合征（溶血、肝功能和低血小板）有明确的相关性，通常直到妊娠中期才被诊断出来，因为库欣综合征的许多症状通常都归因于妊娠。

病史

- 库欣病以往的诊断。
- 之前使用皮质激素的情况。
- 特征性的临床表现，如导致体重有关的问题、面部多毛症或精神症状等。

体格检查

- 脂肪异常沉积与满月脸。
  - 水牛背。
  - 中心性肥胖与消瘦四肢。
  - 锁骨上脂肪沉积：
  - 上述发现应提高警觉：
    - 在患者有应激的情况下有潜在发展为艾迪生病（肾上腺皮质功能不全）危象的可能。
- 心血管系统：
  - 不能控制的高血压。
  - 动脉粥样硬化。
- 神经系统：
  - 动脉粥样硬化或脑栓塞。
  - 假脑瘤（主要是摄入外源性糖皮质激素）：
    - 检查眼底。
- 脊髓脂肪瘤伴神经根或脊髓压迫。
- 消化系统：
  - 消化性溃疡。
  - 胃肠道出血。
  - 胰腺炎（主要是外源性糖皮质激素摄入引起）。
  - 脂肪肝。
- 精神病：
  - 中毒性精神病。
  - 心境障碍（40%）。
  - 抑郁。
  - 记忆障碍。
  - 兴奋。
  - 易怒。
  - 焦虑。
- 肌肉骨骼：
  - 肌病（近端肌无力）。
  - 骨质疏松。
  - 椎体压缩性骨折。
  - 病理性骨折。
  - 肱或股骨头无菌性坏死（主要是由外源性糖皮质激素引起）。
- 内分泌系统：
  - 葡萄糖不耐受。
  - 高脂血症。
  - 月经异常（80%）：月经过少、闭经。
  - 男性秃顶或多毛的女性。
- 血液系统：
  - 中性粒细胞增加。
  - 淋巴细胞和嗜酸性粒细胞减少。
  - 机会性感染。
- 视觉系统：
  - 白内障（主要是由外源性糖皮质激素摄入引起）。
  - 青光眼（主要是由外源性糖皮质激素摄入引起）。
- 皮肤附件：
  - 紫纹直径>1 cm。
  - 色素沉着：尤其是颊黏膜（过多的促肾上腺皮质激素导致）。
  - 多血质外貌。
  - 皮肤萎缩（可看到潜在血管）。
  - 伤口愈合不佳。
  - 瘀斑。
  - 痤疮。
  - 多汗症。

基本检查

- 在急诊室不能确诊。
- 预测到即将发生的艾迪生病（肾上腺皮质功能不全）危象：
  - 库欣综合征最常见和一般的问题是意识到它的并发症并预防急性肾上腺皮质危象。
- 寻找危及生命的情况：
  - 心肌梗死。
  - 卒中。
  - 脓毒症。
  - 病理性骨折。
  - 不能控制的糖尿病。
  - 需要入院的精神科急症。

诊断检查与说明

实验室检查

- 电解质、尿素氮、肌酐、血糖：
  - 低钾血症。
  - 代谢性碱中毒 10%的患者有代谢性碱中毒。
  - 葡萄糖耐量减少（75%）。
  - 20%显性的糖尿病。
- 尿液分析：
  - 50%有糖尿。
- 白细胞：
  - 白细胞计数升高。
  - 嗜酸性粒细胞下降。

影像学检查

- 心电图检查心肌缺血。
- 胸部 X 线片检查肿瘤引起的异位 ACTH。
- 如果怀疑骨龄延迟引起的病理性骨折行 X 线平片检查。

诊断步骤/外科

择期检查：

- 垂体肿瘤的磁共振成像。
- 肾上腺癌、腺瘤或增生的 CT 检查。
- 深夜唾液皮质醇（2 次测量）、24 h 尿游离皮质醇（UFC）或地塞米松抑制试验。
- 地塞米松抑制试验：
  - 如果怀疑内源性库欣综合征存在。
  - 低剂量（筛选试验）：在 23:00 使用 1 mg，早上 8:00 皮质醇水平下降：
    - 特异性低。
- 以下的因素可导致假阳性结果：酒精（乙醇）、雌激素、螺内酯、苯妥英钠、巴比妥类和利福平：
  - 高剂量地塞米松抑制试验用来确认诊断：
    - 2 mg 地塞米松 q6 h 测皮质醇水平。
    - 2 日后测尿游离皮质醇和 17-羟类固醇与基线水平比较。

鉴别诊断

- 酒精引起的假性库欣综合征。
- 肥胖。
- 精神状态：
  - 抑郁。
  - 强迫性障碍。
  - 惊恐障碍。
- 生理状态：
  - 慢性应激。
  - 妊娠。
  - 慢性剧烈运动。
  - 糖尿病控制不佳。

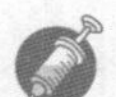

治疗

院前

- 应激引起的急性艾迪生病（肾上腺皮质功能不全）危象可能发展为医源性库欣综

合征。

• 患者可能有带有暴力性的极不稳定的行为。

• 在未经处理的库欣综合征中导致死亡的主要原因：

- 感染。
- 脑卒中(中风)。
- 心肌梗死。

■ 初步稳定/治疗

• 预测到 Addison 病(肾上腺)危象的发生。

• 启动相关并发症的治疗：

- 心肌梗死。
- 脑卒中(中风)。
- 精神稳定。

■ 急诊治疗/程序

• 静脉补液。

• 使用降糖药物治疗高血糖。

• 对可疑感染采取恰当的细菌培养和应用抗菌药物。

• 对于未控制的高血压服用抗高血压药物。

• 如果患者在应激情况下，为防止肾上腺皮质危象使用医源性类固醇(氢化可的松)。

• 手术抗凝，或增加血栓形成风险。

• 降低皮质醇水平的药物(溴隐亭、酮康唑、氨鲁米特、甲吡酮)：

- 等待手术期间有严重症状的患者尽量减少使用。
- 建立一个内分泌专家指导下的机构。
- 确定性的治疗：

• 医源性：

- 尽可能快地给予类固醇减量。
- 如果可能的话，给予补充钙、维生素 D、雌激素。
- 垂体源性库欣：
- 经蝶窦手术。
- 放疗可作为手术失败和一些患者的选择。
- 肾上腺腺瘤/癌：
- 对于不可切除转移灶的可行肾上腺切除术。

• 异位促肾上腺皮质激素：

- 对于转移性灶不可切除的，行肿瘤切除(如果可能的话)。

■ 药物治疗

一线用药

在肾上腺危象中唯有：氢化可的松，100 mg(儿童用药：1～2 mg/kg)，静脉，q6 h。

二线用药

• 与一位内分泌专家讨论。

• 在等待手术或难治的患者的治疗中，对症治疗仅作为附加治疗。

• 类固醇激素合成抑制剂：

- 酮康唑：200 mg，每日 2 次，口服。
- 甲吡酮：0.5～1 g/d，口服 in 4 div. doses。
- 甲苯磺丁脲：250 mg，口服，q6 h。
- 米非司酮：300 mg，口服，每日 1 次。

• 抗肾上腺素的药物：

- 米托坦：口服，500 mg，每日 1 次。

• 促肾上腺皮质激素释放抑制剂：

- 赛庚啶：4 mg，口服，每日 2 次。
- 溴隐亭：2.5～30 mg/d。

• 其他：

- 初始帕瑞肽：0.6 mg，皮下注射。
- 使用螺内酯来缓解高血压和低钾血症的症状。

随访

■ 进一步处理

入院指征

• 如以下并发症需要住院治疗：

- 心肌梗死。
- 脑卒中(卒中)。
- 脓毒症。
- 病理性骨折。
- 不能控制的糖尿病。
- 精神科急症。

• 即将发生的肾上腺皮质肾上腺危象。

出院指征

患者病情稳定，一般情况好，无入院指征。

转诊问题

• 任何疑似库欣综合征的患者需进行进一步的评估。

• 继发于库欣综合征的状况需要处理。

• 偶发肾上腺发现应转诊随访。

■ 随访建议

随访检验以明确诊断。

要点和误区

• 通过病史或身体状态，对生理上有应激的患者保持高度的警觉性，以防止肾上腺皮质危象。

• 当有锁骨上脂肪垫时需怀疑库欣病。

快速节律障碍 Tachydysrhythmias

Andrew P. Pirotte · Matthew J. Pirotte 范浩浩 李文放 译

基础知识

■ 描述

• 任何心脏节律的紊乱导致心室率＞100 次/分。

• 窦性心动过速：

- QRS 波正常规律的节律，速率在 100～150 次/分。
- 最大速率通常为 220 减去年龄(岁)。
- 对所引起的生理压力的功能反应，通过增加儿茶酚胺的口气或减少迷走神经刺激实现。

• 室上性心动过速(SVT)：

- 起源于希氏束之上狭窄的复杂心动过速。

• 常规 SVT：

- 房性心动过速。
- 交界性心动过速：
  ◦ 无先兆去极化波的常规心动过速。

• 不规则的 SVT：

- 心房颤动(房颤)。
- 心房震颤。
- 多发性房性心动过速。

• 室性心动过速(VT)：

- 以连续 3 次连续的心室异位搏动频率在 100 次/分。
- 早期 MI 的患者中猝死最常见的起始节律。

• 尖端扭转：

- VT 的阵发性形式，具有起伏的轴线和基线 QT 间期延长。
- 先天或后天的心室复极异常。
- 通常是药物治疗或电解质紊乱的结果。

• 室颤：

K

- 形态学上为没有离散的 QRST 波证据的波动。
- 占心脏性猝死的 80%～85%。
- 通常为持续的 VT 的结果。

病因

- 窦性心动过速：
- 急性心肌梗死。
- 贫血。
- 焦虑。
- 慢性心力衰竭。
- 药物中毒。
- 甲状腺功能亢进症。
- 血容量不足。
- 缺氧。
- 感染。
- 疼痛。
- 心脏压塞。
- 肺栓塞。
- 房性心动过速：
- 由过早的心房或心室收缩。
- 电解质紊乱。
- 药物毒性。
- 缺氧。
- 交界性心动过速：
- 房室结重新突入。
- 心肌缺血。
- 结构性心脏病。
- 预激综合征。
- 药物和酒精毒性。
- 房颤：
- 甲状腺结节功能亢进。
- 冠状动脉疾病。
- 甲状腺功能亢进症或甲状腺功能减退症。
- 酒精摄入量。
- 二尖瓣疾病。
- 慢性阻塞性肺疾病。
- 肺栓塞。
- 预激综合征。
- 缺氧。
- 地高辛毒性。
- 慢性心包炎。
- 特发性房颤。
- 心房震颤：
- 缺血性心脏病。
- 瓣膜性心脏病。
- 慢性心力衰竭。
- 心肌炎。
- 心肌病。
- 肺栓塞。
- 电解质异常。
- 最近的心脏手术。
- 多发性房性心动过速：
- 慢性肺病的缺氧效应。
- 茶碱毒性。
- VT：
- 扩张型心肌病。
- 心脏缺血。
- 缺氧。
- 心脏瘢痕或纤维化。
- 心脏手术后或先天性异常修复。
- 地高辛毒性。
- 长 QT 综合征。
- 电解质异常。
- 尖端扭转：
- 药物毒性（ⅠA 和Ⅲ类抗心律失常药、抗精神病药、抗生素等）。
- 低钾血症。
- 低镁血症。
- 先天性 QT 延长。
- VF：
- 急性心肌梗死（最常见）。
- 慢性缺血性心脏病。
- 缺氧。
- 酸中毒。
- 过敏反应。
- 电击。
- 休克。
- 低钾血症。
- 奎尼丁治疗。
- 大量出血。

诊断

症状和体征

- 无症状。
- 心悸。
- 头昏、眼花。
- 呼吸困难。
- 出汗。
- 头晕。
- 虚弱。
- 胸部不适。
- 心绞痛。
- 晕厥。
- 突出的颈部静脉。
- 不稳定的迹象：
- 低血压。
- 肺水肿。
- 胸部疼痛。
- 心理状态改变。

病史

- 急性心悸、头晕、全身无力或气短。
- 突然晕厥，通常在几分钟之前有过胸痛。
- 既往有心脏病史（缺血，慢性心力衰竭）。

体格检查

确定患者是否维持在血流动力学稳定：

- 评估心理状态。
- 评估心率。
- 评估血压：正常或低血压。
- 心脏检查。

基本检查

- ABC 管理。
- 确定患者不稳定与稳定。
- 详细的病史。
- 做 12 导联心电图和节律来分类心动过速。

诊断检查与说明

实验室检查

应根据描述进行排序评估潜在的代谢异常或缺血。

诊断步骤/外科

心电图：

- SVT：
- 窄 QRS 波群，通常为 130～160 次/分。
- 极性和幅度一致。
- 没有可见的 P 波。
- AF：
- 不规则，狭窄的 QRS 波群，频率＜150～170 次/分。
- 心房震颤：
- 通常心房率＞300 次/分。
- 周期长度、极性和幅度在波动之间是均匀的。
- 锯齿波扑向上，在导联Ⅱ、Ⅲ、aVF 中最明显。
- 房室阻滞通常为 2∶1，但偶尔会更大或不规则。
- 多源性房性心动过速：
- 与 3 个明显不同的传导 P 波同时伴随变化的脉率间隔。
- VT：
- QRS＞0.12 s，通常＞0.14 s。
- 尖端扭转：
- 复杂的心室率＞200 次/分。
- QRS 结构显示一个起伏的轴，窄 QRS 波形围绕基线发生移位。

K

- 发生时间通常短于 90 s。
- VF：
- 心电图显示没有离散 QRST 形态证据的振荡。
- 振荡通常是不规则的，发生速率为 150～300 次/分。
- 当大多数振荡的振幅是 1 mm 时，使用术语“粗颤”。
- “细颤”用于<1 mm 的振动。

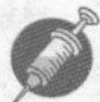

治疗

院前

如果无脉搏行心肺复苏。

初步稳定/治疗

- 建立静脉通路。
- 给予氧气。
- 心脏监护。
- 确定心电图节律。

急诊治疗/程序

- 不规则的窄 QRS 波群(房颤)：
  - 控制频率。
  - β受体阻滞剂或钙通道阻滞剂。
  - 如果发病>24 h，抗凝处理。
  - 严重血流动力学不稳则需要复律。
- 规则的窄 QRS 波群心动过速：
  - Vagal 动作可能会终止此类心律失常：
    - 注意老年人可能的颈动脉疾病。
  - 腺苷：
    - 可能是诊断性的，揭示潜在的房颤/房扑。
- 稳定的宽 QRS 波群心动过速：
  - 确定是否为有异常的 VT 或 SVT。
  - 房室结阻滞剂的管理(维拉帕米、腺苷)可能导致 VF：
    - 合并预激综合征，使用胺碘酮、氟卡尼、普鲁卡因胺或电复律。
  - 机制不明时应使用电复律。
  - 抗心律失常药物包括普鲁卡因胺和胺碘酮。
- 尖端扭转：
  - 镁、超速起搏、胺碘酮。
  - 纠正潜在的电解质紊乱。
  - 考虑补充血清 K^+ 至 4.5 mmol/L。
- 多形性 VT(QRS 形态可变)：
  - 射血分数(EF)正常值：
    - β受体阻滞剂、利多卡因、胺碘酮或普鲁卡因胺。
  - EF 异常：
    - 胺碘酮或利多卡因，然后同步电复律。
  - 治疗局部缺血，纠正电解质紊乱。
- 单形 VT：
  - EF 正常：
    - 普鲁卡因胺优于胺碘酮、索他洛尔、利多卡因；同步电复律。
  - EF 异常：
    - 胺碘酮或利多卡因。
    - 普鲁卡因胺应谨慎使用可能导致低血压，同步电复律。
- VF 或无脉 VT：
  - 按照 ACLS 指南进行治疗。

药物治疗

- 腺苷：6 mg(儿童：0.1 mg/kg 直至 6 mg)迅速静推，如果 1～2 min 后没有反应，那么再次应用 12 mg(儿童：0.2 mg/kg 直至 12 mg)，可以重复 12 mg(0.2 mg/kg)。
- 胺碘酮：
  - 有脉搏的 VT/SVT：在 10 min 内 150 mg 静滴(儿童：在 20～60 min 静脉注射 5 mg/kg，重新达到 15 mg/kg，最大剂量 300 mg)，然后 1 mg/min 6 h 和接下来的 18 h 0.5 mg/min。
  - VF/无脉 SVT：300 mg 静脉推注(儿童：5 mg/kg 静滴)，如果没有好转，可以在 3～5 min 后给予 150 mg 静脉推注(儿童：红糖高达 15 mg/kg，最大剂量 300 mg)，然后如上输注。
- 地尔硫䓬：0.25 mg/kg 静脉注射(通常 10～20 mg) 2 min，随后在 15 min 内以 0.35 mg/kg 静滴，2 min 结束。
- 肾上腺素：1 mg(儿童：0.01 mg/kg)，静推，q3～5 min；2.5 mg(儿童：0.1 mg/kg)气管内给药，q3～5 min。
- 利多卡因：1～1.5 mg/kg(100 mg)(儿童：1 mg/kg)，静推，可每 5～10 min 重复，最大剂量 3 mg/kg。
- 硫酸镁：用 100 ml 5%葡萄糖水溶液稀释 2 g，静滴，超过 2 min(儿童：25～50 mg/kg，最多 2 g，静脉注射，超过 10～20 min)。
- 美托洛尔：在 5 min 时缓慢静脉推注 5～15 mg，总共 15 mg。
- 普鲁卡因胺：
  - VF/无脉室速：30 mg/min(儿童：不推荐)静滴负荷直到节律转复，低血压，QRS 增宽>50%或最大。17 mg/kg，然后 1～4 mg/min，静滴。
  - 多形 VT：20 mg/min(儿童：15 mg/kg，静滴 30～60 min)，静滴负荷，直到转复率低血压，QRS 扩大>50%或最大 17 mg/kg，然后 1～4 mg/min，静滴。
  - SVT：15～17 mg/kg，静滴，20～30 min；或 100 mg，静滴，q5 min。缓慢静滴推，直到节律恢复或最大剂量 1 000 mg(儿童：3～6 mg/kg，静滴，超过 5 min，最大 100 mg，每 5～10 min 可重复，需要总剂量 15 mg/kg)。
- 加压素：40 U(儿童：不推荐)静脉注射一次。

随访

进一步处理

入院指征

- VT 或 VF。
- 可能的心脏缺血事件。
- 持续 SVT。
- 基础代谢异常。

出院指征

没有器官灌注不足的终止的室上性节律。

转诊问题

电生理测试：
- 诊断，但不是紧急需要。
- 确定辅助途径的治疗。

要点和误区

- 始终怀疑 QRS 波群增宽的心室复杂节律，特别是在年长的患者身上。
- 抗心律失常药物可能会增加复律成功率。
- 快速、不间断的胸部按压可能增加无节律的患者除颤的成功率。

K

髋部损伤

Claire T. Wang · Radhika Sundararajan 郇乐 译

基础知识

描述

• 髋部损伤包括由于外伤或过度使用引起的髋部骨折和股骨近端脱位。

• 髋部骨折：股骨近端骨折，分为囊内和囊外。

- 囊内骨折：发生于股骨头或股骨颈，常常伴有股骨颈血管的损伤。股骨头缺血性坏死发病率：
  ◦ 股骨头骨折：常伴有髋关节脱位(前部＞后部)。
  ◦ 股骨颈骨折：通常老年人轻微创伤或者年轻人重伤，症状不一。患者不一定出现行走困难。经常跑步者或新兵有应力性骨折。
- 囊外骨折：发生于髋臼囊以下。通常不影响血供。发病率通常与患者制动有关：如深静脉血栓形成(DVT)和肺栓塞(PE)：
  ◦ 股骨转子骨折：大转子骨折通常由撕脱伤导致，骨折断端插入臀中肌。小转子骨折通常由于髂腰肌剧烈收缩导致，通常见于年轻运动员和儿童。
  ◦ 股骨粗隆间骨折：定义为发生在大小转子间的骨折。在年龄大、骨质疏松的患者跌倒后常见。肢体明显的外旋和缩短。可以是稳定性或不稳定性骨折。患者不能行走。
  ◦ 股骨转子下骨折：通常见于年轻人的严重创伤或老年人的轻度创伤。它是常见的病理骨折，可有大量失血和休克。

• 髋关节脱位：股骨头脱出，分为前脱位、中心脱位和后脱位。

- 髋关节后脱位(最常见)：
  ◦ 通常由于交通事故中膝盖撞击仪表盘所致。
  ◦ 10%存在坐骨神经损伤。
- 髋关节前脱位：占髋关节脱位的10%。
  ◦ 通常见于由创伤导致的大腿极度外展。
  ◦ 多伴有股骨头骨折或者股神经损伤。
  ◦ 可以是前上或者前下脱位。
- 髋关节中心脱位伴髋臼骨折：
  ◦ 通常由于直接碰撞大转子导致。
  ◦ 多伴有明显的出血和坐骨神经损伤。

儿科注意事项

• 髋关节脱位：并不常见，往往自发地减少受伤的时间。通常有其他组织卡在关节腔内。

- 在＜10岁的儿童中，髋关节后部需要的力量小。

• 近端股骨骨折：生长板处断裂，出现缺血性坏死风险高。

• 股骨头骨骺滑脱：通常见于轻度损伤，减少ROM。

• 股骨颈骨折：较常见，年轻运动员中多见病理性骨折。

• 股骨粗隆间骨折：罕见。

• 对于非意外创伤(NAT)都应怀疑是否有骨折。

• 在轻微创伤中要考虑病理性骨折。

病因

参见个人伤害。

诊断

症状和体征

病史

• 腹股沟、臀部、大腿、内侧膝关节痛，外伤导致的行走或负重疼痛。

• 老年人损伤归因于骨质疏松，年轻人中则为高强度创伤。

体格检查

• 明显的创伤标志：

- 畸形或成角，肿胀，开放性骨折或子弹穿透伤。
- 下肢处于舒适的位置。
- 运动范围缩小。

• 髋骨骨折：屈曲，外展，外旋。

• 髋关节后脱位：屈曲，内收，内旋，膝关节弯曲，髋关节固定。

• 髋关节前脱位：屈曲，外展，外旋，大腿缩短，髋关节固定。

儿科注意事项

• 儿童骨折的不同分型与软骨的发育程度有关：

- 评估股骨头骨骺脱位。

• 骨折的分类与处理也各不相同。

> **注意**
>
> 疑似NAT同时不伴有明显的致伤机制。
>
> • 考虑髋部疼痛为单独原因导致(下肢不等长、肌无力或肿瘤骨转移)。

基本检查

• 评估末梢血供，触诊，评估感觉和运动服功能。

• 如果脉搏无法触及或强弱不等，需考虑床旁多普勒超声或血管造影。

• 寻找相关损伤：

- 神经功能缺损。
- 血管损伤。
- 骨盆骨折(包括髋臼骨折)。
- 脊柱骨折。
- 腹部钝性伤。

• X线片如下：

- 检查时去除夹板与衣物。
- 积极检查加上错误的影像学标准可能预示髋部损伤，进一步的影像学检查(CT或MRI扫描)可能发现。
- 髋关节脱位是骨科紧急事件，需要及时的复位(6 h内)。

儿科注意事项

• 在儿童的可疑病例中，使用正确的影像学检查与其他伤害鉴别。

• 评估NAT的标志：

- 延迟出现症状，与伤害不相符合的病史及受伤机制。
- 大腿部的独立损伤、相关的烧伤、擦伤、线性擦伤。

诊断检查与说明

全血细胞计数(CBC)，血型与交叉配型，国际标准化比值(INR)及合适的影像学检查：

• 标准图像：AP骨盆和真实的髋部侧方，倾斜视角。

• 股骨颈骨折：AP骨盆同时伴有骨盆内旋15°～20°。

• 耻骨支和髋臼骨折：骨盆入口和出口视角。

• 髋臼骨折：Judet视角(骨盆斜视图)。

• 高度怀疑无阳性影像学表现的病例：CT、MRI或骨扫描。通常MRI最敏感。

• 复位后需行X线和/或CT扫描。

诊断步骤/外科

• 关节穿刺有或无透视下关节造影，如化脓性关节炎、异物或关节积血，尤其是枪伤应高度怀疑髋部损伤。

• 手术修复或清洗。

■ 鉴别诊断

- 耻骨支骨折。
- 髋臼骨折。
- 化脓性关节炎。
- 大腿、膝盖、踝部或足部损伤。
- 大粗隆滑囊炎。
- 髂胫束肌腱炎。
- 骨盆挫伤。

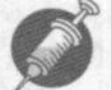

治疗

■ 院前

- 行神经与血管检查。
- 尽量固定在患者感觉舒适的位置。

■ 初步稳定/治疗

- 优先处理气道、头部、胸部或腹部损伤。
- 保持骨盆与髋部稳定。
- 保持血压稳定。
- 注意事项：
  - 不要使用牵引。
  - 密切注意发生失血性休克，因为大腿可以包含 4～6 U 血液。

■ 急诊治疗/程序

- 保持骨盆与髋部稳定。
- 移除夹板和衣物。
- 疼痛控制：
  - 单纯髋部损伤：注射用药物镇痛。
  - 多发伤或儿童患者：股神经阻滞。
- 整形咨询：
  - 适用于所有的骨盆骨折与脱位。
  - 一旦出现神经与血管的损伤，情况紧急。
  - 开放性损伤必须直接送至手术室行冲洗与清创术。
  - 1～2 步急诊室快速处理后可以减少手术室的时间。
- 需要骨折的手术：
  - 头孢唑林，静脉注射。
- 伴有广泛的软组织损伤、撕裂或污染的开放性骨折：
  - 加入庆大霉素或妥布霉素，预防破伤风。
- 如果伤口高度污染：添加青霉素来覆盖梭菌。
- 枪伤：
  - 碘敷料填塞弹道。
- 髋关节脱臼。
  - 真正的骨科急症。
  - 随着时间的延长，缺血性坏死和退行性关节病变的发病率呈线性增长：
- 理想情况下，在发病的 6 h 内减少髋关节脱臼。
- 许多成功的还原技术已经被描述，包括 Allis、Stimson 和“Captain Morgan”方法。
  - 镇静镇痛方案建议氯胺酮、依托咪酯或巴比妥＋咪达唑仑，异丙酚＋芬太尼。
  - 骨折复位后寻找影像学依据（X 线平片、CT）。
  - 在可能需要接受人工髋关节置换术的患者中，可以通过镇痛镇静及适当的监测来减少髋关节置换术的发生。

■ 药物治疗

- 抗生素。
  - 头孢唑林：1 g，肌内注射或静脉注射，q6～8 h[儿童：25～50 mg/(kg・d)，肌内注射或静脉注射，q6～8 h，最大剂量 1 g]。
  - 庆大霉素/妥布霉素：3～5 mg/(kg・d)，肌内注射或静脉注射，q8 h（儿童：2～2.5 mg/kg，q8 h）。
  - 青霉素：200 万 U，静脉注射，q4 h[儿童：10 万～40 万 U/(kg・d)，静脉注射，q4～6 h。24 h 最大剂量 2 400 万 U]。
- 适度镇静：
  - 依托咪酯：0.1～0.3 mg/kg，单次静脉注射(12 岁以下不推荐)。
  - 芬太尼：1～4 μg/kg，静脉注射 1～2 min 1 次(儿童：>6 岁 1～2 μg/kg，单次静注)。
  - 氨胺酮(克他命)：由于出现反应，不推荐给成人(儿童：1～2 mg/kg，静脉注射；4 mg/kg，单次肌内注射)。
  - 美索比妥：1～1.5 mg/kg，单次静脉注射(儿童：不推荐)。
  - 咪达唑仑：0.07 mg/kg，肌内注射；或每 2～3 min 微泵 1 mg，最高可达 2.5 mg(儿童：单次口服 0.25～1 mg/kg，最大剂量 15 mg；6 个月至 5 岁：0.05～0.1 mg/kg 静脉注射，最大剂量 0.6 mg/kg；6～12 岁：0.025～0.05 mg/kg，静脉注射，最大剂量 0.4 mg/kg)。
  - 异丙酚：40 mg，静脉注射，q10 s 直到诱导；5～10 μg/(kg・min)持续静脉微泵。
- 镇痛：
  - 氢吗啡酮：0.5～2.0 mg，皮下注射、肌内注射或慢推，q4～6 h。长期使用需镇痛滴定[儿童：长期使用 0.015 mg/(kg・min)，静脉注射，q4～6 h]。
  - 吗啡：2～10 mg，静脉注射，q4 h，镇痛滴定(儿童：0.1 mg/kg，静脉注射，q4 h，镇痛滴定，最大用量 15 mg)。
    - 儿科用药需使用无防腐剂制剂。

一线用药

- 抗生素：头孢唑林，静脉注射。
- 疼痛：吗啡。
- 镇静：成人用依托咪酯；儿童用氨胺酮(克他命)。

二线用药

- 抗生素：头孢曲松＋庆大霉素。
- 镇痛：氢吗啡酮、芬太尼、神经封闭。
- 镇静：美索比妥、咪达唑仑和异丙酚。

随访

■ 进一步处理

入院指征

- 髋部骨折。
- 化脓性关节炎。
- 怀疑隐匿性骨折。
- 儿童怀疑与遗传性相关。
- 所有儿童髋部骨折和脱位。

出院指征

- 其他原因引起的髋部疼痛。
- 排除骨折(X 线平片＋临床检查阴性)。
- 患者在髋关节脱位复位成功后可在骨科会诊后考虑出院，并采取适当的随访措施。
- 胯部应力性骨折，随访时进行骨扫描或定期 X 线检查。

转诊问题

- 慢性疼痛可能需要主治医师和疼痛专家。
- 儿科患者和老年人可能需要物理治疗。

■ 随访建议

- 非骨折/脱位所致的髋关节疼痛应及时就医。
- 应力性骨折，非负重：骨科随访 2～3 日。

要点和误区

- 骨折位置决定了发病的危险因素，如股骨头坏死和出血。
- 髋关节脱位是骨科急症，需及时复位并多次尝试。
- 对隐匿性骨折应保持警惕，因为 X 线可能对 10%的骨折检测不到。需要 CT 或 MRI 随访，并可能住院。

K

狂犬病 Rabies

Herbert Neil·Wigder. Juliet Evans 郑金浩 毛恩强 译

基础知识

描述

- 由哺乳动物引起的严重中枢感染性疾病。
- 是已知感染性疾病中死亡率最高的感染。

病因

- 流行病学：
- 每年全世界有35000～59000人死于狂犬病。
- 尤其在南亚、菲律宾、非洲、南美洲和印度半岛较常见。
- 美国每年有2～3例。
- 美国的临床病例大多来源于国外旅游和蝙蝠暴露。
- 在美国，蝙蝠是最常见的宿主(30.9%)，还有浣熊(29.4%)、臭鼬(24.8%)、狐狸(5.9%)、猫(4.4%)、牛(1.5%)和犬(1.2%)。
- 在世界范围内，犬咬是最常见的媒介。
- 松鼠、大鼠、小鼠、豚鼠、仓鼠、沙鼠、花栗鼠、兔子也可以感染狂犬病病毒，但没有向人类传播的病例报道。
- 在移植病人中很少有狂犬病病例报告。
- 病理生理学：
- 其核酸为单链RNA病毒，弹状病毒科，狂犬病病毒属。
- 感染发病过程：
- 病毒在局部组织中繁殖。
- 病毒进入末梢神经并进入中枢神经系统。
- 一旦进入中枢神经系统，病毒的快速复制和传播就会引起神经功能障碍。
- 病毒沿着周围神经扩散回唾液腺、皮肤、角膜和其他器官。

诊断

症状和体征

一旦患者出现临床症状，基本全部死亡。

- 5个阶段：潜伏期、前驱症状、脑炎、昏迷和死亡。
- 潜伏期：几日至几年(平均1～2个月)：
- 在周围组织病毒复制增殖并转移至中枢神经。
- 时间取决于病毒数量和侵入位置与中枢神经系统的距离，对于成人及儿童伤口接近中枢神经系统，因此潜伏期短。
- 前驱症状期1～10日：
- 无特异性症状：发热、头痛、乏力、肌肉疼痛、纳差、咽喉痛、恶心、呕吐。
- 咬伤部位感觉异常或肌束震颤为正确诊断提供线索。
- 急性神经症状期(经典型)：2～7日。
  - 焦虑、躁动、幻觉或精神错乱、肌肉痉挛、角弓反张、强直。
  - 畏风(症)：风刺激可引起喉痉挛。
  - 恐水症：咽喉和辅助呼吸肌在试图吞下水时，膈肌不自主的强烈收缩(可在半数以上患者出现)。
  - 心律失常、心肌炎、自主神经功能异常、发热。
  - 脑干受累：复视、面瘫。
- 昏迷：
  - 窒息来源于呼吸中枢受累、血管塌陷、弛缓性麻痹、成人呼吸窘迫综合征、不当利尿激素综合征呼吸暂停。
- 死亡(或痊愈)。
  - 多数于2周内死亡。
  - 罕有存活病例报道。
  - 已知的幸存者有部分神经功能障碍。
- 3种疾病的表现：
- 经典狂犬病或脑炎性狂犬病：占总数的80%左右。
- 麻痹性狂犬病(大约20%)：上行性麻痹，和吉兰-巴雷综合征相似。
- 非典型狂犬病(<1%)：特点是神经性疼痛、感觉或运动障碍、舞蹈病样运动、肌阵挛和癫痫发作。

病史

- 咬伤或其他所知的暴露。
- 在房间发现蝙蝠的人不能提供病史(如小孩，睡眠或者醉酒者)：假设暴露。
- 至流行区域旅游并与犬接触。
- 移植患者。
- 不被认为有传播风险：完整的皮肤情况下，抚摸患狂犬病的动物，或接触患狂犬病动物的血液、尿液或粪。

体格检查

- 体格检查不具有诊断学，除非发现咬伤口。
- 蝙蝠咬伤处不易通过体检发现。

基本检查

- 多种测试可用于诊断人类狂犬病，但单一的测试是不够的。

诊断检查与说明

实验室检查

- 唾液：
- 通过反转录链式反应(RT-PCR)监测狂犬病病毒RNA。
- 独立病毒的细胞培养。
- 血清：
- 若未接种疫苗，检测狂犬病病毒抗体。
- 脑脊液：
- 白细胞和蛋白质轻度升高，糖正常。
- 病毒存在。
- 脑脊液中发现狂犬病病毒或者狂犬病病毒抗体即使免疫也可诊断。
- 皮肤活检。
- 病毒抗原免疫荧光染色。
- 其他实验室工作用来排除其他原因引起的症状。

影像学检查

- 影像学的作用主要是排除可能的病因。

诊断步骤/外科

- 腰椎穿刺，皮肤活检。

鉴别诊断

- 引起脑炎的其他疾病：
- 疱疹病毒：HSV1、VZV。
- 肠道病毒(柯萨奇其病毒、埃可病毒、脊髓灰质炎病毒)。
- 虫媒病毒(西尼罗病毒、东部/西部马脑炎、圣路易斯病)。
- 破伤风。
- 震颤性谵妄。
- 精神病。
- 吉兰-巴雷综合征。
- 脊髓灰质炎。
- 蜱麻痹。
- 免疫介导的多发性神经病。
- 肉毒毒素。

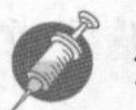

治疗

院前

- 用肥皂和水彻底冲洗伤口。
- 保证自身安全的前提下，捕捉到相应动物予以观察或者处死动物并进行检测。

K

■ 初步稳定/治疗

• 高级生命支持用于稳定期咬伤后的创伤。

• 伤口护理。

- 用肥皂和清水冲洗伤口 15 分钟。

- 如可获得，应使用抗病毒剂(例如聚乙烯吡咯酮碘)。

■ 急诊治疗/程序

- 确定是否需要接触后预防：狂犬病接触是一种医疗紧急情况，而不是紧急情况。如有疑问，请向当地或州卫生官员咨询建议：

- 圈养动物咬伤(犬、猫、雪貂)。

◦ 观察动物 10 日。

◦ 如果动物没有患病的征象，患者不需要暴露后预防。

◦ 如果动物表现出狂犬病的迹象，给予暴露后预防。

- 野生动物咬伤(浣熊、臭鼬、狐狸、大多数其他食肉动物、蝙蝠)：

◦ 牺牲动物进行狂犬病试验。

◦ 是否进行暴露后预防，依据检测结果确定。

◦ 如果未能抓获动物，行暴露后预防治疗。

- 家畜、马、啮齿动物、兔子、其他哺乳动物咬伤：

◦ 向公共卫生局咨询建议。

• 暴露前/后预防：

- 给予人狂犬病免疫球蛋白(HRIG)被动免疫。

◦ HRIG：20 IU/kg：大多数聚集在伤口及周围，剩余的远端肌内注射。

- 主动免疫，注射狂犬病疫苗。

◦ 1 ml 肌内注射：第 0、3、7、14 日，如果免疫缺陷追加第 28 日。

◦ 给药部位：成人为三角肌，儿童和婴儿为大腿前外侧

- 有暴露前预防后者狂犬病暴露史的患者。

◦ 不需要 HRIG。

◦ 在暴露当日和第 3 日需要使用疫苗加强。

- 如果狂犬病毒暴露后就诊较迟：

- 疫苗应当常规注射。

- 如果在第一次接种疫苗时没有疫苗，HRIG 可在第一次接种疫苗后的第 7 日使用

• 暴露前预防：

- 狂犬病疫苗注射：第 0、7、21、28 日。

- 易感人群：兽医、动物管理员、病毒实验室工作人员、在流行地区的旅游者。

• 确保破伤风免疫接种得到更新。

• 预防伤口感染建议使用预防性抗生素

儿科注意事项

和成人相同处理。

妊娠注意事项

孕妇治疗过程中多注意安全。

随访

■ 进一步处理

狂犬病毒暴露后，确定可以获得足量的狂犬病疫苗。

入院指征

患者有狂犬病的症状。

出院指征

• 病情平稳的患者。

• 对狂犬病疫苗无不良反应。

转诊问题

可疑病例转诊至公共卫生中心或 CDC。

■ 随访建议

• 确保后续疫苗按时按量接种。

• 如果源动物死亡或仍在观察，患者应继续关注动物的相关情况。

要点和误区

• 只在确定暴露后给 PEP 治疗。

• 在高暴露风险人群，不应考虑时间问题，都应给予 PEP。

• 任何在海外旅行时被犬咬伤的行为都应该被认为是潜在的接触，直到有证据证明。

• 与美国其他地区相比，美国-墨西哥边境地区的犬更容易患狂犬病。

• 成人疫苗只应注射在三角肌：有臀部皮下注射治疗失败的报道。

眶后血肿 Retrobulbar Hematoma

Chao Annie Yuan • Michael J. Holman　袁晓伟　童朝阳 译

基础知识

■ 描述

• 又称眼球后血肿。

• 眼眶创伤和面部手术的少见并发症。

• 眼球后血液堆积导致眶后压增加和组织缺血。

• 90 min 内可发生视力丧失，如果不及时诊断和治疗，120 min 后将发生不可逆损伤。

• 外侧眦切开术可挽救视力通常需要在急救室中进行。

• 进行彻底检查，因为许多有眶后血肿的患者可能是无意识的。

• 必须进行重复检查，观察血肿进展。

■ 流行病学

• 发病率很难评估，由于眶后血肿病因较多，包括创伤性和医源性：

- 0.45%～3%钝性或穿透伤

- 0.45%～0.6%合并眶壁骨折。

- 0.005 2%由眼睑成形术造成。

- 0.3%由于面部骨折外科修复。

- 0.006%由于窦内镜手术。

• 发病率受争议，因为只有稍微超过一半的眶后出血可通过之前 CT 扫描或血肿的临床表现而诊断。

■ 病因

• 眼球或眶壁和神经丛的外伤。

• 继发于血肿形成的眶后压力迅速升高，阻塞了视网膜及视神经静脉流出和动脉血流入，引起眶间隔综合征。

• 患者眼球不断突出，也可牵拉视神经造成视敏度降低。

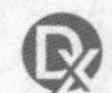

诊断

■ 症状和体征

病史

• 眼眶穿透或钝挫伤。

- 最近面部、眼眶手术。
- 眼痛。
- 视觉丧失。

体格检查

- 视敏度降低。
- 眼压(IOP)升高。
- 眼球突出。
- 复视。
- 疼痛。
- 下降的眼外肌(EOM)。
- 瞳孔直接对光反射消失，间接对光反射保留。

基本检查

- 有受伤史。
- 高度怀疑。
- 全身检查。
- 评估是否立即进行外科手术减压。
- 眼科紧急会诊。
- 影像学检查。

诊断检查与说明

实验室检查

无诊断性或提示性检查。

影像学检查

- CT扫描是金标准，但在影像学检查过程中不要延误视觉挽救性治疗。
- 超声(尽可能床旁)：敏感度和精确度未知。Guitar-pick征。

鉴别诊断

患者在创伤后面部可表现为以下任何症状：

- 视力下降。
- 视力模糊。
- 眼痛。
- 眼分泌物。
- 异位妊娠。
- 畏光。
- 眼压。
- 恶心和呕吐。

患者可在经以下治疗后出现症状：

- 面部骨折复位。
- 眼睑手术。
- 内镜下窦外科手术。
- 球后注射局部麻醉。
- 泪囊切除术

必须考虑以下鉴别：

- 眼眶骨折。
- 眶后水肿。
- 眶后气肿。
- 击入性骨折。
- 眶顶骨折合并脑疝。
- 颅内出血。
- 其他跟较大损伤有关的创伤。

治疗

院前

- 气道、呼吸、循环(ABC)支持。
- 院前外眦切开术具有很大争议。

初步稳定/治疗

- ABC管理。
- 快速转入一级创伤中心。
- 如果错过了90～120 min治疗窗，应由有经验医师行外侧下侧眦切开术。

急诊治疗/程序

手术治疗：

- 适应证：IOP＞40，无意识的眼球突出患者。
- 禁忌证：眼球破裂。
- 唯一的确定性治疗：外侧及下方眦切开术。
- 用5%聚烯吡酮碘准备场所。
- 眼角外侧皮下或深部组织局麻。注意避开眼球和眼眶。
- 止血钳穿过并钳夹外眦1 min。
- 用钝性剪刀沿着钳夹标记从眼睑外侧角到眶缘切开。
- 通过拉下下眼睑暴露外眦腱的上下脚。
- 用钝性剪刀将下脚插入下眼睑并结扎。下眼睑应向下松弛。

药物治疗

- 甲泼尼龙。
  - 30 mg/kg。
  - 15 mg/kg，q6 h。
- 甘露醇：
  - 1.5～2 g/kg 30 min内注射完，首次12.5 g在3 min内注入。
- 乙酰唑胺：500 mg，静脉注射(如果对磺胺类药物过敏或镰状红细胞病)。
- 高压氧。
- 硝苯地平：30 mg，口服，每日1次。
- 昂丹司琼(枢复宁)：4 mg(儿童：0.1 mg/kg)，肌内注射或静脉注射，不能超过8 mg/剂量，静脉注射。
- 丙氯拉嗪(甲哌氯丙嗪)：5～10 mg，肌内注射或静脉注射，q4～6 h；25 mg，栓剂，灌肠。
- 异丙嗪(非那根)：12.5～25 mg(儿童：0.25～1 mg/kg不超过25 mg)，肌内注射、静脉注射或灌肠，q4～6 h。
- 坦索罗辛(flomax)：0.4 mg，口服，每日1次，持续4周。

随访

进一步处理

入院指征

- 所有怀疑ROH的患者应入院在手术室行针对性治疗和观察。
- 所有患者需眼科医师进一步检查。
- 所有患者需要检查以防有其他外伤。

出院指征

患者不能出院。

转诊问题

- 在急诊室请眼科医师紧急会诊。
- 不能因为会诊延误而延误减压术。
- 急诊医师在有经验医师的观看下行紧急外眦切开术。

要点和误区

- 眶后血肿的延误诊断由于：
  - 体格检查不仔细。
  - 缺乏警觉。
  - 缺乏装备，如Tono-Pen：
  - 无意识的患者。
- 等待CT等影像学检查延误了视觉挽救治疗。
- 会诊医师到达延误。

K

眶周和眼眶蜂窝织炎 Periorbital and Orbital Cellulitis

Shari Schabowski · Lotiffa Colibao 钱斌斌 译

基础知识

描述

眼眶周围蜂窝织炎

• 一种影响眼睑的炎症性、典型的感染性疾病。

• 根据位置进行解剖学上的区别，分离前组织到眶隔：

- 眶隔是眶骨膜在上、下眼睑上的结缔组织延伸。

- 延伸到深层组织是罕见的，因为隔膜几乎是一个不可逾越的屏障，但是它可能并不完整。

• 最常见的表现为上呼吸道感染(URTI)和鼻窦炎的并发症：

- 肿胀是由血管和淋巴管阻塞引起的炎性水肿。

• 可能会出现在眼睑或相邻结构的局部炎症或感染的并发症：

- 睑缘炎。

- 睑腺炎。

- 泪囊炎。

- 周围皮肤破损。

• 内部损伤。

• 轻微创伤。

• 脓疱病或其他皮肤疾病。

眼眶蜂窝织炎

• 眶隔结构中的炎症过程。

• 通常继发于相邻结构的扩展：

- 鼻窦炎：

◦ 最常见的筛窦炎穿透薄层纸板。

- 牙脓肿。

- 外体在轨道上保留。

- 穿刺伤。

- 眼眶骨折。

- 术后感染。

- 因无眶静脉远端的血源性传播。

- 罕见原因，眼眶蜂窝织炎的直接延伸。

病因

眼眶周围蜂窝织炎

• 肺炎链球菌。

• 金黄色葡萄球菌。

• 化脓性链球菌。

• 卡他莫拉菌。

• 流感嗜血杆菌。

• 淋球菌，少见。

• 考虑非细菌性原因。

眼眶蜂窝织炎

• 目前链球菌和金黄色葡萄球菌感染是最常见的原因：

- 肺炎链球菌、草绿色链球菌、化脓性链球菌、咽峡炎链球菌、金黄色葡萄球菌。

- 厌氧菌、拟杆菌和革兰阴性菌也可能被看到。

• 一个真正的紧急情况是所有形式的眼眶蜂窝织炎有严重的发病率和可能死亡的风险：

- 永久性视力丧失可能发生。

- 可以延伸到骨膜下间隙，形成脓肿。

- 海绵窦血栓形成和中枢神经系统感染可能危及生命。

• 真菌感染是一种不常见但更致命的形式，特别是在免疫功能低下时：

- 脑鼻眶藻菌病(CROP)。

- 75%的病例迅速致命：

◦ 80%的病例发生在近期患有糖尿病酮症酸中毒的患者。

◦ 易感因素：严重的代谢性酸中毒和免疫功能低下。

◦ 开始于鼻窦，并且在血管中增殖，引起血栓和坏死。

◦ 常见血性鼻分泌物。

◦ 可能存在关于腭和/或鼻黏膜坏死的证据。

儿科注意事项

• 常规疫苗包括乙型流感嗜血杆菌和肺炎球菌，可显著减少眶周和眼眶蜂窝织炎，但是感染仍可能发生在年轻孩子及接种乙型流感嗜血杆菌疫苗的人。

• 眼眶周围蜂窝织炎在 5 岁以下的发生率为平时的 5 倍，而眼眶蜂窝织炎在 5 岁以上的发生率更高。

诊断

症状和体征

眼眶周围蜂窝织炎和眼眶蜂窝织炎

• 同时具备一个单侧、红色、肿胀的眼睛：

- 盖肿胀可能两者都很严重。

• 不同点包括：

- 刺激感染源。

- 单个与两个盖参与。

- 毒性、系统性和神经系统症状。

眼眶蜂窝织炎

病史

• 60%～90%的患者之前患有鼻窦炎、口腔感染、创伤、穿刺伤或近期手术。

• 肿胀与眼周红肿加剧了眼睛疼痛、视觉障碍、色视力丧失，限制眼球运动。

• 头痛、假性脑膜炎和全身性疾病的症状可能会发生。

• 识别复杂的医疗问题：

- 免疫功能低下。

- 糖尿病。

体格检查

• 外观毒性：

- 发热＞39℃。

• 受限的，眼外肌运动疼痛(EOM)。

• 瞳孔传入缺陷。

• 结膜充血。

• 结膜水肿。

• 视力下降。

• 复视。

• 眼球突出。

• 假性脑膜炎和神经刺激症状可能被发现。

眼眶周围蜂窝织炎

病史

• 之前有局部皮肤损伤、昆虫叮咬、上呼吸道感染(URTI)或浅表性眼部感染。

• 询问年轻孩子的疫苗注射情况。

• 低热。

• 亚急性表现。

体格检查

• 眼睑红肿。

• 经常结盖。

• 常见结膜充血。

• 常见低热：

- 罕见全身症状。

• 正常视觉灵敏度：

- 没有严重的眼部受累症状。

基本检查

• 完成眼睛检查：

- 外观检查。

- 视觉灵敏度。

- 受限的，眼外肌运动疼痛(EOM)。

- 瞳孔检查。

- 眼底检查。

- 眼内压测量。

K

- 完成神经系统检查。

诊断检查与说明

实验室检查

支持但不用于诊断：

- 全血细胞计数：
  - 白细胞<15 000 眼眶周围蜂窝织炎。
  - 白细胞>15 000 可能建议菌血症、眼眶周围蜂窝织炎或眼眶蜂窝织炎。
- 血液培养。
- 对化脓性组织进行革兰染色和培养：
  - 当怀疑淋病时准备巧克力琼脂平板。

影像学检查

CT 扫描比对：

- 可能：
  - 中枢神经系统或全身体征。
  - 视觉障碍。
  - 眼球突出，受限的或眼外肌运动疼痛(EOM)。
  - 眼肌瘫痪。
  - 双侧水肿。
  - 24 h 内没有改善或恶化。
- 显示范围：
  - 眼眶蜂窝织炎。
  - 鼻窦炎。
  - 眼眶肿胀。
  - 骨膜下脓肿。
  - 存在异物。
  - 海绵窦血栓症。

诊断步骤/外科

腰椎穿刺：

- 排除由中枢神经参与的出现中毒或假性脑膜炎的患者。
- 外科手术：
  - 清除脓肿。
  - 缓解鼻窦炎。
  - 视神经减压。

鉴别诊断

- 过敏反应。
- 泪腺炎。
- 泪囊炎。
- 格雷夫斯病。
- 睑腺炎。
- 眼眶炎。
- 昆虫叮咬。
- 眼眶横纹肌肉瘤。
- 眶周瘀斑。
- 球后出血。

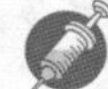

治疗

初步稳定/治疗

静脉输液注入抗生素治疗呕吐、脱水、中毒现象。

急诊治疗/程序

- 解热镇痛药。
- 需要时应用止痛药物。
- 抗生素。

眼眶周围蜂窝织炎

- 通常应口服抗生素，除非出现菌血症或有毒：
  - 力百汀：500 mg[儿童：45 mg/(kg · 24 h)]，口服，每日 3 次。
  - 头孢氨苄：500 mg[儿童：100 mg/(kg · 24 h)]，口服，每日 4 次。
  - 克林霉素：300 mg[儿童：30 mg/(kg · 24 h)]，口服，每日 4 次。
  - 双氯西林：500 mg[儿童：100 mg/(kg · 24 h)]，口服，每日 4 次。
- 注射用抗生素：
  - 头孢噻肟：1～2 g[儿童：150 mg/(kg · 24 h)]，静脉注射，q6～8 h。
  - 克林霉素：600 mg[儿童：40 mg/(kg · 24 h)]，静脉注射，q6 h。

眼眶蜂窝织炎

- 早期应用注射用抗生素。
- 任何眼内表现到眼科会诊。
- 如果鼻窦炎是病源，考虑耳鼻喉会诊，并且在治疗时使用减充血剂。
- 急诊手术干预可能是必要的：
  - 有可疑微生物时应用杀菌药物：
    - 外科清创术。
    - 万可霉素。
    - 在适当的时候使用破伤风疫苗。
- 如果眼球突出使眼角膜暴露：
  - 湿润液(润滑液：2 滴，q2～4 h，需要时使用)。
- 如果怀疑是脑鼻眶藻菌病(CROP)：
  - 最高允许剂量静脉注射两性霉素 B。
  - 局部两性霉素 B 冲洗(1 mg/ml)或鼻腔填塞。
  - 局部清创。

药物治疗

一线用药

- 头孢曲松钠：1～2 g[儿童：100 mg/(kg · 24 h)]，静脉注射，q12～24 h。
- 红霉素眼药膏：q4 h 减少死角。

二线用药

根据可疑的微生物：

- 庆大霉素：5 mg/(kg · 24 h)，静脉注射。
- 甲硝唑：15 mg/kg，静脉注射，然后 7.5 mg/kg，q6 h。
- 萘夫西林：1～2 g[儿童：100 mg/(kg · 24 h)]，静脉注射，q4 h。
- 万可霉素：1 g[儿童：40 mg/(kg · 24 h)]，静脉注射，q12 h。

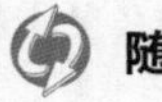

随访

进一步处理

眼眶周围蜂窝织炎

出院使用口服抗生素并且做好随访记录，除非：

- 全身毒性、神经系统、视觉或眼眶调查的证据。
- 不能使用口服类抗生素。
- 口服抗生素感染的进展。
- 在 24～48 h 不能安排随访。
- 高风险 B 型流感嗜血杆菌。
- 复杂医学问题。

眼眶蜂窝织炎

允许：

- 静脉注射抗生素。
- 观察进展。
- 专家会诊。
- 手术切口引流。

要点和误区

- 任何出现眼睛红肿的患者都应考虑眼眶蜂窝织炎。
- 注意以下病史：
  - 近期的鼻窦炎。
  - 近期穿刺、创伤或手术史。
  - 近期口腔感染，特别是犬齿间隙脓肿。
  - 免疫功能低下或近期有糖尿病酮症酸中毒症状。
  - 确定儿童疫苗的注射情况。
- 注意排除：
  - 全身性中毒。
  - 眼睛疼痛或者视觉障碍。
  - 眼睛运动受限。
  - 神经介入的标记与征兆。

莱姆病 Lyme Disease

Morgan P. Eutermoser 王胜云 段立伟 译

 基础知识

描述

• 北美最常见的蜱传播疾病。
• 在东北部呈地方性分布，西北部、中西部为高发地区。

病因

• 高峰期为 4—11 月，80%～90%在夏季发生。
• 硬蜱产生的包柔螺旋体。
- 肩胛硬蜱(鹿蜱)最常见。
- 传播无浆体病的蜱虫病，巴贝虫病。
• 发病机制：
- 机体介导的炎性反应。
- 因子释放。
- 自身免疫。
• 未见人与人感染。

诊断

症状和体征

第一阶段(早期)：
• 被咬后数日至 1 个月。
• 30%～50%的患者能回忆有被咬经历。
• 慢性游走性红斑：
- 特征性病变：
◦ 牛眼征。
- 斑丘疹、环形红斑：
◦ 单发或多发。
◦ 中心区有红色边界。
◦ 直径＞5 cm。
◦ 通常无痛无痒。
• 地区腺病。
• 间断发热。
• 头痛。
• 肌肉疼痛。
• 关节痛。
• 疲劳。
• 萎靡。
第二阶段：
• 被咬后数日到数周。
• 间歇性和波动性症状消失。
• 心脏：
- 心动过速。
- 心动过缓。
- 房室传导阻滞。
- 心肌炎。
• 无菌性脑膜炎、神经炎、神经根炎：
- 面瘫，最常见的症状。
- 可能无皮疹。
- 预后多较好。
• 眼科(视神经炎、角膜炎、上巩膜炎、结膜炎)。
• 淋巴细胞性脑膜炎。
• 第一阶段的症状经常出现。
第三阶段(后期)：
• 发病 1 年后。
• 神经症状：班沃思综合征：神经痛，运动或感觉功能受损，莱姆病脑病。
• 慢性游走性红斑：
- 四肢伸肌面。
- 初始水肿至后期萎缩。
- 类似硬皮病。
• 关节炎：
- 短暂的关节炎发作。
- 单关节。
- 少关节炎。
- 偶尔会迁徙。
- 常见受累关节：
◦ 膝关节。
◦ 肩关节。
◦ 肘关节。
其他：
• 消化系统：
- 肝炎。
- 右上腹痛。
• 眼：
- 角膜炎。
- 葡萄膜炎。
- 虹膜炎。
- 视神经炎。
• 赫氏反应：
- 初始治疗数小时后症状加重。
- 在多发慢性游走性红斑患者中常见。

儿科注意事项

• 较成人患者常见发热。
• 仅约 50%的儿童患者有关节痛表现。
• 1/3 的无菌性脑膜炎患者可有面瘫表现。
• 心电图表现异常。
• 经治疗后患儿预后多较好。
• 未治疗患儿可有角膜炎表现。

妊娠注意事项

未见明显证据表明孕妇患莱姆病会对胎儿造成损害。

病史

• 在疾病流行区域有蜱虫咬伤史。
• 疫区旅行史。
• 夏季类似感冒症状。

体格检查

• 皮疹。
• 关节、心脏、神经系统可有相应表现。

基本检查

• 临床诊断：
- 有慢性游走性红斑时应做血清学检查。
• 寻找咬痕。
• 有脑膜刺激症状时做腰椎穿刺检查。
• 有关节炎时可做关节穿刺。
• 心电图。

诊断检查与说明

实验室检查

• 全血细胞检测：
- 白细胞增多。
- 贫血。
- 血小板减少。
• 红细胞沉降率：
- ＞30 mm/h。
- 最常见的实验室检测异常表现。
• 生化、尿素氮、肌酐、血糖。
• 肝功能：
- 肝酶升高。
• 培养：
- 阳性率低。
- 无特异性。
• 中枢神经系统：
- 细胞数增多。
- 蛋白质水平升高。
- 螺旋体抗体阳性。
• 特殊检测：
- 血清：
◦ 未见特异性慢性游走性红斑时可考虑 ELISA、免疫组化、western-blot。
◦ 抗体存留时间数月到数年。
- PCR：
◦ 高特异性、高敏感性。
◦ 非常规检测。

L

- 关节液：球蛋白水平 5 倍于血浆。
- 关节 X 线平片可能显示软组织、软骨、骨质改变。

■ 鉴别诊断

- 其他蜱咬疾病：
  - 鹿蜱(1 cm)较 ixodid 蜱大(1～2 mm)。
  - 落基山斑疹热。
  - 兔热病。
  - 回归热。
  - 科罗拉多壁虱热。
  - 蜱源性麻痹。
  - STARI：南方蜱类相关皮疹病。
  - 乙型脑炎。
  - 埃立克体病。
- 风湿热：
  - 环形红斑。
  - 颌下关节炎较莱姆病常见。
  - 心脏瓣膜损害。
  - 可见舞蹈症。
- 病毒性脑膜炎：
  - 梅毒。
  - 化脓性关节炎。
  - B19 病毒感染。
  - 感染性心内膜炎。
  - 类风湿关节炎。
  - 瑞特综合征。
  - 褐皮花蛛咬伤。
  - 纤维肌痛症。
  - 慢性疲劳综合征。

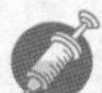

治疗

■ 初步稳定/治疗

- 开通静脉通道。
- 心电监护。
- 重度房室传导阻滞者考虑临时起搏器。

■ 急诊治疗/程序

- 移除蜱虫：
  - 如果蜱虫附着时间少于 36 h，则不太可感染/传播。
  - 消毒咬伤部位。
  - 用钝器轻轻挤压咬伤部位。
  - 确保蜱虫都被清除。
- 第一阶段：
  - 阿莫西林、多西环素[>8 岁患者，头孢呋辛(21 日)]。
  - 阿奇霉素(14～21 日)。
  - 孕妇胃肠外给予。
- 第二阶段：
  - 口服治疗面瘫及轻症患者：
    - 阿莫西林＋丙磺舒(30 日)，多西环素(>8 岁患者，孕妇除外)。
  - 静脉药物治疗症状严重患者：
    - 头孢曲松、头孢噻肟(14～21 日)、青霉素(14～28 日)。
  - 面神经麻痹治疗 14～21 日。
  - 关节炎治疗 28 日。
  - 房室传导阻滞或心脏炎治疗 14～21 日。
  - 脑膜炎/脑炎治疗 14～28 日。
- 第三阶段：
  - 静脉药物治疗：
    - 青霉素、头孢噻肟(14～21 日)、头孢曲松(14～28 日)。

儿科注意事项

儿科严重受伤情况不常见，但是对于有手腕部疼痛的患者应及时明确检查，排除骨折情况。

■ 药物治疗

一线药物

- 阿莫西林：500 mg，口服，每日 3 次(适用于 8 岁以上患者或不能耐受多西环素者)。
- 多西环素：100 mg，口服，每日 2 次，持续 14～21 日(>8 岁患者，孕妇除外)。
- 头孢曲松：2 g，静脉滴注，每日 1 次。

二线药物

- 阿奇霉素：500 mg，口服，每日 1 次。
- 头孢呋辛：500 mg，每日 2 次。
- 头孢噻肟：2 g，静脉滴注，每日 3 次。
- 青霉素：20 万～24 万 U，静脉滴注，q4～6 h。
- 阿司匹林作为心脏受累的辅助治疗。
- 非甾体抗炎药治疗关节炎或关节痛。

随访

■ 进一步处理

入院指征

- 脑膜脑炎。
- 心肌炎患者入住 ICU 监护。

出院指征

口服治疗者。

预防

- 防护服：浅色，裤子塞进袜子，穿长袖。DEET 喷雾。当人/动物返回室内时，进行蜱虫检查。
- 预防莱姆病疫苗：
  - 重组表面蛋白。
  - 适用于高/中度风险地区的人员或前往流行地区的旅客。
  - 2002 年因自身免疫副作用而退出美国。未被证实。

要点和误区

- 在 28 日之外没有临床证据可以治疗。要注意无浆体病和巴贝斯虫病的共同感染。
- 5%的患者会出现疲劳、关节痛等慢性症状。这现在被称为治疗后莱姆病综合征(以前称为慢性莱姆病)。没有进一步抗生素治疗的证据。

阑尾炎

Colleen N. Hickey 李岩 王瑞兰 译

基础知识

■ 描述

- 阑尾炎是最常见的腹部急症。
- 阑尾管腔急性梗阻导致其扩张，随后出现器官缺血、细菌过度生长，最终发生脏器穿孔。
- 疼痛转移：
  - 脐周疼痛：阑尾扩张刺激牵张感受器，并通过内脏痛觉传入纤维将疼痛传递至第 10 胸神经节。
  - 右下腹疼痛：炎症延伸到周围组织，由于腹壁神经纤维受到刺激而出现疼痛，并定位在阑尾的位置。

儿科注意事项

• <12 岁的患者误诊率为 28%～57%（<2 岁的患者几乎为 100%）。

• 幼儿（<4 岁）的穿孔率为 70%～90%。

• 穿孔与延误诊断有很强的相关性。

老年注意事项

• 炎症反应减少。

• 由于解剖结构的变化，穿孔的概率增加 3 倍多。

• 由于表现不典型，往往延误诊断。

妊娠注意事项

• 妊娠第 2 个月与第 1 个月、第 3 个月及产后期相比，发生率略高。

• 穿孔率增加（25%～40%），在第 3 个月最高。

• 右下腹疼痛是最常见的症状。

• 7%～10%会流产，在穿孔性阑尾炎中高达 24%。

病因

• 阑尾管腔梗阻。

• 阑尾管腔变得肿胀，抑制淋巴和静脉回流。

• 肠壁细菌浸润，伴随水肿和动脉血流堵塞。

• 穿孔及泄漏的内容物进入腹腔，引起腹膜炎（通常在发病 24～36 h）。

• 肠壁可脱落，形成脓肿。

• 革兰阴性杆菌和厌氧微生物占主导地位。

诊断

症状和体征

病史

• 腹痛：原发症状：
- 正常位置：
  ◦ 右下腹疼痛。
  ◦ 35%的患者阑尾位于“常见”的位置 5 cm 之内。
- 盲肠后位阑尾（28%～68%）：
  ◦ 背部疼痛。
  ◦ 侧腹痛。
  ◦ 睾丸疼痛。
- 盆腔附件（27%～53%）：
  ◦ 耻骨上疼痛。
  ◦ 泌尿系统或直肠症状。
- 长阑尾（0.2%）：
  ◦ 发炎阑尾头部可能引起右上腹或左下腹疼痛。
  ◦ 厌食症。
  ◦ 呕吐。

• 大便习惯改变：腹泻（33%），便秘（9%～33%）。

• 典型表现（<75%成人）：
- 最初，脐周疼痛。
- 其次是厌食症（95%为第一症状）和恶心。
- 定位于右下腹（发病后 1～12 h）。
- 最后，呕吐伴随发热。

儿科注意事项

• 表现往往无特异性和难以定位（<50%为典型表现）。

• 厌食、呕吐和腹泻比较常见（在抱怨疼痛前的几小时吃半饱，可能会更准确地显示症状的持续时间）。

• 在做局部炎症的细微指标检查前先观察儿童：
- 跛行步态。
- 移动或爬行之前犹豫。
- 右髋关节屈曲。

体格检查

• 生命体征：
- 通常正常。
- 发热：最初正常至轻度升高（<1℃），体温随着穿孔而增加。

• 腹部检查：
- 麦氏点压痛（右髂前上棘到脐连线的中外 1/3）。
- 肌卫：
  ◦ 早期由于肌肉对触诊的抵抗产生主动防卫。
  ◦ 随着炎症的进展和发生穿孔产生被动防卫（板状腹）。
- 反跳痛：
  ◦ 任何快速移动的腹膜会（例如，撞击担架）会产生疼痛。
- 特异性体征：
  ◦ 罗夫辛征：触诊左下腹时，疼痛位于右下腹。
  ◦ 腰大肌征：患者取左侧卧位，右大腿后伸，疼痛加重，是由于发炎的阑尾接触髂腰肌。
  ◦ 闭孔内肌试验：右髋关节屈曲，被动内旋，产生疼痛。

• 直肠检查：
- 价值有限：可定位压痛或肿块的位置。

• 盆腔检查：
- 重要的是鉴别妇科疾病。
- 阴道分泌物和/或附件压痛或肿块，提示妇科疾病。
- 宫颈摇摆痛提示盆腔炎，但可见于大约 25%的女性阑尾炎患者。

• 患者体位：
- 仰卧或用腿支撑的侧卧（尤其是右腿）。
- 不愿动。

• Shuffling 步态被称为阑尾切除术步态。

儿科注意事项

几乎所有的儿童都有一定的伴随腹部僵硬的广泛性腹部压痛。

妊娠注意事项

• 扩大的子宫向上和横向移动。

• 妊娠剧吐及呕吐的其他非手术因素不应该造成腹部压痛。

老年注意事项

老年人可能无腹膜炎的典型体征。

基本检查

• 有提示意义的病史和体格检查足以建立术前诊断及保证外科会诊。

• 下面列出的测试可用于协助诊断。

• 不典型病例：重复测试并结合以下一些测试是有效的，并且降低阴性阑尾切除率而无穿孔率的增加。

诊断检查与说明

实验室检查

• CBC：
- 白细胞>10 000/mm^3，核左移（80%）。
- 白细胞正常不能排除诊断。

• C 反应蛋白：
- 总的敏感性为 62%，特异性为 66%。
- 可能早期不会升高（<12 h）。
- 增加了灵敏度。

• 尿液分析：
- 一般正常。
- 轻度脓尿、菌尿或血尿（25%～30%）。
- 如果发炎的阑尾靠近输尿管或膀胱会出现脓尿。

• 育龄期女性需做妊娠试验。

影像学检查

• 当诊断明确时，无需做。

• 生育年龄的女性患者诊断不明确时最有用。

• 腹部 X 线平片，不推荐。

• 超声：敏感性 86%～90%，特异性 92%～95%：
- 阑尾直径超过 6 mm。
- 阑尾粪石的存在。
- 阑尾周围液体/固体。

L

- 受肥胖、肠道气体、盲肠后位阑尾和操作者限制。
- 排除诊断。

• CT：敏感性 91%～100%，特异性 94%～97%：
- 口服及灌肠造影剂，聚焦阑尾从盲肠上方 3 cm 向远端延伸 12～15 cm 的薄层扫描。
- 脂肪间隙(100%)。
- 阑尾直径 6 mm(93%)。
- 局灶性盲肠顶端增厚。
- 定义阑尾周围组织(蜂窝织炎和脓肿阑尾肿块)。
- 寻找替代诊断的最佳研究。
- 看不到阑尾不能排除阑尾炎。

• MRI：敏感性 97%～100%，特异性 92%～94%。
- 阑尾的直径为 7 mm。
- 阑尾周围脂肪间隙。
- 优点：无辐射，钆造影剂有良好的安全性。
- 缺点：成本高，可用性有限，检查时间长，放射科医师缺乏熟悉阑尾炎的相关知识。
- 无用于妊娠早期的钆(C 类药物)。

儿科注意事项

美国放射学会建议在疑似阑尾炎需要检查时，先做超声之后再做 CT。

诊断步骤/外科

• 腹腔镜：
- 诊断性与治疗性应用。
- 大体病理可能无阳性镜检结果。

• 开腹阑尾切除术。
• 经皮引流。

鉴别诊断

• 胃肠炎。
• 梅克尔憩室。
• 肠脂垂炎。
• 克罗恩病。
• 憩室炎。
• 肠扭转。
• 腹主动脉瘤。
• 肠梗阻。
• 尿路感染。
• 盆腔炎。
• 异位妊娠。
• 卵巢囊肿/扭转。
• 输卵管卵巢脓肿。
• 子宫内膜异位症。
• 肾结石。
• 睾丸扭转。
• 镰刀形细胞病。
• 肠系膜淋巴结炎。
• Henoch-Schönlein 紫癜。
• 糖尿病酮症酸中毒。
• 链球菌性咽炎(儿童)。
• 胆道疾病。

治疗

初步稳定/治疗

• ABC 管理。
• 使用林格液或生理盐水液体复苏。

急诊治疗/程序

• 静脉输液，纠正电解质异常。
• 为了有说服力的病史和体格检查立即外科会诊：
- 腹腔镜与开腹手术。
- 男性阴性阑尾切除率为 10%，女性为 20%。
- 阑尾脓肿 6～8 周需经皮穿刺引流、静脉注射抗生素、肠道休息和可能的择期阑尾切除术。

• 围手术期应用抗生素。
• 禁食。
• 如果右下腹有可触及的肿块，需做 CT 明确是蜂窝织炎或脓肿。
• 如果诊断是不确定的，进一步实验室检查，观察并重复测试(通过观察实验报告，可有 6%～10%的阴性阑尾切除率)。
• 镇痛药：
- 管理止痛药，包括麻醉药，不会对腹部检查产生不利影响以及影响病理结果。

药物治疗

• 氨苄西林-舒巴坦：3 g[儿童：100～200 mg 氨苄西林(kg·24 h)]，静脉给药，q6 h。
• 头孢西丁：2 g[儿童：80～100 mg/(kg·24 h)]，静脉给药，q6 h。
• 头孢曲松钠：1 g(儿童：50～100 mg/kg)，静脉给药，q24 h。
• 环丙沙星：400 mg(儿童：20～40 mg/kg)，静脉给药，q12 h。
• 厄他培南：1 g，肌内注射/静脉给药，q24 h。
• 甲硝唑：500 mg[儿童：30～50 mg/(kg·24 h)]，静脉给药，q8～12 h。
• 硫酸吗啡：3～5 mg(儿童：0.1～0.2 mg/kg，q2 h～q4 h)每 15 min 滴注，滴定至产生效应。
• 哌拉西林-他唑巴坦：3.375 g[儿童：＜6 个月，150～300 mg/(kg·d)；＞6 个月，240～400 mg/(kg·d)]，静脉给药 q6 h。

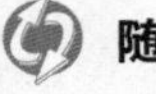

随访

进一步处理

入院指征

• 急性阑尾炎的外科干预。
• 如果诊断不确定，需观察或进一步的诊断检查。

出院指征

如果符合以下标准，有腹痛而不认为是阑尾炎的患者可出院：

• 症状已缓解或正在缓解。
• 腹部压痛极小或无。
• 无实验室或影像学异常。
• 能耐受经口进食。
• 如果症状恶化，有足够的社会支持并能够及时返回医院。

转诊问题

确诊或疑似阑尾炎的外科会诊。

随访建议

从急诊出院的不明的腹痛患者需在 24～48 h 复查。

要点和误区

• 儿童和老年患者表现不典型，穿孔率增加。
• 急性阑尾炎的典型表现不需要影像学检查。
• 如果阑尾不可见，任何成像方式都不能排除阑尾炎。

滥用大麻 Marijuana

Nathan Ansbaugh · Adam Z. Barkin 段立伟 译

基础知识

描述

- 在世界范围内，大麻是最常被滥用的物质。
- 根据美国联邦法律是非法的。
- 在美国9个州和哥伦比亚特区合法化。
- 在29个州和哥伦比亚特区允许用于医疗。
- 在制定了医用大麻法律的州，非法使用大麻的情况显著增加。
- 青少年日常使用量正在上升。
- 又名：线麻、白麻、胡麻、野麻或大麻。
- 大麻叶和花的类烟草制剂。
- 活性成分包括：
  - 反式-19-四氢大麻酚(19-THC)。
    - 介导脑内CB1受体部分激活作用。
  - 大麻二酚(CBD)
    - CBD是非精神病药物，使CBD衍生物在诸如老年痴呆症、癫痫、焦虑症、精神病、炎症过程、癌症、疼痛管理等领域具有治疗意义。
- 代谢：高度亲脂性，所以消除半衰期在25～36 h很长。
- 通过肝脏细胞色素氧化酶，CUP2C9和3A4进行代谢，最终通过粪便(65%)和尿液(20%)排出体外。
- 确凿的证据表明大麻：
  - 有效治疗成人慢性疼痛。
  - 是治疗化疗所致恶心呕吐的有效止吐药。
  - 导致机动车碰撞(MVC)风险增加。
  - 导致婴儿出生体重降低。
  - 导致精神分裂症或其他精神病的风险增高，在频繁使用的人群中风险最高。
  - 较早的年龄使用是导致长期使用大麻的危险因素。
- 适度证据表明大麻：
  - 导致药物依赖或药物滥用的发展。
  - 导致自杀意念和自杀未遂的发生率增加。
  - 导致学习、记忆和注意力受损。

病因

- 吸入：
  - 用纸卷。
  - 汽化装置。
    - 又名“juuling”或“juling”。
    - 通常非常高效。
  - 水管(桶)。
  - 水烟袋。
  - 大麻浓缩液。
    - 从大麻植物中提取的杂碎油被提炼成蜡状。
    - 使用烟管。
    - 非常有效。
- 摄入
  - 药剂。
    - 快速。
    - 酒精通常是溶剂。
    - 滴在舌头下方。
  - 可食油脂。
    - 可以以胶囊的形式吃或吞下。
  - 食品。
    - 任何含有大麻的食物。
    - 起效时间较长。
    - 经常引起全身，精神反应。
    - 经常被注入高脂肪成分中(黄油、橄榄油)。
  - 饮料。
    - 注入大麻或大麻油的饮料。
- 局部使用：
  - 神经影响最小。
- 鼻吸入(THC晶体)。
- 大麻合成素(SCB)：
  - 尽管受到越来越多的法律限制，但通过互联网广泛提供。
  - 主要并发症包括心血管事件(心肌梗死、缺血性中风和栓塞)、急性肾损伤(AKI)、全身强直、阵挛发作、精神症状(包括首发精神病、偏执、自残/自杀意念)和呕吐过度。
  - 最常见的症状是心动过速、烦躁和恶心，只需对症治疗。
  - 研究表明，与部分激动剂性质相比Δ(9)-THC通常在体外观察到，SCB作为CB1和CB2受体激动剂在细胞分析和动物研究中都起作用。
- 湿法：
  - 大麻烟(联合)浸有苯环己定(PCP)和/或甲醛。
  - 症状包括幻觉、迷失方向、协调能力受损、偏执、性抑制、严重攻击、暴力行为、视觉障碍、呼吸衰竭、癫痫、呕吐过度。

诊断

症状和体征

- 中枢神经：
  - 欣快感和烦躁。
  - 惊恐。
  - 自杀倾向。
  - 精神错乱。
- 眼：
  - 视力模糊。
- 消化系统：
  - 食欲增加。
  - 口干。
  - 剧烈呕吐。
- 心血管系统：
  - 心悸。
  - 胸痛。
- 呼吸系统：
  - 支气管痉挛。

病史

- 通常由快递员、朋友、家人提供。
- 询问是否使用合成的大麻。
- 询问其他人是否有类似症状。
- 是否第一次用。
- 共同服用。
  - 其他药物。
  - 酒精。
- 外伤史。

体格检查

- 中枢神经：
  - 可从严重的躁动到严重的昏睡或昏迷。
  - 运动失调。
  - 运动功能亢进。
- 眼：
  - 结膜充血。
  - 眼球震颤。
- 消化系统：
  - 黏膜干燥。
  - 全腹部不适。
- 心血管系统：
  - 高血压、心动过速。
  - 镇静剂：低血压，心动过缓。
- 呼吸系统：
  - 支气管痉挛。
  - 胸部起伏和两侧呼吸音相等(注意气胸)。

L

■ 基本检查

• 考虑精神状态改变的其他病因。
• 评估创伤程度。
• 监测生命体征。
• 放置心电监护。

■ 诊断检查与说明

实验室检查

• 全血细胞计数。
• 电解质、血尿素氮、肌酸酐和葡萄糖水平。
• 肌钙蛋白。
- 如果心电图异常。
- 如果出现胸痛，在吸食大麻的 1 h 内，心肌缺血的风险会增加到正常值的 4.8 倍。
• 对乙酰氨基酚水平。
- 存在一起吸食。
• 水杨酸水平。
- 考虑合并存在阴离子间隙代谢性酸中毒或患者是否出现呼吸性碱中毒。
• 毒理学筛查和使用 AMS 的 EtOH 标准，以及是否与合成有关。

影像学检查

• 拍胸部 X 线片。
- 对于呼吸急促的人。
• 神经影像学(头颅 CT)。
- 如果有局灶性神经系统检查结果，严重的精神状态抑郁，严重的头痛，或者患者出现头部外伤，考虑神经影像学检查。

诊断步骤/外科

• 心电图：
- 如果出现胸痛，生命体征异常，或其他并发症。

■ 鉴别诊断

• 低血糖。
• 电解质紊乱。
• 中枢神经感染。
• 创伤性脑损伤。
• 药物中毒。
- 阿片类。
- 苯二氮䓬类。
- 酒精。
- 可乐定。
- 抗组胺药。
- 精神类药物。
• 一氧化碳。
• 惊厥。
• 脓毒症。

注意

• 大麻过量呕吐综合征：
- 与大麻使用相关的周期性呕吐综合征。
- 在系统回顾中 14 个诊断特征：
◦ 任何时期的常规大麻接触史(100%)。
◦ 周期性恶心、呕吐(100%)。
◦ 停止吸食大麻后症状的缓解(96.8%)。
◦ 强迫性热水浴缓解症状(92.3%)。
◦ 男性占比多(72.9%)。
◦ 腹痛(85.1%)。
◦ 至少每周使用大麻(97.4%)。
- 治疗：
◦ 静脉输液支持，多巴胺拮抗剂，外用辣椒素乳膏。
◦ 在急性发作时，避免使用麻醉药品已显示出一些益处。
◦ 停止吸食大麻是最好的治疗方法。

治疗

■ 院前

• 建立静脉注射通路。
• 心电监护。
• 控制出血。
• 如果精神状态严重抑郁，考虑纳洛酮。
• 如有必要，可考虑使用苯二氮䓬、氟哌啶醇、氯胺酮控制。

■ 初步稳定/治疗

• ABC 管理。
• 建立静脉注射通路。
• 使用心电监护。
• 如果精神状态低落，考虑纳洛酮。
• 检测葡萄糖，低血糖纠正。

■ 急诊治疗/程序

• 静脉输液。
• 如果更多的交感神经表现，考虑苯二氮䓬类药物。
• 止吐药。
• 抗多巴胺药。

■ 药物治疗

• 氟哌啶醇：0.5～10 mg，肌内注射或静脉给药，q1～4 h。
• 氯胺酮：躁动明显时，1～4 mg/kg，肌内注射；0.5～2 mg/kg 静脉给药。
• 劳拉西泮：0.5～4 mg，静脉给药或肌内注射。
• 奥氮平：5～20 mg，肌内注射；或 2.5～10 mg，静脉给药。

一线用药

• 劳拉西泮。
• 氟哌啶醇治疗大麻过度呕吐综合征。

二线用药

• 奥氮平。
• 氯胺酮。

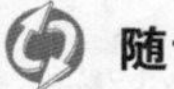

随访

■ 进一步处理

入院指征

• 如果出现以下情况，予以入院：
- 导致精神状态的其他毒性或抑郁需要额外观察。
- 躁动或谵妄需要额外的镇静剂和治疗。

出院指征

大多数单纯性大麻中毒的急诊患者在观察后和临床上清醒后可以出院。

随访

为成瘾性使用者提供的药物康复。

孕妇注意事项

• 9.5%的育龄妇女有过吸食大麻。
• THC 可穿过胎盘。
• 可能影响胎儿神经发育。

儿童注意事项

• 患者在吸食或吸食大麻后可能出现嗜睡、共济失调或呼吸功能不全。
• 食物是常见的来源。
• 可能导致大量检查和入院治疗。
• 如果怀疑的话，考虑及时送毒理学检查。
• 毒物控制中心报告显示，儿童接触大麻的人数从 2005 年到 2011 年增加了 30%。

要点和误区

• 观察数据表明，在易患冠心病的个体中，使用大麻可能会加速心肌梗死的风险。
• 尽管数据有限，但胎儿在子宫内时，大麻有可能干扰胎儿的神经发育。
- 应鼓励妇女在怀孕期间减少或停止使用所有类似药物。
- 即使在大麻合法的环境中，孕妇最终也参与 CPS。
• 合成大麻素常表现为躁动性谵妄。
• 使用大麻素会增加 MVC 的风险。
• 反复出现周期性呕吐综合征的患者应考虑大麻过度呕吐综合征。

肋骨骨折

Charles W. O'Connell 何融冰 译

基础知识

描述

• 严重或轻微胸部外伤所致的结果。

• 可分为创伤性或病理性。

病因

• 钝性胸部外伤：

- 单纯跌倒、高处坠落。
- 车辆碰撞。
- 袭击。
- 子弹。
- CPR 相关。

• 穿透伤是较少见的原因：

- 肋骨通常在着力点或后角处碎裂，即结构薄弱区。

• 上中部肋骨的压力性骨折可由于反复的强力动作导致：

- 体育活动：高尔夫、划船、投掷运动。
- 剧烈咳嗽。

• 与轻微外伤或明显基础疾病相关的病理性骨折：

- 年龄大、骨质疏松、肿瘤。

儿科注意事项

• 相对有弹性的胸壁使肋骨骨折在儿童中较少见。

• 婴幼儿如果没有适当作用机制应考虑非意外创伤。

• 如果怀疑婴幼儿受虐待，应进行骨骼检查来评估是否有其他骨折。

老年人注意事项

• 老年人更易患肋骨骨折以及肺不张、肺炎、呼吸衰竭和其他相关并发症。

• 发病率和死亡率是年轻人群的 2 倍。

诊断

症状和体征

病史

• 任何机制的胸部钝挫伤。

• 机制由患者、父母或院前急救人员描述：

- 安全带使用。
- 方向盘损伤。
- 气囊展开。

• 深呼吸、咳嗽和运动时局部胸部疼痛加剧。

• 胸膜性胸痛。

• 呼吸困难、呼吸短促。

体格检查

• 压痛点。

• 触诊累及肋骨周围时与骨折部位相关的疼痛。

• 骨性错位。

• 捻发音。

• 局部水肿。

• 红斑。

• 淤血：

- 由与机动车事故相关的安全带（称为“安全带征”）或方向盘引起。

• 肋间肌肉痉挛。

• 夹板固定的呼吸运动。

• 缺氧、心悸、呼吸衰竭。

• 听诊表现为呼吸音正常或减低，偶尔在骨折处可闻及喀喇音。

• 胸壁局部反常运动提示连枷胸，表明有多处的游离的肋骨骨折。

基本检查

• 根据临床表现做出初步诊断，由影像学检查确诊。

• 评估基础结构的损伤。

注意

• 前 3 肋相对受保护且需要显著的冲击力才能骨折，可能提示有胸腔内损伤。

• 9～12 肋相对活动，此处骨折提示腹内损伤的可能。

• 多处肋骨骨折可能伴随连枷胸和肺挫伤。

• 发病率与基础结构的损伤程度、骨折数量及年龄有关。

诊断检查与说明

实验室检查

ABGs 可提示低氧血症或肺泡-动脉梯度增高：

• 单处，无并发症的肋骨骨折不需要进行。

• 多处肋骨骨折或之前患有肺部疾病的患者可考虑使用。

影像学检查

• 前后位及侧位胸片常规用于肋骨骨折诊断。

• 胸部平片可用于排除相关胸腔内损伤，但可能遗漏达 66%的肋骨骨折：

- 可揭示相关胸腔内病理学病因：
  ◦ 气胸。
  ◦ 血胸。
  ◦ 纵隔气肿。
  ◦ 肺挫伤。
  ◦ 肺不张。
  ◦ 纵隔影增宽。
- 肺挫伤在受损后 6～12 h 可显现：
  ◦ 从片状肺泡浸润影到明显实变。

• 肋骨片系列提供了更高的灵敏度，但它们的实用性是有争议的，而且通常是低灵敏度的。

• CT 对于发现肋骨骨折和内部损伤更具敏感性。

• 胸部 CT 能够排除胸腔内损伤。

• CT 或超声可用于排除相关腹内伤。

• 如果血管神经方面的症状和体征出现，血管造影可用于探查血管损伤：

- 第 1 肋和第 2 肋的损伤可引起血管损伤，尤其是后移位。

• 超声是一项对于评估肋骨骨折，甚至软骨损伤很有前景的诊断工具。

鉴别诊断

• 肋骨挫伤或肋间肌扭伤。

• 气胸。

• 肋间软骨分离。

• 胸骨骨折和脱位。

• 胸痛的非创伤性原因：

- 心血管性：
  ◦ 心肌缺血或梗死。
  ◦ 心包炎。
  ◦ 主动脉夹层。
  ◦ 肺栓塞。
- 肺部：
  ◦ 栓塞。
  ◦ 感染。
  ◦ 炎症。
  ◦ 气压伤。
- 肌肉骨骼的：
  ◦ 肋软骨炎。
  ◦ 颈椎或胸椎疾病。
- 胃肠道：
  ◦ 食管反流或痉挛。
  ◦ Mallory-Weiss 撕裂。
  ◦ 胆绞痛或肾绞痛。

◦ 消化性溃疡。
◦ 胃炎、胰腺炎、肝炎。
- 皮肤疾病：
◦ 带状疱疹。
◦ 胸壁肿瘤。

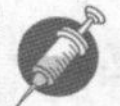

治疗

院前

重点在呼吸道维持、镇痛和供氧。

初步稳定/治疗

• 单纯性骨折，通常无需特殊治疗。
• 评估合并的头部、四肢、腹部和钝性心脏损伤。
• 多处骨折，老年患者或明显的基础肺疾病：
- 根据需要控制呼吸道进行复苏。
- 气管内插管用于有严重低氧血症的患者(PaO_2＜60 mmHg 给予空气，＜80 mmHg 给予 100% O_2)或即将发生呼吸衰竭。

急诊治疗/程序

• 单纯性骨折：
- 控制疼痛：
◦ 关键在于维持合适的肺功能，避免肺不张和继发的肺炎。
- 用 0.5%布比卡因行肋间神经阻滞是安全有效的：
◦ 持续 6～12 h 的疼痛缓解。
◦ 肋间神经阻滞应在脊椎正中线后 2～3 指宽处进行。
◦ 在神经血管束所在的肋骨下缘注射 0.5～1 ml。
◦ 先抽吸确保未刺到肋间血管。
- 深呼吸及诱发性肺量测定法应在适当控制疼痛的情况下进行。
- 头抬高至 30 度，除非有禁忌。
- 避免绑缚或绑扎胸壁以免限制通气及促使肺不张。
• 多处骨折、年长患者或明显的基础肺疾病：
- 控制疼痛和肺清洗。
- 检查并发伤，治疗加重的基础肺疾病。
- 多处骨折的肋间神经阻滞是安全且有效的，可维持 6～12 h，疼痛缓解。
- 对于住院患者，胸部硬膜外镇痛或患者自控镇痛苦(PCA)是有效的，且对呼吸动度限制最小。
- 对于严重肋骨骨折(例如，右胸、多发性移位骨折)可采用手术固定。

药物治疗

• 一线：非甾体抗炎药和/或对乙酰氨基酚加或不含阿片类药物。
- 布洛芬：600 mg，口服，q6 h(儿童：5～10 mg/kg，口服，q6～8 h)。
- 萘普生：250～500 mg，口服，q12 h[儿童：10～20 mg/(kg·d)，口服 div.，q12 h]。
- 对乙酰氨基酚：325～1 000 mg，口服，q4～6 h，最多 4 g/d(儿童：婴儿 10～15 mg/kg，口服，q4～6 h，最多 75 mg/kg，12 岁及以上儿童 325～650 mg，口服，q4～6 h，最多 4 g/d)。
• 阿片类镇痛药，使用最低有效剂量，提倡低起始剂量。
• 多种对乙酰氨基酚/阿片类镇痛药制品；如以下“Men”：
- 对乙酰氨基酚：300 mg/可待因 30 mg(儿童：0.5～1 mg/kg 可待因)，口服，q4～6 h。
- 对乙酰氨基酚：325 mg/氢可酮 2.5～10 mg，口服，q4～6 h。
- 对乙酰氨基酚：325 mg/羟考酮 2.5～10 mg，口服，q4～6 h。
• 二线药物：针对不耐受口服或更严重的疼痛：
- 氢吗啡酮：2～8 mg，口服，q3～4 h(儿童：0.03～0.08 mg/kg，口服，q4～6 h)。
- 氢吗啡酮：0.5～4 mg，静脉注射、肌内注射或皮下注射，q4～6 h(儿童：0.03～0.08 mg/kg)。
- 硫酸吗啡：2.5～10 mg，静脉注射、肌内注射或皮下注射，q2～6 h(儿童：0.1～0.2 mg/kg)。
- PCA 使用氢吗啡酮或硫酸吗啡有效。
- 0.25%～0.5%布比卡因：肋间神经阻滞每次 5 ml。
- 小剂量氯胺酮：0.1～0.3 mg/kg 静脉缓慢推注(次相关剂量)，最大累积剂量 0.3 mg/kg 或 50 mg，仅限成人。

注意
• 多系统和局部镇痛提高疗效。
• 使用胸部硬膜外镇痛：
- 有顽固性疼痛的患者。
- 过度镇静。
- 麻醉镇痛剂导致换气不足。
• 当肾功能不全或胃肠道出血时避免使用 NSAIDs。
• 对乙酰氨基酚/麻醉性镇痛药因对乙酰氨基酚可造成肝中毒的潜在副作用所限制。
- 成人对乙酰氨基酚至多不能超过 4 g/24 h，儿童对乙酰氨基酚不能超过 5 次剂量，10～15 mg/(kg·24 h)。

随访

进一步处理

入院指征

入院通常应该交给创伤专家。
• 顽固性疼痛。
• 无法咳嗽和清理分泌物。
• 肺功能受损。
• 多发骨折，双侧肋骨骨折，第 1、第 2 肋骨骨折。
• 骨折移位。
• 合并气胸、血胸、纵隔气肿、肺挫伤、腹内或胸腔内疾病。
• 老年患者和有明显基础肺疾病的患者：
- 慢性 COPD、CHF、肺纤维化、哮喘。
• 口服药无法适当控制疼痛。
• 有 6 根以上肋骨骨折的老年患者应送入 ICU。
• 主要创伤机制相关的肋骨骨折。

出院指征

• 有正常肺功能的患者、无潜在肺损伤、口服药可适当控制疼痛。
• 在出院前与患者协商严格的回访标准：
- 呼吸短促。
- 疼痛加重。
- 疼痛控制不良。
- 发热。

注意
肋骨骨折与肺炎、ARDS、气胸、误吸、脓胸的发生有关。

随访建议

• 大多数肋骨骨折在 6 周内痊愈，但患者应能更快地恢复规律日常活动。
• 不推荐规律胸部 X 线随访。

要点和误区

• 警惕与肋骨骨折相关的潜在胸腔内和腹腔内损伤。
• 确保合理控制疼痛，通气在治疗中占首位。
• 肋骨骨折转运会增加致病率和病死率。
• 儿童肋骨骨折提示严重外力作用，应怀疑非意外性创伤。

L

泪囊炎和泪腺炎 Dacryocystitis and Dacryoadenitis

Shari Schabowski · Daniella C. Lucas 许磊 译

基础知识

描述

• 泪腺炎和泪囊炎是由于特定条件影响导致眼泪系统的炎症：

- 泪腺炎是泪腺感染或炎症，泪腺为分泌眼泪的腺体。
- 泪囊炎是排泪管道发生的感染。

• 泪腺炎是一种常见的炎症状态或感染过程，可以经由其他部位蔓延或全身感染导致。

• 泪囊炎是泪管和泪囊阻塞引起的化脓性感染。

流行病学

泪腺炎是不多见的疾病，左侧多见：

• 获得：

- 罕见。

泪囊炎是一种更常见的疾病，多发生于大于 30 岁成年女性，但也可见于婴儿，通常在出生后不久。

病因学(泪腺炎)

• 最常由系统性感染引起：

- 自身免疫性疾病。
- 干燥综合征。
- 结节病。
- 克罗恩病。
- 肿瘤。

• 传染为主要原因，也可继发于持续蔓延的细菌性结膜炎或眶周蜂窝织炎。

• 急性化脓性：

- 细菌是成年人感染的最常见原因：
  ◦ 金黄色葡萄球菌。
  ◦ 链球菌。
  ◦ 沙眼衣原体。
  ◦ 淋病奈瑟菌。

• 慢性泪腺炎：

- 鼻腔菌群>眼菌群。

儿科注意事项

• 病毒是儿童感染的最常见病因：

- 流行性腮腺炎。
- 麻疹。
- EB 病毒。
- 巨细胞病毒。
- 柯萨奇病毒。
- 水痘-带状疱疹病毒。

• 缓慢增大的肿块可能是皮样囊肿。

病因学-泪囊炎

• 正常情况下，排泪经过泵动作将泪由泪腺管挤入泪囊，然后进入中鼻甲、鼻窦。

• 当排泪部分或完全阻滞在泪腺管到泪囊中则可出现症状：

- 由慢性筛窦炎引起的泪囊炎很常见，但许多与鼻炎和系统性炎症均可能相关。
  ◦ 也可继发于创伤、泪石、鼻或鼻窦手术或任何可能导致阻塞的原因。
- 通道阻滞可以导致细菌大量增生和感染。
- 感染可能反复发作而演变成慢性：
  ◦ 最常见的细菌：鼻窦>眼菌群。
  ◦ 金黄色葡萄球菌是最常见微生物。

并发症包括瘘管形成、复发性结膜炎甚至脓肿或者眼眶蜂窝织炎。

儿科注意事项

• 先天性的，婴儿期发病常继发于小儿泪囊囊肿，而新生儿发病多由于保留的羊水。

• 以下可导致高发病率和死亡率：

- 全身性的感染扩散或细菌在局部阻塞的腺管大量生长。

• 最常见的微生物为肺炎链球菌。

诊断

两者均可表现为单侧的、红色、疼痛的眼睛。

症状和体征

泪腺炎

多表现为急性或无痛的肿胀，以及上眼睑红疹。

• 肿胀和压痛以下眼睑眶缘最明显：

- S 形眼睑。

• 肿块可触及。

• 可能与以下相关：

- 广泛的蜂窝织炎。
- 结膜充血和流液。
- 产泪增加或减少。
- 同侧结膜感染和水肿。
- 同侧耳前淋巴结肿大。
- 可能出现全身中毒。

• 正常视力敏锐度、裂隙灯检测和眼底镜检查。

• 可能会导致全眼球压力或位移：

- 可能出现视觉失真。

• 慢性型：缓慢进展，无痛，肿胀。

> **注意**
>
> 迅速确定是否有淋病结膜炎的临床传染的可能性：
>
> • 发病率非常高：
>
> - 可能失明。
> - 可能有全身疾病。
>
> • 治疗可随其他原因而有差异。

泪囊炎

表现为急性的炎症，从内眦延伸至鼻中隔和内侧的受限的肿块：

• 泪溢或过度排泪：标志性的症状。

- 眼泪流出受阻。

• 泪腺排出物：

- 按压发炎肿块可以从泪腺中挤出脓性物质。
- 可以作为诊断依据。

• 蜂窝织炎可蔓延到下眼睑。

• 可出现低热，但患者极少出现中毒。

基本检查

完整的眼部检查，包括视力、眼外肌运动、裂隙灯和眼底镜检查：

• 翻转眼睑。

• 检查鼻通道。

儿科注意事项

仔细检查是否有蔓延导致眼眶蜂窝织炎和脑膜炎的证据是必要的。

诊断检查与说明

实验室检查

• 流出物检测(用于协助特异性抗生素治疗)。

- 革兰染色。
- 培养和药敏试验。
- 怀疑淋球菌时做巧克力琼脂平板试验。

• 全血细胞计数和血培养。

影像学检查

• 眶部、鼻窦 CT 扫描评估组织深层可能的泪腺炎病症，尤其是儿童复发案例需要考虑来自泪囊炎的眼眶蜂窝织炎。

• 超声可通过比较回声来区分正常泪囊和慢性泪囊炎。

鉴别诊断

• 泪腺炎：

- 自身免疫性疾病。
- 泪腺肿瘤。
- 麦粒肿。
- 眶周蜂窝织炎。
- 严重的睑缘炎。
- 眼眶蜂窝织炎。
- 昆虫叮咬。
- 创伤性损伤。
- 眼眶或泪腺肿瘤。

• 泪囊炎：
- 昆虫叮咬。
- 创伤性损伤。
- 急性筛窦炎。
- 眶周蜂窝织炎。
- 急性结膜炎。

治疗

■ 急诊治疗/程序

• 早期诊断和初期治疗将减少相邻结构和系统感染的风险。

• 可以考虑局部外用抗生素治疗或避免结膜炎。

泪腺炎

• 冷敷减轻炎症和使用非甾体类药物。

• 4～6 周症状消失。

• 病毒性病因：
- 典型的自限性炎症。

• 细菌性病因：
- 抗生素。
- 轻度感染时口服：
  ◦ 头孢菌素。
  ◦ 阿莫西林-克拉维酸。
- 严重感染时经静脉给药：
  ◦ 头孢唑林。
  ◦ 羟基噻吩青霉素-克拉维酸。

• 如必须予破伤风类毒素。

• 除了非常严重的情况，很少需要切开排出。
- 进行面部手术或眼科咨询服务。

儿科注意事项

• 冷敷。

• 镇痛剂。

• 如原因不明，则同成人一样给予抗生素治疗。

泪囊炎

• 泪囊感染灶的引流是十分必要的：
- 热敷和轻揉以缓解梗阻。
- 收缩剂的推出可能有助于阻塞鼻道的引流。
- 只有严重的病例需切开引流：
  ◦ 通常由眼科来完成。
  ◦ 如果可能，在急诊应尽量避免。
  ◦ 可能导致瘘管形成。
- 急性期不需要置入泪管帮助引流：
  ◦ 如果有需要的话，非急性期备用泪管。
  ◦ 管道发炎的同时进行操作可能导致管道损伤和永久性梗阻的瘢痕和狭窄。
- 局部眼用抗生素滴剂预防继发性结膜炎。

• 全身抗生素治疗控制感染及预防感染蔓延至相邻结构。
- 轻度感染时口服抗生素。
- 发热或严重的感染时静脉使用抗生素。

• 镇痛剂。

儿科注意事项

• 新生儿病例中 95%对轻揉和局部外用抗生素反应良好。

• 如果 1 年内没有解决，可能需要由眼科探测管道。

• 小于 4 岁的泪囊炎患儿：
- 如果没有免疫接种，可增加流感嗜血杆菌感染的风险。
  ◦ 早期报告中提到在典型年龄段完成免疫接种是不太可能的。
  ◦ 推荐免疫接种时间为 2 个月、4 个月、6 个月和 12～15 个月。

• B 型流感嗜血杆菌感染有发生菌血症、败血症和脑膜炎的高风险。

• 对于无发热、表现良好的患儿且有负责任的家长，可口服氯氨苄西林或者阿莫西林-克拉维酸治疗。

• 急性感染可静脉给予头孢呋辛。

■ 药物治疗

• 阿莫西林-克拉维酸（奥格门汀）：500 mg［儿童：阿莫西林 20～40 mg/(kg · 24 h)］，口服，q8 h。

• 氯氨苄西林：500 mg［儿童：20～40 mg/(kg · 24 h)］常释，口服，每日 3 次。

• 头孢唑林：500～1 000 mg［儿童：50～100 mg/(kg · 24 h)］，静脉给药，q6～8 h。

• 头孢呋辛：750～1 500［儿童：50～100 mg/(kg · 24 h)］，静脉给药，q8 h。

• 头孢氨苄：500 mg［儿童：25～100 mg/(kg · 24 h)］，口服，每日 4 次。

• 红霉素眼药膏：2 滴于感染的眼睛，每日 4 次。

• 丁卡因和肾上腺素溶液单剂量鼻腔喷雾剂。

• 替卡西林-克拉维酸：3.1 g［儿童：200～300 mg 替卡西林/(kg · 24 h)］，静脉给药，q4～6 h。

• 复方多黏菌素软膏：2 滴于感染的眼睛，每日 4 次。

随访

■ 进一步处理

入院指征

• 成人：
- 发热或中毒表现。
- 伴随内科问题，包括糖尿病或免疫抑制。
- 广泛的蜂窝织炎。
- 怀疑传播至邻近组织和牵连深部组织或脑膜炎或脑膜炎奈瑟菌感染。

• 儿童：
- 急性病症。
- 伴随内科问题。
- 广泛的蜂窝织炎。
- 流感嗜血杆菌感染高风险（未接种的）。
- 不能安排 24 h 可靠的随访。

转诊问题

泪腺炎和泪囊炎应当及时请教眼科：

• 泪囊炎患者要求进一步检查以确认泪囊已完全引流以及评估是否需要进一步的干预以防止复发。

• 确定有效的随访以及出院前完成眼科会诊。

要点和误区

• 对于眼睛红肿的病例，要特别检查泪腺结构以找出其受感染的证据。

• 皮肤切口和泪囊炎的引流应该尽可能避免瘘管形成。
- 鼻腔血管收缩剂主要用于促进引流。

锂中毒

Sean M. Bryant 王胜云 译

基础知识

描述

- 胃肠道吸收迅速：
  - 规则释放：2～4 h 达血浆峰浓度。
  - 缓慢释放：4～12 h 达血浆峰浓度。
- 半衰期为 24 h。
- 慢分布(至少 6 h)。
- 分布容积 0.6～0.9 L/kg。
- 消除：
  - 不通过新陈代谢。
  - 肾脏排泄(非交换)。
  - 重吸收通过钠转运机制在近端肾小管进行。
  - 消除半衰期为 20～24 h，伴慢性病者延长。
- 治疗及毒性指数：
  - 锂在细胞内才有治疗及毒性作用。
  - 治疗剂量和中毒剂量差距小。
  - 治疗剂量 0.6～1.2 mmol/L。
  - 分子量小，肾脏转运机制同钠、钾、镁离子。
- 危险因素：
  - 急性因素：
    - 脱水。
    - 药物过量。
  - 慢性因素：
    - 高血压。
    - 糖尿病。
    - 肾衰竭。
    - 充血性心力衰竭。
    - 高龄。
    - 剂量变化。
    - 药物间作用。
    - 正在使用锂剂治疗。
    - 低盐饮食。
  - 伴随肾脏清除率降低可能导致血浆锂浓度升高的因素：
    - 非甾体药物。
    - 噻嗪类利尿剂。
    - ACEI 类药物。
    - 苯妥英钠。
    - 三环类抗抑郁药。
    - 吩噻嗪类药物。

病因

- 影响锂清除的急慢性因素。
- 药物过量。

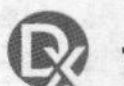

诊断

症状和体征

- 急性中毒：
  - 较慢性中毒少见。
  - 神经系统(较轻)：
    - 虚弱。
    - 频细震颤。
    - 眩晕。
  - 神经系统(中度)：
    - 共济失调。
    - 口齿不清。
    - 视物模糊。
    - 耳鸣。
    - 粗大震颤。
    - 自发性收缩。
    - 反射亢进。
    - 冷漠。
  - 神经系统(严重)：
    - 精神错乱。
    - 神志不清。
    - 癫痫。
    - 抽搐。
    - 锥体外系症状。
  - 胃肠道：
    - 非常常见。
    - 恶心与呕吐。
    - 腹泻。
    - 腹痛。
  - 心脏：
    - QT 延长，ST 段压低。
    - T 波低平。
    - U 波。
    - 恶性心律失常(少见)。
- 慢性中毒：
  - 神经系统：
    - 最常见。
    - 与急性中毒相同症状。
    - 严重中毒症状包括帕金森、精神错乱、记忆障碍等。
  - 肾脏：
    - 肾性尿崩症。
    - 间质性肾炎。
    - 肾小管酸中毒。
    - 直接细胞损害。
  - 皮肤：
    - 皮炎。
    - 溃疡。
    - 局部水肿。
  - 内分泌：
    - 甲状腺功能减退症。
  - 血液系统：
    - 白细胞增多。
    - 再生障碍性贫血。

病史

- 最后摄入锂剂量的时间。
- 摄入史：
  - 急性(一次过量)。
  - 慢性(持续剂量)。
  - 慢加急(在持续摄入锂剂的情况下过量)。

体格检查

基本为神经系统检查。

基本检查

向目击者或施救者明确受伤原因。

诊断检查与说明

实验室检查

- 锂浓度水平：
  - 由于其慢分布特性，应每 2 h 复测一次观察变化趋势。
- 根据患者情况将其分类(急性、慢性或慢加急中毒)：
  - 急性中毒：
    - 以前未服用锂剂者超剂量服用。
    - 锂剂剂量与症状之间无明显量效关系。
    - 毒性水平可能出现在无症状患者中。
    - 锂剂浓度＞4 mmol/L 可能会导致后遗症。
  - 慢加急中毒：
    - 锂剂治疗患者有意或偶然的过量摄入。
    - 锂剂浓度＞3 mmol/L 一般会出现伴随症状。
  - 慢性中毒：
    - 正在接受锂剂治疗的患者因为药物蓄积逐步发展成慢性中毒。
    - 症状与锂剂浓度水平明显相关。
    - 锂剂浓度＞1.5 mmol/L 可有中毒表现。

诊断检查与说明

实验室检查

- 电解质、尿素氮、肌酐和血糖水平，评估有

L

无电解质紊乱及肾功能情况。
• 监测精神病患者丙戊酸和卡马西平浓度。
• 阿司匹林和/或对乙酰氨基酚水平。
• 尿液分析：
- 尿比重。

■ 鉴别诊断

• 与意识状态改变及肌束震颤原因鉴别。
• 内分泌方面：
- 低血糖。
• 毒物方面：
- 胆碱能药物。
- 重金属中毒。
- 安定类药物过量。
- 马钱子中毒。

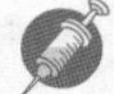

治疗

■ 院前

• 将现场所有药瓶带到医院。
• 开通静脉，吸氧，心电监护。

■ 初步稳定/治疗

• ABC 管理。
• 静脉输注生理盐水。
• 心电监护。
• 神志不清者给予葡萄糖、纳洛酮、维生素 B_1 治疗。
• 癫痫发作者给予苯二氮䓬类药物。

■ 急诊治疗/程序

• 纠正电解质紊乱。
• 保持充足水分。
• 持续心电监护。
• 观察神经功能变化。
• 阻止吸收：
- 误服 1 h 以内考虑洗胃，并且保持呼吸道通畅。
- 活性炭：
◦ 锂几乎不能被活性炭吸收。
◦ 一个剂量的活性炭与山梨醇共同摄入则可能被吸收。
- 全肠道灌洗：
◦ 聚乙二醇溶液。
◦ 通过肠道冲洗排出毒物。
◦ 胃管打水冲洗直至直肠流出物清亮。
◦ 禁忌：肠梗阻、穿孔、低血压及约束体位未做气道保护患者。
• 促进排出：
- 静脉输液：
◦ 快速纠正容量不足（生理盐水 150～300 ml/h）。
◦ 充足水化提高肾小球滤过率，减少近端肾小管重吸收。
◦ 维持尿量在 1～2 ml/(kg·h)。
◦ 当肾小球滤过率达最大后注意控制液体量。
◦ 碳酸氢钠与常规液体相比未见优势。
- 噻嗪类利尿剂、渗透性利尿剂不推荐使用：
◦ 脱水可能加深中毒程度。
◦ 锂主要在近端小管重吸收。
- 降钾树脂：
◦ 动物和临床试验提示有一定效果。
◦ 并发症主要包括低钾血症、高钾血症、容量负荷过重、心律失常。
- 透析：
◦ 腹膜透析不推荐。
◦ 血液透析必要时可以应用。
• 血液透析推荐用于严重中毒及急性摄入高剂量锂剂患者：
- 适应证：
◦ 严重或进行性加重神经功能障碍。
◦ 肾功能不全。
◦ 精神状态变化。
◦ 心律不齐、心源性休克。
◦ 既往有心力衰竭或肺水肿。
◦ 急性摄入锂剂，浓度 4～5 mmol/L 及以上。
◦ 慢性摄入锂剂，浓度 2.5～3 mmol/L 及以上。
- 治疗目标是锂浓度 < 1 mmol/L。
- 血液透析后 6 h 内复查锂浓度（以防锂重新分布）。
- 可能需要反复血液透析。
- 可能可以减轻慢性中毒患者永久性神经功能损害的风险。

■ 药物治疗

• 右旋糖。
• 地西泮（安定）：用于控制癫痫。
• 聚乙二醇。
• 维生素 B_1。

随访

■ 进一步处理

入院指征

• 有中毒症状患者。
• 需要血液透析患者。
• 锂浓度水平未下降或升高 > 2 mmol/L 者。
• 中重度中毒患者伴锂浓度水平 > 4 mmol/L 者应收入 ICU 治疗。
• 有故意摄入锂剂倾向者。

出院指征

无症状且复查血浆锂水平逐步下降并 < 2 mmol/L 的患者（非自杀患者）。

■ 随访建议

精神病慢性中毒患者应随访及时调整药物用量。

要点和误区

• 不要将无症状或既往无药物过量史的患者锂浓度重新分布现象错误理解为中毒。
• 对于有肺水肿、肾功能不全或神志改变患者应积极脱水。

粒细胞减少症 Granulocytopenia

Richard E. Wolfe 祝各亮 译

L

基础知识

■ 描述

• 外周血中的粒细胞数量显著减少。
• 3 种类型的中性粒细胞：
- 中性粒细胞或多形核细胞（PMN）和带状中性粒细胞。
- 嗜酸性粒细胞。
- 嗜碱性粒细胞。
• 以中性粒细胞为主，粒细胞减少和中性粒细胞减少两个词经常被互换使用，因为几乎所有粒细胞减少的类型都是中性粒细胞。

• 白细胞计数：
- 正常范围 4 500～11 000/mm^3。
• 引起粒细胞减少的 4 个基本机制：
- 产生减少。
- 无效造血。
- 中性粒细胞转化为血管内皮细胞。
- 周围破坏增加。
• 随着中性粒细胞绝对计数（ANC）水平的下降，粒细胞减少并发症的风险显著增加。
• 中性粒细胞：
- 临床中通常定义 ANC＜1 400/mm^3。
- ANC＝WBC×（多形核细胞＋带状中性粒细胞）百分比。
- 现代自动化仪器经常计算和报告 ANC。
- 一旦中性粒细胞计数降至 1 000/mm^3 以下，感染风险迅速增加。
- 美国国家癌症研究所（NCI）药物不良血液事件标准采用 4 级系统。
◦ NCI 1 级：正常值下限至 1 500/mm^3。
◦ 轻度中性粒细胞减少症或 NCI 2 级：1 000～1 500/mm^3。
◦ 中度中性粒细胞减少症或 NCI 3 级：在 500～1 000/mm^3。
◦ 严重中性粒细胞减少症或 NCI 4 级：＜500/mm^3。
- 粒细胞缺乏症：
◦ ANC＜100/mm^3。
◦ 最常见的原因是药物反应。
- 感染的风险也受到中性粒细胞减少症的潜在原因、骨髓储备和感染的危险因素的影响。
- ANC 水平＜1 000/mm^3 但近期快速下降的患者，要比＜500/mm^3 但近期在上升的患者感染的风险更大。
- 骨髓增生异常综合征患者应在较高的中性粒细胞计数情况下考虑粒细胞减少，因为其中包括了有缺陷的中性粒细胞。
• 如果不治疗，发热伴中性粒细胞减少的死亡率高达 50%。
- 死亡率与中性粒细胞减少的持续时间、严重程度及第一次抗生素使用前的持续时间有关。
• 治疗后，住院患者死亡率为 6.6%。
• 16%接受化疗的患者至少会出现发热性中性粒细胞减少症。
• 不明原因发热是发热性中性粒细胞减少症的最常见表现：
- 只有 20%～30%的急诊室有临床可检测到的感染。
• 21%的癌症伴中性粒减少性发热的患者会发生严重的并发症。

儿科注意事项

• 严重先天性中性粒细胞减少症：
- 异质性遗传病。
- 严重者表现为口炎或复发性细菌感染。
• 新生儿中性粒细胞计数在出生的几日内会有生理性的升高，即使＞1 500/mm^3，也有粒细胞减少的可能。
• 超过 3 个月的儿童，如果出现单纯中性粒细胞减少症而无免疫缺陷或中心静脉导管，则严重细菌感染的风险较低。

▪ 病因

• 肿瘤的骨髓抑制药物治疗或放射治疗
• 最常见的化疗后 5～10 日。
• 药物不良反应（第二常见原因）：
- 停药通常会在 30 日内解决问题。
- 非化疗药物：
◦ 氯氮平。
◦ 氨苯砜。
◦ 羟基氯喹。
◦ 英夫利希马。
◦ 拉莫三嗪。
◦ 甲基咪唑。
◦ 苯唑西林。
◦ 青霉素。
◦ 普鲁卡因酰胺。
◦ 丙基硫氧嘧啶。
◦ 奎尼丁/奎宁。
◦ 美罗华。
◦ 磺胺吡啶。
◦ 甲氧苄啶-磺胺甲噁唑。
◦ 万古霉素。
- 风险最高的药物：
◦ 抗精神病药：氯氮平。
◦ 抗生素：柳氮磺胺吡啶。
◦ 抗甲状腺药物。
- 抗血小板药。
- 抗癫痫药物。
- 非甾体抗炎药。
• 骨髓抑制药物：
- 甲氨蝶呤。
- 环磷酰胺。
- 秋水仙碱。
- 硫唑嘌呤。
- 更昔洛韦。
• 化学制剂。
• 细菌感染：
- 伤寒。
- 志贺菌肠炎。
- 布氏杆菌病。
- 土拉菌热。
- 结核。
• 寄生虫感染：
- 黑热病。
- 疟疾。
• 立克次体感染：
- 立克次体痘。
- 埃立克体病。
- 落基山斑点热。
• 病毒感染。
• 感染后中性粒细胞减少症：
- 大部分严重和长期的病例与艾滋病病毒、乙型肝炎和 EB 病毒感染有关。
• 免疫相关：
- 原发性免疫性粒细胞减少：
◦ 由于抗中性粒细胞抗体。
- 克罗恩病。
- 系统性红斑狼疮。
- 类风湿关节炎。
- 肺出血肾炎病。
- 韦格纳肉芽肿病。
- 胸腺瘤。
- 补体激活。
• 骨髓浸润。
- 骨髓抑制。
- 门静脉高压症脾大患者的脾隔离。
• 脾功能亢进最常见的原因是肝病伴门静脉高压。
• 输血反应。
• 酒精中毒。
• 维生素缺乏（维生素 B_{12}、叶酸、铜）。
• 慢性特发性中性粒细胞减少。
• 纯白细胞再生障碍性贫血。

儿科注意事项

• 先天性中性粒细胞减少：
- 中性粒细胞减少伴异常免疫球蛋白。
- 网状组织发育不全。
- 重型先天性中性粒细胞减少症或科斯特曼综合征。
- 周期性中性粒细胞减少。
• 慢性良性中性粒细胞减少症。
• 新生儿同种免疫性中性粒细胞减少症。
• 儿童胰腺功能不全伴中性粒细胞减少综合征。
• 软骨毛发发育不全。
• 先天性角化不良。
• 巴特综合征。
• 先天性白细胞颗粒异常综合征。
• 骨髓粒细胞缺乏症。

L

- 懒惰白细胞综合征。
- 科恩综合征。
- 海-普综合征 2 型。

诊断

症状和体征

- 细菌或真菌感染体征：
  - 发热。
  - 局部红斑或波动感。
- 全血细胞减少体征：
  - 疲劳。
  - 苍白。
  - 瘀点。
  - 鼻出血等自发性出血。

病史

- 中性粒细胞减少症的严重程度和持续时间。
- 近期感染性并发症。
- 尝试获得过去的 ANC 水平来评估慢性。
- 应审查致病药物的医疗清单：
  - 询问非处方药、草药和非法药物。
- 新生儿和儿童粒细胞减少症家族史。
- 询问患者发热、寒战、头晕、呕吐，以判断是否存在潜在的严重感染。
- 询问感染非局部症状，如咳嗽、气短、胸部疼痛、排尿困难、尿潴留、尿急或尿频、腹痛及直肠疼痛。
- 询问导致细胞减少的潜在原因的症状：
  - 全身炎症性疾病：
    - 关节炎。
    - 皮疹。
    - 光敏性。
  - 恶性肿瘤：
    - 体重减轻。
    - 发汗。
  - 肝脏疾病：
    - 肝炎史。
    - 黄疸。

体格检查

关注感染的体征：

- 口腔检查：鹅口疮、溃疡、牙周病等口腔黏膜炎。
- 肺：啰音、干啰音。
- 腹部：脾大。
- 皮肤：皮疹、溃疡、脓肿。
- 肛周：检查脓肿和黏膜病变，抗生素开始使用前直肠检查是相对禁忌的。
- 留置导尿管评估。

基本检查

- 对潜在的感染和粒细胞减少症的原因进行全面仔细的病史和体格检查。
- 如果潜在原因不明，由病理学家或血液学家检查外周血涂片。
- 血培养和尿培养。
- 胸片。
- 计算支持癌症的跨国协会癌症风险指数（MASCC）：
  - 发热性中性粒细胞减少症的负担：
    - 一般临床状况。
    - 无或轻微症状(5)。
    - 中度症状(3)。
    - 严重症状(0)。
  - 分数：
    - 无症状或轻微症状的发热性中性粒细胞减少症负担(5)。
    - 无低血压(收缩压＞90 mmHg)(5)。
    - 没有 COPD(4)。
    - 无真菌感染的实体瘤或血液恶性肿瘤(4)。
    - 无需肠外液体脱水(3)。
    - 中度症状发热性中性粒细胞减少症负担(3)。
    - 门诊状态(3)。
    - 年龄＜60 岁(2)。
  - MASCC≥21 时，发生医疗并发症的风险较低。

诊断检查与说明

实验室检查

- 血常规及分型：
  - 粒细胞绝对计数。
- 肝功能检测。
- 在抗生素使用前进行 2 个不同部位的血培养，如果存在静脉置管，则作为 1 个培养部位。
- 尿常规和尿培养：
  - 可能不表现出白细胞数量或白细胞酯酶异常。
- 如果需要，可进行痰培养。
- 如果需要，可进行粪培养。
- 留置导管培养。
- 有精神状态改变或脑膜刺激症，进行脑脊液检测。

影像学检查

胸部 X 线平片可以找到肺部感染的证据。

鉴别诊断

- 实验室误差。
- 肿瘤与化疗。
- 药物反应。
- 化学暴露。
- 感染(病毒、细菌、立克次体)。
- 自身免疫综合征。
- 遗传病因。
- 输血反应。
- 营养缺乏。
- 肿瘤溶解综合征。
- 脾功能亢进。
- 美国黑种人正常情况下 ANC 值也可能较低，可低至 $1\,000/mm^3$。

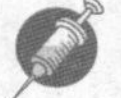

治疗

初步稳定/治疗

对于休克患者：

- 输注 1 L 生理盐水(儿童：20 ml/kg)。
- 如果对静脉补液无反应，需要用升压药维持血压。
- 考虑开始目标导向治疗。

急诊治疗/程序

- 如果可行，应严格隔离在无空气流通的房间内。
- 发热患者的经验性抗生素：
- 如果在某些情况下未提示入院，则口服氟喹诺酮(如环丙沙星)进行预防：
  - 中性粒细胞减少症不发热 10 日以上。
  - 预期中性粒细胞减少持续时间＞7 日的恶性血液病。
- 在可疑感染部位取样后，应用广谱抗生素抗感染：
  - 亚胺培南-西司他丁或氟喹诺酮类。
  - 头孢他啶单独或与氨基糖苷类抗生素联用(丁胺卡那霉素、妥布霉素、庆大霉素)。
- 单独使用头孢吡肟。
  - 与碳青霉烯类药物相比，低剂量方案副作用小，但死亡率高。
- 氨基糖苷类＋抗假单胞菌 β-内酰胺类(美洛西林、哌拉西林或替卡西林)。
- 如果患者存在携带 MRSA 的风险，则用万古霉素。

药物治疗

- 丁胺卡那霉素：15 mg/(kg・24 h)[儿童：15～30 mg/(kg・24 h)]，静脉滴注，q8～12 h。
- 头孢吡肟：0.5～2 g，q12 h。
- 头孢他啶：1～2 g(儿童：30～50 mg/kg，q8 h)，q8～12 h，静脉注射。

• 环丙沙星：500 mg，口服，每日 2 次。
• 庆大霉素：1 mg/kg（儿童：2～2.5 mg/kg），q8 h；或 5 mg/kg，q24 h。
• 亚胺培南-西司他丁：250～1 000 mg，q6～8 h。
• 左氧氟沙星：500 mg，静脉注射，每日 4 次。
• 美洛西林：3 g，q4 h，超过 30 min。
• 妥布霉素：1 mg/kg，q8 h，静脉注射（儿童：2～2.5 mg/kg，q8 h，静脉注射）。
• 万古霉素：15 mg/kg，q8～12 h，静脉注射。

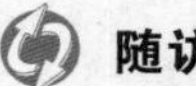

随访

进一步处理

危险分级

MASCC 评分：评估发热性中性粒细胞减少的患者发生并发症的风险。

入院指征

• MASCC<21 时入院。
• MASCC≥21 且：
- 不可靠的中性粒细胞减少症患者。
- 不能密切随访的患者。

出院指征

• 发热化疗患者 MASCC≥21，可靠患者，急诊肿瘤会诊，随访及家庭情况可靠。
• 之前就诊断为粒细胞减少。
• 可以保证密切随访。
• 稳定的患者。

转诊问题

所有粒细胞减少的患者应当咨询他们的家庭医师或血液科专家。

随访建议

• 患者一旦发热，需立即会急诊室就诊。
• 与患者的家庭医师进行 48 h 的密切随访。

要点和误区

• 由于粒细胞减少症患者免疫应答受损，感染常见的症状可能会被掩盖。
• 直肠指检和直肠测温对中性粒细胞减少患者是相对禁忌的，但是在开始应用抗生素后应进行以避免遗漏肛周脓肿。
• 发热且 ANC<500/mm³ 的患者需要立即进行积极的广谱抗生素和补液治疗。
• 肝脾念珠菌病：
- 治疗中性粒细胞减少的并发症。
- 随着 ANC 的上升而形成脓肿。
- 可用两性霉素治疗。

连枷胸 Flail Chest

Stephen L. Thornton 万健 译

基础知识

描述

• 胸壁游离部分：
- 2 处或更多处出现 3 根或更多根相邻肋骨的骨折。
- 肋骨骨折连同胸骨骨折或者肋软骨分离。
• 胸壁游离部分出现吸气时内陷、呼气时外鼓的反常运动。
• 病理改变以与连枷胸相关的肺挫伤为主：
- 游离部分失去通气力学改变。

病因

• 闭合性胸外伤。
• 高处坠落伤。
• 车祸伤。
• 袭击伤。
• 火器伤。
• 肋骨常在撞击处或后角处断裂：
- 第 4～9 肋最易骨折。
- 肋骨与胸骨间 60°旋角处最薄弱。
• 外伤动能传导引起相邻肺实质的损伤：
- 破坏肺泡毛细血管膜及导致肺挫伤。
- 动静脉瘘。
- 通气血流比例失调。
- 低氧血症。
- 可能导致呼吸衰竭。

儿科注意事项

• 富有弹性的胸壁使儿童较少发生肋骨骨折。
• 肋骨的骨折能吸收较高的能量。

老年人注意事项

极易发生肋骨骨折。
• 低代谢状态。
• 合并骨质疏松症。

诊断

症状和体征

病史

• 导致闭合性胸外伤的机制。
• 由患者本人、患儿父母或者院前急救人员描述致伤机制：
- 安全带是否使用。
- 方向盘是否致伤。
- 安全气囊是否打开。
• 局部的胸壁疼痛随着深吸气、咳嗽、活动而加重。
• 肋膜性胸痛。
• 呼吸困难。
• 咯血。

体格检查

• 连枷胸出现吸气时内陷、呼气时外鼓的反常运动。
- 可能会因为肌肉痉挛和夹板固定而消失。
- 在切向光下检查可能更有效。
• 多根肋骨骨折。
- 骨连续中断。
- 瘀斑。
- 捻发音。
- 水肿。
- 红斑和压痛与以下有关：
◦ 夹板固定呼吸。
◦ 肋间肌痉挛。
◦ 呼吸困难，呼吸急促。
- 初期隐匿，随后进展。
• 发绀，心动过速，高血压。
• 起初听诊闻及正常呼吸音之后进展可闻及湿啰音或者呼吸音消失。

基本检查

最初诊断依靠临床依据，由影像学加以证实。

诊断检查与说明

实验室检查

动脉血气分析：

• 可能提示低氧血症。
• 提高肺泡动脉血氧分压差。

影像学检查

• 胸部 X 线辅助诊断和预报：
- 可以显示胸内的相关病理改变：
◦ 气胸。
◦ 血胸。
◦ 纵隔气肿。
◦ 肺挫伤。
◦ 纵隔影增宽。
- 肺挫伤在受伤后 6～12 h 出现：
◦ 范围从片状肺泡浸润发展到 Frank 整合。
• 胸部 CT 能用于识别未被胸部 X 线发现的胸腔内损伤：
- 胸部 CT 相较于胸部 X 线平片能平均多发现 3 处肋骨骨折。

鉴别诊断

• 胸壁挫伤、肋间肌肉拉伤。
• 肋软骨分离。
• 胸骨骨折和脱位。
• 影像学鉴别诊断包括：
- 急性呼吸窘迫综合征(ARDS)。
- 肺裂伤、肺梗塞和肺梗死。
- 充血性心力衰竭(CHF)。
- 肺炎、肺脓肿和其他的感染过程。
- 非心源性肺水肿。

治疗

院前急救

• 将患者伤侧位置朝下可以稳定受伤侧胸壁。
- 改善健侧胸部的通气。
• 严重的胸部外伤或合并既往有肺病疾病者应就近送至最近的创伤中心。

初始稳定/治疗

• 管理气道及必要时复苏。
• 开通静脉，吸氧，持续心电及指末氧监测。
• 维护气道：
- 气管插管。
- 表明患者合并严重低氧血症(PaO_2 < 60 mmHg 吸入空气，< 80 mmHg 吸入纯氧)。
- 重要的基础肺疾病。
- 即将发生的呼吸衰竭。

急诊治疗/程序

• 维持充分的氧合和通气。
• 监测氧饱和度和呼吸频率。
• 意识清醒的患者首选面罩给养。
• 如果通过高流量给氧不能保持 PaO_2 > 80 mmHg，可考虑通过面罩持续正压通气或者经鼻双水平气道正压通气。
• 如果以上措施无效时考虑尽早行气管插管和机械通气：
- 连枷段的生理性内固定。
• 连枷段的内固定和稳定化未被指明。
• 适当的镇痛治疗对保持充分的肺功能很关键：
- 可避免夹板固定、肺不张和肺炎。
• 搜寻相关的受伤部位并治疗潜在的肺部疾病。
• 以下操作执行后使用 0.5%布比卡因进行肋间神经阻滞是安全有效的：
- 提供 6～12 h 的止痛。
- 打肋间神经阻滞时距椎中线后方 2～3 个指宽。
- 在神经椎管束所在肋骨的下表面注射 0.5～1 ml。
- 及时回抽以确定未穿刺进肋间血管。
• 预防性使用抗生素未被指明。

> **注意**
> 避免补液过多。
> • 在肺挫伤的情况下，使用晶体液复苏必须权衡引发肺水肿的风险。

药物治疗

• 多种对乙酰氨基酚/阿片类镇痛剂联合用药是可行的，参阅以下要点。
• 对乙酰氨基酚 300 mg/可待因 30 mg(儿童：0.5～1 mg/kg 可待因)，口服，q4～6 h。
• 对乙酰氨基酚 500 mg/氢可酮 5 mg，口服，q4～6 h。
• 对乙酰氨基酚 750 mg/氢可酮 7.5 mg，口服，q4～6 h。
• 对乙酰氨基酚 325 mg/氢可酮 10 mg，口服，q4～6 h。
• 对乙酰氨基酚 325 mg/羟考酮 5 mg，口服，q6 h。
• 0.5%布比卡因：0.5～1 ml/次注射或肋间神经阻滞。
• 氢可酮：2～8 mg(儿童：0.03～0.08 mg/kg)，口服，q4～6 h。
• 氢可酮：1～4 mg(儿童：0.015 mg/kg)，静脉注射、肌内注射或皮下注射，q4～6 h。
• 硫酸吗啡：0.05～0.1 mg/kg，静脉注射、肌内注射或皮下注射，q2～6 h。
• 使用芬太尼、氢可酮或硫酸吗啡让患者自控镇痛是有效的。

> **注意**
> • 对合并难治性疼痛、过度镇静或通气不足的患者来说，采用胸硬膜外镇痛次要于阿片类药物。
> • NSAIDs 因为有引起胃出血的风险而使用受限。
> • 对乙酰氨基酚/阿片类镇痛剂联合用药的剂量受限于药物的肝毒性。
> • 对乙酰氨基酚的最大剂量是 1 g 每剂和 4 g/d(儿童：15 mg/kg 每剂，不能超过 5 剂/24 h)。

随访

进一步处理

入院指征

所有连枷胸的患者均应收入重症监护室进行严密监测和充分的疼痛管理。

出院指征

凡存在连枷胸的患者无论是否合并肺挫伤都不应出院。

要点和误区

• 早期的疼痛管理是关键。
• 谨防肺挫伤和气胸等继发性损伤。
• 老年患者预后很差。

镰状细胞病

Steven H. Bowman 周健 潘曙明 译

基础知识

描述

• 镰状细胞病(SCD)是常染色体隐性血红蛋白病,其特征在于异常血红蛋白(HbS)在压力下聚合并使 RBC 变形,导致溶血,血管闭塞和随后的组织缺血/梗死。
• 血红蛋白基因中单个氨基酸取代后的 HbS 产生。
• 发生在非洲、地中海、中东和亚洲血统的人中;疟疾流行地区。
• 即使表现相同,也存在各种分类。
• 非裔美国人的基因型和严重程度:
- HbSS,严重。
- HbSC,轻度至中度。
- HbS β 地中海贫血,轻度至中度。
- HbAS,镰状细胞特征:
◦ 无疾病表现。
◦ 极度劳累,严重缺氧,严重脱水或产妇有猝死危险。
• 与系统性和肺动脉高压、胆石症、腿部皮肤溃疡、阴茎异常勃起相关的与进行性血管病相关的慢性溶血性贫血。
• 慢性溶血性贫血伴有进行性血管病变,表现为几乎所有器官系统的疾病。
• SCD 的临床特征是急性发作性疼痛。
• 基本上任何器官系统都可能发生急性血管闭塞性危象(VOC):
• 骨/关节危象:
- 骨骼微血管的血管阻塞导致梗死。
- 长骨、肋骨、胸骨、脊柱和骨盆受到影响。
- 乳腺炎或手足综合征发生在 6~24 个月。
• 急性胸综合征:
- 肺血管的血管闭塞。
- 梗死性骨髓的脂肪栓塞和/或感染(病毒或细菌)可能会导致。
- 痰和肺炎链球菌菌血症中分离出的肺炎衣原体和肺炎支原体。
- 高死亡率(2%~14%)。
- 50%的镰状细胞患者将经历至少 1 次发作。
- 影像学表现为肺部浸润伴发烧和呼吸道症状,难以与肺炎区分开。
- 多见于儿童。
• 脾隔离:
- 脾窦堵塞,流出道阻塞。
- 估计有 SCD 死亡的 6%~17%。
- 循环系统崩溃可能会迅速致死。
- 在 5 岁以下的儿童中更常见。
• 再生障碍危象:
- 骨髓抑制通常继发于病毒感染,最常见的是细小病毒 B19。
- Hallmark 急性贫血,网织红细胞计数低。
- 急性骨髓抑制显著加重慢性贫血。
- 普遍骨髓自身抑制。
- 多见于儿童。
• 脑血管意外/短暂性脑缺血发作(CVA/TIA):
- 分别由儿童和老年患者的镰状细胞和血栓栓塞继发于血管闭塞。
- 患有 SCD 的儿童患 CVA/TIA 的风险增加了 300 倍。
◦ 大多数事件发生在 10 岁之前和 29 岁之后。
• 细菌感染:
- 败血症是 SCD 患者死亡的主要原因。
- 增加菌血症、脑膜炎和骨髓炎的风险。
- 脾功能受损会削弱抵抗包囊生物的能力。
- 肺炎、流感嗜血杆菌、金黄色葡萄球菌、大肠杆菌和沙门菌是主要生物。
◦ <5 岁的儿童肺炎球菌感染增加了 400 倍。
• 阴茎异常勃起:
- 疼痛,持续,不想要的勃起>3 h。
- 高流量(非缺血性)比低流量(缺血性)阴茎异常多。

儿科注意事项

• 儿童急性镰状细胞并发症的发病率很高,应积极筛查。
• 感染通常会引发危象。
• 确认免疫史(肺炎球菌和 B 型流感嗜血杆菌)。
• 确定儿童是否正在接受预防性青霉素,通常在 5 岁以下儿童中使用。
• <3 岁儿童的压倒性感染率最高。

妊娠注意事项

• 危机事件发生频率可变,发生频率增加并不罕见。
• 贫血更为严重。
• 妊娠高血压疾病、无症状细菌感染、泌尿道感染和肾盂肾炎导致败血症的发生率增加。
• 自然流产、产前出血和胎膜早破的风险增加。
• 早产、子宫内生长受限和低出生体重的风险增加。

病因

常见的严重感染因素:
• 感染(细菌和病毒)。
• 脱水。
• 低氧血症。
• 酸中毒。
• 情绪压力。
• 手术或创伤。
• 天气变化。
• 妊娠。
• 毒素。

诊断

症状和体征

• 可能与以下任何一个一起出现:
- 疼痛危象。
- 疾病的并发症。
- 结合以上。
• 通常可能不会显示出急性疼痛的自主神经症状。
• 镰状细胞疼痛危象:
- 四肢、背部、胸骨或关节疼痛。
- 肢体变化和关节肿胀/温暖。
- 婴儿手足综合征;手足肿胀,不愿走路或动手。
• 腹部危象:
- 腹痛无腹膜炎。
- 恶心,呕吐,腹泻。
- 阴茎异常勃起:长时间的痛苦勃起。
• 急性胸部综合征:
- 胸痛。
- 发热。
- 胸部 X 线片上出现新的肺部浸润。
- 呼吸道症状。
- 低氧血症。
• 脾固存危象:
- 腹痛、脾大。
- 疲劳、嗜睡、面色苍白。
- 低血压、心动过速、晕厥、休克。
• 再生障碍危象:
- 发热、头痛、恶心、呕吐。
- 疲劳、面色苍白、心动过速。
• CVA/TIA:
- 局部神经功能缺损。

L

- 精神状态改变。
- 发作。

病史

- 基因型。
- 当前症状发作。
- 以前的危象。
- 免疫接种。
- 手术史。
- 确定典型与非典型危象。

体格检查

进行彻底的身体检查：

- 生命体征：血压、心率、温度、氧饱和度。
- 一般外观：黄疸、面色苍白。
- 心肺检查：
  - 啰音、喘息、呼吸急促。
  - 周围水肿、JVD升高。
  - 奔马律，低语。
- 腹部检查：
  - 睾丸肿大、压痛、腹膜炎。
- 肌肉骨骼检查：
  - 红斑。
  - 儿童手足温暖、肿胀。
- 神经系统检查：
  - 局灶性神经功能缺损。
  - 颅神经麻痹。

基本检查

进行彻底的身体检查，重点检查感染或局部缺血的迹象。

诊断检查和说明

实验室检查

- CBC：
  - 将Hb与先前的值比较（如果有）。
  - 白细胞增多症很常见，并不一定表示感染。
- 网状细胞计数通常在SCD患者中升高，并在再生障碍性疾病中降低。
- 全身机体代谢(CMP)：
  - 要注意，尽管基线慢性肾功能不全，但肌酐可能看起来正常。
  - 总胆红素水平升高可能提示血管内溶血。
- 溶血标记物（总胆红素、触珠蛋白和LDH）可能以不同程度存在。
- 一系列动脉血气和Aa梯度有助于急性胸腔综合征。
- 微生物培养：血液、尿液、咽拭子、脑脊液。
- 分型和筛选（交叉筛选）
- 女性尿液妊娠试验。

影像学检查

- 射线照相应指导确认诊断：
  - 如果怀疑有肺炎或急性胸腔综合征，应进行胸片检查。
  - 怀疑是骨髓炎的四肢X线摄片。
- 静脉造影剂可能加剧疾病。
- 头部CT/MRI评估脑中风。

诊断程序/手术

- 如果怀疑中枢神经系统感染或蛛网膜下腔出血，则进行腰椎穿刺。
- 关节穿刺术治疗急性关节炎。

鉴别诊断

- 镰状细胞危象可能复制或隐蔽了更严重的潜在病理（如急性腹部、MI、PE、肾结石症）。
- 如果疼痛更严重或不典型，应进行其他诊断。

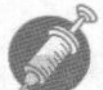

治疗

初步稳定/治疗

- 识别和治疗高发病率并发症。
- 建立静脉通路。
- 评估疼痛并开始治疗。

急诊治疗/程序

- 根据患者表现的严重程度和先前的药物选择镇痛药：
  - 经常（例如，每15～30 min）重新评估一次疼痛，并逐步调整直到疼痛好转。
  - 静脉阿片剂（如吗啡、氢吗啡酮、芬太尼）为一线用药，考虑使用辅助药物。
  - 辅助药：对乙酰氨基酚、非甾体抗炎药（肾功能受损的患者慎用）。
  - 以哌替啶为代谢物时可能会累积并引起癫痫发作风险。
  - 如果没有静脉通路，则口服和皮下镇痛药优于肌内注射。
- 水化作用。
  - 如果患者耐受水化作用，可口服。
  - 胃肠外静脉注射液，成人和儿童为0.45%盐水或婴儿为0.2%盐水。
  - 避免过度补水，有以下危险：
    - 高氯血症代谢性酸中毒，促进红细胞镰刀病变。
    - 肺不张导致急性胸综合征。
- 并发症特异性疗法：
  - 急性胸综合征：
    - 氧气，支气管扩张剂，肺活量计。
    - 呼吸道症状加重，低氧血症和Aa梯度增加时，考虑换血疗法。
  - 脾隔离：
    - 纯输血，促进红细胞的转运。
    - 注意提高血红蛋白水平后会沉淀VOC的风险。
    - 理想的治疗方法是预防：慢性输血，脾切除。
  - 再生障碍危象：
    - 纯输血。
    - 与孕妇医护人员隔离。
  - 阴茎异常勃起：
    - 一线用药：肾上腺素受体激动剂（如肾上腺素、特布他林）冲洗术。
    - 二线用药：如果抽吸失败，请交换输血。
  - 经验性抗生素：败血症、肺炎和骨髓炎。
  - 对于脑血管意外和阴茎持续勃起症等并发症可能需要换血疗法。
- 咨询：
  - 血液科，特别是如果需要换血。
  - 神经内科/神经外科，如果有急性中枢神经系统事件。
  - 泌尿外科阴茎持续勃起。

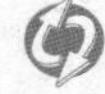

随访

进一步处理

入院指征

- 难治性疼痛。
- 并发症：急性胸腔综合征、隔离症、再生障碍性疾病、CVA/TIA、难治性阴茎异常勃起。
- 细菌感染或病因不明的发热迹象。
- 症状性贫血。
- ICU入院是因为血液动力学不稳定，急性胸腔综合征中的低氧血症加重以及严重的急性中枢神经系统事件。

出院指征

- 解决疼痛危机。
- 没有入院治疗。
- 血液科医师安排了随访。

转诊问题

细致的初级保健可以限制疼痛危机的发生频率和严重程度。

随访建议

如果出院，患者应在1～2日去看PCP或血液科医师。

要点和误区

- 区分典型的镰状细胞危象与危及生命的

急性并发症。

• 使用适当选择和给药的镇痛药积极治疗疼痛。

• 急性疼痛患者可能未表现出典型的症状，如心动过速或发汗。

链球菌病

Scott C. Sherman 江伟伟 李文放 译

基础知识

描述

• 20 世纪 80 年代出现的侵袭性肺炎球菌性坏死性皮肤感染的频率增加，并被称为“食粉菌”。

• 20～50 岁且没有潜在疾病的健康患者多见。

• 快速进展至休克和多器官功能障碍，死亡发生在 1～2 日。

• 工业化国家的发病率为(3～4)/10 万。

• A 群链球菌引起的侵袭性感染(GAS)包括：

- 坏死性筋膜炎(NF)：
  ◦ 快速进展的软组织感染，位于深筋膜和皮下脂肪内。
- 链球菌毒素休克综合征(STSS)：
  ◦ 可能发生在伴有 GAS 相关 NF 的患者中。
  ◦ 进入链球菌的渠道包括阴道、咽、黏膜和皮肤。
  ◦ 50%的患者原因不明。
- “其他”侵入性疾病：从正常无菌身体部位分离 GAS(脓毒症、肺炎相关性菌血症、化脓性关节炎等)。

• 偶尔发生，偶尔在长期护理机构和医院暴发。

• 侵袭性 GAS 发病率是脑膜炎球菌疾病的年发病率的 6 倍。

STSS 定义

• 从无菌或无菌身体部位分离 GAS。

• 低血压。

• 以下两项或多项：

- 肾功能不全。
- 凝血功能障碍。
- 肝脏异常。
- 急性呼吸窘迫。
- 广泛的组织坏死(NF)。
- 红斑的皮疹。

病因

• NF：

- 在 10%的情况下，GAS 是致病的。钝性创伤是危险因素。
- 70%的患者混合厌氧和需氧微生物。
- 金黄色葡萄球菌、梭菌属和其他肠道生物。

• 链球菌毒素休克综合征：

- 易感宿主感染毒性强的菌株时发生。
- 1、3、28 类型 M 蛋白是最常见的。
- 致热外毒素(A、B 和 C)通过激活肿瘤坏死因子和白细胞介素产生发热和休克。
- 非甾体抗炎药会掩盖病情。
- 危险因素：
  ◦ 年龄<10 岁或>60 岁。
  ◦ 癌症。
  ◦ 肾衰竭。
  ◦ 白血病。
  ◦ 严重烧伤。
  ◦ 长期使用激素。

诊断

症状和体征

病史

• 疼痛：

- NF 最常见的初始症状：
  ◦ 发生在 85%的情况下。
- 与体格检查不符。
- 经常突然发作和严重。
- 通常需要静脉使用止痛药缓解。
- 通常涉及手足。
- 可能与腹膜炎、盆腔炎、肺炎、急性 MI 或心包炎相似。

体格检查

• 发热是最常见的：

- 如果患者处于休克状态，可能会出现低体温。

• 目前 55%的病例出现心理状态改变。

• 80%存在软组织感染(红斑和肿胀)：

- 边界不清的水疱、大疱。
- 无淋巴管炎或淋巴结肿大。

• 20%有流感样综合征：

- 发热。
- 发冷。
- 肌痛。
- 恶心、呕吐。
- 腹泻。

• 休克：

- 在所有患者中，发生在入院时或 4～8 h。
- 尽管使用液体、抗生素和血管升压药，但仍然持续存在。

• 肾衰竭：

- 在许多情况下，发生在休克之前。
- 透析往往是必要的。
- 幸存者 4～6 周内肾功能恢复正常。

• ARDS：

- 发病率 55%。

基本检查

• 当疼痛与体格检查不成比例时，怀疑 NF。

• X 线平片以检查软组织中是否有气体。

• 抽血培养。

诊断检查与说明

实验室检查

• 血常规及分类：

- 白细胞增多伴核左移。

• 电解质、尿素氮和肌酐。

• 钙水平：

- 低钙血症与 NF 的脂肪坏死相关。

• 尿液检查：

- 如果存在肾脏受累、血红蛋白尿。

• 血清肌酸磷酸激酶：

- 升高与 NF 或肌炎相关。

• 有氧和厌氧血培养。

• 伤口分泌物培养。

• 凝血功能检测。

影像学检查

• X 线平片：

- 在 25%～75%的 NF 病例中，软组织中有气体，但并不常见于 A 组溶血性链球菌感染。
- 在混合厌氧菌感染中更常见。

L

- CT 扫描：
  - 深筋膜不对称增厚。
  - GAS。
- MRI：
  - T_2 加权图像中筋膜的高信号强度与 NF 有关。

诊断步骤/外科

对有关部位的革兰涂片染色和培养可能是有用的。

■ 鉴别诊断

- 脓血症。
- 蜂窝织炎。
- 丹毒。
- NF 或继发于另一种病原体感染的肌炎。

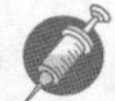

治疗

■ 院前

稳定病情。

■ 初步稳定/治疗

- 保持生命体征。
- 根据需要用液体和血管升压药治疗休克：
  - 低血压往往难以纠正，可能需要 10～20 L/d。
- 插管和机械通气：
  - ARDS。
  - 严重的休克。
  - 无自主呼吸。

■ 急诊治疗/程序

- 在 GAS 存在的情况下，立即进行培养，然后予以广谱抗生素：
  - 克林霉素是 GAS 细菌的有效抑制剂，并能抑制 M 蛋白质合成。
- 早期探讨是否行手术，大多数患者需要手术操作(如筋膜切开术、手术清创术、探查性剖腹手术、眼内抽吸术、截肢术或子宫切除术)：
  - 如果有以下情况立即手术：
    - 广泛性坏死或气体。
    - 房室综合征。
    - 严重的全身中毒表现。
- 注意第一个 24 h 的抗生素治疗的静滴情况。
- 关于静脉使用免疫球蛋白的成功报道。
- 高压氧治疗有争议。

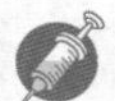

治疗

- 由于侵袭性链球菌病引起的 NF(注意：在急诊治疗中，经验性治疗应开始直到由 GAS 引起的单一生物体 NF 已被证实)：
  - 克林霉素：900 mg 静滴[儿童：40 mg/(kg · d)]和青霉素：400 万 U 静滴(儿童：250 000 U/d)；或如果患者青霉素过敏，则万古霉素：15 mg/kg 静滴(儿童：10 mg/kg，q6 h)。
- 经验治疗 NF 需考虑所有病因(产气荚膜梭状芽孢杆菌、GAS、耐甲氧西林金黄色葡萄球菌 MRSA、混合厌氧菌/需氧菌)：
  - 哌拉西林-他唑巴坦 3.5 g 静脉注射和克林霉素 900 mg 静脉注射和万古霉素 1 g 静脉注射。青霉素过敏患者使用氨曲南 2 g 静脉注射，克林霉素 900 mg 静脉注射，万古霉素 1 g 和甲硝唑 500 mg 静脉注射。

随访

■ 进一步处理

入院指征

所有疑似侵袭性链球菌感染患者均需入住 ICU，NF 的死亡率为 20%，NF 合并 STSS 的死亡率上升到 70%。

出院指征

没有。

要点和误区

- 低血压和休克可能需要大量补液和血管升压药。
- 应该给予广谱抗生素，直到确认 GAS 的存在。
- 应进行手术以进行清创。

淋巴管炎

John Mahoney · Dolores Gonthier　王胜云　段立伟 译

基础知识

■ 描述

- 淋巴管炎是由于淋巴管感染导致的炎症。
- 组织学上来说，淋巴管系统是充满淋巴液和组织细胞的宽大管道系统。

■ 病因

- 急性淋巴管炎：
  - 多由于细菌感染造成。
  - 绝大多数为 A 组 β 型链球菌。
  - 其次，可由于其他链球菌种引起，偶尔也可由金黄色葡萄球菌造成，其他还有链球菌属、甲氧西林敏感金黄色葡萄球菌(MSSA)和耐甲氧西林金黄色葡萄球菌(MRSA)：
    - 葡萄球菌感染的危险因素(MSSA 和 MRSA)：
      - 近期住院或长期住院。
      - 近期手术史。
      - 儿童。
      - 军人。
      - 囚犯。
      - 运动员。
      - 通过静脉注射吸毒人员。
      - 同性恋者(男性)。
      - 透析患者。
      - 有贯穿伤史。
    - MRSA 感染的其他危险因素：
      - 既往 MRSA 感染。
      - MRSA 定殖。
      - MRSA 发病率高的地区。
      - 与 MRSA 患者接触密切。
  - 其他病原菌：
    - 出血败血性巴斯德菌(猫、犬咬伤)。
    - 念珠状链球菌(鼠咬热)。
    - 班氏吴策线虫(丝虫病)：特别是来自非洲、东南亚、热带南美洲来的有下肢症状的移民。
- 慢性(结节性)淋巴管炎：
  - 通常由霉菌、分枝杆菌和丝虫感染导致。
  - 申克孢子丝菌(美国慢性淋巴管炎最常见的原因)：
    - 在园艺或农场干活时接触(玫瑰刺)。
    - 病原体在一些植物和泥炭藓中存在。
    - 淋巴管沿途出现多发的小结节。
    - 传统的抗生素治疗和局部治疗无效。
  - 分枝杆菌感染：
    - 非典型分枝杆菌。

L

◦ 在 25～32 ℃的鱼缸或游泳池中生长。
◦ 可产生慢性单发的疣状结节，在磨损处可产生或溃疡性损伤。
◦ 其他损伤分布同孢子丝菌病类似。
- 巴西诺卡菌。
- 堪萨斯分枝杆菌。
- 班氏吴策线虫。

诊断

症状和体征

• 急性淋巴管炎：
- 自感染部位出现温暖、质软的红斑条纹，在近期不断扩展。
- 区域淋巴结通常扩大，质软(淋巴结炎)。
- 相关区域外周性水肿。
- 系统性临床表现：
◦ 发热。
◦ 寒战。
◦ 心动过速。
◦ 头痛。
• 慢性(结节性)淋巴管炎：
- 红斑性小结、下疳样溃疡或疣状皮肤损害，出现在病原菌接触部位组织。
- 通常不伴有疼痛或系统性感染的征兆。
- 可沿淋巴管行走区域出现多发性损害。

病史

• 职业、居住地和环境暴露。
• 存在感染源。
• 症状的持续和复发的时间。
• 葡萄球菌：病情进展较为缓慢，与外伤有关。
• 链球菌：急性。

体格检查

• 发热，以及其他全身症状。
• 确定感染部位或感染源。
• 从感染源向区域淋巴结寻找红斑、条纹或结节。
• 如果葡萄球菌的病因：来源更有可能有脓疱存在。

基本检查

淋巴管炎属于临床诊断。

诊断检查与说明

实验室检查

• 白细胞检查不必要，但通常升高。
• 伤口或脓疱抽吸后培养：
- 脓疱内脓液。
- 怀疑是一种不常见的或耐药的病原体。
- 初始治疗不成功。
• 组织活检可能有助于确定特定病因。
• 如果怀疑孢子丝菌或海分枝杆菌，伤口处病原体的培养确定对于诊断尤其重要。
• 血液培养可能发现病原体。
• 丝虫病可以用血涂片(夜间)或血清学技术来诊断。

影像学检查

• 如果体格检查不明确或有大面积蜂窝织炎，超声诊断脓肿很有用。
• X线平片可提示脓肿、胃肠胀气或异物存在的可能。
• 特殊情况下，血管多普勒超声可帮助排除深部静脉血栓出现的可能。

鉴别诊断

• 血栓性静脉炎：深部或表浅静脉。
- 同淋巴管炎的鉴别诊断：
◦ 没有原发伤口或感染灶。
◦ 不伴有局部淋巴结病。
• 静脉通道漏出：
• 天花疫苗接种，以及其他疫苗接种后的多样反应。
• 植物日光性皮炎：
- 线状炎症反应，类似淋巴管炎。
- 绿黄色外皮、青柠汁及特殊植物的接触可作为光敏来源。

治疗

初步稳定/治疗

如果患者出现脓毒血症，按照说明进行气道管理和复苏。

急诊治疗/程序

• 在后续治疗中首先进行抗生素治疗。
• 一般治疗：
- 抬高患肢。
- 镇痛。
- 热敷。
• 一般原则：
- 如果将A组β溶血性链球菌作为病因，则建议积极治疗，因为疾病进展很快。
- 在常见原因的基础上，考虑该局部地区MRSA或其他耐药菌种出现的可能性。
- 门诊治疗通常为：7～10日。
- 在48～72 h连续评估改善情况。
- 如果怀疑葡萄球菌可能是致病因素，抗生素应同时覆盖MSSA和MRSA。
◦ 这种怀疑应该基于临床检查、病史和危险因素评估。
• 急性淋巴管炎，经验治疗：
- 门诊患者：
◦ 口服头孢氨苄。
◦ 头孢氨苄的替代药物：可口服双氯西林、克林霉素。
- 住院患者：
◦ 静脉注射纳夫西林或静脉注射头孢唑林。
◦ 替代品：静脉注射克林霉素。
• MRSA：如果怀疑MRSA是病原体。
- 门诊患者：
◦ TMP-SMX。
◦ 替代品：多西环素。
- 住院患者：
◦ 静脉注射万古霉素。
◦ 替代方案：静脉注射利奈唑胺。
• 狗或猫咬伤后的淋巴管炎：
- 静脉注射氨苄西林-舒巴坦。
• 孢子丝菌病：
- 伊曲康唑。
• 海分枝杆菌：
- 常伴发局部肉芽肿。
- 只在特别严重的感染中使用抗生素治疗：
◦ 联合使用药剂应当控制在有限时间段内。

药物治疗

• 氨苄西林-舒巴坦：1.5～3 g[儿童：<40 kg，100～300 mg/(kg·24 h)；>40 kg，给予成人剂量]，静脉给药，q6 h。
• 头孢唑林：1～1.5 g[儿童：50～100 mg/(kg·24 h)]，最大剂量6 g/24 h，静脉给药，q8 h。
• 头孢氨苄：500 mg[儿童：25～50 mg/(kg·24 h)]，口服，每日4次。
• 克林霉素：300～450 mg[儿童：30～40 mg/(kg·24 h)]，口服，q6 h；或600 mg[儿童：25～40 mg/(kg·24 h)]，静脉给药，q8 h。
• 双氯西林：250～500 mg[儿童：12.5～25 mg/(kg·24 h)]，口服，q6 h。
• 盐酸强力霉素：100 mg，口服，每日2次(成人)。
• 伊曲康唑(成人)：200 mg，口服，每日1次，连续用药至损伤全部消失后2～4周(通常3～6个月)。儿童：3～5 mg/(kg·24 h)口服，q12 h。

注意

药物相互作用，以及孕妇。

L

• 利奈唑胺：600 mg，口服或静脉给药，q12 h。
• 萘夫西林：1～2 g，静脉给药，q4 h；最大剂量 12 g/24 h。
• TMP-SMX：2 DS tabs，口服，q12 h。
• 万古霉素：1 g，静脉给药，q12 h（<5 岁儿童用药剂量需调整），血清水平血药浓度监测。

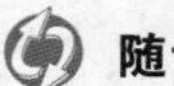

随访

进一步处理

入院指征

• 出现中毒迹象（毒血症或脓毒症）。
• 出现严重全身症状。
• 免疫抑制病史。
• 并发慢性疾病。
• 无法口服药物。
• 依从性差患者。
• 门诊治疗失败患者。

出院指征

• 轻微感染，不伴有中毒症状的患者。
• 没有慢性病或免疫抑制病史。
• 24 h 内可随访。

随访建议

• 随访 24～48 h 观察治疗效果。
• 如果症状加剧如、淋巴结炎加剧或新发、淋巴结局域变红或红色范围扩大、患者发热家中等情况，需要立即到医院接受治疗。
• 在办理出院前，标注出红斑范围，有助于随后质量效果的评估。

要点和误区

• 急性淋巴管炎：
- 链球菌是最常见的原因。
- 可能会发生迅速发展为菌血症的情况。
- 疑似 MRSA 感染较缓慢或存在反复感染。
- 利用临床经验和超声检查，避免漏诊。
• 慢性淋巴管炎：
- 如果适当的抗菌治疗没有改善，可以考虑慢性感染。

淋巴结炎 Lymphadenitis

John Mahoney · Dolores Gonthier 王胜云 段立伟 译

基础知识

描述

• 淋巴结可因感染所致全身系统性反应出现肿大，质地柔软。
- 内部充满淋巴细胞和巨噬细胞。
- 可为初次感染（造成）。
• 按淋巴结肿大的部位和程度分类。
- 急性区域。
◦ 远端感染可导致近端腺炎。
◦ 急性化脓性淋巴结炎可在咽部或皮肤感染后出现。
- 慢性区域性和全身性淋巴结炎的病因在本章中有所提及，但在特定疾病中会有更充分的讨论。

病因

• 颈部：
- 病毒性：常见，通常是双侧腺炎。
◦ EB 病毒。
◦ 巨细胞病毒。
◦ 腺病毒。
- 细菌性：常见，双侧或单侧，更可能为化脓性的。
◦ 皮肤来源：金黄色葡萄球菌：甲氧西林敏感金黄色葡萄球菌（MSSA）和耐甲氧西林金黄色葡萄球菌（MRSA），A 组 β 溶血性链球菌。
◦ 咽部来源：A 组 β-溶血性链球菌。
◦ 牙周来源：A 组 β-溶血性链球菌和厌氧菌。
◦ 结核分枝杆菌，非典型分枝杆菌，罕见。
◦ 亨氏巴尔通体：猫抓病。
• 腋窝部：
- 化脓性链球菌（A 组 β 溶血性链球菌）。
◦ 发热，腋窝疼痛，手臂和胸部的急性淋巴水肿，无蜂窝织炎或淋巴管炎的特征；同侧胸腔积液；主要来源于手臂或手部。
- 皮肤来源：金黄色葡萄球菌和 A 组 β 溶血性链球菌。
- 亨氏巴尔通体：猫抓病。
◦ 最常见的淋巴结受累。
• 腹股沟部：
- 皮肤来源：通常是单侧的。
◦ 金黄色葡萄球菌：甲氧西林敏感金黄色葡萄球菌（MSSA）和耐甲氧西林金黄色葡萄球菌（MRSA），A 组 β 溶血性链球菌。
◦ 性传播疾病：可以是单侧的，也可以是双侧的。
◦ 梅毒（一期、二期）。
◦ 性病淋巴肉芽肿（LGV）：沙眼衣原体。
◦ 软性下疳。
◦ 原发性生殖器疱疹。
- 亨氏巴尔通体：猫抓病。
◦ 通常是单侧的。
- 鼠疫耶尔森菌：腺鼠疫：
◦ 在美国西部，见于啮齿动物或兔子身上的跳蚤。
◦ 在猎人、旅客、农村工人身上都能看到。
• 金黄色葡萄球菌危险因素：
- 葡萄球菌（MSSA 和 MRSA）更常见于化脓性腺炎和/或脓肿形成。
- 葡萄球菌感染的危险因素（MSSA 和 MRSA）：
◦ 近期住院或长期住院。
◦ 近期手术史。
◦ 儿童。
◦ 军人。
◦ 囚犯。
◦ 运动员。
◦ 通过静脉注射吸毒者。
◦ 同性恋者（男性）
◦ 透析患者。
◦ 有贯穿伤史。
- MRSA 感染的其他危险因素：
◦ 既往 MRSA 感染。
◦ MRSA 定殖。
◦ MRSA 发病率高的地区，与 MRSA 患者接触密切。
• 全身性淋巴结炎/淋巴结病：
- HIV。
- EB 病毒，巨细胞病毒。
- 弓形虫。
- 粟粒性肺结核。
- 继发性梅毒。
- 钩端螺旋体病。

L

儿科注意事项

急性单侧颈部化脓性淋巴结炎：

- 常见于 6 岁以下儿童。
- 常见原因为：A 组链球菌、金黄色葡萄球菌、厌氧菌。
- 来源是咽部或头皮。
- 可能出现急性斜颈。

诊断

症状和体征

• 淋巴结炎性肿大伴疼痛。

• 常常伴有急性蜂窝织炎症或脓肿。

病史

• 职业。

• 宠物接触。

• 性行为。

• 药物使用。

• 旅行史（有无疫区暴露）。

• 伴随症状：

- 咽痛。
- 咳嗽。
- 发热。
- 盗汗。
- 乏力。
- 体重减轻。
- 关节痛。

• 淋巴结疾病持续时间。

体格检查

• 发热，其他全身疾病的症状。

• 淋巴结病的范围（局部还是全身）。

• 淋巴结大小：

- 异常大小标准：
  - ◦ 一般淋巴结：>1 cm。
  - ◦ 肱骨内上髁淋巴结：>0.5 cm。
  - ◦ 腹股沟淋巴结：>1.5 cm。

• 淋巴结质地。

• 淋巴结上游区域炎症标志（是否有炎症病灶）。

• 局部有波动或其他化脓或脓肿的迹象。

• 皮肤损害。

• 咽部或牙龈感染的情况。

• 脾大。

• 锁骨上和斜角肌缘淋巴结处的增生通常为异常标志。

基本检查

• 急性局部淋巴结肿大是临床诊断，通常是大的临床综合征中的一部分（如蜂窝织炎）。

• 通过病史和体格检查发现感染原。

诊断检查与说明

实验室检查

• 白细胞检查不必要。

- 白细胞可能升高伴或不伴有白细胞左移。

• 病原学检查：全血细胞计数（CBC）、EB 病毒（EBV）、巨细胞病毒（CMV）、人类免疫缺陷病毒（HIV）及其他基于临床症状的血清学检查。

• 血培养可发现病原体。

影像学检查

• 使用超声和 CT 诊断脓肿，如果出现以下情况：

- 不可明确诊断的。
- 正确治疗后缺乏改善的。
- 进展为化脓的。

• CT 可用于评估深部淋巴结的受累情况。

诊断步骤/外科

• 考虑经皮穿刺抽吸或手术引流，如果存在以下情况：

- 正确治疗后未改善。
- 化脓性感染症状进展。
- 出现脓肿。
- 明显的全身症状或败血症。
- 怀疑有异常或耐药的病原体。

鉴别诊断

• 传染性疾病：

- 炭疽。
- 登革热。
- 白喉。
- 丝虫病。
- 真菌。
- 带状疱疹。
- 传染性肝炎。
- 风疹。
- 猩红热。
- 孢子丝菌病。
- 伤寒。
- 水痘。
- 西尼罗热。

• 非传染性疾病：

- 假体植入。
- 苯妥英钠
- 恶性肿瘤。
- 风湿病。
- 系统性红斑狼疮。
- 类肉状瘤病。
- 淀粉样变性。
- 硅胶植入物。

儿科注意事项

• 川崎病。

• PFAPA 综合征（周期性发热、口疮口腔炎、咽炎、颈部淋巴结炎）。

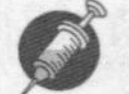

治疗

初步稳定/治疗

• 保持气道通畅，呼吸，循环及血流动力学稳定。

急诊治疗/程序

• 一般治疗：

- 抬高患侧。
- 热敷。
- 镇痛。

• 基本原则：

- 基于原发器官或可疑病原体的抗生素治疗（同时见于蜂窝织炎）。
- 在常见原因的基础上，考虑该局部地区 MRSA 或其他耐药菌种出现的可能性。
- 门诊治疗通常至少为 10 日。
- 治疗可能需要覆盖 MRSA，基于：
  - ◦ MRSA 危险因素的存在，尤其是本地区 MRSA 的患病率。
  - ◦ 全身症状严重程度。
  - ◦ 脓肿的一直无改善。
  - ◦ 疑似存在 MRSA。

• 如果出现脓肿，则进行手术排脓：

- 排脓后进行细菌培养，对鉴定耐药菌种具有特殊意义。

• 颈部：

- 皮肤来源（感染）：
  - ◦ 门诊患者：口服头孢氨苄，头孢氨苄的替代药物：可口服双氯西林、大环内酯类药物或左氧氟沙星。
  - ◦ 住院患者：静脉滴注纳夫西林或静脉注射头孢唑林。
- 咽部或牙龈来源（感染）：
  - ◦ 门诊患者：口服青霉素，替代药物：口服克林霉素或阿莫西林-克拉维酸。
  - ◦ 住院患者：静滴青霉素联合静滴甲硝唑。替代药物：氨苄西林-舒巴坦或克林霉素。

• 腋窝淋巴结炎：

- 链球菌（A 组 β 溶血性链球菌）：
  - ◦ 门诊患者：口服青霉素。替代药物：口服克林霉素或阿莫西林-克拉维酸。
  - ◦ 住院患者：青霉素静滴。替代药物：氨苄

L

西林-舒巴坦。
- 皮肤来源：
◦ 门诊患者：头孢氨苄；替代品：双氯西林、克林霉素。
◦ 住院患者：静脉注射纳夫西林或静脉注射头孢唑林。
• 腹股沟部：
- 皮肤来源：
◦ 门诊患者：头孢氨苄；替代品：双氯西林、克林霉素。
• 住院患者：静脉注射纳夫西林；或静脉注射头孢唑林。
• 急性单侧颈部化脓性淋巴结炎：
- 门诊患者：
◦ 口服青霉素。
◦ 替代品：克林霉素或阿莫西林-克拉维酸。
• MRSA：
- 院内：
◦ 静脉或口服万古霉素；或静滴利奈唑胺。
- 门诊：
◦ 口服：TMR SMX、克林霉素或盐酸强力霉素。

药物治疗

• 阿莫西林-克拉维酸：500～875 mg，口服，每日 2 次；或 250～500 mg，口服，每日 3 次。
• 氨苄西林-舒巴坦：1.5～3 g，静脉注射，q6 h。
• 头孢唑林：1～1.5 g，静脉注射，q8 h。
• 头孢氨苄：500 mg，口服，每日 4 次。
• 克林霉素：450～900 mg，口服或静脉注射，q6 h。
• 双氯西林：125～500 mg，口服，q6 h。
• 盐酸强力霉素：100 mg，口服，每日 2 次(成人)。
• 利奈唑胺：600 mg，口服或静脉注射，q12 h。
• 萘夫西林：1～2 g，静脉注射，q4 h，最大剂量 12 g/24 h。
• 青霉素 VK：250～500 mg，口服，q6 h。
• 青霉素 G：200—400 万单位，静脉注射，q4～6 h。
• TMP-SMX：2 DS tabs，口服，q12 h。
• 万古霉素：1 g，静脉注射，q12 h(<5 岁儿童用药剂量需调整)，监测血药浓度。

随访

进一步处理

入院指征

• 出现中毒迹象(毒血症或脓毒症)。
• 全身疾病症状。
• 淋巴结明显肿大。
• 免疫抑制病史。
• 并发慢性疾病。
• 无法口服药物。
• 依从性差患者。
• 门诊治疗失败。

出院指征

• 轻微感染，不伴有中毒症状的患者。
• 可口服抗生素。
• 没有慢性病或免疫抑制病史。
• 24 h 内可随访。

转诊问题

• 如果在急性感染情况下抗生素治疗效果差或无效，需要考虑更严重的潜在原因(如恶性肿瘤)。
• 淋巴结活检有助于以下情况的判定：
- 与传染源没有明确的关系。
- 临床症状高度怀疑恶性肿瘤的最终鉴定。
- 淋巴结直径>1 cm。
- 锁骨上淋巴结肿大。

随访建议

• 随访 24～48 h 观察治疗效果。
• 如果症状加剧如、淋巴结炎加剧或新发、淋巴结局域变红或红色范围扩大、患者发热家中等情况，需要立即到医院接受治疗。

要点和误区

• 葡萄球菌属感染是导致急性细菌性区域性淋巴结炎最常见的原因。
• 化脓性淋巴结炎和脓肿儿童的葡萄球菌(MSSA 和 MRSA)风险较高。
• 无症状的感染患者也要警惕 MRSA。
• 高度重视颈部深处感染的患者。

淋病 Gonococcal Disease

Roger M. Barkin 祝各亮 译

基础知识

描述

• 美国上报的第二常见的性传播疾病：
- 每年大约有 20000 的新发病例。
- 上报的不到 50%。
- 15～24 岁的黑种人中发病率最高。
- 男同性恋(MSM)者中发病率上升。
◦ HIV 阳性患者中发病率更高。
- 人是目前所知的唯一宿主。
• 常合并沙眼衣原体感染。
• 影响尿道、直肠、宫颈管、咽、女性上生殖道和结膜。
• 男性常表现为尿道炎。
• 女性常无症状。

病因

淋病奈瑟菌：
• 革兰阴性需氧菌。

诊断

症状和体征

• 宫颈炎：
- 定义：
◦ 子宫内膜黏液化脓性分泌物。
◦ 易导致子宫内膜出血。
- 最常见的感染部位。
- 多达 80%无症状。
- 多为非特异性症状：
◦ 阴道分泌物。
◦ 月经过多。
◦ 盆腔疼痛。
◦ 性交疼痛。
◦ 尿频和排尿困难。
• 盆腔炎(PID)：
- 未处理情况下，多达 20%会发展成盆腔炎症。
- 下腹部疼痛：最常见的主观症状。
- 其他常见的症状和体征：
◦ 性交疼痛、异常出血、宫颈或阴道分泌物异常。

- 症状常出现在月经期。
- 发热(50%)。
- 2/3 的患者有轻微的症状，但可能未察觉。
- 菲茨-休米-柯蒂斯综合征(淋球菌性肝周炎)：
  - 发生率为 4%。
  - 最常见的与沙眼衣原体有关。
  - 右上象限的疼痛或压痛。
- 可能会发生不孕症。
- 前庭大腺脓肿。
- 尿道炎。
- 潜伏期为 2~5 日。
- 症状：
  - 尿道分泌物。
  - 排尿困难。
- 前列腺炎：继发于未经治疗尿道炎。
- 附睾炎：
- 急性，单侧睾丸疼痛和肿胀。
- 直肠炎：
- 通常无症状。
- 男同性恋患者中只占 40%。
- 35%~50%的女性子宫内膜感染患者会出现直肠炎。
- HIV 感染者的风险增加 3 倍。
- 症状：
  - 肛周瘙痒，黏液脓性分泌物，轻度直肠出血，严重的肛门疼痛，里急后重，便秘。
- 咽炎：
- 喉咙痛。渗出性扁桃体炎。
- 结膜炎：
- 主要发生在新生儿感染儿童。
- 成人可自行接种。
- 播散性淋菌性感染(DGI)。
- 淋菌性菌血症。
- 关节炎和皮炎综合征：
  - 发生于 0.5%~3%未治疗的黏膜感染。
  - 腱鞘炎、皮炎和多关节痛三联征。
  - 发热、寒战和不适。
- 皮炎：
  - 红斑基础上出现压痛的坏死性脓疱，损伤较少，从远端开始。
- 急性单关节或寡关节炎：
  - 膝关节最常见。
  - 温暖、红斑、关节运动范围内的积液和疼痛。
- 女性>男性，比例为 3∶1。
  - 危险因素：近期月经或近期妊娠。
- 罕见表现：
  - 肝炎。
  - 心肌炎。
  - 感染性心内膜炎。
  - 脑膜炎。

体格检查

- 宫颈炎：
- 宫颈水肿，充血，脆性。
- 盆腔炎：
- 子宫压痛，附件区压痛或宫颈举痛。
- 尿道炎：
- 黄宝色黏性渗出，尿道红斑。

基本检查

- 男性淋球菌病的临床诊断：
- 革兰染色：95%的敏感性。
- 核酸扩增试验(NAAT)检测是常见的，如果可能的话。
- 女性淋球菌病，子宫分泌物培养。
- 同样需要做衣原体和梅毒检查。艾滋病毒筛查。

诊断检查与说明

实验室检查

- NAAT：
- 使用聚合酶链反应(PCR)的 DNA 或 RNA 序列。
- 在泌尿生殖道和非生殖解剖部位检测淋病奈瑟菌的敏感性优于培养，但因 NAAT 类型而异。
- 许多人还检测衣原体。
- 用于尿道、宫颈、阴道和尿液标本。
- 对直肠、口咽或结膜标本不常用。
- 细菌培养(金标准)：
- 塞耶马丁培养基。
  - 支持血液和关节液。
- 革兰染色：
- 细胞内存在革兰阴性的双球菌：
- 方法对有症状的男性 100%敏感。多形核白细胞的存在有助于诊断。
- 在高危人群中出现局部症状可行咽、直肠培养。
- 播散性淋菌性感染：
- 滑膜液分析：
  - 中性粒细胞>50 000/mm^3。
  - 培养结果阳性>80 000/mm^3。
- 2 处以上进行血培养。
- 滑膜、皮肤、尿道或宫颈、直肠培养：
- 塞耶马丁培养基。
- 脑脊液分析可能是必要的。
- 女性盆腔炎和下腹部疼痛：
- 血常规。
- 尿常规。
- 妊娠试验。
- 输卵管卵巢脓肿考虑盆腔超声。
- 快速血浆反应素试验(RPR)：相关的梅毒。

鉴别诊断

- 尿道炎：
- 衣原体。
- 滴虫。
- 泌尿系统感染。
- 梅毒。
- 播散性淋菌性感染：
- 细菌性关节炎：
  - 脑膜炎双球菌(皮疹)。
- 乙型肝炎。
- 结缔组织病：
  - 赖特综合征。
  - 类风湿关节炎
  - 银屑病关节炎。
- 急性风湿热：
  - 链球菌感染后关节炎。
- 感染性心内膜炎。
- 其他：
  - 艾滋病。
  - 二期梅毒。
  - 病毒感染。
  - 莱姆病(皮疹)。
  - 痛风(关节炎)。

治疗

急诊治疗/程序

- 对恶心与呕吐患者进行补液(生理盐水)。
- 性伴侣的治疗。
- 淋病患者通常应考虑衣原体感染的治疗。双重治疗通常用于确保使用不同的机制以及全覆盖。
- 宫颈、尿道及肛门直肠感染：
- 头孢曲松钠 250 mg，肌内注射 1 次。
  - 头孢克肟治疗咽部淋病疗效有限。
- 衣原体治疗：
  - 阿奇霉素：1g，口服，1 次。
  - 多西环素：100 mg，口服，每日 2 次，持续 7 日。
- 盆腔炎：
- 门诊患者：
  - 头孢曲松(250 mg，肌内注射)或头孢西丁(2g，肌内注射 1 次)+丙磺舒(1g，口服，1

次)或第三代头孢菌素(头孢唑肟或头孢噻肟)加多西环素(100 mg,每日 2 次)持续 14 日,伴或不伴甲硝唑(500 mg,口服,每日 2 次)持续 14 日。
- 住院患者:
◦ 头孢西丁(2 g,静脉注射,q6 h)或头孢替坦(2 g,静脉注射,q12 g)+多西环素(100 mg,口服或静脉注射,q12 h)。
◦ 克林霉素(900 mg,静脉注射,q8 h)+庆大霉素负荷剂量 2 mg/kg;接着 1.5 mg/kg,q8 h(或 5 mg/kg, q24 h)。
• 咽炎:
- 头孢曲松(250 mg,肌内注射,1 次)+衣原体的治疗(阿奇霉素 1 g,口服,1 次)。
• 附睾炎:
- 头孢曲松(250 mg,肌内注射,1 次)+多西环素(100 mg,每日 2 次)持续 10 日。
• 性伴侣的治疗。
• 播散性淋菌性感染:
- 头孢曲松:1 g,肌内注射或静脉注射,每日 1 次(推荐)+阿奇霉素 1 g 口服(1 次)
- 替代品(含阿奇霉素):
◦ 头孢噻肟:1 g,静脉注射,q8 h+阿奇霉素:1 g,口服;或头孢唑肟:1 g,静脉注射,q8 h 加阿奇霉素,1 g,口服。
- 改善后 24~48 h,可改用口服治疗,总疗程至少为 7 日:
◦ 头孢克肟:400 mg,口服,每日 2 次。
◦ 头孢泊肟:400 mg,口服,每日 2 次。
- 新生儿淋球菌,包括头皮脓肿:
◦ 头孢曲松:25~50 mg/(kg · d),静脉注射或肌内注射,持续 7 日,如果出现脑膜炎,持续时间为 10~14 日。
◦ 如果存在高胆红素血症:头孢噻肟 25 mg/kg,静脉注射或肌内注射,q12 h,持续 7 日,如果是脑膜炎,持续 10~14 日。
• 结膜炎:
- 成人:
◦ 头孢曲松:1 g,静脉注射,1 次+阿奇霉素和盐水洗眼。
- 新生儿淋菌性眼炎:
◦ 头孢曲松:25~50 mg/kg,静脉注射或肌内注射,1 次,一次最大剂量 125 mg。
◦ 生理盐水冲洗,住院治疗。
• 脑膜炎和心内膜炎:
- 头孢曲松:1~2 g,静脉注射,q12 h:
◦ 脑膜炎持续 10~14 日。
◦ 心内膜炎持续至少 4 周。
• 严重头孢菌素过敏者:
- 传染科会诊。
- 使用脱敏后的头孢菌素进行替代是最好的选择。
- 阿奇霉素,2 g,口服,治疗没有并发症的淋球菌感染:
◦ 限用于阻止疾病发展。

儿科注意事项

• 新生儿淋菌性眼炎:
- 预防性治疗是红霉素眼膏,在所有婴儿出生后立即使用。
- 母亲生殖道感染可传播给新生儿。
- 产后 2~5 日出现双侧结膜炎:
◦ 如果不治疗会导致眼球穿孔。
◦ 用头孢曲松 25~50 mg/kg,肌内注射或静脉注射,最大剂量 125 mg。
• 母亲患有未经治疗的淋病奈瑟菌感染而无症状的新生儿:
- 头孢曲松 25~50 mg/kg,肌内注射或静脉注射,单次剂量不超过 125 mg。
• 体重<45 kg 的儿童合并单纯淋病(外阴阴道炎、尿道炎、咽炎)。
- 头孢曲松 25~50 mg 静脉滴注至 125 mg。
• 体重>45 kg 的儿童无并发症感染。
- 头孢曲松 50 mg/kg 静脉注射至 1 g(见成人)。
• <45 kg 的儿童菌血症或关节炎:
- 头孢曲松 50 mg/kg(最多 1 g),坚持 7 日。
• >45 kg 的儿童患有菌血症或关节炎。
- 每日 1 g 静脉注射,持续 7 日。
• 发现有淋菌感染的儿童应进行沙眼衣原体、梅毒和艾滋病毒检测。应该对潜在的滥用行为进行筛查。

妊娠注意事项

• 并发症包括绒毛膜羊膜炎、胎膜长时间破裂、早产、低出生体重儿、自然流产。
• 30%~50%的病例将淋病传播给婴儿。
• 淋病:头孢曲松 250 mg,肌内注射 1 次,阿奇霉素 1 g,口服 1 次。
- 大观霉素是过敏患者的替代品,但价格昂贵,在美国没有生产。
• 衣原体:红霉素。

随访

进一步处理

入院指征

• 盆腔炎:CDC 建议:
- 病情严重(如出现恶心、呕吐和高热)。
- 妊娠。
- 口服药物无效果。
- 输卵管及卵巢脓肿。
- 其他外科急症可能(如阑尾炎)。

出院指征

• 无并发症的生殖道、咽或结膜感染。
• 与常规检查、接触评估和治疗、减少危险行为和接种人乳头瘤病毒疫苗有关的基本教育。
• 对于简单的泌尿生殖道或直肠淋病感染,一般不需要随访。

转诊问题

• 不孕不育。
• 多次治疗后反复感染。

要点和误区

• 附睾炎:排除睾丸扭转。
• 播散性淋菌性感染:年轻性生活活跃者存在非外伤性寡关节炎或腱鞘炎时需高度怀疑。

流感 Influenza

Kahra Nix · Philip Shayne 倪沁赟 译

基础知识

描述

• 急性,常常为自限性,病毒感染。
• 传播:通过打喷嚏、咳嗽和说话产生的分散的小颗粒气溶胶进行传播。
• 病毒在呼吸道上皮沉积和吸收。
• 潜伏期:1~4 日(平均 2 日)。
• 成人平均持续时间:4 日。
• 季节性暴发,2 月份最常见。
• 新型甲型 H1N1 流感在 2009 年秋季和早冬时间流行。儿童和孕妇的并发症发生率

L

特别高。

• 并发症：

- 原发性流感病毒性肺炎。
- 继发性细菌性肺炎。
- 慢性阻塞性肺疾病急性加重。
- 儿童中耳炎和鼻窦炎。
- 反应性气道疾病。
- 罕见并发症：肌炎、心肌炎、心包炎、急性炎症性脱髓鞘性多发性神经病、无菌性脑膜炎。
- 急性呼吸窘迫综合征和多系统器官衰竭。

• 主要特点：

- 在免疫功能低下的儿童，季节性流行病传播攻击率高。
- 间歇性的不可预知的流行病。
- 死亡主要源于肺部并发症。

儿科注意事项

• 儿童呼吸道表现更少见低（喉炎、支气管炎、毛细支气管炎、肺炎），体温高于成人。

• 儿童特别容易发生甲型 H1N1 流感病毒感染的并发症。

• 小腿肌肉疼痛。

• 5 岁以下流感感染的儿童约 10%发生热惊厥。

• Reye 综合征：

- 流感可能是一个诱发因素。
- 使用水杨酸盐的罕见严重并发症（建议服用阿司匹林的儿童接种疫苗）。
- 急性肝脏和脑损害。

病因

• 通常由 2 种流感病毒类型 A 或 B 中的一种引起，后者通常严重程度较轻。

• A 型流感病毒亚型分为血凝素抗原 H1、H2 或 H3 和不重要的神经氨酸酶亚型。

• 疫苗的目标是亚型抗原，这也是自然免疫的目标。

• 每年的流行病是季节性的：

- 由抗原移位，表面蛋白微小变化而产生的新变种引起。
- 流行持续时间<6 周。

• 流行病：

- 不可预测。
- 因抗原移位引起病毒结构重大变化。

• 水禽流感病毒库。

• 禽流感已经被证明很难传染给人类，很难在人与人之间传播，但是如果发生感染往往很严重。

诊断

• 由其他呼吸道病毒引起的相似的急性感染可能与之类似。

• 疾病预防控制中心（CDC）定义流感样疾病（ILI）为：咳嗽或咽痛，体温高于 100 ℉（37.8℃），并且无其他诊断。

症状和体征

• ILI 患者最重要的预测因素为当地的流行病学结果（CDC 每周更新于官网）。

• 虽然不具有特征性的症状，ILI 发病的数量急剧增长也能预示季节性流感。

病史

• 无单个特异性诊断因素。流感可表现为无症状亦或致死性症状。

• 患者发热和咳嗽同时出现对流感的诊断具有一定特异性，但敏感性不够。

• 特异性诊断还依赖于其他病毒的确定。比如，流行性 RSV 往往同时伴有高频率的发热。

体格检查

• 发热：ILI 患者的随机试验证明，发热程度与发生流感的可能性有关。

• 多项研究表明，体格检查结果与流感无持续相关性，但是目前几乎没有基于急诊科患者的研究。

• 多数患者有气管收缩等气道反应性疾病。

老年人注意事项

老年患者可表现为与肺部疾病无关的高热、疲惫以及意识混乱。

基本检查

在流感暴发的冬季阶段，临床诊断基于流感的症状和体征。

诊断检查与说明

实验室检查

• 全血细胞计数（可选）：

- WBC：正常至轻度下降。

• 肺部症状明显的患者监测指脉氧饱和度/动脉血气分析。

影像学检查

下呼吸道症状或体征突出的患者行胸片检查：

• 正常（50%～90%）。

• 双肺间质浸润。

诊断步骤/外科

• 鼻咽拭子或抽吸物的培养比咽部分泌物的培养更敏感。

• 随着症状的持续时间越长，分泌物量或培养阳性率下降。2 日以后不常表现为阳性。

• 流感快速诊断试验和直接荧光抗体试验廉价、快速且具特异性，但是敏感性低。有些可以区分 A 型和 B 型，但是无法区分 A 型亚型。

• 聚合酶链反应（PCR）试验周期时间短，且同时具备特异性和敏感性，可以区分 H1 和 H2 抗原；H1 和 H2 阴性对 2009H1N1 来说非常特别。

• 病毒培养：对急诊应用来源周期太长，但是对于地方监察是可以的。

鉴别诊断

• 其他呼吸道病毒。

• 军团菌或支原体或其他非典型肺炎。

• 支气管炎。

• 非典型肺炎。

• EB 病毒感染（传染性单核细胞增多症）。

• 炭疽是非常罕见的，且呼吸困难和恶心更常见。

• 急性艾滋病毒感染。

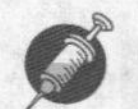

治疗

院前

在暴发期间，环境管理人员需要进行疫苗接种和呼吸卫生管理。

初步稳定/治疗

根据临床情况决定给予积极液体复苏、补充氧气和正压通气。

急诊治疗/程序

• 支持和对症治疗：

- 退烧药（对乙酰氨基酚或非甾体类解热镇痛药）：避免使用阿司匹林。
- 止咳药物（很少使用）。
- 补液。

• 症状发作的 48 h 内使用抗病毒药物是有效的：

- 抗病毒耐药模式各不相同。在 CDC 更新页面进行确认。
- 神经氨酸酶抑制剂扎那米韦（吸入）和奥司他韦（口服）通常对 A 型和 B 型是有效的。
- 金刚烷类化合物金刚烷胺和金刚乙胺是对抗 A 型流感唯一有效的，但是目前使用仍有阻力（目前不推荐使用）。
- 1 日内使用抗病毒药物减少症状的持续时间。严重疾病有效的间接证据。

- 价格昂贵。
- 推荐：
  ◦ 重症患者。
  ◦ 年龄大于6个月的儿童。
  ◦ 免疫功能低下患者。
  ◦ 并发症高危患者。
  ◦ 孕妇及产后2周以下者。
• 预防：
- 多价灭活流感疫苗推荐以下人员每年接种：
  ◦ 成人>50岁。
  ◦ 居住在疗养院和需要长期护理的人员。
  ◦ 6个月至5岁的儿童。
  ◦ 年龄为6岁或18岁的儿童患有流感和慢性阿司匹林并发症的风险增加。
  ◦ 6个月至8岁的儿童如果以前服用的剂量少于2剂，则需要服用2剂(间隔4周)。
  ◦ 9～18岁的儿童需要1剂。
  ◦ 高风险个体(哮喘、COPD、心血管疾病、免疫功能低下、糖尿病)。
  ◦ 健康护理工作者。
  ◦ 病态肥胖(体质指数>40 kg/m^2)。
  ◦ 北美印第安人和阿拉斯加当地居民。
  ◦ 照顾不到6个月的儿童的人员。
  ◦ 在流感季节妊娠的妇女。
- 灭活流感疫苗目前被证明是有效的。鼻喷雾剂疫苗可能对流感感染提供类似的保护。关于流感减毒活疫苗的使用，有不同的建议。人们一致认为，如果孩子对接受肌内注射犹豫不决，应该考虑使用鼻喷雾剂疫苗。在美国以外的一些国家，鼻喷雾剂疫苗是主要的疫苗。最重要的目标是为6个月以上的儿童进行免疫接种。目前的建议必须每年审查一次。
- 灭活疫苗禁忌证：
  ◦ 孕妇。
  ◦ 严重免疫缺陷患者的密切接触者和卫生保健人员。
  ◦ 5岁以下儿童出现反复喘息。
  ◦ 儿童、青少年服用阿司匹林。
  ◦ 对鸡蛋严重过敏。
  ◦ 患有合并症的人，将他们置于流感并发症的高危人群中。
- 以下情况下进行药物预防：
  ◦ 暴露的家庭成员进行暴露后预防，特别是高风险人员。
  ◦ 在A型流感暴发期间没有接受疫苗接种的高危患者进行短期预防。
  ◦ 除了对疫苗反应不佳的患者，高风险患者(包括HIV感染的患者)联合使用疫苗。
  ◦ 高危人群使用疫苗存在禁忌时使用替代疫苗。
  ◦ 为高危人群提供护理的人员。
  ◦ 健康护理人员的长期预防是有效的，但是消耗储备药物的量很大。
  ◦ 例外：
    ▪ 可干扰活病毒疫苗。
    ▪ 接种后至少2周不要开始。
• 支气管狭窄和呼吸音减低的患者使用支气管扩张剂如沙丁胺醇是有效的。

妊娠注意事项

• 在流感季节，建议孕妇接种灭活疫苗。
• 减毒活疫苗禁用于孕妇。

▪ 药物治疗

• 奥司他韦：75 mg，口服，每日2次，持续3～4日：
- 暴露预防：75 mg，口服，1次/日，持续7～10日。
• 扎纳米韦：10 mg，吹鼻(吸入2次)，q12 h，持续3～5日。
• 不再推荐金刚烷胺和金刚乙胺。
• 沙丁胺醇：2.5 mg 3 ml，使用喷雾器或计量吸入器间隔使用。

随访

▪ 进一步处理

入院指征

• 低氧(肺炎或气道反应性疾病)。
• 严重脱水。
• 精神状态改变。

出院指征

大部分患者会经历一个短期的自限性的病程，可以耐受液体和退热药治疗。

转诊问题

当地方疾病状况不明确、诊断不明确、地方抗病毒耐药机制，联系传染病专家会诊。

▪ 随访建议

电话通知患者告知其PCR监测结果。

要点和误区

• 熟悉网络CDC每周的更新，因每个季节流感都会改变。
• 近期旅行的患者应考虑虫媒病毒或SARS与MERS。
• 有高危行为的患者考虑HIV。
• 如果在体检中发现虱子，对于居住在拥挤环境中的无家可归的患者，认为巴通体是流感的模拟物。
• 在大部分患者，可不行检测或抗病毒治疗。
• 有呼吸系统疾病或低氧的患者，考虑并发气道反应性疾病。
• 急诊政策：呼吸卫生协会：
- 宣传海报并提供酒精洗手液。

颅脑穿透伤 Head Trauma, Penetrating

Gary M. Vilke · Siri Shastry　刘雪峰 译

基础知识

▪ 描述

穿透伤易累及颅脑内实质。

• 高速穿透伤：弹道伤常见，直接损伤脑实质，同时在穿透路径周围形成震荡伤。
• 低速穿透伤：常由刀具、鹤嘴锄及其他尖锐物体造成，直接损伤局部的脑实质。

▪ 病因

• 外物穿透颅骨直接进入颅腔：
- 脑实质直接的局限性损伤。
- 颅内出血，包括硬膜下、硬膜外及脑实质出血。
• 子弹击中颅骨后即使未造成颅骨骨折，也会引起明显的弹着点下方脑组织损伤。

诊断

▪ 症状和体征

• 意识状态变化程度和神经系统异常体征

L

与致伤物体及打击部位有密切关系。

• 颅内压升高表现：

- 意识状态恶化。

- GCS 评分降低。

- Cushing 反应：心动过缓、血压升高及呼吸频率减慢。

- 瞳孔扩大，伴有去皮质或去大脑姿势。

• 颅脑穿透伤、颅底骨折及盲管伤：

- 熊猫眼：颅底骨折所致双侧眼眶瘀斑。

- Battle 征：耳后乳突部位皮下瘀斑，伴有颅底骨折。

- 鼓室积血。

- 脑脊液耳鼻漏。

病史

• 确定现场的武器类型及口径。

• 遗忘受伤过程。

• 是否有抗凝药物使用史。

• 头痛、视力改变或听力丧失。

• 局部神经症状。

体格检查

• 头部穿透性损伤及损伤位点。

• GCS 评分。

• 完整的神经系统检查。

• 致伤物和致伤位置对意识状态和神经系统体征有影响。

• 头部穿透损伤的表现。

基本检查

• 通过病史和体格检查评估损伤范围。

• 影像学研究。

诊断检查与说明

实验室检查

• 全血细胞计数。

• 血小板计数。

• 凝血功能（PT、INR、APTT、血小板功能测定）。

• 血型鉴定，交叉配血。

• 血电解质，尿素氮，肌酐。

影像学检查

• 头颅 CT 能够显示损伤部位和损伤范围。

• 颅骨 X 线片能够显示损伤的深度、游离骨折碎片在颅内的位置。

• 颈椎评估：

- 螺旋 CT 或者前后位、侧位及齿状突位的 X 线平片。

鉴别诊断

• 钝性颅脑外伤。

• 颅底骨折。

• 任何可能导致精神状态改变的情况均可引起患者跌倒，从而继发引起穿透性颅脑损伤。

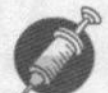

治疗

院前

• 固定异物（如刀具），但不要拔除。

• 确定武器的类型及口径。

• 保持气道通畅避免低氧血症。

• 避免过度通气。

• 保护颈椎。

• 转送至创伤中心。

• 避免低氧血症（氧饱和度＜90%）：

- 必要时可吸纯氧。

• 避免血压过低（SBP＜90 mmHg）：

- 使用晶体液扩容维持血压。

初步稳定/治疗

• 外伤救护 ABC 管理。

• 快速气管插管：

- 如 GCS 评分＜8 分，不能保持气道通畅，或出现低氧血症，均需快速行气管插管。

- 给予甲苄咪酯或芬太尼作为诱导剂，琥珀胆碱（小剂量预处理）、罗库溴铵或者维库溴铵作为肌松剂；吗啡持续镇静。

- 血流动力学不稳定的患者慎用芬太尼。

- 维持正常的二氧化碳分压，避免过度通气或通气不足。

• 输注晶体液，维持收缩压＞90 mmHg。

• 减少喉部操作和交感反射反应。

• 处理与创伤有关的其他问题。

• 警惕颈椎损伤。

急诊治疗/程序

• 早期神经外科会诊。

• 合并脑疝时需要尽快降低颅内压：

- 适当过度通气：成人 20 次/分，儿童 25 次/分，1 岁以下幼儿 30 次/分，以维持呼气末二氧化碳分压处于 30～35 mmHg。

- 升高床头 20°～30°。

- 高渗治疗：患者收缩压＞100 mmHg 且予以充分的液体复苏后可给予甘露醇脱水降颅压。考虑 3% 的生理盐水治疗低血压患者。

• 静脉注射苯妥英钠或左乙拉西坦，预防早期创伤后癫痫。

• 防治低凝状态：考虑使用维生素 K、新鲜冷冻血浆（FFP）、凝血酶原复合浓缩液（PCC）、鱼精蛋白硫酸盐或其他基于凝血病变程度和患者使用抗凝剂的靶向逆转剂。

• 考虑血小板减少患者输注血小板。

• 低颅压的头部创伤患者不推荐使用糖皮质激素。

• 初期急诊治疗不推荐使用巴比妥类药物。

• 必要时可输血，维持血细胞比容＞30%。

• 在确定性脑外科手术前进行颅骨钻孔减压可能挽救患者生命：

- 钻孔减压术在损伤或血肿侧进行，仅用于对过度通气和甘露醇治疗无反应的并且呈去皮层/大脑姿势的昏迷患者。

• 避免低温治疗，因为没有强有力的证据支持常规使用低温治疗。

• 广谱抗生素预防。

• 手术：

- 手术应基于临床及影像学阳性发现以及脑外科会诊。

药物治疗

气管插管，颅内高压，癫痫，高凝状态，止痛。

一线药物

• 甲苄咪酯：0.2～0.3 mg/kg，静脉推注。

• 芬太尼：如 SBP＞100 mmHg，3～5 μg/kg 静脉使用。

• 3% 高渗盐水：3～5 ml/kg，超过 10～15 min。

• 左乙拉西坦：每次静脉推注 1 g（20 mg/kg）。

• 甘露醇：0.25～1 g/kg，静脉滴注。

• 咪达唑仑：0.04～0.2 mg/（kg·h）。

• 苯妥英钠：15～20 mg/kg，静脉推注，最大剂量为 1 000 mg。

• 异丙酚：10～80 μg/（kg·min）。

• 罗库溴铵：0.6 mg/kg，静脉推注。

• 琥珀胆碱：1～2 mg/kg，静脉推注。

• 维库溴铵：0.1 mg/kg，静脉推注：

- 小剂量预处理：0.01 mg/kg，静脉推注。

• 维生素 K：

- 因服用香豆素出现颅内出血的患者可给予维生素 K。

- 10 mg 加入 50 ml 生理盐水缓慢推注，持续 30 min。

• 硫酸鱼精蛋白：

- 使用低分子肝素合并颅内出血时。

- 如 8 h 内使用过低分子肝素，则按 1 mg 低分子肝素：1 mg 鱼精蛋白的剂量缓慢静脉推注，静脉推注时间超过 3 min。

- 如 8 h 前使用过低分子肝素，则按 1 mg 低分子肝素：0.5 mg 鱼精蛋白的剂量缓慢静脉推注，时间超过 3 min。

L

随访

进一步处理

入院指征

所有患者应送入 ICU 或直接进行手术。

出院指征

穿透伤患者不应安排出院。

随访建议

所有颅骨穿透伤患者均应被收入院。

要点和误区

- 遗漏抗凝药物服用史的询问以及未给予适当的影像学检查。
- 未积极纠正低凝状态。

卵巢囊肿/扭转 Ovarian Cyst/Torsion

Reneé A. King · Brittany L. Catanach 王虑 译

基础知识

描述

- 卵巢囊肿：
  - 平常没有症状，直到出现出血、扭转、破裂、感染等并发症才发现。
  - 卵泡囊肿。
    - 最为常见，从胎儿期到更年期都可能出现。
    - 单房直径：3～8 cm。
    - 薄壁的易于破裂，并常造成轻微的出血，有时也不会出血。
    - 破裂常发生在排卵中期，导致月经期疼痛。
  - 黄体囊肿：
    - 最为常见。
    - 直径＞3 cm，但通常＜10 cm。
    - 囊内快速出血导致破裂。
    - 由于血管增多，月经前破裂最为常见。
    - 常导致严重的腹膜内出血。
    - 出血速度较慢或卵巢膨胀，只会疼痛而没有出血。
- 附件扭转：
  - 第五常见的妇产科急诊手术。
  - 卵巢血管、输卵管、管周囊肿发生扭转。
  - 致附件缺血坏死。
  - 会导致不孕不育。
  - 淋巴管静脉回流受阻，导致附件迅速膨胀。
  - 8～12 cm 的囊肿患病风险最大。

风险因素

附件扭转。

- 生育期妇女。
- 卵巢囊肿，特别是直径＞5 cm。
- 卵巢过度刺激。
- 肿瘤：严重的囊腺瘤最为常见，畸胎瘤（良性囊肿＞恶性囊肿）。
- 盆腔手术：输卵管结扎、子宫切除。
- 妊娠。
- 盆腔炎症。

妊娠注意事项

扭转（扭转的 10%～22%）常发生在妊娠的头 3 个月，体外受精或卵巢诱导是其高发风险因素。

儿科注意事项

15%的附件扭转病例是儿童（月经前肾盂漏斗韧带拉长）。

> **注意**
> - 抗凝治疗患者风险增高：
>   - 出血的黄体囊肿。
>   - 破裂囊肿的严重出血。

病因

- 卵巢囊肿：
  - 由未破裂的成熟卵泡或畸形未成熟卵泡生成的卵泡囊肿。
  - 妊娠早期过度生长或排卵后正常的数日的囊内出血，形成黄体囊肿。
  - 其他囊肿：
    - 卵泡膜叶黄素。
    - 畸胎瘤囊肿。
    - 巧克力囊肿。
- 附件扭转：
  - 右侧＞左侧。
  - 最高发于生育期妇女。

> **注意**
> 若囊肿见于绝经后妇女常提示肿瘤。

诊断

症状和体征

病史

- 卵巢囊肿：
  - 腹痛。
    - 单侧，剧烈。
    - 间断 *vs*. 持续。
    - 转移性。
    - 可能发生在运动、性生活、外伤或盆腔体检时。
  - 极少发热。
  - 月经不规律（提示多囊卵巢综合征）。
  - 不孕。
  - 妊娠状态。
  - 性病史。
  - 乳腺癌或胃肠肿瘤病史（转移可能）。
- 附件扭转：
  - 病史多样。
  - 腹痛。
    - 突然，剧烈，绞痛。
    - 局限性和弥漫性。
    - 可能会因为位置的改变而恶化。
    - 腹股沟或腰部放射痛。
    - 可能变为慢性或再发，与扭转、再扭转相关。
  - 发热。
  - 恶心、呕吐。
  - 阴道出血。

体格检查

- 卵巢囊肿：
  - 腹部压痛（随腹膜炎加重压痛加重）。
  - 附件压痛。
  - 盆腔肿块。
  - 失血性休克可能。
    - 常见于黄体囊肿破裂出血。

◦ 体位性、低血压、心动过速。
• 附件扭转：
- 腹部压痛（逐渐加重）。
- 附件压痛。
- 附件肿块。

■ 基本检查

• 妊娠试验以排除宫外孕（异位妊娠）。
• 快速血红蛋白或血细胞比容检测

■ 诊断检查与说明

实验室检查

• 血或尿绒毛膜促性腺激素检测。
• 血细胞计数。
• 尿常规。
• 若严重出血，需做血型鉴定和交叉配血。
• 宫颈分泌物培养以排除盆腔炎。

影像学检查

• 经阴道超声。
- 附件囊肿或肿块。
◦ 非绝经期妇女，<5 cm 的囊性肿块通常是良性的。
◦ 在月经末期要重新评估。
- 盆腔积液。
- 膨胀水肿的卵巢（提示扭转）。
• 多普勒：
- 若是扭转则表现为低回声。
- 在急诊超声记录到正常的血流波形非常重要，但是不能完全排除近期曾发生过的扭转或静脉阻断。
• MRI：
- 对于右下腹痛而阴道超声和多普勒超声无法给出明确诊断时可考虑行 MRI 检查。
• CT：
- 能发现囊肿、腹腔积血或扭转，也可为其他可能的诊断提供证据。
- CT 检查能为因卵巢异常或其他原因引起腹痛的患者的腹腔镜手术提供充分的影像学信息。
- 带蒂扭曲的子宫可移位至扭转附件的一侧，或喙状突起。
- 腹水。

> **注意**
> 阴道超声对于诊断卵巢扭转的敏感性还不是很高，若临床上高度怀疑，其他相关检查继续完善。

诊断步骤/外科

• 穹窿穿刺。
- 不常用。
- 引出破裂囊肿释放的浆液。
- 血细胞比容>15%提示腹腔积血。
• 腹腔镜检查是诊断附件扭转的金标准，然后进行治疗。

儿童注意事项

• 目前推荐通过腹腔镜处理早期出现的附件扭转，这将有利于保护卵巢功能。
• 接下来还需要持续随访监测，以防止恶变出现。

■ 鉴别诊断

• 宫外孕（异位妊娠）。
• 盆腔炎或附件脓肿。
• 圆韧带痛。
• 子宫内膜异位。
• 赘生物。
• 子宫扭转。
• 阑尾炎。

■ 随访建议

卵巢囊肿：
• 如果疼痛缓解，囊肿在 4～5 cm 或以下，妇产科医师应密切随访。

要点和误区

附件扭转：
• 扭转是临床诊断。
• 症状多样，不典型。
• 附件扭转始终要和其他腹痛鉴别。
• 在孕妇和儿科患者中考虑扭转。

落基山斑疹热 Rocky Mountain Spotted Fever

Roger M. Barkin　何融冰 译

 基础知识

■ 描述

立克次体侵犯小血管：
• 直接造成血管损伤。
• 免疫系统引起的叠加血管损伤、血管炎。

■ 病因

• 立克次体通过蜱媒介造成的急性感染：
- 美国西部地区的安氏落基山壁虱（安氏革蜱）。
- 美国东部地区的变异革蜱（犬蜱）。
• 所有州均有报道，1/2 的病例发生于 5 个州（北卡罗来纳州、南卡罗来纳州、田纳西州、俄克拉何马州、阿肯色州），以及美国中部和南部的部分地区。
• 4—9 月份较常见，但任何月份都有可能发生。
• 40～64 岁的男性更常见。

诊断

■ 症状和体征

病史

• 60% 的患者被蜱虫叮咬后 14 日内有皮疹。
• 潜伏期 2～14 日不等，平均 7 日。
• 蜱虫暴露史，通常在农村。

体格检查

• 皮疹：
- 皮疹初发（3～5 日）：
◦ 斑点状，红色，扁平。
◦ 按压可变白。
◦ 直径 1～4 mm。
- 数小时至数日内：
◦ 变深，丘疹，变暗，明显可触及。
- 2～3 日后：
◦ 瘀点性或紫癜性。
◦ 鲁-雷试验阳性。
◦ 可融合或溃疡。
- 在严重病例中，可发生周围区域的坏死。
- 部位：
◦ 起始于腕和踝的屈肌表面，快速播散到掌和足底。
◦ 向心性播散涉及四肢；可波及躯干和面部。
◦ 15%离心性播散至手掌和足底。
◦ 10%的患者无皮疹。

◦ 患者初发就医时通常诊断不明确。
• 肺部：
- 无分泌物性咳嗽。
- 胸痛。
- 呼吸困难。
- 啰音。
• 胃肠道：
- 通常与致命性落基山斑疹热相关。
- 仅次于血管炎。
- 恶心、呕吐。
- 腹痛、腹胀。
- 肠梗阻。
- 肝脾大。
• 神经系统：
- 2/3 患者有局部或全身性神经系统表现。
- 假性脑膜炎。
- 严重的不间断头痛。
- 脑炎。
• 其他：
- 全身性水肿。
- 脱水。
- 全身性乏力。
- 肌痛。
- 视网膜出血和结膜炎。
• 并发症：
- 弥散性血管内凝血(DIC)。
- 非心源性肺水肿。
- 急性肾衰竭。
- 老年人、男性、非裔美国人、慢性酒精滥用者或葡萄糖-6-磷酸脱氢酶缺乏者更常见的严重或致命疾病。

基本检查

临床诊断辅以验证性实验室检查，如低钠血症、贫血和血小板减少。

诊断检查与说明

实验室检查

• 血清学：
- 通过单滴度>1∶64 或升高 4 倍。症状出现的初始几日内抗体可能不被发现。
- 方法：
◦ 免疫荧光抗体(敏感度 95%)。
◦ 补体结合。
◦ 间接血凝试验。
◦ 间接免疫荧光分析是参考标准。
• CBC：
- 正常 WBC 计数。
- 血小板减少症。
- 贫血。
• 电解质、BUN/肌酐、葡萄糖：
- 低钠血症<130 mEq/L。
• 肝功能：
- 天冬氨酸氨基转移酶。
- 乳酸脱氢酶。
• 动脉血气分析：
- 低氧。
- 呼吸性碱中毒。
• 如果怀疑 DIC 则行凝血功能检查。
• 微生物学：
- 皮肤活组织免疫组化抗体染色。
- 立克次体分离(费时/昂贵)。
- 聚合酶链反应分析。
• CSF：
- 脑脊液细胞增多，蛋白质增加。

影像学检查

• 肺水肿、肺炎行胸片检查。
• 超声心动图：
- 左心室收缩能力下降。

诊断步骤/外科

如可进行免疫组化抗体检测，行皮肤组织活检确诊。

鉴别诊断

• 其他蜱传播疾病：
- 埃里希体病，年长患者。
- 回归热。
- 莱姆病：慢性游走性红斑。
- 野兔病。
- 巴贝虫病。
- 科罗拉多蜱热。
• 传染性疾病：
- 脑膜炎球菌血症：见于晚冬、早春；斑丘疹或瘀点疹。
- 麻疹：晚冬、早春，症状严重。
- 野兔病：播散至掌面，足底。
- 水痘：在四肢无皮疹。
- 病毒性皮疹。
- 感染性单核细胞增多症：播散至掌面、足底。
- 弥散性淋球菌感染：脓疱性损害。
- 斑疹伤寒：皮疹从躯干开始，离心性播散。
- 二期梅毒。
- 猩红热和链球菌败血症。
- 川崎病：红色，口唇皲裂。
- 中毒性休克综合征。
- 胃肠炎。
- 葡萄球菌脓血症。
• 炎症性病因：
- 过敏性血管炎。
- 血栓性血小板减少性紫癜。
- 胶原血管病。
- 青少年类风湿关节炎。
• 心脏疾病。

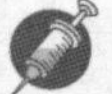

治疗

院前

适当稳定情况。

初步稳定/治疗

• ABC 管理。
• 如果脱水，生理盐水静脉液体输注。
• 低氧的供氧治疗。

急诊治疗/程序

• 纠正液体和电解质缺乏。
• 基于临床和流行病学检查结果迅速开始抗生素治疗。不要延误至获得实验室证据。
- Doxycydine：首选药物。
- 妊娠或过敏患者使用氯霉素。
- 磺胺类药使感染加重。
• 发热使用对乙酰氨基酚。
• 严重病例伴有广泛血管炎、脑炎或脑水肿患者，考虑使用大剂量激素(有争议)。
• 儿童如果在患病第 5 日前开始治疗则预后较好。
• 治疗并发症：
- DIC。
- 成人呼吸窘迫综合征。
- CHF。
• 药物治理。
• 移除蜱虫的临床医生应戴上手套，使用细镊子将其尽可能靠近附着点抓取。轻轻地向外拉，避免扭曲或挤压。伤口取出后清洗消毒。

儿科注意事项

• 5～9 岁发病率最高。
• 2/3 的病例发生于<15 岁的儿童。
• 强力霉素用于存在死亡可能的儿童患者，相比氯霉素短期牙齿褪色的风险小，不良反应少。

妊娠注意事项

尽管存在固有的风险，大多数专家还是建议孕妇使用多西环素。在这一人群中，氯霉素有显著的并发症。

L

▪ 药物治疗

一线用药

强力霉素：100 mg(儿童：2 mg/kg 用于＜45 kg)口服或静脉注射每日 2 次持续 5～7 日。患者在无发热后应继续治疗 2～3 日。

- 对于危重的成人患者，考虑服用 200 mg，q12 h，持续 72 h，通常通过静脉途径给予。

二线用药

- 对乙酰氨基酚：500 mg（儿童：10～15 mg/kg)，口服 q4 h；不能超过 5 剂/24 h 或 4 g/24 h。
- 氯霉素：75 mg/(kg · 24 h)，口服或静脉注射，q6 h，持续 5～7 日，以及退热后 48 h。
- 甲泼尼龙：125 mg(儿童：1～2 mg/kg)，静脉注射。

随访

▪ 进一步处理

入院指征

中度到重度症状。

出院指征

- 经早期治疗的轻微早期疾病。
- 告知家人潜在的聚集和暴露可能。

转诊问题

明确的并发症。

▪ 随访建议

持续存在的并发症。

要点和误区

- 需要进行基于临床表现和流行病学的早期治疗。
- 强力霉素不是儿童的禁忌证。

L

麻疹 Measles

Austen-Kum Chai 段立伟 译

基础知识

描述

• 可用疫苗预防，主要发生于儿童，传染性疾病以发热、咳嗽、感冒、结膜炎和红色斑丘疹为主要表现。
• 又称为风疹。
• 由于广泛免疫，美国发病率低。
• 在美国，死亡率为(1～3)/1 000。
• 在世界许多地方仍然很常见，旅行者可以传播这种疾病。

病因

• 麻疹由麻疹病毒引起，是一种 RNA 副黏病毒。
• 人类是唯一已知宿主。
• 高度传染性。当怀疑麻疹时应开始呼吸道隔离。在没有免疫或免疫状态下均可大暴发。

诊断

症状和体征

• 皮疹出现之前的潜伏期(8～12 日)：
- 通过直接接触或传染唾沫吸入传播。
- 儿童通常不完整或没有免疫。
- 患者在皮疹出现前 4 日和出现皮疹后 4 日是具有传染性的。
• 前驱期(1～7 日)：
- 发热、继发轻度呼吸道疾病、结膜炎、发热。
- Koplik 斑：
◦ 颊黏膜处针尖大小灰色斑点，周围环绕红晕。
◦ 麻疹的特异性表现。
◦ 瞬态：在皮疹发生前 1～2 日出现然后 48 h 后消失。
• 活动性疾病：
- 咳嗽、感冒、结膜炎(三“C”症状)。
- 发热 38.3℃(101℉)，通常更高。发热超过 3～4 日提示麻疹相关并发症。
- 皮疹在第 3～7 日出现，持续 4～7 日。
◦ 皮疹首先出现于头部，然后离心向下蔓延。
◦ 斑丘疹可融合。可能有瘀点。手掌和足底很少累及。
◦ 临床症状改善见于 48 h 内出现皮疹的患者。
◦ 皮疹 3～4 日消除，皮疹按照发生的顺序逐渐脱皮消失。

• 并发症：
- 并发症的高风险人群为 5 岁以下的儿童、20 岁以上的成人、孕妇和免疫功能低下者。
- 呼吸：
◦ 麻疹感染后咳嗽可能持续 1～2 周。
◦ 免疫抑制患者的肺炎(6%)常见。
◦ 是麻疹最常见的死亡原因。
◦ <2 岁患者可发生喉气管支气管炎。
• 中枢神经系统：
◦ 癫痫发作<1%。
◦ 脑炎。
◦ 脑脊髓炎：
▪ 皮疹发生后 1～14 日。由于感染后发生自身免疫反应。
▪ 发热、头痛、呕吐和颈强直。
▪ 嗜睡、昏迷和昏迷后癫痫发作。
◦ 亚急性硬化性全脑炎(SSPE)：
▪ 非常罕见但严重的并发症，发生于感染后 7～10 年。
▪ 中枢神经系统功能逐渐退化。
▪ 人格改变、智力减退、运动和视觉障碍、癫痫发作、昏迷和死亡。
• 心血管：
◦ 短暂性心肌炎、心包炎和传导异常。
◦ 很少有临床意义。
◦ 老年患者可见充血性心力衰竭。
- 血小板减少性紫癜。
- 中耳炎(7%)。
- 鼻窦炎。
- 腹泻(8%)，最常见。
- 由于摄入不足或丢失过多，可能会导致脱水。

儿科注意事项

• 麻疹、腮腺炎和风疹±水痘(MMR 或 MMRV)疫苗应在儿童 12 个月或 12 个月后接种。第二次剂量应该在 4～6 岁(即开始上学前)接种。
• 后续剂量的疫苗接种应至少 4 周分开接种。
• 需要国际旅行的婴儿，应在旅行前进行麻疹免疫。
- 6～11 个月的儿童应在出发前接受 MMR，12～15 个月的儿童应接受第二次剂量的 MMR，4～6 岁的儿童应接受第三次剂量。
- 12～15 个月的儿童应在 4～6 岁时接受第一次和第二次 MMR。
- 12 个月或 12 个月以上的儿童，如果去疫区，应在出发前接受第 2 次 MMR。

妊娠注意事项

• 在妊娠期间感染，自然流产和早产风险增加。
• 不会导致出生缺陷。
• 妊娠期间不应该接种疫苗 MMR 和 MMRV。

老年人注意事项

那些出生在 1957 年前的人一般被认为是免疫的。然而，如果血清学检测显示阴性滴度则应该接受疫苗接种。

基本检查

• 诊断基于临床所见。
• 咳嗽、感冒和结膜炎伴发热和随后的皮疹。

诊断检查与说明

实验室检查

• 疑似脑炎行脑脊液分析。
• 从血液、咽喉、鼻和尿液中分离病毒，用于流行病学监测。
• 麻疹 IgM 和 IgG 滴度血清学试验、麻疹 RNA 病毒 PCR 监测用于明确诊断。

影像学检查

怀疑肺炎的患者行胸部影像学检查。

鉴别诊断

• 风疹：
- 病程较轻、耳后淋巴结、皮疹扁平、无结膜炎。
• 猩红热：
- 砂纸样纹理皮疹、草莓舌、咽喉痛。
• 传染性单核细胞增多症：
- 可行血清学试验。
• 玫瑰疹：
- 热退疹出。
• 传染性红斑(“第五病”)：
- 无前驱症状，无发热。
- 面颊发红伴消退时花边样皮疹。
• 肠道病毒：
- 无呼吸系统症状。
• 川崎病：
- 手掌和足底皮疹。
• 二期梅毒。
• 中毒样休克综合征。
• 药物反应：

- 通常没有发热和上呼吸道感染症状。

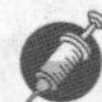

治疗

院前

没有免疫的院前急救人员应被告知上面描述的潜在风险。

- 如果接触，在 72 h 内接种 MMR 疫苗或在 6 日内给予免疫球蛋白。
- 第一次接触后 5 日和最后一次接触后 21 日不可上班。

急诊治疗/程序

- 预防接种是治疗的基础。
- 解热镇痛药。
- ABC 管理：
  - 供氧和气道保护：
    - 肺炎。
    - 脑炎。
  - 如有必要，行静脉补液。
- 隔离疑似病例。
- 如果怀疑麻疹，请上报当地卫生部门。
- 对非免疫患者进行暴露后预防：
  - 暴露后 72 h 给予 MMR 疫苗。
    - 妊娠或免疫抑制者避免使用。
  - 按照 0.25 ml/kg 肌内注射免疫球蛋白，最大剂量 15 ml：
    - 如果在暴露 6 日内给予，可能预防或改善症状的严重性。
    - 易受感染的家庭或其他密切接触者，有指征地给予，特别是 <1 岁的儿童、妊娠妇女或免疫功能低下患者。
    - 定期接受静脉注射免疫球蛋白(IGIV)的患者，在暴露发生接受 IGIV 的 3 周内，常规剂量 400 mg/kg 应该足够用于麻疹预防。
    - 接受免疫球蛋白治疗的患者，如果没有禁忌，不超过 5～6 个月随后接受疫苗治疗。

药物治疗

世界卫生组织建议给予麻疹患儿维生素 A，每日 1 次，共 2 日，当维生素 A 缺乏普遍存在时。这可能降低麻疹死亡的风险：

- <6 个月给予 50 000 IU。
- 6～12 个月给予 100 000 IU。
- >12 个月给予 200 000 IU。
- 在美国肠外及口服制剂可使用。

随访

进一步处理

入院指征

- 严重肺炎。
- 脱水。
- 脑炎。
- 亚急性硬化性全脑炎(SSPE)。
- 免疫功能低下患者：
  - 获得性免疫缺陷综合征(AIDS)。
  - 免疫抑制治疗。
  - 老年患者有合并症的情况。

出院指征

感染持续时间：

- 症状发生前 4 日和皮疹发生后 4 日。
- 在疾病持续期间，免疫功能低下的患者仍具传染性。
- 并发症监测的相关教育。

要点和误区

- 具高度传染性的传染病之一，在美国每 1 000 例患者中有 1～3 例发生死亡。在卫生保健机构呼吸道隔离是必需的。
- 严重免疫功能低下接受免疫治疗的患者和妊娠患者不应接受 MMR 或 MMRV 疫苗接种治疗。
- 免疫抑制患者可能不会发生特征性皮疹。
- 接种疫苗是预防麻疹的基础。

马尾综合征 Cauda Equina Syndrome

Daniel F Morris　彭沪 译

基础知识

描述

马尾区腰骶神经纤维受压：

- 脊髓圆锥神经纤维。
- 纤维在 L_1～L_2 间隙终止。

高危因素

- 肿瘤。
- 静脉药物的应用。
- 免疫功能低下状态。
- 创伤。

病因

- 最常见的椎间盘突出位置：
  - L_4～L_5 椎间盘>L_5～S_1>L_3～L_4。
  - 最常见于 50～60 岁。
- 占位效应来自：
  - 骨髓瘤、淋巴瘤、肉瘤、脑膜瘤、神经纤维瘤、血肿。
  - 脊椎转移(乳腺癌、肺癌、前列腺癌、甲状腺癌、肾癌)。
  - 硬膜外脓肿(特别是静脉吸毒者)。
- 闭合性损伤。
- 穿透伤。
- 腰麻。
- 其他罕见原因：
  - 先天性异常、多发性硬化症、脊髓 AVM、神经结节病、IVC 血栓形成。

诊断

症状和体征

病史

- 腰背痛。
- 坐骨神经痛、神经根痛(单侧或双侧)。
- 下肢麻木或无力。
- 由于无力或疼痛行走困难。
- 膀胱或直肠功能障碍：
  - 尿潴留或尿失禁。

体格检查

- 腰骶部(LS)压痛。
- 下肢感觉或运动障碍：
  - 可能是不对称的。
- 足背屈力量减弱。
- 股四头肌肌力减弱。
- 深腱反射减退。
- 鞍区痛觉减退或麻木。
- 肛门括约肌张力减弱。

基本检查

- 神经系统检查是最基本的：

M

- 直举腿。
- 直腿抬高试验征：
  ○ 患者仰卧，弯曲髋关节和足部背屈。
  ○ 大腿后侧疼痛或痉挛提示神经受刺激。
- 会阴部感觉。
- 肠鸣音。
- 肛门指检：温柔抚摸肛门外侧皮肤诱使肛门外括约肌的反射性收缩。

• 残余尿：
- 通过膀胱导尿或使用超声评估。
- 50～100 ml 及以上被认为是不正常的。
- 残留量随年龄增加。
- 如果正常，诊断的可能性不大。

■ **诊断检查与说明**

实验室检查

• 在鉴别诊断的基础上。

• CBC、尿液分析、ESR 和 C 反应蛋白(CRP)。

影像学检查

• 脊柱 X 线片。

• 脊柱 MRI 是明确诊断的方法。

• 如果无法行 MRI，进行 CT 脊髓造影。

■ **鉴别诊断**

• 骨性关节炎、腰骶部劳损、坐骨神经痛。

• 椎体骨折(病理性和非病理性)。

• 骨髓炎。

• 脊髓硬膜外脓肿。

• 脊髓圆锥或其以上脊髓受压。

• 强直性脊柱炎和椎管狭窄。

• 腹主动脉夹层。

• 血管性跛行。

• 髋关节病变。

• 急性横贯性脊髓炎。

治疗

■ **院前**

• 按要求管理气道和创伤性损伤。

• 如果有外伤的证据，患者转运时需全脊椎固定。

> **注意**
>
> 即使非创伤的患者，考虑到不稳定病变的可能性，应给予脊椎固定。

■ **初步稳定/治疗**

• 如果疑似外伤或脊柱不稳定时给予脊柱固定。

• 镇痛。

• 神经外科评估前予以禁食。

■ **急诊治疗/程序**

• 重复的神经系统检查以检测病情进展。

• 对于急性脊髓损伤(<8 h)，开始大剂量甲泼尼龙治疗。

• 在所有情况下立即神经外科会诊。

• 神经外科会诊后，硬膜外脓肿应给予抗生素治疗。

• 有关减压术的紧迫性存在争议：
- 建议发病 6～24 h 进行。

■ **药物治疗**

甲泼尼龙(大剂量类固醇治疗)：30 mg/kg 静脉推注，然后在接下来的 23 h 5.4 mg/(kg·h)输液。应在受伤 8 h 内开始。

随访

■ **进一步处理**

入院指征

• 所有急性马尾综合征的患者必须收入神经外科。

• 经过快速减压手术的患者具有良好的预后。

• 治疗不应拖延。

• 患者接受延迟手术减压(>48 h)也将获益。

出院指征

患者确诊马尾综合征，先前有完整的评估，并没有新的神经功能障碍出现即可出院，但需与他们的神经外科医师保持紧密联系。

要点和误区

• 理想的情况下，尽可能在患者进展到不可逆的神经功能障碍之前早期确诊。

• 不对称的腰痛。

• 发热和背部疼痛。

• 高危人群发生腰痛，出现疑似感染时检查 ESR 和 CRP。

慢性阻塞性肺疾病 Obstructive Pulmonary Disease

Adam Z. Barkin 陈奇通 译

基础知识

■ **描述**

• 是美国的第三大死因。

• 由以下几个进程导致气道梗阻为特征的疾病：
- 肺气肿：不可逆的肺泡破坏与气道弹性回缩力缺失。
  ○ 标志着肺老化加速。
- 慢性支气管炎：无肺泡破坏的气道炎症。
- 气道反应性疾病：可逆的支气管痉挛、黏液栓塞、黏膜水肿。

• 慢性阻塞性肺疾病(COPD)影响因素 10%的人群，其中 50%为吸烟者。

• 慢性阻塞性肺疾病(COPD)患者高血压、糖尿病、心力衰竭和冠心病发病率增加。

• 急性加重频繁发作导致：
- 更高的死亡率。
- 更快的肺功能下降。
- 更差的生活质量。
- 住院风险增加。

• 改良医学研究委员会(mMRC)呼吸困难量表：
- 0 级，仅仅于剧烈运动后呼吸困难。
- 1 级，快步行走或爬小山坡时气短。
- 2 级，由于气短，平地行走时要比同龄人速度慢，或者需要停下来休息。
- 3 级，平地步行 100 m 即有气短需停下喘息。
- 4 级，因呼吸困难不能离开家，或者穿/脱衣即能引起气急。

• 慢性阻塞性肺疾病全球倡议(GOLD)指南：
- A 组：
  ○ 急性加重不超过 1 次/年。
  ○ 1 s 用力呼气容积(FEV_1)>80%预计值。

M

◦ mMRC 0 或 1 级。
- B组：
◦ mMRC 2 级以上。
◦ 1 s 用力呼气容积（FEV_1）50%～80%预计值。
- C组：
◦ mMRC＜2 级。
◦ 急性加重≥2 次/年。
◦ 1 s 用力呼气容积（FEV_1）30%～49%预计值。
- D组：
◦ 高症状负担。
◦ mMRC≥2 级。
◦ 急性加重的风险高。
◦ 1 s 用力呼气容积（FEV_1）＜30%预计值。

危险因素

遗传学

α_1-抗胰蛋白酶缺乏。

病因

• 吸烟是首要的原因：
- 15%的吸烟者发展为 COPD 患者。
• 空气污染。
• 气道高反应性。
• α_1-抗胰蛋白酶缺乏。
• 自身免疫可能起到了重要的作用。
• 急性发作：
- 病毒感染：
◦ ＞50%急性发作与近期的感冒症状有关。
◦ 免疫功能下降使机体更易受到影响以致 COPD 急性发作。
◦ 鼻病毒。
◦ 呼吸道合胞病毒。
- 细菌感染：
◦ 在急性发作期，40%～60%的患者痰液中分离出细菌。
- 最常见：
◦ 流感嗜血杆菌。
◦ 莫拉克斯菌属。
◦ 肺炎链球菌。
- 更可能出现：
◦ 呼吸困难加重。
◦ 痰液量增加。
◦ 脓性痰。
- 污染物质：
◦ 改变免疫功能。
◦ 增加气道炎症。
- 季节变化：
◦ 冬季更常见并且更严重。

诊断

症状和体征

病史

• 劳力性呼吸困难。
• 咳嗽。
• 咳痰。
• 疲劳。
• 喘息。
• 端坐呼吸。
• 精神状态改变。

体格检查

• 气急。
• 回缩。
• 气流减少。
• 发绀。
• 呼气相延长。
• 桶状胸。
• 下肢水肿。
• 颈静脉怒张。
• 第三心音和第四心音奔马律。
• 神志改变继发于二氧化碳麻醉。

诊断检查与说明

实验室检查

• 全血细胞计数。
- 血细胞比容增高提示可能慢性缺氧。
- 中性粒细胞和白细胞增加提示可能感染。
• 动脉血气：
- 二氧化碳潴留。
- 酸中毒。
- 氧合情况。
• β-利钠肽：
- 鉴别慢性阻塞性肺疾病（COPD）与充血性心力衰竭（CHF）。
• 痰标本检查。
• 必要时检测茶碱水平。

影像学检查

• 胸部 X 线片：
- 气胸。
- 肺炎。
- 慢性充血性心力衰竭。
- 肺叶萎陷。
• 胸部 CT 扫描：
- 需要评估肺栓塞可能或者进一步的疾病特征时。

诊断步骤/外科

• 脉搏氧饱和度仪。
• 心电图（ECG）。
• 肺功能检查。
• 超声心动图：
- 诊断左或右心室衰竭或损伤。

鉴别诊断

• 气胸。
• 充血性心力衰竭。
• 肺炎。
• 肺栓塞。
• 上呼吸道阻塞。
• 哮喘。
• 限制性肺疾病。
• 急性呼吸窘迫综合征。
• 胸腔积液。
• 急性冠状动脉综合征。
• 心包积液。
• 代谢紊乱。

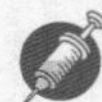

治疗

院前

增加氧供。
• 100%通过非循环呼吸器。
• 不要担心二氧化碳潴留而不使用。
• 启动支气管扩张剂的雾化治疗。

初步稳定/治疗

• 氧疗：
- 维持氧饱和度 90%～92%。
- 呼吸缓慢有二氧化碳潴留风险患者。
- 密切监测的通气抑制患者。
• 无创机械通气：
- 是高碳酸血症呼吸衰竭需辅助呼吸时的治疗选择。
- 可能避免气管插管。
- 可能有助于解决高碳酸血症。
• 气管插管：
- 呼吸肌疲劳。
- 精神状态改变。
- 无法配合紧急治疗。
- 无效通气。
- CO_2 麻醉。

急诊治疗/程序

• 持续心电图和脉搏血氧监测。
• 支气管扩张剂治疗。
• β受体激动剂：
- 沙丁胺醇。
• 抗胆碱能类：
- 异丙托溴铵。

• 糖皮质激素：
- 抗感染。
- 减少复发。
- 甲泼尼龙或泼尼松。
• 抗生素：
- 发热、痰液量增加和/或呼吸困难。
- 大环内酯类抗生素也可能具有与它们抗菌作用不相关的抗感染效果。
• 甲基黄嘌呤：
- 茶碱。
• 呼吸机设置：
- 允许足够的呼气时间以最减小气道压力，防止气压伤。
- 允许性高碳酸血症。

药物治疗

• 沙丁胺醇：2.5 mg，雾化，q10～30 min。
• 阿奇霉素：一次 500 mg，口服/静脉注射，然后 250 mg/d，口服 4 日。
• 头孢曲松钠：1 g，静脉注射，q24 h。
• 异丙托溴铵：0.5 mg，雾化，q6 h。
• 左氧氟沙星：500 mg，口服/静脉注射，q24 h。
• 甲泼尼龙：125 mg，静脉注射，q6 h。
• 泼尼松：40～60 mg/d(1～2 mg/kg)，口服 5 日。
• 特布他林：0.25 mg，皮下注射，q30 min。

一线用药

• 沙丁胺醇。
• 异丙托溴铵。
• 泼尼松或甲泼尼龙。

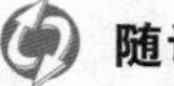

随访

进一步处理

入院指征

• 入重症监护室指征：
- 插管患者。
- CO_2 潴留及氧饱和度<90%。
- 在急诊室的呼吸肌疲劳。
- 严重的酸中毒。
- 伴随心脏或肺部疾病。
- 急性冠状动脉综合征。
- 心律失常。
- 充血性心力衰竭。
- 肺栓塞。
• 普通病房：
- 慢性阻塞性肺疾病患者有额外肺损伤：
◦ 肺炎。
◦ 肺叶萎陷。
◦ 呼吸管增加。
• 运动不耐受。
• 急诊室内病情无改善。
• 门诊患者治疗失败。
• 预测住院死亡率的 3 个条件：
- 年龄>70 岁。
- 严重临床症状：
◦ 发绀、辅助呼吸肌使用等。
- 基线呼吸困难。

出院指征

• 症状减轻。
• 急诊室内病情改善。
• 动态血氧饱和度>92%。

随访建议

• 戒烟。
• 确保疫苗是最新的(流行性感冒疫苗每年一次，肺炎链球菌疫苗至少一次)。
• 确定和避免触发物(如冷空气、香水)。
• 情况允许可行肺减容术。
• 长效毒蕈碱拮抗剂和长效 β_2 受体激动剂在慢性阻塞性肺疾病的长期治疗中显示出了希望。
• 其他新兴的治疗方法已经被证实可以减缓疾病的进展。

要点和误区

• 在最佳的药物治疗仍不能达到理想时选择无创正压通气。
• 激素雾化将会更多地用于急性加重的 COPD 患者。
• COPD 患者患糖尿病、高血压、心脏病的风险增加。
• 认为 COPD 患者应常规接种流感疫苗和肺炎链球菌疫苗。

毛滴虫病 Trichomoniasis

Herbert Neil Wigder · Erin Nasrallah 张晟 林兆奋 译

基础知识

描述

• 性传播疾病(STD)。
• 与其他性传播疾病的高度流行相关。
• 导致泌尿生殖系感染。
• 后遗症：
- 可能导致胎膜早破或早产。
- 可能导致低出生体重新生儿。
- 促进 HIV 传播。
• 流行病学：
- 美国每年 300 万～500 万新发病例。
- 女性在性传播疾病门诊接受治疗的人群有 35%患病。
- 总体发病率为 3.1%(黑色人种女性发病率为 13.3%)。
- 潜伏期为 4～28 日。
- 可以无症状。

病原学

阴道毛滴虫：
• 鞭毛原虫：
- 常分布于尿道、膀胱、斯凯恩腺。

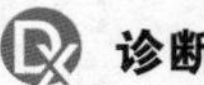

诊断

症状和体征

其他

• 阴道炎症：
- 少于 30%患者出现阴道分泌物。
- 起泡的黄绿色至灰白色。
- 外阴瘙痒刺激不适。
- 阴道异味。
- 同细菌性阴道炎(由阴道加德纳菌导致)和外阴阴道假丝酵母病(由白色假丝酵母菌引起)一样的症状。
- 排尿困难和尿急。
- 性交痛。
- 常无症状(50%)。
• 宫颈：
- 弥漫性红斑(10%～33%)。
- 点状出血：红斑性阴道炎或"草莓样宫颈"。
• 腹痛少见。

男性

• 常无症状(75%)或呈自限性。

- 同性传播少见。
- 非淋病性尿道炎：
- 占非特异性尿道炎的20%。
- 分泌减少。
- 排尿困难和尿道急症。
- 并发症：
- 前列腺炎。
- 附睾炎。
- 可逆性不育。

体格检查

- 女性：
- 阴道分泌物(黄绿色至灰白色泡沫样)。
- 气味。
- 红色溃疡(阴道壁和宫颈)。
- 男性：
- 分泌减少。

基本检查

如果临床怀疑程度足够高，进行经验性治疗。

- 女性：湿片法。
- 60%～70%有症状的患者敏感。
- 阴道穹隆分泌物盐水湿装。
- 需要立即滴镜下检查。
- 分叶核白细胞增多。
- 梨形带鞭毛滴虫运动(比白细胞稍大，可见于60%患者)。
- 中段尿敏感性不高。
- 未发现滴虫不能排除阴道毛滴虫感染(仅60%～70%阳性)。
- 许多急诊室没有设备进行湿装。
- 常见阴道pH升高，不具有特异性。
- 男性：湿片法不敏感。
- PCR诊断可靠，但应用不广。

诊断检查与说明

实验室检查

- 培养：
- 95%敏感性(前列腺按摩后收集分泌物，敏感性高)。
- 镜检未发现滴虫但高度怀疑时送培养。
- 即时检验：特异性高(>97%)，敏感性不稳定。
- PCR检查费用高。

鉴别诊断

- UTI。
- 淋病。
- 衣原体
- 细菌性阴道炎。
- 念珠菌阴道炎。
- 非特异性阴道炎。

治疗

急诊治疗/程序

- 普通女性：
- 甲硝唑2g，单次口服(治愈率90%～95%)。
- 甲硝唑250mg，每日3次，连服7日(尿道炎症)。
- 替硝唑2g，单次口服(治愈率86%～100%)。
- 甲硝唑凝胶，疗效不佳(不推荐)。
- 孕妇：
- 有症状：用甲硝唑(FDA B类)。
- 无症状：
- 治疗有争议，因为它不能降低胎膜早破或早产的发生率。
- 甲硝唑治疗。
- 男性：
- 甲硝唑2g，单次口服。
- 替硝唑2g，单次口服。
- 甲硝唑250mg，每日3次，连服7日。
- HIV阳性：
- 考虑7日疗法，有证据表明增加单药剂量治疗仍失败。
- 治疗性伴侣以防再感染。
- 双方无症状及治疗完成至少1周后才允许性生活。
- 使用乳胶避孕套。
- 服用甲硝唑期间避免同时饮酒。
- 最后一剂甲硝唑服用后至少24h内禁酒，因酒精可沉淀药物。

随访

进一步处理

出院指征

全体患者。

要点和误区

- 非淋病性尿道炎症经典药物(如阿奇霉素、多西环素)不能治疗滴虫性阴道炎。
- 细菌性阴道炎治疗用药无效的女性阴道炎症可能是阴道毛滴虫感染。
- 阿奇霉素、多西环素治疗无效的男性非淋病性尿道炎可能是阴道毛滴虫感染。

毛细支气管炎

Suzanne Schuh 张晓彬 译

基础知识

描述

经呼吸道引起的下呼吸道感染与支气管狭窄合并喘息、气促、呼吸窘迫和上呼吸道前驱症状。

病因

- 85%～90%的患者有呼吸道合胞病毒。
- 流感。
- 副流感病毒。
- 腺病毒。
- 通常发生在冬季。

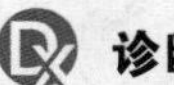

诊断

症状和体征

- 毛细支气管炎常见于≤12个月的儿童，首次发病主要以合并上呼吸道感染、咳嗽和呼吸窘迫为主要表现。
- 鼻塞，经常有明显的流鼻涕。
- 咳嗽，有时伴有呕吐。
- 喘息。
- 湿啰音，干啰音。
- 呼吸窘迫表现为呼吸急促、鼻翼扇动、三凹征、鼾音。
- 发热，通常<39.5℃。
- 可能存在低氧血症(一般为轻度)，发绀少见。
- 通常有液体摄入减少，严重脱水少见。

M

• 可能发生呼吸暂停，尤其出现在有早产史的幼儿。

• 单抗，一种呼吸道合胞病毒特异性免疫球蛋白，在冬季每月给有高风险的孩子肌内注射。这样可以减少呼吸道合胞病毒的感染风险。

基本检查

• 临床诊断。
• 评估临床通气。
• 脉搏血氧饱和度：
- 确认在持续基础情况下的氧合情况。无法依据指脉氧结果来预判轻症细支气管炎的病程，但其与临床情况结合起来有助于患者病情评估。
- 确保在有任何气急症状时或在吸氧过程中维持适当的氧合。

诊断检查与说明

实验室检查

• 大多数患者无需特殊检查，除了血氧饱和度。
• 鼻咽分泌物、冲洗：
- 病毒培养。
- 荧光抗体。
- 可用的商业试剂盒。
- 以下情况考虑此检查，不只是例行公事。
 ◦ 临床症状提示其他原因(百日咳、衣原体)。
 ◦ 危重患儿。
 ◦ 小于3个月的毛细支气管炎发热患儿(考虑合并尿路感染引起的发热)。
 ◦ 合并明显细菌感染(没有合并细菌感染时细菌涂片阳性是比较少见的)。
 ◦ 肺支气管发育不良或慢性肺疾病。
 ◦ 合并心脏疾病。
 ◦ 早产儿。
 ◦ 其他情况需要抗病毒治疗(罕见)。

影像学检查

胸部X线：
• 通常充气过度、气道疾病、肺不张、浸润改变：
- 婴幼儿肺不张提示更严重疾病。
• 少数气道＋气腔疾病，肺炎通常为病毒感染：
• 急性期少有变化。
• 以下情况考虑此检查：
- 需要排除其他诊断，如慢性充血性心力衰竭、误吸、先天性气道异常(罕见)。
- 2～3周鉴别不清的慢性过程。
- 危重症新生儿严重的呼吸衰竭。
- 非典型表现在中毒或进行性恶化的儿童。
- 典型临床表现不经常出现的。

诊断步骤/外科

• 呼吸状态允许的小于28日的感染性发热性细支气管炎。
• 1～3个月的发热婴儿，考虑行尿培养。
• 有明显气急患者需持续监测血氧饱和度。
• 血氧饱和度和密切的临床监测在对病情的持续评估中非常重要。
• 氧饱和度＜90%的患者，氧饱和度的读数变异度较大。

鉴别诊断

• 哮喘、复发性病毒诱导的喘息：需要住院的重症细支气管炎及过敏家族史是将来发生哮喘的危险因素。
• 百日咳：咳嗽痉挛之间没有呼吸窘迫，没有喘息。
• 细菌性肺炎：通常有毒性表现，没有喘息，孤立的空腔疾病(合并)胸腔没有气道异常表现。
• 异物：症状发作突然，通常不发热。
• CHF：先前有临床预警[发育停滞(FTT)，喂食问题]。

治疗

院前

注意

• 婴幼儿的呼吸储备有限会出现毫无征兆的快速失代偿。
• 监测心肺功能状态和氧合情况。
• 吸氧情况下氧饱和度＜90%～92%(海平面)和/或严重窘迫。
• 观察呼吸暂停：
- 儿童＜7周，体重＜4 kg，呼吸频率＞80次/分，心率＞180次/分，是高危因素。
- 如果反复呼吸暂停使用面罩通气。

初步稳定/治疗

• 儿科高级生命支持：建立气道，通气和水化。
• 监测氧饱和度并评估呼吸做功情况。
• 如反复呼吸暂停、严重的呼吸衰竭，立即行紧急气管插管。
• 鼻导管吸氧可能有用。

急诊治疗/程序

• 如果氧饱和度＜90%～92%(海平面)予以补充氧气。
• 后鼻道吸痰可改善鼻腔通畅和氧气供给。
• 经鼻高流量鼻给氧的标准虽然尚未建立，但其对严重呼吸窘迫的婴儿很有用，可通过补充氧气以维持一个合适的氧饱和度。
• 静脉水化如果脱水或严重呼吸窘迫。
• 许多细支气管炎患儿无法从药物治疗中受益。
• 支气管扩张剂(沙丁胺醇、消旋肾上腺素、肾上腺素、左旋沙丁胺醇)：
- 不应该单独使用疗效不确定。
- 在中度至重度的患者中一些临床医师在试验的基础上，连续2～3次治疗，并继续作为管理的一部分，如果出现明显的呼吸做功减弱。
- 经常使用在症状显著不改善的孩子中。一般来说，不会改变整体的疾病结局。
- 高渗盐水没有好处。
• 类固醇：
- 对于大多数没有复发性毛细支气管炎、特异性反应史或过敏性家族史的患者，类固醇本身不会改善其临床病程或住院率。
• 抗生素：
- 一般不用于病毒引起的病例。
- 局灶性细菌性疾病(中耳炎、局灶性肺炎)，X线影像学检查为单独的肺大叶病灶而没有气道病变影像学依据(通常为细菌性肺炎而不是细支气管炎)，有显著的毒性反应，脓毒症，可以考虑使用。
• 利巴韦林：
- 不在急诊室中使用，住院患者少有使用。

药物治疗

• 对于小于12月龄的首发轻症毛细支气管炎患者，一般不推荐药物治疗。
• 支气管扩张剂和皮质类固醇常用于1岁左右反复出现细支气管炎样发作的儿童，特别是有哮喘家族史的儿童。如果呼吸做功有改善，可以考虑进行治疗试验并继续用药。
• 沙丁胺醇：2.5 mg/3 ml，2～3支雾化吸入或400 μg通过MDI吸入，在急诊室间隔20～30 min使用一次。只有在呼吸状态明显改善的情况下可以连续使用，不改变总体的治疗结果。
• 肾上腺素：3 ml(1∶1 000稀释)在急诊室每隔30 min给予2支雾化吸入。
• 2.25%消旋肾上腺素0.25～0.5 ml加入2.5 ml生理盐水中行雾化治疗。
• 泼尼松龙(15 mg/5 ml)：1～2 mg/(kg·d)，每日2次，口服3～5日。

• 地塞米松：每次 1 mg/kg 在急诊室口服，然后 0.15 mg/kg 每日口服，持续 5 日。

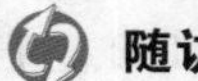

随访

进一步处理

入院指征

• 需要补充氧气（在海平面室内氧饱和度<90%～92%）。

• 需要肠外营养。

• 呼吸时如有明显的吸气凹陷征、鼻音、呼噜声，无论氧饱和度高低均应收入院。

• 呼吸暂停。

• 严重的慢性肺部疾病与心脏病。

• 显著的合并症、怀疑其他诊断、潜在的系统性疾病、免疫缺陷或免疫抑制治疗。

• 小于 7 周的婴儿，体重小于 4 kg，呼吸频率>80 次/分，心率>180 次/分，有合并症或早产儿，强烈建议住院。

• 看护不合规定或无法密切监护孩子。

出院指征

• 相当好的喂养。

• 室内空气可维持氧饱和度（海平面）。

• 没有严重的呼吸窘迫。

• 24 h 内保持随访。

• 适应家庭环境。

• 出院后的居家氧疗方案正在修订中。

- 符合所有入选标准：
  - 伴有喘息或湿啰音的上呼吸道感染者。
  - 2 个月到 2 岁（妊娠>44 周）。
  - 首次出现喘息者。
  - 在 12 月和 4 月之间来急诊就诊者。
  - 具备进行吸痰等气道管理的能力者。
  - 具备无烟家庭环境。
  - 有可靠的家庭条件，包括已接入 EMS，可实现 24 h 随访。
  - 居住环境的海拔≤6 000 ft。
- 不符合以下排除标准：
  - 有毒血症状或细菌感染的证据。
  - 有与疾病相关的 ALTE（明显威胁生命事件）。
  - 存在心脏疾病、慢性肺疾病或神经肌肉疾病。
  - 氧需求处于基线水平。
  - 免疫缺陷。
  - 最近 7 日内曾入院或入急诊救治。
- 在吸氧后和临床观察≥4 h，证实疾病症状轻微者。
  - 婴儿反应、活动良好，喂养情况良好。
  - 无任何吸气凹陷征。
  - 呼吸频率 50 次/分。
  - 吸氧≤0.5 L/min 时氧合良好（清醒状态下在海平面水平的氧饱和度测量值≥90%）。

• 出院说明：

- 症状可能持续 2～3 周。
- 少量频繁喂食。少吃多餐，注意观察容量状况和尿量情况。

• 喂食前经鼻腔吸痰。

• 须在 24～48 h 预约随访。

- 出院后使用支气管扩张剂不是都有效的。

随访建议

• 患儿的进食能力和日常行为能力正常是重要保证。

• 如出现嗜睡、进食不佳或尿量异常均为不良信号，需要立即评估。

• 最重要的是要告诉父母，需要保持鼻腔通畅，经常喂食，同时告知其哪些是病情恶化的标志。24～48 h 安排随访非常重要。

要点和误区

• 血氧饱和度（正常和异常读数）都需要在临床中给予关注。

• 有明显呼吸窘迫、合并症、年龄过小和早产的婴儿通常需要积极的心肺功能的干预和监测，这类患者可能发生病情迅速恶化。

• 如果有明显的充血症状，经鼻吸氧可能是有用的。

• 对于第二次发生上呼吸道感染、咳嗽和呼吸窘迫，或≥18 个月的儿童的第一次发病，则提示病毒感染诱发的喘息可能大（详见哮喘）。

玫瑰糠疹 Pityriasis Rosea

Benjamin S. Heavrin　瞿金龙 译

基础知识

描述

• 原因不明的自限性皮疹性疾病，主要见于儿童和年轻人。

• 最初表现为独立的“前驱斑”，后在躯干和四肢出现卵圆形红斑性皮损。

• 随后继发的皮疹出现在躯干皮纹线和四肢末端形成对称的“圣诞树图形”。

• 约 80%的症状在 2 个月内自行缓解。

病因

• 病因不明，有弱证据和病毒感染有关，如疱疹病毒 6 和 7。

• 很多药物和糠疹性皮疹反应有关：

- 巴比妥类药物。
- 卡托普利。
- 可乐定。
- 金。
- 异维 A 酸。
- 甲硝唑。
- 铋剂。
- 乙肝疫苗。
- 格列卫。
- 干扰素。

• 湿疹、哮喘和潜在的恶性肿瘤有弱相关性。

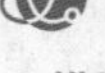

诊断

症状和体征

前驱症状和特征性的皮疹将在下面讨论。

病史

60%～70%的患者有前期症状：

• 心神不安。

• 消化系统症状。

• 呼吸系统症状。

体格检查

皮肤病学表现：

• 前驱斑：

- 孤立的、红斑的、轻微突出皮肤表面的丘疹，直径 2～10 cm。
- 见于 50%～90%的患者。

• 继发性出疹：

- 广泛分布的浅橙色、椭圆形、微小的刮鳞丘疹。
- 常呈“圣诞树形”沿皮纹线对称分布。
- 通常在前驱斑出现 7～14 日后出现。

- 皮损集中出现在躯干和四肢末端。
- 瘙痒常见。

• 皮损集中在面部和四肢的远端和少量躯干皮肤，特征性逆糠疹。

儿科注意事项

• 逆糠疹，皮损多见于面部和四肢远端，特征性的逆糠疹比成人更为常见。

• 极少见口腔损害，多为点状出血和溃疡。

基本检查

排除其他疾病诊断，特别是没有发现前驱斑的情况下：

• 二期梅毒有类似的皮肤表现。对有性病风险因素的患者可行 RPR 检查进行筛查。

• KOH 检测可用于诊断皮肤癣病。

诊断检查与说明

实验室检查

没有需要的检查：

• KOH 检测和 RPR 检查可用于与其他皮肤病鉴别。

鉴别诊断

• 前驱斑：
- 圆形湿疹。
- 体癣。

• 继发皮疹：
- 二期梅毒。
- 药物疹。
- 点滴状牛皮癣。
- 卡波西肉瘤。
- 扁平苔藓。
- 潜在的恶性肿瘤。
- 疥疮。
- 脂溢性皮炎。
- 花斑癣。
- 皮肌炎。
- 侵犯皮肤的淋巴瘤。
- 红斑狼疮。

治疗

初步稳定/治疗

不需要。

急诊治疗/程序

• 糠疹是自限性的。

• 类固醇激素、抗组胺和红霉素治疗后瘙痒症缓解。

药物治疗

• 苯海拉明：成人：25～50 mg，口服，每日 3 次[儿童：5 mg/(kg·d)，每日 3 次]。

• 红霉素：400 mg(10 mg/kg)，口服，每日 3 次。

• 氢化可的松：1%乳膏，每日 3 次。

• 泼尼松：15～40 mg(0.25～0.5 mg/kg)，每日 1 次。

一线用药

• 苯海拉明：成人：25～50 mg 口服，每日 3 次[儿童：5 mg/(kg·d)，每日 3 次]。

• 氢化可的松：1%乳膏，每日 3 次。

二线用药

• 泼尼松：15～40 mg(0.25～0.5 mg/kg)，每日 1 次。

• 红霉素：400 mg(10 mg/kg)，口服，每日 3 次。

随访

进一步处理

入院指征

玫瑰糠疹是一种自限性疾病，不需要住院治疗。

出院指征

若明确诊断是玫瑰糠疹患者即可出院。

转诊问题

严重的难治的瘙痒症需要皮肤科医师随诊。

随访建议

• 根据需要给予必要的护理。

• 症状通常在 1～2 个月缓解。

要点和误区

• 糠疹通常局限在四肢远端和躯干。还应考虑其他诊断，除非患者除了糠疹还包括黏膜和四肢远端受累。

• 当患者有中毒或一些不典型表现时，应考虑其他疾病的可能。

玫瑰疹 Roseola

Roger M. Barkin 何融冰 译

基础知识

描述

• 幼儿急诊。

• 潜伏期为 5～15 日。

• 传播模式未知：
- 可能为口腔排菌的水平播散。
- 在人与人之间播散，但感染性不是很强。
- 人类是唯一的宿主。

• 病理生理学：
- 复杂免疫应答(细胞因子、抗体应答、T 细胞反应)。

病因

• 人疱疹病毒 6 型(HHV-6)：
- 较大的双链 DNA。
- 与人巨细胞病毒密切相关。

• 发病高峰在 6～12 个月的小儿，90%发生在 2 岁以内。

• 晚春和初夏发生率最高。

诊断

症状和体征

• 经常为自限性。

• 腹泻。

• 易激惹。

• 很少引起严重或致死性散播性疾病。
- 肝炎传染性单核细胞增多综合征。

• 并发症：
- 发热性惊厥(5%～35%)。
- 无菌性脑膜炎/脑病。
- 血小板减少性紫癜。

• 在免疫受损个体中易发，表现为发热、皮疹、肝炎、骨髓抑制、肺炎和脑炎。

儿科注意事项

• 大部分新生儿因为经胎盘获得的抗体对 HHV-6 呈血清阳性。

• 1～2 岁时，>90%的婴儿呈血清学阳性。

病史

• 典型病史是突然起病，高热 39.4～41.2℃，随后热退疹出。

• 体格检查无异常：

- 儿童看上去状态良好。
- 体温在 3～4 日趋于正常。
- 可表现为易激惹和厌食。
- 可注意到前囟隆起。

体格检查

• 淋巴结肿大。

• 体温正常后出现从躯干到手臂和颈部的斑丘疹。

• 在 3 日内皮疹消退。

• 咽部红斑丘疹(Nagayama 斑)。

• 中耳炎常见。

• 颈部和枕后部淋巴结病。

基本检查

临床诊断：

• 表现正常的儿童出现高热。

诊断检查与说明

实验室检查

• 全血细胞计数：

- 起初白细胞升高，随后趋于正常伴随淋巴细胞增多；白细胞可在起病后 3～5 日下降。
- 血小板可能下降。

• HHV-6 DNA：

- 通过聚合酶链反应检测。
- 可应用于研究水平。
- IgM 早期出现并且在 IgG 产生时下降。
- 可以使用血液和 CSF。

• 如果怀疑脑膜炎可查脑脊液。

• 尿液检查：可能出现无菌性脓尿。

鉴别诊断

• 原因不明的发热。

• 猩红热：

- 砂纸样皮疹、帕氏线和草莓舌。

• 麻疹(rubeola)：

- Koplik 斑、咳嗽、鼻炎、结膜炎和发热。

• 落基山斑点热：

- 皮疹从踝和腕部开始。

• 风疹：

- 皮疹后发热。

• 传染性红斑(第五病)。

• 登革热。

• 肺炎球菌血症。

• 脑膜炎，特别是伴随前囟隆起的。

治疗

院前

无。

初步稳定/治疗

ABC 管理。

急诊治疗/程序

• 支持性措施。

• 退热治疗：

- 对乙酰氨基酚。
- 布洛芬。

药物治疗

• 对乙酰氨基酚：500 mg(儿童：15 mg/kg，口服，q4 h)；24 h 给药不超过 5 次或 24 h 总量不超过 4 g。

• 布洛芬：200～600 mg(儿童：5～10 mg/kg，口服，q6～8 h)；混悬液 100 mg/5 ml；口服滴剂 40 mg/ml。

随访

进一步处理

入院指征

中毒性发热且对初始支持治疗无反应的儿童。

出院指征

通常所有患者都可以出院。皮疹消退后可以不用返回日间住院病房。

随访建议

3～4 日后发热持续需重新评估。

要点和误区

• 儿童看起来状况较好。

• 免疫功能正常儿童不推荐抗病毒治疗。

• 发热性惊厥需适当评估。

梅毒 Syphilis

Jessica Freedman　范浩浩　李文放 译

基础知识

描述

• 性传播疾病。

• 在 2016 年，全美有新发梅毒 88 042 例。

• 2016 年有 27 814 例原发性或继发性梅毒，较 2015 年增加 17.6%。

• 超过一半的新发梅毒见于男男性行为者。

• 全球每年确诊 1 200 万新病例。

• 通过黏膜、破损的皮肤获得。

• 分为 3 个阶段：

- 一期梅毒：
  ◦ 无痛硬下疳或溃疡。
- 二期梅毒：
  ◦ 病毒复制和血源性传播。
  ◦ 原发病灶开始后 3～6 周。
  ◦ 皮疹，皮肤黏膜损害，淋巴结病变。
  ◦ 继发潜伏晚期。
  ◦ 延迟潜伏期。
- 三期或晚期梅毒：
  ◦ 非常罕见。
  ◦ 心血管和神经系统症状。

病因

梅毒螺旋体：

• 螺旋体细菌。

诊断

症状和体征

一期梅毒

• 有 21 日的潜伏期。

• 没有原发性症状。

• 硬下疳：

- 接触部位的无痛丘疹。
- 底部清洁、圆形、界限清晰：
  ◦ 孤立性病变。
  ◦ 通常在阴茎、外阴和直肠。
  ◦ 双侧区域性淋巴结肿大。

M

- 3～6 周后自发愈合。
• 直肠硬下疳：
- 痛苦或无痛。
- 直肠刺激症状。
- 淋巴结无痛性肿大。

二期（早期）梅毒

• 原发病灶后 3～6 周发生。
• 传播阶段。
• 皮疹（最常见）：
- 对称，弥漫性、多形性、丘疹性或斑丘疹。
- 皮疹可能是多样的，非单一模式。
- 开始于躯干和屈肌四肢。
- 蔓延涉及手掌和足掌：
◦ 离散，红色或红棕色，直径为 0.5～2 cm。
• 尖锐湿疣：
- 大的灰色或白色病变，无痛，潮湿。
- 黏膜：
◦ 口腔和会阴。
◦ 非常具有传染性。
◦ 糜烂部位。
◦ 直肠扁平疣。
• 全身症状：
- 发热、头痛、不适、厌食、喉部疼痛、肌肉痛和体重减轻。
• 弥漫性淋巴结病：
- 腹股沟、腋窝、后部可触及淋巴结。
- 宫颈、股骨和/或滑车前区域。
- 无痛，固定和有弹性。
• 不常见：
- "虫蚀"样脱发。
- 梅毒性脑膜炎。
- 巩膜炎。
• 失去侧面的 1/3 眉毛。
• 无痛黏膜病变（黏液斑）。
• 二期阶段在 1～2 个月自发缓解。

潜伏性二期梅毒

• 主要和次要症状开始后解决。
• 无症状但血清学阳性的时期：
- CSF 正常。
• 除了在孕妇和胎儿中传播，晚期潜伏期不具感染性。
• 终身持续或发展为三期梅毒。

三期（晚期）梅毒

• 约 15% 潜伏性二期梅毒的未治疗患者发生。
• 可能出现在初次感染后 10～20 年。
• 神经系统和心血管受累：
- 疾病的破坏性阶段。
• 神经梅毒（最常见）：
- 无症状：
◦ 脑脊液阳性：性病研究实验室（VDRL）。
◦ 脑脊液细胞增多（10～100 个淋巴细胞）。
◦ CSF 浓度升高 50～100 mg/dl。
- 脑膜炎：
◦ 无菌，CSF 阳性，蛋白质水平较高和葡萄糖水平低（与上述相比）。
◦ 脑神经麻痹，包括单独的第Ⅷ神经麻痹。
- 一般麻痹症：
◦ 皮质功能丧失。
◦ 阿盖尔罗伯逊瞳孔（瞳孔缩小固定）对强光不能做出反应，但能做出集合反射。
- 脊髓结核（周围神经病）。
• 后柱变性、后部或脊髓背根。
• 痴呆症。
• 感觉异常，步态异常和（突然、严重）肢体、躯干疼痛。
• 反射，振动、位置感觉逐渐丧失。
• 闭目难立征阳性。
• 视力：视神经萎缩。
• 瞳孔：阿盖尔罗伯逊瞳孔。
• 尿失禁。
• 树胶样肿：
- 晚期良性梅毒皮肤或内脏：
◦ 骨骼、大脑、腹部脏器等。
• 肉芽肿性细胞超敏反应：
- 圆形，不规则或匐行状。
- "梅毒"。
• 心血管：
- 胸主动脉瘤（升主动脉最多见）：
◦ 扩张的主动脉和主动脉瓣反流。
◦ 主动脉瓣关闭不全。
◦ 冠状动脉血栓形成。
◦ 骨骼结构或皮肤的破坏性损伤。
• 艾滋病病毒感染者：
- 与梅毒密切相关。
• 神经梅毒的发病率增加。

先天性梅毒

• 宫内感染：
- 年龄＜2 岁：
◦ 肝脾大、皮疹、尖锐湿疣、鼻炎（鼻塞）、黄疸（非病毒性肝炎）、骨软骨炎。
• 年龄较大的儿童（梅毒疹）：
- 间质性角膜炎、神经性耳聋、胫骨前屈、额部隆起、桑白齿、哈钦森牙齿、马鞍鼻等。
- 评估有无遭受性侵害的可能。

基本检查

快速血浆反应素（RPR）。

诊断检查与说明

实验室检查

• 血清学：
- 非梅毒螺旋体血清抗体检查：
◦ 快速血浆反应素（RPR）VDRL。
◦ 硬下疳出现后 14 日阳性。
◦ 早期假阴性，特别是一期硬下疳＜7 日后。
◦ 在 2 周重复阴性测试并与疾病活动相关。
◦ 1%～2% 的普通人群出现假阳性。
◦ 滴度的 4 倍变化具有临床意义。
◦ 二期梅毒敏感性为 100%。
◦ 成功治疗后无反应。
- 螺旋体抗体测试：
◦ 荧光密螺旋体抗体吸收（FTA - ABS）。
◦ 抗体的血凝反应测定。
◦ 梅毒螺旋体（MHA - TP）。
◦ 更敏感和更具体。
◦ 1% 的假阳性率。
◦ 确诊测试。
◦ 患者终身有反应。
◦ 更昂贵和更难执行。
- 逆向筛选算法：先进行密螺旋体试验（EIA），如果阳性则反过来行非密螺旋体试验；此方式可增加对潜伏梅毒患者的敏感性。
- 暗视野显微镜：
◦ 识别原发性和继发性螺旋体病变。
◦ 可疑病变和阴性血清学可疑的早期病变（早期原发性梅毒）。
◦ 应用药膏后的假阴性。
◦ 口腔标本不适合。
- 对三期神经梅毒的脑脊液分析：
◦ 三期梅毒阳性。
◦ VDRL/RPR 阳性。
◦ 淋巴细胞＞5/ml。
◦ 蛋白质＞45 mg/dl。
◦ 葡萄糖减少。

鉴别诊断

• 生殖器溃疡：
- 软下疳（疼痛）。
- 生殖器疱疹：
◦ 疱疹，多发病灶。
- 性病淋巴肉芽肿。
- 腹股沟肉芽肿。
- 浅表真菌感染。
- 癌。
• 二期和三期梅毒：
- 玫瑰糠疹。

M

- 药物引起的皮疹。
- 急性热疹。
- 银屑病。
- 扁平苔藓。
- 疥疮。
- 传染性单核细胞。
- 病毒性疾病。
- 菌血症。
- 三期梅毒:
- 精神病。
- 痴呆症。
- 多发性硬化症。
- 脑膜炎。
- 脑炎。
- 谵妄。
- 未知的药物过量。

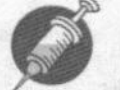

治疗

初步稳定/治疗

降低血压并建立主动脉夹层的静滴通路。

急诊治疗/程序

- 青霉素以外的治疗增加了复发率:
- 对青霉素过敏的人进行脱敏治疗。
- 妊娠:
- 即使在潜伏期梅毒中也用青霉素治疗。
- 如果患者对青霉素过敏,进行脱敏治疗。
- 吉海反应:
- 对治疗的短暂发热反应。
- 可能是由于螺旋体抗原释放或补体级联的激活。
- 8 h 达到峰值,24 h 内缓解。
- 症状:
  - 发热、头痛、不适、皮疹恶化。
- 使用退热药治疗。
- 没有严重的后遗症。
- 推荐的检测:
- 性伴侣。
- 伴随的性传播疾病,包括艾滋病。
- 6 个月和 12 个月重复血清学测试。

药物治疗

- 一期、二期、早期潜伏期(<1 年):
- 苄星青霉素:240 万 U,肌内注射。
- 请注意,这是长效青霉素的 L-B 方案而非 C-R 方案。
- 多西环素,100 mg,口服,2 次/日,持续 14 日。
- 四环素 500 mg,口服,4 次/日,持续 14 日。
- 阿奇霉素:2 g,口服,1 次,在特定地区有效,但不适用于男男性行为者;且已有治疗失败报道。
- 晚期潜伏期(>1 年),除了神经梅毒:
- 苄星青霉素 G:240 万 U 肌内注射 3 次。第 0、7 和 14 日超过 2 周。
- 若两次注射间隔超过 14 日应重新开始用药,所以孕妇均应重新开始用药。
- 多西定:100 mg,口服,持续 4 周。
- 四环素:500 mg,口服,每日 1 次,持续 4 周。
- 神经梅毒:
- 青霉素:300 万~400 万 U,静滴,q4 h,持续 10~14 日。
- 普鲁卡因青霉素:240 万 U,肌内注射,每日 1 次。
- 丙磺舒:500 mg,口服,每日 1 次,持续 10~14 日。
- 先天性梅毒:
- 青霉素:50 000 U/kg,肌内注射,q8~12 h,持续 10~14 日;普鲁卡因青霉素:每日 5 万 U/kg,肌内注射,持续 10~14 日。

随访

进一步处理

入院指征

- 神经梅毒需要静脉注射抗生素。
- 对青霉素过敏需要脱敏的孕妇。

出院指征

后续护理:
- 测量治疗后 6 个月和 1 年后的滴度下降。
- 三期/潜伏(>1 年):
- 测量治疗后 3、6、12 和 24 个月的滴度下降。

转诊问题

- 二期和三期梅毒、先天性和性传播疾病神经梅毒的传染病咨询。
- 有神经系统表现者应转诊眼科进行评估。

随访建议

- 必须监测滴定度。
- 往初级医疗健康机构继续行性病/HIV 检测。

要点和误区

- 梅毒被称为“伟大的模仿者”。
- 对于出现未知皮疹的患者,请考虑梅毒并询问相关生殖器病变的病史。
- 务必检查所有出现皮疹的患者的黏膜。
- 对于病因不明的患者,应注意三级梅毒有神经症状。

梅克尔憩室 Meckel's Diverticulum

Galeta C. Clayton 段立伟 译

基础知识

描述

- 先天性胃肠道畸形最常见。
- 因卵黄管不完全闭塞导致。
- 真性憩室(包含所有层):
- 50%包含正常肠黏膜。
- 50%包含肠(最常见)、胰腺、十二指肠、结肠、子宫内膜或肝胆黏膜。
- “2”的规则:
- 在一般人群中患病率为 2%。
- 发生终身并发症的风险为 2%,随诊年龄增长而发病减少。
- 症状通常发生在 2 岁左右:
  - <2 岁的患者 45%有症状。
- 平均长度为 2 in。
- 在回盲瓣 2 ft 处发现。
- 男女比例大致相等,但在男性症状更多见。
- 合并症:
- 成人可发生梗阻和憩室炎。
- 儿童可发生出血和梗阻。
- 平均年龄为 10 岁。
- 目前病死率为 0.000 1%。
- 在男性中多发。
- 梗阻:
- 附于脐、腹壁、其他脏器的憩室是游离或者独立的,导致:

◦ 肠套叠：憩室在前缘。
◦ 肠扭转：纤维韧带至肠扭转。
• 憩室炎：
- 无梗阻表现。
- 阑尾炎表现(最常见的术前诊断梅克尔憩室)。

儿科注意事项

• 儿童低位胃肠道出血是最常见原因。
• 5 岁以下患儿发作性无痛、肠蠕动活跃和亮红色直肠出血。

病因

残余卵黄管通道在妊娠 7 周退化。异位胃黏膜可分泌酶，导致黏膜壁糜烂，导致出血。

诊断

症状和体征

• 3 种不同表现类型：
- 因直肠出血导致失血，可导致异位胃黏膜溃疡形成。
- 继发于肠扭转、肠套叠或腹腔带引起梗阻从而导致呕吐。
- 因炎症或憩室穿孔导致腹痛(类似于阑尾炎)。
• 一般情况：
- 发热。
- 不适。
- 虚弱。
- 疲劳。
• 胃肠道：
- 经典的无痛性直肠出血。
- 腹痛：
◦ 腹痛位置取决于病因。
◦ 类似于阑尾炎。
- 呕吐。
- 扩张。
- 肠蠕动改变。
- 便血或黑便(取决于憩室的活动和位置)。
- 腹膜炎和感染性休克(晚期并发症)。
• 心血管：
- 心动过速(因疼痛或失血导致)。
- 低血压和休克(因失血导致)。

基本检查

• 可能导致各种症状和体征：
- <10%的患者在术前诊断。
- 对患者需要考虑到非特异性腹痛、恶心、呕吐或直肠出血。
• 病史和体格检查可使诊断范围缩小，但是对梅克尔憩室不会给出具体结果。
• 强制性直肠检查。
• 留置鼻胃管排除上消化道出血。
• 注意老年患者的心电图以排除导致腹痛的心脏原因。

诊断检查与说明

实验室检查

• 全血细胞计数：
- 因出血导致血红蛋白下降。
- 很少是慢性失血的原因。
- 憩室、穿孔或坏疽导致白细胞计数升高。
• 电解质、尿素氮、肌酐、凝血功能。
• 显著出血时行血型及交叉配血。

影像学检查

• 腹部、盆腔 CT：
- 怀疑炎症(阑尾炎、憩室炎)或肠梗阻。
• 腹部 X 线平片：
- 明确有无肠梗阻。
- 不能诊断梅克尔憩室。
• ^{99m}Tc 放射性同位素扫描(Meckel 扫描)：
- 诊断梅克尔憩室的无创性扫描。
- 敏感性：儿童约为 90%，成人约为 60%。
- 特异性：儿童和成人均为 95%。
• 小肠灌肠：
- 准确性为 75%。
- 钡/甲基纤维素通过鼻胃管到远端十二指肠或近端空肠。
- 增加梅克尔憩室在成人的诊断能力。
- 憩室可能短且宽，使诊断变得困难。
• 肠系膜动脉造影可能对快速出血的病例有用，可直接看到造影剂外渗。
• 放射性同位素扫描及灌肠正常时，可做 CT 血管造影对梅克尔憩室进一步评估。
• 超声评估在非出血性表现时可用。
• 胶囊内镜或双气囊小肠镜可能有助于诊断。
• 腹腔镜评估可以提供诊断和明确治疗。

鉴别诊断

• 成人：
- 肠粘连。
- 阑尾炎。
- 动静脉畸形。
- 肠梗阻。
- 痔。
- 炎症性肠病。
- 内疝。
- 肠息肉。
- 肠套叠。
- 消化性溃疡。
- 假膜性小肠结肠炎。
- 肠扭转。
• 儿童：
- 肠粘连。
- 肛裂。
- 阑尾炎。
- 闭锁。
- 胃肠炎。
- 溶血性尿毒症综合征。
- 过敏性紫癜。
- 肠息肉。
- 肠套叠。
- 扭转不良。
- 牛奶过敏。
- 肠狭窄。
- 肠扭转。

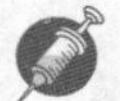

治疗

院前

直肠出血或腹痛患者建立静脉通道。

初步稳定/治疗

• 稳定生命体征，早期手术评估。
• 低血压：
- 液体复苏。
- 活动性直肠出血患者输注红细胞(儿童常见)。
- 感染性休克使用升压药。

急诊治疗/程序

• 胃肠道出血：
- 液体复苏，有指征时输注红细胞。
- 留置导尿，记尿量。
- 留置鼻胃管，排除活动性上消化道出血。
- 有指征时给予外科手术干预。
• 梗阻：
- 鼻胃管。
- 导尿管。
- 外科手术。
• 憩室炎或穿孔：
- NPO。
- 术前应用抗生素。
- 外科手术。
• 外科介入：
- 有症状的梅克尔憩室应切除。
- 儿童剖腹探查术偶然发现梅尔克憩室时应切除。

药物治疗

• 氨苄西林-舒巴坦：3 g[儿童：100～200 mg

氨苄西林/(kg · 24 h)],q8 h,静脉注射。

• 头孢西丁：1～2 g[儿童：100～160 mg/(kg · 24 h)],q6 h,静脉注射。

• 泮托拉唑：20～40 mg,静脉滴注。

随访

进一步处理

入院指征

推断为梅克尔憩室伴随憩室炎、梗阻、肠套叠、出血或肠扭转需要入院和手术评估。

出院指征

无。

随访建议

术后随访。

要点和误区

• 婴儿无痛性活动性直肠出血通常由梅克尔憩室导致。

• 并发症范围较广,如梗阻、肠套叠和出血。

• 常在疑似阑尾炎接受手术中被诊断。

• "2"的规则：

- 在一般人群中患病率为 2%。

- 发生终身并发症的风险为 2%。

- 症状通常发生在 2 岁以下。

- 平均长度为 2 in(1 in=2.54 cm)。

- 在回盲瓣 2 ft 处发现。

梅尼埃病 Meniere Disease

Konstantina A. Papathomas · Charles V. Pollack, Jr. 段立伟 译

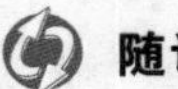

基础知识

描述

• 内耳性疾病。

• 一般为单耳病变(40%的病例可累及双耳)。

• 特点为：复发性偶发性眩晕、感觉神经性听力丧失、耳鸣和耳闷。

• 美国发病率约为 15/10 万。

• 男女比例为 1.3 : 1。

• 阳性家族史达 20%。

• 可在任何年龄：

- 40～60 岁为发病高峰。

• 北欧白种人后裔发病率高于非洲人或黑种人后裔。

• 良性病变,无法治愈。

• 与严重疾病状态相关。

病因

• 特发性。

• 膜迷路积水：内淋巴囊或内淋巴管阻塞,导致内淋巴液外流受阻和内淋巴系统压力增高：

- 压力增高导致内淋巴液(富钾细胞内液)和外淋巴液(贫钾细胞外液)之间的隔膜破裂。

- 化学混合液浸泡前庭神经受体,导致其去极化受阻和短暂性失功能。

• 可能与结构异常相关,如内淋巴囊萎缩、前庭管发育不全、内淋巴管狭窄、侧窦前移位导致压迫和内淋巴囊阻塞。

• 自身免疫：免疫复合物沉积在淋巴囊或自身抗体直接拮抗内淋巴囊功能。

• 认为存在基因易感性：发病年龄越小,症状越重。

• 其他机制：亚临床病毒感染可在数十年后导致迷路水肿、内淋巴囊和内耳缺血。

• 需将梅尼埃病与其他干扰正常内淋巴液产生和吸收的疾病(甲状腺疾病、梅毒导致的内耳炎症、药物)区分开。

诊断

• 依据临床症状和神经科评估进行诊断。

• 尽管 MRI 为明确诊断提供了可能,但确诊只能通过尸体检验获得。

• 诊断标准《美国耳鼻咽喉科学会指南》1995 年版)：

- 至少 2 次自发性偶发性眩晕,时间≥20 min。

- 至少 1 次听力图测试显示听力丧失。

- 受累耳出现耳鸣或耳闷感。

- 确诊为梅尼埃病：明确疾病+组织病理确认。

- 明确为梅尼埃病：至少 2 次明确的伴有听力丧失的眩晕发作,并且有耳鸣或耳闷症状,或两者都有。

- 很大可能为梅尼埃病：1 次明确的眩晕发作伴随其他症状和体征。

- 可能为梅尼埃病：明确的眩晕发作不伴有听力丧失,或听力丧失伴随不确定的前庭失衡。

症状和体征

病史

• 典型四联征：

- 眩晕。

- 听力丧失。

- 耳鸣。

- 耳闷。

• 眩晕可持续数分钟到数小时不等,常伴有恶心和呕吐症状(96.2%)。

• 感觉神经性听力丧失一般呈波动性和渐进性：

- 发作频率低的比发作频率高(87.7%)的受影响更重。

- 经常发作可导致永久性听力丧失。

• 耳鸣一般为低音性。

• 耳闷感表现为单侧耳的压力感、不舒适感和闷胀感。

• 发作后可在数分钟内达到最大强度,而后要数小时缓慢减退。

• 急性发作后,患者一般会感到劳累,不能保持平衡和恶心,可持续数小时到数日。

• 在发作间期,患者可完全无症状。

• 在不伴有意识丧失或眩晕的情况下,可以发生突然性无明显原因的摔倒。

• 患者的临床表现变异性很大。

- 听觉和前庭症状可能不会同时发生,特别是在疾病早期。

• 可能会出现频繁发作。

体格检查

• 检查结果存在变异,其具体结果取决于疾病程度。

• 急性发作期,患者往往会表现为极度的痛苦、大汗和面色苍白。

• 首要体格检查应该是血压、脉搏和呼吸功能的评估。

• 水平眼球震颤。

• 听力损伤。

• 气动耳镜检查可以诱发症状或引起眼球

M

震颤。

• Weber 音叉试验通常横向远离患侧耳。

• Rinne 试验阳性提示气传导要优于骨传导。

• Romberg 试验阳性伴有站立不稳，特别是在闭眼的情况下。

• 必须排除中枢神经系统病变，耳周病变(鼓膜破裂、胆脂瘤、耵聍堵塞等)。

基本检查

• 完整的病史和神经系统检查。

• 患者存在中枢性眩晕或局灶性神经系统症状时，需要进行神经影像学检查。

• 局灶性神经系统症状包括新的单侧听力丧失，通常伴有耳鸣。

诊断检查与说明

实验室检查

当有指征时：

• 全血细胞计数。

• 红细胞沉降率(血沉)。

• 甲状腺功能。

• 快速血脂全套。

• 快速血糖，糖化血红蛋白(HbA_1c)。

• 梅毒螺旋体抗体吸收试验。

• 生化检查。

• 蛋白尿血尿检查。

影像学检查

• 鼓室 MRI 检查和内耳道视图(一般用于门诊患者)。

• 颞骨 CT 扫描。

• 标准侧乳突 X 线。

诊断步骤/外科

• 听力评估。

• 双温热量测试。

• 经鼓膜耳蜗电图。

• 眼球震颤电图。

• 前庭诱发肌源性电位。

鉴别诊断

耳科：

• 慢性化脓性中耳炎。

• 良性位置性眩晕。

• 听神经瘤。

• 前庭神经元炎。

• 前庭阵发症。

• 耳硬化症。

• 听囊发育不良。

• 淋巴周围瘘。

• 迷路炎。

全身：

• 椎基底动脉供血不足。

• 短暂性脑缺血发作或脑卒中(中风)。

• 基底动脉血栓。

• 颅内出血。

• 头部创伤。

• 中枢神经系统病变(肿瘤)。

• 癫痫。

• 多发性硬化症。

• 佩吉特病。

• 糖尿病。

• 脑震荡综合征。

• 假性脑瘤。

• 复杂性或前庭性偏头痛。

• 甲状腺疾病。

• 毒品/药品。

• 自身免疫性疾病(如系统性红斑狼疮)。

• 病毒性脑膜炎/脑炎。

• 来姆病。

• 神经性梅毒。

• 电解质紊乱。

• 恐慌发作。

• 科根综合征。

治疗

院前

• 眩晕+神经系统症状提示脑卒中(中风)。

• 快速转运到急诊。

• 防跌落。

• 保持舒适的姿势。

• 呕吐患者静脉给予等渗液。

• 监测心律失常。

初步稳定/治疗

• 静脉给予等渗液。

• 静脉给予苯二氮䓬。

• 静脉给予止吐药。

急诊治疗/程序

支持治疗。

药物

• 缓解症状药物：

- 美其敏：12.5～25 mg，口服，q8 h。
- 地西泮：5～10 mg，口服、吸入或静脉注射。
- 劳拉西泮：0.5～2.0 mg，口服、静脉或肌内注射。
- 茶苯海明：12.5～50 mg，口服。
- 昂丹司琼：4～8 mg，口服、静脉或肌内注射。
- 甲氧氯普胺(胃复安)：10 mg，静脉或肌内注射。
- 异丙嗪：10～25 mg，口服、吸入、静脉或肌内注射。
- 丙氯拉嗪：10 mg，静脉注射。
- 倍他司汀：8～16 mg，口服，q8 h。
- 氯沙利酮：50～100 mg，口服。

• 治疗药物：

- 氢氯噻嗪：25～50 mg，口服，每日 1 次。
- 氨苯蝶啶：100 mg，口服，每日 1 次。
- 乙酰唑胺：250 mg，口服，每日 1 次。
- 呋塞米(速尿)：20 mg，口服，每日 1 次。
- 泼尼松：1 mg/kg，口服，每日 1 次，7～14 日后减量。

一线药物

• 地西泮或劳拉西泮。

• 昂丹司琼治疗恶心、呕吐。

• 静脉补液。

二线药物

• 美其敏。

• 丙氯拉嗪。

随访

进一步处理

入院指征

对急性控制眩晕和其他相关症状(如长时间呕吐导致的脱水)的治疗产生抵抗的患者。

出院指征

• 口服液体可耐受。

• 步态平稳。

• 神经系统功能检查正常。

• 有跌倒的预防措施。

• 再发症状典型。

• 饮食限制：钠盐、咖啡因、巧克力，限制吸烟和饮酒。

• 患者应避免驾车、操作危险设备和高空作业，直到发作得到缓解和镇静药物已停药。

转诊问题

• 持续性/顽固性症状发作，药物治疗无效。

• 存在耳部疾病。

• ENT 可以提供：

- 地塞米松鼓室注射。
- 庆大霉素经鼓室灌注。
- 压力脉冲处理。
- 外科手术(外科迷路切除术、前庭神经切除术及球囊切开术)。

- 梅尼特装置。

■ 随访建议

• 就饮食控制和相关避免发作知识进行教育指导是有用的。

• 教患者应对眩晕和身体失衡可有益于前庭功能恢复。

• 因疾病发作的不可预测性，应了解工作的跌倒风险，避免进行危险工作。

• 门诊患者需进行听力和眼震电图描记检查时，可转诊给神经学专家、耳科专家和耳鼻咽喉科专家。

要点和误区

• 梅尼埃病一般表现为典型的四联征：眩晕、听力丧失、耳鸣和耳闷。

• 治疗主要是为缓解症状，不是治愈。

• 出院患者应去神经科专家、耳科专家和耳鼻咽喉科专家门诊就诊。

• 一般不需住院治疗，但对急性控制疾病症状或相关不良效应（如呕吐和脱水）的治疗产生抵抗的患者应考虑住院治疗。

• 症状顽固且药物治疗无效的患者可考虑手术治疗。

孟乔森综合征做作性障碍 Munchausen Syndrome(Factitious Disorder)

Sophie W. Galson　伍力学　段立伟 译

基础知识

■ 描述

• 该病是一种故意假作某种疾病的症状或体征从而获得同情和照顾的心理疾病，发生该行为的患者机体并非处于生理疾病状态，也非出于现实利益诉求。

• 在 DSM－5 中称为人为障碍。

• 易患人群尚不明确，但可能的危险因素包括：

- 男性。
- 未婚。
- 年龄在 40～50 岁。
- 性格异常者。
- 有受虐待或遗弃经历者。
- 童年患有慢性疾病者。
- 有医学领域工作史。

■ 病因

• 做作性障碍：

-《精神障碍诊断和统计手册》诊断标准（DSM－5）：

◦ 佯装的机体表现或心理表现。

◦ 患者表现为生病、功能受损或受伤。

◦ 无外部诱因。

◦ 该行为不能由另一种精神障碍更好地解释。

• 发病通常是在年轻的成人中，通常是在因精神障碍或疾病住院之后。

• 临床综合征：

- 自身诱导的感染。
- 模仿特定疾病症状，但无实质病变。
- 慢性损伤。
- 自服药物。

儿科注意事项

• 代理性孟乔森综合征：

- 患者的疾病由照顾者而非患者所造成。
- 照顾者的行为动机是其假设被照顾者处于疾病状态。
- 照顾者对其所照顾的对象（常为儿童）制造伤害或诱导疾病发生。
- 行为人一般是孩子的父母（尤其是母亲）。

• 以各种方式模仿伤害或疾病表现：

- 制造伤害。
- 诱发疾病。
- 编造症状。
- 夸大孩子的疾病症状从而引发过度的医疗干预。

• 为恶者常拒绝承认其欺诈行为。

• 当照顾者和患者分开后症状即停止。

老年人注意事项

患有代理性孟乔森综合征的老年人照顾者也可能对老年人造成伤害。

诊断

■ 症状和体征

病史

• 急诊就诊时行为怪异或失当。

• 频繁就诊。

• 游走就诊：从一个医院到另一个医院。

• 有谎言和幻想症状：

- 善于讲述各种情节复杂的故事。

• 修改病历的信息：

- 使用别名。
- 修改出生日期。

• 对诊断性检查和治疗措施的需求不断增加。

• 当其行为受到医护人员质疑时会对医护人员产生敌意。

• 对与主诉相关的疾病细节闪烁其词。

• 提供大量的既往病历资料。

• 有受虐待的痛苦经历。

• 较之于所述疾病应有的痛苦症状，患者表现得更轻松自然。

• 患者能阐述异常丰富的医学知识。

• 经常无家可归并游走于各个省市。

• 没有密切的人际关系。

• 自行服药。

• 因反复的腹痛主诉而有多次无阳性结果的剖腹探查手术史。

• 故意伪造伤病的方式，包括：

- 违规服药以诱发疾病表现。
- 向体内注射污染物（如粪便、细菌、痰液、腐蚀性物质等）。
- 自伤。
- 吞服血液佯装消化道出血。
- 割脉放血。
- 改动检测仪器使结果失真。

体格检查

• 发热：

- 测量体温时故意作假而显示发热。
- 因注射污染物而致热。

• 自伤。

• 慢性损伤。

• 多发瘢痕。

• 体表及外耳道、尿道等部位损伤。

■ 基本检查

• 需要细致认真的采集病史信息，包括：

- 查阅外院病历。
- 通过患者家属了解既往病史有无自相矛盾之处，以及过量用药史等。
- 联系家庭医师了解背景资料以辨别疾病相关信息。
- 检查患者的房间及随身物品以了解其佯装患病的途径和方法。

• 做出诊断时需要有患者佯装患病的确切依据。

■ 诊断检查与说明

实验室检查

• 行辨别性检测试验过程中需要对患者进行密切监测。

• 常见的实验室结果作假方式，如：

- 粪便潜血阳性。
- 血尿（故意往尿样中滴入血液）。
- 低血糖（自行注射胰岛素）。

• 自行用药导致的结果异常，如：

- 血细胞比容降低（自服华法林或自行放血）
- INR升高（自服华法林）。
- 甲状腺功能检测（自服甲状腺素）。
- 低血糖（自行使用胰岛素或服用降糖药）。

• 鉴别是否装病的证据：

- 以酚酞试剂检测粪便可检测出是否滥用泻药。
- 对高血糖者行C肽检测：
  - C肽水平降低者：提示使用外源性胰岛素。
  - C肽水平升高者：提示本身存在低血糖或服用磺脲类降糖药。

影像学检查

切勿依据患者携带的影像学资料做出诊断。

诊断步骤/外科

慎用外科治疗措施，除非有客观证据证明其必要性。

■ 鉴别诊断

• 真实疾病：

- 原发疾病与精神异常症状无关。

• 继发于某些有假作性行为异常的合并症：

- 继发于痴呆、精神分裂或智能低下等疾病的自毁行为。
- 继发于某些诊断和治疗手段。

• 装病：

- 有明显的牟利取向。

• 转换障碍：

- 自主运动和感觉功能缺陷而出现的不自在行为。

• 躯体化障碍：

- 过度就医，但没有欺骗性的伪造症状。

治疗

■ 初步稳定/治疗

该阶段的处理措施应仅限于维持生命或防治损伤躯体的自伤行为。

■ 急诊治疗/程序

• 明确客观存在的疾病并给予适当的处理。

• 回顾病历资料并查找对假作性行为有提示意义的信息。

• 将患者所使用过的所有别名、地址、生日等信息记录在案。

• 总结患者常用的行为方式（主要是其曾使用过的假作行为方式）。

• 确保这些信息能被所有与该患者有接触的医师所了解。

• 不推荐在急诊室开展诊治工作，除非已收集到确切的证据。

• 向儿童保护机构报告代理性孟乔森综合征患者的信息。

随访

■ 进一步处理

入院指征

• 因自伤导致的外伤或疾病。

• 代理性孟乔森综合征：

- 已疑诊孟乔森综合征但尚无足够证据使儿童保护机构取代其监护权者。

• 密切观察以收集佯病证据：

- 可能同时发现某些罕见的器质性疾病。

• 制定防范自伤和医源性不良事件的长期方案。

• 收入精神科有利于诊治，但很少被患者所接受。

出院指征

• 病情平稳。

• 无明显自伤倾向。

• 已安排好转诊流程，可实施后续临床及精神科随访者。

转诊问题

• 应转诊至精神科以缓解疾病所致的精神压力。

• 若精神科直接设在临床中心（如首诊的内科诊区）则更为理想。这是一种预后不良的慢性疾病。

■ 随访建议

与患者及一位已确认的监护人保持联系。

弥散性血管内凝血 Disseminated Intravascular Coagulation

Steven H. Bowman 谭美春 译

基础知识

■ 描述

• 正常凝血：血管、血小板和凝血因子之间的一系列局部反应。

• 弥散性血管内凝血（DIC）是由其他原发性疾病过程引起的凝血和纤溶系统激活。

• 凝血系统激活导致凝血酶和纤溶酶进入系统循环。

• 凝血酶在DIC中的作用：

- 组织因子/因子Ⅷ(a)激活外源性途径，导致凝血酶形成。
- 凝血酶进入循环，并将纤维蛋白原转化为纤维蛋白单体。
- 纤维蛋白单体在循环中聚合成纤维蛋白（血凝块）。
- 血凝块引起微血管和大血管血栓形成，导致外周缺血和终末器官损伤。
- 血小板聚集成血凝块，导致血小板减少。

• 纤溶酶在DIC中的作用：

- 纤溶酶系统循环将纤维蛋白原转变为纤维蛋白降解产物（FDP）。
- FDP与纤维蛋白单体的结合。
- FDP-单体复合物干扰正常聚合并影响止血。
- FDP也干扰血小板功能。

• 抗凝受损在DIC中的作用：

- 生理性抗凝缺乏是DIC发生的必要条件。
- 抗凝血酶Ⅲ、蛋白C系统和组织因子途径抑制物都受损。

• 急性DIC非代偿形式：

- 凝血因子的消耗比机体生成更迅速。
- 以出血为主要临床特点，易掩盖正在进行

M

的血栓形成。

- 慢性DIC代偿形式：
- 机体能够跟上凝血因子消耗的速度。
- 以血栓形成为主要临床特点。

病因

- 由许多疾病引发。
- 妊娠并发症：
- 胎儿滞留。
- 羊水栓塞。
- 胎盘早剥。
- 流产。
- 子痫。
- HELLP综合征。
- 脓毒症：
- 革兰阴性（内毒素介导的脑膜炎球菌血症）。
- 革兰阳性（黏多糖介导的）。
- 其他微生物（如病毒、寄生虫）。
- 外伤：
- 挤压伤。
- 严重烧伤。
- 严重的头部损伤。
- 脂肪栓塞。
- 恶性肿瘤：
- 实体瘤或转移性疾病。
- 血液系统恶性肿瘤（如白血病）。
- 血管内溶血：
- 输血反应。
- 大量输血。
- 器官破坏：
- 重症胰腺炎。
- 重度肝衰竭。
- 血管畸形：
- 卡-梅利特综合征。
- 大血管动脉瘤。
- 血小板减少症：
- 血栓形成性血小板减少性紫癜。
- 特发性血小板减少性紫癜。
- 其他：
- 蛇咬伤。
- 娱乐毒品。

诊断

体征和症状

- 过度出血：
- 瘀斑。
- 过敏性紫癜。
- 血疱。
- 伤口出血。
- 静脉、动脉干路出血。
- 鼻出血。
- 咯血。
- 胃肠出血。
- 过度血栓形成：
- 大血管。
- 微血管血栓形成及终末器官。
- 功能障碍。
- 心、肺、肝、肾、中枢神经系统。
- 血栓性静脉炎。
- 肺栓塞。
- 无菌性血栓性心内膜炎。
- 坏疽。
- 肾、肝、中枢神经系统、肠的缺血性梗死。
- 急性DIC：
- 出血性并发症占主导地位。
- 慢性DIC：
- 血栓形成并发症占主导地位。

病史

- 既往有出血性疾病史。
- 妊娠、末次月经。
- 恶性肿瘤史或免疫功能低下。

体格检查

- 神经系统：
- 精神状态（MS）改变，意识错乱，嗜睡。
- 心血管：
- 低血压，心动过速。
- 呼吸系统：
- 呼吸急促，干啰音，湿啰音。
- 胃肠道：
- 上消化道或下消化道出血，腹胀。
- 泌尿生殖系统：
- 少尿，血尿。
- 皮肤：
- 瘀斑，紫癜，黄疸，坏疽。

基本检查

- 取决于诱发疾病。
- 一般不在急诊室做出诊断。

诊断检查与说明

实验室检查

- 血小板计数：
- 应重视快速下降。
- $<100\,000/mm^3$。
- 慢性DIC可能正常。
- PT、APTT：
- 增加。
- 慢性DIC可能正常。
- 纤维蛋白原：
- 减少。
- <150 mg/dl者占70%。
- 灵敏度低，可保持在正常水平。
- 慢性DIC可能正常。
- FDP：
- 增加。
- >40 μg/ml。
- D-二聚体升高。
- 全血细胞计数、外周血涂片：
- 红细胞碎片。
- 血小板偏低。
- 外周血涂片证实慢性DIC疾病。
- 电解质、尿素氮、肌酐、葡萄糖：
- 由于肾功能不全引起的尿素氮、肌酐升高。
- 动脉血气：
- 氧、酸碱状态。
- ISTH评分系统：
- 并发DIC的潜在疾病：
  - 否=0，是=2分。
- 血小板计数：
  - >100=0，<100=1分，<50=2分。
- 纤维蛋白标志物（D-二聚体，FDP）：
  - 正常=0，中度增加=1分，显著增加=2分。
- PT延长：
  - <3=0，>3～6=1分，>6=2分。
- 纤维蛋白原：
  - 1 g/L=0，<1 g/L=1分。
- >5分为显性DIC，与死亡率增加有关。

影像学检查

- 怀疑肺炎者查胸部X线平片。
- 精神状态改变者查头颅CT。
- 妊娠患者查产科超声。

鉴别诊断

- 遗传性凝血功能障碍：
- 因子缺乏。
- 其他获得性凝血功能障碍：
- 抗凝治疗。
- 药物。
- 肝脏疾病。
- 维生素K缺乏。
- 大量失血。
- 血小板功能障碍：
- 血栓性血小板减少性紫癜（TTP）、溶血性尿毒症综合征（HUS）。
- 肝素诱导血小板减少症（HIT）。
- 特发性血小板减少性紫癜。

M

治疗

初步稳定/治疗

- 气道管理和复苏措施：
  - 控制出血。
  - 建立静脉通路。
  - 恢复和维持循环血容量。
- 开始治疗诱发疾病：
  - 抗生素治疗脓毒症。
  - 清除子宫内的胚胎遗留物。
  - 恶性肿瘤者进行化疗。
  - 清理创伤失活组织。

急诊治疗/程序

- DIC 治疗有争议，应基于以下因素个体化治疗：
  - 年龄。
  - 血流动力学状态。
  - 出血的严重性。
  - 血栓形成的严重性。
- 在开始具体的 DIC 治疗前进行入院检查。
- 补充耗尽的血液成分：
  - 新鲜冰冻血浆(FFP)：
    - PT 延长者。
    - 提供凝血因子和容量补充。
    - 剂量：10～15 ml/kg。
  - 血小板：
    - 如果血小板计数<20 000/mm^3，或血小板计数<50 000/mm^3 的持续出血。
    - 剂量：1 U/10 kg。
  - 冷沉淀：
    - 比全血浆的纤维蛋白原含量高。
    - 对于严重的低纤维蛋白原血症(<50 mg/dl)，或纤维蛋白原<100 mg/dl 的活动性出血。
    - 剂量：8 U。
  - 重组因子Ⅶa：
    - 有成功使用的报道，受益和安全性未知。
  - 洗涤浓缩细胞。
  - 白蛋白。
  - 非凝血扩容剂。
- 用肝素抑制血管内凝血：
  - 使用有争议。
  - 当血栓形成占主导时考虑。
  - 轻度至中度 DIC 可能有效。
  - 在严重 DIC 疗效不确定。可能的适应证：
    - 暴发性紫癜(手指、足趾、四肢坏疽)。
    - 急性早幼粒细胞白血病。
    - 死亡胎儿综合征——胎儿宫内死亡后数周。
    - 大血管的血栓栓塞并发症。
    - 转移癌手术前。
  - 注射活化蛋白 C(有争议)：
    - 无生存率改善。
  - 抗凝血酶：
    - 同时接受肝素的患者未发现生存率改善。
    - 目前缺乏证据支持此时使用。
- 抑制纤溶：
  - 阻断 DIC 合并继发性代偿纤溶。
  - 并发严重血栓形成时使用。
  - 只在 DIC 合并原发性纤溶时使用：
    - 早幼粒细胞白血病。
    - 巨大血管瘤。
    - 中暑。
    - 羊水栓塞。
    - 前列腺转移癌。
  - 仅在极端情况下开始：
    - 大出血对替代治疗无反应。
    - 纤溶亢进出现(快速全血裂解、短优球蛋白溶解时间)。
    - 6-氨基己酸(EACA)。
    - 氨甲环酸。

药物治疗

具体的 DIC 治疗通常不在急诊室开始，应首先治疗潜在的诱发疾病。

- 肝素：
  - 低剂量：5～10 U/(kg·h)静脉注射，应用于血栓形成占主导的病因。

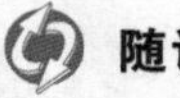

随访

进一步处理

入院指征

合并 DIC 的严重疾病需要入住 ICU。

出院指征

无。

随访建议

随访包括跟踪血小板和凝血因子。

要点和误区

- 把 DIC 当作严重危及生命疾病的一个并发因素。
- 因为 DIC 的后遗症可能是毁灭性的，应建立早期临床怀疑。
- 当病程中的血栓栓塞和出血并发症是主要临床表现时，记得要考虑治疗 DIC 的潜在诱因。

蜜蜂蜇伤 Sting, Bee

Daniel T. Wu 江伟伟 李文放 译

基础知识

描述

- 由膜翅目昆虫毒液引起：
  - 生物胺的释放。
  - 局部或全身过敏反应。
- 反应：
  - 通常 IgE 介导的Ⅰ型超敏反应。
  - 很少发生Ⅲ型过敏反应。

病因

- 膜翅目：节肢动物门。
- 包括蜜蜂(Apidae 家族)、胡蜂和黄蜂(Vespidae 家族)、火蚁(蚁科)。

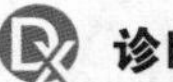

诊断

体征和症状

病史

病史和体格检查是诊断的关键。

体格检查

5 种反应：

- 局部反应：
  - 最常见的反应类型。
  - 刺痛部位局部疼痛、红斑和水肿。
  - 症状立即发生，并在 1～2 h 缓解。
- 大范围局部反应：
  - 与局部反应类似，但影响较大区域或整个肢体。
  - 高峰在 48 h，可持续数日。

M

- 轻度至中度发热。
• 系统反应：
- 全身过敏性反应。
- 可能是致命的(通常是由于呼吸衰竭)。
- 呼吸系统：
◦ 喘息。
◦ 咳嗽。
◦ 喘鸣。
◦ 呼吸急促。
◦ 嘶哑。
◦ 血管性水肿。
- 消化系统：
◦ 恶心。
◦ 呕吐。
◦ 腹泻。
◦ 腹痛。
- 心血管系统：
◦ 低血压。
◦ 胸部疼痛。
◦ 心动过速。
◦ 休克。
- 其他：
◦ 荨麻疹。
◦ 瘙痒。
◦ 脸红。
- 症状在 15～20 min 发生，并持续＜72 h。
• 毒性反应：
- 多次蜇伤和大剂量毒液的结果。
- 症状与过敏反应类似。
• 罕见反应：
- 由于不寻常的免疫反应。
- 血管炎。
- 肾病。
- 血清病。
- 神经炎。
- 脑炎。
- 反应延迟(刺伤后数日至数周)。

基本检查

• 病史和体格检查是诊断的关键。
• 影像学或实验室检查不能证实膜翅目昆虫毒液引起或全身过敏反应。

诊断检查与说明

实验室检查

• 血常规、电解质、尿素氮、肌酐、葡萄糖、动脉血气(ABG)：
- 非常规。
- 当有全身严重反应时需完善。

诊断步骤/外科

心电图：
• 当患有心血管疾病风险的患者出现全身严重反应时。

鉴别诊断

• 昆虫叮咬有时会引起疼痛，蜇伤总是会引起疼痛。
• 蜂窝织炎：
- 很难区分大局部反应和蜂窝织炎。
- 膜翅目昆虫蜇伤罕见，通常是由黄蜂蜇伤造成的。
- 局部反应可能与周围蜂窝织炎相似。
• 痛风。
• 软组织创伤。
• 全身毒性反应：
- 肺栓塞。
- 不同药物的过敏反应。
- 过度通气综合征或焦虑症。
- 急性冠状动脉综合征。

治疗

院前

由于呼吸阻塞或过敏反应导致心血管和呼吸系统衰竭，大多数死亡发生在 1 h 内。

早期治疗

急性全身反应/过敏性休克

• 基础生命体征：
- 有喉头水肿迹象时行气管插管。
- 吸氧。
- 建立静脉通路，给予生理盐水。
• 肾上腺素：皮下或静脉推注。
• 抗组胺药：静脉推注。
• 激素。
• 当有全身性系统反应：
- 评估气道。
- 建立静脉通路。

急诊治疗/程序

• 全身性系统反应：
- 肾上腺素用于呼吸系统症状/低血压。
- 抗组胺药：H_1 受体阻滞剂(苯海拉明)和 H_2 受体阻滞剂(西咪替丁、雷尼替丁或法莫替丁)。
- 激素(泼尼松、甲泼尼龙或地塞米松)。
- 吸入 β 受体激动剂用于喘息、呼吸急促。
- 对于持续性低血压：
◦ 生理盐水静滴复苏。
◦ 血管活性药物(肾上腺素)静滴用于顽固性低血压。
• 通过刮擦，而不是挤压，去除毒液部位(蜜蜂可能会留下带有毒囊)残留的毒刺。
• 局部反应：
- 冷敷。
- 抬高患肢。
- 去除紧身的衣服或珠宝。
- 根据需要局部使用抗组胺药/外用激素。
- 根据需要口服抗组胺药或激素。

药物治疗

• 沙丁胺醇，β 受体激动剂(吸入)：2.5～5 mg 加入 5 mg 生理盐水中，雾化给药(儿童：0.1 mg/kg，5 mg/ml 浓度)。
• 苯海拉明：25～50 mg(儿童：1 mg/kg)，静脉注射或口服，治疗荨麻疹或瘙痒。
• 肾上腺素：
- 0.3 mg：0.3 ml 1：1 000 稀释液(儿童：0.01 mg/kg，最大剂量 0.5 mg)，皮下或肌内注射用于严重反应。
• 法莫替丁：40 mg，静脉滴注[儿童：1 mg/(kg·d)，分 2 次静脉滴注]。
• 甲泼尼龙：125 mg(儿童：1～2 mg/kg)，静脉滴注。
• 泼尼松：60 mg(儿童：1～2 mg/kg)，口服。
• 雷尼替丁：50 mg，静脉滴注或肌内注射[儿童：2～4 mg/(kg·d)，q6～8 h，静脉滴注或肌内注射]。

随访

进一步处理

入院指征

• 症状恶化，累及气道。
• 持续不稳定的生命体征需要 ICU 入院。
• 危及生命的反应需要 24 h 观察。
• 全身反应需要至少 6 h 的观察。

出院指征

• 很小孤立的局部反应。
• 在 6 h 的观察期内，系统性反应缓解，并且不会再发生。

转诊问题

随访：
• 如果患者出现危及生命的反应，启动过敏反应抢救盒(肾上腺素)和相关治疗流程(医疗警报)。
• 全身性反应需要随访以进行可能的免疫治疗。

■ 随访建议

过敏症患者进行全身反应的随访。

要点和误区

• 对叮咬后存在全身反应的患者进行治疗。

• 出院患者提供肾上腺素处方，防止出现威胁生命的反应。

免疫 Immunizations

Garth D. Meckler 倪沁赟 译

 基础知识

■ 描述

• 免疫增强或启动，用于抵抗感染性疾病。

• 免疫保护通过以下几种机制实现：

- 被动免疫：纯化抗体使用或被动母婴转移。

- 主动免疫：刺激免疫系统，7～10 日产生 IgM 抗体，继而产生 IgG 抗体，在 2～6 周达峰值。

• 口腔和鼻疫苗使黏膜分泌 IgA 抗体，肠外疫苗则不会。不正当使用（路径、剂量、不良存储等）会导致免疫功能下降。

■ 病因

• 几种可用疫苗的类型：

- 减毒活疫苗[如水痘-带状疱疹（VZV）、麻疹、流行性腮腺炎、风疹（MMR）、轮状病毒]在宿主复制，同时诱导免疫应答：

◦ 免疫功能低下的患者可能会导致严重感染。

- 灭活疫苗[如脊髓灰质炎（IPV）、甲型肝炎（HepA）、流感、百日咳]对于免疫系统受损的患者是安全的。

- 类毒素、亚单位疫苗、结合疫苗[如白喉、破伤风、B 型流感嗜血杆菌、人乳头瘤病毒（HPV）、肺炎球菌、脑膜炎双球菌]使用毒素的抗原部分、蛋白质、来源于病毒/细菌的碳水化合物，诱导免疫反应。

- 乙型肝炎（HepB）疫苗使用重组 DNA 技术。

• 几种联合疫苗亦可以使用，但是费用增加：

- Pediarix（白喉、破伤风毒素、百日咳、乙型肝炎和脊髓灰质炎灭活疫苗组合）。

- Comvax（B 型流感嗜血杆菌和乙型肝炎联合疫苗）。

- Pentacel（百日咳、脊髓灰质炎灭活疫苗、B 型流感嗜血杆菌联合疫苗）。

- Twinrix（甲型肝炎和乙型肝炎）。

- MMRV（风疹和水痘）。

■ 流行病学

• 因广泛免疫制剂的使用，严重危及生命的疾病的发生率已经显著下降：

- 在西半球，由野生型病毒导致的小儿麻痹症已经消除。

- 在北美的儿童中，B 型流感嗜血杆菌、白喉和破伤风疫苗已经几乎消除了这些传染性/蔓延性疾病。

- 麻疹、风疹和水痘的发生率同样在下降，在未经免疫的社区和去美国的旅行者中散在发生。

- 7 价结合肺炎球菌疫苗（2000 年推出）及其 13 价替代品（2010 年）减少了疫苗血清型（脑膜炎、肺炎、菌血症）＞90% 的侵袭性疾病。

- 自从对婴儿进行常规疫苗接种以来，美国的轮状病毒感染率下降了 58%～90%。

- 全球流感活动的监控需要考虑到对抗季节性流感疫苗的年生产量。灭活疫苗可通过肌内注射，减毒活疫苗可通过鼻道给药。

• 免疫推荐和计划应基于流行病学、疾病和暴露的个体风险和疫苗的安全性及有效性：

- 婴儿和年轻儿童接种疫苗以防儿童时期的常见疾病，但一些疫苗没有免疫原性（如肺炎球菌荚膜多糖抗原疫苗），可能对于婴儿来说有一定的风险（如风疹和水痘-带状疱疹）。

- 其他风险组患者包括国际旅行者、老年患者、卫生保健工作者和免疫功能低下的个体，对于这些患者有具体的推荐意见。

- 呼吸道合胞病毒可用于高危患者。

诊断

■ 症状和体征

• 疫苗相关不良事件：与接种疫苗（牛痘）相关的最常见不良事件比较轻微，有局部反应（疼痛、肿胀、红斑）和/或发热（通常在 7～10 日）。

- 大部分接种疫苗会发生局部反应，在破伤风、白喉和百日咳（特别是重复剂量接种后）、B 型流感嗜血杆菌（婴儿可出现无菌性脓肿）、VZV、HPV 和肺炎球菌疫苗特别常见。

- 免疫接种轮状病毒（40%～43%）、肺炎双球菌（24%～35%）、HPV（10%～13%）、MMR 或 MMRV（后者更常见）、脑膜炎球菌疫苗后可能会出现发热。流感疫苗使用后可能会出现发热 6～24 h。

- 皮疹是 VZV 和 MMRV 疫苗接种后的罕见副作用，MMRV 可能在接种后出现一过性皮疹或发热 6～12 日。

- 神经系统症状少见，但 DTP 疫苗接种后较常见（哭闹、伤心的哭泣、嗜睡、短暂癫痫发作不伴发热、低渗低反应症状、脑病、吉兰-巴雷综合征）。乙肝疫苗和脑膜炎双球菌疫苗接种后可能会出现头痛症状；儿童接种 MMR 和 MMRV 疫苗后可能会出现热惊厥，脑病报道较少。吉兰-巴雷综合征见于成人接种流感疫苗后。

- 婴儿接种轮状病毒疫苗后，罕见呕吐和腹泻不良反应。

- 成年女性使用 MMR 疫苗后会出现关节痛表现，血液系统不良反应如血小板减少症少见。

- 成年人使用流感减毒活疫苗会出现轻度呼吸系统症状，基础有哮喘的儿童会出现哮喘加重。

■ 基本检查

• 任何原因就诊的急诊患者应提供回顾免疫状态的机会，并提供合适的随访。记录免疫状态的病史：

- 既往免疫功能没有得到处理的原因可以归结为病史采集的不完善。

• 接种疫苗的明确禁忌证：

- 对既往使用的疫苗剂量有过敏反应或：

M

◦ 对面包酵母过敏是接种乙肝疫苗的禁忌证。
◦ 对鸡肉或鸡蛋白过敏是接种流感疫苗的禁忌证，但是灭活疫苗应该在医疗环境中使用。
◦ 对新霉素或明胶过敏是接种 MMR 疫苗的禁忌证。
◦ 对新霉素、链霉素或多黏菌素过敏是接种 IPV 疫苗的禁忌证，在一些流感疫苗中也发现了这些物质的微量。
◦ 乳胶过敏是轮状病毒和脑膜炎 B 疫苗的相对禁忌证。

- 48 h 内接种疫苗的具体反应：
◦ 严重无法忍受的痛苦的尖叫持续 3 h。
◦ 大声哭泣。
◦ 低渗低反应症状。
◦ 体温＞40.5 ℃，没有其他原因。
◦ 注射肢体周围的严重的局部反应包括，除非不经意皮下注射了疫苗。
- 接种疫苗 7 日内出现脑病：
◦ 严重急性神经系统疾病表现为癫痫持续发作和/或无意识和/或局部体征。
- 进行性神经系统疾病包括癫痫。

• 推迟使用疫苗的原因：
- 不论是否发热，发生中度至重度急性疾病。
- 先天性或获得性免疫缺陷（如 HIV、恶性肿瘤或化疗相关）：减毒活疫苗（如 VZV、MMR 和流感）带来的可能风险。与免疫功能低下的患者有密切接触的健康个体，当使用这些疫苗时需要引起重视。
- 妊娠对于使用减毒活疫苗（包括 VZV 和 HPV）是禁忌证。灭活病毒（流感病毒）和结合疫苗（DTaP）被认为是安全的。
- 近期有抽搐发作病史是百日咳注射的相对禁忌证。
- 近期使用免疫球蛋白可能降低疫苗的有效性。

• 疫苗可能会在下述伴随情况下使用：
- 急性轻症伴或不伴发热。
- 轻度至中度局部反应（如肿胀、发红、酸痛），低度或中度发热。
- 目前在接受抗生素治疗。
- 疾病恢复期。
- 早产（乙肝疫苗除外）。
- 近期有过感染性疾病。
- 青霉素过敏史、其他感染源过敏、与过敏相关、接受变应原提取物免疫治疗。
- 儿童 HIV 感染患者，无临床表现或没有严重的免疫功能低下，应接种疫苗。

治疗

院前

重点关注气道、呼吸和循环。

初步稳定/治疗

对疫苗过敏的处理药物治疗包括肌内注射或静脉注射肾上腺素、喘息时使用沙丁胺醇和静脉补液纠正低血压。

急诊治疗/程序

• 使用肾上腺素、抗组胺药、沙丁胺醇和静脉补液治疗过敏反应。
• 根据主动或被动免疫的具体指南，治疗感染性病变的潜在暴露因素或污染伤口。
• 根据不同的症状治疗各种不良反应：
- 注射部位的局部反应可给予冷敷、镇痛药物或止痒。使用加压包扎控制出血。
- 使用对乙酰氨基酚或布洛芬治疗发热、头痛、肌痛和关节痛。
- 使用苯二氮䓬类治疗癫痫持续状态。
• 注射疫苗时和 4～8 h 后考虑预防性使用对乙酰氨基酚：
- 接种水痘疫苗的儿童，在接种疫苗 6 周内避免使用水杨酸类药物，因水痘感染可能与水杨酸类药物引起的 Reye 综合征有关。
• 需要与父母具体讨论接种破伤风疫苗的风险及好处，特别是经常发生创伤并需要提供被动和主动免疫治疗时：
- 风险及好处已在图表中进行了彻底的讨论。在某些情况下会使用正式的知情同意书。
-《国家儿童疫苗伤害法案》要求在使用任何剂量的疫苗之前提供一个关于疫苗信息的副本。

药物治疗

• 对乙酰氨基酚：15 mg/kg，q4～6 h，口服，24 h 不超过 4 g。
• 布洛芬：10 mg/kg，q6～8 h，口服。

随访

进一步处理

入院指征

• 免疫接种后出现严重不良反应的患者应收治入院。
• 有过敏反应、脑病及格林-巴利综合征的患者需进儿科 ICU 治疗。
• 不可预测的不良反应应上报疫苗不良事件报告系统。

出院指征

接受常规免疫接种后的患者可出院回家，除非突发不良事件。至关重要的是，安排初级保健医师完成后续的免疫接种。

要点和误区

• 对某些疫苗（如 DTaP）的局部反应可在注射部位产生显著的肿胀、温暖和触痛。这些局部反应不应被误认为是感染或过敏反应。
• 对鸡蛋过敏不再是流感免疫的禁忌证，但建议在监测环境下服用。
• 轻度发热和服用抗生素不是推迟接种疫苗的理由。

免疫抑制 Immunosuppression

Lara K. Kulchycki 倪沁赟 译

基础知识

描述

对抗感染的能力先天性或获得性缺陷：
• 抗体生成（B 细胞）。
• 细胞免疫（T 细胞）。
• 吞噬功能缺乏。
• 补体缺乏。
• 皮肤/黏膜屏障破坏。

病因

• 先天性异常。

M

• 免疫抑制药物。
• 高龄：
- 免疫衰老。
- 循环差和伤口愈合。
• 慢性(肺脏、肾脏或心脏)疾病。
• HIV 感染：
- CD4 计数受该病原体影响。
• 糖尿病：
- 高血糖影响免疫应答。
- 血管条件下降。
• 营养不良：
- 贫穷。
- 酗酒和药物滥用。
- 进食障碍。
• 无脾：
- 功能性无脾(镰状细胞疾病)或外科脾切除后会增加芽孢(如肺炎链球菌和流感嗜血杆菌)感染的风险。
• 器官移植：
- 抗排异药物抑制免疫反应。
- 感染可能是供体来源、受体来源或医源性。
- 病毒感染的风险增加，如巨细胞病毒、EB 病毒和人肝炎病毒。
- 移植后的时间间隔很关键，在移植的早期、中期或晚期，感染的形式不同。
• 恶性肿瘤。
• 化疗：
- 细菌和真菌的感染风险增加。
- 感染风险与粒细胞缺乏的时间和严重程度相关。
• 粒细胞缺乏：
- 定义为绝对中性粒细胞计数<500/mm^3 或<1 000/mm^3 伴预期最低值<500/mm^3。
- 在美国，感染的主要病原体是革兰阴性菌。
- 革兰阴性菌相对来说不常见，但是通常是致命性的。
- 多种病原体混合感染的概率增加。
- 厌氧菌感染相对少见。
- 粒细胞缺乏时间长(>1 周)、早期使用广谱抗生素和强烈的化疗会导致真菌感染的风险增加。

诊断

症状和体征

病史

• 在免疫抑制宿主，威胁生命的感染临床可能仅仅表现为发热。
• 认真做好系统的检查以明确任何局部的症状。
• 明确院内感染的危险因素，如近期住院或家庭护士常驻。
• 询问有无传染性疾病的亲密接触史，如流感。
• 回顾近期免疫抑制药物的使用史，如类固醇激素。
• 关注预防性药物的使用，如甲氧苄胺-磺胺甲噁唑或氟康唑，可能改变可疑病原体的抗菌谱和耐药性。

体格检查

• 从头至足趾给患者进行体格检查。
• 一些临床医师建议，避免对有发热的粒细胞缺乏患者行直肠指检。
• 炎症可能较轻微或无炎症：
- 腹部手术而不伴有腹膜体征。
- 脑膜炎不伴有颈强直。
- 感染伤口或留置内置物不伴有硬结、红斑或化脓。

基本检查

• 所选择的研究必须适用于患者和目前的主要不适。
• 实验室结果解释可能比较困难，因为对于免疫抑制的患者炎症反应较迟钝：
- 肺炎不伴有 X 线片上浸润影。
- 尿路感染不伴有脓尿。
- 脑膜炎不伴有中枢神经系统脑脊液细胞异常增多。

诊断检查与说明

实验室检查

• 不同的全血细胞计数：
- 明确的白细胞增多，核左移，杆状核粒细胞增多，或中性粒细胞减少。
- 一旦粒细胞绝对计数(ANC)<1000/mm^3，感染风险增加。
• 血培养：
- 2 套细菌血培养。
- 如果存在留置物，则从该处留取。
- 如果有征象，留取真菌血培养。
• 尿液分析或尿培养：
- 需要通过无菌方法获取，因为插管可能导致感染。
• 血乳酸：
- 在脓毒症患者明确有无隐匿性低灌注时有意义。
• 动脉血气分析：
- 对怀疑肺孢子菌感染的患者，明确有需使用类固醇激素时可进行动脉血气分析。
• 生育年龄的女性需要行妊娠试验。

影像学检查

• 如果患者中性粒细胞减少、低氧或存在异常肺部体征，可行胸片检查。
• 进一步的影像学检查如 CT 或 MRI，可根据患者的目前情况和相关危险因素决定是否进行。

诊断步骤/外科

• 如果临床怀疑脑膜炎，则需要行腰椎穿刺检查：
- 如果怀疑血小板减少症或凝血功能障碍，行腰椎穿刺前需要明确血小板计数和凝血功能。
- 即使不存在脑脊液细胞增多，亦需要考虑行隐球菌抗原检测。

鉴别诊断

• 感染：
- 口咽。
- 鼻窦。
- 肺部。
- 胃肠道。
- 会阴、肛门。
- 泌尿道。
- 皮肤、软组织。
- 骨。
- 内置物或导管。
• 非感染源性发热：
- 药物发热。
- 移植排斥反应。
- 恶性肿瘤。
- 血管炎。
- 风湿性疾病。
- 肺栓塞。
- 甲状腺功能异常。
- 血制品输注。

治疗

院前

• 建立静脉通道。
• 静脉液体输注。

初步稳定/治疗

• 对低血容量的患者行液体复苏。
• 脓毒症患者行目标导向治疗。
• 除了检查恶性心脏压塞外，亦可使用超声检查评估患者的容量状态。
• 若对液体复苏无反应，针对低血压可使用血管活性药物：
- 多巴胺 5～20 μg/(kg · min)。

- 去甲肾上腺素 2～12 μg/min。

▪ 急诊治疗/程序

• 制定合适的感染控制预防措施，如中性粒细胞减少症或接触预防措施。
• 快速收集合适的病原学培养，同时给予广谱抗生素治疗。
• 大部分发热性中性粒细胞减少的患者需要住院治疗，但是一些发热的低风险患者可能仅作为门诊患者进行治疗。
• 低风险：
- 年龄＜60 岁。
- 发热的时候，在门诊就诊。
- ANC(中性粒细胞绝对值)＞100/mm³。
- 预计中性粒细胞减少的缓解时间＜7 日。
- 一般情况良好。
- 生命体征平稳。
- 没有精神状态的改变。
- 没有脱水。
- 没有基础疾病或缺乏并发疾病的证据：
◦ 慢性肺脏疾病。
◦ 糖尿病。
◦ 器官衰竭。
- 疾病在缓解期。
- 没有真菌感染的病史。
- 胸片正常。

▪ 药物治疗

• 在可能的情况下，应为患者制定合适的治疗方案。
• 对于发热性中性粒细胞减少或脓毒症的患者，立即使用广谱抗生素开始经验性治疗。
• 口服抗生素治疗：
- 适用于低风险的发热性中性粒细胞减少患者。
- 环丙沙星 750 mg，口服，每日 2 次＋阿莫西林-克拉维酸 875 mg，口服，每日 2 次。
• 肠外单药治疗选择：
- 头孢他啶：2 g，静脉注射，q8 h(儿童：50 mg/kg，静脉注射，q8 h)。
- 头孢吡肟：2 g，静脉注射，q8 h(儿童：50 mg/kg，静脉注射，q8 h)。
- 亚胺培南-西司他丁：500 mg，静脉注射，q6 h(儿童：根据年龄和体重调整剂量)。
- 美罗培南：1 g，静脉注射，q8 h(儿童：根据年龄和体重调整剂量)。
- 哌拉西林-他唑巴坦：(在中性粒细胞减少的患者研究较少)4.5 g，静脉注射，q6 h(儿童：根据年龄调整剂量)。
• 对于高风险患者，考虑增加氨基糖苷类药物进行协同治疗：
- 庆大霉素：根据肌酐清除率调整剂量(儿童：根据年龄调整剂量)。
- 使用氨基糖苷类抗生素可能会增加不良事件发生的风险，如急性肾损伤和耳毒性。
• 通常没有指征给予经验性万古霉素治疗：
- 如果怀疑脓毒症或有耐甲氧西林的金黄色葡萄球菌感染的病史，则可加用万古霉素治疗。
- 万古霉素：1 g，静脉注射，q12 h(儿童：根据年龄和体重调整剂量)。
• 如果考虑口腔、腹腔或肛周感染，需要覆盖抗厌氧菌治疗：
- 克林霉素：600～900 mg，静脉注射，q8 h(儿童：根据年龄调整剂量)。

随访

▪ 进一步处理

入院指征

• ANC(中性粒细胞绝对值)＜100/mm³。
• 免疫功能低下的感染患者，且没有达到低风险的标准。
• 在门诊治疗还不够的患者。
• 入院标准较低的患者：
- 老年患者。
- 糖尿病患者。
- 儿科患者。

出院指征

• 低风险患者表现良好，可接受口服抗生素和液体治疗。这种情况下可作为门诊患者进行后续的管理。
• 有多种有效的风险分层工具可帮助识别低风险患者：
- 美国临床肿瘤学会(ASCO)和美国传染病学会(IDSA)在 2018 年指南更新中回顾了这些工具。
• 出院之前，血液科、肿瘤科、传染病科或移植科医师对患者的病情进行讨论。

▪ 随访建议

为了重新评估患者和监测培养结果，必须进行 24 h 的随访。

要点和误区

• 不了解该区域的感染和抗生素耐药的具体情况。
• 没有意识到对于免疫功能低下的宿主，一个模糊不清的临床症状或发热可能是严重感染的唯一警告征象。
• 对于发热性中性粒细胞低下或脓毒症患者没有第一时间使用广谱抗生素治疗。
• 没有回顾患者既往的微生物学结果。
• 无法提供合适的处理保健，当患者的家人中有专业医师时可以提供治疗方案并确保随访。

面部骨折 Facial Fractures

David W. Munter 单怡 译

基础知识

▪ 描述

• 一般由机动车事故、直接暴力袭击或高处坠落造成的钝性创伤。
• 枪击伤也是常见原因。
• 要想到是否有身体攻击和家庭暴力，尤其是妇女和儿童。
• 通常有开放性的骨折。
• 许多面部骨折比较复杂，不易归类。

▪ 病因

• 最常见的是鼻骨、眶底颧骨、上颌窦。
• Le Fort 骨折累及上颌骨，分类如下。
- Le Fort Ⅰ型：上颌骨鼻部以下牙齿以上经上颌窦侧壁到翼突内侧板侧面的横断骨折。
- Le Fort Ⅱ型：从鼻骨到筛骨经颧上颌缝和上颌骨的锥形骨折，通常累及上颌窦和眶下缘。
- Le Fort Ⅲ型：经颧额缝、眼眶、鼻底和筛

M

骨的骨折引起颅面关节分离,使面部变得长而扁平。

- Le Fort Ⅳ型:在 Le Fort Ⅲ型骨折之外还累及额骨的骨折。

- 同一位患者可在面部的两侧分别存在不同程度的 Le Fort 骨折。

• 颧弓通常有 2 处或 3 处骨折,可累及眼眶和上颌骨(三角区骨折)。

• 额窦内板骨折可导致脑脊液漏和视觉损害。

• 眼眶骨折最常累及眶底(爆裂性骨折)并常引起视觉损害,可累及中部和侧面的眶壁。

老年人注意事项

• 高处坠落是常见受伤原因。

• 颧骨是最常累及的骨折部位。

• 注意并发颈部和颅内损伤。

儿科注意事项

• 6 岁以下儿童罕见因非事故原因导致的上颌面骨折。

• 高处坠落和机动车事故是最常见的受伤原因。

• 超过 50%合并有其他严重损伤,发生率最高的是头部损伤。

• 眼眶骨折(除鼻部外)是儿童骨折最常见部位。

诊断

症状和体征

• 大多数创伤后,面部畸形提示有潜藏的骨折。

• 疼痛、水肿、瘀斑和畸形。

• 脑脊液鼻漏、面部出血、鼻出血和熊猫眼。

• 神经压迫或损伤引起的面瘫。

• 合并损伤:牙齿、下颌、眼、泪腺、颅骨和颈部。

• 覆盖于鼻中隔的蓝色液囊提示鼻中隔血肿,需要及时发现。

病史

• 损伤机制。

• 合并损伤。

体格检查

• 立即评估气道。

• 要点:

- 触诊整个面部的硬度、错位情况、凹陷和捻发感。

- 熊猫眼-眼眶周瘀斑,有时需要数小时才能发展,涉及颅底骨折或眼眶骨折。

- 耳后有瘀斑,与乳突或基底骨骨折有关。

- 检查是否存在颚部损伤或咬合不正。

- 鼻窥镜检查是否有鼻中隔血肿或脑脊液漏。

- 评估面瘫的区域。

- 仔细的眼部检查包括眼底镜检查了解视觉敏感度;评估是否有内眦距增宽(眼距宽度在 30~35 mm 及以上),向上的不良共轭凝视(提示眶底爆裂性骨折引起的眼部肌肉受压)。

• 将一只手的拇指和示指放在鼻梁上,用另一只手拉拔上排牙齿来评估是否有 Le Fort 骨折。

- Le Fort Ⅰ型:仅有硬颚和上颌牙列的活动(将手放在鼻部感觉不到活动)。

- Le Fort Ⅱ型:有硬颚、上颌牙列和鼻部的活动(将手放在鼻部能感觉到活动)。

- Le Fort Ⅲ型:整个面中部的活动。

儿科注意事项

可能需要使用镇静剂来协助完成彻底检查。

基本检查

• 气道保护后,面部骨折后检查其他伤情。

• 所有怀疑面部骨折的患者均需行 X 线检查。

诊断检查与说明

实验室检查

评估合并伤或需要术前准备时行相关实验室检查。

影像学检查

• 颌面骨 CT 重建是可疑面部损伤的显像模式。

• X 线平片如 Waters 位片并不适用。

- 可提示鼻窦骨折、不对称或出血,上颌窦出面典型的不透明泪滴提示眶底爆裂性骨折。

• 颏底部的不对称位片可发现颧弓骨折。

• 疑似颌骨骨折行 Panorex 检查。

鉴别诊断

• 鼻骨骨折。

• 颧骨骨折(颧弓或颧骨三角区骨折)。

• Le Fort 骨折。

• 颅骨骨折包括额窦骨折和筛状板骨折。

• 鼻额筛骨复合骨折。

• 颚部骨折。

• 包括爆裂性骨折在内的眼眶骨折。

• 牙齿、颈部和大脑的合并损伤。

• 骨折以外的挫伤或撕裂伤。

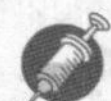

治疗

院前

注意

• 优先保证气道通畅:

- 首先举头抬颏,托颌和气道吸引。

- 潜在的损伤可能使得这些开放气道的手法和面罩球囊通气失败。

- 严重的面部骨折可妨碍口腔吸引。

- 大范围的面部或鼻部损伤禁忌经鼻气管插管。

- 快速顺序气管内插管(RSI)失败时给予环甲膜穿刺。

• 若存在合并伤,需保护颈髓。

初步稳定/治疗

• 积极保护气道,患者需要保护气道以免进行性的水肿或出血阻塞气道。面部损伤时首先给予快速顺序气管内插管(RSI);RSI 时应用依托咪酯、咪达唑仑、维库溴胺、罗库溴胺或琥珀胆碱。

• RSI 失败时需要外科手法建立气道(环甲膜穿刺术或针刺环甲膜穿刺)。

• 大多数面部骨折禁忌经鼻气管插管。

• 保护颈髓直到临床或 X 线检查排除颈髓损伤。

• 一旦保护了气道后,优先处理其他比面部损伤更重要的伤情。

• 若直接压迫止血仍难以控制出血时,可能需要后鼻道填塞止血。

急诊治疗/程序

• 复杂的骨折,包括所有的 Le Fort 骨折,请五官科、整形科或口腔外科医师会诊,累及后壁的额窦骨折请神经外科会诊。

• 开放性骨折和脑脊液漏时使用抗生素(头孢唑林,青霉素过敏患者选用克林霉素)存在争议,穿透性创伤或咬伤的证据最为充分,钝性外伤的证据最为薄弱,尤其是在脑脊液漏的情况下会诊后应使用。

• 预防性应用破伤风抗毒素。

• 口服止痛药物(吗啡或芬太尼)。

• 鼻中隔血肿需及时在急诊室行引流。

- 麻醉后,用 18~20G 针头抽吸,凡士林纱布填塞双侧鼻孔。

- 24 h 内使用氨苄西林或红霉素,并请五官科医师会诊稳定后出院。

• 无颧骨骨折移位者使用止痛剂后(对乙酰

氨基酚或布洛芬)后可以出院;提示颧骨和三角区移位骨折者,经门诊减压处理水肿消退 2～3 日后病情稳定可出院。

• 单纯骨折合并撕裂伤的可在急诊室缝合;患者出院后需要继续给予氨苄西林或阿奇霉素。

• 面部骨折合并鼻窦出血者出院后需要继续给予氨苄西林或阿奇霉素。

儿科注意事项

• 最常见的原因是跌倒、运动和机动车事故。

• 鼻骨和下颌骨最常见骨折。

• 8 岁以下儿童不应行开放性环甲膜穿刺手术:

- 可行针刺环甲膜穿刺后喷射通气。

• 儿童并发损伤的风险较高。

• 面部骨折的修复不应晚于伤后 3～4 日(尽快修复面部骨折,降低骨折畸形愈合和面貌畸形的风险)。

■ 药物治疗

• 对乙酰氨基酚:500 mg(儿童:10～15 mg/kg,24 h 不超过 5 次),q4～6 h,口服,24 h 不超过 4 g。

• 氨苄西林:250 mg[儿童:40～80 mg/(kg·24 h)],q8 h,口服。

• 阿奇霉素:首日 500 mg 口服,接下来 2～4 日 250 mg 口服(儿童:首日 10 mg/kg 口服,接下来 2～4 日 5 mg/kg 口服)。

• 头孢唑林:1 g[儿童:50～100 mg/(kg·24 h)],静脉注射或肌内注射。

• 克林霉素:600～900 mg[儿童:25～40 mg/(kg·24 h)],q8 h,口服。

• 地西泮:5～10 mg(儿童:0.1～0.2 mg/kg)静脉注射。

• 依托咪酯:0.2～0.3 mg/kg(儿童:0.2～0.3 mg/kg),静脉注射(10 岁以下儿童不建议使用)。

• 芬太尼:2～10 μg/kg(儿童:2～3 μg/kg),静脉注射。

• 布洛芬:600～800 mg[儿童:20～40 mg/(kg·24 h)],每日 3～4 次,口服。

• 氯胺酮:1～2 mg/kg(儿童:1～2 mg/kg),静脉注射。

• 咪达唑仑:2～5 mg(儿童:每剂 0.02～0.05 mg/kg,最大总量 0.4 mg/kg,不超过 10 mg),2～3 min 静脉注射。

• 硫酸吗啡:0.1～0.2 mg/kg(儿童:0.1～0.2 mg/kg),q1～4 h,静脉滴注。

• 罗库溴胺:0.6～1.2 mg/kg(儿童:0.6 mg/kg),静脉注射。

• 琥珀胆碱:1～1.5 mg/kg(儿童:1～2 mg/kg),静脉注射。

• 维库溴胺:0.1～0.3 mg/kg(儿童:0.1～0.3 mg/kg),静脉注射。

随访

■ 进一步处理

入院指征

• 明显存在的并发损伤。

• 累及气道。

• Le Fort Ⅱ型和Ⅲ型骨折。

• 脑脊液漏。

• 额窦后壁骨折。

• 除单纯鼻骨撕裂骨折外的大多数开放性骨折。

出院指征

• 无明显存在的头部、颈部或其他部位损伤。

• 颧骨、眼眶、鼻窦或额窦前壁的闭合骨折,24～36 h 需观察随访。

• 鼻中隔血肿在急诊室引流后 24 h 内需观察随访。

• 涉及颧骨移位和颧骨三角区骨折,经门诊减压处理水肿消退 2～3 日后病情稳定者。

转诊问题

耳鼻咽喉科、整形科或神经外科都可处理面部骨折,取决于各个医疗机构的实际情况。如无脑脊液漏或累及额窦后壁时,一般请耳鼻咽喉科会诊即可。

要点和误区

• 面部骨折和损伤表面上会显得非常严重。

- 总是首先保护气道,避免经鼻气管插管。

- 必要的气道保护后,首先评估其他重要伤情,不要忽略危及生命的损伤。

◦ 颈椎骨折。

◦ 肺部或胸廓。

◦ 腹腔内损伤。

• 面部骨折的 CT 指征放宽,以便于评估面部损伤。

• 面部骨折通常合并有视觉损害,需行全面的眼部检查。

• 视力丧失是一个重要的发现,意味着眼球或视神经受损。

• 评估鼻中隔血肿。

• 找出牙齿缺失的原因,行胸部 X 线检查排除误吸可能。

拇指骨折 Thumb Fracture

Daniel R. Lasoff · Leslie C. Oyama　范浩浩　李文放 译

基础知识

■ 描述

• 远端指骨骨折:

- 钝性创伤,拇指过度伸展,轴向负载和挤压伤害。

- 簇绒骨折是其他拇指中类似的骨折,远端指骨被压和/或碎裂。

- 它可能会是开放性或闭合性损伤,并与甲床受伤相关。

- 严重甲床损伤、关节内移位/成角骨折或肌腱损伤,这些情况应请骨科会诊。

- 非复杂的簇状骨折可以固定处理,视为软组织损伤。

• 近端指骨骨折和拇指掌骨骨折:

- 拇指钝挫伤:

◦ 拇指轴向负重的掌指关节(MP)部分弯曲,手握拳,否则掌指关节是稳定的。

- 贝内特骨折(Ⅰ型):

◦ 在掌骨基部关节内骨折/脱位,且在掌骨的尺骨侧保持其连续性。

- 罗兰多骨折(Ⅱ型):

◦ 粉碎的 Y 形或 T 形关节内第 1 掌骨基部骨折。

◦ 类似于粉碎性贝内特骨折,这些可以是更复杂的多个粉碎性骨折。

- Ⅲ型骨折。

◦ 关节外掌骨骨折,倾向于横向较少斜形骨折。

■ 病因

- 跌倒，超屈曲，过度伸展。
- 机动车事故。
- 运动，特别是下坡或高山滑雪。
- 篮球。
- 棒球。
- 足球。
- 橄榄球。

诊断

■ 症状和体征

- 拇指疼痛，肿胀和畸形。
- 检查应该包括最痛处或畸形部位。
- 拇指远端可能相对于骨折部位发生旋转。
- 拇指底部可能会出现相对于手在休息位时的其余部分呈放射状偏移。
- 偶尔可能会损伤拇指手神经。

儿科注意事项

- 拇指骨折有时会发生在儿童身上。
- 考虑非事故性的创伤。
- 不要忽视儿童适当的疼痛管理。

体格检查

- 固定拇指等待确定性的评估。
- 两点辨别觉进行神经血管检查。

■ 基本检查

如下所述的影像学检查。

■ 诊断检查与说明

影像学检查

- 受影响区域的 X 线平片。
- 除非完成所有的 X 线平片，否则应避免测试拇指掌指关节的压力，就像在测试游戏的拇指一样。

■ 鉴别诊断

- 拇指根部和掌骨的关节外骨折。
- 舟骨骨折。
- 游戏拇指：尺骨侧副韧带伤。

治疗

■ 院前

- 包扎开放性伤口。
- 将手、腕和拇指固定在自然休息位。
- 抬高，冰敷以减轻肿胀。
- 适合年龄的社会管理。

■ 初步稳定/治疗

固定拇指等待确定性评估。

■ 急诊治疗/程序

- 在自然休息位下进行拇指夹板固定，手的位置好像拿着一个饮料罐。
- 应向患者说明夹板如何使用。
- 第 1 掌指关节关节外成角骨折需要减小角度，可以容忍高达 30°的角度。角度＞30°时需要尝试减小角度或骨科会诊。
- 远端指骨骨折需要 DIP 夹板伸展固定 3～4 周。

■ 药物治疗

口服止痛制剂控制疼痛。

随访

■ 进一步处理

入院指征

开放性骨折，存在多处创伤或其他更严重的伤害。

出院指征

- 告知患者有很大的可能性第 1 掌骨需要手术修复受伤。
- 闭合性损伤：转诊、夹板和解释需要手术固定的可能。

■ 转诊建议

72 h 矫形转诊。

要点和误区

由于肌腱插入，骨折在拇指基部常常不稳定并且经常需要手术固定。

N

囊性纤维化 Cystic Fibrosis

Joseph H. Kahn 陈奇通 译

基础知识

描述

• 囊性纤维化的跨膜传导调节器功能缺陷(囊性纤维化跨膜传导调节因子)。

• 囊性纤维化跨膜传导调节因子是一种ATP调控的氯离子通道,用于调节细胞表面氯离子和钠离子通道的活性:

- 外分泌腺和分泌性上皮细胞的异常电解质转运。
- 胰腺分泌功能降低导致吸收不良。
- 增厚的黏液、反复的肺部感染和进展性的阻塞性肺损伤。
- 鼻窦疾病复发。

• 白种人新生儿中发生概率为 1/3 600,在非洲裔美国人中为 1/29 000,在西班牙裔美国人中为 1/6 500。

• 30%的病例由新生儿筛查时确诊。

• 75%的病例在出生后前 2 年被诊断。

• 美国约 30 000 个儿童和青年人有囊性纤维化。

• 在美国囊性纤维患者的平均寿命约为 40 岁。

• 约有 40%囊性纤维化患者在 18 岁以上。

• 1 000 万美国人可能为无症状的缺陷基因携带者。

• 美国有 16%肺移植是由于 CF。

危险因素

遗传学

与位于第 7 对染色体长臂上 *CFTR* 基因有关的隐性遗传病:

• 不同的突变;多变的表型。

• 经典疾病:纯合子 Phe508de 突变。

• 美国最常见的致死性遗传病。

病因

肺炎患者常见的病原菌是多种药物抵抗:

• 金黄色葡萄球菌:

- 甲氧西林敏感金黄色葡萄球菌、耐甲氧西林金黄色葡萄球菌。

• 铜绿假单胞菌:

- 患病率随年龄增长而增加,>70%成人为慢性感染。

• 流血嗜血杆菌。

• 嗜麦芽寡养单胞菌。

• 洋葱伯克霍尔德菌:

- 约占 3%。
- 临床进展迅速恶化。

• 木糖氧化无色杆菌。

• 分枝杆菌(非结核性):鸟分枝杆菌复合体、分枝杆菌脓肿。

• 曲霉。

诊断

症状和体征

• 一般情况:

- 发育不良。
- 反复的呼吸道感染。
- 婴儿期水肿。
- 皮肤含盐。

• 头、耳、眼、鼻和喉(五官):

- 鼻息肉、鼻窦炎导致的严重头痛、中耳炎。

• 肺:

- 持续性咳嗽。开始为干咳,然后为分泌性的。
- 第 1 年内反复的肺炎或支气管炎。
- 气喘。
- 咯血。
- 肺炎。
- 慢性支气管炎。
- 支气管扩张。
- 呼吸困难。
- 气胸。
- 纵隔气肿。
- 囊性纤维化住院的最常见原因。

• 心脏:

- 心力衰竭。
- 肺心病、肺动脉高压。

• 胃肠:

- 腹痛。
- 胎粪性肠梗阻。
- 远端肠道阻塞性综合征(DIOS)或"胎粪性肠梗阻"。
- 胃食管反流。
- 胆石症。
- 胰腺炎、胰腺功能不全。
- 回盲部肠套叠。
- 恶臭、脂肪粪。
- 黄疸、肝硬化。
- 直肠脱垂。
- 咯血。
- 小肠菌群过度生长。

• 四肢:

- 骨痛。
- 水肿、关节积液。
- 骨密质降低。

• 反复静脉血栓形成。

• 心肺功能衰竭是最常见的死亡原因。

基本检查

• 汗液氯测试。

• 如果汗液氯测试难以确定则进行 DNA 分析。

• 如果 DNA 分析无果则做鼻电位差。

诊断检查与说明

实验室检查

• 汗液氯测试:

- 氯浓度>60 mEq/L。
- 具有典型症状和体征且检测阳性可确诊。

• 粪便检测:

- 弹性蛋白酶、胰蛋白酶或糜蛋白酶降低。
- 72 h 排泄物中脂肪含量增加。

• 免疫反应性胰蛋白酶(IRT):

- 确定风险增加和/或诊断。
- 可能出现假阳性或阴性。

• DNA 分析:

- 症状明显具有指导意义,但汗液测试阴性。
- 90%囊性纤维化由染色体检测确定。
- 如果检测到两个异常基因则为阳性。
- 基因分型检测不能确诊。
- 已列出 1 300 种囊性纤维化跨膜传导调节因子突变。
- 可能出现二次改善或中和的基因突变。

• 全血细胞计数:

- 血小板减少。

• 血清电解质:

- 低钠、低氯性碱中毒。

• 血糖:

- 青少年和成人中高血糖和新发糖尿病多见;酮症酸中毒罕见。

• 肝功能检测和凝血酶原时间:

- 呕血或咯血或具有其他肝功能衰竭指征。

• 动脉血气分析:

- 低氧血症、代谢性碱中毒。

• 痰培养:

- 可能有假单胞菌定植。

• 对不明诊断的高危患者进行研究：
- 鼻电位差检测：
◦ 复杂而耗时的研究。
- 精液分析：
◦ 无精子症。

影像学检查

• X线片：
- 过分充气。
- 支气管周围增厚。
- 肺不张。
- 肺门淋巴结肿大。
- 气胸或纵隔积气。
- 支气管扩张。
- 肺大疱。
- 胸部CT明确肺大疱、支气管扩张。
- MRI可以描述囊性纤维化的形态学特征。
• 腹部X线平片和/或CT：
- 如有腹痛、呕吐或腹胀则可提示。
- 远端肠梗阻综合征。
- 肠套叠。
• 钡餐：
- 如有可疑的肠套叠。
• 鼻窦摄片：
- 由于常规的摄片难以分辨而限制检测。
- 如果需要手术则需CT评估鼻窦。
• 心电图评估心脏传导阻滞。

诊断步骤/外科

支气管肺泡灌洗：
• 高比例的中性粒细胞和中性粒细胞绝对计数。
• 如有明显的肺部症状则不必要。

鉴别诊断

• 呼吸系统：
- 哮喘。
- 复发性肺炎。
- 支气管扩张。
- 百日咳。
- 免疫缺陷。
- 异物吸入。
- α_1-抗胰蛋白酶缺乏。
- 纤毛发育不良。
• 胃肠：
- 慢性腹泻。
- 肠胃炎。
- 牛奶过敏。
• 汗液中电解质水平增高：
- 岩藻糖苷贮积症。
- 1型糖原贮积症。
- 黏多糖贮积症。
- 甲状腺功能减退。
- 抗利尿激素抵抗性尿崩症。
- 肾上腺功能不全。
- 家族性胆汁淤积症。
- 家族性甲状旁腺功能减退。
- 营养不良。
- 外胚层发育不良。
- 过敏性皮炎。
- 前列腺素E灌注。

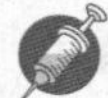

治疗

院前

• 不稳定性二度Ⅱ型或三度传导阻滞经皮起搏。
• 阿托品：
- 二度Ⅱ型传导阻滞应避免使用，因为有可能造成三度传导阻滞。

急诊治疗/程序

• 稳定气道、呼吸和循环系统：
- 纠正体液、呼吸、电解质和血糖紊乱。
- 如有哮喘使用支气管扩张剂、类固醇。
• 气胸：
- 如果小于5%～10%则观察。
- 胸腔闭式引流术。
• 咨询囊性纤维化主治医师或肺科专家。
• 右心衰竭：
- 利尿剂。
• 咯血：
- 血液制品(检查国际标准化比值)。
- 通气支持。
• 远端肠道阻塞性综合征：
- 通常需要外科手术。
• 呕血：
- 浓缩红细胞。
- 对于凝血异常可使用血液制品。
- 早期咨询内镜医师。
• 肠套叠：
- 钡/空气灌肠纠正。
- 可能需要外科手术。
• 直肠脱垂：
- 手法复位。
- 考虑外科意见。
• 呼吸治疗：
- 呼吸道清理/物理疗法。
- 黏液稀释吸入剂。
• 抗生素治疗肺炎：
- 以培养和药敏试验为依据。
- 金黄色葡萄球菌(MSSA)：
◦ 头孢菌素或乙氧萘青霉素。
- 金黄色葡萄球菌(MRSA)：
◦ 万古霉素或利奈唑胺。
- 铜绿假单胞菌：
◦ 哌拉西林-他唑巴坦或头孢他啶或头孢吡肟或亚胺培南-西司他丁或美罗培南或替卡西林-克拉维酸＋环丙沙星或左氧氟沙星或妥布霉素或阿米卡星或结肠杆菌素。
- 金黄色葡萄球菌(MSSA)和铜绿假单胞菌：
◦ 与单独使用铜绿假单胞菌相同的抗生素，但不应使用头孢他啶。
- 金黄色葡萄球菌(MRSA)和铜绿假单胞菌：
◦ 万古霉素或利奈唑胺＋单独覆盖假单胞菌。
- 洋葱伯克霍尔德菌：
◦ 甲氧苄啶-磺胺甲噁唑和/或多西环素和/或头孢他啶和/或美罗培南。
- 流感嗜血杆菌：
◦ 头孢曲松或阿莫西林-克拉维酸盐。
- 鼻窦炎。
- 基于敏感性。
• 囊性纤维化跨膜传导调节因子调控：Ivacaftor。
- 修复蛋白功能。
- Ivacaftor：CFTR电位器。
- Lumacaftor：CFTR校正器。
- Tezacaftor：研究性CFTR校正器。
• 恢复气道表面液体：
- 雾化吸入高渗性盐水。
• 黏液改变：
- 脱氧核糖核酸酶α稀释肺部黏液。
• 未来方向：
- 基因治疗：稳定DNA。
- 抗炎：高剂量布洛芬。
- 抗感染药物：
◦ 吸入妥布霉素、氨曲南、多黏菌素。
◦ 持续万古霉素输注。
- 移植：吸入环孢素。
- 睡眠时无创通气。
- 高剂量维生素D_3。
- 益生菌。
- 营养和锻炼。

药物治疗

• 阿米卡星：30～35 mg/kg，q24 h。

N

• 氨曲南：50 mg/kg，q8 h。
• 头孢唑林：100 mg/(kg · d)，分 3 或 4 剂(最大剂量 6 g/d)。
• 头孢吡肟：150 mg/(kg · d)，静脉给药，分 3 剂(最大剂量 6 g/d)。
• 头孢他啶：150～200 mg/(kg · d)，分 3 或 4 剂(最大剂量 8 g/d)。
• 环丙沙星：40 mg/(kg · d)，口服(分 2 剂)或 30 mg/(kg · d)，静脉给药(分 3 剂)。
• 多黏菌素：2.5～5 mg/(kg · d)，分 3 剂，静脉注射(最大剂量 300 mg/d)。
• 亚胺培南：15～25 mg/kg，静脉注射，q6 h。
• 亚胺培南-西司他丁：60～100 mg/(kg · d)，分 4 次服用(最大剂量 4 g/d)。
• 左氧氟沙星口服和静脉注射：6 个月至 4 年：16～20 mg/(kg · d)，分 2 次服用；5～16 岁：8～10 mg/(kg · d)，q24 h。
• 利奈唑胺：30 mg/(kg · d)静脉或口服，3 剂(3 岁以下儿童)。
• 美罗培南：120 mg/(kg · d)，分 3 次服用(最大剂量 6 g/d)。
• 纳夫西林：100～200 mg/(kg · d)，分 4 或 6 剂(最大剂量 12 g/d)。
• 哌拉西林-他唑巴坦：350～450 mg/(kg · d)，分 4 次，静脉注射(最大剂量 16 g/d)。
• 替卡西林-克拉维酸盐：400 mg/(kg · d)，分 4 或 6 剂(最大剂量 18 g/d)。
• 妥布霉素：10 mg/kg，q24 h。
• TMP - SMX：5 mg/kg TMP 组分静脉给药，q6 h。
• 万古霉素：60 mg/(kg · d)，分 3 或 4 剂(最初最大剂量 1.25 g)。
• 注意：由于许多患者未营养不良状态，抗生素的药物代谢动力学(尤其是氨基糖苷类、青霉素类和头孢菌素类)可能会改变，要求仔细监测。

随访

进一步处理

入院指征

• 肺部恶化伴基本情况差、低氧血症、耐药菌、门诊治疗失败的患者。
• 气胸。
• 咯血。
• 呕血。
• 肠套叠或无法解释的腹痛或肠梗阻。
• 高血糖。

出院指征

• 密切随访确认培养结果和药敏试验，必要时改变治疗。
• 避免热天气。
• 大量出汗时经口补盐。

转诊问题

所有患者在急性加重期需要咨询儿科肺病中心。

随访建议

• 专家团队。
• 呼吸治疗，胸部 PT，锻炼计划，抗生素，胰酶替代。

要点和误区

• 具有呼吸窘迫的囊性纤维化患者一定要考虑到气胸：胸部 X 线检查。
• 伴随腹痛、呕吐的囊性纤维化患者一定考虑远端肠道阻塞性综合征和肠套叠。

脑出血 Intracerebral Hemorrhage

Atul Gupta · Rebecca Smith-Coggins 倪沁赟 译

基础知识

描述

脑实质出血：
• 脑组织压迫。
• 继发性损伤：
- 脑水肿。
- 颅内压增高。
- 脑疝的潜在可能性。

病因

脑出血可自发性或由创伤导致：
• 控制不佳或急性高血压(最常见病因)。
• 血管畸形：
- 动静脉畸形。
- 静脉血管瘤。
- 脑动脉血管瘤破裂。
• 肿瘤(尤其是黑色素瘤和神经胶质瘤)。
• 抗凝药物(华法林、肝素)。
• 溶栓药物。
• 毒品(可卡因、苯丙胺)。
• 出血性疾病(血友病)。
• 脑淀粉样血管病。
• 继发于钝性或穿透性损伤的继发性出血。

诊断

症状和体征

病史

• 剧烈头痛，典型症状为突然起病。
• 癫痫发作。
• 有颅脑损伤的证据。
• 颈强直。
• 呕吐。
• 抗凝治疗。
• 不同水平的意识状态(可能昏迷)：
- 颅脑损伤后最迟 24～48 h 可能发生精神状态的改变。

体格检查

• 高血压。
• 颈强直。
• 精神状态改变。
• 不同的神经功能缺损表现取决于脑出血的部位：
- 壳核出血(35%)：
◦ 对侧偏瘫。
◦ 对侧偏身感觉缺失。
◦ 偶发吞咽困难。
◦ 偶发遗忘。
- 脑叶出血(30%)：
◦ 不同的区域临床征象不同。
- 小脑出血(15%)：
◦ 呕吐。
◦ 共济失调。
◦ 眼球震颤。
- 丘脑出血(10%)：
◦ 与壳核出血相似，但是可能出现眼球运动异常。
- 尾状核出血(5%)：
◦ 意识混乱。

◦ 记忆丧失。
◦ 偏瘫。
◦ 凝视麻痹。
- 脑桥出血(5%)：
◦ 四肢瘫痪。
◦ 针尖样瞳孔。
◦ 共济失调。
◦ 感觉丧失。

■ 基本检查

• 管理气道。
• 立即行头颅 CT 平扫：
- 急性出血表现为高密度病变。

■ 诊断检查与说明

实验室检查

• 全血细胞计数。
• 凝血功能(PT、APTT、INR、血小板)。
• 电解质、尿素氮、肌酐。
• 育龄妇女行妊娠试验。
• 心电图。
• 毒理学检查。

影像学检查

• 头颅 CT 平扫。
• 头颅 MRI 可能有用，但是不如 CT 上表现快速。

诊断步骤/外科

• 血管造影：
- 在急性条件下，被越来越多接受的一种诊断工具。
- CTA 检查后可发现高达 15%的患者有潜在的血管病变，可能改变患者急性期的管理。
- 造影剂外溢表示持续性出血。
◦ 血肿扩大风险极高，最终结局差，病死率高。

■ 鉴别诊断

• 癫痫发作：
- 托德瘫痪。
• 中枢神经系统感染。
• 中枢神经系统占位。
• 电解质紊乱或酸碱平衡失调。
• 中毒。
• 韦尼克脑病。
• 偏头痛。
• 短暂性脑缺血发作。
• 非出血性急性脑血管意外。
• 空气栓塞。
• CT 上出血的不同诊断：
- 自发性脑出血。
◦ 高血压性脑出血。
◦ 动静脉畸形。
◦ 肿瘤。
- 创伤性脑出血：
◦ 蛛网膜下腔出血。
◦ 硬膜下血肿。
◦ 硬膜外血肿。

儿科注意事项

增加不同的诊断包括：
• 烟雾病。
• 急性小儿偏瘫。

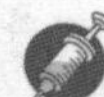

治疗

■ 院前

• 如果怀疑头部或颈部损伤，给予颈椎的预防措施。
• 颈椎保护的情况下抬高头部。
• 院前急救者必须确定神经系统损害的情况，这样才能注意到症状是否进展。

■ 初步稳定/治疗

• 在需要时进行气道管理和复苏：
- 意识水平呈抑制状态的患者，需立即气管插管给予控制通气。
• 早期神经外科咨询。

■ 急诊治疗/程序

• 及时手术和/或神经内科会诊。
• 血压管理：
- 谨慎控制血压，因为在颅内压增高的情况下将血压迅速降至正常水平可能会降低脑灌注。
- 使用拉贝洛尔、尼卡地平、艾司洛尔、依那普利使收缩压初始降低 10%。
- 应在 12～24 h 后降至正常血压水平。
- 可使用硝普钠、硝酸甘油或肼屈嗪作为替代药物。
• 颅高压治疗：
- 控制通气是动脉二氧化碳分压<35 mmHg。
- 液体限制，床头抬高 30°。
- 甘露醇：渗透性利尿。
- 使用呋塞米(速尿)作为替代药物。
• 纠正凝血功能障碍：
- 考虑输注新鲜冰冻血浆。
- 艾达司珠单抗。
- 血小板。
- 凝血酶原复合物、维生素 K。
• 考虑使用抗惊厥药物：
- 左乙拉西坦。
- 苯妥英。
- 磷苯妥英。

■ 药物治疗

• 艾司洛尔：首剂 0.5～1 mg/kg，静脉推注，然后 50～150 μg/(kg · min)，静脉维持。
• 依那普利：1.25～5 mg，q6 h(血压骤降风险，试验剂量 0.625 mg)。
• 新鲜冰冻血浆：10～20 ml/kg，静脉注射。
• 磷苯妥英：15～20 mg/kg，以 100～150 mg/min 的速度静脉注射或肌内注射。
• 呋塞米：20～40 mg(儿童：0.5～1 mg/kg)，静脉注射；必要时重复用药。
• 肼屈嗪：10～40 mg(儿童：0.1～0.2 mg/kg，最大剂量单次 20 mg)，静脉注射；必要时重复用药。
- 艾达司珠单抗：5 g 静脉注射。
- 左乙拉西坦：每日 500 mg(儿童：10 mg/kg，静脉注射；最大剂量 3 000 mg/d)，静脉注射。
• 拉贝洛尔：20 mg(儿童：0.3～1 mg/kg；最大剂量单次 20 mg)静脉注射；可给予额外的 40～80 mg，q10 min，最大剂量为 300 mg。
• 甘露醇：1 g/kg，静脉注射。
• 尼卡地平：5～15 mg/h，静脉注射。
• 硝普钠：开始 0.25～10 μg/(kg · min)，静脉注射[最大剂量 10 μg/(kg · min)]；滴定至合适的剂量。
• PCCs(人凝血酶原复合物)：25～50 U/kg，静滴；最多 5 000 U。
• 苯妥英：15～20 mg/kg(儿童：15 mg/kg)，速度 40～50 mg/min 或以下。
• 血小板：在神经外科会诊后，1～2 U，血小板静脉输注。
• 维生素 K：5～10 mg，静脉注射至少 30 min。

随访

■ 进一步处理

入院指征

• 如果有手术指征则去手术室。
• 如果行气管插管、意识状态改变或静脉药物控制血压则去 ICU。
• 观察神经系统改变，直到神经系统检查没有进一步出血的证据，同时血流动力学稳定。

出院指征

所有脑出血患者均需要住院。

N

转诊问题

康复是关键。

随访建议

• 非急性状态下治疗高血压是降低脑出血风险的最重要的一步。

• 停止吸烟、饮酒和使用可卡因，来预防脑出血的复发。

要点和误区

• 头痛、高血压和/或意识状态改变的患者，大脑影像学检查是急诊评估最重要的组成部分。

• 谨慎控制血压，因为在颅内压增高的状态下血压急性降至正常会降低脑灌注，甚至出现脑缺血。

• 有头部外伤并接受抗凝治疗的患者，需要考虑迟发性脑出血可能。

脑动脉瘤 Cerebral Aneurysm

Veronique Au · Rebecca Smith-Coggins 庄育刚 译

基础知识

描述

• 脑血管壁局部异常膨出或者破裂，人群发生率为5%～10%。

• 5%～15%脑卒中(中风)为囊状血管瘤破裂。

• 其中，40%发生在前交通动脉，30%发生在颈内动脉，20%发生在大脑中动脉，5%～10%发生在椎-基底动脉系统。

病因

• 3.2%的人群无症状。

• 先天性、囊状或脑底动脉瘤常见，大约占90%。

- 由脑动脉壁局部薄弱点和脑血管分叉处进展而来。
- 年龄越大发生率越高。
- 复合发生率为20%～30%。
- 发生率增加因素。
  - 多囊肾。
  - 脑动静脉畸形。
  - Ⅲ型胶原缺乏。
  - 肌纤维发育异常。
  - Ehler's-Danlos综合征。
  - 马方综合征。
  - 弹性假黄色瘤。
  - 神经纤维瘤病。
  - 烟雾病。
  - 主动脉缩窄。
  - 结节性脑硬化。
  - 镰状细胞(贫血)病。
  - Osler-Weber-Rendu综合征。
  - α_1-抗胰蛋白酶缺乏。
  - 系统性红斑狼疮。
  - 糖皮质激素治疗型醛固酮增多症。

• 动脉硬化，梭形或长短膨出(7%)。

- 外周血管更常见。

• 炎症(真菌)。

- 10%的患者存在细菌性内膜炎。

• 合并头部闭合伤的创伤。

• 肿瘤血栓。

• 家族史：直系亲属发生动脉瘤的可能性加大1倍。

儿科注意事项

• 尽管发生率很低，更容易发生巨大动脉瘤(>25 mm)。

• 发生于后循环。

诊断

症状和体征

• 动脉瘤破裂前一般无特殊。

• 30%～60%的破裂有前哨性头痛。

- 可能是单侧的。

• 癫痫、昏厥或不同程度的神志改变。

病史

• 头痛。

• 家族史。

• 精神状况改变。

• 局部神经功能缺失。

• 蛛网膜下腔出血后改变。

- 迅速出现的剧烈的头痛。
  - 有别于以前头痛发作。
  - 通常没有定位体征。

• 脑脊液出血导致的颈项强直(常见)。

体格检查

• 邻近的压迫可能导致神经系统症状：

• 前交通动脉破裂：

- 视束：视野缩小或者同侧偏盲。
- 视交叉：双颞侧偏盲。
- 视神经：单侧弱视。

• 颈内动脉破裂——后交通动脉：

- 动眼神经：瞳孔放大固定，眼睑下垂，复视，眼球颞侧偏移，向上、向内、向下运动不能。

• 大脑皮质动脉瘤可产生的神经系统缺陷包括：

- 轻偏瘫。
- 半身感觉丧失。
- 视觉障碍。
- 失语。
- 癫痫。

基本检查

- 完整的神经系统检查。
- 急诊头部CT能发现90%～95%的蛛网膜下腔出血。
- 若CT不能进行，腰椎穿刺进行脑脊液检查。

诊断检查与说明

实验室检查

• 凝血功能检查。

• 带血小板的血常规检查。

• 电解质。

• 肝肾功能。

• 血气分析。

影像学检查

• 胸部X线检查观察肺水肿。

• 血管颅内血管造影仍旧是金标准。

• 螺旋CT有助于发现>3 mm的动脉瘤。

• 经颅多普勒超声有助于发现血管痉挛。

诊断步骤/外科

头部CT检查怀疑动脉瘤破裂可行腰椎穿刺。

鉴别诊断

• 脑肿瘤。

• 动静脉畸形。

• 视神经炎。

- 偏头痛。
- 脑膜炎。
- 脑炎。
- 高血压脑病。
- 高血糖或低血糖。
- 颞血管炎。
- 急性青光眼。
- 硬膜下出血。
- 硬膜外出血。
- 颅内出血。
- 脑血栓形成。
- 空气栓塞。
- 鼻窦炎。

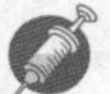

治疗

院前

- 注意：
  - 神经系统检查有极其重要的意义，评估内容：
  - 昏迷程度。
    - 格拉斯哥昏迷评分。
    - 运动缺陷。
    - 语言异常。
    - 步态异常。
    - 面部不协调。
    - 其他定位缺陷。
- 蛛网膜下腔出血患者可能迅速出现意识障碍导致紧急气管内插管。
- 患者必须入院行 CT 检查并进入 ICU 治疗。

初步稳定/治疗

- ABC 管理：
  - 吸氧。
  - 若因气道保护或者控制通气，则迅速气管内插管。
  - 持续心电和 SPO_2 监测。
- 对于精神状态改变的患者：
  - 迅速检查血糖，必要时给 50% 葡萄糖溶液。
  - 纳洛酮。
  - 维生素 B_1。
- 逆转抗凝作用。
- 急性颅内压升高导致呕吐、止吐。
- 静脉使用苯二氮䓬类药物和/或苯妥英钠处理癫痫。
- 癫痫预防治疗有争议，不推荐使用。

急诊治疗/程序

初始治疗后，急诊对于动脉瘤破裂出血的治疗目的主要是防止再次破裂、防止脑血管痉挛或处理脑水肿（参见“蛛网膜下腔出血”）。

外科/其他流程

- 造影和外科手术时机仍有一定争议，但是倾向于早期手术减少再出血和血管痉挛。
- 早期部分合适患者进行脑室造瘘引流，可进行颅内压监测并有助于降低收缩压。
- 已经设计了 2 个评分系统来帮助做出治疗决定：
  - 阶段（人种、高血压、年龄、动脉瘤的大小、较早于另一动脉瘤的 SAH、动脉瘤的部位）：
    - 可以预测自然病史，并且可以与治疗风险进行比较。
  - 颅内动脉瘤破裂治疗评分（UIATS）：
    - 临床决策工具。

儿科注意事项

脑动脉瘤患儿出血概率增大。应该早期迅速处理。

药物治疗

一线用药

- 拉贝洛尔：20～30 mg 静脉负荷量，然后 40～80 mg，q10 min，最大剂量 300 mg；随后 0.5～2.0 mg/min 持续静脉泵入。
- 尼莫地平：60 mg 口服或胃管入，q4 h。
- 昂丹司琼：4 mg，口服或静脉输注，q4 h 或需要时用；幼儿 0.1 mg/kg，静脉输注，最大剂量每次 4 mg。
- 甲哌氯丙嗪：5～10 mg，静脉输注或肌内注射，q6～8 h，最大剂量 40 mg/d；儿童 0.2 mg/(kg·d)。

二线用药

- 地西泮：5～10 mg，静脉注射，q10～15 min，最大剂量 30 mg；儿童 0.2～0.3 mg/kg，q5～10 min，最大 10 mg。
- 多库酯钠：100 mg，口服，每日 2 次。
- 磷苯妥英：15～20 mg/kg，速率为 100～150 mg/min，肌内注射或静脉输注。
- 肼屈嗪：10～20 mg，静脉注射，q30 min。
- 劳拉西泮：2～4 mg，静脉注射，q15 min 或需要时用；儿童每次 0.03～0.05 μg/kg，最大剂量每次 4 mg。
- 尼卡地平：5 mg/h，每 5～15 min 增加 2.5 mg/h，最大剂量 15 mg/h；儿童无推荐。
- 苯妥英钠：15～20 mg/kg 负荷量静脉注射 50 mg/min，最大剂量 1.5 g（成人和儿童）。维持剂量：4～6 mg/(kg·d)，静脉注射或肌内注射。

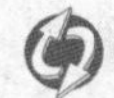

随访

进一步处理

入院指征

- 任何动脉瘤破裂蛛网膜下腔出血患者必须入院，优先 ICU 治疗。
- 有症状未破裂动脉瘤患者必须入院，并紧急神经外科会诊，告知有极大破裂的风险。

出院指征

- 偶然发现的无症状的脑动脉瘤患者可以出院，后期神经外科严密随访。
- 鉴于每年 1%～2% 破裂的风险，因此对于 10 mm 以下（可能 4～8 mm）患者的外科手术仍存在争议。

随访建议

- 神经外科。
- 神经内科。
- 基础护理。

要点和误区

- 不能单凭 CT 扫描排除蛛网膜下腔出血。
- 出血后或术后 3 日脑血管痉挛常见。
- 尼莫地平能防止和治疗血管痉挛，但是不能静脉给予。
- 硝酸甘油和硝普钠可增加颅内血容量，进而导致颅内压升高，因此要避免使用。

N

脑积水 Hydrocephalus

Richard S. Krause 巩博 译

基础知识

描述

• 颅腔内脑脊液(CSF)量增加。

• 脑萎缩也可引起颅内 CSF 增加,但是 CSF 压力不增加。

• 梗阻性脑积水可引起颅内压(ICP)快速上升,迅速导致死亡或永久性脑损伤。

• 非梗阻性脑积水引起亚急性症状,并且是可治疗痴呆的一种形式。

• 也描述为"交通性"和"非交通性":

- 交通性脑积水:当 CSF 流出脑室,CSF 的流动被阻断(脑室内是"交通性")。

- 非交通性脑积水:CSF 在 1 个或多个连接脑室的通道内流动被阻断(脑室内不是"交通性")。

病因

• 梗阻性脑积水:

- 梗阻:

◦ 中脑导水管(最常见,双侧侧脑室和第三脑室扩大,第四脑室不扩大)。

- 中脑导水管狭窄可为先天性或后天性(肿瘤、蛛网膜下腔出血、脑膜炎后遗症、特发性)。

◦ 室间孔(侧脑室扩大,通常为双侧,但也可能为单侧)。

◦ 第四脑室外侧孔和正中孔(第四脑室梗阻继发第三脑室、侧脑室扩大)。

◦ 脑干旁的蛛网膜下腔空间(感染后或蛛网膜下腔出血后全部脑室扩大)。

- 急性症状常继发于 CSF 分流障碍、蛛网膜下腔出血或严重脑外伤。

• 非梗阻性脑积水:

- 正常压力脑积水:

◦ 颅内 CSF 量增加,没有颅内高压。

◦ CT 上脑室体积增加(像脑萎缩,没有量减少)。

◦ 有时叫慢性"脑积水"。

◦ 通常因为中枢神经系统吸收不正常引起。

• 儿童脑积水:

- 先天性脑积水多由于新生儿出现、先天性畸形或获得性脑膜炎后继发脑干周围蛛网膜瘢痕形成。

诊断

症状和体征

• 梗阻性脑积水:

- 头痛。

- 恶心与呕吐。

- 意识水平下降。

- 尿失禁。

- 眼麻痹。

- 视神经乳头水肿,视力下降。

- 瞳孔扩大。

- 库欣反应:

◦ 因为 ICP 增高,出现收缩压升高及心动过缓。

◦ 儿科患者:囟门饱满、易激惹、嗜睡。

- 血压常升高。

- 如果梗阻发展缓慢,症状可能类似于非梗阻性脑积水。

• 非梗阻性脑积水:

- 进行性痴呆或嗜睡。

- 步态失常。

- 尿失禁。

- 向上凝视麻痹。

- 普遍体弱或嗜睡。

- 常常逐渐出现痴呆,伴随智力衰退呈亚急性进程。

- 无头痛或者视神经乳头水肿。

儿科注意事项

• 婴儿通常表现为进行性大头畸形,而 2 岁以上儿童一般表现为颅内压升高的体征和症状:

- 头颅扩大。

- 缺陷、发育迟缓。

- 头皮静脉突出。

- 向上凝视麻痹(落日征)。

- 视神经乳头水肿。

- 恶心、呕吐。

- 嗜睡。

病史

• 出现症状。

• CSF 分流病史。

• 恶心与呕吐。

• 头痛。

• 体弱。

• 意识混乱。

• 视力改变。

• 尿失禁。

体格检查

• 彻底的神经系统检查:

- 运动。

- 感觉。

- 深部腱反射。

- 步态。

- 脑神经检查。

- 可能看到视神经乳头水肿。

• 意识混乱。

• 意识水平下降。

• 通过触摸判断 CSF 引流。

- 引流障碍暗示着不能按下(远端引流障碍)或者充盈障碍(近端引流障碍)。

• 儿童前囟门饱满:

- 标注在"症状和体征"的其他表现。

基本检查

头颅 CT 扫描 w/o 对比可以评估脑室体积和对称性。

• 帮助诊断脑水肿、占位性病变和出血。

诊断检查与说明

实验室检查

腰椎穿刺常在头颅 CT 后实施(非梗阻性原因):

• 腰椎穿刺压力反映非梗阻性脑积水 ICP 上升情况。

• 如果怀疑感染,CSF 应当送检例行检查。

- 革兰染色、培养、蛋白质、葡萄糖和细胞计数。

影像学检查

• CT 可以评估心室大小。

• MRI 显示脑室大小和对称性,可能比 CT 更好地显示肿块。

• 在可行的情况下,MRI 是首选检查(可能需要镇静)。

诊断步骤/外科

如果怀疑有中枢神经系统感染且排除了肿块,则可能提示 LP。

鉴别诊断

• 急性脑梗死或出血。

• 颅内感染。

• 快速生长的肿瘤或出血引起的占位效应。

• 痴呆或谵妄或其他原因。

• 中毒性或代谢性脑病。

儿科注意事项

• 如果婴儿头围增长过大、进行性嗜睡、持续性呕吐、向上凝视麻痹,应怀疑脑积水。
- 先天异常：
- Dandy-Walker 畸形。
- Arnold-Chiari 畸形。
- 脊髓脊膜突出。
- 脉络丛乳头状瘤。
- 发育不良或蛛网膜绒毛功能障碍。

• 感染：
- 风疹。
- 巨细胞病毒。
- 弓形虫。
- 梅毒。
- 细菌性脑膜炎。
- 室管膜细胞瘤。

• 出血：
- 脑室内。
- 蛛网膜下。

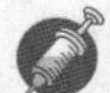

治疗

院前

注意：

• ICP 升高/脑积水无法在院外确诊。

• 如果怀疑脑积水，根据病情需要予以吸氧、管理气道。

• 转运患者时，应抬高头部 0～30°。
- 如果患者有高血压，担心降低脑灌注，不应当抬高床头。
- 高血压初始治疗通常增大剂量和生理盐水一起使用。

初步稳定/治疗

• 有即将形成脑疝的体征：
- 快速插管。
  ◦ 硫喷妥钠或依托咪酯作为诱导。
  ◦ 麻醉的选择是有争议的。
  ◦ 去极化药（琥珀胆碱）可能一过性增加 ICP，这种效果可能不具有临床意义。
  ◦ 非去极化药（罗库溴铵、维库溴铵）可能更好。
- 机械通气，维持 $PaCO_2$ 在 0～35 mmHg。
- 补液或者使用升压药物维持收缩压＞100 mmHg(成人)。
- 甘露醇。

• 如果需要 CSF 分流并且有即将形成脑疝的体征：
- 按压分流阀：
  ◦ 使用 1 ml 盐水冲洗，去除远端堵塞。
  ◦ 缓慢抽出 CSF，达到 ICP＜20 cmH_2O。

急诊治疗/程序

• 脑积水一般不需要急诊治疗，除非出现以下情况：
- 即将形成脑疝的体征。
- 急性引流功能障碍。

• 确定性治疗包括分流装置替代或潜在病因（如肿瘤）的治疗。

• 有神经系统症状（步态失常）或严重头痛而颅内压正常的脑积水，通过腰椎穿刺引流出 CSF(20～30 ml)可能有效。

• 如果脑室内出血（通常来源于创伤或蛛网膜下腔出血）引起急性梗阻性脑积水，可在侧脑室行脑室造瘘术。

• 焦虑或插管的患者应接受镇静治疗。

• 可以使用甘露醇。

• 考虑使用磷苯妥英预防癫痫。

药物治疗

• 阿托品：0.05 mg/kg(最大剂量 0.1 mg)。

• 依托咪酯：0.2～0.3 mg/kg。

• 利多卡因：1 mg/kg，静脉注射。

• 甘露醇：0.5～1.5 g/kg。

• 罗库溴铵：0.6 mg/kg，静脉注射。

• 琥珀胆碱：1～1.5 mg/kg，静脉注射。

• 维库溴铵：0.1 mg/kg。

• 磷苯妥英：15～20 mg/kg 负荷剂量。

随访

进一步处理

入院指征

有 ICP 升高或 CSF 引流障碍的症状需要入院。

出院指征

压力正常的脑积水患者可以出院，继续随访。

转诊问题

在急性梗阻性脑病或急性引流障碍可能需要神经外科会诊。

• 如果当前医院没有神经外科医师，考虑转院。

• 在紧急情况，和转院相比，应优先考虑气道管理。

随访建议

如果患者稳定可以出院，神经科医师和/或神经外科医师随访是必需的。

要点和误区

• 在梗阻性脑积水患者，不应实施腰椎穿刺（有形成脑疝的风险）。

• 儿童头围快速增大，应怀疑脑积水。

• 有脑脊液分流障碍和任何神经系统症状的患者应考虑脑积水。

脑膜炎 Meningitis

Austen-Kum Chai 段立伟 译

基础知识

描述

中枢神经系统感染伴有软脑膜炎症，可表现为脑脊液中白细胞数增高，通常有发热、颈背僵硬、头痛和精神状态改变等症状。

病因

• 细菌：
- 新生儿：B 组链球菌、大肠杆菌或其他肠道杆菌、李斯特菌感染。
- 儿童和成人：肺炎链球菌、脑膜炎奈瑟菌、B 组链球菌和革兰阴性杆菌(＜3 岁)。
- 老年人和饮酒者：肺炎链球菌、革兰阴性杆菌、李斯特菌感染。
- 神经外科手术患者：葡萄球菌和革兰阴性杆菌。
- 移植和透析患者：李斯特菌感染的发病率不断上升。
- AIDS：如上，再加上结核杆菌和梅毒。

• 病毒。

• 真菌。

- 化学、药物或毒素引起的。

诊断

症状和体征

- 一般症状：
- 发热。
- 颈背僵硬：
  - Kernig 征：膝盖弯曲时发生伸展抵抗（双侧）。
  - Brudzinski 征：颈部前屈导致屈曲髋关节。
  - Kernig 征和 Brudzinski 征：对诊断脑膜炎既不敏感也不特异。
- 精神状态改变，头痛。
- 畏光。
- 视乳头水肿。
- 局灶性中枢神经系统异常。
- 癫痫发作，非简单性。
- 瘀点状和紫癜样皮疹（脑膜炎球菌感染）。
- 相关感染：鼻窦炎、中耳炎、肺炎。
- 婴儿和儿童：
- 发热或体温过低。
- 昏睡。
- 吮吸无力。
- 呕吐。
- 脱水。
- 呼吸窘迫。
- 窒息。
- 发绀。
- 囟门膨出。
- 肌张力减退。
- <1 岁儿童通常不会发生脑膜炎。
- 老年人和免疫力低下人群。
- 意识模糊，伴或不伴发热。
- 总体症状不明显。

病史

- 新生儿：早产，分娩并发症，如发热、破膜延长、抗生素使用、B 组链球菌感染。
- 成人：近期旅行史。
- 老年人：肺炎球菌疫苗接种情况。
- 反复感染提示免疫功能缺陷。
- 近期外伤史或耳鼻喉部面部神经系统手术史。
- 分流手术史。

基本检查

- 临床上考虑疑似病例时，立即开始治疗。
- 应在血培养后给予抗生素治疗，如果患者情况不稳定，抗生素治疗应优先于其他的诊断操作。
- 腰椎穿刺（LP）之前的常规 CT 检查是没有必要的，以下情况除外：
- 免疫缺陷/AIDS。
- 中枢神经系统疾病史（脓肿、出血、肿块）。
- 癫痫发作史<7 日。
- 局灶性神经功能缺失。
- 意识水平变化。
- 年龄超过 60 岁。
- 视乳头水肿。
- LP：每个怀疑脑膜炎的患者都要进行检查，除非有禁忌证：
- 有以下情况时可延缓 LP：
  - 存在脑疝风险。
  - 患者状态不稳定。
  - 血小板减少或出血状态。
  - 硬膜外脓肿。
  - 表面软组织感染。
- 脑脊液分析：
- 管 1：细胞计数和分类。
- 管 2：蛋白质和糖。
- 管 3：革兰染色，培养。如果有需要，增加抗酸染色，结核菌培养，墨汁染色和真菌培养，VDRL，隐球菌抗原检测可提高诊断敏感性。
- 管 4：重复细胞计数或存储以便其他检测。
- 检测压力：正常情况下可达 200 mmH_2O。
- 乳胶凝集反应（选择性）：
  - 如果其他检查无诊断意义可进行此项检查。
  - 血液和尿液最好都检查。
  - 可发现的病原体：脑膜炎双球菌、肺炎球菌、B 组链球菌、流感嗜血杆菌、大肠埃希菌、隐球菌。
- PCR 检测（选择性）：
  - 用于病毒（特别是单纯疱疹病毒）和细菌（肺炎链球菌、脑膜炎奈瑟球菌、流感嗜血杆菌 A 和流感嗜血杆菌 B）检测。
- 脑脊液检测结果解读：
  - 培养结果具有诊断性价值。
  - 革兰染色可在培养结果可用前提示细菌感染。
  - 年龄>3 个月的人群，脑脊液中 WBC>4/ml 时，诊断脑膜炎高度敏感。年龄在 20～90 日龄的婴儿，脑脊液中 WBC>9/ml 时诊断敏感性高。
  - 艾滋病患者细胞计数可正常。
  - 新生儿：有些情况下，细胞高达 25 WBC/ml，蛋白质高达 150 mg/dl，早产儿蛋白质高达 100 mg/dl 时也可能是正常现象。
- 典型的细菌性脑膜炎：
  - 脑脊液糖含量<40 mg/dl，糖含量脑脊液/血液<0.6。
  - WBC>500/ml（通常为 1 000～20 000/ml），然而，在疾病早期，WBC 数值可以很低。
  - 多形核中性粒细胞>80%时有提示意义。
  - 脑脊液蛋白质>200 mg/dl，正常<50 mg/dl。

诊断检查与说明

实验室检查

- 在抗生素使用前抽血培养（2 个部位）。
- 尿液培养和尿液分析。
- 血常规，分类计数加血小板。
- 电解质/糖含量检测：
- 计算糖含量脑脊液/血液。
- 代谢性酸中毒评估，抗利尿激素分泌异常综合征评估。
- 根据尿素/肌酐调整药物剂量。
- PT、APTT 和血小板：特别是对于有瘀点和紫癜的患者。
- 存在严重脓毒症或 DIC 时，在 LP 检查前进行。
- 有需要时进行毒物检测。

影像学检查

- CT：参见基本检查部分。
- 胸部 X 线：怀疑肺炎或结核时可考虑。

鉴别诊断

- 脑炎。
- 脑、脊髓、硬膜外脓肿。
- 热性惊厥。
- 中枢神经系统和系统性红斑狼疮脑炎。
- 颅内出血。
- 原发性或转移性中枢神经系统恶性肿瘤。
- 脑卒中（中风）。
- 静脉窦血栓性静脉炎。
- 外伤。
- 毒物/代谢因素。

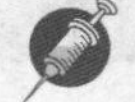

治疗

院前

- 建立静脉通道，吸氧，转运，ABC 管理。
- 对流行性脑脊髓膜炎患者的任何接触者，预防性应用抗生素：
- 成人：
  - 利福平：600 mg，口服，每日 2 次，使用 2 日；或环丙沙星：500 mg，口服，单次，或头孢曲松：250 mg，肌注（如果妊娠）。
- 儿童：

N

◦ 利福平：如果<1月龄，5 mg/kg，如果>1月龄，10 mg/kg，每日2次。

■ 初步稳定/治疗

• 合理的患者隔离。
• ABC管理，治疗癫痫发作。
• 开通静脉通路。
• 根据需要补充葡萄糖。

■ 急诊治疗/程序

• 理想情况下，立即进行LP并给予抗生素±激素治疗。
• 如果LP需要延迟，经验性给予抗生素±激素治疗。
• 如果CT检查可以先于LP进行，应在CT检查前经验性给予抗生素±激素治疗。
• 激素：如果有需要，应先于抗生素治疗或与抗生素治疗同步。
• 抗生素：
- 使用抗生素前先获得血培养结果。
- 除非在十分必要的情况下，不要因为LP或CT检查而延迟抗生素治疗。
• 考虑细菌性脑膜炎的患者，应经验性地给予静脉(或肌内注射)抗生素治疗：
- 新生儿：
◦ 氨苄西林75～100 mg/kg，q6～8 h；+庆大霉素2.5 mg/kg，q8 h或头孢噻肟100 mg/kg，q8 h。
◦ 怀疑单纯疱疹病毒性脑炎的患者加用阿昔洛韦(20 mg/kg，q8 h)。
- >1月龄儿童：
◦ 头孢曲松[100 mg/(kg·d)或50 mg/kg，q12 h]或头孢噻肟(50 mg/kg，q6 h)+万古霉素(15 mg/kg，q8 h)±地塞米松(0.15 mg/kg，q6 h，用4日)。
◦ 免疫缺陷者：另加庆大霉素(2.5 mg/kg，q8 h)或阿米卡星(7.5 mg/kg，q12 h或5 mg/kg，q8 h)。
◦ 中枢神经系统手术患者：万古霉素(15 mg/kg，q8 h)；+美罗培南(40 mg/kg，q8 h)或头孢他啶(50 mg/kg，q8 h)或头孢吡肟(50 mg/kg，q8 h)。
◦ 头部贯通伤：万古霉素(15 mg/kg，q8 h)；+头孢吡肟(50 mg/kg，q8 h)或头孢他啶(50 mg/kg，q8 h)或美罗培南(40 mg/kg)；+庆大霉素(2.5 mg/kg，q8 h)或阿米卡星(5～10 mg/kg，q8 h)。
- 成人：
◦ 头孢曲松(2 g，q12 h)或头孢噻肟(2 g，q4～6 h)+万古霉素[15～20 mg/kg，q8～12 h，最大不超过2 g/次或60 g/(kg·d)]+地塞米松(15 mg/kg，直到10 g，q6 h，静脉注射，如果病原菌为肺炎链球菌则用4日)。
◦ >50岁患者：再加氨苄西林(2 g，q4 h)以覆盖李斯特菌。
◦ 免疫受损患者：万古霉素(15～20 mg/kg，q8～12 h)+氨苄西林(2 g，q4 h)+美罗培南(2 g，q8 h)或头孢吡肟(2 g，q8 h)。
◦ 中枢神经系统手术，分流术，头部外伤：万古霉素(15～20 mg/kg，q8～12 h)+美罗培南(2 g)。
◦ 肾功能正常患者的万古霉素剂量：50～89 kg(1 g，q12 h)，90～130 kg(1.5 g，q12 h)，>130 kg(2 g，q12 h)。
• 其他考虑使用的药：
- 地塞米松：
◦ 有无受益尚无定论。
◦ 可能使患流感嗜血杆菌脑膜炎的儿童受益，也可能使患肺炎链球菌脑膜炎的>6周龄的儿童和成人受益。
◦ 患者有精神状态改变，局灶性神经功能丧失，视乳头水肿或中枢神经系统创伤，手术，或占位性病变时，应提前或与抗生素同时使用。当脑脊液颜色昏暗，存在革兰染色阳性菌，或WBC>1 000/mm^3时，应使用地塞米松。
- 青霉素过敏(严重)：
◦ 氨曲南或氯霉素可用来代替头孢菌素类。
◦ 不要拖延治疗较轻的过敏史。
- 万古霉素：
◦ 考虑为青霉素耐药的肺炎链球菌感染时，应使用万古霉素。
- 当怀疑为单纯疱疹病毒性脑炎时，应使用阿昔洛韦。

■ 药物治疗

• 阿昔洛韦：30 mg/(kg·d)，q8 h，静脉注射[新生儿：20 mg/(kg·d)，q8 h，静脉注射]。
• 阿米卡星：儿童7.5 mg/kg，q12 h或5 mg/kg，q8 h，静脉注射。新生儿首次10 mg/kg，后7.5 mg/kg，q12 h，静脉注射。
• 氨苄西林：2 g(儿童：30 mg/kg)，q6～8 h，静脉注射，最大剂量6～8 g/d。
• 氨曲南：2 g，q4 h(儿童：50～100 mg/kg，q6～8 h)静脉注射，最大剂量12 g/d。
• 复方新诺明：5～10 mg/kg，甲氧苄啶，q12 h，静脉注射。
• 头孢吡肟：2 g，q8 h，静脉注射，最大剂量6 g/d。
• 头孢噻肟：2 g(儿童：50 mg/kg)，q6 h，静脉注射，最大剂量8～12 g/d。
• 头孢他啶：2 g，q8 h，静脉注射，最大剂量6 g/d。
• 头孢曲松钠：2 g(儿童：50～75 mg/kg)，q6 h，静脉注射，最大剂量4 g/d。
• 氯霉素：1～1.5 g(儿童：12.5 mg/kg)，q6 h，静脉注射，最大剂量4～6 g/d。
• 地塞米松：10 mg(儿童：0.15 mg/kg)，q6 h，静脉注射，用4日。
• 庆大霉素：儿童2.5 mg/kg，q8 h，静脉注射。
• 美罗培南：2 g(儿童：40 mg/kg)，q8 h，静脉注射，最大剂量6 g/d。
• 妥布霉素：儿童：2.5 mg/kg，q8 h，静脉注射。
• 万古霉素：1～2 g，q8～12 h，静脉注射，(儿童：12 mg/kg，q8 h)。
• 万古霉素和氨基糖苷类药物：肾功能和血清浓度水平调整。
• 剂量仅供参考，假设肝肾功能正常。

随访

■ 进一步处理

入院指征

• 已知或疑似细菌感染。
• 免疫力低下宿主。
• 任何中毒症状表现的患者。

出院指征

• 清除病毒感染，症状控制良好。
• 症状得到控制。
• 深入和具体的出院指导。
• 在出院前与初级保健医师仔细探讨并建立详细的随访计划。

要点和误区

• 脑膜炎在儿童一般不表现为简单的热性惊厥。
• 诊断失误或治疗不及时会对患者造成灾难性后果，而且并不罕见，很可能给医师带来医疗纠纷。
• 决策要果断，及时询问专家的意见，药房及时发药，医院感染控制及时跟进。

N

脑膜炎球菌血症 Meningococcemia

Brian D. Euerle 段立伟 译

基础知识

描述

• 脑膜炎奈瑟菌导致的细菌感染。
• 可表现为多种疾病形式。
• 轻度脑膜炎球菌血症。
• 严重脑膜炎球菌脓毒症。
• 脑膜炎球菌性脑膜炎。
• 慢性/潜伏性脑膜炎球菌血症。
• 化脓性关节炎。
• 通过与感染者或无症状携带者的亲密接触获得。
• 亲密的接吻和吸烟行为是患病的独立危险因素。

病因

• 脑膜炎奈瑟菌：
- 血清型 A、B、C、D、H、I、K、L、X、Y、Z、29E 和 W135。
- 在美国，血清 B 型最常见。
- 大多数感染是由血清型 A、B、C、Y 和 W135 引起的。
• 细菌附着并进入鼻咽部上皮细胞。
• 细菌从鼻咽进入血管内皮细胞，进而通过血流播撒。
• 循环中的大多数脑膜炎球菌被脾脏清除。
• 脑膜炎球菌可产生内毒素(脂聚糖)：
- 参与皮肤病变、肾上腺表现和血管塌陷的病理过程。
• 人类的口咽、鼻咽部是唯一的细菌存储库。
• 携带者通常会产生针对特定血清亚型的抗体(不能对所有血清型免疫)：
- 年龄<5 岁：1%的携带率。
- 年龄 20～40 岁：30%～40%的携带率。
- 儿童免疫率较低，进而表现为感染率较高。
• 常见于春季和秋季。
• 在军营、密集的居住条件下发病率增加。
• 容易发生流行感染的人群，其年龄大多在 5～9 岁或更早。

诊断

症状和体征

• 轻度脑膜炎球菌血症：
- 最常见的。
- 继发于上呼吸道感染。
- 发热、寒战、肌痛、关节痛、全身乏力。
- 通常为自限性，数日后缓解。
- 可以发展为脑膜炎(死亡率为 2%～10%)或不伴有脑膜炎的严重脓毒症。
• 严重脑膜炎球菌脓毒症：
- 占总脑膜炎球菌血症病例的 10%。
- 高死亡率(20%～60%)。
- 大多数死亡事件发生在第一个 48 h。
- 突然发病，病程进展快。
- 初期表现可能较轻：
◦ 轻度心动过速。
◦ 轻度呼吸急促、呼吸道症状。
◦ 轻度低血压。
- 发热、寒战、呕吐、头痛、皮疹、肌肉触痛。
- 中毒表现。
- 婴幼儿：嗜睡、拒食、囟门膨出。
- 皮疹：
◦ 紫癜/瘀斑混合出现。
◦ 受累皮肤此后可能会表现出聚结、坏死/脱落(暴发性紫癜)。
◦ 瘀斑(皮肤、黏膜、结膜)可见于 50%～60%病例。
◦ 斑疹。
◦ 丘疹(丘疹刮除后用革兰染色可见病原体)。
- 数小时内迅速恶化：
◦ 低血压或休克。
◦ 酸中毒。
◦ 急性呼吸窘迫综合征(ARDS)。
◦ 弥散性血管内凝血(DIC)。
- 可伴或不伴脑膜炎。
- 沃-弗综合征：
◦ 双侧肾上腺出血性破坏。
◦ 血管舒缩崩溃。
- 急性肾衰竭：
◦ 长期低血压导致(肾脏低灌注导致急性肾小管坏死)。
• 慢性脑膜炎球菌血症：
- 罕见。
- 温和出现。
- 反复发热、寒战、关节痛迁延数周到数月。
- 间歇性皮疹：四肢部位皮疹疼痛。
- 游走性多关节炎。
- 脾大(20%)。
- 脑膜炎球菌性脑膜炎(25%)：
- 头痛。
- 发热。
- 颈部僵硬。
- 意识模糊。
- 昏睡。
- 反应迟钝。
• 化脓性关节炎：
- 发生于脑膜炎球菌血症活动期。
- 涉及多个关节。
- 关节疼痛、发红、肿胀、积液、发热、畏寒。
- 四肢运动受限或无法运动。
• 其他脑膜炎球菌感染类型：
- 发生在其他部位的脑膜炎球菌感染。
- 结膜炎：可单独出现。
- 鼻窦炎。
- 全眼球炎。
- 尿道炎。
- 输卵管炎。
- 前列腺炎。
- 肺炎。
- 心肌炎和心包炎：
◦ 发生在发病后期。
◦ 通常与血清 C 型相关。

病史

疾病进展存在变异性，可分为轻度、重度和慢性这几类。

体格检查

• 心动过速。
• 低血压，疾病初期可为轻度的。
• 进展性，快速恶化。
• 表现为 ARDS 特征的呼吸衰竭。
• 瘀斑样皮疹可见于 50%～80%病例。
- 累及腋窝、肋下、腕部、膝部。

基本检查

• 不可因检查操作(包括腰椎穿刺)推迟对疑似脑膜炎球菌血症的患者使用抗生素。
• 存在一系列戏剧性的临床表现时应怀疑诊断的正确性。
• 革兰染色和培养：
- 外周血、脑脊液(CSF)、痰液、尿液、关节抽吸物或瘀斑/丘疹刮出物。
- 革兰染色：出现在细胞内或细胞外的革兰阴性双球菌。

诊断检查与说明

实验室检查

• CBC：

- 疾病初始白细胞升高，在严重病例后期可能会抑制。
- 当发生大面积紫癜、瘀斑或 DIC 时，血小板计数会减少。

• 电解质、BUN、肌酐、葡萄糖。
• CSF：
- 革兰染色、培养、蛋白质和葡萄糖、细胞分类计数。
- 与细菌性脑膜炎表现一致。
• 动脉血气检查明确酸中毒、缺氧情况。
• 如果怀疑 DIC，查纤维蛋白原水平、纤维蛋白降解产物、PT、APTT。
• 喉/鼻咽拭子：
- 检测阳性时尚不能诊断脑膜炎球菌血症。
• 如果怀疑脓毒症，应进行外周血红细胞沉降率棕黄色涂层分析。
• 血培养：
- 在慢性脑膜炎球菌血症常为阴性。
- 在轻度和严重脑膜炎球菌血症阳性。
• 免疫分析(注意假阴性)。
• 聚合酶链反应(PCR)，特别适合在标本采集前已给予抗生素的病例。

影像学检查

胸部 X 线：ARDS/肺炎。

诊断步骤/外科

可能有必要进行四肢和/或坏死组织的截肢和清创。

鉴别诊断

• 病毒疹。
• 血管炎。
• 支原体。
• 落基山斑疹热。
• 中毒性休克综合征。
• 过敏性紫癜。
• 特发性血小板减少性紫癜(ITP)。
• 骨痛热症。
• 播散性淋球菌感染。
• 流感。
• A 组和 B 组链球菌感染。
• 血栓性血小板减少性紫癜。

治疗

院前

与患者密切接触的个人需要暴露后预防。

初步稳定/治疗

• 戴上口罩和手套，警惕飞沫。
• 通知卫生管理部门。
• ABC 管理。
• 严重酸中毒、缺氧或意识状态下降时立即气管插管：
- 过度通气以治疗酸中毒(PCO_2 目标值为 25 mmHg)。
• 治疗低血压：
- 给予生理盐水，20 ml/kg，急性呼吸窘迫综合征和充血性心力衰竭患者应谨慎补液。
- 如果在静脉注射 2 L 液体后仍低血压，开始给予多巴胺和去甲肾上腺素(如无反应，给予肾上腺素)。
• 意识状态改变患者给予纳洛酮、硫胺素、葡萄糖。
• 初始静脉使用抗生素：
- 一线：大剂量青霉素(确诊为脑膜炎球菌血症患者)或第三代头孢菌素(对于待确诊患者，覆盖范围更广)。
- 二线：氨苄西林。
- 三线：氯霉素(青霉素过敏患者)。

急诊治疗/程序

• 严重脑膜炎球菌性脓毒症。
• 严重酸中毒(pH 7.0～7.1 及以下或血清 HCO_3^- 8～10 mmol/L 及以下)。
- 静脉给予 $NaHCO_3$ 并予以过度换气。
• 插入导尿管监测尿量。
• 呼吸道隔离。
• 大剂量的激素：
- 在持续感染情况下防止脑神经损伤(有争议)。
- 存在肾上腺损伤情况下。
• DIC 治疗：
- 新鲜冰冻血浆和血小板输注。
- 除非有明显的血栓并发症临床表现(如发绀或足趾冰冷，尽管容量充足血压正常，但尿量少)，一般不使用肝素。
• 密切接触者的预防措施：
- 理想情况下，预防药物应第一个 24 h 之内给予。
- 10 日的观察窗口期。
- 亚型特异性疫苗只作为辅助措施。
• 疫苗：
- 推荐在军营、流行地区的旅客、补体缺陷或无脾脏患者，住宿舍的大学一年级新生使用疫苗。
- 年龄在 11～18 岁的人群常规推荐注射疫苗。

妊娠注意事项

孕妇使用脑膜炎球菌疫苗的安全性不明确。

药物治疗

一线用药

• 头孢噻肟：2 g(儿童：50 mg/kg)，静脉注射，q6 h。
• 头孢曲松：2 g(儿童：50 mg/kg)，静脉注射，q12 h。
• 青霉素：400 万 U[儿童：25 万 U/(kg·d)]，静脉注射，q4 h。

二线用药

• 氨苄西林：2～3 g[儿童：200～400 mg/(kg·d)]，静脉注射，q6 h。
• 氯霉素：50～100 mg/(kg·d)，静脉注射，q6 h，最大剂量 4 g/d。
• 预防性药物：
- 单剂量头孢曲松：
◦ 年龄<15 岁，125 mg，肌内注射。
◦ 年龄>15 岁，250 mg，肌内注射。
- 环丙沙星：500 mg，口服(成人)。
- 利福平：600 mg(儿童：5～10 mg/kg)，口服，2 次/日，用 2 日。
- 阿奇霉素：单剂 500 mg，口服(不常规使用)。
• 地塞米松：小儿脑膜炎患者 0.15 mg/kg，静脉注射。
• 多巴胺：5～20 μg/(kg·min)，静脉注射，根据血压调整。
• 肾上腺素：2～10 μg/(kg·min)，静脉注射，根据血压调整。
• 肝素：首剂 3 000～5 000 U(儿童：80 U/kg)，静脉推射，后 600～1 000 U/h[儿童：18 U/(kg·h)]静脉滴注。
• 氢化可的松：肾上腺皮质功能不全患者 100 mg(儿童：2 mg/kg)，静脉推注，q8 h。
• 脑膜炎球菌多糖：0.5 ml，肌内注射 1 次。
• 脑膜炎球菌疫苗：0.5 ml，皮下注射 1 次。
• 去甲肾上腺素：0.5～30 μg/min，静脉注射，根据血压调整。
• 碳酸氢钠：2～5 mmol/kg(儿童：0.5～1 mmol/kg)，静脉注射，持续时间 30 min 到 4 h。

随访

进一步处理

入院指征

• 严重脓毒症伴呼吸道隔离患者入住 ICU。
• 轻度脑膜炎球菌血症患者行呼吸道隔离。

出院指征

和患者有密切接触者要给予预防性药物

N

治疗。

转诊问题

• 因出现多器官衰竭较常见，应考虑转诊到三级治疗中心。

• 后续出现的神经科、心血管科和骨科并发症可能需要相应专家指导治疗。

▪ 随访建议

• 完成足够疗程的抗生素治疗。

• 24 h 后不再需要呼吸道预防。

• 所有密切接触者均需使用预防性药物进行治疗。

要点和误区

• 出现任何疑似病例均需通知卫生管理部门。

• 警惕迟发性心脏压塞的发生。

• 抗生素治疗不容迟疑。

脑室腹膜分流 Ventricular Peritoneal Shunts

Richard S. Krause 吴昊 李文放 译

 基础知识

▪ 描述

• 脑室腹膜(VP)分流通常用于脑积水：

- 脑脊液和腹腔(或右心房 VA 分流)之间的导管。

• 需要翻修的并发症很常见。

• 梗阻：分流术失败者行脑脊液引流：

- 增加颅内压(ICP)。
- ICP 的增长率决定了严重程度。
- 第一年有 30%～40%的概率出现装置机械故障。

• 过度排水综合征：

- 直立姿势增加 CSF 流出。
- 降低 ICP。
- 产生姿势性头痛和恶心(如腰椎穿刺后)。

• 感染：

- 分流管路是异物。
- 表皮葡萄球菌等和其他葡萄球菌占感染的 75%。
- 也含有革兰阴性菌。
- 耐多药金黄色葡萄球菌(MRSA)已有报道。
- 大多数发生在放置后不久。
- 通常需要去除分流器。

• 狭窄脑室综合征：

- 长期过量引起脑室大小减少。
- 由于近端阻塞导致 ICP 间歇性增加。

儿科注意事项

• 并发症在儿童中尤其常见，特别是新生儿。

• 如果颅缝是开放的，CSF 可能会积聚，ICP 增加很少。

• 产生相对非刺激性反应和症状：

- 昏昏欲睡。
- 头痛。
- 恶心和呕吐。

▪ 病因

• 由于以下原因可能需要分流来治疗 ICP 升高：

- 先天性畸形。
- 特发性颅内高压症(假性脑肿瘤)。
- 脑血管意外后。
- 肿瘤或其他肿块病变。
- 头部创伤。
- 蛛网膜下腔出血。
- 细菌性脑膜炎后脑部基部的瘢痕。

诊断

▪ 症状和体征

• 分流阻塞：

- 头痛。
- 恶心。
- 心神不安，全身无力，烦躁不安。
- 意识水平下降(LOC)。
- 头部增大或囟门膨胀。
- 癫痫发作：新发或增加发作频率。
- 自发不稳定。
- 向上凝视减少。
- 窒息。
- 视乳头水肿，罕见。

• 过度排水综合征：

- 头痛、局灶性神经系统体征、不适、癫痫发作、昏迷。
- 体征和症状通常和姿势有关。

• 快速过度引流可能导致脑干向上移位，导致脑疝症状和体征：

- 呼吸暂停。
- 心动过缓。
- LOC 降低。

• 分流感染：

- 发热(也可能没有)。
- 脑膜刺激征。
- 局部感染迹象(红斑、肿胀、压痛)。
- 腹膜炎(可引起逆行 CSF 感染)。
- 分流后很快会发生感染(约 80%：6 个月后)。
- 感染是分流功能不全的一个原因，可随着颅内压增高而出现。

• 狭窄脑室综合征：

- 连发性头痛。
- 正常行为和嗜睡的交替出现。
- 头痛、恶心和呕吐。

病史

• 分流布置的时机。

• 分流原因。

• 最近的安置导管/修正。

体格检查

• 精神状态改变。

• 局灶性神经缺陷。

• 发热。

• 红斑或轻度分流。

▪ 基本检查

• 怀疑分流故障：

- 增压室的操作：
  ◦ 增压室应该在 3 s 内完成补充和补充。
  ◦ 压力不足意味着失去作用梗阻。
  ◦ 未能弥补近端障碍。
  ◦ 多达 40%的故障分流器正常压缩/填充。
- 头部 CT。
- 分流相关检查：
  ◦ 颅骨、胸部、腹部的 X 线片。
  ◦ 有助于诊断分流、错位或分流组件的扭结。

• 可疑感染：

- 来自分流脑室的脑脊液(与神经外科医师协商)：
  ◦ 可以使用无菌技术和 23G 蝴蝶针进行。
  ◦ 慢慢地抽取 5～10 ml 脑脊液以进一步

N

研究。

■ 诊断检查与说明

实验室检查

• 电解质、肾功能和葡萄糖。
• 抗惊厥分级。
• CBC。
• 怀疑感染：
- 来自分流储器的 CSF 分析：
◦ 送培养、细胞计数、革兰染色、葡萄糖和蛋白质水平分析。
◦ CSF 分析早期结果可能是正常的，尤其是在事先进行抗生素治疗情况下的血培养。

影像学检查

• 头部 CT：比较脑室大小并评估导管位置。
- 脑室扩大：分流泵故障。
- 小脑室：过度引流。
- 与以前的扫描结果对比分析最有用。
- 诊断硬膜下血肿。
• 美国：用于开放囟门的儿童抽取分流尖端的位置并评估脑室大小。

诊断步骤/外科

• 如果出现分流故障症状，但 CT 扫描无法判断，则下一步可以检测分流头：
- 分流术：高压＞20 cmH$_2$O 意味着分流阻塞。
- 也试图评估中枢神经系统感染。

■ 鉴别诊断

• 癫痫（特发性、中毒性、代谢性）。
• 感染：
- 中枢神经系统感染与分流无关。
- 全身感染。
• 代谢异常：
- 低血糖低钠血症。
- 缺氧。
• 中毒。
• 头部外伤。

治疗

■ 院前

• 分流功能障碍的患者有呼吸暂停和呼吸停止的风险。
• 应密切监测呼吸状况，应用氧气。
• 怀疑增加 ICP 时，头部抬高至 30°的运输患者。

■ 初步稳定/治疗

• 即将发生疝的症状：
- 快速序列插管和控制通气至 P_{CO_2} 约 35 mmHg。
- 考虑用利多卡因预处理（儿童＜5 岁：加阿托品）。
- 硫喷妥钠或依托咪酯用于诱导。
- 琥珀胆碱可使 ICP 增加几毫米汞柱，但这可能并不具有临床意义。
- 如果选择去极化剂，只使用非脱敏剂的预处理剂量。
- 非去极化剂（罗库溴铵）可能是优选的。
• 分流室的强制泵送：
- 用 1 ml 盐水溶液冲洗装置以去除远端阻塞物。
- 允许从储器中缓慢排出 CSF 以实现＜20 cmH$_2$O 的压力。
• 静脉给甘露醇降低 ICP。
• 脑室穿刺和脑脊液引流是创伤较小的手术，若不成功则神经外科手术就不可避免。
• 癫痫持续状态：用苯二氮䓬类（劳拉西泮）。

■ 急诊治疗/程序

• 早期向神经外科医师咨询。
• 分流故障：
- 将床头抬高至 30°。
- 在某些轻度病例中，应用利尿剂（甘露醇、呋塞米）进行医学管理可能适用。
• 过度排水综合征：
- 保持患者的仰卧位。
- 补充容量。
• 分流感染：
- 全身性抗生素：
◦ 万古霉素加头孢噻肟，如果怀疑为革兰阴性则用庆大霉素。

■ 药物治疗

• 成人和小儿剂量：
- 阿托品：0.02 mg/kg，静脉注射（最小 0.1 mg）。
- 头孢噻肟：1～2 g（50 mg/kg），静脉注射或肌内注射，q8～12 h。
- 呋塞米：1 mg/kg，静脉注射。
- 庆大霉素：2～5 mg/kg，静脉注射。
- 利多卡因：1 mg/kg，静脉注射。
- 甘露醇：1 g/kg，静脉注射。
- 罗库溴铵：1 mg/kg，静脉注射。
- 琥珀胆碱：1.5 mg/kg，静脉注射。
- 万古霉素：15 mg/kg 负荷剂量，静脉注射。
- 维库溴铵：0.08～0.1 mg/kg，静脉注射。

随访

■ 进一步处理

入院指征

• 分流并发症患者通常需要神经外科会诊和住院。
• 经常需要 ICU 或其他监测设置。

出院指征

当能排除分流故障时，则取决于替代诊断和患者状况。

要点和误区

• 避免分流患者的“隧道视力”，并考虑其他原因。
• 严重的便秘可能会增加。
• 在腹腔压力和减少排水导致增加 ICP：
- 便秘的治疗可以改善明显的“分流故障”。

脑血管意外 Cerebrovascular Accident

Veronique Au · Rebecca Smith-Coggins 庄育刚 译

基础知识

■ 描述

血流中断进入特定脑区域：
• 受影响区域有明确的神经检查异常。
• 突然、断断续续或者间歇发生和结束。
• 美国每年有 795 000 例卒中。

■ 危险因素

• 糖尿病。
• 吸烟。

N

• 高血压。
• 冠心病，心律失常。
• 心律失常。
• 外周血管病变。
• 口服避孕药。
• 真性红细胞增多症。
• 镰状细胞贫血。
• 抗血栓Ⅲ、蛋白C、蛋白S缺乏症。

病因

• 可能是缺血（血栓、栓塞、继发于剥离/低灌注）或者出血。
• 由于血管堵塞导致血栓性脑卒中：
- 最常见于溃疡性动脉粥样硬化部位的斑块形成。
- 血流淤滞（镰状细胞贫血、真性红细胞增多症、蛋白C缺乏）。
• 急性脑血管堵塞引起的栓塞性脑卒中是由于小片颅外物质堵塞脑血管引起的，包括：
- 二尖瓣狭窄、房颤、心肌病、慢性心功能不全或心肌梗死导致的心室壁血栓。
- 人工瓣膜或瓣膜异常。
- 主动脉或者颈内动脉粥样硬化斑块。
- 心房黏液瘤。
- 心室瘤样扩张的血栓。
• 动脉异常：
- 颈动脉夹层。
- 动脉炎（巨细胞、大动脉炎）。
- 肌纤维发育异常。
• 脓毒血症、出血或休克导致的收缩压下降引起的全身缺血或者低灌注。
• 出血性脑卒中。
- 颅内出血。
- 蛛网膜下腔出血。

儿科注意事项

• 通常是某些疾病的表现，如镰状细胞贫血、白血病、感染或血质不调。
• 幼儿通常表现为癫痫和/或精神状态改变。

诊断

症状和体征

病史

• 起病时间（或发现疾病的时间）。
• 药物史。
• 精神状态改变、昏迷。
• 头痛。
• 眩晕、头晕。
• 神经定位缺陷。

体格检查

• 一般生命体征：
- 潮式呼吸、窒息。
- 高血压。
- 心律失常。
• 大脑前动脉：
- 对侧偏瘫（下/上）。
- 半身感觉缺失。
- 运动障碍。
- 昏迷。
- 定向障碍。
• 大脑中动脉：
- 对侧偏瘫（上/下）。
- 半身感觉障碍。
- 同侧偏盲。
- 中枢性言语障碍。
- 构音障碍。
- 失认症。
- 失语症。
• 大脑后动脉：
- 皮质视野半盲。
- 视觉失认症。
- 神志改变。
- 记忆力受损。
- 动眼神经麻痹。
- 偏侧投掷症（舞蹈动作）。
• 椎基底动脉系统：
- 视力受损，视野缺失，眼球震颤，复视。
- 眩晕，头晕。
- 交差功能缺陷：同侧脑神经受损，对侧运动感觉受损。
• 基底动脉：
- 四肢麻痹。
- 闭锁综合征。
- 昏迷。
• 分水岭区域（各前中后循环交界区）：
- 皮质视野盲。
- 近端四肢乏力，一侧肢体肌力下降，中枢性面瘫。

基本检查

• 根据NHISS进行细致的神经功能检查。
• 急诊头颅CT区分脑出血或者缺血。
- 可能在24～48 h无异常。
- 目标：达到后25 min内行CT检查，45 min内由放射科医师读片，60 min内开始溶栓。
• 若CT检查正常或怀疑蛛网膜下腔出血，则有腰椎穿刺指征。
• 心电图评估有无心律失常或心肌梗死。
• 氧饱和度测定。
• 快速血糖测定。

诊断检查与说明

实验室检查

• 血常规、电解质、肝肾功能、PT、APTT。
• 尿液检查：血尿有助于发现亚急性细菌性心内膜炎引起的栓塞。
• 红细胞沉降率：有助于发现亚急性细菌性心内膜炎、血管炎和高血黏综合征。
• 可选的检查：心肌酶、尿妊娠试验、药物测定、酒精浓度测定、动脉血气分析、血培养。

影像学检查

• 头颅CT。
• 头颈CT血管造影或CT灌注研究。
• 脑MRI±弥散加权成像或灌注加权成像。
• MRI血管造影。
• MRI可发现2 h内缺血。
• 胸部X线检查。
• 颈动脉超声。

诊断步骤/外科

• 心电图评估心律失常。
• 怀疑蛛网膜下腔出血行腰椎穿刺。

鉴别诊断

• 颅内实质出血。
• 低血糖。
• 癫痫发作。
• 惊恐发作、抑郁、反常反应。
• 一过性遗忘。
• 脑膜炎。
• 周围神经病。
• 偏头痛。
• 空气栓塞。
• 一过性缺血发作。
• 脑病。
• 脑肿瘤。
• 巨细胞、大血管炎。
• 多发性硬化。
• 脊髓压迫。
• 前庭炎。
• 药物影响/中毒。

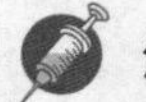

治疗

院前

• 患者可能移动和交流困难。
• 必要的神经系统检查：
- 昏迷程度、格拉斯哥评分、运动评分、言语异常、步态改变、面部不协调和其他神经功能缺陷。

• 末梢血糖。

• 必须验证发病时间或"上次见正常时间"。

• 已经设计了多个院前评分来早期识别 LVO：

– FAST – ED 量表（紧急目的地的现场评估卒中分类）。

– 辛辛那提院前卒中量表（CPSS）和辛辛那提院前卒中量表（CPSSS）。

– 洛杉矶院前卒中量表（LAPSS）。

– 快速动脉闭塞量表（RACE）。

– 认识急诊室脑卒中（ROSIER）。

– 对 NIHSS 的修改。

■ 初步稳定/治疗

• 气道管理。

– 吸氧 2～4 L。

– 气道保护机制受损或进行机械通气降低颅内压，迅速气管内插管。

• 神志改变可考虑给纳洛酮和维生素 B_1 并测定血糖。

■ 急诊治疗/程序

• 溶栓：

– 仅适用于缺血性卒中；在症状出现 4.5 h 内进行。

• 静脉溶栓治疗的禁忌证。

– 头颅 CT 平扫显示出血。

– 之前 3 个月内有脑血管意外病史。

– 之前 3 个月内有严重颅脑外伤、椎管内手术、颅内手术史。

– 颅内出血病史。

– 轴内的颅内肿瘤。

– 临床表现与蛛网膜下腔出血相一致。

– 已知的结构性消化道肿瘤。

– 21 日内的消化道出血。

– 可能的脓毒性栓子；怀疑感染性心内膜炎。

– 主动脉弓夹层。

– 无法控制的高血压，血压水平＞185/110 mmHg。

– 已知的出血体质，比如

◦ 血小板计数小于 100 000/mm^3（如果没有血小板减少病史可以启动溶栓，但如果检验结果回报血小板数量低则应停止溶栓）。

◦ 过去 24 h 内使用过低分子肝素。

◦ 使用华法林抗凝（除非 INR≤1.7 和/或 PT＜15 s）。

◦ 之前 48 h 内使用过直接凝血酶抑制剂或因子Ⅹ抑制剂（除非药物特异活性检测结果正常）。

◦ 使用了血小板膜糖蛋白Ⅱb/Ⅲa 受体抑制剂。

– 血糖＜50 mg/dl（2.8 mmol/L），除非低血糖纠正后症状依然持续。

– CT 上显示超过 1/3 大脑半球存在低密度灶。

• 发作 6 h 内的大血管闭塞性卒中，合适的患者可以考虑血栓切除术。

– 一些卒中中心会延长该干预时间窗至最多 24 h。

• 颅内压升高和脑水肿的治疗：

– 床头抬高 30°。

– 控制通气保持二氧化碳分压在 35～40 mmHg。

– 甘露醇。

• 由椎基底动脉卒中或出血导致的脑干受压可能需要紧急神经外科减压。

• 完全性脑卒中和轻微卒中患者，口服阿司匹林可能预防复发。

> **注意**
>
> 美国 FDA 给 Altepline 开的最新处方信息取消了对既往脑卒中、癫痫发作、特定化验值、特定血压测量、脑卒中严重程度（包括轻微症状）的标准。

■ 药物治疗

一线用药

• 阿替普酶（t – PA）：0.9 mg/kg，静脉注射，最大剂量为 90 mg。超过 1 h：

– 在 1 min 内单次给予 10%的剂量。

– 紧随其后，在随后的 59 min 内输注。

• 拉贝洛尔：10 mg 静脉注射 1～2 min；然后，如果需要：

– 重复或加倍剂量 q10～20 min 至最大 300 mg；或开始以 2～8 mg/min 的速度滴注。

• 阿司匹林：81～325 mg 口服或灌肠。

二线用药

• 氯吡格雷：75 mg/d，口服。

• 氯维地平：滴注 1～2 mg/h；滴定向上的每 2～5 min 加倍剂量至最大剂量 21 mg/h。

• 地西泮：5 mg，静脉注射，q5～10 min，最大 20 mg。

• 依那普利：0.675～1.25 mg，静脉注射。

• 肼屈嗪：10～20 mg，静脉注射，q30 min。

• 甘露醇（15%～20%溶液）：0.5～2 g/kg，静脉注射，5～10 min，然后 0.5～1 g/kg，q4～6 h。

• 尼卡地平：5 mg/h，每 5～15 min 增加 2.5 mg/h，最大 15 mg/h。

• 硝普钠：0.25～10 μg/(kg · min)，静脉注射。

• 阿方那特：1～4 mg/min，静脉注射。

儿科注意事项

• 儿童缺血性脑卒中常用肝素或低分子肝素。

随访

■ 进一步处理

入院指征

• 所有患者必须入院。

• 收住 ICU 指征：

– 意识水平严重下降。

– 血流动力学不稳定。

– 致命性心律失常。

– 颅内压显著增高。

– 接受阿替普酶治疗。

出院指征

• 患者经过数日或者数周治疗后若功能恢复或者有足够的社会支持，可考虑出院。

• 既往有类似发作而且新发症状轻微患者可做门诊治疗，或者本次脑卒中恢复达到上述标准也可考虑出院。

■ 随访建议

• 神经内科。

• 基础护理。

• 语言治疗、康复治疗。

要点和误区

• 始终注意院前报告。

• 早期症状对使用阿替普酶至关重要，包含在 3～4.5 h 注意事项。

• 注意积极的降压处理可能带来的脑低灌注。

• 从进入医院到开始治疗＜60 min。

• 考虑动脉内治疗 LVO。

N

脑炎 Encephalitis

Roger M. Barkin · Mary Saunders 单怡 译

基础知识

描述

- 脑部的急性炎症。
- 美国每年发病 2 000 例。
- 死亡率：10%。
- 脑实质的炎症反应伴随神经元的破坏、脑实质水肿和点状出血。
- 中枢神经系统的感染途径通常是出血。
  - 呼吸道或消化道。
  - 血液传播。
  - 器官移植。
- 狂犬病病毒、单纯疱疹病毒（HSV）和水痘-带状疱疹病毒（VZV）侵犯神经发生脑炎。

病因

- 病毒感染最常见。
- 非感染性：
  - 自身免疫、附肿瘤性、胶原血管病。
- 50%的病例病因不明。

特殊病毒

- 单纯疱疹病毒（HSV）：
  - 占所有脑炎的 10%～20%。
  - 原发或继发。
  - 早期治疗可以改善预后。
- 虫媒病毒：
  - 占所有脑炎的 10%～15%。
  - 在温暖的季节，以动物传播（蚊子、蜱）为主。
  - 东部马脑炎病毒可以导致暴发性脑炎。
    - 聚集于海马区。
    - 暴发性的头痛、发热、呕吐和进行性昏迷。
  - 西部马脑炎病毒大多发生在美国西部 2/3 区域：
    - 早期多有非特异性上呼吸道、消化道症状。
  - 日本，在全世界最广泛流行的虫媒病毒性脑炎：
    - 顽固性的发热、头痛、肌痛和疲劳，继而出现意识障碍、谵妄、面具脸和震颤麻痹、抽搐、脑干功能障碍、水肿，最终死亡。
- 黄病毒属：
  - 西尼罗病毒，在北美的发生率有所增加：
    - 存在于蚊子和鸟类。
    - 为发热性疾病，通常伴随皮疹。
    - 头痛。
    - 淋巴结肿大。
    - 多关节病。
    - 老年人的发病率、病死率增加。
  - 弛缓性瘫痪可以导致呼吸衰竭，致死率可达 50%。
- 肠道病毒：
  - 主要发生在<10 岁的儿童。
  - 病程相对较轻，很少或几乎不遗留长期的后遗症。
- 风疹性脑炎：
  - 首次感染出现皮疹后几日至 2～3 周后发病，或者经过几年的潜伏感染后发病。
  - 迅速发病并且快速进展至昏迷。
  - 癫痫常见（50%～60%）。
  - 接种疫苗后的发生率为 1/100 万。
- 艾滋病性脑炎：
  - CD4 计数低易发生脑炎。
  - 典型表现包括运动痉挛状态和痴呆。
  - 侵犯白质的广泛神经元变性。
- 棒状病毒：狂犬病病毒。
  - 表现为中枢神经系统的感染而缺少全身感染症状。

非病毒性

- 肺炎支原体。
- 刚地弓形虫。
- 立克次体。
- 结核分枝杆菌。
- 伯氏疏螺旋体。
- 巴尔通体。

免疫低下者/艾滋病患者

- 组织胞浆菌属。
- 新型隐球菌。
- 水痘-带状疱疹病毒。
- 单核细胞增生李斯特菌。
- 巨细胞病毒（CMV）。
- 弓形虫。
- 人类疱疹病毒 6 型（HHV-6）。

自身免疫性

- 抗 LGI1 型脑炎。
- 抗-N-甲基-D-天冬氨酸受体（anti-NMDAR）脑炎。

诊断

症状和体征

- 最初的几日会出现感冒样症状：
  - 轻度头痛、发热、咽喉痛、食欲下降、肌痛。
- 意识改变，困倦，昏迷。
- 认知能力受损，性格改变，幻觉，精神错乱。
- 坐立不安，躁动，易怒，谵妄。
- 皮疹：
  - 莱姆病。
  - 落基山斑疹热。
  - 水痘。
  - 带状疱疹。
- 癫痫。
- 发热、头痛、呕吐，可能出现脑膜刺激征。
- 局灶性神经损害，震颤，共济失调，脑神经麻痹（比脑膜刺激征更常见）。
- 眼底检查可见视神经乳头水肿：
  - 自主神经功能障碍可导致低血压和心律失常。
- 临床表现多样，从轻度头痛和轻度认知/情感障碍到严重的肌痛、癫痫、昏迷、永久性神经后遗症甚至死亡。
- 临床病程可呈缓慢或快速进展。

既往史

当蚊虫活跃时，虫媒病毒（东部马病毒、西部马病毒、圣路易斯脑炎病毒和西尼罗病毒）可导致脑炎发病，而 HSV 全年都可以致病。

体格检查

- 脑炎患者的精神状态改变可以从轻度缺陷至完全无反应不等。
- 其他可以反映神经损害的发现。

基本检查

- 腰椎穿刺。
- 细胞计数与生化检查：
  - 白细胞升高，淋巴细胞升高最明显。
  - 蛋白质水平升高。
  - 血糖（病毒性脑炎可以正常）。
  - 对怀疑/确诊的 HIV 感染行革兰染色。
- 病毒和细菌培养（如果有真菌感染史也可做真菌培养）。
- 抗原检查：
  - HSV。
  - 隐球菌。
  - 弓形虫。
  - 如果条件允许可做其他病毒抗原和抗体检查（肠道病毒、腺病毒、CMV、麻疹病毒、水痘-带状疱疹病毒）。

N

诊断检查与说明

实验室检查

• 全血细胞计数：
- 白细胞通常升高，但是白细胞正常也不可排除感染。

• 电解质、血糖、尿素氮、肌酐。
• 细菌和病毒的血培养。
• 肝功能检查，如果怀疑肝衰竭查血氨。
• 如果怀疑 CO 中毒，查碳氧血红蛋白水平。
• 必要时行毒理学检测。

鉴别诊断

• 聚合酶链反应(PCR)：
- 确定脑脊液中病毒核酸。
- HSV、水痘病毒、肠道病毒等。
- 西尼罗病毒 IgM 血清学检查。

影像学检查

• CT：
- 排除创伤、出血和肿块。
- 脑水肿可能是符合脑炎诊断的唯一发现。
- HSV 病毒性脑炎可能会在额叶和颞叶的水肿区出现微小出血区。

• MRI：
- HSV 病毒性脑炎会出现颞叶的低密度影。

诊断性步骤/外科

行 EEG 协助确诊可疑的癫痫。

鉴别诊断

• 脑膜炎。
• 脑脓肿。
• 脓毒血症。
• 脑卒中(出血或缺血性)。
• 头部损伤。
• 蛛网膜下腔出血。
• 脑病(肝性、尿毒症性)。
• 癫痫。
• 急性播散性脑脊髓炎(ADEM)。
• 代谢性疾病：
- 电解质紊乱(Na^+、K^+、Cl^-、Ca^{2+}、Mg^{2+}、磷酸盐)。
- 低血糖。
- 高血糖酮症性昏迷。

• 肿瘤。
• 药物或毒物。
• CO 吸入。

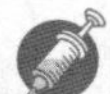

治疗

院前

稳定病情，处理癫痫。

初步稳定/治疗

• ABC 管理：
- 反应迟钝、昏迷、咽反射消失的患者气管插管。

• 对精神状态发生变化的患者应用纳洛酮、硫胺素，监测葡萄糖(或者血糖仪)。
• 对有颅内压升高征象者行眼底检查或者做 CT 检查：
- 过度通气致 PCO_2 到 25～30 mmHg。
- 给予甘露醇。
- 怀疑脑积水者及时神经外科会诊及颅内压监测。

• 开通静脉通路以保持静脉开放，或半开放以避免脑水肿。

急诊治疗/程序

• 控制癫痫。
- 禁用劳拉西泮(氯羟去甲安定)或地西泮(安定)。
- 如果癫痫发作超过 1 次则给予抗癫痫药物(应用磷苯妥英或苯巴比妥)。

• 大多数病毒性脑炎无特殊治疗。
- 激素应用仍有争议。

• 阿昔洛韦静脉注射治疗 HSV 脑炎。
- 如果根据临床表现，CT 和 CSF 检查考虑 HSV 脑炎，可以开始应用阿昔洛韦。

• 怀疑免疫低下相关性感染(CMV、HHV-6)，开始应用更昔洛韦和磷酸盐治疗。
• 如果诊断不明确，尤其是当皮疹出现时(比如脑膜炎球菌血症、立克次体感染)给予对脑炎有效的抗生素治疗。

药物治疗

• 阿昔洛韦：10 mg/kg，静脉注射，q8 h，分 3 次，最大剂量 30 mg/(kg · d)(儿童：12 岁以下 10～15 mg/kg，静脉注射，q8 h，分 3 次)，疗程 14～21 日。
- 阿昔洛韦的替代方案(成人)。
  ◦ 更昔洛韦 5 mg/kg，静脉滴注，q12 h。
  ◦ 膦甲酸 90 mg/kg，静脉滴注，q12 h；或 60 mg/kg，静脉滴注，q12 h。

• 劳拉西泮(氯羟去甲安定)：2～4 mg/每剂，缓慢静脉注射(儿童：0.05～0.1 mg/kg 每剂)。
• 地西泮(安定)：5 mg/每剂，静脉注射(儿童：0.1～0.2 mg/kg，静脉注射；或 0.2～0.5 mg/kg，灌肠)。
• 磷苯妥英钠：负荷剂量 20 mg/kg，静脉注射，最大剂量 1 g。
• 甘露醇：20%甘露醇 0.5～1 g/kg，静脉注射，时间大于 20～30 min。
• 苯巴比妥：15～20 mg/kg 至 300～800 mg 以 25 mg/min 的速度静脉注射。注意呼吸抑制。

随访

进一步处理

入院指征

所有患者均需住院。

要点和误区

只要发现患者有不能解释的脑炎表现，需尽快经验性应用阿昔洛韦治疗 HSV-1 感染，以降低发病率和病死率。

脑再灌注治疗 Reperfusion Therapy, Cerebral

Kama Z. Guluma　袁晓伟　童朝阳 译

基础知识

描述

• 缺血性脑血管意外(CVA)，或阻滞，是一种急性的、突发或渐发的大脑局部血液供应中断现象。
• 大脑再灌注治疗包括：
- 重组组织纤溶酶原激活剂(t-PA)，阿替普酶静脉溶栓。
- 血管内机械性栓塞切除术与支架回收。

病因

• 血栓性 CVA：血栓性病变、高凝状态、淤塞形成的血栓。

• 栓塞性 CVA：由其他部位的栓子引起的急性阻塞，如心脏附壁血栓、主动脉斑块、心脏瓣膜假体。

• 其他闭塞原因包括：解剖因素、血管痉挛。

诊断

症状和体征

病史

• 急性的局灶性神经系统症状在 24 h 内发作。

• 症状出现时间很重要：

- 如果发作时间不能明确，患者最后表现正常的时间可作为替代。

• 病史内容可提示病因而非一般性血栓性脑卒中。

- 颈部损伤导致颈动脉或脊椎夹层。
- 主动脉夹层有撕裂性背部疼痛。
- 药物滥用导致血管痉挛阻塞。

体格检查

• 检查符合低灌注的大脑血管区域时，考虑再灌注治疗(见“脑血管意外”)。

• 美国国立卫生研究院卒中量表(NIHSS)能够用于描述 CVA 的严重程度(亚分类得分总和)：

1a. 意识水平(LOC)：清醒＝0；嗜睡＝1；昏睡＝2；昏迷＝3。

1b. LOC 问题：回答全部正确＝0；1 个正确＝1；均不正确＝2。

1c. LOC 命令：反应都正确＝0；1 正确＝1；均不正确＝2。

2. 注视能力：正常＝0；部分凝视麻痹＝1；被迫偏离＝2。

3. 视力：无视力丧失＝0；部分偏盲＝1；全偏盲＝2；双侧偏盲＝3。

4. 面瘫：正常，对称＝0；轻微麻痹＝1；部分麻痹＝2；完全麻痹＝3。

5～8. 运动能力(计算每条手和腿)：无移动＝0；平移＝1；稍抗重力＝2；无法抗重力＝3；无运动＝4。

9. 共济失调：无＝0；表现在 1 肢体＝1；表现在两个或更多肢体＝2。

10. 感觉(针刺)：正常＝0；部分丧失＝1；高度丧失＝2。

11. 语言能力：无失语＝0；轻到中度失语＝1；严重失语＝2；完全失语＝3。

12. 构音困难：正常发音＝0；轻到中度构音困难＝1；模糊难懂＝2。

13. 忽视/不注意：不会忽视＝0；部分忽略＝1；完全忽略＝2。

基本检查

• 快速床旁血糖检测：

- 在所有患者开始静脉溶栓之前唯一必要的实验室检查。

• 快速无造影剂头部 CT 扫描：

- 所有患者在开始静脉溶栓前必须进行的唯一影像学检查：
  ◦ 如果诊断缺血性 CVA 是不明确，紧急弥散加权(DW)MRI 也可以诊断。
- 可成为多模式成像方案的一部分。
- 可以呈现症状的其他病因(如出血、肿瘤)。

诊断检查与说明

实验室检查

• CBC、INR、PT、APTT：

- 实验室结果不应延迟静脉溶栓，除非怀疑有明显异常。

• 血清电解质、BUN、肌酐：

- 在 0～6 h 的时间窗内，等待肌酐不应延迟急诊 CT 血管造影。

• 尿妊娠试验。

• 尿毒理学检查。

• 针对容易出现肝功能障碍的患者进行肝功能检查。

影像学检查

• 考虑专科会诊和/或转到更高水平的护理，以促进高级神经影像学决策。

• 目标 1：通过再灌注治疗确定出血性转换的显著易感因素：

- 头部 CT 平扫：低密度区。

• 目标 2：确定适合栓塞切除的大血管闭塞(LVO)：

- 不应该延迟静脉溶栓。
- CT 血管造影或 MRI 血管造影。
- 评估颅外颈动脉和椎动脉，以及颅内循环。

• 目标 3：明确栓子切除术增加颅脑挽救的可能性。

- 随 OTT 时间和严重程度(NIHSS)而变化。
- 在 0～6 h OTT 窗口内，不应该延迟静脉溶栓或机械栓塞切除术。
- OTT＝0～6 h，所有 NIHSS：
  ◦ ASPECT 评分。
  ◦ CT 平扫中检查 10 个特定脑区域的缺血性改变。
  ◦ 每有一个受影响区域，从 10 分中减去 1 分。
  ◦ 得分≥6 表示可挽救性增加。
- OTT＝6～24 h；NIHSS≥10：
  ◦ CT 或 MRI 灌注，弥散加权 MRI。
  ◦ 不匹配意味着可挽救性增加，核心病变小于灌注或神经缺陷的预期损伤。

诊断要点

心电图评估节律异常、心包炎、心肌梗死。

鉴别诊断

• 脑血管意外可能的鉴别诊断。

• 在检查和影像学上可能出现血栓栓塞特点的疾病：

- 血管痉挛。
- 脑动脉或椎基底动脉夹层。
- 空气栓塞或减压病。
- 脑静脉窦血栓。

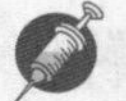

治疗

院前

• 经过验证的院前筛查试验可用于识别中风患者：

- 运送到最近的有能力进行静脉溶栓的医院。

• 院前量表可提示大血管闭塞(LVO)(尽管存在假阳性和阴性)。

• 患者应被送至有能力进行血管内治疗的综合卒中中心(CSC)。

- 怀疑大血管闭塞。
- 最近可用的 CSC 距离最近的脑卒中中心或急性脑卒中准备医院不超过 15 min。

• 通知及调动急诊室和医疗资源。

• 测血糖：

- 低血压可能与 CVA 表现相似。
- 用葡萄糖治疗低血糖。

初步稳定/治疗

• 补充氧气：纠正缺氧。

• RSI：针对气道保护和通气量不足。

• 静脉输液和生理盐水丸：纠正低血压或低血容量。

• 心脏和脉搏血氧监测。

急诊治疗/程序

• 排除需鉴别的其他诊断。

• 再灌注治疗受 OTT 时间的影响。

• OTT＝0～6 h：静脉溶栓(0～4.5 h)和机

械栓塞切除术(0～6 h)。
- 静脉溶栓(t-PA)纳入标准:
◦ 年龄>18 岁。
◦ 能够在症状出现 4.5 h 内开始治疗。
- 机械栓塞切除术纳入标准:
◦ 年龄>18 岁。
◦ 脑卒中前修正 Rankin 量表(mRS)得分为 0～1。
◦ 颈内动脉(ICA)或 MCA 第 1 节(M1)的病因性闭塞。
◦ NIHSS≥6。
◦ ASPECTS≥6。
◦ 能在症状出现后 6 h 内开始治疗(腹股沟穿刺)。
- 对于有下列情况的患者,考虑专科会诊进行机械栓塞切除术:
◦ 不适合静脉溶栓。
◦ 大脑中动脉(MCA)远端闭塞较多。
◦ 除大脑中动脉外的动脉闭塞。
◦ NIHSS 及 ASPECTS 评分较低。
◦ 年龄<18 岁。
• OTT=6～24 h: 选择患者行机械栓塞切除术:
- 晚期机械性栓塞切除术的入选标准。
◦ 年龄: 18～90 岁。
◦ 脑卒中前修正 Rankin 量表(mRS)得分为 0～1。
◦ ICA 或 MCA 第 1 节(M1)的病因性闭塞。
◦ NIHSS≥10(NIHSS≥6 也可以考虑)。
◦ 能够在症状出现 24 h 内开始治疗(腹股沟穿刺)。
◦ 核心病变与灌注区域不匹配或神经缺陷,如 DAWN 或雷迪 3 试验标准。
• 静脉溶栓治疗的禁忌。
- CT 平扫显示脑出血。
- 3 个月内存在脑血管意外。
- 3 个月内严重头部外伤、椎管内手术或颅内手术者。
- 颅内出血(ICH)史。
- 颅内肿瘤。
- 临床表现与蛛网膜下腔出血一致。
- 已知的胃肠道结构性恶性肿瘤。
- 21 日内消化道出血。
- 假定脓毒性栓子,疑似感染性心内膜炎。
- 主动脉夹层动脉瘤。
- 不可控的高血压>185/110 mmHg。
- 已知的出血性因素,例如:
◦ 血小板计数<100 000/mm^3(如果无血小板减少史,可在血小板计数结果前开始溶栓,但如果检查提示血小板水平低,应停止)。
◦ 在 24 h 内应用低分子肝素。
◦ 华法林使用(除非 INR≤1.7 和/或 PT<15 s)。
◦ 在 48 h 内使用直接凝血酶抑制剂或Ⅹa 因子抑制剂(除非药物特异性活性测定正常)。
◦ 糖蛋白Ⅱb/Ⅲa 受体抑制剂的使用。
- 血糖<50 mg/dl,除非症状持续纠正。
- 大脑>1/3 半球 CT 表现为低密度。
• 专科会诊以评估在 6～24 h 时间窗内栓塞切除术潜在禁忌证:
- 包括 NIHSS<6 的快速改善、严重过敏、出血、血管异常(多发性闭塞、血管炎、感染)、CT 中线移位的肿块效应或 ASPECTS 评分<6、早期使用 t-PA。
• 在再灌注治疗前,用 1～2 剂量的拉贝洛尔、尼卡地平或克利夫地平滴注或其他适当的药物治疗 BP>185/110 mmHg。
- 不积极地使 BP 正常化。
- 患者可能依赖于较高平均动脉压来增加脑灌注。
• 美国 FDA 最新关于阿替普酶的处方信息已经取消了先兆脑卒中、癫痫发作、特定实验室值、特定血压测量、脑卒中严重程度(包括轻度症状)的标准。
- 如有需要,给予静脉注射 t-PA;阿替普酶。
• 如果患者符合条件,立即进行机械栓塞切除术:
- 不要等着看 t-PA 是否有效。
- 24 h 内避免使用抗血小板药物和抗凝剂。
• t-PA 治疗后 24 h 监测动脉血压,收缩压>180 mmHg 或舒张压>105 mmHg:
- 最初 2 h 每 15 min 检查一次,随后 6 h 每 30 min 检查一次,随后 24 h 每小时检查一次。
- 控制血压<180/105 mmHg。
- 考虑用硝普钠治疗对其他药物无反应的高血压,或用于 DBP>140 mmHg。
• 监测脑出血症状:
- LOC 降低。
- 乏力加重。
- 头痛。
- 急性高血压或心悸。
- 恶心或呕吐。
• 如果怀疑脑出血,急查头部 CT 来明确诊断:
- 如果明确,治疗如下:
◦ 如果仍在注射,终止 t-PA。
◦ 采血样测 CBC、PT(INR)、APTT、血小板计数、纤维蛋白原水平。血型及交叉匹配。
◦ 准备冷沉淀、氨甲环酸(或氨基己酸)和血小板,并根据需要注射。
◦ 请神经外科会诊。

注意

• 对于发病 3～4.5 h 的患者;静脉 t-PA 有附加的排除标准:
- 年龄>80 岁。
- NIHSS>25 或>1/3MCA。
• 症状改善但仍然有明显障碍的患者可能有持续的严重闭塞,并可能受益于静脉注射 t-PA。
• 脑卒中发作时的癫痫发作不能排除静脉注射 t-PA 的使用,但要警惕假性脑卒中。
• 葡萄糖>400 mg/dl 不排除静脉注射 t-PA 的使用,但应警惕类似高血糖性脑卒中。
• 在 NIHSS>20 的患者中使用 t-PA 时发生 ICH 的风险超过 6%。
• 虽然不是绝对禁忌证,但要仔细考虑静脉注射 t-PA 对以下患者的风险和益处:
- 主要身体(非颅骨)创伤或 14 日内手术。
- 颅内动脉瘤<10 mm。
- 颅内轴外肿瘤(如脑膜瘤)。
- 颅外动脉夹层。
- 最近 3 个月内有急性心肌梗死。
- 妊娠。
- 眼出血病史。

▪ 药物治疗

一线用药

• 阿替普酶(t-PA): 0.9 mg/kg,静脉注射,最大剂量为 90 mg,给药时间为 1 h:
- 1 min 内快速推注 10%的剂量。
- 随后立即输注剩余剂量,59 min 内输注完毕。
• 拉贝洛尔: 10 mg 静脉注射,给药时间为 1～2 min;随后根据需要给药。
- 重复给药或双倍剂量 q10～20 min 最大剂量为 300 mg。
- 起始滴注速度 2～8 mg/min。
• 尼卡地平: 静滴 5 mg/h;每 5 min 边观察边增加 2.5 mg/h 的剂量,直至最大剂 15 mg/h。
• 氯维地平: 每小时滴注 1～2 mg;每 2～5 min 增加 1 倍剂量,最高 21 mg/h。

二线用药

• 硝普钠: 0.5～1 μg/(kg · min),持续静脉

滴注，根据血压参数调整。

• 冷沉淀：10 U，滴注 10～30 min。

- 1 h 后起效，高峰于 12 h。

- 对于纤维蛋白原＜200 mg/dl，给予的额外剂量。

• 氨甲环酸：静脉注射 1 000 mg，超过 10 min；或氨基己酸：4～5 g，持续 1 h 以上，随后静脉注射 1 g，直到出血得到控制（峰值出现在 3 h）。

• 血小板：6～8 U，静脉注射。

随访

进一步处理

入院指征

所有进行再灌注治疗的 CVA 患者应送入重症监护病房反复做神经系统检查和生命体征评估。

转诊问题

不适用。

要点和误区

• 发病时间要精确，患者及家属可把卒中初始发现的时间作为“发病时间”。

• t-PA 血浆半衰期＜5 min；快速注射和输注之间的延误，或输注时的停顿，都会导致血浆浓度和效果的下降。

• “时间就是大脑”（出血也同样）；尽快开始治疗，即使患者在临床症状早期。

内耳迷路炎

Shruti Chandra · Charles V. Pollack Jr.　何超　段立伟 译

基础知识

描述

• 又名听力损失的前庭神经炎。

• 内耳的炎症性改变。

• 常为前庭 CN Ⅷ的病毒性炎症。

• 炎症降低了迷路的声音传入功能。

- 中枢神经对于病态内耳减低的传入信号的解读为头部的旋转感觉。

- 迷路传入信号的不对称导致眼球自发性震颤并向患侧偏斜。

• 良性的，自限性的。

• 单侧前庭功能障碍。

• 非对称性前庭功能障碍造成平衡感觉异常和眩晕感，甚至听力障碍或耳鸣。

• 高发年龄位于 30～60 岁。

• 50%的患者与上呼吸道感染密切相关。

• 头部运动时症状明显，但是在静止状态下症状也会持续存在。

• 恢复期持续数周到数月。

病因

• 造成周围性眩晕的 3 个主要因素：良性发作性位置性眩晕（BPPV）、梅尼埃病和迷路炎。

• 迷路炎：

- 浆液性：病毒或细菌感染。

- 化脓性：细菌感染。

- 自身免疫性：魏格纳或结节性动脉炎型肉芽肿。

- 血管缺血。

- 头部损伤或耳部创伤。

- 药物性：氨基糖苷类抗生素、利尿剂、抗癫痫药物。

- 过敏性。

- 慢性。

• 良性发作性位置性眩晕：

- 耳石位置的改变：

◦ 特发性：49%。

◦ 创伤后：18%。

◦ 迷路炎后遗症：15%。

儿科注意事项

• 化脓性或浆液性迷路炎：

- 通常继发于中耳炎、发汗、共济失调和呕吐。

• 良性发作性位置性眩晕：

- 初发于 1～5 岁。

- 症状：婴儿突发啼哭、眼球震颤、发汗、呕吐、共济失调。

- 3 岁以后会出现症状的复发。

- 偏头痛性：良性发作性位置性眩晕综合征是婴儿眩晕的最主要病因。

• 美尼埃病：10 岁前发病罕见。

诊断

症状和体征

病史

• 眩晕：

- 周围性眩晕。

- 突发。

- 与头部位置的改变相关。

- 感觉房间在旋转或上下颠倒。

• 恶心与呕吐。

• 发生听力障碍：

- 非对称性或对称性。

- 轻度的或持续性的。

- 耳鸣（考虑梅尼埃病）。

- 耳漏（考虑中耳炎、鼓膜穿孔）。

• 相关的近期感染或与相关患者的接触史。

• 诱因包括耳部的手术、糖尿病、卒中、偏头痛和创伤。

• 头部或颈椎的创伤也是内耳损伤的直接原因之一。

• 相关的家族性耳聋病史。

体格检查

• 完整的头颈部检查。

• 内耳的检查（红斑、肿胀、手术痕迹），耳道的检查（耳溢液、瘘管）和中耳的检查（穿孔、胆脂瘤、中耳渗出或中耳炎）。

• 乳突触痛。

• 眼部检查包括眼球的活动范围、瞳孔反射、眼底检查是否存在视乳头水肿。

• 眼球震颤：

- 由于头部的活动或快速的摆头运动而加重。

- 位置性。

- 随旋转运动出现的水平震颤。

- 震颤方向恒定。

- 位置固定后震颤减轻。

- 震颤具有可变性。

• 完整的神经系统和心脏系统检查：

- 评估是否存在引起相同症状的其他疾病。

- 脑神经、Romberg 测试、串联步态、小脑功能。

- 颈部的杂音。

• 可能伴随面部肌无力或不对称表现（考虑卒中或 Ramsay Hunt 综合征）、颈部疼痛或强直（考虑脑膜炎），伴随视力的改变（考虑中枢性损伤产生的眩晕)。

• 头部冲击试验/头部推力试验：

- 阳性标志：头部快速转向病变侧，患者无法保持视觉固定。

- 迷路炎时呈阳性。

• 热量测试：

- 以凉水冲洗外耳道 20 s(检查确认是否存在鼓膜穿孔)。

- 正常表现为水平震颤并且在快速震颤时偏离受刺激耳的一侧。

- 迷路炎会表演为对该刺激部分或完全无反应。

- Dix-Hallpike 试验：检查是否存在良性发作性位置性眩晕。

基本检查

• 仔细的神经系统检查排除眩晕的中枢性原因。

• 排除一些重要的感染：

- 急性中耳炎、脑膜炎、乳突炎、Ramsay Hunt 综合征。

• 患者直立。

• 前庭功能的评估。

诊断检查与说明

• 只有在评估中枢性眩晕或一些少见病因的周围性眩晕患者时考虑该病。

• 当存在反复发生的严重恶心、呕吐时检测电解质。

• 当怀疑脑膜炎或蛛网膜下腔出血时可行腰椎穿刺检查。

实验室检查

• 末梢血糖。

• 梅毒。

• 类风湿因子。

• 电解质。

影像学检查

• 提示：

- 提示存在中枢性眩晕。

◦ 急性或逐渐发病。

◦ 非位置性，但会因头部运动加剧。

◦ 方向性：垂直、水平或扭转的。

◦ 震颤方向可能改变。

- 心血管高位因素。

• 头部 CT：

- 贯穿小脑的细锉纹。

• MRI 或 MRA：

- 评估颅后窝、CN Ⅷ和脑脊液的循环。

- 对于怀疑中枢性眩晕患者的影像学检查手段。

注意

对于>45 岁的患者、儿童或存在心血管危险因素的患者考虑进行颅脑的影像学检查。

鉴别诊断

• 周围性眩晕：

- 中耳炎。

- 前庭神经炎。

- 良性发作性位置性眩晕。

- 听神经瘤。

- 自身免疫性内耳疾病。

- 胆脂瘤。

- 梅尼埃病。

- 耳毒性药物(襻利尿剂、氨基糖苷类、链霉素、水杨酸、乙醇)。

- 带状疱疹(Ramsey Hunt 综合征)。

- 耳膜穿孔。

- 外淋巴漏(鼓膜充气法检测时症状加重)。

- 创伤后的前庭震荡。

- 化脓性迷路炎。

- 颞骨骨折。

• 中枢性眩晕：通常会存在一些不能与周围性眩晕完全区分的症状，因为迷路与脑干之间存在单突触性连接。

- 脑干缺血。

- 小脑出血。

- 小脑前部缺血。

- 中枢神经系统损伤(肿瘤)。

- Chiari 畸形。

- 多发性硬化(感觉异常、视神经炎)。

- 颞叶癫痫部分性发作。

- 前庭-咬肌综合征。

- 前庭偏头痛(30%的患者仅表现为眩晕而无头痛)。

- Wallenberg 综合征(与 Horner 综合征相关，交叉感觉征)。

• 心律失常(存在晕厥前症状)。

• 低血糖(与位置无关，逐渐出现症状)。

• 颈部先天性疾病(首发症状多由颈部的旋转运动引起)。

• 甲状腺功能减退。

• 酒精或药物因素引起的眩晕。

治疗

院前

• 心律失常患者进行心电监测。

• 末梢血糖检测排除低血糖。

• 评估是否存在急性休克。

• 使用止吐药物治疗恶心与呕吐。

• 静脉使用脱水剂。

• 预防跌倒。

初步稳定/治疗

• 卧床休息和进行水化。

• 预防跌倒。

急诊治疗/程序

• 避免长期使用(最多 48 h)，从而导致前庭代偿的发展。

• 缓解症状的药物治疗：

- 前庭抑制剂：地西泮(安定)、氯苯甲嗪、莨菪碱。

- 止吐药：昂丹司琼、普鲁氯嗪、异丙嗪。

- 糖皮质激素：少量证据提示有效。

• 一些增强前庭功能的锻炼。

• 对于药物和物理治疗无效的患者进行手术：

- 后耳道的封堵。

- 神经离断术。

药物治疗

• 地西泮(安定)：2～10 mg 静脉使用，5～10 mg 口服使用，q6～12 h。

• 茶苯海明(乘晕宁)：5 mg/(kg · 24 h)，口服、肌内、静脉或皮下给药。

• 氯苯甲嗪：25 mg(对于 12 岁以上患者 50 mg/24 h)，口服给药，q6 h。

• 劳拉西泮(氯羟去甲安定)：0.5～2 mg 静脉、肌内或口服给药，q6 h(儿童：0.05 mg/kg，静脉或口服给药，q4～8 h)。

• 昂丹司琼：4～8 mg，静脉、肌内或口服给药，q8 h(儿童：1 个月至 12 岁或体重<40 kg：0.1 mg/kg 静脉给药；>12 岁同时体重>40 kg：4 mg 静脉给药)。

• 普鲁氯嗪：12.5～25 mg[儿童：1.5～2 mg/(kg · 24 h)]静脉或口服给药，q4～6 h。

• 莨菪碱(抗胆碱类药物)：0.4 mg，口服，q4～6 h；1.5 mg 透皮贴剂，q3 h。

儿科注意事项

细菌性迷路炎：

• 第四代抗生素。

• 清创术。

一线用药

• 氯苯甲嗪。

• 昂丹司琼止吐。

二线用药

• 地西泮或劳拉西泮。

• 普鲁氯嗪或异丙嗪。

随访

进一步处理

入院指征

- 出现急性休克症状或中枢性病因所引起的眩晕。
- 难治性恶心或呕吐。
- 严重的脱水。
- 步态不稳。

出院指征

- 能够耐受口服液体。
- 步态稳定。
- 神经系统体检正常。
- 避免开车、登高或操作危险的仪器。
- 防跌倒。
- 进行神经内科或耳鼻喉科的随访。

转诊问题

- 症状复发。
- 注意胆脂瘤。
- 对于病情潜在危险因素如椎基底动脉的缺血、脑干肿瘤需要神经外科和神经内科会诊。

随访建议

- 对于由于周围性前庭病变造成的慢性眩晕和持续性前庭症状推荐前庭复位治疗。
- 对于年龄尚小的儿童推荐听性脑干反应测试。
- 对于反复性眩晕可以使用手术治疗，包括迷路切除术、后耳道封堵、前庭神经离断术等。

要点和误区

- 给予患者职业方面的建议，避免高危职业和驾驶工作。
- 避免遗漏威胁生命的病情，如脑膜炎、脑血管缺血和颅脑肿瘤等。
- 良性阵发性位置性眩晕避免暴力性的体格检查，因为颈椎的暴力性过伸会导致椎动脉的离断。

内脏穿孔 Perforated Viscus

Rosaura Fernández　赵铭 译

基础知识

描述

- 器官壁穿孔、破损，内容物渗入腹腔。
- 炎症、感染。
- 溃疡。
- 创伤时的剪切、挤压或冲击。
- 梗阻。
- 由胃或肠道破损导致的化学和/或生物性腹膜炎。

病因

- 消化性溃疡：
  - 主要由非甾体抗炎药和幽门螺旋杆菌导致。
- 食管。
- 小肠：
  - 缺血、异物、新生物、炎性肠病。
- 大肠：
  - 憩室病、异物、新生物、炎性肠病。
- 阑尾炎
- 穿透或钝挫伤。
- 医源性：
  - 内镜、结肠镜检查。
- 放射性小肠炎和直肠炎。

儿科注意事项

- 一般由创伤导致：
  - 难产、虐童、车祸、跌落。
- 破裂的最常见部位是空肠。

诊断

症状和体征

- 突然腹部剧痛：
  - 最初是局部的。
  - 由于腹膜炎而迅速扩散。
  - 因脓肿、蜂窝组织形成而持续疼痛。
- 强直。
- 保护。
- 反跳痛。
- 无肠鸣音。
- 全身炎症反应综合征(SIRS)。
- 低血容量性或感染性休克：
  - 低血糖。
  - 心动过速。
  - 呼吸急促。

老年人注意事项

- 1/3 患者没有主诉消化性溃疡。
- 检查时可能没有明显疼痛或腹膜损伤：
  - 腹壁肌肉组织减少，弹性和保护作用减弱。
  - 慢性者使用疼痛药物。
- 可能出现精神状态变化。
- 体温过低，抑制性心动过速。

基本检查

直立位 X 线胸片：

- 有效诊断气腹。
- 保持直立状态 5～10 min，可能在膈膜下方发现 1～2 ml 游离气体。

诊断检查与说明

实验室检查

- CBC。
- 电解质、尿素氮/肌酸酐、葡萄糖。
- 脂肪酶。
- 尿液分析。
- 肝功能检测、凝固操作盘。
- 动脉血气(ABG)。
- 乳酸盐。
- 血型和交叉配血。

影像学检查

- 直立位胸部 X 线检查：
  - 检查膈膜下方气体。
  - 灵敏度为 50%～85%。
- 腹部 X 线检查：
  - 左侧卧位比仰卧位更有帮助。
  - 内脏穿孔的双壁征：
    - 肠腔和腹腔中的气体能使肠道表面形成可视的浆膜(一般不常见)和黏膜。
- 腹部 CT：
  - 能观测到少量游离气体。
- 心电图。

鉴别诊断

- 纵隔气肿、腹膜胀大。
- 阑尾炎、胆囊炎、胰腺炎。

N

• 肺炎。
• 糖尿病酮症酸中毒(DKA)。
• 腹内脓肿。
• 消化性溃疡。
• 下壁心肌梗死。
• 梗阻。

老年人注意事项

非典型性疼痛,发热,由免疫力下降导致的白细胞减少,常见疾病。

• AAA。
• 急性肠系膜缺血。
• DDx 中所列的非典型表现。

妊娠注意事项

排除异位妊娠。

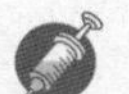

治疗

院前

呕吐病史或生命体征异常的患者,给予静脉补液。

初步稳定/治疗

• 辨别存在全身炎症反应、脓毒症或脓毒性休克的患者。
• 采用积极的支持性措施纠正低氧血症、低血压和低灌注。
• 使用晶体液进行积极的液体复苏。
• 早期广覆盖的使用抗生素或者手术或同时采取这两种措施。
• 如果补液不耐受或者不足以保持生理指标稳定,考虑使用血管活性药物。
• 如果需要,考虑进行气管内插管和机械通气。

急诊治疗/程序

• 鼻胃管。
• 导尿管。
• 给予广谱抗生素覆盖革兰阳性球菌、革兰阴性肠杆菌科细菌和专性厌氧菌。
- 青霉素-β-内酰胺酶抑制剂。
- 基于头孢菌素的疗法。
- 抗厌氧菌药物。
- 单酰胺菌素类药物。
- 碳青霉烯类药物。
- 抗肠球菌和金黄色葡萄球菌类药物。
• 高危的成人和年龄大于 1 个月的儿童患者,给予哌拉西林-他唑巴坦。
• 对于β-内酰胺酶抑制剂过敏的患者。考虑以下三类药物:
- 氨曲南 1～2 g,静脉注射,q8 h(大于 9 个月的儿童:30 mg/kg,静脉注射,q6～8 h)。
- 万古霉素 10～20 mg/kg, q12 h,静脉注射(儿童:10 mg/kg,静脉注射,q6 h)。
- 甲硝唑 1 g 静脉注射[儿童:22～40 mg/(kg·d)的剂量静脉滴注,分 3 次给药,q8 h]。
• 立即请外科会诊考虑手术干预。

药物治疗

• 青霉素-β-内酰胺酶抑制剂:
- 哌拉西林-他唑巴坦 3.375～4.5 g,静脉注射,q6 h[儿童:240～300 mg/(kg·d),静脉注射,分 3～4 次给药]。
• 碳青霉烯类:
- 亚胺培南-西司他丁 0.5～1 g,静脉注射,q6～8 h[儿童:15～25 mg/(kg·d),静脉注射,q6 h]。
- 美罗培南 1～2 g,静脉注射,q8 h[儿童:30～120 mg/(kg·d)静脉注射,分 3 次给药,q8 h]。
• 头孢菌素类药物联合抗厌氧菌药物:
- 头孢吡肟 1～2 g,静脉注射,q12 h[儿童体重小于 40 kg:50 mg/(kg·d)静脉注射,q12 h]联合甲硝唑 1 g,静脉注射;之后 0.5 g,静脉注射,q6～8 h。
• β-内酰胺酶抑制剂过敏的患者。
- 氨曲南 1～2 g,静脉注射,q8 h(儿童大于 9 个月月龄:30 mg/kg 静脉注射,q6～8 h)。
- 万古霉素 10～20 mg/kg,静脉注射,q12 h(儿童:10 mg/kg 静脉注射,q6 h)。
- 甲硝唑 1 g,静脉注射[儿童:22～40 mg/(kg·d)静脉注射,分 3 次给药,q8 h]。
• 硫酸吗啡:2～4 mg(儿童:0.1 mg/kg,静脉注射,q2～3 h)。

随访

进一步处理

入院指征

疑似或确诊穿孔患者需及时手术会诊。

出院指征

由于急性穿孔为外科急诊,此情形不适合出院。

转诊问题

• 为手术治疗进行普通外科会诊。
• 根据情况进行创伤咨询或转诊。

随访建议

术后外科随访。

要点和误区

• 疑似内脏穿孔患者需进行直立位胸部 X 线检查和腹部 X 线检查。
• 胸部 X 线检查未发现气体并不能排除穿孔。
• 若临床高度疑似穿孔但 X 线平片显示正常,应进行腹部 CT 检查以检测微小穿孔。
• 尽早为手术治疗进行外科会诊。

拟交感神经药中毒 Sympathomimetic Poisoning

Sean Patrick Nordt 江伟伟 李文放 译

基础知识

描述

• 直接或间接刺激交感神经和中枢神经系统中的肾上腺素能受体。
• 通常在剂量和毒性之间没有相关性。
• 咖啡因阻断心肌细胞的钠通道,导致Ⅰa 型心律失常。

儿科注意事项

• 儿童拟交感神经中毒可能与脑膜炎或其他全身性疾病相似。
• 尿毒理学筛查可能是患有精神状态障碍的儿童发现拟交感神经中毒的唯一方法。
• 哌甲酯(利他林、专注达)和用于 ADHD 的其他拟交感神经药可能与精神状态改变有交叉反应。

病因

• 交感神经毒性可以由使用任何具有交感神经活性的药物产生,包括:
- 所有苯丙胺、甲基苯丙胺和衍生品(摇

N

头丸)。
- 可卡因。
- 合成卡西酮。
- 苯环已哌啶(PCP)。
- 麦角酰二乙胺(LSD)。
- 消肿剂(罕见)。
• 药物吸收途径：吸入、注射或摄入。

诊断

体征和症状

• 生命体征：
- 心动过速：
◦ 可卡因和其他一些消肿剂可能导致心动过缓。
- 血压升高：
◦ 严重中毒的患者可能会出现低血压。
- 呼吸急促。
- 高热：
◦ 经常出现，可能是严重的，而且经常被忽视。
• 神经系统：
- 焦虑。
- 头痛。
- 烦动。
- 意识状态改变。
- 出汗。
- 癫痫发作。
- 休克。
- 肌张力障碍(罕见)。
• 心血管系统：
- 心悸。
- 胸部疼痛。
- 心肌缺血或梗死。
- 心动过速。
- 心血管衰竭。
- 杂音(如心内膜炎)。
• 其他：
- 瞳孔散大。
- 干燥的黏膜。
- 尿潴留，可能导致膀胱肿大。
- 在四肢找针眼或脓肿。
- 肠鸣音亢进或减弱。
- 出汗和肠鸣音，可能有助于区别抗胆碱能中毒引起的不同的拟交感神经毒性。

病史

• 评估既往可能接触拟交感神经药物的记录：
- 处方苯丙胺。
- 娱乐药物使用。
• 评估可能的合用。
• 评估最终器官损伤的症状：
- 胸部疼痛。
- 呼吸急促。
- 头痛、意识混乱和呕吐。

体格检查

• 常见的症状：
- 烦躁。
- 心动过速。
- 发汗。
- 瞳孔散大。
• 严重中毒的特点：
- 心动过速。
- 高血压。
- 高热。
- 谵妄。
- 癫痫发作。
- 多汗。
• 低血压和呼吸窘迫可能先于心血管病变。
• 评估相关条件：
- 蜂窝织炎和软组织感染。
- 舒张期心脏杂音或脉搏短绌。
- 仔细检查是否有创伤。
- 吸入性损伤引起的气胸。
- 局灶性神经缺陷。

基本检查

• 监测生命体征：
- 温度升高[>40°(可能)]：
◦ 核心温度记录必不可少。
◦ 外周温度低。
◦ 紧急降温。
◦ 不良预后的表现。
- 血压：
◦ 严重的高血压可导致心脏和神经系统异常。
◦ 随后可能出现低血压。
• 心电图：
- 心脏缺血的表现。
- 室性快速性心律失常。
- 反应性心动过缓。

诊断检查与说明

实验室检查

• 尿液检查：
- 红细胞。
- 肌红蛋白。
• 电解质、尿素氮/肌酐、葡萄糖：
- 低血糖可能导致精神状态改变。
- 酸中毒可伴有严重的毒性。
- 横纹肌溶解症可导致肾衰竭。
- 高钾血症：危及生命的急性肾衰竭后果。
• 监测凝血功能，可能出现弥散性血管内凝血(DIC)：
- INR、PT、APTT、血小板。
• 肌酸磷酸激酶(CPK)：
- 横纹肌溶解时明显升高。
• 尿毒理学筛检：
- 对于其他具有相似效果的毒素(如可卡因)。
- 一些苯丙胺类物质(如合成卡西酮、MDMA)可能不会被检测到。
• 检测水杨酸盐和对乙酰氨基酚水平，因为可能自杀或治疗咳嗽、感冒用药。
• 静脉血气，动脉血气。

影像学检查

• X线：
- 成人呼吸窘迫综合征。
- 非心源性肺水肿。
• 头部CT：
- 严重头痛。
- 精神状态改变。
- 局灶性神经系统体征。
- 蛛网膜下腔出血、脑出血。

诊断步骤/外科

腰椎穿刺：
• 怀疑脑膜炎(头痛、精神状态改变、高热)。
• 疑似蛛网膜下腔出血，但CT正常。

鉴别诊断

• 脓毒血症。
• 甲状腺危象。
• 5-羟色胺综合征。
• 神经阻滞剂恶性综合征。
• 嗜铬细胞瘤。
• 蛛网膜下腔出血。
• 导致谵妄的药物：
- 抗胆碱能药物。
- 三环类抗抑郁药。
- 拟交感神经药。
- 乙醇戒断。
- 镇静、催眠戒断。
- 致幻剂。
- PCP。
• 引起高血压和心动过缓的药物：
- 拟交感神经药。
- 抗胆碱能药物。
- 乙醇戒断。
- PCP。
- 咖啡因。
- 单胺氧化酶抑制剂。
- 茶碱。

N

- 尼古丁。
• 引起癫痫发作的药物：
- 莰酮。
- 卡马西平。
- 一氧化碳。
- 氯化烃。
- 胆碱。
- 氰化物。
- 乙醇戒断。
- 降糖药。
- 异烟肼。
- 铅。
- 锂。
- 局麻药。
- 吩噻嗪。
- 丙氧芬。
- 水杨酸。
- 镇静、催眠药停药。
- 士的宁。
- 拟交感神经药。
- 茶碱。
- 三环类抗抑郁药。

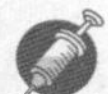

治疗

院前

• 患者可能不合作或有暴力行为。
• 建立静脉通路。
• 防止自我伤害。

初步稳定/治疗

• 监测生命体征。
• 建立静脉通路。
• 心脏功能监测。
• 如果精神状态改变，使用纳洛酮、葡萄糖和硫胺素。

急诊治疗/程序

• 清除毒物：
- 不建议洗胃：
◦ 活性炭不常规推荐使用。
◦ 体内藏毒者需使用活性炭。
• 聚乙二醇溶液灌肠。
• 高血压危象：
- 如果烦躁，最初给予苯二氮䓬类药物，可能需要较高剂量。
- 对苯二氮䓬类药物无反应的严重高血压，静脉使用尼卡地平或硝酸甘油。
- 硝普钠也可用于严重、对苯二氮䓬类药物无反应性的高血压。
- 避免使用β受体阻滞剂，这可能会加剧高血压。
• 激越，急性精神病：
- 苯二氮䓬类药物。
- 谨慎使用丁酰苯（如氟哌啶醇）来控制激动：
◦ 可能降低癫痫发作阈值并可能延长 QT 间期。
• 心律失常：
- 碳酸氢钠静脉推注治疗是指导钠通道阻滞的室性心律失常（宽大 QRS 波群）的治疗选择。
- 如果使用碳酸氢钠、苯二氮䓬类药物和支持治疗，难以纠正室性心律失常，则考虑使用利多卡因。
• 高热：
- 如果激动，使用苯二氮䓬类药物。
- 温度>40℃时给予物理降温：
◦ 微弱的水雾。
◦ 用风扇加快蒸发。
◦ 冰袋置于腋窝和腹股沟降温。
◦ 用非去极化肌松药如维库溴铵行紧急气管插管。
• 瘫痪：
- 肌肉强直和过度运动，则使用热疗法。
- 去极化麻痹首选。
• 横纹肌溶解：
- 苯二氮䓬类药物。
- 含生理盐水的水合物。
- 尿量维持在 1～2 ml/min。
- 血液透析（如果发生急性肾衰竭和高钾血症）。
• 癫痫发作：
- 保持呼吸道。
- 使用苯二氮䓬类药物。
- 如果对苯二氮䓬类药物无反应，则使用苯巴比妥。
- 行头颅 CT 排除可疑的颅内出血。

药物治疗

• 活性炭：1～2 g/kg 至 100 g 口服。
• 右旋糖：$D_{50}W$ 1 安瓿：50 ml 或 25 g（儿童：1～2 ml/kg $D_{25}W$；婴儿：2.5～5.0 ml/kg $D_{10}W$）静脉注射。
• 地西泮（苯二氮䓬）：5～10 mg（儿童：0.2～0.5 mg/kg）静脉注射，不建议<6 个月儿童使用。
• 劳拉西泮（苯二氮䓬）：2～6 mg（儿童：0.03～0.05 mg/kg）静脉注射。
• 尼卡地平：以 5 mg/h 滴注 2.5 mg/h，q5 min 至最大剂量 15 mg/h。
• 硝普钠：0.5～10 μg/(kg·min)静脉注射（根据血压调节滴定）。
• 苯巴比妥：25～50 mg/min，15～20 mg/kg 直至癫痫发作活动停止；监测呼吸，在<6 岁儿童的安全性未确定。
• 苯丙胺：在 5 min 内 1～5 mg（根据血压调节滴定）。
• 碳酸氢钠：1 或 2 安瓿（50 mmol/安瓿）（儿童：1～2 mmol/安瓿）静脉注射。

注意
行气管插管时可能需要应用较大剂量的苯二氮䓬和苯巴比妥。

随访

进一步处理

入院指征

• 体内藏毒者入院。
• 床旁监测毒性表现：
- 癫痫发作。
- 心律失常。
- 高热。
- 横纹肌溶解。
- 严重高血压。
- 精神状态改变。
• 缺血性胸痛。

出院指征

轻度中毒的患者可以在急诊观察和治疗，直到临床表现缓解。

随访建议

患者可能需要药物依赖戒毒和戒毒的转诊。

要点和误区

• 严重或持续症状的患者收入院。
• 40℃以上的高热可能会危及生命：
- 治疗积极镇静和物理降温。
• 认识横纹肌溶解和高钾血症。
• 尽可能避免限制激动患者的身体。
• 以下需紧急情况：
- 胸痛。
- 急性冠状动脉综合征。
- 发热患者的感染和静脉吸毒史。
- 甲胺苯胺滥用引起的创伤性损伤。
• 苯二氮䓬为症状性拟交感神经中毒的一线治疗药物。

N

溺水 Drowning

Colleen N. Hickey　姜颢　张连东 译

基础知识

描述

• 定义：
- 溺水：因淹没或沉浸在液体介质中导致首发呼吸损害的过程。
◦ 致命溺水：由溺水引发的在任何时间的死亡。
◦ 非致命溺水：在肺内吸入液体或喉部痉挛窒息后一段时间之后存活。
- 水上救援：任何淹没或浸泡事故，不伴呼吸损害。
• 溺水的情景：
- 现在认为所有的溺水者都吸入一定量的液体。
- 以前分类为"湿"和"干"溺水：
◦ 湿性溺水(90%)：少量液体吸入肺中。
◦ "干"溺水(10%)：喉痉挛继发于咽或喉存在液体。
- 最后的结果：缺氧。
- 淡水和咸水淹没之间无显著差异。
• 病理生理学：
- 异物吸入：
◦ 少量的水。
◦ 肺顺应性降低造成通气/灌注不匹配和肺内分流。
◦ 没有明显的电解质变化。
◦ 严重污染的水：肺部感染的危险。
- 低氧血症：
◦ 乳酸代谢性酸中毒。
◦ 多器官功能障碍。
◦ 非心源性肺水肿心肌功能障碍(心律失常)。
◦ 凝血异常(弥散性血管内凝血)。
◦ 肾衰竭(通常为急性肾小管坏死)。
◦ 脑缺氧：脑水肿，颅内压增加。

儿科注意事项

• 低体温：
- 在幼儿中比较常见。
- 较大的表面积质量比。
- 代谢率降低。
- 完全恢复的生存是可能的(神经保护)。
• 跳水反射：
- 年幼孩子更容易受到影响。
- 脸浸没在冷水中诱发。
- 心动过缓引起：血流向心脏和大脑的再分配。
- 缺氧相关损伤延迟发作。

> **注意**
>
> 危险因素：
> • 缺乏适当的监管。
> • 酒精或其他药物滥用。
> • 游泳能力有限或疲劳。
> • 创伤。
> • 癫痫。
> • 危险行为。
> • 既往存在或伴随健康问题。
> • 自杀倾向。
> • 缺乏教育。

诊断

症状和体征

• 心肺骤停。
• 发绀。
• 窒息。
• 大量肺部分泌物。
• 意识丧失。
• 脑水肿、损伤。
• 创伤的证据：
- 颅内出血。
- 颈椎损伤罕见(0.5%)。
• 低体温。

基本检查

• 现场目击者或紧急医疗接触人员提供的信息。
• 早期气道管理和心肺复苏术。
• 测直肠温度监测体温。

诊断检查与说明

实验室检查

• 动脉血气(pH)。
• 全血细胞计数。
• 电解质、尿素氮、肌酐、葡萄糖：
- 通常为正常值(>85%)。
- 高钠血症或低钠血症。
• 酒精和药物筛查。

影像学检查

• 胸部X线检查：
- 弥漫性或局灶性浸润，急性呼吸窘迫综合征。
- 最初可能正常。
• 心电图：
- 长QT间期。
- 窦性心动过缓。
- 窦性心动过速。
- 心房颤动。
• CT：
- 脑：在住院期间，任何时候的异常都与不良神经系统结果相关。
- 颈椎：外伤。

鉴别诊断

• 考虑沉溺原因：
- 心律失常(长QT间期综合征、家族性多形性室性心动过速)。
- 心肌梗死。
- 惊厥。
- 晕厥。
- 外伤。
- 自杀企图。

儿科注意事项

考虑虐待、忽略儿童。
• 特别是在浴缸附近溺水的婴儿。

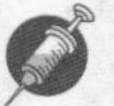

治疗

院前

• 注意基础治疗：
- 避免进一步吸入。
- 安全气管插管。
- 早期心肺复苏。
• 如果怀疑颈椎受伤或相关机制，采取颈椎预防措施。
• 尝试早期复温。
• 适当干预可有90%生存率。
• 所有溺水的受害者需要急诊评估。
• 不推荐压腹排水：
- 仅当异物在气道中时有效。
- 增加吸入的风险。
- 延迟有效心肺复苏。

初步稳定/治疗

• 基础治疗。
• 核心体温：
- 复温(同低体温的处理)。
- 去除湿的衣物。

N

■ 急诊治疗/程序

• 纠正低氧血症：
- 测定氧饱和度。
- 插管提供呼气末正压机械通气。
• 评估和治疗外伤创伤。
• 纠正酸中毒。
• 心肺骤停：
- 开始高级心脏生命支持措施。
- 继续复温：
◦ 被动：毛毯、绝缘体。
◦ 外部主动：温暖的毛毯、辐射热、温暖的沐浴。
◦ 内部主动：胸膜或腹膜灌洗、体外循环。
- 继续复苏，直到核心体温>32 ℃或自主脉搏和呼吸恢复。
• 类固醇类药物使用无效。
• 不良预后迹象：
- 长时间浸泡。
- 严重酸中毒(pH≤7)。
- 需要心肺复苏术。
- 低血氧饱和度。
- 低格拉斯哥昏迷评分(GCS)。

■ 药物治疗

• 肾上腺素：1 mg(儿童：0.01 mg/kg)，静脉推注。
• 加压素：40 U，静脉推注。
• 利多卡因：1 mg/kg，静脉推注。
• 碳酸氢钠：1 mEg/kg，静脉推注。

儿科注意事项

• 低温可以是保护的：
- 积极的复温。
- 积极的复苏。
• 评估虐待、忽视。
• 家族史：突然死亡，类似的事件：
- QT 间期延长综合征。
- 家族性多形性室性心动过速。
• 预防是治疗的关键：
- 监管周围的水域。
- 空提桶和空水桶。

> **注意**
> 争议：治疗性低温。
> • 在成人心搏骤停后自发性循环恢复中广泛接受，在儿科仍有争议。
> • 优化神经系统结局。
> • 抑制再灌注损伤。

随访

■ 进一步处理

入院指征

• 延迟症状发生：
- 肺水肿(12 h 后)。
- 神经系统异常。
• 重症监护病房：
- 需要心肺复苏术或人工通气的患者。
- 胸片异常。
- 动脉血气异常。
- GCS<13 分。
• 入院观察情况：
- 所有有症状的患者。
- 淹没时间超过 1 min。
- 发绀或呼吸暂停史。
- 需要短暂辅助通气的患者。

出院指征

• 可疑沉溺病史：
- 在急诊室中观察 8 h：
◦ 无呼吸窘迫。
◦ 无神经功能损害。
• 出院到可靠家庭。
• 回家指导：
- 出现呼吸急促或精神状态变化返回医院。

■ 随访建议

所有从急诊出院的患者建议密切基础护理随访。

要点和误区

• 所有溺水患者需要至少 8 h 的观察。
• 预后不良的标志：
- 酸血症(显示 pH<7.1)。
- 年龄<3 岁。
- 淹没>5 min。
- 基本生命支持护理时间>10 min。
- 到急诊前运输时间长。
- 持续无呼吸或需要在急诊行心肺复苏术。
- 复苏时间>25 min。

尿崩症 Diabetes Insipidus

Sar Medoff · Melissa H. White 谭美春 译

基础知识

■ 描述

• 一种对精氨酸加压素(AVP)异常反应引发大量稀释性尿液排出(多尿)的疾病。
• 多尿定义为 24 h 内尿液>3 L。
• 通常以大量饮水为特征(烦渴)。
• 2 种类型：
- 中枢性尿崩(DI、CDI、衰竭或 AVP 释放障碍)：
◦ 4 种类型：
▪ 无 AVP 释放(垂体后叶神经元功能障碍或缺失)。
▪ 渗透压感受器缺陷(仅在严重脱水时释放 AVP)。
▪ AVP 释放阈值提高。
▪ AVP 释放量低于正常。
◦ 据报道有家族性病例(常染色体显性遗传)。
- 肾源性尿崩(肾脏对 AVP 缺乏反应)：
◦ 与原发性多尿鉴别。
◦ 一些病例是男性 X 连锁隐性遗传。
• 必须与精神障碍或异常口渴引起的原发性多饮症区分。

■ 病因

• 中枢性尿崩：
- 任何可损害渗透压感受器-下丘脑-垂体轴的状况：
- 在 10～20 岁发病率最高。
◦ 创伤(骨折、出血)。
◦ 垂体或下丘脑手术。
◦ 中枢神经系统(CNS)肿瘤，尿崩可以看作肿瘤的标志。
▪ 垂体腺瘤。
▪ 颅咽管瘤。
▪ 生殖细胞瘤。
▪ 松果体瘤。
▪ 脑膜瘤。
◦ 转移性肿瘤：

■ 白血病、淋巴瘤。

○ 肉芽肿：

■ 组织细胞增生症。

■ 结节病。

○ 先天性中枢神经系统缺陷。

○ 中枢神经系统感染(如脑膜炎、脑炎)。

○ 妊娠(席汉综合征)。

○ 特发性(自身抗体、隐匿性肿瘤)。

○ Wolfram 综合征(尿崩、糖尿病、视神经萎缩、耳聋)。

○ 乙醇。

• 肾源性尿崩：

- 任何损害肾脏对抗利尿激素反应性的疾病：

○ 先天性肾脏病。

○ 阻塞性尿路病变。

○ 肾发育不良。

○ 多囊肾病。

○ 肾脏受累的全身性疾病。

○ 镰刀细胞病。

○ 结节病。

○ 淀粉样变性病。

○ 药物：

■ 两性霉素 B。

■ 苯妥英钠。

■ 锂(最常见且停药后仍持续存在)。

■ 氨基糖苷类抗生素。

■ 甲氧氟烷。

■ 去甲金霉素。

○ 电解质紊乱：

■ 高钙血症。

• 低钾血症。

妊娠注意事项

• 通常出现在妊娠中期：

- 病因不清，但血管加压素酶增加。

- 导致 AVP 降低和一过性尿崩。

- 在麻醉和禁水期间密切观察患者。

- 通常分娩后 2～6 周清除。

- 可用去氨加压素(DDAVP)治疗，通过拮抗血管加压素酶。

• 席汉综合征可导致尿崩。

诊断

症状和体征

病史

• 多尿(尿量多达 16～24 L/d)：

- 注意排尿频次。

• 烦渴(经常渴望冷的液体)：

- 注意每日摄入的口服液体量。

• 药物摄入。

• 下丘脑肿瘤症状和体征：

- 头痛。

- 视觉障碍。

- 生长障碍。

- 肥胖。

- 高热。

- 睡眠障碍。

- 性早熟。

- 情感障碍。

体格检查

• 脱水。

• 恶病质。

• 头部外伤。

• 视野缺损。

• 癫痫。

儿科注意事项

• 多尿和烦渴可能在脱水症状进展后才能被看护者发现。

• 新生儿：

- 常在出生时出现。

- 如未被发现，脱水和高钠可引起永久性中枢神经系统损害。

• 婴幼儿：

- 烦躁。

- 营养不良、体重减轻。

- 便秘。

- 生长障碍。

- 间歇性的高热。

- 异常行为(多动、躁动不安、哭闹不休)。

• 儿童：

- 遗尿。

- 如厕训练困难。

基本检查

• 在急诊室临床诊断。

- 血钠浓度升高。

- 大量稀释性尿液。

• 病史：

- 通常每日口服摄取液体量增加。

- 排尿频繁。

- 药物治疗史。

• 体格检查。

• 实验室检查。

诊断检查与说明

实验室检查

• 尿检：

- 特定的比重降低。

• 血和尿渗透压：

- 血浆渗透压高。

- 尿渗透压低。

• 电解质、尿素氮、肌酐和血糖：

- 高钠血症。

- 高钙血症。

- 低钾血症。

• 全血细胞计数：

- 贫血可能是肿瘤的一个征象。

• 血和尿 AVP 试验昂贵，并且没必要在急诊室检查。

影像学检查

• 评估创伤和查找肿瘤时需要。

• 胸部 X 线检查。

• 头颅 CT。

• 垂体轴 MRI 通常用于门诊患者。

诊断步骤/外科

水剥夺试验(脱水试验)：

• 没必要用于急诊。

• 在低血压时或对年幼儿童可能有危险。

• 作为确诊试验，用于接受治疗患者。

• 限制液体后测量尿和血浆渗透压。

- 尿渗透压＜300 mOsm/L 对尿崩有意义。

○ 应用去氨加压素。

■ 中枢性尿崩——尿渗透增加＞50%。

■ 肾源性尿崩——尿渗透增加＜50%。

- 如果尿渗透压在 300～800 mOsm/L 范围需要进一步测试。

- 如果尿渗透压＞800 mOsm/L，是原发性烦渴。

鉴别诊断

• 原发性缺水：

- 缺乏自由水。

- 非显性失水增加(例如，早产儿)。

- 母乳喂养不足。

• 原发性钠过量：

- 复苏过程中碳酸氢钠过量。

- 高钠灌肠。

- 摄入海水。

- 使用高渗盐水。

- 婴幼儿奶粉中的葡萄糖意外用盐(氯化钠)替代。

- 故意食盐中毒。

- 母乳高钠。

• 原发性烦渴(精神性烦渴)：

- 溶质引起的多尿。

- 使用利尿剂。

- 治疗急性肾衰竭。

- 渗透性利尿。

- 未控制的糖尿病。

N

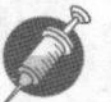

治疗

院前

- 基本生命体征。
- 可疑创伤时制动。
- 血清血糖测定。
- 脱水迹象存在时开放静脉通道及输液。
- 参照医疗指导原则控制癫痫。

初步稳定/治疗

- 基本体征管理。
- 相应的外伤管理。
- 高度怀疑头部创伤。

急诊治疗/程序

- 纠正低血压：
  - 使用0.9%氯化钠，适用于休克。
  - 血管内失液仅占总水量损失的1/12。
- 中枢性尿崩（抗利尿激素缺乏）：
  - AVP（水溶加压素）：
    - 半衰期过短，如果用于治疗需要持续静脉输注。
    - 可能诱发冠状动脉痉挛。
    - 仅用于脱水试验。
  - AVP（lypressin）：
    - 可鼻内给药。
    - 通常需滴注。
  - DDAVP：
    - 用来控制症状的药物。
    - 可以鼻内、皮下、静脉注射或口服给予，根据需要控制多尿或烦渴给予2种不同剂量。
    - 慎用于术后患者，可加重脑水肿。
  - 氯磺丙脲（diabinese）：
    - 增强血管加压素在肾小管的作用。
    - 可能刺激AVP释放。
    - 只对部分CDI有用。
  - 安妥明。
    - 可刺激内源性血管加压素释放。
  - 治疗目标：
    - 24 h排尿量为20～30 ml/（kg·d），24 h尿渗透压为400～800 mOsm/L。
- 肾源性尿崩：
  - 利尿剂：
    - 引起尿钠排泄。
    - 一线药物噻嗪类。
    - 阿米洛利常常与噻嗪类结合使用以降低低钾血症的发生。
  - 限制钠的摄入。
  - 限制溶质和避免过度饮酒，防止水中毒。
  - 避免酒精（尤其是啤酒）的摄入。
  - 每日测体重。
  - 非甾体类抗炎药（吲哚美辛）。
- 在无法口服的病例，肠外给予初始的水分缺失：
  - 通常只用于症状性高钠血症的病例。
  - 液体替代疗法，参照“高钠血症”。

药物治疗

- AVP（水溶加压素）：5～10 U，皮下用于头部外伤或术后的昏迷患者。
- 阿米洛利：2.5～10 mg，口服，每日2次。
- 氯磺丙脲：200～500 mg，口服，每日1次。
- 氯贝丁酯（安妥明）：500 mg，口服，q6 h。
- DDAVP：10～20 μg/d；1～3 μg/d，皮下或静脉注射；0.1～1.2 μg/d，口服。
- 氢氯噻嗪（HCTZ）：50 mg，口服，每日（儿童：2～4 mg/kg，每日1～2次）。
- 赖氨酸加压素喷鼻剂：1～2喷按需，每日3～4次，喷鼻。

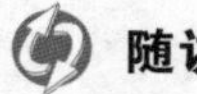

随访

进一步处理

入院指征

- AMS。
- 癫痫。
- 严重脱水。
- 电解质异常。
- 相关创伤。
- 要求去氨加压素测试或水剥夺试验的患者。

出院指征

- 尿崩诊断明确。
- 电解质稳定。
- 充分补水。

随访建议

根据尿崩的病因至专科医师处随访。

要点和误区

- 多尿时监测尿渗透压并考虑尿崩诊断。
- 中枢性尿崩典型表现为对去氨加压素有反应。
- 肾源性尿崩对ADH无反应：
  - 治疗潜在的电解质异常，停用有关药物，并咨询肾脏专科进一步治疗。

尿布疹 Diaper Rash

Cristiana Benucci · Francesco Mannelli 谭美春 译

基础知识

描述

- 婴儿期常见的皮肤病。
- 通常发生在出生后第1个月，9～12个月还会复发。
- 1岁内，可能占到医疗机构皮肤科门诊的25%以上。
- 据报道，该病的发病率在成人尿失禁患者中为5.7%～42%，并且与年龄有显著相关性。
- 主要的刺激性、接触性皮炎：
  - 表皮层被分解，导致炎症，正常皮肤菌群损害，保护屏障功能丧失。
  - 增加皮肤湿度有利于皮肤表面微生物的滋生。
  - 继发的真菌或细菌感染将导致更严重的状况。
- 又称尿布皮炎。

病因

- 刺激物：
  - 水分：
    - 由于不经常换尿布而致皮肤表面长期水分过多，吸收力差的尿布或布尿布，成人大小便失禁。
  - 摩擦：
    - 尿布在皮肤上摩擦或过于宽松的尿布。
  - 化学品：

◦ 皮肤长期暴露于粪便酶和尿环境中。
◦ 在抹布或肥皂上的气味或润肤霜，具有腐蚀性的，如强酸或强碱。
◦ 固定尿布用的材料或黏合剂。
• 感染：
- 白色念珠菌感染：
◦ 高达80%的婴儿尿布中可分离出白色念珠菌。
◦ 通常全身性应用抗生素后大量繁殖。
- 细菌感染：
◦ 常见皮炎并发症的其他原因：金黄色葡萄球菌、链球菌、大肠杆菌是常见的；也会出现消化链球菌和拟杆菌。
◦ 肛周链球菌性皮炎。
- 病毒性的(最常见的是单纯疱疹病毒和肠道病毒)。
• 过敏性尿布皮炎(接触性皮炎)。
• 银屑病。
• 特应性尿布皮炎(接触性皮炎)。
• 危险因素：
- 鹅口疮。
- 尿布疹的早期发作次数。
- 使用尿布的时间。
- 腹泻。

诊断

诊断通常是基于皮疹的表现进行经验性判断。

症状和体征

病史

儿童常在换尿布或擦拭尿布区时哭闹，也可以表现为烦躁。

体格检查

• 刺激性：
- 发红、起疱、脱皮、肿胀，通常保留皮肤皱褶。
• 传染性：
- 念珠菌感染：伴随红斑皮疹，边界常出现卫星脓疱或小丘疹，通常包括皮肤皱褶。
- 细菌感染：浅表糜烂与黄痂，偶尔出现大疱。
- 肛周链球菌性皮炎：持续性、边界分明、肛周皮疹、瘙痒和灼热。
• 脂溢性尿布皮炎：
- 病变常为基底部红斑，表面伴有黄色或灰色的剥脱。
- 婴儿身体的其他部位也会发生类似的病变，尤其是头皮。
• 银屑病：易与脂溢性皮炎混淆，如持续发作至1岁后，尤其是有银屑病家族史的儿童，应考虑银屑病。
• 过敏性、脂溢性尿布皮炎。
- 其他体表，如面部也有边界清楚的瘙痒性红斑皮疹，通常伴有肺泡损伤。
• 变异包括：
- Jacquet形：糜烂伴随溃疡或糜烂边缘高出皮面，通常出现在持续性腹泻或成人尿失禁。
- 婴儿臀部肉芽肿：臀部的紫色斑丘疹及结节，在腹股沟处呈现自限性病程，在数周或数月消失，常残留瘢痕。

基本检查

• 询问换尿布的习惯、排尿及排便习惯。
• 检查其他身体部位，以确定相关的皮疹。
• 考虑儿童虐待或忽视：
- 儿童的整体卫生。
- 烧伤或其他创伤。

诊断检查与说明

实验室检查

• 通常没有必要为尿布皮炎进行实验室评估。
• 除外某些特殊情况，细菌培养通常不说明什么。
• 皮肤表面的碎屑用氢氧化钾准备和/或培养，可以帮助鉴别念珠菌和非典型性脂溢性皮炎：
- 寻找酵母菌和/或假菌丝。

鉴别诊断

• 儿童虐待或忽视。
• 感染：
- 脓疱疮。
- 疥疮。
- 单纯疱疹。
- 水痘。
- 先天性梅毒。
• 牛皮癣。
• 过敏性皮炎。
• 脂溢性皮炎。
• 丘疹性荨麻疹。
• 大疱性类天疱疮。
• 大疱性表皮松解。
• 肠病性肢端皮炎。
• 肠病性肢端皮炎样皮疹。
• 肿瘤：
- 血管瘤。
- 朗格汉斯细胞增生症。

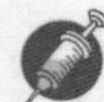

治疗

急诊治疗/程序

尿布皮炎的干预应包括降低尿布区域的湿度，尽量减少皮肤与粪便和尿液的接触，根除感染性微生物。

• 环境的调整：
- 对父母和看护人的教育十分必要。
• 经常使用棉球和清水清洗皮肤。
• 不推荐使用湿巾和滑石粉。
- 频繁换尿布，新生儿每1h一次，婴儿和成人每3～4h一次。
- 用温开水或生理盐水冲洗患处。
- 避免用刺激性的肥皂或酒精擦拭。
- 尽量不去拿尿布覆盖，自然晾干。
- 高吸湿纸尿布的发疹率比布尿布低。
- 刺激性尿布疹患者使用布尿布是不利的。
- 现已证明"透气"尿布或包含的氧化锌/石油硬脂醇衬里顶片的尿布可降低尿布疹的发病率。
• 隔离霜：
- 许多添加物都含有氧化锌、石油、羊毛脂。
- 应在每次更换尿布后应用，持续至皮疹消退，以减少复发。
- 隔离霜的使用和尿布皮炎的早期发作次数呈负相关。
- 如果存在念珠菌感染，则应使用抗真菌药物。
• 糖皮质激素：
- 只用于中度至重度的病情，不应对其他治疗。
- 氢化可的松的浓度不应该超过1%：过高的浓度可能会导致严重的副作用。
- 3～5日后停用。
• 抗真菌药：
- 制霉菌素霜、粉末或软膏：
• 预计1～2日可改善。
• 浸渍皮肤对软膏的耐受最好。
- 克霉唑在换尿布后局部应用。
- 达克宁在换尿布后局部应用。
- 乳液是擦烂区域的优选药物。
- 霜剂应谨慎应用，以避免皮肤浸渍。
- 环吡酮胺在换尿布后局部应用。
- 一般在皮疹消退后再持续使用1～2日。
- 抗真菌剂也具有一定的抗菌活性和抗感染效果。
- 如果并发皮肤或口腔念珠菌病，且病情顽固则可以考虑口服剂，因为粪便可以发生白色念珠菌定植。

N

• 抗菌药物：

- 如果怀疑存在细菌感染，通常情况下与其他疗法联用。

- 2%莫匹罗星在尿布更换后用。

- 很少需要全身应用抗生素。长期口服阿莫西林治疗肛周链球菌性皮炎可能有用。

■ 药物治疗

• 环吡酮胺 0.77%乳剂、凝胶或混悬液：换尿布后局部应用，每日 2 次。

• 克霉唑 1%乳膏：换尿布后，局部应用，每日 2 次。

• 氢化可的松 0.5%～1%药膏：局部应用，每日 2 次。

• 达克宁 2%乳膏：换尿布后外用，每日 2 次。

• 硝酸咪康唑 0.25%软膏：换尿布和洗澡后使用。

• 莫匹罗星 2%软膏或霜剂（百多邦）：更换尿布后局部应用 3～5 次/日（婴幼儿＞3 月龄）。

• 制霉菌素：10 万 U/g，霜剂、粉剂或软膏：换尿布后外用，每日 2 次。

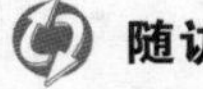

随访

■ 进一步处理

入院指征

• 虐待或忽视儿童的证据。

• 脓毒症的迹象。

尿道创伤 Urethral Trauma

Amanda Lamond Holden　张晟　林兆奋 译

基本内容

■ 描述

• 尿道出血、膀胱肿胀、无法排尿和/或肉眼尿血是尿道创伤的常见表现。

• 发现于 14%的盆骨骨折。

• 与双侧耻骨支骨折（也成为骑跨骨折）密切相关。

• 女性：由于其尿道短、未暴露而且是活动的，尿道损伤较为罕见。

• 女孩＜17 岁：因更灵活的盆骨环损伤风险更高。

• 膀胱颈是最常见的损伤位置。

• 男性：尿道分为两部分。

• 后尿道：

- 更易损伤（～90%）。

- 前列腺部。

- 尿道膜部。

• 前尿道：

- 损伤较少。

- 球部。

- 阴茎。

• 尿道损伤分类如下：

- 第一种：尿道伸展但未破裂。

- 第二种：前列腺/膜部分穿孔（部分或完全），泌尿生殖道隔膜完好无损。

- 第三种：泌尿生殖隔膜近和远端的尿道断裂。

■ 病因

• 女性：

- 骨盆骨折罕见。

- 骑跨伤。

- 分娩或阴道手术。

- 性创伤、性虐待。

• 男性：

- 骨盆骨折常见。

- 骑跨伤常见。

- 穿透伤，切割伤。

- 性活动/器械。

诊断

■ 症状和体征

• 男性：

- 尿道出血。

- 肉眼尿血。

• 女性：

- 阴道穹窿出血。

- 肉眼血尿。

病史

骨盆区创伤。

体格检查

• 再次手术期间检查身体和骨盆可能引起骨盆疼痛。

• 尿道外伤三联征，出血、无法排尿、肿胀膀胱。

• 50%的病例均有尿道出血。

• 肉眼血尿能预测泌尿损伤（尿液不清澈，非黄色尿液）。

• 直肠检查："高位前列腺"，其灵敏度＜50%。如果检测到，请不要用这一发现排除尿道损伤。

• 除超声波外：FAST 超声检测，耻骨上的视图可以揭示膀胱四周出血。

■ 基本检查

• 女性：

- 行包括阴道裂伤和其他出血病因在内的详细阴道检查。

- 如果检测到损伤，应行尿道完整性放射检测导尿管。

- 如果不可能，应该进行耻骨弓穿刺引流术和膀胱造口术。

• 男性：

- 如果检测到损伤，应在导尿管置换前行尿道完整性放射检测导尿管，以防止部分尿道撕裂转变为完全撕裂。

- 如果不可能，应该进行耻骨联合上穿刺和膀胱造口术。

儿科注意事项

• 如果男性和女性生殖器的检测很难实施，可采用麻醉后检测。

• 除更好地让患者能够承受，镇静麻醉下或手术室内的检测允许医生排除性虐待，并确认该损伤与病史前后一致。

■ 诊断检查与说明

实验室检查

尿液分析、血细胞比容、血尿素氮、肌酐。

影像学检查

• 逆行尿道造影(RUG)。

- 水溶性造影剂通过带导管的注射器在尿道口注射。

- 应注意造影剂外渗及其与膀胱前间隙和泌尿生殖隔膜的关系。

- 应对溢出处和尿道及膀胱的距离做出评估。

- 如果尿道全部撕裂，膀胱内则不会出现造影剂，将会出现明显的溢出。

- 部分撕裂将显示膀胱内的造影剂有不同程度的外渗。

N

- 应进行排泄性尿道造影以确定近端尿道撕裂。
• 膀胱造影。
• 40%的尿道损伤伴随膀胱损伤。

诊断步骤/外科

尿道创伤需要紧急泌尿科会诊。

■ 鉴别诊断

• 会阴阴道损伤。
• 膀胱损伤。
• 输尿管及肾脏损伤。

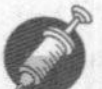

治疗

■ 院前

院前创伤方案。

■ 初步稳定/治疗

危及生命的创伤应该放在首要位置。

■ 急诊治疗/程序

• 最好由有经验的泌尿科医师处理尿道挫伤、撕裂和撕脱。
• 膀胱解压是极为重要的最初预防手段。如果尿道 Foley 尿管置换术不可能实现，应该实施耻骨联合上穿刺术和膀胱造口术。

■ 药物治疗

适当的镇痛。

一线用药

阿片类：
• 根据疼痛创伤方案的需要如吗啡、地乐定或芬太尼。

随访

■ 进一步处理

入院指征

• 并发创伤性损伤。
• 尿道、阴茎和膀胱损伤需紧急手术治疗。
• 部分撕裂：
- 经尿道或耻骨联合上引流处理。
• 完全撕裂：
- 经手术治疗或单独耻骨联合上引流处理：
• 有些通过端端吻合术修复。

出院指征

单独尿道创伤通常能在恰当的导尿术和耻骨联合上膀胱造口术后，通过隔日的泌尿科随访在门诊处理。

转诊问题

如果患者从急诊出院，那么随访是必要的。

■ 随访建议

对所有尿道创伤的患者而言，随访都是有必要的。

要点和误区

• 怀疑患者有尿道创伤的创伤患者在尝试插入 Foley 尿管之前咨询泌尿科。
• 通过 Foley 尿管抵抗阻力能将部分撕裂转变为完全撕裂。
• 未能辨识尿道创伤能导致尿失禁和性功能障碍。

尿道瘘 Urinary Tract Fistula

Patrick G. Meloy　张晟　林兆奋 译

基础知识

■ 描述

尿道瘘可以在泌尿道的任何部分和胸腔、腹腔、盆腔、皮肤之间形成。

■ 病因

• 结肠膀胱瘘：
- 常见于原发性胃肠道疾病的并发症，如憩室、克罗恩病和结肠癌。
- 医源性(术后或放疗后并发症)。
- 创伤性尿道口破裂。
- 男性更见。
• 膀胱阴道、尿道阴道和输尿管阴道瘘：
- 膀胱阴道瘘是尿道后天获得性瘘最常见的。
- 在不同地区(发达国家和发展中国家)病因学不同。
◦ 在发达国家多见于因手术所致的创伤、盆腔的病理状态、放疗后、恢复过程中的损伤。辐射诱发的瘘管可能在照射后数月至数年内不会出现。
◦ 发展中国家多见于难产和产科创伤引起。

诊断

■ 症状和体征

• 结肠膀胱瘘。
- 慢性或反复发作的尿路感染。
- 耻骨联合上疼痛。
- 排尿异常：气尿、粪尿、血尿、尿恶臭、尿杂质。
• 膀胱阴道瘘。
- 如果在术后发生，表现为拔除导尿管后仍有尿液渗出。
- 常无痛。
- 尿持续性从阴道渗漏(可能和尿失禁混淆)。
- 会阴皮肤因持续尿渗漏而受刺激。
• 尿道阴道瘘。
- 症状主要和瘘的位置及大小相关。
- 可以表现为无症状或持续性阴道尿渗漏。
• 输尿管阴道瘘。
- 常有近期手术史，特别是复杂手术史。
- 上或侧腹部疼痛、发热和肠梗阻。如有上述症状则尿囊肿或肾梗阻可能性大。
- 间断性阴道尿渗漏。

病史

• 通过既往用药、手术、妊娠病史了解危险因素。
• 要了解尿渗漏持续的时间和位置：间歇性的或体位性的多见于输尿管膀胱瘘；持续性的多见于膀胱阴道瘘。
• 尿渗漏的特点。
• 伴随症状。

体格检查

• 结肠膀胱瘘：
- 往往伴随胃肠道疾病一起发现。体格检查常没有特殊体征。
- 可以表现为无症状或持续性阴道尿渗漏。
• 膀胱阴道瘘、尿道阴道瘘和输尿管阴道瘘：
- 镜下检查可发现瘘管开口处有一小块肉芽肿组织变红，也可能在阴道穹窿出现尿池。

N

基本检查

必须评估尿路感染、肾脏梗阻情况和一些与原发病相关的急症（如肿瘤或克罗恩病的并发症）。

诊断检查与说明

实验室检查

• 尿分析：
- 结肠膀胱瘘：
◦ 白细胞、细菌、残渣。
- 膀胱阴道瘘、尿道阴道瘘和输尿管阴道瘘：
◦ 白细胞、细菌。
• 尿素和肌酐：
- 如果有尿路梗阻，结果可能有异常。

影像学检查

• 通常不需要做紧急影像学检查，可以和专科医师讨论。
• 结肠膀胱瘘：
- 腹部和盆腔 CT 检查。
• 膀胱阴道瘘、尿道阴道瘘和输尿管阴道瘘：
- 膀胱镜、逆行肾盂造影或静脉肾盂造影。

诊断步骤/外科

• 通常见于门诊。
• 结肠膀胱瘘：口服活性炭能在尿中发现黑色微粒，可以确诊。
• 膀胱阴道瘘、尿道阴道瘘和输尿管阴道瘘：
- 双染料：①卫生棉置于阴道；②口服非那吡啶；③亚甲基蓝或蓝胭脂红缓慢注入膀胱；④如果 1 h 后卫生棉顶端变成橘黄色，输尿管阴道瘘可能性大；若中部变蓝色则可能是膀胱阴道瘘；尾端变色则可能是尿道阴道瘘。

鉴别诊断

• 结肠膀胱瘘：
- 反复的尿路感染。
- 其他原因导致气尿。
◦ 产气的病原体引起的尿路感染，如梭形芽孢杆菌。
◦ 糖尿病尿发酵。
◦ 最近有过经尿路器械检查。
• 膀胱阴道瘘、尿道阴道瘘和输尿管阴道瘘：
- 尿失禁。
- 正常阴道分泌物。
- 阴道炎。

治疗

初步稳定/程序

• 对症治疗。
• 酌情使用静脉补液、升压药和静脉抗生素治疗尿路感染的脓毒症。

急诊治疗/程序

• 结肠膀胱瘘：
- 评估患者的并发症。
- 有尿路感染，取分泌物行培养。
- 有感染征象及早使用抗生素。
- 及早泌尿科转诊以进一步诊治，必要时行外科手术。
• 膀胱阴道瘘、尿道阴道瘘和输尿管阴道瘘：
- 考虑放置导尿管。
- 有感染征象及早使用抗生素。
- 紧急转诊泌尿科和妇科医生进一步治疗。

随访

进一步处理

入院指征

• 脓毒症。
• 需要抗感染又无法口服抗生素的患者。
• 胃肠道疾病或肿瘤的急症。

出院指征

• 脓毒症（经治疗后）无没有感染征象。
• 有尿路感染但可以口服抗生素的患者。

随访建议

泌尿生殖专家（泌尿科或妇科）医师的随访是很有必要的。

要点和误区

• 在有危险因素（通常是复杂的近期盆腔手术）和复发性尿路感染的患者中发现尿路瘘。
• 如果有发现尿道瘘，肿瘤是需要首先考虑的情况。
• 阴道尿渗漏和尿失禁往往不易区分。

尿道炎 Urethritis

Hany Y. Atallah 张晟 林兆奋 译

基本知识

描述

• 尿道炎是指任何原因导致的尿道炎症（通常感染）。
• 大多数病例发生在性行为频繁的年轻男性。
• 伴随尿道分泌物和排尿困难。
• 在与患有性传播疾病、细菌性阴道病及泌尿道感染的伴侣暴露后可能导致尿道炎。
• 尿道炎也可能在性交后发生。

病因

• 性传播疾病，最常见的原因如下：
- 淋病奈瑟菌（35%）。
- 沙眼衣原体（25%～50%）。
- 生殖器支原体和尿素分解尿素原体（30%）。
• 少见原因：
- 阴道滴虫。
- 念珠菌。
- 单纯疱疹病毒。
- 梅毒螺旋体。
- 流感嗜血杆菌。
- 腺病毒。
- 生殖器疣。
- 肠道细菌（如插入肛交）。
- 酒精。
- 系统疾病。
- 尿道异物。

诊断

• 淋菌性尿道炎的症状通常在暴露后 4～7 日出现，非淋菌性尿道炎的症状通常在暴露后 5～8 日出现，在许多患者中基本上很少或没有症状。

N

• 多数患者初期只有细微甚症状至没有症状。

■ 症状和体征

• 尿道分泌物，排尿困难。
• 第一段尿液浑浊。
• 瘙痒。
• 脓尿。
• 可能出现腹股沟区淋巴结肿大。

病史

• 尿道分泌物的颜色、浓度和数量。
• 伴随排尿困难、尿急、尿频、血尿和血性精液的相关症状。
• 性传播疾病的风险因素：
- 新伴侣或性伴侣多。
- 伴侣症状。
- 肛交或口交。
- 青年。
- 社会经济地位低。

体格检查

• 尿道分泌物。
• 内衣上的污渍。
• 尿道结痂。
• 生殖器病变。
• 淋巴结病。
• 触诊睾丸、附睾、精索：
- 肿块或触痛。

■ 基本检查

• 尿道拭子：用于淋病奈瑟菌和衣原体的确诊。
• 脱氧核糖核酸扩增、脱氧核糖核酸探针和通过聚合酶链式反应对尿液样本的检测显示出良好的灵敏度，都是可接受的检测。
• 行快速血浆反应素试验或者性病研究实验室，因为性传播疾病常同时发生。
• 还应向患者提供 HIV 检测。
• 如果无法进行检测，可以根据病史和身体状况做出尿道炎的推定诊断。

■ 诊断检查与说明

• 治疗后患者再次被他(她)的医师评估时复查尿道拭子的革兰染染色和培养。
• 首次排空或在尿道拭子行 DNA 扩增(连接酶链反应)或者聚合酶链反应：
- 对诊断奈瑟菌和衣原体的诊断也同样有效。
• 诊断建议：检测当日首次尿的白细胞酯酶阳性或白细胞计数≥10 高倍镜。

■ 鉴别诊断

• 肥皂和杀精子剂的化学刺激。
• 附睾炎。
• 睾丸炎。
• 盆腔炎。
• 前列腺炎。
• 反应性关节炎(曾称莱特尔综合征)。
• 尿道硬下疳(起源于梅毒)。
• 尿路感染。

儿科注意事项

• 儿童患尿道炎应该怀疑是否有虐待儿童。
• 青春期前奈瑟菌感染整个阴道穹隆，因此不需要进行内镜检查：
- 外部检查和细菌培养就可以了。
• 潜在并发症：
- 反复感染。
- 上行性尿道感染，包括盆腔炎性疾病及附睾睾丸炎。
- 输卵管受损和不孕。
- 关节炎。
- 结膜炎、葡萄膜炎及失明。

治疗

■ 初步稳定/疗法

多数患者生命体征平稳。

■ 急诊治疗/程序

• 基于可能的病因，可凭经验治疗。
• 奈瑟菌和衣原体感染都应被治疗。

■ 药物治疗

• 淋病奈瑟菌：
- 降低药物敏感性已促使建议采用联合疗法治疗淋球菌感染。
- 阿奇霉素：口服 2 g，一次。
- 头孢噻肟：肌内注射 500 mg(同时每次口服 1 g 丙磺舒)，一次。
- 头孢西丁：肌内注射 1 次(同时每次口服 1 g 丙磺舒)，一次。
- 头孢唑肟：肌内注射 500 mg，一次。
- 头孢曲松：250 mg(儿童：25～50 mg/kg)，肌内注射或静脉注射，一次。
- 奇霉素：肌内注射 2 g，一次。
• 衣原体：
- 阿奇霉素：口服 1 g(儿童：第 1 日 10 mg/kg；2～5 日：5 mg/kg)，一次。
- 多西环素：口服 100 mg，每日 2 次，7 日。
- 红霉素成分：500 mg[儿童：40 mg/(kg·d)，分 4 次]口服，每日 4 次，7 日。
- 琥乙红霉素：800 mg[儿童：30～50 mg/(kg·d)，分 4 次]口服，每日 4 次，7 日。
- 左氧氟沙星：500 mg，口服，每日 1 次，7 日。
- 氧氟沙星：300 mg，口服，每日 2 次，7 日。
• 生殖道支原体：
- 阿奇霉素：口服，1 g(儿童：第 1 日 10 mg/kg；2～5 日：5 mg/kg)，每日 1 次。

妊娠注意事项

• 孕妇禁用氟喹诺酮类和多西环素。
• 阿奇霉素有效安全。
• 为确保治愈治疗 3 周后重新检测。

> **注意**
> 全球范围内耐喹诺酮类奈瑟菌的发生率上升。

随访

■ 进一步处理

入院指征

除非患有其他疾病或感染，否则尿道感染患者无需留院。

出院指征

所有患者应该出院，并安排门诊外的随访或者安排家庭医师。

转诊问题

• 如果疑似存在虐童现象，必须采取孩童保护服务；应该确认孩子是否处于安全的家庭状态下。如果不能保证安全的家庭环境，就应该让孩子住院。
• 应该评估性伴侣。
• 在美国很多州，性传染疾病需要上报。

■ 随访建议

• 应该以初级护理随访所有患者，确保对感染治疗足疗程。
• 所有疑似或确定患有尿道炎的患者应该进行 HIV 测验。应向患者提供有关安全性行为的信息。

要点和误区

• 对疑似尿道炎，应同时治疗奈瑟菌和衣原体感染。
• 越来越多的证据表明，患反复尿道炎的患者应该评估其他非典型感染(多西环素耐药的解脲脲原体或生殖道支原体、阴道毛滴虫)。
• 始终考虑尿道炎患者其他性传染疾病。
• 确保患者将通知他们的性伴侣，便于他们同时治疗。

尿路感染(成人) Urinary Tract Infections, Adult

Paul A. Szucs · Barnet Eshin 张晟 林兆奋 译

基础知识

描述

• 尿液中出现病原菌或病菌侵入泌尿道。

• 泌尿系症状伴镜下细菌数 $>10^2\sim10^5$ CFU/ml 和白细胞 $>10/mm^3$。

• 女性一生中患尿路感染的概率>50%。

• 无并发症膀胱炎:

- 女性,年龄在 13~50 岁。
- 症状持续时间少于 2~3 日。
- 未孕。
- 无发热(体温低于 38 ℃)。
- 无腰痛。
- 无肋脊角压痛。
- 前 1 年尿路感染少于 4 次。
- 最近未做过泌尿生殖系统有创检查和手术。
- 没有功能性或结构性泌尿系统功能异常。
- 没有免疫系统功能异常。
- 神经系统功能完整。

• 复杂膀胱炎:

- 不符合上述诊断条件。
- 男性。
- 有功能性或结构性代谢性的泌尿系统功能异常。
- 尿残余。
- 有导尿管。
- 耐药菌。
- 最近有抗生素使用史。

• 简单肾盂肾炎:

- 肾脏薄壁组织的感染。
- 排尿困难、尿频、尿急。
- 高热、寒战、肌肉疼痛、恶心、呕吐。
- 腰背部、腹部疼痛。
- 肋脊角压痛。
- 白细胞增多。

• 复杂肾盂肾炎:

- 肾脏薄壁组织的感染体温>40 ℃。
- 尿脓毒症伴脓毒性休克。
- 糖尿病或其他免疫抑制性情况。
- 妊娠(妊娠期后期)。
- 伴随尿路梗阻或结石。
- 无症状(难以解释)。

病因

• 机制:

- 微生物在尿道周围定植,随后感染泌尿系统。

• 风险因素:

- 人群。
  ◦ 新生儿、青春期女孩、年轻男孩。
  ◦ 性生活频繁女性。
  ◦ 绝经妇女,老年男性。
- 行为。
  ◦ 性生活、杀精剂、隔膜。

• 老年绝经期女性。

• 膀胱排空效率低下、膀胱下垂、膀胱防御系统被破坏。

• 阴道 pH 升高。

• 大小便失禁引起污染(肠杆菌科)。

• 仪器。

- 老年男性多因为前列腺肥大或有创检查。

• 微生物。

- 埃希杆菌(80%~85%)。
- 腐生葡萄球菌(10%)。
- 其他(10%):克雷伯杆菌、变形杆菌、肠杆菌、铜绿假单胞菌、D组链球菌。

诊断

症状和体征

• 下尿路感染:膀胱炎。

- 排尿困难、尿频、尿急、尿等待。
- 耻骨联合上疼痛。
- 血尿。

• 上尿路感染:肾盂肾炎。

- 膀胱炎的症状。
  ◦ 发热、寒战。
  ◦ 腰痛,肋脊角压痛。
  ◦ 恶心、呕吐、厌食。
- 白细胞增多。
- 高达 50%膀胱炎的患者可能伴有肾盂肾炎。
  ◦ 症状持续>5 日,并有反复尿路感染史,均是上尿路感染的危险因素。
- 老年虚弱患者。
  ◦ 精神异常。
  ◦ 厌食。
  ◦ 社交活动减少。
  ◦ 腹痛。
  ◦ 夜尿、尿失禁。
  ◦ 晕厥或头晕。

基本检查

• 尿液分析(试纸检测、显微镜检测)。

• 女性:排除妊娠、尿道炎、阴道炎、盆腔炎。

• 男性:排除尿道炎、附睾炎、前列腺炎,询问是否有肛交史或 HIV 感染。

• 年轻健康男性一般不推荐首先做尿路感染的泌尿系评估。

诊断检查与说明

实验室检查

• 快速尿液筛查:

- 试纸法(白细胞酯酶+亚硝酸)检测效率高,特别是当数量 $>10^5$ CFU/ml。
- 如果已经确定是脓尿或菌尿,就不需实验室检测尿液。
- 白细胞酯酶:阳性比例(LR+)~5,阴性比例(LR−)~0.3。
- 亚硝酸:阳性比例(LR+)~30,阴性比例(LR−)~0.5。

• 尿液分析/镜检:

- 如果无法做快速尿液筛查,或筛查结果是阴性又高度怀疑有尿路感染。
- 中段尿白细胞 $>10\ mm^3$ 提示有感染。
- 细菌 $>10^5$ CFU/ml[阳性比例(LR+)~20,阴性比例(LR−)~0.1]。

• 尿培养:

- 复杂的尿路感染。
- 快速尿液筛查或镜检阴性,但怀疑有尿路感染。
- 治疗 2~3 日症状未有改善的。
- 复发患者。
- 最近住过院的患者。
- 院内感染。
- 肾盂肾炎。

• 尿液颜色:

- 白色、浑浊或模糊的:
  ◦ 结晶、脓尿。
- 红色或粉色:
  ◦ 甜菜、黑莓、大黄。
  ◦ 氯丙嗪、非那吡啶、酚酞、利福平、塞纳、硫咪嗪。
  ◦ 血。
- 褐色:
  ◦ 芦荟、蚕豆、大黄。

N

◦ 咖啡豆外皮、氯喹、左旋多巴、甲硝唑、呋喃妥英、伯氨喹、番泻叶。
◦ 胆红素、肌红蛋白。
- 橘色:
◦ 胡萝卜、维生素C。
◦ 非那吡啶、利福平、磺胺吡啶。
- 蓝色或绿色:
◦ 芦笋、食用染料、B族维生素。
◦ 阿米替林、西咪替丁、吲哚美辛、异丙嗪、丙泊酚、氨苯蝶啶。
◦ 家族性良性高钙血症。
- 紫色(罕见):
◦ 朴啉病。

老年人注意事项

• 无症状的菌尿可见于 20%＞65 岁和 50%＞80 岁的女性,常不需要治疗。
• 对于有症状患者通常治疗 7～10 日以防止复发和持续性菌尿的风险。
• 氟喹诺酮药物会影响中枢系统的副作用。

影像学检查

• 用于复杂的上尿路感染。
• 当怀疑有结石或梗阻时可行 CT、肾脏超声或静脉肾盂造影检查。

诊断步骤/外科

患者有严重的血尿,因同种病原体所致的反复发作的尿路感染,或有梗阻表现,需要泌尿科医师评估结构功能异常情况。

鉴别诊断

• 阑尾炎。
• 憩室炎。
• 附睾炎。
• 肾结石。
• 宫颈炎。
• 前列腺炎
• 肾盂肾炎。
• 尿道炎。
• 外阴道炎。

治疗

初步稳定/治疗

尿脓毒症/脓毒性休克:
• 气道管理和复苏。
• 早期目标导向治疗。
• 静脉补充晶体液(30 ml/kg)。
• 早期抗感染治疗。
• 必要时使用血管活性药。

急诊治疗/程序

稳定的患者

• 选择抗生素需考虑的因素包括:临床疗效、副作用、耐药率、成本、药物可用性。
• 根据患者特点(过敏、耐受性、费用、依从性)和当地社区耐药性流行情况制定个性化的治疗方案。
• 各年龄段的成年女性的最佳抗生素治疗时间(3～7 日)都是相似的。
• 对于不是复杂尿路感染的女性患者,通常进行 3 日抗生素治疗。
- 优于单剂疗法。
- 临床根据效果常用 5～10 日疗法,很少有副作用。
- β-内酰胺类抗生素应当连续使用 7 日。
• 耐药菌因社区而异,随时间而变化。
- 在北美地区,40%～50%的大肠杆菌对氨苄西林耐药,3%～17%对氟喹诺酮类药物耐药。
- 对甲氧苄啶-磺胺甲噁唑耐药率已上升至 30%。
- 一些研究发现对呋喃妥因耐药要少于一些被广泛使用的抗生素。
- 细菌培养的耐药性和临床相关性不大,因为尿的血药浓度大大高于试验时的药浓度,相比耐药菌。
- 避免使用社区耐药率高于 20%的抗生素。
• 蔓越莓汁或片剂/产品:
- 证据表明治疗无效。
- 防止特定大肠埃希菌黏附尿上皮细胞,但可能不降低复发性尿路感染妇女的复发率。
• 上尿路疾病的经典治疗——2 s 规则:
- 2 L 静脉晶体液。
- 2 片羟考酮/对乙酰氨基酚。
- 1 g 头孢曲松或 2 mg/kg 庆大霉素。
- 如果发热下降 2℃,患者可以保持(每日)2 杯水。
- 出院后继续服用喹诺酮类药物 2 周。
- 2 日内跟进。
• 抗生素的选择:
- 呋喃妥因。
◦ 如果肌酐清除率＜30 ml/min 避免(使用)。
◦ 如果怀疑早期肾盂肾炎,则不适用。
- 甲氧苄啶-磺胺甲噁唑。
- 磷霉素。
◦ 如果怀疑早期肾盂肾炎,则不适用。
- β-内酰胺是二线药物。
◦ 疗效逊色于甲氧苄啶-磺胺甲噁唑及氟喹诺酮类。
- 口服头孢菌素在某些特定情况使用是合理的:
◦ 需要 7 日治疗方案。
- 由于氨苄西林或阿莫西林耐药率高,不得用于经验性治疗。
- 阿莫西林-克拉维酸盐的疗效不如环丙沙星,可能是由于未能根除阴道大肠杆菌。
- 氟喹诺酮。
◦ 对妇女用于二线治疗。
◦ 用于简单的尿路感染风险大于收益。
◦ 肌腱断裂,中枢神经系统的副作用。
◦ 所有氟喹诺酮类药疗效相近(约 95%的敏感率),但副作用有所不同。
◦ 抗生素耐药高流行。
◦ 所处地区耐药性不明,＞20%的概率对甲氧苄啶-磺胺甲噁唑耐药。
- 糖尿病的女性患者感染克雷伯杆菌的风险大。
- 非那吡啶治疗排尿困难。
- 用合适的镇痛药止痛。

妊娠注意事项

• 无症状菌尿者给予抗生素 4～7 日:
- 呋喃妥因。
◦ 妊娠期前 3 个月使用可能致婴儿畸形。
◦ 对 6-磷酸葡萄糖脱氢酶缺乏者禁用。
- 阿莫西林(非一线用药,耐药率高)。
- 磷霉素(高效安全)。
- 甲氧苄啶-磺胺甲噁唑。
◦ 磺胺甲噁唑要防止用于妊娠晚期,以避免新生儿红素脑病。
◦ 甲氧苄啶避免用于妊娠期前 3 个月。
- 氟喹诺酮类应避免使用于以下情况。
◦ 中枢神经系统反应。
◦ 恶病质。
◦ 影响胶原形成。

药物治疗

• 阿莫西林-克拉维酸:口服 875 mg,q12 h。
• 头孢羟氨苄:1～2 g,口服,q24 h。
• 头孢地尼:600 mg,口服,q24 h。
• 头孢克肟:400 mg,口服,q24 h。
• 头孢泊肟:400 mg,口服,q12 h。
• 头孢他啶:1～2 g,静脉滴注,q8～12 h。
• 头孢曲松:1～2 g,静脉注射/肌内注射,q24 h。
• 头孢呋辛:250～500 mg,口服,q12 h。
• 头孢氨苄:250～500 mg,口服,q6 h。
• 环丙沙星:500 mg,口服,q12 h。
• 多立培南:500 mg,静脉滴注,q8 h。
• 磷霉素:3 g 单剂量。

• 庆大霉素：2 mg/kg，静脉注射或肌内注射，q8 h。
• 左氧氟沙星：250～500 mg，口服，q24 h。
• 呋喃妥因：100 mg，口服，q12 h。
- 可用于排尿困难对症治疗。
- 可能会使尿液、泪液、隐形眼镜变为橙色。
• 甲氧苄啶-磺胺甲噁唑：口服 160～800 mg，q12 h；或静脉注射 10 mg/(kg·d)，q6～8～12 h。

随访

进一步处理

入院指征

• 不稳定及无法口服药物的患者。
• 中毒表现及生命体征不稳定。
• 肾盂肾炎。
- 难治的患者。
- 年龄极大患者。
- 免疫抑制。
- 尿路梗阻。
- 考虑合并尿路结石。
- 合并其他严重疾病。
- 门诊治疗无效。
- 妊娠晚期。

出院指征

• 生命体征正常。
• 能规律地应用口服药物。
• 没有严重合并症。
• 若有必要，可以 48～72 h 随访。
• 未合并肾盂肾炎的健康患者，按 2 s 规则治疗有反应。
• 妊娠早期肾盂肾炎妇女能做到很好随访，可以作为门诊患者治疗。

转诊问题

对于反复的尿路感染需要团队研究是否有潜在的其他病理因素。

随访建议

尿路感染患者需要基层内科医师随诊。

要点和误区

• 如果女性在 6 个月患 2 次以上急性膀胱炎，或 1 年内患 3 次以上急性膀胱炎，可考虑预防性服用抗生素，或采取性交后预防。
• 妊娠妇女需做无症状菌尿的筛查和治疗，因为有 20%～40%会进展为肾盂肾炎。
• 有无症状菌尿孕妇会增加早产、低体重、围生期死亡率的风险。
• 肾移植患者、最近接受过泌尿系统手术的患者和中性粒细胞减少的患者需治疗无症状菌尿。
• 男性急性膀胱炎风险因素：年龄大、HIV 感染、未割包皮、解剖学异常(前列腺肥大或尿道狭窄)、性活动(尤其是肛交)。
• 25%的男性尿路感染患者患有前列腺炎，甲氧苄啶-磺胺甲噁唑和氟喹诺酮是一线治疗药物。
• 对于留置尿管患者，脓尿和尿路感染相关性弱于非留置尿管者。

尿路感染(儿童) Urinary Tract Infections, Pediatric

Roger M. Barkin · Suzanne Z. Barkin 张晟 林兆奋 译

基础知识

描述

• 直肠和会阴的细菌侵袭入泌尿系统：
- 婴儿，常见血源播散。
- 儿童，膀胱输尿管反流。
• 通过导尿管或耻骨联合上穿刺获得的标本，培养出单一细菌数＞50 000/ml，可诊断为尿路感染，其他的标本收集方法并不常规用于儿童的最终诊断。
• 6 岁人群中，2%的男孩和 8%的女孩患有尿路感染
• 对于 0～3 个月婴儿，30%的尿路感染伴有脓毒症。
• 发病诱因：
- 会阴部卫生差。
- 女性尿道短。
- 女性大于男性。
- 排尿次数过少。
- 便秘。
- 性行为。
- 男性行包皮环切术可以降低患病风险。
- 膀胱输尿管反流(VUR)、尿路阻塞。
- 膀胱功能障碍。
- 高钙尿。

病因

• 发热的婴儿中有 4%～7%患有尿路感染。
• 细菌种类：
- 大肠杆菌(占 80%)。
- 肺炎克雷伯菌。
- 金黄色葡萄球菌。
- 肠杆菌。
- 变形杆菌。
- 铜绿假单胞菌。
- 肠球菌。

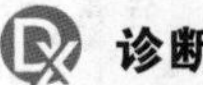

诊断

注意

若没有实验室检查，儿童尿路感染比较难诊断。

症状和体征

病史

• 通常没有什么特殊性。
• 婴儿：
- 脓毒症表现。
- 喂养困难。
- 易激，精神萎靡。
- 发热，低体温。
• 1 个月到 3 岁的幼儿：
- 易激。
- 发热。
- 呕吐，腹泻。
- 腹痛。
- 喂养困难，成长缓慢。
• 血尿。
• ＜2 岁女孩，≥3 危险因素(＜12 个月，白色人种，体温＞39 ℃，持续时间＞2 日，无其他原因的发热)，患病风险增加。
• ＞3 岁儿童：
- 排尿困难。
- 尿频。
- 遗尿。
- 新出现的尿失禁。
- 疼痛：腹部、耻骨上、背部、肋脊角。
- 发热。
- 血尿。

N

- 尿恶臭浑浊。
- 全身中毒表现：高温、颤抖、肋区敏感。
- 并发症：
- 复发尿路感染。
- 肾盂肾炎。
- 慢性肾衰竭：
  - 尽管有证据表明硬化是先天性的，但早发现于预瘢痕可能会减小。
- 肾周脓肿。
- 菌血症或脓毒症。
- 尿石形成。

体格检查

- 重要体征、温度和血压。
- 中毒体征。
- 发育情况。
- 腹部：尤其是肋脊角压痛。
- 生殖器。

基本检查

- 镜检红细胞、白细胞，细菌革兰染色。
- 仅镜检检测在婴儿诊断敏感性低。
- 脓尿的原因包括尿路感染、化学(沐浴液)或物理(手淫)刺激、脱水、肾结核、创伤、急性肾小球肾炎、呼吸道感染、阑尾炎、盆腔炎、胃肠炎。
- 稀释尿液可能会对试纸的可靠性产生不利影响。
- 白细胞酯酶和存在脓尿相关。
  - 有细菌尿的假阴性。
  - 链球菌感染或剧烈运动引起假阳性。
- 亚硝酸盐试验阳性表明存在能固定硝酸盐的细菌。常见的假阴性测试。
  - 需要尿液在膀胱 4 h 转化。
  - 如果阳性对诊断有帮助(假阳性少见)。
- 尿沉渣的革兰染色优于试纸法和传统镜检。
- 患有尿路感染新生儿镜检可以是正常的。在年龄小于 60 日的发热婴儿中，UA(白细胞酯酶、亚硝酸酯或脓尿)阳性对诊断≥50 000 CFU/ml 的尿路感染是敏感和特异性的。
- 尿液培养：
- 一般来说，单致病菌 50 000 CFU/ml 被用来作为感染存在的分界线。较低的菌落计数可用于耻骨联合上取标本。
- 样本需培养 30 min 或冷冻保存。
- 假阴性结果可能由于稀释、不合适培养基、最近有抗生素治疗、难培养菌种、尿液有抑菌剂、尿道完全梗阻。
- 清洁的容器和袋装标本。
  - 配合良好的男孩可做清洁获取标本。
  - 塑料袋收集足够尿液做分析(70%污染率)。如果培养阴性，以下措施很有用：
    - 留取前清洗龟头(男性)或清洁会阴部(女性)。
    - 可以作为筛查工具，排除没有经过经验性抗生素治疗的患者。如果评估感染可能性大，可以做尿培养。
- 置入导管是最佳获取尿液的方法，因为袋子收集清洁收集常会污染标本。
- 膀胱导管插入术。
  - 适用于所有婴儿。
  - 成功率比耻骨联合上穿刺吸引术高。
  - 注意无菌原则。
  - 放弃前面的 1～2 ml 尿液，以避免污染。
- 耻骨上穿刺吸引术用得较少，也能取得高质量的标本。
- 膀胱充盈最优。
- 适用于大部分婴儿。
- 膀胱充盈。
- 不常用。
- 超声可以辅助操作。

诊断检查与说明

实验室检查

- 对发热但又没有特殊体征，体格检查也正常的儿童适合做全血细胞计数和血培养。
- 电解质、尿素、肌酐。
- 如果有脱水、肾盂肾炎或复发的感染可做上述检查。

影像学检查

- 儿童需要影像学行评估：
- 小于 3 个月的婴儿。
- 第一次发生尿路感染的男孩。
- 症状和体征符合肾盂肾炎的诊断。
- 临床证据有肾脏疾病。
- 有人建议女孩＜3 岁且第一次发生尿路感染，也应做检查。
- ＞3 岁女孩。
- 首次感染患者伴有家族尿路感染史、排尿模式异常、发育异常、高血压、尿道异常，治疗效果不佳。
- 再次尿路感染。
- 排尿性膀胱尿道造影：
- 尿路感染患者常伴有膀胱输尿管反流和泌尿生殖道异常，需要排尿性膀胱尿道造影确诊。关于排尿性膀胱输尿管造影确诊的重要性还有争议。
- 提示是否有肾积水或明显的瘢痕。
- 肾脏膀胱超声：
- 超声检查在排除梗阻性病变和确定孤立肾、异位肾的儿童，以及判定肾脏适度的损害和恢复中发挥作用。
  - 超声能用于提示泌尿道解剖异常。需要超声检查的情况有，＜2 岁幼儿首次尿路感染、复发的尿路感染伴有泌尿系感染家族史、发育异常、高血压且对抗生素治疗不敏感的患者。
  - 核素膀胱造影(^{99}Tc DMSA 扫描)：有助于记录瘢痕形成和反流性肾病。
- 进一步的核医学研究评估取决于 VUR 的级别和治疗反应。

鉴别诊断

- 感染：
- 外阴道炎。
- 病毒性膀胱炎。
- 尿道炎(淋病奈瑟菌或沙眼衣原体)、肾小球肾炎。
- 阑尾炎。
- 创伤：
- 化学品刺激、膀胱炎。
- 会阴部。
- 性虐待。
- 手淫。
- 异物。
- 肾结石。
- 糖尿病。

治疗

初步稳定/治疗

- ＜3 个月的婴儿，若伴有发热或全身中毒者症状，按脓毒症治疗直到血或其他培养结果回报。
- 呼吸驱动力下降的患儿进行气道干预。
- 对因脱水、低血容量或脓毒血症的患儿予以 20 ml/kg 的 0.9%氯化钠，可能会重复给药。

急诊治疗/程序

- 对所有发热＜3 个月合并尿路感染的婴儿使用静脉注射抗生素。
- 新生儿用阿莫西林和庆大霉素。
- 出生后 4～8 周后使用头孢菌素。
- 门诊患者给予口服抗生素 7～14 日，单日或单剂量疗法似乎并不够，根据当地的耐药性选择药物，一旦药敏结果回报，抗生素可能需要更改。
- 阿莫西林。

N

- 阿莫西林-克拉维酸。
- 头孢氨苄。
- 甲氧苄啶-磺胺甲噁唑。
- 因为其耐药模式发生了变化，许多人建议将第三代头孢菌素(头孢克肟、头孢地尼)作为治疗无 GU 异常儿童的一线药物。尽管密切随访对于监测临床反应和病原体的敏感性至关重要，但口服治疗通常是足够的。
- 最近的尿路感染治疗可能提供了与复发性尿路感染儿童的敏感性相关的信息。
- 无发热尿路感染患儿的治疗时间可缩短至5日，对于>2岁的患儿，短期疗程通常仍不推荐给发热的尿路感染患儿。

• 中毒儿童和不能耐受口服治疗的儿童可能需要注射头孢曲松等非肠道抗生素。
• 如果病原体易感，患者一般应在 24～48 h 做出反应。如果反应不佳，请重新评估患者。
• 如果存在 VUR，一般会对每个 UTI 进行治疗。小剂量预防性抗生素或手术矫正的益处未得到证实。

■ 药物治疗

一线用药

• 阿莫西林：口服，40 mg/(kg·24 h)，q8 h。
• 阿莫西林-克拉维酸：口服，40 mg/(kg·24 h)，q8 h。
• 阿莫西林：静脉注射，100 mg/(kg·24 h)，q6 h。
• 头孢地尼：口服，14 mg/(kg·24 h)，每日1次。
• 头孢克肟：口服，16 mg/(kg·24 h)，第1日后 8 mg/(kg·24 h)，每日1次。
• 头孢曲松钠：静脉或肌内注射，50～75 mg/(kg·24 h)，q12～24 h。
• 头孢氨苄：口服，50 mg/(kg·24 h)，q6～12 h。
• 庆大霉素：2.5 mg/kg，静脉滴注，q8 h，如果足月和年龄>7日；2.5 mg/kg，静脉滴注，q12 h，如果足月和年龄 0～7日(小于 36 孕周产新生儿特殊给药剂量)。
• 甲氧苄啶-磺胺甲噁唑：口服，5 ml 液体(40/200，每 5 ml)10 kg，每日2次。

 随访

■ 进一步处理

入院指征

• 3个月以内婴儿。
• 脱水、中毒症状。
• 脓毒症表现。
• 怀疑肾盂肾炎。
• 尿路梗阻。
• 呕吐无法口服用药。
• 免疫功能不全。
• 肾功能不全。
• 异物(留置导管)。
• 孕妇。

出院指征

• 充分水化。
• 患脑膜炎或脓毒症风险低。
• 无中毒表现。
• 能遵医嘱口服药物治疗。

转诊问题

• 患者入院需要儿科、泌尿科、感染科医师意见；若有膀胱输尿管反流、肾脏异常、肾功能受损、复发感染或高血压也需入院。
• 要严格执行随访制度。

要点和误区

• 临床怀疑尿路感染时需要实验室检查确认。症状和体征常无特异性。
• 伴发热的尿路感染可以是菌血症。
• 有尿路感染的新生儿尿检可能正常。

尿潴留 Urinary Retention

Denise S. Lawe 张晟 林兆奋 译

 基础知识

■ 描述

• 急性尿潴留。
- 突然不能自发排尿。
- 多发生在年龄>60岁的男性。
- 急性尿潴留常见于因良性前列腺增生所致的后续治疗患者。

■ 病因

• 多种诊断考虑因素，以下的并非全部。
• 解剖因素。
- 阴茎：
◦ 包茎。
◦ 尿道口狭窄。
◦ 异物狭窄。
- 尿道：
◦ 肿瘤。
◦ 盆腔肿块。
◦ 盆腔器官脱垂。
◦ 结石。
◦ 尿道炎。
◦ 狭窄。
◦ 管腔狭窄。
◦ 血肿。
◦ 自然分娩后外阴水肿。
- 前列腺：
◦ 良性前列腺肥大。
◦ 肿瘤。
◦ 前列腺炎。
◦ 膀胱颈痉挛。
◦ 前列腺梗死。
• 神经因素。
- 运动神经麻痹。
◦ 脊髓休克。
◦ 脊髓综合征。
- 感觉神经麻痹。
◦ 糖尿病。
◦ 多发性硬化。
◦ 脊髓综合征。
• 药物。
- 抗组胺类。
- 抗胆碱能类。
- 解痉药。
- 三环抗抑郁类药。
- α受体激动剂。
- 麻醉剂。
- 非甾体抗炎药。

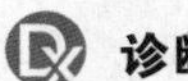 诊断

■ 症状和体征

• 轻度的腹部和耻骨联合上不适。
• 患者表现为坐立不安或痛苦。

• 慢性尿潴留常是无痛的。

病史

• 既往病史：

- 既往尿潴留病史。
- 前列腺增生还是前列腺癌。
- 其他肿瘤病史。
- 放疗病史。
- 骨盆创伤。

• 任何感染的征象包括脓肿。

• 任何结石的征象。

• 任何神经系统体征。

• 既往或现在静脉药物滥用史。

• 有无背部疼痛。

• 所有的药物治疗清单。

体格检查

• 重点(任何感染或休克的证据)。

• 腹部检查。

• 直肠检查。

• 泌尿生殖器检查，对所有女性行盆腔检查。

• 创伤患者应评估尿道的损伤。

基本检查

由于急性尿潴留的多种原因，全面的病史和体格检查是必要的，并将决定进一步的检查。

诊断检查与说明

实验室检查

• 只有在考虑发生急性肾功能不全时才去评估肾功能(这在急性尿潴留患者中少见)。

• 急性尿潴留 PSA 指标通常上升，对后续治疗患者 PSA 检查意义不大。

• 根据病史和体格检查酌情行尿常规检查。

影像学检查

• 如果考虑前列腺增生为病因，往往不需要影像学检查。

• 床旁超声可以快速确诊。

• 当考虑有肿块、肿瘤、脓肿膀胱颈结石时可考虑腹部盆腔 CT。

• 考虑有急性神经过程，可行脊髓影像学检查。

诊断步骤/外科

残余尿量：超过 200 ml 考虑异常。

鉴别诊断

• 慢性尿潴留。

• 考虑到根本原因，急性尿潴留通常是一个替代诊断，即前列腺增生，解剖梗阻。

治疗

院前

解决任何危及生命的征象。

初步稳定/治疗

• 首先识别和处理任何危及生命的情况。

• 膀胱减压。

- 尝试放置 14～18F 导尿管。
- 若放置不了，且有既往经尿道手术史或已知狭窄史，可改用 10～12F 导尿管。
- 若男性患者无法放置又未使用过其他器械，可考虑用带导丝 20～22F 导尿管。
- 若实在无法放置导尿管，可暂时用耻骨联合上穿刺作为临时措施或放置耻骨联合上导尿管。

• 对于创伤患者若考虑有尿道损伤，可以做尿道逆行造影术后再行置入导尿管。

急诊治疗/程序

• 膀胱排空测定尿量。

- 尝试放置导尿管快速减轻膀胱压力，可能产生暂时性肉眼血尿，少有临床意义。
- 去除梗阻后利尿。
  - 急性尿潴留可能会是长期放置尿管患者的并发症。
  - 没有随机试验比较过快速或间歇性膀胱减压这两种方法的优劣。
  - 快速膀胱降压总体是安全的，前提是如果出现低血压可提供支持治疗。

• 膀胱减压后最好观察 2～3 h 以保证去除梗阻后利尿不会带来一些临床恶化。

• 如果导管仍然留置在排尿时可使用腿式导管袋。

• 教导患者和家属进行正确的导管护理。

• 虽然常规使用预防性抗生素，但对于没有感染证据的留置导尿管的患者，并不推荐预防性使用抗生素。

• 良性前列腺肥大的患者可以使用 α 受体滞剂治疗。

• 停用一切可能导致尿潴留的药物。

• 治疗便秘。

药物治疗

• 盐酸哌唑嗪：治疗良性前列腺增生，1 mg，口服，每日 2～3 次，逐步加量到 20 mg/d。

• 坦索罗辛嗪：是一种常用来治疗良性前列腺肥大的 α_1 受体阻滞剂：0.4 mg 同一餐后口服，每日 1 次，逐步加量到 0.8 mg/d。

• 阿夫唑嗪：一种常用于治疗良性前列腺增生的 α 受体阻滞剂：10 mg 同一餐后口服。

• 特拉唑嗪：促进前列腺增生患者的尿流，起始每小时 1 mg 口服，最大剂量 20 mg/d。

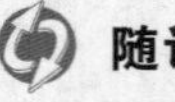

随访

进一步处理

入院指征

• 去除梗阻后，需要静脉补液或者升压药。

• 脓毒症。

• 梗阻由脊髓压迫导致。

• 因肿瘤或肿块压迫导致的梗阻。

• 需要泌尿外科手术或外科手术干预。

出院指征

大部分患者均能出院。

随访建议

• 大部分患者都需要对导管管理和急性尿潴留进行经常性评估。

• 如果是良性前列腺增生，大多数患者需要在 3～7 日进行泌尿外科门诊随访，进行自发排尿试验。

要点和误区

• 积极寻找肿瘤或肿物的证据很可能是急性尿潴留的原因。

• 积极寻找脊髓压迫的证据很可能是急性尿潴留的原因。

• 在找不到明确原因时多分析用药史，包括非处方药。

N

颞下颌关节损伤/综合征 Temporal-Mandibular Joint Injury/Syndrome

Benjamin W. Osborne · Chad B. Farr 范浩浩 李文放 译

基础知识

描述

• 肌筋膜疼痛引起颞下颌关节(TMJ)的功能障碍。
• 颞下颌关节紊乱征兆的发生率为40%～75%。
• 18～44岁的人最常见。
• 女性发病率较男性高1.5倍。
• 40%的患者症状能自己缓解。
• 颞下颌关节是一个滑膜关节。
- 允许铰链和滑动的动作。
- 正常范围为35～55 mm(上下颌门齿之间)。
• 关节疾病:
- 先天性或发育性。
- 退行性关节疾病:
◦ 炎症性(风湿性关节炎)。
◦ 非炎症性(骨关节炎)。
- 创伤。
- 颞下颌关节过度活动:
◦ 松弛。
◦ 脱位。
◦ 半脱位。
- 颞下颌关节活动受限:
◦ 牙关咬紧。
◦ 纤维化。
- 感染。
- 肿瘤。
• 咀嚼肌疾病:
- 局部肌痛。
- 肌炎。
- 肌痉挛。
- 挛缩。
- 肌筋膜疼痛疾病。
• 颞下颌关节弹响:
- 可能是正常表现;40%～60%发病人群中是一过性的表现。
- 颞下颌关节活动:关节粘连限制或关节盘移位或肌肉痉挛引起的牙关咬紧。
- 关节内关节盘功能紊乱:
- 前移脱位伴缩短:
◦ 闭口位的脱位。
◦ 张口时会有弹响及变异性疼痛。
◦ 时间延长症状会加重。
- 前移脱位不伴缩短:
◦ 关节盘是张口的机械性障碍。
◦ 最大开口限度可被限制在20～25 mm。
◦ 通常难以复位。

病因

颞下颌关节功能障碍知之甚少。
• 多因素所致:
- 磨牙症。
- 创伤。
- 错位闭合。
• 可能由于应激发生。

诊断

症状和体征

病史

• 耳前疼痛:
- 强度不等的持续性疼痛。
- 钝性疼痛。
- 可能累及同侧的耳、头部、颈部或眶周部。
- 下颌运动会使症状加重(特征诊断性病史)。
- 夜间更明显,常伴有失眠。
- 一天下来症状通常会加重。
• 夜间更明显,常伴有失眠。
• 舌、唇或面颊部疼痛。
• 耳痛。
• 耳胀。
• 耳鸣。
• 头晕。
• 颈痛。
• 头痛。
• 眼痛。

体格检查

• 关节声响:
- 关节出现刺痛或弹响。
- 张口和闭口时可触及或听到的弹响。
◦ 如果不伴有疼痛或其他功能障碍不足以诊断。
• 不对称和活动度受限:
- 牙槽骨坏死或侧向偏移。
- 下颚开口或闭口锁止。
• 咀嚼肌和颞下颌关节的压痛:
- 咬肌最常被累及。
• 动态负荷引起疼痛(咬合纱布)。

基本检查

• 基于病史和体格检查做出诊断。
• 排除其他原因引起的头痛和面部疼痛。

诊断检查与说明

实验室检查

除非存在其他病理改变,如通过红细胞沉降率区分颞下颌关节功能障碍中存在的巨细胞大动脉炎,否则不需要进行血液检验。

影像学检查

• 曲面体层X线机检查是首选的筛选X线检查:
- 可能表现出骨折或关节内病理学(即肿瘤或退行性关节疾病),但通常不明显。
• CT:最适合评估骨性结构的骨折、错位等。
• MRI:非还原位关节盘移位的最佳成像:
- 可以更好地观察关节。

鉴别诊断

• 急性冠状动脉综合征。
• 颈动脉夹层。
• 颅内出血(蛛网膜下腔出血)。
• 炎症性疾病:
- 巨细胞(颞)动脉炎。
- 类风湿关节炎。
• 三叉神经或舌咽神经痛。
• 血管性头痛。
• 口腔科相关疾病。
• 带状疱疹。
• 唾液腺疾病。
• 中耳炎、外耳炎。
• 鼻窦炎。
• 茎突疼痛。
• 颌骨创伤(骨折或脱位)。

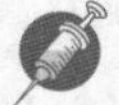

治疗

院前

提供舒适和安心的环境。

初步稳定/治疗

确保气道通畅是首要工作。

急诊治疗/程序

• 急性治疗选择:
- 向患者解释病情和患者健康教育,通常温和自我限制。
- 休息。
- 热疗。

N

- 镇痛药和抗焦虑药。
- 紧急减少打开或关闭锁定的 TMJ。
- 减少 TMJ 错位:
  ○ 错位通常是双侧的。
  ○ 静滴肌肉松弛剂可能有帮助。
  ○ 通常需要手术镇静。
  ○ 监测气道。
  ○ 可以面对患者或从后面执行。
  ○ 用纱布和/或压舌板保护拇指。
  ○ 拇指靠在下颌骨的口腔表面。
  ○ 手指环绕下颚。
  ○ 稳定的,向下的压力,当颚被引导第一在尾部方向,然后向后。
- 理疗:湿热敷或冰袋。
- 类固醇/利多卡因的混合物于疼痛部位注射。
• 门诊管理:
- 联合药物治疗:
  ○ 非甾体抗炎药。
  ○ 肌肉松弛剂。
  ○ 抗抑郁药。
  ○ 镇静催眠药。
- 家庭理疗;湿热敷或冰袋,机械性软食。
- 注意不要张口>2 cm 坚持 2 周。
- 避免嚼口香糖等触发动作。
- 在睡眠期间佩戴咬合器具。
- 转诊给口腔科或口腔颌面外科医师。

■ 药物治疗

一线用药

• 萘普生:250～500 mg,口服[儿童:10 mg/(kg·d)分次口服,q12 h]。

• 环苯扎林:5～10 mg,口服,每日 3 次(儿童:5～10 mg,如果>15 岁,口服,每日 3 次);肝功能障碍谨慎使用。

• 地西泮:2～10 mg,口服,每日 2～3 次[儿童:<12 岁,0.12～0.8 mg/(kg·d),口服,q6～8 h];单独使用时疗效差。

• 布洛芬:600 mg(儿童:10 mg/kg),口服,q8 h;比萘普生更有效。

二线用药

• 去甲替林:10～50 mg,口服,睡前。

• 麻醉止痛剂。

• 镇静催眠药。

随访

■ 进一步处理

入院指征

• TMJ 综合征可以在门诊患者的基础上进行管理。

• 除非锁定或脱位的关节不能缓解。

出院指征

用止痛药、肌肉松弛剂和热敷门诊治疗。

■ 随访建议

颞下颌关节综合征患者可能需要转诊至耳鼻喉科、口腔外科医师或其他口腔医师进一步护理。

要点和误区

• TMJ 锁定必须紧急处理。

• 如果没有耳源性耳痛,评估 TMJ。

• NSAIDs、休息和热敷是一线治疗。

凝血病逆转(非华法林药物所致) Coagulopathy Reversal(Nonwarfarin Agents)

Susanne M. Hardy　陈奇通 译

基础知识

■ 描述

• 服用抗凝药物的患者出现少许、较大或临床症状显著的出血,需要密切监测±抗凝逆转药物。

• 抗凝药物:
- 凝血酶间接抑制剂:
  ○ 肝素(UFH)。
  ○ 低分子肝素(LMWH):
    ■ 依诺肝素。
    ■ 达替帕林。
    ■ 亭扎肝素。
- 抗血小板药物:
  ○ 血小板聚集抑制剂:
    ■ 阿司匹林。
    ■ 氯吡格雷(波立维)。
    ■ 康格雷尔(肯格雷尔)。
    ■ 西洛他唑。
    ■ 双嘧达莫(潘生丁)。
    ■ 普拉格雷(高效)。
    ■ 噻氯匹定(噻氯匹啶)。
    ■ 替卡格雷(布里林塔)。
  ○ 糖蛋白血小板抑制剂(GP Ⅱb/Ⅲa):
    ■ 阿布西单抗(雷奥普)。
    ■ 乙替巴肽(整合素)。
    ■ 替罗非班(侵略者)。
  ○ 蛋白酶激活受体 1 拮抗剂:
    ■ 沃拉帕沙尔。
  ○ 血小板减少的未知机制:
    ■ 阿格雷利德(阿格里林)。
- 凝血因子Ⅹa 抑制剂:
  ○ 磺达肝癸钠(arixtra)。
  ○ 利伐沙班(xarelto)。
  ○ 阿皮沙班(eliquis)。
  ○ 依多沙班(savaysa)。
  ○ 倍他滨(bevyxxa)。
- 凝血酶直接抑制剂(DTI):
  ○ 阿加托班(acova)。
  ○ 比伐卢定(angiomax)。
  ○ 达比加群酯(pradaxa)。
  ○ 水蛭素衍生物:
    ■ 地西卢定(iprivask)。
    ■ 来匹卢定(refludan)。

儿科注意事项

• 肝素和低分子肝素是除华法林外最普遍使用的抗凝药物。

• DTI 的常规应用正在研究中,目前正在用于肝素诱导的血小板减少症(HIT)的设置。

老年注意事项

凝血因子Ⅹa 抑制剂主要通过肾脏排泄,达比加群酯和水蛭素衍生物用于肾功能不全的患者时需引起注意。

■ 流行病学

发病率和患病率估计

• 凝血酶间接抑制剂:
- 有 1/3 的患者发生出血并发症。
- 2%～6%的患者出血较多。

• 抗血小板药物:
- 300 多种 OTC 药物中含有阿司匹林。
- 关于血肿范围和死亡率增加的研究结果存在冲突。

• 凝血因子Ⅹa 抑制剂:
- 未知。

• 凝血酶直接抑制剂。

- 未知。

病因

- 凝血酶间接抑制剂：
  - 抗凝血酶Ⅲ灭活已活化的凝血因子Ⅹa，其同时抑制凝血酶。
  - 低分子肝素有较弱的灭活凝血酶的能力。
  - 半衰期呈剂量依赖性(30～150 min)，低分子肝素可长达 8 h。
- 抗血小板药物：
  - 环氧合酶 1(COX-1)抑制剂(阿司匹林)：
    - 使 COX-1 失活，阻止血小板失活的血栓素 A_2 的形成。
    - 单剂量抑制时间达到 1 周。
    - 新血小板形成可以每日 10%的速度恢复血小板功能。
    - 即使仅有 20%的血小板表现为正常 COX-1 活性时，患者仍可能表现出正常的凝血功能。
    - 阿司匹林的半衰期为 15～30 min。
  - ADP 拮抗剂(噻吩吡啶类)：
    - 抑制 ADP 依赖的血小板活化途径。
    - 氯吡格雷(波立维)的半衰期为 8 h。
  - 磷酸二酯酶抑制剂：
    - 双嘧达莫。
    - 抑制腺苷摄取和环 GMP 磷酸二酯酶活性，从而降低血小板聚集性。
  - GP Ⅱb/Ⅲa 抑制剂：
    - 防止血小板交联。
- 凝血因子Ⅹa 抑制剂：
  - 与抗凝血酶Ⅲ结合，催化凝血因子Ⅹa 的抑制。
  - 对凝血酶无直接抑制作用。
  - 正常肾功能时，半衰期为 5～21 h。
- DTI：
  - 竞争性靶点为凝血酶活性部位±外结合位点(配体结合位点)。
  - 达比加群酯的半衰期长(14～17 h)，其他药物半衰期较短(20～45 min)。

诊断

- 服用抗凝药物的患者出现活动性出血。
- 逆转指征：
  - 严重或危及生命的出血：
    - 外伤。
    - 胃肠道出血。
    - 颅内出血(ICH)。
  - 医学操作。

症状和体征

病史

- 抗凝药物的类型。
- 最后一次服用抗凝药物的时间。
- 接受抗凝治疗的疗程时间。
- 近期损伤或外伤。
- 出血部位。
- 症状(乏力、头重脚轻、头痛、腹痛)。

体格检查

- 生命体征±直立性。
- 寻找出血部位/创伤体征。
- 全面的神经系统检查。
- 直肠肛诊检查。

基本检查

- 血生化全套。
- 全血计数。
- PT/INR。
- APTT。
- 大便愈创木脂测试。
- ±纤维蛋白原/DIC 全套。

诊断检查与说明

- 凝血酶间接抑制剂：
  - APTT。
  - 抗凝血因子Ⅹa。
    - 大于 0.8 U/ml 为增高。
- 抗血小板药物：
  - 出血时间。
- 凝血因子Ⅹa 抑制剂：
  - 抗凝血因子Ⅹa(测量抑制 FⅩa 的抗凝剂浓度)。
  - PT、APTT 帮助小。
  - 磺达肝癸钠水平(有该项检查的医疗机构)。
- DTI：
  - APTT 帮助小。
  - 达比加群酯即稀释凝血酶时间(有该项检查的医疗机构)。

鉴别诊断

- 弥散性血管内凝血。
- 遗传性凝血功能障碍。
- 血小板功能不全：
  - 微血栓性血小板减少症、溶血性尿毒症综合征。
  - 肝素相关性血小板减少症。
  - 免疫性血小板减少症。

治疗

院前

- 压迫止血(如果可能)。
- 2 个大孔径静脉通道。
- 静脉输液。

初步稳定/治疗

- 与院前处理相同。
- 停用抗凝药物。
- 输注洗涤红细胞或启动大量输血方案。
- 考虑血小板减少性或服用抗血小板药物的患者的血小板。

急诊治疗/程序

- 凝血酶间接抑制剂：
  - 出血分级：
    - 小出血：观察 APTT、抗凝血因子Ⅹa。
    - 大出血：鱼精蛋白(类型Ⅱ用于肝素，类型Ⅲ用于低分子肝素)。
  - 鱼精蛋白：
    - 静脉使用 1 mg 中和 100 U 在 3～4 h 前使用的肝素。
      - 肝素使用少于 30 min，使用 1 mg/100 U 肝素。
      - 肝素使用在 30～120 min，使用 0.5 mg/100 U 肝素。
      - 肝素使用大于 120 min，使用 0.25 mg/100 U 肝素。
    - 缓慢静脉注射需大于 1～3 min，每 10 min 内不得大于 50 mg。
    - 短半衰期药物可能需要反复使用。
    - 鱼精蛋白逆转的有效性在于低分子肝素的特异性结构(无法完全逆转依诺肝素，lovenox)。
    - 低分子肝素在 8 h 内使用，1 mg 中和 1 mg/100 U 低分子肝素。
    - 低分子肝素在 8～12 h 使用，0.5 mg 中和 1 mg/100 U 低分子肝素。
    - 低分子肝素使用大于 12 h，不需要使用鱼精蛋白。
    - 对于低分子肝素，如果 APTT 持续延长，可反复使用首次剂量的半量。
    - 高或过大的剂量可引起反常的抗凝效果。
    - 快速使用可导致低血压、窦性心动过缓和过敏。
    - 过敏更易出现于对鱼类过敏或有鱼精蛋白接触史的患者。如果有过敏考虑，可在用药前使用皮质激素或抗组胺药物。

N

◦ andexanet alfa。
◦ 当前不可用。
◦ 作为诱导,靶向并隔离口服和可注射的凝血因子Ⅹa 抑制剂[包括可注射:依诺肝素(lovenox)、磺达肝素(arixtra)]。

• 抗血小板药物:
- 出血分级:
◦ 小出血:观察出血。
◦ 大出血:去氨加压素±血小板输注(类型Ⅲ)。
- 去氨加压素(DDAVP):
◦ 导致血管性假血友病因子和凝血因子Ⅷ释放。
◦ 0.3 μg/kg 静脉注射超过 15 min,限制 2 次静脉注射剂量,可以做皮下注射。
◦ 药效即刻出现。
◦ 多次使用与快速抗药反应、低钠血症和癫痫相关。
- 血小板:
◦ 输注至血小板到达 50 000/μl(平均 1 U 增加血小板计数 10 000/μl)。
◦ 可能需要每日反复输注。
◦ 风险包括输血相关的感染、急性肺损伤和过敏反应。

• 凝血因子Ⅹa 抑制剂:
- 出血分级:
◦ 小出血:观察出血。
◦ 大出血:4 个 F-PCC,如果利福沙班(沙雷托)/阿皮沙班(eliquis)/伊多沙班(savaysa)引起,考虑使用活性炭透析;如果可用,考虑使用氨甲环酸(TXA)、DDAVP 和 andexanet alfa,考虑使用磺达肝素(arixtra)进行血液透析(HD)。
- 浓缩凝血酶复合物(PCC):
◦ 4 因子型(八倍体):包括凝血因子Ⅱ、Ⅸ、Ⅹ和活化的凝血因子Ⅶ。
◦ 剂量为 25~50 U/kg,不超过 2 ml/min,不超过 5 000 U,仅限单次剂量。
◦ 作用时间少于 30 min。
◦ 远期安全尚未评估。
◦ 有血栓形成的风险。
◦ 可能出现过敏反应。
- 活性炭:
◦ 如果是利伐沙班(沙雷托)8 h 内摄入。
◦ 如果是阿皮沙班 6 h 内摄入。
◦ 如果是服用依多沙班后 2 h 内摄入。
◦ 100 g 口服或经胃管。
- DDAVP:
◦ 0.3 μg/kg 静脉注射超过 15 min,限制 2 次静脉注射剂量,可以做皮下注射。
◦ 成本和总体风险低。
- TXA:
◦ 25 mg/kg 静脉注射。
◦ 无疗效研究。
◦ 成本和总体风险低。
- andexanet alfa:
◦ 目前不可用。
◦ 对于阿哌沙班(eliquis),以 30 mg/min 的速度静脉注射 400 mg,然后以 4 mg/min 的速度持续输注 120 min。
◦ 对于利伐沙班(沙雷托),以 30 mg/min 的速度静脉注射 800 mg,然后以 8 mg/min 的速度持续输注 120 min。
◦ 作为诱导饵靶向和分离具有高特异性的口服和注射 FⅩa 抑制剂。
◦ 目前制造商正在寻求美国 FDA 批准,并进入第 4 阶段。
◦ 超滤/透析。
◦ 对于磺达肝癸钠(arixtra),可能会去除 20%,因此可能不会使用。

• DTI:
- 出血分级。
◦ 小出血:观察出血(除达比加群酯的半衰期为 14~17 h 外,其他凝血酶直接抑制剂的半衰期短),静脉输液以提高肾脏清除。
◦ 大出血:4F-PCC,考虑 DDAVP,如果在 1~2 h 摄入达比加群,则考虑使用活性炭,考虑伊达鲁珠单抗(praxbind),如果达比加群则考虑透析。
- PCC:
◦ 剂量为 25~50 U/kg,大于 2 ml/min,不超过 5 000 U,仅限单次剂量。
◦ 伊达鲁珠单抗。
◦ 用于达比加群。
◦ 5 g 总剂量(按 2.5 g 分次给药,间隔 15 min)。
◦ 美国 FDA 批准。
◦ 与高亲和力达比加群结合。
◦ 几分钟内效果明显。
◦ 研究表明止血效果得到改善,无明显血栓形成风险。
◦ 患者预后改善不明确。
- DDAVP:
◦ 剂量 0.3 μg/kg 静脉使用,大于 15 min,限制 2 次静脉注射,可以做皮下注射。
◦ 成本和总体风险低。
- 超滤/血液透析:
◦ 达比加群酯所致出血早期及大出血时考虑。
- 活性炭:
◦ 如果在达比加群 2 h 内摄入。
◦ 100 g 口服或经胃管。

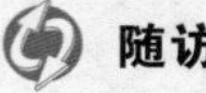

随访

进一步处理

入院指征

• 临床显著的出血。
• 逆转药物的使用。

出院指征

• 不显著的出血未经抗凝剂逆转药物治疗得到控制。
• 与出院后的血液科医师或首诊医师讨论是最为理想的后续进一步处理。

转诊问题

• 血库关于逆转药物的可用性。
• 外科/放射介入专科医师关于出血控制的可行性。

随访建议

密切随访和监测是最为重要的。

要点和误区

• 预防性肝素使用常不增加大出血的风险。
• 鱼精蛋白并非总是逆转低分子肝素,其有成分特异性。
• 如果低分子肝素使用已超过 12 h,鱼精蛋白可能并非是必要的。
• 单剂量阿司匹林可抑制 COX-1 长达 1 周。
• 使用凝血因子Ⅹa 抑制剂,达比加群酯,或者水蛭素衍生物时,需注意肾功能损害。
• 作为一线替代品的新鲜冷冻血浆(FFP)必须与大量的容量负荷进行权衡。
• TXA 疗效尚未证实,但成本低,总体风险低。
• 伊达鲁珠单抗现在美国 FDA 批准用于拮抗达比加群。
• andexanet alfa 目前不可用,但有望逆转 FⅩa 抑制剂和注射用间接因子(依诺肝素和磺达肝素)。
• 重组人因子Ⅶa(rFⅦa, NovoSeven)已在标签外使用,但考虑到所需的高剂量和血栓形成后遗症的可能性,不建议使用。
• 除非没有其他可用的或正在大量输血方案中使用的药物,否则不建议使用新鲜冰冻血浆(非华法林抗凝剂不会抑制非活性凝血成分的总体生成,但只与特定的活性因子结合,因此不会以替代治疗为目的)。

N

脓毒性关节炎

Amin Antoine Kazzi · Stephen R. Hayden · Mohamad Kanso 俞芸 王海嵘 潘曙明 译

基础知识

描述

• 细菌可通过以下途径进入关节：
- 血源性播散(最常见)。
- 侵袭性操作。
- 邻近部位的感染(如骨髓炎、蜂窝织炎)。
- 直接刺入，如植物刺或钉子。
• 急性炎症过程导致白细胞迁移至关节。
• 关节液增生，软骨破坏，并形成脓性渗出。
• 多达50%的患者关节出现不可逆功能丧失。
• 有资料显示死亡率高达11%。

儿科注意事项

• 髋关节感染最常见：
- 常见于患有中耳炎、上呼吸道感染或有股静脉穿刺病史的患者。
- 儿童化脓性髋关节炎的并发症有：缺血性坏死、骨骺分离、病理性脱位、关节炎。
- 50%的儿童患者<3岁。
- 婴儿患者表现为易怒、发热、纳差。
- 年龄大一点的孩子表现为发热、跛行、拒绝负重或活动关节。

病因

• 危险因素：
- 老年人、婴幼儿。
- 风湿病或关节退行性变的患者。
- 静脉注射毒品者(IVDU)、心内膜炎患者。
- 免疫抑制者(AIDS、糖尿病患者、正在接受化疗或激素治疗者)。
- 反复关节内注射，既往有关节疾病、创伤、义肢。
- 皮肤感染，皮肤溃疡。
• 现已证实，10%～20%的患者找不到病原菌。
• 常见病原菌：
- 成人髋关节感染(80%)、风湿性关节炎和糖尿病患者的病原菌为金黄色葡萄球菌。
- 一些研究发现，社区起病的成人关节炎中最常见的是多重耐药金黄色葡萄球菌(MRSA)。
- 健康的年轻患者中，淋球菌最常见，但近10年的发生率下降，这得益于黏膜传播感染发生率的下降。
• 其他病原菌：A组β溶血性链球菌，B组、C组和G组链球菌：
- 10%患者为革兰阴性杆菌(如铜绿假单胞菌、大肠杆菌)。
- 12%合并脑膜炎的患者为脑膜炎奈瑟菌。
• 假单胞菌常见于老年人、婴幼儿、免疫抑制者及静脉注射毒品者。
• 厌氧菌：见于糖尿病患者、人工关节。
• 分枝杆菌和真菌：不典型(如HIV感染进展期)，多为无痛性。

诊断

症状和体征

• 突发一侧关节疼痛、水肿、皮温升高、僵硬。
• 常见表现：
- 发热。
- 其他部位的感染(如皮肤)。
- 所有方向的关节运动均有剧烈疼痛。
- 关节腔积液(骶髂关节、髋关节、肩关节少见)。
• 任何关节均可受累：
- 典型的是单关节受累。
- 最常见于膝关节、髋关节、肩关节及踝关节。
• 骶髂软骨和胸锁关节在IVDU患者中常见。
- 可能累及椎骨如腰椎。
• 人或动物咬伤、植入钢钉、局部激素治疗及创伤等可导致局部症状不典型。
• 10%～20%的患者可累及多关节。
- 多合并风湿性关节炎；由于可能性低而延误诊断，更多的是临床表现轻微(只有50%的患者发热)。
- 脓毒症患者。
• 淋球菌性化脓性关节炎的特点：
- 见于1%～3%未治疗的淋病患者及42%～85%的播散性淋球菌感染。
• 典型的为单关节炎，常见的是多关节炎。
• 游走性多关节疼痛、腱鞘炎(20%合并关节炎)、皮炎。
- 累及小关节(如指间关节、腕关节、肘关节、踝关节)。
• 可能有尿路或阴道淋球菌感染的临床表现。
• 在躯干、上臂、下肢及受累关节周围可见无痛性斑丘疹。

基本检查

关节腔穿刺术

• 在所有可疑患者中均应行关节腔穿刺。
• 穿刺液送检，包括蛋白质及葡萄糖的含量测定、细胞计数、革兰染色、培养。
• 典型的化脓性关节炎表现：
- 浑浊的脓性或血性液体。
- 白细胞增多(50000～150000/mm^3)，分叶核细胞为主(>75%)。
- 通常葡萄糖量降低，蛋白质量升高。
• 晶体形成不能排除化脓性关节炎的诊断。
• 必要时使用特殊染色或特殊培养皿(如淋球菌、厌氧菌、真菌、分枝杆菌等)。
• 关节腔内注射利多卡因会降低之后培养结果的敏感性，立即将穿刺液转至培养瓶能提高敏感性。
• 非淋球菌性化脓性关节炎中，革兰染色和培养的阳性率分别为50%和90%。
- 在淋球菌性化脓性关节炎中，阳性率则分别下降为10%和50%。
• 许多培养阴性的穿刺液，实时PCR可以检测病原菌的DNA。
• 技术难度较大的穿刺可在荧光镜检、超声或CT引导下进行。
• CT及MRI检查有助于关节炎部位的诊断，如骶骨关节。
• 若有潜在人工关节或皮肤感染，则不宜行关节穿刺：
- 如果存在蜂窝织炎，选择经正常皮肤的路径穿刺。

诊断检查与说明

实验室检查

• 常见的有非特异性的白细胞升高(儿童中更常见)、核左移、C反应蛋白(CRP)和ESR升高。
• 降钙素原更有助于诊断化脓性关节炎，而不是排除诊断。
• 尿培养可以找出泌尿系统来源的病原菌。
• 血培养可能有助于诊断：非淋球菌性SA

N

中阳性率为 50%～70%。

• 对所有感染的可能来源均进行培养(咽部、尿道、宫颈或肛门)，尤其是怀疑淋球菌感染时。

影像学检查

• X线平片可以发现：

- 积液。
- 关节基本情况。
- 连续性骨髓炎。
- 并发风湿性疾病。
- 骨折或异物。
- 关节松弛(晚期非特异性表现)。

• 超声、CT 和 MRI 特异性更高：

- 超声可以用于引导穿刺某些关节(如髋关节)，还可以检测关节腔积液。

• 核素扫描诊断化脓性关节炎具有较好的敏感性及特异性，但是急诊室一般不能进行。

• 其他检查：

- 细菌 DNA 扩增技术用于快速检测及鉴定病原菌。

鉴别诊断

• 病毒性关节炎。
• 风湿性关节炎。
• 痛风或假性痛风。
• HIV 相关性关节炎。
• 反应性关节炎。
• 莱姆病。
• 骨髓炎。
• 心内膜炎。
• 化脓性滑囊炎。
• 创伤。
• 儿童中还有：

- 幼年特发性关节炎。
- 股骨头骨骺滑脱症。
- 雷卡佩病。
- 干骺端骨髓炎。
- 一过性滑膜炎。

儿科注意事项

• 因为疫苗接种，流感嗜血杆菌不再是最常见的病原菌。

• 金黄色葡萄球菌最常见。

• B组链球菌、肠杆菌和革兰阴性杆菌在新生儿常见。

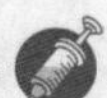

治疗

院前

没有特殊治疗。

初步稳定/治疗

• 患者可能是脓毒症，需要复苏。

• 如果患者病情严重，即使没有穿刺报告，也不要延误抗感染治疗。

急诊治疗/程序

• 及时行关节腔穿刺。

• 进行培养。

• 基于革兰染色结果(如果能够获得)、年龄分组或危险因素等，开始经验性抗感染治疗，考虑覆盖金黄色葡萄球菌、链球菌、革兰阴性菌；在特定患者中还要考虑 MRSA。推荐治疗周期是 2～4 周。禁止关节腔内注射抗菌药物。

• 没有不典型病原菌相关的危险因素：

- 静脉注射氟氯西林等抗生素，可能考虑增加静脉注射庆大霉素。
- 如果青霉素过敏，则可静脉注射林可霉素，或者第二代或第三代头孢菌素。

• 革兰阳性菌所致脓毒症的高危患者(包括高龄、虚弱、复发的 UTI、近期腹部手术史)：

- 第二代或第三代头孢菌素，如静脉注射头孢呋辛，可能考虑第三代头孢菌素联合氟氯西林。
- 革兰染色结果可以指导抗生素的选择。

• MRSA 危险因素(已知 MRSA 感染、近期住院患者、长期住护理医院、下肢溃疡或留置导尿或其他局部地区明确的危险因素)：

- 万古霉素＋第二代或第三代头孢菌素静脉注射。

• 疑诊淋菌或脑膜炎球菌：

- 静脉注射头孢曲松或类似药物。
- 取决于当地流行病学证据。

• IVDU 患者：与微生物学家讨论决定。

• ICU 患者已知其他部位定植(如囊性纤维化)：与微生物学家讨论决定。

• 早期整形咨询，评估是否可行手术引流。

• 止痛：镇静剂，适当夹板固定。

• 免疫治疗是经验性的。

• 人工关节：患者可尝试保留肢体，除非 X 线平片上提示关节已松弛。

• 患者应保持关节最佳姿势，休息，防止进一步损害。

药物治疗

• 头孢唑林：1～2 g，静脉滴注，q6 h。
• 头孢他啶：1～2 g，静脉滴注，q8 h。
• 头孢噻肟：2 g，静脉滴注，q8 h；儿童：50 mg/kg，q12 h。
• 头孢曲松：2 g，静脉滴注，每日 1 次；儿童：50 mg/kg。
• 环丙沙星：400 mg，静脉滴注，q12 h。
• 氟氯西林：2 g，静脉滴注，每日 1 次。
• 庆大霉素：2～5 mg/kg 负荷量，静脉滴注。
• 萘夫西林：2 g，静脉滴注，q4 h；儿童：25 mg/kg，q6 h。
• 妥布霉素：1 mg/kg，静脉滴注，q8 h；儿童：2.5 mg/kg，q8 h。
• 万古霉素：1 g，静脉滴注，q12 h；儿童：10 mg/kg，q6 h。

儿科注意事项

• 在儿童化脓性髋关节时，可选择开放式手术引流。

• 如果之前未预防接种，应覆盖流感嗜血杆菌 B 型。

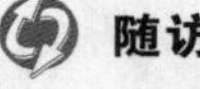

随访

进一步处理

入院指征

• 所有疑诊化脓性关节炎的患者均应住院，直到排除化脓性关节炎。

• 若有指征，进行关节炎引流，方式有持续吸引、关节镜检查或关节切开术。

出院指征

患者疑诊化脓性关节炎，但已明确排除。

要点和误区

• CRP 和 ESR 可用于随访治疗效果。

• 化脓性关节炎有时很难与中毒性滑膜炎及结晶性关节病鉴别，关节穿刺的指征较低。

N

脓毒症 Sepsis

Annette M. Ilg · Nathan I. Shapiro 周健 潘曙明 译

基础知识

描述

• 存在与相关的全身炎症反应相关的感染。
• 全身炎症反应综合征（SIRS）由 4 个标准组成：
- 温度>38 ℃或<36 ℃。
- 心脏率>90 次/分。
- 呼吸率>20 次/分或 $PaCO_2$<32 mmHg。
- 白细胞>12 000/mm^3 或<4 000/mm^3，或未成熟细胞>10%。
• 脓毒症≥2 SIRS 标准的感染：
- 化学信使的释放，炎症反应。
- 大循环衰竭，心脏输出减少或降低灌注压力。
- 微循环衰竭，受损的血管自动调节机制和功能分流。
- 细胞缺氧和线粒体功能障碍。
• 炎症反应导致血流动力学改变：
- 血管扩张引起的心脏输出量增加。
- 晚期心脏低灌注。
• 多器官功能障碍综合征（MODS）：
- 成人呼吸窘迫综合征（ARDS）。
- 急性肾小管坏死和肾衰竭。
- 肝损伤和衰竭。
- 弥散性血管内凝血。
• 败血症应被视为从炎症反应到器官功能障碍和组织灌注不足的一个连续的严重程度：
- 严重脓毒症：脓毒症至少有 1 个器官功能障碍：
◦ 酸中毒。
◦ 肾功能障碍急性精神状态变化。
◦ 肺功能障碍低血压。
◦ 血小板减少症或凝血功能障碍。
◦ 肝脏功能障碍。
- 败血性休克：脓毒症引起的低血压，尽管液体复苏：
◦ 收缩压<90 mmHg 或减少>40 mmHg 从基线。
• 败血症是导致死亡的第十大原因：
- 对感染性休克患者的住院死亡率约为 30%。

病因

• 革兰阴性菌最常见：
- 大肠杆菌。
- 铜绿假单胞菌。
- 立克次体。
- 军团菌属。
• 革兰阳性细菌：
- 肠球菌。
- 金黄色葡萄球菌。
- 肺炎链球菌。
• 真菌（念珠菌属物种）。
• 病毒。

儿科注意事项

• 轻微感染的儿童可能有很多 SIRS 的发现。
• 小儿细菌性脓毒症的主要原因：
- 脑膜炎双球菌。
- 链球菌肺炎嗜血杆菌。
- 流感嗜血杆菌。

诊断

症状和体征

病史

• 关于感染迹象和全身炎症反应的问题：
- 发热。
- 呼吸困难。
- 心理状态改变：
◦ 精神状态改变。
◦ 嗜睡。
◦ 神志昏迷。
- 恶心和呕吐。
• 寻找感染源：
- 咳嗽，呼吸急促。
- 腹痛。
- 腹泻。
- 排尿困难/频繁。
• 过去的病史应该突出风险因素和免疫抑制状态：
- 晚期疾病。
- 近期化疗。
- 恶性肿瘤。
- 脾切除术史。
- HIV。
- 糖尿病。
- 养老院居民。

体格检查

• 呼吸率升高是脓毒症的早期预警信号，没有潜在的肺病理或酸中毒。
• 在脓毒症早期，血压通常是正常的。
• 发生脓毒性休克时的低血压。
• 尽管有低血压，但四肢经常发热和发红。
• 寻找感染源：
- 腹部检查。
- 直肠检查评估脓肿。
- 胸部检查肺炎体征。
- 任何皮疹都很重要：
◦ 局部红斑与淋巴管炎（链球菌或葡萄球菌蜂窝织炎）。
◦ 皮疹手掌的手和底脚（立克次体感染）。
◦ 瘀点分散在躯干和四肢（脑膜炎球菌血症）。
◦ 坏死性脓疮（假单胞菌败血症）。
◦ 圆的、固化的、无痛的病变与周围红斑和中央坏死黑色焦痂。
- 压疮性溃疡。
- 留置导管。
• 中枢神经系统感染：
- 昏迷。
- 颈项强直（脑膜炎）。

基本检查

• 血清乳酸应在课程的早期进行，以评估其严重程度和目标指导治疗的需要。
• 抗生素之前的血培养：
- 广泛的实验室检查和影像学研究，以确定感染源和评估 MOF。
- 位置的中央线 $ScvO_2$ 导管可用于调整治疗。

诊断检查与说明

实验室检查

• 血清乳酸：
- >4 mmol/L 定义为严重脓毒症。
- 正常乳酸不排除脓毒性休克。
• 白细胞减少：
- 白细胞减少是不敏感的，非特异性。
- 中性粒细胞计数<500/mm^3 应在化疗患者中提示隔离和经验静脉抗生素。
- 外周血涂片上的>5%是不完全的感染指标。
- 血细胞比容：
◦ 患者应该保持一个血细胞比容>30%，血红蛋白>100 g/L。
- 血小板：
◦ 可能升高的感染或诱发感染体积损耗。
◦ 低血小板计数是菌血症和死亡的一个重要预测。

N

• 电解质、BUN、肌酐、葡萄糖：
• Ca^{2+}、Mg^{2+}的 pH。
• C 反应蛋白。
• 皮质醇水平。
• INR、PT、APTT。
• 肝功能检查。
• ABG 或 VBG。
- 混合酸碱异常：呼吸碱中毒与代谢性酸中毒。
- VBG 与 ABG 密切相关，SaO_2 除外。
• 血培养。
• 尿液分析。

影像学检查

• 胸部 X 线：
- 确定肺炎是否是感染源。
- 斑片状的双侧浸润可能表明 ARDS 已经存在。
- 横膈膜下的自由空气表明腹腔内感染源，必须进行手术干预。
• 软组织素膜：
- 如果肢体出现红斑或严重疼痛，说明软组织中与坏死性或气体形成感染有关的空气。
• 通过影像学研究来定位感染源。
- 腹部和骨盆 CT。
- 腹部超声检查胆囊疾病。
- 经胸或食管超声心动图。

诊断步骤/外科

• 腰椎穿刺：
- 脑膜标志或精神状态改变。
• 中心静脉监测：
- 监测中心静脉压(CVP)，并持续中心静脉氧含量测定。

鉴别诊断

• 胰腺炎。
• 创伤。
• 出血。
• 心源性休克。
• 中毒性休克综合征。
• 速发型过敏反应。
• 肾上腺功能不全。
• 药物或毒素反应。
• 重金属中毒。
• 肝衰竭。
• 神经源性休克。

治疗

院前

积极液体复苏治疗低血压。

初步稳定/治疗

• ABC 管理。
• 补充氧气来维持 $PaO_2>60$ mmHg。
• 有休克或缺氧时插管和机械通气。
• 使用生理盐水静脉输入。

急诊治疗/程序

• 早期目标导向治疗：
- 500 ml 生理盐水至 1～2 L。
- 建立中心静脉通路。
- 继续 500 ml 盐水快速扩容，直至 CVP＞8 cmH_2O。
- 如果平均动脉压＜65 mmHg，CVP＞8 cmH_2O，则启动前体：
◦ 去甲肾上腺素和多巴胺提高血压。
◦ 去甲肾上腺素是首选，如果心动过速或心律失常。
◦ 肾上腺素强心。
◦ 如果 $ScvO_2$＜70 和血细胞比容＜30，输血 2 U PRBC。
◦ 如果 $ScvO_2$＞70 和血细胞比容＞30 和 MAP＞60(然后添加多巴酚丁胺)。
• 根据最可能的有机体或感染部位，尽早使用抗生素。
• 如果来源被确认或高度怀疑，治疗最可能的有机体：
- 如果有危险因素——肺源性，则覆盖 MRSA、VRE 和假单胞菌。
◦ 第二或第三代头孢菌素和庆大霉素。
- 腹腔内来源：
◦ 氨苄西林、甲硝唑和庆大霉素。
◦ 头孢西丁和庆大霉素泌尿道来源：
◦ 氨苄西林、哌拉西林和庆大霉素或左氧氟沙星。
• 如果近期使用类固醇或肾上腺皮质功能不全，考虑使用压力剂量氢化可的松。

儿科注意事项

• 基于年龄的抗生素治疗：
- ＜3 个月(2 种药物)：氨苄西林、庆大霉素或头孢噻肟[50～180 mg/(kg · d)，静脉滴注，q4～6 h]。
- ＞3 个月：头孢噻肟或头孢曲松[50～100 mg/(kg · d)，静脉滴注，q12～24 h]。
• 在 60 ml/kg 静脉滴注液体没有反应后，启动血管升压剂。
• 避免低钠血症和低血糖。
• 地塞米松治疗细菌性脑膜炎儿童：
- 0.15 mg/kg q6 h，服用 4 日。

药物治疗

• 氨苄西林：1～2 g[儿童：50～200 mg/(kg · 24 h)]，静脉滴注，q4～6 h。
• 头孢西丁：1～2 g[儿童：100～160 mg/(kg · 24 h)]，静脉滴注，q6～8 h。
• 头孢噻肟：1～2 g[儿童：100～150 mg/(kg · 24 h)]，静脉滴注，q8～12 h。
• 多巴胺：1～5 μg/(kg · min)(肾剂量)；5～10 μg/(kg · min)(升压剂量)。
• 庆大霉素：1～1.5 mg/kg(儿童：2～2.5 mg/kg)，q8 h。
• 氢化可的松：100 mg，静脉滴注，q6～8 h。
• 甲硝唑：装入 1 g(儿童：15 mg/kg)，静脉滴注，然后 500 mg(儿童：7.5 mg/kg，q6 h)。
• 青霉素：1～2 g 静脉滴注，q4 h[儿童：50 mg/(kg · 24 h)，div，q4～6 h]。
• 去甲肾上腺素：2～8 μg/min。
• 哌拉西林：3～4 g，静脉滴注，q4～6 h。
• 万古霉素：500 mg(儿童：10 mg/kg)，静脉滴注，q6 h。

一线用药

• 没有可识别来源的正常免疫功能：
- 第二代或第三代头孢菌素和庆大霉素。
- 青霉素和庆大霉素。
- 如果有耐甲氧西林史，就加入万古霉素。金黄色葡萄球菌，或患者居住在护理机构，或有近期住院史。

二线用药

免疫缺陷宿主，无可识别来源：
• 哌拉西林和庆大霉素。
• 头孢他啶和青霉素或万古霉素和庆大霉素。

随访

进一步处理

入院指征

脓毒症几乎总是需要住院治疗。

出院指征

• 感染较轻的患者(如链球菌咽炎)符合脓毒症的标准。
• 生命体征稳定。

转诊问题

• 脓毒性败血症、败血症或败血症性休克。
• 要求进入 ICU。

要点和误区

• 一旦怀疑脓毒症就开始使用抗生素。
• 在脓毒症最初出现时，不能识别多器官衰竭并开始积极的液体复苏是一个缺陷。

脓疱病 Impetigo

Sandra A. Deane　倪沁赟 译

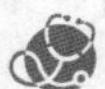

基础知识

描述

• 脓疱病是一种表皮细菌感染。
• 原发性感染：
- 原正常皮肤直接细菌侵入而引起的感染。
• 继发性感染：
- 轻微皮肤外伤或先前有皮肤损伤的部位感染。
• 多在 2～5 岁儿童中流行。
• 多发生在夏季和温暖潮湿的气候。
• 易感因素：
- 轻微的创伤，特别是在鼻周围的区域。
- 烧伤。
- 昆虫咬伤。
- 人类免疫缺陷病毒(HIV)感染。
- 糖尿病。
- 基础皮肤病。
- 水痘感染。
• 并发症：
- 急性链球菌感染性肾小球肾炎。
◦ 1%～5%的患者有非大疱性脓疱病。
- 脓毒症。
- 蜂窝织炎。
- 感染性心内膜炎。
- 中毒性休克综合征。
- 葡萄球菌皮肤烫伤样综合征(SSSS)。

病因

• 经典的脓疱病(非大疱)：
- 细菌通过皮肤上的伤口进入，如皮肤划痕、皮肤磨损或昆虫咬伤。
- 最常见的形式。
- 由金黄色葡萄球菌、A 组 β 溶血性链球菌或两者引起。
- 通常与卫生不良有关。
- 针对金黄色葡萄球菌和 A 组 β 溶血性链球菌进行治疗。
• 大疱性脓疱病：
- 由金黄色葡萄球菌、噬菌体Ⅱ组引起。
- 表皮分裂由表皮剥脱毒素 A、B 和 D 引起，该毒素是结合和切割桥粒芯糖蛋白 1 的丝氨酸蛋白酶，属于一种桥粒细胞间的黏附分子。

妊娠注意事项

妊娠期间目前对锌元素的补充可能会降低婴儿的发病率。

诊断

症状和体征

• 经典的(非大疱性)脓疱病：
- 起始表现为单独的直径 2～4 mm 的红斑或丘疹，可能演变成水疱或脓疱。
- 通常在 24 h 内水疱破裂，留下蜂蜜色、深棕色或红黑色渗出性外皮。
- 通常位于面部和四肢。
- 高度传染性。
- 通常瘙痒明显，可能通过抓原来的感染部位出现感染的播散。
- 轻度淋巴结肿大，通常不发生淋巴结炎。
- 全身表现较少见。
- 链球菌皮肤感染不会出现风湿热。
- 致肾炎的 A 组链球菌菌株导致的皮肤感染是链球菌感染后肾小球肾炎主要的早期表现。
• 大疱性脓疱病：
- 大部分发生于新生儿，但是在任何年龄均可发生。
- 由水疱起病，然后发展为松弛性大疱，内含干净黄色液体。
- 尼科利斯基征是不存在的。
- 大而脆弱的大疱很快破裂，留下亮且红的皮肤基底，可见剥脱的皮肤边缘。
- 通常位于躯干。

病史

发热和全身症状不常见。

体格检查

• 常见感染部位：
- 面部。
- 四肢。
- 头皮。
• 诊断基于体格检查的发现，特别是外观和分布。

基本检查

使用传统的治疗方案效果不佳的病例或在疾病暴发期特别怀疑耐甲氧西林的金黄色葡萄球菌感染，可考虑将大疱或脓疱内的液体进行培养。

诊断检查与说明

实验室检查

• 通常不能检测出。
• 链球菌脓疱病后抗链球菌溶血素 O 的反应较弱，所以检测链球菌抗体是没有用的。
• 抗去氧核糖酸酶 B 反应容易发生。90%的肾炎合并链球菌皮肤病的患者滴度会升高。
• 行尿液分析来评估有无血尿或蛋白尿，可提示链球菌感染后肾小球肾炎的发生。

影像学检查

不是经常需要做的检查。

诊断步骤/外科

• 诊断通常不需要进行活检。
• 如果进行活检：
- 角层下表皮裂解平面。
- 在真皮层上中性粒细胞和淋巴细胞炎性浸润。
- 角层下水疱内偶见棘细胞。
• 对水疱内液体进行革兰染色可表现为数串或数群中性粒细胞或革兰阳性球菌。

鉴别诊断

• 单纯疱疹。
• 水痘-带状疱疹(带状疱疹)。
• 特应性皮炎。
• 接触性皮炎。
• 皮肤癣菌病。
• 丹毒。
• 念珠菌病。
• 疥疮。
• 毛囊炎。
• 虱病。
• 寻常型天疱疮。
• 大疱类型天疱疮。
• 脂溢性皮炎。
• 热烧伤。
• Stevens-Johnson 综合征。
• 大疱性多形红斑。
• SSSS，在敏感个体通过表皮的播散引起。
• 新生儿天疱疮(Ritter 病)或新生儿 SSSS。
• 中毒性表皮坏死松解症。
• 皮肤炭疽。

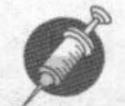

治疗

院前

• 转运时给予皮肤覆盖。
• 必须戴手套，因为可在人与人之间传播。
• 注意事项：
- 保持普遍的预防措施。
- 在一起生活的受到影响的兄弟姐妹应检查病灶。

N

■ 初步稳定/治疗

在健康成人或儿童，经典的或大疱性的脓疱病并不威胁生命，不需要进行复苏措施。

■ 急诊治疗/程序

• 非大疱性的小病灶可仅给予局部治疗。
• 播散性的大病灶，或存在大疱性脓疱病或存在淋巴结肿大，应给予全身治疗。
• 全身治疗包括耐β-内酰胺酶的青霉素、头孢菌素或大环内酯类抗生素，疗程为10日：
- 如果没有效果，检查是否存在MRSA，同时调整抗生素覆盖MRSA。
• 在急性链球菌感染后肾小球肾炎流行期间或广泛的MRSA存在的社区，需要全身使用抗生素。
• 局部治疗应该包括清洗、去除表皮和在损伤区域湿敷。

■ 药物治疗

• 所有治疗方案均需要7～10日，除非局部治疗仅需要5日而且局部治疗可提供依从性，5日后可开始口服阿奇霉素，持续9日。
• 因链球菌和金黄色葡萄球菌对红霉素耐药率高，避免使用红霉素治疗。
• 口服治疗：
- 阿莫西林-克拉维酸：250 mg，口服，q8 h[儿童：30 mg/(kg·d)，口服，q8 h]。
- 阿奇霉素：第1日500 mg，口服；第2～5日250 mg，口服(儿童：第1日10 mg/kg，口服；第2～5日5 mg/kg，口服)。
- 头孢氨苄：500 mg，口服，每日4次[儿童：25～50 mg/(kg·d)，口服，q8～12 h]。
- 克拉霉素：250 mg，口服，q12 h(儿童：15 mg/kg，口服，q12 h)。
- 克林霉素：150 mg，口服，每日3次(儿童：5 mg/kg，口服，每日3次)。
- 双氯西林：250 mg，口服，q6 h[儿童：25～50 mg/(kg·d)，口服，q6 h]。
- 多西环素：当怀疑MRSA感染时，100 mg，口服，q12 h[8岁以上及45 kg以下的儿童，给予4.5 mg/(kg·d)，q12 h]。8岁以下儿童不推荐使用。
- 琥乙红霉素：250 mg，口服，q6 h[儿童：40 mg/(kg·d)，口服，q6 h]。
- 甲氧苄啶-磺胺甲噁唑DS：1片，口服，每日2次，共10日(儿童：＞2个月；4 mg/kg，口服，q12 h，共10日)；对怀疑MRSA感染时使用同样有效。
- 利奈唑胺：600 mg，口服，每次2日，昂贵，仅用于过敏患者或MRSA(儿童：不适用)。
• 局部治疗：
- 莫匹罗星：成人和儿童：局部使用，每日3次，共10日(仅非大疱性脓疱病使用)。
- 瑞他莫林软膏：成人和＞9个月的儿童：局部使用，每日2次，共5日。

一线用药

• 局部治疗：
- 莫匹罗星：在美国，300株携带基因编码的社区获得性MRSA，高达46％对莫匹罗星耐药。

二线用药

• 局部治疗：
- 瑞他莫林软膏：因为没有足够的案例研究，说明书没有说适用于MRSA，但是对莫匹罗星耐药的MRSA治疗上可见其有效。
• 口服抗生素：
- 阿莫西林-克拉维酸。
- 头孢菌素。
- 双氯西林。
- 红霉素。
- 多西环素。

随访

■ 进一步处理

入院指征

• 单纯的脓疱病很少需要住院。
• 如果疾病分布较广，特别是广泛的大疱存在，或者有大面积裸露的皮肤、脱水或门诊治疗难以治愈。
• 中毒、全身不适或免疫功能低下的患者需要住院治疗，怀疑脓毒症的新生儿亦需要住院。
• 如果临床表现延迟＞4～5日，在患者接受护理治疗之前肾炎可能已经存在。
• 更典型的是，肾炎一般发生在皮肤链球菌感染后2～4周。

出院指征

• 患者没有中毒表现。
• 患者/照顾者有能力遵循推荐的治疗方案。
• 随访时进行重新评估。
• 开始抗菌治疗后，儿童可在24 h内返回学校。
• 引流性病变应保持覆盖。

转诊问题

眶周水肿、下肢肿胀或血尿或蛋白尿提示链球菌感染后肾小球肾炎，转诊至肾内科。

■ 随访建议

• 初级保健医师随访时应确保患者无并发症的发生。
• 病变治疗失败需重新返回治疗。
• 出现血尿、眶周水肿或下肢肿胀需重新返回治疗。

要点和误区

• 存在大疱性脓疱病或淋巴结肿大的患者，接受全身抗生素治疗。
• 继续限制使用历史标准的抗生素协议，则抗生素耐药性会进一步增加。
• 因莫匹罗星存在耐药性，在治疗失败时需考虑到这一点同时调整为使用瑞他莫林软膏。
• 对于顽固性病变需要进行培养和药物敏感试验。
• 没有在同一时间进行治疗的其他家庭成员可能发生复发或再次感染。

疟疾 Malaria

Roger M. Barkin·Jordan Moskoff 王胜云 段立伟 译

基础知识

■ 描述

• 通过按蚊原生动物感染传播。
• 潜伏期为8～16周。
• 发病周期因疟原虫生活周期而定：
- 红细胞外期：未成熟孢子体迁移至肝脏，随后大量复制产生成熟个体(裂殖子)。
- 红细胞内期：裂殖子释放入血，在血液循环中侵袭红细胞。
- 红细胞内复制期：48～72 h后，红细胞破裂，大量裂殖子被释放进入循环，侵袭新的红细胞，如此反复。

- 随着红细胞周期性裂解，出现周期性发热。

• 恶性疟原虫：

- 多数病例的病因，多导致死亡。
- 通常急性发病，暴发性感染。
- 可感染所有阶段的红细胞：
  ◦ 导致严重的溶血和贫血。
- 导致广泛的毛细血管功能障碍：
  ◦ 导致末端组织缺氧，功能障碍。
- 对于正在接受或刚刚停止疟原虫预防措施的患者，感染要轻很多。
- 创伤后免疫功能障碍可导致疫区患者疟疾复发。

• 间日疟原虫性疟疾和卵形疟。

- 可以急性发热症状出现。
- 肝脏休眠阶段的孢子体可在初次病原体暴露后的6～11个月后引起复发。

• 三日疟：

- 可以较低水平在血液中存在长达30年。

▪ 病因

• 通常经雌性按蚊叮咬传播。

• 北美的传播途径可能通过：

- 东海岸和西海岸的雌性按蚊。
- 使用带有病原体的血液制品或共用针头也可导致疾病的传播。

儿科注意事项

• 镰刀形红细胞的个体对疟疾具有一定抵抗力。

• 儿童更易出现脑型疟疾。

• 在缺少实验室检查条件的疟疾高发区，所有出现发热的患儿均应接受疟疾治疗。

妊娠注意事项

孕妇，特别是初孕妇，属于高危人群。

诊断

▪ 症状和体征

• 时间特点：

- 恶性疟原虫在接触后8周内发病。
- 间日疟可延迟至数月后。
- 多数症状在1年内出现。

• 一般症状：

- 烦躁。
- 寒战(特别是感到冷)。
- 发热通常超过38℃。
- 经典的疟疾发病周期：
  ◦ 15 min到1 h的寒战。
  ◦ 随后出现2～6 h无汗的高热(<39～42℃)。
  ◦ 热退后，大量出汗。
  ◦ 每个48 h(间日疟)或72 h(三日虐)周期性出现。
  ◦ 发热周期多变，较少出现典型的发热周期。
- 直立性低血压。
- 肌痛关节痛。

• 血液学：

- 溶血：
  ◦ 黑尿热：因恶性疟导致暴发性溶血，患者出现黑色尿液得名。
- 黄疸。
- 脾大：
  ◦ 可导致脾破裂。
  ◦ 在慢性病例中更常出现。

• 中枢神经性疟疾：

- 头痛。
- 局部神经症状。
- 精神状态改变。
- 昏迷。
- 痉挛。

• 腹型疟疾：

- 呕吐。
- 腹泻。
- 腹痛。

• 肺部症状：

- 呼吸短促。
- 肺湿啰音。
- 肺水肿。

• 重型疟疾：

- 出现以下至少1条：
  ◦ 在理想管理状况下仍有高于20%的死亡率。
  ◦ 平卧状态下无法独自坐起。
  ◦ 意识障碍。
  ◦ 呼吸困难或肺水肿。
  ◦ 惊厥。
  ◦ 循环障碍。
  ◦ 异常出血。
  ◦ 黄疸。
  ◦ 血红素尿。
  ◦ 严重贫血。

• 可能会发生复发和再感染。

▪ 基本检查

油镜下吉木沙染色剂涂片检查：

• 红细胞内疟原虫检查。

• 不能在没有48 h内涂片阴性结果的情况下排除诊断。

• 只有高度寄生虫病的情况下才会直接在标准血涂片中找到证据。

▪ 诊断检查与说明

实验室检查

• 全血细胞计数：

- 贫血：25%。
- 血小板减少症：70%的人<150×10^9/L。
- 白细胞减少。

• 电解质、尿素氮、肌酐、葡萄糖：

- 肾衰竭。
- 低血糖(极少)。
- 乳酸酸中毒。
- 低钠血症。

• 尿液检查。

• 肝功能：

- 升高25%。
- 胆汁酸和乳酸脱氢酶升高，提示红细胞的溶解。

影像学检查

胸部X线检查以排除肺水肿。

诊断步骤/外科

• 免疫荧光检测、酶联免疫吸附试验或DNA探针：

- 不同类型疟原虫的区别。
- 5%～7%的患者属于混合感染。

• 吉姆萨染色剂涂片找到病原虫后。如果最初为阴性，可能需要在接下来的72 h内重复。

• 腰椎穿刺/脑脊液检查：

- 以区分脑型疟和脑膜炎。
- 脑脊液蛋白因感染疟疾升高。
- 脑脊液细胞数量通常不会因疟疾感染升高。
- 诊断快速。结果准确。基于抗原的检测可以区分种类。

• 分子学检测用来研究流行病学。为CDC提供PCR结果。

▪ 鉴别诊断

• 脑膜炎。

• 脑炎。

• 脑卒中(中风)。

• 急性肾功能障碍。

• 急性溶血性贫血。

• 败血症。

• 肝炎。

• 病毒性腹泻。

• 低血糖昏迷。

• 中暑。

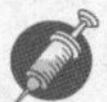

治疗

初步稳定/治疗

- 气道、呼吸、循环。
- 如果出现低血压，进行生理盐水液体复苏。
- 体温高于 40℃需要即刻进行降温。
- 对乙酰氨基酚。
- 物理降温。
- 纳洛酮，D_{50} W，如果出现精神改变，加用维生素 B_1。

急诊治疗/程序

- 根据疟疾的发病类型和疫区情况，明确诊断。
- 在未被证明前，假设其为耐药型。
- 青蒿素和其他抗疟疾药物联合使用，是治疗耐药疟疾的一线药物。
- 基于青蒿素的联合治疗：具体差异依据疫区不同，可由 WHO 数据库中查到：
  - 青蒿素＋苯芴醇。
  - 青蒿素＋阿莫地喹。
  - 青蒿素＋甲氟喹。
- 奎宁：
  - 成人每日 542 mg 基础剂量，持续 3～7 日。
- 奎尼丁静脉给药。如果青蒿琥酯不可用，可以考虑。
  - 与 QT 间期延长有关。
  - 对于严重的病例。
- 阿托伐醌(250 mg)-百忧解(100 mg)(马龙酮)。4 片，每日 1 次，连续服用 3 日；小儿片剂是成人剂量的 4 倍。
- 对非严重氯喹敏感的感染可立即用 600 mg 氯喹治疗，然后在 6 h、24 h 和 48 h 用 300 mg 治疗(成人)。
- 严重的恶性疟：静脉滴注药物治疗。
  - 青蒿素可静脉滴注或肌内注射。
- 并发症的支持治疗。
- 化学预防：必须依据旅行的地区，可在 WHO 数据库中查得：
  - 所有前往疟疾地区的旅行都应遵守避蚊措施。
  - 在疟疾只偶尔发生且风险较低的地区，应避免蚊虫叮咬，而不必进行化学预防。
  - 玛拉隆：
    - 每日服用。
    - 人体耐受性好。
    - ＞5 kg 的儿童可安全使用。
    - 妊娠期使用不安全。
    - 250/100 mg，口服，每日 1 次。
    - 在进入疫区前 1～2 日开始服用，直到离开疫区后 7 日。
  - 氯喹：
    - 适合那些倾向于每周服用药物的旅行者。
    - 妊娠期可安全使用。
    - 每周口服 300 mg。
    - 进入疫区前 2 周开始服药至离开疫区后 4 周。
  - 甲氟喹：
    - 每周服药。
    - 妊娠期服用安全，但不适合用于特定精神疾病患者。
    - 每周 250 mg 口服。
    - 进入疫区前 2 周开始服药至离开疫区后 4 周。
  - 盐酸强力霉素：
    - 每日服药。
    - 最便宜。
    - 妊娠期使用不安全。
    - 8 岁以下儿童使用不安全。
    - 日光照射下存在风险，服药后不宜长时间接受太阳照射。
    - 每日 100 mg 口服。
    - 进入疫区前 1 日开始服药至离开疫区后 4 周。
  - 伯氨喹：
    - 每日服药。
    - G-6-PD 缺乏症患者不能使用。
    - 妊娠期使用不安全。
    - 每日 30 mg 口服。
    - 进入疫区前 1 日开始服药至离开疫区后 1 周。
- 目前还没有疫苗，但有几种正在进行试验。
- 正在研究新药和杀虫剂。
- 青蒿素方案与杀虫剂处理的蚊帐联合使用，可显著降低发病率。

药物治疗

- 对乙酰氨基酚：500 mg，口服，q4～6 h；每日服药不能超过 5 次，总量不能超过 4 g。
- 青蒿素(40 mg)＋苯芴醇(240 mg)：6 个疗程，口服，每日 2 次×3 日。
- 阿托喹酮(250 mg)＋氯胍(100 mg)：成人每日 4 片，口服×3 日。
- 青蒿琥酯(100 mg)＋阿莫地喹(270 mg)：成人每日 1 次，口服×3 日。
- 青蒿琥酯(100 mg)＋甲氟喹(220 mg)：3 个疗程，2 片，口服每日 1 次×3 日。
- 葡萄糖：25 g，静脉注射。
- 纳洛酮：2 mg，静脉注射或肌内注射。
- 硫胺素(维生素 B_1)：100 mg，静脉注射或肌内注射。
- 其他药物治疗方案可考虑与 CDC 协商，需要准确反映疾病的敏感性和严重性。

随访

进一步处理

入院指征

- 严重的恶性疟感染需要收入 ICU。
- 疑似急性恶性疟感染。
- 严重脱水。
- 不能耐受口服药剂的患者。
- 超过 3%的红细胞受到侵染。
- 儿童和免疫功能低下患者。

出院指征

- 明确非恶性疟感染者。
- 可耐受口服药物。
- 需要密切随访。

要点和误区

当考虑疟疾时，应进行传染病咨询。由于不同种类的治疗药物方案不同，在确诊时应咨询当地专家或 CDC，必须准确反映疾病的严重程度。

虐待(儿童,非意外性创伤) Abuse, Pediatric (Nonaccidental Trauma, NAT)

Jody A. Vogel · Suzanne Z. Barkin 马林浩 林兆奋 译

基础知识

描述

• 虐待儿童每年影响 1 400 万美国儿童,占 2%～3%。

• 美国每年有 1 200～1 400 名儿童死于虐待。其中 80%<5 岁,40%<1 岁。

• 涉嫌虐待或忽视的案例包括所有卫生保健工作者。

• 风险因素:

- 孩子:通常<4 岁,大多存在残疾、智力障碍或有特殊需要("弱势儿童"),早产,多产。
- 虐待型父母:低自尊,童年时受虐待,脾气暴躁,有精神病史,对孩子有严格和不切实际的期望,或年轻母亲。
- 家庭:经济问题、被孤立或流动的或婚姻不稳定。
- 糟糕的亲子关系,意外妊娠。
- 虐待可存在于所有宗教和社会经济群体。

诊断

症状和体征

病史

• 以开放式的问题询问损伤和受伤原因。

• 不存在包含所有虐待迹象的清单。

• 从入院前接触的人中寻找周围环境的信息。

• 外在表现的模式应该提高对虐待或忽视问题的警惕。

- 与损伤或疾病不一致的经历和机制:

• 不明原因的死亡、呼吸暂停和伤害。

• 不明原因的摄入或毒素接触。

- 复发性损伤。
- 父母、看护人不愿提供的信息或否认有关受伤发生的原因。
- 不同照顾者之间的矛盾陈述。
- 损伤事件随时间发生改变的情况。
- 与孩子生长发育不相关的伤害。
- 护理人员对伤病的不恰当反应,延迟寻求就医。

• 代理人的夸张表述:

- 医学无法解释的经常发生的疾病。
- 原因不明的怀疑中毒的代谢性疾病。

• 未能茁壮成长:

- 糟糕的亲子关系、忽视所导致的能量摄入不足。
- 回顾过去的遭遇,与患者的初级保健医师联系可能会有所帮助。

体格检查

• 与病史不相符的损伤。

• 非意外性创伤导致的损伤一般比意外性创伤严重。

• 皮肤瘀伤/青肿:

- 在小孩可以自己动之前,如果没有创伤的话,5 岁之前少见瘀伤。
- 规则的图案,笔直的分界线,规则的角度,手指拍打的痕迹,浸润性的烧伤,袜子、手套烧伤,臀部环状烧伤,咬伤,捆绑伤,扣伤,香烟烧伤。
- 部位:臀部、臀部、面部(非额头)、手臂、背部、大腿、生殖器或耳郭。
- 不同时间段的挫伤。
  ◦ 瘀伤的时间常不相同。
  ◦ 黄色的瘀伤通常超过 18 h。
  ◦ 红色、蓝色、紫色或黑色的瘀伤可能发生在损伤 1 h 后。
  ◦ 红色的瘀伤可能存在于伤后各个阶段。
  ◦ 同一时间段的损伤在同一个人身上可能有不同的表现。

• 骨创:

- 通常是多个、不明原因的、不同阶段的愈合。
- 干骺端(典型干骺端病变)骨折(病理)。
- 交叉缝合线的颅骨骨折。
- 后肋骨骨折(心肺复苏中婴儿几乎从未发生肋骨骨折)。
- 长骨螺旋骨折。
- 骨膜下新生骨形成。
- 无明显机制的罕见骨折(椎骨、胸骨、肩胛骨、棘突)。

• 中枢神经系统:

- 精神状态的改变或癫痫。
- 脑外伤是被虐待儿童死亡的主要原因。
- 颅骨骨折:必须考虑 1 岁以下儿童的虐待。
- 硬脑膜下血肿、蛛网膜下腔出血。
- 剪切和旋转损伤所致的摇晃婴儿综合征。

• 眼部损伤:

- 视网膜出血或脱离:
  ◦ 65%～90%的虐待性头部损伤伴有视网膜出血(通常发生在双侧),而 0～10%的该损伤只出现在严重的意外创伤。
  ◦ 在没有头部创伤和正常神经影像学证据的情况下很少见。
- 眼前房积血。
- 角膜擦伤或结膜出血。
- 小于 3 岁的小孩在怀疑被虐待时建议进行眼科检查。

• 口腔损伤。

• 腹部损伤:

- 肝、脾、肾或胰腺损伤。
- 壁内血肿(十二指肠最常见)。
- 腹膜后血肿。

• 肛门生殖器或性虐待:

- 可行常规泌尿生殖器检查。
- 青肿、红斑、开放性伤口、瘢痕或异物(毛发碎屑或精液)。
- 儿童疾病或怀孕的时间<12 岁。

• 死亡:

- 不能解释的死亡。

基本检查

• 向合适的儿童福利机构提供正式的口头和书面报告。

• 家庭和环境评估,通常与负责的儿童福利机构合作。

• 详尽的检查发现的报告记录。

• 瘀伤的图解或照片是有帮助的。

> **注意**
>
> 当怀疑时,卫生专业人员有法律义务向相关部门报告。

诊断检查与说明

实验室检查

• 有复发性瘀伤史或瘀伤为突出表现;通常可以选择:CBC、血小板、PT、APTT 或出血时间(或 PFA 胶原肾上腺素)。

• 如果钝挫伤严重,可以选择 CBC、LFT、淀粉酶和尿液分析。

• 伴有精神状态改变的儿童可以做毒理学、化学和代谢筛查。

• 考虑其他鉴别诊断的因素。

影像学检查

• 评估没有确定的意外性创伤,不一致的病史,隐匿的骨骼状况不佳或明显的出生创伤史的小儿骨骼状况。

- 0～23 个月伴以下任一联合损伤:
  ◦ 众所周知的虐待。

◦ 家庭暴力的损伤史。
◦ 玩具导致的损伤或其他物体导致的骨折。
◦ 延迟就医时间超过24小时。
◦ 在大于12个月的小孩儿没有明确的创伤病史来解释骨折,除了以下的情况:远端的尺桡骨巴氏骨折或远端的胫腓骨,螺旋形或巴氏骨折,且他们的致伤因素都是一致的。

- 0～11月龄如果没有其他额外的考虑,且有任何一种骨折类型,如下所示:
◦ 大于9个月的无创伤病史的学步小孩有远端尺桡骨骨折或学步导致的胫腓骨骨折。
◦ 明确高处坠落史的大于6个月的小孩儿有线性的或单边的颅骨骨折。
◦ 出生时导致的锁骨骨折。
- 12～13个月大小伴以下任一种骨折:
◦ 肋骨骨折。
◦ 典型的干骺端骨折。
◦ 复杂性的或乒乓球颅骨骨折。
◦ 3楼以下的坠落导致的肱骨骨折伴远端分离。
◦ 高处坠落导致的股骨干骨折。
- 在临床需要的时候检查骨骼情况是适宜的。

• 整体评估:
- 小于2岁的小孩儿排除了损伤,但怀疑虐待的时候。
- 2～5岁的儿童,在强烈怀疑受到身体虐待行为时需要排除。
- 年龄较大的儿童,临床上涉嫌受伤的个别伤口部位需借助以下检查:
- 骨骼成像:
◦ 头骨的正侧位。
◦ 颈椎的侧位片。
◦ 胸腰椎的正侧位片。
◦ 胸部的正位和斜位片。
◦ 骨盆的正位片。
◦ 肱骨、前臂和双手的正位片。
◦ 股骨、胫骨和双足的正位片。
- 如果发现骨折,至少需要2张成像,原始成像和90°成像。
- 可能需要关节的椎束视图(一种投射方式)来观察在典型的干骺端损伤。
- 如果怀疑存在骨骼之外的损伤可以应用骨骼闪烁成像作为辅助筛查。

• 内脏成像:
- 疑似胸腹的损害:
◦ 腹部CT扫描伴静脉和可能的口服造影剂对比。

• 神经影像:
- 头颅CT平扫,脑部、硬膜下和骨窗。
- MRI:
◦ 用于急性、亚急性和慢性颅内损伤的辅助评估,适用于剪切伤、出血、挫伤或继发性缺氧/缺血损伤。

鉴别诊断

• 一般情况:
- 创伤:分娩时意外。
• 皮肤:
- 烧伤:意外。
- 感染。
- 脓疱、蜂窝织炎。
- 葡萄球菌所致的烫伤样皮肤综合征。
- Henoch-Schonlein紫癜。
- 暴发性紫癜、脑膜炎球菌血症。
- 脓毒症。
- 皮炎:接触。
- 血流系统肿瘤(特发性血小板减少性紫癜、白血病)。
- 自发性出血、血友病。
- 营养不良:维生素C缺乏病(坏血病)。
- 特殊的文化治疗方案(压印、拔火罐)。
• 骨骼:
- 成骨不全症。
- 营养不良(佝偻病、缺铜或坏血病)。
- Menkes综合征。
- 周围感觉障碍(对疼痛的感知力差)。
• 眼部:
- 结膜炎。
• 腹部和肠道:
- 肠道疾病(梗阻、腹膜炎或炎症性肠病)。
- 肠道感染/异常。
• 中枢神经系统:
- 中毒,摄入(CO、铅或汞)。
• 感染:
- 代谢:低血糖。
- 癫痫。
• 死亡:
- 婴儿猝死综合征(SIDS)和危及生命的疾病(ALTE)。

治疗

院前

• 诊断依赖于与儿童病史与发病机制不相符合的体格检查证据。
• 对场景的检查可能有用:
- 评估机制的有效性。
- 家庭的一般外观。
- 由多个照顾者提供的病史的一致性。
- 亲子互动的评估。

初步稳定/治疗

根据具体的损伤而定。

急诊治疗/程序

• 根据需要进行医疗和创伤管理。
• 如果当地有儿童虐待咨询的团队或专家机构,及时尽早向他们征询进行评估。
• 强制性要求向当地儿童福利机构报告任何疑似虐待儿童的行为,以确定适当的社会倾向。
- 这并不意味着或要求100%确定存在虐待(只是流程性质的筛查是否存在虐童行为)。
- 迅速地对家庭、环境和社会进行评估。
- 要做到不带偏见。
• 与家庭成员就儿童福利的责任进行沟通。
- 需要保障儿童和工作人员的安全。
• 必须在适当的时间内对兄弟姐妹和其他家庭子女进行调查。

随访

进一步处理

入院指征

• 创伤性损伤的观察与干预。
• 如果需要的话,关注儿童福利接收地点的可用性。
• 目标必须始终是确保孩子和其兄弟姐妹的安全。

离院指征

• 充分的评估和医疗随访。
• 儿童安全设置决定其后续处置。
• 受虐儿童很有可能进一步受到虐待,因此必须与社会服务合作及对家庭的评估来确定后续进一步处理。
• 孩子(和兄弟姐妹)可能需要寄养。

转诊问题

• 所有患者都需要转介到适当的儿童福利机构。
• 在决定进一步处理前,需要对其他家庭成员进行评估。

要点和误区

• 与体格检查结果不一致的病史即可怀疑。
• 特定的损伤是和虐待儿童联系在一起的,并且需要进一步的调查。
• 当怀疑虐待儿童时,必须报告。
• 医疗和创伤的管理必须及时进行。

虐待(老年人)

Helen Straus 马林浩 林兆奋 译

 基础知识

描述

虐待老年人,包括:
- 情感虐待:
  - 辱骂。
  - 羞辱。
  - 送养老院或遗弃的威胁。
- 身体虐待或性虐待:
  - 殴打。
  - 掌掴。
  - 推搡。
  - 烧伤。
  - 不适当的限制。
  - 强迫性性行为。
- 物质侵占:
  - 偷窃或限制患者的财富。
- 忽视:
  - 患者或看护者的行为损害患者的健康或安全。
  - 未能提供足够的食物、住所、卫生和/或医疗服务的行为。

流行病学

发病率和患病率

- 估计患病率为10%(可能是由于从认知功能受损的老年人团体取样,这一人群有更高的可能遭受虐待和剥削,而低估了总体患病率)。受害人的绝对人数可能随着美国高龄人口的增长,近期内将会继续增加。
- 60岁以上的老年人受到各种形式的虐待的数量(缺乏全球数据支持):
  - 忽视:4.2%。
  - 身体虐待:2.6%。
  - 财政剥夺:6.8%。
  - 情感虐待:11.6%。
  - 性虐待:0.9%。
- 家庭成员,包括伴侣和成年子女,都是作恶者。
- 在一个纽约的研究中,每报告1例虐待案,就有24例未被报道。
- 财政剥夺的1年发生率为2.7%,终身剥夺为4.7%。
- 虐待老年人会导致300%的死亡风险(及300%的住院风险),同时还会增加其他健康问题的发生率,如慢性疼痛、骨关节、消化或心理障碍(与未受虐待的老年人相比)。

病因

- 照顾者的压力,依赖关系,病理心理。
- 对受害者的依赖或其进行日常生活活动能力的减退。
- 受害者认知损伤或社会绝缘的情况会增加虐待和忽视的风险。
- 长期住在养老机构的老年人有更高的风险承受来自员工的虐待及同机构其他老年人的虐待。

诊断

体征和症状

异常的、不相符合的病史或体格检查。

病史

- 不愿意或不能获得足够的食物、服装、住所。
- 不提供个人卫生、安全。
- 延误就医、既往无治疗。
- 未处理的疼痛(可能由照顾者提供医疗史)。
- 含糊的(或不合理的、不恰当的)解释。
- 由患者和护理人员所提供病史之间的差异。
- 坚持提供患者病史的护理人员。
- 药物治疗困难:
  - 错误的剂量。
  - 药物的缺失。
  - 处方的不完善。
- 人际互动的改变:
  - 孤僻。
  - 冷漠。
  - 低落。
  - 恐惧。
  - 药物滥用。
- 照顾者:
  - 对患者的经济依赖。
  - 药物虐待、精神或暴力史。
  - 控制行为(拒绝让老年人单独与医生相处)、知识的匮乏。
  - 生活压力。
  - 关系问题。
  - 财政困难。
  - 法律问题。

体格检查

- 不一致的发现:
  - 不同年龄的瘀伤、烧伤、割伤/擦伤。
    - 考虑以下情况:面部、右胳膊、背部、胸部、腰部或臀部侧面的瘀伤(这些发现不能单纯指向虐待,但可以引起进一步调查)。特殊的瘀伤部位(内臂、躯干、臀部、头皮)。
  - 与创伤导致的瘀伤面积不符的大面积瘀伤。
  - 不卫生(皮肤、指甲、牙齿护理不足)。
- 防御导致的伤害:
  - 胳膊表面伸肌的瘀伤。
- 难以解释的伤情:
  - 生殖器或直肠区域瘀伤或出血。
  - 腕部或踝关节损伤。
- 在寻求/获得医疗帮助过程中被忽视或被延迟处理而发生的相应的结果:
  - 脱水。
  - 体重的减少。
  - 压疮。
  - 营养不良。
    - 低白蛋白。
    - 贫血。

诊断检查与说明

- 根据患者情况进行任何检查、实验室或放射学研究。
- 考虑不足或过量医疗或无法解释的非法药物使用(医疗或药物检测水平)作为可能的忽视或故意伤害(不治疗或下毒)。

基本检查

- 在没有家人或照顾者在场的情况下取得病史:
  - 如果受虐的长者举报照顾者,可能会害怕被送进福利院。
  - 很多人可能觉得尴尬,并因此对虐待负责。
  - 通常不会主动提供信息。
  - 询问患者有关虐待或被忽视的具体情况(私下)。
- 患者的身体状况可能会影响病史的获得。
- 通过照顾者、亲戚、朋友、邻居获得病史。
- 记录1份清晰详细的调查结果,如使用老年虐待可疑指数(EASI)6个问题,包括以下内容:
  - 与虐待有关的患者陈述。
  - 心理历程:
    - 家庭和其他社会关系。
    - 照顾者负担、应对机制。
    - 药物、乙醇应用史。
    - 先前的成人保护服务报告。
  - 皮肤和其他身体发现:
    - 影像记录。

N

◦ 安全评估。

■ 诊断检查与说明

根据身体状况酌情决定。

影像学检查

根据身体状况酌情决定。

诊断步骤/外科

根据身体状况酌情决定。

■ 鉴别诊断

• 患者可能出现的主诉：

- 潜在的鉴别诊断是非特异性的。
- 在护理人员、家庭成员之外直接询问患者，并与风险因素和提供者的调查结果相关，这是诊断虐待的最佳方法。

• 区分与虐待/忽视所导致的相同结果的其他疾病：

- 脱水。
- 不合适的义齿。
- 烧伤。
- 瘀斑。
- 失眠。
- 治疗的不依从。
- 痴呆。
- 抑郁。

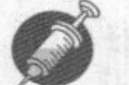

治疗

■ 院前

观察患者的环境细节，这些细节可能不能立即用于医院护理团队，包括：

• 现场的人际互动：

- 窘迫。
- 羞愧。
- 对报复、遗弃、住福利院的恐惧。

• 存在潜在危险的物理环境条件。

■ 初步稳定/治疗

• ABC 管理。

• 酌情治疗危及生命的疾病、创伤性疾病。

■ 急诊治疗/程序

• 可能要求患者与护工或家庭成员隔离。

• 可能的话利用专家和多学科的团队。

• 社会工作转介：

- 安全计划。
- 护工的暂缓计划。
- 成人防护服务转介。

• 有能力的老年患者可以自由接受或拒绝治疗和进一步处理，但是他们这样做可能会有风险。

• 适用于明确的医疗/创伤状况的一般措施：

- 液体。
- 药物。
- 外科。
- 饮食。
- 活动。
- 护理。
- 物理疗法。

随访

■ 进一步处理

入院指征

由医疗状况和家庭环境决定的相应处理。

• 入院的身体状况。

• 虐待或忽视使家庭环境不安全。

• 需要更多的信息或时间来加强客观决策和患者管理。

出院指征

• 已解决的身体状况。

• 可用的安全的环境。

• 社会服务和/或法律成功干预虐待或疏忽行为。

转诊问题

• 美国许多州都有强制性的报告要求：

- 符合当地法律要求。

• 适当的乙醇、药物治疗。

• 通知成人防护服务。

■ 随访建议

根据身体状况酌情决定。

要点和误区

• 考虑到老年患者可能受到虐待或忽视，这为诊断和成功干预提供了最好的可能性。

• 在过去 1 年里，只有 1/3 的医疗服务提供者发现了虐待老年人的案例。

• 目前的数据还不能确定干预措施对于减少老年人虐待复发的有效性。

• 如果一个弱势且有能力的长者试图拒绝有关虐待/忽视长者的调查，应寻求社工、患者信任的医师，甚至是道德顾问的协助。

呕吐(成人)

Mattew. M. Hall 吴昊 李文放 译

O

 基础知识

描述

• 咽肌一种不自主的、完整的咽和胸腹平滑肌的综合运动,以排出胃内容物。
• 三个阶段:
- 恶心:呕吐前的不愉快感觉。
- 反胃:横膈膜、腹部肌肉肋间肌的节奏性收缩,使胃内容物反流至食管。
- 呕吐:驱使胃内容物通过口腔的强有力的逆行运动。
• 呕吐中枢:位于延髓,通过依次兴奋迷走神经、膈神经及脊神经。
• 呕吐反射:来自胃肠道、咽部、前庭系统、心脏、生殖器的刺激,或药物、毒素或体内循环的激素通过对颅后窝的化学感受器触发区(CTZ)的刺激。
• 受体:CTZ 反应由多巴胺 D2、5-羟色胺($5-HT_3$)、胆碱能与组胺受体调控:
- 对症处理的止呕药物通过拮抗上述受体。

病因

• 胃肠道:
- 阑尾炎。
- Boerhaave 综合征。
- 肠梗阻或局部缺血。
- 胆囊炎、胆绞痛。
- 胃出口梗阻,胃轻瘫。
- 胃炎。
- 胃肠炎(例如,感染性)。
- 胃肠道出血。
- 肝炎。
- 炎症性肠病。
- 胰腺炎。
- 消化性溃疡、消化不良。
- 穿孔。
- 腹膜炎。
• 神经系统:
- 颅内压(ICP)增高。
- 颅内出血。
- 迷路炎、眩晕。
- 脑膜炎。
- 偏头痛。
- 脑卒中。
- 肿瘤。
• 内分泌:
- 肾上腺功能不全。
- 糖尿病酮症酸中毒(DKA)。
- 甲状旁腺功能减退、甲状旁腺功能亢进。
- 甲状腺功能减退、甲状腺功能亢进。
- 尿毒症。
• 妊娠:
- 妊娠剧吐。
- 妊娠期恶心/呕吐。
• 药物毒性:
- 对乙酰氨基酚。
- 阿司匹林。
- 地高辛。
- 茶碱。
• 治疗性药物使用:
- 抗生素。
- 阿司匹林。
- 化疗药物。
- 布洛芬。
• 滥用药物:
- 麻醉/麻醉品戒断。
- 酒精。
- 大麻素性呕吐。
• 泌尿生殖道:
- 性腺扭转。
- 肾石病。
- 肾盂肾炎。
• 其他:
- 急性冠脉综合征。
- 一氧化碳或有机磷中毒。
- 电解质紊乱。
- 青光眼。
- 晕动病。
- 疼痛。
- 术后(麻醉后)。
- 自我诱导(进食障碍)。
- 脓毒症/休克。

诊断

症状和体征

病史

• 症状持续时间、频率、严重程度:
- 急性、复发性、慢性、反复性。
• 呕吐的特点:时间、性状、呕吐物的内容。
• 相关症状:疼痛、发热、腹泻、神经系统。
• 过去的外科手术或胃肠道病史。
• 服药史。
• 末次月经。
• 完整的既往病史。

体格检查

• 重要体征:
- 发热:盲肠炎、肠胃炎、胆囊炎、肝炎、肠穿孔。
- 心动过速:脱水。
• 头、耳、眼睛、鼻、喉:
- 异常前房:青光眼。
- 粘膜干燥:脱水。
- 眼球震颤:内耳炎、脑卒中、肿瘤、颅内出血。
- 视神经乳头水肿:颅内压升高。
• 腹部:
- 大便或呕血:消化性溃疡、食管黏膜撕裂症。
- 肠鸣音减少:肠梗阻。
- 腹胀,高亢的肠鸣音、瘢痕或疝、肠梗阻。
- 压痛:阑尾炎、胆囊炎、胰腺炎、穿孔、卵巢扭转。
- 睾丸疼痛:扭转。
• 神经系统:
- 异常精神状态、小脑异常、脑神经异常:病理性中枢神经系统。

基本检查

这项工作的目的是确定呕吐的根本原因,排除危险的结果。

诊断检查与说明

实验室检查

• CBC:
- 白细胞升高:感染过程(如盲肠炎、肠胃炎)。
- 血细胞比容升高:脱水。
- 血细胞比容减少:胃肠道溃疡出血。
• 电解质/肾功能:
- 长时间的呕吐可能导致低氯低钾代谢性碱中毒。
- 尿素/肌酐>20 表示脱水。
- 脱水可能导致肾损害。
• 肝/胰腺功能:
- 淀粉酶和脂肪酶升高:胰腺炎。
- AST/ALT 升高:肝炎。
- 碱性磷酸酶升高:胆囊病变。
• 尿常规:
- 白细胞,亚硝酸盐,白细胞酯酶,细菌:尿

O

路感染。
- 酮体：脱水、酮症酸中毒。
- 育龄妇女的妊娠试验。
• 毒理学筛查/血药浓度：
- 对于疑似药物毒性或过量服用。

影像学检查

• 腹部系列(肾、输尿管、膀胱/立位片)：
- 疑似肠梗阻或穿孔。
• 腹部或骨盆 CT：
- 怀疑阑尾炎、梗阻、肾结石。
• 头颅 CT/MRI：
- 怀疑颅内病因。
• B超：
- 疑似胆道病变、性腺扭转、肾结石。

诊断步骤/外科

• 心电图。
- 怀疑 MI。
• 内镜检查：
- 消化性溃疡导致严重的胃肠道出血。

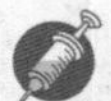

治疗

院前

• 目的是稳定患者直到到达急诊，能够判断呕吐的病因。
• 建立静脉通路，吸氧，心脏监护。
• 开始对疑似脱水输注等渗液。
• 对精神状态变化或已知糖尿病患者，检测指脉血糖。
• 对于晕动症或者其他特定呕吐原因可能应用止吐剂。

初步稳定/治疗

• ABC 管理。
• 低血容量休克：紧急液体复苏。
• 紧急止吐疗法可使患者感到舒适并降低误吸风险。
• 必要时采用止痛疗法。

急诊治疗/程序

• 急诊室治疗的 3 个原则：
- 纠正液体、电解质和呕吐导致的营养缺乏。
- 识别和治疗潜在的原因。
- 抑制或消除症状。
• 抗生素使用：尿路感染、阑尾炎、细菌性肠胃炎(罕见)。
• 其他药物：
- 5-羟色胺拮抗剂通常是一线治疗：
◦ 奥坦西隆、多拉司琼、盐酸格拉司琼。
◦ 用于化疗所致恶心。
◦ 昂丹司琼可作为口服溶解剂对于不能耐受药片的患者。
◦ 会导致 QT 间期延长。
- 多巴胺 D2 拮抗剂(在大多数呕吐中很有用)。
◦ 普鲁氯嗪、异丙嗪、甲氧氯普胺(胃复安)、氟哌利多。
◦ 副作用(例如，静坐不能、肌张力障碍)较 5-羟色胺拮抗剂更常见。
◦ 注意使用的氟哌利多黑箱警告[潜在的 QT 间期延长和/或尖端扭转]和异丙嗪(静脉给药导致组织损伤)。
- 抗胆碱能和抗组胺剂适用于迷路炎，位置性眩晕和晕动症。
◦ 氯苯甲嗪、苯海拉明、莨菪碱。
- 苯二氮䓬类和糖皮质激素具有温和的止吐作用，可作为止吐剂使用。
• 根据病因咨询其他专科(如外科、妇科、消化科)。

药物治疗

• 苯海拉明：25～50 mg，肌内注射、静脉注射或口服。
• 多拉司琼(dolasetron)12.5 mg，肌内注射或静脉注射。
• 多西他明/吡哆醇：10 mg/10 mg 至每日 3 次口服。
• 氟哌利多：0.625～1.25 mg，肌内注射或静脉注射。
• 盐酸格拉司琼(granisetron)：1 mg，静脉注射；或 2 mg 口服。
• 羟嗪：25～100 mg，肌内注射。
• 氯苯甲嗪：25～50 mg，口服。
• 甲氧氯普胺：10 mg，肌内注射、静脉注射或口服。
• 奥坦西隆：4～8 mg，肌内注射、静脉注射或口服。
• 丙氯哌嗪：5～10 mg，肌内注射、静脉注射或口服；或 25 mg 灌肠。
• 异丙嗪：12.5～25 mg，口服、灌肠或深部肌内注射。
• 莨菪碱：旅行前 4 h 在耳后应用 1.5 mg 的贴片。

老年人注意事项

多巴胺拮抗剂类止吐药有潜力心脏的副作用：
- 在老年人使用时应该减少剂量。
• 5-羟色胺拮抗剂在这些人群中更安全：
- 仍然考虑使用低剂量的药物，使用行心电图检测是否存在 QT 间期延长。

儿科注意事项

• 儿童呕吐可能是由其他病因引起的，如结构、解剖疾病、感染及代谢紊乱：
- 因此儿童的诊疗需要特别对待。

妊娠注意事项

• 妊娠期间呕吐的发生率>25%。
• 妊娠剧吐需要酮症和减肥。
• 多巴胺 D2 拮抗剂(如异丙嗪、氯丙嗪、甲氧氯普胺)或 5-羟色胺拮抗剂(如奥坦西隆、盐酸格拉司琼是常用的药)。多西拉明-吡哆醇也可以是有用的。

一线用药

• 5-羟色胺拮抗剂。
• 多巴胺 D2 拮抗剂。

二线用药

• 抗胆碱能类。
• 抗组胺药。
• 苯二氮䓬类药物。
• 糖皮质激素。

随访

入院指征

• 由潜在的病因决定。
• 需要密切观察或手术治疗的重大潜在疾病或症状。
• 导致无法进食的不受控制的呕吐。
• 严重脱水需要继续静脉输液。
• 严重电解质紊乱。
• 不明原因的呕吐与无法门诊随访的患者。

出院指征

• 排除严重的潜在病因。
• 患者足够的水分含量。
• 患者能耐受口服。
• 密切跟踪安排(最好是在内部 24～36 h)。

随访建议

• 所有在家中无法进水的患者应该回到急诊室。
• 呕吐的病因是未知或有电解质紊乱的患者应随访。

要点和误区

• 呕吐是一种症状，而不是诊断：
- 熟悉呕吐的不同病因诊断并排除危险的病因是很重要的。
• 许多抗吐药有显著的副作用，包括从肌张力障碍及心律失常。
- 了解使用这些药物前的禁忌和不良反应的治疗。
• 口服溶解药片和栓剂利于家庭护理并避免了静脉给药。

呕吐(儿童) Vomiting, Pediatric

Rajender K. Gattu 吴昊 李文放 译

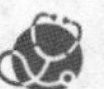

基础知识

描述

• 由于腹部肌肉、膈肌、幽门和胃窦的持续收缩引起的,通过强力而协调的动力促使胃内容物通过口腔,其特征是恶心、反胃、呕吐。干呕指无胃内容物排出。

• 呕吐源于中脑的化学敏感触发区(CTZ)的激活。

病因

呕吐的原因因年龄而异,从非常温和到严重危及生命。

• 新生儿(<2 个月):

- 肠道因素:
  ◦ 喂食问题,如喂食过量、反刍、吮吸和吞咽困难、技巧或姿势不当。
  ◦ 其他严重的胃肠道疾病包括:
    ▪ 胎粪性肠梗阻、新生儿坏死性小肠结肠炎、肥厚性幽门狭窄、旋转不良伴中肠扭转、先天性肠梗阻(闭锁、狭窄和网)、嵌顿疝。
- 非肠道因素:
  ◦ 神经系统:中枢神经系统出血(常因产伤)、脑积水、出生窒息。
  ◦ 感染性:急性肾盂肾炎、肺炎、败血症、胃肠炎、脑膜炎/脑炎、宫内感染(Torches)。
  ◦ 代谢/内分泌:先天性代谢错误(氨基酸尿、半乳糖血症、脂肪酸氧化障碍、尿素循环缺陷)、先天性肾上腺增生、胆红素脑病。

• 婴儿期(2 个月至 2 岁):

- 肠道因素:
  ◦ 胃食管反流病(GERD)、牛奶不耐受或牛奶过敏、饭后呕吐、病毒性胃炎或胃肠炎、食物中毒。
  ◦ 胃肠道梗阻——幽门狭窄、肠套叠、旋转不良伴中肠扭转和嵌顿疝、异物/牛黄、外伤。
- 非肠道因素:
  ◦ 代谢/内分泌:先天性代谢错误(氨基酸尿、脂肪酸氧化紊乱、尿素循环缺陷)。
  ◦ 神经学:硬膜下血肿、闭合性脑损伤、非意外伤害、脑积水引起的颅内压升高。
  ◦ 感染:急性胃肠炎、尿路感染、肺炎、中耳炎。潜在严重感染,如败血症、脑膜炎或脑炎。
  ◦ 慢性器官疾病:肝胆疾病、慢性肾脏疾病、胰腺炎。
  ◦ 其他:中毒性摄入。

• 儿童(3~12 岁):

- 肠道因素:
  ◦ 急性胃肠炎。严重的病因包括食管异物、嗜酸性食管炎和肠梗阻,如肠套叠、旋转不良伴中肠扭转、腹部手术粘连、腹股沟嵌顿疝、麻痹性肠梗阻、外伤。
- 非肠道因素:
  ◦ 高反应性气道疾病、肾盂肾炎、链球菌性咽炎、中耳炎和上呼吸道感染引起的呕吐。
  ◦ 代谢:糖尿病酮症酸中毒(DKA)。
  ◦ 神经学:肿瘤、脑假瘤、硬膜下血肿引起的颅内压增高,严重头部损伤。
  ◦ 中毒摄入:意外或故意过量用药。
  ◦ 周期性呕吐。
  ◦ 其他:化疗后。

• 青春期(13~18 岁):

- 肠道因素:
  ◦ 急性胃肠炎、消化性溃疡、阑尾炎、肠梗阻、肠梗阻、外伤。
- 非肠道因素:
  ◦ 妊娠、假性肿瘤、药物滥用/戒断、饮食失调、精神性疾病。
  ◦ 潜在慢性器官疾病(慢性胰腺炎、终末期肾病、肝胆疾病)。
  ◦ 药物滥用、药物诱发、毒素或过量。

诊断

症状和体征

• 一般情况:

- 外观取决于根本病因。
- 脱水表现,包括心动过速、呼吸急促、脸色苍白、灌注减少、休克。
- 表明严重疾病的警告标志和症状。

• 呕吐:

- 胆汁性(绿色)呕吐提示十二指肠壶腹部以下梗阻;在婴儿中,胆汁呕吐与更严重的潜在疾病(旋转不良、扭转、肠套叠、肠梗阻)有关;也可能是由于麻痹性肠梗阻或脓毒症。
- 非胆汁性呕吐是由近端幽门病变引起的。
- 呕血提示病变通常靠近 Treitz 韧带;鲜血不伴有或伴有少量胃液通常提示活动性出血点位于或在贲门之上。
- 咖啡色样呕吐物:由被还原胃分泌物还原的血红色导致。
- 呕吐未消化的食物:提示食管病变在或贲门之上。
- 恶臭:提示低位的阻塞或腹膜炎。

• 神经系统症状:

- 肿瘤、震颤婴儿综合征、出血和脑膜炎/脑炎引起的颅内压增高可能继发于持续性剧烈头痛或颈项僵硬或小脑角膨出。
- 在肠套叠或中毒或其他颅内病变(如出血、肿瘤或脑膜炎/脑炎)时,可看到精神状态的改变。

• 腹部:

- 突然发作伴有严重持续性腹痛和腹胀,提示肠梗阻、肠缺血或肠梗阻。
  ◦ 病情发展迅速,与疾病持续时间不成比例。
  ◦ 腹部肿胀和压痛与旋转不良伴中肠扭转、肠套叠、坏死性小肠结肠炎有关。
- 腹膜征象提示腹胀和可能的穿孔。
- 肥厚性幽门狭窄在 2~6 周龄时开始隐匿发作,并在喂食后变得越来越强(射弹)。
- 直肠出血和阵发性腹痛与肠套叠有关。也可能改变了精神状态。

• 高热及中毒症状:肺炎、肾盂肾炎、脑膜炎。

- 并发症:误吸、食管黏膜撕裂症、Boerhaave 综合征。

病史

• 首发症状:

- 发热。

• 呕吐特点:评估颜色、成分、起病、进展、频率。

- 发病时间,持续时间。
- 演变特征——间歇性、后发性、持续性或持久性。
- 模式——喂食后,清晨。
- 胆小?
- 血性?

• 伴随症状:

- 腹泻。
- 厌食。
- 腹痛。
- 排尿困难。

- 腹股沟肿胀。
- 神经系统症状(头痛、精神状态改变)。

• 既往史:
- 类似发作史。
- 手术史。

体格检查

• 一般情况:
- 一般的外观、生命体征、液体容量。

• 心血管疾病:
- 心音。
- 脉搏、灌注压。

• 腹部:
- 柔软度、腹胀程度、包块、肠鸣音、腹膜刺激症状。

• 泌尿生殖器:
- 阴囊肿胀程度、压痛、包块。

• 直肠:
- 有血,肿块,柔软度。

基本检查

需排除危及生命的呕吐原因。

诊断检查与说明

实验室检查

• 根据病史和体征的结果:
- 代谢评估(葡萄糖、电解质)。
- 感染评估(CBC、尿培养)。
- 育龄妇女做妊娠检查。
- 粪便显微镜检查和隐血。

影像学检查

• 根据不同表现进行考虑。

• 腹部X线片(平片、直立位和卧位)有助于评估梗阻或穿孔。

• 骨盆和腹部超声评估肥厚性幽门狭窄、肠套叠、盲肠炎及盆腔或阴囊病理性改变。

• 腹部CT扫描有助于评估鉴别阑尾炎、肿块和肿瘤。

诊断步骤/外科

• 鼻胃管:
- 胃出血的位置、特征和严重程度。

• 食管胃十二指肠镜可用于上消化道活动性出血、食管异物清除及复发性持续性呕吐等特殊情况。

鉴别诊断

• 新生儿/婴儿:
- GERD表现为不费力的呕吐。
- 蛋白质引起的肠病可表现为发育不良、呕吐和便血;幽门狭窄出现在2~6周龄,喂食后呕吐越来越强烈。
- 肠梗阻——表现为胆汁性呕吐和腹胀。
- 先天性代谢障碍,包括器质性酸血症,表现为嗜睡、进食不良、呕吐和代谢性酸中毒。
- 食管异物阻塞表现为进食后呕吐,有时伴有流口水和吞咽困难。
- 肠套叠发生在6~36个月,伴有偶发性呕吐,有时伴有血便或精神状态改变。

• 儿童/青春期:
- 急性阑尾炎表现为呕吐并伴有右下腹部疼痛和腹部检查的腹膜征。
- 妊娠。
- 偏头痛。
- 周期性呕吐。
- 进食障碍。
- 假性肿瘤。
- 呕吐与头痛相关。
- 化疗引起的呕吐。
- 术后呕吐。

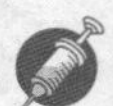

治疗

院前

无特殊治疗,除非脱水需要紧急复苏。

初步稳定/治疗

• 液体复苏,静脉给予生理盐水;如考虑出现颅内压升高,须引起注意。

• 需进行床边末梢血糖监测。

急诊治疗/程序

• 继续进行液体复苏,如果存在电解质失衡,给予纠正。

• 如腹胀或呕吐持续存在,鼻胃管胃肠减压。

• 评估潜在的病因。

• 必要时使用止吐剂药物。

• 如果出现急腹症,考虑急诊手术;如出现腹膜炎体征或其他系统性感染症状,给予抗生素。

药物治疗

- 一旦确定了呕吐的症状,止吐药可能会有帮助。

一线用药

昂丹司琼:4~8 mg:(儿童:0.1 mg/kg),静推或口服,q6 h。

二线用药

• 甲氧氯普胺:10 mg(儿童:1 mg/kg),口服,q6 h。

• 丙氯哌嗪:2.5~5 mg(儿童:每次0.1 mg/kg),静脉、肌内注射或耳用,q6 h。

• 异丙嗪:12.5~25 mg(儿童:每次0.25 mg/kg),口服、耳用或肌内注射,q6 h。

• 考虑使用其他5-HT3受体拮抗剂,如阿瑞匹坦或格拉司琼用于化疗引起的呕吐或术后呕吐。

随访

进一步处理

入院指征

• 不稳定的生命体征,包括持续的心动过速或低血容量。

• 存在严重的病因或不能排除。

• 难治性呕吐或无法耐受口服补液。

• 不良社会性因素及随访困难者。

出院指征

• 病情稳定的,能够忍受口服补液。

• 被认为最可能是良性病因或者已排除严重或者潜在的重要的病因。

• 父母了解如何缓慢给予清液,并且患儿出现持续呕吐、腹胀、排尿减少、发热、嗜睡或异常行为时即使就诊。

转诊问题

慢性或复发性呕吐以及腹部疼痛:查询儿科胃肠病学。

随访建议

PCP在1~2日。

要点和误区

• 明确呕吐物中是否胆汁或血液。

• 新生儿的胆汁性呕吐通常提示解剖异常如扭转,直到排除此情况。

• 需鉴别胃肠道以外的呕吐原因(参见鉴别诊断)。

帕金森病 Parkinson Disease

Ryan Circh 王虑 译

基础知识

描述

- 中老年人出现的渐进性的神经系统失调。
- 黑质多巴胺能神经元的变性。
- 剩余的多巴胺神经元内路易体增多。
- 大脑皮质萎缩加速。
- 有的是单侧起病,但大多是双侧。
- 生命周期风险:男性占2%,女性占1.3%。
- 平均发病年龄为60岁。
- 可能在确诊前20年就出现症状:
  - 非特异性:
    - 疲劳。
    - 便秘。
    - 嗅觉减退。

病因

- 不定时性和自发性。
- 帕金森病的异常表现:
  - 药物诱导:
    - 帕金森高热症状(服用多巴胺能药物退热)。
    - 两性霉素B。
    - 化疗类药物。
    - 抗精神病类药物诱导。
  - 毒物:
    - 一氧化碳。
    - 甲醇。
    - 氰化物。
    - 有机磷类药物。
    - 1-甲基4-苯基-1,2,3,6四氢吡啶。
  - 脑损伤:
    - 基底神经节梗死。
    - 中脑损伤。
    - 脑积水。
  - 感染:
    - 支原体。
    - 病毒性脑炎。
  - 其他:
    - 中脑桥脂肪髓磷脂化。
    - 流行性脑炎(抗基底神经节自身抗体)。

诊断

症状和体征

- 非运动和运动型症状:
  - 非运动:
    - 直立性低血压。
    - 便秘。
    - 延迟性胃排空。
    - 吞咽困难。
    - 疼痛感觉障碍。
    - 沮丧。
    - 幻觉。
    - 痴呆。
    - 睡眠紊乱。
  - 运动型症状:
    - 搓丸样静息颤抖。
    - 肌张力增高"齿轮"样强直。
    - 驼背和行动不稳。
    - 动作徐缓,尤其是在行动时。
    - "面具脸"表现。

病史

- 突然出现的运动平衡和精神状态的改变。
  - 可能是系统性疾病(如感染)的唯一表现。
- 突然停多巴胺类药可能会导致出现帕金森高温综合征:
  - 强直,发热,意识模糊。
  - 并发症:
    - 急性肾衰竭。
    - 静脉血栓。
    - 弥散性血管栓塞。
    - 横纹肌溶解。
    - 自主神经失调。

体格检查

- 齿轮样强直:
  - 移动时震颤,肌肉被动伸展。
- 弯腰姿势。
- 搓丸样颤抖。

基本检查

- 病史最为重要:
  - 诊断是以临床症状为基础的。
- 重要的病史信息包括:
  - 症状何时出现,是渐渐出现还是突然出现。
  - 帕金森样症状可能的病因。
  - 确诊的帕金森病患者:
    - 运动平衡突然出现改变。
    - 精神系统改变。
    - 需加强对传染性方面的工作。

诊断检查与说明

实验室检查

- 没有明确的特异性实验室诊断指标。
- 对也有帕金森病的异常症状的可疑患者,需通过实验室检查排除。
- 如果怀疑患有帕金森高热综合征,可通过实验室检查明确。

影像学检查

- CT和MRI不用于帕金森病的诊断,但常作为评估痴呆症的手段。
- X线胸片可以帮助诊断呼吸系统感染征兆。

鉴别诊断

- 良性遗传性颤抖。
- 重度抑郁。
- 威尔森病。
- 亨庭顿病。
- 老年痴呆症。
- 海绵状脑病。
- 一氧化碳中毒。
- 维生素 B_{12} 缺乏。
- 脑积水。
- 多发性脑梗死性痴呆。
- 特发性震颤。
- 甲状腺功能减退。
- 路易体痴呆。

治疗

急诊治疗/程序

- 服用抗帕金森药治疗控制症状可能引发勃起功能障碍。
- 根据神经科医师建议规律服药,并持续监测。
- 病情较轻的不需要药物治疗。
- 病情中等的患者可以服用抗胆碱类药和多巴胺能类药。
- 治疗潜在的感染。
- 治疗帕金森高热综合征:
  - 用左旋多巴或溴隐亭替代。
  - 支持治疗。
  - 治疗并发症。

药物治疗

- 帕金森病:
  - 金刚烷胺:100 mg,口服,每日2次。
    - 刺激多巴胺的分泌。
  - 苯托品:0.5~1 mg,口服,每日3次。
    - 抑制副交感神经。
    - 仅用于颤抖型帕金森病患者。

P

- 甲基多巴/左旋多巴：25/100 mg，口服，每日 3 次。
  - 甲基多巴增加前左旋多巴的药物生物利用度，还能减轻其副反应。
  - 左旋多巴是多巴胺的前体。
- 恩替卡朋：200 mg，口服，每日 2 次。
  - 辅助治疗；应与卡比多巴/左旋多巴同时使用。
  - 提高中枢神经系统左旋多巴的生物利用度。
- 单胺氧化酶抑制剂：
  - 司来吉兰：5 mg，每日上午和中午服用。
- 雷沙吉兰：1～2 mg，每日 1 次。
- 多巴胺激动剂：
  - 年轻患者选择的一线治疗。
  - 普拉克索：0.125 mg，口服，每日 3 次。
  - 罗匹尼罗：0.25 mg，口服，每日 3 次。
  - 阿扑吗啡：0.2～0.6 ml，必要时皮下注射。
- 帕金森综合征-高热综合征：
  - 左旋多巴：50～100 mg，静脉滴注，超过 3 h。
  - 溴隐亭：7.5～15 mg，口服，每日 3 次。

P

随访

进一步处理

入院指征

- 先前已确诊的帕金森病患者，患有感染、创伤、心血管急症、脑血管急症、消化系统急症、电解质紊乱、精神状态改变或其他医疗问题的。
- 抑郁有自残倾向的。
- 确诊帕金森病但对左旋多巴治疗无效的。
- 并发症(帕金森高热综合征)。
- 症状波动，运动困难。
- 因被虐待不能回家生活的。
- 大脑深度刺激引起的并发症(如头痛、感染、精神状态改变)。
- 不活跃的。

出院指征

- 不需要治疗的轻中度患者。
- 需服药治疗的中重度患者，紧急时可门诊随访。

随访建议

讨论疾病管理的预防策略。

要点和误区

- 帕金森病的诊断常常比较困难，要常考虑那些可能被误诊为帕金森病的疾病。
- 突然停多巴胺能类药可能会致帕金森高热综合征，这是一临床急症。

膀胱损伤 Bladder Injury

Mohannad F. Allehyani · Gary M. Vilke 宋振举 童朝阳 译

基础知识

描述

- 钝性外伤是最常见的机制。
- 10%的骨盆骨折有严重的膀胱损伤。
- 80%～90%的膀胱破裂有骨盆骨折。
- 总体死亡率为 80%～90%。
- 如果联合腹腔内/腹腔外的尼尔断裂为 60%。

病因

- 机制。
- 创伤：82%。
- 钝性创伤：机动车事故(MVA，87%)、跌倒(7%)和袭击(6%)。
- 穿透伤：枪伤(85%)和刺伤(15%)。
- 医源性：14%，前列腺切除术和泌尿外科操作、妇科手术、产科程序、腹部手术、疝修补、宫内节育器(IUD)、骨科髋关节手术、活检、留置导尿管。
- 中毒：2.9%。
- 自发性：<1%。
- 分类。
- 腹膜外膀胱破裂(62%)。
  - 伴有骨盆骨折。
  - 由钝力或骨折碎片引起。
- 腹膜内膀胱破裂。
  - 直接压缩充盈的膀胱。
  - 由膀胱穹窿破裂所致。
- 腹膜外腹膜内联合破裂(12%)。
  - 因相关损伤造成的死亡率最高。
- 膀胱挫伤。
  - 膀胱壁完整的内皮层或肌层的损伤。
  - 过度体力活动后的严重血尿(长跑)。
  - 影像学检查正常，肉眼血尿。
  - 通常不用治疗。

儿科注意事项

- 在儿童中，膀胱是腹腔内脏器官，在 20 岁时下降到骨盆。
- 相比成人，腹腔内破裂在儿童中更常见，因为膀胱是一个腹部器官。
- 儿童中的膀胱损伤比成人更常见，因为小儿骨盆不太坚硬，并且会向邻近结构传递更多力量。

诊断

症状和体征

三联征

- 肉眼血尿。
- 耻骨上疼痛。
- 排尿困难。

病史

存在潜在诱因。

体格检查

评估尿道口，如果有血液存在，直到进行逆行尿道造影前不要插入导尿管(RUG，10%～29%的患者伴随尿道和膀胱损伤)。

基本检查

- 创伤史或手术史。
- 评估尿道口的血液。
- 尿液分析(UA)。
- 逆行膀胱造影。

诊断检查与说明

实验室检查

- UA。
- 95%～100%的膀胱或尿道创伤患者出现肉眼血尿。
- 5%的患者为显微镜下血尿。
- BUN 和肌酸酐。
- BUN 可以通过腹膜内尿液的再吸收而升高。

- 电解质。
- 高钾血症和高钠血症可能是由于尿液在腹膜内吸收造成的。

影像学检查

- 逆行膀胱造影和逆行CT。膀胱造影是诊断膀胱破裂的首选方法。两项研究分别报道了95%和100%的敏感性和特异性。
- CT细胞成像在鉴别膀胱内骨性碎片、膀胱颈损伤及其他腹部损伤方面具有优势。
- 如果怀疑有尿道损伤，膀胱造影是在RUG后进行的。
- 膀胱造影。
- 肾-输尿管-膀胱摄影。
- 通过导尿管将100 ml稀释对比剂注入膀胱。对比剂需要稀释：30%或6∶1盐水；否则浓度过高。
- 如果初始影像正常，请用稀释的造影剂填充膀胱的其余部分：
  - 最小值：成人300～350 ml。
  - 对于无法耐受者或儿童患者为3～5 ml/kg(或60 ml)+[年龄(岁)×30]。
- 有一个完整显影的膀胱对于诊断是非常重要的，仅以正向方式放置对比并夹紧导尿管是不够的。
- 除非已经行膀胱CT造影，否则应该排空膀胱，获得排空后影像。
- 如果没有膀胱CT造影，10%的膀胱破裂仅在排空后膀胱影像上可见；充盈的膀胱可能会隐藏外渗。
- 膀胱造影解读。
- 腹膜外破裂：泪滴状或星状形状。
- 腹腔内破裂：与结肠肠腔相反的显影。

■ 诊断步骤/外科

- 创伤重点超声评估(FAST)。
- 盆腔积液应注意有无膀胱损伤。
- 诊断膀胱损伤仅有超声检查是不够的。

■ 鉴别诊断

- 腹膜创伤。
- 尿道外伤。
- 肾或输尿管损伤。

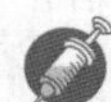

治疗

■ 院前

不要尝试在院外导尿。

■ 初步稳定/治疗

- ABC管理。
- 早期泌尿科会诊。

■ 急诊治疗/程序

- 确诊膀胱破裂时需要泌尿科会诊。
- 腹膜外非穿透性破裂可以通过导管引流来控制。
- 20F以上导尿管或留置14日。
- 80%的伤口会在3周内愈合。
- 如果患者因其他损伤正在进行腹部或盆腔手术，建议进行手术修复。
- 腹膜内破裂需要手术探查。
- 对于伴有严重神经损伤(头部和脊髓)或骨折而瘫痪的患者，可以考虑行耻骨上造瘘。

- 膀胱挫伤不需要任何特定的干预措施。

■ 药物治疗

如有腹膜破裂应用广谱抗生素。

随访

■ 进一步处理

入院指征

- 需要入院或观察的合并的重大创伤。
- 需要手术干预。

出院指征

- 膀胱挫伤、没有破裂或合并需要住院重大创伤。
- 膀胱破裂的大多数病例需要入院，通过泌尿科会诊排除无其他相关的伤害。

转诊问题

作为门诊患者处理的任何膀胱损伤应该有泌尿系统转诊。

■ 随访建议

安排泌尿科随访：

- 用导尿管治疗腹膜外膀胱破裂应在14日内拔除导尿管。

要点和误区

- CT或超声检查中的积液都应怀疑是否有膀胱损伤。
- 反应迟钝、意识改变及过度兴奋的患者应仔细检查。
- 腹部穿透性损伤患者任何程度的血尿都值得膀胱造影。

佩吉特病 Paget Disease

Matthew C. Kostura · Anna L. Waterbrook 王虑 译

基础知识

■ 描述

- 佩吉特病表现包括正常骨组织吸收及被纤维和硬化组织替代。
- 也被认为是畸形性骨炎。
- 通常是局灶性，骨组织最常受累。
- 骨盆(70%)。
- 股骨(55%)。
- 颅骨(42%)。
- 胫骨(32%)。
- 脊柱(53%，腰椎)。
- 扁骨。
- 通常在偶然情况下发现，平时没什么症状。
- 55岁以上老年人群发病率为1%～2%。
- 随年龄增加，发病率增高。
- 发生在溶骨期，破骨细胞进入正常骨组织。
- 易导致血肿和骨折。
- 吸收的骨被无序、密集的硬化骨小梁替代，经过成骨期显示成“马赛克图案”。
- 恶性变很少见：
- 骨肉瘤恶性程度高。
- 通常恶变率在1%。
- 男性多见。
- 欧洲地区高发。
- 亚洲和斯堪的纳维亚地区少见。
- 典型的一般仅侵犯一块骨(单骨性)。
- 也可以侵犯多根骨(多骨性)。

■ 病因

- 不明。
- 基因构成：

- *SQSTM1* 突变见于许多病例，但不是所有病例。
• 环境因素也很重要。
- 发现风疹病毒、犬瘟热病毒、副黏病毒和呼吸合胞病毒核衣壳提示此病和病毒也有关。
- 可能与农村生活和密切接触牲畜有关。
• 继发炎症反应可致血管增生。
• 显微镜观察破骨细胞可以发现细胞核仁增加和核内包含物。

儿科注意事项

通常此病未见于儿童。

诊断

症状和体征

• 许多患者平时无症状，偶然影像学检查或碱性磷酸酶检查才发现。
• 到晚期出现剧烈的骨痛。
• 若股骨或胫骨受累则表现为负重痛。
• 非负重骨在休息时疼痛反而更剧烈。
• 急性期(再吸收/溶骨期)：
- 病理性骨折。
- 疼痛源于细胞溶解、骨折和关节炎。
- 高血钙或肾结石。
- 血管过度增生导致骨折后严重出血。
- 普遍疾病：
◦ 增加的血管和血流将导致高排性心力衰竭。
• 第二期(硬化/成骨期)：
- 长时间导致长骨肿胀畸形，步态异常。
- 长时间导致颅骨变形和头痛。
- 长时间颅骨脊柱受累会导致中枢神经压迫症状。
- 听力丧失可能和神经压迫及听小骨受累有关。

基本检查

• 通常通过影像学检查做出诊断。
• 当脊柱或骨盆受累时，需行详细的全身神经系统检查。

诊断检查与说明

实验室检查

• 碱性磷酸酶是该病活动期最敏感的标志物。
• 血钙和磷酸盐水平应一起检测，但通常在正常范围。
• 血钙增高多见于活动受限或骨折患者，若是行动正常患者则应考虑是否有甲状旁腺功能亢进。
• 若怀疑有高钙血症或高排性心力衰竭，行心电图和胸部X线片检查。
• 骨再生行成将导致尿羟脯氨酸上升或血骨钙素和骨胶原片段增加。
• 甲状旁腺素水平变化发生在再吸收/溶骨期(低甲状旁腺素)和硬化/成骨期(高甲状旁腺素)。

影像学检查

• X线平片：
- 在再吸收期，溶骨病变不容易看见，但在颅骨可以看见界限清晰的病变区(局限性骨质疏松症)。
- 长骨随着吸收和应力的缺失会出现弯曲。
- 新生骨促使表现为不规则和斑点状，后来演变为均匀紧密(象牙图案)。
- 多余骨质顺着应力线沉积，使骨皮质不规则及增厚。
• CT或MRI检查协助鉴别肿瘤和血肿：
- 螺旋CT检测肾结石。
• 放射性核素检查可用于评估疾病累及范围和活动度。
• X线平片最经常用于诊断骨折。

鉴别诊断

• 甲状旁腺功能亢进症。
• 多发性骨髓瘤。
• 霍奇金病变异。
• 肢端肥大症。
• 骨肉瘤。

治疗

院前

• 院前医务人员应收集伤情的相关信息和病理性骨折可能的致病因素。
• 充分的制动能有效减轻患处出血。

初步稳定/治疗

• 气道管理和复苏。
• 高排性心力衰竭应按照慢性心力衰竭治疗指南进行。
• 及时的制动能有效减轻患处出血。

急诊治疗/程序

• 对因溶骨、骨折或关节炎引起疼痛可予以对乙酰氨基酚或麻醉剂止痛治疗。
• 骨折的治疗通常比较保守，因为易于出血，复位比较困难。
• 严重的关节炎和明确需处理的骨折应请骨科会诊。
• 高钙血症可以通过静脉补液、降钙素和双膦酸盐类药物治疗。
• 若出现中枢神经压迫症状需紧急求助脑外科医师，必要时减压治疗。

药物治疗

药物治疗的指征为有症状的患者，或无症状但病变在可能发生并发症的部位。

一线用药

• 含氮双膦酸盐类药物治疗：
- 氨羟二磷酸二钠：30 mg，静脉注射，每日1次，持续3日；注射时间需超过4 h。
- 阿仑膦酸钠：40 mg，口服，每日1次，持续6个月。
- 利塞膦酸钠：30 mg，口服，每日1次，持续2个月。
- 唑来膦酸：5 mg，静脉注射1次，注射时间不少于15 min。

二线用药

• 简单的双膦酸盐类药物和降钙素：
- 依替膦酸钠：5 mg/kg，口服，每日1次，持续6个月。
- 替鲁膦酸钠：400 mg，口服，每日1次，持续3个月。
- 降钙素：50～100 U，皮下注射；不超过6个月。
• 放射治疗和简单的双膦酸盐类药物不作长期的推荐。
• 使用降钙素和简单的双膦酸盐类药物限于那些不能耐受或对含氮双膦酸盐类药物过敏的患者。
• 双膦酸盐类药物的副作用主要是类流感症状和颌骨骨坏死。
• 治疗期间需要补充维生素D和钙剂以维持血钙水平。

随访

进一步处理

入院指征

• 严重的外伤或大量的出血。
• 骨科手术。
• 高血钙。
• 中枢神经压迫症状，神经截断需要手术治疗。

出院指征

• 没有严重出血、神经压迫或高血钙，并且疼痛得到有效控制。
• 骨折得到适当的固定制动和有骨科医师

随访。

转诊问题

• 任何急性的外伤。

• 出院后 1～2 周可考虑转诊至内分泌科。

■ 随访建议

• 随访通常在急性外伤后经放射检查做出佩吉特病诊断后。

• 随访了解通过药物治疗使血碱性磷酸酶水平恢复正常的情况。

• 如果血碱性磷酸酶水平再次升高，临床症状再出现，或影像学发现疾病有进展，需要重新药物治疗。

要点和误区

• 佩吉特病通常都是偶然通过影像学检查发现的。

• 积极对骨折处制动能有效控制骨折处的出血。

• 目前认为佩吉特病和血碱性磷酸酶水平升高有关。

P

盆腔炎 Pelvic Inflammatory Disease

Adam Z. Barkin 王虑 译

基础知识

■ 描述

• 骨盆炎症疾病(PID)是一种急性社区获得性通过性传播的上尿路感染，包括子宫、输卵管、卵巢或其他组织。

• 急诊最常见的妇科疾病的原因(350 000/年)。

• 代表一系列感染：

- 没有单一的诊断金标准。
- 骨盆炎症需降低诊断标准和开始经验性抗生素治疗。

• 疾病进展至输卵管卵巢脓肿。

• 盆腔感染综合征是与盆腔炎相关的肝囊性炎症反应：

- 剧烈的右上腹疼痛。
- 当呼吸、移动或咳嗽时疼痛加重。

■ 病因

• 风险因素：

- 年龄＜25 岁。
- 多个性伴侣或患病的性伴侣。
- 既往盆腔炎病史。
- 口服避孕药。
- 无避孕措施。
- 非洲美洲人。

• 盆腔炎的致病菌大多是沙眼衣原体和淋球菌。

• 其他致病菌包括 A 型链球菌、葡萄球菌、革兰阴性杆菌(克雷伯杆菌属、埃希杆菌属、变形杆菌)和厌氧菌。

诊断

■ 症状和体征

• 下腹部疼痛，通常双侧。

• 阴道分泌物。

• 尿路异常出血。

• 痛经。

• 排尿困难。

• 性交困难。

• 恶心和呕吐。

• 寒战、发热。

• 直肠炎。

• 下腹部触痛。

• 肠鸣音减弱。

• 双侧附件触痛。

• 宫颈触痛。

• 子宫颈脓性分泌物。

• 附件肿块。

• 右上腹触痛。

病史

• 下腹疼痛是最常见的盆腔炎症状，程度从轻度到严重疼痛都有。

• 腹痛且在性交或月经期加重往往提示盆腔炎。

• 腹痛常为双侧，持续时间＜2 周。

• 新的阴道分泌物、尿道炎、发热和寒战是最常见症状。但对于诊断盆腔炎，上述表现特异性和灵敏性都不够。

妊娠注意事项

盆腔炎在妊娠期比较少见，如果发病，常发生在妊娠前 3 个月，因为后期随着激素水平改变，黏液栓可以保护子宫免受细菌侵袭。

体格检查

• 仅有 50%的盆腔炎患者有发热。

• 腹部触痛尤其是下腹部，并不总是对称。

• 反跳痛和肠鸣音减低较常见。

• 右上腹触痛提示肝周炎。

• 宫颈脓性分泌物，子宫颈触痛或附件触痛。

• 如果子宫和附件的触痛不明显，需考虑其他疾病诊断。

■ 基本检查

• 询问病史和体格检查，包括骨盆检查。

• 妊娠检测以排除异位妊娠和宫内孕的并发症。

• 宫颈分泌物培养淋球菌和衣原体。

• 临床诊断基本标准：

- 下腹部触痛。
- 子宫/附件触痛。
- 子宫颈触痛。

• 诊断辅助标准：

- 体温＞38.3℃。
- 反常宫颈/阴道分泌物。
- 子宫颈革兰染色，革兰阴性双球菌阳性。
- 白细胞增多＞10 000/mm^3。
- 红细胞沉降率和 C 反应蛋白升高。
- 后穹窿穿刺或腹腔镜所得腹腔液中白细胞增多或发现细菌。

■ 诊断检查与说明

实验室检查

• 全血细胞计数。

• 子宫颈内膜革兰染色。

• 尿聚合酶链反应检测衣原体和淋球菌。

• 显微镜检查阴道分泌物。

• 盆腔感染综合征会有肝酶升高。

• 尿粪潜血阳性的盆腔炎概率不高。

• 红细胞沉降率和 C 反应蛋白升高，但不做常规检查。

影像学检查

• 影像学检查发现附件肿大或肿块，还需做经阴道超声以排除输卵管卵巢脓肿。

• 门诊患者经抗生素治疗效果不好或因疼痛或肥胖检查不彻底的，考虑行盆腔超声检查。

诊断步骤/外科

腹腔镜对怀疑盆腔炎或门诊治疗效果不佳患者的明确诊断有帮助。

鉴别诊断

P

- 异位妊娠。
- 急性阑尾炎。
- 附件扭转。
- 子宫内膜异位症。
- 膀胱炎。
- 尿路结石。
- 卵巢肿瘤。
- 子宫腺肌病。
- 慢性盆腔疼痛。
- 良性卵巢囊肿。
- 肠憩室炎。
- 炎症性肠炎。
- 肠系膜血管病。
- 肠易激综合征。

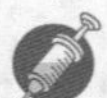

治疗

院前

- 院前没有特别注意事项。
- 适度的疼痛控制。

初步稳定/治疗

- 极少需要复苏。
- 疼痛控制。

急诊治疗/程序

门诊患者

- 头孢曲松钠-丙磺舒＋多西环素：当考虑有厌氧菌时使用甲硝唑治疗。
- 供选择的治疗方案还有头孢曲松钠＋阿奇霉素。
- 同时要对性伴侣进行检查和治疗。

住院患者

- 多西环素＋头孢西丁或头孢替坦。
- 供选择的治疗方案还有庆大霉素＋克林霉素、氨苄西林-舒巴坦＋多西环素。
- 持续静脉用抗生素抗感染，临床症状改善后改口服抗生素14日。
- 腹腔镜可以用于盆腔感染综合征急性期和慢性期的粘连松解。
- 考虑有厌氧菌时使用甲硝唑治疗。

药物治疗

- 氨苄西林-舒巴坦：3 g，静脉注射，q6 h。
- 阿奇霉素：1 g，口服，每日1次，持续服用2周。
- 头孢替坦：2 g，静脉注射，q12 h。
- 头孢西丁：2 g，肌内注射(门诊患者)；2 g，静脉注射，q6 h(住院患者)。
- 头孢曲松钠：250 mg，肌内注射。
- 克林霉素：450 mg，口服，每日3次，持续服用14日(门诊患者)；900 mg，静脉注射，q8 h(住院患者)。
- 多西环素：100 mg，口服，每日2次，持续服用14日(门诊患者)；100 mg，静脉注射或口服，q12 h(住院患者)。
  - 因静脉注射的疼痛原因，口服更为患者接受。
  - 口服和静脉用药生物利用度相似。
- 庆大霉素：先2 mg/kg负荷量后1.5 mg/k，q8 h；也可以每日1次。
- 甲硝唑：500 mg，口服，每日2次，持续服用14日(门诊患者)；500 mg，静脉注射，q8 h(住院患者)。
- 丙磺舒：1 g，口服，每日1次。

一线用药

- 门诊患者：
  - 头孢曲松钠或头孢西丁-丙磺舒＋多西环素。
    - 考虑有厌氧菌时使用甲硝唑治疗，尤其怀疑阴道滴虫感染。
    - 女性患者最近有骨盆固定病史的。
- 口服头孢菌素已不作为淋球菌感染的推荐治疗方案(疾病预防控治中心推荐肌内注射头孢曲松钠＋口服阿奇霉素或多西环素)。
- 住院患者：
  - 多西环素＋头孢西丁或头孢替坦。

二线用药

- 门诊患者：
  - 头孢曲松钠＋阿奇霉素联用或不联用甲硝唑。
- 住院患者：
  - 庆大霉素＋克林霉素或氨苄西林-舒巴坦＋多西环素。

随访

进一步处理

入院指征

- 诊断不明确并有中毒表现。
- 怀疑有骨盆，包括输卵管卵巢脓肿。
- 孕妇。
- 免疫功能缺陷。
- 症状严重(呕吐或严重疼痛)。
- 门诊患者治疗效果不佳。
- 无法遵循门诊治疗方案(如儿童)。
- 患者无法随访可以收入院。

出院指征

- 盆腔炎患者没达到入院条件可以门诊治疗的。
- 最近研究表明对于轻中度盆腔炎妇女，门诊治疗和住院治疗相比最终的生育情况没有明显区别。

转诊问题

输卵管卵巢脓肿除了抗生素治疗还需引流和手术干预。

随访建议

- 门诊患者治疗后48～72 h后要评估临床治疗效果。
- 如果患者72 h体温没有下降，需考虑住院治疗和进一步病情评估。

要点和误区

- 盆腔炎代表了一系列疾病从简单的子宫内膜炎到严重的腹腔脓毒症。
- 在美国口服喹诺酮和头孢菌素已不被推荐用来治疗淋球菌感染的盆腔炎，因为耐药率越来越高。
- 盆腔炎患者需做性传播疾病的相关检查和咨询，包括艾滋病。
- 女性盆腔炎患者的男性性伴侣，如果和患者出现症状前60日有过性接触，那他也要接受治疗。

皮肤或软组织脓肿 Abscess，Skin/Soft Tissue

Neal P. O'Connor 马林浩 林兆奋 译

 基础知识

描述

- 局部的脓液聚集并以被炎症组织包围起来：
  - 脓肿可以出现于身体的任何部位。
- 疖：
  - 由感染的毛囊引起。
  - 多常见于后背、腋下和下肢。
- 痈：
  - 比疖更大，累及范围更广。
- 猫/犬咬伤：
  - 通常是多种微生物致病。
- 乳房：
  - 产褥期。
    - 通常在泌乳期间。
    - 位于周边的楔形。
    - 通常由葡萄球菌引起。
  - 乳管扩张。
    - 由扩张的乳管导致。
    - 位于乳晕部位。
    - 通常由多种致病菌所致。
- 化脓性汗腺炎：
  - 顶泌汗腺的慢性脓肿。
  - 腹股沟和头皮。
  - 金黄色葡萄球菌和草绿色链球菌常见。
  - 慢性疾病中也可见大肠杆菌和变形杆菌。
- 毛囊脓肿：
  - 臀沟至尾骨的上皮细胞破坏。
  - 葡萄球菌属最为常见。
  - 可能是多种微生物致病。
- 巴多林脓肿：
  - 前庭大腺导管阻塞。
- 直肠周围脓肿。
  - 由肛周隐窝起病并通过坐骨直肠间隙扩散。
  - 炎症性肠病和糖尿病是易患因素。
  - 脆弱拟杆菌和大肠杆菌最为常见。
  - 需要手术引流。
- 肌肉(脓性肌炎)：
  - 在热带典型。
  - 金黄色葡萄球菌最常见。
- 静脉药物滥用：
  - 葡萄球菌属最常见。
  - 甲氧西林耐药的金黄色葡萄球菌常见。
  - 可能是无菌的。
- 甲沟炎：
  - 指甲褶皱周围的感染。
  - 通常是金黄色葡萄球菌。
- 脓性指头炎：
  - 手指末节闭合间隙内的脓肿。
  - 通常是金黄色葡萄球菌。

病因

- 典型的脓肿形成是由于皮肤的破损、皮脂腺或汗腺阻塞，或者毛囊炎症引起的。可以分为细菌性和无菌性：
  - 细菌性：大多数的脓肿由细菌及其代谢产物影响身体部分所致。
    - 金黄色葡萄球菌是最常见的致病微生物。
    - 社区获得性的甲氧西林耐药金黄色葡萄球菌(CA-MRSA)常见。
- 无菌性：多与静脉药物滥用和注射刺激性化学物质有关。
- 脓肿形成的危险因素：
  - 免疫抑制。
  - 软组织创伤。
  - 哺乳动物/人咬伤。
  - 组织缺血。
  - 静脉注射药物。
  - 克罗恩病(直肠周)。

诊断

症状和体征

- 局部：
  - 红。
  - 痛。
  - 热。
  - 肿。
  - 波动感。
  - 可能存在周围蜂窝织炎。
  - 可能出现区域性的淋巴结病和淋巴管炎。
- 全身性：
  - 经常不存在。
  - 大范围皮肤软组织受累，坏死性筋膜炎或者经受菌血症的患者可能表现出脓毒症样症状：
    - 发热。
    - 寒战。
    - 低血压。
    - 意识状态改变。

病史

- 之前的病史：警惕 CA-MRSA。
- 免疫抑制。
- 用药史。
  - 慢性激素治疗史、化疗史。
- 静脉注射吸毒者。
- 哺乳动物咬伤史。

体格检查

- 感染的部位和范围。
- 有无以下表现：
  - 邻近的蜂窝织炎。
  - 皮下积气。
  - 累及深部组织。
- 涉及专科检查的部位：
  - 直肠肛周。
  - 手部。
  - 面部、颈部。

基本检查

- 病史和体格检查。
- 健康患者的普通脓肿无须进行革兰染色。
- 创面培养：
  - 不出现于单纯性脓肿中。
  - 如果计划进行系统治疗，可能有助于指导治疗。
  - 可能有助于证实复发性脓肿患者是由于 CA-MRSA 所致。
  - 可指导对受损宿主、中央面部或手的脓肿和治疗失败的特定治疗。

诊断检查与说明

实验室检查

- 常规实验室检查通常不适用。
- 在以下情况下，葡萄糖测定可能很有用：
  - 潜在的未确诊糖尿病是一个令人担忧的问题。
  - 可能与糖尿病酮症酸中毒的影响有关。
- 对于出现脓毒症、全身疾病或最近有 IVDU 的发热患者，建议进行以下实验室检查：
  - 血培养。
  - 乳酸测定。
  - 肾功能。
  - 如果怀疑为肌炎，则为 CK。

影像学检查

- 床旁超声有助于区分蜂窝组织炎和脓肿。
- CT/MRI 有助于确定深层组织受累。
- X 线平片可能显示组织平面内的气体。

鉴别诊断

- 蜂窝织炎。

- 坏死性筋膜炎。
- 动脉瘤(尤其是静脉吸毒者)。
- 囊肿。
- 血肿。

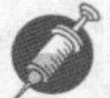

治疗

院前

注意：脓毒症患者需要快速静脉滴注液体和容量复苏。

初步稳定/治疗

脓毒症患者：

- 立即建立静脉通路。
- 吸氧。
- 晶体液容量复苏。
- 血培养/乳酸。
- 早期抗生素疗法——覆盖 MRSA 的广谱抗生素。
- 快速控制病因(脓肿引流)。
- 若患者容量复苏后持续性低血压：
  - 中心静脉压检测。
  - 混合静脉血取样。

急诊治疗/程序

- 切开和引流是主要的治疗措施。
  - 切开要足够深以保证引流充分。
  - 切口要够宽以防皮肤闭合。
  - 椭圆形切口防止早期闭合。
  - 轻柔探查来突破局部脓肿部位。
  - 引流充分后灌洗空腔。
    - 推荐灌洗但可能应用没那么广泛。
- 填塞是有争议的，且小的研究在小脓肿(<5 cm)的有效性上提出质疑。
  - 以下推荐填塞：
    - 大于 5 cm。
    - 存在其他疾病。
  - HIV。
  - 糖尿病。
  - 恶性疾病。
  - 长期使用激素。
  - 免疫抑制。
  - 脓肿部位：面部、颈部、头皮、手足、肛周、直肠周围、生殖器。
- 抗生素：
  - 最近的研究说明短期和中期治疗对小脓肿的患者有治疗价值。
  - 决定使用抗生素治疗时要考虑治疗的费用和潜在副作用。
  - 建议告知患者治疗决定。
- 一般使用抗生素的指征包括：
  - 脓毒症、系统性疾病。
  - 面部脓肿引流入颈静脉窦。
  - 同时存在蜂窝织炎。
  - 哺乳动物叮咬。
  - 宿主免疫受抑制。
- 肛周脓肿需要在手术室治疗。
- 手感染需要手术干预。
  - 深部脓肿。
  - 咬伤脓肿。
  - 联合腱鞘炎、深筋膜感染。
- 从小的研究结果来看，环状引流技术仍是一个选择。
  - 更少的侵入。
  - 简化伤口护理。
  - 流程。
    - 局麻。
    - 沿脓肿外缘切开。
    - 使用止血钳来突破并手动排脓。
    - 使用止血钳定位脓肿边界以指导二次切开。
    - 用止血钳抓住硅质环并套入轻柔固定。
    - 患者应每日移开环以促进引流。
    - 通常不需要频繁去急诊换药。
  - 7～10 日去环是无痛的。

儿科患者的考虑

切开和引流是痛苦的过程常需要震惊和麻醉。

药物治疗

注意

- 了解当地敏感病原体。
- 口服抗生素(中毒蜂窝织炎)。
  - 阿莫西林-克拉维酸盐：
    - 用于：哺乳动物叮咬、MSSA、链球菌。
    - 成人剂量：500～875 mg[儿童：40～80 mg/(kg · d),静脉滴注,q12 h],口服,q12 h。
  - 甲氧苄啶-磺胺甲噁唑：
    - 用于：MRSA。
    - 成人剂量：160/800 mg[儿童：4～5 mg/(kg · d)],口服,q12 h。
  - 氯林可霉素：
    - 用于：MRSA。
    - 成人剂量：300～450 mg(儿童：4～8 mg/kg),口服,q6 h。
  - 脱氧土霉素：
    - 用于：MRSA。
    - 成人剂量：100 mg(儿童：大于 8 岁，1.1 mg/kg),口服,q12 h。
  - 头孢氨苄：
    - 用于：MSSA、链锁状球菌。
    - 成人剂量：250 mg,口服,q6 h;或 500 mg,口服,q12 h[儿童：25～50 mg/(kg · d),静脉滴注,q12 h]。
  - 红霉素：
    - 用于：MSSA、链锁状球菌。
    - 成人剂量:250～500 mg(儿童：10 mg/kg),口服,q6～8 h。
- 静脉抗生素(系统性疾病或广泛蜂窝织炎)。
  - 安比西林-舒巴坦：
    - 用法：人或哺乳动物咬伤及广泛蜂窝织炎。
    - 成人用量：1.5～3 g(儿童<40 kg, 75 mg/kg; ≥40 kg,成人用量),静脉滴注,q6 h(最大 12 g/d)。
  - 万古霉素：
    - 用于：MRSA。
    - 成人用量：15 mg/kg，静脉滴注，q12 h[儿童：10～15 mg/(kg · d),静脉滴注,q6～8 h](最大 2 000 mg/d)。
  - 达托霉素：
    - 用于：MRSA。
    - 成人用量：4 mg/kg,静脉滴注,q24 h。
  - 利奈唑胺：
    - 用于：MRSA。
    - 成人用量：600 mg/kg,静脉滴注或口服，q12 h[儿童：30 mg/(kg · d), div, q8 h]。
  - 氯林可霉素：
    - 用于：MRSA。
    - 成人用量：600 mg/kg(儿童：10～15 mg/kg), div, q8 h。

随访

进一步处理

由脓肿类型和感染严重程度决定。

入院指征

- 脓毒症、系统性疾病。
- 免疫损伤宿主伴中或大范围蜂窝织炎。
- 累及肛周。
- 任何需要在手术室切开和清创的患者。

出院指征

大多数非复杂性脓肿患者可在切开引流后闭合切口出院后随访。

- 24～48 h 重复检查填塞物的移除和损伤处。
- 移除填充物后温暖浸泡 2～3 日。

要点和误区

在复发的脓肿要考虑 CA - MRSA。

- 脓肿切开和引流时有必要止痛。
- 警惕腱鞘炎和深部筋膜感染。

皮肤癣 Tinea infections, cutaneous

Aaron J. Monseau 范浩浩 李文放 译

基础知识

描述

- 表面真菌感染的头发、皮肤或指甲：
  - 通常局限于角质层。
  - 世界范围内最常见的疾病。
- 需要角质增长，所以不涉及黏膜。

病因

- 皮肤癣菌：
  - 小孢子菌。
  - 毛癣菌。
  - 表皮癣菌。
  - 马拉色菌属，一种酵母菌，是该病的病原体(不是真正的癣)。
- 皮肤创伤或浸软可能会导致真菌感染进入皮肤。
- 传染可能是人对人、动物对人或土壤对人。

儿科注意事项

- 真菌可以从玩具和刷子传播。
- 甲癣在儿童中很罕见，并与以下相关：
  - 唐氏综合征。
  - 免疫抑制。
  - 足癣或头痛。

诊断

症状和体征

- 头癣：
  - 主要是儿童受到影响。
  - 大多数传染性皮肤癣菌病。
  - 脱发、头皮屑样结垢。
  - 脓癣：
    - 散发脓液的炎症性肿块，且引起颈部淋巴结肿大。
  - 从头皮感染的头发上脱落的"黑点"。
- 体股癣("癣")：
  - 手臂、腿和躯干。
  - 边缘清晰，环状病变伴有边缘凸起，中央清楚。
  - 毛囊受累可能会产生硬结丘疹和脓疱。
  - 病变可能是单处的、多重的或同心的。
  - 宠物往往是一种载体。
- 股癣：
  - 会阴、大腿和臀部的红斑、鳞屑、边缘斑块。
  - 与热量、潮湿和紧身内衣有关。
  - 与念珠菌病疱不同，阴囊和阴茎不受侵犯。
- 足癣("运动员足")。
  - 缩小，浸软，趾间裂开。
  - 危险因素：
    - 年龄增加。
    - 免疫受损状态。
    - 炎热潮湿的气候。
    - 不经常更换袜子。
  - 成人比儿童更常见。
  - 美国最常见的癣感染。
  - "癣菌疹"反应：
    - 远离感染的水疱疹破裂。
    - 涉及双手，汗疱疹。
- 灰指甲：
  - 1种类型的甲癣。
  - 黄色或棕色变色，增厚和指甲下的碎片。
  - 甲剥离：指甲从甲床上松开。
  - 可能涉及足底的足底表面。
- 花斑癣(不是真癣)：
  - 在温暖的月份最常见。
  - 圆形或椭圆形浅棕色，黄色或可能会合并的低色素斑。
  - 上身、胳膊和颈部。
  - 面部表现在儿童中很常见。

病史

- 从接触发病到可见皮肤变化的时间大约2周。
- 主要症状是瘙痒：
  - 脱发伴头癣。
- 参与接触性运动或与类似患者接触。

体格检查

- 头癣：脱发、头皮表面头发剥离。
- 体癣：典型的皮肤环状鳞状斑块，边缘凸起，可能有脓疱和囊泡。
- 股癣：腹股沟、耻骨区域和髋部有中央清楚，边缘凸起红斑病变。
- 足癣：结痂、浸软和趾裂开，往往只有1只脚受影响。
- 癣油灰指甲：指甲分离，断裂，甲床变厚，变色。

基本检查

- 通过临床检查进行诊断。
- 如果诊断有疑问，在开始口服抗真菌剂之前镜检，因为抗真菌药可能有副作用。

诊断检查与说明

实验室检查

真菌培养生长缓慢，不能常规进行。

影像学检查

一般没有必要。

诊断步骤/外科

- 普通染色不敏感：
  - 毛癣菌、癣感染最常见的原因，不发出荧光。
  - 小孢子菌发出绿色荧光。
  - 马拉色菌(花斑癣)发出黄色至黄绿色荧光。
  - 红癣(非棒状杆菌感染)会发出珊瑚红色荧光。
- 显微镜：
  - 用70%乙醇清洁感染区。
  - 用10号或15号手术刀片刮除活动的病变边缘。
  - 将碎屑放在载玻片上，加入一滴10%～20%氢氧化钾溶液，并盖上盖玻片。
  - 隔膜菌丝的存在证实皮肤癣菌感染。
  - 发芽酵母和短菌丝证实了马拉色菌属。

儿科注意事项

- 获得培养或培养真菌成分的方法或显微镜检查：
  - 用刷子刷头发。
  - 湿棉签滚动蘸取。
  - 用透明胶带收集皮肤细胞。

鉴别诊断

- 头癣：脓疱疹、虱病、斑秃、脂溢性皮炎、特应性皮炎和银屑病。
- 体股癣：脓疱病、单纯疱疹、莱姆疾病、寻常疣、牛皮癣、钱币湿疹、环状肉芽肿、先驱补丁玫瑰糠疹、多形红斑、荨麻疹、脂溢性皮炎和继发性梅毒。
- 股癣：脓疱病、脂溢性皮炎、牛皮癣、念珠菌感染、刺激性和过敏性接触性皮炎和红癣。
- 足癣：疥疮、红癣、念珠菌、过敏和接触性皮炎，以及牛皮癣。
- 甲癣：牛皮癣、皮炎、地衣扁平癣和先天性指甲营养不良。
- 花斑癣：白癜风、继发性梅毒。

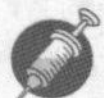

治疗

院前

保持通用的预防措施。

初步稳定/治疗

只限于免疫力低下或脓毒症患者。

急诊治疗/程序

- 改善通常在 1～2 周发生治疗，头癣和甲癣需要 3～6 个月。
- 外用抗真菌剂不能穿透头发/指甲：
  - 与全身用药一起用于头癣或甲癣。
- 头癣：
  - 特比萘芬现在由大多数人被认为是首选药物：
    - 丸剂可能会在食物中粉碎。
  - 较新的口服抗真菌剂，包括特比萘芬、伊曲康唑和氟康唑是优选的：
    - 保留在组织中更长的时间。
    - 允许缩短治疗过程，而不降低功效。
    - 改进依从性。
  - 硫化硒或酮康唑洗发水降低传播。
  - 加入泼尼松可能会对癣脓肿效果更好(儿童：1 mg/kg，口服，每日 1 次 2 周)。

注意

特比萘芬对针对引起头癣的小孢子菌种可能不如灰黄霉素有效；然而，毛癣菌属是主要的儿童致病微生物：

- 体股癣、足癣和足癣：
  - 局部特比萘芬或咪唑(酮康唑、咪康唑和克霉唑)为一线药物：
    - 外用特比萘芬已被证明和咪唑类一样有效，且疗程更短。
  - 对于耐局部治疗或免疫力低下的病例可能需要口服治疗。
  - 保持该区域干燥(滑石粉)并经常换袜子和内衣。
- 甲癣：
  - 需要口服治疗，较其他癣感染疗程较长。
  - 在 meta 分析中，特比萘芬的治愈率略高于咪唑类(酮康唑、咪康唑和克霉唑)或灰黄霉素。
  - 环罗匹斯 8%指甲油可用于治疗但治愈率低：
    - 可以加强口腔治疗。
- 花斑癣：
  - 外用药是一线疗法：
    - 硫化硒 2.5%洗发剂和局部酮康唑一样有效。
  - 口服酮康唑、伊曲康唑或氟康唑治愈率高达 97%，但不像局部用药那么安全。

药物治疗

- 环罗匹斯 8%指甲油：每日涂于指甲，最长 48 周；每 7 日用乙醇去除(儿童：相同)。
- 克霉唑：在受影响区域每日 2 次涂抹 1%乳膏 4～6 周(儿童：相同)。
- 氟康唑：甲癣 150～300 mg/周，脉冲疗法 3～6 个月用于指甲，6～12 个月用于趾甲；股癣、股骨和足部：150 mg/周，口服 4～6 周；花斑癣 400 mg，口服，单剂量(小儿头癣：每日 6 mg/kg，3～6 周)。
- 灰黄霉素：头癣、体癣、股癣，500 mg，口服，每日 1 次，4～6 周(儿童：10～20 mg/kg) 500 mg 口服每日 1 次直到头发再生，通常 6～8 周。
- 伊曲康唑：头癣，成人和小儿：3～5 mg/kg 口服每日 1 次 2～4 周；甲癣，200 mg 口服每日 1 次，3 个月；花斑癣，400 mg 口服每日 1 次 3～7 天；禁用于充血性心力衰竭。
- 酮康唑：2%局部用乳膏每日 1 次，4～6 周；头癣、体癣、小腿、足部，200 mg 口服每日 1 次，4 周(儿童：3.3～6.6 mg/kg，口服，每日 1 次，4 周)；花斑癣，400 mg 口服×1 或 200 mg 每日 1 次，7 日(禁忌与特非那丁和阿司咪唑同用)；苏打水增加吸收 65%。
- 咪康唑：将乳剂涂抹在患病区域 4～6 周(儿童：相同)。
- 硫化硒：2.5%香波到受影响的区域持续 10 周，持续 1～2 周(儿童：相同)。
- 特比萘芬：1%外用乳剂，每日 2 次，4～6 周足癣，每日 1 次，用于股癣和股癣；甲癣：250 mg，口服，每日 1 次，6 周用于指甲，12 周用于趾甲(儿童：<20 mg，67.5 mg/d；20～40 kg，125 mg/d；>40 mg，250 mg/d，与成人相同)；足癣，每周 250 mg 口服，2 周；头癣，250 mg/d，持续 4 周(按重量计剂量，甲癣用药 4 周)。
- 托萘脂：将 1%乳剂、粉末、溶液涂抹在牙齿上受影响的区域每日 2 次为 4～6 周(儿童：同)。

注意

口服抗真菌剂可能很少引起肝毒性，在开始治疗前考虑检查肝脏转氨酶。

儿科注意事项

如果可能的话，局部制剂是优选的。

妊娠注意事项

- 几乎没有人类妊娠期间使用抗真菌药物的相关研究。
- 一些咪唑已在动物中显示出不利影响：C 类(氟康唑、伊曲康唑、酮康唑)。
- 克霉唑、咪康唑和特比萘芬是 B 类药物。
- 重视风险：有利于作为选择，抗真菌治疗一般不推荐。

一线用药

- 头癣：特比萘芬。
- 股癣、股癣、足癣：局部用特比萘芬或咪唑类(酮康唑、咪康唑和克霉唑)。
- 花斑癣：硫化硒洗发水和局部酮康唑。

随访

进一步处理

入院指征

- 免疫功能低下宿主的侵袭性疾病。
- 继发细菌感染的癣脓肿。

出院指征

- 大多数患者可以作为门诊患者进行管理。
- 孩子可以在适当的治疗已经开始后回到学校。

转诊问题

口服抗真菌剂的患者应注意监视疗效和伴发的肝炎症状。

随访建议

- 监测细菌超感染、蜂窝织炎、广泛侵袭性感染：
  - 尤其是免疫功能低下(糖尿病患者、HIV 感染患者)皮疹和瘙痒症。
- 头癣是最常见的儿童皮肤病感染。
- 瘙痒是大多数癣的发作表现，与头癣相关的有脱发。
- 蜂窝织炎常常伴有足癣。
- 足癣、股癣复发常见。
  - 患者应清洗或更换污染的袜子、毛巾、鞋袜。

皮肌炎和多肌炎 Dermatomyositis/Polymyositis

Sean-Xavier Neath 谭美春 译

P

基础知识

描述

• 皮肌炎(DM)和多肌炎(PM)是系统性炎症性肌肉疾病,它们是引起骨骼肌无力的最大的获得性和潜在性的原因。

• 患者经历明显进展的肌无力超过几周至几个月。

• 呼吸肌无力可导致呼吸衰竭。

• 由于咳嗽功能减弱、咽肌功能障碍和食管运动功能障碍可发生吸入性肺炎。

• 心脏表现包括心肌炎、传导缺陷、心肌病和充血性心力衰竭(CHF)。

• 右美沙芬患者出现手、腕、膝和肩关节病变,并伴有明显相关的皮肤症状。

• 眼肌不受累,但是在进展病例中可见到面部肌肉无力。

病因

• 尽管自身免疫机制被认为是主要原因,但确切的原因未知。

• 发病率约为 1/10 万,女性多见。

• 多肌炎通常与某些病毒、细菌和寄生虫感染有关。

• 皮肌炎和多肌炎约 20%的时间并发胶原血管疾病。

• 在皮肌炎中,累及体液免疫机制,导致微血管病变和肌肉缺血。

• 在多肌炎中,提出一个 T 细胞介导的细胞毒机制。

– CD8 受体 T 细胞连同巨噬细胞破坏身体健康,异常表达的未坏死肌肉纤维主要为组织相容性复合体(MHC)分子。

• 补体沉淀物是最早和最特殊的病变,随后发炎、局部缺血、微梗死、坏死和破坏肌纤维。

儿科注意事项

• 尽管皮肌炎在儿童和成人中都能看到,但多肌炎在儿童中是很少见的。

• 与成人多肌炎相似,青少年多肌炎(JDM)主要累及皮肤和骨骼肌。

• 青少年型可能包括血管炎、异位性钙化(钙质沉着)和脂肪代谢障碍。

• 青少年型可能和柯萨奇病毒有关。

诊断

症状和体征

病史

• 多肌炎区别于皮肌炎的是无皮疹。

• 一种变体称为无肌病性皮肌炎(ADM)表现为皮疹,无明显的肌病。

• 多肌炎的患者表现为肌肉疼痛和近端肌无力。

• 皮肌炎表现为皮疹、肌肉疼痛和无力。

• 全身症状包括体重减轻、发热、厌食、晨僵、肌痛和关节痛。

• 患者经常提出日常活动中感到疲劳:

– 梳头、爬楼梯、手举过头、自椅子上起身。

– 也可能提出吞咽困难、呼吸困难和咳嗽。

• 早期表现为进行性加重的近端肢体和腰肌的无力;疾病晚期出现远端肌无力。

体格检查

• 常规:

– 疲劳。

– 发热。

– 体重减轻。

• 吞咽困难。

• 进行性肌无力:

– 主要累及近端肌。

– 对称性的。

• 皮肌炎的皮肤表现:

– 皮疹伴随或先于肌无力出现。

– 在上眼睑上的紫红斑(淡紫色变色)与水肿相关。

– 戈特勒征:在关节,尤其是指关节、膝盖和肘部的伸肌表面的紫罗兰色或红斑状丘疹。

– 披肩征:V 形红斑状皮疹出现在背部和肩部。

– 甲周毛细血管扩张:甲床毛细血管变化包括不规则增厚和扭曲的角质层。

– "机械师手":变黑的水平线穿过手掌外侧的手指。

基本检查

• 评估气道和呼吸状况,查找误吸或损伤的征象。

• 评估心脏受累或并发症的征象。

诊断检查与说明

实验室检查

• 血清肌酶:

– 肌酸磷酸激酶(CPK)增高,其他肌酶如醛缩酶、肌红蛋白,也能增高。

– 尿肌红蛋白。

– 自身免疫抗体。

– 80%的患者抗核抗体阳性。

– 30%~40%的患者肌炎特异性自身抗体阳性。

• 自 2017 年以来,诊断标准的共识指南发生了变化:

– EULAR/ACR 标准根据评分和相应的患病概率将患者分为"明确""可能"和"可能"。

– 有两种不同的评分系统,取决于是否进行了肌肉活检。

– 亚群的分类树使用皮肤病学特征和肌肉检查结果对亚群进行进一步分类。

• 使用自身抗体(抗 Jo-1、抗 SRP、抗 Mi-2)或免疫组织学特征可能有助于特异性疾病亚群的更特异性诊断。

影像学检查

• 胸片检查可以显示间质性肺病、吸入性肺炎、充血性心力衰竭或心肌病。

• 肌电图测定显示肌病电位,可以支持诊断,但对于皮肌炎和多肌炎无特异性。

• MRI 在确定炎症最适合活检区域中的作用在增加。

诊断步骤/外科

• 肌肉活组织检查是确诊性试验:

– 在多肌炎、炎症性浸润主要侵及肌内膜,虽然它们也可能在血管周围。

– 在皮肌炎、炎症性浸润主要侵及血管周围组织,包括高百分比的 B 细胞。

• 患者肾活检可以显示局灶性增生性肾小球肾炎。

• 肺功能测定对进展性间质性肺病的诊断是有帮助的。

鉴别诊断

• 胶原血管疾病。

• 肌肉萎缩症。

• 脊髓性肌萎缩。

• 重症肌无力。

P

• 肌萎缩性侧索硬化症。
• 脊髓灰质炎。
• 吉兰-巴雷综合征。
• 甲状腺功能减退症。
• 甲状腺功能亢进症。
• 库欣综合征。
• 药物引起的：
- 秋水仙碱。
- 青霉胺。
- 吐根。
- 乙醇。
- 氯喹。
- 皮质类固醇。
- 他汀类药物。
• 感染：
- 弓形体病。
- 毛线虫病。
- 柯萨奇病毒。
- 艾滋病、流行性感冒。
- EB 病毒。
• 电解质紊乱：
- 低钾血症。
- 高钙血症。
- 低镁血症。
• 血管炎。
• 副癌神经肌病。
• 高嗜酸性粒细胞肌痛综合征。

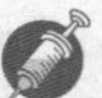

治疗

院前

• ABC 管理。
• 抬高床头转运。

初步稳定/治疗

• 根据需要插管和机械通气。
• 鼻胃管(NG)抽吸预防误吸。
• 气胸在儿童皮肌炎的患者中罕见发病。

急诊治疗/程序

• 抬高床头预防误吸。
• 开始大剂量皮质类固醇治疗抑制炎症和改善肌无力。
• 避免用曲安奈德和地塞米松，因为它们可能引起药物关联性肌病。
• 泼尼松的功效客观增加了肌肉强度，不改变 CK 水平。
• 一些临床医师在发病时开始给糖皮质激素，不应用免疫抑制剂，另一些医师把这些药剂保留给对皮质类固醇无效的患者。
• 多肌炎患者比皮肌炎患者对糖皮质激素产生反应的可能性低。
• 由于不良反应，咪唑硫嘌呤和甲氨蝶呤应用有一定局限性。
• 环孢素和单克隆抗体治疗方法已经被应用，但成效甚微。
• 严重(危及生命的)病情可以用静脉注射免疫球蛋白(IVIG)治疗。
• 不要单独依据 CPK 水平决定治疗策略。

药物治疗

一线用药

• 泼尼松：60 mg/d，口服[儿童：1～2 mg/(kg·d)，口服]，在危重症考虑甲泼尼龙冲击 1 000 mg/d，连续 3 日：
- 治疗的时长和个体化逐步减量依据临床反应和肌酸激酶的正常化决定。

二线用药

• 甲氨蝶呤：每周 15～25 mg，口服[儿童：每周 15 mg/m^2，口服，不超过 25 mg]。
• 咪唑硫嘌呤：开始 50 mg/d，然后 2 周增加 50 mg，直到 1.5 mg/(kg·d)的一个剂量。
- 3 个月后，如果能耐受可以增加剂量至 2.5 mg/(kg·d)。
• 有些风湿病学家也应用静脉注射免疫球蛋白(IVIG)、血浆置换和环孢素。

随访

进一步处理

入院指征

• 呼吸衰竭。
• 吸入性肺炎。
• 深度肌无力。
• 咳嗽机制减弱。
• 咽功能障碍。
• 充血性心力衰竭。

出院指征

• 患者情况良好，没有呼吸功能障碍和没有吸入风险。
• 作为门诊患者，患者能口服糖皮质激素和免疫抑制剂。

转诊问题

当诊断不明确需要获得帮助来决定诊断和进一步治疗时，应该咨询风湿病学家。

随访建议

• 与普通人群相比较，在皮肌炎患者中恶性疾病的发病率似乎有增加(但不在多肌炎患者中)。
• 一份完整的年度体检包括骨盆检查、乳房检查、直肠检查、尿液分析、全血细胞计数，血液化学测试和胸部 X 线检查经常被推荐给有皮肌炎病史的患者进行肿瘤监测。

要点和误区

• 炎性肌病的诊断主要基于选择的实验室检查和肌肉活检的临床支持。
• 大多数患者治疗后改善，很多人功能完全恢复，这通常由维持疗法保持。
• 多达 30% 的患者可能遗留一些残余肌无力。
• 最重要的是，切记尽管成功治愈，但随时可能复发。

皮疹 Rash

Richard E. Wolfe · Peggy A. Wu 袁晓伟 童朝阳 译

基础知识

描述

• 使用适当的术语对未知皮疹进行分类：
- 基本形态。
  ◦ 直径。
  ◦ 平坦或凸出。
  ◦ 固态或含液体。
- 颜色。
  ◦ 色素过度型。
  ◦ 色素减退型。
  ◦ 红斑。
- 形状。
  ◦ 盘状。
  ◦ 椭圆形。

◦ 环形。
◦ 弯曲型。
◦ 靶型。
- 分布。
◦ 外周型或者中央型。
◦ 对称性。
◦ 不连续性(相互分离)。
◦ 线性。
◦ 皮区。
◦ 波状。
◦ 网状。
◦ 串状。
◦ 图片分布型。
- 相关症状。
◦ 瘙痒。
◦ 疼痛。
◦ 柔软性。
◦ 烧灼感。
◦ 系统症状。
- 皮疹的演变。
◦ 初发及持续时间。
◦ 严重性及加剧情况。
• 皮疹的形态:
- 囊泡性病变:充满液体的皮肤肿胀或由于表皮/真皮完整性的破坏而导致的剥脱。
- 紫癜和瘀点:由正常血管的完整性或止血机制病理性改变导致,触诊不褪色。
- 红斑:
◦ 红皮病(皮肤表面覆盖>90%)。
◦ 浅血管的血管扩张导致红黄斑病变。
◦ 触诊褐色。
- 固定形状红斑:由其特定的环形或弧形形状分类。
- 鳞屑样丘疹:
◦ 皮肤丘疹和鳞状脱屑。
◦ 病变也可能是红色和黄斑。
◦ 分为牛皮癣样、糠秕状、苔藓样变、环形、湿疹。
- 肉芽肿病变:
◦ 有浸润性丘疹和斑块,无鳞片。
◦ 苹果酱状(按压载玻片)。
- 结节:继发于慢性炎症反应、囊肿或渗出性病变。
• 潜在紧急情况的警告信号:
- 红皮病。
- 起疱/脱皮。
- 紫癜。
- 伴有全身症状的皮肤疼痛。

病因/鉴别诊断

• 水疱性损伤:
- 中毒性表皮坏死松解症(黏膜及>30%体表面积)。
- 史-约综合征(黏膜和<10%体表面积)。
- 寻常天疱疮。
- 大疱性类天疱疮。
- 播散性单纯疱疹。
- 带状疱疹。
- 水痘。
- 天花。
- 牛痘。
- 变应性接触性皮炎。
• 紫癜和瘀点:
- 脑膜炎球菌血症。
- 淋球菌血症。
- 紫癜、暴发性/弥散性血管内凝血(DIC)。
- 落基山斑疹热(RMSF):明显的前驱症状、发热、头痛、肌痛、皮疹、外周转移至手掌/足底。
- 坏死性脓疮:严重假单胞菌感染及免疫缺陷患者。
• 巴贝虫病:
- 类似于 RMSF、少量皮疹,常合并莱姆病感染。
- 血管炎。
- 多种系统性疾病(见紫癜)。
• 红皮病:
- 中毒性休克综合征。
- 药物引起的。
- 牛皮癣。
- 脂溢性皮炎。
- 蕈样真菌病。
- 皮肤淋巴瘤。
• 红斑性皮疹:
- 局限性:蜂窝织炎、早期坏死性筋膜炎伴皮肤疼痛,风团。
- 弥漫性:葡萄球菌烫伤皮肤综合征、中毒性休克综合征、药物诱导,包括嗜酸性粒细胞和全身症状的药物反应(DRESS)、病毒疹、荨麻疹:由药物、食物、感染、压力、热或冷引起的过敏反应。
• 花纹状红斑:
- 慢性移行性红斑(蜱虫咬伤周围出现的较大红色环形红斑)、莱姆病。
- 多形性红斑:支原体肺炎、单纯疱疹、药物反应导致史-约综合征。
• 鳞屑性丘疹:
- 银屑病:牛皮癣、脂溢性皮炎、药物引起的。
- 糠疹:玫瑰糠疹、二期梅毒、花斑糠疹。
- 苔藓样:扁平苔藓、药物引起。
- 环状:癣、花纹状红斑(见下文)。
- 湿疹:特应性皮炎、过敏性接触性皮炎、刺激性皮炎。
• 结节性:
- 肉芽肿疾病:肉瘤、环形肉芽肿、感染性、麻风病、肺结核、真菌感染。
- 脂膜炎:结节性红斑。
- 皮肤淋巴瘤。
- 囊肿。
- 肿瘤和转移性疾病。

诊断

症状和体征

病史

• 年龄。
• 免疫状态(HIV、化疗、糖尿病、类固醇)。
• 病程及机体变化。
• 既往发作、既往史、反应。
• 相关症状:
- 瘙痒。
- 发热。
- 腹部疼痛肌痛、关节痛。
• 前驱症状:
- 发热。
- 头痛。
- 咳嗽。
- 吞咽痛。
- 鼻漏。
• 环境暴露:
- 蜱虫咬。
- 不寻常的植物。
- 饮食史。
- 旅行史。
- 物理创伤史(寒、热、晒)。
• 近期药物接触病。
• 家族史。

体格检查

• 相关体征及症状。
- 感染性发热、药物反应、系统性炎症反应。
- 与临床表现不一致的皮肤疼痛提示可能即将发生皮肤坏死。
- 淋巴结病可能是 DRESS 的一个表现。
- 全身和接触过敏反应引起的瘙痒。
• 评估系统性体征的严重性:
- 生命体征异常、呼吸窘迫、血流动力学不稳定。
• 主要病变外观:
- 水疱:小,隆起,充满澄清液体(<5 mm)。
- 大疱:大,隆起,充满澄清液体(>5 mm)。

P

- 斑疹：无隆起，局限性颜色改变。

- 丘疹：隆起，皮损直径<5 mm，而不充满液体。

- 脓疱：与水疱及大疱相似，但含有脓性积液。

- 结节：固体，隆起>5 mm，病变位于在深层皮肤和组织。

- 皮疹的分布：描述为中心、边缘，支流、分散，黏膜或非黏膜，手掌、足底。

• 继发性改变：

- 鳞屑、苔藓样变、剥落、裂隙（由于操作、抓伤导致或表皮细胞增殖/脱落所致的）。

- 侵蚀、溃疡（由于血管供应、组织完整性的丧失而造成的不同程度的组织损失造成的）。

基本检查

• 识别系统性疾病。

• 局部感染源的迹象/症状。

• 对病变形态和分布进行分类。

诊断检查与说明

• 如果出现发热、全身症状或可能的感染，应进行血液检查：

- CBC 及分型、电解质、BUN/肌酐。

- 血液培养、病毒培养。

- 革兰染色及脓性病灶培养。

- 疑似病灶的聚合酶链反应（PCR）或直接荧光抗体（DFA）。

• 疑似梅毒。

- 快速血浆反应素试验（RPR）或荧光密螺旋体抗体试验（FTA）。

• 疑似自身免疫性疾病：

- CBC。

- ESR、CRP。

- ANA，抗中性粒细胞质抗体（风湿免疫专家评估协商）。

• 瘀斑/紫癜：

- CBC 及血小板。

- 部分凝血活酶时间、凝血酶原时间、INR；DIC 筛选：纤维蛋白原、纤维蛋白裂解产物、钩珠蛋白、LDH。

- 尿常规：对怀疑侵犯肾脏血管炎。

诊断步骤/外科

• 在发热和重症患者中，可疑的脓毒症需要被切开、排干并送去培养。

• 尼氏征试验：大疱性病变在侧压作用下扩张，导致表皮与基底层分离，表明表皮内缺乏内聚力。

• 刮伤：排除局部真菌感染和寄生虫。

- 病灶边缘氢氧化钾制剂显示菌丝。

- 用普通矿物油排除手部瘙痒病损处线性疥疮。

• 在皮肤科会诊下进行活检以鉴别过敏、自身免疫、感染过程。

鉴别诊断

见病因。

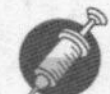

治疗

院前

综合性预防，使用口罩，如果怀疑感染性病因。

初步稳定/治疗

对潜在致命的病情进行积极的、有依据的管理：

• 瘀斑的病变。

• 弥漫性红斑或囊泡性病变。

• 有全身症状的紫癜。

• 有全身症状的红皮病。

急诊治疗/程序

• 根据潜在原因进行治疗。

• 急性经验性抗生素：针对脑膜炎球菌血症和 RMSF 的不稳定的发热和紫癜患者。

• 严重热烧伤后播散性大疱性或脱落性疾病的治疗。

• 瘙痒的对症治疗（苯海拉明或羟嗪）。

• 类固醇疗法用于明确的过敏反应、已知类固醇反应性疾病的复发，或咨询皮肤科医师。

• 过敏反应：H_1 受体阻滞剂、H_2 受体阻滞剂、类固醇、肾上腺素（如呼吸功能损害）。

药物治疗

• 泼尼松：1 mg/kg（最大剂量 60 mg/d）。

• 羟嗪：25～100 mg，口服，q6 h。

• 苯海拉明：25～50 mg，口服、肌内注射或静脉注射，q6 h。

• 泼尼松龙：125 mg，静脉注射，q24 h。

• 局部类固醇：根据部位和严重程度分为 3～5 类。

随访

进一步处理

入院指征

• 大疱性、脱落性疾病患者。

• 相关的系统性症状。

出院指征

• 病灶有限。

• 病毒疹病，表皮内缺乏内聚力。

• 稳定，慢性表现。

转诊问题

出院后随访初级保健医师、皮肤科医师。

随访建议

• 让患者放心，在急诊中不能诊断的皮疹通常是由于轻微的病毒感染或过敏反应引起的。

• 要强调随访他们的初级保健医师或皮肤科医师，以获得最佳结果的重要性。

• 患者应尽快看门诊医师，或在病情恶化时返回急救室：

- 红疹扩散。

- 皮疹引起的疼痛增加。

- 关节疼痛。

- 皮疹伴皮屑播散。

- 发热。

- 严重头痛。

- 神志不清。

- 危及生命的过敏反应迹象：感到头晕或头晕、呼吸或吞咽困难、舌肿。

要点和误区

• 有全身症状的皮疹的快速发展可以提示皮肤病的急症。

• 用经验性抗生素迅速治疗紫癜和发热患者，以覆盖脑膜炎球菌血症和 RMSF。

• 用经验性抗生素迅速治疗红皮病、发热和低血压患者，以涵盖中毒性休克综合征。

• 手掌和足底上的鳞状丘疹需要排除继发性梅毒。

疲乏 Fatigue

Richard E. Wolfe 万健 译

基础知识

描述

• 一种强烈的持续存在的主观疲劳感觉，对体力和脑力工作的能力下降，且休息后不能缓解。
• 疲乏可有或没有体格检查异常。
• 无论有无全身疾病的人群均可主诉疲乏，这给医师带来了一定的诊治难度。
• 高水平的疲劳与一般人群的死亡率有关。

病因

• 疲乏的确切机制目前未知。
• 血液系统：
- 贫血。
- 白血病。
• 内分泌系统：
- 甲状腺功能异常。
- 肾上腺功能减退。
- 妊娠。
• 恶性肿瘤：
- 副癌综合征。
• 精神病学的：
- 慢性疼痛。
- 情感障碍。
- 抑郁。
- 进食障碍。
- 药物依赖。
- 戒断症状。
• 睡眠障碍：
- 失眠。
- 睡眠呼吸暂停。
• 心肺功能障碍。
• 急性和慢性感染。
• 风湿病和自身免疫功能异常。
• 营养缺乏，包括电解质紊乱。
• 运动不足和适应力下降。
• 药物。
• 慢性疲乏综合征：
- 疾病预防控制中心定义为复杂的综合征。
- 严重的慢性疲乏持续>6个月。
- 不能用药物或精神性原因诊断。
- 下列8种症状持续≥4个月：
◦ 头痛。
◦ 关节痛。
◦ 睡眠紊乱。
◦ 淋巴结病。
◦ 运动耐力下降。
◦ 肌痛。
◦ 记忆力及注意力损害。
◦ 咽喉痛。

诊断

症状和体征

• 疲乏是一种干扰正常生活的疲劳主观感觉，且症状不因睡眠而缓解。
• 疲乏没有特异性的表现，但体格检查通常能提示可能的病因。

病史

• 疲乏的起病时间、形式及持续时间。
• 相关的症状：发热、夜间盗汗、无力、呼吸困难、体重减轻或增加、睡眠节律变化。
• 既往药物史及手术史。
• 精神疾病史：情感和精神应激、抑郁。
• 个人史：乙醇、药物使用、主要的生活事件。
• 药物。
• 全面的系统回顾。

体格检查

• 全面的体格检查应能根据患者的症状发现可能的病因。疲乏没有特异性的体征。
• 提示可能病因的体格检查结果应包括：
- 生命体征。
- 头、眼、耳、鼻和喉：
◦ 瞳孔变化提示中毒。
◦ 巩膜黄染提示肝脏疾病。
◦ 结膜苍白提示贫血。
◦ 甲状腺肿大、疼痛或结节提示功能异常。
- 心脏：心脏杂音或第三心音提示左心室功能障碍。
- 肺：肺动脉直径异常或呼吸音异常可提示慢性或急性肺疾病。
- 腹部：注意腹肌紧张或包块。
- 皮肤：皮疹可提示感染或自身免疫疾病，皮肤弹性下降提示脱水，皮肤色素沉着提示艾迪生病。
- 神经系统：肌力下降或反射消失提示神经肌肉疾病，所有新出现的局部肌力下降均应进一步检查。
- 肌肉与骨骼：出现电解质紊乱或隐匿性的血流感染应检查静脉留置针或透析管路。

基本检查

由于疲乏是一种主观感觉，因此关键性的检查有助于确认可能的病因。

诊断检查与说明

• 根据病史和体格检查做相应的实验室检查。
• 全血细胞计数：
- 用于筛查贫血或白血病。
• 血糖：
- 高血糖和低血糖都能表现为疲乏。
• 检测是否妊娠。
• 电解质、肌酐和尿素氮。
• 甲状腺刺激素：
- 用于筛查甲状腺功能减退。
• 尿液药物筛查。
• 炎症标志物如ESR和CRP可能有助于发现隐匿的炎症状态。

影像学检查

在异常体格检查或病史的基础上行影像学检查进一步评估病情。

诊断步骤/外科

在异常体格检查或病史的基础上行诊断性操作进一步评估病情。

鉴别诊断

• 感染：
- 菌血症。
- 尿路脓毒症。
- 肺炎。
- 病毒感染。
- 脓肿。
- EB病毒感染、传染性单核细胞增多症。
- 巨细胞病毒尿。
- 人类免疫缺陷病毒感染。
- 人类疱疹病毒6感染。
• 免疫系统及结缔组织病：
- 风湿病（风湿性关节炎、系统性红斑狼疮、青少年风湿性关节炎）。
- 骨关节炎。
- 纤维肌痛。
- 重症肌无力。
- Lambert-Eaton肌无力综合征。
• 肿瘤：
- 实体或血液系统肿瘤。

P

• 代谢病：
- 电解质紊乱。
- 线粒体疾病。
- 溴中毒。
• 血液系统：
- 贫血。
- 低血容量。
- 血红蛋白病。
• 内分泌：
- 甲状腺功能亢进或甲状腺功能减退。
- 肾上腺功能减退。
- 糖尿病。
- 低血糖。
• 神经系统：
- 多发性硬化症。
- 脑血管意外。
- 脊髓侧索硬化症。
• 心血管系统：
- 心肌梗死。
- 心肌病。
- 充血性心力衰竭。
• 肺：
- 肺炎。
- 慢性阻塞性肺疾病。
- 哮喘。
- 睡眠呼吸暂停。
• 消化系统：
- 食管反流。
- 消化性溃疡病。
- 肝脏疾病。
• 自主神经功能紊乱。
• 生活方式：
- 运动过度或运动不足。
- 肥胖。
• 精神疾病：
- 抑郁。
- 焦虑。
- 悲伤。
- 紧张。
• 药物相关性：
- 药物相互作用。
- 常见于高血压、心血管、精神类和麻醉药物。
• 脱水。

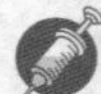

治疗

院前

生命体征评估：
• 通过相关的信息进行社会心理评估。

初始稳定/治疗

• ABC 管理。
• 缺氧时给予氧气。
• 有脱水表现时给予静脉补液。

急诊治疗/程序

• 治疗应旨在发现疲乏的可能病因。
- 识别和处理各种感染。
- 纠正代谢和血液系统异常。
- 诊断进展性的神经疾病和急性精神心理危机。
- 行内分泌和肿瘤相关检查。
- 停止违规用药或毒物。
• 大多数病例没有确定性的病因，因此需要反复评估检查和密切随访。
• 推荐合理的节食、运动方案和规律的睡眠节律。
• 建议随访门诊健康维护和适龄癌症筛查。

药物

一线用药

使用能够治疗可能病因的药物。

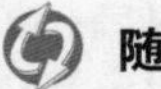

随访

进一步处理

入院指征

• 可能的疾病需要静脉用药或监测。
• 门诊处理不了。
• 生活无法自理的患者。

出院指征

• 能够生活自理者。
• 排除了严重的功能异常者。
• 能够予以全面的随访者。

转诊问题

大多数急诊诊断疲乏的患者应咨询：
• 当患者疲乏的病因已明确时，直接请合适的专科医师会诊。
• 当患者疲乏的病因不太明确时，建议给予基本的医学咨询。

要点和误区

• 疲乏是一种复杂的主观症状，需要全面了解病史和体格检查。
• 注意患者的病史和体格检查结果不一定可信。高龄、儿童、中毒和精神心智下降的患者都可能有危及生命的疾病而出现疲乏的临床表现。

脾脏损伤 Splenic Injury

Albert S. Jin　江伟伟　李文放 译

基础知识

描述

• 脾脏由网状和淋巴组织形成，是最大的淋巴器官。
• 脾脏位于胃底和膈肌之间的左上象限后侧。

病因

• 脾脏是最常见的受伤的腹内器官：
- 在近 2/3 的病例中，它是唯一受损的腹膜结构。
- 钝器更常见。
• 机动车事故（自动撞自动、自动撞行人）是主要原因（50%～75%），其次是腹部打击（15%）和高处坠落（6%～9%）。
• 损伤和运动机制是评估可能的脾脏损伤患者的重要因素。
• 脾脏的医源性损伤可由手术或胃、胰腺、肾脏或近端腹主动脉等脏器的内镜操作引发。
• 脾脏损伤按伤害类型和严重程度分级[美国创伤外科学会（AAST）标准]：
- Ⅰ级：
◦ 血肿：静止性被膜下血肿<10%表面积。
◦ 撕裂：被膜撕裂深达实质<1 cm，无腹腔出血。
- Ⅱ级：
◦ 血肿：静止性被膜下血肿占 10%～50%表面积，静止性实质内血肿直径<5 cm。

◦ 撕裂：或被膜撕裂出血，实质撕裂深 1～3 cm，但未累及小梁血管。

- Ⅲ级：

◦ 血肿：被膜下扩张性或实质内血肿，出血性被膜下血肿或被膜下血肿>50%表面积。

◦ 撕裂：实质内撕裂深达 3 cm 或累及小梁血管。

- Ⅳ级：

◦ 裂伤：撕裂累及段或脾门造成游离的无血管脾块>25%总体积。

- Ⅴ级：

◦ 裂伤：完全粉碎或脾脏撕脱。

◦ 血管：脾门撕裂全脾无血管。

儿科注意事项

• 由于肌肉组织发育不良、前后径相对较小，损伤的风险增高。

• 肋骨架非常柔软，不易断裂，但仅提供部分保护以防止脾脏损伤。

• 儿童脾囊比成人厚，脾脏实质似乎比成人含有更多的平滑肌。

• 仅约 5% 的儿童虐待案件发生严重腹部损伤，但是脾脏损伤仅次于头部受伤，是第二大常见的死亡原因。

诊断

体征和症状

既往史

• 在钝性创伤中，请注意任何撞击力的类型和方向（水平或垂直）：

- 损伤是由前腹壁和胸廓后椎骨压迫脾脏引起的（如安全带束缚）。

• 在穿透伤中，注意武器的特性（类型和口径）、与武器的距离、刀具或刺穿物体的类型和长度：

- 伤害是由动能和剪切力引起的。

体格检查

• 急性失血症状：

- 晕厥、头晕、无力、萎靡。

- 低血压或休克。

• 阳性体征：

- 腹部压痛。

- 可触及脾脏（正常位置）。

- 提到左肩疼痛（Kehr 症状）。

- 腹胀、僵硬、反跳痛、肌卫。

• 胸部、侧腹或腹部的挫伤、擦伤或穿透伤，需怀疑潜在的脾脏损伤。

• 脾脏损伤时常伴左下肋骨骨折。

儿科注意事项

与年龄有关的交流困难、恐惧引起的不合作行为或伴随头部损伤使得检查不太可靠。

基本检查

• 既往史和体格检查对脾脏损伤既无特异性也无敏感性。

• 辅助影像学检查是必需的。

诊断检查与说明

实验室检查

• 没有专门用于诊断脾脏损伤的血液学实验室研究。

• 获得基础血红蛋白、血型和交叉配血，以及生化。

影像学检查

• 腹部 X 线片：

- 特异性不高，意义不大。

- 胸片结果提示脾脏损伤：

◦ 左下肋骨骨折。

◦ 左侧膈肌的抬高。

◦ 胃泡内侧移位（正常位置）。

◦ 左胸腔积液。

• 超声：

- 床旁超声检查，作为重点评估的一部分。

- 主要作用是检测腹腔内血液，这可能提示脾脏损伤。

- 无法显示实质脏器的损伤。

- 不合作的患者、肥胖、大量肠道气体和皮下空气患者干扰检查。

• CT：

- 稳定的患者首选 CT 检查，由于其快速和可及性。

- 能提示脾脏和邻近器官（包括腹膜后）的损伤和严重程度。

- 提供患者最全面的信息，稳定患者应该行 CT 检查。

• MRI：

- 可能适用于不能进行 CT 扫描的血流动力学稳定的患者。

• 血管造影：

- 可用于部分患者的诊断和治疗。

诊断步骤/外科

• 诊断性腹膜腔灌洗（DPL）：

- 对腹腔出血诊断非常敏感，但无法确定出血点，并且无法评估腹膜后出血。

- 在大多数创伤中心被超声检查取代。

鉴别诊断

• 腹腔器官损伤，特别是肝脏。

• 腹膜后损伤。

• 胸部损伤。

治疗

院前

• 获取损伤的过程。

• 建立静脉通路。

• 开放性伤口或内脏脱出应该用无菌敷料覆盖。

初步稳定/治疗

• 气道护理（包括颈椎固定）。

• 标准的高级创伤生命支持（ATLS）复苏措施：

- 根据患者的血流动力学状态，建立适当的静脉通路，包括中心静脉和静脉切开术。

- 最初使用 2 L 晶体液（盐水或乳酸林格溶液）进行液体复苏，然后根据需要使用血液制品。

急诊治疗/程序

• 急性损伤并血流动力学不稳定的患者，怀疑为腹腔积血和脾脏损伤，立即行剖腹手术。

• 大多数急性脾脏损伤患者血流动力学稳定或经少量液体复苏后稳定。

• 补充完善体格检查，有阳性诊断后行剖腹手术。

• 在手术室中常规探查前腹部枪伤。

• 当怀疑腹膜穿刺伤时，刺伤可局部伤口探查，然后行 B 超和腹腔灌洗。

• 手术与非手术指征：

- 有腹腔内出血症状和体征的患者，影像学/诊断程序有手术指征者和保守治疗失败的患者应进行剖腹手术。

- 在血流动力学稳定的患者中，血管造影栓塞是一种选择。

- 脾脏切除术与脾脏挽救取决于脾脏损伤的程度。

- 稳定患者中 70% 以上不需行手术治疗：

◦ 血液动力学稳定。

◦ 腹部检查阴性体征。

◦ CT 上没有造影剂外渗。

◦ 没有其他探查性剖腹手术指征。

◦ 有出血风险患者（如凝血功能障碍、肝功能衰竭、抗凝血药物使用、凝血因子缺乏症）。

◦ 脾脏损害Ⅰ～Ⅲ级患者。

老年人注意事项

• 因为对创伤性损伤（随年龄增长的脾囊膜）的生理耐受力下降以及生理储备下降，

P

55 岁以上的患者行手术治疗。

• 55 岁以上患者，栓塞是相对禁忌，这些患者的失败率较高。

儿科注意事项

• 脾脏损伤的非手术治疗被认为是安全的：

- 担心脾脏切除后的感染和败血症。

随访

进一步处理

入院指征

所有脾脏损伤患者都需要住院接受剖腹手术，监测腹部体格检查，测定血细胞比容，卧床休息。

出院指征

只有无症状的患者，各项检查均提示无脾脏或其他外伤可以出院。

P

蜱咬伤 Tick Bite

Joiathan A. Edlow 范浩浩 李文放 译

基础知识

描述

即使在蜱传疾病的高流行地区，蜱传病原体感染的风险也很低。蜱咬后，病人相关表现包括：

• 蜱虫移动。

• 蜱咬的局部效果。

• 获得蜱传疾病的可能性：

- 害怕染上莱姆病。

- 欲检验或治疗莱姆。

病因

• 特定的蜱传感染见其他章节。

• 蜱咬可以来自 2 种主要不同类型的蜱：

- 软蜱（Omithodoros）：

◦ 导致蜱传性反复发热。

◦ 吸血只要数分钟，因此患者几乎不会去急诊治疗。

- 硬蜱：尤其是 Ixodes 和 Dermacentor。

◦ 吸血数日至 1 周，更有可能被患者注意到并导致患者去急诊治疗。

• 莱姆病传播：

- 蜱种类、发育阶段、持续接触时间和地理可能都在莱姆病发生起作用。

- 莱姆的大多数病例都与蜱螨肩胛蜱叮咬有关。

- 莱姆的大部分病例只是在经过虱虫接触后 24～48 h 才传播：

◦ 充血程度是持续时间的标志。

诊断

症状和体征

蜱虫附在皮肤上。

病史

• 患者通常自己已经做出诊断，虽然有时他们错误地将其当作皮肤标志或其他皮肤损伤。

• 询问有关蜱虫接触的持续时间，因为这一点可能会影响开预防性抗生素的使用。

体格检查

直接检查皮肤和蜱：

• 尝试识别蜱虫种类。

• 估计充血程度。

> **注意**
>
> • 一些蜱传感染可能致命。因为没有确定的实时可用的诊断测试，必须根据病史、体格检查和流行病学进行诊断。
>
> • 因这些感染的可选药物多西环素并不常用于急性发热患者的经验性治疗，在病史中询问发热患者是否有虱咬并考虑在合适的情况下使用这一药物。

基本检查

准确的病史和体格检查查找蜱的存在。

诊断检查与说明

实验室检查

• 没有标明莱姆病的检测结果：

- 这种抗体测试只会反映过去暴露于伯氏疏螺旋体。

- 对治疗目前咬伤无任何影响。

诊断步骤/外科

• 不建议测试蜱虫本身。

• 参考蜱虫清除。

鉴别诊断

• 北美蜱传疾病：

- 莱姆病。

- 其他类似莱姆病的疾病，如南方人蜱相关的皮疹疾病（STARD）和包柔螺旋体感染。

- 巴贝虫病。

- 无形体病（以前称埃里希体病）。

- 落基山斑疹热（RMSF）。

- 复发性发热。

- 兔热病。

- 科罗拉多蜱热。

- Q 热。

- 蜱传脑炎（鲍桑热）。

- 蜱瘫痪。

• 欧洲发现的额外蜱传疾病：

- 传播脑炎。

- 南欧斑疹热（Rickettsia conorii）。

- 其他斑点热立克次体。

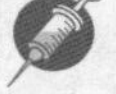

治疗

初步稳定/治疗

清除蜱虫：

• 提早清除会降低蜱传感染传播的可能性。

急诊治疗/程序

• 蜱虫清除方法：

- 用非常细的镊子抓住蜱虫，尽可能靠近皮肤，并轻轻地抬起来 30～120 s 及更长时间。

- 大多数蜱虫会自动出来。

- 不要挤压，蜱可注射传染性物质进入患者的皮肤。

- 如果口腔部分留在皮肤中，虽然这可能导致局部感染或异物反应，它不会传播蜱传疾病。

• 另一种有记载的方法：

- 在蜱虫下皮内注射利多卡因和肾上腺素。

- 蜱虫可能会自行爬出。

• 不使用的方法包括：

- 用火柴燃烧蜱虫。

- 用凡士林或其他有毒物质覆盖。

• 莱姆病预防：

- 若在虫咬伤的 72 h 内发现症状，或医师决定预防，怀疑是充盈的肩胛型蜱幼虫。
- 多西定 200 mg，1 次剂量。
- 对于儿童，没有研究单剂量给药：
  - 阿莫西林(25～50 mg/kg)10 日剂量。
  - 没有数据支持其他蜱传疾病的预防性抗生素治疗。

儿科注意事项

- 几项研究涉及 10 日的阿莫西林治疗来预防儿童莱姆病。
- 治疗组没有患者发生莱姆病或血清感染。
- 蜱麻痹是一种罕见的疾病，但通常发生在儿童，特别是长发女孩；决不能不做整个身体的彻底检查尤其是头皮蜱咬而诊断为吉兰-巴雷综合征。

妊娠注意事项

虽然没有关于抗生素预防孕妇莱姆病的高质量数据，一些学者建议有一个非常低的药物治疗阈值用于治疗孕妇蜱叮咬(使用阿莫西林)。

- 阿莫西林：25～50 mg/kg，每日 3 次，治疗 14～21 日。
- 多西定：1 剂量 200 mg 口服。

随访

进一步处理

入院指征

- 蜱叮咬有蜱麻痹症状或已发生严重的蜱传疾病(如低血压或败血症)。
- 叮咬导致全身感染，严重到需要入院[例如，RMSF、无形体病、巴贝虫病(特别是在脾切除患者)]。

出院指征

所有其他患者，绝大多数，都是安全的。

随访建议

- 如果有关于蜱咬伤的当地感染(蜂窝织炎)的问题，或以上列出的蜱传疾病的症状体征时，寻求当地基层内科医师的帮助。
- 有持续发热的患者应就医并告知医师蜱咬伤病史。
- 蜱咬伤患者应询问预防再次咬伤的建议，包括可能的 DEET 在皮肤的使用和经氯菊酯处理的衣服。

要点和误区

- 提前清除蜱减少了传播蜱传感染可能性。
- 如果蜱是饱满的肩胛骨若虫，则需要预防莱姆病。
- 脾切除患者出现发热，考虑巴贝虫病。

P

偏头痛 Headache, Migraine

Benjamin W. Friedman 刘雪峰 译

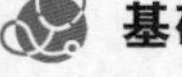

基础知识

描述

- 慢性阵发性疼痛疾病。
- 神经血管的病理生理：
  - 异常的三叉神经传导冲动发送。
  - 脑干的痛感神经通路激活。
  - 血管扩张是一系列刺激因素作用的结果，而不是原因。
  - 不再认为是血管性头痛。
  - 无序的感觉处理及自主神经功能障碍。
  - 偏头痛预兆的基础是大脑皮质活动信号扩散受到抑制。
- 每年有 100 万人发病。
- 大部分急诊头痛为偏头痛。
- 女性的发病率是男性的 3 倍。
- 发病高峰在 40 岁。
- 发作预兆不是确诊标准：
  - A. 5 次符合 B、C、D、E 的发作。
  - B. 发作持续 4～72 h。
  - C. 具有下列 4 项中的 2 项：
    - 单侧。
    - 搏动性疼痛。
    - 中重度疼痛。
    - 身体活动可加重症状。
  - 恶心、呕吐、畏光或畏声。
  - 其他原因无法解释。
- 偏头痛预兆：
  - 不太常见。
  - 头痛发作之前有可逆的神经系统体征。
  - 也有患者表示预兆与疼痛同时出现，或在疼痛之后。
  - 更加少见的偏头痛亚型：
    - 基底型偏头痛。
    - 构音障碍、眩晕、共济失调、复视、意识障碍。
    - 偏瘫型偏头痛。
    - 可逆性的运动无力。
    - 视网膜型偏头痛。
    - 反复发作的单眼视力障碍。

儿科注意事项

- 常见双侧疼痛，发作持续时间较短。
- 伴发症状不易出现，可从动作行为中推断。
- 可伴随顽固性的呕吐。
- 安慰剂有效率高。

病因

不同外显率的遗传性疾病，与环境因素的影响有关。

诊断

症状和体征

病史

- 可被食物、乙醇、病毒性疾病或压力等诱发。
- 月经偏头痛可能比月经早几日。
- 前驱症状可出现在疼痛之前的几日：
  - 包含认知和情绪改变、打哈欠、困倦。
- 预兆出现在头痛发作 1 h 之前：
  - 常见的预兆包括视觉与感觉障碍：
    - 视觉盲点的闪烁。
      - 通常是闪烁的灯光。
      - 不同程度的视觉损伤。
    - 闪光、暗点。
      - 一种可能具有曲折图案的光弧。
    - 麻木或刺痛。
- 单侧，搏动性疼痛。
- 影响活动。
- 可以双侧发作。
- 通常伴发嗅觉恐怖(嗅觉的敏感性)、畏光、畏声、恶心或呕吐。
- 一半逐渐开始加重。
- 之前的病史中多有类似的头痛发作。

体格检查

- 触摸痛意味着难治性偏头痛。
- 其他方面的体格检查无异常。
- 体格检查应包括眼底与视域评估。
- 血压升高不能排除偏头痛诊断。
- 鼻窦压痛不能排除偏头痛诊断。

基本检查

- 详细的病史和体格检查能确认诊断。
- 有新头痛症状的患者可能需要影像学及脑脊液检查。

诊断检查与说明

实验室检查

无要求。

影像学检查

无要求。

诊断步骤/外科

临床诊断,无要求。

鉴别诊断

- 冲击性头痛。
- 药物过量所致头痛。
- 紧张性头痛。
- 过敏性或病毒性鼻窦炎。
- 先天性颅内压增高。
- 可逆性的脑血管收缩综合征。

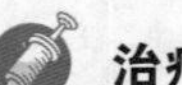

治疗

院前

- 将患者安置在安静、避光的环境。
- 吸氧可能有所帮助。

初步稳定治疗

- 排除继发性头痛。
- 快速有效的止痛。

急诊治疗/程序

- 大多数患者可通过详细的病史排除继发性原因。
- 提供非麻醉性阵痛。
- 静滴生理盐水常常有帮助。
- 告知患者偏头痛的诊断,教育其如何避免诱发偏头痛。
- 在繁忙的轮班期间,坚持使用阿片类药物治疗的频繁来访者很难管理。针对这些病人的治疗计划可以由跨学科委员会制定,然后由所有急救人员统一实施。

妊娠注意事项

甲氧氯普胺(胃复安)、普鲁氯嗪对孕妇是比较好的治疗手段。

药物治疗

- 急诊的顿挫疗法:
  - 多巴胺拮抗剂:
    - 普鲁氯嗪(10 mg,静脉注射)联合苯海拉明(25 mg,静脉注射)预防静坐不能。
    - 氟哌啶(2.5 mg,静脉注射)联合苯海拉明(25 mg,静脉注射)预防静坐不能。
    - 甲氧氯普胺:10 mg,静脉注射。
  - 曲坦类:
    - 舒马曲坦:6 mg,皮下注射,高危心脏风险患者禁用。
    - 依立曲坦:40 mg,口服。
  - 麦角生物碱:
    - 双氢麦角胺:1 mg,静脉注射,联合止吐剂(心脏病风险患者、正在使用大环内酯类抗生素及抗反转录病毒药物者禁用)。
  - 非甾体抗炎药:
    - 酮洛酸:30 g,静脉注射。
  - 糖皮质激素:
    - 地塞米松:10 mg,静脉注射或肌内注射。
    - 泼尼松逐渐减量。
  - 抗癫痫药:
    - 丙戊酸钠 500 mg,静脉滴注。
    - 左乙拉西坦 1 000 mg,静脉滴注。

治疗策略

- 止吐药、曲坦类、地塞米松、非甾体抗炎药可用顿挫疗法。
- 对上述药物无反应时可选用阿片类药物。
- 糖皮质激素可避免离开急诊后头痛的复发。
- 0.5%布比卡因枕大神经阻滞对难治性患者可能有一定作用。

随访

进一步处理

入院指征

- 顽固的剧烈头痛或局部神经损害。
- 顽固性呕吐,电解质紊乱,无法进食水。
- 与药物过量同时存在。

出院指征

- 头痛缓解。
- 除外病理原因所致的头痛。

转诊问题

慢性偏头痛或频繁发作的阵发性偏头痛需要推荐给有相关经验的临床医师。

随访建议

- 记录详情,以确定诱因,避免诱发。
- 坚持随访以确定有效的口服治疗药物。

要点和误区

- 阿片类药物不应作为急诊的一线治疗药物。
- 患者应携带药物处方回家。
- 区分慢性反复发作的偏头痛与新发的渐进性头痛。

贫血 Anemia

Stevan A. Vuckovic · Paul J. Allegretti 李岩 王瑞兰 译

基础知识

描述

- 减少或低于正常水平红细胞的数量。
- 检测一个或多个主要的红细胞成分:
  - 血红蛋白:在全血中主要携带氧气物质的浓度。
  - 血细胞比容(HCT):全血红细胞占用体积百分比。
  - 红细胞计数:全血中红细胞的数量。
- 成年女性:血红蛋白＜120 g/L 或血细胞比容＜37%。
- 成年男性:血红蛋白＜140 g/L 或血细胞比容＜42%。
- 正常人血液中的计数值取决于年龄:
  - 新生儿:血红蛋白 165 g/L,血细胞比容 51%。
  - 1 岁:血红蛋白 120 g/L,血细胞比容 36%。

- 6岁：血红蛋白125 g/L,血细胞比容37%。
- 成年男性：血红蛋白140 g/L,血细胞比容42%。
- 成年女性：血红蛋白120 g/L,血细胞比容37%。
• 血红蛋白/血细胞比容取决于氧分压。
- 生活在4 000 ft高度之上的新生儿和居民会增加。
• 血红蛋白、血细胞比容和红细胞计数是浓度：
- 依赖于红细胞的数量和血浆量。
- 如果红细胞数量减少或血浆量增加导致值下降。
- 贫血是一个潜在的病症或不足的表现。

病因

• 从来不是一种正常变异：
- 可能是全身性疾病的第一表现。
- 需要不断寻找原因。
• 失血过多(最常见的原因)：
- 创伤。
- 消化道出血。
- 经血。
• 溶血(红细胞增多破坏,红细胞寿命<100日)：
- 脾功能亢进。
- 免疫性溶血性贫血。
- 机械性损伤[假体心脏瓣膜、血管炎、血栓、血小板减少性紫癜(TTP)、溶血性尿毒症综合征(HUS)或弥散性血管内凝血(DIC)]。
- 毒素。
- 感染(疟疾、巴贝虫病)。
- 细胞膜异常。
- 红细胞内异常(G-6-PD、镰状细胞性贫血、珠蛋白生成障碍性贫血)。
• 红细胞减少合成：
- 通过红细胞大小的测量分类。
- 小细胞低色素。
◦ 铁缺乏。
◦ 珠蛋白生成障碍性贫血。
◦ 铁粒幼细胞。
◦ 慢性疾病。
- 正色素/大细胞：
◦ 甲状腺功能减退症。
◦ 叶酸缺乏。
◦ 维生素 B_{12} 缺乏症。
◦ 肝病。
◦ 骨髓增生异常。
◦ 某些白血病。
- 正色素/正常红细胞：
◦ 再生障碍性贫血。
◦ 慢性肾衰竭。
◦ 恶性肿瘤。
◦ 肾上腺皮质功能不全。
◦ 甲状旁腺功能亢进症。
◦ 酗酒。
◦ 急性失血。

诊断

体征和症状

依赖于以下因素：
• 快速发作：
- 急性贫血会导致低血容量。
- 轻度和慢性贫血可以无症状。

病史

• 基础疾病。
• 贫血的严重程度和类型。
• 疲劳。
• 减少运动耐量。
• 呼吸急促。
• 呼吸困难。
• 胸痛/心绞痛。
• 晕厥。
• 黑便或血便。
• 月经不规则或量多。
• 容易挫伤或出血过多病史。

体格检查

• 心血管系统：
- 心动过速、心脏肥大或杂音。
- 体位性低血压。
• 皮肤病：
- 皮肤：
◦ 冷。
◦ 苍白。
◦ 黄疸。
◦ 紫癜。
◦ 毛细血管扩张。
◦ 瘀点。
◦ 淤斑。
- 匙状指甲(反甲)。
• 神经系统：
- 神经病。
- 精神状态改变。
• 骨(特别是胸骨)或关节痛(镰状细胞病)。
• 肝大,脾大。
• 淋巴结肿大。
• 调查结果反映了潜在的疾病。

基本检查

• 全血细胞计数。
• 生命体征。
• 确定有无：
- 出血。
- 增加红细胞破坏。
- 骨髓抑制。
- 缺铁。

诊断检查与说明

血型和交叉匹配或类型和扫描：
- 取决于严重性。
• 全血细胞计数：
- 红细胞指数：
◦ 平均红细胞体积(MCV,正常：80～100 μm^3)。
◦ 平均红细胞血红蛋白含量(MCH,正常：27～34 pg/细胞)。
◦ 平均红细胞血红蛋白浓度(MCHC,正常：33%～36%)。
- 血小板计数：
◦ 血小板增多表明：
▪ 缺铁。
▪ 骨髓增殖性疾病。
▪ 炎症。
▪ 感染。
▪ 肿瘤。
◦ 血小板减少表明：
▪ 骨髓恶性肿瘤。
▪ 脾功能亢进。
▪ 脓毒症。
▪ 维生素 B_{12} 或叶酸缺乏。
▪ 自身免疫性疾病。
• 网织红细胞计数：
- 普通0.5%～1.5%(网织红细胞/1 000红细胞)。
- 增加的网织红细胞计数：持续失血或溶血增加红细胞生成。
- 低网织红细胞计数的稳定性贫血：红细胞生成受损。
- 活动溶血或低网织红细胞计数性失血：并发疾病。
- 低网织红细胞计数与全血细胞减少：再生障碍性贫血。
- 低网织红细胞计数与正常白细胞和血小板：纯红细胞再生障碍性贫血。
• 网织红细胞指数(RI)：网织红细胞计数(%)×(患者血细胞比容/正常血细胞比容)：
- RI<2%意味着红细胞生产不足。
- RI>2%,意味着增加红细胞的生成与红细胞过度破坏或失利。
- 白细胞差分和外周血涂片。
• 白细胞减少症伴贫血表明骨髓抑制、脾功能亢进或缺乏维生素 B_{12}/叶酸。

• 粪便隐血。

• 电解质、BUN、肌酸酐、葡萄糖：

– 慢性肾衰竭。

• 尿液分析：

– 血尿。

– 溶血性贫血的血红蛋白尿。

• 后处理策略：

– 小细胞低色素性贫血：

◦ 铁。

◦ 总铁结合力。

◦ 转铁蛋白饱和度。

◦ 铁蛋白。

– 大细胞性贫血：

◦ 叶酸。

◦ 维生素 B_{12}。

◦ LFT。

◦ 甲状腺功能检查。

– 溶血性贫血：

◦ 快速下降的血红蛋白。

◦ 网状细胞。

◦ 破碎的红细胞。

◦ LDH 增加。

◦ 增加间接胆红素。

◦ 血清结合珠蛋白降低。

◦ 库姆斯试验阳性。

• 特殊检查：

– 外周血涂片：

◦ 头盔细胞/裂，微血管病性溶血。

◦ 泪滴状红细胞，骨髓纤维化。

◦ 球形红细胞，自身免疫性溶血。

◦ 白细胞增生，骨髓移植。

◦ 咬细胞氧化溶血。

◦ 红细胞的寄生虫、疟疾或巴贝斯虫病。

◦ 靶细胞、肝脏疾病。

◦ 伯尔细胞尿毒症。

◦ 铁粒幼细胞、酗酒或骨髓增生异常。

◦ Howell-Jolly 小体，无脾。

– 血红蛋白电泳镰状细胞/地中海贫血。

– 铁，铁结合力，转铁蛋白饱和度，铁蛋白：

◦ 缺铁。

◦ 铁减少。

◦ 铁结合能力提高。

◦ 转铁蛋白饱和度下降。

◦ 铁蛋白下降。

– 慢性疾病：

◦ 铁减少。

◦ 铁结合能力下降。

◦ 转铁蛋白饱和度降低/正常。

◦ 铁蛋白正常/升高。

– 珠蛋白生成障碍性贫血：

◦ 铁正常。

◦ 铁结合力正常。

◦ 铁蛋白正常。

– 铁粒幼细胞性贫血：

◦ 铁增加。

◦ 铁结合力正常。

◦ 铁蛋白增加。

诊断步骤/外科

骨髓活检评估：

• 再生障碍性贫血。

• 骨髓增生异常。

• 骨髓恶性肿瘤。

• 骨髓增殖性疾病。

▪ 鉴别诊断

• 后天与遗传性贫血。

• 慢性病贫血。

• 失血。

• CHF。

• 稀释性贫血。

• 溶血。

• 恶性肿瘤。

• 营养缺乏症/吸收不良。

• 骨髓抑制。

儿科注意事项

• 新生儿溶血性贫血。

• 当 Rh 阴性的母亲怀有 Rh 阳性的孩子 Rh 抗体穿过胎盘。

妊娠注意事项

• 生理或稀释性贫血的晚期妊娠。

• 增加红细胞量的 25%，增加血浆量的 50%。

老年注意事项

• 在健康老年人血红蛋白/血细胞比容的一般比在年轻的成人低。

• 这种较低的"正常"必须是排除诊断。

治疗

▪ 院前

继续失血，需要密切评估和快速运输：

• 控制出血。

• 建立多条快速静脉通路。

▪ 初步稳定/治疗

• ABC 管理，吸氧。

• 如果持续亏损/低血压用生理盐水静脉液体复苏。

▪ 急诊治疗/程序

• 取决于贫血的严重程度。

• 具有不稳定生命体征的出血输血，对晶体复苏无反应。由于持续大量失血，仅 PRBC 的输血不足。考虑输血（血浆、血小板和红细胞的比例为 1∶1∶1）。

• 急诊大部分贫血是慢性的，不需要立即进行干预。

• 治疗具体贫血：

– 缺铁：

◦ 硫酸亚铁：300 mg，口服，每日 3 次。

◦ 调查根本原因。

◦ 预计在 2～3 周血红蛋白增加。

– 肾衰竭：

◦ 内源性促红细胞生成素减少。

◦ 替换为重组促红细胞生成素。

– 自身免疫性溶血性贫血：

◦ 皮质类固醇（泼尼松 60 mg/d，直到响应）。

◦ 免疫抑制剂。

◦ 血浆置换。

◦ 脾切除。

– 药物性溶血性贫血：停用该药。

– 慢性病贫血：治疗潜在疾病。

– 维生素 B_{12} 缺乏：

◦ 维生素 B_{12}：1 000 μg 每日肌内注射，持续 1 周，然后每周到 1 个月，然后是每月使用。

◦ 血液学指标在 2 个月恢复正常。

◦ 神经系统症状，口服>6 个月可能是永久性的。

– 叶酸缺乏症：

◦ 叶酸：1 mg 每日口服。

– 再生障碍性贫血。

– 抗胸腺细胞球蛋白。

– 骨髓移植：

◦ 镰状细胞性贫血。

◦ 支持治疗用氧，补液，镇痛。

◦ 治疗突发原因。

– 白血病：

◦ 骨髓移植。

▪ 药物治疗

• 补铁。

• 补充促红细胞生成素为肾衰竭患者。

• 皮质类固醇的自身免疫性。

• 维生素 B_{12}。

• 叶酸。

随访

▪ 进一步处理

入院指征

• 生命体征不稳定。

• 继续失血。
• 贫血症状，心绞痛、呼吸困难、晕厥。
• 全血细胞减少。
• 需要输血。
• 积极的评估。
• 严重贫血：
- 最初，原因不明的血红蛋白小于 80 g/L。
- 在获得门诊治疗的患者，其血红蛋白的主要问题是显著降低或合并症时存在。

出院指征

门诊后处理的绝大多数治疗稳定的患者。

■ 随访建议

新确诊的贫血患者需要进行后处理：
• 如果稳定从急诊科出院，提供后续选项后处理。

要点和误区

• 贫血是一个潜在的病症或不足的表现。
• 严重或危及生命的情况下，需要通过输血立即改正。
• 在急诊遇到的大多数情况下是慢性和不需要立即干预的。

P

破伤风 Tetanus

Daniel T. Wu 范浩浩 李文放 译

基础知识

■ 描述

• 美国罕见的疾病，但仍在第三世界国家流行。
• 美国每年约有 30 例。
• 一半的案件涉及年龄＞50 岁的人。
• 美国大多数病例发生在未接种疫苗或自上次增强免疫或静滴类毒素＞10 年的人群。
• 全球有 500 000～1 000 000 例。
• 即使接受治疗，死亡率也很高。
• 潜伏期：
- 感染后到第一次临床症状的出现。
◦ 48 h 至 3 周或更长时间。
- 发病期。
• ＜7 日，预后差。
• 如果症状到初始反射痉挛＜48 h，预后极差。
• 新生儿破伤风：
- 由于感染脐带残端。
- 产妇第 2 周出现症状抗体减少。
- 在美国很少见，但在第三世界国家很普遍。
- 在全球范围内，占所有破伤风感染的一半以上。

■ 病因

• 破伤风梭菌。
- 细长、活动、热敏、无氧、革兰阳性杆与末端球形孢子。
- 孢子特征。
- 耐氧，耐潮湿，耐极端温度。
- 可以无限期地存活直到它萌发。
- 土壤和排泄物中无处不在。
• 当接种到伤口或失活组织或作为滥用药物的污染物静脉注射时，孢子在厌氧条件下发芽并产生 2 种毒素。
• 毒素。
- 破伤风溶血素。
◦ 损伤组织。
◦ 不会引起破伤风感染临床表现。
- 破伤风痉挛毒素。
◦ 强大的神经毒素。
◦ 扰乱作为神经递质的 γ-氨基丁酸(GABA)的释放。
◦ 引起临床表现。
• 肌肉痉挛。
• 自主神经不稳定。
• 不受控制的运动。

诊断

■ 症状和体征

一般型

• 最常见类型，约占病例的 80%。
• 初始表现：
- 肌肉僵硬和疼痛。
- 牙关紧闭(初始时)。
- 苦笑面容(特征面部症状)。
• 全身症状：
- 易怒。
- 不安。
- 出汗。
• 后期表现：
- 肌群僵硬。
- 紧张性肌肉收缩突然发作：
◦ 角弓反张。
◦ 手臂的屈曲和内收。
◦ 拳头握紧。
◦ 下肢过伸。
- 膈肌痉挛或瘫痪：
◦ 可能会危及呼吸。
• 交感过敏状态(最常见的死亡原因)：
- 在第 2 周开始。
- 心律失常。
- 血压变化。
- 出汗。
- 高热。

局部型

• 不太常见的疾病形式，约占所有病例的 17%。
• 典型的局部痉挛发生在可能感染的初始区域：
- 症状较轻。
- 缓解之前持续数月。
- 转换为一般型(13%)。

头部型

• 罕见的疾病变种。
• 头部受伤或中耳炎。
• 颅底和面部肌肉痉挛：
- 脑神经(CN)麻痹，第 7 脑神经最常见。
• 可能会发展为普遍性破伤风。

新生儿

• 出生后第 1 周发生的一般形式的破伤风。
• 通常由脐部残端感染引起。
• 临床表现：
- 易怒。
- 吮吸无力。
- 面部表情异常。
- 触摸处肌肉痉挛。
• 非常高的死亡率(50%～100%)。
• 潜伏期 1～2 周。

病史

• 调查感染源。
• 急性皮肤伤口不是感染所必需的。
• ＞25%的感染发生在没有已知的急性创

伤感染的情况下。

• 感染可能发生于脓肿、溃疡和脓肿、坏疽。

• 引发破伤风免疫状态改变。

基本检查

• 进行完整的体格检查，重点集中在心血管系统和呼吸状态、周围神经和中枢神经检查。

• 破伤风是临床诊断：

- 所有的牙关紧闭患者均应该怀疑。
- 1/5 的病例没有伤口。
- 完全破伤风免疫的患者几乎可以排除诊断。

诊断检查与说明

通常对诊断无效或无益处，但有助于排除其他病因或评估疾病并发症。

实验室检查

• 血常规。

• 电解质、血尿素氮、肌酸酐、葡萄糖、钙：

- 低钙血症。

• 士的宁水平。

• 动脉血气分析，指脉氧：

- 检测氧合状态。

• 破伤风梭菌的培养：

- 只有大约 30%的概率。

• 破伤风杆菌效价：

- 回顾性诊断才有用。

• 脑脊液分析：

- 破伤风正常。
- 排除脑膜炎/脑炎。

影像学检查

精神状态改变的患者行头颅 CT 检查：

• 破伤风正常。

鉴别诊断

• 马钱子碱中毒。

• 士的宁中毒患者下颚肌肉通常在早期不表现。

• 多巴胺阻断的肌张力障碍反应。

• 感染：

- 脑膜炎。
- 狂犬病。
- 脑炎。
- 腹膜炎。
- 肺脓肿。

• 黑寡妇蜘蛛蜇伤。

• 肉毒中毒。

• 血清素综合征。

• 低钙血症。

• 贝尔麻痹(头痛形式、牙关紧闭前)。

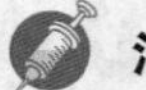

治疗

院前

• 仔细评估气道：

- 牙关紧闭、声带麻痹及面部、颈部僵硬可致气管插管困难。

• 避免过度刺激，因为它可能会引发手足肌肉组织的抽搐。

初步稳定/治疗

• 检查气道、呼吸、循环：

- 预防性插管。
- 由于牙关紧闭需要神经肌肉阻滞。
- 建立静脉通路输生理盐水。
- 监测血压和心律(自主神经不稳定)。

• 排除肌张力障碍反应后给予阿托品或苯海拉明。

急诊治疗/程序

• 重点关注 3 个目标：

- 稳定患者和支持性护理。
- 中和毒素。
- 去除任何剩余的有机毒素。

• 稳定和支持性护理：

- 气道保护：
  ◦ 可能需要预防性插管。
- 牙关紧闭可能需要麻痹剂：
  ◦ 由于乙酰胆碱受体上调导致的高钾血症的风险，应谨慎使用琥珀胆碱。
- 用苯二氮䓬治疗肌肉痉挛；如果大剂量无效，可以给予丹曲林。

• 自主神经不稳定疗法：

- 症状发作后几日至几周发生。
- 快速心律失常和高血压：
  ◦ 没有普遍有效的治疗方法。
  ◦ 可以尝试 α 和 β 受体阻滞剂，但可能会导致症状恶化(由于拉贝洛尔的 α 和 β 受体阻滞效果，可应用拉贝洛尔)。
  ◦ 可乐定、镁、吗啡、芬太尼也可以尝试硬膜外麻醉。
- 低血压：
  ◦ 排除败血症和血容量不足。
  ◦ 心输出量低时应用多巴胺或多巴酚丁胺。
  ◦ 毒素的中和。

• 人类破伤风免疫球蛋白(TIG)：

- 成人和儿童的 3 000～6 000 单位，即时肌内注射。
- 清创前给药。
- 中和未结合的毒素。
- 对 CNS 中已经结合的毒素没有影响。

• 去除剩余的生物体：

- 限制感染的严重程度。
- 清创可清除任何坏死组织。
- 当与清创一起使用时，抗生素可有效消除破伤风梭菌。
- 甲硝唑是可选择的抗生素。
- 青霉素是一个可行的选择。

• 预防：

- 首次系列疫苗接种应该在 18 个月之内完成；儿童在 4～11 岁时进行加强，然后每 10 年加强一次。
- 儿童＜7 岁接受白喉，百日咳和破伤风疫苗。
- 破伤风白喉疫苗(Td)可用于＞7 岁儿童或大人。
- 如果以前没有接种过，＞11 岁都应给予 1 剂百白破疫苗，以解决百日咳发病率的增加。
- 临床破伤风感染不赋予免疫力。
- 对于干净轻微的伤口：如果事先未知疫苗接种情况或最后一次加强＞10 年，应给予 Td。
- 对于破伤风倾向的伤口：
  ◦ 如果未知疫苗接种病史最后一次加强＞5 年应给予 Td。
  ◦ 如果未知的疫苗接种史应给予人破伤风免疫球蛋白。

药物治疗

• 苯托品：1～2 mg，静脉注射。

• 氯丙嗪：10～50 mg，静脉注射。

• 地西泮(苯二氮䓬类)：5～10 mg(儿童：2～0.4 mg/kg)，静脉滴注。

• 苯海拉明：50 mg，静脉注射。

• 多巴酚丁胺：2.5～15 μg/(kg·min)，静脉滴注。

• 多巴胺：2～20 μg/(kg·min)，静脉滴注。

• 多西定：100 mg，静脉滴注，q12 h。

• 红霉素：500 mg，静脉滴注，q6 h。

• 拉贝洛尔：20 mg(儿童：每次 0.3～1 mg/kg)静脉滴注 q10 min 至 300 mg，必要时，开始输注 2 mg/min[根据需要，儿童：0.4～1 mg/(kg·h)，最大剂量 3 mg/(kg·h)]。

• 甲硝唑：1 g(儿童：15 mg/kg)负荷，其次 500 mg(7.5 mg/kg)，静脉滴注，q6 h。

• 青霉素：1 200 万 U/d[儿童：10 万 U/(kg·24 h)]，静脉滴注，q6 h，持续 10 日。

• 普萘洛尔：0.5～1 mg(儿童：0.01～

0.1 mg/kg)静滴。
- TIG：
  - 250 U 肌内注射。
  - 与破伤风分开给药。
  - 应用于未完全免疫的破伤风倾向伤口。
- Td 0.5 ml 肌内注射。

随访

处置

入院指征

所有患者都应该入住 ICU。

出院指征

未见广泛性破伤风。

要点和误区

易发破伤风伤口的积极治疗。

葡萄球菌烫伤样皮肤综合征 Staphylococcal Scalded Skin Syndrome

Roger M. Barkin 江伟伟 李文放 译

基础知识

描述

- 由金黄色葡萄球菌产生的可溶性表皮外毒素的作用的结果：
  - 由远离感染或定植部位产生。
  - 血液传播。
  - 浅表表皮颗粒细胞的桥粒裂解。
  - 导致广泛表皮剥脱。
- 通常会影响<6 岁的婴幼儿：
  - 成人具有特定的葡萄球菌抗体，能够定位、代谢和排泄葡萄球菌毒素。
  - 婴儿和儿童不能有效地代谢和排泄毒素。
  - 3～7 日龄的婴儿，可有发热，出现弥漫性的烫伤样红斑和松弛样水泡，伴尼氏征阳性。
  - 免疫功能低下的成人和严重肾功能不全的人也容易感染。
- 按年龄和皮疹范围分类：
  - 经典葡萄球菌烫伤皮肤综合征。
  - 天疱疮新生儿。
  - 大疱性脓疱病。
  - 新生儿：里特病。
- 典型的凝固酶阳性噬菌体Ⅱ群葡萄球菌：
  - 噬菌体Ⅰ群和Ⅲ群。

病因

- 定植处通常没有明显的感染。
- 并发感染或皮肤屏障破坏：
  - 鼻、咽。
  - 尿道。
  - 轻微的皮肤擦伤。
  - 包皮环切部位。
  - 结膜炎。
  - 脐炎。
  - 脓疱疮。
  - 心内膜炎和败血症。
- 往往没有确定部位。
- 可能与链球菌感染相似，虽不常见。革兰染色可能有用。

诊断

体征和症状

- 全身中毒症状：
  - 萎靡。
  - 发热。
  - 易怒。
  - 孩子可能出现生病或携带病毒。
  - 突然发作。
- 猩红热样红斑(砂纸样)类似于"晒伤"红皮病。
- 异样的皮肤。
- 好发部位：
  - 围绕颈部的屈肌部位。
  - 易摩擦部位，特别是腋窝和腹股沟。
  - 靠近眼睛和唇。
  - 皮肤皱纹增加，皮肤红肿。
- 面部水肿，眼睛、鼻和口周围有结痂裂。
- 松弛大疱：
  - 在皮疹发生后 1～3 日。
  - 最初在弯曲部位(腋窝、腹股沟、身体孔)。
  - 大疱通过侧压力在表皮转移，表皮分离(尼氏征)。
  - 在数小时内破裂。
  - 轻微的创伤造成表皮分离。
  - 表皮是大块脱落。
  - 裸露的区域湿润、敏感、疼痛。
  - 在 2 周内完成愈合，无瘢痕。
- 脓性结膜炎。
- 黏膜不受影响。
- 罕见并发症：
  - 体温低。
  - 水电解质平衡紊乱。
  - 继发感染。
  - 肺炎。
  - 败血症。
  - 蜂窝织炎。
  - 骨髓炎。

基本检查

- 临床表现可诊断。
- 确定毒素产生的位置和来源。
- 评估全身的感染。

诊断检查与说明

实验室检查

- 血常规和尿液分析：
  - 如果来源不明显则评估败血症。
- 电解质：
  - 提示是否有脱水或广泛皮疹。
- 血培养(很少阳性)。
- 可能与链球菌感染相似，虽不常见。革兰染色可能有用。

影像学检查

可指导确定感染的位置/来源。

诊断步骤/外科

- 吸取大疱里液体：
  - 在葡萄球菌性烫伤样皮肤综合征中无菌。
  - 与血行播散的毒素一致。
- 从水疱以外的部位分离葡萄球菌：
  - 通常结膜、鼻咽或血液。
- 皮肤活检或冷冻组织切片：
  - 确定表皮/真皮分离的水平(卵裂在真皮颗粒层中)。
  - 指导>6 岁儿童和合并多种临床表现的用药。

P

■ **鉴别诊断**

- 感染：
  - 猩红热：
    - 涉及黏膜。
    - 草莓舌。
    - 不会发生痛苦的脱屑。
- 大疱性脓疱疮：
  - 浑浊或混浊的大疱性液体。
- 大疱性水痘：
  - 病毒培养基见巨型细胞。
  - 在水痘出现5日后。
- 中毒性休克综合征：
  - 临床症状和症状的快速发展。
  - 黏膜和多器官受累。
- 中毒性表皮坏死松解或药疹：
  - 成人更常见。
  - 黏膜损伤重。
  - 全层表皮坏死。
- 皮肤病：
  - 红斑多形性。
  - 表皮松解角化过度。
  - 大疱性表皮松解症。
  - 寻常型天疱疮。
- 烫伤。
- 潜在病症的次要皮疹：
  - 淋巴瘤。
  - 曲霉病。
  - 辐射病。
  - 移植免疫反应。
  - 川崎病。

治疗

■ **院前**

- 如果存在脱水，输注盐水。
- 初始烧伤治疗。

■ **初步稳定/治疗**

- 管理类似于广泛的二度烧伤：
  - 有大体积表面区域损伤的需要静脉输液。
- 提供足够的镇痛药。
- 脱下衣服并将孩子放在无菌亚麻上。
- 少接触孩子。
- 应用潮湿的无菌敷料。
- 避免多余的热量损失。

■ **急诊治疗/程序**

- 局部烧伤膏证实对病情无改善。
- 禁止使用激素。
- 使用对耐甲氧西林金黄色葡萄球菌有效的抗生素：
  - 头孢唑林。
  - 乙氧萘青霉素。
  - 万古霉素，如果怀疑耐甲氧西林金黄色葡萄球菌(MRSA)。
- 轻度受累的口服抗生素：
  - 双氯西林。
  - 红霉素。
  - 头孢氨苄。

■ **药物治疗**

- 头孢唑林：50～100 mg/(kg·24 h)，静脉滴注，每日2次。
- 头孢氨苄：25～100 mg/(kg·24 h)，口服，每日2次。
- 双氯西林：12～25 mg/(kg·24 h)，口服，每日2次。
- 红霉素：30～50 mg/(kg·24 h)，口服，每日2次。
- 乙氧萘青霉素：1～2 g，静脉滴注，q6 h；新生儿，50～100 mg/(kg·24 h)静脉滴注 q6 h；儿童，100～200 mg/(kg·24 h)，静脉滴注，q6 h。
- 万古霉素：40 mg/(kg·24 h)，静脉滴注，q6 h。

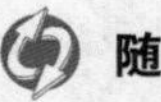

随访

■ **进一步处理**

入院指征

- 儿童<1岁。
- 所有中毒性表现的儿童。
- 广泛的皮肤病变。
- 脱水和/或电解质紊乱。

出院指征

- 年龄较大，轻微受累的表现良好的儿童。
- 口服抗生素7日。
- 在48 h内进行随访。

转诊问题

- 传染科会诊。
- 咨询外科医师是否需要引流。

葡萄胎 Hydatidiform

Johanna E. Kreafle · Joshua W. Loyd　巩博 译

基础知识

■ **描述**

- 一种起源于胎盘的妊娠滋养细胞疾病(GTD)，可局部侵及子宫或转移。
- 肿瘤起源于妊娠组织而不是母体组织。
- 发展成恶性肿瘤的可能性：
  - 妊娠滋养细胞瘤(GTN)。
- 完全性葡萄胎。
  - 发病率为1/1500孕妇。
  - 不出现胎儿组织。
  - 弥漫性绒毛肿胀。
  - 弥漫性滋养细胞增生。
  - 15%～20%发生恶变，常常转移至肺。
  - 遗传学：
    - 染色体：46，XX(90%)；46，XY(10%)。
    - 表达父系DNA。
    - 空卵受精2个单倍体精子或受精1个单倍体精子再自身复制。
- 部分性葡萄胎：
  - 发病率为1/750孕妇。
  - 存在胎儿或胚胎组织。
  - 局部绒毛膜肿胀。
  - 局部滋养细胞增生。
  - 4%～12%发生恶变。
  - 遗传学：
    - 染色体：90%是三倍体，常为69，XXX；69，XXY；很少为69，XYY。
    - 包含母系和父系DNA。
    - 单倍体卵子复制并受精正常精子或单倍体卵子受精2个精子。
- 正常妊娠双胎可能有部分胎：
  - 孕妇罹患持续性疾病和转移的风险较高。
  - 有可能有一个正常的婴儿。

病因

- 大部分未知。
- 风险因素：
  - 极端产妇年龄的最佳估计风险因素：
    - ＞35 岁的携带 2～7.5 倍的风险。
    - 15 岁以下儿童。
  - 既往葡萄胎妊娠在未来妊娠中有 1%～2% 的风险（一般人群的 10～15 倍）。
  - 缺乏动物脂肪和维生素 A。
  - 吸烟（>15 支/天）。
  - 母系血型 AB、A 或 B。
  - 不孕和/或自然流产史。
- 因地理而异：
  - 亚洲国家的风险最高。
  - 美国和西欧的风险最低（每 1 000～1 500 例中活产 1 例）。
  - 据报道在其他国家每 12～500 名活产婴儿中有 1 名。
- 在 600 例治疗性流产中发现了 1 例。

诊断

症状和体征

- 经常夸大妊娠的主观症状。
- 完全性葡萄胎：
  - 阴道流血：
    - 最常见的症状。
    - 由于分离的白齿绒毛从下面的蜕膜。
    - 晚期妊娠前 3 个月。
    - 通常无痛，像"李子汁"。
  - 通常有阴道排出物：
    - 通常描述为葡萄样小泡。
    - 常发生在妊娠中期，<20 周。
  - 高水平 β-HCG 引起剧烈呕吐。
  - 先兆子痫：
    - 视觉变化。
    - 妊娠期高血压。
    - 蛋白尿。
    - 反射亢进。
    - 可能出现惊厥。
  - 甲状腺功能亢进：
    - 标志性心动过速、震颤。
    - 可能是由于高剂量的 β-HCG（>100 000 mIU/ml）或甲状腺刺激物质（促甲状腺素）。
  - 急性呼吸窘迫：
    - 呼吸急促、弥漫性啰音、心动过速、精神状态改变。
    - 可能出现滋养层组织栓塞。
    - 也可能是因为先兆子痫、甲状腺功能亢进或医源性补液引起的心肺改变。
- 部分性葡萄胎：
  - 通常不表现出完全性葡萄胎的临床特点。
  - 常常出现和先兆流产、自发性流产类似的症状。
    - 阴道出血。
    - 可能会有胎心。
  - 多出现在较晚的妊娠期。

病史

与妊娠类似：

- 月经周期消失。
- 妊娠检查阳性。
- 恶心、呕吐、阴道出血。

体格检查

- 50%～66%出现子宫大小和孕龄不一致。
  - 完全性葡萄胎大小通常比孕龄推测的大。
  - 部分性葡萄胎会比孕龄推测的小。
- 卵巢肿块：
  - 常见于完全性葡萄胎，部分性葡萄胎很少见。
  - 通常是因为卵巢肿大。
  - 高水平 β-HCG 导致双侧多发卵泡膜黄素囊肿，通常被超声检查发现。

基本检查

- HCG：
  - 完全性葡萄胎 β-HCG＞100 000 mIU/ml，但是也可能在正常范围。
  - 部分性葡萄胎：通常低于正常妊娠水平。
  - β-HCG>40 000 mIU/ml 通常预后不良。
- 超声检查：
  - 完全性葡萄胎：
    - 特点是"落雪"样水疱。
    - 缺少胎儿组织，绒毛水肿且无回声。
    - 没有羊水。
    - 卵泡膜黄素囊肿。
    - 增大的子宫。
- 部分性葡萄胎：
  - "瑞士奶酪"样外表。
  - 形成孕囊，胎盘出现扇贝形囊泡。
  - 可能有胎儿。
  - 存在羊水，但容量可能减少。
- β-HCG>100 000 mIU/ml 胎儿正常出现。
  - 1 周内重复 β-HCG 和超声。
  - 可能是双胎妊娠或部分葡萄胎妊娠。

诊断检查与说明

实验室检查

- β-HCG。
- 血型、Rh 及交叉配血。
- 全血细胞计数评估有无贫血及血小板减少。
- 凝血检查评估弥散性血管内凝血。
- 电解质、尿素氮及肌酐。
- 如果怀疑甲状腺功能亢进检查促甲状腺素和甲状腺素（游离 T_4）。
- 如果怀疑先兆子痫，检查尿蛋白。

影像学检查

- 超声检查：
  - 可以在床边检查。
  - 经阴道比经腹部更敏感。
- 胸部 X 线：
  - 在急性呼吸窘迫的患者中评估肺水肿情况。
  - 筛查转移性疾病。
  - 基础调查。

诊断步骤/外科

病理/病史：

- 所有排出物应该进行正式评估。
- 排出物可能是诊断部分性葡萄胎的唯一方法。
- 完全性葡萄胎：
  - 绒毛水肿。
  - 滋养层增生。
- 部分性葡萄胎：
  - 胎儿组织和血管。
  - 羊膜。
  - 绒毛水肿。

鉴别诊断

- 异位妊娠。
- 子痫/子痫前期。
- 甲状腺危象/甲状腺功能亢进。
- 先兆流产。
- 稽留流产。
- 不全流产。
- 妊娠剧吐。
- 非极性怀孕。

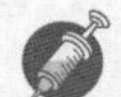

治疗

院前

- 保证气道通畅，吸氧。
- 建立静脉通路。
- 用合适的苯二氮䓬类药物治疗抽搐。
- 保存排出组织进行组织学评估。

初步稳定/治疗

- 保证气道通畅。
- 建立静脉通路。

• 心电监测。
• 查血型及交叉配血，尤其是患者需要子宫切除术时。

急诊治疗/程序

• 急性呼吸窘迫：
- 胸部X线检查可显示浸润。
◦ 可能与滋养层栓塞、甲状腺危象或医源性液体复苏有关。
- 可能需要NIPPV或插管。
• 甲状腺功能亢进：
- β受体阻滞剂：
◦ 推荐普萘洛尔。
◦ 清除葡萄胎前给予。
◦ 麻醉或手术应激可能诱发甲状腺危象。
• 先兆子痫/子痫：
- 抽搐：
◦ 解决妊娠的治疗问题。
◦ 给予苯二氮䓬类药物（地西泮）。
◦ 给予硫酸镁。
- 高血压：
◦ 给予肼屈嗪或拉贝洛尔。
• 凝血功能障碍：
- 按需输血液制品。
- 抗D人免疫球蛋白(RhoGAM)：
◦ 尽管胎血不出现在完全性葡萄胎，但可能延迟出现在部分性葡萄胎。
• 抽吸刮除术：
- 由产科医师完成，可以在急救室操作。
- 80%有效。
- 妇女选择能保存生育能力的方法。
- 注射催产素诱导子宫平滑肌收缩，可能需要其他子宫收缩剂。
• 药物预防：
- 非常有争议。
- 产科医师只能给可随访观察的患者开具处方。
- 通常用在高风险的完全性葡萄胎或无法监测激素水平时。
• 子宫切除术：
- 高龄患者。
- 患者对保持生育能力不感兴趣。
- 高风险疾病。
- 不能阻止转移可能。

药物治疗

• 地西泮：0.2～0.4 mg/kg，静脉注射；或0.3～0.5 mg灌肠，多达5～10 mg，最大剂量30 mg。
• 肼屈嗪：每20 min 5～10 mg，静脉注射，累计60 mg。
• 拉贝洛尔：20 mg，静脉注射，每10 min双倍剂量，最多300 mg。
• 硫酸镁：4～6 g，静脉注射，超过15～20 min，然后维持1～2 g/h。
• 催产素：产后出血，10 U，肌内注射。
• 普萘洛尔(心得安)：1 mg，静脉注射，每2 h调整剂量。
• RhoGAM：72 h内300 μg。

随访

进一步处理

入院指征

• 子宫增大至大约妊娠16周。
- 子宫越大，抽吸刮除术时子宫穿孔、出血、肺栓塞的风险越大。
• 有先兆子痫、甲状腺功能亢进、呼吸窘迫的症状。
• 子宫切除。
• 部分性葡萄胎。
• 血流动力学不稳定。

出院指征

• 低风险和较小的葡萄胎行非复杂的宫颈扩张和刮除术的可信赖患者。
• 强调随访的重要性。
• 子宫排空后休息4～6周。
• 推荐12个月内暂停妊娠。
• 由于将来妊娠时意外风险增大，应在妊娠早期进行超声评估。

随访建议

• 妇产科医师密切随访。
• 连续监测HCG水平：
- 每周1次至少连续4周，然后每月1次。
- 应该持续下降并且无上升趋势。
- 如果出现上升，应评估转移性疾病。
• 避孕。
• 超声检查：
- 将来妊娠时早期检查。
- 将来妊娠时出现葡萄胎的风险增加(第二次增加1%～1.5%，2次葡萄胎后增加20%)。

要点和误区

• 和误诊相关：
- 正常妊娠。
- 先兆子痫，尤其<24周孕龄。
- 正常妊娠剧烈呕吐。
• 必须强调随访的重要性：
- 如果不监测HCG，可能导致转移性疾病漏诊。
- 20%可发展为恶性肿瘤。

气喘 Wheezing

stephen K. Epstein 吴昊 李文放 译

基础知识

描述

- 由于湍流气流：
- 高频率的声音，频率在400Hz：
◦ 气体通过类似于振动簧片的狭窄气道。
- 当气流速度达到临界值时，支气管壁共振振动。
- 由2～5 mm的狭窄气道引起的。
- 喘息的时间很低，气道直径为5 mm。
- 气道<2 mm的气道不能传输声音，因为能量会随着摩擦而失去。
- 气道狭窄通常是由以下多个因素造成的：
- 收缩(如反应性呼吸道疾病)。
- 支气管旁间质水肿。
- 炎症。
- 阻塞。

病因

- 肺部(小气道)：
- 哮喘。
- 急性呼吸窘迫综合征。
- 速发型过敏反应。
- 吸入性肺炎：
◦ 随着吸入异物后，由于强烈的支气管痉挛，在起病的早期会发生气喘。
- 棉纤维吸入性肺炎。
- 暴露于棉粉尘的纺织工人的职业性肺病。
- 药物：
◦ 会导致血管性水肿或过敏反应。
◦ 血管紧张素转换酶抑制剂。
◦ β受体阻滞剂。
◦ 阿司匹林和NSAIDs。
- 在正常的患者中强制呼气。
- 过度通气。
- 慢性阻塞性肺疾病。
- 慢性肺源性心脏病。
- 化学性肺炎。
- 类癌肿瘤。
- 阵发性夜间呼吸困难。
- 肺水肿。
- 肺栓塞：
◦ 很少出现气促。
◦ 局灶性。
- 肺炎。
- 睡眠呼吸暂停综合征。
- 肺部(大气道)：
- 声带功能障碍(瘫痪、拮抗运动)。
- 异物。
- 会厌炎：
◦ 在10%的病例中会出现喘鸣。
- 白喉。
- 烟尘吸入。
- 支气管肿瘤。
- 气管肿瘤。

儿科注意事项

- 3岁以下患者的病毒性细支气管炎。
- 哮喘。
◦ 感染：
- 格鲁布性喉头炎。
- 鼻病毒。
- 会厌炎。
- 胃食管反流。
- 异物吸入。
- 先天性异常。
- 气管软化。
- 气管狭窄。
- 血管环。
- 囊性纤维化。
- 心脏病。
- 心因性呼吸窘迫。
- 以吸气时声带内收异常为特征的反常声带功能障碍。

诊断

症状和体征

- 在呼吸时发出的一声哨鸣音：
- 弥漫性。
◦ 与反应性呼吸道疾病或肺水肿一样。
- 局灶性：
◦ 类似肺炎或肺栓塞。
- 呼吸困难。
- 呼吸窘迫。
- 胸部疼痛。
- 咳嗽。
- 咳痰。
- 泡沫样痰(肺水肿)。
- 喘鸣。
- 发热。
- 发绀。
- 呼吸急促。
- 心动过速。

病史

- 目前的上呼吸道感染。
- 与反应性呼吸道有关的鼻病毒。
- 最近的检查：
- 运动诱发的哮喘、声带功能障碍。

体格检查

- 精神状态：
- 在呼吸窘迫的环境中，嗜睡、困惑和疲劳是气道管理的主要因素。
- 肌肉收缩。
- 肺部听诊。

基本检查

- 脉搏血氧测量：
- 用于评估严重程度，但不适用于预测住院治疗。
- 峰流量：
- 在评估住院治疗需求方面很有用。
- 胸部X线检查。

诊断检查与说明

实验室检查

- 动脉血气：
- 通过观察氧合下降，二氧化碳升高和酸中毒来判断患者是否呼吸衰竭。
- 对于是否需要气道管理，临床评估是一个更可靠的指标。
- 白细胞：
- 升高的白细胞并不能区分感染和其他疾病，因为血压会导致脱水。
- 在未感染的患者服用类固醇时，白细胞也升高了。
- 正常的白细胞不排除潜在的肺炎。

影像学检查

- 最大呼气流量(PEF)：
- 评估小气道的功能。
- 用于确定病情严重程度，并跟踪治疗反应性气道疾病患者的治疗进展。
- 胸部X线检查：
- 评估肺部疾病的诊断：
◦ 肺炎。
◦ 异物吸入。
- 评估肺水肿。
- 心电图：
- 适用于对于具有心脏缺血的风险时。
- 适用于所有由喘息引起肺水肿的病例。

Q

• 颈部软组织：
- 用于评估异物或阻碍肿块。

诊断步骤/外科

• 喉镜检查/支气管镜检查：
- 适用于梗阻性病变。
- 用于检查吸入异物或诊断潜在肿瘤。

■ 鉴别诊断

见病因。

治疗

■ 院前

• 吸氧。
• 指脉氧监测和心电监测。
• 对潜在条件进行初始治疗：
- 哮喘。
- 肺水肿。
• 对于呼吸衰竭或预期呼吸衰竭患者行气管插管。

■ 初步稳定/治疗

• 气道/呼吸/循环管理。
• 对即将发生的气道故障进行气管插管：
- 为可能的气道异物做好准备。
- 预测困难气道。

■ 急诊治疗/程序

• 纠正低氧血症：吸氧。
• 初步评估病情严重性：
- 中度：PEF≥40%。
- 重度：PEF<40%。
• 治疗原发病。
• 气流纠正气道梗阻：
- 支气管扩张药：
◦ 使用短效的β受体阻滞剂，如舒喘宁等短效药后，症状改善提示反应性呼吸道疾病。
- 抗胆碱能类：异丙托溴铵。
• 对于重度病情加重此类药物。
• 减少复发的可能性：
- 如果气喘是由支气管痉挛或非传染性炎症引起的，类固醇的使用能减少复发。
• 辅助治疗：
- 氦氧混合气：
◦ 比空气或氧气的密度更小。
◦ 减少呼吸功。
◦ 对于大呼吸道疾病更加有效。
◦ 对小气道疾病没有那么有效。
- 硫酸镁：
◦ 只对在中度到重度哮喘患者有疗效。
- 氯胺酮：
◦ 对哮喘患者行插管。

■ 药物治疗

一线用药

• 舒喘宁：2.5～5 mg＋2.5 ml 生理盐水 q20 min 吸入×3 剂量(儿童：每次 0.15 mg/kg，q20 min×3 剂；最小剂量 2.5 mg)。
• 左沙丁胺醇：0.63 mg，q8 h(儿童：6～12 岁 0.31 mg，q8 h；8～12 岁 0.63 mg，q8 h)通过喷雾装置。
• 泼尼松：40～80 mg，口服[儿童：1 mg/(kg·d)，分两次用，最大剂量 60 mg/d]。
• 泼尼松龙：儿童：1～2 mg/(kg·d)，分两次用，口服，在儿童剂量加入异丙托溴铵(儿童：12 岁 0.25～0.5 mg)。
• 外消旋肾上腺素：儿童 0.25～0.5 ml 对于喉头炎者雾化吸入。

二线用药

• 异丙托溴铵：0.5 mg，q20 min×3 剂量(儿童：0.25～0.5 mg，q20 min×3 剂)，可能与沙丁胺醇混合。
• 甲泼尼龙：40～80 mg，静脉注射[儿童：1～2 mg/(kg·d)静脉注射或口服，分 2 次]。剂量最大：对于不能口服患者，60 mg/d。
• 特布他林：0.25 mg，皮下注射，q0.5 h，2 剂(儿童：0.01 mg/kg，最大剂量 0.3 mg)：
- 在气溶胶疗法方面没有明显的优势。
• 硫酸镁：0.1 ml/kg 50%溶液静脉注射大于 20 min，然后是 0.06 mg/(kg·h)。

随访

■ 进一步处理

入院指征

• 缺氧。
• 喘息持续或恶化。
• 一般情况需要住院。

出院指征

• 喘息症状改善或解决。
• PEF>70%预测。
• 足够的氧化。

转诊问题

哮喘：
• 应提交一份书面的哮喘行动计划。
• 考虑开始吸入皮质类固醇。

■ 随访建议

患者若出现气短、发热、咯血或胸痛等症状即使返回到急诊室就诊。

要点和误区

如果使用抗焦虑的治疗，就要准备好气道管理。

气道辅助装置 Airway Adjuncts

David W. Schoenfeld 马林浩 林兆奋 译

基础知识

■ 描述

• 气道辅助装置是用于管理上呼吸道的装置。
• 在无法使用标准技术进行插管及难以进行面罩通气时经常用作救援技术或设备。
• 口腔和鼻咽气道：
- 减轻舌后坠。
- 在开放气道时配合定位辅助装置。
- 鼻咽反射正常时可以使用鼻咽通气道。
- 口咽部气道放置适用于鼻咽反射消失者。
• Extraglottic 设备(EGD)：
- 声门上(SGD)类(即 LMA、PAXpress、CobraPLA、iGel 等)。
- 这些装置在声门上面并包绕着声门。
- 声门后(RGD)或声门下(IGD)类(即 Combitube、King tube、Ruch EasyTube 等)。
- RGD/IGD 在下咽部通气并使食管闭塞。
• 盲插技术(限于特定设备)。
• 与 ET 管相比，减少了对误吸的保护。
• 放置 EGD 的成功率很高。

■ 流行病学

• 第一种气道管理方法成功率达 95%。

• 插管总体成功率为 98%。
• 4%的急诊室气道管理很困难。

诊断

■ 症状和体征

体格检查

• 难以面罩通气的预测因子(MOANS)。
- M：面罩密封(胡须/结构异常)。
- O：肥胖或阻塞。
- A：高龄(>55 岁)。
- N：没有牙齿。
- s：顺应性差。
• 喉镜检查和气管插管困难的预测因子(LEMON)。
- L：外形。
◦ 小颌畸形。
◦ 龅牙。
◦ 舌大。
◦ 颈部短。
- E：评估(3-3-2)。
◦ 嘴巴张开<3 指宽。
◦ 下颌骨水平长度<3 指宽。
◦ 甲颏距离<2 指宽。
- M：Mallampati 得分(难度阶梯式增加)。
◦ 一级：软腭、悬雍垂、咽门(喉头)、双侧颚弓可见。
◦ 二级：软腭、悬雍垂、喉头可见。
◦ 三级：可见软腭。
◦ 四级：只有硬腭可见。
- O：障碍物。
◦ 声音变化、声音听不清。
◦ 气道分泌物多。
◦ 喘鸣。
- N：颈部活动(受限)。
• 难以行环甲膜切开术的预测因子(SHORT)。
- S：手术或气道离断。
- H：血肿或感染。
- O：肥胖(通路问题)。
- R：放射物沾染。
- T：肿瘤。
• EGD 困难的预测因子(RODS)。
- R：张口受限。
- O：障碍物。
- D：气道解剖结构中断或扭曲。
- S：肺部顺应性差或颈椎损伤。

■ 诊断检查与说明

• 气道管理成功时脉搏血氧仪数值应升高或保持在高水平。
• 确认正确的位置。
• 纤维支气管镜检查(金标准)。
• 结束呼吸二氧化碳浓度测定/二氧化碳图(可靠率>99%)。
• 体格检查(常用但不可靠)。
• 胸廓起伏。
• 呼吸音的听诊未闻及上腹部声音。
• ETT 内部凝结。
• 一旦气道建立，动脉血气用于指导呼吸机参数设置。

影像学检查

胸部 X 线检查(CXR)：仅适用于气管内插管的患者以排除管插入主干支气管或气胸，并调整管的位置。

> **注意**
> CXR 无法排除气管插管误入插管。

治疗

■ 院前

• 需要院前气道管理的患者的选择因地区而异，包括：
- BVM 通气±OPA 或 NPA。
- 经口气管插管(±RSI)。
- 经鼻气管插管。
- EGD 放置。
- 手术开放气道。

■ 初步稳定/治疗

• 创伤患者保持颈椎固定在一条线。
• 氧气(通过可以回吸呼吸器或 BVM 的高流量)。
• 血管通路(用于液体复苏和药物管理)静脉注射或 IO。

■ 急诊治疗/程序

• 快速有序插管。
• 准备。
- 负压吸引，BVM，ETT，基础气道管理，救援气道管理，用药。
• 预氧合。
- NRB 或 BVM，FiO_2 100%，持续 3 min。
• 预处理。
- 尽量减少气道管理的不良反应。
- 怀疑 ICP 升高。
- 缺血性心脏病或主要血管离断、破裂。
- 成人患有明显的反应性气道疾病。
- 儿童年龄不超过 10 岁。
• 诱导麻痹。
- 诱导剂的给药。
- 快速有序地给予麻醉药。

> **注意**
> 在预期开放困难的气道，瘫痪是麻醉的相对禁忌证。
> • 体位。
> - 头部伸展(环状软骨压力)。
> • 放置管。
> • 插管后。
> - 确认 ETT 安置合适。
> - 使用苯二氮䓬类药物、阿片类药物、丙泊酚(异丙酚)或其他药剂。
> - 根据需要继续麻痹并结合充足的镇静作用。
> • 插管失败。
> • 失败后考虑其他插管技术或使用气道辅助。
> • 手术开放气道作为最后的手段。

■ 药物治疗

• 诱导：
- 依托咪酯：0.3 mg/kg，静脉注射。
- 氯胺酮：1～2 mg/kg，静脉注射；或 4～7 mg/kg，肌内注射。
- 咪达唑仑：0.07～0.3 mg/kg，静脉注射。
- 丙泊酚：2～2.5 mg/kg，静脉注射。
- 硫喷妥钠：3 mg/kg，静脉注射。
• 麻醉：
- 琥珀胆碱：1～1.5 mg/kg(儿童：2 mg/kg)，静脉注射；2.5 mg/kg，肌内注射或皮下注射。
- 罗库溴铵：1 mg/kg，静脉注射(麻醉剂量)；0.1 mg/kg，静脉注射(肌纤维收缩剂量)。
- 泮库溴铵：0.1 mg/kg，静脉注射(麻醉剂量)；0.01 mg/kg，静脉滴注(肌纤维收缩剂量)。
- 维库溴铵：0.1 mg/kg，静脉注射(麻醉剂量)；0.01 mg/kg，静脉滴注(肌纤维收缩剂量)。

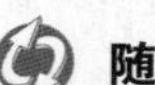

随访

■ 进一步处理

入院指征

几乎所有插管患者都应该入住 ICU 或在抢救室。

■ 出院指征

很少见，插管的急诊患者可能会在急诊室观察一段时间后拔管出院。

要点和误区

• 呼吸衰竭是一种危及生命的情况。

• 评估每位患者是否存在面罩通气或插管的困难。

• 在发生失败的尝试时始终制定备用计划。

• 不要固定插管，除非成功通气和氧合良好。

• 转向替代气道管理技术及考虑手术开放气道如果使用了气道辅助装置仍无法成功插管或进行通气。

儿科注意事项

• 口咽和鼻咽气道可用婴儿+尺寸。

• LMA 有婴儿+尺码可供选择。

• 联合导管仅适用于体长>48 in(1.2 m)的患者。

• 鼻气管插管在 10 岁以下的儿童是禁忌的。

气道管理 Airway Management

Thomas L. Knorr · Carlo L. Rosen 马林浩 林文放 译

Q

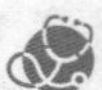

基础知识

■ 描述

• 确保充分氧合和通气的技术。
• 口腔和鼻咽气道：
- 抬高咽部舌后坠。
- 促进 BVM 通气。
- 咽反射消失时插入。
• 快速诱导插管(RSI)：
- 急诊口腔插管的优选方法(最小化吸入风险)。
- 快速诱导麻醉和麻醉维持。
- 禁忌证同普通麻醉。
- 具有替代方案的预先制定的备份气道技术至关重要。
- 使用纤支镜技术可最大限度地提高成功率。
• 口腔清醒插管：
- 仅行镇静进行口腔插管。
◦ 麻醉是有禁忌证时使用。
- 最常用的是氯胺酮。
◦ 与苯二氮䓬类药物一起使用。
• 口香糖弹性探针：
- 当声带可视性不佳时使用的气道辅助装置。
- 通过感觉探头撞击气管环确认放置位置。
- 在探条上滑动气管导管(ET 管)然后移除探条。
• 替代气道装置：
- 声门外的设备：
◦ 盲插入口咽并充气。
◦ 喉罩气道(LMA)在下咽部的声门结构周围形成密封。
◦ LMA 比 ET 管提供较少的防吸入保护。
◦ 插入 LMA 可用于放置 ET 管。
◦ 食管-气管导管(如 Combitube、King LT)闭塞食管并使下咽部通气。
- 视频喉镜：
◦ 喉镜刀片上的光纤摄像头(如 Glidescope、C-MAC)或 LMA 可视化管路放置。
- 纤支镜插管探针：
◦ 在探针尖端的光纤摄像头带有 ET 管(如 Shikani)。
• 经典纤支镜插管：
- ET 管放在支气管镜上。
- 鼻气管或口气管入路。
- 适应证：
◦ 声门可视化的解剖学限制。
◦ 下颌骨或颈椎活动受限。
◦ 颈椎损伤不稳定。
- 禁忌证：
◦ 需要立即进行气道管理。
◦ 明显的口咽出血。
• 鼻气管插管：
- 适应证：
◦ 口腔通路受损。
◦ 口腔插管不成功。
◦ 麻醉禁忌。
◦ 颈椎活动受限。
- 禁忌证：
◦ 呼吸暂停(唯一绝对禁忌证)。
◦ 抗凝。
◦ 面部、鼻腔或头部严重创伤。
◦ 上呼吸道脓肿。
◦ 会厌炎。
◦ 贯穿性颈部创伤。
• 环甲膜切开术：
- 对气道开放失败进行限定性的治疗。
- 环甲膜下的切口。
- 经皮造口气管切开插管。
- 适应证：
◦ 其他气道开放尝试失败时快速开放气道。
◦ 巨大的面部创伤。
◦ 上呼吸道完全阻塞。
- 禁忌证：
◦ 喉部挤压伤。
◦ 气管离断。
◦ 相对禁忌证：扩大Ⅱ区或Ⅲ区血肿。
• 无创正压通气：
- 不使用有创人工气道的通气支持。
- 通常通过口罩或鼻梁。
- 适应证：
◦ 合作患者。
◦ 院前无呼吸困难。
◦ 对于对治疗快速反应的疾病(COPD 和 CHF)最有效。
- 禁忌证：
◦ 顽固性呕吐。
◦ 上呼吸道阻塞。
◦ 无法保护呼吸道或清除分泌物。
◦ 血流动力学不稳定。
◦ 精神状态或昏迷改变。
◦ 心脏呼吸停止。
• 高流量鼻氧：
- 与常规鼻插管相比，加热，加湿的高流量氧气可提供更高的舒适度。
- 以 60 L/min 的速度提供高达 1.0 的 FiO_2。
- 提供最小的呼气末正压。
- 适应证：
◦ 低氧性呼吸衰竭，无高碳酸血症。
- 禁忌证：
◦ 鼻出血。
◦ 鼻阻塞。
◦ 基底部颅骨骨折。
• 经皮经喉通气(PTV)：
- 经皮通过环甲膜放置 12G 或 14G 导管。
- 用高压氧气进行间歇性通气。
- 适应证：
◦ 直至环甲膜切开术完成，经口腔或鼻腔插管失败。

- 禁忌证：
  ◦ 上呼吸道阻塞，阻碍呼气。

诊断

症状和体征

需要气道管理的临床情况：

• 未能维持或保护气道：
- 口咽肿胀。
- 咽反射消失。
- 无法清除分泌物，血液。
- 喘鸣。

• 缺氧或通气障碍：
- 呼吸急促。
- 精神状态改变。
- 意识状态改变（癫痫状态）。

• 预期的临床情况：
- 头部受伤或三环类药物过量的通气控制。
- 诊断或治疗程序的镇静。
- 如果气道情况可以，早期管理。

基本检查

• 在开始程序之前始终准备好困难的气道开放步骤。

• 识别开放困难的气道（LEMON）：
- 了解解剖学因素：
  ◦ 短领骨，颈部粗，口窄，大舌和突出的牙齿。
  ◦ 先天性综合征，肢端肥大症，肥胖。
- 评估 3-3-2 规则（遇到开放困难的气道）：
  ◦ 嘴巴张开<3 指宽。
  ◦ 下颌骨水平长度<3 指宽。
  ◦ Thyromental 距离<2 指宽。
- MALLAMPATI 标准（梯次增加难度）：
  ◦ 一类：完全显露声门。
  ◦ 二级：软腭、悬雍垂、喉头可见。
  ◦ 三级：软腭可见。
  ◦ 四级：仅硬腭可见。
- 来自潜在疾病状态的阻塞：
  ◦ 血管神经性水肿。
  ◦ 甲状腺肿
  ◦ 喉气管肿瘤。
  ◦ 颈部放射治疗史。
  ◦ 感染（会厌炎、声门上炎、格鲁布性喉头炎、口内或咽后脓肿、脓性颌下炎）。
  ◦ 大量上消化道出血。
  ◦ 创伤（面部、颈部、颈椎、喉-气管、烧伤）。
- 颈部移动限制：
  ◦ 类风湿关节炎和其他关节病降低颈椎活动度。
  ◦ 脊柱制动用于创伤。

• 验证正确的置管位置：
- 可视管路通过声门。
- 气管导管深度（管尖至上切牙）：
  ◦ 21 cm（女）。
  ◦ 23 cm（男）。
  ◦ 年龄（年）/2+12（儿童）。
- 呼气末 CO_2 比色装置：
  ◦ 如果存在 CO_2，则颜色改变，表示管放在气管。
  ◦ 心搏骤停时可能看不到颜色变化。
- 在胃、腋窝和前部肺野听诊。
- 观察胸壁运动。
- 通气期间管中冷凝。

诊断检查与说明

实验室检查

• 气管插管后脉搏血氧饱和度会升高。

• 连续二氧化碳图用作辅助手段。

• 插管后用动脉血气管理呼吸机参数。

影像学检查

CXR：

• 排除主干支气管插管或气胸。

• 不排除食管插管。

诊断步骤/外科

直接可视 ET 管通过声带是金标准。

鉴别诊断

• 插管进入食管。

• 右侧或左侧主干支气管插管。

• 通过梨状窦或气管撕裂口将管插入气管外。

• 气胸。

治疗

院前

呼吸停止患者的高级生命支持提供选择：

• 急救时进行确定的气道管理，随后进行袋式阀管理（BVM）。

• 气管插管。

• 食管-气管导管。

• LMA。

初步稳定/治疗

• 创伤患者颈椎制动成一直线。

• 氧气，监护，静脉给药。

急诊治疗/程序

• RSI：
- 同时给予镇静剂（诱导剂）和麻醉药为紧急气道管理提供最佳条件。

• 准备设备：
- 负压吸引、BVM、各种尺寸的 ET 管和喉镜刀片、导丝、药物和备份设备。

• 预氧合：
- 诱导和麻痹之前 3 min 内 1.0 的 FiO_2。
- 通过无呼吸器和鼻导管麻痹后的呼吸性充氧。

• 预处理：
- 预防插管的生理后遗症。
- 在麻醉前 3 min 进行。
- 非去极化剂量的肌松药。
- 芬太尼和利多卡因可以最小限度地使 ICP 升高和降低头部受伤患者行气管插管的血流动力学反应。
- 利多卡因和沙丁胺醇在反应性气道疾病中的作用。

• 诱导麻醉：
- 诱导剂的给药（如依托咪酯、硫喷妥钠、咪达唑仑、氯胺酮）。
- 快速跟进麻醉药（如琥珀胆碱、罗库溴铵）。
  ◦ 琥珀胆碱相对禁忌。
- 预期困难的口腔插管，开放的球部损伤，有机磷中毒，烧伤>3 日，去神经支配综合征，肌病和疑似高钾血症。
  ◦ 非去极化剂（如罗库溴铵）可以用作琥珀胆碱的替代品。

• 体位：
- 头部伸展，如果是创伤患者保持中线颈椎稳定。
- 环形压力（Sellick 策略）是有争议的和可选的。

• 放置管：
- 肌肉张力消失后（琥珀胆碱给药 45～60 s 后）。
- 使用 ET 管的导丝。
- 通过声带置管。
- 气囊充气。
- 开始通气。
- 确认正确的 ET 管放置。

• 插管后：
- 用于治疗的苯二氮䓬类药物，阿片类药物或丙泊酚持续镇静。
- 维库溴铵可用于麻醉维持。

儿科注意事项

• 估计 ET 管尺寸：4+年龄/4。

• 8 岁以下的患者可使用无气囊 ET 管。

• 直接米勒刀片适用于<3 岁的患者。

• 环甲软骨切开术禁用于<12 岁的患者，PTV 是首选的。

• 使用阿托品作为预处理以减少分泌物并减弱迷走神经的影响。

Q

· 神经肌肉阻滞剂对于＜5 岁的孩子来说是不必要的。

用药治疗

· 阿曲库铵：0.4～0.5 mg/kg，静脉注射。
· 阿托品：0.02 mg/kg，静脉注射。
· 地西泮：2～10 mg（儿童：0.2～0.3 mg/kg），静脉注射。
· 依托咪酯：0.3 mg/kg，静脉注射。
· 芬太尼：3 μg/kg，静脉注射。
· 氯胺酮：1～2 mg/kg，静脉注射；或 4～7 mg/kg，肌内注射。
· 利多卡因：1.5 mg/kg，静脉注射。
· 咪达唑仑：1～5 mg，静脉注射（0.07～0.30 mg/kg）用于麻醉诱导。
· 丙泊酚：2～2.5 mg/kg，静脉注射。
· 泮库溴铵：0.01 mg/kg，静脉注射（肌松剂量）；0.1 mg/kg，静脉注射（麻醉剂量）。
· 罗库溴铵：1 mg/kg，静脉注射。
· 琥珀胆碱：1.5 mg/kg（儿童：2 mg/kg），静脉注射；2.5 mg/kg，肌内注射或皮下注射。
· 硫喷妥钠：3 mg/kg，静脉注射。
· 维库溴铵：0.01 mg/kg，静脉注射（肌松剂量）；0.1 mg/kg，静脉注射（麻醉剂量）。

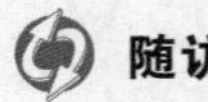

随访

进一步处理

入院指征

几乎所有插管患者都应该入住 ICU。

出院指征

很少见，紧急患者已经进行插管用于气道保护或便于诊断检查，可能会在急救室观察一段时间后拔管出院。

要点和误区

重视呼吸道管理。插管和通气失败是危及生命的情况：

· 评估每位患者是否有插管困难。
· 准备并熟悉所需的一切设备和药物（包括禁忌证和副作用）。
· 开始操作前始终制定备份计划应对气道崩溃或标准的经口插管失败的情况。

气胸 Pneumothorax

William A. Porcaro 瞿金龙 译

基础知识

描述

· 胸腔内存在游离气体。
· 自发性气胸是指非外伤引起的支气管、肺泡等破裂引起气体进入胸膜腔。
· 原发性自发性气胸（2/3）：
- 无潜在的肺病存在。
- 胸膜下肺泡破裂。
- 年轻健康的患者（20～40 岁），高瘦体型多见。
- 高危因素：吸烟、家族史、马方综合征、同型胱氨酸尿症、胸腔内子宫内膜异位症等。
· 继发性自发性气胸：有原发性肺脏疾病史。
· 张力性气胸：
- 气体持续进入胸膜腔通过支气管肺泡的损伤处，胸膜腔压力越来越大。
- 胸膜腔压力增大。
- 静脉回流右心血减少，导致心排血量减少。
- 纵隔摆向无气胸侧。
- 通气/血流值不协调导致缺氧，低氧血症发生。

病因

· 自发性。
· 气道疾病：
- COPD。
- 哮喘。
- 囊性纤维化。
· 感染：
- 坏死性细菌感染性肺炎。
- 结核。
- 肺部真菌感染。
- 卡氏肺孢子病。
· 肺部肿瘤，新生物形成。
· 间质性肺疾病：
- 结节病。
- 自发性肺纤维化。
- 淋巴管肌瘤病。
- 结节性硬化。
- 尘肺。
· 结缔组织病。
· 肺梗死。
· 子宫内膜异位症。
· 钝性胸部创伤。
· 颈部或躯干穿透性创伤。
· 操作失误：
- 中心静脉置管。
- 其他血管置管。

诊断

症状和体征

病史

· 严重程度与气胸大小有关。
· 患侧胸痛：
- 锐利的胸膜痛。
- 突然发生。
- 钝痛持续存在。
· 气短。
· 很少咳嗽，全身乏力。

体格检查

· 呼吸困难。
· 自发性单纯气胸，一般心率＜120 次/分。
· 颈静脉怒张。
· 心肺检查：
- 双侧呼吸音不对称，呼吸音减低。
- 叩诊鼓音。
· 张力性气胸：
- 低血压。
- 心动过速＞120 次/分。
- 出汗。
- 发绀。
- 心血管系统异常。
- 双肺叩诊不对称。

基本检查

· 影像学检查是主要的手段。
· 如果血流动力学不稳定或有明显的临床证据，及时处理。

实验室检查

动脉血气提示低氧血症。

影像学检查

· CXR。

- 胸部正位片。
• 如果患者不能耐受立位片，可以拍卧位。
- 外侧见肺缺损，外周明显看出胸膜线。
- 纵隔偏移。
- 呼吸深凹症。
• 前位看，肋膈角比健侧增大。
• 膈可以往反的方向打的凹陷：
- 评估气胸大小，决定临床治疗方法。
• 呼气片：
- 可以提示小的气胸，但是并不能提高气胸的检出率。
• 胸部 CT：
- 对小的气胸也能敏感地提示。
• 超声：
- 需要有经验的医师。
- 床边快速诊断。
- 缺乏肺的移动和气胸彗尾症。
- M 模式可以确认气胸的胸膜界。
- 对于有经验的医师，敏感性超过胸片。

诊断步骤/外科

心电图。
• 用来排除胸痛的心脏方面的因素。
• T 波非特异性的改变，心电轴左偏，R 波减低。

■ 鉴别诊断

• 急性腹部疾病。
• 主动脉瘤或夹层。
• 哮喘加重。
• 胸壁痛。
• COPD 急性加重。
• 心肌梗死。
• 心包炎。
• 胸膜炎。
• 纵隔积气。
• 肺栓塞。

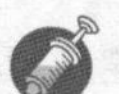

治疗

■ 院前

注意

不平稳的患者如果怀疑张力性气胸，需紧急行胸膜腔穿刺术。

■ 初步稳定/治疗

• 心电监测。
• 氧饱和度监测。
• 面罩吸氧。
• 静脉通路建立。
• 张力性气胸要求尽快行胸膜腔穿刺术。
• 胸腔穿刺术：
- 张力性气胸患者尽快行胸腔穿刺术置管。
- 14～18 号导管在第 2 肋间或者第 4 或第 5 肋间腋前线。
- 提醒：标准导管在部分患者太短可以选择长的导管。

■ 急诊治疗/程序

• 非创伤性气胸肺压缩<15%，无明显心血管和呼吸系统症状。
- 吸氧支持，观察 4～6 h。
- 复查胸片，如果无明显变化可予以出院。
• 单纯吸出：
- 指征：
◦ 简单的气胸，肺压缩 15%～30%。
◦ 在观察中气胸的变化。
- 留置带有三通的导管排气(8F)。
- 单纯吸出，一般不超过 3 L。
- 如果连续 2 次超过 4 h 的胸片未见气胸，可将导管拔除。
- 如果拔除导管后 2 h，患者胸片正常，可予以出院。
- 如果气胸仍未吸收，可以第二次抽出气体。
• Heimlich 翼瓣引流管：
- 吸出失败后。
- 连接 Heimlich 翼瓣引流管至导管或胸管。
• 吸引：
- Heimlich 翼瓣引流管失败。
- 20 cmH_2O 压力持续吸引。
- 急诊室观察 1 h。
• 胸腔闭式引流：
- 指征：
◦ 张力性气胸。
◦ 胸部枪击伤。
◦ 胸部钝击伤或贯通伤。
◦ 正压通气呼吸机支持患者，对于任何大小的气胸。
◦ 气胸肺压缩>30%。
◦ 继发性气胸。
◦ 张力性气胸穿刺针治疗后的最终治疗方法。
- 导管尺寸：
◦ 自发性气胸 7～14 号导管。
◦ 继发性自发性气胸 20～28 号导管。
◦ 胸腔积液或机械通气患者选择 28 号的导管。
- 导管打折可以通过旋转导管实现。
- 导管所有的侧孔必须全部放入胸腔。
- 导管需连接水封瓶。
- 在病情稳定的患者 Heimlich 翼瓣引流管可取代水封瓶。
- 防止发生肺复张性肺水肿。
• 可能的并发症：
- 肋间血管损伤出血。
- 引流不充分：
◦ 导管打折。
◦ 导管堵塞。
◦ 胸腔漏气。
- 复张性肺水肿：
◦ 液体复苏。

■ 药物治疗

• 局部麻醉：
- 1%利多卡因和 1∶100 000 肾上腺素。
- 7 mg/kg 最大剂量 500 mg。
• 稳定患者，镇静治疗。
• 干净伤口无需使用抗生素。

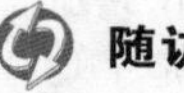

随访

■ 进一步处理

入院指征

• 张力性气胸。
• 需要留置胸管。

出院指征

• 气胸量<15%，未见明显增大，在急诊室内已经充分成功地抽出气体。
- 出院后 24 h 和 1 周复查胸片。
• 可靠的患者无通气障碍，并且成功抽出气体或带有安全的导管和 Heimlich 翼瓣引流管。
- 出院后 24～48 h 随访。
- 48 h 的随访：
◦ 夹管，观察 2 h，复查胸部 X 线片。
◦ 如果气胸明显吸收或者改善予以拔管。
◦ 观察 2 h，复查胸部 X 线片。
◦ 如果没有增加，可以出院后 24 h 和 1 周复查胸部 X 线片。
• 如果出现新的胸痛或呼吸困难，及时急诊就诊。
• 1 周后复查无明显增加或气胸明显减少，急诊就诊时需要胸外科医师会诊。

转诊问题

药物或胸部引流治疗。

Q

要点和误区

• 如果患者不稳定不及时处理可能引起血流动力学不稳定。

• 避免使用劣质的导管，包括出现打折、过深等等，避免二次留置导管。

• 避免过低留置管，可能出现腹部损伤。

• 不要漏诊下颈部或纵隔损伤。

• 如果出现纵隔积气，需要考虑食管的穿孔。

气压伤 Barotrauma

Nicole L. Lunceford 宋振举 童朝阳 译

基础知识

描述

气体在封闭的空间扩张或收缩造成的损伤。

病因

• 当充气空间不能用外部压力平衡其压力时会导致组织损伤。
• 波义耳定律：在恒定的温度下，压力(P)与体积(V)成反比：
- PV=K(常数)或 $P_1V_1=P_2V_2$。
- 随着压力的增加/减少，体积减小/增加。
• 固体和液体充满的空间压力是平均分配的。
• 体积变化在离表面最近的几英尺处最大。
• 身体内的充气腔体会发生膨胀或收缩：
- 外部物体：
◦ 潜水服，面罩里的气袋会膨胀和收缩。
- 副鼻窦：
◦ 下潜的气压伤。
◦ 压力平衡受到鼻腔的影响，导致窦腔负压。
◦ 额窦最常受影响。
- 外耳：
◦ 下潜的气压伤。
◦ 外耳道的堵塞使空气不能进入，导致真空。
- 中耳：
◦ 下潜的气压伤。
◦ 是最常见的气压伤部位。
◦ 发现于 30% 的经验不丰富的潜水员和 10% 的经验丰富的潜水员。
◦ 咽鼓管为中耳提供唯一的压力平衡路径。
◦ 通过咽鼓管排气不足，导致跨鼓膜(TM)的负压力梯度逐渐增大。
- 内耳：
◦ 下潜的气压伤。
◦ 由于中耳和内耳的压力差快速增大(Valsalva、Frenzel 动作、快速下降)。
◦ 内耳压力增加可能导致圆形或椭圆形窗口破裂。
◦ 常伴有中耳气压伤。
- 牙齿：
◦ 在牙齿内部或周围有封闭气腔。
- 胃肠道：
◦ 上浮的气压伤。
◦ 由于外部压力下降，胃肠道中的吞入的气体膨胀。
- 肺：
◦ 上浮的气压伤。
◦ 肺部气体扩张(声门闭塞、支气管痉挛)导致肺泡膨胀。
◦ 可导致肺泡破裂。
◦ 最常见的是纵隔症。
◦ 可导致动脉气体栓塞(AGE)(见“动脉气体栓塞”)。
◦ 潜水员的肺顺应性下降、肺容积增大的风险增加[慢性阻塞性肺疾病(COPD)、哮喘]。

诊断

症状和体征

• 面部：
- 封闭的潜水面罩：结膜出血，面部水肿和肿胀。
• 四肢：
- 紧身潜水服：气袋位置的皮肤水肿和红斑。
• 鼻旁窦(气压鼻窦炎)：
- 鼻窦充血，疼痛，鼻出血。
- 上颌牙痛。
- 来自第五对脑神经失常的头晕、嘴唇麻木。
• 外耳：
- 可能因紧身的头罩、耳塞或耳垢堵塞导致。
- 耳道黏膜变得水肿，然后出血，最终撕裂。
• 中耳(气压炎症导致)：
- 开始于堵塞感。
- 随着跨越鼓膜的压差不断增加，疼痛越来越严重。
- 进展至撕裂鼓膜。
- 鼓膜外观：
◦ 从正常表现到水肿到出血到鼓膜撕裂，逐步进展(Teed 分类)。
• 内耳：
- 耳鸣，听力下降和眩晕。
- 类似症状以内耳减压病(通常较少眩晕)。
• 牙齿(气压性牙痛)：
- 严重的牙齿疼痛：可能是空气被困在填塞物中。
• 胃肠道(气体性消化道痛)：
- 大量嗳气。
- 胀气。
- 腹胀。
• 肺[肺气压伤(PBT)或肺超压综合征]：
- 局限性肺损伤。
◦ 胸痛，咳嗽，咯血。
- 皮下气肿。
- 纵隔积气。
◦ 胸部疼痛，颈部胀满。
- 气胸。
◦ 胸痛(胸膜炎性的)，呼吸困难。
- 延迟症状包括颈部外观饱满，吞咽困难，语音变化。

病史

详细了解潜水史和与潜水有关的症状时间(上升，下降，延迟)。

体格检查

• 鼓膜损伤、破裂的耳鼻喉科检查。
• 胸壁、颈部检查皮下气肿。
• 肺的气胸检查。
• 内耳病变特征性的失平衡、共济失调的神经科检查。

基本检查

临床诊断：细致的体检(如上)和详细的病史应指导各项检查。

■ 诊断检查与说明

实验室检查

血气分析用于存在肺部症状的患者。

影像学

• 鼻窦成像：
- CT。
- X线平片。
• X线胸片用于鉴别肺气压伤。
• 腹部系列(立位、卧位)鉴别内脏破裂释放的游离气体。

■ 鉴别诊断

• 减压病。
• 中耳炎。
• 外耳炎。
• 鼻窦炎。

治疗

■ 院前

• 对于下潜的气压伤，除非存在含气腔破裂，预计回到正常气压下疾病不会进展。
• 如果患者需要排出气体，将舱内压力保持在1个大气压或飞行高度在1 000 if 以下，以避免气压伤。

■ 初步稳定/治疗

ABC管理：
• 对于出现不适的患者用纯氧。
• 颈部皮下气肿患者需插管。
• 如有张力性气胸的证据，需据立即用针进行胸腔造瘘。

■ 急诊治疗/程序

• 为不稳定的患者建立静脉补液通路。
• 控制耳或鼻的出血。
• 严重气胸需胸腔置管。
• 减充血剂治疗中耳或鼻窦充血。
• 鼓膜或鼻窦撕裂需用抗生素。
• 止痛药。

■ 药物治疗

• 阿莫西林：250～500 mg[儿童：40 mg/(kg·24 h)]，口服，每日3次。
• 甲氧苄啶-磺胺甲噁唑(复方新诺明)：

复合剂型(160 mg/800 mg)[儿童：40 mg/200 mg/5 ml，5 ml/(10 kg·剂)]，口服，每日2次。
• 羟甲唑啉(阿弗林)0.05%：每鼻孔2或3滴/喷雾，每日2次，持续3日。
• 伪麻黄碱(苏达菲)：60 mg[儿童：6～12岁，30 mg；2～5岁，15 mg/剂]，口服，每4～6 h。

随访

■ 进一步处理

入院指征

• 肺气压伤。
• 伴有圆窗破裂或严重眩晕的内耳气压伤。

出院指征

• 大多数非肺气压伤。
• 耳鼻喉科随访严重鼓膜或鼻窦病患。

■ 随访建议

有鼓膜或内耳相关破裂征象转诊耳鼻喉科。

要点和误区

• 密切关注有气压伤的患者的减压病发展。
• 针对气胸征象仔细进行肺部检查。
• 对患者有肺气压伤的患者进行详细的病史记录，任何神经系统症状史表明有动脉气体栓塞。

憩室病 Diverticulosis

Joseph S. Palter 谭美春 张连东 译

基础知识

■ 描述

• 由于结肠肌肉功能障碍，通常为获得性单(憩室)或多(憩室)肠壁膨出。
• 次序：
- 膳食纤维量不足引起粪便体积减小。
- 为推动粪便通过结肠，结肠收缩力增加，导致肠腔内压增高。
- 压力增加使黏膜和黏膜下层在固有肌层的最弱点膨出，形成直肠憩室。

■ 病因

• 本病见于全消化道，以结肠最常见：
- 左侧95%(西方国家)。
- 右侧70%(亚洲国家)。
- 最常见的部位是乙状结肠。
• 假憩室：
- 只有黏膜和黏膜下层膨出。
- 最常见的形式是结肠憩室。
- 真正的先天性憩室(罕见)包含所有肠壁层。
• 在西方社会中常见，主要由于精细的饮食和纤维摄入不足。
• 患病率与年龄相关：
- 60岁时为50%，80岁时为70%。
- 对男性和女性的影响相同。
• 并发症：
- 70%无症状。
- <5%发展为憩室炎。
- 5%～15%发生出血，肥胖是一个危险因素。
  ◦ 75%的病例出血自行停止。
- 炎症(憩室炎)。
- 大动脉出血通常见于右结肠：
  ◦ 粪石(干燥、坚硬的硬粪便)侵蚀大动脉分支。
- 穿孔。
- 脓肿。
- 梗阻。

诊断

■ 症状和体征

病史

• 慢性或间歇性腹痛。
- 通常与进食有关。
- 有时因胀气或肠蠕动缓解。
• 排便模式的改变。
- 便秘(50%)或腹泻(25%)。
• 消化不良。
• 无痛血便；75%自限性。
- 来源于左结肠：鲜红色。
- 来源于右结肠：黑色或栗色，与粪便混合在一起。

- 憩室炎和憩室出血多独立存在，很少同时起病。

体格检查

- 不发热。
- 腹部检查通常为良性，但是表现多变：
  - 左下腹压痛。
  - 左下腹可触及坚硬的乙状结肠。
- 直肠检查表现多样：
  - 便血阴性。
  - 如果憩室出血则出现血便。

基本检查

全面的病史和必要的体格检查，避免过度检查。

诊断检查与说明

- 实验室检查：
  - 无症状憩室。
  - 不需要检查，经常是偶然发现的。
- 当前症状无并发症的憩室病(SUDD)：
  - 不需要检查。
- 新发单纯疼痛疾病：
  - 需要排除恶性肿瘤(如B症状和/或粪隐血阴性)。
  - 血细胞计数检测白细胞增多或贫血。
  - 尿检排除血尿或脓尿。
- 出血性憩室：
  - 血细胞计数。
  - 电解质、尿素氮、肌酐、血糖、钙。
  - 血型及4单位浓缩红细胞交叉配血。
  - 凝血酶原时间、部分凝血酶时间及国际标准化比值。
  - 心电图。

影像学检查

- 当前症状无并发症的憩室病(SUDD)：
  - 腹部和骨盆的CT或CT结肠镜检查：
    - 急诊诊断的标准。
    - 极好的敏感性和特异性。
    - 比结肠镜检查或乙状结肠镜检查更容易漏诊。
  - 结肠镜检查：
    - 憩室病是常规检查中最常偶然发现的。
    - 如果考虑到急性憩室炎有穿孔的风险，一般应避免。
  - 灵活的乙状结肠镜检查。
- 出血性憩室病：
  - 结肠镜检查。
    - 憩室出血诊断和治疗的首选初始方法。
    - 能够直接观察出血。
    - 对于大量/快速出血不太成功，因为无法观察出血部位。
  - 放射性核素显像。
    - 安全，不需要肠道准备。
    - 出血部位定位能力差。
    - 由于放射性同位素的半衰期长(24～36 h)，检测间歇性出血较理想。
    - 没有治疗干预的可能，但对血管造影有帮助。
  - 传统的血管造影。
    - 对结肠镜检查不能确定出血部位，且出血速度至少0.5 ml/min的活动性出血有帮助。
    - 定位出血部位(在放射性核素扫描后更准确)。
    - 可以治疗。
    - 有肠梗死风险。
  - CT血管造影术：
    - CT血管造影术的作用可能会越来越大，尤其是在其他成像方式不可用的情况下。
    - 如果需要的话可以帮助指导外科手术治疗。
  - 钡餐灌肠：
    - 钡灌肠曾经是诊断标准，现在由于检查时间长、并发症风险和辐射暴露，通常不主张使用。

鉴别诊断

- 疼痛性憩室病：
  - 肠易激综合征(几乎相同的临床表现)。
  - 憩室炎。
  - 结肠癌。
  - 克罗恩病。
  - 泌尿系统(肾绞痛)。
  - 妇科病(破裂或扭转的卵巢囊肿)。
- 出血性憩室病：
  - 痔。
  - 肛裂。
  - 直肠炎。
  - 结肠炎。
  - 恶性肿瘤。
  - 息肉。
  - 缺血性肠炎。
  - 血管畸形。
  - 淀粉样变性。
  - 血管性肠内瘘。
  - 上消化道出血。

治疗

院前

- 当腹痛原因不明时避免使用阿片类药物。
- 建立静脉通路。
- 大量出血或低血压：
  - 1～2 L(20 ml/kg)0.9%氯化钠注射液。
  - 头低足高位。

初步稳定/治疗

- 出血憩室病(大量)：
  - 评估气道、呼吸和循环。
  - 放置两个大口径静脉导管或额外的中心静脉导管通路进行大容量复苏。
  - 如果低血压，初始晶体液输注是合适的。
  - 考虑通过机构大量输血方案使用血液制品；理想情况下，红细胞：血小板：血浆的比例为1：1：1。
  - 如果类型和交叉尚未确定，则使用O阴性血(女性)和O阳性血(男性)。
  - 如果患者接受了抗凝治疗，可能需要适当的拮抗剂。
  - 必要时放置鼻胃管以排除上消化道出血。
  - 导尿管以监测尿量。
  - 对于持续出血即将发生的出血性休克患者请消化内科和外科医师会诊(大多数憩室出血会自动停止)。

急诊治疗/程序

- 有症状无并发症的憩室病：
  - 常推荐高纤维饮食，但几乎没有高质量的证据支持。
  - 解痉药可能对部分肠易激综合征和突发性腹泻患者有作用。
  - 美沙拉嗪可能会控制症状，但应由消化专家开具。
  - 益生菌被认为有助于胃肠蠕动和降低管腔内压力。
  - 腹部热敷。
  - 安慰患者。
  - 避免使用通便泻药。
- 出血性憩室病(大量)：
  - 初始症状稳定(见上文)。
  - 结肠镜检查是诊断和潜在的手段。
  - 放射性核素扫描；敏感且无创，但只针对活动性出血。
  - 选择性血管造影与注射血管加压素控制出血。
  - 栓塞术、介入放射术，可予以手术前选择应用。
  - 手术干预部分结肠切除术。

药物治疗

- 双环胺：20 mg，口服或肌内注射，每日4

次(不静脉注射)。

• 丙胺太林：15 mg，口服，30 min，饭前或睡前。

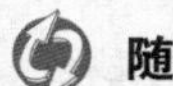

随访

进一步处理

入院指征

• 大量出血且生命体征不稳定的憩室病患者收入ICU。

• 轻度或间歇性憩室病，病情稳定从而可以确定出血部位通过评估选择明确的治疗。

出院指征

• 无并发症的症状性憩室病。

• 病情稳定粪微量隐血，胃吸取物阴性，无贫血，并且无其他并发症。

转诊问题

结肠镜检查后应消化科消随诊。

随访建议

• 病情初步稳定患者在48 h内行结肠镜检查。

• 停止抗凝药物、阿司匹林和非甾抗炎药。

• 没有证据支持禁食坚果、玉米、爆米花。

要点和误区

• 10%便血有上消化道来源。

• 大多数病例(75%～95%)可自行缓解或保守治疗。

• 9%～19%的患者出现大量失血，特别是那些伴发疾病或年龄大者。

• 结肠镜检查是病情稳定患者的首选诊断程序。

Q

憩室炎 Diverticulitis

Joseph S. Palter 谭美春 译

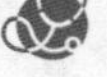

基础知识

描述

• 微小或巨大的憩室穿孔：

- 单纯性(75%)与复杂性。

• 发病率增加：

- 憩室疾病增加=憩室炎增加。
- 西方饮食习惯的增加导致发病率增加。

病因

• 憩室内的粪便变硬，形成粪石，增加腔内压力。

• 侵蚀憩室壁导致炎症反应。

• 局灶性坏死导致穿孔。

• 微小穿孔：单纯性憩室炎。

- 结肠壁增厚。
- 炎性改变(CT上的脂肪间隙)。

• 巨大穿孔：复杂性憩室炎。

- 脓肿。
- 肠梗阻。
- 反复发作后的瘘。
- 结肠膀胱瘘(最常见)出现排尿困难、尿频、尿急、气尿和粪尿。
- 腹膜炎。

诊断

症状和体征

病史

• 典型症状通常在几日内进展：

- 几乎50%之前有过疼痛发作。

• 西方国家70%的病例有左下腹疼痛：

- 最初是模糊的，然后局限化。
- 75%的亚洲患者有右下腹疼痛。

• 恶心、呕吐、便秘、腹泻、泌尿系统症状(按递减顺序)。

体格检查

• 轻度发热或无发热伴无并发症憩室炎。

• 并发憩室炎引起的高热伴腹膜炎或败血症。

• 左下腹压痛偶伴触及蜂窝织炎(20%)：

- 蜂窝织炎，肠袢发炎或脓肿。

• 腹胀。

• 肠鸣音变化。

• 直肠触痛伴粪隐血阳性：

- 大量直肠出血(罕见)。

• 腹膜炎(肌卫、板状腹)伴穿孔或脓肿破裂。

• 如果有以下情况，查体不易发现阳性结果：

- 老年人。
- 免疫功能低下。
- 服用糖皮质激素。

基本检查

• 全血细胞计数。

• 尿酸。

• 血培养和乳酸：

- 如果出现脓毒症的迹象。

• 腹部、骨盆CT：

- 首选诊断方法。
- 口服和静脉造影剂对比检查对憩室的诊断有97%的敏感性，99%的特异性。
- 能诊断引起腹痛的非憩室性原因。
- 首选胃泌素造影剂(水溶性)；避免钡剂造影，特别是考虑到可能有穿孔时。

诊断检查与说明

实验室检查

• 全血细胞计数：

- 白细胞增多常见，但没有时不能排除诊断。

• 尿常规：

- 可能有无菌脓尿。
- 结肠菌群(细菌)提示结肠膀胱瘘。

影像学检查

• 腹部(卧位和立位)和胸部X线平片：

- 游离气体提示穿孔。
- 气-液平面提示梗阻。

• CT：

- 诊断标准包括：
    - 肠壁增厚>4 mm。
    - 憩室的存在。
    - 结肠周围脂肪炎。
    - 代替静脉的软组织肿块。
    - 结肠周围积液/脓肿。
- 复杂憩室炎的诊断标准：
    - 小的结肠周围脓肿。
    - 大的结肠周围脓肿。
    - 穿孔性憩室炎伴腹膜炎。
    - 自由穿孔伴粪性腹膜炎。

• 内镜/结肠镜检查：

- 诊断急性疾病无需使用。
- 硬式乙状结肠镜检查有助于诊断腹痛的非憩室性病因(痉挛、狭窄、水肿、脓或憩室周围红斑)。

• 超声检查：
- 诊断结肠壁增厚、炎症、肿块、脓肿或瘘。
- 极大地依赖于操作者。
- 肠道存在气体时不可靠。
• 钡剂灌肠：
- 曾经是诊断的标准，现在由于检查时间长、并发症的风险和辐射暴露而普遍不提倡。

■ 鉴别诊断

• 结肠癌伴穿孔。
• 缺血性结肠炎。
• 细菌性结肠炎。
• 急性阑尾炎：
- 如因阑尾破裂致腹膜炎，有左侧疼痛。
- 右侧憩室疼痛伴盲肠憩室（罕见）或乙状结肠冗长。
• 炎症性肠病。
• 缺血性肠病。
• 肠梗阻。
• 肠易激综合征。
• 卵巢囊肿破裂或扭转。
• 胰腺疾病。
• 盆腔炎性疾病。
• 消化性溃疡疾病。
• 肾绞痛。

治疗

■ 院前

• 当病因不确定时，避免在腹痛中使用阿片类制剂。
• 重新建立静脉通道。
• 建议静脉注射晶体液。

■ 初步稳定/治疗

• 用生理盐水液体复苏。
• 肠道休息：
- 禁食或无渣流质饮食。
- 如持续呕吐或怀疑肠梗阻者使用鼻胃管（NG管）。

■ 急诊治疗/程序

• 复发性无并发症/轻度憩室炎：
- 与前几次憩室炎有类似症状的稳定患者给予有限的评估。
- 使用广谱口服抗生素的预防性药物治疗（见下文）。
- 密切随访以评估症状缓解情况。
• 新的无并发症/轻度憩室炎或诊断不明确：
- 通过影像学明确诊断（急诊时首选的CT检查）。
- 广谱抗生素（见下文）。
- 保守治疗有90%的成功率。
- 抗生素可能不会缓解症状，但可能会减少复发和以后的并发症。
- 新的憩室炎的确诊病例应转至消化科进行缓解后结肠镜检查。
• 复杂的憩室炎：
- 广谱抗生素。
- 入院治疗。
- 外科会诊（见下文）：
◦ CT引导经皮脓肿引流。
◦ 治疗感染和并发症的外科手术。
• 镇痛：
- 抗胆碱能药（双环胺）：
◦ 减少结肠痉挛。
◦ 不掩盖潜在的病因。
- 用于更积极的疼痛管理的阿片类药物（理论上增加腔内压力，导致穿孔）。
◦ 注意是否血流动力学不稳定。
• 应谨慎进行外科治疗：
- 伴有脓肿的非穿孔性憩室炎：
◦ CT或超声引导下经皮脓肿引流通常是成功的，并限制了并发症和额外手术的需要。
◦ 微脓肿通常仅用保守疗法治疗。
- 穿孔性憩室炎伴腹膜炎：
◦ 需要紧急手术。
◦ 分2阶段手术，切除结肠病变部分和近端结肠造口术，随后进行再吻合术。
- 择期手术：
◦ 多次反复发作（>2次）、无广泛性腹膜炎时使用（有争议）；瘘形成；难治性疼痛；未消退的梗阻；内科治疗失败；<50岁的患者单次严重发作（有争议）。
◦ 内科治疗炎症消退后的一阶段手术。
◦ 复杂性憩室炎可考虑非手术治疗。
- 憩室周围脓肿引流术：
◦ 如界限清楚、容易进入时使用。
◦ 通过CT或超声引导下经皮穿刺完成。
• 门诊治疗：
- 无渣流质，2～3日随访。
- 当急性状况已消退：
◦ 高纤维、低脂肪饮食，以减少发反复发作。

■ 药物治疗

轻度疾病门诊用药方案（治疗7～14日）：
• 甲氧苄唑：500 mg，口服，q8 h加左氧氟沙星：750 mg，口服，q12 h；或环丙沙星：500 mg，口服，q12 h；或甲氧苄啶-磺胺甲噁唑DS：1片，口服，q12 h。
• 阿莫西林-克拉维酸：500/125 mg，q8 h；或875/125 mg，口服，q12 h加左氧氟沙星：400 mg，口服，q12 h。
• 莫西沙星：每日400 mg，口服。

中度疾病住院患者用药方案：
• 莫西沙星：500 mg，静脉注射，q8 h加头孢曲松：每日1 g，静脉注射；或环丙沙星：400 mg，静脉注射，q12 h；或左氧氟沙星：每日750 mg，静脉注射；或氨曲南：2 g，静脉注射，q8 h。
• 厄他培南：每日1 g，静脉注射。
• 替普瑞林-他唑巴坦：4.5 g，静脉注射，q8 h。
• 红霉素：400 mg，静脉注射，q12 h。

严重/复杂疾病住院用药方案：
• 替普瑞林：500 mg，静脉注射，q6 h。
• 红霉素：1 g，静脉注射，q8 h。
• 替普瑞林-他唑巴坦：4.5 mg，静脉注射，q8 h。
• 拉米西林：2 g，静脉注射，q8 h加甲硝唑：500 mg，静脉注射，q8 h加环丙沙星：400 mg，静脉注射，q12 h或左氧氟沙星：750 mg。

门诊预防药物：
• 膳食纤维：旨在降低管腔内压力。
• 双环胺：旨在降低管腔内压力的目标，减少疼痛。
• 利福昔明：旨在减少结肠淤滞。
• 美沙拉嗪：旨在减少可能类似IBD的结肠炎症。
• 益生菌：旨在恢复正常结肠菌群和减少致病性炎症的目标。

随访

■ 进一步处理

入院指征

• 难治性疼痛和/或呕吐。
• 高热。
• 腹膜炎。
• 对门诊治疗无反应。
• CT扫描上提示严重疾病。
• 显著白细胞增多。
• 免疫低下或激素依赖患者。
• 反复发作。
• 合并症：肾功能不全、肝功能障碍、慢性阻塞性肺病，伴靶器官损害的糖尿病。
• 处于年龄两极。

• 诊断不明确。

出院指征

• 已知的轻度憩室疾病(低热、轻度不适)。

• 轻微合并症。

• 耐受口服。

转诊问题

巨大憩室出血或需要消化科或外科会诊。

■ **随访建议**

• 无渣流质。

• 3日内应看到临床症状改善,之后可增加进食。

• 建议患者疼痛加重、发热或不能耐受口服时呼叫求助。

• 初次发作消退后应该行结肠镜(或软式乙状结肠镜对照钡剂灌肠X线)。

• 患者不需忌食种子类和坚果类食物。

要点和误区

• CT扫描将憩室炎分为复杂性和简单性:

- 用于对复杂病例保留手术,但非手术治疗越来越普遍。

• 大多数简单性憩室炎病例很少进展成复杂性疾病:

- 多次发作似乎并未导致并发症的增加。

• 憩室炎似乎并非一个逐步恶化的过程:

- 急性发作可在任何阶段。

• 首次CT扫描提示的严重疾病:

- 内科治疗失败的风险增加。

- 继发并发症的风险高。

Q

铅中毒 Lead Poisoning

Vinodinee L. Dissanayake 何超 译

基础知识

■ **描述**

• 铅有多种毒性:

- 能够与巯基结合从而影响多种酶的活性。

- 结构与钙离子相似,因此能够干扰钙离子依赖的各种过程,如信号传导。

- 具有诱变作用,因此对人体有一定的致癌性。

• 分布:

- 在摄入后99%的铅会聚集在细胞内。

- 最终会重分布进入骨内。

- 血清中高浓度的铅会透过血脑屏障进入大脑产生神经毒性。

• 当合并存在铁离子缺乏时,胃肠道对于铅的吸收会增加。

• 损伤造红细胞,导致红细胞游离原卟啉增加,这些复合物与锌结合后形成锌卟啉。

• 可能会导致智商的下降和一些暴力性行为的发生。

■ **病因**

• 急性毒性:

- 大部分是由于吸入含有铅的空气或摄入含有铅的相关物质:

◦ 陶釉。

◦ 一些偏方。

◦ 化妆品。

◦ 宝石。

◦ 砝码。

◦ 家庭酿造的一些饮料。

◦ 弹药或底漆产生的粉尘。

• 慢性中毒:

- 职业性暴露。

◦ 电池工厂或回收机构。

◦ 架桥涂装油漆。

◦ 建筑工人。

◦ 电子废弃物回收。

◦ 电焊工。

◦ 采矿和炼钢。

- 家庭性暴露:

◦ 来源于玩具和墙面的富含铅的涂层散发的铅。

◦ 老旧水管里的水。

◦ 父母从事相关职业后经衣服带回家的粉尘。

◦ 食物。

◦ 假药。

诊断

■ **症状和体征**

病史

• 神经系统:

- 癫痫(可能会反复发作)。

- 脑病。

- 学习能力下降。

- 心理异常。

- 脑水肿。

- 周围运动神经病变,但是在慢性中毒中少见。

• 消化系统:

- 腹部绞痛。

- 肠梗阻。

- 恶心与呕吐。

- 伯顿线(在牙龈出现的蓝线)的出现,提示长期暴露。

- 肝炎或胰腺炎。

• 心血管系统:

- 高血压(通常继发于肾脏损伤)。

- 心肌炎。

• 肾脏:

- 长期暴露导致慢性肾衰竭。

• 血液系统:

- 贫血。

- 红细胞脆性增加导致红细胞的半衰期缩短。

• 骨骼肌肉系统:

- 导致钙离子沉积在骨骺线处。

- 缩短了骨骼的长度和生长。

■ **基本检查**

血铅浓度。

■ **诊断检查与说明**

实验室检查

• 全血铅浓度:

- 没有血铅浓度的正常值。

◦ 对于儿童,当血铅浓度≥10 μg/dl时会对学习能力产生影响。

◦ 儿童血铅浓度≥45 μg/dl时进行螯合治疗。

◦ 成人血铅浓度≥70 μg/dl时进行螯合治疗。

- 血铅浓度达到100 μg/dl时会出现脑病,随着浓度的进一步提高出现意识的改变。

- 采取一定的治疗后由于铅的重分布也会造成血铅浓度的升高。

• 全血细胞计数:

- 判断是否存在贫血。

- 红细胞的相关指标和铁离子的指标。

• 电解质、肌酐、尿素氮、血糖:

- 检查是否有肾功能不全。
• 转氨酶,在开始螯合治疗之前检查肝功能。
• 红细胞游离原卟啉和锌卟啉。

影像学检查

• 腹部X线平片检查是否存在异物。
• 对于儿童观察长骨骨骺线情况。
• 根据患者情况选择进行头部CT。

鉴别诊断

• 急性中毒:
- 急性阑尾炎、胃肠炎和结肠炎。
- 腹腔疾病。
- 霍乱。
- 分布异常性休克。
- 脑病。
- 中毒。
◦ 伞形毒菌蘑菇中毒。
◦ 三环类抗抑郁药物或其他抗抑郁类药物中毒。
◦ 有机磷酸酯类。
• 慢性中毒。
- 艾迪生病。
- Guillain-Barre综合征或其他神经病变。
- 维生素缺乏(B_6、B_3、B_{12})
- Wernicke-Korsakooff综合征。

Q

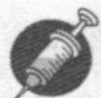

治疗

院前

• 呼吸道和循环的支持治疗。
• 心电监测。
• 治疗癫痫。

> **注意**
> • 在怀疑存放过量毒物或中毒的地方时,确保足够安全。
> • 对皮肤进行消毒,防止明显的皮肤暴露。

初步稳定/治疗

• ABC管理:
- 心电监测。
- 输注等张晶体液纠正低血容量,对于难治性低血压选用血管加压素。
• 纳洛酮、硫胺素、葡萄糖治疗能够改善大脑功能。
• 心血管:
- 输注等张晶体液维持血压。
- 针对难治性低血压选用血管加压素。
• 神经系统。
- 使用苯二氮䓬类药物纠正癫痫。
- 对于由于神经肌肉无力导致的呼吸衰竭进行机械通气。
• 肾脏:
- 出现肾衰竭时进行血液透析。
• 饮食:
- 输注葡萄糖或进行肠内、半肠内营养对于患者的恢复有益。

急诊治疗/程序

• 排除污染:
- 若在腹部X线平片上观察到斑片影,立即使用聚乙二醇1~2 L/h进行全肠道灌洗直至腹部X线平片变得干净。
- 活性炭无效。
• 评估是否需要螯合疗法。
- 血铅浓度。
- 暴露剧烈程度。
- 临床症状。
- 咨询医学毒理学家或毒物中心。

成人注意事项

• 多数暴露是通过吸入或职业性暴露或种族产物。
• 成人伴有脑病或血铅水平:>100 mg/dl需要螯合治疗。
- 起始使用二巯基丙醇(BAL),持续5日。
- 第二剂BAL后开始乙二胺四乙酸钙二钠($CaNa_2$ EDTA)。
• 无症状、血铅水平70~100 μg/dl的患者可使用口服螯合剂二巯琥珀酸(DMSA)治疗。
• 血铅水平<70 μg/dl的无症状患者无需螯合治疗。

儿科注意事项

• 当前,BLL≥10 μg/dl需要调查和教育介入:
- 调查暴露原因和重复监测。
- 应进行家长教育。
• BLL≥45 μg/dl:
- 开始螯合治疗。
- 无症状患儿使用DMSA治疗。
- 有症状或BLL≥70 μg/dl的患儿使用BAL和$CaNa_2$ EDTA治疗。
- 如考虑螯合治疗时,咨询医学毒理学家/毒物中心。

妊娠注意事项

• 对胎儿铅中毒存在争议。
• 对BLL升高的孕妇,咨询产科新生儿科和医学毒理学家或毒物中心。

药物治疗

• 螯合剂:
- 二巯基丙醇(BAL),症状中度者3 mg/kg,深部肌内注射,q4 h,持续3~5日;症状重者(癫痫、脑病)4 mg/kg,深部肌内注射,q4 h,持续5日:
◦ 注意:对花生过敏者禁用。
- 乙二胺四乙酸钙二钠($CaNa_2$ EDTA),50 mg/(kg·d)持续静脉输注(成人或儿童)或1 g/(m^2·d),持续静脉输注。
◦ 治疗5日,BAL后4 h开始。
- 二硫琥珀酸(DMSA):
◦ 成人:10 mg/kg经口每8 h持续5日,然后每12 h给药14日。
◦ 儿童:350 mg/m^2 每8 h给药5日,然后每12 h给药14日。
• 50%葡萄糖:25 g(50 ml;儿童:0.5 g/kg 25%葡萄糖),静脉治疗低血糖。
• 地西泮:5~10 mg(儿童:0.1 mg/kg),静脉给药控制癫痫。
• 劳拉西泮:2~4 mg,静脉或肌内注射。
• 纳洛酮:0.4~2 mg(儿童:0.1 mg/kg),静脉给药。
• 硫胺素:100 mg(儿童:0.1 mg/kg),肌内注射或静脉给药。

随访

进一步处理

入院指征

• 有症状的铅中毒。
• 在患儿的环境中有高再暴露风险的患儿。
• 不能耐受DMSA的患儿。
• 血铅水平升高的孕妇,咨询产科和毒理学家。

出院指征

• 无症状患者不需要静脉使用螯合治疗。
• 慢性暴露患者不需要收治,需门诊随访评估。
• 首先要保证家庭环境是安全的才能出院。
• 首先要保证患儿能耐受口服螯合治疗才能出院。

随访建议

医学病理学家或首诊医师随访。

要点和误区

• 足跟采血会导致BLL假性升高,重复血检验阳性验证。
• 安全社工保证家庭环境安全后才能出院。
• 当一位患者铅中毒时,询问并检查其兄妹或家庭成员。
• 若患者对花生过敏,不要使用BAL。

前臂骨干/远端骨折 Forearm Fracture, Shaft/Distal

Joseph R. Brown · Christopher J. Coyne 万健 译

基础知识

描述

- 前臂骨干骨折(单发或成对)经常会因手臂肌肉收缩而产生移位,有时伴发的(关节)脱位:
  - 盖氏(Galeazzi)骨折:
    - 桡骨远端骨折桡尺关节脱位。
  - 孟氏(Monteggia)骨折:
    - 尺骨近端骨折合并桡骨头脱位。
  - Essex-Lopresti 骨折:
    - 桡骨头粉碎性骨折伴桡尺骨远端脱位。
  - 远端骨折分类包括过伸、屈曲和关节内型:
  - Colles 骨折:
    - 过伸性桡骨远端骨折。
    - 远端向桡背侧移位。
    - 径向偏差。
    - 往往涉及尺骨茎突和桡尺远端关节。
  - Smith 骨折:
    - 桡骨远端屈曲型骨折。
    - 骨折远端掌桡侧移位。
  - Barton 骨折:
    - 桡骨远端背侧关节内骨折。
    - 常伴腕关节脱位。
  - Reverse Barton 骨折:
    - 桡骨远端腹缘关节内骨折。
    - 常伴有腕骨脱位。
  - Hutchinson 骨折:
    - 桡骨茎突关节内骨折。

儿科注意事项

- 骨干骨折:
  - 螺旋骨折:
    - 单侧或双侧骨皮质压缩(屈曲)。
  - 青枝骨折:
    - 单侧骨皮质离断伴对侧(骨皮质)完整。
  - 畸形:
    - 桡骨或尺骨弯曲未伴有明显的骨皮质破坏。
    - 多发小骨折。
- 远端骨折:
  - Salter-Harris 型骨折(见 Salter-Harris分类)。

病因

- 前臂直接受到打击。
- 纵向受力:
  - 砸到伸出的手。
  - 水平方向受力。
- 过度旋前、旋后、过伸或屈曲。

诊断

症状和体征

- 畸形。
- 疼痛、肿胀、瘀斑。

病史

- 相关事件和外伤史。
- 既往有骨疾病或陈旧骨折史。
- 前臂重复性受力的运动史。
- 职业。
- 优势手。

体格检查

- 体检时需特别注意皮肤完整性、畸形、神经血管状况。
- 前臂疼痛、捻发音、触痛、畸形、前臂短缩。
- 前臂肿胀、瘀斑、肘或腕关节积液。
- 肘、腕、手功能异常或丧失功能。
- 神经系统异常。
- 血管损害。

> **注意**
>
> 注意可能出现的骨筋膜室综合征。

基本检查

疑似前臂骨折,需要进行包含受伤部位上下关节(手、腕、肘)的后前位、侧位X线摄片检查。

诊断检查与说明

实验室检查

如有必要完善术前检查。

影像学检查

- 部分关节内骨折可能需要CT扫描。
- 在评估前臂远端骨折时考虑使用超声心动图(95%的特异性,97%的敏感性)。

诊断步骤/外科

如怀疑骨筋膜室综合征则需进行骨筋膜室压力测定。

鉴别诊断

- 上肢肌肉拉伤和韧带损伤。
- 肘或腕关节脱位,包括小儿保姆肘。
- 前臂挫伤、血肿。
- 蜂窝织炎、脓肿、软组织肿块。
- 前臂骨肿瘤。
- 骨髓炎。
- 上肢血管或神经损伤。
- 肘或腕关节炎、关节积液。
- 小儿骨骺,滋养血管可能被误诊为骨折。

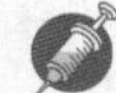

治疗

院前

- 所有怀疑前臂骨折的患者需抬高患肢,夹板固定,固定时需包含肘腕关节。
- 所有开放性骨折在固定前需使用无菌敷料覆盖。
- 不要将开放的骨折断端复位。
- 如患者仅有创伤所致的疼痛,可考虑使用镇痛药物。

急诊治疗/程序

- 骨干骨折,无移位:
  - 长上肢夹板。
  - 转诊至骨科。
- 骨干骨折,移位:
  - 骨科会诊。
  - 通常需要切开复位,内固定。
- 远端骨折,无移位:
  - 前臂 Sugar-tong 或后前位夹板固定。
  - 转诊至骨科。
- 远端骨折:Colles 骨折或 Smith 骨折:
  - 简单,非粉碎性,关节外的 Colles 骨折和 Smith 骨折可以考虑在急诊进行复位。
    - 夹板固定(长上肢 Sugar-tong 夹板)。
    - 悬吊。
    - 建议骨科就诊。
  - 复杂的 Colles 骨折和 Smith 骨折需要骨科会诊。
- 远端骨折:Barton 骨折或 Hutchinson 骨折:
  - 非粉碎性 Barton 骨折和 Hutchinson 骨折。
    - 夹板固定(后前位或 Sugar-tong 夹板)。
    - 悬吊固定。
    - 建议骨科就诊。
  - 复杂的骨折需要骨科会诊。
- 开放性骨折:
  - 无菌敷料覆盖。
  - 肌内注射或静脉注射抗生素。
  - 破伤风免疫接种(如有)。

- 夹板固定。
- 紧急骨科会诊。

• 前臂骨折合并骨筋膜室综合征或者神经血管损伤的患者，均需紧急请骨科会诊。

儿科注意

• Torus骨折和青枝骨折伴<10°的成角畸形，可与长上肢夹板固定，悬吊，并转诊至骨科。

• 生长畸形，需要骨科会诊：
- 部分小的错位的畸形可被长夹板固定或悬吊而消失。

• Slater-Harris型骨折需要骨科会诊。

Q

药物治疗

• 对乙酰氨基酚：325～1 000 mg，口服，q4 h（儿童：10～15 mg/kg，q4 h，口服）。

• 抗生素：
- 开放性骨折需要肌内注射或静脉注射抗生素。
- 头孢唑林：1～2 g肌内注射或静脉注射或等效剂量的第一代头孢菌素；如有伤口污染，加用一种氨基糖苷类抗生素。

• 酒石酸二氢可待因酮：5～10 mg口服，q4 h。

• 布洛芬：200～800 mg，q4～8 h（儿童>6个月，5～10 mg/kg，q6 h）。

• 硫酸吗啡：2～10 mg静脉或肌内注射；滴定用药（儿童：0.1 mg/kg每次静脉或肌内注射）。

• 破伤风：0.5 ml，肌内注射，每10年一次。

随访

进一步处理

入院指征

• 开放性骨折。

• 骨折伴骨筋膜室综合征或神经血管损伤。

• 骨折需要紧急手术或全麻下复位。

• 怀疑为非意外受伤。

出院指征

• 已妥善复位和固定的患者。

• 已安排骨科随访。

• 已有妥善的疼痛控制。

• 患者已知晓出院后夹板相关护理知识。

• 急诊治疗后有血管神经功能状态完好。

转诊问题

所有从急诊出院的骨折（或怀疑骨折）的患者，都需建议由骨科医师密切随访。

随访建议

所有患者都建议至骨科或手外科医师处随访。

要点和误区

• 遗漏其他骨折。

• 遗漏伴发的关节脱位或半脱位。

• 可能会出现的骨筋膜室综合征。

前房积血 Hyphema

Sami H. Uwaydat · Jamil D. Bayram 巩博 译

基础知识

描述

• 眼睛前房（AC，在虹膜和角膜之间）有血。

• 前房积血：很明显可以看到血液沉积。

• 微量前房积血：只能通过裂隙灯看到悬浮红细胞。

• 遗传学：
- 遗传易患性与遗传性血液恶病质相关。

病因

• 钝挫伤：最常见（70%～80%）。

• 眼球前后收缩的同时眼球赤道扩张，引起虹膜基质/睫状体血管破裂。

• 穿透伤：直接损伤基质血管或突然眼部减压。

• 自发性：少见，并发症的发病率低：
- 肿瘤：
  ◦ 黑色素瘤。
  ◦ 视网膜母细胞瘤。
  ◦ 黄色肉芽肿。
  ◦ 转移瘤。
- 血液恶病质：
  ◦ 血友病。
  ◦ 白血病。
  ◦ 血小板减少症。
  ◦ 血管性血友病。
- 血液稀释剂：阿司匹林、香豆素、肝素。
- 虹膜新血管形成：糖尿病视网膜增殖性病变，视网膜静脉闭塞，颈动脉狭窄。
- 术后：白内障摘除术、小梁切除术和平坦部玻璃体切除术。

> **注意**
> 如果儿童没有外伤史出现前房积血，怀疑虐待儿童。

诊断

症状和体征

• 畏光。

• 视力模糊。

• 视敏度下降。

• 眼部疼痛。

• 恶心与呕吐。

病史

• 以前视敏度。

• 先前眼部手术。

• 先前青光眼治疗。

• 过去用药史（血液病包括镰状细胞疾病）。

• 受伤机制。

• 受伤的准确时间和视力下降的准确时间。

• 受伤后有无大量流泪。

> **注意**
> 大量流泪可能暗示着开放性眼球损伤。

体格检查

• 通用体检，重视相关的身体损伤。

• 眶周瘀斑。

• 眼睑撕裂伤。

• 眼球内陷（眼球压进眼眶内）。

• 眼球活动受限伴复视（可能提示眼眶底骨折）。

• 眼球突出（可能提示球后出血）。

• 眼部检查：
- 视敏度。
- 排除开放性眼外伤（赛德尔征阳性、角膜撕裂、弥漫性结膜下出血、眼球运动度下降、眼内结构脱垂）。
- 瞳孔对光反射（使用扩瞳药前检查瞳孔传入障碍）。

- 测量眼内压(IOP)。

> **注意**
> 测量眼压前排除开放性眼球外伤。
> • 裂隙灯检查,在 AC 寻找积血:
> - 根据前房积血占前房容积的百分比分为4级:
> ◦ Ⅰ级:<1/3。
> ◦ Ⅱ级:1/3~1/2。
> ◦ Ⅲ级:>1/2。
> ◦ Ⅳ级:全部(血呈暗红色,充满前房)。
> - 高等级前房出血:
> ◦ 更可能再出血(Ⅰ级 25%,Ⅲ级 67%)。
> ◦ 更容易出现青光眼和角膜血染。
> ◦ 步态可能恢复视敏度。
> - 眼底扩张试验(避免对眼球施压)。

诊断检查与说明

实验室检查

• 根据情况,实验室检查应当个体化。
• 如果怀疑出血性疾病或者患者在进行抗凝治疗,检查血小板计数、PT、APTT、出血时间。
• 如果使用氨基己酸(见下文),检查尿素氮、肌酐和孕检。
• 如果有家族性血友病,进行Ⅷ因子分析。
• 在非裔美国人和地中海后裔人群中进行镰状细胞筛查。

影像学检查

• 如果怀疑开放性眼球损伤、眼内异物、眶壁骨折,行眼眶 CT 检查(层厚 1 mm)。
• 如果前房全部积血,眼内组织不能形象化,行超声生物显微镜检查。

> **注意**
> 如果怀疑开放性眼球外伤不要行超声检查(检查过程中施压可能会挤出眼内容物)。

基本检查

• 体格检查:视敏度、眼球状态、眼内压、相关的眼部/身体外伤。
- 实验室检查:血小板计数、PT、APTT,如果有提示进行镰状细胞筛查。
- 影像学检查:如果有提示,进行超声扫描或眶周 CT。

鉴别诊断

• 葡萄膜炎。
• 眼内炎。

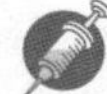

治疗

院前

如果出现角膜穿孔或可疑开放性眼球外伤,放置眼罩。

初步稳定/治疗

• 保持头部正直,让前房血液向下沉积。
• 限制活动,避免弯腰、用力、剧烈活动。
• 在患侧眼部放置金属和塑料护眼罩,直到确认眼球完整。
• 不要完全遮住患侧眼睛(如果眼睛被遮住,患者无法发现突发的视力下降)。
• 注意金属和塑料眼罩应有孔,可以让患者看到外界,而不是完全阻挡患者的视野。

急诊治疗/程序

• 轻度止痛药(因为抗血小板作用,避免使用非甾体抗炎药)。
• 止吐药(可能会增加房内压,加重前房积血)。
• 睫状肌麻痹剂减轻虹膜引起的疼痛:
- 1%阿托品或 1%环喷托酯滴眼液:2 次或 3 次/日,直到前房积血症状消失。
• 局部使用类固醇可减轻虹膜炎症:
- 醋酸泼尼松龙:1%滴眼液(或等效)每日 4~8 次直到前房积血症状消失(一般 7~10 日)。
• 氨基己酸(抗纤维蛋白溶解):
- 在眼科医科会诊后使用:
◦ 因为频繁全身副作用,一般不推荐使用。
- 稳定前房纤维蛋白凝块,降低再出血风险,但是对最终的视力恢复没有效果。
- 50 mg/kg,口服 8 日(不要超过 30 g/d)。肾衰竭患者调整剂量。
- 可能引起体位性低血压、恶心、呕吐、腹泻。
- 新型局部制剂未通过 FDA 认证。
- 孕妇或有血栓倾向的患者禁止使用。血友病患者使用,可能会引起急性肾衰竭。
• 口服泼尼松:
- 适应证:
◦ 血友病。
◦ 不配合的儿童。
◦ 前房全部积血。
◦ 有血栓性疾病史。
- 剂量:0.6~0.75 mg/(kg·d)分次口服,最多 60 mg/d,连续 5 日。
• 眼压升高:
- 非镰状细胞患者,如果 IOP>30 mmHg 需要治疗。
- 镰状细胞患者,如果 IOP>24 mmHg 需要治疗。
- 开始只使用 1 种药物。如果降压失败再增加另外一种:
◦ β受体阻滞剂——首选药物:0.5%噻吗洛尔或 0.5%左布诺洛尔,2 次/日。
◦ α受体激动剂:0.2%溴莫尼定或 0.5%阿可乐定,3 次/日。
◦ 局部碳酸酐酶抑制剂(CAI):2%多佐胺或 1%布林佐胺,3 次/日。
◦ 口服 CAI:乙酰唑胺 500 mg,口服,q12 h(儿童每日 8~30 mg/kg,q6 h);或醋甲唑胺 50 mg,q8 h。
◦ 当所有其他滴眼液不能降压至可接受水平,使用甘露醇(1~2 mg/kg 静脉注射,时间超过 45 min,q24 h)。
◦ 镰状细胞病患者避免使用 CAI 和甘露醇,因为它们可能引起酸中毒和诱发镰状变形。
- 每种滴眼液要 20~30 min 发挥作用。如果使用所有的滴眼液和甘露醇后,IOP 仍高,开始血凝块外科消除(前房穿刺或冲洗)。
• 用药避免:
- 匹鲁卡品:缩瞳并且阻止视网膜和晶体成像。
- 前列腺素滴眼液(如拉坦前列素):加重炎性反应。

> **注意**
> • 约 5%的外伤性前房积血患者需要手术治疗。
> • 急诊室内需要紧急眼科会诊的标准(有条件的话,会诊应安排在 24 h 内):
> - 视敏度差于 20/200。
> - 镰状细胞病/伴有高眼压。
> - 大面积前房积血(充满>1/3 前房)。
> - 药物不能控制的眼压。

药物治疗

一线用药

• 阿托品:1%,每日 3 次。
• 醋酸泼尼松龙:1%,每日 1 次。

二线用药

• 0.5%噻吗洛尔或 0.5%左布诺洛尔,每日 2 次。
• 2%多佐胺或 1%布林佐胺,每日 3 次。
• 乙酰唑胺:500 mg,口服,q12 h。

随访

进一步处理

• 出院患者携带阿托品、醋酸泼尼松龙和任何合适的降眼压药物。

• 如果在急诊室决定开始用氨基己酸，继续使用。

• 视病情需要予以止吐治疗。

• 使用通便药，排便时尽量少用力。

入院指征

• 前房积血面积不是入院或者出院的标准，控制眼压是最重要的因素。

• 药物不能控制的眼压需要外科干预。

• 眼球破裂。

• 依从性差的患者。

• 相关眼睛或眶周外伤。

• ＜7 岁的儿童：

- 此年龄段有弱视的风险（不可逆的视力下降，继发于幼童时的视觉剥夺）。

• 可能出现的并发症（镰状细胞病、血友病）。

出院指征

没有入院指征，且非镰状细胞病患者 IOP ＜30 mmHg，镰状细胞病患者 IOP＜24 mmHg。

随访建议

安排眼科医师随访：

• 初次受伤后每日 1 次裂隙灯检查，连续 3 日，监测再出血、角膜穿孔和高眼压。

• 随访检查决定阿托品、氨基己酸和降眼压滴剂的治疗时间。

要点和误区

• 在检查眼压和初步治疗前排除眼球破裂。

• 控制眼压不是立即起效的。给任何治疗预留至少 30 min 发挥作用：

- 在非裔美国人中检查镰状细胞病。

- 限制身体活动至少 1 周。

前列腺炎

Nicole M. Franks 郑金浩 毛恩强 译

基础知识

描述

• 急性（细菌性）前列腺炎：

- 急性发热疾病。

- 局部尿路症状出现前出现全身症状。

- 患者可能出现中毒症状并且经常并发膀胱炎。

• 前列腺脓肿：

- 急性前列腺炎后常常出现，在免疫力低下患者中基本全部发生。

- 治疗后仍有发热、直肠疼痛、白细胞增多。

- 直肠指检有波动感。

• 慢性细菌性前列腺炎：

- 占前列腺炎总数的 10%左右。

- 大多数病因是反复尿路感染。

- 前列腺按摩液可能有白细胞和细菌。

• 慢性非细菌性前列腺炎（也称为前列腺病）：

- 和慢性细菌性前列腺炎有相同的症状，但是不能从尿液及前列腺按摩液（EPS）中培养出细菌。

• 慢性盆腔疼痛综合征（CPPS）：

- 症状由前列腺引起。

- 无炎细胞浸润。

- 尿液及前列腺按摩液细菌培养为阴性。

病因

• 常常为前列腺感染单一细菌。

• 急性前列腺炎：

- 年龄＜35 岁。

◦ 淋病奈瑟菌和沙眼衣原体是常见致病菌。

- 年龄＞35 岁：

◦ 肠杆菌科或大肠杆菌（常见）、克雷伯杆菌属、假单胞菌、肠球菌、变形杆菌属。

- 沙门菌、梭菌属、结核杆菌、真菌不常见。

- 新型隐球菌可见于获得性免疫缺陷综合征的患者。

• 慢性细菌性前列腺炎：

- 肠杆菌科（80%）、肠球菌（15%）和铜绿假单胞菌。

• 慢性非细菌性前列腺炎：

- 可能为衣原体、解脲支原体、阴道毛滴虫及人支原体感染。

诊断

症状和体征

病史

• 尿路刺激症状。

- 尿频、尿急、排尿困难。

• 腰部疼痛。

• 会阴、耻骨弓上或睾丸疼痛。

• 膀胱出口梗阻或尿潴留。

• 射精症状，如血性精液。

• 急性前列腺炎：

- 发热、寒战。

- 乏力。

- 关节肌肉疼痛。

• 慢性前列腺炎的主要症状是反复发作性的排尿困难。

体格检查

• 急性前列腺炎：

- 强烈的前列腺压痛。

- 红肿。

- 前列腺触诊硬或韧。

- 急性前列腺炎禁忌前列腺按摩，因为病原体可能出现血行播散。

• 慢性前列腺炎患者行前列腺常规检查。

诊断检查与说明

实验室检查

• 尿常规（包括镜检）和尿培养。

• 急性前列腺炎：

- 血常规、电解质、血培养：对于急性患者可能有意义。

- 如果患者＜35 岁或怀疑由性传播引起，重点检查梅毒：

◦ 性传播疾病研究实验室或快速血清反应素监测。

• 慢性前列腺炎/慢性盆腔疼痛综合征。

- 若尿常规中细菌培养阴性白细胞正常范围，可经直肠前列腺按摩获取前列腺液进行革兰染色和培养。

影像学检查

• 急性前列腺炎无特征表现。

• 如果怀疑前列腺脓肿，经直肠超声或盆腔 CT 联合直肠内造影将确认诊断。

诊断步骤/外科

此疾病无需有创操作。

■ 鉴别诊断

• 良性前列腺增生。
• 膀胱炎。
• 附睾炎。
• 睾丸炎。
• 直肠周/肛周脓肿。
• 直肠炎。
• 前列腺癌。
• 前列腺梗死。
• 肾盂肾炎。
• 精囊炎。
• 尿道炎。
• 尿结石。
• 膀胱结石(vesicular calculi)。
• 其他引起腰痛的疾病(扭伤、椎间盘疾病、骶髂关节疾病等)。

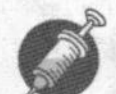

治疗

■ 初步稳定/治疗

开始恢复措施作为指导。

■ 急诊治疗/程序

• 前列腺脓肿需泌尿外科急会诊及超声引导下穿刺引流。
• 应当开始抗感染治疗(参考药物治疗)。
• 避免使用经尿道的仪器设备。
- 急性前列腺炎患者若有尿潴留伴疼痛,应考虑行耻骨联合上经皮穿刺引流术或穿刺置管。
• 静脉补液对大多数患者有益。
• 必要时可使用非甾体抗炎药或麻醉性镇痛药止痛。
• 保持大便通畅。
• 卧床休息。
• 抗感染治疗后膀胱刺激症可能持续数月,可以使用非甾体抗炎药治疗。

■ 药物治疗

• 止痛:
- 麻醉类止痛混合制剂;如氨酚氢可酮:1~2粒,口服,q4 h。
- 非甾体类解热镇痛抗炎药;如布洛芬:800 mg,口服,3次/日。
• 急性前列腺炎的肠外抗生素使用:
- 左氧氟沙星:750 mg,静脉滴注,每日1次。
- 氨苄西林:2 g,静脉滴注,q6 h。
- 头孢噻肟:2 g,静脉滴注,q8 h。
- 头孢曲松:2 g,静脉滴注,每日1次。
- 环丙沙星:400 mg,静脉滴注,每日2次。
- 氧氟沙星:200 mg,静脉滴注,每日2次。
- 哌拉西林-他唑巴坦:3.375 g,静脉滴注,q6 h;或4.5 g, q8 h。
- 羟基噻吩青霉素:3.1 g,静脉滴注,q6 h。
• 门诊患者(<35岁)抗生素治疗急性前列腺炎,病原学疑似淋病奈瑟菌或沙眼衣原体:
- 头孢曲松钠:250 mg,肌内注射,继而口服脱氧土霉素100 mg,每日2次,持续10~14日。
- 左氧氟沙星:每日500 mg,口服10~14日。
- 氧氟沙星:400 mg,口服一次,继而300 mg每日2次,持续10~14日。
• 门诊患者(>35岁)抗生素治疗急性前列腺炎,病原学疑似肠杆菌科(大肠杆菌);部分专家推荐疗程3~4周。
- 环丙沙星:500 mg,口服,每日2次,持续14日。
- 左氧氟沙星:500 mg,口服,每日1次,持续14日。
- 氧氟沙星:200 mg,口服,每日2次,持续14日。
- 甲氧苄啶-磺胺甲噁唑:1片强效或2片常效口服,每日2次,持续28日。
• 慢性盆腔疼痛综合征:
- 坦索罗辛:0.4 mg,口服,每日1次。
- 多沙唑嗪:1 mg,口服(迅速吸收),每日1次。
- 外周β受体阻滞剂对部分患者有效,请泌尿科医师会诊。
- 哌唑嗪:1 mg,口服,每日2~3次。
- 特拉唑嗪:1 mg,口服,睡前1次。

随访

■ 进一步处理

入院指征

• 急性前列腺炎:
- 出现不适或中毒症状。
- 低血压。
- 尿潴留。
• 慢性前列腺炎:
- 一般不收入院治疗,除非患者有急性前列腺炎的症状与体征。

出院指征

• 急性前列腺炎:
- 中毒症状消失。
- 可以饮水,可口服药物(止痛药和抗生素)。
- 无排尿困难。
- 免疫力正常。
- 并发症相对独立。
- 有住院相似的护理条件。
• 慢性前列腺炎:有住院相似的护理条件即可院外治疗。

转诊问题

需泌尿科医师确诊患者为急性前列腺炎还是慢性前列腺炎。

要点和误区

完整病史及抗生素的使用时间有助于区分急性和慢性前列腺炎。
• 在性生活正常的青年男性也要考虑到前列腺炎。
• 无论有无免疫力低下,急性患病男性经正规抗生素治疗失败后均应检查有无前列腺脓肿。

前庭大腺脓肿 Bartholin Abscess

Steven P. Gohsler 宋振举 童朝阳 译

基础知识

■ 描述

• 前庭大腺位于阴道开口的下部。在4点和8点的位置。
• 这些腺体在女性生殖系统中起着重要的作用。
• 主要功能是分泌黏液,提供润滑。
• 导管开口于阴唇前庭。
• 导管的梗阻形成无痛的囊肿。
- 囊肿的感染导致脓肿的形成。

Q

■ 流行病学

发病年龄

通常女性发病年龄在 20～40 岁。

■ 病因

• 在阴道里通常会发现厌氧菌和需氧菌：
- 大肠埃希菌最常见。
- 拟杆菌属。
- 金黄色葡萄球菌。
- B 组链球菌。
- 消化链球菌属。
- 大肠埃希菌属。
- 其他革兰阴性菌。
- 偶尔会有淋病奈瑟球菌和沙眼衣原体。

■ 危险因素

• 巴塞林腺(前庭大腺)囊肿史。
• 多性伴侣史。
• 性传播疾病史。
• 外阴创伤史。

诊断

■ 症状和体征

• 阴唇的肿胀和疼痛。
• 阴道的后外侧角柔软，有波动。
• 红色皮疹形成。

病史

急性起病。
• 单侧阴唇疼痛。
• 坐位或者行走时疼痛。
• 性交疼痛。

体格检查

• 前庭大腺脓肿：
- 质软、有波动感的单侧阴唇包块。
- 外阴不对称。
- 阴道分泌物。
- 蜂窝织炎可表现为周围红斑和水肿。
- 发热不常见。
• 前庭大腺囊肿：
- 无痛性单侧阴唇上的肿块。

■ 基本检查

诊断基于在前庭大腺区域找到柔软、局限、有波动的区域。

■ 诊断检查与说明

实验室检查

• 脓肿的常规培养应包括淋病和衣原体的检测。
• 培养来源于带有淋病奈瑟菌与衣原体的脓液。
• 培养子宫颈的淋病菌和衣原体。

影像学检查

影像学检查一般无明显提示作用，但是超声检查有可能提供确证依据。

■ 鉴别诊断

• 前庭囊肿。
• 不同类型的囊肿：包涵囊肿、加特内囊肿(Gartner)、尿道旁腺囊肿(Skene)和前庭黏膜囊肿。
• 前庭大腺的原位癌。
• 会阴部疝。

治疗

■ 急诊治疗/程序

• 主要治疗是手术引流，必要时辅以抗生素。
• 患者取截石位，局部麻醉行切开引流。
• 麻醉止痛。
• 可供选择的办法：
- 切开引流。
- 导管引流。
- 荷包缝合。
• 简单切开引流：
- 患者取截石位。
- 在局部浸润麻醉前可行胃肠外镇静、镇痛或程序性镇静。
- 局部麻醉后，用拇指和示指固定脓肿。
- 将外阴分开，在脓肿处的黏膜表面纵行切开 1 cm，使切口平行于处女膜环。
- 将切口延伸至脓腔内。
◦ 有脓液流出表明穿透了脓肿壁。
- 用纱布包扎伤口。
- 随后 24～48 h 移除纱布。
- 24 h 后坐浴。
- 考虑转诊，避免袋装缝合复发。
• Word 导管法：1964 年由 Buford Word 博士首次提出。
- 该导管直径 5 cm，由乳胶制成，尖端为 10 Fr。
- 尖端含有一个 5 ml 的气球。
- 可能避免疾病复发，以及没必要使用造袋术。
- 患者的准备类似于切开引流技术。
- 在前庭的黏膜表面刺入脓腔：
◦ 它应该足够大，可以很容易植入导管，以便当气囊膨胀起来时不易滑脱。
- 当导管植入否，用 2～4 ml 的生理盐水使气囊膨胀起来。
◦ 过度充气可能使患者感到不适。
◦ 补救的方式就是在气囊里回抽一点水。
- 坐浴必须在 24 h 以后。
- 后续跟进 2～4 日。
- 导管植入至少 6～8 周直到表皮完全形成，等导管移除后，腺体就能恢复其正常的功能了。
- 如果出现导管过早的脱落。
◦ 假如出现这样的情况，那么只能重新植入导管，或者是脓肿通过简单的切开引流愈合。
• 造袋术：
- 手术过程允许永久性瘘管缝合伤口到阴唇。
◦ 对于专科医师来讲这项技术具有挑战性。
- 切除覆盖在囊肿/脓肿腔上的椭圆形前庭黏膜。
- 插入一个牵引器将黏膜拉开并观察囊壁。
- 外翻脓肿的边缘，应用可吸收缝线将它们缝合到阴唇的表面。
◦ 敞开将会使其收缩，并保持原有的状态。
◦ 不需要包裹。
- 24～48 h 后坐浴。
- 随后跟进 1 周。
• 切开引流后不需要抗感染治疗：
- 假如出现中度蜂窝织炎或者免疫功能低下的患者，可以应用广谱抗生素。
- 如果有性传播疾病，可以考虑抗感染治疗。

■ 药物治疗

一线用药

广谱抗生素覆盖。
• 阿莫西林-水杨酸类：500～875 mg，每日 2 次，口服 5 日；联合甲硝唑 500 mg，q8 h，口服 5 日。
• 环丙沙星 500 mg，每日 2 次，口服 5 日；联合甲硝唑 500 mg，q8 h，口服 5 日。

二线用药

如果有性传播疾病，也需要治疗。

转诊问题

患者需要跟进随访。
• 24～48 h 换 1 次药。
• 导管植入需要 2～4 日随访 1 次。

■ 随访建议

持续坐浴至少 72 h。

要点和误区

• 不要误诊前庭大腺囊肿，它不需要立刻处理。

• 此部位的肿物也要考虑肿瘤性疾病，特别是年龄>40 岁的女性。

• 必须从脓肿表面的黏膜切开。

前置胎盘 Placenta Previa

W. Bryson Bendall · Katherine Hiller 瞿金龙 译

基础知识

描述

• 胎盘组织覆盖或接近内宫颈口。

• 子宫增大和宫颈扩张导致靠近宫颈的胎盘血管破裂，引起阴道出血。

• 90%以上的前置胎盘在妊娠 20 周前诊断时存在，但将迁移并在足月时具有正常的胎盘位置。

• 占所有产前出血病因的 20%。

• 分类：

- 前置胎盘：内宫颈口完全或部分被胎盘覆盖（以前分别称为完全前置或部分前置）。
- 低置胎盘：胎盘植入在下段子宫壁，并且边缘未达到内口，并且保持在 2 cm 的范围之外。

病因

• 发病率：3～5/1 000 出生人口。

• 孕妇死亡率：0.03%。

• 围产期发病率和死亡率：由于早产会增加 3 倍。

• 影响着床位置的因素：

- 由自然流产或人工流产引起的刮宫次数增加。
- 子宫内膜血管异常。
- 排卵延迟。

• 危险因素：

- 多产（高龄多产孕妇患者 5% *vs* 初产妇 0.2%）。
- 多胎妊娠（双胎妊娠时风险增加 30%～40%）。
- 先前剖宫产（增加 3 倍，随着先前剖宫产次数的增加而增加）。
- 增加的孕妇年龄（12～19 岁 0.1%，≥35 岁 0.9%）。
- 先前发生过前置胎盘（4%～8%的复发率）。
- 吸烟（增加 2～4 倍）。
- 男性胎儿（增加 14%）。
- 辅助受精。

• 相关情况：

- 胎盘植入、侵袭、穿透（胎盘生长到子宫壁内）在胎盘前置症患者中发生率为 5%～10%；持续出血可能需要剖宫产子宫切除术。
- 早产前羊膜破裂。
- 血管前置：胎儿血管穿过羊膜覆盖宫颈口。
- 先天畸形。
- 胎儿异常。

• 高出血风险：

- 妊娠晚期子宫颈长度过短。
- 胎盘边缘静脉窦。
- 剖宫产时母亲年龄较大。
- 先前剖宫产。

诊断

症状和体征

• 妊娠 20 周后出现无痛性阴道出血，需要首先考虑宫底前置胎盘。

• 注意：如果患者同时处于分娩过程中，可能会伴有疼痛。

病史

• 70%～90%的患者出现无痛性鲜红色阴道出血。

• 20%的患者子宫收缩，第一次出血通常发生在妊娠 27～32 周。

• 出血程度可能从轻微到大量不等；出血次数与胎盘前置的程度无关。

• 诱发因素：通常没有，近期的性行为或剧烈运动可能会有所促进。

• 初次出血通常是自限性的，不致命，但常常会复发。

• 在妊娠中期的超声检查中常见的偶然发现（16～18 周时占 6%）。

体格检查

• 在排除前置胎盘之前，妊娠中期阴道出血不轻易做直肠指检或器械探查。

• 低血压和心动过速可能表明出血性休克。

• 应监测胎心音和孕妇的子宫收缩，以及其他生命体征。

基本检查

超声检查是首选的诊断程序。

诊断检查与说明

实验室检查

• 全血细胞计数。

• 血型检测；如果需要输血，则升级至交叉配型。

• Rh 血型。

• 如果怀疑凝血功能障碍（罕见）：凝血酶原时间/部分凝血活酶时间、纤维蛋白分解产物、纤维蛋白原（<300 mg/dl 为异常）。

影像学检查

• 腹部超声：93%～98%准确：

- 在执行超声检查前排空膀胱。
- 假阴性：肥胖、胎盘后置或侧置、胎头位于宫颈口上方。
- 假阳性：膀胱过度充盈。

• 经阴道超声：安全且最准确：

- 比经腹部超声更准确。
- 正确操作时，不会加重出血。
- 被认为是诊断的金标准。

• 彩色多普勒超声：用于确定胎盘植入。

• MRI：在紧急情况下不用于确认此诊断：

- 在门诊评估诸如植入胎盘和前置胎盘异常时可能有用。

鉴别诊断

• 胎盘早期剥离（可能同时发生）。

• 子宫破裂。

• 胎儿血管破裂。

• 宫颈/阴道损伤。

• 宫颈/阴道病变。

• 出血性疾病。

• 自发流产。

• 胎儿足月或早产时的“带血提示”。

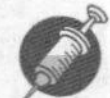

治疗

院前

• 孕妇出现大于 24 周的阴道出血应被送往能够处理高危和早产孕妇的医疗机构。

• 如果妊娠后期出现低血压，应将患者放置于左侧卧位。

• 给氧，心电监护，建立两条大的静脉通路进行静脉输液(晶体液输注)。

• 如果患者出血严重，专科会诊干预(产科、外科、血库等)应尽早进行。

初始稳定/治疗

• 与任何原因导致的出血一样，对失血性休克进行复苏，包括凝血功能异常时输注新鲜冰冻血浆。

• ABC(气道、呼吸、循环)＋FHT(胎心率监测)(＜120 次/分或＞160 次/分为异常)。

• 使用生理盐水或乳酸钠林格液进行复苏，建立两根大的静脉输液通路。

• 如果妊娠后期出现低血压，应将患者放置于左侧卧位。

• 对出现活动性出血的患者进行紧急产科会诊。

急诊治疗/程序

• 立即进行产科会诊。

• 输血以维持血细胞比容＞30%。

• 如果母亲 Rh 阴性，应注射 Rho(D)免疫球蛋白。

• 胎儿监测。

• 在产科医生认为稳定之前，保持禁食和卧床休息。

• 与产科医生协商使用硫酸镁，以发挥其对可能需要早产剖宫产患者的神经保护作用。

• 在妊娠 24～34 周时使用产前类固醇(倍他米松)促进胎儿肺部成熟。

• 对持续出血或胎儿受损的患者进行紧急剖宫产或分娩。

药物治疗

• Rho(D)免疫球蛋白：如果在 28 周时尚未给予，肌内注射 1 瓶(300 μg)；如果 KB 指示胎儿 RBS＞15 ml，则可能需要多于 1 瓶。

• 硫酸镁：20 min 内静脉注射 6 g，然后 2～4 g/h，根据宫缩情况进行调整。

• 倍他米松：肌内注射 12 mg，q24 h，给予 2 个剂量。

随访

进一步处理

入院标准

胎盘前置引起的活动性出血是一种潜在的产科急症，所有患者应接受产科会诊并入院监测和治疗。

出院标准

经产科会诊后，如果出血得到缓解，可选择患者在门诊基础上进行管理。

随访建议

• 无症状患者：

- 不需要卧床休息。
- 避免剧烈的体力活动。
- 盆底休息(妊娠 28 周后或任何时间若发现胎盘前置伴有出血时，不要进行性交或在阴道使用卫生棉条)。
- 报告出血或宫缩。
- 若妊娠＜32 周发现胎盘前置或低置胎盘，应重复进行超声检查，并应在 32 周安排产科随访。

• 70%的患者将出现第二次出血。

要点和误区

• 妊娠 20 周后出现无痛性阴道出血，首先考虑是前置胎盘，直到证实是其他原因。

• 前置胎盘可能会引起疼痛，并被误认为是胎盘早期剥离。

• 在妊娠中期后可疑阴道出血前进行超声检查，避免直肠指检。

• 前置胎盘导致的出血性休克应该输注至较高的目标红细胞比容(30%)。

强直性脊柱炎 Ankylosing Spondylitis

Daniel R. Lasoff · Brian K. Snyder 李岩 王瑞兰 译

基础知识

描述

• 为炎症性疾病，主要侵犯脊柱，普遍累及骶髂关节(SI)：

- 骶髂关节 100%受累。
- 颈椎 75%受累。
- 胸椎 70%受累。
- 脊柱 50%受累。
- 髋关节 30%受累。
- 肩关节 30%受累。

• 强直性脊柱炎(AS)椎骨的炎症开始于椎骨纤维环(肌腱)外部纤维的附着点。

- 骨化(骨赘形成)可能导致椎骨的完全融合、僵硬。
- 广泛的脊髓受累会产生僵硬的"竹节样脊柱"的影像学表现。

• 15～35 岁发病。

• 男女比例为 3∶1。

> **注意**
>
> 与普通人群相比，AS 患者的骨折和瘫痪风险高 4 倍。他们患脊髓损伤的可能性高 11 倍。

危险因素

遗传学

有很强的遗传成分，HLA－B27 基因 HLA－B27 存在于 80%～90%的 AS 患者中。

病因

疾病可能是由环境因素作用于遗传易感性个体所引起的，如外伤或感染。

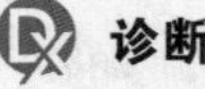

诊断

症状和体征

• 脊柱：下腰痛和骶髂关节炎是最常见的表现：

- 炎性背痛，通过运动和锻炼得到改善。
- 轻度创伤机制造成严重伤害的风险更高。

• 脊柱外炎症(可能出现脊柱症状)：

- 眼部(最常见)：
  ◦ 葡萄膜炎(25%～40%)。通常起病为急性和单侧，可以交替眼睛发生。

- 心脏：
  - 轻微增加CAD风险。
  - 随着AS病程延长，瓣膜功能不全的风险增加。
- 肺：
  - 限制性扩张和纤维化导致进展性限制性肺疾病。
- 胃肠道：
  - 5%～10%的炎症性肠病患者。
- 泌尿生殖系统：
  - IgA肾病或淀粉样变性病的风险。使用抗炎药也会增加NSAID肾病的风险。
- 肠炎（肌腱或韧带插入时发炎）：

经常发生跟腱炎或足底筋膜炎。

• 颈椎损伤：
- 高受伤率。
- 极易受到低能机制的严重伤害。
- 普通胶片通常不足以识别骨折。

病史

• <40岁以下患者的隐匿性下腰痛发作>3个月，从SI区域放射到臀区域，并逐渐累及整个脊柱区域：
- 休息时更严重，轻度运动可改善病情。下半夜疼痛，将患者从睡眠中唤醒。
- 女性可能比男性具有更多的颈椎和脊柱外表现。

• 葡萄膜炎、限制性肺疾病、炎症性肠炎、附着点炎、迁徙性或多关节炎的可能的既往史。

体格检查

• 同时在两个患者的ASIS上施加直接压力导致SI关节变软。
• 牙根炎或肠炎。
• 正常腰椎前凸变扁平胸椎后凸畸形。
• 脊柱运动受限胸部扩张减少。

儿科注意事项

• 幼年强直性脊柱炎（JAS）可以类似于一个伴随发热和全身症状的炎症过程。
• JAS发病于童年晚期或青春期（在8～12岁，在20岁之前），主要是男孩。
• JAS对脊柱外关节和下肢骨质的偏爱更大。除SI压痛外，请检查：
- 下肢不对称性关节炎。
- 踝、膝或跗骨的附着点炎。足底筋膜炎和跟腱炎通常是常见的表现。

基本检查

• 任何新出现的脊柱疼痛（即使没有创伤）而怀疑为强直性脊柱炎的患者都需排除骨折或神经损伤。
• 如有临床表现，排除脓毒症或脓性关节。
• 通过骨盆摇摆试验（加压）或帕特里克试验（骶髂关节牵引）来评估骶髂关节炎。

诊断检查与说明

实验室检查

• CBC可显示轻度白细胞增多而忽视中度贫血和血小板增多症。
• 尿素氮、肌酐、电解质可能对评估肾脏受累有用。
• 红细胞沉降率（ESR）、C反应蛋白（CRP）可能升高，但在急诊中作用有限。
• HLA-B27测试可以由专家执行。阴性结果并不排除AS。

影像学检查

• 骨盆正位X线片：任何疑似强直性脊柱炎而未确诊的成年患者均应做。
- 骶髂关节炎对于强直性脊柱炎的诊断是必不可少的，这最初被视为骶髂关节髂侧软骨下骨侵蚀，后来表现为骨质增生和硬化。

• 对于腰椎、胸椎、颈椎新出现的有或无创伤的疼痛，X线片可以排除骨折。
• 应做CT进一步评估X线片上可能发生的骨折。
• 任何神经功能损伤的患者都应立即做MRI。
• 胸片可能显示斑片状炎性浸润。

诊断步骤/外科

• 心电图指征：
- 急性冠状动脉综合征（高危）。
- 症状性心律失常：
  - 房室传导阻滞（20%）。

• 超声心动图显示：
- 严重的急性心瓣膜炎。
  - 伴有严重AR或MR的急性心力衰竭。

鉴别诊断

• 幼年强直性脊柱炎：
- 20岁前发病。
- 肠炎和脊柱外关节受累。

• 反应性关节炎（原Reiter综合征）：
- 关节炎、尿道炎和结膜炎大约在尿道炎或肠炎1个月后开始产生。

• 肠病性关节炎：
- 克罗恩病或溃疡性结肠炎。
- 主要涉及膝、肘、踝关节或腕关节，通常因肠道疾病的暴发而加剧。

• 银屑病性关节炎：
- 银屑病皮疹。
- 常见于手和足。

• 化脓性关节炎：
- 如果临床怀疑单关节受累，需关节穿刺排除。

• 机械性腰痛：
- 在没有系统性感染过程的情况下，休息会好转而运动会加剧。

• 感染性腰痛：
- 更持续稳定，通常伴随发热。IVDA病史或免疫抑制有关。

• 肿瘤性腰背痛：
- 通常发生在40岁以上的患者，更为稳定持续，夜间更典型。

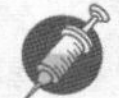

治疗

院前

注意

• 小的创伤有更高的脊柱损伤的风险。
• 脊柱固定必须避免造成进一步的伤害。
- 舒适的垫子和铲板是比颈托和/或背板更好的方法。

• 插管困难。
- 颈椎和颞下颌关节的限制可能会导致插管成功率下降，但是纤维光学技术可以使插管变得容易。
- 在插管成功之前，考虑替代气道方法如喉罩或带储气袋的面罩。

• 通气困难。
- 胸壁畸形限制与肺纤维化。

• 心肺复苏术，虽然不可避免的，但可能会带来更高的肋骨骨折的风险。

初步稳定/治疗

• 创伤：在良好固定前提下进行心肺复苏。
• 急性创伤性瘫痪：立即大剂量甲泼尼龙静脉注射以及神经外科评估。

急诊治疗/程序

• 如果临床怀疑，需排除脊髓压迫（磁共振是首选）。
• 任何新出现的脊柱疼痛均需排除脊柱骨折（CT可能是必要的）。
• 如果临床怀疑需采用实验室分析或关节穿刺术来排除感染。
• 非甾体抗炎药控制疼痛和炎症。
• 电视喉镜检查可以降低插管的难度和与插管相关的颈椎损伤的风险。

药物治疗

• 非选择性非甾体抗炎药：

- 布洛芬：35 mg/(kg·d)，每日 4 次，最大剂量 50 mg/(kg·d)(成人：300～800 mg，口服，每日 3～4 次)。
- 吲哚美辛：1～2 mg/(kg·d)，每日 2 次或每日 4 次，最大剂量 4 mg/(kg·d)(成人：25 mg，口服，每日 2～3 次)。

• 耐药性差，尤其是在高剂量时，因为会影响消化道和中枢神经系统。

- 萘普生：10 mg/(kg·d)，每日 2 次，最大剂量为 1 000 mg/d(成人：250～500 mg，口服，每日 2 次)。

• COX-2 抑制剂：

- cefelocoxib(成人：100～200 mg，口服，每日 2 次)。

• TNF-α 抑制剂：

- 阿达木单抗：成人 40 mg，皮下注射，2 周 1 次。
- etanercept：成人 50 mg，皮下注射，每周 1 次。

妊娠注意事项

• 妊娠期应避免使用非甾体抗炎药。

- 对乙酰氨基酚是一线用药。
- 阿片类药物是二线用药。

老年注意事项

• 非甾体抗炎药可能会增加老年人心血管疾病、胃肠道出血、肾功能减退、高血压的风险。虽然对特定患者有效，但是密切随访是有必要的。

注意

• 急性瘫痪需大剂量类固醇：

- 甲泼尼龙：30 mg/kg，然后 24 内总共需 5.4 mg/(kg·h)。

• 非甾体抗炎药：

- 胃肠道出血的风险：
  ◦ 老年人、PUD 史、同时使用糖皮质激素、抗凝治疗、低剂量阿司匹林(<325 mg/d)、吸烟、饮酒及更高的剂量。
  ◦ 如果患者胃肠道出血的风险较高，考虑塞来昔布或添加 H_2 受体阻滞剂或质子泵抑制剂。

二线用药

如果非甾体抗炎药或对乙酰氨基酚在合适的剂量是无效的，需考虑：

• 阿片类镇痛药、肌肉松弛剂或低剂量类固醇。

随访

进一步处理

入院指征

• 急性神经功能损伤。

• 难以治疗的疼痛。

• 不能排除脓毒症或脓性关节。

出院指征

• 无严重损伤或神经功能缺损。

• 疼痛对于患者来说是易于控制的。

转诊问题

• 应鼓励患者获得医疗提醒。

• 风湿病学：

- 延误诊断仍然是一个挑战。有新诊断强直性脊柱炎充分证据的患者应考虑早期转诊到风湿病专科医师。
- 对某些患者 β 受体阻滞剂是有效的辅助治疗，当涉及进一步的门诊治疗时可以考虑。

• 物理医学与康复医学：

- 发炎的关节可采用夹板。
- 矫形器治疗附着点炎(如插入足跟垫让跟腱休息)。

随访建议

• 1～2 周进行再评估，来评价疗效。

• 非甾体抗炎药不良反应风险较高的患者应早期随访：

- 老年人、高血压患者和有较高胃肠道出血风险的患者。

要点和误区

• 插管可能很困难，应避免颈部复位。

- 考虑气道辅助(如喉罩)直到最终的气道插管(通常是纤维支气管镜辅助)是安全的。

• 固定时必须避免造成额外的损伤。

- 在舒适程度上，优先考虑垫子、胶带固定而不是颈托和背板。

• 强直性脊柱炎患者微小的损伤就可导致脊柱骨折和脊髓损伤。要保持高度的临床怀疑。

鞘膜积液 Hydrocele

Jessica L. Ostrman　巩博 译

基础知识

描述

• 大部分起因于无痛性阴囊肿胀。

• 分为先天性和后天性(继发性)：

- 先天性鞘膜积液源于鞘突未闭，腹腔内液体与鞘膜囊内液体相通。
  ◦ 一般自动发生，大部分在 2 岁前鞘突关闭。
- 后天性鞘膜积液常继发于阴囊内感染、新生物、腹股沟或阴囊手术、局部或全身性疾病。

• 交通性鞘膜积液：

- 鞘突未闭。
- 体位和腹腔内压力决定腹腔液体充满阴囊或流出阴囊。

• 非交通性鞘膜积液是某种疾病过程中产生浆液的产物或阴囊自身吸收功能受损。

病因

• 鞘膜和白沫间的空间内，液体产生和重吸收不平衡。

• 引起非交通性鞘膜积液的疾病包括：

- 附睾炎。
- 低蛋白血症。
- 结核。
- 创伤。
- 腮腺炎。
- 精索静脉结扎术。
- 在发展中国家，鞘膜积液主要由感染引起，如班氏线虫或罗阿丝虫(世界范围内丝虫病是大部分鞘膜积液的病因)。
- 少数恶性肿瘤(Ⅰ度睾丸肿瘤或淋巴瘤)。

• 因为受压，少数腹阴囊鞘膜积液可能引起输尿管积水或单侧肢体水肿。

- 超声检查可以显示单个阴囊通过腹股沟

深环突入腹腔的情况。

儿科注意事项

- 6%的新生男孩出现先天性鞘膜积液。
- 通常在新生儿病房诊断出。
- 由鞘突未闭引起，85%的新生男孩出生时未闭合。
- 阴囊因为体位或者哭闹表现出不同的大小：
  - 患者可能存在已解决的阴囊肿块病史。
- 大部分在2岁时闭合。

诊断

症状和体征

无痛性阴囊肿胀，伴随拖拉感或下坠感。

病史

病史和检查尤其注意鉴别睾丸扭转。

体格检查

- 肿块可为柔软的、面团似的或坚硬的，取决于目前的液体量。
- 初步评估包括患侧透照法（寻找没有内部阴影、均匀性透光区域）。
  - 作为诊断性检查的方法，很快被床旁超声代替。

基本检查

- 床旁超声：
  - 使阴囊积水视觉化，同样适用于睾丸。
  - 无回声聚集表现为睾丸周围的黑色液体。
  - 最常见于阴囊前外侧。
  - 尤其在大量积液的患者，应行床旁超声作为诊断性检查。
  - 可能有助于鉴别潜在的肿块。
- 因为成人可能出现肿瘤引起阴囊积水，睾丸必须完全触诊检查。

诊断检查与说明

实验室检查

没有特别的实验室检查，除非潜在的病因需要实验室检查（如尿酸、甲胎蛋白、HCG）。

影像学检查

超声是诊断性检查，并且使睾丸解剖视觉化：

- 表现为大量无回声的液性区域，围绕在睾丸的前外侧。

鉴别诊断

- 附睾炎。
- 腹股沟斜疝。
- 睾丸炎。
- 睾丸肿瘤。
- 睾丸扭转。
- 精索静脉曲张。

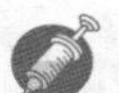

治疗

初步稳定/治疗

治疗应关注基本病因（如创伤）。

急诊治疗/程序

恰当的睾丸检查以排除原发性肿瘤及相关疾病。

药物治疗

治疗根本病因。

随访

进一步处理

入院指征

继发性鞘膜积液患者可能需要入院，进一步评估根本病因（如肿瘤、创伤）。

入院指征

- 健康人没有并发症可被转诊至泌尿科，进一步评估。
- 如果为了美观或者由于鞘膜积液引起不适，鞘膜积液通常被修复。
- 修复：
  - 外科手术：
    - 水囊肿切除术后选择抽吸术或硬化治疗。
  - 药物：
    - 抽吸阴囊水肿内容物，并且硬化治疗阻止复发。

儿科注意事项

- 大部分有鞘膜积液的婴儿将在12个月时自愈。
  - 一旦确诊，可考虑转诊和观察。
- 12～18个月后，转诊外科修复治疗，因为交通性鞘膜积液常常有需要修复的疝气。

随访建议

患者应转诊至泌尿科。

要点和误区

因为鞘膜变厚，肿块可能透照失败。

- 床旁超声可以使充满液体的肿块和睾丸视觉化。

青光眼 Glaucoma

Yasuharu Okuda · Lisa A. Jacohson 祝各亮 译

基础知识

描述

以眼压升高、视神经病变、视力逐渐丧失为特征的疾病。

病因

- 原发性青光眼：
  - 开角型青光眼：
    - 正常前房角。
    - 起病隐匿伴眼内压持续上升。
    - 最常见的青光眼类型，占90%。
    - 美国黑种人失明的主要原因。
    - 危险因素包括非洲人、年龄>40岁、家族史、近视、糖尿病和高血压。
  - 急性闭角型青光眼：
    - 前房角的狭窄或闭合，妨碍了房水通过小梁网的滤过部分从后房向前房的自然流动。
    - 通常急性发作的伴眼内压的突然增加。
    - 危险因素包括亚洲人、因纽特人、远视、家族史、年龄和女性。
- 继发性青光眼继发于其他疾病，包括眼部疾病、创伤和药物：
  - 可以是开角型和闭角型。
  - 药物：皮质激素、舍曲林、支气管扩张剂和托吡酯。

- 疾病：神经纤维瘤病、葡萄膜炎、新生血管形成和眼内肿瘤。
- 创伤。
- 血糖的快速变化。

诊断

症状和体征

经典表现：

- 开角型青光眼：
  - 无痛和视力逐渐丧失。
- 闭角型青光眼：
  - 疼痛、视力丧失与瞳孔固定中度大小。

病史

- 原发性开角型青光眼：
  - 周围视野逐渐缺失或夜间失明。
  - 通常双侧受累。
  - 无痛。
- 原发性闭角型青光眼：
  - 重度深眼痛和同侧头痛，常伴有恶心及呕吐。
  - 视力的下降通常被描述为视力模糊，与周围的光源出现光晕。
  - 与腹部疼痛相关，会误导诊断。
  - 药物：
    - 散瞳剂：东莨菪碱、阿托品。
    - 拟交感神经药：伪麻黄碱、沙丁胺醇。
    - 抗组胺药：苯海拉明、氯苯甲嗪。
    - 抗精神病药物：氟哌啶醇。
    - 吩噻嗪类药物：氯丙嗪、异丙嗪。
    - 三环类抗抑郁药：阿米替林。
    - 磺胺类药物：托吡酯。

体格检查

- 原发性开角型青光眼：
  - 视力下降。
- 原发性闭角型青光眼：
  - 视力下降。
  - 瞳孔中度扩张和无反应。
  - 角膜水肿伴朦胧感。
  - 结膜充血，睫状体潮红。
  - 触诊眼球坚硬。

基本检查

- 详细的眼部检查。
- 视力检查：
  - 通常都可以看见手动。
- 测眼压：
  - 正常眼压为 10～21 mmHg。
  - 原发性开角型青光眼：
    - 升高的程度可以变化，25%～30%的患者眼压可能正常。
  - 原发性闭角型青光眼：
    - 任何的升高都是不正常的，通常>40 mmHg。
- 裂隙灯检查：
  - 评估前房角。
  - 用于排除其他可能性，包括角膜擦伤和异物。

诊断检查与说明

实验室检查

直接进行检查和鉴别。

影像学检查

直接进行检查和鉴别。

诊断步骤/外科

前房角镜检查：

- 直接测量前房角是否关闭。

鉴别诊断

- 海绵窦血栓形成。
- 急性虹膜炎和葡萄膜炎。
- 视网膜动脉或静脉阻塞。
- 颞动脉炎。
- 视网膜脱离。
- 结膜炎。
- 角膜擦伤。

治疗

院前

- 送达医院前无需特殊眼部干预措施：
  - 可能需要进行止痛处理。
  - 创伤性病因，需稳定其他损伤。

初步稳定/治疗

- 第一步需降低闭角型青光眼的眼内压：
  - 如果是创伤性病因，解决创伤的其他影响因素。
  - 如果是药物性病因，停止药物的刺激。

急诊治疗/程序

- 原发性开角型青光眼：
  - 识别和及时进行眼科咨询。
  - 局部维持 β 受体阻滞剂或前列腺素类似物降低眼压。
- 原发性闭角型青光眼(眼科急症)：
  - 降低眼压：
    - 局部 β 受体阻滞剂，马来酸噻吗洛尔，减少房水生成。
    - 局部 α_2 受体激动剂，安普尼定，减少房水生成。
    - 碳酸酐酶抑制剂，乙酰唑胺，减少房水的生成。
    - 高渗剂，甘露醇，引起房水经玻璃体入血(病情严重时)。
  - 将虹膜与小梁网分离：
    - 一旦眼压<40 mmHg，局部应用拟副交感神经药、盐酸毛果芸香以收缩瞳孔。
  - 减少炎症反应：
    - 外用皮质激素，醋酸泼尼松龙。
  - 如果药物治疗无效，紧急眼科咨询以明确是否需要手术治疗，如激光虹膜切除术。
  - 需要适当的麻醉镇痛和止吐药。

药物治疗

- 乙酰唑胺：500 mg，静脉注射或口服。
- 20%甘露醇：1～2 g/kg，静脉注射，超过 30～60 min。
- 1%～2%盐酸毛果芸香碱溶液：1 滴，q15～30 min 直到缩瞳反应出现，然后 1 滴 q2～3 h。
- 1%醋酸泼尼松龙溶液：1 滴，q15～30 min，总共 4 次。

一线用药

- β 受体阻滞剂：
  - 0.25%或 0.5%噻吗洛尔：
    - 1 滴，滴眼，每日 2 次。
  - 0.25%或 0.5%左布诺洛尔：
    - 1 滴，滴眼，每日 2 次。
  - 1%盐酸卡替洛尔：
    - 1 滴，滴眼，每日 2 次。
  - 0.25%或 0.5%倍他洛尔：
    - 1～2 滴，滴眼，每日 2 次。

二线用药

- 肾上腺素受体激动剂：
  - 0.5%或 1%阿普尼定：
  - 1～2 滴，滴眼，每日 3 次。
  - 溴莫尼定：
    - 1 滴，滴眼，每日 3 次。
- 碳酸酐酶抑制剂：
  - 乙酰唑胺：
    - 125～250 mg，口服，每日 4 次。
  - 醋甲唑胺：
    - 50～100 mg，口服，每日 4 次。
  - 盐酸多佐胺：
    - 1 滴，滴眼，每日 3 次。
  - 布林佐胺：
    - 1 滴，滴眼，每日 3 次。

• 前列腺素衍生物：
- 拉坦前列素：
◦ 1滴，滴眼，睡前用。
- 0.03%比马前列素：
◦ 1滴，滴眼，睡前用。
- 曲伏前列素：
◦ 1滴，滴眼，睡前用。
- 乌诺前列酮：
◦ 1滴，滴眼，每日2次。

■ 处方

• 由于对前列腺素衍生物副反应的不断认识，它已成为原发性开角型青光眼的标准用药。
• 因为花费原因，β受体阻滞剂仍作为最初用药。

随访

■ 进一步处理

入院指征

• 严重的疼痛、恶心或呕吐。
• 接受肠外给药的患者必须进行副反应的观察。
• 症状不改善或眼压不下降的患者应持续监测眼压、药物治疗，必要时进行手术干预：
- 激光治疗比手术更容易进行。
- 白内障摘除也可以考虑。

出院指征

• 眼压显著升高但症状轻微的患者，可在眼科专家会诊允许后出院，并进行24 h的密切随访。

转诊问题

如果没有眼科专家，应当进行初始治疗并请邻近医院的眼科专家进行会诊。

■ 随访建议

• 开角型青光眼患者需要紧急眼科处理和有效的医疗管理。
• 闭角型青光眼患者需要立即干预。

要点和误区

• 眼压升高可引起血管功能不全，视力下降的治疗延迟可能会造成永久的视力丧失。
• 眼痛、头痛可与严重的腹部疼痛相关，不要因为忽视了眼部而误诊漏诊。
• 使用β受体阻滞剂的开角型青光眼患者可能会出现全身性副反应，包括直立性低血压、心动过缓或晕厥。

Q

氰化物中毒 Cyanide Poisoning

Kirk L. Cumpston 陈奇通 译

基础知识

■ 描述

• 通过吸入、胃肠道吸收或注射产生毒性。
• 通过中断氧化磷酸化抑制有氧代谢的细胞内毒素。
- 会降低氧的利用和ATP产生。
• 内在解毒：
- 硫氰酸酶：肝线粒体酶负责以下的代谢过程：
◦ 以含硫共价键（限速步骤）结合氰化物（含氰）形成毒性较低的水溶性硫氰酸盐（T-CN）。
◦ CN清除速率需要足够的含硫化合物的生物利用度[硫代硫酸盐（TS）]。

■ 病因

• 火灾：
- 天然和合成产品燃烧形成的副产品。
• 工业：
- 金属电镀，微芯片制造。
- 化学合成。
- 塑料制造。
- 农药。
• 溶剂：
- 人工钉器（乙腈）。
- 金属抛光剂。
• 硝普钠的代谢产物（非酶化反应）。
• 苦杏仁苷（由肠道菌群转化成CN），含氰化物的植物（杏仁、桃核、苹果、梨和木薯）。
• 珠宝首饰制作。

诊断

■ 症状和体征

• 心脏和大脑：最敏感的器官，最先出现临床症状。
• 中枢神经系统：
- 头痛。
- 意识混乱。
- 晕厥。
- 癫痫发作。
- 昏迷。
• 心血管系统：
- 心律失常。
- 胸痛。
- 心肺衰竭而死亡。
• 其他：
- 恶心、呕吐。
• 口服：可为腐蚀性，50 mg就可引起死亡。
• 吸入：
- 50 ppm：导致焦虑、心悸、呼吸困难、头痛。
- 100～135 ppm：吸入时间<1 h是致命的。

■ 基本检查

• 暴露史：
- 密闭空间内的烟雾吸入。
- 工业暴露。
- 故意自杀。
- 故意杀人。
• 临床线索：
- 特殊的苦杏仁味（可变感知）。
- 鲜红色的（动脉化）视网膜血管。
- 突然发作和/或毒副作用。
- 酸中毒。
- 高的静脉血氧饱和度（继发于细胞内氧耗的阻断），动脉化的静脉血液气体。

■ 诊断检查与说明

实验室检查

• 全血细胞计数。
• 电解质、尿素氮、肌酐、葡萄糖：
- 阴离子间隙酸中毒。
• 肝功能。
• 磷酸肌酸激酶（CPK）。
• 碳氧血红蛋白（COHgb）水平。
• 高铁血红蛋白水平（MIH）水平。
• 氰化物水平：
- 在临床相关时间段，实验室检测通常不可用。

- 浓度水平>0.5～1 mg/ml：中毒。
- 浓度水平在 2.5～3 mg/ml：致命。

• 血气测定：
- 动静脉血氧分压差下降：AVO_2 下降（正常在 3～4.8 ml/dl）。

• 乳酸水平：
- 乳酸升高（>8 mmol/L）是一种替代标志物，它与适当的病史和体格检查一起表明了氰化物的存在。

影像学检查

胸部 X 线检查。

鉴别诊断

• 一氧化碳。
• 硫化氢。
• 高铁血红蛋白血症。
• 硫化血红蛋白血症。
• 惰性气体"窒息"。
• 高阴离子间隙代谢性酸中毒的其他原因。

治疗

院前

• 脱离氰化物的污染源。
• 防止他人受到污染。
• 如果是液体污染，请脱掉所有受污染的衣物，并用肥皂和水大量清洗受影响的区域。
• 如果蒸汽污染，可能需要将患者从氰化物环境中移除。

初步稳定/治疗

• 基本步骤：
- 吸 100%氧气。

• 如果在 1 h 内由口腔摄入，胃净化措施如下：
- 如果摄入固体氰化物或含有氰化物的产品且无禁忌证，则服用活性炭（AC）。
- 不要催吐。

• 皮肤暴露：标准去污染。

急诊治疗/程序

• 羟钴胺（维生素 $B_{12}a$）Cyanokit：
- 如果有明显的氰化物中毒表现，持续性高阴离子间隙代谢性酸中毒和高乳酸血症，伴有晕厥、癫痫、心律失常、低血压，立即使用。
- 管理者通常制定经验性的治疗流程，氰化物水平浓度不是立即可检测的。
- 结合氰化物：
  ◦ 形成氰钴维生素（维生素 B_{12}），从肾脏排出。
- 优势：
  ◦ 无高铁血红蛋白形成。
  ◦ 导致高血压。
  ◦ 分细胞内再分布。
- 局限性：
  ◦ 成本。
- 在同一个静脉输液管道内不相容的（药物）：
  ◦ 地西泮（安定）。
  ◦ 多巴酚丁胺。
  ◦ 多巴胺。
  ◦ 芬太尼。
  ◦ 硝酸甘油。
  ◦ 戊巴比妥。
  ◦ 异丙酚。
  ◦ 硫代硫酸钠。
  ◦ 亚硝酸钠。
  ◦ 维生素 C。
  ◦ 血液制品。
- 羟钴胺的副作用：
  ◦ 高血压。
  ◦ 红色的皮肤和排泄物。
  ◦ 对用比色法测定的碳氧血红蛋白、天冬氨酸氨基转移酶、丙氨酸氨基转移酶、总胆红素、肌酐、镁、铁等的干扰。
  ◦ 由于检测到机器内的红色而导致血液透析失败。

• 使用氰化物解毒剂的套装：
- 解毒药：如果有明显的氰化物中毒表现，持续性高阴离子间隙代谢性酸中毒和高乳酸血症，伴有晕厥、癫痫、心律失常、低血压，立即使用。
- 管理者通常制定经验性的治疗流程、氰化物水平浓度不是立即可检测的。
- 内容：亚硝酸异戊酯、亚硝酸钠和硫代硫酸钠。
- 戊基和亚硝酸钠作用：
  ◦ 通过氧化血红蛋白（Fe^{2+} 到 Fe^{3+}）诱导产生一种清除氰化物的高铁血红蛋白，而吸引了细胞外氰基脱离线粒体形成毒性小的氰化高铁血红蛋白。
  ◦ 不要经验性或预防性应用。
- 硫代硫酸钠的作用机制：
  ◦ 硫氰酸酶的底物。
  ◦ 结合氰基形成毒性小的硫氰酸盐。

药物治疗

活性炭：1 g/kg，口服。

一线用药

羟钴胺素：

• 70 mg/kg，静脉或骨髓腔注射，最大剂量为 5 g。
• 该套件包 5 g/瓶的 1 瓶。管理药瓶。
• 用注射用水加入粉剂中轻轻滚动药瓶，后加入 100 ml 生理盐水中。
• 1 瓶 5 g 超过 15 min。5 g 的剂量可以重复。

考虑加用硫代硫酸钠。

二线用药

• 氰化物解毒剂套装：亚硝酸异戊酯、亚硝酸钠和硫代硫酸钠。
• 亚硝酸异戊酯的使用要点：
- 在纱布中冲上 1～2 安瓿，紧贴鼻、面膜唇部或安瓿袋内。
- 吸气 30 s 至 1 min，直到获得静脉通路。

• 亚硝酸钠（$NaNO_2$）：10 ml（300 mg）（儿童：0.15～0.33 ml/kg），3%溶液静脉注射 5～20 min：
- 可在 30～60 min 内重复一次，剂量减半。
- 保持高铁血红蛋白（MH）水平<30%。
- 稀释；低血压时缓慢输注。

• 硫代硫酸钠：50 ml：12.5 g（儿童：0.95～1.65 ml/kg），静滴 10～15 min，25%溶液。
- 可在 30～60 min 后给予 1/2 的首剂。

孕妇注意事项

• 羟钴胺为 C 类。
• 亚硝酸戊酯为 X 类。
• 亚硝酸钠未知。
• 硫代硫酸钠为 C 类。

老年患者注意事项

• 约 50 名年龄在 65 岁或以上的已知或疑似氰化物中毒患者接受羟钴胺治疗，其安全性和疗效与年轻患者相似。
• 羟钴胺在肾脏排泄时不会随尿液变化，因此肾损害可延长排泄半衰期。
• 羟钴胺治疗肝损害的安全性和有效性尚不清楚。
• 硫代硫酸钠在肝脏代谢，由肾脏排出。任何一个器官的损伤都可能延长清除时间。
• 亚硝酸盐是短效的。肝或肾损害可延长清除时间。

儿科注意事项

羟钴胺在儿童中的安全性和有效性尚未确定，但已使用 70 mg/kg 剂量。

注意

• 亚硝酸钠对儿童的剂量是以体重为基础的。
• 当临床情况不需要在实验室测试前给予解毒剂以挽救生命时，亚硝酸钠剂量可基于血清血红蛋白。

血红蛋白	亚硝酸盐 (mg/kg)	亚硝酸盐 (ml/kg)
7	5.8	0.19
8	6.6	0.22
9	7.5	0.25
10	8.3	0.27
11	9.1	0.30
12	10.0	0.33
13	10.8	0.36
14	11.6	0.39

随访

进一步处理

入院指征

所有有症状的暴露史都应进入ICU治疗。

出院指征

- 无症状患者至少观察4 h。
- 急性暴露4 h后的存活率通常与完全恢复有关。

转诊问题

故意过量服用和自杀的患者转诊至精神科。

要点和误区

- 对于低血压、高阴离子间隙代谢性酸中毒、高乳酸血症、癫痫、晕厥、精神状态改变的患者，在鉴别诊断中考虑氰化物中毒，并经验性进行治疗。
- 使用血清乳酸作为氰化物暴露的替代标志物。
- 吸入烟雾的受害者可能有以下几种情况：
  - 氰化物毒性。
  - MH。
  - 一氧化碳毒性。
  - 如果COHgb浓度极高，也可认为是伴随氰化物暴露。
  - 避免氧转运进一步减少；最初用羟钴胺或硫代硫酸钠治疗，不含亚硝酸钠，以避免高铁血红蛋白血症。

桡骨小头半脱位(保姆肘) Nursemaid's Elbow

Roger M. Barkin 朱妍 译

基础知识

描述

＜5 岁儿童最常见的肘部损伤。发病高峰在 2～3 岁。据报道,在 9 岁大的儿童中也有这种情况。

病因

• 桡骨远端突然的牵拉导致部分环状韧带在桡骨头上下滑动,从而被卡在桡骨和肱骨小头之间。肘关节旋前和伸展时的纵向牵引可通过摆动儿童、摔跤和抬起儿童的手臂而导致半脱位。

• 当孩子到 5 岁以后,环状韧带粗壮和强大足以对抗撕裂和/或位移。

• 通常称为"肘部拉伤"或桡骨头半脱位。

诊断

症状和体征

• 孩子拒绝使用手臂。

• 肘部略弯曲,前臂紧贴躯干。

• 肘部的弯曲导致疼痛。

• 前臂疼痛,通常为内旋。

• 无压痛点。

• 极轻微或不肿胀。

病史

• 孩子不敢活动患侧手臂。

• 50%曾报告有牵拉手臂的经典病史。

• 也可以由摔倒、肘部轻微外伤或前臂的扭转所致。

• ＜6 个月的孩子滚动手臂也可能引起。

体格检查

• 患侧手臂靠近躯干。

• 手臂通常将手掌向下或向后转动。

• 肘部充分扩展或轻微弯曲。

• 儿童不会伸展或弯曲肘部。

• 前外侧桡骨头可有轻微压痛,但是其余的手肘无痛感。

• 被动活动无痛感。

• 旋后产生疼痛感。

基本检查

临床诊断:

• 典型病史、被动的手臂姿势体格检查足以明确诊断。

诊断检查与说明

影像学检查

X 线摄片:

• 通常没有表现。

• 如果以下任一情况存在可排除或诊断为其他伤情:

- 压痛点。
- 软组织肿胀。
- 畸形。
- 肘部瘀斑。
- 复位失败。
- 手法复位后孩子仍喜欢制动。
- 如果出现明显的疼痛、肿胀、畸形或瘀斑,可在复位前提示。

• 在不典型的表现和复位后确认的情况下,床旁超声检查可能是有用的。在关节间隙可见环状韧带,形成由环状韧带移位到关节间隙形成的病理性"钩征"。

鉴别诊断

如果多次尝试后仍未减少,则必须考虑。

• 肱骨、桡骨、尺骨或锁骨骨折。

• 肘关节脱臼。

• 关节感染。

• 骨髓炎。

• 肿瘤。

治疗

院前

注意:

• 冰敷受伤的肘部,以减少疼痛和肿胀。

• 固定在吊腕带或夹板上以便于运输,并防止进一步损害。

• 评估远端血管神经状态。

初步稳定/治疗

评估远端运动、感觉和血管功能。

急诊治疗/程序

• 旋后、屈曲技巧:

- 更常用。
- 以握手的姿势抓住孩子的手并温和地轴向牵引。
- 用另一只手来稳定受伤的手肘并以拇指对桡骨头施加适当压力。
- 以一个流畅、迅速的动作使掌心充分向上并翻转手肘。

• 高度内旋、伸展技巧:

- 一些人认为不那么痛苦。
- 以握手的姿势抓住孩子的手并温和地轴向牵引。
- 用另一只手来稳定受伤的手肘并以拇指对桡骨头施加适当压力。
- 高度内旋手臂,并将未伸展的手臂伸展。

• 将检查者的拇指放在桡骨头上可以进行点击触诊。

• 孩子可能在复位的过程中哭叫,但很快活动手臂时就会感到疼痛消失。如果复位延迟,制动时间可能会延长。

- 如果半脱位超过几小时,手臂可能在长时间不能恢复正常功能。

• 如果尝试第一次复位后的 15 min 内儿童仍不能活动手臂,则可尝试第二次复位。

• 如果第一次尝试失败,请考虑第二次减少尝试的替代技术,因为没有关于两种技术的相对有效性的明确数据。

• 影像学检查研究表明,如果第二次复位仍未成功,则应评估有无骨折。

• 进行复位后血管与神经的评估。

药物治疗

• 对乙酰氨基酚:10～15 mg/kg,口服,q4 h;不超过 5 次剂量/24 h 或 4 g/24 h。

• 布洛芬:10 mg/kg,口服,q6～8 h。

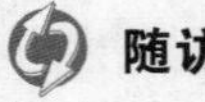

随访

进一步处理

入院指征

无。

出院指征

• 当孩子完全恢复,能够自由使用手臂时即可出院。

• 患者指导:

- 告知父母不要牵拉或提升孩子的手、手腕或前臂。
- 5 岁前复发率高达 39%。
- 很少需要止痛药。

转诊问题

复位失败或儿童不使用正常功能手臂:

• 如果 X 线检查也阴性,则需要把孩子转至骨科。

• 将手臂置于后夹板中，肘部保持 90°，前臂旋后，以便门诊随访。

• 没有证据表明稍微延期复位有长期后遗症。

随访建议

• 成功复位后无需其他治疗。

• 复位失败后需要在 24 h 内转至骨科。

要点和误区

• 如果有经典病史则需考虑桡骨小头半脱位。

• 影像学检查不是必需的，除非肘部有局部压痛或肿胀，或者病史中未提示桡骨小头半脱位。

• 早期服用止痛剂可以促进功能恢复。

• 复位尝试应至少包括一次使用超旋内翻方法。

• 两次复位不成功应促使放射学评估。

• 复位失败的患者，在把手臂固定在吊腕带或安置夹板后需要将其转至骨科。

人类免疫缺陷病毒/获得性免疫缺陷综合征 HIV/AIDS

Ankia Backster · Martine Lory Camille 陈奇通 李文放 译

基础知识

描述

• 获得性免疫缺陷综合征(AIDS)是因人类免疫缺陷病毒(HIV)感染致 $CD4^+$ 细胞＜200/mm^3 或 AIDS 相关性疾病，如感染(隐孢子虫)、恶性肿瘤(卡波西肉瘤、宫颈癌)或其他疾病(HIV 消瘦综合征、HIV 脑病)。

• 机会性疾病：

- $CD4^+$＜500/mm^3。
  ◦ 食管念珠菌病。
  ◦ 肺炎球菌感染。
  ◦ 毛状白斑。
  ◦ 免疫性血栓局部减少性紫癜。
- $CD4^+$＜200/mm^3。
  ◦ 肺孢子菌肺炎(PCP)。
  ◦ 隐球菌感染。
  ◦ 播散性肺结核。
  ◦ 隐孢子虫病。
  ◦ 等孢子虫病。
  ◦ 弓形虫病。
  ◦ 组织胞浆虫病。
- $CD4^+$＜50/mm^3。
  ◦ 中枢神经系统淋巴瘤。
  ◦ 禽分枝杆菌疾病。
  ◦ 结核性心包炎或脑膜炎。
  ◦ 巨细胞病毒。
  ◦ 胆管相关疾病：常见于微小隐孢子虫感染。

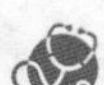

诊断

症状及体征

• 感染急性期(感染 HIV 后 2～6 周)：90%的患者无明显症状，少数患者出现发热、不适、咽炎、腹泻、面部及躯干有皮疹、伴有淋巴结病和肝脾大的流感样症状。

• 晚期 HIV 疾病(CD4＜200/mm^3)：疲乏、发热和盗汗、消瘦、脱发、慢性腹泻、咳嗽、呼吸困难、咯血、慢性头痛、精神状态、癫痫、痴呆、精神病变、无痛性视力丧失、皮肤病变。

病史

• 危险因素：
- 性行为混乱，多名性伴侣。
- 静脉毒品滥用。
- 男性同性行为者。
- 1985 年前输血者。
- 与危险性伴侣无保护性行为。
- 未受割礼者。

• 近期 CD4 计数和病毒载量、最低 CD4 计数。

• 抗反转录病毒药物的历史或现状。

• 服药依从性。

• 诊断及病程时间。

• 机会感染既往史。

• 住院及 ICU 住院既往史。

基本检查

• 诊断测试可能呈阴性的窗口期取决于所使用的诊断测试：
- DNA 扩增在 1～2 周为阳性。
- 15 日内可检测到 P24 蛋白。
- 血清抗体检测至少需要 20 日的时间进行检测。
- POCT/快速 HIV 检测：使用口腔拭子或手指棒血液：
  ◦ 实验室血清检测对急性 HIV 感染更敏感。

• 血清学检查：原发性感染及血清学转化之间存在潜伏期，持续约 24 周，在此期间检测可能为阴性。

• HIV 核酸检测：在感染后 1～2 周可呈阳性，但在急诊室可能不可行，需要密切随访和咨询。

• 呼吸系统：胸部 X 线检查、动脉血气、痰革兰染色，AFB 及培养、卡氏肺囊肿虫肺炎中 LDH 升高、血培养。

• 循环系统：血清心脏标志物、电解质、胸部 X 线检查、可疑心包炎、积液或压塞的心电图；如果怀疑心内膜炎，进行血液培养；对可卡因和苯丙胺进行药物筛选。

• 神经系统症状：头颅 CT、腰椎穿刺减压、CSF 检查葡萄糖、蛋白质、革兰染色及培养、细胞计数与鉴别、AFB 涂片，印墨染色、单纯疱疹、隐球菌抗原和 VDRL。

• 胃肠道症状：粪便卵细胞及寄生虫、革兰染色、培养、艰难梭状芽胞杆菌分析、尿妊娠试验(对于女性)、盆腔体液检测、淋病/衣原体检查、肝功能检查、淀粉酶、脂肪酶、肝炎血清学、低剂量盆腹腔 CT、超声(存在胆道症状)、降低外科剖腹探查指征(HIV 感染患者可能不存在典型急腹症体征)。

• 发热：包括需氧/厌氧菌、真菌、抗酸染色和 MAC 血液培养。

• 眼部症状：裂隙灯荧光染色检查。

诊断实验检查与说明

实验室检查

• ELISA：检测 HIV 抗体 IgG，检查敏感性和特异性为 99%，但窗口期可以是负值。

• 抗原检测：CDC 不再推荐作为检查的一部分。

• 初步检测应采用第四代抗原-抗体结合试验来筛选感染：
- 可检测 HIV-1、HIV-2 抗体和 HIV-1 p24 抗原。

- 可以更早发现。
- 阴性无须进一步检测。
- 如果阳性，使用抗体免疫分析来区分 HIV-1 和 HIV-2。
- 抗体分化免疫测定无反应或不确定者，应进行核酸检测确认。

• 绝对淋巴细胞计数：白细胞与淋巴细胞百分比的乘积，如计数＞2 000，则 CD4 细胞可能＞200；如计数＜1 000，则 CD4 细胞可能＜200。

影像学检查

• 胸部 X 线：
- 双侧间质浸润：PCP。
- 网状结节浸润：TB、KS 或真菌性肺炎。
- 感染性肺门淋巴结病：结核、隐球菌病、组织胞浆菌病、肿瘤。
- 大叶实变：细菌性肺炎。
- 空洞：结核、坏死性细菌性肺炎球虫样真菌病。
- 正常 X 线并不排除 PCP 或 TB。

• 头部 CT 平扫及增强：
- 基底神经节或皮层水肿的多发环增强病变：弓形虫病或中枢神经系统淋巴瘤。
- 皮质下非增强病灶：PML。

• 脑梗死腹部/盆腔 CT：
- 脾大：巨细胞病毒，TB。
- 肠穿孔或肠梗阻：巨细胞病毒性结肠炎、淋巴瘤、组织浆菌病、MAC、阑尾炎、溃疡性疾病、卡波西肉瘤。
- 胆囊炎或胆管炎：隐孢子虫、微孢子虫、巨细胞病毒。
- 胰腺炎：医源性、肿瘤性、感染性。

鉴别诊断

• 肺部症状：肺栓塞、肺动脉高压、肺结核、肺炎（细菌、真菌、病毒）、肺恶性肿瘤、淋巴细胞间质性肺炎。

• 中枢症状：神经梅毒、巨细胞病毒或单纯疱疹病毒性脑炎、弓形虫脑、脑膜炎（细菌性、球孢子菌等）、蛛网膜下腔出血、脑梗死、HIV 感染或代谢性脑炎、进行性多灶性白质脑病。

• 心血管症状：心肌病、心包炎、心肌炎、心内膜炎、急性冠状动脉综合征、心包积液。

• 口腔症状：真菌感染（念珠菌等）、病毒感染（HSV、CMV、毛状白斑）、细菌感染（结核、牙周病）、自身免疫性疾病（唾液腺疾病、口腔溃疡）、肿瘤（卡波西肉瘤、淋巴瘤）。

• 食管症状：感染性食管炎（假丝酵母、CMV、HSV）、反流性食管炎。

• 腹泻症状：药物副作用、寄生虫（隐孢子虫、鞭毛虫等孢子球虫属）、细菌、病毒（CMV、HSV、HIV）、真菌（组织胞浆菌、隐球菌）、HIV 相关性肠病。

• 肝大：肝炎、机会性感染（CMV、MAC、TB）。

• 肾脏疾病：药物肾毒性、HIV 肾病、血管炎、梗阻性。

治疗

治疗方案及流程

• 抗生素治疗：伴随细菌感染、中毒或症状迅速加重患者应给予抗生素治疗。

• 抗 HIV 治疗：CD4 水平低（＜300）或病毒载量高、怀孕、AIDS 相关性疾病或 HIV 相关性肾病（一般情况下，有记录的原发性 HIV 感染患者在确诊后也会进行耐药性检测）。

• 高效抗反转录病毒疗法（HAART）：1 个非核苷反转录酶抑制剂（NNRT）和 2 个核苷反转录酶抑制剂（NRTI）、1 和 2 个 NRTIS、3 种 NRTI。

• 暴露后预防：在感染后 2 h 内开始治疗，并持续 4 周；两种药物联合：齐多夫定＋拉米夫定（康比韦）；拉米夫定＋司他夫定；司他夫定＋地达诺辛；3 种药物联合用于高风险感染的情况。

• 弓形虫病：（乙胺嘧啶）磺胺嘧啶、四氢叶酸、激素（脑水肿）、治疗持续至少 6 周。

• 隐球菌脑膜炎：两性霉素 B，氟胞嘧啶，治疗持续 2 周；氟康唑治疗 8 周。

• 巨细胞病毒视网膜炎：更昔洛韦。

• 食管念珠菌病：氟康唑 14～21 日；病情严重可加用利福平。

• 卡氏肺囊肿虫肺炎：甲氧苄啶-磺胺甲噁唑、喷他脒或氨苯砜（磺胺类药物过敏者）、如 PaO_2＜70 mmHg 或者 A-a 压力差＞35 mmHg，则加用泼尼松 40 mg，口服，每日 2 次，持续 5 日。

• 口腔念珠菌病：克曲马唑。

• HIV 相关急性脱髓鞘性多发性神经病：血浆置换。

药物治疗

• 常见药物并发症：
- 过敏反应：阿巴卡韦。
- 胰腺炎：二脱氧肌苷、二脱氧胞苷、二达诺辛、拉米夫定、复方新诺明、戊咪定、利托那文、斯塔夫定、扎尔西他滨。
- 周围神经病变：地达诺新、异烟肼、利奈唑胺、司他夫定、扎西他滨。
- 肾结石：地达诺新。
- 史蒂文斯-约翰逊综合征：奈韦拉平、阿扎那韦、地拉夫定、依法韦仑、甲氧苄啶-磺胺甲噁唑。
- 溶血性贫血：氨苯砜、齐多夫定。
- 精神病：依法韦仑。
- 低血糖：喷他脒。
- 体位性低血压、躯干性肥胖、动脉粥样硬化：司他夫定。
- 扩张性心肌病：齐多夫定。
- 间接胆红素良性增生：阿扎那韦、茚地那韦。
- 巨红细胞性贫血：齐多夫定。
- 许多药物都能引起血液改变、胃肠不适及皮疹。

随访

入院指征

• 不明原因发热伴中枢神经系统受累或疑似心内膜炎。
• 中性白细胞减少的发热。
• 低氧血症：PaO_2＜70 mmHg。
• 提示 ACS 的心脏症状。
• 心包积液。
• 怀疑细菌性肺炎或肺结核。
• 神经状态改变。
• 新发癫痫。
• 血流动力学不稳定。
• 不能走动或不能忍受口服。
• 顽固性腹泻伴脱水。

出院指征

能维持口服足量药物，提供自我护理和走动。

转诊问题

• 患者应转诊到主要的 HIV 感染护理场所，以便开始接受 HAART 治疗方案和相关护理。

• 警惕抑郁症的迹象，并咨询心理咨询或精神治疗，因为这可能会抑制治疗依从性。

• HIV 患者在许多恶性肿瘤中有更高的风险——将那些有相关症状的患者作为随访对象。

随访建议

• 免疫重建炎症综合征通常在 HAART 治疗后 8 周内出现，表现出机会性或自身免疫性疾病的症状。

• 对于职业暴露，血清转化的风险较低（显著的经皮和经皮血清转化的风险为 0.3%，黏膜暴露为 0.09%)。

• 接受 HAART 治疗的 HIV 感染患者胰岛素抵抗和急性冠状动脉综合征的风险较高，不受其他风险影响。

• 通过检测运动后氧饱和度结合胸片及肺炎症状有助于诊断 PCP。

• HIV 是 COPD、肺动脉高压、脑血管意外、静脉血栓栓塞、血栓性血小板减少性紫癜、骨质疏松症及髋关节坏死的独立风险因素。

妊娠(无并发症) Pregnancy, Uncomplicated

Patricia De Melo Panakos · Ivette Motola 郑金浩 毛恩强 译

基础知识

描述

• 妊娠不是病理过程而是生理过程。由于要促进胎儿生长发育，孕妇有严重的新陈代谢压力。

• 所有生育期妇女甚至有不孕史的妇女出现腹部疼痛均应考虑妊娠的可能，除非明确有其他原因。

• 妊娠期出现的变化主要是由于胎盘分泌大量的激素：

- 胎盘孕酮和雌激素。

儿科注意事项

• 美国人初次月经在 11～15 岁。

• 被送至急诊的妊娠少女可能不知道自己有身孕或不愿承认：

- 不要因为各方面压力忽视了少女妊娠的情况。

- 少女妊娠增加难产的风险。

病因

• 出现的症状与体征可以通过多种激素水平的升高、妊娠解剖结构的改变进行解释。

• 胎盘分泌的人绒毛膜促性腺激素(HCG)：

- 阻止月经周期末黄体素的降低。

- 促进黄体分泌大量的雌激素和孕激素。

- 人绒毛膜促性腺激素水平的升高是引起妊娠期恶心、呕吐的主要原因。

• 胎盘源性的孕酮：

- 促进子宫内膜的蜕膜细胞继续发育，为早期胚胎提供营养。

- 减少妊娠期子宫的宫缩，降低自发流产。

- 对雌激素促进乳房发育准备哺乳起帮助作用。

• 胎盘源性雌激素：

- 促进子宫、乳房、乳腺导管的生长。

- 扩大女性外生殖器，松弛骨盆、耻骨联合、骶髂关节。

诊断

诊断妊娠及妊娠综合征需借助以下 3 种诊断方法。

• 病史及体格检查。

• 激素试验。

• 超声。

症状和体征

• 近期有性生活的妇女出现停经伴恶心、呕吐。

• 停经：

- 在生育年龄的继发性停经最常见的因素为妊娠。

• 恶心、呕吐(清晨较重)。

• 乳房疼痛(乳腺痛)。

• 尿频。

• 头痛。

• 腰背痛。

• 异食癖。

• 足踝水肿。

• 体重增加。

• 极易疲劳、全身不适。

• 腹围增长。

• 便秘。

• 胃痛。

• 长时间膈肌痉挛。

• 皮肤变黑。

病史

• 明确末次月经的首日(FDLMP)。

• 约 40%的妇女不能明确提供末次月经的首日。

体格检查

• 骨盆检查。

• 通过测量宫高估计妊娠时间。

• 妊娠 16 周后耻骨到子宫底的距离(以 cm 为单位)近似等于妊娠时间。

• 尽早发现病理性骨盆疼痛以及肿块。

诊断检查与说明

实验室检查

• 早孕检测：

- β-HCG。

- 定量检测 HCG，6～7 周前每 2 日 HCG 升高 1 倍。

- 孕酮。

• 监测 β-HCG：

- 大多数尿早孕测试的敏感度在 25 mU/ml：

◦ 尿被稀释或摄入维生素 C 过多会引起结果假阴性。

- 家用的早孕试纸结果不准确：

◦ 特别是妊娠 9～12 日时检测。

- HCG 水平可能在流产 60 日内均保持在较高水平。

• 血清孕酮水平提示胚胎的变化也可以作为评估妊娠预后的参考：

- 血清孕酮水平<5 ng/ml 预示着胚胎不能存活(自发流产、宫外孕)。

- 孕酮水平在 25 ng/L 表示适合继续妊娠。

影像学检查

• 腹痛、阴道流血或其他产科疾病时使用超声确诊妊娠：

- 可以估测妊娠时间。

- 可以鉴别宫内妊娠和异位妊娠。

- 可以评估胎儿发育情况。

- 可以确诊胎儿畸形。

• 经腹部超声与经阴道超声：

- 经阴道超声更加敏感，但难于操作。

- 经阴道超声在妊娠 4～5 周即可观察到子宫内妊娠。

- 胚胎在妊娠 5.5～6 周后才能被经复超声检测。

- 经阴超声的禁忌是羊膜早破和妊娠晚期阴道流血。

• 超声联合血清 HCG 水平诊断病理性妊娠更有价值。

• MRI：没有证据表明 MRI 对于孕妇有副

R

作用。

- 在孕妇中，研究所选的人群多数是为了评估阑尾炎而行 MRI。

• X 线平片和 CT：

- X 线致畸剂量依赖。

- 比较小的增加胎儿幼儿时期肿瘤的发生率。

- 胎儿目标剂量为不超过 5 000 mrad。

  ◦ 腹部穿防辐射服，胸部 X 线检查：<1 mrad。

  ◦ 腹部 X 线平片：240 mrad。

  ◦ 胸部 CT：<10 mrad。

  ◦ 头颅 CT：<10 mrad。

  ◦ 胸部 CT 平扫：1 000 mrad 增强 2 000 mrad。

  ◦ 心内科介入：1 300 mrad。

  ◦ VQ 扫描：<50 mrad。

▪ 鉴别诊断

待妊娠期妇女性生活正常提供停经的病史应当考虑妊娠，除非有明确患其他疾病的证据。

治疗

▪ 院前

• 怀疑患者妊娠。

• 注意避免使用致畸药物，对于穿透胎盘屏障的药物谨慎使用。其他药物依据病情调整。

• 如果妊娠>24 周，孕妇保持左侧卧位。

▪ 急诊治疗/程序

治疗目的为优化孕妇的妊娠条件，改善胎儿的发育环境。

▪ 药物治疗

• 妊娠前期是胚胎器官形成的时期。

• 若妊娠前期胚胎发育出现畸形，中后期将会一直存在。

• 在使用药物以前参考 FDA 孕妇安全分级：

- 分级目录把药物分为 A、B、C、D、X。目录中 A 级药物为最安全的药物，X 级为对于孕妇副作用最大的药物。

• 镇痛：对乙酰氨基酚是最适合孕妇使用的非处方镇痛药。

• 阿司匹林和非甾体抗炎药没有致畸作用，但是使用前最好咨询产科医师。

• 氢可酮、可待因、氧可酮、哌替啶及吗啡没有发现有致畸的作用，可以短期用于孕妇剧烈的疼痛(3～4 日)。

• 抗生素：妊娠期妇女选择正确的抗生素基于以下几个因素：

- 孕妇的药物过敏史。

- 妊娠时长。

- 感染类型及引起感染可能的病原体。

• 给孕妇产前适量补充维生素。

• 疼痛治疗：

- 对乙酰氨基酚：500 mg，口服，q6 h，极量 4 g/d。

• 止吐药物：

- 昂丹司琼：40 mg，肌内注射/静脉注射，q8 h。

- 维生素 B_6：25 mg，每日 3 次或服用姜汤可以起辅助治疗作用。

随访

▪ 进一步处理

入院指征

• 有以下产科并发症的孕妇应当收入院进一步治疗：

- 呕吐、子痫不能耐受口服药物。

- 复杂性尿道感染。

- 异位妊娠或葡萄胎。

- 脓毒症性流产。

- 早产。

- 胎盘早破引起早产。

- 子痫前期/子痫。

- 严重的妊娠相关性高血压。

妊娠注意事项

患有疾病的孕妇可能会根据病情决定是否终止妊娠。

出院指征

没有上述疾病的孕妇可以考虑出院。

▪ 随访建议

孕妇出院后应当每 6～8 周做一次产检。

要点和误区

• 所有的妇女均考虑妊娠，除非有明确的证据没有妊娠。

• 在按规定分类前，所有的患者均认为妊娠是安全的。

• 胎儿射线暴露最小剂量设为<5 000 mrad。

妊娠剧吐 Hyperemesis Gravidarum

David Della-Giustina · Alina Tsyrulnik　巩博 译

基础知识

▪ 描述

• 妊娠剧吐是妊娠时持续恶心、呕吐最严重的形式。

• 也叫恶性妊娠呕吐。

• 以不明原因的难治性呕吐和脱水为特点。

• 妊娠期发生率为 0.3%～2%。

• 排除性诊断。

▪ 病因

• 具体原因未明。

• 可能的原因如下：

- 妊娠期激素水平上升：如人绒毛膜促性腺激素(HCG)和/或雌激素。

- 甲状腺功能亢进。

- 上消化道运动功能紊乱。

- 肝脏功能异常。

- 自主神经系统功能紊乱。

- 心理因素。

- 幽门螺杆菌感染。

- 遗传易感性。

诊断

▪ 症状和体征

• 妊娠期恶心、呕吐的发生率在 50%～90%。

• 妊娠 4～10 周出现症状，第 20 周消失。

- 妊娠 20 周后仍有症状，应怀疑其他疾病。

- 症状高峰期在第 8～12 周。
- 妊娠剧吐是一个临床诊断，根据以下来定义：
  - 顽固性恶心、呕吐。
  - 脱水。
  - 减去妊娠前体重的 5%。
  - 随着体重减轻，每日出现大于呕吐 3 次或体重减少 3 kg 或妊娠前体重的 5%。
  - 实验室检查：
    - 增加尿液比重。
    - 酮尿。
    - 电解质紊乱。
    - 酮血症。

症状

- 出现呕吐。
- 妊娠史：
  - 多见于未产妇女。
  - 在先前的妊娠史，有类似的症状。
- 末次月经。
- 经口进食。
- 排尿。
- 血性或胆汁性呕吐。
- 腹痛。
- 阴道出血。
- 危险因素：
  - 晕动症病史。
  - 年轻孕妇。
  - 偏头痛。
  - 一日中较早时间出现症状。
  - 妊娠期体质指数低。
  - 更常见于未生育过的妇女。
  - 如果在先前妊娠时出现，再发的概率是 15%。

体格检查

- 观察脱水的体征。
- 腹部压痛。
- 多涎（流涎）。

基本检查

- 病史和体格检查尤其注意脱水状态，腹部检查注意排除与呕吐有关的其他诊断（阑尾炎、胆囊炎）。
- 获得一份未被污染的尿液检查。
- 如果患者不间断呕吐>24 h，检查全血细胞计数、电解质、肾功能、肝酶、胆红素及脂肪酶。

诊断检查与说明

实验室检查

- 尿液分析：
  - 尿比重和尿酮升高。
  - 出现尿糖，检查血糖排除糖尿病。
  - 出现尿胆红素，查找引起呕吐的肝胆病因。
- 全血细胞计数：
  - 因为脱水，可能出现血细胞比容上升。
  - 白细胞通常正常。
- 电解质：
  - BUN 上升暗示着容量不足。如果出现肾衰竭，肌酐上升。
  - 呕吐时 HCl 丢失，可能出现低钠血症、低钾血症、低氯血症或代谢性碱中毒。
- 肝功能检测：
  - 可能出现胆红素轻度升高，应<4 mg/dl。
  - AST 和 ALT 也可能轻度升高，但是不应该>100 U/L。
  - 隆起的程度与呕吐的严重程度有关。
- 淀粉酶/脂肪酶：
  - 在一项研究中，淀粉酶在 24%的妊娠剧吐患者中升高，但是淀粉酶可能来源于唾液。使用脂肪酶而不是淀粉酶来评估胰腺炎。
- TSH：
  - 30%～70%的妊娠剧吐女性在妊娠早期有甲状腺功能异常。
  - 轻度甲状腺功能亢进，可能是由于血清 HCG 水平高，具有促甲状腺活性。
  - TSH<0.4 mU/L，游离 T_4 略有升高。
  - 无典型 Graves 特征（甲状腺肿、眼病、热耐受、震颤）。
- 如果已知宫内妊娠，不需要检查血清 HCG 水平。

影像学检查

- 妊娠早期行超声检查以评估：
  - 葡萄胎。
  - 多胎妊娠。

鉴别诊断

- 肾盂肾炎，常常被漏诊。
- 肠胃炎、胃轻瘫、肠梗阻、食管黏膜撕裂症。
- 肝胆疾病：肝炎、胆囊炎、妊娠脂肪肝、失弛缓症。
- 胰腺炎。
- 阑尾炎。
- 甲状腺功能亢进和甲状旁腺功能亢进。
- 尿毒症：严重肾衰竭可出现持续恶心与呕吐。
- 假性脑瘤。
- 大麻素剧吐综合征。
- 妊娠相关条件：
  - 多胎妊娠。
  - 葡萄胎。
  - 子痫前期/HELLP 综合征（非妊娠早期）。
  - 妊娠期急性脂肪肝（非妊娠早期）。

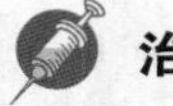

治疗

院前

- 建立静脉通路，如果出现严重容量不足的体征，监测生命体征。
- 静脉补液。

初步稳定/治疗

静脉补液使用一种晶体溶液（乳酸林格液或生理盐水）。

急诊治疗/程序

- 静脉补液使用乳酸林格液或生理盐水。
- 可以添加葡萄糖有助于打破酮体循环。
- 治疗患者一直到血容量不足的症状消失。
- 静脉使用止吐药物，打破呕吐循环。
- FDA 妊娠类（A、B、C、D 和 X）已经被基于现有数据的“风险叙述性总结”所取代。
- 在发布时，这个更改还没有完全实现。
- 急诊室最常用的初始药物：
- 常用的药物治疗：
  - 甲氧氯普胺（B 类）。
  - 丙氯拉嗪（原 C 类）：
    - 目前的风险总结：在妊娠期间使用丙氯拉嗪的安全性尚未确定。因此，不建议在孕妇中使用丙氯拉嗪，除非出现严重且难以处理的恶心和呕吐，医师认为需要药物干预，且潜在的好处大于可能的危险。
  - 异丙嗪（C 类）。
  - 昂丹西酮（前 B 类）。
    - 当前风险总结：现有数据不能可靠地告知不良胎儿结局的关联。
    - 避免患者先天性长 QT 综合征。
    - 心电图监测，注意电解质异常（如低钾血症或低镁血症）。
    - 之前的担忧，在更大的研究中有关胎儿心脏畸形和腭裂已确定不是一个问题。
  - 止吐药可能有加重酮症和血容量不足的风险。
- 在急诊室予以初步的液体复苏和止吐药后，口服补液。
- Wernicke 脑病需要静脉补液、硫胺素 100 mg，静脉注射、肌内注射或口服。
- 抗组胺药已经证明有效。

R

• 甲泼尼龙可能对妊娠剧吐有效。

- 最后手段。

如果妊娠期<10 周，避免使用。

■ **药物治疗**

一线用药

• 茶苯海明：25～50 mg，口服，q4～6 h（如果患者也服用多西拉敏，不超过 200 mg/d）；50 mg，静脉注射（在 50 ml 生理盐水中，20 min 内缓慢注射），q4～6 h。

• 甲氧氯普胺（B 类）：10～20 mg，静脉注射。

• 昂丹司琼（B 类）：4～8 mg，静脉注射；或者 4 mg，口服；或者口腔崩解片（ODT），q8 h。

• 丙氯拉嗪（C 类）：5～10 mg，静脉注射，不超过 40 mg/d。

• 异丙嗪（C 类）：12.5～25 mg，肌内注射。

• 出院患者药物治疗：

- 氯苯甲嗪（B 类）：25 mg，口服，q6 h，需要时使用。

- 甲氧氯普胺（B 类）：10 mg，口服，q6～8 h，需要时使用。

- 丙氯拉嗪（C 类）：5～10 mg，口服 q6 h；或肛门塞剂 25 mg，q12 h，需要时使用。

- 异丙嗪（C 类）：12.5～25 mg，口服或肛门塞剂，q4～6 h，需要时使用。

- 吡哆醇（维生素 B_6，A 类）：25 mg，口服 3 次/日（非处方药）。

- 姜黄：500～1 500 mg 分次，分 2～3 次服用。

- Diclegis（A 类）：多西拉敏和吡哆醇的联合制剂，10 mg/10 mg，每晚睡前服 2 片。

- 硫胺素：妊娠期>3 周有症状者 50 mg，每日口服。

二线用药

甲泼尼龙（C 类）：16 mg，静脉注射或口服，q8 h，3 日后逐渐减量。应当请产科医师会诊后开具处方。

随访

■ **进一步处理**

入院指征

• 治疗后不能耐受口服。

• 尽管治疗不能控制呕吐。

• 严重的电解质紊乱或代谢紊乱。

• 妊娠<8 周的最高风险期间。

出院指征

• 大多数患者只要能耐受口服并且有合适的随访，就可以出院。

• 纠正脱水相关症状。

• 尿酮下降。

• 使患者放心：他们的症状很常见并且是自限性的。

• 应当建议患者频繁、少量进餐可能有帮助：

- 食物应包含碳水化合物，并且是低脂的。

- 避免刺激性或辛辣食物。

• 如果有适应证，可以安排家庭输液治疗。

■ **随访建议**

• 所有诊断明确的患者应每日至少口服 3 mg 硫胺素以防止 Wernicke 脑病。推荐每日补充 50 mg。

• 在妊娠早期，有剧烈呕吐症状的孕妇流产风险较小。

要点和误区

• 妊娠 9 周后仍存在恶心与呕吐，应当考虑以恶心与呕吐为首发症状的其他疾病。

• 和使用鼻胃管或者单独药物治疗的患者相比，使用 PICC 被证明明显增加孕妇死亡率。

• 低钠血症患者补钠时，应小心脑桥中央髓鞘溶解。

• Wernicke 脑病是最严重的妊娠期并发症：

- 患者可能没有经典的三联征：共济失调、眼球震颤及痴呆。注意任何冷漠或混乱的症状。

- 任何出现冷漠或者混乱的患者，一定要给予硫胺素 100 mg 静脉注射。

妊娠期阴道出血 Vaginal Bleeding In Pregnancy

Paul Ishimine　周秋香　毛恩强 译

基础知识

■ **描述**

• 是孕妇和婴儿发病和死亡的主要原因。

• 妊娠早期（≤20 周）出血：

- 孕妇中发生率为 30%。

- 50%会发展为自然流产。

• 妊娠晚期（≥20 周）出血：

- 孕妇中发生率为 3%～5%。

• 风险因素：

- 大龄孕妇。

- 药物滥用。

- 盆腔炎。

- 先前有剖宫产史。

- 先前有终止妊娠史。

- 先前有过扩宫刮宫术史。

- 先前有宫外孕史。

- 多胎妊娠。

- 多次妊娠。

- 子痫前期。

- 高血压。

- 创伤。

- 使用辅助生殖技术。

• 遗传学：

- 50%～60%流产是因为染色体异常。

■ **病因**

• 阴道。

• 子宫颈。

• 子宫。

• 子宫胎盘接触面。

• 血流动力学不稳定。

诊断

■ **症状和体征**

病史

• 大量和持续出血。

- 量大（血块，多块卫生棉）。

- 颜色（暗红色或鲜红色）。

- 疼痛或无痛。

- 水性微带血性黏液。

- 卫生棉吸纳 5 ml。

- 棉垫能吸纳 5～15 ml。

- 在有威胁生命的条件下表现的可能仅仅是少量出血。

• 最近一次月经周期。

• 评估妊娠时间。

- 妊娠次数。
- 发热。
- 最近一次性交。
- 子宫避孕环。
- 最近妇产科就诊过程。
- 晕厥。
- 自发流产：痉挛，盆腔放射痛。
- 宫外孕：盆腔侧边剧烈疼痛。
- 前置胎盘：典型的无痛性出血。
- 胎盘早剥：典型的疼痛伴暗红色出血。

体格检查

- 重要体征：
  - 心率快。
  - 低血压。
  - 直立位的改变。
  - 没有出现血流动力学不稳的征象，可能和妊娠使全身血容量增加的生理因素有关。
- 胎心：
  - 经阴道超声能在妊娠 6.5 周闻及胎心音。
  - 多普勒超声要在妊娠 10 周后可以听见。
  - 正常的胎心在 120～160 次/分。
- 重要体征：
  - 子宫大小：
    - 12 周在下腹部可触及。
    - 20 周在脐可触及。
  - 腹水征。
- 盆腔检查，仅在妊娠早期。
  - 分析出血量和频次。
  - 确定子宫颈口开发程度(指诊仅在妊娠期 3 个月)。
    - 先兆流产(子宫颈口闭合)。
    - 进行性流产(子宫颈口开发)。
    - 不完全流产(子宫颈口开发或闭合)。
    - 完全流产(子宫颈口闭合)。
    - 胚胎死亡(子宫颈口闭合)。
  - 完全或不完全流产后的滞留物需要引起重视。
    - 滞留物在子宫颈口引起持续出血。
  - 评估子宫大小和柔软度。
  - 评估子宫肌瘤和附件肿块。
  - 妊娠晚期：外部检查可以，除非在受控或环境中，否则不要进行盆腔检查。
    - 随后可能出现严重出血。
    - 严重的出血需要确认，此时超声优于盆腔检查。

基本检查

- 全血细胞计数。
- 血型和 Rh。
- 妊娠早期 HCG 定量。
- 尿液检查。
- 超声：
  - 妊娠早期阴道超声优于腹部超声。

诊断检查与说明

实验室检查

- 全血细胞计数：
  - 稀释性贫血是正常生理改变。
    - 总血容量增加 45%。
- β-HCG 定量检测。
  - 不和超声检查结果完全吻合。
  - 可在排卵后 9～11 日检测到。
- 血型和 Rh。
  - 如果出血严重需做交叉配血。
- 若有胚胎死亡或胎盘早剥可做 DIC 方面检测。
- 感染性流产需要做血培养。
- 怀疑产后滞留物的，可送实验室鉴别是否是绒毛膜绒毛。

影像学检查

- 超声检查：
  - 对于有任何 β-HCG 水平的有症状的患者应进行 B 超检查。
    - 确认为子宫内孕。
    - 在第 5 周检查妊娠囊(通常 β-HCG≥1 000～2 000 U)，卵黄囊在第 6 周，胎心在 5～6 周可闻及。
    - 需要确认宫内孕，排除宫外孕。
    - 通过妊娠囊在子宫外，确诊宫外孕。
    - 通过发现穹隆处或附件有液体，确诊宫外孕。
    - “暴雪征”提示妊娠滋养细胞疾病。

诊断步骤/外科

- 后穹隆穿刺术：
  - 限制使用。
  - 确认有液体在穹隆处。
- 负压吸引术：
  - 如果怀疑不完全或脓毒性流产、死胎、妊娠滋养细胞疾病，可促进残留物排出。
- 腹腔镜检查/腹腔镜手术：
  - 用于不稳定患者。
  - 可用于宫外孕的诊断和治疗。

鉴别诊断

- 妊娠早期(<20 周)：
  - 着床出血。
  - 先兆流产。
  - 完全流产、不完全流产、死胎、脓毒性流产。
  - 宫外孕。
  - 妊娠滋养细胞疾病。
  - 绒毛膜下出血。
  - 感染。
  - 创伤。
  - 子宫和阴道损伤。
  - 出凝血功能紊乱。
- 妊娠早期(>20 周)：
  - 胎盘早剥(30%)。
  - 前置胎盘(20%)。
  - 见红(和子宫功能异常及劳累有关)。
  - 前置血管。
  - 子宫阴道外伤或病理因素。
  - 子宫破裂。
  - 感染。
  - 创伤。
  - 子宫阴道损伤(息肉、外翻、肿瘤)。
  - 出凝血功能紊乱。

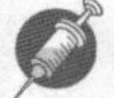

治疗

院前

- 生命体征不平稳的应积极复苏。
- 在妊娠晚期，孕妇取左侧卧位以减轻子宫对下腔静脉的压缩。
- 优先考虑将孕妇转运到有妇产科的医疗机构诊治。

初步稳定/治疗

- 气道管理。
- 心电监测。
- 给氧。
- 脉氧监测。
- 两路静脉通道。
- 必要时输血。
- 妊娠晚期持续的胎心监测。

急诊治疗/程序

- 所有的妊娠早期孕妇阴道出现流血都要排除宫外孕(经阴道超声)。
- 如果是 Rh 阴性患者予以抗 Rh 的免疫球蛋白。
- 疑似宫外孕：
  - 不稳定：超声检查，并请急诊妇产科医师会诊，安排腹腔镜检查或手术。
  - 稳定：先超声检查。
    - 如果确诊宫外孕，急诊妇产科医师会诊并安排腹腔镜检查或手术。
    - 如果不能确定，急诊妇产科医师会诊并 2 日后复查 β-HCG。
- 先兆流产：

- 出血严重的需要急诊妇产科医师会诊。
- 少量出血时，安排妇产科医师随诊。
• 难免流产、不完全流产、死胎：
- 有残留物在子宫口会引起持续出血。
- 如果残留物不易取出，请急诊妇产科医师会诊。
• 完全流产：
- 出血严重的需要急诊妇产科医师会诊。
- 少量出血时，安排妇产科医师随诊。
• 感染性流产：
- 使用广谱抗生素。
- 安排急诊妇产科医师会诊。
• 妊娠晚期阴道出血：
- 血流动力学稳定。
◦ 补液。
◦ 孕妇取左侧卧位以减轻子宫对下腔静脉的压缩。
- DIC。
◦ 和妊娠晚期出血有关。
◦ 多见于胎盘早剥。
◦ 输注血制品。
- 立即请产科医师会诊并转入产科病房。

药物治疗

一线用药

• 抗 Rh 的免疫球蛋白：妊娠＜12 周，50 μg 肌内注射；妊娠＞12 周，300 μg 肌内注射。
• 甲氨蝶呤：
- 不同剂量给药方法不同。
- 仅建议给血流动力学稳定且未破裂的宫外孕患者小剂量 β-HCG。
- 给药前应咨询妇产科医生。
• 针对感染性流产的抗生素。
- 能选择的抗生素种类很多。
- 需选择抗菌谱广的。

二线用药

米索前列醇已用于完全流产，有助于子宫排空。

随访

进一步处理

入院指征

• 妊娠早期阴道出血：
- 生命体征不稳，出血严重。
- 宫外孕破裂。
- 不完全流产(宫口开)。
- 感染性流产。
• 所有妊娠晚期有阴道出血者都需入院。

出院指征

• 病情稳定的先兆流产、完全流产、死胎的患者。
• 无小未破裂宫外孕且症状血流动力学稳定，需妇产科医师会诊。
• 阴道子宫出血得到控制。
• 对于在美国不明部位妊娠的患者，请咨询妇产科。

随访建议

• 出院指导：
- 不要干重体力活，不使用卫生棉，不做灌洗，不进行性生活。
- 出现疼痛、出血、发热等及时就医。
• 所有妊娠期阴道出血患者从急诊出院后都需要随访。
• 孕妇有先兆流产或怀疑宫外孕需反复做 β-HCG 检查，并在 2 日后复查。

要点和误区

• 对出血孕妇没有做 Rh 检测。
• 对 Rh 阴性患者没有予以抗 Rh 的免疫球蛋白。
• 无论 β-HCG 水平如何，妊娠早期症状孕妇未进行盆腔超声检查。
• 对于前置胎盘或血管，在妊娠晚期患者应首先考虑行超声检查而不是盆腔检查。

肉毒中毒 Botulism

Betty B. Dean · Philip Shayne　　陆晓烨　朱长青 译

基础知识

描述

• 在美国比较少见，每年发病率小于 200 例。但是它有潜在的恐怖袭击风险。
• 由一类不耐热肠毒素肉毒梭菌产生。
- 非常强的毒性。
• 毒素阻断胆碱能神经纤维的神经肌肉传递。
• 通过抑制突触前神经膜乙酰胆碱的释放而产生症状：
- 损害是永久性的。
- 恢复通过从轴突发芽形成新的突触。
• 暴露后 12～72 h 开始发病，可能持续 1 周以上：
- 出现症状 24 h 后可导致死亡。
• 恢复缓慢，症状常持续存在数月。
• 死亡率：
- 未经治疗：60%～70%。
- 治疗：3%～10%。
• 3 种主要类型：食源性肉毒中毒、伤口肉毒中毒和婴儿肉毒中毒(见儿科注意事项)。通过黏膜或不完整的皮肤吸收。
• 食源性肉毒中毒：
- 从不正常的灌装食物、冷冻食品中摄取。
- 致病条件：
◦ 肉毒梭菌或芽孢污染的食品。
◦ 繁殖的条件。
◦ 食用前有时间及条件产生毒素。
◦ 加热不足而没有破坏毒素。
◦ 含毒素的食物进入易感人群。
• 伤口肉毒中毒：
- 创伤后形成感染伤口而出现肉毒杆菌中毒症状，没有食源性中毒的临床依据。
- 占肉毒杆菌中毒的 50%。
- 伤口常被土壤污染。
- 在美国，大多数病例是由于静脉注射毒品导致的。
• 其他类型：
- 成人肠源性肉毒中毒：
◦ 发生在消化系统结构或功能异常、免疫功能受损、长时间抗生素治疗的成人患者。
◦ 人群易感性。
◦ 可以有少数或复发的未知来源的肉毒杆菌感染，甚至在肉毒杆菌免疫球蛋白治疗后。
- 医源性肉毒中毒：
◦ 化妆品中的剂量不足以引起全身症状。
◦ 最近的一些不明确的病例都经过医疗环节。
◦ 典型的肉毒杆菌中毒症状。

- 吸入性肉毒中毒：
  - 生物恐怖袭击中使用雾化毒素。最近的报道发生于1962年处理动物遗体时。

儿科注意事项

- 婴儿摄入肉毒杆菌孢子，在肠道产生毒素而中毒。
- 占肉毒中毒的50%～76%。
- 90%发生在6个月以下的婴儿。
  - 患者或家人可能接触土壤、尘埃或农业产品。
  - 也可能与断奶有关，断奶导致肠道菌群失调，该病和梭状芽胞杆菌感染的易感性增加。
- 通常表现为粪便形状改变或便秘，进一步影响延髓导致肌无力症状，然后出现下降型弛缓性麻痹。
- 摄入较低剂量导致发病缓慢。
- 蜂蜜中可分离出肉毒杆菌：
  - 不推荐对1岁以下的儿童服用蜂蜜。

病因

- 肉毒杆菌是革兰阳性菌，严格的厌氧菌，以大孢子形式在大自然中无处不在。
- 根据菌株毒素抗原性不同，分为A～G类型：
  - A、B、E和少数F型在人类中最为常见。

诊断

症状和体征

既往史

- 4～5日前有异常饮食史：
  - 家庭自产的水果或蔬菜。
  - 监狱中摄入"pruno"(囚犯利用剩下的食物酿成的一种酒)。
- 免疫抑制状态(AIDS、肿瘤、慢性疾病)。
- 静脉注射毒品。

体格检查

- 食源性肉毒中毒(典型的肉毒杆菌中毒)：
  - 在早期延髓功能减弱，表现可多种多样：复视、吞咽困难、构音障碍和发音困难。
  - 随后出现对称性下肢乏力及瘫痪(疾病的典型表现)。
  - 无感觉障碍。
  - 深反射逐渐变弱。
  - 患者清晰/警觉；心理状态受到影响。
  - 呼吸肌无力导致通气不足。
  - 自主神经功能障碍(交感和副交感神经)：
    - 口干。
    - 视力模糊。
    - 体位性低血压。
    - 便秘。
    - 尿潴留。
  - 恶心和呕吐只出现在食源性肉毒杆菌中毒。
  - 不发热。
- 伤口型肉毒中毒：
  - 表现同食源性肉毒杆菌中毒。
  - 软组织感染可以导致发热。
- 婴儿肉毒中毒：
  - 便秘。
  - 虚弱。
  - 吸奶无力。
  - 哭泣无力。
  - 嗜睡。
  - 肌张力低下。
  - 面部表情淡漠。
  - 呼吸困难。
- 吸入性肉毒中毒：
  - 同食源性肉毒杆菌中毒，但缺乏消化道症状。

基本检查

- 诊断完全是临床性的。
- 检查的重点是鉴别其他原因导致的全身瘫痪。
- 对于疑似病例，可通知国家健康部门或是疾控中心。

诊断检查与说明

实验室检查

- 血常规。
- 电解质、尿素氮、肌酐、血糖：
  - 低钾血症。
- 动脉血气分析(ABG)：
  - 呼吸功能不全。
- 确诊试验是相关部门和美国联邦实验室通过老鼠试验进行的，标本来自：
  - 血液。
  - 粪便。
  - 胃内容物。
  - 可疑的食物或污染物。
  - 6～96 h可出结果。
- 厌氧菌血培养：
  - 可能发现致病菌。
- 鼻拭子ELISA测试。
  - 对于吸入性肉毒中毒的病例有用，而在其他形式的肉毒中毒病例中不可靠。
  - 标本在暴露后24 h内进行采集。

影像学检查

头颅CT/MRI：

- 正常。

诊断程序/外科

- 脑脊液检查：
  - 正常。
  - 与吉兰-巴雷综合征鉴别(脑脊液蛋白明显升高)。
- 电生理检查：
  - 神经传导正常，但肌肉诱发动作电位减弱。
- 腾喜龙试验阳性，与重症肌无力鉴别。

鉴别诊断

- 重症肌无力(非急性期)。
- 兰伯特-伊顿肌无力综合征(非急性期)。
- 脊髓灰质炎(发热和不对称瘫痪)。
- 吉兰-巴雷综合征(感觉异常和脑脊液蛋白升高)。
- 蜱瘫痪。
- 镁中毒。
- 低钾血症周期性麻痹。
- 白喉神经炎。
- 罕见的基底节、延髓卒中。

儿科注意事项

- 常误诊为脱水、败血症或Reye综合征。
- 其他诊断包括先天代谢缺陷病、吉兰-巴雷综合征和脊髓肌萎缩。

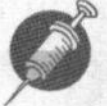

治疗

注意

进行性呼吸衰竭导致死亡：

- 呼吸衰竭时或根据动脉血气情况选择气管插管。
- 可能需要数周机械通气。

院前

- 对于不稳定的二度及三度房室传导阻滞(AVB)需要安装起搏器。
- 阿托品：
  - 避免在二度AVB时使用，因为会导致完全性AVB。
  - 在宽QRS综合波的三度AVB患者中禁止使用。
- 防止迷走神经张力过高。

初步稳定/治疗

- 存活的关键在于早期气管插管及机械通气。

R

• 呼吸困难进展迅速。

■ **急诊治疗/程序**

• 肉毒杆菌毒素拮抗剂：
- 静脉给药，一旦确诊，并收集初步样本，无需等待实验室确认。
- 使用前先用马血清或抗毒素做皮试。
- 推荐剂量为小于1%，具有较好的敏感性。

• 伤口肉毒中毒彻底清创，即使它可能愈合。

• 对于有感染并发症的患者使用抗生素。

• 积极的预防措施，没有人传染人的依据。

• 假如是在环境中暴露，用肥皂水将衣服及皮肤洗净。

■ **药物治疗**

ABE抗毒药物不再被使用。

一线用药

• A和B的肉毒素抗体治疗婴儿肉毒中毒，由美国FDA授权，由加拿大公共卫生部发放。

• 对于非婴儿肉毒中毒，七价抗毒素是试验阶段药物，只能在紧急情况下使用，可从疾控中心获取。

儿科注意事项

• 婴儿住院时间为3～6周：
- 成年马抗毒药不能用于小儿。

• 抗生素：
- 清除肠内微生物是无作用的。
- 细菌在肠道中破坏，其毒素释放可能会加重神经症状。

二线用药

五价类毒素还在试验阶段。

随访

■ **进一步处理**

入院指征

对于疑似肉毒中毒的患者需要安置在观察床位：

• 对于所有呼吸功能受损的患者都需要入住ICU。

出院指征

肉毒中毒的临床进程是不可预知的，它会迅速或进行性导致死亡的发生：

• 经过长时间逐步恢复、症状逐步消失的患者才能出院。

■ **随访建议**

• 物理治疗及康复：
- 乏力可持续1年以上。

• 心理健康：
- 对于长时间的康复过程，患者及他们的家属会感到沮丧及抑郁。

要点和误区

• 肉毒中毒属于公共卫生安全事件；美国州政府及联邦卫生部门要求尽早上报。

• 发病大于2例需考虑肉毒中毒可能，其他疾病不会暴发。

• 抗毒素不改善瘫痪但停止其进展。因此，一旦怀疑该诊断则需要立即使用抗毒素，不要等到出现呼吸功能不全的症状。

• 有瘫痪继发的呼吸窘迫在早期其临床表现可不明显。

• 延髓麻痹的临床表现被错误地认为是精神状态的改变。

乳突炎 Mastoiditis

Jonathan Fisher · Christopher J. McCabe 段立伟 译

基础知识

■ **描述**

• 颞骨的乳突细胞炎症，一般由急性化脓性中耳炎直接蔓延引起。

• 中耳和乳突是乳突窦的共同入口。

• 因中耳炎分泌的液体积聚造成感染。

• 临床表现从乳突轻微的炎症到乳突感染和骨破坏。

• 急性乳突炎：
- 在中耳炎病例中有一定程度的发生。
- 早期体征和症状是急性中耳炎的表现。
- 继发于乳突中的感染性材料，由中耳到乳突通道的炎症梗阻引起。

• 急性乳突炎伴骨膜炎：
- 感染进展涉及乳突骨膜，引起骨膜炎。
- 骨膜下脓肿可能存在。

• 急性乳突骨炎（又称融合性乳突炎）：
- 乳突气房内的感染进展导致乳突骨小梁破坏，造成骨小梁贯通。
- 乳突积脓或引流瘘可能存在。
- 如果不治疗可能进展为严重的头部和颈部并发症。

• 隐匿性乳突炎：
- 乳突感染，在急性中耳炎治疗后可持续存在。
- 可进展为急性或融合性乳突炎。

• 慢性中耳乳突炎：
- 感染持续超过3个月。

• 乳突炎可能是其他原发疾病的并发症：
- 白血病。
- 单核细胞增多症。
- 颞骨肉瘤。
- HIV感染。
- 川崎病。

• 较急性中耳炎而言，乳突炎更加普遍使用抗生素。

• 幼儿和婴儿更加常见。

■ **病因**

• 引起急性乳突炎的病原体类似于急性中耳炎，但频率不同：
- 肺炎链球菌。
- A组链球菌。
- 金黄色葡萄球菌。
- 流感嗜血杆菌。

• 慢性中耳乳突炎以革兰阴性肠道细菌最常见：
- 铜绿假单胞菌。
- 大肠埃希菌。
- 变形杆菌。
- 拟杆菌属。

• 其他少见病因：
- 结核分枝杆菌。
- 曲霉（免疫抑制状态下）。

儿科注意事项

• 儿童人群中更常见，与中耳炎明显相关。

• 肺炎是儿童最常见的病因。

诊断

■ **症状和体征**

病史

• 耳痛。

- 耳溢液。
- 中重度听力损失。
- 发热。
- 头痛。
- 儿童过敏史。
- 复发性中耳炎病史。

体格检查

- 乳突压痛、水肿和红斑。
- 侧面及下耳郭位移。
- 耳后折痕损失。
- 耳后壁和上耳道壁肿胀。
- 鼓膜异常伴重度中耳炎。
- 耳脓液引流术。
- 鼓膜膨出。
- 第 3 对脑神经(CNⅢ)麻痹,罕见。

基本检查

乳突炎是临床诊断。

诊断检查与说明

实验室检查

- 全血细胞计数:
  - 白细胞增多。
- 因微生物的多样性,引流液的培养很重要:
  - 自发性引流或手术后引流。
  - 如果患者出现毒样反应给予血培养。

影像学检查

- 乳突 X 线检查:
  - 疾病早期表现较朦胧或称云雾状,乳突结构完整。
  - 乳突表现较浑浊时提示疾病进展。
  - 因灵敏度低,临床较不可靠。
- CT 扫描:
  - 更有用,尤其当脓肿形成时。
  - 可以确定骨小梁破坏是否存在和破坏程度,同样可评估中耳乳突炎的并发症。
- MRI:
  - 如果怀疑颅内侵犯,但 CT 未确诊。

儿科注意事项

- 儿童患者使用 CT 扫描要谨慎。
- 诊断多以临床为依据,避免辐射。
- 无造影剂的 MRI 是 CT 的一个很好的替代。

诊断步骤/外科

腰椎穿刺:

- 通过脑脊液评估脑膜炎征象。

鉴别诊断

- 中耳炎。
- 蜂窝织炎。
- 外耳中耳炎。
- 头皮感染伴耳后淋巴结炎症。
- 风疹:耳后淋巴结肿大。
- 耳郭或耳后区域创伤。
- 脑膜炎。

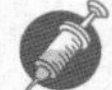

治疗

院前

- ABC 管理。
- 气道管理。
- 低血压/容量丢失时静脉输注生理盐水。

急诊治疗/程序

- 首先静脉给予抗生素。
- 咨询耳鼻喉科医师关于手术引流:
  - 急性或融合性乳突炎时需要行引流治疗。
  - 如果患者出现毒性表现,需急诊行引流术。
  - 外科手术类型:
    - 鼓膜切开引流和鼓膜置管。
    - 对严重病例,行乳突根治术及引流术(约 50%病例需要)。

药物治疗

- 首先静脉注射抗生素:
  - 因金黄色葡萄球菌感染比例增加,在有培养结果之前治疗上覆盖抗葡萄球菌药物。
  - 患者体温正常 36～48 h 后可以考虑调整为口服抗生素。
  - 合适的时候考虑覆盖假单胞菌。
- 疼痛药物管理:
  - 非甾体类解热镇痛药物。
  - 口服或静脉使用麻醉类药物。

一线用药

- 头孢曲松:1～2 g[儿童:50～75 mg/(kg·24 h)],静脉注射,q12～24 h。
- 头孢噻肟钠:1～2 g[儿童:50～180 mg/(kg·24 h)],静脉注射,q4～6 h。

二线用药

- 氨苄西林-舒巴坦:1.5～3 g,静脉注射,q6 h。
- 氯霉素:50～100 mg/(kg·24 h),静脉注射或口服,q6 h。
- 克林霉素:600～2 700 mg/d,静脉注射,q6～12 h;或 150～450 mg,口服,q6～8 h[儿童:20～40 mg/(kg·d),肌内注射/静脉注射,q6～8 h;或 10～25 mg/(kg·d),q6～8 h]。
- 替卡西林-克拉维酸:3.1 g,静脉注射,q4～6 h。
- 哌拉西林-他唑巴坦:3.375 g,静脉注射,q6 h。
- 万古霉素:1 g,q8 h[儿童:40 mg/(kg·24 h)],静脉注射,q6～8 h。

随访

进一步处理

入院指征

- 临床怀疑急性或融合性乳突炎。
- 骨膜下脓肿。
- 出现中毒症状。

出院指征

急性或融合性乳突炎患者不宜出院。

转诊问题

- 咨询耳鼻喉科是否需要行手术引流。
- 乳突炎缓解后通过测听术评估听力损失。

随访建议

出院后随访耳鼻喉科医师。

并发症

- 颈部脓肿:
  - 通过乳突尖腐蚀,感染扩大至颈部胸锁乳突肌旁或后软组织。
- 颞骨岩部炎:
  - 感染扩散至岩空细胞。
- 颅骨骨髓炎。
- 颅内并发症:
  - 骨膜下脓肿。
  - 硬膜下积脓。
    - 感染扩散至中枢神经系统伴骨幕周围积脓。
- 窦内血栓形成。

儿科注意事项

虽然中耳炎保守治疗,一项 10 年的分析并没有显示急性乳突炎病例增加。

要点和误区

- 在中耳炎持续存在或没有治疗的情况下,需要对乳突炎保持高度怀疑。
- 需要注意识别脑膜炎和颅内侵犯,这在临床上要求更加积极的管理。
- 引流是权威的治疗方法。

R

乳腺炎 Mastitis

Sean N. Fling · Kathryn West 段立伟 译

基础知识

描述

- 乳腺感染会导致疼痛、肿胀和红斑。
- 哺乳期的女性，最常见的原因是长时间的充血或排乳不畅。
- 非哺乳期，由于乳突下导管炎症（导管周围乳腺炎）或特发性肉芽肿性大叶乳腺炎（不太常见）。
- 常伴随全身症状：
  - 萎靡不振。
  - 发热。
- 哺乳期女性的发生率高达 33%。
- 发病通常在产后 1～6 周。
- 并发症：
  - 母乳喂养停止（最常见）。
  - 复发。
  - 脓肿。
  - 脓毒症。
  - 坏死性筋膜炎。
  - 皮肤瘘。
  - 母乳量持续性降低。

儿科注意事项

可发生在 2 个月内的足月婴儿。

R

病因

- 金黄色葡萄球菌常见。
- 少见病因：
  - 凝固酶阴性的金黄色葡萄球菌。
  - 链球菌属。
  - 大肠杆菌。
  - 流感嗜血杆菌。
  - 白色念珠菌。
- 危险因素：
  - 哺乳期：
    - 乳头破裂。
    - 与婴儿问题有关。
    - 局部乳汁淤积。
    - 乳头穿孔。
    - 产妇营养不良。
    - 既往有乳腺炎病史。
    - 初产妇。
    - 使用手动吸奶器。
    - 高龄产妇。
    - 产妇糖尿病。
    - 产妇使用抗生素。
  - 非哺乳期：
    - 皮肤破裂。
    - 静脉吸毒。
    - 吸烟。
    - 外伤。
    - 湿疹或其他皮肤疾病。
    - 全身性疾病。

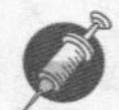

诊断

症状和体征

病史

- 流感样症状：发热、头痛、不适、发冷和肌肉酸痛。
- 通常体温＞38.3℃（101℉）。
- 乳房红肿、疼痛和肿胀。
- 母乳流出减少。

体格检查

- 乳房：
  - 温度高。
  - 柔软。
  - 有硬结。
  - 红斑，通常呈楔形。
- 通常单侧乳房发病。
- 腋窝淋巴结可增大。
- 乳头外伤。
- 典型的症状是发热和心动过速。

基本检查

体格检查时需特别注意脓肿和严重脓毒症的表现。

- 脓肿常常较难触及，但是多见于乳晕区域。
- 触诊见化脓性乳头溢液。

儿科注意事项

- 新生儿：
  - 通常为单侧。
  - 50%～63%发生脓肿。
  - 新生儿发热或生病的败血症检查。
  - 如小于 2 个月，需静脉使用广谱抗生素。

诊断检查与说明

实验室检查

在复发或难治病例中考虑母乳培养。

影像学检查

超声检查：明确是否脓肿或 48 h 后无改善。

鉴别诊断

- 乳房肿胀：
  - 短暂发热（＜38.3℃），持续 4～16 h。
  - 产后 48～72 h 出现。
  - 双侧非红斑性肿胀。
- 乳腺癌。
- 乳腺脓肿。
- 乳性鞘膜积液。
- 乳腺管堵塞。

治疗

院前

一般不需要院前治疗。

初步稳定/治疗

无特殊稳定治疗。

急诊治疗/程序

- 通过直接母乳喂养或吸奶继续排空乳房。
- 按摩。
- 热/冷治疗。
- 改善母乳喂养技术：
  - 可能需要一位哺乳期顾问。
- 保持良好的母体水化。
- 如果症状出现＞24 h、严重症状或伴有发热，则使用抗生素。
- 如果有脓肿的证据，可请外科会诊。
- 用退热药和非甾体抗炎药控制症状。

> **注意**
>
> 有乳腺炎的母亲，HIV 感染（母亲或婴儿）的垂直传播可能会增加。

药物治疗

- 头孢氨苄：500 mg，口服，q6 h，治疗 10 日。
- 克林霉素：300 mg，口服，q6 h，治疗 10 日。
- 双氯西林：500 mg，口服，q6 h，治疗 10 日（一线治疗方案）。
- 甲氧苄啶-磺胺甲噁唑（TMP - SMX）：160/800 mg，口服，q12 h。
  - 缺乏抵抗力的婴儿和＜2 个月的健康婴儿避免使用。
- 如果严重需要静脉注射抗生素：万古霉素 1 g，静脉用药，q12 h。

• 口服乳酸菌可有效预防复发。

一线用药

双氯西林。

二线用药

• 头孢氨苄。
• 克林霉素(严重青霉素过敏)。
• TMP - SMX。

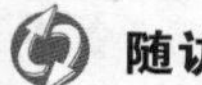

随访

■ 进一步处理

入院指征

• 全身麻醉下行切开引流的患者需要入院治疗。
• 免疫功能低下或有败血症证据。
• 新生儿乳腺炎需要入院治疗。

出院指征

• 大部分患者需要门诊治疗。
• 48 h 内经过治疗大部分症状可缓解。
• 家庭护理包括频繁的乳房排空、按摩/振动疗法、乳房支撑、温敷和非甾体抗炎药。
• 确保母亲得到适当的社会支持。

■ 随访建议

• 患者应至初级保健医师处随访。
• 如果在 48～72 h 没有改善,则应进行超声检查,以评估乳腺炎症的其他原因
• 哺乳顾问可能会有帮助。

要点和误区

• 大部分病例可以哺乳和热敷。
• 如果症状严重或 24 h 后没有改善,则应使用抗生素。
• 向产妇告知直接母乳喂养是安全的。
• 最常见的乳腺炎并发症是母乳喂养停止。
• 如果患者需要入院,建议婴儿一同入住,以鼓励继续母乳喂养。

软下疳 Chancroid

Robert Kregg Laundon · Dalton Cox 庄育刚 译

基础知识

■ 描述

• 性传播性生殖器溃疡性疾病。
- 增加 HIV 感染的风险。
• 非洲、东南亚和拉丁美洲常见生殖器溃疡的病因。
- 美国不常见。美国性病传播为:单纯疱疹病毒＞梅毒＞＞软下疳(译者补充:中国也极为罕见)。
- 新鉴定为在热带太平洋岛屿儿童下肢皮肤慢性溃疡的病原体。

■ 病因

• 致病菌:杜克雷嗜血杆菌。
• 高传染性细菌。

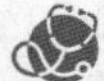

诊断

■ 症状和体征

• 在接触病原体后,感染部位出现一个小炎性丘疹或脓疱。
- 迅速变为痛性下疳。
- 质地软,易出血,表面不光滑,边界不规则。
• 早期容易破溃形成溃疡。
• 基底潮湿,表面颗粒状。
• 脓性或血性分泌物。
• 部位:
- 男性:
◦ 阴茎、龟头、包皮内侧、肛周。
- 女性:
◦ 宫颈、阴道、阴唇、会阴、肛周。
• 接触后 4～7 日(中位数)发病。
• 潜伏期平均为 3～10 日(1～35 日)。
• 腹股沟淋巴结增大:
- 50%的男性存在,女性少见。
- 初起溃疡后 3～14 日发病。
- 通常为单侧。
- 疼痛。
- 巨大脓性淋巴结炎。
- 可自然破溃流脓,形成溃疡和窦道。
• 因为接触破溃处可出现排尿困难和性交困难。
• 其他形式:
- 崩蚀性溃疡:
◦ 二次感染(尤其是螺旋体感染),迅速出现巨大组织缺损。
- 巨大软下疳:
◦ 非常巨大的单个溃疡。
- 匐行性溃疡:
◦ 腹股沟区或大腿部位出现迅速蔓延的无痛的条索状溃疡。
- 毛囊破坏:
◦ 多发的毛囊周围破坏。

■ 基本检查

临床诊断依赖于临床表现,往往不够精确,实验室检查有一定困难或不能进行,所以需要考虑:

• CDC 诊断:
- 确诊:杜克雷嗜血杆菌培养阳性。
- 可疑:软下疳的典型症状和体征＋暗视野苍白螺旋体检查阴性＋梅毒血清学检查阴性＋单纯疱疹病毒培养阴性(或疱疹临床表现不典型)。

■ 诊断检查与说明

实验室检查

• 革兰染色可信度不高(阳性率 50%～80%):
- 革兰阴性杆菌:
◦ 线性或鱼群样图案。
• 培养相当困难(阳性率 0～80%),需要符合培养基。
- 从溃疡基底或腹股沟淋巴结穿刺(经过皮下隧道以免形成窦道)获取标本。
• 聚合酶链(PCR)反应:敏感性和特异性强,但是尚未广泛应用。
• 快速血浆反应素试验(RPR):
- 常见合并梅毒感染。
- CDC 指南关于软下疳可能临床诊断的部分。
• 单纯疱疹病毒(HSV)培养:
- CDC 指南关于软下疳可能临床诊断的部分。
• HIV 检测。

■ 鉴别诊断

• 感染性疾病:
- 梅毒(苍白螺旋体):无痛性、无感觉、无

渗出的硬下疳。

- HSV：小疱疹，多发、反复发作。
- 腹股沟肉芽肿（杜诺凡病，肉芽肿荚膜杆菌）：边缘隆起、硬化。
- 淋巴肉芽肿（性病肉芽肿，衣原体感染）：单个损害，疼痛，有波动感，单侧的淋巴结炎。

• 非感染性疾病：
- 药物损伤。
- 少见：
  ◦ 坏疽性脓皮病。
  ◦ Behcet 病。

治疗

■ 初步稳定/治疗

接触患者和标本时要注意安全。

■ 急诊治疗/程序

抗生素：

• 阿奇霉素：单剂口服。
• 头孢曲松：单剂量肌内注射（孕妇首选）。
• 环丙沙星：口服 3 日，孕妇和哺乳期禁用。
• 红霉素：口服 7 日，在孕妇中为二线用药。
• 脓肿细针穿刺（5 cm 以上）。
- 防止自发破裂引起慢性窦道形成。
- 18G 细针，从一侧完整皮肤穿刺。
- 可能需要重复穿刺。

同步行梅毒、HSV、HIV 检测，初次阴性需要连续测 3 次。

■ 药物治疗

一线用药

• 阿奇霉素：1 g，顿服。
• 头孢曲松：250 mg，肌内注射，一次。

二线用药

• 环丙沙星片：500 mg，每日 2 次，持续 3 日。
• 红霉素：500 mg，每日 4 次，持续 7 日。

随访

■ 进一步处理

入院标准

• 损伤恢复前禁止性交或使用避孕套。
• 以下情况入院：
- 治疗 2 日后症状加重。
- 3～7 日溃疡进展。
- HIV 阳性患者未能及时治疗或者未做包皮环切术。

■ 随访建议

• 发病 10 日内有性接触的伴侣建议同步检查和治疗。
• HIV 阳性患者接受单剂量治疗的应密切随访（治疗失败率高）。

要点和误区

• 符合 CDC 可疑诊断即可开始治疗，不能等培养结果。
• HIV 感染患者治疗失败率高。
• 性接触患者的治疗。
• 治疗失败：考虑耐药、药物依从性差，合并感染（梅毒）。
• 2016 年在美国有 7 例个案报道。

瑞氏综合征 Reye Syndrome

Brian D. Euerle 何融冰 译

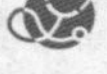

基础知识

■ 描述

• 病因不明的可逆性临床病理综合征。
• 主要为线粒体损伤。
• 酶活性降低：
- 三羧酸循环。
- 糖原异生。
- 尿素生成。
• 脂肪浸润：
- 肝：
  ◦ 由于氨转化为尿素减少引起的高氨血症。
  ◦ 最终导致肝肾综合征。
  ◦ 幸存患者肝功能可迅速恢复。
- 大脑：
  ◦ 不明原因的脑病。
  ◦ 细胞毒性水肿。
  ◦ 意识水平恶化反映颅内压（ICP）增加。
  ◦ 脑疝是死亡最常见的原因。
  ◦ 幸存患者神经功能可恢复正常。
- 骨骼肌和心肌。
- 脂肪浸润和线粒体畸形。
• ＜10%在 1 岁以前发生：
- 平均年龄是 7 岁。
- 好发年龄是 4～11 岁。
- 年龄＞18 岁极少见。
• 种族差异：
- 中西部地区发病率最高。
- 东南和极西部地区发病率低。
• 在白种人中比黑种人中更常见。
• 发病高峰在冬季和早春。
• 类瑞氏综合征：
- 导致尿素和脂肪酸代谢缺陷、中毒性损伤和糖原异生受损。

■ 病因

• 至今不确定。
• 流行病学涉及多种因素：
- 发病前病毒感染征象。
- 流感 A 型或 B 型。
- 水痘。
- 腹泻疾病。
- 遗传学易感性。
- 水杨酸盐暴露史。
- 其他不明确因素。

诊断

■ 症状和体征

病史

• 患者通常无发热。
• 心动过速。
• 换气过度。

体格检查

• 双相病史包括感染期（病毒性疾病或前驱症状）之后为脑病期。
• 大量反复呕吐：
- 通常起始于病毒性疾病发病 4～5 日。
- 明显的行为改变，包括谵妄、好胜、定向障碍和幻觉。

■ 基本检查

• 无局部神经学体征。

- 40%病例有肝大。
- 胰腺炎。
- Lovejoy 分类法：
  - 0期：
    - 清醒的。
  - Ⅰ期：
    - 呕吐。
    - 昏睡。
    - 嗜睡。
  - Ⅱ期：
    - 定向障碍。
    - 谵妄。
    - 好斗、木僵。
    - 过度换气。
    - 反射亢进。
    - 伤害性刺激可做出适当反应。
  - Ⅲ期：
    - 迟钝。
    - 昏迷。
    - 过度通气。
    - 对伤害性刺激不能做出适当反应。
    - 去皮质体位。
    - 瞳孔对光反射保留。
    - 眼前庭对光反射保留。
  - Ⅳ期：
    - 深昏迷。
    - 去大脑强直。
    - 眼前庭反射消失。
    - 扩大的固定的瞳孔。
    - 对冷热刺激有无关联的眼球运动。
  - Ⅴ期：
    - 癫痫。
    - 深反射消失。
    - 呼吸停止。
    - 迟缓性麻痹。
    - 瞳孔反射消失。
- 新生儿：非典型表现。
  - 气促。
  - 呼吸暂停。
  - 易激。
  - 癫痫。
  - 低血糖。

基本检查

- 证实有脑病和肝异常的表现。
- 实验室检查评估特征性生物化学指标异常。
- 肝活检可明确诊断。

诊断检查与说明

实验室检查

- 肝功能检查：
  - 天冬氨酸氨基转移酶，丙氨酸氨基转移酶升高超过3倍。
  - 血氨水平>正常值的1.5～3倍：
    - 精神状态改变后24～48 h一过性改变。
    - >300 μg/dl 提示预后不良。
  - 血清胆红素正常或轻微增高。
- 可能出现低血糖，尤其是新生儿。
- BUN升高。
- 酮尿症。
- 凝血酶原时间可由于肝依赖性凝血因子（Ⅱ、Ⅷ、Ⅸ、Ⅹ）减少而延长。
- 血小板计数和血涂片正常。
- 毒理学筛查阴性。

影像学检查

头部CT扫描：

- 可显示弥散性脑水肿。
- 水肿弥散且腰椎穿刺不是禁忌的：

诊断步骤/外科

- 腰椎穿刺：
  - 头部CT后进行。
  - 测量开放液压力。
  - 白细胞<8/mm³。
- 经皮肝活检：
  - 对非典型表现的患者有用（1岁，复发，有家族性）。

鉴别诊断

- 先天性代谢性疾病：
  - 尿素循环障碍。
  - 脂肪酸氧化障碍。
  - 系统性肉毒碱缺乏。
  - 有机酸血症。
  - 电子传递链紊乱。
- 低血糖。
- 毒物暴露：
  - 不伴有肝功能丧失的中毒性脑病（Gall综合征）。
  - 铅。
  - 烃类。
- 药物中毒：
  - 对乙酰氨基酚。
  - 水杨酸盐类。
  - 乙醇。
- 感染：
  - 脓毒症。
  - 脑膜炎。
  - 脑炎。
  - 水痘性肝炎。
- 头部外伤。

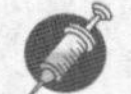

治疗

院前

- 精神状态改变：
  - 葡萄糖。
  - 盐酸纳洛酮。
- 昏迷：
  - 球囊面罩辅助呼吸。

初步稳定/治疗

- 心肺功能监测。
- 供氧。
- 如需气道管理则行快速序贯气管内插管。
- 如果精神状态改变则应用葡萄糖：
  - 10%葡萄糖溶液静脉注射。
  - 脱水纠正后给予2/3维持剂量。
  - 每小时测血糖；维持血糖在125～175 mg/dl。
- 避免早期液体过多。

急诊治疗/程序

- 在肝活检前开始治疗。
- 维生素K：
  - 凝血酶原时间升高时使用。
- 冷冻血浆。
  - 控制出血。
  - 纠正严重凝血病。
- 针对低ICP的干预措施：
  - Ⅲ期或更严重。
  - 伴有血氨>300 μg/L的Ⅱ期：
    - 快速序贯插管。
    - 过度通气。
    - 限制液体。
    - 巴比妥酸盐性昏迷。
- 渗透压活性剂：
  - 甘露醇。
  - 呋塞米。
- 监测ICP：
  - 蛛网膜下腔栓。
  - 心室内置管。

药物治疗

- $D_{50}W$：1～2 ml/kg（0.5～1 g/kg），静脉注射，年龄>3岁。
- $D_{25}W$：2～4 ml/kg（0.5～1 mg/kg），静脉

R

注射，年龄<3岁；以2/3维持剂量持续输注10%葡萄糖溶液。

• 冷冻血浆：10 ml/kg，q12～24 h，静脉注射或必要时使用。

• 呋塞米：1 mg/kg，静脉注射。

• 甘露醇：0.25～1 g/kg，静脉注射，q4～6 h。

• 戊巴比妥：3～5 mg/kg边监测血压边缓慢静脉注射；持续输注1～2 mg/(kg · h)；检测药物水平。

• 维生素K：1～2 mg，缓慢静脉注射（新生儿和儿童）；2～10 mg，静脉注射（青少年）。

随访

进一步处理

入院指征

• 通过合适的咨询，所有怀疑瑞氏综合征的儿童应送入ICU。

• 初次住院进行院内ICP监测。

出院指征

出院标准依患者情况而定。

• 精神状态和实验室指标好转并稳定。

转诊问题

胃肠道疾病（肝病）及神经病学专家密切随访。

随访建议

长期精神病学和神经心理学方面测试。

要点和误区

• 很多药物和联合药物产品中有阿司匹林和水杨酸类，以及天然药物，如柳树皮草药茶。

• 对怀疑瑞氏综合征的患者必须全力确定其他可能病因。

• ICP的监测和控制是治疗的重要组成部分。

腮腺炎 Mumps

Auten-Kum Chai 伍力学 段立伟 译

基础知识

描述

• 该病是一种以唾液腺尤其是腮腺肿大为特征的传染性疾病，可通过疫苗预防。

• 其他并发症可能包括睾丸炎、无菌性脑膜炎、感音神经性耳聋、胰腺炎、卵巢炎。

• 最近在大学校园等人群密切接触的环境中发病率有所增加。

病因

• 是一种腺病毒，为单链 RNA 病毒，属于多黏病毒家族。

• 人类是其唯一宿主。

儿科注意事项

• 满 1 岁的儿童应行首次腮腺炎疫苗和麻疹、水痘三联疫苗(简称 MMR 或 MMRV)预防接种。第 2 次接种应在 4～6 岁，即学龄前完成。

• 追加免疫，两次免疫注射时间间隔至少 4 周。

• 相比成年感染者，儿童感染者的全身症状和严重并发症较少见。

妊娠注意事项

• 如感染发生在妊娠期前 3 个月内，自发性流产发生率明显增加。

• 虽然腮腺炎病毒可透过胎盘屏障，但尚无证据表明其具有致畸作用。

老年人注意事项

• 目前认为，1957 年以前出生者已有腮腺炎暴露史，对该病具有免疫力。

• 但是，如处于该病的暴发流行期，1957 年前出生的医护人员，以及未经实验室检测证实具有免疫力者，均应接受 2 次 MMR 疫苗接种。

诊断

症状和体征

• 潜伏期计算，从暴露时起到起病时止(14～18 日)：

- 病毒通过飞沫、唾液及接触被污染物品而传播。
- 病毒在鼻咽部和淋巴结内复制。
- 经血行播散到达各唾液腺、胰腺、睾丸、卵巢及脑膜。

• 被感染者从起病前 1～7 日前到起病后 6 日均有传染性。

• 被感染者多为未行或未完成免疫接种人群。

• 活跃期(1～10 日)：

- 前驱症状无特异性，起病前有低热、头痛、精神萎靡、肌痛、厌食、耳痛、下颌疼痛等，持续可达 48 h。
- 约 20%的感染者无症状但仍有传染性。
- 约 50%的病例有上呼吸道感染症状，伴低热、精神萎靡、厌食和头痛等，但无明显腮腺肿大。
- 腮腺炎表现(占 30%～40%)：
  ◦ 最常见的腮腺炎症状，发生于 95%有症状的腮腺炎患者中。
  ◦ 单侧或双侧(占 90%)腮腺肿大伴疼痛。
  ◦ 疼痛可能以耳痛或下巴疼痛开始。
  ◦ 其他的唾液腺也可能受牵连。
  ◦ 腮腺导管红肿并有清亮液体渗出。
  ◦ 位于皮下的肿大唾液腺无发红症状。
  ◦ 症状在 7～10 日缓解。
  ◦ 在水肿消退前仍应注意其传染性。
- 睾丸炎(发生于 20%～50%成年男性)：
  ◦ 这是发生在后青春期男性患者最常见的并发症。
  ◦ 可能但最为常见，在腮腺炎后。
  ◦ 单侧或双侧发病(双侧占 30%)。
  ◦ 起病急骤，表现为疼痛、睾丸肿胀，伴恶心、呕吐及发热症状。
  ◦ 疼痛及肿胀症状在 1 周内缓解。
  ◦ 超过 50%的患者出现睾丸萎缩。
  ◦ 不育罕见。
- 卵巢炎(发生于 5%的成年女性)：
  ◦ 发生在右侧时症状与阑尾炎相似。
  ◦ 对生育能力没有影响。
- 胰腺炎(发生率为 2%～5%)：
  ◦ 发生时可不伴随其他腮腺炎表现。
  ◦ 发热、恶心、呕吐和上腹痛。
  ◦ 可有暂时性血糖升高。
  ◦ 可并发假性囊肿和休克。
- 中枢神经系统受累：
  ◦ 无菌性脑膜炎(发生于 10%～15%的患者)。
  ◦ 多在 3～10 日好转，无后遗症。
  ◦ 脑炎(罕见)。
  ◦ 感音神经性耳聋(80%为单侧)并有永久性听力损害。
  ◦ 小脑共济失调。
  ◦ 横贯性脊髓炎。
- 其他：
  ◦ 心肌炎(很少有症状)。
  ◦ 肾小球肾炎。
  ◦ 多关节痛。
  ◦ 血小板减少性紫癜。
  ◦ 眼部症状。
  ◦ 甲状腺炎。
  ◦ 乳腺炎。

基本检查

诊断依靠临床症状、相关体征和并发症。

诊断检查与说明

实验室检查

• 实验室检查为必需检查。

• 有中枢神经系统症状者需留取脑脊液(CSF)标本送检。

• 淀粉酶升高多因腮腺炎所致，是支持该病诊断的依据。

• 对急性期和康复期的标本可行腮腺炎 RNA 序列的 PCR 测定、腮腺炎病毒培养或 IgM 抗体的免疫酶学测定，以及测定 IgG 效价是否明显升高：

- 可提供确诊依据。
- 病毒培养标本可取自血液、咽拭子、唾液腺分泌物、脑脊液或尿液。PCR 技术可快速诊断脑脊液中的腮腺炎病毒感染。

鉴别诊断

• 细菌性腮腺炎：

- 金黄色葡萄球菌最常见。
- 腮腺可出现发红和肿胀表现。
- 多见于老年人或免疫抑制患者。

• 腮腺结石：

- 结石可触及或 CT 扫描可见。

• 颈部淋巴结炎。

• 肿瘤：

- 老年患者。
- 病程中出现无痛性的肿块者。

• 睾丸扭转。

• 细菌性附睾-睾丸炎。

• 其他所致的腮腺炎：如甲型流感病毒、副流感病毒、巨细胞病毒、柯萨奇病毒、HIV 等。

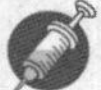

治疗

■ 院前

- 凡有腮腺炎病毒暴露史的所有未接种过疫苗的院前救护人员均有潜在感染风险。
- 不建议感染后使用预防措施。

■ 初步稳定/治疗

在呕吐和脱水时给予静脉补液。

■ 急诊治疗/程序

- 免疫接种阻断腮腺炎病毒传播是防治腮腺炎的基石。
- 支持治疗：
  - 退热药物。
  - 镇痛药：
    - 可选用对乙酰氨基酚、非甾体类解热镇痛药和麻醉药物(对疼痛剧烈者)。
  - 针对呕吐和脱水给予止吐药和静脉补液。
  - 使用冰块物理降温。
  - 并发睾丸炎者可予以睾丸悬吊并卧床休息。
- 对感染者行隔离，预防飞沫传播。

随访

■ 进一步处理

住院指征

- 病情严重需要支持治疗者。
- 呕吐剧烈和脱水者。
- 并发脑炎、脑膜炎者。
- 严重的胰腺炎。
- 需要住院隔离者。

出院指征

- 几乎所有患者均可痊愈出院。
- 该病的传染性可持续到发病后1周。

要点和误区

- 腮腺炎病毒是导致流行性腮腺炎的唯一病原体。
- 腮腺炎疫苗安全高效，正确接种后免疫率达90%以上。孕妇、免疫抑制或免疫功能不全者不宜接种。
- 麻风腮三联疫苗(MMR)不应该给孕妇或严重免疫抑制或免疫受损的患者服用。
- 腮腺炎病毒在世界上分布广泛，未行疫苗接种的旅游者具有感染风险。

S

三叉神经痛 Trigeminal Neuralgia

Joel Kravitz 张晟 林兆奋 译

基础知识

■ 描述

- 三叉神经经通过感觉纤维支配面部、口腔黏膜、鼻黏膜和角膜。
- 三叉神经为第5对脑神经(CNV)。
- 同义词：Tic douloureux：
  - Tic：抽筋的肌肉收缩或移动。
  - Douloureux：疼痛。
- 多发生于年龄>50岁者。
  - 最常见的年龄是50～60岁。
- 女性多于男性。
- 仅凭病史即可辨认的面部疼痛综合征。
- 典型。
  - 单侧发作性痛(少见双侧)，影响一支或多支三叉神经。
  - 有以下特征之一：
    - 表面的、尖锐的刺痛。
    - 由触发区域或因素引发。
  - 持续时间短，1 s到2 min以下。
  - 每位患者的发作都是刻板性重复动作。
  - 没有临床症状明显的神经功能缺损。
  - 排除其他病因导致。
- 神经症状：
  - 同上但是病因明确(不是血管压迫)。

■ 病因

- 疼痛产生的机制仍然存在争议，目前所公认的理论认为：
  - 中枢神经脱髓鞘导致异位刺激和疼痛。
  - 脱髓鞘是由于神经根的营养血管受压迫或异常弯曲。
  - 80%～90%典型的三叉神经痛有血管受压。
  - 小脑上动脉受压最多见(70%)。
  - 小脑前下动脉(10%)。
  - 其次原因。
  - 带状疱疹。
  - 多发性硬化。
  - 占位性病变。
    - 小脑桥脚肿瘤。
    - 动脉瘤。
    - 动静脉畸形。

诊断

■ 症状和体征

- 明确的、剧烈的反复发作的锐痛。
- 阵发性和扁平性疼痛。
- 常被描述为“像过电一样”，渐强然后灼热。
- 单侧三叉神经分支分布的区域：可发生于3支神经中任一支，上颌支>下颌支>眼支。
- 常发生于右侧面部。
- 常无明显诱因，但可由以下因素激发：说话、笑、咀嚼、刷牙、刮脸或触摸面部。
  - 触摸和震动是最常见诱因。
- 可很少发作，亦可每日百余次。
- 发作间隙疼痛消失，但慢性患者可能主诉持续性疼痛。

病史

- 排除具有以下非典型特征引起症状的可能性：
  - 神经学检查异常。
  - 口腔、牙齿检查异常。
  - 听力异常或失聪。
  - 昏睡、眩晕、视力改变、麻木的症状。
  - 疼痛持续>2 min。
  - 不在三叉神经支配区域内。

体格检查

- 体格检查正常，如有异常，考虑其他原因。
- 详查头颈部，重点检查脑神经。
- 患者报告的触发点刺激后疼痛是病理性的。

■ 基本检查

- 主要结合临床进行诊断。

• 根据临床特征来鉴别典型的三叉神经痛和症状性疾病：
- 年龄<50 岁。
- 感觉缺失。
- 单侧发病。

■ 诊断检查与说明

实验室检查

无，只有在怀疑其他原因的情况下才适用。

影像学检查

• 有典型病史和神经学检查正常者无需进一步影像学检查。
• 如果提示牙齿问题，牙齿 X 线片可能有用。
• 如果怀疑多发性硬化或肿瘤，颅脑 MRI 或 CT 可能有用：
- 在病变初期可能有用。

■ 鉴别诊断

• 多发性硬化。
• 颞下颌关节综合征。
• 吞咽神经痛。
• 三叉神经根受肿瘤压迫。
• 牙痛。
• 丛集性头痛。
• 带状疱疹后遗神经痛。
• 鼻窦炎。
• 中耳炎。
• 颞关节炎。

治疗

■ 急诊治疗/程序

• 适当缓解疼痛。
• 药物疗法。
- 卡马西平最常用。
- 其他抗癫痫药对难治性疼痛显示出辅助作用。
• 可能需要神经手术的治疗及相关探索。

■ 药物治疗

一线用药

• 卡马西平 200～800 mg/d，口服，每日 2 次。通常需要 600～1 200 mg/d。

二线用药

• 加巴喷丁：启始 300 mg，口服，每日 1 次。
• 拉莫三嗪：启始 25 mg，口服，每日 1 次。
• 奥卡西平：450～1 200 mg，口服，每日 2 次；启始 300 mg，口服，每日 2 次。
• 苯妥英钠：300～400 mg/d，div. 每日 1～3 次。
• 丙戊酸：启始 250 mg，口服，每日 2 次。

随访

■ 进一步处理

入院指征

• 三叉神经痛伴随其他紧密相关神经存在的问题。
• CT/MRI 阳性结果可能需要急诊神经内科或神经外科的会诊意见。
• 难治性或复发性三叉神经痛治疗与门诊疼痛管理和抗惊厥疗法不同。可能需要入院接受手术干预和三叉神经消融术。

出院指征

没有任何神经症状并且疼痛改善的患者可以转至门诊处理。

转诊问题

• 药物治疗失败的可以手术治疗。
- 疼痛缓解率在 85%～90%。
• 转诊至疼痛控制中心也许对难治性疼痛的患者有帮助。
• 麻醉阻断三叉神经节也许有帮助。

■ 随访建议

• 寻求 PCP 或神经病学专家进行治疗。
• 转诊至神经外科也许有帮助。
- 经皮或开放性手术。

要点和误区

• 单侧、阵发性、尖锐/刺激性面部疼痛遵循 CNV 分布的一部分。
• 触发点是病理性的。
• 不要忽视导致神经受压的替代(非血管性)原因，如中枢神经系统肿块或动脉瘤。
• 卡马西平是最常用治疗药物。

S

三环类抗抑郁药中毒 Tricyclic Antidepressant Poisoning

Arkady Rasin · Steven E. Aks 张晟 林兆奋 译

基础知识

■ 描述

• 一类具有相似三环结构的药物。
• 治疗剂量的作用机制。
- 抑制 5-羟色胺再摄取。
- 抑制去甲肾上腺素再摄取。
• 主要用于抗抑郁药。
- 减少用于抗抑郁，因为具有更安全的替代药物防止过量服用。
• 越来越多地用于慢性和神经性疼痛。
• 也用于强迫症、遗尿症和注意缺陷多动障碍。

■ 病因

• 三环类抗抑郁药(TCA)毒性的主要机制：
- 钠通道阻滞效应(奎尼丁样效应)。
- 抑制去甲肾上腺素再摄取。
- 阻滞外周 α 受体。
- 抗胆碱能作用。
• 三环类抗抑郁药。
- 阿米替林。
- 去甲替林。
- 丙咪嗪(米帕明)。
- 多赛平(多虑平)。
• 更新一代抗抑郁药(非三环类)。
- 选择性 5-羟色胺再摄取抑制剂(SSRIs)：
◦ 比 TCA 安全范围更宽。
◦ 中枢/心血管毒性。
- 非选择性 5-羟色胺再摄取抑制剂：
◦ 5-羟色胺和去甲肾上腺素再摄取抑制剂(SNRI)。
◦ 较少的中枢/心血管毒性。
◦ 可导致心律失常或癫痫。
◦ 万拉法新(Effexor)。
- 请参考抗抑郁药中毒。

诊断

■ 症状和体征

• 可能发生快速恶化。
• 典型 TCA 族(丙咪嗪、阿米替林、去甲替林)：更强的心血管毒性。
• 中枢神经系统。
- 刺激作用或抑制作用。
- 刺激作用。

◦ 震颤。
◦ 兴奋。
◦ 抽搐。
◦ 癫痫发作(酸中毒会进一步加重心血管毒性)。
- 抑制作用。
◦ 睡意(意识模糊)。
◦ 昏睡。
◦ 昏迷。
• 心血管系统。
- 低血压。
- 心动过速。
◦ 期前收缩,由于去甲肾上腺素重摄取被阻断和抗胆碱能效应阻断。
- 心动过缓。
◦ 迟,由于儿茶酚胺耗竭。
- 心电图改变。
◦ QRS 波群增宽(＞100～120 ms)。
◦ 额面轴末梢 40 ms 电轴右偏(aVR 导联 R 波＞3 mm)。
- 心律失常。
◦ 室上性心动过速(SVT)。
◦ 室性心律失常。
• 抗胆碱能效应(少见)。
- 瞳孔散大。
- 肠鸣音减弱。
- 尿潴留。

病史

TCA 中毒患者摄入的物质。

体格检查

• 中枢神经系统:
- 兴奋或抑制。
• 心血管系统:
- 心动过速。
- 瞳孔中度扩大或散大。
- 肠鸣音减弱。
- 皮肤黏膜干燥。
- 尿潴留(罕见)。

■ 基本检查

• 心电图:与 TCA 中毒相关的因素。
- 窦性心动过速(基本总是出现在中毒后)。
- QRS 波群增宽。
◦ 与癫痫发作相关＞100 ms。
◦ 与室性心律不齐相关＞160 ms。
- QT 间期延长。
- PR 间期延长。
- 额面后 40 ms 电轴右偏。
- aVR R 波振幅＞3 mm。
• 持续心电监测。
• 血气分析。
- 酸中毒增强了 TCA 的毒性。

■ 诊断检查与说明

实验室检查

• 全血细胞计数。
• 电解质、尿素氮、肌酐、血糖。
• ABG。
• 尿液毒理学筛查:排除其他毒物。
- 评估暴露于其他毒素。
- 定性筛查,与毒性程度相关性不大。
• TCA 水平。
- 无用。
- 与毒性大小相关性低。
- 必要时定性筛查来确定摄入。

影像学检查

胸部 X 线检查有无吸入性肺炎、肺水肿。

■ 鉴别诊断

• 可致昏迷的药物。
- 酒精。
- 酒精戒断。
- 抗胆碱能药物。
- 含锂药物。
- 苯环己哌啶。
- 阿片类。
- 吩噻嗪。
- 镇静催眠类。
- 水杨酸制剂。
• 心脏毒性药物。
- 抗心律失常类(ⅠA类)。
- 地高辛毒性作用。
- 交感神经兴奋药。
- 抗胆碱能。
• 导致癫痫发作的药物。
- 酒精戒断。
- 抗胆碱能药物。
- 樟脑。
- 异烟肼。
- 含锂药物。
- 吩噻嗪。
- 交感神经兴奋药。
- 酒精中毒。

治疗

■ 院前

• 不要被外观良好的患者产生安全的错觉麻痹。
- 快速进展的意识障碍、癫痫发作、心律失常发生。
• 有任何病情加重需要实施气管插管。
• 建立静脉通路。
• 有任何 QRS 波群增宽(＞100～120 ms)的证据,服用碳酸氢钠。
- 成人 1 安瓿。
- 小孩 1～2 mEq/kg。
• 丙哌酸禁忌证(有神志不清加重伴吸入性肺炎或癫痫发作风险)。

■ 初步稳定/治疗

• ABC 管理。
- 精神状态不稳定者插管指征可放宽。
• 静脉注射生理盐水。
• 吸氧。
• 心电监测,宽大的 QRS 波群(QRS＞100～120 ms)给 $NaHCO_3$ 单次快速静脉注射。
• 精神状态不稳定者用纳洛酮、硫胺素、糖水(罗康全)。
• 有 TCA/苯二氮䓬超剂量者禁忌使用氟马希尼。

■ 急诊治疗/程序

心脏毒性

• 可积极治疗心脏毒性症状以防恶化。
• QRS 波群增宽(＞100～120 ms)。
- $NaHCO_3$ 单次快速静脉注射 1 安瓿(儿童:1～2 mEq/kg),如 QRS 波群突然增宽可重复给药。
- 在服用碳酸氢钠的同时运行心电图机以评估对碳酸氢钠的反应。
- 在如果插管,过度通气以维持动脉 pH 于 7.35～7.45。
- 如单纯高通气量不能达到预期 pH,给 $NaHCO_3$ 输注。
• 心律失常。
- 窦性心动过速不需治疗。
- 节律突变给 $NaHCO_3$ 单次快速静脉注射 1～2 安瓿(儿童:1～2 mEq/kg)。
- 根据高级心脏生命支持共识增加 $NaHCO_3$ 单次快速静脉注射给药量,利多卡因是 $NaHCO_3$ 后二线用药。
- 禁用经典ⅠA类(普鲁卡因胺)、ⅠC类和毒扁豆碱。

低血压

• 生理盐水单次快速静脉注射。
• 去甲肾上腺素。
- 首选的升压药(超过多巴胺)。
- 拮抗"α 受体阻断"效应更加。

- 多巴胺要用更大剂量。

清除药物

• 使用活性炭。

• 禁忌催吐。

癫痫发作

• 地西泮作为一线用药，效果不佳则用苯巴比妥。

• 难治性癫痫发作（监测脑电图）的神经肌肉震颤使用速效药（罗库溴铵/维库溴铵）。

• $NaHCO_3$ 单次快速静脉注射防止酸中毒。

药物治疗

一线用药

• 碳酸氢钠：1～2 安培（50～100 mEq）静脉推注（儿童：1～2 mEq/kg）。

• 活性炭浆：1～2 g/kg 至 90 g，口服。

二线用药

• 葡萄糖：$D_{50}W$（50% 葡萄糖液），1 安瓿：50 ml 或 25 g（儿童：$D_{25}W$，2～4 ml/kg），静脉注射。

• 地西泮（苯二氮䓬）：5～10 mg（儿童：0.2～0.5 mg/kg），静脉注射。

• 多巴胺：2～20 μg/(kg·min)，静脉注射，滴注至预定效应。

• 20% 脂肪乳剂：1.5 ml/kg，静脉注射，随后 0.25 ml/(kg·min)（对 $NaHCO_3$ 抵抗者行试验性治疗）寻求毒药控制中心的指导。

• 劳拉西泮（苯二氮䓬类）2～6 mg（儿童：0.03～0.05 mg/kg），静脉注射。

• 纳洛酮（narcan）：2 mg（儿童：0.1 mg/kg），静脉注射或肌内注射，初始剂量。

• 去甲肾上腺素：4～12 μg/min［儿童：0.05～0.1 μg/(kg·min)］，静脉注射，滴定至预定效应。

• 高渗盐水：7.5% 盐水，200～250 ml（适用于 pH>7.55 的碳酸氢盐难治性心律失常患者实验）。致电毒物控制中心寻求指导。

随访

进一步处理

入院指征

• 观察到有症状的患者>6 h。

• 神志状态改变。

• 心律失常或传导阻滞。

• 癫痫发作。

• 服药 6 h 后心率>100 次/分。

• 合并服他药要求延长观察。

出院指征

• 观察 6 h 后无症状。

• 神志状态无改变。

• 心电图正常，心率<100 次/分。

• 肠鸣音活跃，可耐受时用活性炭。

• 如果有自杀企图或行为，需排除精神病学疾病。

转诊问题

咨询毒理学或毒物控制中心以获知清楚服药情况。

随访建议

精神病学分析自杀原因。

要点和误区

• TCA 中毒的临床特点是病情快速恶化。

• 预警性监测 QRS 波群增宽超过 120 ms 是必要的。

• TCA 过量患者，插管并过度通气以达到预期 pH。

• 苯二氮䓬类药物为一线用药，然后苯巴比妥二线用于癫痫。

S

瘙痒 Pruritus

Christine Tsien Silrers 郑金浩 毛恩强 译

基础知识

描述

• 可激起爪挠欲望的不适感。

• 皮肤上部经 C 型无髓神经纤维介导传输：

- 传入脊髓后角。
- 通过脊髓丘脑束传入大脑皮质。

• 周围介质（组胺和多肽，如 P 物质释放组胺）刺激 C 型神经纤维引起瘙痒。

• 前列腺素（PGE_2、PGH_2）可以降低瘙痒的阈值。

• 阿片类物质通过激活中枢受体引起瘙痒。

• 瘙痒的机制不同，没有一种药物可以治疗所有瘙痒。

• "痒-挠-痒"循环：

- 瘙痒引发抓挠。
- 挠损伤皮肤刺激神经末梢引起更严重的瘙痒。

病因

• 皮肤病病因。

• 神经系统原因：中枢神经系统或三叉神经系统损害。

• 心理原因。

• 系统性原因。

诊断

症状和体征

病史

• 开始：

- 开始淡水浴后迅速产生游泳者瘙痒。
- 晚上瘙痒更强力并出现疥疮。
- 瘙痒呈阵发性并伴多重硬化。
- 真性红细胞增多症患者温度迅速改变。

• 特点：阵发性，炙热感，刺痛感。

• 发生时间与持续时间。

• 严重程度：影响生活质量。

• 有没有皮损。

• 组织区域（如仅为暴露皮肤部分）。

• 加重或缓解因素（如水、热、干燥、潮湿、寒冷）。

• 药物。

• 新产品（如肥皂、化妆品、洗衣粉、衣服柔软剂）。

• 年龄。

• 过敏性皮炎或皮肤病的家族史。

• 个人的过敏史，以及是否患哮喘。

• 家人是否有相同的瘙痒。

• 全身性相关症状（如夜间流汗、发热、寒战、体重减轻、疲劳、黄疸、贫血、神经症状）。

• 冶游史、HIV 或 AIDS 病史。

• 个人史：职业，兴趣，有无宠物接触史，近期有无至外地。

体格检查

• 皮肤病学：

- 出现皮疹。
- 分散或局限性的皮疹。
- 局限的部位：生殖器、指缝间、腋窝、腕关节等。
- 广义的麻疹样暴发。
- 离散泡状的泪滴样斑块。
- 皮肤干燥。
- 黄疸。
- 囊泡(毛发周围)。
- 无囊泡(如昆虫叮咬、疥疮)。
- 原发灶：
  ◦ 丘疹、脓疱、荨麻疹或形态多样的疹。
- 继发性病变。
  ◦ 表皮脱落。
  ◦ 苔藓样硬化。
  ◦ 色素沉着。
  ◦ 丘疹样痒疹：不断摩擦抓挠使生疹区皮肤增厚。
- 精神性因素：患者可以触摸到的区域不断挠抓。

S

基本检查

- 病史是进一步检查的重点。
- 体格检查可以获取皮肤病变的特点。
- 寻找全身性病变的依据。

诊断检查与说明

实验室检查

临床表现结合特殊检查(如血常规、红细胞沉降率、C反应蛋白、肌酐、尿素氮、血糖、肝功能、甲状腺功能、HIV、梅毒抗体、肿瘤标志物、腹部超声、CT、MRI)进行鉴别，检查结果应当结合临床进行分析。

诊断步骤/外科

- 疥疮和皮癣进行皮肤刮诊。
- 进一步检查时有皮肤科专科医师进行皮肤活检。
- 皮肤培养细菌、真菌等病原体。

鉴别诊断

皮肤病学

- 干燥症(皮肤干燥)。
- 虫侵袭：
  - 疥疮：皮损区囊泡和隧道。
  - 虱病(虱子)。
- 虫咬伤：局限咬伤部位丘疹。
- 皮炎：
  - 特发性皮炎。
  - 接触性皮炎(如接触毒性常春藤)。
  - 钱币状皮炎：圆形湿疹或暴发水疱。
- 药物疹(无疹时需考虑)。
  - 阿片类药物及其衍生物。
  - 阿司匹林、非甾体抗炎药。
  - 奎尼丁、胺碘酮。
  - 部分抗生素、抗真菌药物、抗疟疾药物。
  - 吩噻嗪。
  - 雌激素类、孕激素类、睾酮。
  - 他汀类。
  - 其他。
- 扁平苔藓：苔藓样硬化，色素沉着，皮肤增厚。
- 风疹。
- 大疱类天疱疮。
- 嗜酸性毛囊炎。
- 银屑病。
- 疱疹样皮炎：灼烧感。
- 晒伤。
- 水源性瘙痒症。
- 玻璃纤维皮炎。
- 脂溢性皮炎：承重区皮肤的皮脂腺出现皮屑斑。
- 游泳者瘙痒、血吸虫尾蚴性皮炎及血吸虫病：
  - 重复湖水暴露。
  - 瘙痒起始点位于接触水的部位。
  - 数小时后出现高度瘙痒性丘疹。
- 汉疹(痱子)。

妊娠注意事项

- 孕妇暴发不同形态的。
- 妊娠期类天疱疮。
- 妊娠期肝内胆汁淤积。
- 妊娠期遗传性过敏症的暴发。

感染

- HIV。
- 寄生虫：
  - 钩虫病(钩虫)。
  - 盘尾丝虫病(线虫)。
  - 蛔虫病(蛔虫)。
  - 旋毛虫病(蛔虫)。

胆汁淤积

- 胆管梗阻性疾病。
- 原发性胆汁性肝硬化。
- 药物性胆汁淤积症。
- 妊娠相关性胆汁淤积。
- 肝外胆管梗阻。
- 慢性肝炎，尤其是丙型肝炎。

血液病

- 真性红细胞增多症。
- 缺铁性贫血。
- 副蛋白血症。
- 瓦氏巨球蛋白血症。
- 肥大细胞增多症。

肿瘤

- 淋巴瘤，包括霍奇金淋巴瘤。
- 蕈样肉芽肿病。
- 白血病。
- 中枢神经系统肿瘤。
- 多发性骨髓瘤。
- 良性肿瘤。
- 内脏恶性肿瘤(乳房、胃、肺)。

内分泌代谢疾病

- 尿毒症。
- 甲状腺功能亢进症。
- 甲状腺功能减退症。
- 甲状旁腺功能亢进症。
- 糖尿病。
- 良性肿瘤。

神经病

- 多发性硬化：阵发性瘙痒。
- 感觉异常性背痛：后背肩胛骨内侧轴瘙痒。
- 脑脓肿。
- 中枢神经系统感染。
- 脑肿瘤。

肾脏疾病

- 慢性肾衰竭。
- 慢性血液透析。

风湿免疫疾病

- 干燥综合征。
- 皮肌炎。

精神性

- 紧张、焦虑、神经症性表皮剥脱。
- 妄想症。
- 精神性瘙痒症。

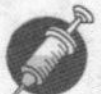

治疗

急诊治疗/程序

- 未确定病因的瘙痒，首先使用抗组胺药物。
- 干燥皮肤使用润滑剂。
- 降温剂可缓解瘙痒，用于神经调节：薄荷醇(1%～5%)、樟脑、桉树油、炉甘石液、冰、局麻药。
- P物质减少剂(辣椒素)，阻断C型神经纤维传导。
  - 初期使用时有炙热感。
  - 可以先使用麻醉药。
- 局部使用糖皮质激素治疗接触性皮炎。
- 皮疹提示可能为疥疮和虱疮，可给予氯菊酯乳霜治疗。

• 湿疹、风疹、蚊虫咬伤，可使用局部抗组胺药（如多虑平）。
• 游泳者瘙痒：
- 使用抗组胺药控制、冷敷、炉甘石液。
- 局部使用糖皮质激素：抑制强烈的炎症反应。
- 预防方法：离开水后立即用毛巾擦干。
• 停止用药可能引起过敏反应。
• 紫外线治疗尿毒症性瘙痒。
• 治疗引起瘙痒的原发病。

■ 药物治疗

• 口服抗组胺药：
- 氨苯那敏 4 mg 口服，q4～6 h，按需给药，最大剂量为 24 mg/24 h[儿童：0.35 mg/(kg·24 h)，4～6 h 给药 1 次，或按需给药；2～6 岁最大剂量 4 mg/24 h；6～12 岁最大剂量 12 mg/24 h]。
- 苯海拉明：25～50 mg，口服，q4～6 h，按需给药，最大剂量为 400 mg/24 h[儿童：5 mg/(kg·24 h)，q6 h，按需给药；2～5 岁最大剂量 37.5 mg/24 h；6～11 岁最大剂量 150 mg/24 h；>12 岁最大剂量 400 mg/24 h]。
- 羟嗪：25～100 mg，口服，6～8 h，按需给药；最大剂量 600 mg/24 h[儿童：2 mg/(kg·24 h)，q6 h，按需口服]。
• 局部治疗：
- 0.025%、0.075%辣椒素乳霜：每日 3～4 次。
- 5%多虑平乳霜：每日 4 次持续 8 日（最大使用面积为体表面积的 10%）。
- EMLA（2.5%利多卡因＋2.5%普鲁卡因）：在辣椒素之前使用。
- 0.5%、1%、2.5%氢化可的松：最多每日 4 次。
- 5%氯菊酯乳霜（用于疥疮）：
◦ 洗澡后从颈部向下涂抹。
◦ 8～12 h 后用水彻底清洗。
◦ 可在 7 天后重复使用。
- 1%氯菊酯洗剂冲洗（用于虱疮）：
◦ 洗发，冲洗，擦干，充分浸湿头发和头皮（以及其他相关部位），静待 10 min，冲洗。
◦ 7 日重复使用 1 次。
- 白色凡士林：短时温水（不要用热水）清洗后使用。
• 其他对于特殊疾病的治疗。

 随访

■ 进一步处理

入院指征

• 过敏反应。
• 全身剥脱性病变。
• 需要住院的全身表现的疾病。

出院指征

病因不同。

转诊问题

• 推荐皮肤病变的患者就诊于初级保健师或皮肤科医师。
• 建议没有皮肤病变、病情稳定伴有皮肤瘙痒的患者，经过止痒药物治疗后就诊于内科医师，进一步排除全身性疾病。

■ 随访建议

• 日常生活中保持皮肤干燥：
- 使用小苏打、沐浴油或胶态燕麦片沐浴。
- 沐浴后立刻使用保湿霜并保持日常使用。
• 避免：
- 干燥的空气（湿度<40%）。
- 刺激物接触（如羊毛物制品、清洁剂）。
- 碱性肥皂，辛辣食物。
- 过度暴露于热水。

要点和误区

• 在急诊过程中详细的病史是诊疗关键。
• 全身性疾病也会引起瘙痒。
• 单一药物不可能治疗所有原因引起的瘙痒。

S

闪电击伤 Lightning Injuries

Tarlan Hedayati 王胜云 译

 基础知识

■ 描述

• 闪电是能量释放的一种方式，包括云间放电（90%）和云对地放电（10%）。
• 闪电特点：
- 发生时间短（1～100 ms）。
- 多发生在户外活动时。
- 夏季 15:00—18:00 是高发时刻。
- 死亡率为 8%～10%。

■ 病因

• 受伤机制——电流：
- 直接击伤（5%）。
- 接触电势放电（15%～25%）：
◦ 电流通过接触物品击伤人体。
- 边缘放电（20%～30%）：
◦ 电流从附近物体跳跃击伤人体。
- 接地电位升高（40%～50%）：
◦ 电流通过地表可能导致多人受伤。
◦ 电流通过电话线、金属管道等可能导致电击伤。
• 受伤机制——创伤：
- 气压伤。
- 钝性受伤：
◦ 肌肉收缩可导致伤者跌倒。
- 热灼伤。

诊断

■ 症状和体征

病史

• 户外环境无目击者的心跳呼吸骤停，以及不明原因的昏迷，要考虑闪电击伤。
• 意识清楚患者可能出现的症状：
- 肌肉酸胀、疼痛。
- 胸痛。
- 呼吸短促。
- 剧痛。
- 烧伤。
- 神经功能障碍：
◦ 感觉异常。
◦ 感觉迟钝。
◦ 麻木无力。
◦ 视觉障碍或失明。
◦ 头痛。
◦ 失忆。
◦ 听力丧失或减弱。
◦ 头晕。

体格检查

• 头面部：

- 头部外伤。
- 骨膜破裂(50%以上)。
- 眼睛损伤:
  ◦ 白内障。
  ◦ 角膜溃疡。
  ◦ 眼内出血。
  ◦ 视网膜剥离。
• 颈部:
- 颈椎损伤。
• 心肺损伤:
- 首次心跳骤停:
  ◦ 心脏停搏。
  ◦ 直流电直接损伤。
  ◦ 心脏正常电生理受干扰。
- 高血压:多为一过性。
- 肺挫伤及出血。
- 呼吸骤停:
  ◦ 呼吸中枢受抑制。
  ◦ 可能比心跳停止时间长,产生低氧血症,导致二次心跳停止和脑损伤。
• 四肢:
- 骨折、脱臼。
- 肌肉撕裂、挫伤。
- 骨筋膜室综合征。
- 四肢花斑、湿冷:
  ◦ 血管自动舒张功能异常。
  ◦ 一般数小时后自动缓解。
• 皮肤:
- 灼伤:
  ◦ 一般在受伤数小时后出现。
  ◦ 闪电击伤皮肤入口一般不明显。
  ◦ 多为浅表组织灼伤,深部组织罕见。
  ◦ 由于直流电短促,直接的热烧伤少见。
  ◦ 热烧伤可由皮肤表面的水分、着火的衣物和随身的金属物件引起。
• 中枢神经系统损伤:
- 认知或记忆障碍。
- 意识不清(>70%的病例)。
- 迟缓性运动麻痹。
- 癫痫。
- 脑血管意外。
- 严重脑外伤或中枢神经系统受损引起的瞳孔扩大。
• 休克:
- 神经源性休克(脊髓休克)。
- 低容量性休克(外伤)。

基本检查

向目击者或施救者明确受伤原因。

诊断检查与说明

实验室检查

• 全血细胞计数。
• 尿液查肌红蛋白(少见)。
• 电解质。
• 肌酐、尿素氮。
• 凝血功能检查。
• 肌钙蛋白、心肌酶。

影像学检查

• 胸部X线平片:
- 肺水肿。
- 肺栓塞、出血。
- 肋骨骨折。
• 颈椎X线平片。
• 头颅CT检查以明确有无颅脑外伤。
• 其他相关伤情检查。

诊断步骤/外科

心电图:
• QT延长(最常见)。
• 非特异性ST段改变。
• 室性期前收缩(早搏)。
• 心房颤动。
• 室性心动过速。
• 急性心肌梗死(少见)。

鉴别诊断

主要与其他原因导致的昏迷、心律失常、外伤鉴别:
• 低血糖。
• 中毒、醉酒。
• 药物过量。
• 心血管疾病。
• 脑血管意外。
• 癫痫。
• 晕厥。

治疗

院前

• 对于在事发现场意识不清及心跳呼吸停止的患者,应快速给予呼吸支持:
- 阻止原发的心跳骤停进展为缺氧导致的二次心跳骤停。
- 意识清楚患者死亡风险较低。
• 颈椎固定:
- 心跳呼吸骤停患者(怀疑外伤导致者)。
- 明显的机械损伤。
- 怀疑意识丧失者(任何时候)。
• 无菌生理盐水纱布覆盖表面烧伤部位。
• 固定四肢。
• 迅速离开事发地点以免二次电击。
• 心律失常时行心电监测。

初步稳定/治疗

• ABC管理。
• 心跳骤停患者给予标准心肺复苏治疗。
• 对创伤及其他原因导致的损伤进行仔细询问、检查以防漏诊:
- 颈椎始终采取保护措施直至排除损伤可能。
• 给予葡萄糖、纳洛酮、维生素 B_1 治疗意识障碍。
• 低血压患者给予扩容、血制品及升压药物支持。

急诊治疗/程序

• 开通静脉通路。
• 心电、血氧监测。
• 烧伤处清创。
• 破伤风预防性注射。
• 肌红蛋白尿治疗(如果出现):
- 利尿剂(呋塞米或甘露醇)。
- 静脉输注碳酸氢钠碱化尿液。
• 扩容:
- 不要依据烧伤治疗进行补液,因为闪电击伤通常不是体液丢失的原因。
- 与其他类型电流损伤相比,闪电击伤导致深度烧伤比较少见。
- 根据尿量管理静脉液体。
- 液体负荷过重比较危险(如果患者合并头部损伤)。
• 骨筋膜室综合征:
- 与血管痉挛、自主神经失调、瘫痪麻痹等自限性疾病鉴别。
- 筋膜切开术很少有必要。
• 非甾体及高剂量类固醇类药物被推荐用于减轻神经及角膜损伤。

药物治疗

• 呋塞米:1 mg/kg,静脉慢滴,q6 h。
• 甘露醇:0.5 mg/kg,静脉滴注,必要时重复。
• 碳酸氢钠:1安瓿,静脉注射(儿童:1 mEq/kg),在2~3安瓿/L的静脉补液之后。

随访

进一步处理

入院指征

• 心肺复苏术后患者。

• 意识状态有变化的患者。
• 既往有胸痛、心律失常、心电图变化的患者：
- 不能自发缓解。
- 观察 24～48 h 排除不稳定性病变。
- 肌红蛋白尿。
- 酸中毒。
- 伴有骨筋膜室综合征损伤的患者。

出院指征

无症状的患者。

随访建议

• 安排专科医师密切随访以防迟发性后遗症：
- 中枢神经系统随访。
◦ 记忆障碍。
◦ 注意力缺陷。
◦ 失语症。
◦ 睡眠障碍。
◦ 感觉障碍及迟钝延长。
- 眼科随访。
- 五官科随访。
• 心理/精神方面：
- 焦虑。
- 抑郁。
- 个性变化。
- 创伤后应激障碍。

要点和误区

• 不要按照烧伤治疗原则来治疗闪电击伤。
• 主要完善检查以防漏诊。
• 对于有心肺不适主诉患者应尽早心电监测 24～48 h，以防不良事件发生。

疝 Hernias

Sean P. Dyer 陈奇通 译

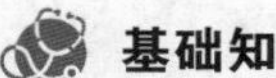

基础知识

描述

• 机体的结构或器官穿过组织的薄弱部位形成突出物。
• 由于腹壁肌纤维层的薄弱或破裂造成的腹壁疝。
• 分为外疝、内疝和交界性疝。外疝肉眼可见，而内疝突出物位于身体内部，交界性疝疝囊包含腹壁。
• 腹股沟区的疝包括股疝、腹股沟直疝和腹股沟斜疝。
• 腹部的疝包括腹壁疝、脐疝和半月线疝。
◦ 外观：
- 腹股沟斜疝：
◦ 由于持续性的腹压升高。
◦ 腹膜通过腹股沟环脱出。
◦ 右侧多于左侧。
◦ 男性修复后有 27%，女性仅有 3%。
- 腹股沟直疝：
◦ 由于股疝三角横纹肌缺陷而导致。
◦ 腹股沟韧带位于内侧。
◦ 疝囊是从腹壁下动脉的内侧穿出。
◦ 一般位于腹直肌外侧。
- 股疝：
◦ 疝囊通过股环、经股管向卵圆窝突出的疝。
◦ 难以回复原位。
◦ 疝囊内有大网膜、网膜孔。
• 腰部：
- 腰疝：发生在后腹壁上、下腰三角(嵌顿 25%)常见于中年人，合并有腰背痛。
• 骨盆：
- 闭孔疝：疝囊通过闭孔膜，位于耻骨肌下方。
• 腹侧：
- 切口疝：外科手术史。
- 上腹部疝：剑突和脐之间的中线。
• Spigelian 疝：突出通过斜筋膜外侧的腹直肌。
- 脐疝：
◦ 先天性失败的脐带环关闭。
◦ 突出通过纤维肌肉脐带环/脐。
◦ 常见于成人，但很少见于婴儿(通常自发闭合)。
◦ 20%～45%的复发率。

流行病学

• 疝修补术极其常见，美国每年有 75 万多的病例。
• 患病率：5%的人群。
• 腹股沟疝和股疝占 85%，脐疝和切口疝占 10%。

病因

• 易复性疝：突出物能够回纳。
• 嵌顿性疝：疝内容物无法回复。
• 绞窄性疝：嵌顿性疝合并有血运障碍，极其危险。有肠梗阻的症状和体征，并可出现恶心和发热。

诊断

症状和体征

病史

• 疼痛和肿块：疝囊的位置。
• 持续性疼痛、恶心和发热：提示有可能是嵌顿性疝、绞窄性疝或者肠梗阻。

体格检查

• 生命体征：
- 大多数正常。
- 疼痛、脱水或者感染时可有心动过速。
- 脱水、绞窄性疝或感染时可有高血压。
- 感染和败血症时会出现发热。
- 脱水时皮肤颜色发生变化。
• 腹股沟疝：
- 疼痛：
◦ 腹股沟区疼痛。
◦ 用力时疼痛加重。
◦ 休息时疼痛缓解。
- 肿块：
◦ 男性肿块可进入阴囊。
◦ 女性肿块可越过腹股沟韧带至阴唇。
- 精索、阴囊或睾丸处可有肿块。
- 进行瓦氏动作可用手指触碰到内环。
• 股疝：
- 疼痛和肿块。
◦ 位于腹股沟韧带下方的卵圆窝。
• 切口疝：
- 疼痛和肿块：
◦ 位于之前的切口或瘢痕部位。

• 闭孔疝：
- 非特异性腹痛。
- 间歇性肠梗阻。
- 体重减轻。
- 疼痛：
◦ 闭孔疝压迫闭孔神经导致疼痛，豪-罗二氏征。
◦ 疼痛沿着股内侧，放射至臀部。
◦ 大腿屈曲时疼痛减轻。
◦ 臀部肌肉紧张，内旋或外展时疼痛加重。
• 半月线疝：
- 疼痛，肿块位于前腹壁。
- 腹内压增加的相关运动可致疼痛加重。
- 间歇性肠梗阻。
- 沿半月线可见明显突出的肿块：沿着腹直肌由肋弓至耻骨结节。

儿科注意事项

• 诊断通常较为困难：
- 父母描述腹股沟处出现肿块，但是体格检查时消失。
- 嵌顿性疝可能同时伴有腹痛，间歇性呕吐。
• 嵌顿和绞窄的概率为 10%～20%：50%以上的患儿年龄小于 6 个月。
- 男孩嵌顿可能性高于女孩。
• 脐疝：
- 少有绞窄或嵌顿的可能性。
- 大部分能够自行愈合。
- 手术时机要等到 4 岁以后，但是目前手术时机仍存在争议。
• 腹股沟疝(考虑鞘膜积液)：
- 如果鞘膜积液，颈部狭窄外腹股沟管没有延伸到腹股沟管。

妊娠注意事项

• 妊娠期间极其少见。
• 腹股沟疝发病率在 1/(1 000～3 000)，75%为经产妇。
• 嵌顿性疝和绞窄性疝的诊断和处理较为困难。
• 妊娠期难复性疝的治疗尚未达成共识。妊娠期并发症的处理比择期疝修补术更为重要。

老年人注意事项

• 年龄>65 岁的嵌顿疝的老年进行肠切除的风险较高。
• 术后心肺并发症的概率较大。

基本检查

• 仔细询问病史和进行体格检查。
• 触诊腹股沟和股区有压痛、肿块。
• 如果疝不明显尝试让患者站立或用力(Valsalva 动作)。
• 女性需进行盆腔检查，分析腹股沟疼痛的病因。

诊断检查与说明

实验室检查

• 血常规。
- 发生绞窄会有白细胞增多。
• 发生呕吐或脱水时，电解质、肌酐、血糖会出现异常。
• 腹股沟疼痛可能是泌尿系统的原因。

影像学检查

• 腹部 X 线平片：
- 出现嵌顿和绞窄时可有肠梗阻的征象。
• 超声：
- 区分肿物位于腹股沟区还是腹壁。
- 肥胖患者难以分辨。
• CT：
- 诊断闭孔疝和半月线疝。
- 身体状况不适合超声时考虑使用。

鉴别诊断

• 鞘膜积液。
• 精索静脉曲张。
• 淋巴结炎。
• 睾丸肿瘤。
• 隐睾。
• 肾结石。
• 尿路感染。
• 卵巢蒂扭转。
• 淋巴肉芽肿。
• 腹壁血肿。
• 腹壁肿瘤。
• 腹壁脓疡。

治疗

初步稳定/治疗

• 出现脱水、绞窄、肠梗阻或者败血症时，应用生理盐水补液。
- 成人：1 L。
- 儿童：20 ml/kg。

急诊治疗/程序

• 绞窄性疝：
- 肠外营养。
- 鼻胃管进行胃肠减压。
- 外科会诊。
- 广谱抗生素的使用仍存在争议。
• 疝复位手术：
- 阵痛(吗啡)，镇静(地西泮)。
- 患者取屈曲位。
- 观察 20～30 min，能够自发复位。
- 人工复位：
◦ 在肿块位置轻轻压迫疝囊。
◦ 腹股沟疝需要把 1 个手指向内环轻轻拉，并压迫外环远端。
- 疝囊无法减小，复位失败时及时手术。
- 复位禁忌证：
◦ 发热。
◦ 白细胞增多。
◦ 合并绞窄性疝。
- 肠发生绞窄进入腹腔。
- 临床症状并无改善或进一步发生缺血坏死。
- 女性如果卵巢位于疝囊内，则复位更加困难。

药物治疗

• 镇痛药：
- 硫酸吗啡：每次 2～10 mg(儿童：0.1～0.2 mg/kg，2～4 h 可重复使用)。
• 镇静药：
- 地西泮(安定)：1～2 mg。
- 咪达唑仑：2.5～5 mg(儿童：0.07 mg/kg)。

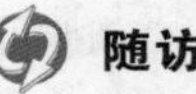

随访

进一步处理

入院指征

• 绞窄性疝需要立即手术治疗。
• 嵌顿疝需要紧急手术干预入场。
• 肠梗阻。
• 腹膜炎。
• 呕吐与脱水。
• 严重的疼痛。

出院指征

复位成功，患者无症状。

转诊问题

持续性疼痛、发热或者呕吐应及时转诊进行手术治疗。

随访建议

普通外科的转诊。

要点和误区

• 不能辨别嵌顿性和绞窄性疝的症状和体征。
• 腹股沟疝强迫复位。
• 腹腔内肠绞窄。

烧伤 Burns

Gabriel Wardi · Anthony J. Medak 沈黎蔚 译

基础知识

描述

烧伤是一种皮肤的急性损伤，最常见的是暴露在高温或火焰下。

病因

烧伤可以分为 7 种类型。
• 烫伤：热的液体、油脂或蒸汽。
• 接触伤：热的或冷的表面。
• 热烫伤：火或火焰。
• 放射性烧伤。
• 化学性烧伤。
• 电烧性烧伤。
• 擦伤：道路摩擦、绳索摩擦。

诊断

症状和体征

• 大部分烧伤皮肤表面都有明显的外伤特征。
• 吸入性损伤若出现下列症状则可能危及生命，须警惕：
- 颜面部烧伤、喉头水肿。
- 烧焦的鼻、头发、睫毛。
- 碳化的痰液。
- 呼吸力学的改变(喘鸣、咳嗽、气促)。
- 声音变化，声音沙哑，喘鸣。
• 电烧伤及化学烧伤的表面损伤很小(入口伤、出口伤)。

病史

• 大量的事实，火源(塑料、木头、化学品等)、场所和环境、爆炸。
• 医学、手术、社会史、用药情况、变态反应、破伤风用药状态。
• 暴露于以木头为基础引起的火灾或者燃烧中所引起的一氧化碳(CO)中毒(火灾中引起死亡的最常见原因)。
• CO 中毒的患者指脉氧是不可靠的。
• 羊毛、蚕丝、尼龙燃烧引起的氰化物中毒，以及家具/纸燃烧引起的聚氨基甲酸酯中毒。

体格检查

• 首先检查气道，然后检查其他的损伤。
• 评估颜面部、口咽及鼻孔的损伤作为化学性吸入伤的体征。
• 评估是否需要颈椎固定(爆炸或坠落中)。
• 角膜烧伤的眼部检查。
• 通过评估烧伤的大小及深度估计局部和全层烧伤的严重程度。

儿科注意事项

损伤的具体模式可能表示非意外伤害(浸泡伤、香烟烧伤等)。

基本检查

• 通过烧伤的面积和深度评估烧伤的严重程度。
• 通过以下 3 种方法中的 1 种确定烧伤占全身体表面积(TBSA)的百分比：
• 9 分法(仅适用于成人)：
- 将人体体表面积按照 9%的倍数分配。
- 成人体表面积百分比的分配：
◦ 头和颈部：9。
◦ 手臂：右侧 9；左侧 9。
◦ 腿：右侧 18；左侧 18。
◦ 躯干：前 18；后 18。
◦ 会阴，手掌：1。
- 婴幼儿头占全身体表面积的百分比更多，腿所占比例更少。
- 婴儿/儿童：
◦ 头和颈部：18。
◦ 手臂：右侧 9；左侧 9。
◦ 腿：右侧 14；左侧 14。
◦ 躯干：前 18；后 18。
• Lund-Browder 计算法：基于年龄划分身体区域以及分配体表面积的百分比，可以得出比 9 分法更加可靠的结果。
• 手掌表面积：患者的手掌及手指占全身体表面积的 1%，这点对于评估不规则或散在烧伤的损伤程度是很有帮助的。
• 浅表伤或 1 度烧伤(仅伤及表皮)：局部红斑，轻度肿胀或疼痛，无水疱(可能会在 2～3 日出现)，几日内痊愈，不留瘢痕。
• 部分皮肤层烧伤或 2 度烧伤(表皮和真皮层损伤)：表面皮肤层或者深部皮肤层的烧伤。
- 表面皮肤层烧伤(表皮和浅层真皮)：
◦ 常见于烫伤。
◦ 形成广泛的水疱，创面红润、潮湿，有疼痛感，毛细血管填充，感觉完整。
◦ 通常 14～21 日愈合，不形成瘢痕。
- 深部皮肤层的烧伤(表皮和深层真皮)：
◦ 皮肤从白色到黄色真皮膨胀，缺乏毛细血管填充和疼痛感。
◦ 在 3～12 周通过上皮增殖愈合，通常会形成严重的瘢痕并且需要手术治疗。
• 全层或 3 度烧伤(从表皮到真皮)：
- 皮肤烧焦、皮革状、灰白色，不形成水疱，没有感觉。
- 不能自行愈合，需要实施手术以及植皮。
• 全层皮肤烧伤或 4 度烧伤(损伤皮肤下组织)：
- 全层皮肤损伤，包括皮肤下软组织、肌肉、骨骼和其他组织。
- 需要广泛的清创及移植。
- 导致残疾。

诊断检查与说明

实验室检查

• 严重烧伤：CBC、血清电解质、血糖、尿素氮、肌酐、凝血酶原时间、血型鉴定和交叉配血、妊娠试验。
• 密闭空间里的患者或有可疑吸入性暴露的患者血气中 CO 水平。
• 氰化物水平(如果有接触可能的话)。

影像学检查

胸部 X 线检查。

诊断步骤/外科

• 评估吸入性损伤的支气管镜检查。
• 心电图，尤其是电烧伤、老年患者。

鉴别诊断

• 电损伤。
• 化学损伤。
• 中毒相关损伤。

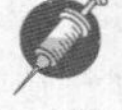

治疗

院前

• 脱离热源，扔掉易燃、污染的衣服和首饰。
• 将患者移至温暖、干燥的开阔地方。
• 建立通畅的气道，持续评估，给予 100%氧气吸入。
- 呼吸窘迫的患者早期插管。
• 早期静脉输液治疗，特别是烧伤面积超过 20% TBSA 的患者。
• 缓解疼痛，必要时可使用麻醉剂。
• 使用干净的床单保护损伤部位。
• 如果运输时间少于 30 min，将患者运去烧

S

伤中心(对于烧伤患者较多时)。
• 脊椎固定,如果机制涉及的话。

■ 初步稳定/治疗

• 首先要保持气道通畅:
- 对于上呼吸道损伤的患者早期予以气管插管,特别是对于鼻唇部烧伤或颈周烧伤的患者有特殊意义。
• 开放静脉通路,提供100%氧气吸入、心电监测及血氧监测。
• 评估同时发生的其他损伤。
• 提供足够的镇痛。
• 阿片类药物是主要药物:
- 对乙酰氨基酚、非甾体抗炎药、氯胺酮(亚解离剂量)可作为辅助用药。
• 早期液体复苏是必要的。

■ 急诊治疗/程序

• 液体复苏:部分及全层皮肤烧伤患者(>20% TBSA)。
- 派克兰烧伤公式(不适用于儿科患者):每千克体重每BSA的百分比予4 ml乳酸林格液(首选)或生理盐水(NS)。
- 第一个8 h补充全部液体的1/2,接下来16 h补充剩下的1/2。

例如:一个70 kg烧伤面积达到40% TBSA的患者超过24 h需要4 ml×70 kg×40%=11 200 ml液体,第一个8 h内需要5 600 ml液体或每小时补充700 ml液体。

- 在初始的液体复苏后,烧伤面积超过20% TBSA的患者需要依据侵入性血流动力学监测或尿量结果继续予以静脉输液治疗。
- 需要保持成人0.5 ml/(kg·h)以及儿童1 ml/(kg·h)的尿量。
• 焦痂切开术:
- 环形烧伤焦痂会引起血管或气道塌陷。
◦ 适应证:通过抬高患肢不能改善的肢端循环障碍,或者胸壁烧伤中引起的气道塌陷。
◦ 四肢:四肢的切口应该沿着肢体的长轴位于内侧或外侧,并且通过整个焦痂位于皮下脂肪的表面。
◦ 胸壁:从第2肋到第12肋沿着腋前线做纵切口,沿着胸壁用2条横切口连接。
• 伤口护理:
- 使用多链丝霉素或杆菌肽软膏及非黏附性敷料覆盖在伤口上。
- 在污染/肮脏的伤口上涂磺胺嘧啶银(避免如果转运至烧伤中心而干扰后续的烧伤评估)。
- 新型银基敷料对MRSA有更好的抑制作用,且有文献显示其有利于在烧伤创面恢复。

此外,这类敷料可以持续留置数日,既提高了患者的舒适度,也减少了总耗费。

• 为了伤口护理的进行不要延误转运至烧伤病房的时间。
• 预防性使用抗生素没有明确的指征。
• 轻微烧伤的门诊患者的处理:
- 清洁和清创的消毒技术。
- 止痛通常是需要的。
- 去除松脱、坏死的皮肤,清除坏死、紧缩或感染的水疱。
- 局部使用抗生素(如磺胺嘧啶银、杆菌肽、醋酸磺胺米隆)仅推荐用于深度烧伤或者全层烧伤患者。
- 目前在有焦痂形成的部分厚度伤口表面使用胶原酶(胶原蛋白),3度烧伤伤口不需使用,这个缺乏抗生素属性。
- 需使用3层敷料以保持创面湿润及吸收渗出物:
◦ 内层应该使用饱含非石油基润滑油的多孔网状纱布,或者在不粘连的多孔纱布覆盖下使用温和的药膏(杆菌肽或多链丝霉素)。
◦ 第二层应使用软毛粗纱布。
◦ 最外层覆盖的敷料应无收缩性。
◦ 敷料应该保持每日更换1次。
- 银伤口敷料(Silverlon和Acticoat):
◦ 针织物的背面覆有金属银薄涂层。
◦ 需要敷料保持创面潮湿。
◦ 需要放置于伤口表面超过3日。
- 如果有指征的话,轻微烧伤也需使用破伤风。

儿科注意事项

• 派克兰公式低估了儿童的液体需要;加尔维斯顿公式更合适,5 000 ml/m² BSA烧伤面积+2 000 ml/m²。
• 第1个24 h内使用乳酸林格液和5%葡萄糖静脉注射,第1个8 h内输入总液体的1/2,剩下的1/2液体在接下来的16 h内使用。
- 输液的目标是尿量要达到1 ml/(kg·h)。
• 考虑非意外性创伤,特别是烧伤在手、足、臀部、会阴及大腿背面时。
• 避免低温:
- 儿童有更大的体表面积/质量,散热更快。
• 避免低血糖:
- 由于糖原储备有限,儿童更容易出现低血糖。

孕妇注意事项

• 是母亲和孩子重要的年患病率。
• 液体需要量超过估算量。
• 建议胎儿检测和早期产科咨询。

■ 治疗药物

• 杆菌肽软膏:每日4次。
• 醋酸磺胺米隆软膏:每日1次或2次。
• 阿片类药物:尤其适用于水疱的创面和更大的严重烧伤。
• Acticoat、Aquacel AG、Mepilex AG:这几种敷料可依据烧伤面积大小进行裁剪,敷盖前可能需用无菌水润湿敷料。
• 破伤风类毒素或免疫球蛋白:0.5 ml肌内注射;与类毒素一起250 U肌内注射。
- Santyl:每日1次涂在焦痂/烧伤表面。

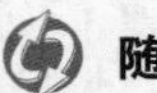

随访

■ 进一步处理

入院指征

• 需要收入院的创伤:
- 成人非关键部位的部分厚度烧伤(除外眼睛、耳、脸、手、足或会阴)达到10%~20% BSA(>10岁和<50岁)。
- <10岁的儿童非关键部位的部分厚度烧伤达到体表面积的5%~10%。
- 怀疑非意外性创伤的患者。
- 不能在院外护理和照顾的烧伤患者(如无家可归的患者)。
• 需要转入烧伤中心的创伤:
- 部分厚度烧伤或者全层烧伤≥10% BSA。
- 全层烧伤>5% BSA。
- 脸、手、足、生殖器、会阴或主要关节的部分或全层烧伤。
- 电烧伤,包括雷击伤。
- 典型的化学烧伤。
- 吸入性损伤。
- 患者患有需要系统管理的其他疾病。
- 有其他伴发的创伤或社会障碍的患者。

出院指征

成人部分厚度烧伤面积<10% BSA(儿童或老人<5% BSA)包括仅有非关键部位烧伤的患者。患者必须有院外管理创伤的能力,并应随访。

转诊问题

当对于烧伤部位的美容需求较大时,应降低收入烧伤中心的标准,包括手、脸、眼、会阴部位的烧伤,或者烧伤叠加到关节部位时。

■ 随访建议

创伤后的1～2日评估早期抗感染、敷料浸润情况及疼痛管理。

要点和误区

• 早期静脉输液、水化是必要的。早期静脉补液对严重烧伤(体表面积大于15%～20%)的治疗至关重要。

• 有呼吸窘迫迹象患者的早期插管,必须识别出呼吸窘迫的可能性。

• 早期镇痛是所有烧伤处理的基本要求。

Parkland公式低估了儿科患者的液体需求。

蛇毒液螫伤 Snake Envenomation

Patrick M. Lank · Timothy B. Erickson 周健 潘曙明 译

基础知识

■ 描述

• 蝮蛇毒:

- 蛋白水解酶和凝血酶样酯酶的混合物:
  ◦ 酶引起局部肌肉和皮下组织坏死。
  ◦ 酯酶具有去纤化抗凝血作用,在严重中毒时可导致毒性消耗性凝血病(VICC)。

• 咬位置:

- 极端咬最常见。
- 头部、颈部或躯干的咬伤比四肢的咬伤更严重。

• 表面变质严重:

- 直接咬入动脉或静脉。
- 神经毒性表面变质。

• 咬痕的意义:

- 蝮蛇咬:经典包括1或2个刺伤。
- 无毒蛇和袋尾蛇:一排多齿的马蹄形痕迹。

• 25%的蝮蛇咬伤是干燥的,不会导致中毒。

■ 病因

毒蛇原产于人类。

• 蝰蛇(Crotalinae):

- 占所有表面变质的95%。
- 水蝮蛇、响尾蛇、铜斑蛇。

• 珊瑚蛇(眼镜蛇科):

- 神经毒性。
- 西部珊瑚蛇,发现于亚利桑那州和新墨西哥州。
- 更毒的东部珊瑚蛇,发现在卡罗来纳州和海湾国家。

国际外来毒蛇

出现在动物园或外来蛇的主人。

儿童注意事项

• 30%的蛇咬伤发生在20岁以下人群,12%的蛇咬伤发生在9岁以下儿童。

• 由于体重较轻,较小的儿童和婴儿更容易出现全身症状的严重中毒。

诊断

■ 症状和体征

• 本地(响尾蛇的):

- 典型的皮肤变化:
  ◦ 1个或2个刺伤。
  ◦ 部位疼痛和肿胀。
- 涉及肢体肿胀和水肿:
  ◦ 严重中毒1h内。
  ◦ 近端淋巴结软化。
- 瘀斑、瘀点和出血性囊泡在几小时内发育。

• 全身(响尾蛇):

- 虚弱,头晕。
- 发汗。
- 恶心。
- 头皮感觉异常。
- 眶周的束状震颤。
- 金属的味道。
- 严重咬伤会导致:
  ◦ VICC。
  ◦ 低血压。
  ◦ 肺水肿。
  ◦ 血尿。
  ◦ 横纹肌溶解。
  ◦ 肾衰竭。
  ◦ 心功能不全。
- 累及的肢体潜在间隔室压力升高。

• 症状(响尾蛇的):

- 主要神经毒性,导致虚弱、复视、混乱,推迟呼吸抑郁症:
  ◦ 局部影响可能小得令人迷惑。

病史

• 描述的蛇的类型。

• 咬伤的地理位置。

体格检查

寻找上述咬伤的表现。

■ 基本检查

• 仔细检查伤口部位和受累肢体:

- 表面变质的重要判断严重程度。
- 标记伤口边缘发展。

• 评估过敏反应。

■ 诊断检查与说明

■ 实验室检查

• CBC。

• 凝血。

• 纤维蛋白原,肺动脉栓塞。

• 电解质/肌酐、葡萄糖。

• 肌酸磷酸激酶(CPK)。

• UA。

• 类型和交叉匹配,中度至重度中毒。

影像学检查

如怀疑有异物,应做X线平片检查。

■ 鉴别诊断

• 无毒蛇(美国):

- 狭窄的头。
- 圆的瞳孔。
- 不摇铃。

• 蝰蛇:

- 三角形或箭头状的头。
- 垂直或椭圆的头。
- 热敏感凹仅次于面前的鼻孔和眼睛。
- 摇铃。

• 珊瑚蛇(仅适用于美国,不适用于其他国家):

- "红黄相间,杀死同伴"。
- "红黑相间,缺少毒液"。

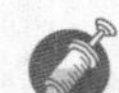

治疗

■ 院前

• 撤退到蛇的攻击范围之外。

S

• 将肢体固定在心脏水平的功能位置。
• 尽量少运动。
• 取下戒指、手表和所有紧绷绷的衣物。
• 出于鉴定的目的，将蛇送到医疗机构是不明智的：
- 如果你离得足够近，可以用相机或手机拍一张好照片，那么你离一条潜在的毒蛇太近了。
- 即使是被砍下的头也会产生毒液。
• 争议：
- 不建议进行院前局部伤口手术，因为它们会造成更严重的局部组织损伤，增加感染的风险。这些包括：
◦ 切开及引流。
◦ 机械吸引装置。
◦ 口吸。
◦ 止血带。
◦ 冷冻疗法。
◦ 电刑。
◦ 压力固定。
◦ 无经验的切口会导致严重的肌腱、神经和血管损伤。

儿科注意事项

• 中毒更严重。
• 严重程度：由于幼童体重较轻，且毒液量相同。

■ 初步稳定/治疗

• ABC 管理。
• 用生理盐水（NS）维持高血容量，以维持肾血流量。
• 伤口监测。
• 固定被咬肢体。

■ 急诊治疗/程序

• 支持性护理。
• 筋膜室综合征监测：
- 每 15～20 min 重复测量肢体周长，直到局部进展/肿胀消退。
- 响尾蛇中毒后不太可能出现真正的筋膜室综合征。
- 更多的抗蛇毒血清可治疗升高的腔室压力，因为筋膜切开术的外科干预会对该区域造成更大的损害。
- 外科治疗被认为只有在非常罕见的情况下，只应考虑咨询区域中毒中心和医学毒理学家。
• 静脉阿片类镇痛药。
• 必要时预防破伤风。
• 广谱抗生素没有常规指示。
• 除对抗蛇毒血清有反应外，未使用类固醇（见下文）。
• 常规使用血液制品未注明。
• 伤口严重程度：
- 最小：
◦ 局部肿胀和压痛。
- 中度：
◦ 肢体肿胀。
◦ 全身系统性毒性。
- 严重：
◦ 明显中毒。
◦ 不稳定的生命体征。
◦ 凝血功能障碍。
◦ 毒蛇表面变质。
◦ 实验室检查异常。

抗蛇毒血清

• 抗蛇毒血清治疗指标：
- 超过最小的肢体肿胀。
- 肢体肿胀正在进展。
- 全身毒性的临床症状。
- 不稳定的生命指征。
- 凝血病（低血小板或纤维蛋白原，PT 升高）。
• CroFab：更新的 F(ab′)2 抗蛇毒血清：
- 北美蝮蛇毒中毒的基本治疗。
- 高亲和纯化羊 Fab 抗体片段抗蛇毒血清。
- Fab 抗蛇毒血清比旧的多价抗蛇毒血清引起更少的频繁过敏反应。
- 儿童抗蛇毒血清剂量＝成人抗蛇毒血清剂量。
- 剂量：4～6 瓶。
- 用 25 ml 无菌水重新装瓶，用 250 ml 生理盐水稀释，注入 1 h 以上。
- 如有低血压或严重活动性出血，初始剂量为 8～12 瓶。
- 抗蛇毒血清输注后 1 h 评估中毒控制情况。控制的定义是稳定的伤口外观，改善凝血研究和血流动力学稳定性。
- 如果在第一次注射抗蛇毒血清后中毒得到控制，可能需要 2 瓶、q6 h ×3 剂的抗蛇毒血清维持治疗。
- 如果在第一次注射抗蛇毒血清后仍未达到中毒控制，则重复第一次注射并重新评估。与当地毒物中心或医学毒理学家讨论。
• 对抗蛇毒血清产生过敏反应的中毒受害者：
- 停止注射抗蛇毒血清。
- 给予抗组胺药、皮质类固醇和液体。考虑肾上腺素的严重反应。
- 应与当地毒物中心或医学毒理学家讨论重新使用抗蛇毒血清的风险/益处。
• 珊瑚蛇抗蛇毒素：
- 已不再生产，但在适当地点储存。
- 对东方珊瑚蛇有效，但对西方珊瑚蛇无效。
- 在适当的皮肤测试后，建议 3～5 瓶抗蛇毒血清。
- 治疗并发症包括过敏反应和血清病。
- 珊瑚虫的毒液具有神经毒性；注意呼吸抑制，控制气道。
• 国际外来毒蛇：
- 抗蛇毒血清可通过抗蛇毒血清指数在当地动物园获得。

儿童注意事项

• 按体重比例增加抗蛇毒血清。
• 所需标准成人剂量。

妊娠注意事项

• 如果母亲有全身中毒的迹象，胎儿也有危险；及时抗蛇毒血清治疗仍有必要。
• 咨询产科医师。

治疗援助

• 联系当地毒物中心、医学毒理学家、当地动物园或地区爬虫科医师。
• 查询抗蛇毒血清指数，请求协助治疗非本地的外来蛇类咬伤。

随访

■ 进一步处理

入院指征

• 蝮蛇咬伤后需要抗蛇毒血清的患者在毒液进展控制后 24 h 观察。
• 24 h 观察无症状的毒蛇咬伤患者。
• ICU 住院：
- 接受抗蛇毒血清的患者。
- 中度至重度中毒的证据，特别是儿童。
- 所有被蛇咬伤和有症状的外来毒蛇中毒的受害者。

出院指征

可疑咬伤，6～8 h 无中毒症状，实验室检查正常：
• 如果局部毒性没有发展，实验室检查正常，可以观察干咬 8 h 后出院。
• 轻微的中毒应观察 12～24 h，并在出现后 6 h 重复实验室检查，然后在出院前再次检查。
• 出院后 24 h 随访。

S

■ 随访建议

抗蛇毒血清治疗后1周进行PCP或毒理学随访，以评估可能的血清疾病或毒性伤口感染。

要点和误区

• 避免过度积极的院前护理干预。最好快速运送到最近的医疗中心。

• 临床需要时，应及时给予适当剂量的抗蛇毒血清。

• 用于复发性凝血病的后期治疗。

社区获得性耐甲氧西林金黄色葡萄球菌感染 MRSA, Community Acquired

Benjamin S. Heavrin　伍力学 译

基础知识

■ 描述

• 耐甲氧西林金黄色葡萄球菌(MRSA)多发生在医疗机构中，常感染老年人和慢性疾病患者，因此又被称为医疗机构相关性耐甲氧西林金黄色葡萄球菌(healthcare-associated MRSA, HA-MRSA)。

• 在最近10余年，在青年人和无医疗机构暴露史的人群中发生的MRSA感染不断增加。这一类MRSA被称为社区获得性耐甲氧西林金黄色葡萄球菌(community-acquired MRSA, CA-MRSA)。

• CA-MRSA是急诊最常见的皮肤和软组织感染。

• CA-MRSA不仅可以引起皮肤和软组织感染，还可能诱发多系统疾病，包括脓毒症和坏死性肺炎。

老年人注意事项

HA-MRSA作为MRSA另一基因亚型，在老年人中发病率较高，尤其是居住在养老院或有医疗机构暴露史的老年人。

■ 病因

• 金黄色葡萄球菌是一种好发于皮肤的革兰阳性菌。

• MRSA是金黄色葡萄球菌中对包括甲氧西林在内的多数抗生素具有耐药性的类型。

• 囚犯、运动员、军人、幼儿园的儿童、静脉吸毒者、此前接受过抗MRSA治疗者及有MRS暴露史的人群是发生MRSA定植和后续感染的高危人群。

诊断

■ 体征和症状

病史

• 皮肤和软组织感染：

- 局部发红。
- 疼痛。
- 肿胀。
- 发热。
- 寒战。
- 精神萎靡。

• 脓毒症及肺炎：

- 乏力。
- 呼吸困难。
- 发热。
- 寒战。
- 咳嗽、咳痰。
- 胸痛。

• 仔细询问既往有无MRSA感染史，有无MRSA暴露史，以及家人或周围的人有无MRSA近距离接触史，有上述病史接触史者为CA-MRSA感染的高危人群。

体格检查

• 皮肤和软组织感染：

- 脓肿：表现为局部隆起的质软包块，皮下可有硬结和波动感。
- 蜂窝织炎：病灶局部发红、皮温高且有伴淋巴管走行红线征。

• 脓毒症：

- 生命体征不平稳，包括心动过速、低血压、呼吸衰竭、神志改变、皮肤出血点、全身毒症状。

• 肺炎：

- 心动过速、肺部啰音、胸闷、低氧血症。
- 胸片提示肺野实变影。

儿科注意事项

MRSA是急诊收治的儿童患者皮肤和软组织感染的主要病因。

■ 基本检查

• 脓肿：

- 切开引流后包扎伤口，嘱患者随访是脓肿痊愈的保障。
- 微生物学培养可能提示病原体对抗生素耐药谱常发生改变。

• 脓毒症：

- 液体复苏治疗开始的同时需明确感染源(包括血/尿培养、胸片等)。

• 肺炎：

- 需要行胸部X线检查和持续生命体征监测。

■ 诊断检查与说明

实验室检查

• 皮肤和软组织感染：

- 需要行微生物学培养以监测菌群的耐药性。

• 脓毒症和肺炎。

- 血、尿和体液培养。行CBC、CMP以评估脏器衰竭程度。

影像学检查

• 床旁超声：

- 脓肿：表现为液性无回声区。
- 蜂窝织炎：软组织内呈"鹅卵石样"改变。

• 胸部X线检查：

- 对可疑的肺脓肿、全身疾病或肺炎有提示意义。

诊断步骤/外科

常常需要对皮肤和软组织感染灶的标本进行培养，结果以明确微生物的种类及耐药性分布，进而判断治疗方案是否有效。

■ 鉴别诊断

• 其他皮肤和软组织感染：

- 需要考虑有无除MRSA以外的可引发脓肿和蜂窝织炎的病原体感染(如链球菌)。

• 坏死性筋膜炎。

• 接触性皮炎。

• 深静脉血栓。

• 蜘蛛、昆虫叮咬。

• 药物反应。

S

注意

针对皮肤和软组织感染的经验性抗感染治疗还应覆盖 MRSA 以外的常见的皮肤病原菌（如链球菌）。

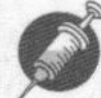

治疗

院前

• 对所有怀疑有 MRSA 感染者应防范接触传播。

• 对可能存在脓毒症者建立静脉通路并实施液体复苏。

初步稳定/治疗

开始复苏并早期经验性应用抗生素，如有肺炎、筋膜炎或考虑有脓毒症者：

• 包括早期使用覆盖 MRSA 的抗生素。

急诊治疗/程序

• 皮肤和软组织感染：

- 脓肿：

◦ 切开引流。

◦ 如果没有深部组织感染或蜂窝织炎的证据，不必使用抗生素。

- 蜂窝织炎：

◦ 对于一般情况良好的健康人群，发生 CA-MRSA 蜂窝织炎后，可选择在门诊使用口服抗生素治疗。

◦ 一般状况差、有潜在的基础疾病及门诊治疗无效者需要静脉使用覆盖 CA-MRSA 的抗生素。

• 脓毒症和肺炎：

- 对有 CA-MRSA 感染风险者应早期预防性使用对 MRSA 有效的广谱抗生素。

药物治疗

注意

在选择特定抗生素治疗方案前，请回顾所在社区的 CA-MRSA 耐药谱，因为下列许多抗生素未必对 CA-MRSA 有效。

一线用药

• TMP-SMX：

- 成人：Bactrim DS 800/160；1～2 片，口服，每日 2 次。

- 儿童：10 mg，口服，每日 2 次。

• 克林霉素：

- 成人：150～450 mg，口服，每日 4 次。

- 儿童：5 mg/kg，口服，每日 3～4 次。

- 对克林霉素的耐药率正在上升。

• 多西环素：

- 成人：100 mg，口服，每日 2 次。

- 儿童：2.2 mg/kg，口服，每日 2 次。

• 万古霉素：

- 成人：1 g，静脉注射，q8～12 h。

- 儿童：15 mg/kg，静脉注射，q8～12 h。

二线用药

• 利福平：

- 不应单药使用以免出现耐药。

- 成人：10～20 mg/(kg·d)，静脉使用 2 日；口服疗程为 5 日，每日不超过 600 mg。

• 达托霉素 6 mg/kg，静脉滴注，每日 1 次。

• 利奈唑胺：

- 成人：600 mg，口服或静脉使用，q12 h。

- 儿童：10 mg/kg，口服或静脉使用，q8 h。

妊娠注意事项

妊娠期应避免使用四环素。

随访

进一步处理

入院指征

• 有菌血症的症状和体征者，以及进展性的感染或系统性疾病者：

- 发热、寒战、淋巴管炎。

• 具有糖尿病或免疫功能缺陷等并发疾病者。

• 门诊治疗无效者应收入院并静脉使用对 MRSA 有效的抗生素治疗。

出院指征

体健且一般情况良好的单纯皮肤和软组织感染者可在门诊治疗随访。

转诊问题

多药治疗无效的难治性 MRSA 感染则需要会诊。

随访建议

• 所有的皮肤和软组织感染患者均应在 24～48 h 再次评估以了解病情有无好转。

• 门诊治疗无效者应收入院并静脉应用抗生素。

要点和误区

• 在流行病学中，CA-MRSA 是皮肤和软组织感染最常见的病因。

• 由 CA-MRSA 引起的侵袭性肺炎和脓毒症虽不多见，一旦发生就非常严重。

• 抗生素耐药谱会动态变化而且地区差异巨大。

• 避免在儿童中长时间应用四环素类抗生素。

砷中毒 Arsenic Poiso

Vinodinee L. Dissanayake 李岩 王瑞兰 译

基础知识

描述

• 急性毒性：

- 可能是故意摄入、投毒或用药错误。

• 最低致死摄入剂量为 2 mg/kg。

• 慢性毒性：

- 可能是职业暴露、饮用污染的水或食品，或使用含砷的民间偏方。

• 主要途径是口服摄入。

• 也可能是吸入毒性的砷化氢气体所致。

病因

• 急诊室中见到的砷中毒大多是故意摄入或恶意中毒。

• 砷酸钠，在杀蚁药中发现，在美国是最常见的急性暴露原因。

• 总体而言，世界范围内受污染的食品/水供应是最常见的原因。

• 三氧化二砷最近已被批准用于急性髓细胞性白血病（AML）的化疗。

• 美拉胂醇在发展中国家作为抗锥虫剂使用。

• 在农药、某些民间偏方（草药球）、木材的防腐剂中发现。

• 也可能是作为含锌或含砷化合物燃烧时产生的砷化氢气体释放。

机制

• 砷存在的几种形式：气态（砷化氢或路易试剂）、有机物形式、单质和无机物形式。

• 无机形态的砷是最常遇到的毒性接触。

• 无机的砷存在于三价（亚砷酸盐）或五价（砷酸盐）的形式：

- 大多数的五价砷在身体中转化为毒性更强的三价砷。
- 三价砷与巯基结合干扰血红蛋白的产生。
- 某些三价砷可能被甲基化成毒性不同的物种。
- 更具反应性的物种是 DNA 破坏和遗传毒性。

诊断

症状和体征

• 心血管系统：

- QT 间期延长。
- 低血压（急性）或高血压（慢性）。
- 心律失常，主要是室性的。
- 非特异性 ST 段改变。
- 非心源性肺水肿。

• 中枢神经系统：

- 精神状态改变/脑病。
- 儿童神经发育缺陷。
- 周围神经病变：
  ◦ 急性：感觉神经病变。
  ◦ 亚急性：感觉运动神经病变。
- 外周感觉迟钝：
  ◦ 肌肉无力到麻痹。
- 头痛。
- 癫痫发作。

• 呼吸系统：

- 吸入暴露会增加肺癌风险和呼吸系统疾病死亡率。
- 大量急性摄入（8 mg/kg）可能导致严重的呼吸窘迫。
- 肺水肿、出血性支气管炎和支气管肺炎。

• 消化系统：

- 恶心、呕吐：
  ◦ 病程较长并且常规剂量的止吐药可能难以治愈。
  ◦ 可有出血性肠胃炎；对胃肠道有腐蚀性。
- 米汤样腹泻。
- 腹痛。
- 呼吸、呕吐、粪便有大蒜味。
- 引起急性肝炎，慢性可引起门静脉高血压。
- 慢性暴露可能与糖尿病有关。

• 其他：

- 急性横纹肌溶解。
- 台湾的黑脚病：由于血液循环障碍至四肢坏疽。
- 皮肤炎，如中毒性红皮病和角化过度、色素沉着过度。
- 溶血性贫血（暴露于砷气中更为明显）。
- 甲状腺功能减退（拮抗甲状腺激素）。
- 增加患癌的风险（肝、基底细胞、皮肤鳞状细胞、支气管癌）。
- 白细胞减少症（几日后）。
- 米斯线（由于砷引起的生长停滞，指甲上出现白色条带）。
- 斑秃。
- 雷诺现象和血管痉挛。

基本检查

• 急诊尿砷水平检测。

• 全血细胞计数。

诊断检查与说明

实验室检查

• 尿液中砷浓度>1 000 μg/L，可确诊。

- 摄入后 10～50 h 达高峰。

• 确诊检测是收集 24 h 尿液并分析其中含砷有机物和无机物的形成。

• 由于血清中半衰期短（约 2 h），所以血液水平经常无用。

• 全血细胞计数：

- 贫血。
- 白细胞减少症。
- 嗜碱性颗粒。

• 电解质、尿素氮、肌酐和葡萄糖。

• 尿沉渣分析：寻找溶血/横纹肌溶解的证据。

• 肝功能试验。

• 总肌酸激酶（CPK）用于横纹肌溶解。

• 头发和指甲砷含量：

- 难以解释和不能立即有效。
- 可能有助于确定特定人群的慢性暴露。

影像学检查

• 腹部 X 线平片寻找不能透过 X 线的异物。

• 根据患者病情做头部 CT 或其他检查。

鉴别诊断

• 急性中毒：

- 急性阑尾炎、结肠炎和胃肠炎。
- 腹腔疾病。
- 霍乱。
- 分布性休克。
- 脑病。
- 有毒物质的摄入。
  ◦ 鹅膏菌蘑菇中毒。
  ◦ 环状抗抑郁药或其他诱发癫痫的毒素。
  ◦ 有机磷酸酯慢性毒性：

• 艾迪生病。

• 吉兰-巴雷综合征或其他神经病。

• 雷诺现象。

• 血栓闭塞性脉管炎或其他血管炎。

• 维生素缺乏症（维生素 B_3、维生素 B_6 或维生素 B_{12}）。

• Wernicke-Korsakoff 综合征。

S

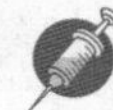

治疗

院前

> **注意**
>
> • 如果能做到尽可能的安全，将怀疑过量/中毒的容器带走。
>
> • 净化皮肤。
>
> • ABC 管理。
>
> • 心电监测。

初步稳定/治疗

• ABC 管理：

- 心电监测。
- 低血压所需的等渗液。
- 如果出现顽固性低血压使用升压药。

• 纳洛酮、硫胺素和葡萄糖（$D_{50}W$）用于精神状态改变。

• 心血管：

- 升压药，如果存在难治性低血压。
- 监测中心静脉压以防止肺/脑水肿。
- 避免使用ⅠA 类抗心律失常药。
  ◦ 加重 QT 间期延长。
- 连续监测，因为 QT 间期延长很常见。

• 神经系统：

- 用苯二氮䓬类治疗癫痫发作。
- 由于神经肌肉无力导致的呼吸功能不全，需要辅助通气。

• 肾：

- 碱化尿液治疗横纹肌溶解。

- 血液透析治疗肾衰竭。
• 饮食：
- 葡萄糖，肠内或肠胃外喂养可能有益。

■ 急诊治疗/程序

• 去除污染：
- 假如患者处在摄入后第 1 h 内，试着经口灌洗/抽吸。
- 活性炭：不结合砷。
- 如果在腹部立位片可见混浊，用聚乙二醇 1～2 L/h 全肠灌洗，直到腹部平片变清楚。
- 如果皮肤接触，将净化皮肤作为治疗的第一步。
• 确保没有其他人被污染并且环境已被评估过。
• 基于接触和症状的水平、剧烈程度，评估螯合疗法的需要：
- 向医学毒理学专家咨询建议：
- 药品：
◦ 二巯基丙醇。
◦ DMSA(二巯丁二酸)。
• 清除：
- 血液透析不常有效。
◦ 肾衰竭患者考虑用。
◦ 必须通过血液透析(HD)继续螯合。

S

■ 药物治疗

• 二巯基丙醇：3 mg/kg，24 h 内，q4 h 肌内注射；接下来 24 h 中 q6 h；然后每 12 h 一次，直到能够口服。
- 注意：如果患者有花生过敏，不能使用。
• 右旋糖 50%：25 g(50 ml)(儿童：0.5 g/kg D_{25}W)，静脉注射，用于低血糖。
• DMSA：10 mg/kg，口服，q8 h，共 5 日；然后每 12 h 一次，14 日。
• 碳酸氢钠：1 mmol/kg 静脉推注，随后将 150 mmol 溶于 1 L D_5W 中输注，150 ml/h：
- 用于治疗横纹肌溶解。
• 纳洛酮：0.4～2.0 mg(儿童：0.1 mg/kg)，静脉注射，怀疑阿片中毒可能会重复至最大剂量 10 mg。
• 硫胺素：100 mg，肌内注射或静脉注射(儿童：1 mg/kg)。
• 充足液体后的血管加压药：
- 多巴胺 5 μg/(kg · min)，增加 5～10 μg/(kg · min)(q10～30 min)最大剂量：20 μg/(kg · min)。
- 去甲肾上腺素 0.01～3 μg/(kg · min)，开始于 2 μg/min，滴定至 MAP 65～90 mmHg；最大剂量：20 μg/min。

随访

■ 进一步处理

入院指征

有症状的砷暴露应收入 ICU。

出院指征

• 尿液中砷浓度＜50 μg/L 的无症状患者可出院。
• 可疑的慢性暴露而不需要住院时，应转到门诊进行评估并收集 24 h 尿。
• 在出院前要确保患者的家庭环境是安全的。

■ 随访建议

患者故意过量的需精神病性随访。

要点和误区

• 砷中毒会导致多种体征和症状：
- 当患者出现胃肠道不适和神经系统症状时，怀疑是急性砷中毒。
- 怀疑患有神经功能缺损，非特异性消耗和角化过度的皮肤病变的患者出现慢性砷中毒。
• 请教医学毒理学专家关于螯合治疗的需要。

深静脉血栓形成 Deep Vein Thrombosis

Sarah K. Flaherty 许磊 译

基础知识

■ 描述

• 血管内凝血点和溶血点保持平衡状态，当凝血大于溶血时，血块形成。
• 血块可能是肤浅的(去筋膜)或深的，后者被称为深静脉血栓形成(DVT)。
• 肺栓塞(PE)和深静脉血栓是同一疾病的不同临床结果(深静脉血栓栓塞)。
• 深静脉血栓形成可以是上肢或者下肢，以及远端或者近端(腘静脉)。上肢 DVT 深静脉血栓占所有诊断深静脉血栓者的 4%。
• 发病率是每年 1 000 个人中有 21 个有深静脉血栓。
• 随着年龄的增长发病率也增加。
• 常见于医疗和住院手术患者。
• 诊断更准确是使用主动监测而不是临床怀疑。

儿科注意事项

深静脉血栓的儿童是不常见的，但当疾病发生时，应该寻找高凝状态的根本原因。此外，上肢深静脉血栓与中央静脉有关。

■ 病因

• 血凝块的形成、溶解是一个复杂的平衡系统，这个系统受多因素的影响，必须考虑这一点。
• Virchow 三要素：高凝状态，血流缓慢，血管内皮损伤。
• 高凝状态(通常多个伴随)：
- 癌症(特别是肺、胰腺、结肠直肠癌、肾和前列腺)。
- 骨髓增生性疾病。
- 肾病综合征。
- 脓毒症。
- 炎性疾病：
◦ 溃疡性结肠炎、克罗恩病。
- 增加雌激素：
◦ 妊娠。
◦ 外源激素(有机氯农药、HRT)。
◦ 睾丸激素补充剂。
- 抗磷脂综合征。
- 蛋白 S、C 和抗凝血酶缺乏，因子 V 莱顿突变，凝血酶原基因突变，狼疮，其他。
• 静止：
- 长期卧床。
- 不动(如演员)，或长时间坐着，比如在工作环境中。
- 长时间乘坐飞机、汽车、火车。
- 神经系统疾病，瘫痪。
- CHF。

- 肥胖。
- 血管损伤/伤害：
- 创伤。
- 手术，尤其骨科手术。
- 静脉注射吸毒。
- 透析。
- 解剖异常（May-Thurner 综合征、先天性心脏病、Paget-Schroetter 病）。
- 中心静脉导管/放置起搏器：
  - 尤其是上肢 DVT。
- 多因素的问题：
- 年龄增加。
- 合并症（糖尿病、高脂血症、高血压）。
- 其他药物（肼屈嗪、普鲁卡因胺、吩噻嗪、他克莫司、糖皮质激素、贝伐珠单抗，还有一些抗抑郁药物）。
- 烟草使用。
- DVT 或 PE 病史。
- 遗传学：
- DVT/PE 家族史是独立危险因素，应询问家族凝血史。
- VTE 遗传凝血测试。

妊娠注意事项

妊娠、包括产后 6 周，是深静脉血栓的一个危险因素。由于解剖因素，容易累及左侧，且有可能累及盆腔静脉。妊娠期治疗手段更有限。

老年人注意事项

年龄本身就是 DVT（和 PE）的危险因素。与许多疾病一样，这种症状在老年人中可能不典型。由于合并症、跌倒风险等，治疗方面的考虑更复杂。

诊断

症状和体征

- 腿肿：最常见于小腿后部。
- 腿部发热和发红。
- 腿部疼痛和压痛。
- 可触及条索状静脉，表浅静脉扩张。
- 在浅表血栓性静脉炎，可看到并触及一根。
- 手臂肿胀，发热，压痛：
- 牵涉上肢或锁骨下静脉，可以看到手或手指发绀。
- 炎症因素：
- 冷，一触即痛，肿胀，腿部发蓝（继发性动脉供血不足，静脉性坏疽）。
- 在炎症刺激下：
- 冷，一触即痛，腿部发白（继发性动脉供血不足）。

基本检查

- 患者的临床（预测）风险的确定是检查深静脉血栓形成的重要一步。Wells 评分（或改良的 Wells 评分）最常用。
- 详细的病史和体检，解释风险因子分布的情况下，是随诊的重要一步。评估作为个体的临床研究结果是一种孤立的预测。
- 考虑进一步评估潜在的损害，深静脉血栓形成可能是最初的表现。

诊断检查与说明

实验室检查

D-二聚体检测：

- D-二聚体，内源性血凝块形成的副产物，在评估深静脉血栓和肺栓塞患者中很有用。
- 仅当结果是阴性时是有用的（排除 DVT）。阳性 D-二聚体不做出诊断，它仅提示需进行更深入的检查（高度敏感性但是特异性不强的测试）。
- 低或中度怀疑的患者可以用 D-二聚体筛查，高度怀疑的患者建议优先做影像学检查。
- 测定 D-二聚体水平的方法不同（取决于测试机构）：
- 胶乳凝集（第一代测试）和微胶乳凝集（第二代）是不够的。
- 全血乳胶凝集（SimpliRED）只有在低概率患者中是有价值的（使用 Wells 标准）。
- 酶联免疫吸附试验（ELISA）给出了一个定量的结果，并已经在急诊患者中大量的临床研究中证实，特别是结合预测概率评估时。

影像学检查

- 静脉造影术：
- 以前常用的成像试验，现在很少用了，因为它是有创的，昂贵的，并且有并发症。
- 涉及注射造影剂到腿部静脉，在患者进行这种操作时，可能会导致血栓性静脉炎、造影剂反应和可能的肾损害。
- 压缩超声：
- 标准一线诊断方法。
  - 近端（股总静脉、股静脉、腘静脉）或全腿。
- 静脉研究。正常的静脉压缩，那些血块没有。
- 彩色多普勒可用于识别血供正常的静脉，但基本上不增加精度。双面扫描指的是压缩 B 超和彩色多普勒组合。
- 灵敏度达 90%以上。
- 对于高危患者，即使超声阴性，建议 48～72 h 应重复。
- 其他测试包括 CT、MRI，放射性核素造影和阻抗体积描记法，然而这些在临床实践中并不常用。
- 上肢血管病例需要完善胸部 X 线检查。

鉴别诊断

- 血栓性浅静脉炎。
- 蜂窝织炎。
- 肌肉和/或韧带撕裂（包括跖和腓肠肌撕裂）。
- 贝克破裂囊肿（双边）水肿继发于心脏、肝脏或肾脏病。
- 静脉瓣膜关闭不全。
- 药物引起的水肿（钙通道阻滞剂）。
- 腹部（单侧）包块（妊娠子宫或肿瘤）或淋巴水肿。
- Postphlebitic 综合征（从以前的血栓性静脉炎）。

S

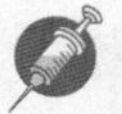

治疗

初步稳定/治疗

在股青肿、股白肿或较大凝血负担情况下：

- 建立静脉通路。
- 氧气支持。
- 应该考虑尽快外科或血管外科会诊。

急诊治疗/程序

- 全身抗凝：
- 在无禁忌证的情况下，50%未经治疗的深静脉血栓患者，将会发生肺栓塞，所以偶然发现的深静脉血栓也要治疗。
- 可以使用普通肝素或低分子量肝素（LMWH）、磺达肝癸或口服抗凝药。
- 许多患者最初可以在门诊治疗。
- 不管用完形/风险分层（如 HAS-BLED 评分），如果出血风险降低至合理的低，可接受系统的治疗。
- 华法林（维生素 K 拮抗剂）：
- 开始后不久，肝素已经可以使用。
- 不久前，因为肝素的理论风险可以诱导瞬间高凝状态。
- 直接口服抗凝剂：
- 达比加群、利伐沙班、阿哌沙班或依多沙班。
- 一般来说首选口服，除非 DVT 与癌症诊断有关，这时低分子肝素可能更有益。
- 腔静脉滤器：

- 主要适用于有全身抗凝禁忌的患者：
  ◦ 如果在充分抗凝基础上发生新的血栓栓塞事件，立即改予低分子肝素或在常规用量基础上增加低分子肝素剂量。
- 腔静脉滤器通常由血管或创伤外科医师、放射科医师放置。
- 经验性滤器置入可能在某些情况下有用。
  ◦ 持续性致病因素，如癌症、多发性损伤。
  ◦ 肺栓塞再发的风险是致命的，因为不良的心肺储备或新近发生的肺栓塞。
- 随机数据表明，过滤器的放置并不比抗凝更有效，而且可能增加继发于血管损伤的深静脉血栓风险。
- 过滤器也可安装在上腔静脉的上肢深静脉血栓处，尽管很罕见。

• 溶栓：
- 很少建议，一般仅适用于股青肿；持续给予全身抗凝药物。
- 大约增加 3 倍的出血并发症。
- 导管给药溶栓治疗多用于上肢 DVT。

S

• 取栓术（手术或经皮）：
- 有时建议用于患有全身性疾病的患者。
- 请血管外科会诊，持续给予全身抗凝药物。

• 腐蚀性血栓性静脉炎：
- 手术切除静脉或静脉抗生素。

药物治疗

• 华法林：5 mg/d 的起始剂量，第 3 日开始检查凝血酶原时间；应持续静脉输注或皮下注射治疗直至 INR 达标连续 2 日。

• 磺达肝素钠：基于体重，给予 5 mg、7.5 mg 或 10 mg 皮下注射，每日 1 次，与华法林重叠使用。

• 肝素（普通）：80 U/kg 负荷剂量之后，18 U/(kg · h) 点滴，活化部分凝血激酶时间(APTT)滴定正常的 1.5～2.5 倍。

• LWMH（依诺肝素）：门诊患者 1 mg/kg 皮下注射，每日 2 次（可选：1.5 mg/kg，皮下注射，每日 1 次）。

• 达比加群：150 mg，口服，每日 2 次，用于初次使用注射用抗凝剂的患者。

• 利伐沙班：15 mg，口服，每日 2 次，服用 21 日；然后每日 20 mg，口服。

• 阿哌沙班：10 mg，口服，每日 2 次，服用 7 日；然后 5 mg，口服，每日 2 次。

• 依多沙班：如果体重＜60 kg，30 mg，口服，每日 1 次；否则 60 mg，口服，每日 1 次；用于非口服抗凝剂治疗的患者。

• 达肝素钠：200 U/(kg · d)，皮下注射，分为 2 次/日，每剂不超过 18 000 U；与华法林重叠。

• 剂量方案是基于总体重。然而，在肥胖患者应考虑替代给药。

• 治疗通常可维持至少 3 个月，总长度是个性化的。

• 注意大多数治疗药物需要根据肾功能调整。

随访

进一步处理

入院指征

• 深静脉血栓的患者中无法接受低分子量肝素或口服药物的门诊或随访不佳的患者。

• 伴发 PE 或其他严重疾病（即肾衰竭）。

• 存在高出血风险的患者。

• 存在髂股疾病或股白肿的患者。

出院指征

• 门诊治疗：
- 无严重的需要住院治疗的合并症，血流动力学稳定，无显著的肾功能不全。
- 患者有必要的沟通手段和交通工具返回医院，以及适当的随访。
- 患者（或家属）愿意并能够注射用药如低分子肝素。

• 有着浅静脉或者远处血栓的患者也可以在出院后密切随访。

转诊问题

• 如果有任何关于动脉供血不足的问题，请咨询血管外科医师。

• 考虑对有充分抗凝禁忌证的患者进行放置下腔静脉滤器。

• 对无诱因的深静脉血栓患者应考虑行高凝血功能相关的检查。

> **注意**
>
> 当临床高度怀疑但是 B 超结果阴性时候，告知患者要找最初治疗的医师进行随诊，并且步随诊，在 1 周内做 B 超检查。

随访建议

• 对于低分子肝素：患者需要 2～3 日检查血细胞比容、血小板计数和 INR。

• 建议步行，不会引起血栓脱落。

• 不常规建议穿弹力袜。

要点和误区

• 阴性的 Homans 征不能排除 DVT 的诊断。

• 使用一些措施（临床完形或正式的评分系统，如 Wells 评分），以确定 DVT 预测概率。

• 在高预测概率患者，不要仅仅依赖 D-二聚体检测。相反，应该行静脉成像检查，一般行压缩超声检查。

• 在中等风险和高风险患者中具有 D-二聚体检查阴性或 B 超阴性，安排或推荐重复检查在 1 周内。

神经阻滞剂恶性综合征 Neuroleptic Malignant Syndrome

Lindsey M. Retterath · Sarah A. Watkins · Nicholas B. Hurst 朱妍 译

基础知识

描述

• 与抗精神病药物（多巴胺拮抗剂）或多巴胺激动剂停药相关的罕见但危及生命的疾病。

• 死亡率可高达 20%。

• 在治疗期间的任意时间内都有可能发生，从数日到数年。

• 最常见于治疗的第一个月，或剂量增加后，或胃肠外（静脉/注射）长效给药。

• 黑质纹状体通路的多巴胺阻断会导致肌强直和震颤。

• 射频消融术、谵妄和/或由于下丘脑多巴胺受体阻滞引起的自主神经失调。

• 可能无法与药物引起的高热（恶性高热、血清素综合征、抗胆碱能或拟交感神经毒性）原因区别。

• 可能会有一个起伏的过程。

• 大多数症状在停止违规用药后 3～14 日消失。

• 诊断标准：
- 与使用抗精神病药物/抗精神病药物相关的发热＋严重肌肉僵硬。
- 以下 2 个或更多：
◦ 出汗。
◦ 吞咽困难。
◦ 震颤。
◦ 尿失禁。
◦ 精神状态改变。
◦ 缄默症。
◦ 心动过速。
◦ 眼球震颤。
◦ 不稳定的高血压。
◦ 白细胞增多。
◦ 肌肉损伤的实验室依据。
- 症状不是由其他疾病引起的。

■ 病因

• 抗精神病药治疗的罕见并发症：
- 吩噻嗪类。
◦ 氯丙嗪（可乐静）。
◦ 氟奋乃静（Modecate）。
◦ 丙氯拉嗪（甲哌氯丙嗪）。
◦ 异丙嗪（非那根）。
◦ 甲氧氯普胺（胃复安）。
- 丁酰苯。
◦ 氟哌啶醇。
◦ 氟哌利多。
- 非典型抗精神病药。
◦ 利培酮（维思通）。
◦ 奥氮平（再普乐）。
◦ 喹硫平（思乐康）。
◦ 氯氮平（可治律）。
◦ 阿立哌唑（安律凡）。
• 约 1/1 000 用抗精神病药物治疗的患者发生本病。
• 也与帕金森病患者突然撤除多巴胺受体激动剂有一定关系。
• 5-羟色胺再摄取抑制剂 SSRI、TCA、卡马西平、甲氧氯普胺和锂也可能导致 NMS 沉淀；然而，很难与血清素综合征区分开来。
• 危险因素：
- 快速撤药。
- 高剂量的抗精神病药。
- 高效力的抗精神病药。
- 静脉注射/肌内注射药物。
- 负荷剂量过量。
- 脱水。
- 有神经阻滞剂恶性综合征（NMS）病史。
- 极端精神运动性亢奋。
- 感染或手术。
- 身体束缚。
- 紧张症的病史。
- 低铁水平。
- 发热。

诊断

■ 症状和体征

• 危及生命的症状。
• 疾病特点：
- 发热［温度可能高达 41 ℃（106～107 ℉）］。
- 意识程度的改变，可能从神志不清到昏迷。
- 严重的肌肉强直：铅管样强直。
- 自主神经不稳定。
◦ 心动过速。
◦ 血压不稳定。
◦ 呼吸急促。
◦ 大量出汗。
◦ 心律失常。

病史

• 使用抗精神病药。
• 停止使用抗帕金森病药物。
• 精神状态改变。

体格检查

• 发热。
• 心动过速、血压不稳定。
• 谵妄。
• 肌强直。
• 发汗。

■ 基本检查

• 准确的病史（特别是当前的药物）和体格检查用来确诊。
• 肌酸磷酸激酶（CK）、白细胞测定、肝功能试验和铁水平。

■ 诊断检查与说明

实验室检查

• 全血细胞计数并进行鉴别。
• 电解质（包括钙、镁）。
• 肌酸激酶。
• AST/ALT、乳酸脱氢酶、碱性磷酸酶。
• 其他旨在排除其他原因的检查。

影像学检查

如果意识状态改变的原因不明确需行 CT 扫描和脑电图检查。

诊断步骤/外科

通过腰椎穿刺来排除其他原因引起的发热或精神状态改变。

■ 鉴别诊断

相关疾病

• 恶性高热。
• 血清素综合征（阵挛，但无强直）。
• 抗胆碱能毒素（无强直）。
• 拟交感神经毒素。
• 锂中毒性脑病（无发热）。
• 致死性紧张症（不含抗精神病药 HX）。
• 热休克（无出汗，无僵硬）。
• 鞘内注射巴氯芬治疗的撤药。

不相关的疾病

• 中枢神经系统感染（脑膜炎、脑炎）。
• 破伤风。
• 中暑。
• 急性肌张力障碍。
• 士的宁中毒。
• 中枢神经系统脑血管事件。
• 甲状腺功能亢进症。
• 狂犬病。
• 酒精戒断。
• 癫痫发作。
• 嗜铬细胞瘤。
• 急性卟啉病。
• 急性脑积水。
• 急性脊髓损伤。
• 全身感染（如肺炎、脓毒症）。

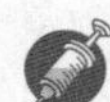

治疗

■ 院前

• 胸壁强直可能导致呼吸困难。
• 如果发作，患者需镇静并治疗癫痫。
• 监测末梢血糖。

■ 初步稳定/治疗

• 根据需要进行气道干预和循环支持。
• 静脉注射，补充氧气，心电监测。
• 静脉注射苯二氮䓬类药物（地西泮、劳拉西泮、咪达唑仑）。
- 可能需要大剂量反复使用。
• 如果症状在几分钟之内没有控制，快速诱导插管（RSI）及神经肌肉阻滞是必要的：
- 非去极化神经肌肉阻滞剂（维库溴铵、罗库溴铵、泮库溴铵）比琥珀胆碱更好。
• 控制过高热的措施：
- 冰袋。
- 喷雾和风扇。
- 冰毯。

S

- 冰水洗胃。
- 防止寒战产热的瘫痪。
- 用晶体液积极的静脉输液治疗。

■ 急诊治疗/程序

- 停止服用违规药物。
- 保持房间凉爽(21～23℃及以下)。
- 尽可能避免身体上的束缚。
- 纠正电解质/pH紊乱。
- 在一线药物治疗方面没有明确的共识。
- 为了缓解肌肉僵硬,可以使用苯二氮䓬类药物,但是可能需要使用麻醉药物。
- 溴隐亭是一种多巴胺激动剂,可在长期治疗中发挥作用。
- 丹曲林是一种直接的骨骼肌松弛剂,在NMS中的使用证据相互矛盾,它可能会引起严重的肝毒性。
- 溴隐亭和丹曲林都不能快速起效,也不能改变预后。
- 金刚烷胺具有多巴胺能和抗胆碱作用,可作为溴隐亭的替代品。
- 识别并发症(横纹肌溶解、呼吸衰竭、急性肾衰竭)。

■ 药物治疗

一线用药

- 地西泮：5 mg,静脉注射,q5 min。
- 劳拉西泮：1 mg,静脉注射,q5 min。
- 咪达唑仑：1 mg,静脉注射,q5 min。
- 罗库溴铵：600～1 200 μg/kg,静脉注射×1次,用于重复性压迫性损伤RSI。
- 泮库溴铵：60～100 μg/kg,静脉注射×1次,用于气管插管。

二线用药

- 溴隐亭：5～10 mg,口服,3～4次/日(开始2.5 mg,每日增加2.5～7.5 mg,每日最多45 mg)。
- 丹曲林：1 mg/kg,静脉注射,q4～6 h,用24～48 h,累计剂量10 mg/(kg/24 h)。
- 金刚烷胺：100 mg,口服,2次/日。

随访

■ 进一步处理

入院指征

NMS患者应进入ICU。

■ 随访建议

患者和家属在未来使用任何可能触发NMS的药物时必须被告知。

要点和误区

- 使用抗精神病药物的患者如发生精神状态变化、强直、发热或自主神经功能异常时,临床需高度怀疑NMS。
- 一定要排除其他导致发热和精神状态改变的病因(如脑膜炎、脑炎)。
- 判断NMS时用药史是必不可少的。
- 停止使用致病药物是治疗的关键。
- 积极的支持治疗是必不可少的。

S

肾病综合征 Nephrotic Syndrome

Patrick G. Meloy 朱妍 译

基础知识

■ 描述

- 疾病导致肾小球滤过屏障缺陷,产生蛋白尿：
  - 24 h内蛋白尿>3 g。
  - 低蛋白血症(血浆白蛋白<3 g/dl)。
  - 低蛋白血症引起外周水肿。
  - 低丙球蛋白血症。
  - 高血脂(空腹胆固醇>200 mg/dl)。
- 尿液中的脂肪(椭圆的脂肪滴、脂肪/蜡样管型)。
- 肾小球基底膜的改变通过：
  - 免疫复合物。
  - 肾毒性抗体。
  - 非免疫机制。
  - 结果：肾小球基底膜渗透性增加,白蛋白和大分子蛋白的排泄增多。

■ 病理生理

- 肾小球滤过率增加产生蛋白尿。
- 钠潴留和低蛋白血症引发水肿。
- 严重的低蛋白血症引发体位性低血压、晕厥和休克。
- 血浆胶体渗透压降低刺激肝脏脂蛋白的合成,引发高脂血症。
- 累积血栓栓塞的风险增加,如果：
  - 低血容量。
  - 低血清白蛋白。
  - 高蛋白质排泄。
  - 高纤维蛋白原水平。
  - 低抗凝血酶Ⅲ水平。

■ 病因

- 由于原发性肾脏或全身性疾病。
- 膜性肾病：
  - 引发成人肾病综合征的主要病因。
  - 其他病因包括慢性感染(乙型肝炎病毒、丙型肝炎病毒、自身免疫性疾病)。
  - 肾活检显示所有肾小球均累及。
  - 女性预后较好。
  - 30%的患者可能会缓慢进展至肾衰竭。
  - 肾静脉血栓导致肾功能突然丧失。
  - 在重症患者使用类固醇和细胞毒性药物治疗。
- 微小病变：
  - 儿童肾病综合征最常见的病因(90%)。
  - 其他病因：特发性、NSAIDs、恶性肿瘤相关的副癌综合征(常见于霍奇金淋巴瘤)。
  - 所有的肾病综合征中预后最佳的类型。
  - 类固醇激素治疗疗效好。
- 局灶性节段性肾小球硬化(FSGS)：
  - 年轻的肾病综合征患者(15～30岁)。
  - 表现为高血压、肾功能不全、蛋白尿、镜下或肉眼血尿。
  - 病因包括HIV感染、海洛因滥用、肥胖、血液系统恶性肿瘤。
  - 原发性FSGS激素治疗有效。
  - 继发性FSGS使用ACEI。
  - 塌陷型FSGS常见于AIDS患者。
- 膜增生性肾小球肾炎：
  - 可能表现为肾病、非肾病或肾脏沉积物。
  - 补体水平持续偏低。
  - 支持治疗：类固醇可能对儿童有疗效。
  - 阿司匹林和双嘧达莫可能减缓病程进展。
- 糖尿病/糖尿病肾病：
  - 成人肾病蛋白尿第二常见的病因。
  - 微量白蛋白尿(30～300 mg/24 h)为肾脏病变的主要指标。

- 5～7年后肾功能恶化。
- 不会引起肾功能快速下降。
- 严格控制血糖和ACEI治疗可减缓病程进展。
• 单克隆丙种球蛋白病：
- 包括淀粉样变、多发性骨髓瘤和轻链肾病。
- 肾脏表现包括蛋白尿、肾病综合征、肾炎综合征和急性肾衰竭。
- 实验室的研究结果包括假低钠血症、低阴离子间隙、高钙血症，以及本周蛋白尿。
- 淀粉样蛋白的刚果红染色在偏振光下呈现苹果绿双折射光。
- 支持治疗：类固醇激素和马法兰有一定疗效。
• 系统性红斑狼疮(SLE)：
- 最初表现为肾炎过程，可发展为肾病综合征。
• HIV相关性肾病：
- FSGS是最常见的肾病类型。
- 塌陷型肾小球疾病在血清反应阳性的HIV病毒携带者伴有超级肾病综合征，导致快速进展至终末期肾衰竭(数月)。
• 其他病因包括先兆子痫、肝炎和药物反应(包括NSAIDs、金盐、青霉胺)。

诊断

症状和体征

• 许多患者无症状。
• 蛋白尿。
• 外周性水肿：
- 轻度凹陷性水肿至全身性水肿伴腹水。
• 高脂血症。
• 脂肪尿(尿脂肪管型和椭圆形脂肪滴)。
• 体位性低血压、晕厥、休克。
• 高血压。
• 血尿：
- 显微镜或肉眼血尿(继发于肾静脉血栓形成)。
• 部分病例肾功能不全转为急性肾衰竭。
• 呼吸急促，心动过速，伴/不伴低血压：
- 急性起病：提示肺栓塞(PE)，继发于肾或深静脉的血栓形成和高凝状态。
- 膜性肾小球肾炎最多30%的肺栓塞发生率。
- 慢性或劳力性呼吸急促是由于：
◦ 肺水肿。
◦ 胸腔积液。
◦ 由于免疫抑制治疗和频繁接触感染源(如肺炎球菌)引发的感染风险。
◦ 腹水。
• 蛋白质营养不良。

病史

• 全身性疾病如糖尿病、系统性红斑狼疮、HIV感染。
• 使用NSAIDs、金盐或青霉胺。
• 不明原因的体重增加史(由于液体潴留)。
• 尿液中出现"泡沫"的病史。

体格检查

不同的表现取决于低蛋白血症的程度，血流动力学状态和肾病综合征的病因：
• 水肿。
• 低血压、高血压。
• 休克。

基本检查

尿液分析：
• 试纸蛋白大部分是阳性的：
- 尿比重>1.025降低蛋白尿的诊断意义。
• 显微分析尿管型和细胞成分的存在：
- 椭圆形脂肪滴。
- 游离的脂肪滴。

诊断检查与说明

实验室检查

• 血常规+鉴别：
- 贫血常见。
- 白细胞增多：感染。
- 白细胞减少症：肿瘤性疾病或脓毒症。
- 血小板减少症：肝脏疾病。
• PT、APTT、INR：
- 凝血状况异常并发于肝脏疾病。
• D-二聚体、纤维蛋白原、抗凝血酶Ⅲ：
- 可疑血栓栓塞事件：
◦ 通常患者发生PE或肾静脉血栓形成时无症状，因此需要临床高度警惕。
• 24 h尿蛋白，总蛋白/肌酐。
• 血清白蛋白：<3 g/dl。
• 血清总蛋白。
• 基础代谢与钙、镁、磷。
• 血脂：升高的总胆固醇、LDL和VLDL。
• 其余的实验室检查可能对诊断系统疾病是必要的：
- 包括抗核抗体、血清和尿蛋白电泳、肝炎、梅毒、冷凝蛋白、补体水平。

影像学检查

肾脏超声：用于疑似继发性肾病综合征。

诊断步骤/外科

• 肾脏活检：
- 用于短疗程糖皮质激素治疗无反应的患者的明确诊断。
- 帮助识别原发或继发的病理类型。
• 怀疑肾静脉血栓形成行肾血管造影、CT扫描或MRI。

鉴别诊断

蛋白尿形成的其他病因：
• 肾实质病变：
- 慢性肾脏疾病。
- 机械性肾病(出口梗阻、反流)。
- 急性肾盂肾炎。
- 镰状细胞病。
• 其他原因：
- 心力衰竭。
- 原发性高血压。
- 急性发热性疾病。
- 妊娠(先兆子痫)。
- 重度肥胖。

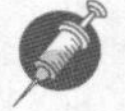

治疗

院前

提供基础支持治疗。

初步稳定/治疗

基础支持治疗：
• 如果呼吸窘迫则予以吸氧。
• 静脉输液：
- 由于血容量减少引起血压下降或体位性低血压。
- 在存在严重低血压，休克时积极液体复苏。

急诊治疗/程序

• 控制水肿：
- 限制钠盐摄入：2 g/d氯化钠。
- 襻利尿剂(呋塞米)：剂量滴定，直至见效。
- 噻嗪类利尿剂和保钾利尿剂。
- 目标：缓慢利尿。
◦ 强化利尿可引起血容量减少，从而诱发急性肾衰竭并增加血栓栓塞风险。
• 血栓栓塞的预防与治疗：
- 肝素：血栓栓塞情况下，80 IU/kg静脉推注，继而18 IU/kg静脉滴注。
- 现在认为当严低蛋白血症时候(<2.5 g/dl)，预防性抗凝可以接受的：目标INR 1.8～2。
- 建议低剂量阿司匹林81 mg。
- 提供弹力袜。

S

• 重症病例血浆置换。

• 糖皮质激素：治疗原发性肾病综合征的主要药物。

• ACEI/ARB：降低蛋白尿，防止肾功能恶化：

- ACEI 的副作用包括肾衰竭和高钾血症。

• 降胆固醇药物/膳食控制（如胆汁酸树脂、他汀类）。

• 在专家指导下可以考虑其他手段：

- 细胞毒剂、环孢素。

- 重组红细胞生成素治疗贫血。

药物治疗

• 依诺肝素（低分子肝素）：30～40 mg（儿童：0.5～0.75 mg/kg），皮下注射，q12 h。

• 呋塞米：20～80 mg（儿童：1～6 mg/kg），口服，每日 1 次或 2 次。

• 肝素：80 IU/kg 静推，继而 18 IU/(kg · h)，静脉滴注。

• 赖诺普利（ACEI）：10～40 mg（>6 岁儿童：0.07 mg/kg），口服，每日 1 次。

• 氯沙坦（ARB）：25～100 mg（>6 岁儿童：0.7 mg/kg），口服，每日 1 次。

• 美托拉宗：5～20 mg（儿童：0.2～0.4 mg/kg），口服，每日 1 次。

• 泼尼松：5～60 mg（儿童：0.5～2 mg/kg），口服，每日 1 次。

随访

进一步处理

入院指征

• 中度至重度心力衰竭、腹水、呼吸窘迫。

• 合并症的迹象，如未确诊恶性肿瘤、控制不佳的糖尿病、免疫功能低下患者。

• 急性肾衰竭。

• 栓塞事件的证据。

出院指征

• 无合并症，生命体征正常，血液循环正常。

• 肾内科密切随访，强制性进一步检查和治疗。

转诊问题

肾内科：

• 常规随访血压和疾病治疗。

• 为合适的患者进行肾活检。

随访建议

• 除了肾脏病，患者应随访风湿病、感染性疾病、血液/肿瘤或内分泌专科（取决于引起肾病综合征的基础疾病）。

• 严格控制血压，在长期的疾病治疗中为获得最佳的预后应注意保持低胆固醇饮食。

要点和误区

• 以蛋白尿、低蛋白血症和外周水肿为特征。

• 在儿童患者和成人糖尿病肾病患者最常见的病因是微小病变。

• 可能沿着从高血压到严重低血压甚至休克的疾病谱出现，所以在适当的情况下应保持高度警惕。

• 考虑血栓栓塞性疾病的相关风险。

S

肾结石 Renal Calculus

Ryan A. Stroder · Connor A. Cohick　何融冰 译

基础知识

描述

• 尿路梗阻。

• 肾盂近端输尿管间歇性扩张产生疼痛。

• 肾脏结石：

- 肾绞痛的最常见原因。

- 结石成分：

◦ 80%：碳酸钙结石（草酸钙>磷酸钙）。

◦ 尿酸。

◦ 其他：磷酸镁胺（玻璃状结晶）、胱氨酸。

- 磷酸铵镁：与尿素分解机制（如假单胞菌属、变形杆菌属、克雷伯菌属）及碱性尿液引起的感染有关。

- 90%的尿结石是不透射线的。

病因

• 在一般人群中有 6%～12%的终身危险。

• 男性发病率是女性的 2 倍。

• 男：女为(1.3～1.6)：1。

• 发病峰值在 40～60 岁。

• 有关结石形成的理论：

- 尿中溶质过饱和继发结晶沉淀。

- 正常尿液中抑制结晶形成蛋白的减少。

- 生理异常、放置导尿管、神经源性膀胱或异物的出现导致的尿停滞。

• 1 年复发率为 15%，5 年复发率为 40%，10 年复发率为 50%，20 年复发率为 75%。

• 与慢性肾脏疾病、高血压、2 型糖尿病、代谢综合征、痛风、胃旁路手术、短肠综合征、频繁尿路炎和冠状动脉疾病危险性增加有关。

儿童注意事项

• 儿童很少见。

• 如果出现，经常是代谢或遗传疾病的指征。

• 60%出现胁腹部部或腹部疼痛，超过 30%仅出现血尿。

• 所有肾结石病例中<16 岁的儿科患者占约 7%。

• 1：1 性别比例。

• 结石形成的原因：

- 代谢异常（50%）。

- 泌尿系统畸形（20%）。

- 感染（15%）。

- 制动综合征（5%）。

诊断

症状和体征

病史

• 突然发作的肋脊角、胁部和/或侧腹部重度疼痛。

• 继发于输尿管和肾包膜扩张的绞痛或持续痛：

- 患者无法找到舒适体位。

- 持续 20～60 min。

• 肉眼/镜下血尿。

- 治疗早期更常见（95%第 1 日 *vs*. 68%第 3～4 日）。

- 1/3 的患者有肉眼血尿。

• 恶心、呕吐。

• 出汗。

• 睾丸和阴囊疼痛。

• 尿频，尿急，一旦输尿管远端出现结石便排尿困难。

• 既往结石形成史。

体格检查

• 生命体征：

- 发热提示潜在感染。
- 低血压伴随精神状态改变提示脓毒症。

• 腹部检查。

- 触诊有压痛、反跳痛或肌紧张，提示更严重的腹内病变。
- 触诊腹主动脉有压痛或搏动范围扩大，提示动脉瘤。

• 泌尿生殖器检查：

- 检查生殖器查找有无疝气、附睾炎、扭转或睾丸肿块。

基本检查

• 尿液分析。

- 表现为显微镜下血尿＞80%。
- 肉眼血尿。
- 10%～30%无血尿。
- 白细胞/细菌提示感染。
- 血尿量和尿路梗阻程度无相关性。

诊断检查与说明

实验室检查

• 全血细胞计数：

- 白细胞＞15 000 提示合并感染。

• 尿培养。

• 电解质、葡萄糖、BUN、肌酐。

• 可疑时可行妊娠试验。

影像学检查

• CT：

- 螺旋 CT 已经代替了经静脉肾盂造影(IVP)成为检查选择。
- 可以发现直径为 1 mm 的结石。
- 直接可见并发症，如输尿管积水、肾积水、输尿管水肿，肾周脂肪绞合。
- 优点：
  ◦ 完成迅速。
  ◦ 无需静脉注射造影剂。
  ◦ 可发现其他导致症状的非泌尿系统因素，如腹主动脉瘤(AAA)。
- 缺点：
  ◦ 不能评估流量和肾功能。
- 非增强螺旋 CT 在肾绞痛的评估中：
  ◦ 敏感性 97%。
  ◦ 特异性 95%。
  ◦ 准确性 97%。
- 增强螺旋 CT 对＞3 mm 结石的敏感性为 95%。当结石小于 3 mm 时，敏感性降低。
- 适应证：
  ◦ 初次诊断。
  ◦ 持续痛。
  ◦ 与肾盂肾炎分辨不清时。

• 超声：

- 二线选择。
- 用于发现大结石和肾积水。
- 仅提供解剖学信息。
- 用于诊断梗阻和定位输尿管近端和远端结石。
- 能发现肾积水：
  ◦ 敏感性：85%～94%。
  ◦ 特异性：100%。
- 局限：
  ◦ 可能无法发现＜5 mm 的结石。
  ◦ 定位结石的灵敏度 54%～57%。
  ◦ 可能看不到肾绞痛早期梗阻。
  ◦ 延迟至出现肾盂肾盏扩张甚至完全阻塞后。

• IVP：

- 95%可明确诊断。
- 显示阻塞的严重程度。
- 示踪片可提前定位可能被染料遮蔽的结石。
- 排泄后片。
- 对鉴别肾盂积水、输尿管囊泡连接处结石或膀胱充盈的输尿管远端结石十分有用。

• 肾脏、输尿管、膀胱(KUB)X 线片：

- 适用于当对 IVP 染料过敏及无法使用肾脏扫描和超声时。
- 区分以碳酸钙为主的结石(不透光)与非碳酸钙结石。
- 协助定位不透光结石并排除非妊娠者的其他疾病。
- 识别不透光体很困难：
  ◦ 静脉石。
  ◦ 肠内容物。
  ◦ 在 KUB 上的泌尿道梗阻。
  ◦ 斜位片有助于定位可疑钙化。

妊娠注意事项

• 尽量减少对胎儿的电离辐射暴露。

• 超声是可选影像模式。

- 如果超声阳性，可以用 MRI 检测出钆。

诊断步骤/外科

输尿管镜检查术、冲击波碎石术、经皮肾石切开术。

鉴别诊断

• 夹层或破裂的腹主动脉瘤。

• 肾盂肾炎。

• 肾乳头坏死(镰刀形红细胞病、NSAID 类止痛剂滥用、糖尿病或感染)。

• 肾梗死(血管夹层或动脉栓子)。

• 异位妊娠。

• 卵巢囊肿/扭转。

• 阑尾炎。

• 肠梗阻。

• 憩室炎。

• 胆囊炎/胆绞痛。

• 胆道疾病。

• 肌肉骨骼劳累。

• 下叶肺炎。

• 诈病或麻醉药品依赖(排除诊断)。

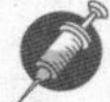

治疗

院前

长时间转运时的疼痛控制可能需要非口服剂型的阿片类药物。

初步稳定/治疗

• 血尿快速试纸检测。

• 阳性测试结果结合临床表现，足以开始止痛治疗。

• 临床表现和实验室结果做出疑似诊断时，可进行适当镇痛。

急诊治疗/程序

• 液体：

- 起始静脉晶体注入，1 L 生理盐水 30～60 min 注入，继以 500 ml 剂量 200～500 ml/h 快速注射给容量受损患者，直至排尿量适当。

• 镇痛药(吗啡、酮咯酸)。

- 联合静脉注射非甾类和阿片类镇痛药降低急诊等待，而且比两者单用效果更佳。

• 止吐药(丙氯拉嗪、昂丹司琼、氟哌利多、羟嗪)。

• 磷酸二酯酶 5 型抑制剂。

• α受体阻滞剂(坦索罗辛)、(西洛多辛)、钙通道阻滞剂(硝苯地平)、磷酸二酯酶 5 型抑制剂(他达拉非)可减少自发排石的时间：

- 对于直径＜5 mm 的结石更有效。
- 有限的数据显示，硅氧烷、坦索罗辛和硝苯地平的结石通径率分别为 83%、64%和 67%。
- 出院时开处方。

妊娠注意事项

妊娠期间避免非甾类药物，尤其是妊娠 3 个月内。

药物治疗

• 氢吗啡酮(盐酸氢吗啡酮)：1～4 mg(儿

童：0.015 mg/kg)，肌内注射、静脉注射或皮下注射，q4～6 h，必要时使用。首次使用阿片类的患者要减少剂量。

• 盐酸羟嗪（羟嗪口服剂）：25～50 mg（儿童：0.5～1 mg/kg），肌内注射（不能静脉注射），q4～6 h。

• 酮咯酸（酮咯酸注射剂）：30～60 mg，肌内注射；或 30 mg［儿童：0.5 mg/kg/剂量至 1 mg/(kg·24～48 h)］，静脉注射（单独或合并阿片类）；如果＞65 岁或＜50 kg 减少剂量至 30 mg（肌内注射）或 15 mg（静脉注射）。

• 硫酸吗啡：2～10 mg（儿童：0.1～0.2 mg/kg，q2～4 h），肌内注射、静脉注射或皮下注射，q2～6 h，必要时使用。如需可更频繁调整剂量。

• 硝苯地平：30 mg，口服，每日 1 次。

• 昂丹司琼（枢复宁）：4 mg（儿童：0.1 mg/kg），肌内注射或静脉注射，不能超过 8 mg 剂量静脉注射。

• 丙氯拉嗪（甲哌氯丙嗪）：5～10 mg，肌内注射或静脉注射 q4～6 h；25 mg 栓剂灌肠。

• 异丙嗪（非那根）：12.5～25 mg（儿童：0.25～1 mg/kg 不超过 25 mg），肌内注射、静脉注射；或灌肠，q4～6 h。

• 坦索罗辛（Flomax）0.4 mg，口服，每日 1 次，持续 4 周。

• 西洛多辛：8 mg，口服，每日 1 次，持续 4 周。

• 他达拉非：10 mg，口服，每日 1 次，持续 4 周。

随访

进一步处理

入院指征

• 梗阻存在感染需要直接泌尿外科干预。
• 顽固性疼痛伴反复恶心、呕吐。
• 严重容量不足。
• 无尿。
• 尿外渗。
• 顽固性恶心或呕吐。
• 高血钙危象。
• 孤立肾合并完全梗阻。
• 相对入院指征（与泌尿外科医师协商）：
- 高度梗阻。
- 原有肾脏疾病。
- 结石＜5 mm 通常可自发排出；＞10 mm 的很少。

出院指征

• 生命体征正常。
• 无合并尿道感染证据。
• 适当镇痛。
• 能耐受术后液体量，维持液体情况。
• 患者依从性好和舒适家庭环境。
• 已安排适当的出院随访。
• 肾脏功能正常。
• 提供收集结石的尿滤过器，将来可能做结石分析。
• 安排泌尿外科随访。

转诊问题

如果在急诊室持续疼痛诊断不明确应做影像学检查。

随访建议

所有患者应进行泌尿科随访，尤其是：
• 肾结石 1 期。
• 大结石＞5 mm。
• 患者保守治疗 4 周后未能排石。

要点和误区

• 不要遗漏类似肾绞痛的血管严重病变。
• 积极控制疼痛及补液可促进结石排出。
• 无血尿不能排除急性肾绞痛的诊断。

肾上腺功能减退症

Terry Singhapricha · Todd A. Taylor 马林浩 译

基础知识

描述

• 不足的糖皮质激素（皮质醇）和/或盐皮质激素（醛固酮）分泌无法满足身体的应激需求。

• 与受损的糖皮质激素和盐皮质激素产生相关的原发性肾上腺功能不全。

• 与仅患有糖皮质激素缺乏的继发性/三级肾上腺功能不全。

• 肾上腺功能不全：
- 皮质醇/醛固酮不足。
- 对促肾上腺皮质激素释放激素（ACTH）刺激无反应。

• 肾上腺危象（Addison 危象）。
- 威胁生命的紧急情况。
- 由以下因素引发：
  ◦ 应激下的类固醇依赖患者（妊娠、手术、创伤、感染或脱水）。
  ◦ 快速停用类固醇。
  ◦ 急性肾上腺出血。
  ◦ 最近垂体/颅垂体瘤切除。
  ◦ 先天性肾上腺增生。
  ◦ 产后垂体腺坏死（希恩综合征）。

病因

原发性肾上腺功能不全：肾上腺功能障碍

• 肾上腺发育不全/类固醇合成受损：
- 先天性发育不全。
- Allgrove 综合征：
  ◦ ACTH 抵抗。
  ◦ 气管食管括约肌失弛缓。
  ◦ 无泪。
- 甘油激酶缺乏症：
  ◦ 精神运动迟缓。
  ◦ 性腺功能减退。
  ◦ 肌肉营养不良。
• 先天性肾上腺增生症：
- 21-羟化酶缺乏占 95%。
• 醛固酮合成酶缺乏。
• 线粒体疾病。
• 肾上腺功能受损。
- 自身免疫：
  ◦ 自身免疫多腺体综合征类型 1 和 2（全脱发、慢性黏膜真菌感染、甲状旁腺功能减退、甲状腺自身免疫、糖尿病、乳糜泻、恶性贫血）。
  ◦ 肾上腺白质脂代谢障碍。
- 感染性：
  ◦ 肉芽肿性：结核病。
  ◦ 原虫和真菌性：组织胞浆菌病、角孢子菌病和念珠菌病。
  ◦ 病毒性：巨细胞病毒、单纯疱疹病毒和人类免疫缺陷病毒。

◦ 细菌性。
◦ 真菌性。
- 转移性肿瘤。
- 浸润：
◦ 结节病。
◦ 血色素沉着病。
◦ 淀粉样变性。
◦ 铁耗竭。
• 双侧肾上腺切除术。
• 出血：
- 脓毒症：尤其是脑膜炎球菌感染(Waterhouse-Friderichsen 综合征)，假单胞菌感染。
- 出生创伤/缺氧。
- 妊娠。
- 癫痫发作。
- 抗凝药物。
- 横纹肌溶解。
• 药物抑制：
- 依托咪酯。
- 苯巴比妥。
- 酮康唑/氟康唑。
- 苯妥英钠。
- 利福平。

继发性肾上腺功能不全：垂体功能障碍(皮质激素分泌素缺乏)

• 垂体功能不全。
• 脓毒症。
• 头部创伤。
• 出血。
• 梗塞(希恩综合征)。
• 浸润：肿瘤、淀粉样变、结节病和血色素沉着症。
• 普拉德-威利综合征。

第三类肾上腺功能不全：下丘脑功能障碍(皮质激素释放激素缺乏)

• 药物抑制：
- 糖皮质激素治疗。
- 米非司酮。
- 氯丙嗪。
- 丙咪嗪。
• 脓毒症。
• 浸润性：肿瘤、淀粉样变、结节病和血色素沉着症。
• 头部创伤(颅底骨折最常见)。

诊断

▪ 症状和体征

• 症状：
- 抑郁。
- 体弱、疲劳。
- 厌食。
- 腹痛(可出现急性腹痛)。
- 恶心或呕吐。
- 渴盐(仅限于原发性肾上腺皮质功能不全)。
- 体位性头晕。
- 肌肉或关节疼痛。
- 脱水(仅见于原发性肾上腺皮质功能不全)。
- 皮肤干燥或瘙痒(女性)。
- 性欲丧失(女性)。
• 体征：
- 发热或低体温。
- 精神状态改变。
- 低血压(收缩压＜110 mmHg)。
- 心动过速。
- 直立位血压变化或明显休克。
- 体重减轻。
- 甲状腺肿。
- 性腺发育不全。
- 高钾血症(原发性)。
- 高钙血症(原发性)。
- 钠丢失。
- 氮质血症。
- 嗜酸性粒细胞增多。
- 皮肤色素沉着增多(仅限原发性)。
- 白癜风。
• Addison 危象(肾上腺危象)：
- 低血压和休克。
- 低钠血症。
- 高钾血症。
- 低血糖。

▪ 基本检查

• 实验室确认诊断可能无法在急诊室内进行。
• 肾上腺危象：威胁生命的疾病。
- 高度怀疑时应在明确诊断之前立即开始治疗。
• 血浆皮质醇水平。
• 甲状腺水平。
• 血液生化检测。
• 带分类的全血细胞计数。
• 核心体温。

▪ 诊断检查与说明

实验室检查

• 带分类的全血细胞计数：
- 贫血。
- 嗜酸细胞增多。
- 淋巴细胞增多。
• 动脉血气/生化检测：
- 低氧血症。
- 酸中毒。
- 高钾血症(仅原发性肾上腺功能不全)。
- 低钠血症。
- 肌酐升高(仅原发性)。
- 葡萄糖下降。
- 高钙血症(仅原发性)。
• 危重患者的皮质醇水平：
- 基础晨间皮质醇小于 3 μg/dl 诊断肾上腺功能不全，但在急诊科不切实际。
- 用于诊疗危重症患者诊断急性肾上腺功能不全的共识：
◦ 随机血清皮质醇＜10 μg/dl(在生理应激情况下)。
◦ 卡曲诺肽(250 μg)注射后 60 min 内皮质醇减少＜9 μg/dl。
• 卡曲诺肽刺激试验如果 60 min 内皮质醇水平＜10 μg/dl 也提示存在问题。
• 寻找潜在的感染。

影像学检查

X 线片：
• 寻找感染或肺水肿。

诊断步骤/外科

心电图：
• 评估电解质紊乱的迹象。

▪ 鉴别诊断

• 脓毒症。
• 休克。
• 低血糖。
• 低体温。
• 急性腹部疾病。

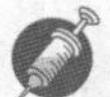

治疗

▪ 初始稳定/治疗

• ABC 管理。
• 心脏监护。
- 低血压支持：生理盐水静脉注射 500～1 000 ml(儿童：20 ml/kg)快速输注。
• 吸氧以满足代谢需求。
• 纠正发热/或低体温。

▪ 急诊治疗/程序

• 糖皮质激素/盐皮质激素替代：
- 立即静脉注射氢化可的松或地塞米松。
- 如果没有静脉通路，使用肌内注射途径。

S

- 地塞米松不会干扰卡曲诺肽刺激试验的结果。
- 氢化可的松剂量＞50 mg 提供足够的盐皮质激素覆盖，地塞米松不具备这一功能。
- 孤立性盐皮质激素缺乏可口服氟氢可的松。

• 扩容。
- 生理盐水或右旋糖酐生理盐水以每小时500～1 000 ml 的速度补充 3～4 h。
- 扩容补液过程中应注意患者的年龄、容积，以及心功能和肾功能。

• 低血糖时：
- 50%葡萄糖注射液。

• 用钙、碳酸氢盐和胰岛素/葡萄糖治疗继发于高钾血症导致的危及生命的心律失常。

• 识别和纠正潜在诱因。

• 治疗后应在 4～6 h 看到血压改善。

药物治疗

• 地塞米松：6～10 mg(儿童：每次剂量 0.15 mg/kg)，q12 h。

• 氢化可的松：50～100 mg(儿童：1～2 mg/kg)静脉注射，q6 h，剂量＞50 mg 足够治疗盐皮质激素缺乏。

• 孤立性盐皮质激素缺乏患者只能口服氟氢可的松(50～100 mg)。

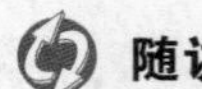

随访

进一步处理

入院指征

• 所有肾上腺功能不全患者。

• 对于不稳定或潜在不稳定患者，入院应收入 ICU。

出院指征

• 肾上腺功能不全经治疗后实验室检测结果正常。

• 对于慢性肾上腺功能不全患者，出院前应咨询内分泌科医师。

随访建议

• 根据症状，应在几周内进行门诊随访。

• 可能从内分泌科转诊中受益。

要点和误区

• 急性肾上腺功能不全是一种危及生命的急症，在急诊室的治疗不应该因为等待确切的实验室诊断而被延迟。

• 原发性肾上腺功能不全患者缺乏糖皮质激素和盐皮质激素。

• 继发性和第三类肾上腺功能不全患者只缺乏糖皮质激素。

• 早晨皮质醇水平检测在急诊室不太实用，但对于一个处于生理应激状态下的患者，随机皮质醇检测水平＜18 μg/dl 可提示存在肾上腺功能不全。

• 卡曲诺肽给药后 1 小时皮质醇增加＜9 μg/dl 或卡曲诺肽给药后 1 h 皮质醇水平＜18 μg/dl 也可提示存在肾上腺皮质功能不全。

• 氢化可的松剂量＞50 mg 能够提供充分的盐皮质激素覆盖。

• 地塞米松可以用于治疗糖皮质激素缺乏，并且不会影响卡曲诺肽刺激试验。地塞米松的盐皮质激素替代作用很小。

• 基础使用类固醇的患者在危重症情况下可能需要增加剂量。

• 感染性休克时使用皮质类固醇是有争议的，但仍然建议在对血管活性药物耐药或长期使用类固醇患者中使用。

• 单剂量依托咪酯用于快速序贯插管的临床后果存在争议。研究显示了药物的肾上腺生化抑制作用，这使得在执行关键的、拯救生命的措施时与其他不良反应的药物必须进行权衡。

肾损伤 Renal Injury

Albert S. Jin　袁晓伟　童朝阳 译

基础知识

描述

• 肾脏位于腹膜后间隙，被脂肪组织和疏松结缔组织包围。
- 由下肋骨、背部肌肉及会阴部脂肪保护。

• 肾脏正对下位 2 个胸椎和第 1～4 腰椎。

• 左肾的位置比右肾稍高。

• 肾脏不是固定的：
- 随着横膈移动，被肾动脉、静脉和肾(Gerota)筋膜的脂肪组织支撑。

病因

• 在泌尿外科损伤中最常见。

• 在所有腹部外伤中发生率为 8%～10%。

• 肾钝挫伤占所有肾损伤的 80%～85%，且其发生率是穿透伤的 5 倍。
- 机制：包括机动车事故、坠落、家庭暴力和运动冲撞。
- 病理生理学：包括快速减速和移位机制。
- 约 20%的病例与腹膜内损伤有关。

• 导致严重肾损伤的机制不仅仅影响到肾脏：
- 经常影响并损伤其他可以导致患者死亡的重要器官。

• 肾损伤通过损伤类型和严重程度分级[外伤手术协会(AAST)标准]。
- Ⅰ级：
  ◦ 挫伤：显微镜下或肉眼血尿，泌尿外科检查正常。
  ◦ 血肿：被膜下不扩张且无实质撕裂伤。
- Ⅱ级：
  ◦ 血肿：不扩张，肾周血肿被限制在腹膜后腔。
  ◦ 撕裂伤：在肾皮质中深度＜1 cm 不伴有尿外渗。
- Ⅲ级：
  ◦ 撕裂伤：在肾皮质中深度＞1 cm 不伴有肾集合系统破裂或尿外渗。
- Ⅳ级：
  ◦ 撕裂伤：肾实质撕裂伤穿过肾皮质，髓质和集合系统。
  ◦ 血管：主要肾动脉或静脉损伤包括出血。
- Ⅴ级：
  ◦ 撕裂伤：肾完全破裂。
  ◦ 血管：肾门撕裂、肾血供中断。

儿科注意事项

• 肾脏是最容易被腹部钝器伤波及的器官。
- 自行车事故是损伤的重要机制之一。

• 促成因素：
- 跟成人相比，肾的体积相对较大。
- 直到 20 余岁第 10 肋和第 11 肋才能完全骨化。

• 严重腹部损伤在非偶然性创伤中发生率为 5%，但是仅次于头部损伤的第二大死亡原因。

• 儿童可能不像成人那样经常表现出低血压伴有肾损伤。

诊断

症状和体征

病史

• 损伤机制和运动学是重要因素。
• 大多数肾损伤合并其他腹部器官损伤。
• 钝器伤中注意任何减速或压力的类型和方向(水平或竖直)。
• 穿刺伤须注意锐器的特点(类型和口径)、武器距离、刀或锐器的类型及长度:
- 伤口是由锐器的动能和剪切力联合造成的。

体格检查

• 血尿是泌尿系统创伤的最佳指征:
- 血尿程度与肾损伤的严重程度不相关。
- 无血尿不能排除肾损伤。
• 显微镜下血尿伴随收缩压＜90 mmHg。
• 胁部肿块或瘀斑。
• 胁部、腹部或背部压痛。
• 下端肋骨或脊柱横突骨折。
• 恶心和呕吐。

基本检查

• 1989 年 Mee 等人发表了标志性文章(10 年的前瞻性研究)建立了肾脏钝器伤的评估与治疗指南。
- 严重肾脏撕裂伤相当于显著的可修复的肾损伤。
- 成年患者出现以下症状时可能存在严重撕裂伤:
◦ 肉眼血尿。
◦ 显微镜下血尿(＞3～5 个红细胞/HPF),当场或抵达急诊室后出现休克(收缩压＜90 mmHg)。
◦ 不伴有血尿或休克的突发撕裂伤病史。
• 静脉造影增强 CT 是明确泌尿系统损伤的程序。
• 上述指南不适用于儿童或肾脏穿透伤。
• 有肾脏钝器伤和血尿,或合并显微镜下血尿及休克的成年患者,需要进行肾脏影像学检查,进一步评估肾损伤。
• 对于有肾脏穿透伤的成年患者来说,明显肾及输尿管损伤可以不出现血尿:
- 穿刺伤位置与泌尿道的关系是决定是否需 X 线摄片的最重要因素。
- 穿刺伤伴有任何程度的血尿均需影像学检查。
- 排除合并伤很重要。

诊断检查与说明

实验室检查

• 尿液分析:肉眼血尿或成年人和儿童＞50 个红细胞/HPF,提示肾损伤。
• 基础实验室检查应该包括血细胞比容、BUN/肌酸。

影像学检查

• 腹部 X 线检查:
- 可以显示下部肋骨或横突骨折,单侧肾影增大或腰大肌模糊。
• 静脉肾盂造影(IVP):
- 24 h 内无法应用 CT 时可选择 IVP 及肾断层造影检查。
- 快速注入 1.5～2 ml/kg 造影剂至最大量 150 ml 或直至获得初始的肾脏、输尿管和膀胱影像。
- 注射造影剂后患者取仰卧位摄片,接着进行 1、2、3 min 仰卧位摄片。
◦ 能够对肾脏活性及功能进行评估。
◦ 尿外渗反映集合系统损伤。
◦ 肾脏不显影可能提示肾蒂损伤或肾实质破裂。
◦ 异常指标通常是非特异性的,需要更明确的检查。
• 超声:
- 在评估肾损伤中的作用是有争议的。
- 常规床旁进行,作为创伤超声检查焦点性评估(FAST)的一部分。
- 可以显示肾周血肿的大小,以及是否扩大或缩小。
- 发现腹膜后积液的敏感度低。
- 检查是非特异性的,不能提供足够信息。
• CT:
- 静脉造影增强螺旋 CT 是诊断性措施。
- 良好地显示解剖学细节,肾损伤诊断的准确度达 98%。
- 是探查微小尿外渗、实质性撕裂伤、血管损伤和非肾脏损伤的敏感指标。

儿科注意事项

• 较大的肾钝器伤发生可无肉眼血尿或休克表现(儿童受创伤后产生大量儿茶酚胺,可以维持血压直至超过 50% 的血容量丢失)。
• meta 分析定义显微镜下低于 50 个红细胞/HPF 可以忽略,且不会漏掉明显损伤。
• CT 是可选的影像学检查方法。

诊断步骤/外科

• 肾实质损伤。
• 肾血管损伤。
• 输尿管损伤。
• 膀胱或尿道损伤。

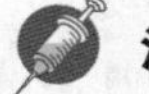

治疗

院前

• 从院前救援者了解受伤细节。
• 建立静脉通路。
• 穿透伤或内脏外露应覆盖无菌敷料。

初步稳定/治疗

• 气道管理(包括颈椎固定)。
• 进展性创伤生命支持标准(ATLS)复苏措施。
- 根据患者的血流动力学状态进行合适的静脉导管置入,包括中心静脉导管置入和切开。
- 液体复苏,起始为 2 L 晶体液(生理盐水或乳酸林格液),随后根据需要输入血液制品。
• 第一步应排除潜在的威胁生命的损伤。

急诊治疗/程序

• 紧急泌尿科会诊。
• 血流动力学不稳定可能有腹腔积血和肾损伤的重伤患者应立即行剖腹手术。
• 只有 5.4% 的肾损伤患者可发现有明显损伤(Ⅱ～Ⅴ级)。
• 98% 的肾钝器伤可以非手术治疗。
• 80%～90% 的肾损伤合并可以影响肾损伤治疗决策的较大器官损伤。
• 相对于剖腹手术,血管造影术和选择性肾栓塞术对于不需要立即手术的患者来说是另一种可选的治疗方法。
• 肾穿透伤:
- 目前肾穿透伤患者的治疗推荐剖腹探查术。
- 采取非手术方法治疗Ⅰ～Ⅲ级肾穿透伤不合并腹内伤或血流动力学不稳定情况的患者,越来越被人们认可。
• 钝性肾损伤:
- 无明显合并伤的单肾损伤更多地发生于钝挫伤,且在大多数情况下可非手术治疗。
- Ⅰ级和Ⅱ级:生命体征稳定且尿路造影肾功能正常的挫伤和小撕裂伤可以非手术治疗。
- Ⅲ级:有尿外渗的肾撕裂伤。
◦ 手术与保守治疗间存在争议。
◦ 治疗应依据 CT 扫描显示的受伤程度。
- Ⅳ级和Ⅴ级:肾破裂或肾蒂损伤且血流

S

动力学不稳定的患者须紧急剖腹手术。
- 所有输尿管损伤均需手术修补。

随访

进一步处理

入院指征

明显肾损伤需要住院行剖腹手术或观察的患者。

出院指征

• 无血尿、休克或无 X 线摄片证实有肾损伤的患者。
• 伴有镜下血尿(＞3～5 个红细胞/HPF)但无休克(收缩压＜90 mmHg)的成年钝性肾挫伤患者。
• 镜下＜50 个红细胞/HPF 且无合并重要器官损伤的小儿钝性肾损伤患者。

转诊问题

• 转诊到泌尿外科的门诊患者需做镜下血尿检查,确保无潜在危险。
• 肾创伤患者最普遍的并发症是尿性囊肿形成(1%～7%)。
• 尿外渗在 76%～87%的病例中可自行缓解。

肾小球肾炎 Glomerulonephritis

Emma K. Sizemore · Melissa H. White 祝各亮 译

基础知识

描述

• 肾炎综合征,特点:
- 血尿。
- 蛋白尿。
- 红细胞管型。
- 高血压。
- 肾功能不全。
• 常见的致病方式是多种疾病导致肾小球内炎症和细胞增殖。
• 危险因素:
- 遗传。
- 感染。
- 风湿性疾病。
- 导致抗体沉积。
  ◦ 抗体附着于肾小球抗原(自身或植入)。
  ◦ 不断进行抗原抗体复合物沉积。
- 引起炎症介质的大量汇聚和激活:
  ◦ 白细胞、补体和细胞因子。
  ◦ 细胞介导的免疫机制。
• 导致肾小球功能障碍。
• 持续性炎症可导致瘢痕和永久性损伤。

病因

• 感染后:
- 链球菌感染后肾小球肾炎(PSGN):
  ◦ 链球菌性咽炎或皮肤感染后 7～21 日发生,但最迟可在皮肤感染后 6 周出现。
  ◦ A 群链球菌释放的外毒素与肾小球结合,激活抗体反应而引起的。
  ◦ 患病率最高的是 2～14 岁的儿童和老年人。
  ◦ 男性占大多数。
  ◦ 症状可从无症状血尿到肾衰竭。
- 可以继发于其他细菌、真菌、病毒或寄生虫感染。
• IgA 肾病(伯杰病):
- 最常见于 30～40 岁的男性。
- 可能与感染后 IgA 合成增加有关,常为上呼吸道感染,遗传易感个体。
- 过敏性紫癜(HSP)会导致 IgA 肾病,但多影响年轻患者,并且有全身症状。
• 急进性肾小球肾炎(RPGN):
- 能在数日内破坏肾小球功能。
- 新月体沉积破坏肾小球功能。
- 微量免疫(小血管炎)。
  ◦ 无免疫沉积的坏死性肾小球肾炎。
  ◦ 通常抗中性粒细胞胞质抗体(ANCA)阳性。
  ◦ 可以涉及其他部位(如肺、皮肤)。
  ◦ 韦格纳肉芽肿病。
  ◦ 显微镜下多血管炎。
  ◦ 施特劳斯综合征。
- 免疫复合物沉积:
  ◦ 感染后。
  ◦ 与心内膜炎相关。
  ◦ 系统性疾病[如系统性红斑狼疮(SLE)、过敏性紫癜]。
- 抗肾小球基底膜(GBM)抗体沉积。
  ◦ 不清楚诱因,但可能是感染后出现。
  ◦ ＞60 岁的老年患者。
  ◦ 肺出血-肾炎综合征。
• 膜性增生性肾小球性肾炎(MPGN):
- 补体沉积于基底膜。
- 丙型肝炎。
- 非霍奇金淋巴瘤。
- 隐匿性感染。

诊断

症状和体征

• 基本体征:
- 血尿。
- 蛋白尿。
• 水肿:
- 钠水潴留。
- 眶部水肿。
- 腹水。
- 胸腔积液。
• 高血压。
• 少尿。
• 氮质血症。
• 充血性心力衰竭。
• 肾衰竭。
• 非特异性表现:
- 疲劳。
- 体重下降。
- 腹部疼痛。
- 恶心与呕吐。
• 自身免疫功能紊乱:
- 关节痛。
- 关节炎。
- 皮疹。
- 发热。
• 肺出血-肾炎综合征:
- 咯血。
• 韦格纳肉芽肿:
- 脓性鼻漏与鼻窦疼痛。
- 关节炎与关节痛。
- 咯血。
• 过敏性紫癜:
- 腹痛。

- 紫癜。
- 关节炎。

儿科注意事项

• 急进性肾小球肾炎在儿童中最常见(血尿、蛋白尿和肌酐升高)。

• 需要紧急诊断和活检,因为它可能会进展为终末期肾病。

• 咨询肾脏病专家关于激素和环磷酰胺的使用,以及血浆置换等问题。

基本检查

尿常规:

• 血尿、蛋白尿、红细胞管型。

诊断检查与说明

实验室检查

• 电解质、血尿氮、肌酐和肾小球滤过率:
- 肾功能。
- 高钾血症。

• 白蛋白和总蛋白:
- 根据临床过程会出现不同程度的低白蛋白血症。

• 血常规:
- 继发于慢性肾脏病、肿瘤和肺出血:肾炎综合征和韦格纳肉芽肿的贫血。
- 伴或不伴白细胞升高的感染。

• PT/PTT:
- 部分类型的肾小球肾炎会有凝血因子的消耗。

• 会诊所需的实验室检查:
- 细菌培养:咽喉、皮肤及血液。
- 24 h 尿液收集:蛋白质及尿电解质。
- 链球菌酶或抗链球菌溶血素 O 滴度。
- 补体水平(C1、C3、C4、CH_{50}):在链球菌感染后肾小球肾炎、膜性增生性肾小球性肾炎、系统性红斑狼疮中会减少。
- 抗核抗体、类风湿因子:结缔组织病。
- 炎性指标:红细胞沉降率和 C 反应蛋白。
- 抗 DNA 抗体(SLE)。
- 乙型肝炎、丙型肝炎系列。
- 艾滋病病毒。

影像学检查

• 肾脏超声(如果肾小球滤过率下降):
- 根据肾脏大小预测疾病潜在的可逆性,以及可能的诊断(如肿瘤、结石)。

• 胸部 X 线片:心脏大小、肺部水肿或出血。

诊断步骤/外科

• 肾活检:鉴别原发性肾小球疾病和其他原因导致的肾脏疾病。

• 膀胱镜检查:如果考虑膀胱肿瘤。

鉴别诊断

• 血液:
- 镰状细胞病。
- 凝血功能障碍。

• 肾脏:
- 感染。
- 畸形。
- 肿瘤。
- 缺血。
- 创伤。
- 血管炎。

• 肾后性:
- 机械性(如结石、反流、梗阻和导尿管)。
- 炎症(如膀胱炎、前列腺炎、附睾炎、子宫内膜异位症、尿道周围炎)。
- 肿瘤。

• 假阳性:
- 食品。
- 药物。
- 色素(如肌红蛋白、卟啉症、血红蛋白)。
- 阴道出血。

治疗

院前

• 支持治疗。

• 心肺复苏,对于体征稳定伴显著水肿的患者需限制液体量。

初步稳定/治疗

气道、呼吸和循环支持。

急诊治疗/程序

• 支持治疗:
- 血压控制:<125/75 mmHg。
  ◦ 襻利尿剂。
  ◦ ACEI 维持。
  ◦ 治疗高血压急症。
- 透析:
  ◦ 液体超负荷。
  ◦ 高钾血症。
  ◦ 尿毒症。

• 链球菌感染后肾小球肾炎:
- 支持治疗。
- 通常具有自限性。
- 抗生素无作用。

• IgA 肾病:
- 支持治疗。
- 如果活检示炎性,则使用免疫抑制剂。
- 转归可变,可以恢复也可以复发。

• 急进性肾小球肾炎:
- 能在数日内不可逆地破坏肾功能。
- 肾内科急会诊,讨论是否开始细胞毒药物治疗。
- 免疫抑制剂和大剂量激素。
  ◦ 甲泼尼松和泼尼松。
  ◦ 环磷酰胺。
  ◦ 利妥昔单抗。
  ◦ 血浆置换,清除抗肾小球基底膜抗体。

• 膜性增生性肾小球肾炎:
- 治疗已知的基础疾病。
- 肾内科急会诊,讨论是否开始细胞毒药物治疗。
- 可能进行血浆置换,环磷酰胺和/或糖皮质激素治疗。

药物治疗

• 苯那普利:5～40 mg,口服,每日 1 次(或其他 ACEI)。

• 环磷酰胺:剂量与肾脏病专家讨论决定。

• 二氮嗪:1～3 mg/kg,静脉注射,最大剂量 150 mg,可重复 q15 min。

• 呋塞米:20～80 mg,静脉注射,最大剂量 2 mg/(kg·d)。

• 甲泼尼松:30 mg/kg,静脉注射,每日 1～3 次,之后口服泼尼松(剂量与肾脏病专家讨论决定)。

• 硝普钠:0.3～10 μg/(kg·min),静脉滴注。

• 泼尼松:0.5～2 mg/(kg·d)。

随访

进一步处理

入院指征

• 生命体征不稳定。
• 少尿,无尿。
• 尿毒症。
• 急性肾衰竭。
• 电解质异常。
• 高血压急症。
• 充血性心力衰竭。
• 感染引起的肾小球肾炎。

出院指征

不伴其他疾病,仅仅表现为轻度血尿、蛋白尿的健康患者。

• 生命体征稳定。
• 没有感染指征。
• 正常的实验室诊断结果。

S

• 密切的随访推荐。

■ 随访建议

所有肾小球肾炎的患者都应进行肾脏病专业随访。

要点和误区

• 如果考虑使用免疫抑制剂，一定要与肾脏病专家进行讨论。

• 血尿、蛋白尿的患者应当密切随访，防止进展为肾小球肾炎。

肾炎综合征 Nephritic Syndrome

Patrick G. Meloy 朱妍 译

 基础知识

■ 描述

• 急性肾小球肾炎（AGN）是肾小球的急性炎症性损害，与以下因素相关：

- 突然发生的血尿，不管有没有红细胞管型。
- 主要表现为血尿、高血压、氮质血症、尿量减少的急性肾功能不全。
- 不同程度的蛋白尿。
- 活动性尿沉渣（红细胞管型）。

• AGN 确切的发病机制尚不明确：

- 对肾脏肾小球特定抗原产生自身免疫反应并结合。
- 其特点是新月体形成继而引起肾小球壁的非特异性损伤。

■ 病因

• 链球菌感染后肾小球肾炎（PSGN）：

- 由于感染 A 组 β 溶血性链球菌引起的急性肾炎综合征。
- 被认为是非化脓性并发症（抗生素治疗不能预防）。
- 当免疫复合物在肾小球上皮下沉积形成驼峰时发生。
- 大部分通常发生于 3～15 岁的患者，但在任何年龄都可能发生。
- 咽炎后肾炎的发生率在 5%～10%，皮肤感染后肾炎发生率在 25%。
- 当有新发蛋白尿、红细胞管型、水肿和近期任何感染发生时应该考虑 PSGN。
- 感染后发生肾炎的潜伏期有助于鉴别 PSGN 和 IgA 肾病（IgA - N）：
  ◦ 咽部感染后 1～3 周。
  ◦ 皮肤感染后 2～4 周。
- 诊断不一定必须做肾脏活检。
- 补体减低（C3）持续 6～8 周。
- 如果潜在感染不治疗持续存在，可能进展到严重肾衰竭。
- 预后：
  ◦ 良好；＞95%的肾功能正常的患者，甚至有些透析患者，在 6～8 周自愈。
  ◦ 血尿常在 3～6 个月缓解。
  ◦ 20%的患者在疾病治疗过程中处于短暂的肾病阶段。
  ◦ 终末期肾病的发生率＜5%。
  ◦ 急进性肾炎（RPGN）罕见，发生率＜1%。
  ◦ 大部分病例自发缓解且没有长期后遗症。

• 其他感染来源的肾小球肾炎（GN）：

- 脓毒症、肺炎、心内膜炎、病毒感染、HIV 感染。
- 肺部、腹腔或皮肤感染。
- 梅毒、麻风、血吸虫病和疟疾。
- 目的：治疗潜在的感染。

• 肝炎病毒相关性的肾小球疾病：

- 可以表现为肾炎或肾病综合征。
- 导致膜增生性 GN。
- 补体持续减低（与 PSGN 相比）。

• 非感染性因素导致的肾小球肾炎（由免疫复合物形成引起）：

- 系统性红斑狼疮、过敏性紫癜、血管炎、韦格纳肉芽肿。
- Goodpasture 综合征。

• IgA 肾病（IgA - N）：

- 全世界 AGN 最常见的病因（＞25%）。
- 抗原-抗体引起 IgA 和 C3 的免疫复合物沉积。
- 补体水平通常正常。
- IgA - N 有不同的临床表现：
  ◦ 上呼吸道（URI）感染后的肉眼血尿。
  ◦ 镜下血尿合并蛋白尿。
  ◦ 病毒感染或运动后出现的血尿。
  ◦ 预后与血清肌酐、血压和蛋白尿有关。
  ◦ 50%的蛋白尿患者可能发展成进展性肾病。
  ◦ ACEI 类或 ARB 治疗可能有效。

• RPGN：

- 某些 AGN 患者可能快速进展至肾衰竭。
- 肾脏活检发现新月体有标志性意义。

• 遗传性肾炎：

- Alport 综合征。

诊断

■ 症状和体征

• 血尿：

- 突然发生的肉眼血尿，占 30%～40%（咖啡色或可口可乐尿）。

• 水肿：

- 眶周水肿。
- 在婴儿和儿童中全身水肿更常见。

• 感染源或近期感染：上呼吸道或皮肤常见，如 PSGN。

• 充血性心力衰竭的症状：

- ＞60 岁患者有 40%的发生率。
- 儿童罕见。

• 关节炎、关节痛和不同类型的皮疹：PSGN、系统性疾病。

• 非特异性临床表现：

- 萎靡。
- 虚弱。
- 纳差。
- 恶心、呕吐。

病史

• 近期有上呼吸道或皮肤或其他部位的感染。

• 尿液颜色改变。

体格检查

• 高血压。

• 水肿。

■ 基本检查

尿沉渣分析检测：

• 红细胞数、蛋白尿和红细胞管型。

• 红细胞管型对活动性肾小球炎症有诊断意义。

■ 诊断检查与说明

实验室检查

• 血常规：

S

- 贫血(多见于慢性肾炎患者或其他系统性疾病)。
- 急性白细胞增多(可能提示感染过程)。

• 基础代谢板:
- 评估肾功能基线。
- 检查有无电解质异常。
- GFR 可能正常或接近正常。

• 尿液分析:
- 红细胞数±,管型,尿蛋白。

• 血清白蛋白。

• 培养(咽拭子、皮肤、尿液、血液):
- 临床疑似感染源。
- 链球菌酶。

• 血清补体水平(C3):在感染性心内膜炎、分流性肾炎和 PSGN 中减少。

• 链球菌抗体:
- 抗链球菌素(ASO)、抗链球菌激酶(ASK)、抗脱氧核糖核酸酶 B(ADNase B)、抗辅酶Ⅰ酶(ANADase)和抗透明质酸酶(AH)。
- ASO 在咽部感染时阳性率更高。
- ADNase B、ANADase 和 AH 在皮肤感染时更高。
- ASK 在近期溶血性链球菌感染后升高。
- 滴度高低与疾病的预后无关。

• 尿渗透压、钠、肌酐。

• 24 h 尿液收集:
- PSGN 患者中 5%的儿童和 20%的成人首先表现为蛋白尿。

影像学检查

• 肾脏超声:肾脏大小异常。

• 胸部 X 线检查:心脏扩大、肺水肿、感染。

诊断步骤/外科

肾脏活检:

• 一般不推荐用于 PSGN,因为症状通常在短暂的疾病状态后缓解。

• 推荐用于症状不典型的 PSGN、持续异常的补体水平、持续高血压和尿蛋白>3 g/d。

• 有利于其他原因肾炎的诊断。

▪ 鉴别诊断

• 其他类型的肾炎更多信息参见“肾小球肾炎”。

• 肾脏:
- 初始的肾脏疾病。

• 系统性:
- Goodpasture 综合征。
- 血管炎。
- 过敏性紫癜。

• 其他(罕见):
- 溶血-尿毒综合征。
- 血栓性血小板减少紫癜。
- 急性过敏性间质性肾炎。
- 血清病。

治疗

▪ 院前

提供基础支持治疗。

▪ 初步稳定/治疗

基础支持治疗。

▪ 急诊治疗/程序

• 针对链球菌感染使用抗生素:
- 青霉素(如果青霉素过敏,选红霉素)。

• 限制盐和液体摄入。

• 使用袢利尿剂(呋塞米)。

• 恢复少尿患者的尿量:
- 甘露醇。

• 治疗肺水肿:
- 吸氧。
- 吗啡。
- 袢利尿剂。

• 控制血压以减少蛋白尿及延缓肾炎进展:
- ACEI、ARB。
- 高血压急症:硝普钠或其他可滴定的降压药。

• 透析指征:
- 严重高血钾。
- 液体超负荷。
- 尿毒症。
- 严重酸中毒。
- 纠正电解质异常。

▪ 药物治疗

• 红霉素:250~500 mg 口服,q6 h,持续 7~10 日[儿童:30~50 mg/(kg·d)]。

• 呋塞米:20~80 mg(儿童:1~6 mg/kg)口服,1 次/日或 2 次/日。

• 赖诺普利(ACEI):10~40 mg(>6 岁儿童:0.07 mg/kg)口服,1 次/日。

• 氯沙坦(ARB):25~100 mg(>6 岁儿童:0.7 mg/kg)口服,1 次/日。

• 甘露醇:12.5~100 g(儿童:0.25~0.5 g/kg),静脉注射:
- 可以单次使用或重复给药;结合 1 st 中做的测试。

• 硫酸吗啡:0.1 mg/kg,静脉注射,q4 h。

• 硝普钠:0.3~4 μg/(kg·min)静脉注射。
- 对高血压急症滴定至目标平均动脉压。
- 青霉素:
- 苄星青霉素:每次 120 万 U(儿童:30 万~90 万 U,根据体重)肌内注射。
- 青霉素 V 钾:250~500 mg[<12 岁儿童:25~50 mg/(kg·d)],口服,q6~8 h,持续 10 日。

• 其他药物在专家会诊后可能会建议使用,包括鱼油(起抗感染作用的 ω-3 脂肪酸)和免疫抑制剂(糖皮质激素、环磷酰胺)。

随访

▪ 进一步处理

入院指征

• 有感染证据的肾炎。

• 少尿、无尿。

• 尿毒症。

• 肌酐升高。

• 水肿。

• 电解质紊乱。

• 严重高血压。

• 慢性充血性心力衰竭。

出院指征

病房肾炎轻症患者有以下情况时:

• 无合并症。

• 严格监督/监测症状、饮食、尿量和药物。

• 密切随访 PMD 和肾内科转诊患者。

转诊问题

肾内科:

• 在 2~3 日。

▪ 随访建议

• 建议坚持使用抗生素和降压药治疗。

• 限制盐和液体摄入。

要点和误区

• 活检发现肾小球特征性新月体形成则诊断明确。

• 必须获得全面的关于持续性或近期感染的病史作为肾炎的可能病因。

• IgA 肾病是肾炎最常见的原因。

• 患者需要积极控制血压和容量状态。

肾盂肾炎 Pyelonephritis

Matthew D. Bitner · William Manning 马林浩 译

基础知识

描述

• 肾盂和肾脏的炎症。
• 疾病的严重程度可以从轻微症状到脓毒性休克不等。
• 通常是下尿路感染的细菌通过向上感染上尿路引起的并发症。
• 主要是临床诊断。
• 男性各年龄组的发病率较低。
• 在一些研究中，女性的终身发病率超过 50%。
• 男女比例：
- 出生后的前几年为 1∶10。
- 儿童时期为 1∶5。
- 生育年龄为 1∶50。
- 50 岁及以上为 1∶1。
• 约 25%的病例为双侧感染。

S

病因

• 细菌学：
- 大肠杆菌(>90%在年轻女性中发生)。
- 泌尿道病原体：
◦ 克雷伯菌属。
◦ 柠檬酸杆菌属。
◦ 肠杆菌属。
- 其他细菌性病原体：
◦ 表皮葡萄球菌 5%～15%。
◦ 奇异变形杆菌。
◦ 沙雷菌属。
◦ 假单胞菌属。
◦ 金黄色葡萄球菌(增加)。
◦ 念珠菌(少见)。
• 易感因素(考虑复杂感染)：
- 最近的仪器检查史：
◦ 导尿。
◦ 膀胱镜检查。
- 尿潴留：
◦ 机械性(可见梗阻)。
◦ 药物(如抗胆碱能药物)。
◦ 其他感染(如单纯疱疹病毒感染)。
- 尿路梗阻：
◦ 狭窄。
◦ 肾结石。
◦ 前列腺肥大。
- 解剖异常：
◦ 尿道下裂。
◦ 输尿管畸位。
◦ 分叉输尿管。
◦ 肾脏瘢痕。
◦ 输尿管膀胱反流。
◦ 后尿道瓣。
- 神经系统疾病。
◦ 神经源性膀胱。
◦ 脊髓损伤。
- 异常尿动力学。
- 儿童时期的先前尿路感染(上一年度>3 次)。
- 最近的肾盂肾炎(1 年内)。
- 糖尿病。
- 免疫抑制。
- 妊娠。
- 高龄(>65 岁)。

诊断

症状和体征

• 关于诊断标准没有共识。
• 通常是局部和全身炎症的结合。
• 局部症状：
- 尿频、尿急。
- 背部、腰部或腹部疼痛。
- 肋脊角/耻骨上区压痛。
• 全身症状：
- 寒战、发热。
- 关节痛、肌肉痛、倦怠。
- 恶心和/或呕吐。
- 病态/中毒表现。
- 脱水。
• 隐匿性肾盂肾炎：
- 上尿路侵袭，但没有临床症状。
- 对于标准治疗无法缓解的下尿路感染，应怀疑此种情况。

儿科注意事项

• 发热、烦躁、呕吐、昏睡、进食不良或黄疸可能是婴儿中唯一的症状。
• 以前训练过的有遗尿病史的儿童。
• 新生儿、幼儿和免疫功能低下者(血行播散)严重细菌感染的常见原因。
• 肾脏瘢痕：比成人更常见的后遗症。
• B组链球菌。
• 新生儿的病因学因素。
• 便秘/肠功能障碍。

老年人注意事项

症状常表现为非典型：
• 缺乏经典的尿道炎、尿频症状。
• 反而以恶心、呕吐、腹泻、发热或精神状态改变为主要症状。

基本检查

• 尿液分析：
- 清洁尿标本或导尿管尿液标本；如果存在以下情况，则使用导尿管尿液标本：
◦ 阴道分泌物或出血。
◦ 污染的标本。
- 脓尿：5～10 个白细胞，外加白细胞酯酶和亚硝酸盐：
◦ 如果不存在，考虑其他诊断。
◦ 亚硝酸盐代表革兰阴性病原体，可以将食物中的硝酸盐转化为亚硝酸盐。
◦ 需要注意，假单胞菌、肠球菌和腐生葡萄球菌等一些尿路病原体不是硝酸盐还原菌。
- 血尿：
◦ 白细胞管型：脓尿的肾脏来源。
• 尿培养和敏感性(确诊金标准)：
- 在以下情况下进行：
◦ 可疑的肾盂肾炎。
◦ 诊断不明确时。
◦ 治疗失败、反复感染。
◦ 临床怀疑但尿检阴性。
- 大于 10 000 个菌落形成单位(CFU)/ml 的尿路病原体结果为阳性。
- 100～10 000 CFU 在以下情况下被考虑为阳性：
◦ 早期感染。
◦ 临床表现与尿路感染一致。
◦ 导尿或耻骨上标本。
◦ 男性患者标本。

诊断检查与说明

实验室检查

• 全血细胞计数：
- 白细胞增多。
- 不能诊断或排除上尿路感染。
• 血培养：
- 除非患者感染严重，否则不需要进行血培养；血培养阳性与疾病的严重程度无关。
- 尿培养更容易鉴定细菌。

• 生化检测：
- 对于存在严重电解质异常风险的患者进行检测（如严重恶心、呕吐或使用药物的患者）。
• 炎症标志物：
与C反应蛋白、白细胞计数和红细胞沉降率相比，血清降钙素原与疾病严重程度评分(SOFA)更相关，有助于区分脓毒症的严重程度。没有任何炎症标志物能够准确预测死亡率。

影像学检查

• 对于患有脓毒症/脓毒性休克、已知/疑似尿路结石/尿液 pH＞7、肾小球滤过率下降＞40 ml/min（提示梗阻）的患者，需要进行影像学检查。
• 需要进行影像学检查以区分肾盂炎（无实质受累）和肾盂肾炎（实质受累）；然而，这通常不会改变急诊治疗。
• 床边超声检查：
- 作用有限，但对有经验的操作者来说比 CT 更敏感，可被用于检测肾积水、脓肿、梗阻。
• 螺旋 CT：
- 在检测异常/特征化疾病范围诊断方面优于肾脏超声检查。
- 一致或需要关注的影像学发现：
◦ 实质的条索状或炎症和水肿。
◦ 肾周积液。
◦ 结石、梗阻。
◦ 肾实质、肾周脓肿。
◦ 实质内气体形成（肾盂肾炎）。
• MRI：
- 适用于：
◦ 妊娠患者（无辐射）。
◦ 肾衰竭患者（无碘造影剂）。
- 成本/可用性限制了 MRI 在急诊科的使用。
- 如果存在以下情况，请进行 MRI 检查：
◦ 同时存在结石/梗阻。
◦ 存在肾盂肾炎、脓肿的风险（糖尿病、免疫受损、老年人）。
◦ 对男性肾盂肾炎进行选择性泌尿生殖道评估。

儿科注意事项

• 获得导尿的标本：
- 绝大多数袋式尿标本会产生阳性培养结果（污染）。
- 清洁获取的标本与导尿或经腹膜获取的标本，敏感性为 75%～100%，特异性为 57%～100%。
- 仅在培养结果为阴性时有助于排除疾病。
• 导尿或经腹膜获取的标本＞1 000 CFU 为阳性。通常在 1 岁以下的儿童进行血培养（由于存在 SBI 的风险）。
• 所有首次患肾盂肾炎的儿童应在后续评估中进行泌尿道成像以评估输尿管膀胱反流情况。
• 肾脏超声：
- 如果没有临床改善，则在 48 h 内进行。
- 如果临床有改善，则在 3～6 周进行。

诊断步骤/外科

耻骨上膀胱穿刺造瘘：
• 当导尿管插入不成功或不可能时（包皮过长、尿道狭窄等）。
• 当存在造瘘部位覆盖性感染、已知解剖异常（肿瘤）、最近完全排空膀胱时禁忌。

鉴别诊断

• 腹主动脉瘤或夹层。
• 阑尾炎。
• 胆囊炎。
• 膀胱炎。
• 结肠憩室炎。
• 子宫颈炎或盆腔炎性疾病。
• 子宫内膜炎或输卵管炎。
• 下叶肺炎。
• 前列腺炎或睾丸炎。
• 肾结石或尿路结石。
• 肾/肾周脓肿。
• 尿道炎。
• 脊肌疾病。

治疗

院前

对于病情危重/中毒表现明显的患者建立静脉通路并进行适当的液体复苏。

初始稳定/治疗

使用生理盐水行抗休克治疗，剂量为 30 ml/kg（儿童：20 ml/kg）静脉液体快速输注。
• 尽管休克需要积极治疗，但需要注意合并症患者（肾衰竭、充血性心力衰竭）可能发生液体超负荷。

急诊治疗/程序

• 静脉抗生素适用于：
- 无法耐受口服治疗。
- 超高龄、免疫抑制、妊娠。
- 口服或门诊治疗失败。
- 尿路梗阻。
• 怀疑抗生素耐药的病原体。
• 经验性使用静脉注射抗生素：
- 氟喹诺酮类（儿童不适合使用）。
- 氨基糖苷类（庆大霉素）加氨苄青霉素。
- 第三代头孢菌素（头孢曲松）。
- 妊娠期间：
◦ 第三代头孢菌素。
◦ 庆大霉素/氨苄青霉素。
◦ 头孢唑林。
◦ 氨曲南。
• 门诊口服抗生素：
- 对于病情稳定和既往身体健康的患者：
◦ 氟喹诺酮：7～14 日为 1 个疗程。
- 可在口服抗生素前给予 1 次静脉抗生素：
◦ 确保及时中止细菌繁殖。
◦ 没有文献证明其有效性。
• 对于门诊治疗的患者，可以考虑使用更窄谱的抗生素（适合于门诊治疗的患者致病菌耐药的可能较低）。
• 止吐剂和镇痛剂。

药物治疗

• 口服抗生素：对于没有泌尿生殖系统异常的患者，可以接受 7～14 日的抗生素疗程，而对于存在泌尿生殖系统异常的患者，建议进行 10～14 日的疗程：
- 环丙沙星：500 mg，口服，每日 2 次（7 日）。
- 缓释环丙沙星：每日口服 1 000 mg。
- 左氧氟沙星：每日口服 750 mg（5 日）。
- 氧氟沙星：200 mg，口服，每日 2 次。
- 阿莫西林-克拉维酸：875 mg/125 mg 口服，每日 2 次（10～14 日）。
- 头孢呋辛：200 mg，口服，每日 2 次（10～14 日）。
- 头孢噻肟：400 mg，口服，每日 2 次（10～14 日）。
- TMP-SMX：大肠埃希菌耐药性一般＞10%，考虑在初始静脉注射剂量后，继续口服剂量 160 mg/800 mg，每日 2 次（10～14 日）。
- 如果怀疑有肾盂肾炎，呋喃妥因、磷霉素不适用。
• 静脉注射抗生素：
- 头孢曲松：静脉注射 1 g，q24 h。
- 环丙沙星：静脉注射 400 mg，q12 h。
- 氨苄西林-舒巴坦：静脉注射 3 g，q6 h。
- 头孢唑林：静脉注射 1～1.5 g，q8 h。
- 庆大霉素：静脉给药 3～5 mg/kg。

S

- 左氧氟沙星：静脉注射 500 mg，每日 1 次。
- 哌拉西林-他唑巴坦：静脉注射 3.375 g，q8 h。

儿科考量

• 儿童口服抗生素剂型：
- 阿莫西林：30～50 mg/(kg · 24 h)，口服，每日 3 次。
- 阿莫西林/克拉维酸：45 mg/(kg · 24 h)，口服，每日 3 次。
- 头孢噻肟：8 mg/(kg · 24 h)，口服，每日 3 次。
- 头孢泊肟：10 mg/(kg · 24 h)，口服，每日 2 次。
- 头孢氨苄：50～75 mg/(kg · 24 h)，口服，每日 4 次。
- 红霉素-磺胺嘧啶：50 mg/(kg · 24 h)，口服，每日 4 次。

• 住院儿童的静脉抗生素：
- 年龄 0～3 个月：
  ◦ 头孢噻肟[50～180 mg/(kg · d)，每日 3 次]＋氨苄西林[50～100 mg/(kg · d)，每日 4 次]。
  ◦ 庆大霉素[1～2.5 mg/(kg · d)，每日 3 次]＋氨苄西林。
- 年龄＞3 个月：

可以用头孢曲松[50～100 mg/(kg · d)，每日 2 次到每日 1 次]来替代头孢噻肟。

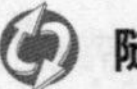

随访

进一步处理

入院指征

• 脓毒症，疾病、中毒表现。
• 不能耐受口服治疗。
• 难以控制的恶心、呕吐。
• 社会因素导致依从性不佳。
• 妊娠。
• 导尿管置入。
• 尿路梗阻、解剖异常。
• 免疫抑制、糖尿病。
• 极端年龄(2～6 个月及以下的婴儿)。
• 门诊治疗失败、最近使用抗生素。
• 需要根据影像学指导进行治疗。

出院指征

• 在急诊科病情改善。
• 能够正常口服药物。
• 用口服镇痛药控制疼痛。
• 正常肾功能。
• 48～72 h 复诊。

随访建议

• 无合并症的非复杂病例可以由其初级保健医生安全的随访。
• 如果进行了培养，患者需要随访结果，一旦了解抗生素敏感性，可能需要改变治疗方案。
• 所有儿科患者都需要随访其儿科医生，进行必要的影像学检查以评估解剖异常。
• 妊娠患者需要重复尿液分析，以评估是否解除/复发，并可能需要抑制性治疗。
• 有反复感染的患者及已识别的不寻常或耐药菌株感染的患者需要密切随访，并行泌尿外科/或感染病科咨询。

要点和误区

• 主要是临床诊断，至少需要进行实验室检查。
• 对于儿童、老年、免疫抑制和孕妇患者需要积极治疗。
• 考虑其他的诊断(例如，妇科病因、腹主动脉瘤)。

生物武器 Biological

Brigham R. Temple　宋振举　童朝阳 译

基础知识

描述

• 可以大范围播散的自然生物体或经过提取的毒物，以期造成较高的发病率、死亡率和社会动荡。
• 生物体包括细菌、病毒和真菌。
• 超过 400 种可能或被确认的冰原物质具有被用作生物武器的可能：
- 与其他大规模杀伤性武器相比成本低，高效且携带隐蔽。
- 其隐蔽性来源于生物体的自然繁殖过程。
• 易隐藏且难以发现。
- 病原体常无色，无味。
• 患者因常见主诉就诊于各医疗机构，这延误了生物武器隐蔽施用的识别。
• 生物武器的受害者可通过直接皮肤接触、吸入雾化介质经呼吸系统传播，接触食物或水源经消化道传播。

病因

• 细菌。
- 炭疽：炭疽杆菌。
- 鼠疫：鼠疫耶尔森菌。
- 霍乱：霍乱弧菌感染。
  ◦ 表现为严重消化道症状并逐渐导致严重脱水。
- 兔热病：土拉热弗朗西斯菌。
- 布鲁菌病：布鲁菌属生物。
- Q 热：贝氏柯克体。
• 病毒：
- 天花：天花病毒。
- 病毒性脑炎：甲病毒属成员(委内瑞拉马脑炎、东部马脑炎和西部马脑炎)。
- 病毒性出血热：来自 4 个家族的病毒，包括埃博拉出血热、马堡热、拉萨热和登革热。
• 毒素：
- 蓖麻毒素。
- 葡萄球菌肠毒素 B。
- 肉毒杆菌毒素。
- 真菌毒素类。

诊断

症状和体征

• 医护人员需要时刻警惕去发现可以提示生物武器播散的疾病模式和诊断线索。
• 生物武器物质故意释放的提示：
- 在一同生活、工作、参加集会的人群中聚集发病(如果在同一办公室工作的许多人感染肺炎，这可能代表呼吸道病原体播散)。
- 常见病的不常见年龄分布(在成人中的水痘样疾病，可能代表天花播散)。
- 大于 2 名患者表现相似，无法解释症状(2 名患者表现出迟缓性麻痹，可能提示肉毒毒素)。
- 不常见介质传播的单一病例(天花、吸入性炭疽)。

- 大量有着相同症状表现的患者，且有着不断增加的发病率和死亡率。

炭疽病

- 吸入性炭疽。
  - 发热。
  - 寒战。
  - 疲倦、全身乏力、昏睡。
  - 咳嗽，通常为干咳或少痰。
  - 恶心、呕吐。
  - 呼吸困难。
  - 出汗。
  - 胸痛。
  - 肌痛。
  - 心动过速。
  - 脑膜刺激征。
- 接触性炭疽。
  - 皮肤损害。
    - 无痛性瘙痒疱疹。
    - 转变为水疱，继而破裂形成坏死性溃疡。
  - 黑色焦痂。
  - 周围环绕胶状非点状水肿。

鼠疫

- 突然起病。
- 发热、寒战。
- 咳嗽、咯血、呼吸困难。
- 头痛。
- 呕吐。
- 淋巴结软性肿胀(腹股沟腺炎)。
- 预防接种处出现皮肤肿胀。
- 精神错乱。
- 腹痛。
- 少尿。
- 反应迟钝。
- 大面积瘀斑。
- 耳坏疽。

兔热病

- 详见“兔热病”。
- 伤寒。
  - 当病原体被武器化且经过气体传播最可能出现的疾病形式。
  - 发热、头痛。
  - 干咳。
  - 经治疗有35%的死亡率。

Q热

- 潜伏期为10～40日。
- 2～10日的感冒样症状和胸膜炎性胸痛。
- 胸部X线正位片示斑片状浸润。
- 最终诊断依赖血清学。
- 未经治疗死亡率<1%。

布鲁菌病

- 潜伏期为3～60日。
- 感冒样症状和神经精神症状(头痛、抑郁、疲惫和易怒)。
- 关节和消化道感染可导致局部疼痛，尤其是背痛。
- 通过血清学、血培养及体液联合诊断。
- 死亡率小于<2%。

天花

- 潜伏期为7～17日(平均12日)。
- 2～3日的感冒样症状(发热、疲惫、肌痛、头痛)，继而出现：
  - 由斑疹变为丘疹，继而转变为脓疱性病变和结痂性病变。
  - 由面部和肢体(包括手掌和足底)继而在1周内蔓延至躯干。
  - 1～2周结痂。
- 死亡率：
  - 未经治疗为30%。

出血热

- 见“出血热”。
- 潜伏期为1～3周。
- 由感冒样症状起病，包括发热、萎靡、肌痛、头痛和咽痛。
- 其后出现传染性胃肠炎症状，皮疹和肝肾功能不全。
- 最终，出血症状在约第5日出现，伴随休克和死亡。
  - 埃博拉出血热未经治疗，死亡率为50%～90%。

基本检查

遇到以下情况需要怀疑生物恐怖：

- 许多相对年轻、健康的患者，表现出感冒样症状且在数日内快速恶化。
- 典型接触性损害出现。
- 一些常见疾病出现在特殊年龄或特殊地理位置。

诊断检查与说明

实验室检查

- 全血细胞计数。
- 电解质、尿素氮、肌酐。
- 动脉血气。
- 脑脊液(CSF)：
  - 炭疽：50%吸入性炭疽发展为出血性脑膜炎。
- 凝血功能检查：
  - 霍乱：弥散性血管内凝血。
- 血培养。
- 伤口培养。
- 提醒实验室人员有关临床医师可能关注的内容。

影像学检查

胸部正位：

- 炭疽：纵隔增宽，肺部浸润/实变，胸腔积液。
- 鼠疫：支气管肺炎。

鉴别诊断

- 炭疽：
  - 流感。
  - 细菌性肺炎，细菌性脑膜炎。
  - 棕色隐遁蛛咬伤。
  - 兔热病。
  - 链珠菌性或葡萄球菌性皮肤感染。
- 鼠疫：
  - 兔热病，猫抓病。
  - 性病淋巴肉芽肿，软下疳。
  - 肺结核。
  - 链球菌性淋巴结炎。
  - 脑膜炎、脑炎、脓毒症。
- 天花：
  - 水痘。
  - 出疹顺序为从躯干向四周播散。
    - 不同进展阶段的皮肤损害。
    - 罕见累及手掌和足底。
    - 播散性传播性软疣。
    - 猴痘，药物性皮炎。
- 毒素：
  - 葡萄球菌肠毒素B：
    - 食物中毒的最常见原因。
    - 可投放于水库，也可经空气传播。
    - 被吸入后，可出现发热症状，并可以进一步发展为脓毒性休克。
  - 蓖麻毒素：
    - 蓖麻子豆中提取的植物蛋白。
    - 导致上呼吸道阻塞继而快速进展为心肺功能衰竭。
    - 食用该毒素危害较小，因为消化道对其吸收一般，但可导致局部细胞死亡，休克甚至死亡。
  - 肉毒素：
    - 最初症状包括脑神经功能不全，表现为进展性麻痹导致呼吸衰竭。
  - 真菌毒素：
    - 特定真菌种类产生的高毒性化合物。
    - 皮肤、呼吸道、消化道受累，继而快速进展至多器官功能衰竭以致死亡。

S

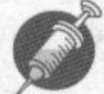

治疗

院前

使用 N95 口罩进行一般性防护。

初步稳定/治疗

- 心肺复苏。
- 低血压患者以生理盐水液体复苏。
- 对缺氧者予辅助给氧。
- 对持续低血压予以升压药。
- 对疑似病例予以呼吸及接触隔离。

急诊治疗/程序

- 所有的治疗均包括：
  - 对乙酰氨基酚控制发热。
  - 对特定疾病进行治疗。
- 炭疽：
  - 初始抗生素：
    - 静脉应用于吸入性或严重接触性患者。
    - 抗生素选择取决于敏感性。
  - 抗生素选择：
    - 环丙沙星：一线药物。
    - 多西环素。
    - 利福平。
    - 氯林可霉素。
    - 万古霉素。
- 鼠疫：
  - 抗生素在 24 h 内应用可降低死亡率。
  - 一线药物：链霉素或庆大霉素。
  - 加用氯霉素，如果有脑膜炎迹象或情况不稳定患者。
  - 预防用药：多西环素或环丙沙星。
- 布鲁菌病：
  - 支持治疗。
  - 起始多西环素 100 mg，每日 2 次，口服持续 6 周，并在第 1 周每日加用链霉素 1 g 肌内注射，或每日利福平 900 mg 持续 6 周。
- Q 热：
  - 2 周内无需治疗可恢复。
  - 多西环素缩短疾病期。
- 天花：
  - 支持治疗。
  - 最初暴露 4 日内给予疫苗降低感染及进展出现严重症状的概率。
  - 在 5～7 日接种疫苗仍可减轻症状的严重程度。
  - 医务人员的免疫接种。
  - 治疗二次细菌感染。
- 结核病：
  - 见结核病。
- 出血热：
  - 见出血热。

S

药物治疗

- 氯霉素：25 mg/kg，静脉滴注，q6 h。
- 环丙沙星：400 mg，静脉滴注，q12 h；或 500 mg，口服，每日 2 次（儿童：15 mg/kg，每日 2 次，口服）。
- 克林霉素：900 mg，静脉滴注，q12 h。
- 多西环素：100 mg（儿童≥45 kg，100 mg；如果体重≤45 kg，2.2 mg/kg，静脉滴注），口服或静脉滴注，q12 h。
- 庆大霉素：5 mg/kg，肌内注射或静脉滴注，q24 h（儿童：2.5 mg/kg，肌内注射或静脉滴注，q8 h）。
- 利福平：10 mg/kg，静脉滴注，不超过 600 mg/d。
- 链霉素：1 g（儿童：20～40 mg/kg），肌内注射，q12 h。
- 万古霉素：1 g，静脉滴注，q12 h。

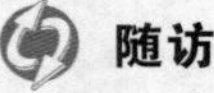

随访

进一步处理

入院指征

- 入院或门诊收治患者的决定取决于总体伤害情况。
- 中毒或缺氧患者需要入院治疗。
- 呼吸隔离。
- 高传染性感染（即埃博拉）。

出院指征

轻症、无传染性疾病。

转诊问题

- 患者或确诊与生物武器相关的疾病时，联系地方或州一级健康管理部门。
- 对可疑疾病进行传染性疾病和毒理学咨询。

随访建议

- 暴露后预防及疫苗接种应当在病原生物体基础上继续进行。
- 遭到暴露的人员应当在职员健康及感染控制部门随访后再返回工作。

要点和误区

- 早期诊断是困难的，高度怀疑是必需的。
- 未能使用个人保护措施进行个人保护时要注意。
- 一同生活、工作、参加集会的患者聚集发病，需要怀疑生物武器。
- 对于怀疑病例早期开始治疗或预防。

生长发育滞缓 Failure to Thrive

Roger M. Barkin 万健 译

基础知识

描述

- 并非单一疾病，而是一组症状的描述。
- 体格生长迟缓：
  - 通常可在 2 岁前被诊断。
- 广义地分为：
  - 器质性（原发疾病）。
  - 非器质性（非原发疾病）。
- 可在所有经济社会阶层中出现。
- 贫穷增加发生生长发育滞后的风险。
- 可能是长期生长、行为和发展障碍的结果，特别是在生命中最初的几个月就有发育迟缓的儿童。

病因

许多患者具有以下一种或多种特征性病因。

- 热量摄入不足。
- 热量吸收不良，吸收障碍。
- 热量消耗过度。
- 继发于原发的慢性疾病。

诊断

症状和体征

- 尚无公认的定义。
- 未达到和保持与年龄相宜的生长速度。

• 体重比相同年龄(修正早产)与性别发育正常的儿童低 2 个标准差以上。

• 体重下降超过标准生长表中的 2 个重要百分位数(重要百分位数指第 5、10、25、50、75 和 90 的对应数)(可查看的附加说明)。

• 有以下 1 种或以上生长速度的指标发生变化,以下 3 种常规监测的生长发育指标可能提示原发性损害。

- 由于热量摄入不足导致的生长身长/身高与最终头围降低,伴发体重降低。
- 原发性身长/身高缩短常与内分泌障碍有关。
- 头围异常通常是由中枢神经系统原发病变所导致的。

• 尽管通常情况下表现为生长速度的逐渐减慢,但也可以出现生长速度突然减慢,通常源于器质性疾病。

• 可表现为:

- 肌肉含量的减少。
- 皮下脂肪的丢失。
- 脱发。
- 皮炎。
- 慢性病。
- 消瘦。
- 恶性营养不良。
- 内分泌功能的异常。
- 神经系统检查异常和发育异常。
- 免疫功能下降及感染概率增加。

病史

• 详尽的喂养史:

- 母乳喂养:
  ◦ 既往母乳喂养史。
  ◦ 喂奶的频率。
  ◦ 喂奶的时长。
  ◦ 母乳喂养的家庭支持。
- 人工喂养:
  ◦ 人工喂养的类型(牛奶、豆浆、元素、早产)。
  ◦ 如何准备配方(随时可使用、粉末、浓缩液)。
  ◦ 喂食的频率。
  ◦ 每次喂食的量。
- 固体食物。
- 与喂养相关的呕吐。
- 尿量和排便量。
  ◦ 有无血便。

• 妊娠史:

- 母亲的并发症。
- 药物或酒精(乙醇)使用情况。

• 生产史:

- 并发症,子宫内发育迟缓,早熟。
- 出生体重。
- 先天性异常。
- 子宫内不良接触史/感染史。

• 发育史:

- 达到合适的生长标准。
- 儿童自身的性格。

• 社会心理史:

- 家庭构成。
- 家庭及社会支持。
- 应激。
- 母亲抑郁。
- 虐待或照顾失职。

体格检查

• 体重、身长/体重和头围:

- 在正常生长发育表中标记:
  ◦ 尽可能多的包含既往的生长发育标记点。

• 异常特征:

- 心脏功能异常。
- 肺功能异常。
- 消化功能异常。

• 皮肤检查包括虐待儿童的各种体征检查。

■ 基本检查

• 详细的病史和体格检查。

• 在正常的生长发育表格上标记生长发育参数。

• 注意家庭儿童之间的关系。

• 直接的喂养观察。

• 白细胞计数、C 反应蛋白、电解质、尿常规和尿培养,如有必要,测定铅含量。

■ 诊断检查与说明

实验室检查

• 白细胞计数:

- 贫血。
- 感染。
- 白血病、恶性肿瘤。
- 血铅水平。
- 铅中毒。

• 生化检查(电解质、尿素氮、肌酐、血糖、肝功能、总蛋白、白蛋白、钙、磷、镁):

- 脱水和酸中毒。
- 代谢和内分泌异常包括甲状腺疾病。经常进行新生儿常规筛查(NBS)是有利的。
- 糖尿病。
- 肾脏病。
- 血气分析。
- 肾小管酸中毒。
- 先天性代谢异常。

• 尿培养:

- 肾脏病。
- 感染。

• HIV 感染。

• 粪便检查:包括隐血、培养、寄生虫及虫卵。

影像学检查

• X 线检查:

- 结核。
- 肺炎。
- 心脏扩大。

诊断步骤/外科

• pH 探针。

- 胃食管反流。

• 汗液氯化物检查:

- 囊性纤维化(可为 NBS 的一部分)。

• 皮肤结核菌素检查。

■ 鉴别诊断

• 器质性疾病:

- 消化系统:
  ◦ 营养吸收不良综合征。
  ◦ 腹部疾病。
  ◦ 囊性纤维化。
  ◦ 食物过敏。
  ◦ 感染性肠病。
  ◦ 肝胆性疾病。
  ◦ 肝炎。
  ◦ 肝硬化。
  ◦ 胆道闭锁。
  ◦ 梗阻性疾病。
  ◦ 幽门狭窄。
  ◦ 肠扭转。
  ◦ 先天性巨结肠。
  ◦ 胰腺炎。
  ◦ 短肠综合征。
  ◦ 胃食管反流。
  ◦ 维生素缺乏。
- 心源性:
  ◦ 先天性心脏病。
  ◦ 发绀。
  ◦ 充血性心脏病。
  ◦ 后天性(获得性)心脏病。
- 肺源性:
  ◦ 支气管肺发育不良。
  ◦ 阻塞性睡眠呼吸暂停。
  ◦ 慢性肺疾病。
  ◦ 囊性纤维化。
- 血液系统:
  ◦ 缺铁性贫血。
  ◦ 地中海贫血(珠蛋白生成障碍性贫血)。

S

◦ 铅中毒。
◦ 白血病。
- 肾脏：
◦ 慢性肾功能不全。
◦ 肾小管性酸中毒。
◦ 反复尿路感染。
- 神经系统和中枢神经系统：
◦ 脑积水。
◦ 高渗性或低渗性。
◦ 广泛肌无力(如脊髓肌肉萎缩)。
◦ 口部运动障碍。
- 免疫系统：
◦ HIV 感染。
- 内分泌系统：
◦ 糖尿病。
◦ 甲状腺、甲状旁腺疾病。
◦ 肾上腺疾病。
◦ 生长激素缺乏。
◦ 垂体功能减退症。
◦ 低磷酸盐血症性佝偻病。
- 感染：
◦ 结核。
◦ 寄生虫。
◦ 尿路感染。
- 遗传病或先天性疾病：
◦ 胎儿酒精综合征。
◦ Smith-Lemli-Opitz 综合征。
◦ 唇腭裂。
◦ 先天性代谢异常。
◦ 一些基因性综合征。
- 中毒。
• 非器质性病因：
- 父母-儿童综合征：
◦ 母亲-婴儿关系问题。
◦ 母亲精神疾病和滥用药物。
◦ 母亲经验缺乏。
◦ 母乳喂养困难。
◦ 人工喂养配方不当。
◦ 人工喂养配方不足。
◦ 混乱的家庭环境。
◦ 虐待儿童或疏忽照顾。
◦ Munchhausen 综合征。

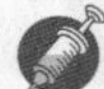

治疗

初步稳定/治疗

• 检查有无低血糖。
• 脱水时给予液体复苏。
• 支持性/无偏见的环境。

急诊治疗/程序

• 识别生长发育迟缓的儿童。
• 除外器质性异常：
- 器质性病因常需要特殊的治疗。
• 社会服务咨询。
• 母乳喂养咨询：
- 给予正确喂养的建议。

药物

取决于潜在的病因。

随访

进一步处理

入院指征

• 器质性病因需要药物治疗。
• 非器质性病因需要儿童照顾者的介入。
• 非器质性病因需要监测摄入量来观察体重。尤其适用于 3～6 个月的婴儿，因为其对认知发展的影响较大。
• 怀疑虐待儿童或照顾不当。
• 严重脱水、营养不良或电解质紊乱。
• 未能达到预期的增长参数。
• 体重增加尽管几个月的门诊治疗。

出院指征

• 经主诊医师妥善治疗后。
• 有条件时密切监测随访摄入量和生长发育情况。
• 安全的家庭环境，合作的父母。

转诊问题

• 专科转诊取决于病因。

生殖器疱疹 Herpes

Benjamin Mattingly · Benjamin Wilks 陈奇通 译

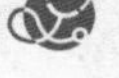

基础知识

描述

• 生殖器疱疹是一种终身复发性感染。
• 两种类型的生殖器单纯疱疹病毒(HSV)可以引起生殖器疱疹：HSV-1 和 HSV-2。
• 大多数复发性生殖器疱疹是由 HSV-2 引起的。
• 有越来越多的比例的 HSV-1 肛门生殖器疱疹感染。
• 在美国，大约有 5000 万人感染了 HSV-2。
• 大多数报道的病例年龄在 16～40 岁。
• HSV 感染被指定为原发性、非原发性首发、复发、无症状。
• 初步 HSV 感染：
- 指患者在感染前没有 HSV-1 或 HSV-2 抗体。
- 暴露后的平均潜伏期为 4 日(范围 2～12 日)。
• 非初步感染第一阶段：
- 指已存在 HSV-2 抗体的患者获得生殖器 HSV-1，反之亦然。
- 与原发感染相比，病灶和症状更少。
- 一种 HSV 的抗体对另一种 HSV 有一定的保护作用。
• 复发性 HSV 感染：
- 指生殖器 HSV 的重新激活，病变处恢复的 HSV 类型与血清抗体相同。
- 病变持续时间比原发感染短(10 日和 19 日)。
- 症状可以不那么严重。生殖器病变可能无症状，数量少，外观不典型。
- 病毒脱落的持续时间比原发感染短(2 日和 9 日)。
• 无症状的 HSV 感染：
- 病毒间歇性传播，通常由无病变或无症状的人传播。
- 无症状地从生殖道排出 HSV 是最常见的感染传播源。

病因

• 70%～90%由 DNA 病毒 HSV-2 引起：
- 其余由 HSV-1 引起。
• HSV-1 感染通常发生在口咽黏膜：
- 三叉神经节定植；潜伏病毒。
- 在生殖道发现 HSV-1 的证据越来越普遍，通常是由于口交。
- 生殖道 HSV-1 复发不常见。

• 获得 HSV-2 感染通常是通过生殖器接触传播的结果：

- 病毒在生殖器官、后生器官或肛门皮肤复制：

◦ 骶神经节潜伏病毒。

- HSV-2 也可感染口腔：

◦ 复发，在这个部位不常见。

• HSV 疫苗至今未成功，研究仍在进行中。

• 与 HIV 和其他性传播疾病有很高的相关性。

注意

• 应保持接触隔离和普遍预防措施。

• 感染 HSV-2 的人感染 HIV 的可能性是其他人的 2～3 倍：

- HSV-2 呈阳性的患者也应进行 HIV 病毒检测。

诊断

症状和体征

• 根据感染是原发、非原发还是复发，差异很大。

• 原发性生殖器感染的潜伏期为 4～7 日：

- 潜伏期过后，生殖器或邻近皮肤可能出现多发病变。

- 有症状的生殖器病变患者约有一半报告头痛、发热、不适、排尿困难、腹股沟淋巴结压痛。

- 初次生殖器疱疹感染的患者也可能完全无症状。

• 非原发感染（原存在 HSV-1 抗体的人的 HSV-2 生殖器感染）的最初表现通常是无症状的。

• 潜伏期 HSV 感染的再激活导致生殖器疱疹症状复发或无症状病毒脱落：

- 复发性感染之前可能会出现瘙痒、灼烧或疼痛等前驱症状，然后才会出现病灶。

- 复发性感染往往症状轻微，很少损伤，或根本没有症状。

病史

初步感染：

• 潜伏期过后，生殖器或邻近皮肤上可能出现多发病变。

• 病变进展为红斑、丘疹、短期的小疱、疼痛的溃疡和结痂。

• 症状会在 2～3 周后消失。

复发性感染：

• 暴发前的局部刺痛、灼烧、瘙痒或疼痛的 1～2 日为前驱症状。

• 病变通常是单侧的，可能是不典型的；以线状裂隙或剥落的形式出现。

• 症状在 5～10 日消失。

• 临床上很难区分原发性和复发性感染，但存在前驱症状。

体格检查

• 外阴、阴道、子宫颈、会阴、臀部的病变；阴茎柄或龟头。

• 成组的小疱在红斑的基底上。

• 在潮湿的黏膜表面，溃疡可能是主要的。

• 不典型特征包括局部水肿、红斑、结痂或裂隙。

儿科注意事项

• 新生儿感染常播散性或累及中枢神经系统，发病率和死亡率较高。

• 没有小疱的新生儿先天性 HSV 可能模仿风疹、巨细胞病毒（CMV）或弓形体病。

• 儿童生殖器 HSV 感染需考虑性虐待。

• 疑似性病患者的培养病变和检测。

基本检查

• 仅根据临床资料做出的诊断可能并不准确。

• 其他细菌感染的症状可能与 HSV 混淆，导致错误诊断。

• 生殖器疱疹可引起非典型症状。

• 准确诊断生殖器疱疹需要病史、体格检查和实验室检查确认。

诊断检查与说明

实验室检查

• 细胞培养和 PCR 是首选的 HSV 检测方法：

- 病毒培养使用生殖器损伤处的拭子。

- 病毒可在组织培养 5 日内生长。

- 病毒培养对复发性病变的敏感性较低，随着病变愈合迅速降低。

- PCR 更快，比病毒培养敏感 4 倍。

- PCR 是检测中心和全身 HSV 感染的首选方法。

- 由于病毒脱落是间歇性的，单纯疱疹病毒培养或 PCR 阴性，特别是没有活动性病变时，并不意味着没有单纯疱疹病毒感染。

• 血清试验也可用于检测 HSV；检测 HSV IgG1 抗体和 HSV IgG2 抗体：

- 敏感性在 80%～98%。

- 在感染早期，假阴性结果更常见。

- HSV 抗体在感染后的最初几周内产生，并在血清中无限期检测到。

- 可以区分 HSV-1 和 HSV-2。

- 可以确认感染是原发感染还是复发感染。

- 如果反复出现生殖器症状或非典型症状，HSV PCR 或培养阴性，可能有用。

• Tzanck 制备是不敏感的，非特异性的。

影像学检查

一般无影像学提示。

鉴别诊断

• 梅毒（梅毒螺旋体）。

• 软性下疳（嗜血杆菌 ducreyi）。

• 性病淋巴肉芽肿（LGV）。

• 腹股沟肉芽肿（肉芽克雷伯菌）。

• 念珠菌病。

• Behcet 综合征。

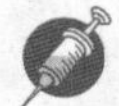

治疗

院前

应保持普遍的预防措施。

初步稳定/治疗

很少需要，除非与需要住院治疗的系统性症状有关：

• 播散性感染。

• 肝炎。

• 肺炎。

• 脑膜脑炎。

急诊治疗/程序

• 治疗可部分控制症状和病变，一旦停止用药不根除潜伏病毒或影响复发。

• 所有首次出现生殖器疱疹的患者都应该接受抗病毒治疗：

- 新获得的生殖器疱疹可引起严重的系统症状的长期疾病。

- 即使是首发疱疹患者，初期症状轻微，也可能发展为严重症状。

• 复发的偶发治疗可缩短病灶持续时间或改善复发。

• 对复发频繁的患者进行每日抑制治疗可使复发频率降低 75%。

• 伐昔洛韦和万乃洛韦是同样有效的药物，使用频率较低，都干扰病毒 DNA 聚合酶。

• 免疫缺陷个体对无环鸟苷的耐药性为 5%～10%：

- 膦甲酸 40 mg/kg，静脉，q8 h 可能有效。

妊娠注意事项

• 妊娠期原发性 HSV 感染的妇女应接受抗病毒治疗：

- 有症状和无症状患者的新生儿发病率

S

较高。

- 在分娩前后感染生殖器疱疹的妇女中，由受感染母亲传染给新生儿的风险为30%~50%。

• 妊娠晚期抑制抗病毒治疗可减少分娩时病变的复发和降低剖宫产率。

■ **药物治疗**

• 需要住院治疗的系统性或严重感染：

- 阿昔洛韦：5~10 mg/kg，静脉，q8 h持续2~7日或直到观察到临床改善，随后口服抗病毒治疗完成至少10日的全面治疗。

- 新生儿/婴儿：如果疾病局限于皮肤和黏膜，口服20 mg/kg，q8 h，持续14日；如果疾病播散性，持续21日。

• 第一阶段(7~10日治疗；延长，如果在10日没有愈合)：

- 阿昔洛韦：400 mg，口服，每日3次；200 mg，每日5次。

- 儿童：20 mg/kg，口服，每日3次；或5 mg/kg，静脉，q8 h。

- 泛昔洛韦：250 mg，口服，每日3次，持续7~10日。

- 缬阿昔洛韦：1000 mg，口服，每日2次，持续7~10日。

• 复发性感染：

- 必须在出现病变的第1日或前驱症状时开始。

- 阿昔洛韦：400 mg，口服，每日3次，持续5日，或800 mg，口服，每日2次，持续5日，或800 mg，口服，每日3次，持续2日。

- 泛昔洛韦：1000 mg，口服，每日2次，口服1日；或125 mg，口服，每日2次，持续5日。

- 缬阿昔洛韦：500 mg，口服，每日2次，持续3日；或每日服用1000 mg，口服，持续5日。

• 抑制治疗(每日)：

- 阿昔洛韦：400 mg，口服，每日2次。

- 泛昔洛韦：250 mg，口服，每日2次。

- 缬阿昔洛韦：500 mg，口服，每日1次，如果>10例每年复发，1000 mg，口服，每日1次。

• 合并HIV感染患者的治疗：

- 复发感染(5~10日治疗)：

◦ 无环鸟苷：每日400 mg。

◦ 泛昔洛韦：500 mg，口服，每日2次，坚持5~10日。

◦ 万乃洛韦：1000 mg，口服，每日2次。

- 每日抑制治疗：

◦ 阿昔洛韦：400~800 mg，口服，每日2~3次。

◦ 万昔洛韦：500 mg，口服，每日2次。

◦ 万乃洛韦：500 mg，口服，每日2次。

随访

■ **进一步处理**

入院指征

• 全身受累(脑炎、脑膜炎)，显著播散。

• 严重局部症状(疼痛、尿潴留)。

• 免疫系统严重受损患者。

出院指征

• 无全身受累的免疫功能患者。

• 出院咨询：

- 在前驱症状期间避免性接触，直到痊愈。

- 即使没有损伤，也要采取安全的性行为。

- 预期未来复发。如果频繁的话，考虑进行抑制治疗。

- 需要时使用止痛剂和止痒剂。

- 通过坐浴或在排尿过程中向病变处温水冲洗可缓解排尿困难和尿潴留。

转诊问题

• 新生儿感染疱疹。

• 儿童性虐待。

• 妊娠期疱疹感染。

要点和误区

• 疱疹是一种终身性感染。

• 治疗原发性感染。

• 虑患有生殖器疱疹的儿童遭受性虐待。

S

失血性休克

Theodore C. Chan 陈奇通 译

基础知识

■ **描述**

• 有效循环血量损失导致灌注不足。

• 失血超过了代偿，组织和器官灌注减少。在组织层面，灌注不足会导致氧合不足，无氧代谢，细胞死亡。

• 出血性休克是创伤所致休克中最常见的原因。

• 代偿性休克：

- 患者的生理储备可以防止生命体征发生剧烈的变化。

• 失代偿性休克：

- 丢失的循环血容量超过了患者生理储备，导致生命体征发生剧烈变化。

• 估计失血量：

- 标准体重的患者丢失总血容量的7%(70 kg的成人约有4900 ml血液)或70 ml/kg。

- 70 ml/kg×体重(kg)×丢失百分比，由此来决定出血的类型。

■ **病因**

• 创伤：钝性伤和穿刺伤。

- 腹部：

◦ 脾脏损伤。

◦ 肝脏损伤。

- 胸部：

◦ 血胸。

◦ 主动脉或大的静脉损伤。

- 骨盆：

◦ 骨盆骨折导致血管损伤。

• 血管畸形：

- 可能导致胸腔、腹腔、腹膜后出血。

- 动脉瘤：

◦ 腹主动脉瘤最常见。

◦ 心内膜炎继发细菌性动脉瘤。

- 主动脉胃瘘。

- 动静脉畸形。

• 流产：完全性，部分或者难免流产。

• 宫外孕(异位妊娠)。

• 鼻出血。

• 骨折(尤其是骨盆和长骨骨折)。

• 胃肠道出血。

• 咯血。

• 恶性肿瘤。

• 贲门黏膜撕裂。

• 前置胎盘。

• 产后出血。

• 腹膜后出血。

- 脾破裂。
- 血管损伤。

诊断

症状和体征

- Ⅰ类出血：丢失最多15%的血容量(在70 kg的患者最多丢失750 ml)。
  - 心率＜100次/分。
  - 收缩压正常。
  - 呼吸频率在14～20次/分。
  - 脉压升高或正常。
  - 轻微焦虑。
- Ⅱ类出血：丢失15%～30%的血容量(750～1 500 ml)。
  - 心动过速：心率＞100次/分。
  - 收缩压正常或者稍降低。
  - 呼吸急促：呼吸频率20～30次/分。
  - 脉压变窄。
  - 轻度焦虑。
  - 尿量稍减少。
- Ⅲ类出血：丢失30%～40%的血容量(1 500～2 000 ml)。
  - 明显心动过速：心率＞120次/分。
  - 低血压：收缩压降低。
  - 明显呼吸急促：呼吸频率30～40次/分。
  - 脉压明显变窄。
  - 精神状态明显变化：意识模糊。
  - 毛细血管充盈时间延长。
  - 尿量明显减少。
- Ⅳ类出血：出血超过40%的血容量(＞2 000 ml)：
  - 心率＞140次/分。
  - 明显低血压：收缩压降低。
  - 呼吸频率＞35次/分。
  - 脉压极窄。
  - 精神萎靡：意识模糊，嗜睡，意识丧失。
  - 无尿。
  - 皮肤湿冷。

注意

单独以收缩压作为休克状态指征，可能会导致对病情的不正确认识。

儿科注意事项

- 儿童通常具有比成人更强大的生理储备，可以保持生命体征平稳更久。
- 儿童患者对于失血产生的全身反应包括：
  - 失血量＜25%：脉搏细速和心动过速；嗜睡、易怒和意识模糊；皮肤湿冷；尿量减少/尿比重增加。
  - 失血量介于25%～40%：心动过速；意识出现明显改变；对疼痛刺激反应迟钝；四肢湿冷，发绀；尿量很少。
  - 失血量＞40%：低血压，心动过速或心动过缓；昏迷；皮肤苍白，皮温低；无尿。

妊娠注意事项

生理上产妇血容量增多，因而需要更大的丢失量才会显示出异常灌注，但这可能导致对胎儿的灌注减少。

老年人注意事项

基础疾病和药物可能会改变出血和失血时的反应。

病史

全面的健康史和既往史：

- 基础疾病、危险因素及年龄。
- 药物治疗。
- 创伤。

体格检查

- 通过全面的体格检查来决定休克的类型和估计出血的来源。
- 生命体征包括心率、呼吸及血压。
- 体温。
- 精神状态(焦虑、意识模糊、嗜睡、反应迟钝及昏迷)。
- 脉搏特征，毛细血管充盈和皮肤灌注。
- 脉压。
- 腹部检查。
- 骨盆/直肠出血检查。

基本检查

- 全面的健康史和既往史。
- 建立静脉通道。
- 血型鉴定与交叉配型。

诊断检查与说明

实验室检查

- CBC。
- 血型鉴定与交叉配型。
- 凝血功能：
  - PT、APTT。
  - INR。
- 其他手段检测组织低灌注：
  - 动脉血气分析。
  - 碱缺失。
  - 血清乳酸水平。
  - 血电解质。
- 妊娠检测。

注意

大量出血有可能仅导致血红蛋白和血细胞比容轻度降低。

影像学检查

- 胸部X线检查：
  - 血胸：
    - 钝性胸部伤。
    - 胸动静脉畸形。
- 骨盆X线检查用来发现隐匿性骨折。
- 重点关注腹部超声检查(快速检查)：
  - 腹部创伤。
  - 可能发现腹主动脉瘤。
  - 非创伤性出血。
  - 液体在墨里森袋意味着有明显的出血或腹水。
  - 阴性结果并不能排除腹腔内出血。
- 阴道超声检查：
  - 阳性妊娠试验。
  - 穹窿部液体。
  - 宫外孕。
- 腹部CT扫描(患者病情稳定)：
  - 可以发现腹腔内与腹膜后出血。
  - 腹主动脉瘤。

诊断步骤/外科

- 导尿：
  - 记录尿量。
- 鼻胃管：
  - 适用于所有的低血容量性休克，用来排除胃肠道出血。
- 诊断性腹腔灌洗：
  - 适用于B超不能发现隐匿性出血的不稳定外伤患者。
- 内镜检查：
  - 用来区分上消化道或者下消化道出血。
- 血管造影：
  - 骨盆骨折。
  - 腹膜后出血。
  - 下消化道出血。
  - 可以对动脉源性的出血实施血管栓塞术。

鉴别诊断

- 心脏压塞。
- 张力性气胸。
- 心源性休克。
- 脓毒症。
- 肾上腺皮质功能不全。
- 神经源性休克。

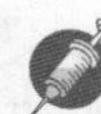

治疗

- 治疗应该在休克开始阶段就实施，同时确定潜在的出血来源。
- 治疗的目标是恢复组织和器官灌注，控制出血源头。

• “平衡”和“控制”复苏：在恢复灌注、再出血的风险和患者的个体差异三者间找到平衡：

- 钝性创伤时血压维持可能优先于降低创伤性脑损伤的风险。
- 贯通伤导致的出血，延缓盲目液体复苏，直到完全控制，可能会降低出血风险。
- 出血或复苏引起的凝血病变必须尽量减少，以减少额外出血的风险。

■ 院前

• 快速评估并转运至恰当的保健中心。

• 建立静脉通道与液体复苏是基础，在穿透性创伤的情况下，可能需要延迟液体复苏。

■ 初步稳定/治疗

• 气道与呼吸：

- 根据患者的呼吸和精神状态决定是否插管。
- 应该给予面罩吸氧，氧浓度为100%。

• 循环：

- 建立两条大口径静脉通路(16G 或者更大)。
- 必要时行中心静脉插管或静脉切开术。
- 可以考虑骨髓腔内输液。
- 液体复苏时将液体加热，使用等渗晶体液。
- 液体复苏的总量由患者对初始静脉液体推注的反应决定。

• Ⅲ级或Ⅳ级休克早期输血全血或平衡血液制品(见下文)：

- 在时间允许的情况下(通常 1 h)优先选择血型与交叉配型成功的血液。
- 血型鉴定通常 10～15 min。
- 在危及生命的情况下，可以立即给予O型血(O型 Rh 阴性血只适用于育龄妇女)。
- 1 h 内需要>4 U pRBC 或>10 U pRBC/24 h 的大量输血方案。

■ 急诊治疗/程序

• 持续心电监测。

• 禁食，卧床。

• 控制出血(加压、骨盆固定、制动)。

• 中心静脉通道可以监测 CVP，但不能影响液体复苏。

• 不断重新评估患者临床反应/恶化：

- 生命体征、精神状态及尿量。
- 根据血气分析、乳酸水平、血红蛋白/血细胞比容。
- 保持尿量达到 50 ml/h。

• 对最初液体复苏的反应是决定后续治疗的关键：

- 快速反应一般表明出血量较小(<20%)。
- 瞬态反应预示着有持续的出血或者复苏不充分；持续液体与血液管理，获取必要的研究和协商。
- 对容量复苏反应不明显或不反应预示着持续大量失血，必须尽快行血管造影或外科手术。

• 使用微波炉或取暖器加热液体(约39℃)。

• 输注全血、红细胞悬液、血小板及其他血液制品。

• 血胸时可以考虑使用自体输血装置接胸廓造口管。

• 在大量输血的患者须密切监测凝血功能。

• 根据出血性休克的原因和来源来指导专业咨询和额外程序(手术)。

儿科注意事项

• 在尝试外周通路失败 1～2 次后，可以考虑骨髓腔内输液。

• 维持儿童尿量 1 ml/(kg·h)，婴儿为 2 ml/(kg·h)。

妊娠注意事项

优化灌注和对孕妇的治疗就是对胎儿最好的选择。

■ 药物治疗

一线用药

• 静脉给药：

- 晶体液：生理盐水或者乳酸林格液。
- 成人：1～2 L 单次快注。
- 小儿：20 ml/kg 单次快注。
  ◦ 根据临床反应/恶化进行再评估。

• 血液制品：血型，交叉配型，O型 Rh 阳性或阴性。

- O型 Rh 阴性血只适用于育龄妇女。
- 成人：初始 4～6 U。
- 小儿：10 ml/kg。

二线用药

• 其他血液制品：

- 血小板。
- 凝血因子，如新鲜冰冻血浆、冷沉淀。

• 抗纤维蛋白溶解药物，基于血红蛋白的氧携带体，全氟化碳。

- 正在研究中，但尚未证明有疗效。

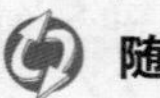 随访

■ 进一步处理

入院指征

所有出血的患者都应得到恰当的医学处置。

出院指征

N/A。

■ 随访建议

N/A。

要点和误区

• 出血性休克的分级和出血量可以通过生命体征和细致的体格检查发现。

• 液体复苏时须在恢复器官灌注和再出血的风险之间进行衡量。

• 机体对液体复苏的反应可以指导后续的治疗。

虱病 Pediculosis

Andrew B. Ziller 王虑 译

 基础知识

■ 描述

• 寄生在宿主的有机体侵染宿主。

• 无痛性叮咬。

• 宿主的症状和体征取决于其在喂食时唾液和注射抗凝剂的反应。

• 通过直接接触和污染物传播。

• 头虱由头和头接触传播：

- 梳子。
- 枕头。
- 帽子。

• 头虱在儿童和女性中常见。
• 阴虱通过性接触传播。
• 以人为宿主的寄生虫在离开宿主 7～10 日后无法再存活。

■ 病因

被感染：
• 头虱：
- 最常见。
- 群体生活。
• 体虱：
- 和贫困、卫生条件差和过度拥挤人群生活有关。
- 存在于衣服里后为喂食转移到人体。
- 离开人体可以存活 30 日。
- 和床虱有关。
• 阴虱。

儿科注意事项

阴虱提示可能有儿童性虐。

诊断

■ 症状和体征

病史

• 头虱：
- 头皮屑。
- 瘙痒。
- 常常无症状。
• 体虱：
- 瘙痒。
- 表皮脱落，皮带处或衣服缝线处明显。
• 阴虱：
- 剧烈瘙痒，尤其在夜晚。

体格检查

• 检查头发有无虱子和卵。
- 虫卵黏合于发干处不容易移出。
- 头虱和体虱感染可以通过虫卵尺寸的不同和头发的管型区分。
- 空的虫卵不能作为活动性感染的证据。
• 头皮和颈后红斑、脱皮、顽固的丘疹：
- 会导致脓皮病、颈后淋巴结肿大和细菌反复感染。
• 体虱只有在非常严重的感染才见到，通过在衣服接缝处发现虫卵确诊：
- 颈部和躯干线性表皮脱落。
- 脓或血的污斑在衣服上。
• 阴虱：
- 突然出现的潮红色风团。
- 感染儿童的睫毛和头皮。
- 特征性的蓝色斑疹偶尔会出现在躯干和股骨。
- 喜欢在会阴区活动。
- 腹股沟腺病。

■ 基本检查

• 详细的病史和仔细的体格检查是对儿童伤情做出全面评估必需的工作。
• 一般防范措施。

■ 诊断检查与说明

实验室检查

• 虫卵可以在低倍显微镜顺着发干发现，大小<1 mm：
- 伍德灯下可见荧光。
- 成熟虱 3～4 mm 长。
- 阴虱约 1 mm 长但比头虱和体虱宽。

影像学检查

没有影像学检查提示。

■ 鉴别诊断

• 疥疮。
• 接触或过敏性皮炎。
• 脂溢性皮炎。
• 床虱(臭虫科)。

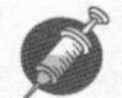

治疗

■ 院前

注意
保持一般的防护措施。

■ 初步稳定/治疗

对一般患者不需要。

■ 急诊治疗/程序

• 口服抗组胺药和局部用类固醇类药对虱感染引起的瘙痒症有一定作用。
• 头虱：
- 局部抗组胺类药物：
◦ 1%苄氯菊酯润丝膏是较理想的药物，毒性低、价格便宜并对虱卵有杀灭效果，但耐药性也越来越常见。
◦ 除虫菊酯毒性也低，效果不佳。
- 如果又发现虱子或虫卵需再使用药物 7～10 日。
- 用细密齿的梳子清除虫卵。
- 对同房间的所有人检查，以确保没有传染其他人。
- 更换衣服并机洗烘干所有衣服、床单、毛巾和帽子等：
◦ 吸尘器清洁地板和家具。
◦ 用热水清洗头梳 10～20 min 或用灭虱药清洗外套 15 min。
- 高于 55 ℃热水能杀死虫卵和虱子。
• 体虱：
- 清洗衣服和床上用品并用机器热烘干。
- 使用灭虱药膏或洗液从下颌一直涂抹清洗到足趾。
• 阴虱：
- 局部外用灭虱药膏涂抹胸部、腋窝和腹股沟等有毛发的部位。
- 使用细密齿的梳子清除虫卵。
- 患者的性伴侣同时接受治疗。
- 清洗衣服和床上用品并用机器热烘干。
- 睫毛处受累使用灭虱药膏涂抹每日 2 次持续 9 日。

■ 药物治疗

一线用药

• 止痒剂：
- 苯海拉明：25～50 mg，口服(儿童：5 mg/kg，每日 1 次)，q6 h。
- 羟嗪：25 mg，口服，q8 h(儿童：12.5 mg/剂，q6 h)。
• 灭虱药：
- 1%苄氯菊酯润丝膏：涂抹头皮头发，10 min 后冲洗掉；如果需要，7～10 日后再用一次。
- 除虫菊酯/胡椒基丁醚：涂抹头皮头发，10 min 后冲洗掉；如果需要，7～10 日后再冲洗用一次；注意使用的患者不能对豚草属过敏。
- 5%苯甲醇洗液：涂抹头皮头发，10 min 后冲洗掉；7 日后再用一次。
- 1%氧化汞眼膏：用于眼睑虱子感染，每日 4 次，连续使用 14 日。

二线用药

• 灭虱剂：
- 0.5%伊维菌素洗剂：涂抹头皮头发，10 min 后冲洗掉。
- 0.9%多杀菌素悬乎剂：涂抹头皮头发，10 min 后冲洗掉，如果需要 7 日后再用一次。
- 伊维菌素片：200～400 μg/kg 口服一次；7～10 日后再服用一次。

S

◦ 在一线灭虱药效果不佳或不能耐受时使用。

• 抗组胺剂：

- 西替利嗪：年龄＞12 岁，5～10 mg 口服(6～11 岁，5～10 mg 口服；2～5 岁，2.5 mg 口服)，每日 1 次。

妊娠注意事项

• 苄氯菊酯是 B 级，哺乳期使用可能是安全的。

• 除虫菊酯是 C 级，哺乳期使用可能是安全的。

• 苯甲醇洗液是 B 级(但需要看说明书)，哺乳期使用安全否还不清楚。

• 伊维菌素是 C 级，哺乳期使用安全否还不清楚。

• 多杀菌素是 B 级(但需要看说明书)，妊娠期使用安全否还不清楚。

随访

进一步处理

入院指征

广泛的细菌多重感染，全身过敏反应伴有心肺功能不佳的。

出院指征

• 轻中度虱感染，且没有严重的多重感染和全身过敏反应。

• 儿童经过最初治疗，后续治疗在 7～10 日后，可以先出院回学校。

• 阴虱常伴有其他性传播疾病，建议仔细体检。

随访建议

• 治疗成功后病情的再评估是有必要的。

• 对于儿童患者适度的社会服务和患者管理是需要的。

要点和误区

• 诊断可以根据直接观察病情做出。

• 大部分外用药在用过后，需要在 7～10 日后再用一次，因为一些未孵化的虫卵未被杀死。

• 衣服和床上用品必须清洗并热风烘干以彻底去除感染源。

• 林丹已不再为推荐用药。

• 对苄氯菊酯和除虫菊酯耐药情况越来越多见。

- 二线用药价格更昂贵。

S

湿疹/特应性皮炎 Eczema/Atopic Dermatitis

James A. Nelson 姜颢 译

基础知识

描述

• 特应性皮炎是湿疹的最常见的原因，往往作为同义术语：

- 与过敏性疾病(如哮喘和过敏性鼻炎)相关。

• 湿疹的字面意思是“煮沸”，指的是海绵层水肿、微泡形成和破裂的过程，留下红斑、水肿、结痂和渗出。

• 瘙痒是高度特征性的：

- 患者刮擦皮肤破裂，致渗出、结痂。

- 长期导致表皮增生和角化过度。

• 90％的患者有金黄色葡萄球菌定植，且易出现二重感染。

危险因素

遗传学

• 过敏家族史(哮喘、过敏性鼻炎)。

• 中间丝蛋白是表皮屏障的组成部分，突变与之密切相关。

病因

特应性皮炎是由于皮肤的完整性不足，外来物质进入和触发免疫反应。

诊断

症状与体征

病史

• 瘙痒和典型皮疹(红斑、丘疹、浆液性渗出)是疾病诊断的关键。

• 英国诊断标准敏感性为 95％，特异性为 97％，包含瘙痒和下述特点中的 3 项：

- 发病年龄小于 2 岁。

- 过敏史(哮喘、过敏性鼻炎)。

- 皮肤干燥史。

- 病史是屈侧分布。

- 此次就诊为屈侧皮炎。

体格检查

位于创伤或运动区域(如手、足和屈侧区域)的急性皮炎：

• 表皮损害：

- 皮肤干燥。

- 漏液。

- 渗出。

- 最后结痂。

• 炎症：

- 红色斑丘疹。

- 水肿。

• 抓挠导致。

- 脱落。

- 开裂。

• 慢性病变：

- 苔藓化。

- 角化过度。

• 特殊表现：

- 手或足皮炎。

- 乳头湿疹。

- 唇炎。

- 丹尼-摩根眶下皱襞。

- 眼眶发黑。

- 面部苍白或面部红斑。

- 毛囊突显。

儿科注意事项

• 婴幼儿患者可见分布于伸肌面及头面部。

• 70％的病例在生命的第一个 5 年期间开始。

• 只有 10％的病例在成年期开始。

• 30％的特应性皮炎儿童发展成哮喘，35％发展成过敏性鼻炎。

基本检查

病史与体格检查。

诊断检查与说明

实验室检查

• 临床诊断。

- IgE 通常升高，但一般不需要检测。

诊断步骤/外科

一般备用于急诊外的环境：

- 放射过敏原吸附试验(RAST)有时用于鉴别过敏性诱因。
- 如怀疑接触性皮炎，则进行斑贴测试。

鉴别诊断

- 接触性皮炎。
- 脂溢性皮炎。
- 神经性皮炎(慢性单纯性苔藓)。
- 银屑病。
- 出汗障碍。
- 鱼鳞癣。
- 疥疮。
- 皮肤淋巴瘤。

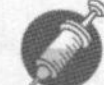

治疗

急诊治疗/程序

- 日常教育：
  - 温水泡澡，尽量不要用热水。
    - 这可以暂时使皮肤湿化。
  - 在洗澡后立即使用保湿剂。
  - 尽量使用含有亲脂成分和可以形成肌肤表面屏障的药膏或乳剂。
  - 洗涤剂可能造成皮肤干燥。
  - 尽量避免碱性或干性肥皂。
- 细菌感染：头孢氨苄、头孢唑林。
  - 考虑耐甲氧西林金黄色葡萄球菌(MRSA)。

药物治疗

- 优色林霜：适用于受影响区域，每日 2 次：
  - 含有羊毛脂醇。
- 头孢氨苄：500 mg[儿童：25～100 mg/(kg·24 h)]，口服，q6 h。
- 苯海拉明：25～50 mg[儿童：5 mg/(kg·24 h)]，口服或静推，q6 h。
- 优色林霜：适用于受影响区域，每日 2 次：
  - 含有羊毛脂醇。
- 0.05%醋酸氟轻松软膏：适用于暴发期间的身体受影响区域(高效力)，每日 2 次。
- 2.5%氢化可的松软膏：适用于暴发期间的身体、面部受影响区域(低效力)，每日 2 次。
- 羟嗪：25～100 mg[儿童：2 mg/(kg·24 h)]，口服，q4～6 h。
- 1%吡美莫司乳膏：适用于暴发期间的受影响区域(2 岁以上儿童)，每日 2 次。
- 0.1%他克莫司软膏(2 岁以上儿童：0.03%)：适用于暴发期间的受影响区域，每日 2 次。
- 0.1%曲安奈德软膏：适用于暴发期间的受影响区域(中等效力)，每日 2 次。

一线用药

- 日常宣教关于泡澡湿化皮肤、使用药膏保湿。
- 2.5%氢化可的松软膏：适用于暴发期间的身体、面部受影响区域(低效力)，每日 2 次。
- 优色林软膏：适用于受影响区域，每日 2 次。

二线用药

- 0.1%曲安奈德软膏：适用于暴发期间的身体受影响区域(中等效力)，每日 2 次：
  - 避免用于面部和眼睑。
- 0.05%醋酸氟轻松软膏：适用于暴发期间的身体受影响区域(高效力)：
  - 避免用于面部和眼睑。
- 0.1%他克莫司软膏(2 岁以上儿童：0.03%)：适用于暴发期间的受影响区域，每日 2 次：
  - 可以用在面部。
- 1%吡美莫司乳膏：适用于暴发期间的受影响区域(2 岁以上儿童)，每日 2 次：
  - 可以用在面部。

随访

进一步处理

转诊问题

疑难病例转诊至皮肤科。

随访建议

- 应告诫患者治疗的不良后果：
  - 高效力的类固醇会导致皮肤变薄。
  - 他克莫司和吡美莫司在治疗第 1 周造成刺痛的感觉。长期使用可增加患癌症的风险。

要点和误区

- 不同部位的各异表现有时往往导致临床医师误诊。
- 有严重皮疹瘙痒的患者应考虑。
- 乳液具有较低的脂肪含量，会导致干燥。
  - 厚的霜或膏是首选。
- 在面部或眼睑不要用醋酸或醋酸氟轻松。

S

史-约综合征 Stevens-Johnson Syndrome

Michael J. Bono　江伟伟　李文放 译

基础知识

描述

- 史-约综合征(Stevens-Johnson 综合征，SJS)是一种损害皮肤黏膜，导致其坏死和表皮剥脱的皮肤疾病，又称重症多形性红斑。
- SJS 可能是药物诱发或与感染相关，也可以是特发的：
  - <10%的体表面积(BSA)起疱。
  - 95%的患者有黏膜病变：
    - 通常在 2 个或更多的部位。
  - 85%有球结膜病变。
  - 常常涉及面部、颈部和躯干部的损伤，在数小时至数日内融合。
- 与中毒性表皮坏死松解症(TEN)相关，但被认为是不同于多形红斑(EM)的独特疾病：
  - SJS：<10%的体表面积。
  - SJS-TEN 重叠综合征：10%～30%的体表面积。
  - TEN：>30%的体表面积，会影响高达 100%的体表面积。
- 发病年龄是任何年龄段，但最常见于 40 岁以上的成人。
- 女性多见，男女比例为 2∶1。

病因

- 最常见的原因包括药物和感染：
  - 皮肤损伤的病理学机制尚未完全明确。
  - 皮肤损伤被认为是由细胞毒性 T 淋巴细

胞和单核细胞介导的,它们作用于角质(与药物有关的),产生抗原:
◦ 导致大片坏死。
- 药物导致了绝大多数的 SJS,通常在治疗开始后的前 8 周。
- 活化的单核细胞的细胞因子可能与细胞破坏和全身表现有关。
• 药物:
- 抗生素(如青霉素、磺胺类药物)。
- 抗惊厥药(苯妥英钠、苯巴比妥、卡马西平、拉莫三嗪等)。
- 非甾体抗炎药。
- 抗肿瘤药(沙利度胺、三苯氧胺及其他)。
- 别嘌醇。
• 感染:
- 肺炎支原体。
- 单纯疱疹。
- 病毒感染。

诊断

S

症状和体征

病史

• 药物暴露史或发热性疾病史。
• 前驱症状:
- 通常在发生皮肤损伤前 1～3 日。
- 发热。
- 头痛。
- 全身不适。
- 上呼吸道感染(URI)症状。
- 关节炎、关节痛和肌痛在黏膜病变之前。
• 皮肤:轻度至中度皮肤压痛,继而出现皮肤疼痛、灼热感和感觉异常。
• 眼睛:结膜灼烧感或瘙痒。
• 黏膜:排尿痛苦,吞咽痛苦。
• 药物暴露通常在症状出现之前 2 周:
- 再次暴露可能导致 48 h 内出现症状。
• 风险因素包括人类免疫缺陷病毒(HIV)、遗传因素、病毒感染和基础免疫疾病。

体格检查

• 皮疹:
- 靶样病变,红斑易于于合并紫癜中心合并。
- 可能是无皮疹的弥漫性红斑。
- 病变往往开始于面部和胸部,然后扩散;通常是对称的。
- 皮肤触感很软。
- 水泡和大疱会随着疾病的进展而形成。
- Nikolsky 征:对未受累部位的皮肤稍加侧向压力即可导致皮肤延展和塌陷。
- Asboe-Hansen 征:"大疱扩散征"是大疱在直接压力下的展两侧延伸。
- 类似于广泛的热损伤。
• 黏膜:
- 90%会有黏膜受累。
- 可能在皮肤损害之后或之前。
- 口腔、咽部、气管、生殖器、尿道或肛门的注入性侵蚀,可能形成假膜。
- 疼痛的口腔病变(口炎、黏膜炎)可能导致经口摄食减少和眼睛脱水:
• 眼睛:
- 80%的人会累及眼睛。
- 伴有脓性分泌物的严重结膜炎。
- 角膜溃疡常见。
- 可发生前葡萄膜炎或全眼炎。
- 可形成假膜。
- 评估眼部病变严重程度的分级标准,包括是否存在结膜炎、角膜或结膜缺损和假膜形成。

基本检查

详细的病史和体格检查,注意黏膜、大疱情况及可能的病因。

诊断检查与说明

实验室检查

• 电解质。
• 肝酶可轻度升高。
• 血常规:贫血和淋巴细胞减少症很常见。
• 尿酸可能轻度升高。
• 红细胞沉降率(ESR)、C 反应蛋白(CRP)。
• 病原学培养:伤口、血液和黏膜区域应进行细菌和真菌培养。
• 儿童患者:应获得肺炎支原体的聚合酶链反应和血清学证据。

影像学检查

如果考虑肺炎,行胸部 X 线平片。

诊断步骤/外科

损伤和黏膜的皮肤活组织检查显示整个表皮层的坏死,基底膜上的表皮分裂。

鉴别诊断

• SJS:＜10%的体表面积。
• SJS-TEN 综合征:体表面积的 10%～30%皮肤分离加广泛的斑块或平坦的非典型靶病变。
• TEN:皮肤脱离＞体表面积的 30%及广泛的斑块或平坦的非典型目标。
• EM。
• 热烧伤。
• 光毒性反应。
• 剥脱性皮炎。
• 脓疱疹药疹。
• 大疱性药疹。
• 副肿瘤性天疱疮。
• 骨髓移植患者中排斥反应。
• 毒性休克综合征。
• 葡萄球菌烫伤样皮肤综合征。

儿科注意事项

葡萄球菌性烫伤样皮肤综合征在小儿严重起疱性皮肤黏膜病的鉴别诊断中的应用。

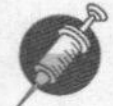

治疗

院前

• ABC 管理。
• 一般预防措施。
• 建立静脉通路。
• 如果身体表面超过 30%,送至烧伤中心。

初步稳定/治疗

• 气管插管和通气支持可能需要用于呼吸衰竭(更常见的是与 TEN 相关)。
• 静脉输液。

急诊治疗/程序

• 停用与病情有冲突的药物。
• 补液:
- 液体损失可能很大,SJS 应按烧伤患者的补液方式处理。
• 认识并治疗潜在感染:
- 脓毒症是导致死亡的主要原因,通常来自革兰阴性肺炎。
- 二次感染的皮肤损伤可以用水疱清创、压迫和全身抗生素治疗。
- 皮肤病变的感染宜采用良好的无菌伤口护理、非黏附性纱布敷料或生物合成皮肤替代品进行治疗。
- 避免全身性使用抗生素。
- 金黄色葡萄球菌、铜绿假单胞菌和肠杆菌感染是死亡的主要原因。
• 不推荐预防性使用抗生素。
• 激素使用存在争议且尚无证据表明可以收获益。
• 如果给予全身性激素,可能需要预防性应用抗生素。
• 静脉注射免疫球蛋白可能有用。
• 环孢素可能有效,因其可抑制 T 细胞激活。

- 其他疗法：血浆置换和肿瘤坏死因子抑制剂也有好处，但尚需大样本的研究。
- 轻度全身症状可以用对乙酰氨基酚或非甾体抗炎药治疗，只要它们不是皮肤黏膜反应引起的。
- 黏膜损伤极其痛苦，可能需要肠胃外镇痛药。
- 应该清创大面积的大疱，理想的是在烧伤部位。
- 绝大多 SJS 患者应入住 ICU 或烧伤科。
  - 皮肤受累有限的 SJS 患者应入院治疗，但不需要烧伤科或 ICU。
  - 中度至广泛皮肤或黏膜受累的 SJS 患者在进入烧伤科或 ICU 治疗可获得更好的预后。

■ **药物治疗**

- 对乙酰氨基酚：500 mg，口服，q4～6 h（儿童：10～15 mg/kg；不超过 5 次/24 h）：不要超过 4 g/24 h。
- 阿昔洛韦：5～10 mg/kg，静脉滴注，q8 h（用于单纯疱疹病毒感染）。
- 布洛芬：300～800 mg，口服（儿童：5～10 mg/kg）。
- 硫酸吗啡：0.1 mg/kg，静脉推注。

一线用药

- 补液。
- 治疗潜在的病因。
- 治疗继发感染。
- 镇痛。

二线用药

- 静脉使用免疫球蛋白。
- 激素。

随访

■ **进一步处理**

入院指征

- 绝大多 SJS 患者应入住重症监护室或烧伤科病房。
  - 皮肤受累有限的 SJS 患者应入院治疗，但不需要烧伤科或 ICU。
- 中度至广泛皮肤或黏膜受累的 SJS 患者在进入烧伤病房/ICU 治疗可获得更好的预后。
- 患有广泛表皮脱落的患者应该进入烧伤科或专门的 ICU。

出院指征

EM 未成年患者可以及时适当的随访。如果有眼部、泌尿生殖道或口腔受累，患者可能需要转诊至眼科、泌尿科、妇科或肠胃科。

转诊问题

必须让患者了解可能的药物（及其类别），并且绝不能再次对其使用。

■ **随访建议**

随访皮肤科。

要点和误区

- SJS 可能会像流行病一样开始，病灶出现在前驱症状后的 1～3 日。
- 诊断需临床和活检支持。
- 肺炎支原体和单纯疱疹是儿童比成人更常见的诱因。

S

十二指肠损伤

Christanne H. Coffey 姜颢 张连东 译

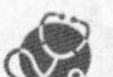

基础知识

■ **描述**

- 十二指肠的特点。
  - 长度 12 in（20～30 cm）。
  - C 形。
  - 从幽门至屈氏韧带。
  - 分为 4 部分：
    - 处于腹膜后的后 3 段与第 1 段远端相连。
  - 大部分位于第 1～3 腰椎。
  - 第 2 段最容易受伤。
- 损伤类型：
  - 十二指肠壁内血肿。
  - 肠壁穿孔。
  - 出血，包括腹膜后。
  - 挤压。
- 十二指肠损伤的发生率为外伤性腹部损伤的 3%～5%。
- 穿透性创伤约占十二指肠损伤的 75%。
  - 死亡率在 13%～28%。
  - 与出血相关。
- 由于力量更大损伤，闭合性十二指肠损伤具有更高的死亡率，并且位置在腹膜后往往延误诊断：
  - 死亡率在 15%～20%。
  - 最后死亡通常由于脓毒症。

儿科注意事项

- 多数继发于娱乐的损伤（例如，由于自行车车把导致受伤）。
- 十二指肠壁内血肿可发生在非意外创伤：
  - 如有可疑，须立即转介至适当的儿童保护机构。
- 在儿童中，血肿最常见于十二指肠的第 1 段。

妊娠注意事项

- 腹膜后出血多见因盆腔和腹部血管增加。
- 大子宫可保护肠道免受损伤。
- 妊娠时腹膜刺激反应迟钝，因此更应提高警惕。

■ **病因**

- 钝性创伤：
  - 剪切应变：在连接点处的突然加速/减速（常见快速减速引起腹膜后损伤）。
  - 拉伸应变：直接压缩或拉伸组织（方向盘伤、击打或车把损伤）。
- 穿透性创伤：
  - 最常见的伤害原因。
  - 空洞性创面，可引起感染。

诊断

■ **症状和体征**

- 主诉可能只有不明确的腹部、腰部和背部疼痛。
- 高位消化道梗阻可见于十二指肠血肿。

病史

腹部穿透性或钝性损伤。

体格检查

- 腹膜后：常细微，右上腹疼痛、恶心、呕吐、心动过速、发热。
- 腹腔：腹膜炎。
- 腹部瘀斑。

▪ 基本检查

- 包括淀粉酶等基础实验室检查。
- 腹部 CT。
- 如果病情不稳定，高度怀疑本病时行诊断性腹腔灌洗(DPL)或剖腹探查。

▪ 诊断检查与说明

实验室检查

- 实验室检查正常不能排除受伤的可能。
- 50%十二指肠损伤患者的血清淀粉酶升高。
- 逐渐增多白细胞可能提示未诊断的十二指肠损伤。

影像学检查

- CT，口服和静脉注射造影剂对比：
  - 最佳的影像学诊断检查，显示少量腹膜后气体和造影剂外渗。
  - 十二指肠壁增厚，周围积液，损伤附近的"哨兵血块"。
  - 十二指肠壁香肠状肿胀，提示血肿。
- 用超声检查集中评估外伤(FAST)：
  - 确认腹腔积血。
  - 对十二指肠损伤不可靠。
  - 1/3 腹膜后损伤可用一般性 FAST。
- 立位胸部和腹部 X 线平片：
  - 腹腔内气体。
  - 腹膜后气体。
  - 胆管内气体。
  - 脊柱右侧侧弯。
  - 腰大肌阴影缺失。
  - 右肾气体。
  - 鼻胃管注入空气可更清楚地显示腹膜后气体。
  - 无泄漏壁内血肿可能有螺旋弹簧样外观。

诊断步骤/外科

- 当其他诊断测试是阴性，但仍然高度怀疑时，腹部探查是最终的诊断性检查。
- DPL：
  - 血液、胆汁或肠内容物通常呈阳性。
  - 阴性灌洗结果不排除损伤(65%假阴性率)。

▪ 鉴别诊断

- 空腹器官损伤(胃、小肠和大肠)。
- 肝脏和胆管损伤。
- 血管损伤(主动脉和肠系膜动脉，以及静脉损伤)。
- 十二指肠手术或损伤修补术的术后并发症，如感染、缝合线撕裂等。

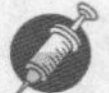

治疗

▪ 院前

- 遵循创伤救治方案。
- 重要的是要有院前急救人员提供受伤途径的明确描述和运送至合适的场所。

▪ 初步稳定/治疗

- 根据需要进行气道管理，液体复苏。
- 如果患者存在低血压，用温热的生理盐水或乳酸林格液积极补液；按指示输液体。
- 如果患者病情不稳定可能需要中心静脉置管。
- 早期创伤外科会诊。
- 可能需鼻胃管减压。

▪ 急诊治疗/程序

- 对穿透性伤口给予破伤风和抗生素预防。
- 低级别(Ⅰ级或Ⅱ级)闭合性十二指肠损伤通常保守治疗，10%失败。
- 决定性的治疗包括剖腹探查十二指肠损伤(建议Ⅲ级及以上，穿透性创伤)。
- 穿孔患者给予广谱抗生素预防脓毒症。

▪ 药物治疗

- 术前使用单一广谱抗生素治疗十二指肠穿透性损伤。
- 如果在剖腹探查时发现空腔内脏穿孔，预防性使用抗生素可持续至 24 h。
- 必要时使用止痛药。
- 必要时使用止吐药。

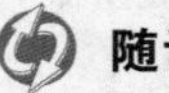

随访

▪ 进一步处理

入院指征

- 所有十二指肠损伤患者均需入院行手术治疗。
- 不需要立即手术的十二指肠小血肿，可能需要鼻胃管减压防止梗阻(大于 7 日)，同时观察血肿扩大或血肿破裂的可能。

出院指征

- 没有确定外伤性十二指肠损伤的患者应从急诊室出院。
- 并发症：腹腔内脓肿、十二指肠瘘、胰瘘、创伤后胰腺炎、脓毒症。

转诊问题

- 美国创伤外科协会十二指肠器官损伤量表(DIS)：

分级	十二指肠损伤描述
Ⅰ	血肿：单一部位 或裂伤：局部增厚，无穿孔
Ⅱ	血肿：大于 1 个部位 或裂伤：撕裂小于 50%圆周，没有胆管损伤
Ⅲ	只有裂伤： - 破坏 50%～75%的周长(D2) - 破坏 50%～100%的周长(D1、D3、D4)
Ⅳ	只有裂伤： - 破坏大于 75%的周长(D2) - 涉及壶腹或胆总管远端
Ⅴ	裂伤：大量破坏胰十二指肠吻合部或血管，十二指肠断流

D1～D4，十二指肠 1～4 段。

- 绝大多数伤害等级为Ⅱ级或Ⅲ级。
- 初期手术缝合 80%。

▪ 随访建议

- 所有诊断为十二指肠损伤的患者应入院。
- 如果诊断试验是阴性的，建议初级保健医师 24～48 h 随诊。
- 饮食：无渣流质，耐受为前提。

要点和误区

- 显著的发病率和死亡率，以及误诊或漏诊。
- 定位在腹膜后时体格检查可被误导。
- 诊断检查阴性仍持续高度怀疑时，请外科会诊。

S

食管创伤 Esophageal Injuries

Susan E. Dufel · Anumeha Singh 单怡 译

基础知识

描述

- 成人食管长度为 25～30 cm，胸膜腔内邻近纵隔。
- 其起于咽后方的咽喉部，相当于环状软骨水平。
- 食管两侧裂隙状结构为梨状隐窝：
  - 易滞留异物。
- 食管狭窄处：
  - 环状咽肌处（食管括约肌上方）。
  - 左主支气管与动脉弓的交叉点。
  - 胃食管连接处（食管括约肌下方）。
  - 病变部位（肿瘤、食管蹼或 Schatzki 环）。
- 食管上 1/3 为横纹肌：
  - 启动吞咽。
- 食管中 1/3 由横纹肌及平滑肌组成。
- 食管远端 1/3 为平滑肌。
- 食管固定，但可受其他组织挤压移位：
  - 甲状腺肿。
  - 增大的心房。
  - 纵隔占位性病变。

病因

机制

- 外力或外因（30%）：
  - 穿透性损伤：导致撕裂：
    - 刺伤。
    - 火器伤。
  - 穿孔性损伤：
    - 外物直接穿透。
    - 压力性坏死。
    - 化学性坏死。
    - 选择性的组织消融致放射性坏死。
    - 器械损伤。
  - 钝挫伤：机动车事故。
- 内力或内因：
  - 摄入腐蚀剂/灼伤：
    - pH＜2 的酸性物，pH＞12 的碱性物。
    - 碱性物质（42%）：液化坏死引起灼伤、气道水肿或狭窄。
    - 酸性物质（32%）：凝固性坏死、热损伤及脱水等引起穿孔、溃疡及感染，相比碱性物质更易于穿孔。
    - 氯漂白剂（26%）：黏膜水肿、表面红斑。
  - 感染：
    - 病毒（巨细胞病毒、人乳头状瘤病毒及单纯疱疹病毒）或免疫功能缺陷患者真菌感染。
  - 药物：
    - 较少见，有部分病例报道；阿仑膦酸钠、多四环素、非甾体抗炎药；吗替麦考酚酯；可能引起食管腐蚀或食管炎。
  - 吞入异物：
    - 食物块的挤压。
    - 硬币、骨块、纽扣、弹珠、大头针、纽扣电池。
  - 最常见的是肉块。
- 成人：囚犯、精神病人、中毒患者或无牙的患者。
- 医源性损伤（55%）：
  - 器械所致的继发性穿孔，最常见为内镜。
- 急诊室最常见的是经鼻气管插管/鼻胃管（NG）。
- 胃内压升高（15%）：
  - 胸腹腔压力差过大：
    - 可能导致撕裂或穿孔。
  - 马-魏综合征：
    - 远端食管黏膜纵行撕裂伴出血。
  - 布哈综合征：
    - 自发性食管破裂。
    - 远端食管全层破裂。
    - 常见于饮酒或暴食后呕吐。

儿科注意事项

- 异物：
  - 占吞咽异物的 75%～80%。
  - 常见于 18～48 个月的婴幼儿。
  - 通常嵌顿于食管上括约肌。
  - 穿孔。
  - 医源性常见于放置鼻胃管、食管狭窄扩张术、气管插管术。
- 腐蚀物摄入：
  - 更常见于 5 岁以下儿童。
  - 如果强碱性的纽扣电池进入食管 4～6 h 需取出。
  - 美国毒物控制中心协会发布安全警告，单独包装的衣物碗碟洗涤剂常导致腐蚀物摄入。

诊断

症状和体征

全身症状

- 吞咽困难：难以吞咽。
- 吞咽痛：吞咽时疼痛。
- 胸痛：类似心绞痛，常为严重持续的胸膜炎性疼痛。
- 声音嘶哑。
- 呼吸困难。
- 撕裂或者穿孔：
  - 出血。
  - 呕血。
- 摄入异物：
  - 大量流涎。
  - 窒息、恶心、呕吐、喘鸣或喘息。
  - 无法进食水。
- 腐蚀物摄入：
  - 口腔疼痛。
  - 腹痛。
  - 呕吐。
  - 流涎。

病史

- 摄入史（种类、时间、数量）。
- 迟发性呕吐的病史。
- 进食后无法吞咽、喉部异物感的病史。
- 穿透性损伤史。
- 肿瘤治疗史。

体格检查

- 撕裂或穿孔：
  - 颈根部皮下气肿。
  - 哈曼征：
    - 存在纵隔气肿时，可听到与心跳一致的噼啪音。
  - 休克。
  - 败血症。
  - 腹膜炎。
- 穿透性创伤：
  - 涉及颈部、胸部或者腹部的损伤。
    - 最常见于气道。
    - 与穿透伤、钝挫伤有关。
- 腐蚀物摄入：
  - 气道水肿引起喘鸣。
  - 口腔灼伤。

基本检查

高度警惕及早期诊断为关键：

- 24 h 内修补穿孔死亡率可小于 5%。如果延误，死亡率升高至 75%。
- 摄入腐蚀剂后早期内镜处理。
- 胸部、颈椎侧位 X 线片。

S

■ 诊断检查与说明

实验室检查

• 胃肠道出血患者行全血细胞检查。
• 存在或可疑大量出血患者应行交叉配血。
• 凝血功能检查。
• 持续呕吐或异物过久残留的患者应查电解质。
• 摄入酸性物患者应行动脉血气分析。

影像学检查

• 异物或穿孔行胸部 X 线检查：
- 纵隔气肿。
- 纵隔增宽。
- 气胸。
- 胸腔积液。
• 异物或穿孔行颈部侧位片检查：
- 咽后气体或液体。
- 颈部气肿。
• 应用纤维鼻咽内镜取出异物。
• 异物或可疑穿孔时行食管 X 线检查。
- 10%～25%假阴性。
- 如可能穿孔，目前首选水溶性造影剂(泛影葡胺)。
- 食管钡剂检查可能限制之后的内镜检查的清晰度。
◦ 若钡剂进入纵隔可加重刺激。
- 水溶性造影剂提供更好的能见度：
◦ 若造影剂进入纵隔刺激相对较小。
◦ 如误吸可能导致化学性肺炎。
- 非离子造影剂可能是最安全的，但相对昂贵。
• 应用内镜判断可疑穿孔、腐蚀物摄入及食管内异物取出。
- 腐蚀物摄入损伤的严重程度分级。
◦ 一度：表浅黏膜损害，局灶或弥散，红斑，水肿脱落，不留瘢痕。
◦ 二度：黏膜及黏膜下损害，溃疡及水疱，肉芽组织及瘢痕形成，狭窄可能。
◦ 三度：透壁性损害，深溃疡，黑色斑点及食管壁穿孔。
• 口服稀释的造影剂后行 CT 扫描可能有助于食管穿孔的诊断。

■ 鉴别诊断

• 肺部：
- 气管损伤。
- 气胸。
- 气道异物
• 心血管：
- 心肌梗死。
- 主动脉夹层。
- 自发性纵隔气肿。
• 其他食管急症：
- 消化性狭窄。
- 食管肿瘤。
- 下食管括约肌环(Schatzki's Ring)。
- 憩室。
- 贲门痉挛。
- 弥漫性食管疼痛。
- 胡桃夹食管。
- 胃食管反流。
- 食管炎：
◦ 尤其是四环素类抗生素所致的食管炎。

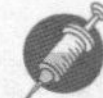

治疗

■ 院前

注意

• 胸痛需与心脏疾病鉴别。
• 气道保护，反复吸除分泌物。
• 如患者出现低血压、呕吐或呕血，需静脉补充晶体液。
• 镇痛。
• 应避免使用中和剂处理腐蚀物摄入，以免可能加重损伤。
• 摄入腐蚀物患者避免反复大量口服补液，以免呕吐。
• 避免接触嫩肉剂，因为可能造成严重食管炎。

■ 初步稳定/治疗

• 必要时气道管理及复苏。
• 建立静脉通路，监测。
• 穿透性颈部及胸部损伤患者应尽早行气管插管。
• 反复吸除分泌物。
• 补液。

■ 急诊治疗/程序

• 异物/食物压迫：
- 80%自行通过食管，20%需要内镜取出，<1%需手术治疗。
- 可尝试应用胰高血糖素：静推 1 mg，20 min 后重复。大部分研究者表明这可能无效。
- 硝酸甘油或硝苯地平可能有效。
- 地西泮对于在上段食管(横纹肌)可能有用。
- 如无缓解，则在消化内科协助下行内镜治疗取出异物。
• 腐蚀物摄入：
- 禁忌催吐及呕吐。
- 立即用牛奶中和。
- 避免应用中和剂以防其所导致的发热反应。
- 消化内科协助早期内镜检查，利于判断预后。
- 糖皮质激素无效，并且可能有害。
• 撕裂和穿孔：
- 局部肌层撕裂通常可自愈。
- 消化内科会诊行内镜检查有助于明确诊断。
- 穿孔需要外科行开胸术及早期修复，部分患者可行保守治疗。
- 穿孔患者需给予广谱口服抗生素治疗。
- 药物包装需要内镜下取出或其他毒物造成的撕裂。

儿科注意事项

• 摄入特定的异物者需要消化内科会诊并内镜取出异物。
- 尖锐物体：鱼骨、直别针、剃须刀片、铅笔。
- 腐蚀性物体：纽扣电池。
• 物体可能会自行排出：
- 硬币、纽扣、弹珠。
- 钝性末端的别针可能自行排出。
• 请儿科消化科专家会诊。

■ 药物治疗

• 异物或食物压迫：
- 胰高血糖素：1～2 mg(儿童：0.02～0.03 mg/kg)，静脉注射，可每 20 min 重复注射一次。
- 硝酸甘油：0.4 mg，舌下含服。
- 地西泮：5～10 mg(儿童：1～2 mg)，静脉注射。
• 穿孔：
- 头孢他啶：1～2 g[儿童：100～160 mg/(kg · 24 h)]，静脉注射，q6～8 h。
- 庆大霉素：1～1.7 mg/kg[儿童：1.5～2.5 mg/(kg · 24 h)]，静脉注射，q8 h。
- 不建议对摄入腐蚀性物质者应用皮质激素。

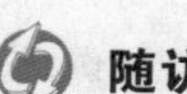

随访

■ 进一步处理

入院指征

• 摄入腐蚀性物质。
• 尖锐异物。
• 气道损伤。

• 贯穿性颈部或胸部创伤。

• 存在脓毒症、纵隔炎或食管穿孔。

• 明显出血。

• 不能耐受口服液体。

出院指征

• 局部食管壁撕裂伤出血已自止。

• 造成压迫的异物或食物已经通过食管下端括约肌。

要点和误区

预测食管损伤预后的因素：

• 确诊及确定性治疗时间：小于 24 h，死亡率可减半。

• 损伤部位：颈段较胸段及腹段少。

• 损伤机制：自发性穿孔死亡率最高达 30%～40%，医源性 15%～20%，直接损伤 5%～10%。

• 嗜酸性粒细胞增多性食管炎应该被认为是异物阻塞的潜在病理表现。

食管异物 Foreign Body, Esophageal

Joanna W. Davidson 万健 译

基础知识

描述

• 食管异物易于停留的 3 个解剖狭窄部位：

- 63%在环咽肌，最为多见（C_6 水平）。
- 20%在胃食管连接处（T_{11} 水平）。
- 10%在主动脉弓（T_4 水平）。

• 90%的消化道异物能自行通过。

• 10%～20%需要在内镜下取出，不到 1%需要通过外科手术取出。

病因

• 造成大多数成人和青少年食管异物的原因是食物团和骨片。

• 风险增加的因素：

- 牙齿脱落的成人。
- 中毒患者。
- 原有食管疾病者：Schatzki B 环或溃疡性狭窄较为多见。

儿科注意事项

• 80%的消化道异物发生在儿童中，峰值年龄为 6 个月至 6 岁，特别是 2 岁以下。

• 硬币最为常见：

- 占食管异物的 80%。

• 另外两个狭窄部位：喉入口（T_1 水平）和气管分叉处（T_6 水平）。

诊断

症状和体征

• 急性摄入症状：

- 吞咽困难。
- 吞咽痛。
- 流涎。
- 呕吐或自诱发的呕吐。
- 哽噎感。
- 窒息。
- 唾液带血。

• 慢性滞留症状：

- 呼吸系统症状（由食管周围组织肿胀导致气管受压影响通气功能）。
  ◦ 咳嗽。
  ◦ 喘鸣。
  ◦ 声音嘶哑。

• 胸痛。

• 感觉异物所在部位通常与异物在食管内的部位相符。

• 食管穿孔。

• 15%～35%的摄入尖锐物体者有以下表现：

- 充血。
- 肿胀。
- 颈部捻发音。
- 腹膜炎。
- 不到 20%的患者没有症状。

儿科注意事项

• 拒绝进食。

• 喘鸣。

• 上呼吸道感染。

• 颈部、喉部疼痛。

病史

• 成人：

- 通常能提供明确的病史。
  ◦ 80%在 1～24 h 出现症状。
  ◦ 5%的患者有呼吸道梗阻症状。

• 儿童：

- 50%没有症状。
- 如果没有目击者，异物摄入史难以明确。
- 流涎，拒食，不能解释的恶心，咳嗽，喘息，憋气。
- 似乎比成人更多表现出呼吸系统症状。

基本检查

• 异物摄入史：包括类型、时间和方式。

• 体检时注意呼吸困难的程度：

- 食管：
  ◦ 梗阻：流涎积聚，叹气样呼吸。
  ◦ 穿孔：捻发音，疼痛，胸膜炎。
  ◦ 出血。
- 口咽：
  ◦ 充血，咽喉过敏感。
  ◦ 上腭破损。
- 肺：
  ◦ 喘鸣和哮鸣音。
- 腹部：
  ◦ 腹膜炎或肠梗阻。

诊断检查与说明

影像学检查

• 包含颈部的胸部 X 线检查，定位异物：

- 食物团通常不需要 X 线检查。
- 通过冠状面成像常可以确定异物所处位置。
- 食管穿孔可见食管后方、颈部软组织及纵隔积气。

• 不到 50%的摄入性损伤性骨片能在 X 线平片上被发现。

• CT 能显示食管对比度，可能发现不被 X 线显影的异物：

- X 线不显影的异物包括玻璃片、骨片、铝片、塑料、木块等。
- 可发现穿孔或感染。

• 内镜是定位异物和取出多数异物的方法。

- 可清楚看见食管黏膜病理情况。
- 可进行诊断和治疗。

鉴别诊断

• 癔症。

• 食管黏膜激惹。

• 食管炎。

• 喉头炎。
• 会厌炎。
• 上呼吸道感染。
• 食管后脓肿。

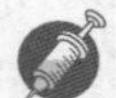

治疗

院前

• 维持呼吸道通畅和预防窒息至关重要。
• 导管吸出分泌物。
• 将患者安放于合适体位。
• 禁忌催吐和导泻。

初步稳定/治疗

• 基本生命支持。
• 预防窒息。

急诊治疗/程序

• 直接喉镜和纤维光镜可用来取出近端的异物。
• 急诊内镜建议：
- 尖锐的或可拉伸的异物。
◦ 在食管>5 cm。
◦ 在胃部>6 cm。
◦ 不规则/锋利的边缘(牙签、汽水罐标签)，高达35%的尖锐物体会穿孔。
◦ 多种类异物，特别是磁铁。
- 穿孔。
- 儿童环咽肌水平有硬币滞留。
- 呼吸道损伤。
- 异物滞留时间>24 h。
- 食物团造成完全性梗阻。
• 留院观察。
• 摄入硬币或光滑物体(非纽扣电池)，位于食管下段且没有症状：
- 观察时间24 h以上，看异物能否下行进入胃内。
- 能到达胃内长度<5 cm、直径<2 cm者，通过肠道多无困难，但建议每日行X线检查。
- 24 h后穿孔的发生率增加。
• 取异物方法：
- 静脉注射胰高血糖素：
◦ 不影响食管收缩的情况下降低食管下段括约肌张力。
◦ 可一定程度上替代内镜。
◦ 对有Schatzki环或狭窄者效果不佳。
◦ 可将食管下端的食物团推入胃内。
◦ 适用于阻塞时间24 h内的患者。
- 荧光镜引导下的Foley导管取异物术：
◦ 应由经验丰富操作熟练而安全的医师实施。
◦ 将Foley导管(10～16F)经鼻插至食管，尖端球囊在荧光引导下推至异物下方。
◦ 向Foley导管球囊中充入对比剂，缓慢回撤导管。
◦ 本法忌用于慢性异物存留、不配合的患者、带有尖头的异物等。
◦ Foley导管或扩张条有助于将异物推入胃内。
- 内镜术：
◦ 是取出急性或慢性异物的最佳方法。
◦ 98%的有效率。
◦ 通常用于异物存留超过2～4日，食管受到刺激和水肿的患者。
◦ 某些困难病例需在气管插管全身麻醉下操作：婴幼儿、精神病患者、难取的异物。
◦ 最好是6～12 h完成，超过24 h则并发症风险增加。
- 外科手术：
◦ 用其他方法无法取出异物。
◦ 占全部病例的1%～2%。
◦ 异物常为牙签和骨片。
• 特殊摄入物：
- 食物团完全性食管阻塞：
◦ 急诊取出。
◦ 不建议使用蛋白分解酶消化食物团块，因其可能造成食管穿孔、高钠血症和误吸并发症。
• 纽扣电池：
- 需紧急取出。
- 电池泄漏：内含氢氧化钾和汞，均为剧毒物质。
- 碱泄漏可致黏膜溶解坏死。
- 4～6 h即可发生黏膜全层灼伤(化学、电流、压迫混合作用)。
- 胃内的电池排出则没有困难，若存留时间3～4日以上，则应设法取出。
- 一旦通过十二指肠，85%可于72 h内排出。
• 麻醉性毒品或苯丙胺包：
- 身体藏毒在毒品流通区高发。
- 毒品包在X线下可显影。
- 包裹破裂或泄漏可能致命。
• 磁铁或“巴克球”：
- 磁铁相吸可导致局部胃、肠挤成一团而发生梗阻。
- 应尽早请消化科会诊取异物或剖腹探查。

药物治疗

胰高血糖素：1～2 mg，静脉注射，需预先行过敏试验。

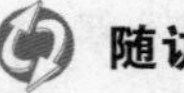

随访

进一步处理

入院指征

• 病情严重和合并并发症，如食管穿孔、异物穿透食管壁、活动性出血等患者。
• 气道受阻。
• 取异物不成功且有症状的患者。

出院指征

• 异物已经除去或推移通过食管远端没有症状的患者。
• 存在于食管远端的光滑异物没有症状者，12～24 h需复诊以确定异物是否自行进入胃腔。

转诊问题

对于食管异物为尖锐或有尖点的病例，这些异物阻塞于食管上段或中段，还有异物为纽扣电池时，应请消化专科会诊。

随访建议

合并食管易梗阻基础疾病者应由消化专科医师随访。

要点和误区

• 应X线检查以明确异物位置。
• 高度警惕食管穿孔。

S

视觉丧失

D. Taylor Gammons · Eric Deutsch 吴昊 李文放 译

基础知识

描述

• 视功能下降(即视力、视野、视力模糊)。

• 视觉丧失有许多病因,可能是由多系统引起的。

病因

• 眼科:

- 泪液膜异常。
- 前段(角膜、前房、虹膜、晶状体)。
- 后段(玻璃体、视网膜、视神经)。
- 眼后段(视神经、交叉、辐射)。

• 外伤性:

• 其他眼外和全身性疾病,包括神经、心血管、免疫、内分泌、感染和毒理学原因。

诊断

症状和体征

病史

• 视力丧失的特征:

- 丧失程度:模糊、完整、特殊区域。
- 急性发作与逐渐发作。
- 暂时性与持续性。
- 单眼与双目。
- 无痛与疼痛。
- 存在重影。

• 外伤史:钝性与穿透性。

• 接触史:化学品、焊接、金属或木工、毒素摄入。

• 矫正镜片的使用:眼镜、隐形眼镜。

• 结膜红斑或分泌物。

• 闪光灯或荧光灯。

• 眼动疼痛。

• 既往眼科手术或问题。

• 相关症状:头痛、神经系统疾病、其他全身症状。

• 相关疾病:

- 动脉粥样硬化性疾病或危险因素。
- 免疫低下状态。
- HIV 感染。
- 慢性类固醇或其他免疫抑制。
- 神经、内分泌或免疫紊乱。
- 凝血功能障碍。

体格检查

• 眼科检查:

- 视力——斯内伦图表,芬格计数,手部运动,光感知。
- 瞳孔检查,传入性瞳孔缺损。
- 对抗性视野检测。
- 眼外肌功能。
- 狭缝灯检查。
- 眼底镜放大瞳孔检查。
- 荧光素检查。

• 心血管系统:杂音、颈动脉挫伤、颞动脉压痛。

• 神经检查:评估其他障碍。

• 一般检查:免疫、内分泌或中毒性疾病的征兆。

基本检查

• 病史与眼科检查。

• 其他的实验室检查和影像学检查都应基于病史和体征。

诊断检查与说明

实验室检查

• 可以获得确定与视力丧失有关的其他共同因素的程度(即糖尿病、心血管疾病)。

• 如果怀疑巨细胞动脉炎,测红细胞沉降率。

影像学检查

• 床旁超声可以检测晶状体或视网膜脱离、玻璃体出血、异物,或测量视神经直径。

• 如果怀疑巨细胞动脉炎,可能需颞动脉活检。

• 脑 CT、MRI、MRA 和经颅多普勒可用于评估神经系统症状和椎基底动脉。

• 如果诊断出视网膜动脉闭塞,则紧急行心脏和颈动脉超声。

• 面部 CT 可用于评估创伤程度。

鉴别诊断

• 短暂性:

- 黑矇症。
- 偏头痛(可出现而不头痛)。
- 持续性原因的早期表现。

• 持续性单眼,无痛:

- 视网膜中央动脉阻塞。
- 视网膜中央静脉阻塞。
- 视网膜脱离或出血。
- 玻璃体出血。
- 颈内动脉阻塞/剥离。
- 巨细胞动脉炎。

• 持续性单眼,疼痛:

- 急性闭角型青光眼。
- 眼内炎。
- 视神经炎。
- 葡萄膜炎。
- 角膜炎。

• 双眼:

- 视乳头水肿。
- 神经系统、感染性、毒性、免疫、心血管和内分泌疾病应考虑为单眼和双眼视觉障碍。
- 慢性疾病。
- 屈光异常、白内障、开角型青光眼、黄斑变性、视网膜病变。
- 功能性视力丧失、装病、癔病。

• 外伤:从前到后。

- 眼睑损伤、水肿。
- 角膜擦伤、水肿。
- 角膜异物。
- 前房积血。
- 外伤性虹膜炎。
- 外伤性散。
- 外伤性白内障。
- 晶状体脱位。
- 视网膜震荡。
- 视网膜脱离。
- 视网膜或玻璃体出血。
- 眼内异物。
- 外伤性视神经病变。
- 眼球破裂。
- 球后血肿。
- 眼眶骨折。
- 中枢神经系统损伤。

• 感染性:眼眶蜂窝织炎、眼内炎、海绵窦血栓形成、HIV 神经病变、CMV 视网膜炎、HSV/带状疱疹、病毒性/细菌性结膜炎。

• 中毒:甲醇、地高辛、胺碘酮、某些抗生素、抗疟药、抗结核药物、化疗药物等。

• 神经性:MS、CVA、偏头痛、肿瘤、后可逆性脑病综合征(PRES)、椎基底动脉功能不全。

• 免疫性:白塞病、狼疮、葡萄膜炎、交感性眼炎、巨细胞动脉炎。

• 心血管性:血栓、栓塞、高血压、解剖因素。

S

• 内分泌：糖尿病、Grave 病。

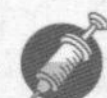

治疗

院前

• 化学灼伤：
- 立即用水或生理盐水大量冲洗。

急诊治疗/程序

• 直接治疗导致视力丧失的病因。
• 对于有严重潜在病因、程度严重或不确定诊断的视力丧失，需进行眼科会诊。
• 必须迅速在急诊室开始识别和治疗的救治时间敏感事件：
- 视网膜中央动脉阻塞。
- 化学灼伤。
- 急性闭角型青光眼。
- 眼球开放。
- 眼后隔血肿。

视网膜中央动脉阻塞

• 临床标准：
- 单方面，无痛，急剧视力下降。
- 传入瞳孔缺陷。
- 淡红色的眼底与樱桃红点（黄斑）。

化学烧伤

• 临床标准：
- 碱比酸更严重。
- 例如：催泪气体、水泥、石膏、溶剂。
• 治疗：
- 局部麻醉。
- 用林格液或生理盐水大量灌注眼睛（普通水也可以接受的，如果其他无法获得）。
- Morgan 镜片（如有），否则鼻插管连接盐水袋或洗眼台。
- 目标：冲洗完后 5～10 min pH 中性，如果 pH 未中和，则重复上述步骤。
- 不要试图用碱中和酸，反之亦然。
- 盖上盖子并使用潮湿的棉签涂抹器清扫炉中残留的化学沉淀剂。
- 与睫状肌麻痹剂（阿托品、环戊烯醇、托吡卡胺）。
- 不要使用去氧肾上腺素；血管收缩剂可能致血管缺血性。
- 红霉素软膏 q1～2 h。
- 人工泪液 qh。
- 检测眼内压。

急性闭角型青光眼

• 体征和症状：
- 单侧，疼痛伴视力丧失。
- 恶心，呕吐，头痛。
- 角膜充血，水肿。
- 中间扩张，呆滞，瞳孔无反应。
- 肿胀，“蒸汽”晶状体。
- 细胞，在浅前房内发光。
- 眼内压增加（＞20 mmHg）。
• 治疗：
- 抬高床头。
- 外用，β 受体阻滞剂。
- 局部用前列腺素。
- 乙酰唑胺。
- 局部用 α_2 受体激动剂。
- 缩瞳剂。
- 如果 1 h 后眼压没有下降，可考虑使用甘露醇。
- 针对的局部类固醇、压缩性角膜炎、周边虹膜切除术，紧急眼科会诊。

眼球破裂

• 临床标准：
- 创伤史——可能不太明显，如无眼部防护的金属加工。
- 疼痛和视力丧失。
- 液体渗漏/塞德征。
- 针尖样瞳孔。
- 360°大疱性结膜下出血。
- 角膜/巩膜全层撕裂伤。
- 怀疑时不要检查眼压。
• 治疗：
- 护眼。
- 眼眶 CT，特别是异物。
- 禁食、卧床。
- 镇痛和止吐。
- 注射破伤风疫苗。
- 静脉抗生素——氟喹诺酮＋万古霉素。
- 紧急眼科咨询或修复。

球后血肿伴眶间隔综合征

• 临床标准：
- 钝挫伤病史。
- 疼痛和视力丧失。
- 水肿和眼球突出。
- 眼球外运动减弱。
- 传入性瞳孔缺损。
- 眼压升高。
- CT 可以确定诊断，但如果有视力下降，成像不应延误治疗。
• 治疗：
- 侧眦切开术。
- 适应证：
  ◦ 视力下降/视神经病变。
  ◦ 眼压＞40 mmHg。
- 禁忌证——眼球破裂。
- 程序：
  ◦ 注射局部麻醉剂并在外眦处应用止血剂 1 min。
  ◦ 使用缝合剪刀切割外眦。
  ◦ 识别并切断下眦肌腱。
  ◦ 如果眼压仍然升高，识别并切断上眦肌腱。
- 如果眼压中度升高而无视神经病变（＞30 mmHg 但＜40 mmHg），可考虑采用药物治疗降低眼压。
- 急诊眼科会诊。

药物治疗

• 抗生素滴剂：
- 0.3％环丙沙星：1～2 gtt，q1～6 h。
- 0.3％庆大霉素：1～2 μg，q4 h。
- 0.3％氧氟沙星：1～2 h，q1～6 h。
- 0.5％左氧氟沙星：1～2 μg，q2 h。
- 多黏菌素（polytrim）：1 gtt，q3～6 h。
- 磺胺醋酰（10％、0.3％）：1～2 gtt，q2～6 h。
- 0.3％妥布霉素：1～2 gtt，q1～4 h。
- 1％三氟尿苷：1 gtt，q2～4 h。
• 抗生素软膏：
- 杆菌肽 3～6 h 中杆菌肽 500 U/g 1/2。
- 0.3％环丙沙星：1/2 in-ribbon，q6～q8 h。
- 0.5％红霉素：1/2 in-ribbon，q3～6 h。
- 0.3％庆大霉素：在第 3～4 h 时为 1/2。
- 新斯波林 1/2 in-ribbon，q3～4 h。
- 多链丝霉素 1/2 in-ribbon，q3～4 h。
- 10％磺胺醋酰：1/2 in-ribbon，q3～8 h。
- 0.3％妥布霉素：1/2 in-ribbon，q3～4 h。
- 阿糖腺苷：1/2 in-ribbon，每日 5 次。
• 散瞳药和散瞳药：
- 阿托品（1％、2％）：1～2 gtt，每日 1～4 次。
- 0.5％环戊酯（1％、2％）：1～2 gtt，必要时。
- 2％后马托品：1～2 gtt，每日 2～4 次。
- 苯肾上腺素（0.12％、2.5％、10％）：1～2 μg，每日 3～4 次。
- 托品酰胺（0.5％、1％）：1～2 gtt，必要时用。
• 皮质类固醇-抗生素药物治疗（与眼科协商）：
- 泼尼松（Blephamide）1～2 gtt，q1～8 h。
- 氢化可的松/新霉素/杆菌肽/多黏菌素 B（Cortisporin）1～2 gtt，q3～4 h。
- 地塞米松/新霉素/多黏菌素 B（Maxitrol）1～2tt，q1～8 h。

- 泼尼松/庆大霉素(Pred - G) 1～2 gtt，q1～8 h。
- 地塞米松/妥布霉素/三氯叔丁醇(TobraDex)1～2 gtt，q2～26 h。
• 青光眼剂(总是与眼科疾病相关)：
- α_2 受体激动剂：
◦ 1%溴莫尼定：1 μg，每日 3 次。
◦ 1%阿拉可乐定：1 gtt，每日 3 次。
- β受体阻滞剂：
◦ 倍他洛尔(0.25%或 0.5%)：1～2 gtt，每日 2 次。
◦ 1%卡替洛尔：1 gtt，每日 2 次。
◦ 左布诺洛尔(0.25%、0.5%)：1 μg，每日 1～2 次。
- 碳酸酐酶抑制剂：
◦ 乙酰唑胺：500 mg，口服或静脉注射，每日 1～4 次。
- 缩瞳剂(拟副交感神经药)：
◦ 匹罗卡品(0.25%、0.5%、1%、2%、3%、4%、6%、8%、10%)：1～2 gtt，每日 3～4 次。
- 渗透剂：
◦ 在 45 min 内静脉注射甘露醇 1～2 g/kg
- 前列腺素类似物：
◦ 1%溴莫尼定：1 gtt，每日 3 次。
◦ 1%阿可乐定：1 gtt，每日 3 次。
- 前列腺素类似物：
◦ 0.005%拉那普斯特：1 gtt，每日 1 次。
• 只有排除闭角型青光眼才可用：
- 噻吗洛尔(0.25%、0.5%)：1 gtt，每日 2 次。

随访

进一步处理

入院指征

• 眼球破裂。
• 明显前房积血。
• 眼内炎、眼眶蜂窝织炎/脓肿、海绵窦血栓形成和其他重要感染。
• 显著的心脏、颈动脉或神经系统疾病。
• 球后血肿伴眼间隔综合征。
• 骨折伴夹闭征原因不明。
• 进行性视力丧失。
• 眼科咨询建议的其他诊断。

出院指征

诊断确定，并且视力丧失将不会进展。

随访建议

• 随访应与眼科讨论紧急问题。
• 细菌性结膜炎、单纯疱疹病毒/带状疱疹感染、复发性结膜下出血、角膜溃疡、前房积血、后玻璃体脱离、视网膜脱离、视神经炎、葡萄膜炎需要紧急转诊。
• 血栓和栓塞性疾病心脏和颈动脉检查的转诊。

要点和误区

• 记录所有有视力改变的患者。
• 局部麻醉将有助于诊断，并有助于进行适当的眼科检查。
• 头痛患者要注意详细眼科检查。

S

视神经炎

Christopher J. Dudley 朱妍 译

基础知识

描述

• 由炎症过程导致的视神经功能障碍，一般与髓鞘受损有关，导致严重视力丧失。
• 与多发性硬化(MS)高度相关：15%～20%的 MS 患者表现出这种特征。
• 根据炎症部位分类：
- 视乳头炎：视盘炎症。
- 球后视神经炎：靠近眼球的视神经炎。
• 临床确诊多发性硬化 5 年内继发视神经炎的风险：
- MRI 正常：16%。
- MRI>3 处病变：51%。
• 35%的患者会复发。

危险因素

基因

• *A23*、*B7*、*DR2 HLA* 等位基因的患者视神经炎高发。
• 特别是已经进展到临床确诊的多发性硬化患者。

病因

• 原发性：
- 最常见。
- 单侧发生。
• 多发性硬化：
- 20%～50%的患者有视神经炎。
- 可能的遗传成分。
◦ 视神经炎患者 *A23*、*B7* 和 *DR2 HLA* 等位基因的高患病率。
• 病毒感染：
- 水痘。
- 风疹。
- 单核细胞增多症。
- 单纯疱疹病毒和带状疱疹病毒。
- 脑炎。
• 病毒感染后视神经炎：
- 通常在非特异性病毒感染 4～6 周后发病。
• 肉芽肿性炎症：
- 结核。
- 梅毒。
- 结节病。
- 隐球菌感染。
• SLE。
• HIV：
- 巨细胞病毒。
- 弓形虫病。
- 组织胞浆菌病。
- 隐球菌病。
• 莱姆病。
• 持续性脑膜、眼眶、鼻窦和眼内炎症。
• 药物，包括：
- 胺碘酮。
- 乙胺丁醇。
- 他莫昔芬。

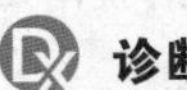

诊断

症状和体征

• 失明和疼痛是最常见的症状。
• 失明在几日后发生(少数几小时)，1～2 周达到高峰：
- 成人多为单侧(90%)。

- 双眼失明多见于儿童。
• 球后疼痛：患眼活动后加重。
• 亮、色觉和深感觉比视敏度丧失更显著。
• 瞳孔传入障碍：几乎总是发生在单侧而另一只眼健康。
• 视野缺损：
- 通常表现为中央暗点型。
- 56%的患者缺损视野在1年内恢复，而10年内73%的患者能恢复。
• 眼底镜检查通常提示水肿（视乳头炎）或正常视盘。
• Uhthoff征：
- 视野缺损在活动或体无温上升时发生。
- 偶尔可见到不寻常的体征。

病史

• 性别（2/3的病例发生在女性）。
• 年龄（特别是20～50岁的女性）。
• 眼运动时疼痛。
• 症状发生的速度。
• 伴随症状。
• 以前是否有发作史。
• 视神经炎和MS的家族史。

体格检查

• 检查血压。
• 完整的眼科和神经科检查，特别是：
- 瞳孔功能。
- 传入瞳孔功能障碍（如果其他眼睛未受影响）。
- 视野缺损。
- 色觉（石原颜色板）。
◦ "红色去饱和度"受试者可以感觉到，当用受影响的眼睛观察时，与他们未受影响的眼睛的感觉相比，红色物体看起来是"褪色的"。
- 裂隙灯检查（葡萄膜炎或前房细胞不常见，建议另行诊断）。
- 加宽视网膜检查（水肿视盘）。

■ 诊断检查与说明

实验室检查

• 全血细胞计数。
• 红细胞沉降率（血沉）。
• 快速血浆反应抗体、荧光密螺旋体抗体吸附试验（FTA-ABS）。
• 莱姆效价。
• 抗核抗体。
• 重组血管紧张素转换酶水平。
• 纯蛋白衍生物。
• HIV。

影像学检查

• 胸部X线检查排除TB、肉芽肿。
• 脑和眶部的CT或MRI扫描：
- 球后视神经炎症在急性期可能出现视神经肿大，会增加视神经肿瘤的误诊。
- 氧化钆增强MRI：可见95%的视神经炎症。
- 视野检查：最好是机械化检查，如Octopus或Humphrey。

■ 鉴别诊断

• 急性视乳头水肿。
• 缺血性视神经病。
• 严重系统性高血压。
• 颅内肿瘤压迫视觉传入通路。
• 眶内肿物压迫视神经。
• 毒性或代谢性神经病变：
- 重金属中毒。
- 贫血。
- 营养不良。
- 乙醇、甲醇。
- 氯喹。
- 乙胺丁醇。
- 异烟肼。
• Leber遗传性视神经萎缩（最常见的遗传性线粒体疾病）。

儿科注意事项

儿童患者，应考虑感染性和感染后的原因。

老年人注意事项

>50岁的患者，缺血性视神经病变（如糖尿病和巨细胞动脉炎）更常见，应进行相应的诊治。

治疗

■ 急诊治疗/程序

• 早期眼科和神经科会诊。
• 静脉使用类固醇激素冲击后口服序贯：
- 推荐MRI发现≥2处脱髓鞘病灶而无多发性硬化、视神经炎，或严重视觉丧失既往史的患者使用。
- 减少2年以上病程的多发性硬化患者复发和进展并缩短视觉障碍的持续时间，但对1年内的视觉恢复和5年内的病变进展率无效。
- 对MRI只有1个病灶的患者应行个体化治疗。
- 警告：单独口服类固醇激素增加复发率，应避免。

■ 药物治疗

甲泼尼龙：250 mg静脉注射，q6 h，持续3日，口服序贯泼尼松[1 mg/(k · d)]持续11日，而后4日内递减停药。

随访

■ 进一步处理

入院指征

• 双侧视觉丧失。
• 其他急性视觉丧失的原因不能排除。
• 需要静脉类固醇激素治疗。

出院指征

• 单侧视觉受损。
• 良好的家庭支持系统。
• 安排神经科和眼科随访。

转诊问题

参照门诊患者使用干扰素β-1a治疗高危患者（MRI发现≥2处脱髓鞘病变）：减缓了多发性硬化症的发展。

■ 随访建议

需眼科转诊。

要点和误区

• 做出视神经炎诊断前应先排除占位性病变。
• 急性双侧视觉丧失伴严重头痛或复视应关注垂体卒中。
• 对视神经炎使用皮质激素治疗的益处仍不明确，急诊医师应咨询相应的专家制定当地实践标准。
• 脑MRI是判断多发性硬化预后最有效的方法。

S

视网膜脱离 Retinal Detachment

Robyn R. Essendrop · Carl G. Skinner 何融冰 译

基础知识

描述

- 3 种导致共同最终结果的视网膜脱离：
- 孔源性视网膜脱离(RRD)。
- 牵拉性视网膜脱离(TRD)。
- 渗出性视网膜脱离(ERD)。
- RRD：
- 最常见。
- 视网膜破裂或撕裂，导致液体进入玻璃体腔内分离了视网膜神经上皮和色素上皮。
- 严重症状，闪光继发于神经纤维撕裂，飞蚊症继发于出血。
- TRD：
- 以前的创伤导致纤维性玻璃体条索的牵拉，使感觉性视网膜与色素上皮脱离。
- 慢性，进展性。
- 无症状，除非发生出血或视网膜脱离。
- ERD：
- 视网膜下液体积聚使视网膜脱离而未分离任何一层。
- 一般无需手术。
- 经常继发于系统性疾病，如严重的重度高血压、肉瘤病、癌症。

病因

- RRD：
- 近视。
- 白内障手术。
- 马方综合征。
- 玻璃体、视网膜神经或色素上皮解剖结构退变。
- 创伤。
- TRD：
- 增生性糖尿病视网膜病变。
- 血管病变。
- 穿孔性损伤。
- 脉络膜视网膜炎：
  - 早产、镰状细胞疾病、弓蛔虫病导致的视网膜病变。
- 创伤。
- ERD：
- 恶性高血压、先兆子痫。
- 脉络膜或视网膜肿瘤(黑色素瘤、视网膜母细胞瘤)。
- 炎症性疾病(Coats 疾病或 Harada 疾病、后巩膜炎)。

诊断

症状和体征

病史

- 闪光症，飞蚊症。
- 片状视觉丧失。
- 周围/中心视觉丧失或其他视野缺损。
- 无症状。

病史

- 症状的发生与进展，描述：
- 可以在数小时或数周内进展。
- 黑幕布或面纱感。
- 经常从周围开始。
- 相关症状：闪光症、飞蚊症、无痛。
- 眼科病史：视力、近视、手术、眼部疾病、外伤。
- 系统性疾病。

体格检查

- 在扩瞳前对诊视敏度，视野：
- 如果黄斑未累及则有正常视敏度。
- 脱离在视野缺损的对侧。
- 可能有传入性瞳孔反应缺陷。
- 可能失去视网膜红反射。
- 眼底镜检查：
- 视网膜苍白，不透光，萎缩。
- 单凭眼底镜不能排除视网膜脱离。
- 裂隙灯检查：
- 玻璃体前色素颗粒("烟草尘")，提示视网膜脱离。

基本检查

- 眼科检查。
- 神经学检查，排除脑血管事件/暂时缺血。

诊断检查与说明

实验室检查

根据需要检查根本病因。

影像学检查

眼部超声：受过训练的 EM 医生检查敏感度达 97%。

- 高回声皮瓣，低活动度动态扫描。
- 残留在视神经和锯齿口。

诊断步骤/外科

- 眼内压(IOP)测量：受感染的眼睛 IOP 通常降低。
- 用短效扩瞳剂扩瞳造成急性闭角型青光眼的风险很低。

鉴别诊断

- 中心视网膜动脉或静脉阻塞。
- 玻璃体出血。
- 有或无先兆的偏头痛。
- 脉络膜脱离。
- 甲醛中毒。
- 视神经炎或缺血性视神经病变。
- 其他视网膜或 CNS 疾病。

治疗

院前

- 卧床休息。
- 入院后随诊神经科或眼科医师。

初步稳定/治疗

如果怀疑 ERD，治疗系统性疾病。

急诊治疗/程序

- 卧床休息：
- 头垫枕头使脱离的一侧朝下，即与视野缺损的一侧相对。
- 紧急请眼科医师会诊。

随访

进一步处理

入院指征

需要手术修补。

出院指征

- 任何患有视网膜脱离的患者应在眼科医师检查并确定安全后回家。
- 慢性视网膜脱离的修复时间与脱离的时间相当。
- ERD 在治疗根本病因后可缓解。

转诊问题

- 症状性"黄斑上"脱离(保留中心视力)通常需要更紧急的修复(≤24 h)。
- 如果在症状出现后 3 日内进行手术修复，视力结果对"黄斑脱离"也可能更好。

随访建议

均建议眼科医生随访。

S

要点和误区

- 检眼镜不能提供足够的证据排除诊断。
- 早期识别视网膜脱离，进行预防：
  - "烟灰尘"征象表明有 90% 的视网膜撕脱危险。
- 不要忽略辨别视网膜中心动脉阻塞(CRAO)。
  - 患有 CRAO 的患者在有颈动脉疾病或颈动脉栓塞性疾病时发生卒中的风险增加。

视网膜中央动脉阻塞 Central Retinal Artery Occlusion

Yasuharu Okuda · Braden HexQm 彭沪 译

基础知识

描述

- 视网膜中央动脉阻塞伴随突发的无痛性视力丧失。
- 通常发生于 50～70 岁年龄患者。
- 眼动脉是颈动脉的一级分支。
- 危险因素包括高血压、动脉粥样硬化性疾病、镰状细胞疾病、血管炎、心脏瓣膜病、狼疮、创伤和冠状动脉疾病。
- 发病率为(1～10)/10 万。
- 经常被描述成"眼卒中"。

病因

- 栓子：
  - 来源于近端的血管内物质引起阻塞：
    - 动脉粥样硬化性疾病(大部分)。
    - 颈动脉狭窄。
    - 心脏瓣膜病(心源性栓子)。
    - 心房黏液瘤。
    - 眼动脉夹层。
    - 颈动脉夹层。
- 血栓形成：
  - 已存在的血管内粥样硬化斑块破裂引起的血流阻塞。
  - 血液高凝状态(镰状细胞)。
- 炎症：
  - 由于颞动脉炎、狼疮、血管炎。
- 灌注减少：
  - 低血流状态比如在严重低血压时，或者在闭角性青光眼或眼球后出血引起的高压情况。

诊断

症状和体征

病史

- 突发无痛的单侧视力丧失。
- 突发视力丧失的前驱阶段：
  - 可能有持续数秒到数分钟的(一过性黑矇)。
  - 由于短暂性血栓现象或眼血流量下降。

体格检查

- 明显下降的视觉敏锐度。
- 经常存在瞳孔传入缺陷。
- 视网膜表现：
  - 视网膜血管树内可见血栓。
  - 血管内表现闪闪发光的白色或黄色斑点(Hollenhorst 斑)。
  - 血流阻断 15～20 min 可见缺血性水肿。
  - 视网膜的中央凹上存在"樱桃红斑"(仅仅在视网膜很薄的位置上使血管脉络膜完全显示)。
  - 累及的动脉为空的或表现黑红静止的或少见的搏动性串珠状隔断。
  - 通常透明的堵塞的视神经分层发生后 1～2 h 出现乳浊化。
- 部分视野缺失：
  - 仅仅发生于视网膜中央动脉分支。

基本检查

- 视觉灵敏度和视野测试。
- 眼底检查。
- 眼压测定。
- 眼科急会诊。

诊断检查与说明

实验室检查

直接评估潜在的血管阻塞病因：

- 全血细胞计数、分类及血小板计数。
- PT、APTT。
- 电解质、尿素氮/肌酐、血糖。
- 电子自旋共振检测巨细胞动脉炎(患者年龄>55 岁)。
- ANA、RF、CRP、ESR。
- 快速血浆反应素环状卡片试验(RPR)。
- 血红蛋白电泳。
- 血清蛋白电泳。

影像学检查

直接评估潜在的血管阻塞病因：

- 颈动脉超声/多普勒超声。
- 可选择超声心动图。
- 荧光素眼底血管造影、视网膜电图确诊。

鉴别诊断

- 急性闭角性青光眼。
- 视网膜中央静脉阻塞。
- 巨细胞动脉炎(颞动脉炎)。
- 视神经炎。
- 视网膜剥离。

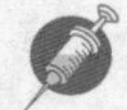

治疗

> **注意**
>
> 初始治疗应立即开始，因为 90 min 后将发生不可逆的视力丧失：
>
> - 只有立即治疗才可能帮助挽救或维持受累侧的视力。
> - 治疗的目标包括去除或溶解栓子，扩张动脉以提高前向流量，降低眼压提高灌注梯度。
> - 目前，没有足够的证据支持任何列出的治疗方法，尽管正在进行多项研究，但没有发现一种方法比观察方法更好或更差。

急诊治疗/程序

- 立即眼球按摩尝试清除血栓：
  - 患者平躺并且应用数字全眼按摩眼球血栓。
  - 闭上睑，施加恒定压力 15 s，然后放松 15 s。重复 5 次循环。
- 立即通过非重复呼吸器行 100% 高流量氧疗：
  - 如果症状发作<24 h，考虑转移到一个能够提供高压氧(HBO)设施的机构。
  - 如果可能，可以使用吸入二氧化碳和氧的混合气。
- 静脉给予四乙酰唑胺降低眼压。

• 应用马来酸噻吗洛尔局部滴眼降低眼压。

• 给予口服阿司匹林和静脉肝素预防血栓的进展。

• 请眼科急会诊：

- 前房穿刺术有助于降低眼压。

- 可能行动脉内溶栓溶解血块。

• 在炎症性动脉炎疑似病例给予高剂量的全身性类固醇。

■ 药物治疗

一线药物

• 乙酰唑胺：500 mg，静脉或口服。

• 卡波金：吸入95%氧气和5%二氧化碳的混合物。

• 肝素：80 U/kg负荷静脉注射，18 U/(kg · h)持续输注(速度的调整基于PT水平)。

• 0.5%马来酸噻吗洛尔溶液：1滴局部滴患眼。

二线药物

• 甲泼尼龙：疑似炎性动脉炎患者静脉给予250 mg。

• 阿司匹林：325 mg，口服。

• 甘露醇。

• 舌下含服硝酸甘油。

随访

■ 进一步处理

入院指征

在急性病例需要检查接近的病因(栓塞来源、血栓形成或炎症性)。

出院指征

慢性视网膜动脉闭塞疾病稳定期可以在门诊治疗。

转诊问题

所有可疑病例必需眼科急会诊。

■ 随访建议

大部分病例需要颈动脉超声排除动脉粥样硬化性疾病。

要点和误区

• 一过性黑矇(短暂的，可能再通的视网膜动脉阻塞)是一个突发事件，可能导致完全闭塞或脑卒中。不要忽视这些症状，需要紧急处理。

• 视网膜动脉闭塞是医学上一种急症，需要立即治疗，以防止视力丧失。

• 重要的是要完成一个完整的眼科检查，包括视力和眼底检查。

S

视网膜中央静脉阻塞 Central Retinal Vein Occlusion

Lisa A. Jacobson · Yasuharu Okuda 彭沪 译

基础知识

■ 描述

• 指因各种病因导致静脉阻塞引起的视力下降而引起的疾病。

■ 病因

• 缺血性CRVO(视网膜中央静脉阻塞)：

- 占病例的20%～25%。

- 阻断了静脉回流导致毛细血管回流、出血和黄斑水肿。

- 筛板内有限的空间由于慢血流和血管壁的变化，容易形成血栓。

- 理论上认为相邻的动脉硬化改变可能侵犯静脉。

- 血黏度也认为发挥作用。

• 非缺血性CRVO：

- 轻度，不完全阻塞。

诊断

■ 症状和体征

典型表现：

• 急性，单侧的，无痛的视力丧失。

• 眼底检查可见视网膜静脉迂曲扩张，呈火焰型。

病史

• 无痛的，单侧视力丧失。

• 如果没有缺血，可能有不完全和间歇的视力丧失。

体格检查

• 视力下降：

- 通常恶化程度超过20/200。

• 瞳孔传入缺陷。

• 曲张静脉扩张。

• 视网膜出血：

- 如果是中央性的，4个象限均可见。

- 广泛出血表现在眼底的经典描述为“血和雷声的出现”。

• 视盘水肿。

• 棉絮状渗出点。

■ 基本检查

• 血压。

• 视力检查：

- 如果是中央性的，4个象限均可见。

- 所有的手部动作通常都是可见的。

• 视野检查。

• 眼压测量：

- 正常压力在10～21 mmHg。

■ 诊断检查与说明

实验室检查

• 全血细胞计数。

• PT、APTT。

• 红细胞沉降率。

• ANA。

• 血清蛋白电泳。

影像学检查

眼底荧光血管造影：

• 眼科医师使用它显示血管无灌注区。

• 可选择超声心动图。

• 鉴别缺血和非缺血原因。

诊断步骤/外科

前房角镜检查：

• 测定虹膜或房角新生血管化。

■ 鉴别诊断

• 糖尿病性乳头炎。

• 一过性黑矇/短暂性缺血发作。

• 海绵窦血栓形成。

• 糖尿病。

• 高血压/高血压性视网膜病。

• 高黏滞综合征：

- 镰状细胞、红细胞增多症、白血病、多发性骨髓瘤。

- 癔症性失明。
- 眼缺血综合征。
- 视神经乳头水肿。
- 视网膜动脉阻塞。
- 视网膜剥离。
- 严重贫血合并血小板减少。
- 颞动脉炎。
- 玻璃体出血。

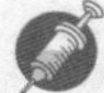

治疗

院前

目前没有具体的干预措施需要在到达医院之前实施。

初步稳定/治疗

- 如果眼压是升高的，采取逐步降低眼压方法。
- 治疗潜在的医学问题。

急诊治疗/程序

- 识别和及时转诊眼科是急诊室治疗的基石。
- 虽然没有证据，以下请眼科医师会诊给予治疗意见：
  - 抗感染治疗。
  - 全身激素。
  - 全身抗凝。
  - 纤溶药物(有争议)。
  - 激光脉络膜视网膜吻合术。

药物治疗

没有可靠实用的药物用于治疗视网膜中央静脉阻塞，眼科医师可能用以下治疗：

- 玻璃体内注射氟羟泼尼松龙。
- 抗血管内皮生长因子：
  - 贝伐单抗。

处方中的注意事项

使用口服避孕药会增加视网膜中央静脉阻塞的风险。

随访

进一步处理

入院指征

患者可入院手术治疗，依赖眼科医师的评估。

出院指征

患者可以从急诊室出院，只要他们有负责的眼科医师可以随访。

转诊问题

- 如果没有眼科医师可以给予治疗，应开始治疗同时把患者转到最近的有眼科医师可以会诊的医院。
- 如果发现新生血管形成，眼科医师经常进行全视网膜光凝术。

随访建议

- 缺血性 CRVO 患者需要长期随访，掌握新生血管和青光眼这些典型的进展。
- CRVO 患者可能有其他血管疾病，需要完整的医疗检查。
- 患者应该找一个内科医师以随访处理合并症及危险因素。

要点和误区

- 新生血管和水肿引起的眼压增加，可以导致血管功能不全，延迟治疗可引起永久性的视力下降。
- 当患者表现为双侧 CRVOS 或为年轻患者 CRVO，治疗组必须寻找有无高血黏度综合征。
- 尽管心血管疾病的危险因素易导致 CRVO，但抗血小板治疗似乎会导致更坏的结果。

室上性心动过速 Supraventricular Tachycardia

Andrew P. Pirotte · Matthew J. Pirotte 江伟伟 李文放 译

基础知识

描述

- 起源于希氏束以上的异位搏动。
- 心率 100 次/分或更高。
- 不规则狭窄复合性室上性心动过速(SVT)：
  - 心房颤动(AF，简称房颤)：
    - 在急诊中看到最常见的病理性 SVT 形式。
    - 10% 75 岁以上的人有房颤。
  - 多形性心房扑动。
  - 多发性房室性心动过速。
- 规律狭窄的复杂的 SVT：
  - 心房扑动(简称房扑)。
  - 房室结折返性心动过速(AVNRT)：
    - 成人 SVT 的 60%，70%是女性。
    - 通常年龄为 30～40 岁。
  - 房室折返性心动过速(AVRT)有旁通路。
- 宽大的复杂的 SVT：
  - 传导是在正常的希氏束浦肯野系统之外。
  - 存在旁路途径。
  - 年轻的无结构性疾病的患者更常见。
  - 宽大复杂的波形需考虑室性节律。
  - 除非绝对确定 SVT，否则视为室性心动过速(VT)。

病因

- 窦性心动过速：
  - 急性心肌梗死。
  - 贫血。
  - 焦虑。
  - 慢性心力衰竭。
  - 药物中毒。
  - 甲状腺功能亢进。
  - 血容量减少。
  - 缺氧。
  - 感染。
  - 疼痛。
  - 心脏压塞。
  - 肺栓塞。
- 房性心动过速：
  - 由于过早的心房或心室收缩所致。
  - 电解质紊乱。
  - 药物毒性(即茶碱)。
  - 缺氧。
  - 心房压力增加。
- 交界性心动过速：
  - 房室结折返。
  - 心肌缺血。
  - 结构性疾病。
  - 预激综合征。
- WPW 综合征：
  - 内在通路。
  - 药物和酒精毒性。
- 心房颤动：

S

  - 高血压。
  - 冠状动脉疾病。
  - 甲状腺功能亢进症。
  - 大量酒精摄入量。
  - 二尖瓣疾病。
  - 慢性肺病。
  - 肺栓塞。
  - 缺氧。
  - 地高辛中毒。
  - 慢性心包炎。
  - 特发性心房颤动。
- 心房扑动：
  - 缺血性心脏病。
  - 瓣膜性心脏病。
  - 慢性心力衰竭。
  - 心肌炎。
  - 心肌病。
  - 肺栓塞。
  - 电解质紊乱。
  - 其他肺部疾病。
- 多灶性房性心动过速。
  - 慢性肺病所致的缺氧影响。
  - 茶碱中毒。

诊断

体征和症状

- 心悸（最常见）。
- 头晕，目眩，头部压力大。
- 呼吸困难。
- 发汗。
- 头晕。
- 乏力。
- 胸闷。
- 昏厥。
- 突出的颈静脉“青蛙标志”。
- 不稳定的体征：
  - 精神状态的改变。
  - 胸痛/局部缺血。
  - 急性肺水肿。
  - 低血压。

病史

- 突然出现心悸、头晕、无力、胸痛：
  - 目前的症状。
  - 以前出现过。
- 全身无力、运动不耐受和不适的隐匿性发作。
- 心脏病既往史。
- 药物：
  - 非处方药、消肿剂。
- 非法药物使用。

体格检查

- 生命体征：
  - 呼吸频率正常或心动过速。
  - 心动过速。
  - 血压正常或低血压。
  - 呼吸频率正常或呼吸急促。
- 心脏：
  - 规则或不规则的节奏。
  - 心力衰竭患者可有颈静脉扩张。
- 肺：
  - 湿啰音可能存在于心力衰竭的情况下。
  - 发现有慢性肺疾病可能提示 MAT。

基本检查

- 生命体征、评估稳定与不稳定。
- 既往史。
- 心电图。

诊断检查与说明

实验室检查

- 血常规。
- 电解质。
- 心肌酶谱、BNP。
- 甲状腺功能（通常低血容量）。
- 如果怀疑贫血需检测肌钙蛋白。
- 如果怀疑慢性心力衰竭需检测 BNP。

影像学检查

- X 线：
  - 评估心脏大小。
  - 评估肺状况。
  - 房颤更有用。

诊断步骤/外科

- 心电图：
  - 房颤：
    - 心房纤颤波没有可辨别的 P 波。
    - 心律不规律，100～220 次/分。
  - 房扑：
    - 常规心房率通常＞300 次/分。
    - 周期、极性和幅度的规律均匀。
    - 锯齿颤动波向上导向，在导联Ⅱ、Ⅲ、aVF 中最明显。
    - 房室传导阻滞，通常为 2∶1，但偶尔较大或不规则。
  - 多形性房性心动过速：
    - 3 种明显不同的 P 波，具有不同的脉率间隔。
  - 房性心动过速：
    - 速率为 100～200 次/分。
    - P 波在 QRS 波群之前，并且在形态上不同于窦性 P 波。
  - 交界性心动过速：
    - 通常 1∶1 传导，心室率等于心房率。
    - 可能是阵发性或持续性的。
    - 成人的心室率＞200 次/分提示 WPW 综合征。
    - 没有先前的 P 波。
    - 隐藏在 QRS 波群中的经常是逆行的 P 波。

鉴别诊断

- 窦性心动过速：
  - 脓血症。
  - 低血容量。
  - 心脏压塞。
  - 急性心肌梗死。
  - 药物中毒。
- 宽大复杂的心动过速：
  - 区分是室上性或室性。

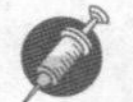

治疗

S

院前

- 吸氧。
- 建立静脉通路。
- 监测。

初步稳定/治疗

- 建立静脉通路。
- 吸氧。
- 监测。
- 血流动力学不稳定的患者实施电复律。

急诊治疗/程序

- 房颤/房扑：
  - 当节律不规则时，AF 被诊断出来。
  - 当生命体征不稳定时，立即同步复律。
  - 稳定时，控制心室率是重中之重：
    - β受体阻滞剂或钙通道阻滞剂，胺碘酮和地高辛。
    - 存在栓塞风险，除非已知为急性心律失常（持续时间＜48 h），否则不应尝试复律。
    - 应考虑使用 CHA2DS2－VASc 评分进行卒中风险分层评估。
- 预激综合征：
  - 考虑直流电复律或胺碘酮、氟卡尼或普鲁卡因胺。
  - 避免 AV 节点阻断剂，如腺苷、β受体阻滞剂、钙通道阻滞剂和地高辛。
- 在常规狭窄的复杂 SVT 中：
  - 刺激迷走神经偶尔会终止心律失常：

◦ 颈动脉按摩(注意颈动脉疾病,尤其是老年人)。
◦ 把冰放儿童脸上(哺乳动物反射)。
◦ 瓦氏法复律。
◦ 仰卧位使腿部抬高可能会提高瓦氏法的成功率。
– 如果不成功,腺苷是首选药物。
– 腺苷 6 mg 转复 60%～80%的 SVT。
• 宽大复杂的 SVT:
– 确定 VT 异常还是 SVT 异常。
– 如果无法确定,必须视为 VT 异常。
– Brugada 标准可能有助于确定 VT(请参阅"室性心动过速")。
– 维拉帕米绝对禁忌。
– 腺苷应该用于 SVT 异常。
– 电复律:
◦ 当机制不明时,比使用抗心律失常药物的并发症少很多。
– 抗心律失常药物:
◦ 静脉注射普鲁卡因胺和静脉注射胺碘酮。
◦ 利多卡因疗效不佳,但有时更容易获得。
◦ 溴苄乙胺缺乏任何有效性证据。

S

儿科注意事项

• 不稳定患者同步复律 0.5～1 J/kg。
• SVT 是年轻人和无心血管疾病的儿童中最常见的心律失常:
– 初始刺激迷走神经手法:
◦ 婴儿:冰/水袋敷前额×15 s。
◦ 孩子:瓦氏动作"吹入稻草"。
• 异常传导:
– WPW 综合征和 AVNRT 是 SVT 在儿童中最常见的两种形式。
• 仅>1 岁儿童使用维拉帕米。

老年人注意事项

• 腺苷被认为是安全的。
• 二线用药静脉注射普萘洛尔或美托洛尔。
• 禁忌使用维拉帕米(产妇低血压)。
• 复律是安全的。

■ 药物治疗

• 腺苷:6 mg(儿童:0.1 mg/kg 至 6 mg)快速静脉注射;如果 1～2 min 后没有反应,则 12 mg(儿童:0.2 mg/kg 直至 12 mg),可以重复 12 mg(0.2 mg/kg)。
• 胺碘酮:在 10 min 内静脉负荷 15 mg/min 静脉内(儿童:5 mg/kg, 20～60 min),然后静脉滴注 1 mg/min 6 h,然后静脉滴注 1 mg/min 6 h,然后静脉滴注 0.5 mg/min,静脉注射 18 h。
• 地高辛:最初 0.5 mg 静脉注射,然后 0.25 mg,静脉注射,q4 h。
• 地尔硫䓬:在 2 min 内 0.25 mg/kg,静脉注射(通常 10～20 mg),然后在 15 min 内以 2 min 内 0.35 mg/kg 静脉注射。
• 艾司洛尔:1 min 内静脉给药 0.5 mg/kg;维持输液,4 min 静脉注射 0.05 mg/(kg·min),然后静脉注射 0.1～0.2(kg·min)。
• 利多卡因:100 mg,静脉注射。
• 美托洛尔:以 5 min 的间隔缓慢推注 5～15 mg,至总共 15 mg。
• 普鲁卡因胺:20～30 mg/min 静脉注射高达 17 mg/kg,对于更紧急的情况可能增加至 50 mg/min。
• 普萘洛尔:0.1 mg/kg,静脉注射,以 2～3 min 的间隔分成等剂量。
• 索他洛尔:静脉注射,10 mg/min,静脉注射,至 1～1.5 mg/kg。
• 维拉帕米:2.5～5 mg 超过 2 min 静脉推注;可以用 5～10 mg, q15～30 min,重复至最大剂量 20 mg。

随访

■ 进一步处理

入院指征

• 可能的心脏缺血。
• 持续存在 SVT。
• 可能预激综合征。
• 其他潜在的代谢异常。

出院指征

终止异常节律,没有器官灌注不足。

转诊问题

如果不存在潜在心脏疾病或代谢紊乱,那么成功治疗的无并发症的 SVT 患者可以出院,接受医生或心脏病专家随访。

■ 随访建议

如果患者感到头晕、麻木或四肢乏力,或视物、说话困难,应该返回急诊。避免高风险活动(游泳、驾驶、潜水等),直到进一步评估。

要点和误区

• 应该在患者平躺时尝试 Valsalva,成功的可能性很小,但操作简单而高效。
• AF 伴有旁路途径,最令人担忧的异常节律如 WPW 综合征,在心室率快时,房颤可能看起来很规则,但不应被误认为良性 SVT。
• 当腺苷没有明显效果时,有时会使用剂量超过 12～18 mg。然而,如果任何较低的腺苷剂量瞬时减慢心脏节律,但很快恢复快速速率,那么增加剂量是不必要的,并且应该使用替代药物。
• 不确定病因的宽大复杂心动过速应视为 VT。通常使用胺碘酮,如果有旁路途径,可使用普鲁卡因胺。
• 由于普鲁卡因胺可以以 50 mg/min 的最高速率给药,至少需要 20 min 来使用 1 g 或 30 min 来使用 1.5 g。因此,要及时给药优化用药时机。如果出现 QRS 波群宽大或低血压,则减慢给药速度或停止用药。

室性心动过速 Ventricular Tachycardia

Emily M. Mills · Rama A. Salhi 吴昊 李文放 译

基础知识

■ 描述

• 广泛复杂的快速性心律失常:
– ≥3 个连续 QRS 波群,心室率>100 次/分,QRS 持续时间>120 ms。
– 独立于心房和正常的传导系统的心室快速、规则的去极化。
– 如果持续时间大于 30 s,出现晕厥或停搏,或需要心脏复律/起搏,则视为持续。
• 单一形态 VT——单一、稳定的 QRS 形态图。
• 多形态 VT——QRS 形态改变:
• 尖端扭转:
– VT 的多形态性形式。

- 交替的电动极性和幅度。
- 基线心电图上出现长 QT。
- 后天性或先天性。
- 双向 VT - QRS 额平面轴上的逐拍交替：
- 洋地黄中毒。
- 儿茶酚胺能多形性 VT(遗传性，罕见，高致命性)。

▪ 病因

- 广泛的复杂心动过速：
- 成为 VT 的可能性为 80%。
- 20% 左束支传导阻滞(LBBB)或异常性 SVT。
- 广泛的复杂性心动过速和心肌梗死的病史：
- >98%可能发展为室速。
- 年龄>35 岁：80%发展为室速。
- 年龄<35 岁：发展为室速的风险为 75%。
- 非持续性室速的发病率：
- 总人口中的 0～4%。
- 高达 60%的扩张型心肌病患者患有室速。
- 与心脏性猝死(SCD)风险增加有关。
- 室速的机制：
- 可重复：
  - 常见于结构性心脏病(扩张型心肌病、缺血、先天性心脏病、心肌梗死、瘢痕形成、手术前)。
  - 单向传导。
  - 固定或功能性传导阻滞。
  - "慢传导"区域。
- 异常自律性：
  - 心室细胞区域加速产生的异常脉冲。
- 触发的活动：
  - 由于去极化后的早期或晚期。
- 多形态室速的原因：
- 获得性(药物诱导或电解质异常)。
- 先天性(长 QT 间期综合征)。
- 缺血。
- 器质性心脏病。
- 不管其机制如何，所有室颤 VT 都可能演变为室颤(VF)。

诊断

▪ 症状和体征

病史

- 无症状。
- 晕厥/接近晕厥。
- 头晕。
- 呼吸急促。
- 心悸。
- 胸部不适/疼痛。
- CHF。

体格检查

- 脉搏缺失，精神状态和生命体征异常。
- 心脏的听诊会发现心动过速。
- 发汗。
- 大炮型 A 波。
- 低血压。
- 收缩压的搏动变异性。
- 心音的变异性，特别是第一心音。

▪ 基本检查

- 心电图是最重要的初步检查。
- 有利于单形性室颤的心电图标准。
- RBBB 的 QRS 波群>140 ms。
- LBBB 的 QRS 波群>160 ms。
- A - V 分离(融合波，节律捕获)。
- 电轴偏转(−90°～+180°)。
- 心前区 R 波一致性进行模式。
- 右束支传导阻滞 RBBB：V_1 具有 R>R′。
- 右束支传导阻滞 LBBB：V_6 具有 Q 或 QS。
- Brugada 标准定义室速(逐步算法，只需要一个来诊断 VT)。
- RS 在所有心前区导联缺席。
- 胸导联 RS 间期>100 ms。
- A - V 分离。
- V_1～V_2 和 V_6 中 VT 的形态学标准(见附加阅读)。
- SVT 伴异常传导的心电图指标。
- 正常轴 QRS<140 ms。
- 无 Q 波。
- V_1 中 RBBB 表现为 rsR 三相模式。
- 房室结阻滞：抗心律失常药物引起的冲动传导速度减慢在更快的速度下更为明显，因此可能导致广泛的复杂 SVT(SVT 伴异常偏离)。
- 尖端扭转。
- 每 10～20 次旋转一次的多形态室速。

▪ 诊断检查与说明

实验室检查

- 心脏酶。
- 电解质、BUN、肌酐、葡萄糖。
- 镁。
- 钙。
- 地高辛浓度，如果怀疑毒性。

影像学检查

胸部 X 线检查：

- 心脏病或其他心脏明显异常。

超声：

- 评估左心室功能。
- 结构性疾病可能被发现。

诊断步骤/外科

食管导管起搏：

- 可能能够检测心房活动以建立房室分离并因此诊断 VT。
- 如果心动过速用抗心律失常药物难控制，导管可以用来调整心率。

▪ 鉴别诊断

- SVT 伴有异常的左束支传导阻滞。
- 继发于抗心律失常药物的心律失常；怀疑是否：
- VT 形态与以前的 VT 发作不同。
- 最近药物改变。
- QT 间隔>440 ms。
- 尖端扭转。
- 如果室速反复发作可考虑电复律。

治疗

▪ 院前

- 注意事项：
- 运送稳定的疑似室速患者而不尝试复律。
- 对脉搏不稳定的患者进行同步心脏复律。
- 无脉搏室颤的除颤。
- 不建议使用预防性利多卡因(Ⅲ类：危害)。

▪ 初步稳定/治疗

ABC 管理，建立静脉通路，监测，心电图。

▪ 急诊治疗/程序

无脉 VT：

- 立即除颤并遵循 ACLS 无脉性室性心动过速(pVT)治疗计划。
- 胺碘酮可用于对 CPR、除颤和血管加压疗法无反应的 pVT(Ⅱb 类)。
  - 利多卡因可作为替代品(Ⅱb 类)。
- 不建议常规使用镁(第三类：无益处)。
- 没有抗心律失常药物被证明可以增加 pVT/VF 引起的心搏骤停后的生存率/神经系统转化率。
- 具有脉搏的 VT 患者。
- 定义：
  - 胸部疼痛。
  - 低血压。
  - 心功能不全证据。
- 如果患者没有反应，立即启动 100 J 的同步心脏复跳，若仍无反应则升至 200 J、300 J 和 360 J。

◦ 如果室速是多形的，则在 200 J 开始复律。

- 在复律之前给患者充分镇静。

- 如果无法终止室速，则应用利多卡因（Ⅱb 类）并继续复律。

◦ 利多卡因可作为替代品（Ⅱb 类）。

- 在窦性心律恢复成功后，开始使用胺碘酮。

- 如果室速对静脉注射镁没有反应。

- 如果不能立即使用除颤器，则考虑心前区重击，以观察、监测、不稳定的 VT（Ⅱb 类）。

- 钙通道阻滞剂对未知来源的 WCT 有潜在危害（Ⅲ类：危害）。

- 不稳定、不规则或 WCT 不应给予腺苷，因为它可能导致室颤（Ⅲ类）。

注意

2017 年 AHA/ACC/HRS 和 2015 年 ESC 指南均推荐普鲁卡因胺使用，最近的研究表明其有效，但胺碘酮是最新 ACLS 指南中列出的用于 pVT 治疗的唯一药物，在美国，胺碘酮是 VT 的首选药物。需要进一步的研究。

S

• 稳定单形性 VT：

- 基线的正常 QT 间隔：

◦ 胺碘酮（Ⅱb 类）：如怀疑为新的 HF 或急性 MI，则输注。

◦ 普鲁卡因胺（Ⅱa 类）：避免使用如果出现心力衰竭、急性心肌梗死或延长 QT（Ⅲ类）。

◦ 考虑索他洛尔（Ⅱb 类）：避免使用如果出现 HF 或 QT 延长（Ⅲ类）。

◦ 利多卡因：效果较差，但考虑是否对其他措施无反应。

- 基线时心功能受损：

◦ 输注胺碘酮。

- 如果抗心律失常治疗不成功，考虑同步心脏复律或专家会诊。

• 稳定多形态 VT/尖端扭转。

- 基线的正常 QT 间隔：

◦ 纠正电解质异常，尤其是 K^+、Mg^{2+}。

◦ 治疗缺血，如果存在。

◦ 胺碘酮可能有效（Ⅱb 类）。

◦ 镁对 QT 正常的患者疗效较差（Ⅱb 类）。

◦ 静脉注射 β 受体阻滞剂对缺血（Ⅱa 类）可能有用。

- QT 延长。

◦ 纠正电解质。

◦ 静脉注射镁。

◦ 超速起搏，如果对镁没有反应。

◦ 如果患者没有冠状动脉疾病史或先天性长 QT 综合征（Ⅰ类），因获得性 QT 延长引起的复发性扭转和静脉镁不能抑制心动过缓，故可采用起搏或异丙肾上腺素治疗。

- 儿茶酚胺能多形态 VT：

◦ 寻求专家咨询。

◦ 如果既往有耐受阻断剂，可能需要联合药物治疗、心脏交感神经去神经术或 ICD（Ⅰ类）。

- 基线时心脏功能受损。

◦ 胺碘酮（或利多卡因），然后同步心脏复律。

妊娠注意事项

• 潜在结构性心脏病患者发生 VT 的风险增加。

• 如果有长 QT 综合征史，妊娠期间应继续使用阻断剂（Ⅰ类）。

• 不稳定时用复律治疗（Ⅰ类）。

• 考虑索他洛尔或普鲁卡因胺在稳定单形 VT（Ⅱa 类）。

• 如果电复律难治、不稳定或对其他药物无反应（Ⅱa 类），可使用胺碘酮。

• 注：妊娠期胺碘酮为 D 类。

• 可以考虑导管消融。

儿童注意事项

• 原发性心搏骤停和 VT 在儿童中罕见。

• 通常继发于缺氧和酸中毒。

• VT 对于儿童较长时期的耐受性高于成人，并且不太可能退化为 VF。

• VT 中最常见的 VT 表现为 CHF。

• 儿童 VT 的结果来自：

- 心肌病。

- Congeital 结构性心脏病。

- 先天性延长的 QT 综合征。

- 继发于血管炎的冠状动脉疾病。

- 毒素、毒药、毒品。

- 严重的电解质紊乱，尤其是钾。

• 胺碘酮或利多卡因可用于治疗休克难治性 pVT（Ⅱb 类）。

• 心脏复律启动能量剂量 0.5～1.0 J/kg，如果失败则增加到 2 J/kg。

• 无脉室速启动能量剂量 2～4 J/kg，如果失败可能增加，但不要超过 10 J/kg 或成人最大剂量。

药物治疗

一线用药

• 胺碘酮：无脉性 VT 静脉注射 300 mg，第二次静脉注射 150 mg，稳定 VT 静脉注射 150 mg，注射 1 mg/min×6 h，0.5 mg/min×18 h。24 h 最大累计剂量 2.2 g［儿童：5 mg/kg 静脉注射/骨髓腔注射超过 20～60 min，最大剂量 15 mg/（kg · d）］。

• 普鲁卡因胺：20～50 mg/min 静脉注射（最大剂量 17 mg/kg）或 100 mg 持续 2 min 以上（每 5 min），直到心律失常被抑制，随后维持输注 1～4 mg/min（儿童：15 mg/kg 静脉注射/骨髓腔注射，超过 30～60 min）。应避免延长 QT、HF 或急性心肌梗死。如需心电图和血压监测，并停止。

• $MgSO_4$：2 g 加入 D_5W，5～10 min，然后输注 0.5～1 g/h 静脉注射，滴定以控制转室（儿童：25～50 mg/kg，静脉注射或骨髓腔注射，最大剂量 2 g）。

二线用药

• 利多卡因：1～1.5 mg/kg 静脉推注第一剂，第二次剂量 0.5～0.75 mg/kg，最大剂量 q5～10 min，为 3 mg/kg；气管给药 2～4 mg/kg；如果转换，维持输液 1～4 mg/min。不建议用于 ACS 诱发的室速［儿童：1 mg/kg 推注，输注 20～50 μg/（kg · min）］。

• 异丙肾上腺素：2～10 μg/min，滴定至心率［儿童：0.1 μg/（kg · min）］。注意：不要给予肾上腺素，可能沉淀 VT/NF（不再是 ACLS 方案的一部分），如果延长 QT 则不给予。

• 索他洛尔：5 min 内 100 mg 静脉注射（儿童：不推荐用于初始管理）。注意：不要延长 QT。

随访

进一步处理

入院指征

• 承认 VT 持续到 ICU。

• 承认非持续性室速和心肌梗死病史或扩张型心肌病的电生理研究。

出院指征

• 罕见的非特发性 VT 患者和以前没有发现结构性心脏病的评估可以出院：

- SCD 的风险较低。

• 具有良好功能的心脏自动心脏起搏器的患者也可以出院。

转诊问题

所有出院的患者应在 48 h 内接受心脏科医师随访。

随访建议

患者应该随访心脏病学专家。

要点和误区

• 寻找毒素、代谢异常、创伤、体温过低、血栓形成等因素。

• 不稳定的 VT 需要重新开始复律。

• 给予复苏后维持用药以防止复发。

• 胺碘酮治疗后注意心动过缓和胃肠道毒性。

• 停止使用任何心律失常药物。

• 针对缺血诱导的 VT 和多形态 VT 考虑 β_2 受体阻滞。

• 延长 QT 时避免普鲁卡因胺和索他洛尔。

嗜铬细胞瘤

Kristen G. Moore　瞿金龙　林兆奋 译

基础知识

描述

• 嗜铬细胞瘤(pheo)是一种可分泌儿茶酚胺、起源于交感神经系统嗜铬组织的肿瘤。

• 起源于肾上腺髓质或交感神经节：
- 80%孤立肾上腺(通常是右方)。
- 10%两侧(通常为遗传)。
- 10%肾上腺外位置：
  ◦ 腹部、肠系膜神经节内(86%)。
  ◦ 胸部(10%)、颈部(3%)、膀胱(1%)。
- 10%为恶性(通常为遗传)。

• 发生率：
- 高血压患者为 0.2%～0.4%，但重度高血压患者的发生率更高。
- 每年每 100 万人口中有 2～8 例。
- 几十年高峰为 3～5 例，10%为儿童。
- 男性同女性。
- 约 50%的病例是死后确诊的。
- 10%为无临床症状的，包括偶尔在 CT 影像上。

• 遗传：
- 25%为常染色体显性遗传。
- 通常与 MEN 2A 相关，与 MEN 2B 或希佩尔-林道综合征(VHL)相关性小些。
  ▪ MEN 2A(甲状腺髓样癌、嗜铬细胞瘤和甲状旁腺功能亢进)。
  ▪ MEN 2B(甲状腺髓样癌、嗜铬细胞瘤、口腔黏膜神经瘤、骨骼瘦小和骨骼畸形)。
  ▪ VHL(视网膜和中枢神经系统的血管母细胞瘤、胰腺和肾囊肿的血管母细胞瘤，以及 PHEO 的血管母细胞瘤)。
- 其他相关疾病：神经纤维瘤病、结节性脑硬化、斯德奇-韦伯综合征、颈部神经节瘤。

病因

• 肿瘤合成及存储儿茶酚胺的方式与正常肾上腺髓质相同。

• 肿瘤主要分泌去甲肾上腺素，也分泌少量的肾上腺素(有些肿瘤有肾上腺素优势，低血压是其特征)。

• 儿茶酚胺的阵发性释放：
- 由于血流量或肿瘤坏死的变化而自发地释放。
- 来自外部压力(损伤、锻炼)的腺体的直接压力。
- 沉淀析出(阿片类药物、类固醇激素、胰高血糖素、甲氧氯普胺、酪胺的食物、碘造影剂)。
- 儿茶酚胺效应增强(TCA、β 受体阻滞剂、拟交感神经药)。

诊断

症状和体征

病史

• 高血压，中度至重度，难治性：
- 40%：正常血压阵发性发作。
- 30%：持续的高血压发作。
- 30%：持续的高血压没有发作。
- 有时血压正常，为家族形式和小肿瘤：<5%。

• 阵发性症状：
- 猝发，逐步解决。
- 持续时间：数分钟至数小时(平均 20 min)。
- 间隔：数小时至数月(平均数周)。
- 随着时间的推移，频率增加、持续时间延长且更加严重。

• 阵发性的临床特征：
- 高血压危象或紧迫感。
- 头痛，突发，搏动，双向。
- 心动过速或心悸。
- 忧虑、焦虑或颤抖。
- 与创伤、手术、分娩、麻醉相关的休克。

• 急性危象：
- 严重阵发性延长(>24 h)。
- 严重高血压或休克，高热。
- 多器官功能衰退或乳酸性酸中毒。
- 由于心肌病(扩张型心肌病、肥大性心肌病或 Takotsubo 心肌)的肺水肿。
- 脑卒中(蛛网膜下腔出血、可逆性后部脑病综合征、RCVS、脑栓塞)。
- 严重头痛或脑病。
- 胸痛(心肌梗死或解剖)。
- 急腹症：
  ◦ 出血性肿瘤坏死。
  ◦ 肠系膜梗死。

• 慢性症状：
- 胸痛或心悸。
- 静态平衡位(血浆容量减少和减弱交感神经反射)。
- 便秘可能严重，导致肠梗阻塞或假梗阻(儿茶酚胺抑制蠕动)。
- 体重减轻或发热(代谢加快)。
- 昏睡，疲乏(儿茶酚胺回退)。
- 多饮、多尿(葡萄糖耐受不良)。
- 焦虑、震颤、热耐受不良。

体格检查

• 中度至重度高血压，经常伴有体位变化。

• 心动过速、发汗、体重减少、低热。

• 苍白、手足冰冷(脸红的人看不到，除了很少的阵发后可见)。

• 震颤、焦虑。

• 瞳孔放大、高血压性视网膜病变。

• 咖啡牛乳色斑、纤维神经瘤、甲状腺结节。

• 无明显的肿块(肿瘤往往比较小)。

基本检查

• 直立时血压测定比较准确。

• 心电图排除缺血或心律失常。

诊断检查与说明

• 诊断过度>20%，来自对边缘生化测试的误解和过度成像。

• 漏诊通常是因为没有考虑过诊断或忽视了 CT 图上的肾上腺肿块。

S

实验室检查

• 计数检查：
- 血红蛋白的升高是由于血浆容量减少。
- 白细胞总数比界限升高。

• 电解液、血尿氮、肌酸酐、葡萄糖：
- 乳酸性酸中毒。
- 肾衰竭继发于高血压肾病。
- 高血糖是由于对胰岛素反应受损及儿茶酚胺作用。
- 高血钙症是由于甲状旁腺激素过量。

• 尿分析：蛋白尿与血尿。

• 血浆游离甲氧基肾上腺素(分次的)：
- 敏感性 96%，特异性 85%。
- 最好的筛选测试。正常水平排除诊断，但有很多假阳性。
- 最不可能被药物或压力干预，而且没有对静脉穿刺特殊准备。

• 24 h 尿液的收集来获得游离的儿茶酚胺和变肾上腺素(总的和分次的)：
- 99.7%的结合特异性和 87.5%的敏感性(确诊的最好测试)。
- 必须包括肌酸酐以证实采集充分。
- 有干扰的药物：左旋多巴、甲基多巴、单胺氧化酶抑制剂(MAIO)、拉贝洛尔、普萘洛尔、放射摄影(对比)造影剂、三环类、咖啡因、尼古丁。

影像学检查

• 肾上腺肿块的 CT 灵敏度要>1 cm(静脉造影可能会引起轻度危险)：
- 5%在 CT 上看到的偶发性肾上腺瘤是嗜铬细胞瘤。

• 磁共振成像或正电子发射断层扫描在鉴别肾上腺嗜铬细胞瘤和肾上腺外肿瘤上敏感性更高。

• 间碘苯甲胍(放射性核素闪烁扫描：定位特异性高，但对排除嗜铬细胞瘤的敏感性还不够)。

• 肺水肿需拍摄 X 线胸片。

• 脑卒中或脑出血需拍摄头部 CT。

诊断步骤/外科

• 如果诊断不确定采用可乐定抑制测试(如果是嗜铬细胞瘤则水平无抑制)。

• 不推荐使用胰高血糖素激发测试。

• 忌用细针穿刺。

• 腹腔镜切除术在许多情况下是可行的。

鉴别诊断

• 戒酒综合征。

• 自主性反射亢进。

• 脑血管病变。

• 可卡因或苯丙胺中毒。

• 高血压危象。

• 偏头痛或蛛网膜下出血。

• 惊恐发作。

• 直立性心动过速综合征。

• 阵发性室上性心动过。

• 后可逆性脑病综合征。

• 5-羟色胺(血清素)综合征。

• 甲状腺毒症。

• 毒血症。

治疗

院前

• 建立静脉通路，给氧。

• 连续心脏或血压监测。

• 对胸痛和高血压用硝化甘油 0.4 mg 舌下含服。
- 头部外伤常见于癫痫人群。

• 收集或运输药瓶和药物来帮助识别和量化摄入。

初步稳定/治疗

• 基本体征。
- 建立静脉通路。
- 心脏监测示波器(伴随静脉注射超剂量)。

• 对精神状态的改变：
- Accu-Chek。
- 使用所示的纳洛酮、葡萄糖和硫胺素。

• 通过静脉输液和头低足高体位治疗低血压。
- 多巴胺治疗顽固性低血压。

• 地西泮治疗反常痉挛。

急诊治疗/程序

高血压疾病的管理

• 酚妥拉明：α 受体阻滞剂：
- 1 mg 静脉注射测试剂量。
- 2.5～5 mg 静脉注射大丸剂给药速度在 1 mg/min。每 5～15 min 重复大丸剂给药来控制血压，随后注入。
- 注入开始速度在 0.1 mg/min 逐渐增加至 1 mg/min。
- 当血管收缩减轻时需要有力的体液复苏。
- 习惯方法，但尼卡地平或硝普盐点滴可能更实用。

• β 受体阻滞剂：
- 添加到 α 受体阻滞剂中进一步控制血压。
- 可能在 α 受体阻滞剂诱导过程中形成心动过速。
- 从不单独使用：没有事先用 α 受体阻滞剂试验而直接用 β 受体阻滞剂的话可能由于抑制了平滑肌中 β 受体介导的血管舒张而加剧高血压。
- 艾司洛尔：前 1 min 负荷量 500 μg/kg，接下来 4 min 为 50 μg/(kg · min)；如果在 5 min 内没有达到足够的治疗效果，重复加药且增加输液流速至 100 μg/(kg · min)；重复加药且输液滴速按需要在 q4～q5 min 50 μg/(kg · min)；一旦接近治疗靶点不用再进一步加药。
- 拉贝洛尔：开始为 10～20 mg 静脉注射；血压在 5 min 内下降，在 10 min 时效果最佳；在 q15～q30 min 内静脉注射双倍剂量药物直到到达靶点(α 受体阻滞剂不足以作为一个单独的药剂)。
- 美托洛尔：q15 min 静脉注射 5 mg 直到有反应。

• 如果对酚妥拉明不敏感会对 α 受体和 β 受体阻滞剂或一线药物产生耐药性：
- 硝普盐：
  ◦ 开始速度在 0.5 μg/(kg · min)。
  ◦ 滴速增量为 0.5 μg/(kg · min)。
  ◦ 最大剂量 10 μg，一般需要 3～4 μg。
- 尼卡地平：
  ◦ 开始输液为 5 mg/h。
  ◦ 滴速每 15 min 增加 2.5 mg/h。
  ◦ 最大剂量至 15 mg/h。
- 如果需要添加 β 受体阻滞剂来扩张血管。

• 心室快速性心律失常：
- 利多卡因：
  ◦ 大丸剂 50～100 mg。开始速度在 0.5 μg/(kg · min)。
  ◦ 重复大丸剂 q5 min(最大剂量 5 mg/kg)。
- 艾司洛尔注射速度为 50～200 μg/(kg · min)。

药物治疗

一线治疗

• 苯氧苄胺：开始口服：一次 10 mg，每日 2 次；之后每日增加 10 mg 直至达到需要的效果(术前至少 7 日开始)。

• 其他 α 受体阻滞剂(首次剂量影响)：
- 多沙唑嗪：1～8 mg/d(开始在 1 mg)。
- 特拉唑嗪：1～10 mg/d(开始在 1 mg)。

• 添加 β 受体阻滞剂来控制反射性心动过速：
- 美托洛尔或阿替洛尔：25～100 mg/d。

二线治疗

• 钙通道阻滞剂：
- 氨氯地平、尼卡地平或硝苯地平。

• 合成儿茶酚胺抑制剂：
- 美替罗星：250～500 mg q6 h。

> **注意**
> 下列药物可在嗜铬细胞瘤中产生高血压危象：
> • β受体阻滞剂(如果没有用α受体阻滞剂前处理)。
> • 胰高血糖素。
> • 糖皮质激素。
> • 碘化造影剂(离子的)。
> • 氯胺酮。
> • 灭吐灵。
> • 阿片类。
> • 拟交感神经药，包括非处方药。

妊娠注意事项

• 可能会与中毒混淆，但通常不伴有蛋白尿。
• MRI 是首选成像方式。
• 硝普钠不宜用于高血压危象，但其他所有血压药物都可接受。
• 自然阴道分娩可能会诱发高血压危象，应该计划剖宫产。

随访

进一步处理

入院指征

• 怀疑嗜铬细胞瘤患者，出现血压波动大、病情严重。
• 急性或高血压危象。
• 心律失常。
• 靶器官损害：充血性心力衰竭、心肌梗死、肾功能不全、脑卒中、腹痛。
• 考虑需要进行内分泌学和全科医学会诊。

出院指征

患者高血压轻度、稳定。

随访建议

• 在高血压发作时检测血浆游离甲氧基肾上腺素。
• 考虑使用多沙唑嗪、特拉唑嗪或钙通道阻断剂来控制血压。
• 安排密切随访。

要点和误区

• 严重的高血压、头痛、紧张出汗、心悸的发作构成了嗜铬细胞瘤的 4 个明显特征。
• 苍白、出汗、不脸红，是典型的嗜铬细胞瘤危象。
• 直立性低血压在嗜铬细胞瘤中很常见，并且在α受体阻滞剂治疗前，除非同时进行容量复苏，否则低血压会进一步加重。
• 在难治性高血压、不明原因休克、多系统器官功能衰竭、心肌病、新发生的葡萄糖耐量不良伴体重减轻和原因不明的焦虑发作中考虑嗜铬细胞瘤。
• 通过间歇性症状、不太可能出现高热、热不耐受和体重减轻，可以将嗜铬细胞瘤与甲状腺危象区分开。
• 在嗜铬细胞瘤患者中不要在使用α受体阻滞剂之前使用β受体阻滞剂(即使是拉贝洛尔)。
• 在发作期间血浆游离甲氧基肾上腺素非常敏感，但不具有特异性。

S

手部感染

Chester D. Shermer 刘雪峰 译

基础知识

描述

• 手部感染是急诊科的常见疾病。
• 其病理范围广泛，包括各种急慢性情况。

> **注意**
> • 因为有可能发展成严重的手部感染，所以需要谨慎处理。
> • 对握紧的拳头伤势保持高度怀疑。
> • 建议转诊至手外科。

病因

• 手部的细菌感染常常与皮肤上寄生的病原体相关：
- 葡萄球菌或链球菌属。
- 局部外伤病史。
• 75%的儿童甲沟炎可归因于吮吸手指或咬指甲导致的厌氧菌感染。
• 白色念珠菌感染可导致慢性甲沟炎。
• 1 型和 2 型单纯疱疹病毒可引起疱疹性指头炎。
• 握拳伤感染可由多种病原菌引起，包括厌氧链球菌属和艾肯菌属。

诊断

症状和体征

• 甲沟炎：
- 近端甲襞侧面部分局限性红肿、疼痛。
- 可存在波动感，扩展至甲缘下。
- 通常无全身症状。
• 化脓性指头炎：
- 因脓液不能扩散通过指关节，出现红肿、局部张力增高。
- 早期出现疼痛，可进展为搏动性疼痛。
- 多无全身症状。
• 疱疹性指头炎：
- 指端肿胀，但无明显张力增高。
- 可累及侧甲襞。
- 指端的搏动性疼痛。
- 指端存在非化脓性水疱，可融合。
- 全身症状，如发热、淋巴结肿大等。
• 屈肌腱鞘炎：
- 卡纳佛尔征：
◦ 指端对称性肿胀，伴有严重疼痛。
◦ 腱鞘区域可由波动感。
◦ 手指被动弯曲。
◦ 感染早期可出现伸指疼痛。
• 握拳伤感染：
- 由于握拳击打物体导致手背跨掌指关节的撕裂伤。
- 任何跨掌指关节的撕裂伤，除非能够证实受伤方式，否则必须假定为人咬伤(患者拳头击打对方口唇部牙齿而受伤)。
• 指蹼间隙脓肿：
- 感染间隙及邻近部位的疼痛、肿胀。
- 手指呈被动的外展状。
• 手掌间隙感染：
- 鱼际间隙感染：
◦ 鱼际疼痛、肿胀，可存在波动感。
◦ 拇指背侧张力增高的水肿。
◦ 拇指处于被动的外展屈曲位，被动外屈引起疼痛。

- 掌中间隙感染：
  - 掌中间隙肿胀疼痛。
  - 指背水肿。
  - 中指、环指（无名指）伸指运动可导致疼痛。
- 小鱼际间隙感染：
  - 小鱼际肿胀疼痛。
  - 手指运动不受限。

病史

参见症状与体征。

体格检查

参见症状与体征。

基本检查

多数手部感染可通过病史和体格检查明确，但是需明确手部神经及血管的状态。

诊断检查与说明

实验室检查

- 多数手部感染通常不需要进行实验室检查，但是疱疹性指头炎可以通过赞克试验证实。
- 革兰染色和细菌培养在化脓性指头炎治疗中可以指导抗生素的选择。
- 必要时可行血培养。
- 红细胞沉降率（ESR）和 C 反应蛋白（CRP）不是急性感染的常规指标。

影像学检查

- 放射线检查通常不必要，除非有外伤或异物。
- 对于化脓性指头炎、屈肌腱鞘炎、手掌间隙感染，放射线检查对是否存在骨髓炎或异物有帮助。
- 在握拳伤中可辅助诊断骨折。

鉴别诊断

- 甲沟炎应与疱疹性指头炎和化脓性指头炎鉴别。
- 各种类型手掌间隙感染的相互鉴别。

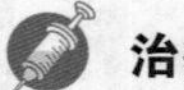

治疗

院前

酌情固定受伤手。

急诊治疗/程序

- 甲沟炎：
  - 早期未化脓的甲沟炎可予以口服抗生素和休息：
    - 阿莫西林-克拉维酸、环丙沙星、多西环素、复方新诺明、头孢呋辛、青霉素 V。
    - 如果与啃咬指甲或口腔接触有关，则使用克林霉素或甲硝唑。
  - 通过在指甲和甲上皮之间插入 11 号的刀片并将甲上皮从指甲上提起来引流浅表感染。
  - 如果需要，可以沿着指甲的曲线切开侧面指甲皱褶。
  - 当邻近指甲的背侧顶部下有脓液时，去掉近端指甲的 1/3。
- 指尖脓肿：
  - 首选侧面切口以避开神经血管束。
  - 但也可以通过在最大肿胀和疼痛区域用 11 号刀片行经皮小切口。
  - 更广泛的指尖脓肿可以通过单侧纵向切口进行引流，不要穿过远端指间关节（DIP）。
  - 不再推荐破坏纤维隔板：
    - 会导致指尖功能的不稳定。
    - 可能需要切开脓肿。
  - 给予口服抗生素以覆盖皮肤病原体，放置引流管，并在 48 h 内复查：
    - 头孢菌素、双氯西林、克林霉素、复方新诺明、阿莫西林-克拉维酸盐。
- 疱疹性指套炎：
  - 通常为自限性疾病；不需要切开和排脓。
  - 对于有全身受累的患者，可以给予口服阿昔洛韦。
- 屈肌腱鞘炎、指蹼间隙脓肿、掌侧间隙感染：
  - 抬高患处，静脉注射抗生素和疼痛控制。
    - 万古霉素、左氧氟沙星、环丙沙星、头孢噻肟。
  - 所有这些感染需要立即向手外科医生求助。
- 握拳伤：
  - 在急诊室抬高患处，静脉注射抗生素，破伤风预防和疼痛控制：
    - 氨苄西林-舒巴坦、头孢噻肟、替卡西林-克拉维酸、哌拉西林-他唑巴坦、甲硝唑。
  - 所有伴有感染证据或关节受累的咬伤需要紧急向手外科医生求助。
  - 如果没有感染迹象和没有关节穿透，患者经过适当冲洗和伤口护理后，可考虑口服抗生素门诊治疗：
    - 氨苄西林-克拉维酸或青霉素 V+头孢氨苄或双氯西林或甲硝唑。
    - 不要直接闭合被人咬伤的裂口；适当延迟初次闭合或次级愈合是合适的。

药物治疗

- 阿昔洛韦：每日口服 400 mg，每日 3 次，连续 10 日（儿童：不推荐用于疱疹性脓肿）。
- 阿莫西林-克拉维酸：每日口服 875/125 mg，每日 2 次（儿童：每日 40 mg/kg 口服，分 4 次，q6 h）。
- 氨苄西林-舒巴坦：静脉注射 1.5～3 g，q6 h（儿童：每日静脉注射 300 mg/kg，分 4 次，q6 h）。
- 头孢西丁：静脉注射 2 g，q8 h（儿童：每日静脉/肌内注射 80～160 mg/kg，分 4 次，q6 h）。
- 头孢氨苄：每日口服 500 mg，每日 4 次，连续 7 日（儿童：每日 40 mg/kg 口服，分 4 次，q6 h）。
- 克林霉素：每日口服 300～450 mg，每日 4 次，连续 7 日。严重病例可静脉使用：600～900 mg，q8 h（儿童：每日口服、静脉或肌内注射 20～40 mg/kg，q8 h）。
- 双氯西林：每日口服 500 mg，每日 4 次，连续 7 日（儿童：每日口服 12.5～50 mg/kg，分 4 次，q6h）。
- 甲硝唑：每日口服 500 mg，每日 3 次（儿童：每日口服或静脉注射 7.5～30 mg/kg，q12 h）。
- 青霉素 V：每日口服 500 mg，每日 4 次（儿童：每日口服 40 mg/kg，分 4 次，q6 h）。
- 替卡西林-克拉维酸：静脉注射 3.1 g，q4～6 h（儿童：每日静脉注射 150～300 mg/kg，q6～8 h）。
- 哌拉西林-他唑巴坦：静脉注射 3.375 g，q6 h（儿童：每日静脉注射 300 mg/kg，q8 h）。
- 复方新诺明：每日口服或静脉注射 10 mg/kg 药物，q12 h。

一线用药

根据病原学调整。

二线用药

根据病原学调整。

随访

进一步处理

入院指征

- 屈肌腱鞘炎、指蹼间隙脓肿、手掌间隙感染：
  - 均需静脉滴注抗生素和切开引流。
- 有感染征象的握拳伤：
  - 需外科清创并静脉滴注抗生素。

出院指征

- 甲沟炎与化脓性指头炎：

- 无并发症的患者给予急诊治疗，48 h 内复查并行切开引流后出院。
• 疱疹性指头炎：
- 给予急诊治疗和必要的复查后出院。
• 伴发感染的握拳伤：
- 口服抗生素，24 h 复查后出院。

转诊问题

建议申请手外科急会诊。

■ 随访建议

通常在有效的治疗后由内科医师安排。

要点和误区

• 诊断不及时。
• 未详细了解握拳伤的病史。
• 未迅速邀请手外科会诊。

手指骨损伤 Injuries, Hand

Vishnu Parthasarathy · Stephen R. Hayden　马林浩 译

基础知识

■ 描述

• 所有外伤中有 1/3 伤及手部。
• 趾(指)骨是骨骼系统中最易骨折的部分，手的远指端最常见。
• 手指近端指间关节的背侧移位是频繁发生的脱臼。

儿科注意事项

儿童受伤可能较难诊断，因为他们不能配合完成全项检查。

■ 病因

• 创伤(一般是和工作、运动有关)。
• 感染后遗症：
- 皮肤菌群：金黄色葡萄球菌和链球菌。
- 猫、犬咬伤：金黄色葡萄球菌和多杀巴斯德菌。
- 人类咬伤：艾肯菌。
- 荆棘植物或木本植物刺伤：真菌。
- 淡水、海水接触：海鱼分枝杆菌和铜绿假单胞菌(绿脓杆菌)。
• 过度使用损伤(例如，猎场看守人的拇指)。

诊断

■ 症状和体征

病史

• 受伤机制：
- 过伸性损伤最常见的是造成韧带受伤(如“杰西指”，指深屈肌腱从其远端附件开始破裂)或切屑断裂。
- 手指浸润部的过伸过屈性损伤可能造成“锤状指”，使远节指骨上的伸指肌腱插入点发生撕脱性骨折。
- 挤压伤最常见的是造成骨折和弥散性软组织损伤。
• 与偏手性有关。
• 与职业或爱好有关。
• 其他可能影响愈合的因素(如年龄、糖尿病、免疫抑制、抗凝血作用)。

体格检查

• 肿胀和/或变形(如切断、扭断、缩短或折断)。
• 皮肤改变(如淤斑、撕裂、烧伤、灰白)或者相关的指甲损伤。
• 手指运动范围减小或无力：肌腱功能。
- 手指外旋、内收功能(骨间肌)。
- 手指伸展功能(常见的伸肌肌腱)。
- 掌指关节屈曲功能(表浅屈肌腱)。
- 近端指关节屈曲功能(深部屈肌腱)。
• 受伤区域疼痛或知觉上的变化。

> **注意**
>
> Kanare 征(感染性屈肌腱鞘炎)：
> • 被动拉伸时沿肌腱疼痛(早期体征)。
> • 受影响的手指对称性放大。
> • 静止态下手指微弯曲。
> • 沿屈肌鞘横向条纹柔软(后期体征)。

儿科注意事项

婴儿发生手指疼痛或肿胀，考虑使用深嵌式头发止血带，不会在表浅检查中遮盖病情。

■ 基本检查

• 特别要注意用于评估个体肌腱状态、神经血管完整性，识别旋转畸形的手段：
- 隔离并评估每一个单独的关节(近侧指间关节、远侧指间关节、掌指关节)、被动活动及自发抗病性的范围。
- 标准两点辨别距离 4～5 mm。
- 可以通过弯曲掌指关节和伸展近侧指间关节即远侧指间关节的方法来定位手指，从而评估旋转不良：
◦ 通常情况下，所有手指指向桡骨后关节应该没有重叠或旋转。
• 首先行功能性评估，然后麻醉，如果需要不带血的区域，最后再使用止血带止血以便对撕裂区进行更好的检查。

■ 诊断检查与说明

实验室检查

如果存在感染体征或考虑屈肌腱鞘炎，考虑伤口组织培养。

影像学检查

• 所涉手指的清晰的 X 线检查应该包括前后位图、侧位图及斜视图。
• 超声对诊断肌腱断裂有所帮助。

儿科注意事项

开放性骨骺会使 X 线检查灵敏度下降。

■ 鉴别诊断

• 肌腱局部、完整的撕裂或破裂。
• 复杂的开放性损伤可能包括多处损伤，整个手部应该仔细检查。
• 当心掌指背部区域的撕裂伤，可能是殴斗性咬伤(人咬伤)。

儿科注意事项

• 儿童的许多骨折是手指骨的隆起(皮带扣形)骨折。
• 儿童的生长板通常比周韧带弱，因而多伴随有 Salter-Harris 骨折的脱臼发生。

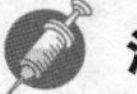

治疗

■ 院前

• 手指骨脱臼不应当考虑现场复位，除非患者运送时间会较长或者患者血管或神经受到损害。
- 现场复位可能会成功，但也会使医师遗漏重要的韧带损伤。

• 伤口流血应该使用适当的定向压力包覆处理。

> **注意**
> • 断掉的手指或组织应该放在干净润湿的生理盐水纱布上，置于塑料袋中，然后再放在一个单独装有冰块的袋子里。不要将断指与冰块直接接触！
> • 适用于断肢再植：
> - 拇指。
> - 近侧指间关节和远侧指间关节之间的单个指节。
> - 多个指节。
> - 儿童断指。

初步稳定/治疗

• 除去损伤手上的所有戒指。

• 通过近侧-远侧指关节间的夹板来固定受伤区域。

• 在头一个 24 h 内使用冰袋进行间歇性的冷敷。

• 会造成血管损伤的脱臼或严重变形的骨折，应该立即复位到空挡位置并固定好。

急诊治疗/程序

• 指节间复位：

- 指背脱臼：
  ◦ 当推动脱臼指骨底部回位时，需提供纵向牵引并轻柔地过渡伸展关节。
- 掌侧脱臼：
  ◦ 当推动脱臼指骨底部回位时，需提供纵向牵引并轻柔地过渡弯曲关节。
- 侧方脱臼：
  ◦ 当纠正尺骨或径向变形时，需提供纵向牵引并轻柔地过渡伸展关节。

• 指节间固定：

- 远侧指间关节背部或手指侧向脱臼：
  ◦ 当近侧指节关节具有全活动度的情况下，将远侧指间关节满张后打夹板。
- 近侧指间关节背部或手指侧向脱臼：
  ◦ 给近侧指节关节背部打夹板，弯曲度为 20°～30°。
- 掌侧手指脱臼：
  ◦ 将近侧指间关节和远侧指间关节满张后打夹板。

• 掌指关节脱臼：

- 手指脱臼：给手指的掌指关节打夹板，弯曲度为 90°。
- 拇指脱臼：给拇指的掌指关节打人字形夹板，弯曲度为 20°。

• 开放性骨折：

- 在创伤后的 4～6 h 立即转诊到手外科处理。
- 针对革兰阳性菌和革兰阴性菌使用的预防性抗生素应该在 6 h 内经非肠道途径来执行。

• 闭合性骨折：

- 远节指骨：
  ◦ 损伤较为稳定可以对远侧指骨关节打一定弯曲度的夹板，而对于近侧指骨关节则不需要打夹板；将夹板的顶端延伸盖过指节末端以增加保护，维持 3～4 周。
- 中节指骨：
  ◦ 无位移式稳定的骨折可以给邻近的指节打石蜡膜带。
  ◦ 位移式或成角骨折可以复位(使用三点压力的纵向牵引让骨碎片对齐)并固定(使用石蜡膜带或尺骨/径向沟形夹板)。
  ◦ 应给腕关节打夹板，扩展度为 20°～30°，掌指骨打夹板弯曲度为 70°～90°，而近侧指间关节和远侧指关节打夹板为 5°～10°。
- 近指节骨：
  ◦ 无位移式的、无成角的、稳定的损伤可以对邻近的手指使用石蜡膜带；尺骨/径向沟形或 Burkhalter 形夹板可能会增加舒适感。
  ◦ 位移式的或成角的骨折可以通过将掌指关节和近侧指间关节弯曲 90°来复位，然后使用三点复位技术来背侧复位近端骨碎片和掌侧复位远端骨碎片。一旦复位，应该扩展近侧指间关节(避免屈曲挛缩)，掌指关节应该保持 70°～90°的弯曲度，而且径向或尺骨沟形夹板应该置于和邻近手指打了石蜡膜带的骨折手指上。

> **注意**
> 不超过 1 mm 或 2 mm 的位移或缩短是可接受的。10°以内的成角是可接受的，但是任何程度的旋转都是不允许的。
> • 锤状指：
> - 当近侧指间关节可以全活动度活动时，满张远侧指间关节然后固定，或者轻柔地过渡伸展(5°～15°)。
> - 不要企图在打夹板前对任何位移式骨折进行复位，因为任何复位都不可能在未经过手术条件下维持；要参考紧急的整形外科意见。
> • “杰西指”：
> - 给近侧指间关节打上铝制夹板，并且将远侧指间关节轻微的弯曲。
> - 应该避免伸展远侧指间关节，直至指节伤情由手外科专家评估(对于肌腱完全破裂的最终治疗是手术)。
> • 扳机指：
> - 使用石蜡膜带对其邻近的手指固定 4～6 周。
> - 如果石蜡膜带固定不成功，使用金属或热塑夹板来固定。
> • 猎场看守人拇指：
> - 对掌指关节使用冰块急冻。
> - 对拇指采用人字形夹板固定(掌指关节弯曲度 20°)3 周。
> • 甲下血肿：
> - 使用加热的回形针、电灼器或 18G 针进行指甲环钻术。
> - 这种损伤没有必要像开放性损伤那样处理，除非有潜在的指端粉碎性骨折。
> • 指甲撕裂：
> - 清创并使用极细(如 6－0)可吸收缝合。
> - 给甲上皮和带有生发基质的撕脱甲打夹板，包上小块纱布或金属薄片，防止组织液黏附。
> • 不带有隆起骨的及<1 cm 的开放式的远侧和掌侧定向指尖伤口，允许二次愈合。

药物治疗

• 评估破伤风状态并按照免疫程序接种疫苗。

• 应该使用不含肾上腺素的麻醉剂进行指神经传导阻滞。

• 抗生素使用：

- 不适用于简单洁净的创伤。
- 对于严重污染的损伤、刺伤或传染性腱鞘炎，其治疗方法要根据伤口所接触的特定病原体来定制(如皮肤菌群、淡水、咬伤)。

随访

进一步处理

患者伤情稳定并打了合适的夹板，在整形外科随访及可能的重复性影像学检查后 1 周就可以出院。

> **注意**
> 下列情况下需要紧急咨询整形外科：
> • 发生断指。
> • 开放性关节损伤或骨折。
> • 指节神经血管损伤。
> • 有关节感染或传染性腱鞘炎的体征。

- 高压喷射损伤。
- 紧急整形外科咨询：
  - 不稳定的骨折(旋转式的变形、倾斜的或成角的骨折、关节骨折、骨骺损伤)。
  - 任何带有肌腱破裂的关节脱臼。
  - 指节脱臼不能复位的。
  - 企图复位脱臼关节后造成的关节不稳定。

要点和误区

- 如果手指是伸直状态，旋转式的变形不能明显看出，此时要求弯曲状态下的检查。
- "杰西指"(指深屈肌腱破裂)常常被误诊为手指夹伤或扭伤，但"杰西指"要求比这些次要的伤情更紧急的处理。
- 务必要通过确认患者的手指活动度并检查复位后的X线来检查复位后的手指骨稳定度。

输血并发症 Transfusion Complications

Darin S. Williams 张晟 林兆奋 译

基础知识

流行病学

- 2007年的一项研究发现，每年有约1460万例输血。
- 2015年，美国有37例死亡完全可归因于输血并发症。
- 2%的输血反应发生在单位输血后的24h内。
- 非感染性并发症：
  - 非溶血性发热反应：最常见，发生在0.1%～1%的输血中，更常见于儿童，血小板1/900。
  - 超敏反应(非过敏性)：常见，1/100～1/33。
  - 过敏性：1/50000～1/20000。
  - 急性溶血反应：1/70000～1/38000，每1000万次输血中有5例死亡。
  - 慢性溶血反应：1/11000～1/4000。
  - 输血相关循环超负荷(TACO)：1/100，在敏感人群中高达10%。
  - 同种免疫：1/100～1/10。
  - 移植物抗宿主反应：1/400000，罕见但死亡率达90%以上。
  - 输血相关肺损伤(TRALI)：1/190000～1/5000；在已报输血相关死亡病例中占13%。
  - 铁超负荷：发病率不明，取决于输血量，多发生于输100单位以上红细胞时。
  - 低血钙：发病率不明。
  - 高血钾：发病率不明。
- 感染性并发症：
  - 细菌污染：红细胞1/500000～1/65000；血小板1/10000～1/1000。
    - 最常见细菌：小肠结肠炎耶尔森菌、假单胞菌属、沙雷菌属、金黄色葡萄球菌。
    - 感染性并发症是导致死亡最主要的原因：17%～22%。
  - 丙型肝炎病毒：1/1600000。
  - 乙型肝炎病毒：1/400000～1/100000。
  - HTLV1型和2型：1/3000000～1/500000。
  - HIV：1/4700000～1/1400000。
  - HAV：1/1000000。
  - B19细小病毒：1/40000；有输血后贫血症的罕见分散报道。
  - 寄生虫：巴贝西亚与疟疾，低于1/1000000。
  - 寄生虫：克氏锥虫，1/42000。
  - 曾有EB病毒、莱姆病、布氏杆菌病、人类疱疹病毒、克雅病病例等报道。

急性输血性血管内溶血反应

- 死亡率和发病率与血型不合有关(当输血量为5～20ml时症状即可出现)。
- 通常是由于实验室错误。
- 以下情况时立即出现。
  - ABO血型排斥(最常见)。
  - 也来自其他抗原不相容，即Kell、JK。
- 血管内溶血激活凝血系统，导致炎症、休克、DIC。
- 炎症反应中介质(细胞因子)释放。
- 临床上可能出现寒战、发热、低血压、血红蛋白尿、背痛和DIC。
- 肾衰竭。
  - 细胞因子导致肾脏内内皮素局部释放，造成血管收缩。
  - 引起实质缺血和急性肾衰竭。
- 肺水肿导致呼吸衰竭/ARDS。
  - 游离血红蛋白引起肺内血管收缩。

其他输血相关并发症

- Rh不合导致的溶血。
  - 轻微，有自限性。
  - 输血1：200U。
- 发热性非溶血性输血反应。
  - 最常见的输血反应，排除性诊断。
  - 6h内体温上升超过1℃，伴寒战。
  - 由血液储存过程中产生的细胞因子引起的。
  - 通常较轻微。
  - 多发生于经产妇和多次输血者。
  - 15%的患者再次发生。
  - 对乙酰氨基酚用于治疗发热，也可用于预防；虽然无害，但其作为输血前用药仍有争议。
- 输血过敏反应。
  - 1%～3%的输血中发生。
  - 可发生在输血前、输血期间或输血后。
  - 常见于IgA缺乏的患者。
  - 只要没有其他过敏反应的迹象，荨麻疹不是停止输血的指征。
  - 抗组胺药可用于治疗或预防性用药。
- 试验显示，对乙酰氨基酚和苯海拉明作为预防用药相对于安慰剂没有明显效果。

慢性反应

- 感染：
  - HIV、HBV和HCV。
    - 血液筛查病毒。
    - 血液病毒灭活处理。
    - 有旅行史或健康状况欠佳的供血者应延缓献血。
  - 细菌。
    - 2015年有5人死亡。
    - 金黄色葡萄球菌最常见病原菌。
- 迟发性血管外溶血反应。
  - 发生于输血后7～10日。
  - 输血后发生的抗原-抗体反应。
  - Coombs试验阳性。

S

- 常无临床症状，但可出现低热、黄疸。
- 血液中心分析检测发现抗体。

• 电解质失衡：
- 低血钙：钙与柠檬酸结合。
- 高低钾血症：柠檬酸代谢为碳酸氢盐，使钾离子进入细胞内，血液延期储存可能导致溶血和高血钾。

• 移植物抗宿主病：
- 90%以上为致命性。
- 有免疫活性的淋巴细胞输入免疫活性宿主体内。
- 宿主无法裂解新的白细胞。
- 供血者的白细胞识别受体为异物并攻击其组织。

• 过敏反应：
- 输血量少于 10 ml 时即可发生。
- 广泛发红、荨麻疹、喉头水肿、支气管痉挛、低血压、休克或心搏骤停。
- 用皮下注射肾上腺素，血流动力学支持和呼吸支持。

• 输血相关的循环超负荷：
- 输血后 6 h 内典型症状出现。
- 由于循环容量增加
- 约 20%的严重急性输血反应，比 AHTR、过敏反应和 TRALI 更常见。
- 可以看到呼吸窘迫和低血压，更常见于充血性心力衰竭患者。
- 治疗包括利尿剂和呼吸机支持，即无创正压通气。

• 输血相关性急性肺损伤：
- 症状通常始于 6 h 的输血。
- 呼吸窘迫急性发作、双肺水肿、发热、心动过速、低血压、心脏功能正常。
- 输血致死的最常见原因。
- 难以与 ARDS 和 TACO 鉴别，经常发生误诊和漏报。
- 提供支持治疗。
- 疾病有典型的自限性，96 h 内。
- 死亡率为 5%～10%。
- 利尿剂禁忌。

儿科注意事项

可在一定压力下(＜300 mmHg)22G 外周导管内输血，达到最小溶血。

诊断

症状和体征

• 全身：
- 发热。
- 寒战。
- 输液部位灼烧痛。
- 荨麻疹、皮肤红斑、瘙痒。

• 肺：
- 呼吸困难。
- 支气管痉挛。
- 呼吸窘迫/衰竭。

• 心血管：
- 心动过速。
- 低血压。
- 胸骨后胸痛/胸闷。

• 胃肠道：
- 恶心。
- 呕吐。
- 腹泻。

• 血液：
- 出血。
- 血红蛋白尿。
- 外科伤口渗出。
- 黄疸。
- DIC。

• 其他：
- 下背部疼痛。
- 肾衰竭(少尿/无尿)。
- 急性溶血反应经典三联征：发热、腰痛和棕红色尿，较罕见。

基本检查

• 辨认输血反应的临床表现。
• 复查血液和患者配型识别信息。
• 正确辨认低血压、休克、严重呼吸困难、脓毒血症、发热和血尿等。

诊断检查与说明

• CBC。
• 电解质、血尿氮、肌酐和葡萄糖：
- 电解质失衡。
• PT、PPT。
• 血钙。
• 纤维蛋白原，纤维蛋白降解产物。
• 胆红素(直接/间接)。
• Coombs 试验(如果怀疑 AHTR)。
• 血红蛋白血症：
- 血清或血浆有粉色或红色上清液表明有溶血。
• 尿常规：
- 血红蛋白尿：微观无红细胞而血液试纸阳性。
• 实验室检查提示 Rh 血性不合导致溶血：
- 血小板减少症(＜100 000)。
- 纤维蛋白原缺乏(＜150 mg/L)。
- 纤维蛋白降解产物。
- APTT 延长。
- 球形红细胞增多症。
• 实验室检查提示 Rh 不亲和性引起的溶血。
- Coombs 试验阳性。
- 间接胆红素升高。
- 输血后血红蛋白未如预期升高。

影像学检查

胸部 X 线：TRALI 时弥散性斑片状浸润不伴心脏肥大。

诊断步骤/外科

心电图示心律不齐，有电解质失衡的症状。

鉴别诊断

• 脓毒血症。
• 过敏反应/药物过敏反应。

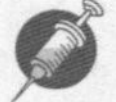

治疗

院前

常规稳定。

初步稳定/治疗

• 立即停止输血。
- 反应的严重程度与输血量成正比。
• 基础生命支持。
• 补充氧气，必要时气管插管和机械通气。
• 复查血液信息、患者手环、血液标签。
• 联系血液中心。
• 开始生理盐水输液 100～200 ml/h。

急诊治疗/程序

• 低血压。
- 建立 2 路静脉通路，输注生理盐水。
- 避免乳酸林格液或溶液含有葡萄糖的溶液。
- 特伦德伦伯格卧位。
• 预防肾衰竭。
- 保持 1 ml/(kg · h)的尿量。
- 补充水分。
- 呋塞米用于 TACO，避免 TRALI 时使用。
• 发热反应。
- 解热镇痛药(对乙酰氨基酚/非甾体类抗炎药)。
- 抗组胺药(苯海拉明＋雷尼替丁)静脉注射。
- 制剂(甲泼尼龙)。
• 过敏反应：
- 抗组胺药(苯海拉明＋雷尼替丁)静脉注射。

- 有呼吸症状时使用肾上腺素。
- 类固醇激素(甲泼尼龙)。
- 重新抽血进行 ABO/Rh 血型检验,直接抗球蛋白试验。
- 用 Foley 导尿管监控尿量。
- 如果低血钙加重则补充钙离子。
- 治疗 DIC。

■ 药物治疗

- 苯海拉明:25～50 mg(儿童:1.25 mg/kg),静脉注射。
- 雷尼替丁:50 mg,静脉注射(儿童:1～2 mg/kg,最多 50 mg)。
- 肾上腺素(1∶1 000):0.3～0.5 ml(儿童:0.01 ml/kg),皮下注射。
- 甲泼尼龙:125 mg(儿童:2 mg/kg),静脉注射。
- 利尿剂:对于 TACO,滴定到尿量至少 1 ml/(kg·h)。

 随访

■ 进一步处理

入院指征

- 急性溶血性输血反应、肺部并发症、过敏反应、脓毒血症:
- 需要入住 ICU。
- 迟发性溶血性输血反应评估或治疗。
- 电解质失衡要求心电监测。

出院指征

非复杂发热或过敏反应。

要点和误区

- 输血严重过度使用,并且有显著的相关风险,如输血反应、病原体的感染和免疫抑制。
- 大量输血过程中保持体温是纠正凝血功能障碍的关键。
- 未能核对患者信息和血液标签或未能等到配型完全吻合的血液将带来很大风险。
- 若患者出现低血压、深色尿或注射部位渗液等,应怀疑急性血管内溶血。

束支传导阻滞 Bundle Branch Blocks

Annette M. Grajny · James Scott 黄聪华 译

S

 基础知识

■ 描述

- 通过左、右束的脑室电脉冲阻滞。
- 完全束支传导阻滞。
- 一束支没有或延迟传导,其他束支正常传导。
- 影响心室肌以缓慢和混乱的方式去极化。
- QRS 波长在 120 ms 或更长。
- 不完全束支传导阻滞。
- 延迟去极化,但比完全束支传导阻滞短。
- QRS 波群时间在 100～120 ms。
- 右束支传导阻滞(RBBB)。
- 右心室延迟去极化。
- 左束支传导阻滞(LBBB)。
- 左心室延迟去极化。
- 左束支传导阻滞可因左主束支延迟或全部左束支传导延迟。
- 室间隔右侧及右室心肌的早期激活(因此在心电图上表现为"室间隔 Q 波"的缺失)。
- 左束支分为 2 束。
  - 左前分支:室间隔初始向下激活,然后向前,向右。
  - 左后分支:单独阻滞罕见,在室间隔中部激活,在下壁和后壁结束。
- 双束支阻滞:
- 右束支传导阻滞伴左前或左后分支阻滞。

■ 病因

- 心肌梗死。
- 心肌病。
- 肺心病。
- 高血压。
- 年龄相关的浦肯野纤维化。
- 心脏瓣膜病。
- 运动性。
- 先天性房间隔缺损。
- Brugada 综合征(RBBB):健康患者发生心源性猝死的原因。
- 沙加斯病(美洲锥虫病)(尤其是中/南美洲)。
- 手术后,即将行心脏外科手术。
- 药物。
- β受体阻滞剂。
- 钙通道阻滞剂。
- 三环类抗抑郁药。
- Ⅰa 类和Ⅰc 类抗心律失常药。
- 洋地黄。

诊断

■ 体征和症状

- 无症状。
- 右束支传导阻滞:呼气时持续存在的分裂 S2。
- 左束支传导阻滞:反向/反常的分裂 S2。
- 晕厥。
- 胸痛。

■ 基本检查

心电图。

- 右束支传导阻滞。
- 完全:QRS 波群≥0.12 s。
- 不完全:QRS 波群时间 0.10～0.12 s。
- 在 V_1 和 V_2 导联表现为 rsr′、rsR′、rSR(M 型)。
- 在 V_5～V_6 导联出现宽而深的 S 波。
- Brugada 综合征:右束支传导阻滞和 ST 段在 V_1～V_3 导联抬高。
- 左束支传导阻滞。
- V_5～V_6、aVL 和Ⅰ导联出现宽大有切迹的 R 波。
- V_1～V_2 导联出现小或缺失的 R 波及深 S 波。
- V_5～V_6 和Ⅰ导联缺少正常 Q 波。
- 左前分支传导阻滞:
- QRS 波群<120 ms,电轴在 45°～90°。
- Ⅱ、Ⅲ、aVF 导联出现深 S 波,aVL 和Ⅰ导联出现 qR 波。
- 左后分支传导阻滞:
- QRS<120 ms,电轴≥120°。
- Ⅰ和 aVL 导联出现 RS 波群,Ⅱ、Ⅲ、aVF 出现 qR 波。
- 排除其他导致电轴右偏的原因(右心室超负荷、右心室肥厚、侧壁心肌梗死)。

■ 诊断检查与说明

实验室检查

- 电解质:如怀疑高钾血症、高钙血症。
- 心肌酶:如果怀疑心肌缺血。

影像学检查

- X线检查：
  - 可显示心脏扩大或心力衰竭。
- 电生理测试。
  - 住院后处理的一部分，特别是因结构性心脏病而出现不明原因晕厥的患者。

鉴别诊断

- 室性心动过速。
- 心肌梗死：
  - 诊断伴有LBBB的心肌梗死的标准（斯加尔博撒标准）包括以下几条。
    - ST段抬高≥1 mm一致的QRS波群。
    - ST段抬高≥5 mm伴有异常QRS波群。
    - V_1～V_3导联ST段压低≥1 mm。
- 高钾血症。
- 心室肥厚。
- 药物影响（见病因部分）。

治疗

院前

注意：

- 监测：单导联难诊断。
- 避免与室性心动过速或心肌缺血混淆。
- 患者处置：束支阻滞不需要特殊的治疗。

初步稳定/治疗

- 对缺血、呼吸困难和晕厥症状的患者行标准治疗。
- 有症状的双束支阻滞、高度房室传导阻滞。
  - 在胸背部应用经皮起搏器。
  - 静脉镇静、镇痛。
  - 逐渐增加电流，直到心室起搏。

急诊治疗/程序

- 无症状：无处理。
- 对症状提示心肌梗死和新发束支传导阻滞的患者行溶栓或心导管检查。
- 经静脉植入心脏起搏器的指征：
  - 双束支阻滞型和二度Ⅱ型或三度房室传导阻滞。
  - 交替存在左束支传导阻滞和右束支传导阻滞。

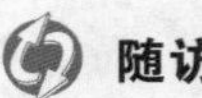

随访

进一步处理

住院指征

- 可疑心肌缺血。
- 晕厥。
- 心律失常。
- 低血压，生命体征异常。
- 心脏衰竭表现。
- 高度房室传导阻滞。

出院指征

- 无症状或偶发的束支传导阻滞。

转诊问题

出院时，患者因潜在心脏病需进行专业评估。

随访建议

- 安抚不需要治疗的患者是必需的。
- 提示患者返院或寻求帮助：
  - 头晕。
  - 昏厥，不省人事。
  - 心悸。

要点和误区

- 应注意所有有新发传导异常的心肌缺血患者。
- 特定的标准可用于诊断伴有束支传导阻滞的心脏缺血患者。

双硫仑样反应 Disulfiram Reaction

Timothy J. Meehan · Sean M. Bryant 谭美春 译

基础知识

描述

- 抑制各种酶及其活性代谢物发挥额外的作用。
- 双硫仑-乙醇反应：
  - 通常发生于服药后8～12 h，不应在给药后超过24 h观察。
  - 使醛脱氢酶竞争性和不可逆性失活。
  - 乙醇代谢受阻，导致乙醛蓄积。
  - 乙醛产物释放组胺导致血管扩张和低血压。
  - 严重反应可发生在50～100 mg/dl乙醇水平饮酒者。
  - 反应的严重程度和持续时间与乙醇摄入量成正比。
- 双硫仑阻断多巴胺β-羟化酶并限制多巴胺合成去甲肾上腺素：
  - 多巴胺相对过量可能导致行为改变。
  - 去甲肾上腺素相对消耗可能导致低血压。
- 双硫仑代谢物（二硫化碳）与磷酸吡哆醛相互作用：
  - 减少可用于中枢神经系统中形成γ-氨基丁酸（GABA）的吡哆醇浓度。
  - 可能降低癫痫发作阈值。
  - 二硫化碳也具有心脏毒性、肝毒性，并抑制细胞色素P450（CYP2E1）。
- 双硫仑代谢物可能螯合各种酶系统中必不可少的重要金属（铜、锌、铁）。
- 双硫仑代谢物可引起剂量和时间依赖性周围神经病变。

病因

- 双硫仑可用于慢性酒精滥用的治疗。
- 许多药物使用者佩戴一个药物警报手环。
- 其他产生双硫仑样反应的药物：
  - 抗生素：
    - 甲硝唑。
    - 头孢菌素类（有nMTT侧链者）。
    - 头孢哌酮、头孢替坦、头孢美唑。
    - 呋喃妥因。
  - 口服降糖药：
    - 磺脲类药物。
  - 工业药物：
    - 二硫化碳。
    - 硫化氢。
  - 蘑菇：
    - 墨汁鬼伞。
    - 棒柄杯伞。

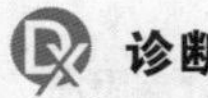

诊断

症状和体征

- 双硫仑-乙醇反应：

- 低血压、心动过速、呼吸急促。
- 面部、颈部、躯干发红。
- 瘙痒、出汗、感觉温暖。
- 恶心、呕吐、腹痛、腹泻。
- 头痛、共济失调、困惑、焦虑、头晕。
- 呼吸困难、肺水肿、胸痛、心律失常、心肌梗死。
- 双硫仑过量：
  - 摄入低于 3 g 者症状罕见。
  - 10～30 g 可能是致命的。
  - 可能类似休克和/或脓毒症。
  - 心动过速、低血压、呼吸急促。
  - 腹痛、腹泻、大蒜或臭鸡蛋味呼气。
  - 激动、烦躁、共济失调。
  - 构音障碍、幻觉。
  - 嗜睡、昏迷、癫痫、乏力。
  - 帕金森病。

病史

双硫仑或以上所列药物的摄入可为诊断提供必要线索。

体格检查

- 生命体征：
  - 低血压、心动过速、呼吸急促。
- 心血管：
  - 心动过速、心律失常。
- 肺部：
  - 肺水肿、呼吸困难。
- 腹部：
  - 弥漫性腹痛、恶心、呕吐。
- 皮肤：
  - 发红、出汗。
- 神经系统：
  - 烦躁、困惑、小脑功能障碍体征、癫痫。

基本检查

伴以下表现应怀疑双硫仑-乙醇反应：

- 存在典型的体征和症状。
- 慢性酒精滥用治疗结合近期乙醇摄入或接触含乙醇的食物或药物，包括漱口水。

诊断检查与说明

实验室检查

- 乙醇水平。
- 电解质、尿素氮、肌酐和葡萄糖。
- 如果怀疑肝炎，查肝功能。
- 如果据癫痫或躁动考虑横纹肌溶解，查肌酸磷酸激酶(CPK)。
- 尿液分析(肌红蛋白)。
- 血清中的违规药物水平无临床意义。

影像学检查

- 心电图评估心肌缺血或心律失常。
- CT 或 MRI：
  - 表明精神状态改变、癫痫。
  - 有报道过基底节缺血和梗死。
- 脑电图：
  - 在急性中毒昏迷的情况下可见到无局灶性异常的弥漫性减慢。

鉴别诊断

- 脓毒症。
- 脑膜炎和脑炎。
- 继发于急性冠状动脉综合征的心源性休克。
- 过敏/过敏反应。
- 胃肠炎、胰腺炎伴脱水。
- 乙醇戒断。

儿科注意事项

- 急性中毒时主要产生严重中枢神经系统毒性。
- 共济失调，无力，嗜睡，癫痫。
- 严重病例可有 Reye 综合征样脑病。
- 成人症状也可能存在。

治疗

院前

- 基础生命支持，建立静脉通路。
- 如果没有肺水肿的体征或症状，开始 IVF 复苏。
- 快速血糖测定(Accu-Chek)。

初步稳定/治疗

- 基本治疗：
  - 必要时气道保护。
  - 补充氧气。
  - 按需进行机械通气。
  - 对低血压者以生理盐水静脉复苏。
- 对顽固性低血压者以去甲肾上腺素升压支持。

急诊治疗/程序

- 治疗主要是积极、适当的支持治疗：
  - 无特定的解毒剂。
- 胃肠道净化：
  - 在双硫仑过量的情况下使用活性炭：
    - 如精神状态抑郁应注意。
    - 如呕吐应注意(可能会吸入)。
    - 不插管仅给予活性炭。
  - 无需洗胃。
  - 无全肠灌洗指征。
- 缓解皮肤发红：
  - 抗组胺(H_1 和 H_2 受体拮抗剂)。
  - 前列腺素抑制剂(吲哚美辛、酮咯酸)。
- 止吐药治疗顽固性呕吐(昂丹司琼、甲氧氯普胺)。
- 癫痫：
  - 地西泮(安定、劳拉西泮)。
  - 吡哆醇(维生素 B_6)。
  - 4-甲基吡唑：
    - 抑制乙醇代谢的乙醇脱氢酶。
    - 常规的双硫仑-乙醇反应或轻度双硫仑过量不应使用。
    - 可改善中至重度过量者的血流动力学。
- 血液透析：
  - 双硫仑和乙醇大量摄入后伴顽固性低血压时考虑。
  - 没有研究证明有获益作用。

药物治疗

- 地西泮：5～10 mg(儿童：0.2～0.5 mg/kg)，静脉注射。
- 苯海拉明：25～50 mg(儿童：1～2 mg/kg)，静脉注射。
- 吲哚美辛：50 mg，口服(儿童：年龄＞14 岁者，0.6 mg/kg，口服)。
- 劳拉西泮：2～6 mg(儿童：0.03～0.05 mg/kg)，静脉注射。
- 甲氧氯普胺：10 mg(儿童：1～2 mg/kg)，静脉注射。
- 去甲肾上腺素：4 ml 加入于 1 000 ml 5% 葡萄糖溶液，以 0.1～0.2 μg/(kg · min)注入。
- 昂丹司琼：4 mg(儿童：＞2 岁者，0.1 mg/kg)，静脉注射。
- 吡哆醇：1 g(儿童：500 mg)，静脉注射，必要时重复。

随访

进一步处理

入院指征

- 需要机械通气、昏迷、需要升压药的顽固性低血压、心肌缺血、难治性癫痫和严重躁动需入住 ICU。
- 持续呕吐、腹痛或皮肤发红。
- 老年患者或已有心脏疾病的患者。

出院指征

- 在 8～12 h 的观察期后支持治疗可消退的轻度反应：

S

- 在最后服用双硫仑或引起双硫仑样反应的药物后，症状可能因酒精激发试验复发长达 7～10 日。
- 戒除乙醇使用，直到距最后服用这类药物至少 2 周后。
- 适当随访以评估肝或神经系统后遗症的进展。

■ 随访建议

- 对故意服用过量双硫仑者进行精神病学随访。
- 双硫仑-乙醇反应患者进行戒瘾随访。

要点和误区

- 教育那些使用有潜在戒酒硫样反应处方药的患者，应避免所有含乙醇物品：
- 包括：漱口水、醇基洗手液、醇基须后水、某些止咳糖浆和酏剂液体药物。
- 建议戒酒时间长于疗程 3 日，以确保反应的低可能性。

双相障碍 Bipolar Disorder

Paul H. Desan · Gary S. Sachs　许磊　郭东风 译

基础知识

■ 描述

- 躁狂：
- 表现形式多样，诊断时可能存在困难：
  ◦ 易烦躁。
  ◦ 情绪高涨。
  ◦ 精神病。
  ◦ 谵妄。
  ◦ 易激。
- 往往只能通过外界表现得到全部的病理学特征。
- 发作过程呈渐进性或急性，持续数周或数月，很少呈慢行病程。
- 轻度躁狂：
- 症状较轻，没有明显症状。
- 情绪混杂：
- 同时出现躁狂和抑郁症状。
- 急诊治疗躁狂症。
- 双相障碍：
- 以前的躁郁症定义为一次或多次轻度躁狂、狂躁或混合情绪发作。
- 可能伴有抑郁情绪发作。
- 双相障碍用于表示病症过程中出现轻躁狂但无躁狂发作的情况。
- 通常开始于十几岁或二十几岁。
- 情绪异常的情节可能是轻微或严重的，短暂的或持续的，低频的或慢性的，主要表现为情绪高涨或主要表现为抑郁的性格。
- 双相障碍可能容易对治疗产生反应，也可能几乎对治疗不产生任何应答。
- 分裂性情感障碍：
- 以情绪改变时出现精神病征为特点，但即使情绪正常时也可存在精神病特征。

■ 病因

- 通常是一种原发性精神疾病，伴有遗传相关性。
- 可能继发于其他疾病（如药物毒性、内分泌、神经疾病过程中伴发）。
- 若出现以下表现则很可能是继发疾病：
- 第一次发作。
- 患者>40 岁。
- 非典型或混合性的表现。
- 感觉异常。

诊断

■ 症状和体征

病史

- 精神病史：
- 躁狂症前出现的症状（通常是病史采集中的重要部分）：情绪升高，膨胀或易怒；体能和活动都增加；对睡眠的需求减少；不负责任，不顾行为的负面后果；多语；注意力分散；思维闪现；过度自信。
- 躁狂症病史或抑郁症病史。
- 对情绪稳定服药不依从。
- 最近开始或停用抗抑郁药。
- 近期药物滥用。
- 双相家族史。
- 疾病史：
- 内分泌、代谢或神经系统疾病。
- 当前或最近服用药物。

体格检查

- 表现：
- 在非激动情绪下多动。
- 多语，经常大声，快速或"施加压力式"的讲话。
- 影响：
- 易怒，喜争论，近期通常有多次争吵或打架发生。
- 较不常见的欣快感或膨胀感。
- 经常处于抑郁或痛苦间歇期的不稳定状态（可能会对诊断造成干扰）。
- 患者可能会将情绪描述为紧张、易怒或抑郁，而不是欣快。
- 神经创伤：
- 体能增强，每日长达数小时从事多项目标指向性活动。
- 思维闪现。
- 睡眠减少。
- 思考过程：
- 快速，不易集中注意力的，可能是不连贯的，神志不清的。
- 思想内容：
- 可能存在精神病症状，情绪一致（例如，夸张或者对力量夸大的妄想）或者情绪不一致（可能与其他精神障碍无法区分）。
- 判断：
- 夸大自尊，以至于到非常夸张甚至精神病的程度。
- 不具备特征性，不负责任的行为，如经济或性方面的轻率行为，无法识别行为的负面后果。
- 躁狂症发作期间频繁滥用药物。
- 感觉中枢：
- 通常正常。
- 可能存在混乱或者谵妄状态。

■ 基本检查

- 身体和神经系统检查，生命体征。
- 躁狂症可能表现为谵妄，需要对谵妄进行全面鉴别诊断所需的检查。

■ 诊断检查与说明

实验室检查

- 毒理学筛选（尿液或血清）。
- 血液乙醇浓度。

- 电解质。
- 血糖。
- CBC。
- TSH。
- 如果存在相关性,需检查锂、卡马西平、丙戊酸血清水平。
- 以往就诊过程或体检所建议的其他测试。

影像学检查

CT检查只在怀疑存在神经系统异常的情况下进行。

鉴别诊断

- 双相障碍或分裂性情感障碍的原发性躁狂症。
- 精神病。
- 激动的抑郁症。
- 人格障碍:
  - 边界线。
  - 自恋。
  - 反社会。
- 注意力缺陷症。
- 行为间歇性暴发性疾病。
- 器质性脑综合征。
- 乙醇、镇静剂中毒或戒酒。
- 用可卡因、苯丙胺、苯环利定或其他拟交感神经药中毒。
- 意外或蓄意的毒剂摄入过量。
- 在易感个体中使用抗抑郁药或电休克疗法。
- 最近停用抗抑郁药物。
- 使用皮质类固醇或甲状腺激素。
- 使用抗胆碱能药。
- 进行帕金森病的治疗。
- 使用环苯扎林(Flexeril)。
- 内分泌或代谢紊乱(特别是甲状腺疾病)。
- 脑炎。
- 全身轻瘫。
- 脑膜炎。
- 发作性疾病后状态。
- MS(多发性硬化症)。
- 脑血管意外后遗症。
- 中枢神经系统肿瘤。
- 中枢神经系统血管炎。
- 一般麻痹。

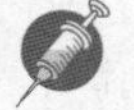

治疗

院前

- 高度的暴力可能性:
  - 安静的环境。
  - 及时评估。
  - 非对抗性的方式态度。
  - 充足的安全保证。
  - 根据需要进行肢体约束和镇静。
- 对于具有协作性但行为激动的患者:
  - 口服精神抑制药(如氟哌啶醇,考虑奥氮平或氯丙嗪作为替代药)或口服苯二氮䓬(例如,奥拉西泮)。
- 不合作的焦虑患者:
  - 广泛使用氟哌啶醇和劳拉西泮的协同用药,给药途径:肌内注射、静脉注射或口服(某些权威机构赞成使用苯二氮䓬类药物或安定类药物进行单药治疗)。
- 当给予苯并二氮䓬类药物时,通常不需要使用苯甲脒预防氟哌啶醇可能产生的急性肌张力障碍反应。
  - 考虑使用奥拉西泮、奥氮平、齐拉西酮或氯丙嗪作为替代方案。

急诊治疗/方法

- 门诊管理:
  - 临时或持续用于症状治疗的精神抑制药。
  - 睡眠药物。
  - 如果与目前的轻度躁狂或躁狂症相关,停用抗抑郁药。
  - 开始或重新开始情绪稳定性药物治疗。
    - 情绪稳定剂的作用需要数日或数周开始发挥,甚至可能会在血清水平完全改变之后。
- 住院治疗:咨询精神科医师后,镇定或开始情绪稳定剂治疗。

药物治疗

- 剧烈情绪激动:
  - 劳拉西泮:2 mg,肌内注射(轻度情绪激动或虚弱或老年患者剂量应较低);q30 min 重复使用一次,一般不超过 12 mg/24 h 的剂量。
  - 氟哌啶醇:5 mg,口服(在轻度情绪激动或虚弱或者老年患者使用较低剂量);q30 min 重复使用一次,通常不超过 20 mg/24 h 的剂量。
  - 根据需要,氟哌啶醇,5 mg,肌内注射、静脉注射或口服+劳拉西泮 1～2 mg 肌内注射、静脉注射或口服,重复 q30 min 给药的协同组合(在老年人或虚弱患者中剂量可以更小)。
  - 奥氮平 10 mg 肌内注射,齐拉西酮 10 mg,肌内注射,阿立哌唑 9.75 mg 肌内注射或氯丙嗪 50 mg 肌内注射可能是有用的胃肠外替代治疗方法,在体质较弱或老年患者当中使用较低剂量(避免低血压患者使用氯丙嗪;齐拉西酮可能比其他抗精神病药物具有更多的 QT 延长作用,但这种效应在该剂量下的临床相关性尚不清楚)。

> **注意**
>
> 肌内注射奥氮平不能与肌内注射苯二氮䓬联用:已导致数起心血管、呼吸不良事件,包括死亡。

- 典型的门诊药物:
  - 阿立哌唑:5～20 mg,口服,每日 1 次。
  - 苯噻啶:1 mg,口服,每日 2 次。
  - 卡马西平:400～2 000 mg/d(通常为分次给药或持续释放剂型)。
  - 氯硝西泮:0.5～2 mg,口服,每晚睡前;或 0.5～2 mg,口服,每日 2 次。
  - 氟哌啶醇:0.5～5 mg,口服,每日 2 次。
  - 拉莫三嗪:25～200 mg/d,一次或者两次分次给药(服用丙戊酸钠的患者通常高达 100 mg/d,服用卡马西平或某些其他细胞色素诱导剂但不服用丙戊酸盐的患者高达 500 mg/d)。

> **注意**
>
> 拉莫三嗪必须遵守药物说明书规定的剂量时间表开始逐渐加量,以避免严重皮肤病学反应的风险增加;如果在停止使用超过 5 个半衰期后复发,则必须再次使用逐渐增加的剂量方案(一些药物的半衰期较短,如某些抗癫痫药、OCP、利福平,请参见处方文献)。

  - 锂:600～3 000 mg/d(常以分次剂量或持续释放剂量形式;在急性躁狂症中,以 300 mg 口服,每日 3 次开始)。
  - 卢拉西酮:20～160 mg/d,必须与食物一起服用(>350 cal)。
  - 奥氮平:1.25～30 mg/d,每晚睡前或分次给药。
  - 奋乃静:4～32 mg/d,口服,每晚睡前或分次给药。
  - 喹硫平:50～400 mg,口服,每晚睡前;或 100～400 mg,口服,每日 2 次;喹硫平 XR 口服 50～800 mg,每晚睡前。
  - 利培酮:0.5～6 mg/d 口服,每晚睡前或以分次给药。
  - 丙戊酸钠(如 Depakote):750～3 000 mg/d(通常以分次给药发放;在急性躁狂症中,以 250 mg 口服,每日 3 次开始)。

S

妊娠注意事项

妊娠期间精神药物的安全性是一个复杂的问题：锂、丙戊酸钠和卡马西平是妊娠用药 D 类，存在特殊风险，在妊娠早期风险最高。使用前须咨询专家意见。

随访

进一步处理

入院指征

- 由于存在自身伤害的风险，即使非患者自愿，收入院也是必要的：
  - 自杀风险，特别是存在混合或不稳定的情绪或精神病。
  - 由于判断力受损导致不安全行为。
  - 病情不稳定。
  - 住院诊断需要。
- 符合下列情况的非自愿也应收入院：
  - 危害他人行为的风险。
  - 无力照顾自己（无法获得食物、衣服或住所等基本需求）。

出院指征

- 如果存在以下情况，症状轻微的患者可出院进行药物治疗：
  - 确保安全的必要支持已到位。
  - 患者病情进展符合治疗计划。
  - 1～3 日可至精神科门诊进行随访。
- 一些在法律上不具有合法性的患者可能会拒绝治疗：向患者和其家属、朋友解释未来可施行的治疗方案。

要点和误区

- 狂躁患者更容易出现焦虑或易怒，而不是“快乐”。
- 应该询问抑郁症的患者是否存在躁狂和轻度躁狂的表现，70%的双相障碍患者以前曾被误诊。
- 双相障碍患者成瘾的风险很高，治疗进一步复杂化。
- 及时识别最早的躁狂症征兆可能有助于预防病情进展。
- 儿童双相障碍常表现为行为抑制或烦躁。

水痘 Varicella

Michael J. Bono 周秋香 毛恩强 译

基础知识

描述

- 俗称水痘。
- 在冬末和早春最为常见。
- 也称水痘-带状疱疹病毒（VZV）。
- 疫苗使发病率降低了 85%。
- 成人的水痘死亡风险比儿童高 15 倍。

病因

- DNA 病毒：
  - 潜伏于性脑神经节神经节、背根神经节和具有周期性再激活的自主神经节中。
  - 在原发感染数十年后，以带状疱疹或单纯疱疹形式发病。
  - 病毒通过飞沫从感染宿主传播到易感患者的呼吸道黏膜。
  - 病毒通过呼吸途径传播或破损皮肤直接接触传播。
  - 也通过直接接触皮肤病变传播。
  - 人类是目前所知的唯一宿主。

诊断

症状

- 水痘引起一系列疾病。
- 儿童经典患病表现：
  - 通常会感染 1～9 岁的儿童。
  - 低热[100～103 ℉（37.7～39.4 ℃）]、头痛、不适的症状通常在出疹前 1～2 日出现。
  - 瘙痒，厌食和无精打采。
  - 潜伏期 10～21 日。
  - 从囊泡形成前 48 h 开始感染，直到所有囊泡结痂，通常在出疹后 3～7 日出现明显症状。
  - 经典皮疹表现：
    - 皮疹最早出现在脸上，后蔓延到躯干和四肢。
    - 表现为红斑丘疹、囊泡或脓疱。
    - 不同发展阶段的皮肤有不同的病变，这是水痘的皮肤病变的特点。
    - 如同“玫瑰花瓣上的露珠”。
    - 囊泡直径为 2～3 mm。
    - 囊泡形成的持续时间为 3～5 日。
    - 可能涉及结膜、口咽部或阴道黏膜。
    - 1%～4%的健康儿童患有 A 组链球菌或葡萄球菌的皮肤超感染。
- 青少年和成人患病表现：
  - 同儿童的患病表现相似，但有更大风险进展为重症：
    - 皮肤真皮 5%～50%损伤，肺炎。
  - 免疫力低下人群。
  - 艾滋病病毒感染者、移植患者、白血病患者是高危人群。
  - 接受化疗、免疫抑制剂和长期皮质类固醇激素治疗的患者也是高风险人群。
  - 过多的皮损可能有出血性风险。
  - 愈合可能需要更长的时间。
  - 这些人群常伴有肺炎。
- 妊娠患者：
  - 在年轻的孕妇中常见。
  - 更严重的疾病表现：
    - 妊娠早期对胎儿威胁最大。
    - 妊娠晚期对母亲的威胁大。
  - 围生期疾病可发生于预先输注后 5 日至输注后 48 h。
- 先天性水痘综合征：
  - 母婴垂直感染。
  - 肌肉骨骼：肢体发育不全或轻瘫。
  - 中枢神经系统：小头、皮质萎缩、癫痫或智力残疾。
  - 眼部缺陷：白内障、脉络膜视网膜炎或霍纳综合征。
- 皮肤外表现：
  - 肺炎。
    - 比成人发病率高 25 倍。
    - 成人吸烟者和免疫力低下儿童的患病风险最高。
    - 在出现皮疹后 3～5 日发病。
    - 体征：持续出现新的病灶和新发咳嗽。
    - 呼吸急促、呼吸困难、发绀、胸膜炎性胸痛和咯血。
  - 小脑性共济失调：
    - 皮疹可能会发展 5 日。
    - 共济失调、呕吐、言语不清、发热、眩晕、震颤。
  - 脑炎：

◦ 在皮疹开始后3～8日发展。
◦ 大约2周的时间。
◦ 头痛、脑膜炎、呕吐、发热、谵妄、癫痫发作。
- 急性脑病综合征。

老年人注意事项

• 真皮外皮损增加风险。
• 较低的免疫力人群带状疱疹复发风险。

儿科注意事项

• 阿司匹林无效的发热，考虑可能伴发Reye综合征：
- 对乙酰氨基酚是推荐的退热药物。
• 父母需要注意避免继发细菌感染和可能进展为败血症风险。

妊娠注意事项

• 童年的没有水痘史和没有水痘-带状疱疹病毒(VZV)抗体的孕妇需要注射水痘-带状疱疹免疫球蛋白(VZIG)。
• 孕妇水痘肺炎急症，有威胁生命的呼吸表现和死亡风险(死亡率可能为10%～45%)。
• 最可能在妊娠晚期出现。

病史

- 发热，全身症状。
- 免疫药物治疗史。
- 免疫活性与免疫力低下。

体格检查

• 全面体检：
- 独特的皮疹和分布范围。
- 评估任何皮肤外表现。
• 一些不复杂的病例，询问病史和查体是非常重要的。
• 表现：
- 显示2～5 mm的皮疹，可能聚结并持续数周。
• 水痘性脑炎。
- 氨水平升高。
- LFT会升高。
- PT、APTT。
- 腰椎穿刺显示淋巴细胞增多，蛋白质水平升高。

实验室检查

• 病毒培养(培养3～5日)、聚合酶链反应(PCR)或直接荧光抗体，使用来自病灶的基底或皮肤刮屑。
• 血清学检测血管内抗体。
• PCR是首选的诊断方法，但无并发症的患者不需要实验室检查。

鉴别诊断

• 脓疱疮。
• 播散性疱疹。
• 传播的柯萨奇病毒。
• 麻疹。
• 立克次体病。
• 昆虫叮咬。
• 疥疮。
• 红斑多形性。
• 药疹(特别是Steven-Johnson综合征)。

治疗

院前

• 非免疫接种人员必须避免与患者呼吸或身体接触。
• 有水痘-带状疱疹的携带者不应该接触免疫功能低下或妊娠的患者。

初步稳定/治疗

• 气道管理和液体复苏。
- 保护气道。

急诊治疗/程序

• 一般来说，对乙酰氨基酚和止痒剂是治疗经典儿童疾病的关键。
• 勤剪指甲和良好的卫生习惯有助于预防继发性细菌感染。
• 婴幼儿或小于12岁儿童：
- 阿昔洛韦：
◦ 建议患儿服用皮质类固醇、长效水杨酸盐治疗慢性皮肤或肺部疾病。
◦ 有适度的益处，减少25%的病变和降温。
◦ 应在症状出现后24 h内给予。
◦ 不推荐用于健康儿童的简单水痘。
- 对易感人群使VZIG的预防治疗：
◦ 免疫功能低下的儿童有高风险并发症和明确接触史。
◦ 作为患有活动性水痘或带状疱疹的患者的同一家庭中易感染儿童。
- 2012年FDA将VZIG给药延长至有接触史10日后。
- VZIG供不应求，难以获得。
• 青少年/成人：
- 阿昔洛韦现推荐在24 h内引发无并发症的水痘，以减少进展为播散性疾病。
- 用退热药和止痒剂进行对症治疗。
• 孕妇：
- 如果暴露于水痘，没有儿童期的水痘病史，没有抗VZV的抗体，则需要VZIG治疗。
- 80%～90%在免疫前感染，需要在使用VZIG之前进行抗体测试。
- 特别是在妊娠中期或晚期，阿昔洛韦或伐昔洛韦预防治疗：
◦ 在妊娠期间是安全的(B类)。
- 静脉阿昔洛韦治疗肺炎并发症：
- 呼吸系统、神经系统、出血性皮疹或持续发热>6日。
• 免疫功能低下患者：
- 推荐静脉注射阿昔洛韦，口服生物利用度较差。
- 口服伐昔洛韦对低风险免疫低下患者具有更好的生物利用度。
- 应在发病后24 h内开始使疗效最大化。
- 膦甲酸钠用于阿昔洛韦抗体耐药患者。
- 用VZIG预防治疗可疑的免疫功能低下患者。
• 皮肤外：
- 如果耐药就选择静脉注射阿昔洛韦或膦甲酸钠。
• 疫苗：
- 儿童：
◦ 12个月及以上的所有易感儿童常规接种疫苗，2次。
- 青少年和成人：
◦ 13岁及以上没有水痘史的人需要接种疫苗。
◦ 注射2次，第2次在4～8周后注射。
◦ 高危人群中推荐接种：
  ▪ 卫生保健工作者。
  ▪ 免疫抑制人员的家庭成员。
  ▪ 育龄妇女易感。
  ▪ 教师。
  ▪ 军人。
  ▪ 国际旅行者。
- 暴露后预防措施：
◦ 易感染的患者12个月或更长时间，72～120 h后给药，间隔适当时间第2次给药。
◦ 如果不感染，会产生免疫力。
- 免疫功能不全患者：
◦ 大多数免疫功能低下者不应进行免疫接种。

药物治疗

• 阿昔洛韦：
- 不复杂的患者：成人，800 mg，口服，每日4次，持续5日；青春期(13～18岁)，剂量为20 mg/kg，每日4次，持续7日；儿童：20 mg/kg悬浮液，口服，每日4次，持续5日(最大剂量：800 mg，口服，每日4次)。

S

- 免疫功能低下：成人，10 mg/kg，静脉注射，q8 h，输注超过 1 h；或 800 mg，口服，每日 5 次，持续 7 日。儿童：10～12 mg/kg，静脉注射，q8 h，输注超过 1 h；或 500 mg/(cm² · d)，静脉注射，q8 h，持续 7～10 日。

• 伐昔洛韦：1 g，口服，每日 3 次，持续 5～7 日。

• 泛昔洛韦：500 mg，口服，每日 3 次，持续 7 日。

• 膦甲酸钠：成人，90 mg/kg，q12 h，静脉注射，维持 90～120 min，2～3 周；儿童：40～60 mg/kg，历时 120 min，历时 7～10 日；膦甲酸钠还未被 FDA 批准。

• 羟嗪（安泰乐）：成人，25～50 mg，肌内注射或口服，q4～6 h。儿童：0.5 mg/kg，q4～6 h 悬浮液（以 10 mg/5 ml 和 25 mg/5 ml 提供）。

• 苯海拉明：成人，25～50 mg，静脉注射、肌内注射或口服，q4 h。儿童：5 mg/(kg · d)。

• VZIG：成人，625 IU，肌内注射。儿童：1 瓶/10 kg，肌内注射。最多用 5 瓶（每瓶含 125 IU）。

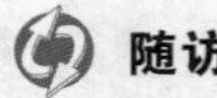

随访

进一步处理

入院指征

• 肺炎患者需要纳入：
- 在 ICU 行呼吸支持的。

• 免疫功能低下的患者：ICU 或病房，取决于疾病的严重程度。

• 所有入选的患者必须保持隔离。

出院指征

• 没有脑炎或继发性细菌感染证据的免疫功能正常的患儿。

• 没有证据表明有皮肤外伤的成人。

随访建议

出院的患者需要 PCP 密切随访，以确保没有并发症。

要点和误区

• 水痘患者在囊泡形成前 48 h 具有传染性，直到所有囊泡结痂。

• 免疫功能低下的患有水痘的患者在大多数情况下需要考虑收入院。

• 水痘肺炎是医疗急症，尤其是在妊娠期间。

S

水杨酸盐中毒 Salicylate Poisoning

Michele Zell-Kanter　何融冰 译

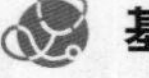

基础知识

描述

• 呼吸性碱中毒和代谢性酸中毒：
- 继发于三羧酸循环受抑制和氧化磷酸化解偶联。

• 脱水、低钠血症或高钠血症、低钾血症、低钙血症：
- 由于出汗、呕吐和气促引起。

• 非心源性肺水肿：
- 因为水杨酸盐对肺内皮的毒性作用导致液体外渗。

• 水杨酸盐在剂量过大时药代动力学从一级改变为零级。例如，小剂量的增加会导致水杨酸盐浓度大幅度升高。

老年人注意事项

• 发病率更高。

• 呼吸窘迫、精神状态改变等严重中毒表现。

• 基础疾病如 CHF 可掩盖症状和体征，从而导致水杨酸盐中毒的诊断延误。

儿科注意事项

• 儿童比成人发病更迅速且症状和体征更严重：
- 由于水杨酸杨可更快地分布到靶器官，如大脑、肾脏和肝脏中。

• 呼吸性碱中毒（成人水杨酸盐中毒的标志）可能不会表现于儿童。

• 低血糖比高血糖更常见。

• 摄入不止“一种味道”的油。

• ＜6 岁的儿童摄入冬绿油（98%水杨酸甲酯）或＞6 岁的患者摄入＞4 ml 的冬绿油必须进行急诊室评估。

病因

水杨酸盐的来源：

• 阿司匹林：
- 摄入＞150 mg/kg 可导致严重中毒。

• 冬绿油：
- 任何暴露都是危险的。

• 次水杨酸铋（双水杨酯）。

诊断

症状和体征

• 胃肠道：
- 恶心。
- 呕吐。
- 上腹部疼痛。
- 呕血。

• 肺部：
- 呼吸急促。
- 非心源性肺水肿。

• CNS：
- 耳鸣。
- 耳聋。
- 癫痫。
- 昏迷。

病史

• 询问是否服用阿司匹林或阿司匹林制品：
- 许多患者未把阿司匹林列入他们的常规用药中，可能未把阿司匹林当作药物。

• 患者或许不知道阿司匹林、对乙酰氨基酚和 NSAIDs 非处方药之间的区别。

基本检查

• 水杨酸盐水平：
- 目前水平然后 q2 h 直至水平开始下降。
- 证实单位是正确的，一般为 mg/dl。

• 注意观察水杨酸盐中毒体征再现以及水平上升，甚至继发于水平下降后，由于肠道对肠衣片和双水杨酯的吸收。

评估水杨酸盐中毒严重性指南

• 快速服用：
- ＜150 mg/kg 或＜6.5 g 阿司匹林等效物：考虑无毒性。
- 150～300 mg/kg：轻度到中度中毒。
- ＞300 mg/kg：有致命可能。

• 慢性服药过量：
- 对症治疗不单单以水杨酸水平为指标。

- 临床表现比血浆水杨酸盐水平能更好显示病情的严重程度。
- 无有效数据图来解释水杨酸盐水平。
- 能达到抗感染效果的水杨酸盐水平(20～25 mg/dl)与中毒水平较接近。
- 阿司匹林肠衣片在小肠吸收,高峰浓度延迟。

诊断检查与说明

实验室检查

- 动脉血气(ABG):
  - 呼吸性碱中毒。
  - 代谢性酸中毒。
- CBC。
- 电解质、BUN/肌酐、葡萄糖:
  - 阴离子间隙代谢性酸中毒。
  - 低钾血症。
  - 肾功能。
- 尿分析:
  - 尿 pH。
- 大量服用后测 PT、APTT。
- 氯化铁试验:
  - 如有水杨酸盐则呈紫色。
  - 服用后 30 min 阳性。
- 存在水杨酸时,Phenistix 变为棕-紫色,最低可检测到浓度为 20 mg/dl。

影像学检查

- 腹部 X 线平片检查凝结物。
- 胸部 X 线检查肺水肿。

鉴别诊断

- 急性水杨酸中毒:
  - 精神状态改变,不明原因的非心源性肺水肿,混合的酸碱平衡失调应考虑该病。
  - 甲醇。
  - 乙二醇。
  - 造成非心源性肺水肿的疾病。
- 慢性水杨酸中毒:
  - 濒临心肌梗死。
  - 戒酒。
  - 器质性重症精神病。
  - 脓毒症。
  - 痴呆。

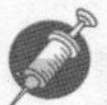

治疗

院前

如果怀疑服药过量,应带回药瓶以供回顾病情。

初步稳定/治疗

- ABC 管理。
- 精神状态改变应用纳洛酮、硫胺素、葡萄糖(或 Accu-Chek)。
- 生理盐水(NS)静脉补液治疗低血压。

急诊治疗/程序

- 慢性水杨酸盐中毒的发病率可能大于急性中毒。
- 全肠灌洗理论上的作用:
  - 腹部 X 线平片可见凝结物。
  - 服用缓释制剂。
  - 如果经适当治疗后水杨酸水平仍持续上升。
  - 已经发生精神状态改变的患者不能使用。

加强排泄

- 碱化。
  - 加强离子状水杨酸盐的排泄。
  - 适应证:
    - 酸中毒。
    - 出现症状。
    - 水杨酸盐水平升高。
  - 1 或 2 安瓿碳酸氢钠,随后静脉注入 D_5W 1 L 加 3 安瓿碳酸氢钠:
    - 目标:尿 pH 7.5～8,维持 3～6 ml/(kg·h)速率。
    - 每升增加 20～40 mEq KCl 以防低钾血症。
    - 避免 CHF 或 CAD 患者药物过量。
    - 密切监测血清钾。
- 血液透析的适应证包括:
  - CHF。
  - 非心源性肺水肿。
  - CNS 损害。
  - 癫痫。
  - 生命体征不稳定。
  - 严重酸碱平衡失调。
  - 肝损伤。
  - 凝血病。
  - 基础疾病影响水杨酸的排泄。
  - 水杨酸盐水平绝对值不是决定是否做透析的唯一标准,应结合患者的临床表现除非急性服用过量>80～100 mg/dl 时。
- 慢性服药过量的患者透析阈值较低。

药物治疗

- 活性炭膏剂:1～2 g/kg 至多 90 g,口服。
- 葡萄糖:$D_{50}W$ 1 安瓿(50 ml 或 25 g)(儿童:$D_{25}W$ 2～4 ml/kg),静脉注射。
- 纳洛酮(盐酸烯丙羟吗啡酮):首剂 2 mg(儿童:0.1 mg/kg),静脉注射或肌内注射。
- 硫胺素(维生素 B_1):100 mg(儿童:50 mg),静脉注射或肌内注射。

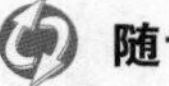

随访

进一步处理

入院指征

- 检测患者水杨酸水平>25 mg/dl 直至水平降至<25 mg/dl 且症状缓解。
- 水杨酸水平在降至接近无毒性水平后再次上升:
  - 在患者服用阿司匹林缓释片、肠衣片和其他吸收延迟的阿司匹林制品后。
- 精神状态改变、代谢性酸中毒、肺水肿的患者入 ICU。

出院指征

反复检查水杨酸盐水平<25 mg/dl 且症状缓解。

随访建议

- 故意服用应转入精神科。
- 慢性服药过量患者应密切重点随访。

要点和误区

- 患者需要维持呼吸驱动来对抗代谢性酸中毒、呼吸性酸中毒:
  - 不要过早插管。
  - 这些患者达到和维持机械通气尤其困难。
- 水杨酸盐中毒可由暴露于水杨酸洗剂、乳膏、直肠栓剂、口服止泻药导致。
- 水杨酸盐水平在有肠药物吸收或肠道中水杨酸盐结石时可发生有下降趋势后水平又上升的情况。

水肿 Edema

Laura J. Macnow 姜颢 译

基础知识

描述

• 由于渗透压和静水压平衡紊乱，临床上见血管外液显著积聚：
- 静脉、毛细血管静水压升高。
- 血浆胶体渗透压降低。
- 间质胶体渗透压升高。
- 毛细血管通透性增高。
- 梗阻所致淋巴压力增加。
- 这些因素相结合：

• 全身性，如伴充血性心力衰竭或肾病综合征。

• 局限性，如伴深静脉血栓形成。

• 静脉静水压增高或胶体渗透压下降导致凹陷性水肿。

• 富含蛋白质的渗出液导致非凹陷性水肿。

• 某些疾病，与 Starling 力没有明显关系：
- 特发性（循环）水肿：
  ◦ 恶化伴发热。
  ◦ 女性更常见。
  ◦ 与月经不一定相关。

病因

• 全身性：
- 心力衰竭。
- 肺心病。
- 心肌病。
- 缩窄性心包炎。
- 肺动脉高压：
  ◦ 睡眠呼吸暂停综合征。
  ◦ 慢性阻塞性肺疾病（COPD）。
- 急性肾小球肾炎。
- 肾衰竭。
- 药物相关（通常为盐潴留）：
  ◦ 类固醇、雌激素、孕激素。
  ◦ 非甾体抗炎药。
  ◦ 抗高血压药（尤其是血管扩张剂）。
  ◦ 米诺地尔。
  ◦ 交感神经抑制剂（可乐定、胍乙啶、甲基多巴）。
  ◦ 锂盐。
  ◦ 胰岛素。
  ◦ 噻唑烷二酮类药物（格列酮类）。
  ◦ 生长激素。
  ◦ 白细胞介素 2。
  ◦ 单胺氧化酶抑制剂。
  ◦ 普拉克素。
  ◦ 多西他赛。
  ◦ 环孢素。
  ◦ OKT3 单克隆抗体。
  ◦ 利尿剂的急性戒断。
- 特发性（循环）水肿。
- 黏液性水肿。
- 肝硬化。
- 肾病综合征。
- 蛋白丢失性肠病/吸收不良。
- 饥饿。
- 妊娠。

• 局限性：
- 深静脉血栓形成。
- 静脉功能不全。
- 血栓性静脉炎。
- 慢性淋巴管炎。
- 蜂窝织炎。
- 贝克囊肿。
- 血管炎。
- 血管性水肿：
  ◦ 过敏性。
  ◦ 获得性。
- 甲状腺功能减退（黏液性水肿）。
- 机械损伤。
- 热损伤。
- 辐射损伤。
- 化学烧伤。
- 偏瘫。
- 反射性肌营养不良。
- 压缩或浸润性肿瘤。
- 淋巴管术后切除。
- 放射治疗。
- 丝虫病。

诊断

症状与体征

• 体重增加（数千克）。

• 受影响部位出现不适。

• 肿胀。

• 压痛。

• 凹陷性水肿：
- 静脉静水压增加，胶体渗透压下降。

• 非凹陷性水肿：
- 富含蛋白质的渗出液。

• 全身性水肿：
- 水肿在坠积区域最为突出：
  ◦ 足。
  ◦ 骶骨。
  ◦ 双侧下肢。
  ◦ 面部、眶周（尤其是早晨）。
- 心脏：
  ◦ 呼吸困难。
  ◦ 端坐呼吸。
  ◦ 夜间阵发性呼吸困难。
  ◦ 颈静脉压力增加。
  ◦ 啰音。
  ◦ S3 奔马律。
- 肾：
  ◦ 厌食。
  ◦ 眼睑肿胀。
  ◦ 泡沫尿。
  ◦ 少尿。
  ◦ 深色尿。
  ◦ 血尿。
  ◦ 高血压。

• 肝脏：
  ◦ 黄疸。
  ◦ 蜘蛛痣。
  ◦ 手掌红斑。
  ◦ 男性乳房发育症。
  ◦ 睾丸萎缩。
  ◦ 腹水。
- 黏液性水肿：
  ◦ 胫前非凹陷性水肿。
  ◦ 皮肤和皮下组织的干蜡样肿胀。
  ◦ 眼眶最常见（眼袋）。
  ◦ 非相关区域。
  ◦ 疲劳。
  ◦ 不耐寒冷。
  ◦ 体重增加。
  ◦ 便秘。
  ◦ 缓慢的腱反射松弛。
- 特发性：
  ◦ 日间体重增加/减少。

• 局限性：
- 慢性静脉功能不全：
  ◦ 慢性凹陷性。
  ◦ 皮肤变色（含铁血黄素沉积）。
  ◦ 皮炎/溃疡。
  ◦ 静脉曲张。

- 创伤史：
  ◦ 机械、热、辐射。
- 感染性、炎症性：
  ◦ 寒战。
  ◦ 发热。
  ◦ 红斑。
  ◦ 温度增高。
- 过敏：
  ◦ 荨麻疹。
  ◦ 瘙痒。
  ◦ 嘴唇和口腔黏膜受累。

妊娠注意事项

- 常继发于激素介导的液体潴留。
- 当涉及手和面，可能是先兆子痫的早期征兆。
- 坠积性水肿：
  - 通常在妊娠晚期。
  - 来自静脉回流受阻。
  - 禁用利尿剂。

基本检查

诊断性检查应针对病史和体格检查所提示的潜在病因。

诊断检查与说明

实验室检查

- 怀疑心脏疾病：
  - BNP 或 NT-proBNP。
- 怀疑深静脉血栓形成：
  - D-二聚体(用于临床排除深静脉血栓的可能性低的患者)。
- 怀疑肾脏疾病：
  - 电解质。
  - 尿素氮和肌酐。
  - 尿液分析。
  - 尿电解质和蛋白质。
  - 血脂。
- 怀疑肝脏疾病：
  - 血清白蛋白。
  - 肝功能试验。
  - 凝血酶原时间和部分凝血活酶时间。
- 怀疑黏液水肿性：
  - 甲状腺功能检查。

影像学检查

- 怀疑心脏疾病：
  - 心电图(EKG)。
  - 胸部 X 线平片。
  - 心电图(ECG)。
- 局限性肢体水肿：
  - 超声(双重扫描)或静脉造影术。
- 高度怀疑腹部或盆腔恶性肿瘤：
  - 腹部、盆腔 CT。

鉴别诊断

- 蜂窝织炎。
- 接触性皮炎。
- 弥漫性皮下浸润过程。
- 淋巴水肿。
- 肥胖。

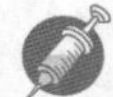

治疗

初步稳定/治疗

见“急诊治疗”。

急诊治疗/程序

- 治疗应针对根本原因。
- 利尿剂通常用于全身水肿的病例，但并非迫切需要。
- 由于快速的体液转移可能导致肝肾综合征，利尿剂可能对肝硬化腹水患者有害。

药物治疗

- 阿米洛利：5～10 mg，口服，每日 1 次。
- 卡托普利：6.25～100 mg，口服，每日 3 次(最大剂量为 450 mg/d)。
- 呋塞米：20～80 mg，静脉推注/口服，每日 4 次(最大剂量为 600 mg/d)。
- 氢氯噻嗪：25～100 mg，口服，每日 2 次。
- 螺内酯：25～200 mg，口服，每日 2 次。

随访

进一步处理

入院指征

- 基于原发病决定收治患者。
- 伴心血管或肺损害。
- 没有足够的家庭支持而无法活动。
- 缺氧。

出院指征

- 应建议患者减少盐摄入量。
- 弹力袜。
- 抬高患肢。

转诊问题

- >45 岁的慢性水肿患者，或其症状提示有心肺疾病需要随访心电图。
- 不明原因的肺动脉高血压患者应做睡眠监测以评估睡眠呼吸暂停。
- 超声阴性有深静脉血栓形成高风险的患者，需在 5～7 日立即复查。

随访建议

慢性水肿患者可与初级保健医师随访持续的检查和治疗。

要点和误区

- 水肿分为全身性和局限性，凹陷性与非凹陷性。
- 凹陷性水肿是由“贫蛋白质”渗出液引起的(静水压力增加或胶体渗透压下降)。
- 非凹陷性水肿是由“富蛋白质”渗出液引起的(淋巴水肿和毛细血管通透性增加)。
- 全身性或双侧下肢水肿需要行全身性疾病检查。
- 急性单侧下肢水肿需要评估 DVT。
- 在妊娠期考虑先兆子痫。

睡眠呼吸暂停

Ajay Bhatt 周健 潘曙明 译

基础知识

描述

- 以睡眠时呼吸停止为特征的紊乱：
  - 定义为呼吸暂停发作>10 s 伴短暂 EEG 觉醒或>3%氧合降低。
- 风险因素：
  - 肥胖。
  - 男性。
  - 大于 40 岁。
  - 上呼吸道异常。
  - 水肿(甲状腺功能减退)。

- 酒精/滥用镇静剂。
- 吸烟。
• 相关疾病：
- 各种心律失常，特别是心颤动和缓性心律失常。
- 左心衰竭、右心衰竭。
- 心肌梗死。
- 大吃大喝。
- 机动车事故。
- 药物治疗不能很好地控制高血压。

流行病学

• 大约 15%的中年男性和 5%的中年女性受到影响。
• 由于肥胖率的提高，患病率也有所上升。
• 80%的中重度病例在中年未确诊。

病因

睡眠呼吸暂停的 3 种分类：
• 阻塞(84%)是由于上呼吸道关闭，尽管完整的呼吸驱动：
- 也被称为 Pickwickian 综合征。
- 咽导气管变窄。
• 中枢性(0.4%)是由于尽管上呼吸道通畅，但呼吸做功不足。
• 复杂性(15%)是由于阻塞性和中枢性睡眠呼吸暂停综合征。

诊断

症状和体征

• 嗜睡(白日过度嗜睡)。
• 打呼噜。
• 易怒。

病史

• 重要的其他呼吸暂停(窒息)记录。
• 入睡困难。
• 注意力下降。
• 沮丧。
• 性欲降低/阳痿。

体格检查

• 高血压，血氧低。
• 肥胖。
• 颅面畸形。
• 巨舌。
• 扁桃体红肿。
• 颈静脉怒张(继发于肺动脉高压)。
• 大脖子(大颈围)。

基本检查

• 脉搏血氧仪。
• 心电图。
• 胸部 X 线检查。

诊断检查和说明

实验室检查

ABG 是证实高碳酸血症和低氧血症的最佳方法。

影像学检查

• 考虑侧颈部软组织 X 线片排除上呼吸道梗阻的其他病因。
• 胸部 X 线检查以评估低氧血症的其他病因。
• 胸部 CT 很少显示。

诊断步骤/外科

• 多导睡眠图(PSG)是诊断所必需的。
• 每小时 5 次。
• 家庭睡眠呼吸暂停测试(HSAT)对无共病者可能足够。
• 不考虑电渗析管理。

鉴别诊断

• 哮喘。
• 潮式呼吸。
• 慢性阻塞性肺疾病。
• 膈肌麻痹。
• 高海拔诱导的周期性呼吸。
• 甲状腺功能减退。
• 左心衰竭。
• 嗜睡症。
• 肥胖过度通气综合征。
• 原发性肺动脉高压。

治疗

急诊治疗/程序

慢性一氧化碳潴留患者注意不要过度通气。

初步稳定/治疗

• 提下颌/推下颌手法，根据需要吸氧，口腔或鼻道人工气道。
• 双人技术，确保密封良好。
• 治疗标准为持续气道正压(CPAP)：
- 作为气动夹板，保持上呼吸道通畅。
- BiPAP 是需要高血压或合并呼吸障碍患者的另一种选择。
- 长期 CPAP 治疗可降低血压、胰岛素抵抗、代谢综合征和心血管疾病的风险。

注意

• 气管插管术。
• 插管困难发生率较高：
- 患者的 Mallampati 评分通常较高。
- 咽侧壁组织过度常阻碍气道暴露。
- 患者整体动脉血氧饱和度较低。
• 计划和考虑几种最终气道控制方法：
- 有替代设备(面罩气道，通气导管)。
- 如有必要，准备行环甲切开术。
• 只有在合理可能的情况下，且易于面罩通气时，才可使用神经肌肉阻滞。
• 通气患者的呼气末正压。

药物治疗

• 没有足够的证据推荐任何药物治疗。
• 有关诱导剂和神经肌肉阻滞的详细信息，请参阅气道管理。
• 促醒剂(莫达非尼和阿莫达替尼)被批准作为过度嗜睡的 CPAP 患者的辅助药物。

注意

• 避免镇静剂使用：
• 放松上呼吸道，加重呼吸道阻塞和打鼾。
• 长期管理：
- 美国医师学会强烈推荐遵守 CPAP 和减肥。
• 手术注意事项：
- 大多数人试图减少或绕过睡眠中出现的咽/气道过度阻力。
- 疗效是不可预测的；没有好的随机试验。
- 不考虑教育管理。
• 口腔科设备：
- 目前由美国睡眠医学学会(AASM)推荐。
- 可用的器具包括舌复位和下颌装置或软腭提升器。

随访

进一步处理

入院指征

• 呼吸困难，尤其是需要插管时。
• 血流动力学不稳定。

出院指征

• 使用患者家中可用的充氧或通气设备，将氧浓度>85%维持数小时。
• 极低的夜间失代偿的可能性。
• 车祸后出现睡眠呼吸暂停的患者。
• 像其他钝器外伤患者一样处理：
- 随后，考虑睡眠呼吸暂停增加的风险，并进行干预以预防未来的事故。

随访建议

• PCP 转诊治疗睡眠呼吸暂停和相关

共病。
- 鼓励遵守，使用 CPAP。
- 怀疑有睡眠呼吸暂停的患者转诊到肺科医院。
- 鼓励减肥和控制饮食。
- 当睡眠呼吸暂停并发心衰或心律失常时，应转诊。

要点和误区

- 睡眠呼吸暂停会增加心血管疾病、脑卒中和糖尿病的风险。
- CPSP 是治疗的标准。
- 避免使用镇静剂。
- 准备是必要的，因为睡眠呼吸暂停会增加插管并发症。
- 初级保健转诊和 CPAP 依从性。
- 教育提高治疗。

撕裂伤处理 Laceration Management

Gordon S. Chew 何超 译

基础知识

描述

- 大多数是由于创伤引起的皮肤完整性的破坏。
- 可以是单层或多层的。

病因

多发性病因。

诊断

症状和体征

撕裂伤同时伴发：
- 流血。
- 组织异物留存。
- 血肿。
- 疼痛或麻木感。
- 运动功能丧失。
- 动脉搏动减弱，毛细血管充盈延缓。

病史

- 受伤机制或环境。
- 受伤时间。
- 是否留有异物（玻璃、牙齿）。
- 破伤风免疫。
- 同时患有的其他疾病或妨碍伤口愈合的药物。

体格检查

- 评估神经和运动功能。
- 记录相关的神经血管损伤。
- 评估是否存在威胁生命的组织损伤、异物残留、骨骼或关节的碎片，以及肌腱损伤。
  - 如果残留异物比较锋利，避免用手指进行探查。

基本检查

- 在急诊室治疗安全性不能保证的情况下，特别是需要进行镇静的儿童患者，可以考虑入手术室进行修复。
- 对于复杂的撕脱伤尤其涉及眼部或面部的情况下进行外科手术修复。

儿科注意事项

对所有非偶然性的损伤进行评估。

诊断检查与说明

实验室检查

- 评估是否有异物存留。
- X 线平片：
  - 软组织可视化成像。
  - 和软组织相同密度的物质可能无法看见（如木头、植物）。
- 超声检查。
- CT。
- MRI（排除金属存在）。

鉴别诊断

- 皮肤撕裂。
- 挫伤。
- 擦伤。

治疗

院前

- 观察出血情况或直接压迫止血。
- 对于血供不良的皮瓣进行修复以恢复血供。
- 必要时以夹板固定。
- 进行全面的预防措施。

初步稳定/治疗

- 气道、呼吸、循环的管理。
- 控制出血。
- 摘除指环、钻石等，因为肿胀的手指会由于指环而缺血坏死。

急诊治疗/程序

- 发生的第一时间：
  - 血供不良区域的撕裂伤在 8 h 以内能够一期缝合。
  - 血供正常区域的撕裂伤在 12 h 内能够一期缝合。
  - 在面部区域的撕裂伤在充分冲洗之后 24 h 内能够一期缝合。
  - 如果没有进行一期缝合，伤口可以在 3～5 日后进行延期缝合。
- 止痛和镇静：
  - 充分的止痛对于伤口的愈合有积极意义。
  - 同时需要清醒状态下的镇静。
- 局部麻醉：
  - 局部：
    - TAC（盐酸丁卡因、肾上腺素、可卡因）。
    - EMLA（共晶混合物、利多卡因、普鲁卡因）。
    - LET（利多卡因、肾上腺素、盐酸丁卡因）。
  - 区域性：
    - 利多卡因、布比卡因。
    - 肾上腺素可以造成血管的收缩从而延长药物的麻醉时间。
    - 在阴茎、手指、足趾、耳、眼睑、鼻尖、坏死皮瓣和严重污染的伤口等处使用肾上腺素。
    - 为了增加患者的舒适度，使用细针进行缓慢注射药物，并且每 9 ml 1%利多卡因使用 1 ml 8.4%碳酸氢钠进行缓冲。
    - 配备 1%苯海拉明用于治疗利多卡因重度患者。
- 检查并去除异物：
  - 能够对肌腱、神经、血管组织造成损伤的异物。
  - 具有毒性的物质。
  - 给患者带来持续性疼痛的异物。
- 冲洗和消毒：

- 损伤周围皮肤以抗菌溶液进行冲洗(洗必泰)。
  - 不要使用抗菌溶液对伤口内部进行冲洗,会造成伤口的进一步损伤。
- 当皮肤存在污染物或微粒时可使用柔软的海绵进行刷洗。
- 使用至少 200 ml 的生理盐水进行冲洗。
- 避免刮除毛发,必要时可以使用镊子夹取。
  - 刮除的过程中会增加皮肤感染的机会。
  - 不要刮除或夹除眉毛,因为它可能不能再长回原来的外观。
- 去除失活或污染严重的组织。

• 创伤的修复:
- 全面的预防措施。
- 不能完全清洁的窗口应做二期缝合或延期缝合。
- 仔细修剪组织边缘。
- 确保组织愈合边缘清洁,张力低。

S

• 单层缝合:
- 单纯间断缝合:
  - 避免由于张力过大产生的创口再次撕裂。
- 水平褥式缝合:
  - 缝合手指或手部伤口。
  - 对于边缘可能发生坏死的皮瓣是比较理想的缝合方式。
- 垂直褥式缝合:
  - 针对张力较大的伤口。
  - 第一针确保足够的深度并且皮肤闭合良好。
- 半包水平褥式缝合:
  - 对于 v 形或 y 形并且可能发生缺血的伤口而言是比较理想的缝合方式。

• 多层缝合:
- 缝合存在无效腔的较深组织。
- 减少表皮的张力,使皮肤愈合更加美观。
- 包埋部分缝合使用可吸收线,表皮连续缝合使用不可吸收线。

• 修整:
- 在伤口处涂抹抗生素药膏并覆盖多层的不黏敷料。
- 告知患者存在瘢痕和感染的风险,并使用光照疗法。
- 必要时使用夹板固定。

• 抗菌药物:
- 不推荐预防性使用抗生素。
- 在进行伤口处理之前使用抗生素或尽可能早地开始使用抗生素。
- 感染高发的撕裂伤:
  - 人或动物咬伤,特别是手部的损伤。
  - 伤口含有不洁的体液或者排泄物。
- 破伤风免疫。

药物治疗

• 破伤风疫苗:0.5 ml 肌内注射。

• 局部麻醉:
- 伤口局部使用纱布或棉花覆盖:
  - EMLA(共晶混合物、5%利多卡因、普鲁卡因):能持续 60 min。注意每克 EMLA 含有 2.5 g 的利多卡因,不要超过 3 mg/kg 剂量的利多卡因。
  - TAC(5%盐酸丁卡因、1∶2 000 肾上腺素、11.8%可卡因):持续 20～30 min,伤口上使用 2～5 ml。
  - LET(4%利多卡因、1∶1 000 肾上腺素、0.5%盐酸丁卡因):持续 20～30 min,使用 1～3 ml。不要超过 3 mg/kg 剂量的利多卡因。

• 注射:
- 布比卡因(最大剂量 2 mg/kg,持续 3～10 h)。
- 利多卡因(最大剂量 4.5 mg/kg,持续 1.5～3.5 h)。

• 缝合材料:
- 可吸收:
  - 用于浆膜面后者包埋的肌肉筋膜的缝合。
  - 自然源性:1 周内吸收,张力强度较弱。
  - 合成编织物:张力能够维持 1 个月,轻度炎症反应,包括聚乙醇酸。
  - 合成单纤维丝:1 个月后能维持 70%的张力,包括聚二噁烷酮或聚葡萄糖酸酯。
- 不可吸收:
  - 张力最强。
  - 单纤维:尼龙、聚丙烯、聚丁烯酯可以用来缝合肿胀伤口,聚乙烯。
  - 多纤维:棉线、涤纶或丝线(会产生局部的炎症反应)。
- 针的类型:
  - 锋利型的多用于表皮伤口的修复。

• 吻合器:
- 用于头皮、四肢和躯干的线性伤口缝合。
- 在手部、面部或者需要进行 CT 或 MRI 检查部位避免使用。

• 黏附的胶布:
- 对于清洁、微小或张力很小的伤口以胶布闭合。
- 对于可能会发生肿胀的伤口避免使用。
- 伤口预先使用安息香酊进行处理来增加黏附性。

• 组织黏合剂:
- 对于张力较小的撕裂伤使用组织黏合剂能够起到美容的作用。
- 除了缝合和吻合器之外的一个选择,特别适用于儿童。

 随访

进一步处理

入院指征

• 大部分的撕裂伤不需要住院治疗,除非需要进一步的清创、静脉注射抗生素、损伤严重复杂需要周密的护理;或重要器官的撕裂伤,如头部损伤、腹部创伤。

出院指征

• 对于感染高发或可能愈合不良的伤口要在 48 h 内进行复查。

• 拆除缝线的时限依据损伤的位置和末梢血供而有所差异:
- 头皮伤:7～10 日。
- 头面部:3～5 日。
- 口腔:7 日。
- 颈部:4～6 日。
- 胸腹部、背部、手足:7～10 日。
- 上肢:7～10 日。
- 下肢:10～14 日。
- 跨越关节:10～14 日。

随访建议

• 对于眼部的撕裂伤怀疑伤及泪管时要立刻进行确认。

• 复杂性的撕裂伤(涉及肌腱损伤)则需要在门诊手术室进行进一步的损伤修复。

• 征询外科医师的建议是否需要进行临时的皮肤缝合和夹板固定。

• 患者出院前进行复查。

四肢穿透伤 Extremity Trauma, Penetrating

Gary M. Vilke · Peter H.D. Solomon 单怡 译

基础知识

描述

四肢的穿透性创伤。

病因

- 捅伤或刺伤。
- 枪伤。
- 撕裂伤。
- 咬伤。
- 高压注射伤。

诊断

症状和体征

- 创口有入口和出口(如果有的话),撕裂伤。
- 高速枪弹伤口:
  - 产生振荡波导致严重的组织损伤。
  - 通常出口的组织损伤比入口更严重。
- 血管损伤:
  - 动脉损伤:
    - 末梢脉搏减弱或消失。
    - 末梢坏死改变。
    - 逐渐增大的血肿。
    - 损伤部位的杂音或震颤。
  - 末梢脉搏存在不能排除四肢血管损伤。
- 神经损伤:
  - 感觉异常。
  - 邻近关节的韧带松弛,提示肌腱损伤。
  - 邻近关节积液,提示骨折或韧带损伤。
- 骨筋膜室综合征:
  - 提示受累的骨筋膜室内严重症的和持续的疼痛。
  - 四肢远端主动和被动的伸直或屈曲都有疼痛。
  - 骨筋膜室内无力或触痛。
  - 骨筋膜室内神经感觉过敏。
  - 迟发性的无脉和苍白。

病史

- 损伤机制。
- 受伤年龄。
- 受伤时的情况:
  - 暴力攻击。
  - 自残。
  - 家庭暴力。
- 合并症:
  - 免疫功能低下或糖尿病。
  - 心脏瓣膜病。
  - 无脾。
  - 外周血管病。

体格检查

- 注意原发伤和出口伤的部位、长度、深度及形态(如果有出口)。
- 血管损伤:
  - 通过触诊和多普勒检查对比末梢的脉搏情况。
  - 评估毛细血管再充盈:
    - 大于 2 s 为异常。
  - 踝-肱指数(ABI):
    - 测量小腿和上臂的血压(包括四肢)。
    - 收缩压差大于 10 mmHg 时提示有血管损伤。
  - 损伤部位扩张性血肿、杂音或震颤也提示血管损伤。
- 神经损伤:
  - 评估损伤远端的运动和感觉功能:
    - 两点辨别觉。
    - 轻触觉。
    - 本体感觉。
- 骨骼肌肉损伤:
  - 注意相关的挤压伤、肌腱、韧带和骨骼畸形。
  - 检查邻近关节的活动范围。
  - 评估骨筋膜室综合征。
- 检查伤口有无异物(FB)。

基本检查

- 体格检查。
- 影像学检查发现骨骼损伤或可能的异物。

诊断检查与说明

实验室检查

- 新鲜伤口不需行培养。
- 血有感染征象的伤口可做细菌培养以指导抗生素的选择。

影像学检查

- X线检查可评估有无不透X线的异物或相关的骨折:
  - 前后位和侧面影像。
- 可透X线的异物,可用荧光镜在X线、超声或CT下定位检查。

诊断步骤/外科

怀疑有血管损伤时建议动脉血管造影,而并不推荐立即行血管手术。

鉴别诊断

任何存在四肢创伤的情况。

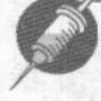

治疗

院前

注意:

- 受伤部位直接压迫控制出血。
- 抬高四肢。
- 评估神经血管情况。
- 把穿刺物保留在伤处并固定于原位。
- 镇痛。

初步稳定/治疗

- 保护气道,必要时给予复苏。
- 彻底暴露伤口,去除紧束的衣物或首饰。
- 直接压迫止血。
- 不建议在伤口内盲目钳夹止血以及长时间使用止血带。

急诊治疗/程序

- 镇痛。
- 在局麻前全面评估神经情况。
- 不宜长时间浸湿伤口,尤其是使用有细胞毒性的制剂。
- 去除肉眼可见的碎屑和失活组织。
- 最重要的是用大量生理盐水高压冲洗。
- 预防破伤风。
- 刺伤或火器伤的患者应在急诊室应用1个剂量的头孢唑林。
- 怀疑有明显血管损伤、肌腱损伤、骨折或关节损伤者,患肢需制动。
- 脉搏消失或末梢缺血者需紧急手术治疗:
  - 勿行动脉造影而延迟手术治疗。
- 撕裂伤在伤后 6~8 h 经充分清创且组织缺失很少者,可一期缝合。
  - 对伤后时间较长或污染伤口,可行延期缝合。
- 穿刺伤或枪伤者不行一期缝合。
- 特殊注意事项:
  - 足底刺伤:
    - 在光线明亮处仔细检查伤口。
    - 去除所有异物。

S

◦ 仔细清洗伤口。

- 伤口核心处理有争议，应仅用于去除失活组织或被包埋的碎片。

◦ 探查或高压冲洗刺伤的伤口只会使微小的异物推向伤口的更深处。

◦ 不推荐预防性使用抗生素（除非患者有糖尿病、免疫功能低下、伤口高度污染或伤后时间较长的伤口）。

- 如不积极的清创，可导致骨髓炎。

- 手部的高压损伤：

◦ 急诊室整形科的评估是非常重要的，因为表面上并不严重的创口可能沿着腱鞘损伤到手的深部。

◦ 某些涂料和其他物质是不透 X 线的，可能过 X 线检查显示其累及的范围。

- 软组织异物：

◦ 伤口中小的惰性异物，包括子弹，很难取出，在远离关节、肌腱、血管或神经时，将异物保留在原处并密切随访。

◦ 手部和足部的异物常会移动位置并且产生相应症状，故应请专科会诊。

◦ 有机材料（刺、木头、脊骨、衣物）很易发生反应，应及时去除。

S

■ 药物治疗

• 预防破伤风：百白破疫苗 0.5 ml 肌内注射（65 岁以上只接种白破疫苗）。

• 受伤超过 12 h，尤其是手部和下肢的损伤，挤压伤伴失活组织以及污染伤口应使用抗生素。

一线药物

• 头孢唑林：1 g，静脉注射或肌内注射（儿童：20～40 mg/kg，静脉注射或肌内注射，在急诊室使用 1 剂）。

• 头孢氨苄：500 mg，口服［儿童：25～50 mg/(kg · d)］，每日 4 次，连续 7 日。

- 阿莫西林/克拉维酸：875/125 mg 口服［儿童：25 mg/(kg · d)］，每日 2 次，连续 7 日。

• 红霉素：333 mg，口服，每日 3 次［儿童：40 mg/(kg · d)］，q6 h，连续 7 日。

• 心脏瓣膜病患者的污染伤口：

- 头孢唑林：1 g，静脉注射或肌内注射，后用头孢氨苄 500 mg，口服，每日 4 次，连续 7 日。

• 有铜绿假单胞菌风险的足部伤口：

- 环丙沙星：500 mg，每日 2 次，连续 7～10 日。

- 左氧氟沙星：500 mg，每日 1 次，连续 7～10 日。

二线药物

如青霉素过敏：

• 琥乙红霉素（EES）：800 mg 口服，后 400 mg 口服，q6 h，连续 7 日。

• 克林霉素：300 mg 口服，q6～8 h，连续 7 日。

随访

■ 进一步处理

入院指征

• 任何伴有血管损伤、骨筋膜室综合征或关节穿透伤的四肢穿透伤患者，均须外科紧急会诊并收住院。

• 高速的穿透性火器伤。

• 糖尿病患者或免疫功能低下者伴伤口污染。

出院指征

不需要外科治疗的四肢穿透伤患者，经过适当的创面处理后可出院，并嘱咐患者抬高患肢，保持创面清洁，在 24～48 h 或有任何感染征象时返院复查。

转诊问题

• 足部穿刺伤：需密切随访以评估是否有不可见的异物所引起的感染。

• 受伤时间过长或污染的伤口需延期缝合。

• 感染风险高的伤口应在 1～2 日密切随访。

■ 随访建议

疼痛加剧、麻木、刺痛、发红、肿胀流液、发热或出现其他临床时应及时返回急诊室就诊。

要点和误区

• 末梢脉搏存在并不排除末梢血管损伤。

• 手部的高压损伤伤口表面上看并不严重但会沿着肌腱进入手的深部。

• 通过鞋子或袜子引起的足部表面的刺伤有存在异物的相对风险，患者应知晓这种可能。

• 刺伤后的伤口感染对抗生素治疗无效时应怀疑存在异物的可能。

酸中毒 Acidosis

Matthew T. Robinson · Catherine D. Parker 马林浩 林兆奋 译

基础知识

■ 描述

呼吸性酸中毒

• 由于肺泡肺换气不足与 $PaCO_2$ 升高降低机体 pH。

• $PaCO_2$ ＞45 mmHg 或超过代谢性酸中毒呼吸代偿范围。

• 分为 3 大类。

- 中枢神经系统衰竭所致的呼吸障碍。

◦ 睡眠呼吸暂停。

◦ 麻醉。

◦ 镇静剂过量。

- 肺泡 CO_2 的排出障碍：

◦ 慢性阻塞性肺疾。

◦ 重症肌无力。

◦ 严重低血钾。

◦ 吉兰-巴雷综合征。

- CO_2 从组织到肺泡的运输障碍：

◦ 严重心力衰竭、肺水肿代谢性酸中毒。

代谢性酸中毒：

• 通过降低血浆碳酸氢盐水平或升高 H^+ 水平来降低血清 pH 的过程。

• 主要原因：

- 固定酸生成增多。

- 排酸减少。

- 丢失碳酸氢根。

• 代谢性酸中毒通主要分为 2 组进行临床评估：

- 高阴离子间隙代谢性酸中毒：

◦ 通过加入的强酸减少碳酸氢盐。

◦ 由于滴定的强酸中包含未测量的潴留的阴离子，阴离子间隙增加。

- 正常阴离子间隙代谢性酸中毒：
  - 肾脏不能重新吸收或再生碳酸氢盐。
  - 胃肠道碳酸氢盐的流失(腹泻)。
  - 摄入或输注含有盐酸的物质。
- 由于不存在任何未滴定的酸根和继发于碳酸氢根的丢失伴氯离子滞留，所以未观测到阴离子间隙。

病因

- 呼吸性酸中毒：
  - 抑制呼吸中枢：
    - 心搏骤停。
    - 药物(阿片类药物、苯二氮䓬类药物等)。
    - 脑膜炎/脑炎。
    - 中枢神经系统病变(肿块、CVA)。
  - 气体交换受损：
    - 肺水肿。
    - 哮喘/COPD。
    - 肺炎。
    - 间质性肺病。
    - 肥胖。
    - 肺挫伤。
  - 神经肌肉疾病：
    - 膈麻痹。
    - 吉兰-巴雷综合征。
    - 重症肌无力。
    - 肌肉萎缩症。
    - 脊髓损伤。
    - 低钾血症、低磷酸盐血症。
    - MS。
  - 阻塞性：
    - 先天性病变(喉软骨软化病)。
    - 异物吸入。
    - 血管环。
    - 传染性(会厌炎、喉炎、脓肿)。
- 代谢性酸中毒：
  - 阴离子间隙酸中毒：记为 *A CAT PILES MUD*。
    - 酒精性酮症酸中毒。
    - 一氧化碳或氰化物。
    - 阿司匹林。
    - 甲苯。
    - 三聚乙醛铁、丙烯乙二醇、二甲双胍。
    - 铁/异烟肼
    - 乳酸性酸中毒。
    - 乙烯乙二醇、乙醇。
    - 饥饿、水杨酸盐。
    - 甲醇、甲福明二甲双胍。
    - 尿毒症。
    - 糖尿病酮症酸中毒。
  - 渗透间隙增加型代谢性酸中毒：记为 *ME DIE*。
    - 甲醇。
    - 乙烯乙二醇。
    - 利尿剂(甘露醇、非酸中毒)。
    - 异丙基酒精(非酸中毒)。
    - 乙醇。
  - 阴离子间隙增加型代谢性酸中毒。
    - 胃肠道丢失碳酸氢根。
      - 腹泻(最常见的病因)。
      - 绒毛状腺瘤。
      - 小肠胰腺或胆汁分泌物。
      - 引流管。
      - 小肠、胰瘘。
    - 阴离子交换树脂(即消胆胺)。
    - 摄取氯化钙或氯化镁。
    - Ⅰ型肾小管酸中毒(远端)：低钾高氯代谢性酸中毒：
      - 分泌氢能力降低。
      - 未经治疗的血清 HCO_3^- <15 mEq/L。
      - 低钾血症。
      - 常见于肾结石。
    - Ⅱ型肾小管酸中毒(近端)：低钾高氯代谢性酸中毒：
      - 近端重吸收 HCO_3^- 能力降低。
      - 近端小管对 HCO_3^- 的再吸收能力控制酸中毒程度。
      - 血清 HCO_3^- 通常为 14～18 mEq/L。
      - 低钾或正常。
    - Ⅳ型肾小管性酸中毒(醛固酮增多症)：
      - 醛固酮缺乏或醛固酮抵抗导致 H^+ 分泌减少。
      - 血清碳酸氢钠>15 mEq/L。
      - 正常或高钾血症。
    - 碳酸酐酶抑制剂。
    - 肾小管间质性疾病。
    - 醛固酮减少症。
    - 静脉营养液。
    - 酸物质增多，例如：
      - 氯化铵。
      - 精氨酸氯化氢。
      - 赖氨酸氯化氢。

诊断

体征和症状

- 非特异性发现。
- 生命体征。
  - 呼吸急促或 Kussmaul 呼吸伴代谢性酸中毒。
  - 呼吸性酸中毒引起的通气不足。
  - 心动过速。
- 嗜睡。
- 意识障碍。
- 精神状态改变(CO_2 麻醉)。
- 心肌传导和收缩功能紊乱(心律失常)。

基本检查

- 电解质、BUN、肌酐和葡萄糖：
  - 减少碳酸氢盐与代谢性酸中毒。
  - 高钾血症和高钙血症伴严重代谢性酸中毒。
- 动脉血气分析：
  - pH。
  - CO_2 潴留呼吸性酸中毒。
  - CO_2 水平。

通过计算期望值并与实验室检测值进行比较，计算补偿程度，如下。

- 呼吸性酸中毒：
  - 急性：$PaCO_2$ 每增加 10 mmHg，HCO_3^- 的预计值会增加 1 mEq/L。
  - 慢性：$PaCO_2$ 每增加 10 mmHg，HCO_3^- 的预计值会增加 4 mEq/L。
- 计算阴离子间隙：$Na^+ - (HCO_3^- + Cl^-)$：
  - 纠正低蛋白血症造成负离子间隙。
    - 当白蛋白每下降 1 g/dl(从 4 g/dl 开始)，阴离子间隙上加 2.5。
  - 在计算明显高血糖导致的阴离子间隙异常时，不要纠正钠的浓度，因为高血糖会影响氯、碳酸氢盐及钠的浓度。
  - 正常范围＝5－12±3 mEq/L。
  - 阴离子间隙>25 mEq/L 仅可出现在：
    - 乳酸酸中毒。
    - 酮症酸中毒。
    - 中毒性酸中毒。
- 计算补偿量：
  - 期望 $PaCO_2 = 1.5[HCO_3^-] + 8$。
  - 若 $PaCO_2$ 过高，患者伴有呼吸性酸中毒和/或补偿不足。
- 评估 delta 间隙(ΔGap)：
  - 在单纯的酸碱紊乱中，阴离子间隙每增加 1，HCO_3^- 应该减少 1 mEq/L。
  - 当分布容量中不可测量的阴离子与血浆中的 HCO_3^- 量不一致时，若 ΔGap>6 则表示有混合型酸碱平衡紊乱。
- 通过比较阴离子间隙(AAG)随 HCO_3^- ($AHCO_3^-$)与正常值的变化来评估 ΔGap。
  - HCO_3^- 降低～AG 增加(ΔGap 0±6)只有 AG 酸中毒。
  - HCO_3^- 降低>AG 增加(ΔGap≤6)，非

AG代谢性酸中毒和呼碱。

- HCO_3^- 降低<AG增加(ΔGap≥6)代谢性碱中毒和呼吸性酸中毒。

诊断检查与说明

实验室检查

- ABG：参见上面的解释。
- VBG：
  - 明显的好处是减少患者的不适和容易获得样本。
  - 当与动脉血气样本相比pH变化<0.04个单位。
  - 与 PCO_2 变化的关系。
  - 在高碳酸血症筛查中的作用有限。PCO_2>45 mmHg是敏感的(但不是特异性的)检测动脉 PO_2>50 mmHg血流流动学稳定的患者。
  - 用于简单的酸碱紊乱。
- 葡萄糖和酮的尿液分析。
- 测量血清渗透压。
  - 计算血清渗透压=2 Na^+ +葡萄糖/18+BUN/2.8+ETOH/4.6。
- 渗透压间隙=计算和测量的渗透压差。
  - 正常≤10。
  - 渗透压间隙升高可能表明毒性酒精是酸中毒的病因。
  - 不应使用渗透压间隙来排除有毒的摄入物。
    - 不严密定义的渗透压间隙。
    - 延迟报告可能正常的差距。
    - 正常患者的差值过大。
- 毒理学原因：
  - 甲醇、乙二醇、乙醇和异丙醇导致的渗透压间隙增加。
  - 怀疑摄入阿司匹林或铁超量。
- CO曝光的一氧化碳测量法。
- 血清酮或β-羟基丁酸水平。
- 血清乳酸。

影像学检查

胸部X部检查：

- 可识别心肌病或CHF。
- 潜在的肺炎。

诊断步骤/外科

心电图：

- 可识别区室壁运动异常或瓣膜功能障碍。
- 评估传导阻滞。

鉴别诊断

- 阴离子间隙酸中毒：
  - 记为 *A CATPILES MUD*。
- 增加渗透压间隙：
  - 记为 *ME DIE*。

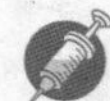

治疗

初步稳定/治疗

ABC管理。

- 早期插管治疗严重代谢性酸中毒，进展/呼吸代偿可能减弱。
- 纳洛酮，D_{50} W(或Accu-Chek)，精神状态改变时使用硫胺素。

急诊治疗/程序

- 呼吸性酸中毒：
  - 治疗潜在的风险。
  - 避免加重高碳酸血症，提供通气支持。
  - 识别和纠正加重因素(肺炎)，尤其是慢性高碳酸血症。
- 代谢性酸中毒：
  - 识别并发渗透压改变。
  - 治疗潜在的风险：
    - 糖尿病酮症酸中毒。
    - 乳酸酸中毒。
    - 酒精酮症酸中毒。
    - 摄入。
  - 纠正电解质异常。
- 静脉输液：
  - 如果患者血容量不足，可使用生理盐水补充水分。
  - 考虑血液透析。

药物治疗

- 葡萄糖：D_{50} W 1安瓿(50 ml或25 g)(儿童：D_{25} W 4 ml/kg)，静脉注射。
- 纳洛酮(Narcan)：2 mg(儿童：0.1 mg/kg)，静脉注射或肌内注射初始剂量。
- 硫胺素(维生素 B_1)：100 mg(儿童：50 mg)，静脉注射或肌内注射。

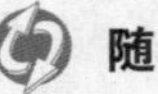

随访

进一步处理

入院指征

考虑入住ICU。

- pH<7.1。
- 精神状态改变。
- 呼吸性酸中毒。
- 血流动力学不稳定。
- 心律失常。
- 电解质异常。

出院指征

阴离子间隙代谢性酸中毒好转或痊愈。

要点和误区

- 不能鉴别混合酸碱紊乱中的酸中毒。
- 未能意识到代谢性酸中毒的呼吸补偿不足和需要通气支持。
- 混合酸碱紊乱的存在的线索是正常pH与异常的二氧化碳分压或 HCO_3^- 浓度和二氧化碳分压时相反的方向移动，或者pH的变化方向与已知的原发性疾病相反。

锁骨骨折

Sean Patrick Nordt 陈奇通 译

基础知识

描述

- 在所有年龄组中锁骨骨折占所有骨折的5%。
- 80%的锁骨骨折发生在锁骨中1/3。
- 15%的发生在外侧1/3。
- 5%的发生在内侧1/3。

分类

- Ⅰ类：中1/3骨折。
- Ⅱ类：外1/3骨折：
  - Ⅰ型：喙锁韧带完整的(无骨折移位)。
  - Ⅱ型：喙锁韧带断裂(锥形韧带)。
  - Ⅲ型：包括肩锁关节关节面受累。
- Ⅲ类：内(近身体端)1/3骨折。

病因

机制

- 锁骨直接损伤。

- 落在侧肩。
- 落在伸出的手上。

儿科注意事项

- 所有的小儿骨折都很常见。
- 可能发生在新生儿出生时的创伤。

老年人注意事项

- 老年患者发生锁骨骨折可能很难进行日常生活活动，应评估患者的社会和生活状况，以确定一个安全的出院计划，家里可能需要额外的帮助。

孕妇注意事项

- 锁骨骨折是直接创伤的结果。
- 对妊娠的患者，应适当地处理其他损伤，但也应接受胎儿监护，以确保胎儿的健康。
- 即使是轻微受伤也会导致胎儿的损伤或危害胎儿。

诊断

症状和体征

病史

- 骨折部位的局部疼痛、压痛和肿胀。
- 捻发音往往出现在锁骨皮下位置。
- 控制手臂内收对抗胸壁对运动的抵抗。
- 肩关节向前方和下方移位。

体格检查

- 触诊锁骨压痛、捻发音和肿胀。
- 检查肱骨和肩关节其他骨折、脱位或半脱位。
- 确定骨折是开放性或闭合性的。
- 评估相关的损伤（通常是严重的和危及生命的），必须排除：
  - 骨骼损伤：
    - 第1肋骨骨折合并主动脉损伤。
    - 胸锁关节分离/骨折（脱位）。
    - 肩锁关节分离/骨折（脱位）。
    - 颈椎损伤。

诊断检查与说明

影像学检查

- 双侧锁骨X线平片都是必需的，并且包括：
  - 肱骨上1/3段。
  - 肩胛带（排除其他骨折）。
  - 上肺野（排除气胸）。
- 倾斜位和向顶部前凸位像：
  - 尤其是对中、远段不易显示的锁骨骨折，可能有助于发现骨折线。
  - 远端锁骨骨折的压力位像（负重）不再常规推荐。
- 血管照影：
  - 如果有任何证据或怀疑血管损伤都应该进行（最常见的锁骨下血管）。

鉴别诊断

- 远端骨折：考虑肩锁关节分离。
- 近端骨折：考虑胸锁关节分离。
- 肩部骨折（脱臼）。

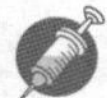

治疗

院前

- 骨折部位冰袋冷敷。
- 使用麻醉或非甾体类药物镇痛治疗。
- 绷带固定患侧。

初步稳定/治疗

- 依病情予以气道管理和复苏。

急诊治疗/程序

- 开放性骨折：不常发生，但通常需要开放清创和内固定（立即转诊骨科）。
- 闭合性骨折：如果严重移位，尝试闭合复位和固定取决于骨折的类型。
  - 中1/3骨折：
    - 如果没有移位，绷带或肩部固定器即可提供足够的支持。
    - 由于即使夹板固定技术解剖对准也不能维持，那么闭合性复位是否还有必要存在争议。
    - 为完成闭合性复位，需要在骨折血肿部位注射1%利多卡因。肩膀向上、向外、向后拉升，使骨折获得复位。
    - 给予镇静剂以缓解疼痛和焦虑。
    - 应用"8"字石膏绷带或肩部固定器固定。
    - 第一个24 h内应使用冰袋。
    - 止痛药（麻醉药或非甾体类药物）镇痛。
  - 外1/3骨折Ⅰ型：
    - 第一个24 h使用冰块。
    - 使用石膏绷带或肩部固定器固定。
    - 骨科会诊。
    - 止痛药（麻醉药或非甾体类药物）镇痛。
    - 早期关节活动范围。
  - 外1/3骨折Ⅱ型：
    - 第一个24 h使用冰块。
    - 使用石膏绷带或肩部固定器固定。
    - 骨科会诊（可能需要手术修复）。
    - 止痛药（麻醉药或非甾体类药物）镇痛。
  - 外1/3骨折Ⅱ型：同Ⅱ型。
  - 内（近身体端）1/3骨折：
    - 第一个24 h使用冰块。
    - 使用石膏绷带或肩部固定器固定。
    - 止痛药（麻醉药或非甾体类药物）镇痛。
    - 骨科随访。
- 石膏夹板固定后再评估神经血管状况。

儿科注意事项

- 不能配合"8"字形石膏固定的患儿应该由骨科医师行肩部"人"字形绷带固定。
- 多数患儿能耐受肩部固定器。

药物治疗

- 对乙酰氨基酚：成人650 mg（儿童：10 mg/kg）口服，q6 h，需要时。成人不超过3 g/24 h，儿童不超过4剂/24 h。
- 布洛芬：600～800 mg进餐时口服，q6 h，需要时（儿童：10 mg/kg口服，q6 h，需要时）。
- 成人：二氢可待因酮/对乙酰氨基酚5 mg/325 mg，1片口服，q6 h，需要时，对乙酰氨基酚24 h不超过3 g。避免同时使用含有对乙酰氨基酚的药物。使用非阿片类药物作为一线药物。
- 避免同时使用包含对乙酰氨基酚的药物二氢可待因酮、羟考酮，并且包含可待因的药物应避免用于儿童患者。

随访

进一步处理

入院指征

- 开放性骨折。
- 有潜在危及生命的联合损伤。

出院指征

- 仅有闭合性锁骨骨折而无其他损伤。
- 家里有适当的支持服务（尤其是老年患者）。
- 骨科随访。
- 充分止痛。

转诊问题

- 开放性骨折、复合性创伤、有神经血管损伤征象需立即转入骨科。

随访建议

骨科医师随访。

- 有任何神经功能、感觉、运动强度改变，均要立即就诊。

要点和误区

- 始终警惕相关的损害，包括危及生命的颈椎损伤、大动脉损伤、心肺损伤。
- 经常评估任何骨折相关的神经系统缺陷。

胎盘早剥 Placental Abruption

Heather L. Groth 瞿金龙 译

基础知识

描述

• 胎盘的蜕膜面出血致胎盘在胎儿分娩前部分或全部分离。
• 发生率/患病率：
- ～1%的孕妇。
- 妊娠期第二阶段约 30%会出现出血。
- 15%的胎儿死亡率。
- 10%～30%的新生儿死亡。
- 6%的孕妇死亡率。
• 同义词：胎盘分离，意外出血(英国)。

病因

• 主要原因不清楚。
• 血管损伤导致血进入蜕膜层，或胎盘和子宫的机械分离致出血和血凝块形成。
• 严重的患者会导致：
- 发展为弥散性血管内凝血(DIC)。
- 产妇和胎儿的取舍。
• 研究显示多数的胎盘早剥是慢性过程：
- 胎盘出现炎性反应。
- 胎盘缺血的表现。
• 急性胎盘剥离的原因：
- 创伤。
- 迅速的子宫减压。
- 胎盘植入异常或子宫肌瘤。
• 多种危险因素：
- 先前发生过早剥(10%～20%的再发风险)。
- 妊娠高血压(＞140/90 mmHg)和子痫前期。
- 高龄孕妇。
- 多胎妊娠。
- 子宫肌瘤或其他子宫胎盘的异常。
- 吸烟。
- 吸食可卡因。
- 创伤。
- 胎膜早破，尤其是伴绒毛膜羊膜炎或羊水过少。
- 子宫快速减压：
◦ 羊水过多伴膜破裂。
◦ 第一胎双胞胎快速分娩。
- 第二胎妊娠产妇血清 α 甲胎蛋白升高。
- 血栓性静脉炎。
- 母亲的种族：
◦ 常见于非洲美洲和白种人。
◦ 发病率在非洲和美洲妇女中上升很快。

诊断

症状和体征

病史

• 妊娠 20 周以上。
• 阴道出血(＞80%，常有疼痛)。
• 腹部或背部疼痛(＞50%)。
• 子宫痉挛、触痛、宫缩频繁或手足抽搐。
• 恶心、呕吐。
• 突发原因不明的未足月产。
• 近期创伤病史。
• 近期服药史，尤其是服用可卡因或其他拟交感类药物。
• 以前有早剥病史或其他风险因素。
• 估计孕龄。
• 产前检查史。

体格检查

• 低血压休克体征。
• 子宫触痛常见。
• 阴道流血(20%～25%可没有)。
• 出血点、出血和其他 DIC 症状。
• 胎心率下降。
• 胎儿心动过缓或胎心不清。

> **注意**
> • 必须行无菌阴道检查避免组织损伤，特别是怀疑前置胎盘时：
> - 评估羊水的性质(硝嗪试纸变蓝色、玻片边缘羊齿状结晶)。
> - 评估阴道和子宫颈撕裂情况。

基本检查

• 建立快速静脉通道。
• 血型、Rh 和交叉配血。
• 快速血红蛋白测定。
• 多普勒超声测定胎心率。
• 胎儿监测早期胎儿窘迫情况。
• 宫缩监测。

诊断检查与说明

诊断主要根据临床、实验室检查。

实验室

• 血型和 Rh。
• 全血细胞计数。
• 凝血时间。
• 纤维蛋白原水平和纤维蛋白裂解产物水平。
• 纤维蛋白原＜200 mg/dl 和血小板＜100 000/μl 高度提示胎盘早剥。
• 如果孕妇是 Rh 阴性，需行胎儿血红蛋白酸洗脱试验检测。

影像学检查

• 超声检查：仅能发现 50%的病例(假阴性常见)。
• MRI：敏感，但不实用。
• 如果下腹部/骨盆 CT：评估孕妇伤情，早剥的征象也能发现。

鉴别诊断

• 前置胎盘。
• 分娩时出血。
• 阴道或子宫颈撕裂。
• 子宫破裂。
• 早产。
• 卵巢囊肿蒂扭转。
• 肾盂肾炎。
• 胆石症。
• 阑尾炎。
• 其他腹部钝性伤和骨盆损伤。

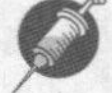

治疗

院前

• 胎盘早剥患者常处于休克状态，需要积极复苏治疗。
• 使患者保持左侧卧位。

初步稳定/治疗

• 保持气道通畅，呼吸循环稳定，吸氧。
• 心电监测。
• 建立快速静脉通道。
• 静脉补充晶体液复苏。

急诊治疗/程序

• 母亲心率和宫缩监测。
• 持续性胎儿监测。
• 输注浓缩红细胞，新鲜冰冻血浆，冷沉淀和血小板。
• 妇产科医师紧急会诊。
• 近距离监测尿量的 Foley 导尿管。

- 抑制宫缩药的应用有争议。
- 如果怀疑因创伤引起早剥,孕妇生命体征的稳定是最重要的:
  - 所有的相关的影像学检查都需完成。

药物治疗

一线用药

- Rh 阴性免疫球蛋白治疗 Rh 阴性孕妇:
  - 300 μg 肌内注射适用于妊娠期大于 12 周孕妇。
  - 大剂量使用需根据胎儿血红蛋白酸洗脱试验检测结果。
- 上面所提到的血液制品。

二线用药

按照产科医师的推荐:

- 如果要使用宫缩抑制剂可使用硫酸镁。
- 妊娠期 24～34 周可使用糖皮质激素促胎儿肺成熟。

随访

进一步处理

入院指征

- 胎盘早剥患者必须入院对孕妇和胎儿进行监测。
- 如果有 DIC 表现,羊水栓塞或严重出血需收入 ICU 治疗。
- 多发伤患者伴有胎盘早剥的需收入院,并处理好和创伤病情处理的协调。
- 如果患者情况稳定而当地没有合适的设备,那么转运到上一级创伤或产科治疗中心是很有必要的。

出院指征

- 创伤患者无胎盘早剥明显的证据,或其他伤情在对孕妇及胎儿 4～6 h 监测正常的可予以出院。
- 出院后注意事项包括骨盆的休息、禁止性生活、不要搬重物、不要过长时间的站立等。
- 出院的决定经妇产科医师会诊后做出,并且保持密切随访。

转诊问题

所有确证或怀疑胎盘早剥的患者都需要紧急产科医师会诊。

要点和误区

- 首先是临床诊断:没有一种可靠的检查能完全确诊或排除胎盘早剥。
- 典型的低血压表现往往比较迟。
- 应早期估计消耗性凝血功能障碍的出现,以在凝血功能障碍出现早期予以血制品治疗。
- 胎盘早剥常伴有子痫前期,这会使低血容量休克的患者血压表现为正常。
  - 对于严重胎盘早剥又无明显诱因的孕妇应高度怀疑有无子痫前期的可能。

糖尿病(青少年) Diabetes Mellitus, Juvenile

Madeline M. Joseph 谭美春 译

基础知识

描述

- 有效循环胰岛素减少。
- 反调节激素增加,包括胰高血糖素、儿茶酚胺、皮质醇、生长激素。
- 高血糖由于:
  - 外周葡萄糖利用降低。
  - 肝脏糖异生增加。
- 因高血糖存在高渗和渗透性利尿。
- 通过增加脂肪分解和酮体(β-羟丁酸、乙酰乙酸乙酯)生成,引发酮症酸中毒,导致酮血症和代谢性酸中毒,这一过程可被组织灌注不良导致的乳酸性酸中毒加强。
- 缺钾:
  - 由于氢离子交换细胞内转移到细胞外。
  - 渗透性利尿丢失。

病因

机制:

- 免疫介导胰岛 B 细胞破坏。
- 过去 20 年,世界总体发病率已经增加了 2%～5%。
- 突发事件导致糖尿病酮症酸中毒(DKA):
  - 感染,通常是轻度急性疾病,如病毒感染、A 组链球菌咽炎或尿路感染。
  - 应激。
  - 内分泌:妊娠、青春期、甲状腺功能亢进。
  - 精神障碍,包括饮食障碍。
  - 用药依从性差,不适当的中断胰岛素泵治疗或错误治疗。
- 与糖尿病酮症酸中毒相关的脑水肿的危险因素:
  - DKA 治疗过程中测量血清钠降低(与容量或静脉输液钠含量或血糖变化率无关)。
  - 应用碳酸氢钠纠正酸中毒。
  - 低碳酸血症。
  - 血清尿素氮增高。
  - 与高血糖程度无相关性。
  - 与脑水肿增加风险相关的人口统计学因素包括年纪轻、症状持续时间较长和新发糖尿病。这些因素也与严重 DKA 的风险增加有关。

诊断

症状和体征

- 多饮。
- 多尿(尽管脱水仍有较大尿量)。
- 夜尿。
- 多食。
- 疲乏,体重减轻。
- DKA:
  - 初步显示在 20%～40%的患者中出现。
  - 通常伴有呼吸急促(Kussmaul 呼吸)、心动过速、体位性血压改变。
  - 恶心。
  - 呕吐。
  - 腹痛,经常在酮症、酸中毒减轻时好转。
  - 喘息。
  - 酮症,继发出现水果味口气。
- 应用胰岛素泵治疗时,如果输液设备或胰岛素输注出现障碍,DKA 可在 7～8 h 急性发病。这是由于缺乏长效胰岛素提供安全保障(>10 岁女性更常见)。
- 更严重的疾病结果。

- 脱水、嗜睡、精神状态改变，并且晚期出现昏迷和休克。
• 与糖尿病酮症酸中毒相关的脑水肿：
- 发病率范围从 0.87%～1.1%。
- 脑水肿占所有 DKA 死亡率的 57%～87%。
- 它通常发生在开始治疗后 4～12 h，但可在治疗开始之前出现(亚临床)。
- 头痛。
- 神经系统状态改变，如嗜睡、烦躁不安，或特定的神经功能缺损，如瞳孔反应或脑神经麻痹。
- 脉搏不适当减慢。
- 血压升高。
- 氧饱和度降低
• 高血糖非酮症高渗性昏迷：
- 葡萄糖水平>600 mg/dl。
- 静脉 pH>15，动脉 pH>7.3。
- 轻微酮尿，未达到轻度酮血症。
- 有效的血清渗透压为 320 mOsm/kg。
- 精神状态改变(畏缩、好斗)或发作。
- 罕见于儿童，成人更常见。

T

基本检查

针对 DKA：
• 国际儿童和青少年糖尿病学会(ISPAD)定义 DKA 为血碳酸氢盐水平<15 mmol/L 或静脉血 pH<7.3 和高血糖(>200 mg/dl)伴有酮症或尿酮。
• 修订的 ISPAD 指南包括了对羟基丁酸盐(BOHB)的定量测量。浓度反映酮体产生的速率，它伴随着等摩尔的氢离子产生。血清 BOHB 值≥3 mmol/L 有助于确诊 DKA。
• DKA 的分类：
- 轻度 DKA：静脉血 pH<7.2～7.3 或 HCO_3^-<10～15 mmol/L。
- 中度 DKA：静脉血 pH<7.1～7.2 或 HCO_3^-<5～10 mmol/L。
- 严重 DKA：静脉血 pH<7.1 或 HCO_3^-<5 mmol/L。
• 每小时的生命体征和神经检查。
• 反复血生化检查。
• 心电图监测(重症 DKA)评估 T 波查找高钾血症或低钾血症的证据。
• 精确的液体出入量。意识障碍患者考虑尿管置入术。

诊断检查与说明

实验室检查

针对 DKA：
• 血清血糖：高血糖。
• 尿液分析：
- 尿糖。
- 尿酮。
- 排除尿路感染。
• 血生化检查每 2～4 h 1 次直到酸中毒改善(在更严重的病例需要更频繁应用的临床指征)。
• 电解质(包括 Mg^{2+} 和 PO_4^{3-})和静脉血 pH。
• 阴离子间隙代谢性酸中毒：
- 血钾——高或正常(细胞外转移造成假象)。
- pH 每减少 0.1 血清钾上升 0.5 mEq/L。
- 血钠——低或正常(可能因高血糖造成)。
- 校正 Na^+ (mEq/L) = [血清钠测量值 (mEq/L) + 血糖(mg/dl) − 100] × 0.016。
- 碳酸氢盐——低。
- 计算：$Na^+ - (Cl^- + HCO_3^-)$。
• 血酮升高。β-羟丁酸(BHOB)试验是一个定量测试，可用于取代经典的硝普钠试验检测血清酮。
• 血清渗透压。
• 全血细胞计数：
- 由于应激或感染白细胞通常升高。
• 钙。
• 磷酸盐(低磷酸盐血症可导致细胞内 2,3-二磷酸甘油酸[DPG]减少，从而增加血红蛋白对氧的亲和力，减少组织中 O_2 的释放)。
• 有指征时培养：A 群链球菌咽拭子、尿液培养等。
• 有指征时做妊娠试验。
• 如果血钾明显异常时心电图检查。

影像学检查

• 如果有任何肺炎表现时做胸部 X 线检查。
• 如果担心脑水肿时行头颅 CT 检查。

鉴别诊断

• 感染(可能突发)：
- 尿路感染。
- 胃肠炎。
- 阑尾炎。
- 脓毒症。
• 摄入(水杨酸酯、乙醇、乙二醇)。
• 尿崩症。

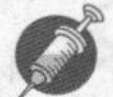

治疗

院前

对 DKA：
• 基础支持治疗。
• 气道保护。
• 开放静脉通道和开始输液治疗。

初步稳定/治疗

对 DKA：
• 吸氧。
• 心电监测。
• 静脉通道和容量复苏。

急诊治疗/程序

• 对 DKA：
- 补液：
- 假定液体损失占体重 10%(估计中度 DKA 为 5%～7%，重度 DKA 为 7%～10%)。
- 初始应用 0.9% 氯化钠或乳酸林格液 10～20 ml/kg 扩容，可重复应用直到血流动力学稳定。
  ◦ 大容量(20 ml/kg)液体复苏可以缩短代谢正常化时间，但不会改变住院治疗的总时间。
- 随后的补液速度应考虑提供维持用的液体需求，目标是在 48 h 内匀速地补充丢失的液体。
- 输液速度不应超过正常日常维持量的 1.5～2 倍。
- 不要在第 1 个 24 h 内补液>3 L/m^2。
• 确认酮症酸中毒并开始补液后开始静脉输注胰岛素。
- 连续输注的初始速率(普通胰岛素)为 0.1 U/(kg · h) 静脉注射[可从较小的 0.03～0.05 U/(kg · h)开始，但对低剂量无反应的患者应通过临床判断来指导所需剂量]。
- 调整速率使血糖下降 50～100 mg/(dl · h)。
- 当血糖<300 mg/dl 添加葡萄糖补液。
- 当无明显酸中毒并开始进食时胰岛素改为皮下注射。
• 一些医师更喜欢肌内注射，通常最初使用普通胰岛素剂量为 0.1～0.2 U/(kg · h)。
• 补充钾和磷酸盐损失：
- 查实尿量充足。
- 加入补液乙酸钾(或如果没有乙酸钾时氯化钾)和等量磷酸钾。
- 大剂量的 K^+ 可能是必需的，通过反复监测 K^+ 指导治疗。
• 监测血清钠：
- 当葡萄糖下降时，如果 Na^+ 不能上升，有脑水肿的风险。
• 碳酸氢盐治疗：
- 在大多数情况下不推荐，因为一般来说它不能改变结果，而且增加了脑水肿的风险。

- 严重酸中毒(pH<6.9)的患者应谨慎使用。它可以扩张外周血管,降低心肌收缩力,可能会进一步损害组织灌注和引起潜在的致命高钾血症。

• 血清 Mg^{2+}<1.0 mEq/L 或严重低钙血症时,用硫酸镁(25 mg/kg)维持静滴 4 h 以上补镁。

• 有症状的低钙(癫痫、抽搐、心律失常),用葡萄糖酸钙(100 mg/kg)静脉滴注 30 min 以上以补钙。注意有无外渗。

• 不论是给药速度还是静脉液体中钠的含量均会影响糖尿病酮症酸中毒患者的神经系统预后。

• 脑水肿:

- 由于高死亡率和发病率,分别为 21%~25%和 10%~26%,一旦怀疑有脑水肿时要立即治疗。

- 降低输液速度。

- 甘露醇(0.25~1 g/kg 超过 20 min):迄今没有大样本的研究表明明确的有益或有害的影响。在有脑水肿的迹象尚未出现呼吸衰竭患者考虑应用。如没有初始反应可在 2 h 内重复剂量应用。

- 3%高渗盐水以 2.5~5 ml/kg 的剂量,注射 10~15 min 以上使用。它可作为甘露醇的替代品,特别是当甘露醇没有初始反应时。

- 将床头抬高到 30°。

- 气管内插管和通气:避免积极的过度换气,通常与 DKA 相关脑水肿的不良预后相关(与头部外伤后果类似)。

药物治疗

• 滴注胰岛素:开始普通胰岛素静注 0.1 U/(kg·h)(一些医师更喜欢肌内注射方式和剂量)。

• 甘露醇:0.25~1 g/kg 静脉注射。

随访

进一步处理

入院指征

对 DKA:

• 入住 ICU:

- 精神状态改变。

- 休克或心律失常。

- 初始葡萄糖>700 mg/dl。

- 初始 pH<7。

- 脑水肿的危险因素(年龄≤5 岁,长期症状,尿素氮高)。

• 住院病房:

- 稳定的新发糖尿病患者需要强化教育。

- 酮症酸中毒患者不符合 ICU 住院指征。

- 依从性相关或其他社会问题。

出院指征

• 已知的糖尿病患者对治疗反应良好并且葡萄糖、pH 和酮症正常。

• 耐受口服药物。

• 可靠的父母。

• 可靠的 24 h 随访,包括适当的教育。

转诊问题

• 危重病。

• 精神状态持续异常。

• 控制不佳的糖尿病。

随访推荐

• 在 DKA 解决后初级保健医师的密切随访仍然重要,可以确保糖尿病患者的适当管理以进一步预防 DKA 复发。

• 许多患有糖尿病的儿童都在综合型糖尿病中心与初级保健医师合作下随访。

要点和误区

• DKA 死亡率主要与脑水肿发病率相关,因此早期和适当的治疗对管理 DKA 儿童非常重要。

• 儿童避免使用胰岛素药丸,因为它增加脑水肿的风险。最近,一些数据表明,起始胰岛素滴注 0.05 U/(kg·h)可以减少液体快速转移风险,因此减轻脑水肿风险。

• 血糖矫正后的钠不上升可能是脑水肿的早期警示症状。

• 尽管脑水肿患者通常在最初 4 h 内接受更多的补液,但这并不以可预见的方式影响血糖矫正后的钠和有效渗透压的时间变化曲线。

• 有必要对 pH、PCO_2 和碳酸氢盐进行初步测量,以确认 DKA 的诊断并判断其严重程度。

• β-羟丁酸(BOHB)的实时监测可能替代 DKA 管理中对这些参数的重复测量。

T

糖尿病酮症酸中毒 Diabetic Ketoacidosis

Stella C. Wong 谭美春 译

基础知识

描述

• 糖尿病酮症酸中毒(DKA):

- 高血糖。

- 酮症。

- 代谢性酸中毒。

• 轻度 DKA:

- 动脉 pH:7.25~7.3。

- 血清碳酸氢盐(mmol/L):15~18。

- 阴离子间隙:>10。

- 精神状态:躁动。

• 中度 DKA:

- 动脉 pH:7.0~7.24。

- 血清碳酸氢盐(mmol/L):10~15。

- 阴离子间隙:>12。

- 精神状态:躁动或嗜睡。

• 重度 DKA:

- 动脉 pH:7.0~7.24。

- 血清碳酸氢盐(mmol/L):10~15。

- 阴离子间隙:>12。

- 精神状态:昏睡/昏迷。

病因

• 胰岛素不足。

• 过多的反调节激素(胰高血糖素、儿茶酚胺、生长激素和皮质醇)。

• 干预不当。

• 感染(脓毒症、泌尿系感染、肺炎)。

• 新发糖尿病。

• 妊娠甲亢。

• 胰腺炎。

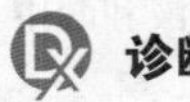

诊断

症状和体征

• 全身不适。

• 多饮。

• 多尿。

• 腹痛、恶心、呕吐。
• 精神状态改变。
• 胸痛。
• 感染时发热。

病史

• 未给药。
• 糖尿病药物的改变(例如,剂量的改变)。
• 饮食或饮食习惯的改变。
• 近期疾病状态。

体格检查

• 容量减少时的低血压。
• 心动过速。
• 口腔黏膜干燥。
• 精神状态异常。
• 呼吸急促。
• 腹痛。

基本检查

• 电解质、尿素氮/肌酐、葡萄糖。
• 红细胞计数。
• β-羟丁酸盐。
• 心电图。
• 静脉血气分析 VBG。
• 尿常规。
• 影像学检查(例如,怀疑肺炎时做胸部 X 线检查)。
• 血培养和怀疑感染时的尿培养。

诊断检查与说明

实验室检查

• 血清葡萄糖:
- DKA:通常<800 mg/dl,如果患者昏迷,可能更高。
- 如果患者处于高渗透压高血糖状态(HHS):>1 000 mg/dl 且尿酮阴性或弱阳性。

• 钠:
- 低钠血症:继发于高血糖导致的水从细胞内转移到细胞外。
- 校正的钠=测量的钠+[1.6(葡萄糖-100)/100]。

• 钾:
- 正常、低或高,但不管血钾水平如何,患者都可能全身衰竭。
- 通常表现为降低,但可以通过补液和酸中毒的纠正迅速纠正。
- 随着患者病情的改善,需要预测即将发生的低钾血症。

• 阴离子间隙:
- $Na^+ - (Cl^- + HCO_3^-)$。
- DKA 时阴离子间隙>12。

• 血清酮:
- β-羟丁酸盐是首选(与丙酮相比更敏感和更具成本效益)。
- 在血糖正常或轻度升高的 DKA 患者中仍可升高(有助于诊断 DKA)。

• 尿酮:
- 敏感(98%敏感性),但不具特异性(35%特异性)。
- 其他原因,如脱水,也会升高尿酮。

• 碳酸氢盐:
- 通常<18 mmol/L。

影像学检查

• 根据临床表现(例如,如果怀疑肺炎,则行胸部 X 线检查)。
• 以下情况做心电图检查:
- 心肌梗死。
- 心律失常。
- 异常间期。
- 异常 T 波形态。
- U 波。

鉴别诊断

不限于以下情况:
• HHS。
• 酒精性酮症酸中毒。
• 脓毒症。
• 水杨酸盐中毒。
• 外科腹部(如阑尾炎)。

治疗

院前

• 监测血糖。
• 静脉大量补液。

初步稳定/治疗

• 气道、呼吸、循环。
• 心电监测。
• 心电图。
• 监测血糖。
• 静脉大量补液。

急诊治疗/程序

• 静脉补液(注意不要使冠心病或肾衰竭患者超负荷):
- 生理盐水:第 1 h 首剂(1~2 L)。
- 2 L 之后:
◦ 如果校正钠低,轻度脱水,使用生理盐水 250~500 ml/h。
◦ 如果校正钠高或正常,轻度脱水,使用 1/2 生理盐水 250~500 ml/h。
- 如果血糖<200 mg/dl。
◦ 5%糖盐水。

• 胰岛素(注意纠正低血钾)。
- 轻度 DKA。
◦ 皮下胰岛素 0.3 U/kg 初始剂量,然后 0.1 U/kg, q1 h。
◦ 遵循自己医院的方案。
- 中度至重度 DKA:
◦ 静注常规胰岛素 0.1 U/kg/h,或
◦ 您机构的方案。
- 血糖<200 mg/dl:
◦ 将静脉常规胰岛素降低至 0.02 U/(kg·h) 至 0.05 U/(kg·h)。

• 钾(公认的正常肾功能):
- 如果钾<5.3 mEq/L,在每升液体中加入 20~30 mEq 的钾,以保持钾在正常范围内。
- 如果钾<3.3 mEq/L,暂停胰岛素,直到钾达到≥3.3 mEq/L,以避免加重低血钾和危及生命的心律失常。
◦ 通过在 1/2 生理盐水中混合 40~60 mEq 的钾,以 20~30 mEq/h 的速度给钾,或遵循您的机构的方案。

• 碳酸氢钠:
- 没有改善临床结果的证据。
- 然而,一些作者建议,如果 pH<6.9,则建议使用碳酸氢钠。

• 镁:
- 用静脉注射硫酸镁纠正低镁血症(<1.2 mg/dl)(通常剂量为 2 g)。

• 磷:
- 在最初的急诊复苏期间不常规补充。
- 如果<1 mg/dl 有症状性肌肉无力,可以补充。
- 作为磷酸钾使用。

儿科注意事项

• 液体:
- 平均液体缺乏 100 ml/kg。
- 最初 10~20 ml/kg 推注生理盐水以恢复血管内容量。
- 严重脱水的儿童可以重复一次。
- 在治疗的前 4 h 内不应超过 40~50 ml/kg 的液体。
- 在 24~36 h 以 1.5~2 倍的维持时间补充剩余的液体。
- 过度积极的液体复苏被认为是导致脑水肿的原因:
◦ 发生在 1%~2%患有 DKA 的儿童中。
◦ 导致 31%的与 DKA 相关的死亡。
◦ 确切的原因不详

T

◦ 可能与昏迷，精神状态异常、心动过缓、HTN、严重头痛、尿量减少或校正的 Na^+ 或渗透压迅速下降至低于正常水平有关。

◦ 甘露醇：应立即给予 0.25～1 g/kg 静脉注射超过 30 min，并可每小时重复使用。

◦ 液体速度应放慢并采取其他相应措施。

▪ 药物治疗

胰岛素输注：生理盐水 100 ml 中加入普通胰岛素 100 U，以 0.1 U/(kg · h)给药。

随访

▪ 进一步处理

入院指征

• 重度 DKA：ICU。

• 生命体征稳定的中度 DKA：常规病房。

• 轻度 DKA：观察室。

出院指征

• DKA 纠正。

• 生命体征稳定。

• 能够接受口服。

▪ 随访建议

与首诊医生和/或内分泌专家密切随访。

要点和误区

• 过度积极的液体复苏可导致儿童和成人的脑水肿。

• 密切监测血钾水平并相应纠正低钾血症。

泰瑟枪损伤

Christian M. Sloane 范浩浩 李文放 译

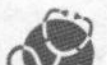

基础知识

▪ 描述

• 泰瑟枪属于传导能源武器(CEW)，是非致死性武器中的一部分。

• 美国最常见的是泰瑟国际公司的产品，这些包括 M - 26、X - 26 和 X2，其他类型的也存在。

• 这些装置使用高电压低电流来降低受试者控制周围神经系统的能力，它们引起疼痛以诱导受试者配合。

• 手持设备(如电击枪)需要使用 2 个暴露的探头接触皮肤(或靠近皮肤)引起局部反应(通常是疼痛)。

• 其他设备，如带刺探头连接到细线可以射到 35 ft(1 ft=30.48 cm)的距离以传输电流。

• CEW 倒钩针的长度不同，但通常≤0.5 in (1 in=2.54 cm)。

• CEW 的效果因类型而异，与正在使用的设备、位置和受试者身体上的探头之间的距离有关。如果探头散布在身体上<5 cm，效果较差。

• 皮肤效应。

- 可能在探头接触点留下痕迹，称为“签名标记”。

- 倒钩小刺伤。

• 骨骼效应。

- 跌倒可能导致骨折。

- 椎骨压缩骨折已被作为泰瑟枪电击的结果报告。

- 倒钩可能穿透骨。

• 对肌肉的影响。

- 可能有细菌感染。

- 重复延长使用可能出现横纹肌溶解症，更可能是由于使用泰瑟枪的潜在原因造成横纹肌溶解(如兴奋性妄综合征)。

• 心血管效应。

- 理论上可能会导致心室颤动，如果一次放电在心动周期的易损期。这个风险不是容易量化，但估计非常低。

- 已报道 1 例泰瑟枪使用后心房纤颤。

- 对健康没有显著影响。不会导致心电图或肌钙蛋白 I 改变。

- 不清楚设备将如何影响心脏起搏器/自动心脏除颤器(AICD)。能量低，理论上不应造成损害。如果 CEW 的电活动被误解为心律失常，可能会引起 AICD 放电。

• 神经系统影响。

- 有颅骨穿透和癫痫发作的病例报道。

- 呼吸效应：并无证据支持最初的观点，CEW 会抑制呼吸。研究表明，受试者在应用过程中实际上增加了通气量。

▪ 病因

这些武器通常用于执法，但也可用于军事、自卫、犯罪分子或持有者意外伤害。

诊断

▪ 症状和体征

> **注意**
>
> 设备暴露的患者可能是处于激动谵妄综合征状态。

病史

通常可以获得使用设备的病史。重要的因素是：

• 设备的类型。

• 使用的模式(探测器或驱动器眩晕)。

• 循环放电的次数。

• 循环使用的持续时间。

• 身体接触的位置。

体格检查

• 特别注意倒刺的位置。皮肤上的倒刺，虽然不太可能，但会对下面的结构造成伤害。

- 眼睛。

- 面部。

- 颈部。

- 腹股沟。

- 生殖器。

- 继发性伤害确实发生。

◦ 跌倒损伤。

◦ 如果设备在水中使用，则可能导致误吸。

◦ 强直性肌肉收缩导致的损伤。

◦ 倒钩刺入导致的损伤。

▪ 基本检查

• 所有暴露于 CEW 激活的人都应该接受医疗评估。评估的范围应该取决于使用者使用的类型和状态。

• 对于一个随后变得顺从、警觉、行为得当和/或 CEW 击中医学上不敏感区域的患者，可在进驻拘留所时移除飞镖进行评估。

• 考虑处于激动谵妄综合征状态患者的风险，无论是否有 CEW 暴露史，这种人均需要急诊评估。

老年人注意事项

上述组需要医疗评估，因为很少有数据来

指导使用的任何权威性声明。

诊断检查与说明

实验室检查应针对这个人被使用泰瑟枪的根本的原因。只是因为这个人使用泰瑟枪可不需要实验室检查。

实验室检查

如果 EXDS 存在：

- 全血细胞检查。
- 生化检查。
- 肌酸激酶。
- UTOX。
- VBG 检查是否有酸中毒。
- 乳酸。

影像学检查

- 不是常规检查。
- 如果意识水平的改变没有明确的原因，行头部 CT。
- 泰瑟枪穿透骨骼时行 X 线。如果它碰到了手指或足趾，或骨靠近皮肤，发生的可能性大(如胫骨、鼻)。
- 如果妊娠行超声检查。
- 以外伤、继发性损伤为导向的其他影像学。

诊断步骤/外科

- 如果患者有起搏器或 AICD，则检查起搏器，因为武器可能损坏起搏器或 AICD 设备或已经引起患者休克。
- 如果有潜在的重大心脏疾病，行心电图。
- 妊娠＞20 周的妇女应该接受胎儿监护治疗。

鉴别诊断

通常不清楚是否使用了装置。

治疗

院前

- 如果患者行为正常，生命体征正常，4 次骨折排查阴性，适当的话，不需要特殊干预。根据倒钩的位置，如果不在敏感区域(面部、眼睛、腹股沟、颈部、生殖器)，倒钩可以被移除。否则，稳定倒钩并将患者运送到医院进行移除。
- 如果患者烦躁不安，按躁动、激动谵妄综合征进行治疗。
- 如果存在心脏不适，启动心电监测，建立静脉通路，给予氧气，在相关指南和监护下治疗。
- 治疗任何继发性创伤性损伤。

初步稳定/治疗

如果兴奋谵妄综合征，然后按相应治疗指南治疗，包括药物治疗。

急诊治疗/程序

- 初始治疗转向潜在的伤害。
- 如果患者行为正常，生命体征正常，4 次骨折排查阴性，无继发性损伤的主诉，无需特殊干预。根据需要处理破伤风。
- 泰瑟针的移除：使用 2 个非优势手的手指，通过按压皮肤来稳定倒刺周围的皮肤。用优势手抓住倒钩轴并拔出倒钩。像其他伤口一样治疗伤口。
- 采用创伤方案治疗继发性创伤性损伤。
- 按照指南治疗嗅觉障碍。
- 如果患者不稳定，考虑和治疗 EXDS。

药物治疗

- 接种破伤风或百白破疫苗：0.5 ml 肌内注射。
- 咪达唑仑：5 mg 肌内注射或静脉注射，用于躁动患者。
- 氟哌啶醇：5 mg 肌内注射或静脉注射，用于躁动患者。

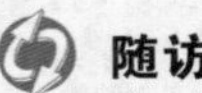

随访

进一步处理

入院标准

有以下征象收入院：

- 心脏不稳定。
  - 兴奋谵妄综合征。
  - 严重继发性损伤。

妊娠注意事项

任何妊娠的妇女都应接受妊娠的医学评估；如果可行，她应该在适当设施下行胎儿监护。

出院指征

患者行为正常，生命体征正常，4 次骨折排查阴性，无继发性损伤的主诉，或继发性损伤治疗和稳定的患者可出院。

转诊问题

伤口护理，受伤后要随访。

要点和误区

- 这些患者可能患有 EXDS，因此强制执法或使用泰瑟枪。
- 如果不积极地治疗这种危及生命的疾病，将会导致不良后果。经常筛查可能发生的继发性损伤。
- 稳定、警觉、适当的受试者只需要简单地去除倒钩(必要时)、破伤风疫苗要接种和伤口护理即可。

特发性颅内高压 Idiopathic Intracranial Hypertension

Martin D. Klinkhammer　江伟伟 译

基础知识

描述

- 脑脊液压力增高，无肿块病变或明确的病因。
- 相似的症状。
- 大脑假瘤。
- 良性颅内高压：
  - 确切机制未知，可能包括：
    - 可能与静脉窦狭窄有关。
    - 脑脊液流出阻力。
    - 肥胖相关的腹部和颅内静脉压升高。
    - 改变了钠和水的保留。
    - 维生素 A 代谢异常。
- 与育龄妇女肥胖有关。
- 青春期前儿童：男女发病率相等。
- 平均发病年龄：30 岁。
- 青春期后＞90％的病例发生在妇女身上。
- 不常见：约 1/100 000。

病因

相关：

- 肥胖。

- 维生素 A 过量。
- 类固醇/类固醇戒断。
- 生长激素补充。
- 四环素类抗生素。
- 口服避孕药。
- 最近体重增加。

诊断

症状和体征

病史

- 头痛：
 - 可以是持续的或间歇性的，双侧，或单侧的。
 - 压力性。
 - 通常位于球后，眼球运动时加重。
- 恶心、呕吐。
- 搏动性耳鸣-典型特征。
- 复视(第Ⅵ脑神经麻痹)。
- 头晕。
- 暗点。
- 持续数秒的短暂视觉模糊。
- 盲点。
- 视野受限。

体格检查

- 视野缺陷(高达 90%)：
 - 典型的是下鼻视野丧失。
- 乳头水肿：
 - 标志性标志，通常是双侧的，但也可以是单侧的。
- 腰椎穿刺可以改善症状
- 第Ⅵ脑神经麻痹：
 - 可以是单边的，也可以是双边的。
- 视力丧失
- 其他神经检查正常，个别脑神经除外。

儿科注意事项

- 在常规眼科检查中可能仅表现为视乳头水肿。
- 通常表现为：
 - 斜视。
 - 颈部僵硬。
 - 易怒。
 - 嗜睡。
 - 头晕。
 - 共济失调。
 - CN 麻痹。
- 一半病例有次要原因：
 - 病毒感染。
 - 头部外伤。
 - 中耳炎。
 - 药物。

基本检查

- 全面的病史和体格检查。
- 详细的神经系统评估和眼底镜检查。

诊断检查与说明

实验室检查

- 腰椎穿刺：脑脊液正常或低蛋白，细胞计数正常。
- 镇静儿童的开启压力＞25 cmH_2O 或＞28 cmH_2O：
 - 检查侧卧位的压力，双腿和颈部伸直。
- 如果使用镇静剂，必须尽量保持二氧化碳水平正常，因为二氧化碳滞留会增加脑脊液压力。
- 腰椎穿刺症状改善。

影像学检查

- 头部 CT/MRI 以排除肿块性病变(腰椎穿刺前)。
- 通常，头部 CT 应正常或显示侧脑室的狭缝状额角。
- MRI/MRV 建议对次要原因进行全面检查(所有非典型或有静脉血栓形成危险因素的患者；男性、苗条女性、儿童、产后)：
 - 可在门诊检查。
 - 脑静脉血栓形成在各个方面与特发性颅内高压(IIH)相似，包括正常头部 CT。

诊断过程

- 修订版 Dandy 诊断标准：
 - 颅内压升高症状。
 - 除第Ⅵ脑神经麻痹外，无局部症状。
 - 患者清醒且警觉。
 - CT/MRI 检查结果正常，无血栓形成迹象。
 - 腰椎穿刺打开压力＞25 cmH_2O(镇静儿童＞28 cmH_2O)。
 - 正常脑脊液成分。
- 腰椎穿刺：
 - 应在侧卧位进行打开压力，颈部和腿部伸直。
 - 观察呼吸变化，确保压力测量准确。
- 腰椎穿刺可改善症状。

鉴别诊断

- 偏头痛。
- 高血压性头痛。
- 缺氧性头痛。
- 紧张性头痛。
- 丛集性头痛。
- 蛛网膜下腔出血。
- 动脉瘤/动静脉畸形。
- 脑膜炎/脑炎。
- 硬膜下血肿。
- 硬膜外血肿。
- 肿瘤。
- 脓肿。
- 三叉神经痛。
- 巨细胞/颞动脉炎。
- 鼻窦炎。
- 青光眼。
- 视网膜中央静脉/动脉阻塞。
- 先天性视神经头抬高。
- 视神经核。
- 迷路炎。
- 视神经炎。
- 脑静脉血栓形成。
- 慢性二氧化碳滞留。

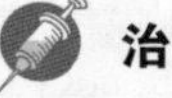

治疗

院前

疼痛控制(视情况而定)。

初步稳定/治疗

- 按指南气道和循环管理。
- 静滴液体水化。

急诊治疗/程序

- 大容量腰椎穿刺 20 ml 脑脊液：
 - 只有在确诊和头部 CT 显示基底池和第四脑室开放的情况下。
 - 未证实和短暂起效(脑脊液在 6 h 内再次累积)。
- 乙酰唑胺。
- 疼痛控制。
- 神经学会诊。
- 眼科会诊。
- 对利尿剂无反应的急性或迫在眉睫的视力丧失的请神经外科会诊(腰腹腔分流术)。
- 视神经开窗术是另一种手术选择。
- 如果存在狭窄，静脉窦支架置入术。
- 减肥。
- 停止使用任何可能引起感染的药物。
- 通常解决自发性。

药物治疗

- 对乙酰氨基酚：500～1 000 mg[儿童：(10～15) mg/kg；不超过 5 次/24 h]，口服，q6 h；不超过 4 g/24 h。

- 乙酰唑胺：每日 1 次服用 500 mg(如果症状持续，逐渐减少到每日 4 g，每日 1 次)用法：25 mg/(kg · d)，每日 3～4 次，口服或静脉注射。
- 布洛芬：400～600 mg(儿童：10 mg/kg)，口服，q8 h。
- 呋塞米：0.5～1 mg/kg，静脉注射或口服。
- 吗啡：0.1 mg/kg，静脉注射或肌内注射。
- 泼尼松：有严重视觉症状时有帮助，建议 5 日疗程(不建议长期治疗)。

一线用药

- 乙酰唑胺。
- 盐和液体限制。
- 肥胖减肥。
- 非甾体抗炎药。

二线用药

托吡酯曾被用作二线药物，但未获得美国 FDA 批准。

随访

进一步处理

入院指征

急性或即将失明。

出院指征

- 神经科和眼科会诊后。
- 随访。
- 耐受口服利尿剂。
- 疼痛得到控制。

转诊问题

及时转诊和转回注意事项：

- 视力下降。
- 局灶性神经功能缺损。
- 头痛加重。

随访建议

建议随访神经内科和眼科。

要点和误区

- 在患有慢性头痛的年轻患者中考虑此诊断。
- 对头痛患者进行眼底镜检查。
- 在进行腰椎穿刺治疗头痛时，考虑测量开启压力。
- 颈部和腿部伸直，侧卧位测量开启压力。
- 视力变化可能预示视力下降。
- 脑静脉血栓形成也有类似的表现。

特发性血小板减少性紫癜 Idiopathic Thrombocytopenic Purpura

Douglas W. Chesson · Matthew T. Keadey　倪沁赟 译

基础知识

描述

- 特发性血小板减少性紫癜(ITP)是原因不明的血小板减少或其他细胞系异常的一种疾病。
- 发病率在(2～5)/(10 万人 · 年)，因未被发现或亚临床的原因，该发病率可能被低估。
- 急性 ITP：
  - 1/2 的病例发生于儿童。
  - 经过或未经过治疗，80%的儿童患者会在 8 周内恢复。
  - 成年患者恢复时间相对延长，且需要特别的治疗获得临床缓解。
- 慢性 ITP：
  - 血小板<150×10^9/L(1×10^9/L=1 000/mm^3)，持续时间>6 个月，诊断 ITP。
  - 成年患者多发。
  - 成年女性最易受感染。
  - 特征性表现为对糖皮质激素反应各异及免疫抑制。
- 慢性难治性 ITP：
  - 血小板计数通常逐渐降低。
  - 对治疗反应差。
  - 没有明确的最佳治疗方法。
- 遗传性：
  - ITP 表现为家族遗传性，对糖皮质激素治疗的反应性各不相同。

病因

- B 细胞和浆细胞产生的自身抗体导致免疫介导的循环血小板破坏。
- 脾脏和肝脏的巨噬细胞通过 IgG 自身抗体导致血小板破坏。
- IgM 和 IgA 很少参与。
- 一些没有自身抗体的患者，提示 T 细胞介导的细胞毒性在该疾病中有一定的作用。
- 一些缺乏自身抗体的患者，提示补体 C3 和 C4 在该疾病中也有一定的作用。
- 血小板生成障碍也对该疾病有一定的影响，特别是针对慢性或难治性 ITP 患者。
- 根除幽门螺旋杆菌有时候与血小板的恢复有一定的关系(机制不明确)。

诊断

症状和体征

病史

- 出血是最常见的不适主诉：
  - 常见：
    - 黏膜：牙龈、鼻出血、结膜出血、月经过多。
  - 少见(凝血功能障碍者常见)：
    - 胃肠道出血、关节积血、血尿、血肿。
- 84%的儿科患者在发病前 2～3 周一般有病毒感染病史。
  - 小部分在接种疫苗后发病。
- 大部分成年患者起病隐匿：
  - 多达 28%的患者缺乏临床症状，诊断基于常规全血细胞计数。
  - <5%的患者可出现危及生命的出血。

体格检查

- 有临床表现的患者常表现为黏膜出血。
- 通常继发于口腔科手术或创伤。
- 瘀斑。
- 紫癜，ITP 与过敏性紫癜的鉴别。
- 与儿童过敏性紫癜(HSP)鉴别。
- 黑便、鲜红色血便或类便隐血阳性。
- ITP 患者脾脏大小正常：
  - 白血病或其他血小板聚集综合征的患者可能会出现脾大。
- 颅内出血(ICH)患者出现神经损伤：
  - 颅内出血是 ITP 患者死亡的最常见原因。
  - ITP 患者发生 ICH 的风险随着年龄的增加而增加：
    - 年龄<40 岁：2%。
    - 年龄>60 岁：48%。

基本检查

• 诊断之前因其他原因导致的血小板减少症应排除，如白血病、再生障碍性贫血和溶血性尿毒症综合征(HUS)。
• 全血细胞计数各不相同。
• 如果存在活动性出血行 PT 和 APTT 检查，同时需排除其他凝血功能障碍疾病。
• 检查尿素氮和肌酐水平来评估肾功能。
• 检查肝功能来排除肝脏疾病。
• 如果活动性出血，需检查血型。
• 生育年龄的患者行妊娠测试。
• HIV 检测。

诊断检查与说明

实验室检查

全血细胞计数和外周血涂片：
• 血小板减少症。
• 评估血小板体积增加。
• 白细胞和红细胞形态及大小正常。
• 肝功能、凝血功能和肾功能应该都在正常范围内。

影像学检查

如果有颅内出血的临床征象(头痛、颅脑外伤等)，可能头颅 CT 检查进行评估。

诊断步骤/外科

骨髓活检：
• 所有>60 岁的成年患者行骨髓活检对恶性肿瘤进行评估。
• 非典型临床表现和难治愈的病例。
• 考虑脾切除的患者。
• 儿童持续血小板减少超过 6 个月。
• 对静脉注射人免疫球蛋白治疗无反应的儿童患者。
• 抗体检测无临床价值的患者。

鉴别诊断

• 骨髓生成功能障碍：
- 骨髓纤维化。
- 因恶性肿瘤导致骨髓浸润。
- 化疗过程中使用细胞毒性药物。
- 先天性或获得性骨髓异常。
• 脾隔离症：
- 门静脉高压症。
- 肿瘤浸润。
- 镰状细胞贫血病。
• 血小板破坏速度增加：
- 血管炎。
- 血栓性血小板减少性紫癜/溶血性尿毒性综合征。
- 弥散性血管内凝血综合征。
- HELLP 综合征。
- 心血管疾病。
• 药物因素：
- 血小板生成降低：
◦ 化疗。
◦ 噻嗪类利尿剂。
◦ 乙醇。
◦ 雌激素。
- 血小板破坏增加：
◦ 阿司匹林。
◦ 肝素。
◦ 氯磺丙脲。
◦ 氯喹。
◦ 氯金酸钠。
◦ 磺胺类药物。
◦ 杀虫剂。

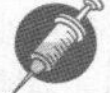

治疗

院前

ABC 管理：
• 严重的口腔或喉部出血可能影响气道。
• 中枢神经系统病变影响对气道的控制能力。
• 立即建立静脉通道。
• 通过直接压迫止血控制出血。

初步稳定/治疗

• ABC 管理。
• 控制危及生命的出血：
- 脑出血：
◦ 气道控制。
◦ 神经外科会诊：除非血小板计数>75×10^9/L，否则一般不考虑行开颅手术。
- 失血性休克：
◦ 建立 2 条大静脉通路。
◦ 直接压迫止血。
◦ 输血及等渗晶体液进行液体复苏。
◦ 急性危及生命的大出血给予药物和血小板治疗：
  ▪ 静脉给予大剂量地塞米松或甲泼尼龙。
  ▪ 静脉注射免疫球蛋白。
  ▪ 血小板输注：正常数量的 2～3 倍。
- 通常在给予激素和/或静脉注射免疫球蛋白后，输注血小板。
- 黏膜出血：
◦ 外用药物。
◦ 其他：
  ▪ 可以考虑静脉使用氨基己酸。
  ▪ 在少数病例中，血浆置换被证明是有效的治疗方式。

急诊治疗/程序

• 针对 ITP 首选的治疗方案基于：
- 血小板减少的程度。
- 病情的严重程度。
- 症状的持续时间。
- 年龄。
- 出血的危险因素(高血压、消化性溃疡、充满活力的生活方式)。
• 治疗的有效性是以血小板恢复时间来证明的，因为没有研究显示任何治疗可以降低发病率/死亡率或降低急性 ITP 进展为慢性 ITP 的可能性。
• 具体治疗方案：
- 观察治疗主要适用于没有出血并发症或严重血小板减少[(20～30)×10^9 L]及以下的儿童。
- 严重血小板减少(<20×10^9/L)：
◦ 大剂量糖皮质激素：75%有效。
◦ 静脉注射免疫球蛋白：80%有效，但是费用高，所以一般在紧急情况下使用。
◦ 抗 D 免疫球蛋白：70%有效(仅适用于 Rh+患者)。
- 脾切除：
◦ 二线治疗方案，适用于使用糖皮质激素治疗一段时间后无效的患者。
◦ 2/3 的成人患者有效，3/4 的儿童患者有效。
◦ 急诊脾切除无具体指征。

妊娠注意事项

• 妊娠期间血小板减少的鉴别诊断：
- 妊娠血小板减少症(75%)：
◦ 通常没有临床意义。
◦ 不引起新生儿血小板减少。
◦ 影响分娩后的 1～2 周。
◦ 血小板计数通常>50×10^9 L。
• HELLP 综合征(溶血、肝酶升高和血小板减少)。
• ITP(15%)：
- 血小板通常<50×10^9 L。
- 产妇血小板计数与新生儿血小板减少无关。
- 使用类固醇激素或静脉注射免疫球蛋白治疗不改变新生儿血小板减少的发病率。
- 血小板减少的程度一般不改变阴道分娩或剖宫产的决定。
- 测量新生儿全血小板计数或行颅脑超声检查明确有无颅内出血。
- 使用类固醇激素和静脉注射免疫球蛋白治疗新生儿血小板减少症。

T

■ 药物治疗

一线用药

• 糖皮质激素(大剂量使用 2～3 周):
- 地塞米松:40 mg,口服,每日 1 次。
- 泼尼松:1～2 mg/(kg · 24 h),口服,每日 1 次。
- 甲泼尼龙:1 g,静脉注射,q8 h[儿童:30 mg/(kg · 24 h)]。

• 静脉注射免疫球蛋白:1～2 g/kg,静脉注射×1 次(24 h 内可重复):
- 适用于严重出血或需要血小板快速升高如急诊手术时使用。

• 抗 D 免疫球蛋白:50 μg/(kg · 24 h),静脉注射:
- 仅适用于脾切除手术前和 Rh+患者。

二线用药

• 慢性长期抑制和类固醇激素治疗。
• 免疫抑制药物治疗:
- 硫唑嘌呤。
- 环孢素。
- 麦考酚酯。
- 化疗药物。
- 长春花碱。
- 环磷酰胺。
- 联合化疗。

• 其他:
- 力妥昔单抗:单克隆抗体直接对抗 B 细胞抗原。
- 达那唑:抗雄激素。

• 试验性药物:
- 其他对抗 B 细胞的单克隆抗体。
- 干细胞移植。
- 血小板生成素和血小板生成素样激动剂。

随访

■ 进一步处理

入院指征

• 危及生命的出血,无论血小板计数多少。
• 任何情况下的出血伴血小板计数＜20×10^9 L。
• 血小板计数＜20×10^9/L 的无症状患者,但存在不遵医嘱或随访差的情况。

出院指征

• 无症状的患者。
• 轻微出血且血小板计数＞30×10^9/L 的患者。

■ 随访建议

所有血液疾病的患者均需要转诊(无论是门诊患者或住院患者)。

要点和误区

• 在低血小板计数纠正之前,应排除假性血小板减少症。
• 血小板计数＜10×10^9/L 的情况下才可能发生自发性出血。

疼痛(原则、药物、舒适护理) Pain (Principles/Meds/Comfort Care)

Vincent Bounes　王虑 译

基础知识

■ 描述

不愉快的感觉和情感经历会对躯体感觉系统产生二次实际和感知性打击,或致心因性功能障碍。

• 个体、主观、多因素经历,受到文化、医疗史、信仰、情绪和应对能力的影响。

■ 流行病学

发病率和患病率预测

• 最常见的理由是寻求健康护理。
• 78%的患者会去急诊。
• 疼痛患者中有 2/3 疼痛较为严重。
• 慢性疼痛的发病率为 35%。
• 在急诊神经痛的发病率是 21.4%。

■ 病因

• 不同的疼痛能出现在同一个患者身上。
• 疼痛感受器疼痛:
- 刺激外周神经纤维(非疼痛感受器)会触发对其他非神经组织实际或威胁性的伤害。
- 内脏痛:
  ◦ 刺激内脏感受器。
  ◦ 发散,难以定位,常感觉遥远,结构表浅。
  ◦ 令人厌恶,深部,压榨性,钝痛。
- 深部躯体痛:
  ◦ 刺激位于韧带、肌腱、骨骼、血管、筋膜和肌肉的疼痛感受器。
  ◦ 钝痛,定位模糊。
- 浅表痛:
  ◦ 刺激位于皮肤和其他浅表组织的疼痛感受器。
  ◦ 刺痛,定义明确,定位清晰。

• 神经性疼痛:
- 正常非疼痛刺激而引起疼痛加剧(触摸痛)。
- 像触电似突然发作。
- 持续性的烧灼或冰冷感、针扎样、麻木、痒等。

• 精神痛:
- 由精神、情绪或行为因素引起,增加或延长的疼痛。

诊断

■ 症状和体征

病史

• 患者的主诉是评估疼痛程度的最好方法。
• 疼痛细节的获取:
- 发作。
- 若因创伤引起,查明受伤的机制。
- 疼痛的定位。
- 疼痛的严重程度。
  ◦ 轻度疼痛＞0 至≤3/10。
  ◦ 中度疼痛＞3 至≤6/10。
  ◦ 严重疼痛≥6/10。
- 疼痛的类型。
- 疼痛持续的时间。
- 疼痛的变化:
  ◦ 每日、每周或每月变化。
  ◦ 因身体运动引起的变化。
- 在就医前服用止痛药的效果。
• 急性疼痛和慢性疼痛的比较。
- 急性疼痛。

◦ 短暂的,通常<30 日。
◦ 疼痛的停止需以有害刺激结束和潜在威胁被治愈为前提。
◦ 治愈迅速。
- 亚急性疼痛。
◦ 持续 1~6 个月。
- 慢性疼痛。
◦ 持续时间 3~6 个月。
◦ 治疗后的疼痛持续时间超预期。
• 数字评价量表(NRS):
- 患者根据疼痛程度从 0~10 打分。
• 视觉模拟评分量表(VAS):
- 患者通过一根 0~10 cm 的横线描述自己的疼痛,0 代表无痛,另一端为 10 代表剧痛。
• 临床上疼痛描述 VAS 通常在 13~19 mm 这段,而 NRS 评分在(1.3~1.9)/10。
• 面部表情量表:
- 为 4~10 岁儿童准备的自我评价疼痛程度量表。
• DN4 测试。
- 神经痛的筛选方法。
- 评分从 0~10。
- 评分 4 分以上可以认为是神经痛而不是伤害痛。
- 疼痛特点:
◦ 灼烧痛(是=1)。
◦ 冰冷刺痛(是=1)。
◦ 电击痛(是=1)。
- 与同一部位疼痛相关的症状:
◦ 刺痛(是=1)。
◦ 针扎(是=1)。
◦ 麻木(是=1)。
◦ 痒(是=1)。
◦ 触摸感觉下降(是=1)。
◦ 刺扎感觉下降(是=1)。
◦ 疼痛是否会因刷牙引起或加重(是=1)。
• 记得对于同一个患者用以前用过的评分量表做评测。

体格检查

• 观察者对不能说话患者疼痛的评估量表:
- 发生如呻吟、幽咽、叹息、哭、悲啼。
- 脸部表情,如看起来紧张、皱眉头、愁眉苦脸、看起来恐惧。
- 使用止痛药的目的是保护身体处于休息位。
- 小心移动,自发或被要求时。
• 需要轻柔地完成全方位的体格检查。
• 姿势、点压痛、挤压痛、被动和主动的移动范围和主动抵抗。
• 检查时在各个部位间移动要轻柔,同时告知患者有关每个阶段的信息。
• 一定要先检查未受伤的组织,避免突然移动。
• 疼痛缓解后复查。

■ 诊断检查与说明

根据患者的实际情况开展实验室检查或影像学检查。

■ 基本检查

• 获得患者完整的疼痛。
• 当患者不能说话或自己讲述病史,应通过其看护人、亲戚朋友邻居等获取。

■ 诊断检查与说明

实验室检查

根据实际的医疗条件而定。

影像学

根据实际的医疗条件而定。

诊断步骤/外科

根据实际的医疗条件而定。

■ 鉴别诊断

• 阿片类药物依赖患者。
- 频繁通过急诊向不同医师索要药物。
- 病史不清,只有不停的主观抱怨(难以客观证实)。
- 患者有强迫表现并缺乏耐心,重复要求使用止痛药。
- 某些方面的检查结果与病情不一致。
- 实验室和影像学检查可以正常。

治疗

■ 院前

• 在院前通过非药物治疗的方法使疼痛有效缓解。
• 一氧化二氮是高效的院前使用止痛剂。
• 吗啡、芬太尼和曲马多都可以在院前使用。

■ 初步稳定/治疗

• 生命体征支持。
• 将可能危及生命的创伤等情况处理妥当。
• 患有严重疼痛的患者需有专门部门优先予以分流以确保疼痛得到迅速控制。

■ 急诊治疗/程序

• 非药物治疗在缓解疼痛方面效果好,需要系统进行:
- 对伤肢予以充分制动。
- 抬高患肢。
- 冰敷。
• 严重疼痛使用阿片类药物。
- 最好使用静脉推注,若条件不允许也可以骨内注射。
- 不同个体对药物剂量反应上有很大差异性,肌内和皮下注射则有吸收的延迟。
- 口服阿片类药物和对乙酰氨基酚对少数严重疼痛有效:
◦ 羟考酮:5~10 mg。
◦ 二氢可待因酮:5~10 mg。
◦ 可待因:30~60 mg。
◦ 曲马多:50~100 mg。
• 非甾体抗炎药:
- 适合中等程度的疼痛。
- 肌肉痛。
- 肾脏和胆源性急腹症。
- 高发的副作用包括胃出血和肾病。
• 对乙酰氨基酚对于轻中度疼痛效果肯定且副作用较小。
• 协同对于焦虑情绪的治疗。
◦ 局麻主要用于急性的局部疼痛,如牙痛、骨折、手足伤。

■ 药物治疗

• 对乙酰氨基酚:500 mg(儿童:10~15 mg/kg,24 h 不超过 5 片),口服,q4~6 h,24 h 不超过 4 g。
• 可待因:30~60 mg,口服,q4~6 h,当需要时。
• 吗啡:
- 初始剂量 0.05~0.1 mg/kg,静脉注射。
- 15~30 mg,口服,q4~6 h。
• 二氢吗啡酮:
- 初始剂量 1 mg,静脉注射。
- 2~4 mg,口服,q4~6 h。
• 羟氢可待因酮:5~10 mg,口服。
• 羟考酮:5~10 mg,口服。
• 曲马多:50~100 mg,口服。
• 羟氢可待因酮/对乙酰氨基酚:5/500 mg,口服,q4~6 h。
• 布洛芬:600~800 mg,口服,q6~8 h(儿童:10 mg/kg,q6 h)。
• 萘普生:250~500 mg,口服,q12 h。

随访

■ 进一步处理

入院指征

经医疗救治疼痛持续不缓解的患者。

• 病情符合入院条件的。
• 疼痛无法控制。

出院指征

• 病情得到控制。
• 最终的疼痛评估≤3/10 和/或比原先疼痛程度减轻 50%，或疼痛缓解到患者能耐受的程度。
• 医师能在急诊通过静脉用药控制疼痛，但离开医院会有通过口服阿片类药物控制疼痛效果不佳的风险。

- 应考虑不同阿片类药物的转化率。
- 应考虑从静脉用药到口服用药的转化。
- 阿片类药物的服用应固定时间间隔，在病情需要时再额外加量。

随访建议

对于持续服用止痛药仍然再发的疼痛或未预期出现的新发疼痛，需要对患者的诊断做出重新的评估并考虑引起疼痛的其他可能原因。

要点和误区

• 对于严重疼痛的患者，疼痛最初缓解同时对病情也有最初的评估。
• 系统规律的疼痛评估有利于日后疼痛的管理。
• 非药物治疗在疼痛缓解方面效果肯定，当条件允许时需始终考虑并使用。
• 滴定大剂量的阿片类药物能达到快速给药并有效缓解疼痛。

体温过低 Hypothermia

Jordan Moskoff　倪沁赟 译

基础知识

描述

• 体温<35℃。
• 危险因素：
- 体温调节功能差。
◦ 年幼。
◦ 年老。
◦ 合并症。
◦ 中毒。
• 病理生理：
- 热量丢失：
◦ 辐射：速度最快，占热量丢失的 50%。
◦ 传导。
◦ 对流。
◦ 蒸发。
◦ 呼吸。
- 产热：
◦ 颤抖。
◦ 非颤抖性产热。
◦ 甲状腺素水平增加。
◦ 肾上腺素水平增加。

病因

• 皮肤疾病：
- 烧伤。
- 剥脱性皮炎。
- 严重银屑病。
• 环境：
- 浸润性。
- 非浸润性。
• 医源性：
- 大量液体置换。
- 热休克治疗。
• 代谢：
- 肾上腺功能减退症。
- 垂体功能减退症。
- 甲状腺功能减退症。
• 神经系统：
- 急性脊髓横断伤。
- 颅脑外伤。
- 休克。
- 肿瘤。
- 韦尼克病。
• 神经肌肉功能下降：
- 年老过小或过大。
- 颤抖不能。
- 环境适应能力低下。
• 脓毒症。

儿科注意事项

婴儿有更大的体表面积。

诊断

症状和体征

• 轻度：35～32.2℃(95～90℉)：
- 早期应激阶段应减轻寒冷：
◦ 高血压。
◦ 颤抖。
◦ 心动过速。
◦ 早期心动过速，而后心动过缓。
◦ 呼吸急促。
◦ 血管收缩。
- 随着时间的推移会出现疲劳：
◦ 冷漠。
◦ 共济失调。
◦ 冷利尿。
◦ 远端肾小管对水钠重吸收障碍。
◦ 判断力下降。
• 中度：32.2～28℃(90～82.4℉)：
- 房性心律失常。
- 心动过缓：
◦ 起搏细胞自发性去极化能力下降。
◦ 对阿托品无效。
- 意识水平下降。
- 呼吸频率下降：
◦ 进行性呼吸抑制致 CO_2 潴留。
- 瞳孔散大。
- 咽反射减弱。
- 颤抖消失。
- 反射减弱。
- 低血压。
- 心电图上 J 波出现。
• 重度：<28℃(<82.4℉)：
- 呼吸暂停。
- 昏迷。
- 异常脑电图表现(脑电活动下降或消失)。
- 瞳孔无反应性。
- 少尿：
◦ 肾血流下降 50%。
- 肺水肿。
- 室性心律失常或心脏停搏：
◦ 心动周期延长。

病史

在冷水中淹没的时间。

体格检查

• 也许无法触及动脉搏动。
• 也许无法测得血压。
• 当体温<26℃时瞳孔散大。

基本检查

- 准确的体核温度可明确诊断。
- 理想的食管探针或膀胱探针。

诊断检查与说明

实验室检查

- 指尖血糖。
- 动脉血气分析：
  - 不需要进行温度校正。
- 全血细胞计数：
  - 因血浆容量降低，导致血细胞比容升高。
  - 白细胞减少并不意味着不存在感染。
    - 高风险患者（如新生儿、免疫功能低下）应该接受经验性抗感染治疗。
- 电解质、尿素氮、肌酐：
  - 复温过程中会发生改变，肌酸磷酸激酶和血钾指标更加需要频繁复查。
- 血乳酸。
- PT、APTT、血小板：
  - 凝血时间延长，血小板减少常见。
- 毒理学筛查：
  - 酒精/药物摄入常见。

影像学检查

- 胸部X线检查：
  - 肺炎是常见的并发症。
- 心电图：
  - 心动过速到心动过缓。
  - 慢心房颤动。
  - 心室颤动。
  - 心脏停搏。
  - PT、QRS、QT间期延长。
  - J波出现。
  - ST段抬高，与急性冠状动脉综合征相似。

鉴别诊断

- 环境因素。
- 脓毒症。
- 原发性中枢神经系统疾病。
- 代谢因素。
- 药物相关。

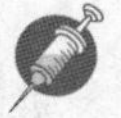

治疗

院前

- 应使用瑞士分期系统 HT1 - HT_4 来指导处理和运输。
  - HT Ⅰ：清醒，颤抖：32～35℃。
  - HT Ⅱ：意识受损，但不发抖：28～32℃。
  - HT Ⅲ：无意识：24～28℃。
  - HT Ⅳ：明显死亡：13.7～24℃。
  - HT Ⅴ：不可逆低温导致死亡：小于13.7℃。
- 消除寒冷压力（尽可能轻柔地）。
- 尽量保持水平。
- 干燥患者（当保护从寒冷的环境）和绝缘与地面。
- 放置在由绝缘层、蒸汽屏障和优选热源组成的低温包裹中。
- 在“复苏和死亡”之前，患者不会死亡：
  - 建议在转运过程中实施CPR。
- 心脏触诊/听诊时间延长：30～45 s。
  - 明显的心血管虚脱可使心排血量下降，往往足以满足代谢需求。
  - 在心搏骤停时应转移到ECMO功能中心。

初步稳定/治疗

- ABC管理：
  - 提供氧气。
  - 经口/鼻气管插管是安全的。
  - 留置鼻胃管。
  - 心电监测。
  - 加热过的葡萄糖或生理盐水优于林格液：
    - 颤抖会消耗糖原。
- 脱去湿衣服，同时开始进行体外复温。
- 给予患者输注纳洛酮、50%葡萄糖溶液和硫胺素，同时监测患者的精神状态。
- 对于肾上腺功能不全或治疗失败的患者，给予负荷剂量类固醇激素（氢化可的松琥珀酸钠注射剂100 mg静脉注射）。
- 监测直肠温度以获得精确的体核温度。

急诊治疗/程序

- 心搏骤停复苏：
  - 单纯通过复温可以纠正大部分的心律失常。
  - 因操作粗暴、胸外按压、低氧血症和酸碱的改变，会诱发心室颤动的发生。
  - 因胸壁弹性下降，会导致胸外按压效率下降。
  - 在体温小于28～30℃的情况下除颤成功率低：
    - 除颤1～3次，然后再立刻进行复温。
    - 当体温>30℃，如果心室颤动持续存在，可给予胺碘酮。
    - 直流电会导致心肌的损伤。
- 心律失常的管理/治疗。
  - 心房纤颤：
    - 一般体温<32℃。
    - 通常可自行转复。
  - 恶性室性心律失常：
    - 选择胺碘酮尚缺乏有效的证据。
- 复温技术：
  - 快速复温（1～2℃/h）相对于缓慢复温（<0.5℃/h）来说，对预后改善更有利。
  - 当核心体温<32℃时，需要主动复温。
    - 自身产热不足以增加体温。
    - 颤抖消失。
- 被动体外复温：
  - 对于大部分健康患者理想的复温技术是亚低温治疗。
  - 必须有完整的体温调节机制、正常的内分泌功能和足够的能量储备。
  - 使用干燥的绝缘材料覆盖患者。
  - 内源性产热必须达到一个可接受的复温速度：
    - 必须增加0.5～2℃/h。
  - 缺点：核心体温升高非常缓慢。
- 主动体外复温：
  - 使热源直接接触皮肤。
  - 既往身体健康、年轻的患者，低体温发病急，使用主动体外复温是安全的。
  - 需要良好及完整的循环功能，将外周循环复温的血液迁移至体内核心。
  - 会出现体温后降（afterdrop）效应。
  - 复温休克：四肢复温后静脉血管床舒张。
  - 优先覆盖躯干。
  - 拜尔充气加温装置可以提供温暖的空气：预防休克或体温后降效应。
- 主动核心复温技术：
  - 气道复温（在40～45℃充分加湿）：
    - 适用于所有患者。
  - 静脉输注加热的（40～42℃）5.9%盐水：
    - 适用于所有患者。
    - 必须保持高流速。
    - 使用血液温热装置或校准过的微波加热装置。
  - 通过鼻胃管或者口胃管，使用加热的液体灌胃：
    - 没有推荐意见。
    - 表面面积小。
    - 如果气道不安全，有误吸风险。
  - 胸腔灌洗（30～42℃生理盐水）：
    - 适用于严重低体温、没有心搏的患者。
    - 1～2根胸管；双侧腋中线和锁骨中线。
    - 心脏节律有问题的患者禁忌，因为胸管可能诱发心室颤动的发生。
  - 腹腔灌洗（40～45℃生理盐水）：
    - 适用于生命体征不稳定的低体温患者，或者复温速度<1℃/h但生命体征平稳的

严重低体温患者。
◦ 1～2 根导管。
◦ 对药物过量或者横纹肌溶解症的患者有利。
• 体外复温：
- 最有效的复温方法。
- 血液透析：
◦ 药物过量或者严重内环境紊乱的患者首选。
- 持续动-静脉复温：
◦ 血压必须>60 mmHg。
◦ 血液通过温热装置进行循环(置管从股动脉至对侧静脉)。
- 体外静-静脉复温：
◦ 血液从中心静脉引出，加热至 40 ℃，通过第二根中心静脉或大外周静脉会输至体内。
- 心肺旁路：
◦ 有心跳骤停的严重低体温患者，可选择该治疗方法。
• 其他治疗：
- 怀疑肾上腺皮质激素缺乏或类固醇依赖的低体温患者可给予甲泼尼龙或氢化可的松治疗。
- 经验性给予左旋甲状腺素，仅适用于黏液性水肿患者。

■ 药物治疗

• 胺碘酮：心室颤动患者予以 300 mg 静脉推注，然后 1 mg/min 静脉维持。
• 葡萄糖：50%葡萄糖注射液 50 ml 或 25 g(儿童：25%葡萄糖注射液 2～4 ml/kg)静脉滴注。
• 氢化可的松：250 mg，静脉推注。
• 左旋甲状腺素：50～500 μg，静脉滴注，至少维持数分钟。
• 甲泼尼龙：30 mg/kg，静脉推注。
• 纳洛酮：初始剂量 2 mg(儿童：0.1 mg/kg)，静脉滴注或肌内注射。
• 硫胺素(维生素 B_1)：100 mg(儿童：50 mg)，静脉滴注或肌内注射。

随访

■ 进一步处理

入院指征

• 中度到重度低体温患者(<32 ℃)。
• 轻度低体温(>32 ℃)、没有合并症、对复温治疗反应较好的年轻健康患者：
◦ 适合在观察室观察。
◦ 无临床症状 8～12 h 且持续没有不适可以出院。

出院指征

• 没有合并症的年轻健康患者。
• 极轻度低体温(>35 ℃)且对复温治疗反应较好的患者。
• 出院后的患者安全且温暖。

■ 随访建议

暴露在寒冷及低温环境下的无家可归的患者需要进行随访。

要点和误区

• 当体温<28～30 ℃的时候除颤成功率低：
- 除颤 1～3 次，然后继续复温治疗。
• 心房纤维性颤动通常是自发性的。
• 快速复温的预后较好。
• 体温后降(afterdrop)效应是复温后核心体温的再次下降：
- 因热传导出现外周复温先于体内核心。
• 复温休克：
- 复温休克继发于复苏过程中纠正容量失败。

体温过高

Michelle J. Sergel · Alexandra Mannix 巩博 译

基础知识

■ 描述

• 因为逐渐增长的大量热应激导致进行性加重的疾病。
• 开始出现脱水、电解质异常，进展至体温调节功能障碍和多系统脏器功能衰竭。
• 机体通过调节产热和散热平衡维持体温在一个小范围内。
• 超过 42 ℃(108 ℉)，体内无法进行氧化磷酸化，酶失去功能。

热射病

• 核心温度>40.5 ℃(105 ℉)。
• 体温调控功能障碍导致严重的中枢神经系统功能障碍和多系统脏器衰竭。
• 传统型热射病(非劳力性)：
- 出现在体温调控功能障碍或者不能从热环境中靠自己散热的人(如高龄、体弱)。
- 通常出现在炎热期，发病时间从数日到数周。
- 严重脱水，皮肤温暖干燥。
• 劳力性热射病：
- 更年轻、健壮的患者伴有环境和运动热性应激综合作用(如军队新兵)。
- 发病时间数小时。
- 尽管患者持续出汗，体内产热大大超过散热。

热衰竭

• 核心温度中度上升，通常<40 ℃(104 ℉)。
• 热应激后出现液体和/或盐丢失。
• 可维持温度调控机制功能，中枢神经系统功能基本正常。
• 多种非特异性症状包括乏力、头痛、疲劳和恶心。
• 如果不治疗，进展为热射病。

■ 病因

• 阻碍人体散热容易出现热相关疾病的因素：
- 高龄。
- 脱水(包括肠胃炎、补液不充分)。
- 心血管疾病(包括慢性心力衰竭、冠状动脉粥样硬化性心脏病)。
- 肥胖。
- 嗜铬细胞瘤、甲状腺功能亢进和糖尿病。
- 发热性疾病。
- 阻碍出汗的皮肤病(包括牛皮癣、湿疹、囊胞性纤维症和硬皮病)。
• 药物因素：
- 拟交感神经药。
- D-麦角酸二乙胺、普斯普剂和可卡因。
- 单胺氧化酶抑制剂、抗精神病药和抗焦虑药。

- 抗胆碱药。
- 抗组胺药。
- β受体阻滞剂。
- 利尿剂。
- 泻药。
- 药物或酒精戒断。
• 环境因素:
- 过热或潮湿。
- 长时间活动。
- 缺乏流动性。
- 没有空调。
- 不适应环境。
- 密闭、无孔的衣服。

儿科注意事项

儿童出现中暑的风险更高,因为儿童出汗更少,并且需要增加体表面积达到相同质量比。

诊断

症状和体征

热射病

• 典型三联征:体温过高、中枢神经系统(CNS)功能障碍、皮肤热(通常无汗)。
• 核心温度>40.5℃(105℉)。
• 中枢神经系统:
- 严重意识混乱或谵妄。
- 嗜睡或昏迷。
- 抽搐。
- 共济失调。
• 心血管:
- 心动过速。
- 脉压增大。
- 外周血管阻力低。
- 传导紊乱。
• 肺:
- 呼吸急促。
- 非心源性肺水肿,水泡音。
- 呼吸性碱中毒(可能引起手足抽搐)。
- 低氧血症(因为误吸、肺炎、肺水肿和高代谢需求)。
• 消化道:
- 恶心与呕吐。
- 腹泻。
• 皮肤:
- 皮肤血管扩张致皮肤发热。
- 通常干燥,如果没有脱水可能出现出汗。
• 因为脱水出现急性少尿型肾衰竭。
• 肝衰竭可能出现转氨酶上升至数万。
• 凝血功能疾病,包括 DIC(预后差的标志)→紫癜、黑便、便血、血尿、中枢神经系统出血。

热衰竭

• 核心温度中度上升,通常<40℃(104℉),从不>40.5℃。
• 中枢神经系统:
- 前额头痛。
- 疲劳与乏力。
- 判断力受损。
- 眩晕。
- 躁动。
- 无严重的中枢神经系统功能障碍。
• 心血管:
- 轻度心动过速。
- 脱水。
• 肺:呼吸急促。
• 消化道:恶心、呕吐。
• 皮肤:通常大量出汗。

热痉挛

• 活动后运动量大的肌肉出现痉挛。
• 常在大量出汗补充低渗液体(如水)后出现。
• 导致低钠血症和低氯血症,不伴有横纹肌溶解或肾功能损害。
• 如果症状较轻,口服盐水溶液治疗,如果症状重,静脉补充生理盐水。

高温性水肿

• 不适应环境的人因为环境湿热出现足部/足踝水肿。
• 因为血管扩张、直立时下肢回流不畅和醛固酮增加。
• 一般适应环境后症状消失。可以通过抬高下肢或弹力袜治疗。

热晕厥

• 在高热环境中长时间站立后出现不能解释的晕厥,尤其是老年人。
• 皮肤血管扩张以加强散热,回心血量下降,晕厥。
• 自限性疾病。当患者平躺后症状消失。

痱子

• 穿紧身衣服大量出汗后,在衣服覆盖的地方出现瘙痒的斑丘疹或水疱。
• 因为毛孔堵塞,可能出现继发性葡萄球菌感染。

基本检查

• 精确的核心温度。
• 高热环境暴露史。
• 热衰竭是一种排除性诊断。
• 核心温度>40.5℃(105℉)和中枢神经系统功能受损需要诊断为热射病。

诊断检查与说明

热射病和热衰竭

• 全血细胞计数:
- 白细胞升高,血液浓缩。
• 电解质、尿素氮、肌酐、血糖:
- 严重脱水时出现高钠血症。
- 如果饮用大量自由水可能出现低钠血症。
- 急性肾衰竭。
• 尿:
- 横纹肌溶解可出现肌红蛋白尿。
• 血和尿培养以排除感染性病因。
• 毒理学筛查。
• 血肌酸激酶以排除横纹肌溶解。
• 动脉血气:
- 酸中毒常见于劳力性热射病,乳酸常常升高。

热射病

• PT、APTT、DIC 检查,凝血功能障碍暗示着预后差。
• 肝功能检查。
• 肌钙蛋白 I,如果升高,预后差。
• 考虑腰椎穿刺以鉴别脑膜炎/脑炎。

影像学检查

• 老年人或者有心脏病风险的患者检查心电图。
• 精神状态改变查头颅 CT。
• ARDS、吸入性肺炎查胸部 X 线,排除感染性病因。

鉴别诊断

• 发热性疾病/脓毒症。
• 甲状腺危象。
• 嗜铬细胞瘤。
• 可卡因/五氯苯酚。
• 抗胆碱类药物。
• 单胺氧化酶抑制剂。
• 脑膜炎/脑炎。
• 脑恶性疟。
• 震颤性谵妄。
• 神经阻滞剂恶性综合征。
• 恶性高热。
• 5-羟色胺综合征。

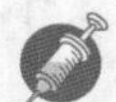

治疗

院前

• 严重中暑患者开始降温治疗。
- 脱离热环境。
- 脱去患者衣物。

- 用湿床单覆盖患者。

■ 初步稳定/治疗

• ABC。

• 使用直肠或者食管探头持续监测核心温度。

• 如果温度>40℃(104℉)快速降温。

• 如果出现低血压,使用生理盐水 500 ml 快速滴注。

• 如果出现精神状态改变,予以葡萄糖(或查血糖)、硫胺素及纳洛酮。

■ 急诊治疗/程序

降温措施

• 体温>40℃(104℉)启动。

• 蒸发散热:

- 非常有效(0.05~0.3℃/min)。

- 向脱去衣物的患者喷洒温水制成的水雾(防止寒战)。

- 风扇降温。

• 传导散热:

- 腹股沟、腋下放置冰袋,联合上述蒸发散热措施使用。

- 冰水或冷水浸浴,有效但是不切实际。

• 难治性病例可以使用冰水腹腔灌洗、体外循环或者使用低温透析液的血液透析,目前缺乏研究。

• 降至 39℃(102℉)时停止降温,避免降温过度和低体温。

• 退热药没有效果,因为根本机制不包括下丘脑体温调定点改变。

• 避免使用酒精擦浴。因为皮肤血管舒张,可能出现中毒。

支持治疗

• 热衰竭/热射病需要补液治疗:

- 开始使用生理盐水 0.5~1.0 L 补液。

- 积极液体复苏直到血压>90/60 mmHg。

- 避免补液过多,可能引起肺水肿和 ARDS。

- 儿童:从 20 ml/kg 开始补液。

- 热射病患者可放置导 Foley 导管监测尿量。

- 如果出现横纹肌溶解,维持尿量>2 ml/(kg·h)。

- 使用生理盐水补液,直至血流动力学稳定,如果需要纠正高钠血症,慢慢予以自由水。

• 癫痫、躁动或控制寒战时:使用苯二氮䓬类药物。

• 可能出现心动过速,通常体温下降后症状消失。在心肌冷却前,避免电刺激和使用 α 肾上腺素能药物。

• 热痉挛:使用镇痛药,口服或静脉滴注含有电解质的液体。

• 热性水肿:下肢抬高+穿弹力袜。

• 汗疹:氯己定(洗必泰)霜/乳液±1%水杨酸,每日 3 次。

■ 药物治疗

• 地西泮:5~10 mg(儿童 0.2~0.4 mg/kg),静脉推注。

• 劳拉西泮(氯羟去甲安定):1~2 mg(儿童 0.05~0.1 mg/kg),静脉推注。

• 纳洛酮:2 mg(儿童 0.1 mg/kg),静脉推注。

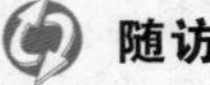

随访

■ 进一步处理

入院指征

• 热射病:入住 ICU。

• 热衰竭:如果出现下列情况进入普通或者监护病房:

- 严重电解质异常。

- 横纹肌溶解出现肾衰竭。

- 老年。

出院指征

除了热射病或者严重热衰竭的其他患者都可以出院。

要点和误区

• 没有温度>40.5℃(105℉)和中枢神经系统功能受损时不能诊断为热射病。

• 治疗热射病需要 ABC 管理和快速降温。

• 直肠或者食管探头持续监测核心温度是治疗标准。

• 蒸发散热是需要选择的降温措施。

天疱疮 Pemphigus

Adam Z. Barkin　王虑 译

基础知识

■ 描述

• 自身抗体(IgG)介导的表皮和黏膜松解的大疱性皮肤病。

- 细胞和细胞间黏附缺失致皮肤棘层松解。

• 年龄中位数为 71 岁。

- 有报道新生儿发病的。

• 较少见,全世界发病率为 0.7/10 万。

• 男性多于女性,66%比 34%。

• 帕菲克斯是希腊语中"泡沫"或"水泡"的意思。

• 天疱疮:是部分皮肤组织的自生免疫性疾病。

• 类天疱疮:是指上皮从皮肤分离的一类皮肤综合征,典型的多为良性。

• 病死率高的多见于皮肤黏膜受累的:

- 如果不治疗,病死率为 60%~90%,治疗则病死率约为 5%。

• 3 个主要的亚型:

- 寻常型:典型的因深部黏膜受累病情更为严重。

◦ 占天疱疮患者的 70%~80%。

◦ 70%的寻常型天疱疮患者有口腔受损,常是患者最经常的主述。

◦ 常侵犯所有人种的中年人和老年德裔犹太人。

- 落叶型:病情较轻和累及皮肤更表浅。

◦ 口腔受损病情预后较好。

- 副肿瘤性天疱疮:常有严重皮肤黏膜受累。

◦ 常见于淋巴恶性肿瘤。

儿科注意事项

• 天疱疮很少见于新生儿和儿童,但见于青少年。

• 早期诊断和治疗对儿童的成长有益。

• 组织病理学和成人相同。

• 新生儿天疱疮由 IgG 经胎盘传播导致。

• 新生儿天疱疮能随着来自母体的 IgG 代谢后自行缓解。

妊娠注意事项

应积极优先治疗孕妇的天疱疮疾病,这能

降低新生儿感染的风险和妊娠期并发症的发生率。

病因

• IgG 自身抗体直接作用于皮肤角质细胞桥粒钙黏蛋白 1 和 3。
• 自身抗体导致皮肤棘层松解、细胞骨架排列错乱和细胞凋亡。
• 大疱的形成是由于角质细胞间黏附和分离功能的丧失。
• 免疫遗传倾向于白细胞抗原 HLA 单倍型包括 DR4 和 DRw6 的人群有更高的发病率。
• 药物青霉胺、甲巯丙脯酸、利福平、吡罗昔康和苯巴比妥能诱发天疱疮的免疫反应。
• 地方流行性落叶型天疱疮，最常见于南美，可能因被飞行昆虫叮咬触发和传播。
• 类天疱疮反应常伴发于肿瘤，常见于淋巴瘤（副肿瘤天疱疮）。

诊断

症状和体征

• 皮肤和黏膜广泛或局部的大疱。
• 皮肤疼痛、糜烂伴有分离的上皮组织碎片。
• 疼痛难治愈的口腔、阴道皮肤黏膜糜烂。
• 大疱破裂后部分愈合的皮肤糜烂、结痂。
• 皮肤肥厚增生糜烂，糜烂区有脓疱（增生型天疱疮）。
• 皮脂丰富的皮肤潮湿、水肿、表皮剥脱糜烂（落叶型天疱疮）。
• 面颊的皮肤红斑鳞状硬皮状损害（红斑型天疱疮）。
• 若不治疗，皮肤损害持续存在：
- 治疗后会有炎症后色素沉淀。

病史

• 特征性的皮肤黏膜大疱和皮肤糜烂。
• 发病最先侵犯黏膜后到皮肤，最常见部位为头皮、胸部、腋窝和腹股沟区。
• 皮肤损害主要表现为疼痛性松弛性大疱，能发生在身体任何部位。

体格检查

• 尼氏征阳性，但不能作为确证依据。
• 灵敏度差。

基本检查

• 疑诊基于临床表现。
• 皮肤活检行组织病理和免疫荧光检查是确诊天疱疮的必须检查。

诊断检查与说明

实验室检查

• 血清抗体滴定度的免疫荧光检查常作为评估天疱疮病情活动度的指标，但急诊医师常不做该项检查。
• 酶联免疫吸附测定可用于区分亚型。

影像学检查

没有能协助诊断的检查。

诊断步骤/外科

彻底去毛和皮肤钻取活组织检查。

鉴别诊断

• 类天疱疮。
• 接触性皮炎。
• 疱疹样皮炎。
• 多形性红斑。
• 丹毒。
• 红皮病。
• 中毒性表皮坏死松解症。
• 表皮松解。
• 手足口病。
• 系统性红斑狼疮。
• 结节性脉管炎。
• 口腔念珠菌病。
• 单纯疱疹龈口炎。
• 扁平苔藓。
• 脂溢性皮炎。

治疗

院前

• 如果病情严重：
- 建立静脉通道，血脉氧监测，心电监测。

初步稳定/治疗

• 如果患者有低血压和脓毒症表现，需静脉补液复苏。
• 如果有脓毒症的表现，则需要广谱抗生素治疗。
• 对于类固醇激素依赖患者，需管理类固醇剂量。

急诊治疗/程序

• 全身用糖皮质激素是核心治疗方案。
• 轻中度患者应口服泼尼松治疗，局部用曲安奈德治疗。
• 重症患者：大剂量糖皮质激素治疗。
- 如果对口服大剂量泼尼松治疗无反应，可考虑使用静脉用糖皮质激素和血浆置换治疗。
• 免疫抑制剂联合大剂量糖皮质激素能减轻症状，若不适合用糖皮质激素治疗也可以用免疫抑制剂治疗。
- 氨苯砜、咪唑硫嘌呤、环磷酰胺、环孢素、甲氨蝶呤、麦考酚酯和静脉输注免疫球蛋白。

药物治疗

一线用药

• 免疫抑制剂：
- 氢化可的松：100～300 mg/d 静脉输注负荷量后再根据患者实际情况调整。
- 甲泼尼龙（静脉输注治疗，成人）：1 g，每日 1 次，静脉输注 3 h 以上。
- 泼尼松：1 mg/(kg · d) 口服，每日 1 次（成人）；中重度患者口服，每日 1 次，服用 5～10 周，后逐渐减量。
- 曲安奈德：可以减少口服糖皮质激素治疗，10 mg/ml 0.1 ml 注射入每个大疱内。
• 疼痛：
- 阿片类、抗炎药、对乙酰氨基酚。
- 合成生物膜敷料。
- 盐酸苯海拉明和抗酸剂或利多卡因漱口液。

二线用药

• 常用于治疗住院的难治患者。
• 免疫抑制剂：
- 静脉注射免疫球蛋白：单剂 400 mg/kg，每日 1 次，连用 5 日。
- 利妥昔单抗。
- 曲安奈德：10 mg/ml 0.1 ml，注射入每个大疱内。
• 疼痛：
- 加巴喷丁起始 300 mg 每日 1 次静脉滴注；后 300 mg，每日 3 次，使用 1 个月。
• 其他注意事项：大剂量使用糖皮质激素患者日常应补充维生素 D 和钙剂、服用质子泵抑制剂或二膦酸盐类药物。

随访

进一步处理

入院指征

• 天疱疮患者需住院治疗的较少，多可以在皮肤科医师随访的情况下口服糖皮质激素治疗。
• 将第一次发病需要立刻治疗并皮肤活检以排除高病死率的大疱性皮肤病的患者收入院。

• 将有广泛皮肤黏膜受累、难治的疼痛，合并皮肤感染或有脓毒症表现的患者收入院。

• 需要静脉用糖皮质激素和血浆置换治疗的患者收入院。

• 如果有休克或脓毒症表现的患者需要收入 ICU 或烧伤病房，因这类患者需积极液体复苏治疗、伤口护理和多样药物治疗。

出院指征

轻中度患者不再需要积极糖皮质激素治疗、血浆置换或积极疼痛控制，可予以出院。

随访建议

• 皮肤科医师需要随访监测患者病情并及时调节治疗方案。

• 大剂量服用糖皮质激素患者行骨扫描风湿病科医师能对患骨质疏松的风险做出适当的评估。

要点和误区

• 皮肤黏膜损害常开始于面部、头/头皮或口腔。

• 确保皮肤科医师长期随访是很有必要的。

• 糖皮质激素是核心的治疗手段。

• 副肿瘤天疱疮常有严重的口腔黏膜受累，考虑可能有淋巴增生性障碍。

• 行免疫抑制治疗包括糖皮质激素和免疫调节剂治疗的患者，患相关并发症的风险很大，如肾上腺危象、严重的脓毒症或继发于 2 型糖尿病的非酮性高渗性酸中毒。

• 低血压患者需要积极的液体复苏治疗。

铁中毒 Iron Poisoning

Sean M. Bryant 倪沁赟 译

基础知识

描述

• 摄入后 2～4 h 达峰浓度。

• 摄入超过 4～6 h 后血清浓度不可靠：

- 肠溶或持续释放。

• 吸收完毕：铁分布到组织中，然后血清铁浓度下降导致细胞内游离铁浓度改变，进而发生细胞损伤。

• 损伤形式：

- 对肠黏膜的腐蚀性损伤可能导致深层液体丢失(休克)、出血和穿孔。

- 因门静脉循环，肝脏所受的铁负荷最大——出血性门静脉周围坏死。

• 游离铁：

- 集中在线粒体，扰乱氧化磷酸化；催化脂质过氧化和自由基的形成，导致细胞死亡，增加无氧代谢和酸中毒。

- 引起心肌抑制、静脉扩张和脑水肿。

• 铁水化释放 3 个质子，导致酸血症。

病因

铁元素摄入：

• 无中毒＜20 mg/kg。

• 中重度＞40 mg/kg。

• 致死可能＞60 mg/kg。

• 铁元素当量：

- 硫酸亚铁，20%(325 mg＝65 mg Fe)。

- 葡萄酸亚铁，12%。

- 富马酸亚铁，33%。

• 产前维生素每片含铁元素 60～90 mg 不等。

• 儿童维生素每片可能含铁元素 5～18 mg。

儿科注意事项

• 历史上臭名昭著的事件，即儿童意外接触(使用成人铁产品)死亡率最高。

• 儿童可拒绝铁剂被证明是安全的。

诊断

症状和体征

• 经典地被分为 5 个阶段：

- 第一阶段：胃肠道(0.5～6 h)：

◦ 腹痛。

◦ 呕吐。

◦ 腹泻。

◦ 吐血。

◦ 便血。

- 第二阶段：潜伏/静态(6～24 h)：

◦ 辨别胃肠道症状。

◦ 欺骗期(持续损伤?)。

◦ 可能出现低血压或酸中毒。

- 第三阶段：休克和器官衰竭(6～72 h)：

◦ 低灌注。

◦ 代谢性酸中毒。

◦ 昏迷。

◦ 凝血功能障碍。

- 第四阶段：肝衰竭(2～3 日)：

◦ 凝血功能障碍。

◦ 低血糖。

◦ 黄疸。

◦ 肝功能(转氨酶)和胆红素升高。

- 第五阶段：梗阻(2～4 周)：

◦ 幽门或小肠梗阻。

◦ 腹痛、呕吐。

• 患者可能出现在或跳过 5 个阶段中的任何一个。

• 如果第一阶段的出现不在 6 h 内，可能提示没有显著摄入。

基本检查

急性铁中毒是一种临床诊断，不论实验室结果如何。

诊断检查与说明

实验室检查

• 血清铁水平(mg/dl)：

- 吸收峰值 2～6 h。

- 4 h 是最常见的达峰时间。

- 肠溶片/缓释片致达峰延迟。

• 电解质、尿素氮/肌酐、血糖：

- 阴离子间隙代谢性酸中毒。

- 早期高血糖。

- 晚期低血糖。

• 动脉血气分析：

- 代谢性酸中毒。

• 全血细胞计数：

- 贫血伴显著失血。

- 白细胞增多。

• 肝功能。

• 凝血功能。

• 乳酸。

• 出血类型及筛选。

• 总铁结合能力没有用，因此不推荐。

影像学检查

腹部放射学检查：

- 片剂(很少见儿童的咀嚼片)。
- 丸片丢失的解释：
  - 患者没有摄入铁。
  - 铁在溶液中或者已溶解。
  - 患者摄入儿童维生素产品。
  - X线阻射性缺乏不能排除重大或致命性的摄取。
- 穿孔/隔下游离气体。

鉴别诊断

- 脓毒症。
- 对乙酰氨基酚中毒。
- 毒物摄入导致阴离子间隙酸中毒：
  - 水杨酸盐。
  - 氰化物。
  - 甲醇。
  - 乙二醇。
- 蘑菇。
- 重金属。
- 茶碱中毒。
- 其他原因导致的胃肠道出血(酒精性肝脏疾病)。

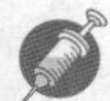

治疗

院前

在急诊室收集处方瓶或处方药物用于鉴定。

初步稳定/治疗

- ABC管理：
  - 如不稳定，及时气管插管。
  - 建立静脉通道补液，纠正低血压。
  - 心功能及脉氧饱和度监测。
- 精神状态改变可使用纳洛酮、硫胺素、葡萄糖。

急诊治疗/程序

- 清除毒物：
  - 活性炭吸附不良。
  - 洗胃未被证明可改善结局。
  - 不推荐使用碳酸氢钠、磷酸钠和口服去铁胺。
  - 如果在X线下可见药片碎片或病史提示显著摄入：
    - 考虑全肠灌洗[使用NG GoLytely：儿童：10～15 mg/(kg·h)；成人：1～2 L/h]，同时通过X线(腹部平片)监测病情进展。
    - 注意胃肠道出血。
  - 大量摄入后通过内镜或胃肠手术可清除胃石(>240 mg/kg)。
- 螯合去铁胺(DFO)：
  - DFO是高度特异的肠外铁螯合剂。
  - 静脉输液可使DFO水平更加恒定，静脉输液是可选择的路径：
    - 尽快在24 h内给予输注。
  - 管理技术：
    - 增加静脉输注速度至15 mg/(kg·h)超过20 min，同时监测有无低血压的发生。
    - 如果发生低血压，减慢输液速度。
    - 可耐受45 mg/(kg·h)的输液速度。
    - 请无视该条制造商的建议：在严重铁暴露情况下每日最大剂量为6 g。
  - 不建议肌内注射DFO。
  - 仔细解读血清水平：
    - 摄入时间必须考虑：某些患者临床表现较晚、摄入超过8 h且血清铁水平<350 mg/dl，仍提示需要进一步治疗。
  - 如果血清铁水平不易获得，根据临床状态决定基础治疗。
  - 输注时间(存在争议)：
    - DFO-铁复合物导致尿液呈玫瑰红葡萄酒颜色，该征象提示持续输注直到尿液恢复正常。
    - 显著中毒的症状和体征的缓解提示可停止输注DFO。
    - 延长DFO治疗超过24～48 h可能导致成人呼吸窘迫综合征。
    - 症状和体征持续不缓解的严重病例，可能需要小剂量持续输注。
  - 争议：
    - DFO输注超过24 h的安全性。
    - 最大输注速度和总剂量。
    - 需要治疗的血清铁浓度水平。
    - 治疗终点(最好的治疗终点是毒性缓解，即酸血症)。
    - 体外清除。
  - 中重度铁暴露联系当地毒物中心。

药物治疗

- DFO 15 mg/(kg·h)，见急诊治疗。
- 葡萄糖：50%葡萄糖注射液1安瓿(50 ml或25 g；儿童患者：25%葡萄糖注射液2～4 mg/kg)，静脉输注。
- 纳洛酮：初始剂量2 mg(儿童：0.1 mg/kg)，静脉或肌内注射。
- 硫胺素(维生素 B_1)：100 mg(儿童：50 mg)，静脉或肌内注射。

随访

进一步处理

入院指征

- 胃肠道症状或脱水。
- 精神状态改变。
- 低血压、嗜睡、代谢性酸中毒或休克。
- 血清铁>500 mg/dl。
- 血清铁>350 mg/dl且在腹部X线平片上看见片剂。
- 血清铁水平升高。
- 接受去铁胺治疗的患者。
- ICU入院指征：昏迷、休克、代谢性酸中毒或血清铁>1 000 mg/dl。

出院指征

- 无症状且影像学上表现阴性。
- 观察6 h后轻微或无症状。
- 轻度胃肠道症状，无代谢性酸中毒表现且血清铁<350 mg/dl。

转诊问题

轻中度中毒联系当地毒物中心。

随访建议

- 有幽门梗阻风险的患者出院后随访。
- 故意过量使用的精神患者。

要点和误区

- 某些患者临床表现较晚、摄入超过8 h且血清铁水平<350 mg/dl，有细胞内中毒征象(如阴离子间隙代谢性酸中毒)，均需要DFO治疗。
- 胃肠道症状缓解并不表明没有持续的毒性，可能会随着时间进展。

T

烃类物质中毒 Hydrocarbon Poisoning

James W. Rhee 巩博 译

基础知识

描述

- 烃类暴露的主要并发症是误吸：
- 吸入烃主要影响中枢神经和呼吸系统。
- 物理特性决定了中毒的类型和程度：
- 黏稠度(流动阻力)：
  - 较低黏稠度的物品误吸的风险更高。
- 挥发性(物质蒸发的能力)：
  - 芳香烃类替换肺泡中的空气引起缺氧。
- 表面张力(在液体表面黏附于自身的能力)：
  - 低表面张力容易从口咽传播至气管，促进误吸(如矿物油、海洋石油)。
- 挥发性物质滥用：
- 通常为溶剂滥用：
  - 打字机修正液。
  - 黏合剂。
  - 汽油。
  - 打火机液。
- 吸入：直接从容器内吸入。
- 吹气：通过浸泡的布吸入。
- 装袋：产品倒入袋中，然后多次从袋里吸入。
- 烃类物质主要分类：
- 脂肪烃：
  - 包括煤油、矿物油、海洋石油、汽油、溶剂、涂料稀释剂。
  - 通过吸入产生肺毒性。
  - 气态甲烷和丁烷取代肺泡氧气引起窒息。
- 卤代烃：
  - 包括四氯化碳和三氯乙烷。
  - 工业用溶剂。
  - 容易被肺和肠道吸收。
  - 高毒性。
  - 吞入可引起肝脏和肾脏衰竭。
- 环状或者芳香族化合物，包括甲苯和二甲苯。
  - 高挥发性且容易被肠道吸收。
  - 据报道，口服 15 ml 苯可引起死亡。
- 萜烯，包括松节油和松树油：
  - 容易被消化系统吸收。
  - 强大的中枢神经系统抑制作用。

病因

- 儿童以意外暴露为特点。
- 滥用挥发性烃类导致吸入。
- 成人和青少年试图自杀。

诊断

症状和体征

- 通常无症状。
- 可闻到烃类物质的气味。
- 早期：欣快症。
- 解除抑制。
- 晚期：烦躁不安。
- 共济失调。
- 混乱。
- 幻觉。
- 吸气性猝死：
- 挥发性物质滥用者出现心跳停止，继发于肾上腺素刺激、心肌高敏感导致恶性心律失常。
- 肺：
- 轻度到严重的呼吸抑制。
- 发绀。
- 误吸(主要并发症)。
- 中枢神经系统：
- 中毒。
- 欣快症。
- 言语不清。
- 嗜睡。
- 昏迷。
- 胃肠道：
- 局部黏膜刺激。
- 胃炎。
- 腹泻。
- 心脏：
- 心动过速。
- 心律失常(挥发性物质滥用者)。
- 皮肤：
- 局部红斑。
- 斑丘疹或小疱疹。
- 慢性皮肤暴露引起脱脂性皮炎。
- 长期滥用者出现面部皮疹。

病史

- 暴露的途径、类型、量和时间：
- 确定意向性。
- 症状：
- 呕吐、呼吸衰竭、精神状态改变或疼痛。
- 旁观者救助或者院前干预。

体格检查

- 对于意识水平下降伴有呕吐的患者，评估气道有无狭窄。
- 呼吸道症状一般在 30 min 内发生，但经常延迟数小时。
- 监测低氧、低血压、心律失常。
- 发绀和低氧暗示呼吸衰竭，但也可能是高铁血红蛋白症。
- 误吸后体温可能上升，并且暗示着肺炎：
- 48 h 后发热提示细菌二重感染。

基本检查

按下文获得信息：

- 产品：标签上准确的名字、制造者及成分。
- 摄入或暴露的原因：意外或者故意。
- 估计吞下的量。
- 在工厂，查找材料安全数据表。

诊断检查与说明

挥发性物质滥用者检查心电图。

实验室检查

- 血氧测定：
- 如果不正常，进行动脉血气分析。
- 电解质、尿素氮、肌酐和葡萄糖水平，肝功能检验。
- 卤化烃和芳香烃暴露。
- 代谢性酸中毒。
- 低钾血症。
- 二氯甲烷暴露检测碳氧血红蛋白水平：
- 在体内二氯甲烷代谢为一氧化碳。

影像学检查

胸部 X 线检查：

- 暴露 20 min 至 24 h(通常 6 h)可见异常。
- 增强的支气管血管纹理和肺底、肺门渗出(特征)。
- 大叶实变(不常见)。
- 气胸、纵隔气肿和胸腔积液(少见)。
- 肺囊肿于数周后消失。
- 如果呼吸症状加重，重复胸片检测。

鉴别诊断

- 腐蚀性液体、杀虫剂或者有毒酒精摄入。
- 偶然还是有意：
- 全部故意摄入者应由精神科医师进行评估。
- 儿童照管不良：

- 监管不力或者不安全的家庭环境。

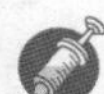

治疗

院前

- 去除衣物、皮肤、头发或者任何暴露处的烃类物质。
- 不要胃排空治疗。
- 因为增加误吸的风险，所以不建议催吐。
- 保持挥发性物质滥用者平静，避免引起焦虑或者忧虑的干预。
- 在家里治疗偶然性烃中毒存在争议：
  - <1%需要医师干预。
  - 对于吞入后无症状或者短期无症状可进行可靠观察者，可采取家庭治疗。
  - 当产品明确、成分清楚，且没有胃净化的适应证，或者迟发性器官毒性的可能。

初步稳定/治疗

- ABC 管理。
- 如果存在低血压或者进行性液体丢失，建立静脉通道，进行液体复苏。
- 吸氧。
- 心电监测。
- 如果精神状态改变，予以纳洛酮、硫胺素、50%葡萄糖(或检查血糖)。

急诊治疗/程序

- 支持治疗。
- 治疗呼吸道症状：
  - 吸氧。
  - 雾化。
  - 支气管痉挛予 β_2 受体激动剂。
  - 呼吸衰竭予以气管插管和机械通气。
  - 类固醇不适用于支气管痉挛。
  - 避免在挥发性物质滥用者使用肾上腺素，它可能导致突发性节律障碍。
- 机械通气：
  - 在发生肺炎患者需要机械通气时，应采用肺保护策略。
  - 高频通气对那些发展为严重肺炎并对常规通气无反应的患者可能是有益的。
- 肺毒性明显的患者可能受益于体外膜氧合(ECMO)，应考虑入院或转到 ECMO 中心。

> **注意**
> - 胃排空不适用于大多数口服烃。
>   - 误吸的风险增加，引起严重的化学性肺炎。
>   - 脂肪烃多数为口服，误吸的风险比全身性吸收的风险高。
>   - 如果出现自发性呕吐，为禁忌证。
>   - 通过小孔鼻胃管吸出胃内容物可能是口服有全身毒性的某些烃(CHAMP)的适应证：
>   - CHAMP：樟脑、卤化烃、芳香烃、金属(如铅、水银)、杀虫剂。
>   - 只对短时间内口服(60 min)。
>   - 从此操作中收益必须考虑误吸和继发性肺炎的风险。
>   - 如果咽反射消失或者精神状态改变，洗胃期间气管插管保护气道。
> - 活性炭不能与烃很好地结合，不适用于烃中毒，除非是严重威胁生命的情况。
> - 导泻不适用：
>   - 烃中毒常常出现腹泻。

药物治疗

- 支气管痉挛使用沙丁胺醇 2.5～5 mg，雾化(儿童：0.15～0.3 mg/kg)。
- 葡萄糖：50%葡萄糖 1 安瓿 50 ml 者 25 g(儿童：25%葡萄糖 2～4 ml/kg)，静脉注射。
- 纳洛酮：2 mg(儿童：0.1 mg/kg)，静脉注射或初始量肌内注射。
- 硫胺素(维生素 B_1)：100 mg(儿童：50 mg)，静脉注射或肌内注射。

随访

进一步处理

入院指征

- 有症状的患者。
- 患者有潜在迟发性器官毒性(四氯化碳或其他有毒添加剂)。
- 对于有明显肺毒性的病人应考虑入院或转到 ECMO 中心。

出院指征

- 观察 6 h 出院：
  - 无症状的患者胸片正常，指脉氧饱和度正常。
  - 无症状的患者胸片异常，氧合和呼吸频率正常，如果有可靠的随访，可以出院。
  - 目前有症状，但症状快速消失。
- 观察挥发性物质滥用者，直到状态正常。

转诊问题

按需要进行精神科会诊。

随访建议

- 最少观察 6 h 后，如果患者仍然无症状，随访 24 h。
- 胸片异常的无症状患者，24 h 内应进行一次复查。

要点和误区

- 烃类暴露的主要并发症是误吸：
  - 误吸的风险直接和挥发性相关，与黏稠度、表面张力相反。
- 去除外部污染物。
- 洗胃很少适合。
- 避免诱导呕吐和腹泻。
- 口服中毒后观察患者至少 6 h。
- 允许有症状的患者住院治疗。
- ECMO 可能对严重肺毒性有益。
- 当有延迟性器官毒性时，住院治疗。
  - CHAMP。

T

痛风和假性痛风 Gout/Pseudogout

Delaram Ghadishah 祝各亮 译

基础知识

描述

- 尿酸沉积在组织中，主要影响中年男性和绝经后女性：
  - 最常见的结晶性疾病。
  - 4 期：
    - 无症状高尿酸血症(血清尿酸>7 mg/dl)。
    - 急性痛风。
    - 间歇发作期。
    - 痛风石病变期(多达 45%的病例)。
  - 危险因素：
    - 年龄>40 岁。
    - 男性与女性比例：<65 岁为 2∶1～6∶1，≥65 岁为 1∶1。

◦ 高血压。
◦ 使用襻或噻嗪类利尿剂。
◦ 大量摄入酒精、肉类、海鲜和果糖等甜饮料。
◦ 肥胖。
– 尿酸结石沉积于泌尿系统可能会导致肾功能障碍。
– 与股骨头缺血性坏死和变形性关节炎有关。
– 最常见于之前被损坏过的关节及组织：
◦ 滑膜。
◦ 软骨下骨（鹰嘴、髌下囊、髌前）。
◦ 跟腱。
◦ 前臂伸肌表面、手指、足趾及耳。
◦ 很少发生于中枢神经系统或心脏（瓣膜）。
• 假性痛风：一种焦磷酸钙沉积引起的代谢失调：
– 最常由单关节炎症引起，常见于 60 岁以上的人群。
– 危险因素：
◦ 高钙血症（如甲状旁腺功能亢进症、家族性高钙血症）。
◦ 血色素沉着症，含铁血黄素沉着症。
◦ 甲状腺功能减退症和甲状腺功能亢进症。
◦ 低磷血症和低镁血症。
◦ 淀粉样变性。
◦ 痛风。

病因

• 尿酸钠晶体从过饱和的细胞外液沉积于组织中，其原因为：
– 排泄（最常见）或尿酸过多。
– 尿酸水平的快速变化：
◦ 开始使用利尿剂或停止使用利尿剂。
◦ 酒精、水杨酸和烟酸。
◦ 环孢素。
◦ 醋酸铅中毒。
◦ 促尿酸排泄药或别嘌醇。
• 假性痛风继发于焦磷酸钙晶体在滑膜中堆积过多。
• 沉淀剂可以导致痛风和假性痛风，包括轻微损伤和急性疾病：
– 手术及缺血性心脏病。

诊断

症状和体征

• 痛风和假性痛风都可表现为急性单关节或寡关节炎：
– 表现为发热、红斑和关节肿胀。
– 早期发作在 3～21 日会自然消退，即使不治疗。
– 晚期发作可能会持续更长的时间，发作更为密集，症状更为严重，累及更多的关节。
• 痛风：
– 发作后 12～24 h 出现症状高峰期。
– 可表现为痛风石和关节脱屑。
– 女性主要发生于绝经后，且累及多关节（70%）。
– 在免疫抑制人群和老年人群中发病较少。
– 最常见于第 1 跖趾关节（75%）＞踝、跗、膝＞手腕。
• 假性痛风：
– 与痛风相比，更易累及大关节。
– 最常见：膝＞腕＞掌、肩、肘、踝＞髋、跗。
– 单关节（25%）。
– 无症状（25%）。
– 假性骨关节炎（45%）：逐步退化，常对称。
– 假性类风湿关节炎（老年）。
• 混合型多关节病变。

基本检查

• 关节穿刺抽吸痛风石：
– 抽吸物结晶，革兰染色，细菌培养，白细胞计数及鉴别。
– 常为黏稠白色液体。
◦ 痛风：白细胞 20000～100000/mm^3，很少的纤维和蛋白凝块，无细菌。
◦ 假性痛风：白细胞最多 50 000/mm^3，无细菌。
• 偏振光显微镜下晶体检测：
– 痛风：
◦ 针形。
◦ 强双折射。
◦ 负延伸率。
– 假性痛风：
◦ 菱形。
◦ 弱双折射。
◦ 正延伸率。

诊断检查与说明

实验室检查

• 血常规常显示白细胞增多。
• 生化项目评估肾脏损害。
• 镁、钙、促甲状腺激素（TSH）和血清铁。
• 尿酸水平。
• 如果考虑感染性关节炎：
– 血、尿培养。
– 尿道、宫颈、直肠或咽部淋球菌培养。

影像学检查

• X 线平片：
– 积液。
– 关节间隙变窄。
– 关节基线状态。
– 邻近处骨髓炎。
– 骨折或异物。
• 急性痛风：软组织肿胀，矿化正常，关节间隙存在。
• 慢性痛风：痛风石钙化，不对称骨侵蚀，悬挂边缘，骨轴逐渐变细。
• 假性痛风：软骨钙化，软骨下骨硬化（腕）或囊肿，软骨、肌腱和韧带不透射性钙化，不投射性骨赘。
• 双能 CT 扫描：肾结石或软组织的尿酸盐结晶。

诊断步骤/外科

• 关节穿刺术。
• 痛风石抽吸术。

鉴别诊断

• 感染性关节炎。
• 创伤。
• 骨关节炎。
• 反应性关节炎。
• 杂结晶性关节炎。
• 无菌性坏死。
• 类风湿关节炎。
• 系统性红斑狼疮。
• 镰刀形细胞。
• 骨髓炎。
• 银屑病关节炎。

治疗

初步稳定/治疗

• 止痛。
• 排除感染因素。

急诊治疗/程序

• 非甾体抗炎药是一线用药。
• 非甾体抗炎药无效或禁忌：
– 糖皮质激素（口服、静脉注射、肌内注射、关节内注射）。
– 秋水仙碱（需限制毒性）。
– 关节抽吸。
– 避免阿司匹林。
• 高尿酸血症的处理，以及痛风和假性痛风的长期管理，不在急诊室治疗的一般范围内：
– 尽量不使用会加重痛风的药物。

- 促尿酸排泄药(如丙磺舒、苯磺唑酮)。
- 别嘌醇减少尿酸合成。
- 增加液体摄入量和尿液碱化以预防肾结石。
- 长期预防性使用秋水仙碱或非甾体抗炎药。

▪ 药物治疗

• 阿那白滞素：100 mg,皮下注射,每日1次。
- 慢性痛风,治疗伴肾衰竭的难治性痛风或假性痛风的超适应证用药。

• 别嘌醇：100 mg,口服,每日1次,逐周增加,最大剂量至800 mg,每日1次：
- 痛风发作期后1～2周开始用药。
- 存在肾脏疾病时需做调整。
- 出现皮疹或发热时需停药。
- 可用于尿酸性肾结石的治疗。
- 剂量>400 mg时应当分次服用。

• 秋水仙碱：痛风发作时1.2 mg,口服;1 h后0.6 mg,口服：
- 大剂量时会引起骨髓抑制。
- 不可进行透析。
- 长期服用可能会造成肌病。
- 根据肝肾功能情况调整剂量。
- 不能防止尿酸盐沉积或慢性痛风造成的关节损伤。

• 糖皮质激素：
- 促肾上腺皮质激素：40 U,肌内注射,q8 h,最多2次。
- 甲泼尼松：40 mg(儿童：1～2 mg/kg),肌内注射或静脉注射,每日1次,持续3～4日。
- 泼尼松：40 mg(儿童：1～2 mg/kg),口服,每日1次,持续3～4日,逐渐减量至7～14日。
- 曲安奈德(10～40 mg)+地塞米松(2～10 mg):关节内注射。

• 非布索坦：40～80 mg,每日1次：
- 第一时间与非甾体抗炎药或秋水仙碱一起使用。
- 抑制尿酸的产生。
- 对轻度或中度肾脏病患者是安全的。

• 非甾体抗炎药在最初3日用最大剂量,接着4日内剂量递减：
- 布洛芬：800 mg(儿童：10 mg/kg),口服,每日4次。
- 吲哚美辛：25～50 mg,口服,每日3～4次[儿童：2 mg/(kg·d),每日3～4次];14岁以下儿童禁用。
- 酮咯酸：15～30 mg肌内注射/静脉注射,可重复进行一次(儿童：1 mg/kg,最大剂量30 mg,肌内注射;或0.5 mg/kg,最大剂量15 mg,静脉注射)。
- 萘普生：500 mg,口服,每日3次(儿童：5 mg/kg,口服,每日2次)。
- 舒林酸：200 mg,口服,每日3次。

• 聚乙二醇尿酸酶：8 mg,静脉注射,每2周1次：
- 用于治疗难治性痛风。
- 优先考虑用抗组胺药和类固醇。
- 可能会导致过敏反应。
- 如果尿酸>6 mg/dl就停药。
- G-6-PD缺乏症者禁忌。

• 丙磺舒250～500 mg,口服,q12 h;最大剂量3 g,每日1次：
- 促进尿酸排泄。
- 在肾脏疾病或阿司匹林或利尿剂使用情况下减效或失效。
- 尿酸肾结石存在时相对禁忌。

• 利洛纳塞：2×160 mg(2×2 ml)同一日内在2个不同部位皮下注射,之后160 mg(1×2 ml)皮下注射,每周1次,急性痛风或预防的超适应证用药。
- 降尿酸治疗开始后可以使用该药。

• 硫氧唑酮：200～400 mg,口服,每日2次,餐时用药;维持剂量400 mg,每日2次：最大剂量800 mg,每日1次。

老年人注意事项

非甾体抗炎药可能会加重肾功能不全、体液潴留、胃病、肝毒性和认知功能,特别是老年人。

儿科注意事项

痛风在儿童中不常见,但在癌症化疗期间仍有可能发生。

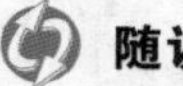

随访

▪ 进一步处理

入院指征

• 怀疑感染性关节炎。
• 急性肾衰竭。
• 顽固性疼痛。

出院指征

• 无感染证据。
• 疼痛已充分缓解。

转诊问题

• 化脓性关节炎。
• 肾衰竭。

▪ 随访建议

• 病情严重或难以控制情况下,进行风湿科随访。
• 出现肾功能不全时,进行肾内科随访。
• 出现尿酸性结石时,进行泌尿科随访。
• 出现化脓性关节炎或明显关节损伤,进行骨科随访。
• 建议患者低嘌呤饮食。

要点和误区

• 急性痛风发作的同时,可发生化脓性关节炎。
• 一般情况下非甾体抗炎药是一线用药。
• 发作往往具有自限性。
• 痛风和假性痛风会导致骨和软骨的损伤。

头部钝性伤 Head Trauma, Blunt

Gary M. Vilke · Heather E. Boynton 刘雪峰 译

基础知识

▪ 描述

外伤中常见头部钝性伤,轻者出现闭合性颅脑伤,重者导致死亡。

▪ 病因

头部钝性伤可引起以下几种类型的闭合性颅脑损伤：

• 脑震荡：短暂的意识丧失或记忆缺失,头颅CT正常。
• 硬脑膜下血肿：硬脑膜下桥静脉撕裂,血液流入硬脑膜下腔隙。
• 硬脑膜外血肿：颅骨骨折常常导致硬脑膜动脉损伤,特别是脑膜中动脉：

- 可出现典型的中间清醒期表现，如处理不及时可迅速导致死亡。

• 蛛网膜下腔出血：创伤后血液流入蛛网膜下腔。

• 脑挫伤：颅脑损伤病灶以损伤区下方局部或远离损伤区的对冲伤为特征。

• 脑内出血：血液流入脑实质引起脑损伤。

• 弥漫性轴索损伤：颅脑广泛分布微损伤，患者处于昏迷状态。

诊断

■ 症状和体征

• 头部创伤的表现：

- 头皮裂伤、头皮血肿或瘀斑。
- 熊猫眼：颅底骨折所致双侧眼眶瘀斑。
- Battle 征：耳后乳突部位皮下瘀斑，伴有颅底骨折。
- 鼓室积血。
- 脑脊液耳鼻漏。

• 颅内高压的表现：

- 意识状态变差，GCS 评分降低。
- 库欣反应：心动过缓，血压升高，呼吸频率减慢。
- 瞳孔扩大，伴有去皮质或去大脑姿势。

病史

• 受伤机制。

• 遗忘受伤过程。

• 是否有抗凝药物使用史。

• 头痛、视力改变或听力丧失。

• 局部神经症状。

• 颈部疼痛。

体格检查

• 评估头皮血肿、Battle 征和熊猫眼。

• 完整的神经系统检查。

• 颈椎的检查。

• 评估其他创伤性损伤（高达 60% 的 TBI 患者）。

■ 基本检查

• 伴有下列任一项症状的患者需行影像学检查：

- 意识或记忆丧失。
- 进行性头痛。
- 酒精或药物中毒。
- 病史不详或危险的受创途径。
- 创伤后癫痫发作。
- 反复呕吐。
- 有颅底骨折的体征。
- 颅骨穿透伤或者凹陷性骨折。
- GCS 评分＜15 分。
- 神经定位体征。

• 服用香豆素、肝素或者其他抗凝药物以及既往有出血性疾病的患者必须进行影像学检查：

- 若伤后 4 h 内头颅 CT 正常，必须在伤后 4～6 h 再次复查 CT，若患者临床症状逐渐恶化可提前复查 CT。

• 嗜酒可增加出血风险，应行头颅 CT 检查。

老年人注意事项

• 60～65 岁及以上的老年患者颅内出血风险增加。

• 许多老年患者长期服用抗凝剂，仔细询问病史。

• 高危因素较多，需尽早行头颅 CT。

■ 诊断检查与说明

实验室检查

• 快速血糖检测。

• 全血细胞计数、血小板计数及凝血功能。

• 血型鉴定，交叉配血。

• 血液电解质、尿素氮及肌酐。

• 血液酒精含量（如有饮酒史）。

影像学检查

• 头颅 CT/MRI。

• 酌情行颈椎 X 线检查或者螺旋 CT。

诊断步骤/外科

CT 显示蛛网膜下腔出血可行腰椎穿刺术。

■ 鉴别诊断

• 穿透性脑外伤。

• 任何可能导致精神状态改变的情况均可引起患者跌倒，继而出现头部外伤表现（如低血糖、癫痫）。

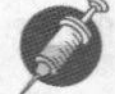

治疗

■ 院前

• 合并颅内损伤风险的头部钝性伤患者必须到创伤中心诊治：

- 包括意识状态改变、有神经定位体征、多发伤或者明显的凹陷性颅骨骨折。

• 中危患者应该就诊于可进行脑外科会诊的医院：

- 包括进行性头痛、酒精或药物中毒、受伤史不明、创伤后癫痫、反复呕吐、伤后记忆丧失、颅底骨折体征。

• 保护气道的通畅，必要时可予以气管插管：

• 不合并脑疝时应避免过度通气。

• 血压正常的患者合并脑疝或者进行性意识状态改变，为了降低颅内压，应当：

- 适当的通气频率以保持呼气末二氧化碳分压处于 30～35 mmHg；
- 升高床头 30°。

• 所有患者均需警惕颈椎损伤。

• 注意：

- 避免血压过低（SBP＜90 mmHg），使用晶体液扩容维持血压。
- 避免低氧血症（氧饱和度＜90%），必要时可吸纯氧。
- 监测血糖，目标维持在 140～180 mg/dl。

■ 初步稳定/治疗

外伤救护 ABC 管理：

• 气道管理：

- 如 GCS 评分＜8 分，不能保持气道通畅，或出现低氧血症，均需快速行气管插管。
- 维持正常的动脉血二氧化碳分压，避免通气不足与过度通气。

• 给予甲苄咪酯或芬太尼作为诱导剂，琥珀胆碱（小剂量预处理）、罗库溴铵或维库溴铵作为肌松剂；吗啡持续镇静。

• 血流动力学不稳定的患者慎用芬太尼。

• 放置静脉导管输注晶体液以避免低血压状态（保持收缩压＞90 mmHg）。

• 警惕颈椎损伤。

■ 急诊治疗/程序

• 早期神经外科会诊。

• 合并脑疝时需要尽快降低颅内压：

- 适当过度通气：成人 20 次/分，儿童 25 次/分，1 岁以下幼儿 30 次/分，以维持呼气末二氧化碳分压处于 30～35 mmHg。
- 升高床头 30°。
- 甘露醇静脉滴注：患者收缩压＞100 mmHg 且予以充分的液体复苏后可给予甘露醇脱水降颅压。否则不要使用甘露醇，考虑 3% 盐水治疗低血压患者。

• 提供足够的镇静和镇痛。

• 早期应用苯妥英或左乙拉西坦预防创伤后癫痫发作，在昏迷患者中获取脑电图。

• 防治低凝状态。

• 低颅压的头部创伤患者不推荐使用糖皮质激素。

• 初期急诊治疗不推荐使用巴比妥类药物。

• 在脑外科手术确定进行之前给予颅骨钻孔减压可能挽救患者生命：

- 钻孔减压术在损伤侧进行，仅用于对过度通气和甘露醇治疗无反应的并且呈去皮质/

大脑姿势的昏迷患者。

• 必要时可输血，维持血细胞比容>30%。
• 避免体温过低，以防增加手术出血风险。
• 禁食。
• 手术：
- 手术应基于 CT 的阳性发现以及脑外科会诊。

■ 药物治疗

用药原因：气管插管、颅内高压、癫痫、高凝状态及止痛。

一线药物

• 甲苄咪酯：0.2～0.3 mg/kg，静脉推注。
• 芬太尼：如 SBP>100 mmHg，3～5 μg/kg，静脉使用。
• 3%高渗盐水：3～5 ml/kg，超过 10～15 min。
• 左乙拉西坦：每次静注 1 g(20 mg/kg)。
• 甘露醇：0.5～1 g/kg，静脉滴注。
• 咪达唑仑：0.04～0.2 mg/(kg·h)。
• 苯妥英钠：15～20 mg/kg，静脉推注，最大剂量为 1 000 mg。
• 异丙酚：10～80 μg/(kg·min)。
• 罗库溴铵：0.6 mg/kg，静脉推注。
• 琥珀胆碱：1～2 mg/kg，静脉推注。
• 维库溴铵：0.1 mg/kg，静脉推注；小剂量预处理：0.01 mg/kg，静脉推注。
• 维生素 K：
- 因服用香豆素出现颅内出血的患者，可给予维生素 K。
- 10 mg 加入 50 ml 生理盐水缓慢推注，持续 30 min。
• 硫酸鱼精蛋白：
- 使用低分子肝素合并颅内出血时。
- 如 8 h 内使用过低分子肝素，则按 1 mg 低分子肝素：1 mg 鱼精蛋白的剂量缓慢静脉推注，静脉推注时间超过 3 min。
- 如 8 h 前使用过低分子肝素，则按 1 mg 低分子肝素：0.5 mg 鱼精蛋白的剂量缓慢静脉推注，时间超过 3 min。

 随访

■ 进一步处理

入院指征

• 头部外伤合并血肿的患者必须送入 ICU 或者接受手术。
• 蛛网膜下腔出血和弥漫性轴索损伤的患者需立即送入 ICU。
• 症状进行性加重的患者，如重复询问、早期记忆丧失、定向障碍的患者应当送入监护病房进行神经系统评估。

出院指征

• 症状缓解，头颅 CT 阴性且无其他因素(如中毒、其他外伤)的患者可以出院。
• 既往抗凝的患者伤后 4～6 h 的头颅 CT 无阳性发现。
• 轻微头部外伤、无意识丧失且神经系统查体正常的患者可在家人陪同下医嘱离院。

儿科注意事项

怀疑非意外造成的创伤必须向有关法律部门报告。

转诊问题

有脑震荡症状的患者需要由心理医师、运动医学医师或神经科医师随访判定合适才能正常运动。

■ 随访建议

如果出现头痛加重、视力变化、意识模糊、神经定位体征或有其他症状的改变，需要立即复诊。

要点和误区

• 遗漏抗凝药物服用史的询问以及未给予适当的影像学检查。
• 未积极纠正低凝状态。
• 未建议脑震荡患者经过心理医师、运动医学医师或神经科医师判定即开始恢复运动。

T

头痛 Headache

Josh W. Joseph 刘雪峰 译

 基础知识

■ 描述

• 包含颅脑、眼眶、上端颈项等部位的疼痛。
• 头颅疼痛可投射于体表：
- 颅内：
◦ 动脉、静脉、硬脑膜及脑膜。
- 颅外：
◦ 皮肤、头皮、筋膜及肌肉。
◦ 鼻窦黏膜。
◦ 动脉。
◦ 颞颌关节，牙齿。
• 三叉神经可传导疼痛。
• 可能由几种机制导致：
- 神经刺激。
- 痛敏血管的收缩。
- 痛敏血管的舒张。
◦ 低氧血症，高碳酸血症，发热，组胺释放，摄入硝酸甘油。
• 占全部急诊的 2%～4%：
- 95%由良性病因导致(50 岁以上人群中此比例下降)。
- 威胁生命的病因较少，且难以确诊。

■ 病因

• 偏头痛：
- 颅内/外痛敏血管的舒张与牵拉。
- 可与皮质抑郁有关。
- 搏动性疼痛。
• 紧张性头痛：
- 类似疼痛发作 10 次以上。
- 病因不明(可能与 5-羟色胺失衡、内啡肽释放减少、痉挛相关)。
- 反复发作性头痛中最常见的类型。
- 可由不良姿势、应激、焦虑、抑郁、颈椎病引起。
- 双侧，非搏动性，束带感。
- 持续 4～13 h。
• 丛集性头痛：
- 由酒精、某种事物、睡眠习惯改变、强烈的情绪波动诱发。
- 可能与脑神经旁的血管痉挛有关。
• 颅内病变(牵拉、压力改变)：
- 占位性病变。
- 特发性颅内压增高。
• 颅外病变(非紧张性)：
- 病变累及头颈部的外周神经引起疼痛。
• 炎性头痛：
- 颞动脉炎。
- 脑内血管炎。
• 血栓性头痛：

- 颅内静脉窦血栓。
• 血管损伤后出现的内皮功能紊乱与自动调节：
- 后部可逆性白质脑病综合征。
- 可逆性脑血管收缩综合征。

儿科注意事项

儿童引起头痛的严重疾病较少见，但因此就诊的患儿都应该接受儿科医师随访。

老年人注意事项

老年人新出现的头痛很可能由某种严重疾病引起，因此应该酌情使用影像学检查进行彻底评估。

妊娠注意事项

孕妇头痛除其他原因外，需要重视静脉窦血栓、子痫、后部可逆性白质脑病综合征，以及可逆性脑血管收缩综合征。

诊断

症状和体征

病史

• 疼痛的属性：PQRST。
- 诱发与缓解的特点：
◦ 头部位置、咳嗽或牵拉(增加颅内压)，以及运动。
- 性质：
◦ 搏动性或持续性。
◦ 深部或表浅部位。
◦ 与之前相比有无变化。
- 范围。
- 严重程度。
- 是否是经历过的最严重的？
- 时机。
- 突发性或规律性？
• 相关检查结果：
- 视力、头晕、恶心与呕吐。
• 附加试验：
- 新发作病例：
◦ 年龄>50 岁。
◦ 艾滋病、移植或肿瘤患者。
- 创伤或跌倒(即使无头部撞击)。
- 顽固性呕吐。
- 任何新的局部神经系统或视觉症状体征。
• 静脉窦血栓的危险因素：
- 恶性肿瘤。
- 妊娠或产后。
- 蛋白质 S/C 缺乏。
- 口服避孕药。
- 溃疡性结肠炎。
- 白塞综合征。

体格检查

• 体温和血压。
• 完整的神经系统检查。
• 视神经检查。
• 皮肤：
- 带状疱疹。
- 紫癜。
- 颞动脉触诊。
• 检查假性脑膜炎。
- 颈强直。
- Kerning 征：
◦ 大腿在 90°在臀部和膝盖处弯曲，随后膝盖的伸展会产生疼痛。
- Brudzinski 征：
◦ 当颈部弯曲时，严重的颈部僵硬会导致患者的臀部和膝盖弯曲。
- 耻骨联合征：压迫耻骨联合导致腿外展，髋关节和膝关节屈曲反射。
- 面颊征：颧骨下方面颊的压力导致前臂的上升和屈曲。

基本检查

• 详细病史询问，详细检查中枢神经系统、五官及颈部。
• 除病史与体格检查以外，指示需要安排排查的因素：
- 严重的舒张压升高。
- 发热。
- 意识状态改变。
- 视神经乳头水肿。
- 异常的神经系统检查或脑膜刺激征。

诊断检查与说明

实验室检查

• 脑脊液：
- 脑膜刺激征可疑阳性及蛛网膜下腔出血患者的基本检查。
• 红细胞沉降率：
- 一过性动脉炎或其他炎性反应失衡：
◦ 见巨细胞动脉炎。

影像学检查

• 头颅 CT：
- 适应证：
◦ 依靠病史和体检无法确诊。
◦ 有颅内压增高的表现。
◦ 首次发作或剧烈疼痛。
◦ 新的异常局部神经定位体征。
◦ 视神经乳头水肿。
◦ 反复发作的晨起头痛。
◦ 顽固性呕吐。
◦ 伴有发热、皮疹及恶心。
◦ 头部外伤伴有意识障碍、局灶性的神经系统异常及昏睡。
◦ 神志状态改变，脑膜刺激征阳性。
- 发作 6 h 内行 CT 并由影像科主诊医师阅片，可明确是否存在蛛网膜下腔出血(SAH)。
- 24 h 内灵敏度>95%(随着时间的延长，灵敏度快速下降，7 日后约为 50%)。
• 静脉窦成像可以显示急性静脉窦炎，慢性静脉窦炎很少引发急性头痛。
• MRI：
- 可用于评估 CT 及 LP 未显示的病因：
◦ 颅后窝病变。
◦ 垂体卒中。
◦ 颅内静脉窦血栓。
• MRA：
- 怀疑蛛网膜下腔出血，CT 显示阴性结果又无法行腰椎穿刺检查者。
- 怀疑由颈动脉及颈椎的问题所致(如近期曾有颈部操作或创伤)。
- 怀疑非偏头痛性血管性头痛。

诊断步骤/外科

腰椎穿刺：
• 首先行 CT 检查：
◦ 新的神经系统阳性发现。
◦ 视乳头水肿。
◦ 神志状态异常。
◦ HIV 阳性或患有其他免疫抑制疾病。
• 检测颅内或脑膜感染。
• CT 不明显时可检测血细胞：
- 红细胞计数没有排除 SAH 的下限阈值，它将随时间变化。
• 脑脊液测压：
- 诊断假性脑瘤静脉窦血栓的必需方法。
- 可以区分真性出血与操作引起的假性出血还是真性出血。
• 黄变症：
- 蛛血发病 12 h 可以观察到。
- 目测是最常用的办法，光谱测定敏感度高，但也有很高的假阳性率。

鉴别诊断

• 注意：下面分组中存在有意义的重叠部分。
• 急性单发性头痛：
- 蛛网膜下腔出血。
- 脑膜炎。
- 血管源性：
◦ 急性颅内出血。

T

    - 高血压脑病。
    - 颅内动脉解剖异常。
    - 静脉窦血栓。
    - 小脑卒中。
  - 视觉相关性：
    - 急性闭角性青光眼。
    - 垂体卒中。
    - 颞神经炎。
  - 外伤。
  - 急性鼻窦炎。
  - 中毒/代谢性。
    - 发热。
    - 低血糖。
    - 高原反应。
    - 一氧化碳中毒。
  - 麻醉药、酒精、苯二氮䓬类药物戒断症状。
  - 腰椎穿刺术后。
  - 冷刺激头痛。
- 急性复发性头痛：
  - 病程几日到几周。
  - 静脉窦血栓。
  - 假性脑瘤。
  - 颞动脉炎。
  - 蛛血(再次出血)。
  - 偏头痛、丛集性头痛及紧张性头痛。
  - 低氧血症。
  - 三叉神经痛。
  - 带状疱疹所致神经痛。
  - 性交劳累性头痛。
- 亚急性头痛：
  - 病程由几周至数月。
  - 慢性硬膜下血肿。
  - 脑肿瘤。
  - 脑脓肿。
  - 慢性鼻窦炎。
  - 颞颌关节综合征。
  - 慢性创伤后头痛。
  - 假性脑瘤。
  - 颞动脉炎。
- 慢性头痛：
  - 病程在数月以上。
  - 慢性紧张性头痛。
  - 镇痛药滥用或戒断症状。
  - 抑郁。
  - 颅外疾病：
    - 三叉神经痛：短暂、电击样面部疼痛。
    - 颞动脉炎：中老年多发、疼痛剧烈、头皮动脉变硬肿胀。
    - 代谢性：中重度贫血。
    - 急性青光眼：恶心、眼痛、结膜充血、眼压增高。
    - 颈椎：椎关节僵硬、外伤、关节炎。

治疗

初步稳定/治疗

- 如神志状态有变化进行急救 ABC 管理。
- 如果考虑细菌性脑膜炎，经验性给予抗生素，如果患者伴有免疫功能低下，需要给予阿昔洛韦。

急诊治疗/程序

- 偏头痛(见头痛、偏头痛)。
- 紧张性头痛：
    - 阿司匹林。
    - 对乙酰氨基酚。
    - 非甾体抗炎药。
    - 非药物疗法(冥想、按摩、生物反馈疗法)。
  - 丛集性头痛(见头痛、丛集性头痛)。
  - 颞动脉炎(见巨细胞动脉炎)。
  - 颅内感染(见脑膜炎)。
  - 颅内出血(见蛛网膜下腔出血)。
- 避免对疑似偏头痛患者使用阿片类药物。

药物治疗

- 氯丙嗪：25～50 mg，肌内注射或静脉注射(儿童：0.5～1 mg/kg，肌内注射或静脉注射或口服)，q4～6 h。
- 地塞米松：10～24 mg，静脉注射。
- 双氢麦角胺：1 mg，肌内注射或静脉注射，1 h 可重复 1 次；最大剂量为 3 mg。
- 麦角胺：首剂 2 mg，口服或皮下注射，之后 1 mg，口服，q30 min；最大剂量 10 mg/周。
- 酮洛酸：30～60 mg，肌内注射；首剂 15～30 mg，静脉注射，此后每 6 h 重复 1 次(儿童：1 mg/kg，静脉注射，q6 h)。
- 4%利多卡因：患侧鼻内给予 1 ml。
- 甲氧氯普胺(胃复安)：50～10 mg，肌内注射、静脉注射或口服，q6～8 h。
- 吗啡：2.5～20 mg(儿童：0.1～0.2 mg/kg)，肌内注射、静脉注射或皮下注射，q2～6 h。
- 普鲁氯嗪：5～10 mg，肌内注射或口服，1～3 次/日；最大剂量 40 mg/d。
- 舒马曲坦：6 mg，皮下注射，1 h 内可重复给药 1 次，最大剂量为 12 mg/24 h。

> **注意**
>
> 药物治疗有效不代表头痛由良性疾病诱发。

随访

进一步处理

入院指征

- 头痛继发于可疑的器质性病变。
- 顽固性呕吐和脱水。
- 门诊止痛治疗无效。
- 入 ICU 标准：
  - 怀疑有症状表现的动脉瘤。
  - 急性硬膜下血肿。
  - 蛛网膜下腔出血。
  - 卒中。
  - 颅内压增高表现。
  - 颅内感染。

出院指征

- 多数的偏头痛、丛集性头痛、紧张性头痛在疼痛缓解后即可出院。
- 局限性或轻微的系统感染。

随访建议

反复发作的头痛患者应由神经科医师随访。

要点和误区

- 24 h之后 CT 对蛛网膜下腔出血的诊断灵敏度快速下降；发病 6 h 后，腰椎穿刺对所有怀疑蛛网膜下腔出血的患者均有必要。
- 不能因神经科会诊而耽搁高风险患者的影像学检查时机。
- 对使用多巴胺的患者需警惕 QT 间期延长和电解质紊乱。合并冠心病的患者需谨慎使用麦角胺和曲坦类药物。
- 多次复诊的慢性头痛患者可以从疼痛门诊管理中受益，但是医师需要警惕他们症状的变化。
- 怀疑脑膜炎可在腰椎穿刺结果回报之前给予经验性治疗。

T

头晕/眩晕 Dizziness/Vertigo

Kiersten L. Gurley · Jonathan A. Edlow 姜颢 张连东 译

基础知识

描述

• 头晕，3%～4%的患者到急诊就诊，每年花费超过 40 亿美元，症状难以诊断，经常被误诊。

• 患者用各种词语来描述他们的经历，包括：

- 眩晕(运动的错觉)。
- 虚弱，昏厥。
- 头晕。
- 不稳定。

• 关键点：患者使用的词(例如，眩晕和头晕)在诊断上并不重要。发作的时间和触发因素推动了评估(见下文)。

• 为了最好地找到原因，而不是专注于患者使用的描述语，请记录一份标准病史，重点是尝试了解患者是否有某种毒性-代谢-感染原因(例如，胃肠道出血、全身感染或心律失常)，50%患有头晕的勃起功能障碍患者就是这种情况。

• 如果没有明显的原因，使用定时和触发器将患者分为三类之一：

- 急性前庭综合征(AVS)：连续眩晕的急性发作。
- 触发性阵发性前庭综合征(T-EVS)：通常由头部或身体运动触发的短暂性眩晕发作。
- 自发性阵发性前庭综合征(S-EVS)：无任何原因触发的较长时间头晕发作。

病因

• 毒性-代谢-感染性原因：

- 毒素和多种药物。
- 电解质紊乱和脱水。
- 全身性感染。
- 节律障碍。

• AVS：

- 最常见的原因。
- 前庭神经炎和迷路炎。
- 后循环卒中。
- 多发性硬化。
- 韦尼克-特里格。

• T-EVS：

- BPPV。
- 直立性低血压。
- 罕见的中枢性阵发性位置性眩晕(CPPV)。

• S-EVS：

- 前庭偏头痛。
- 短暂性脑缺血发作(后循环)。
- 梅尼埃病。
- 惊恐发作。
- 罕见的间歇性低流量状态(如心律失常或肺栓塞)。

诊断

症状和体征

病史

• 询问 HPI、ROS 和既往病史中的标准问题，以尝试确定病因是否为毒性-代谢-传染性：

- 如果病史提示这些问题之一，则应进一步询问病史以确定细节(例如，新药物或胃肠道出血)。

• 如果没有，询问发作、持续时间，以及头晕是持续的还是间歇性的：

- 如果头晕是急性开始并持续存在的，这就是动静脉畸形。
- 动静脉畸形患者通常会出现运动不耐受、恶心、经常呕吐，有时步态不稳。
- 运动会加重头晕，但在休息时头晕仍然存在。

• 如果头晕是间歇性的，询问触发因素：

- 间歇性前庭综合征患者在两次发作之间无症状。
- 如果有强制性触发因素(例如，当患者转动或移动头部时)，这是 T-EVS。
- 如果没有明确的触发因素，这是 S-EVS。

体格检查

• 关键点，3 种前庭综合征的体格检查各不相同：

• 头部脉冲试验、眼球震颤试验和偏斜偏差试验(HINTS)已经过专业医师的验证，但不是常规的急救医学实践。

- 我们认为可以学习，但建议采用不同的顺序，并增加脑神经、小脑和步态试验。
- 大多数动静脉畸形患者都有眼球震颤，其特征很重要。
- 首先测试眼球震颤。在动静脉畸形中：方向固定的眼球震颤通常是周边性的；方向改变的、垂直的或主要是扭转性的眼球震颤是中心性的。
- 如果眼球震颤不存在，前庭神经炎或迷路炎几乎肯定不是正确的诊断。
- 在没有眼球震颤的患者中，步态测试变得更加重要：头部脉冲试验(HIT)尚未被证实是有用的。
- 眼球震颤测试后，进行交替遮盖测试以寻找偏斜偏差。
- 下一步，如果存在眼球震颤，进行头部脉冲试验(HIT)：
  - 如果存在矫正性眼跳(水平眼球运动)，这通常是外周性(前庭神经炎)。
  - 如果没有矫正性眼跳，这与后循环脑卒中一致。
- 测试脑神经是否有任何异常(这意味着颅后窝的结构诊断)。
- 测试小脑功能-手指到鼻和脚跟到胫骨的测试。
- 最后，测试步态：
  - 大多数前庭神经炎患者能够行走，而大多数后循环脑卒中患者不能行走。
  - 对于太恶心而不能行走的患者，可以通过要求患者坐在担架上而不扶着侧栏来测试躯干共济失调。
- 如果这些测试中的任何一项令人担心是中枢原因造成，则假设是脑卒中，直到找到证据排除。

• 阵发性前庭综合征：

- 测量直立性位状态下生命体征，一般有直立性低血压病史。
- 测试小脑功能-手指到鼻和脚跟到胫骨的测试。
- 如果 BPPV 是可能的诊断，首先进行双侧 Dix-Hallpike 操作(以测试后半规管)：
  - 在 BBPV 中，Dix-Hallpike 一侧为阳性(症状和通常向上震颤扭转性眼球震颤)而另一侧为阴性。
  - 如果 Dix-Hallpike 双侧为阴性，通过进行仰卧位头部滚动测试来测试水平管。
  - 在仰卧位头部滚动中，双侧都是阳性，但其中一侧症状更加明显。
- 如果没有眼球震颤，前庭神经炎或迷路炎几乎肯定不是正确的诊断。

• S-EVS：

- 体检在阵发性前庭综合征是无用的，因为根据定义，患者不再有症状，并且不能在床边引发眩晕。

注意

- HIT 仅在伴有眼球震颤的动静脉畸形患者中有意义。
- Dix-Hallpike 试验仅一侧阳性(除了非常罕见的双侧后半规管 BPPV 的情况)。

基本检查

要点:检查取决于体格检查:

- 在动静脉畸形患者中,没有令人担忧的眼震,没有偏斜偏差,正常的 HIT,包括步态在内的正常神经系统检查,可以当前庭神经炎/迷路炎治疗。
- 在 T-EVS 试验中,位置动作试验阳性的患者不需要任何检查,可以当 BPPV 治疗。
- 在 T-EVS 试验中,直立引起的,需要检查直立眩晕的病因。
- S-EVS 的患者,需要进行短暂性脑缺血发作检查,除非怀疑是前庭性偏头痛。

诊断检查与说明

实验室检查

- 对于可能具有毒性-代谢-传染性的头晕患者,实验室检测的用处取决于诊断的可能性。
- 前庭综合征患者,实验室检测用处较少。

影像学检查

- CT 扫描在后循环卒中的患者中用处不大。
- 在最初的 48 h, MRI 可能假阴性。

诊断步骤/外科

- 交替遮盖试验:让患者将注意力集中在检查者的鼻上,交替遮盖一只眼睛和另一只眼睛;寻找一个小的垂直校正(偏斜偏差)来指示中央病变。
- 头部脉冲试验:患者将注意力集中在检查者的鼻上,非常快速地将患者的头部从偏离中心移动 10°~15°,首先在一侧,然后在另一侧。这测试前庭眼反射。在阳性测试中(涉及中枢),患者的眼睛仍然盯着检查者的鼻。在阴性测试中(周围性病变),有一个正确的扫视。
- Dix-Hallpike 和仰卧摆头试验是测试 BPPV 的物理动作。优秀的视频剪辑可以在网上找到。

鉴别诊断

始终寻找引起症状的中毒性-代谢性-感染原因,包括但不限于:

- 糖尿病。
- 甲状腺功能减退。
- 娱乐药物(如酒精、巴比妥酸盐、水杨酸盐)。
- 过度通气。
- 心血管(如心律失常、心肌梗死或晕厥的其他病因),外周血管疾病(如高血压、直立性低血压、血管迷走性)。
- 感染/败血症。
- 急性贫血(如胃肠道出血)。
- 严重电解质异常和低血糖。
- 急性毒性药物:
  - 氨基糖苷类药物。
  - 抗疟药物。
  - 红霉素。
  - 呋塞米。
- 急性神经瘤和其他颅后窝肿瘤:
- 外伤:
  - 鼓膜破裂、圆窗、迷路震荡或外淋巴瘘均可出现严重症状。
  - 震荡后综合征或继发于颅底骨折的迷路或第 8 脑神经损伤。
  - 椎动脉损伤曾在颈椎按摩治疗后出现。
- 中耳炎和伴有渗出的浆液性中耳炎。
- 脑干高血压性脑病。
- 颞叶癫痫:
  - 与幻觉、失语症、恍惚状态或抽搐有关。
  - 更常见于年轻患者。
- 锁骨下动脉盗血综合征:
  - 手臂运动导致血液从椎基底动脉分流至锁骨下动脉,导致眩晕或晕厥。
  - 继发于锁骨下动脉狭窄。
  - 单侧桡动脉脉搏减弱或两臂间收缩血压差异。

治疗

初步稳定/治疗

绝大多数头晕患者不需要稳定,除非他们需要静脉补液治疗脱水。最初的步骤完全基于患者个体的潜在病因。

急诊治疗/程序

- BPPV 患者,可采取有明确治疗效果的各种耳石复位方法(优秀的视频剪辑可在网上获得):
  - 对于后耳道 BPPV, Epley 策略通常是有治疗价值的。
  - 对于水平耳道 BPPV, Lempert 翻滚策略通常是治疗性的。
  - 对于难治性患者存在替代方法。
- 必要时给予药物控制眩晕症状和/或恶心。
  - 抗组胺药。
  - 苯二氮䓬类。
  - 止吐药。
- 静脉注射抗生素治疗急性细菌性迷路炎(罕见)。

药物治疗

- 地西泮(安定):2.5~5 mg,静脉注射,q8 h;或 2~10 mg,口服,q8 h。
- 乘晕宁(晕海宁):25~50 mg,静脉注射、肌内注射或口服,q6 h。
- 苯海拉明(苯那君):25~50 mg,静脉注射、肌内注射或口服,q6 h。
- 氯羟去甲安定(劳拉西泮):1 mg,静脉注射或肌内注射;或 1~2 mg,口服,q4~6 h。
- 氯苯甲嗪(敏克静):25 mg,口服,q6 h,必要时。
- 异丙嗪(非那根):12.5 mg,静脉注射,q6 h;或 25~50 mg,肌内注射或口服,q6 h。

儿科注意事项

同样的鉴别诊断。

孕妇建议

妊娠剧吐的孕妇可能会患 Wernicke 脑病,表现类似动静脉畸形。

随访

进一步处理

入院指征

- 入院取决于病因。
- 患有前庭神经炎或迷路炎的患者通常建议门诊使用类固醇激素。
- 症状太剧烈或持续呕吐,或不安全而无法回家的患者,可能需要入院接受补液治疗和控制症状。
- 患有短暂性脑缺血发作或脑卒中的患者,通常会入院接受进一步的检查和治疗。

出院指征

- 大多数周围神经所致眩晕患者可以安全出院。
- 如果在急诊或急诊留观完成必要的检查,TIA 患者可以出院。

转诊问题

见出院标准。

■ 随访建议

所有因动静脉畸形或 EVS 综合征而出院的患者都应进行密切随访，通常由神经科医师或耳鼻喉科医师进行。

要点和误区

• 基于时间和触发因素来鉴别（动静脉畸形、T-EVS、S-EVS），而不是将患者用来描述其头晕的词（如眩晕与头晕）。

• 动静脉畸形患者，使用物理检查来区分外周原因（前庭神经炎或迷路炎）和中枢原因（后循环脑卒中）。

• 动静脉畸形患者，使用物理检查来诊断和治疗 BPPV 病患者。

• 后循环短暂性脑缺血发作可出现孤立的自发性头晕发作。

透析并发症 Dialysis Complications

Erika Phindile Chowa · Brooks L. Moore 谭美春 译

基础知识

■ 描述

透析并发症有：

• 血管通路相关（感染、出血）。

• 非血管通路相关（低血压、高血钾）。

• 腹膜透析相关。

■ 病因

• 血管通路相关：

- 感染：

◦ 感染（大部分通路相关或者腹膜炎）是透析患者的主要死因。

◦ 常由葡萄球菌引发。

◦ 可表现为局部感染或全身感染。

◦ 血液透析导管的感染风险比房室瘘或移植物高 2～3 倍。

◦ 感染性并发症包括心内膜炎、骨髓炎、脊髓硬膜外脓肿、脓毒性关节炎、脑脓肿和菌栓性肺动脉栓塞。

- 房室置入物/瘘血栓形成或狭窄。

◦ 血栓形成和狭窄是血液透析房室通路最常见的并发症。

◦ 必须尽快处理（24 h 内），以避免血管通路的丧失。

◦ 处理主要是外科手术；然而，介入治疗也被使用。

- 出血：

◦ 动脉瘤形成和/或细菌感染削弱了血管壁，增加了出血的风险。

◦ 导管与房室通道断开后，血液透析后会发生出血。

• 非血管通路相关因素：

- 低血压：

◦ 最常见的血液透析并发症。

◦ 透析后：经常由于循环血液量急性减少所致。

◦ 透析时：低血容量（更常见）或由于容量超负荷矫正后出现突然全身代偿性积液导致心脏压塞。

◦ 心肌梗死、败血症、心律失常和缺氧。

◦ 抗凝治疗继发出血、肾衰竭所致的血小板功能异常。

- 呼吸急促：

◦ 容量负荷过重。

◦ 透析期间呼吸困难的发生常由于心脏压塞、心包积液、出血、过敏反应、肺栓塞、空气栓塞造成。

- 胸痛：

◦ 缺血性：

▪ 有动脉粥样硬化性疾病的透析患者往往存在高风险。

▪ 透析是一个急性生理应激源，伴有一过性低血压和低氧血症，可增加心肌耗氧量。

◦ 胸膜炎：

▪ 心包炎、肺栓塞。

- 神经功能障碍：平衡失调综合征。

◦ 透析过程中血浆渗透压急剧下降使得大脑处于相对高渗的状态。

• 腹膜：

- 腹膜炎：

◦ 液体交换期间由于腹膜透析液或管道的污染造成。

▪ 可能是肠道细菌移位造成的。内脏穿孔可以有类似表现。

◦ 金黄色葡萄球菌或表皮葡萄球菌（70%）。

◦ 大多数接受腹膜透析的患者一生中至少会发生一次腹膜炎。

- 感染或炎症导致纤维蛋白堵塞导管。

诊断

■ 症状和体征

• 血管通路相关因素：

- 穿刺部位出血。

- 瘘管或移植物杂音或震颤消失。

- 局部感染，蜂窝织炎，发热。

- 血管通路远端感觉和力量减退。

- 毗邻血管通路处新生或尺寸增大的包块。

• 非血管通路相关：

- 术前、术中或术后的低血压。

- 心动过速。

- 心悸。

- 晕厥。

- 胸痛：

◦ 缺血性。

◦ 胸膜炎。

- 出血：

◦ 胃肠道。

◦ 胸膜。

◦ 腹膜后。

- 呼吸急促：

- 神经系统症状（平衡失调综合征）：

◦ 头痛。

◦ 不适。

◦ 癫痫。

◦ 昏迷。

• 腹膜：

- 腹痛。

- 浑浊的透析液。

- 恶心、呕吐。

- 在 Tenckhoff 导管插入部位有分泌物或炎症。

■ 基本检查

• 仔细的查体：

- 寻找感染的迹象，感受有无疼痛和在房室管路中明显的震颤消失。

- 一套完整的生命体征，包括血压、脉搏、呼吸频率，精确测量体温、脉搏和血氧饱和度。

- 仔细体检查找隐匿性感染源(牙源性、直肠周围脓肿)。
- 肺部听诊查找感染(干啰音)或容量超负荷的证据(湿啰音)。
- 寻找容量超负荷的其他证据(水肿)。
- 仔细的心脏检查,包括听诊杂音或摩擦音。
• 心电图:寻找电解质紊乱或传导阻滞的征象。
• 感染:
- 血液和创面分泌物的培养。
- 细胞计数,革兰染色,腹水培养。
• 出血:
- 全血细胞计数:评估贫血和血小板计数。
- 凝血功能检查。
• 胸痛或气促:
- 胸部 X 线检查。
- 动脉血气分析。
- 心电图、心肌酶(根据病史适合时)。
• 神经功能障碍:脑 CT 用于检查颅内出血。

诊断检查与说明

实验室检查

• 葡萄糖、电解质、尿素氮和肌酐。
• 全血细胞计数。

影像学检查

• 心电图怀疑有:
- 高钾血症。
- 心包炎。
- 心包积液。
- 心脏压塞。
• 超声评估可能凝固的连接处或瘘口。
• 心脏超声评估心包积液、压塞。
• 腹膜透析管阻塞。
• 肺栓塞及头颅的 CT 扫描:
- 肾功能不全时可给予静脉造影剂。
◦ 造影剂加重肾单元负担,但不需要紧急透析。

鉴别诊断

• 低血压:
- 脓毒症。
- 心源性休克、急性心肌梗死、心脏压塞、心律失常。
- 电解质紊乱,导致心律失常(高血钾和低血钾)。
- 栓塞:空气栓塞或肺栓塞。
- 低血容量。
- 血管不稳定:自主神经病变、药物相关、透析液相关。
• 神经系统并发症:
- 脑血管意外。
- 平衡失调综合征。
- 高血糖或低血糖。
- 高钠血症或低钠血症。
- 低氧血症。
- 颅内出血。
- 脑膜炎或脓肿。
- 尿毒症。
• 腹膜并发症:
- 腹膜炎。
- 疝嵌顿。
- 内脏穿孔。
- 急性腹痛:阑尾炎、胆囊炎。

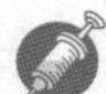

治疗

院前

> **注意**
> • 不要用肢体移植物或瘘管执行静脉内给药和血压测量。
> • 尽可能放慢静脉补液速度,并保持最小速度。
> • 肺水肿使用呋塞米(无尿患者:最高使用剂量≤200 mg)。

初步稳定/治疗

• 检查气道、呼吸及循环。
• 血管通路相关:
- 出血:
◦ 压迫止血。
◦ 不要完全堵塞通道,否则可能导致凝血。
◦ 压迫止血至少需要持续 5～10 min,即使是轻微的出血。
◦ 记录按压后是否有震颤感。
◦ 应用明胶海绵。
• 非血管通路相关:
- 低血压:
◦ 寻找根本原因。
◦ 升压药,补液。
- 呼吸急促:
◦ 用硝酸酯类和 ACEI 类药物减轻心脏前、后负荷。
◦ 如果怀疑体液过多则尝试用利尿剂。
◦ 安排透析。
- 高钾血症:
◦ 在适当的时候静脉使用钙剂、碳酸氢盐、胰岛素和葡萄糖(请参见"高钾血症")。
◦ 监测心脏节律。
◦ 用离子交换树脂(聚苯乙烯磺酸钠)有争议。
◦ 安排紧急透析。
- 神经系统并发症:
◦ 使用纳洛酮、硫胺素、葡萄糖(或 POC 葡萄糖)治疗精神异常。
◦ 用苯二氮䓬类药物控制癫痫发作。

急诊治疗/程序

• 血管通路相关:
- 感染:
◦ 静脉使用抗生素抗葡萄球菌。
- 通路凝血:
◦ 镇痛。
◦ 热敷。
◦ 血管外科会诊。
- 出血:
◦ 控制出血。
◦ 纠正凝血功能障碍。
◦ 静脉输注液体和血液制品。
• 非血管通路相关:
- 电解质失衡:
◦ 初始稳定后,安排透析。
◦ 如果透析不容易获得:
◦ 前、后负荷降低后(硝酸甘油、依那普利)用呋塞米利尿。
◦ 持续监测。
◦ 继续处理电解质异常。
- 容量超负荷:
◦ 尝试用亚硝酸盐和呋塞米利尿。
◦ 必要时进行无创正压通气。
◦ 安排透析。
- 心包积液或心脏压塞:
◦ 对生命体征不稳定的患者进行必要的紧急心包穿刺。
◦ 安排透析。
- 急性心肌梗死:
◦ 依据患者情况选择溶栓或血管成形术。
◦ 硝酸酯类药物减轻心肌负荷。
- 平衡失调综合征:
◦ 排除其他原因造成的精神状态改变。
◦ 一般情况下随着时间推移可以缓解。
• 腹膜:
- 腹膜炎:静脉注射或腹腔内使用抗生素。
- 导管培养或通道感染,可见分泌物:
◦ 口服抗生素(抗葡萄球菌)。
◦ 如果复发或通道感染,可能需要切开。
◦ 细致的局部护理。
- 腹膜穿孔或粘连:
◦ 静脉使用抗生素。

T

◦ 外科会诊。

▪ 药物治疗

• 葡萄糖酸钙：1 g，缓慢静脉注射（高钾血症与 QRS 波群增宽）。

• 头孢唑林：1 g，静脉注射或肌内注射，随后 250 mg/2 L 袋，10 日（腹膜炎）。

• 卡托普利：25 mg，舌下含服。

• 葡萄糖 D_{50} W：1 安瓿 50 ml 或 25 g（儿童：葡萄糖 D_{25} W 2～4 ml/kg）静脉注射。

• 多巴胺：2～20 μg/（kg · min），静脉注射。

• 依那普利：1.25 mg，静脉注射。

• 呋塞米：20～100 mg，静脉注射（慢性肾衰竭影响利尿时可能需要剂量≥30 mg）。

• 胰岛素：5～10 U，常规胰岛素静脉注射（D_{50} 的高钾血症）。

• 纳洛酮（盐酸烯丙羟吗啡酮）：初始剂量 2 mg（儿童：0.1 mg/kg），静脉注射或肌内注射。

• 硝酸甘油：0.4 mg，舌下含服；5～20 μg/min 静脉注射。

• 碳酸氢钠：1 mmol/kg 增量至 50～100 mmol，必要时静脉注射。

• 降钾树脂（聚苯乙烯磺酸钠）：1 g/kg 增量至 15～60 g 口服或 30～50 g 保留灌肠，q6 h，必要时（高钾血症）。

• 维生素（维生素 B_1）：100 mg（儿童：50 mg），静脉注射或肌内注射。

• 妥布霉素：1.7 mg/kg，静脉注射或肌内注射，随后 10 mg/2 L 袋，10 日（腹膜炎）。

• 万古霉素：1 g，静脉注射或肌内注射，随后 50 mg/2 L 袋，10 日（腹膜炎）。

随访

▪ 进一步处理

入院指征

• 入住 ICU：
- 严重高钾血症。
- 严重肺水肿。
- 持续性低血压。
- 不受控制的癫痫发作。
- 急性心肌梗死。
- 心血管意外。
- 心包炎。
- 严重脓毒症。
- 有全身中毒症状的腹膜炎。

• 常规住院：
- 发热。
- 呕吐。
- 无中毒或全身症状的腹膜炎。
- 无致命性的生命的电解质紊乱。
- 非长期卧床的患者进行连续的腹膜透析而不能够自主抗生素治疗的。

出院指征

• 轻微通路感染。

• 一些血栓切除术的日间手术。

• 穿刺部位止血。

▪ 随访建议

大多数透析患者由肾脏专科医师的密切随访。

要点和误区

• 透析患者需考虑心脏压塞，即使他们没有表现出典型症状。

• 透析患者始终需考虑高钾血症。

• 透析患者感染可表现轻微，感染是导致并发病和死亡的常见原因。

• 早期血管外科会诊对通路凝血或破裂非常重要。

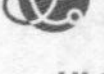

T

兔热病 Tularemia

Scott Bentz　张晟　林兆奋 译

基础部分

▪ 描述

• 兔热病是由需氧的细胞内寄生的多形性革兰阴性土拉热弗朗西斯菌所致急性发热性疾病。
- 传染性强。
- 尚无人传人的报道。

• 人类通过于不同的环境的暴露而被感染。
- 被受感染的蜱、鹿蝇、蚊子或其他昆虫叮咬。
- 与受感染的动物组织或体液直接接触。
- 接触或摄入受污染的食物、水、土壤。
- 吸入受感染的气溶胶（如使用高功率割草机打草可使病菌被气雾化）。
- 预防应以驱虫剂为主，避免接触未经处理的地表水，在接触动物如兔子、土拨鼠、啮齿动物和彻底烹调肉类时应戴手套。

• 该菌的 4 种主要菌株有不同的毒力和地理分布。
- 在北美 2 个亚种可造成人类感染：F. tularensis 亚种 tularensis（A 型，毒性较强）和 F. tularensis 亚种 holartica（B 型，毒力弱）。在欧洲，B 型占主导地位。

• 自然宿主：
- 兔类和其他啮齿动物。
- 发现于野生动物（野兔、蜱、苍蝇、麝鼠、海狸、家鼠）、家畜（羊、牛、猫）、蜱，以及被感染动物污染的土壤和水中。

• 自然带菌者：
- 蜱。
- 苍蝇。
- 蚊子。
- 野兔。
- 啮齿动物。

• 兔热症的生物武器化是在冷战期间完成的。
- 因其毒力强，可以雾化喷洒传播，它仍是潜在性大规模杀伤性生物武器。

• 实验室技术人员培养样本的风险很高。
- 土拉热弗朗西斯菌培养只能在生物安全 3 级实验室进行。

▪ 病因

• 在流行区进行户外活动的个体受感染的风险很高：
- 农民。
- 猎人。
- 林务人员。
- 割草工/园艺师。
- 处理动物尸体的人风险最高（动物标本制作者和屠夫）。
- 那些接触过受污染的水域的人。
- 2/3 的病例是男性。

• 兔热病在世界范围内都有发生，但主要流行于北半球：
- 除夏威夷，在全国（美国）范围内都有报道。
- 发病率最高的州包括密苏里州、阿肯色

州、堪萨斯州、南达科他州、俄克拉何马州。
- 科罗拉多州、内布拉斯加州、南达科他州和怀俄明州发病率增加。
- 保守估计美国每年有数百例病例。
- 高发季节是6—10月。
• 死亡率为5%～15%，接受适当治疗的患者死亡率低至1%。

儿科注意事项

• 25%的病例是1～14岁的儿童。
• 在流行区域的乡村户外活动的儿童感染风险高。

诊断

症状和体征

• 因侵入途径不同，兔热病有不同的表现。
- 主要的入侵途径是经皮肤，最常见的是皮肤溃疡。
• 孵化需要3～5日，常为1～14日，皮损通常始于丘疹，往往伴发热。
• 6种疾病：
- 腺体溃疡：
◦ 最常见的表现(见于70%～80%的病例)。
◦ 经皮入侵(抓痕、磨损、昆虫叮咬)至少需要50个病原体。
◦ 最开始，在病菌侵入的部位形成皮肤丘疹。
◦ 随之出现小区域的腺体病变以及全身症状(包括发热、寒战、肌痛、头痛)。
◦ 在30%的病例与肺炎相关。
- 腺病：
◦ 不常见。
◦ 由不明显的磨损侵入淋巴系统或血流。
◦ 小区域的腺体病变而没有周围病变。
- 眼腺型土拉菌病：
◦ 不常见。
◦ 病原体由受污染的血/液体溅入眼内的或者在处理受感染的材料后揉眼睛(如染病的兔子尸体)。
◦ 水肿、结膜炎、刺痛、耳前、颌下或颈部淋巴结肿大。
- 咽部病变：
◦ 不常见。
◦ 摄入受污染的食物或水。
◦ 严重的喉痛、渗出性咽炎和区域性淋巴结炎。
- 肺炎：
◦ 因吸入病原菌引起。
◦ 见于剪羊毛者、农民、园艺工人、实验室技师。
◦ 发热、干咳和发展为胸膜炎胸痛。
◦ 兔热病溃疡性腺病患者中30%可出现肺炎。
- 伤寒形式：
◦ 过去，伤寒形式被定义为没有皮肤或黏膜受损或者没有明显的淋巴结肿大。
◦ 侵入途径不清楚(或许是经口或经呼吸道)。
◦ 只有当不能确定感染途径时才会考虑伤寒。
◦ 在北美，A型流行，据报道有暴发性，症状，包括严重的脓毒症、脑膜炎、心内膜炎、肝衰竭和肾衰竭。
◦ 与A型兔热病相关的脓毒症常极其严重并有潜在致命性。发热、腹痛和腹泻可发生在疾病早期。

病史

• 暴露史和流行病学危险因素可能会有助于诊断。
• 突发高热、寒战、头痛。
• 疾病进展过程中的症状和体征对诊断疾病类型可能有用。

体格检查

• 发热。
• 触痛，界限清楚的皮肤溃疡。
• 区域淋巴结肿大；淋巴结炎可进展为有波动感并且自发溃烂引流。
• 渗出性咽炎(咽部土拉弗朗西斯菌感染)。
• 球结膜溃疡和明显水肿(眼部土拉弗朗西斯菌感染)。

诊断检查与说明

实验室检查

• 缺乏可靠的快速诊断试验。
• 常规实验室检查缺乏特异性：
- 全血细胞计数可正常。
- 红细胞沉降率可能轻度升高。
- 脑脊液：蛋白质增多或细胞计数轻度升高。
- 肝功能通常不正常。
• 革兰染色涂片，培养及组织活检，常阴性。
• 因要求特殊培养基，血培养常阴性。如果需要血液、皮肤、溃疡、淋巴结的培养，这些材料应该接种在富含半胱氨酸的培养基上。
• 可通过参考实验室，获得直接荧光抗体，酶联免疫吸附试验和多聚链反应(的结果)。
• 血清抗体效价：
- 通常情况下，直到发病10日以后才达到诊断标准。
- 试管凝集试验单抗体滴度至少1∶160才可诊断土拉弗朗西斯菌感染。
- 能在发病11日前可能不会升高，通常在发病第16日才能诊断出来。

影像学检查

• 胸部X线：查看实变进程、胸膜腔积液及肺门结节病变。
• 胸部CT：
- 严重的肺部症状。
- 非典型肺炎的其他可能病因。

鉴别诊断

• 与腺体溃疡性兔热病症状类似的包括：
- 结核。
- 猫抓病。
- 梅毒。
- 软下疳。
- 淋巴肉芽肿。
- 弓形虫病。
- 孢子丝虫病。
- 鼠咬伤热。
- 炭疽。
• 与眼腺体兔热病症状类似的包括：
- 腺病毒感染。
• 与咽部兔热病症状类似的包括：
- 白喉。
- 细菌性咽炎。
- 传染性单核细胞增多症。
- 腺病毒感染。
• 与伤寒兔热病症状类似的包括：
- 沙门菌病。
- 布鲁菌病。
- 军团菌感染。
- Q热。
- 疟疾。
- 传染性真菌或分枝杆菌感染。
• 与肺兔热病症状类似的包括：
- 支原体感染。
- 军团菌感染。
- 衣原体感染。
- 结核。

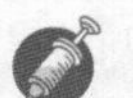

治疗

院前

• 广泛预防。
• ABC管理。
• 对脱水、低血压患者单次快速输入生理盐水。

初步稳定/治疗

• ABC管理。
• 对低氧血症补充性给氧。
• 评估脓毒症/感染性休克的体征并进行相

T

应治疗。

■ 急诊治疗/程序

• 用对乙酰氨基酚控制发热。
• 获得培养结果后，早期应用抗生素治疗。
• 抗生素的选择：
- 一线试剂：链霉素或者庆大霉素连用10日。
- 满18岁患者鉴别诊断社区获得性肺炎时用环丙沙星。
- 四环素、强力霉素或者用氯霉素用于>8岁儿童。
  ◦ 连用14日，因为这些药物只有抑菌作用，三线选择。
  ◦ 比起之前提过的抗生素，治疗失败率更高。
- 土拉弗朗西斯菌对β-内酰胺类和碳青霉烯类抗生素耐药。

儿科注意事项

推荐链霉素或者庆大霉素作一线用药。

■ 药物治疗

一线用药

• 庆大霉素：5 mg/kg，静脉注射或肌内注射，q24 h(儿童：2.5 mg/kg，静脉注射或肌内注射，q8 h)，连用10日。
• 链霉素：1 g，肌内注射(儿童：15 mg/kg，每日不超过2 g)，q12 h，连用10日。

二线用药

• 环丙沙星：400 mg(儿童：15 mg/kg)，静脉注射，q12 h，连用10日。
• 多西环素：100 mg(儿童：如体重≥45 kg，用100 mg；若体重≤45 kg，2.2 mg/kg)，静脉注射，q12 h，至少用14日(因多西环素只是抑菌药，可能需要增加疗程)。
• 氯霉素常有副反应，尽量避免使用。然而，氯霉素因其能穿过血脑屏障并在脑脊液中达到高水平药物浓度，被用于土拉弗朗西斯菌脑膜炎。
• 如果图拉菌被用作生物武器，建议在暴露后预防14日。首选药物是口服环丙沙星和多西环素。

随访

■ 进一步处理

入院指征

• 高龄、中性粒细胞减少、严重的低氧血症、血液动力学不稳或有伤寒免热病表现的患者可进入ICU。
• 轻至中度病情可住院治疗：
- 只有在用于排除其他病原体感染(如结核病)时才需要隔离病床。

出院指征

对病情轻微者紧密跟进治疗可选择口服或肌内注射给药方式并密切随访的门诊管理。

转诊问题

重症监护和传染病科会诊，辅助鉴别诊断和管理威胁生命的并发症。

■ 随访建议

咨询传染病学专家以改进正在进行的治疗方式并降低之后的暴露风险。

要点和误区

• 若患者有高热和区域性淋巴结病变，尤其是有溃疡或球结膜炎，应考虑兔热病的鉴别诊断。
• 病史在指示诊断方面可能有帮助(就业史、接触病或死动物、昆虫叮咬)。
• 最终确诊要以血清学检查为依据，而血清要在感染10日后才呈现阳性。
• 又称“兔子热”或“鹿蝇热”。
• 疫苗目前正在由美国FDA审核，目前在美国并未推广。
• 因其致病性被最新列为A类生物恐怖武器(值得注意的危险种类)，它可通过食物、水或空气传播。隔离是必不可少的。

退行性关节炎 Arthritis, Degenerative

Patrick H. Sweet III · Uziel Sauceda　陈其琪　王海嵘　潘曙明 译

基础知识

■ 描述

• 退行性关节炎或骨关节炎(OA)是最常见的进行性关节疾病，根据CDC国家统计，截至2015年，美国估计患病率为5 400万例。
• 由于人口老龄化和肥胖，预计这一数字将继续增加。
• 几乎只在老年人中发现。

■ 病理学

• 关节滑膜的重复性应力与年龄相关。
• 在年轻患者中可能继发关节创伤。
• 关节软骨的破坏：
- 关节缘骨和软骨下硬化的反应性病变。
• 危险因素包括年龄、肥胖、外伤、遗传、性别和环境。

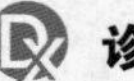

诊断

■ 症状和体征

• 慢性进行性关节疼痛：
- 肢体负重越大越疼痛，休息会缓解疼痛。
• 非对称关节包含：
- 包括手、足、膝、髋关节和脊柱关节。
• 早上关节僵硬时间<30 min。
• 关节畸形表现为活动范围受限。
• 远端指间关节Heberden节点。
• 近端指间关节处的Bouchard节点。
• 缺乏全身症状。
• 常见捻发音。

■ 基本检查

• 将活动范围和功能的检查与评估彻底结合起来。
• 放射线检查：OA典型表现为关节间隙减少、关节边缘的不规则骨及骨刺。
• 设定积液中的滑膜液分析：可能有治疗和诊断作用(见下文)，如果出现红斑和皮肤温度升高，排除感染性关节或痛风是绝对必要的。
• ESR、CRP和CBC：如果感染是在微分关节穿刺术中可以表明，但如果不能排除较浅表的感染(如脓毒性滑囊炎、蜂窝织炎等)。

■ 诊断检查说明

滑液检查典型地显示了如下信息：
• 清除。
• 升高的白细胞计数，但<4 000/mm³。
• 多形核白细胞<25%。
• 类似于血液中的葡萄糖水平(95%～100%)。

影像学检查

- X线片。
- 关节间隙变窄。
- 骨赘形成。
- 边缘骨质侵蚀。
- 软骨下硬化。

鉴别诊断

- 痛风或假性痛风。
- 化脓性关节炎。
- 类风湿关节炎。
- 夏科关节病。
- 关节血肿。
- 覆滑囊炎或软组织感染。

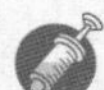

治疗

治疗的总体目标是从症状上缓解。患者可能有疾病的显著的影像学证据，但很少有症状。因此，治疗方案是针对患者的症状而言。

院前

受影响的关节的固定化可以指示直至断裂被排除在外。

初步稳定/治疗

- 敏锐的疼痛管理。
- 开始每日用药，可以让初级保健医师进行管理。
- 适当地加强锻炼。
- 避免不必要的关节固定。

急诊治疗/程序

关节内(IA)的关节穿刺和注射：

- 专业技术和仪器可使用时，建议使用超声(美国)指导。
- 显示了对于具有或不渗液的 OA 的有效低风险干预。
- 虽然在较大的关节比较少见，由于关节和关节周围的软组织(如脂肪垫)的解剖特点可出现干抽。
  - 这种情况下在美国较常用。
- 必须仔细注意无菌操作，在适当位置进行联合，以减轻肌肉紧张，暴露关节间隙。
- 蒸汽冷却剂及 1%或 2%利多卡因用于局部麻醉。
- 在关节穿刺术中通常为 1.5 in 或更大的 22G 或 18G 皮下注射针头应采用 1 注射器在关节穿刺术，而另一个用于 IA 注射皮质类固醇。
- 如果不能排除感染性关节，关节穿刺术后不应服用皮质类固醇。

皮质类固醇的剂量当量：

- 小关节、腕关节和足：
  - 甲泼尼龙 10～20 mg，曲安西龙 10 mg，倍他米松 0.75～1.5 mg。
- 中型关节、肘关节和踝关节：
  - 甲泼尼龙 40～80 mg，曲安西龙 20 mg，倍他米松 3～6 mg。
- 大关节、膝盖和肩膀：
  - 甲泼尼龙 80～120 mg，曲安西龙 40 mg，倍他米松 6～9 mg。
- 有研究表明曲安西龙比其他糖皮质激素更有效，如果有的话建议使用。

药物治疗

一般指导原则：

- 对乙酰氨基酚是首选药物，最初是因为它与非甾体抗炎药相比更安全，在一些患者中已被证明有效。
- 如果一类药物出现问题，可以考虑另一类药物(如水杨酸盐与 COX-2 抑制剂)。
- 最近研究中的 meta 分析表明 2 个替代药物已被证明具有一个小而积极的影响，并可以被认为是辅助剂。
- 所有患者都建议进行餐后管理。胃肠出血加重的患者(如消化性溃疡等的历史)应用 COX-2 抑制剂或质子泵抑制剂与非选择性 COX 抑制剂一起应用。
- 非甾体抗炎药：
  - 塞来昔布(可逆的选择性 COX-2)口服给药间隔 24 h：
    - 注意：禁用于磺胺过敏。
  - 布洛芬(可逆的非选择性 COX)：每 6 h 口服给药 400～600 mg。
  - 萘普生(可逆的非选择性 COX)：每 12 h 口服给药 500 mg。
  - 美洛昔康(可逆的非选择性 COX)：每 12 h 口服给药 7.5 mg 或每 24 h 口服给药 7.5～15 mg。
- 止痛药：
  - 每 24 h 口服对乙酰氨基酚 500 mg(儿童：10～15 mg/kg，不超过 5 剂量/24 h)，不超过 4 g/24 h。
  - 曲马多：每 4～6 h 口服 50 mg：
    - 注意：在老年人慎用，癫痫患者，同时使用抗抑郁药，或肝或肾功能不全患者禁用。
  - 其他阿片类毒品很少使用。
- 替代疗法(单独或组合)：
  - 氨基葡萄糖：每 8 h 口服 500 mg。
  - 软骨素：每 24 h 口服 1 200 mg。
- 改变生活方式：
  - 针对肥胖者减肥。
  - 加强锻炼。

T

随访

进一步处理

入院指征

大多数伴骨折。

出院指征

- 能够走动并能够进行日常生活。
- 活动改善症状(即疼痛)。

运动医学跟进

- 考虑转诊至运动医学诊所进行最终管理。
- 如果髋部或膝盖的晚期 OA，请考虑转诊至关节置换诊所。

吞咽困难 Dysphagia

Daniel A. Willner　姜颢　张连东 译

基础知识

描述

- 吞咽困难。
- 可以是神经肌肉性、机械性、感染性，或是消化道异物。
- 吞咽困难的东西可能是固体、液体，或两者都有。

病因

- 口咽(转移)吞咽困难：
  - 从口中的转移近段食管困难(难以启动

吞咽）。

- 与液体相比更容易吞咽固体。
- 吞咽在几秒钟内。
- 伴有鼻腔或口腔回流、咳嗽或窒息。
- 通常是一个神经肌肉障碍导致延髓肌肉无力或协调受损。

• 食管（传送）吞咽困难：
- 不能正常从食管通过。
- 吞咽后突然感觉胸骨后黏滞感。
- 夜间反流、误吸。
- 流口水或未消化的食物和液体反流（食管梗阻特征）。
- 运动障碍与机械性梗阻相比。

• 功能性吞咽困难：
- 排除诊断。
- 全面检查无机械或神经肌肉病理学证据。
- 症状>12 周。

• 吞咽时痛：
- 吞咽时疼痛。
- 独立的，但通常是相关的，实际存在。
- 原因包括感染、药物诱导和炎症状态。

• 疼痛模式：
- 吞咽困难时疼痛定位整体能力较差，在口咽部稍好。
- 神经纤维位于食管上段，更好疼痛定位。
- 食管下段的内脏疼痛很难定位，难以与急性冠状动脉综合征区分。

儿科注意事项

• 儿童吞咽困难：
- 在婴儿、新生儿常见的原因包括早产、先天性畸形、神经肌肉疾病、感染（例如，念珠菌病）、炎症。
- 儿童吞咽困难通常考虑异物吸入。
- 其他儿童常见的原因包括碱中毒、感染、神经系统疾病（包括头部受伤的后遗症）。
- 儿童获得性气管食管瘘可能由于中毒（磁盘电池、碱中毒）或之前的手术。
- 吞咽困难其他危及生命的原因包括会厌炎、咽后脓肿、中枢神经系统感染、中毒、食管穿孔、白喉。

诊断

症状和体征

• 难以启动吞咽。
• 吞咽后食物梗阻感觉。
• 进食后咳嗽、窒息。
• 咽反射和清咽能力损伤。
• 语音变化、发音困难。
• 流口水。
• 构音障碍。
• 胸痛。
• 呕吐/反流未消化的食物。

病史

• 吞咽固体或液体时有困难，或两者都有困难吗？
- 固体和液体，表明一种神经肌肉疾病。
- 固体或从固体到液体进展，表明一个机械性异常。

• 吞咽后多久出现症状？
- 症状立即发作，表明口咽部原因。
- 延迟（吞咽后数秒），表明食管原因。

• 症状是间歇性的还是渐进的？
- 间歇性症状，表明环状或网状。
- 渐进的症状，表明消化性或恶性狭窄。
- 运动障碍，可以是间歇性的或渐进的。

• 症状持续多久？
- 急性发病与恶性致命性病因更相关。
- 食物的影响是急性发作性吞咽困难的最常见原因。
- 恶性肿瘤也可能进展相对较快。

• 最后一餐吃的什么食物？是什么时候？
- 食物梗阻更可能含有动物蛋白质（牛排、鸡肉、火鸡肉）。
- 鱼刺残留是一种常见的病因。

• 是否有其他相关的症状？
- 例如，鼻腔反流、窒息、心痛、体重减轻。

体格检查

• 常常不显著。
• 口咽检查。
• 对分泌物的耐受情况。
• 发声情况。
• 心肺听诊。
• 神经系统检查重点在脑神经（特别是Ⅴ、Ⅶ、Ⅸ、Ⅹ、Ⅻ）。

基本检查

• 充分气道评估。
• 完整神经系统检查。

诊断检查与说明

心电图：

• 考虑胸部不适的心脏病因。

实验室检查

没有具体检查可用。

影像学检查

• 胸部 X 线检查：
- 贲门失弛缓症：食物扩张食管可被看作纵隔增宽，后纵隔气液平。
- 吸入性肺炎。
- 大量外部肿块压迫。
- 扩张的胸主动脉。
- 异物（纽扣电池、硬币）。

• 颈侧位软组织 X 线。
• 颈部 CT：
- 看不到的异物。

• 改良的吞钡（固体丸）或透视：
- 确定食管解剖。
- 评估功能。
- 如果准备胃镜检查，不进行操作。

• 头颅 CT/MRI。
- 提示新发性神经肌肉性吞咽障碍。

诊断步骤/外科

• 经常在门诊进行：
• 上消化道胃镜：
- 用于解除梗阻或食管解剖。
- 食物嵌顿可以通过取出或将其推进胃里两种方法解除。
- 需要可活检。

• 食管压力测试。
• 纤维喉镜。

鉴别诊断

• 口咽：
- 感染：
  ○ 肉毒中毒。
  ○ 中枢神经系统感染。
  ○ 黏膜炎。
  ○ 莱姆病。
- 机械性：
  ○ 先天性。
  ○ 恶性。
  ○ 咽囊。
- 药物：
  ○ 抗生素（尤其是多西环素）。
  ○ 阿司匹林和非甾体抗炎药。
  ○ 硫酸亚铁。
  ○ 磷酸盐。
  ○ 氯化钾。
  ○ 奎尼丁。
- 神经肌肉：
  ○ 肌萎缩侧索硬化症。
  ○ 脑血管意外。
  ○ 吉兰-巴雷综合征。
  ○ 脑神经麻痹。
  ○ 亨廷顿舞蹈病。
  ○ 多发性硬化症。
  ○ 肌无力。
  ○ 帕金森病。
  ○ 脑外伤。

- 心理/行为。
- 食管：
- 机械的：
  - 憩室。
  - 食管网。
  - 异物。
  - 肿瘤。
  - 消化性食管狭窄。
  - 术后(咽部、脊柱)。
  - 放射损伤。
  - 舍茨基环。
- 动力：
  - 贲门失弛缓症。
  - 恰加斯病。
  - 库欣综合征。
  - 弥漫性食管痉挛。
  - 甲亢、甲减。
  - 胡桃夹食管。
  - 硬皮病。
  - 维生素 B_{12} 缺乏。
- 炎症：
  - 嗜酸性粒细胞性食管炎。
  - 药物性食管炎。
  - 咽下腐蚀剂。
- 外源性：
  - 心血管异常(血管环、胸动脉瘤、左心房扩大、迷走锁骨下动脉)。
  - 颈椎骨赘。
  - 纵隔肿块。

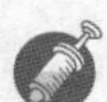

治疗

院前

- 注意气道管理。
- 可呼吸的舒适位置。

初步稳定/治疗

- 注意气道管理。
- 可呼吸舒适的位置。
- 病情不稳定者立即请专家会诊。
- 禁食。
- 明显脱水时，生理盐水 500 ml(儿童：20 mg/kg)静脉滴注。
- 对致命性的吞咽困难进行评估，包括：
- 咽后血肿、脓肿。
- 会厌炎。
- 速发型过敏反应。
- 碱摄入。
- 异物(儿科患者应特别注意食管内有无纽扣式电池)。
- 上呼吸道梗阻，心血管疾病(胸主动脉瘤)。

急诊治疗/程序

- 硝酸甘油用于食管痉挛。
- 胰高血糖素用于异物压紧的。
- 治疗并发症：
- 气道梗阻。
- 误吸、肺炎、肺脓肿。
- 脱水、营养不良。
- 内镜检查。
- 膳食调整：
- 神经肌肉障碍时用黏稠流质。
- 机械性障碍时用稀薄流质。

药物治疗

一线用药

- 食物填塞时用胰高血糖素：1 mg 静推，如果无改善，5 min 后再次静推 1 mg(儿童：0.02～0.03 mg/kg，不超过 0.5 mg)。
- 成功率从 12%到 50%不等，可能与自发的通过率差不多。

二线用药

钙通道阻滞剂和硝酸盐可用于运动障碍(例如，贲门失弛缓症和胡桃夹食管)。

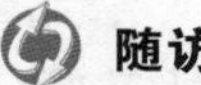

随访

进一步处理

入院指征

- 经治疗食管梗阻仍持续存在。
- 液体或营养状况损害。
- 无法保护气道。
- 无法耐受分泌物。

出院指征

- 体液充足的患者。
- 紧急转诊至神经病学，耳鼻咽喉科或安排进一步评估与治疗。

转诊问题

第 2 日初级保健医师或耳鼻喉、消化科随访。

随访建议

- 在耳鼻喉科随诊之前，给予无渣流质饮食。
- 如果呼吸急促、胸部疼痛或无法耐受自己的分泌物，返回医院。

要点和误区

- 表现为吞咽困难的儿童应考虑到异物吸入。
- 吞咽困难是脑卒中的常见症状。
- 有复发性肺炎患者应考虑。
- 建议患者门诊就诊明确诊断前评估有无危及生命的吞咽困难的病因。

外耳道炎

Assaad J. Sayah　王虑 译

基础知识

描述

- 耳郭、外耳道或鼓膜表面的炎症和感染：
  - 炎症会影响到中耳。
  - 在美国每 1 000 人中就有 4 个患外耳道炎。
- 外耳道炎也被称为游泳耳，该病患者通常有近期游泳史。
  - 偶尔会发生在正常洗澡后。
- 坏死性（恶性）外耳道炎。
  - 感染开始于外耳道，随后进展到耳周组织，最后侵犯颅骨表面。
  - 发病于老年、糖尿病和其他免疫低下患者（化疗、类固醇）。
  - 致病菌为铜绿假单胞菌。
  - 能导致蜂窝织炎、软骨炎、骨髓炎。
  - 死亡率为 20%（如果未经治疗，则为 50%）。
- 慢性外耳道炎：
  - 常见。
  - 由过度操作引起。
  - 外耳道炎治疗不彻底。

病因

- 外耳道长期磨损，或外耳皮肤长期浸渍水中或过于干燥。
- 易感因素包括：
  - 耳手术史或鼓膜穿孔史。
  - 过窄或异常外耳道。
  - 潮湿。
  - 过敏。
  - 湿疹。
  - 肿瘤。
  - 耵聍分泌异常。
- 最常见的细菌：
  - 假单孢菌。
  - 金黄色葡萄球菌。
  - 链球菌。
- 耳霉病：继发于真菌种类，如念珠菌或曲霉。

诊断

症状和体征

病史

- 近期游过泳或者长期暴露于水中。
- 糖尿病史。
- 放射性治疗史、长期使用类固醇激素、HIV/AIDS 或其他一些免疫功能低下的人群。
- 1～2 日出现逐渐加重的疼痛感。
- 外耳道出现分泌物。
- 耳鸣。
- 听力下降。
- 耳内有明显异物堵塞感。

体格检查

- 耳自发痛或牵拉耳郭疼痛。
- 外耳道红肿。
- 外耳道液体流出。
- 听力下降。
- 前耳肿痛。
- 坏死性（恶性）外耳道炎：
  - 前耳区疼痛、触痛、肿胀。
  - 头痛。
  - 耳漏。
  - 脑神经麻痹：
    - 面神经受累最为常见。

基本检查

临床诊断依据典型的症状和体征。

- 耳自发痛或牵拉耳郭疼痛。
- 耳镜检查。
- 外耳道红肿。
- 外耳道液体流出。
  - 白色或灰绿色的干酪状渗出物。

诊断检查与说明

实验室检查

- 以下指标可供参考。
  - 评估全身毒性或感染局部扩散的迹象。
- 实验室检查：
  - 白细胞计数。
  - 红细胞沉降率。
  - 血糖（糖尿病患者）。
  - 微生物培养。

影像学检查

当患者有炎症反应或累及骨质时，可行 CT、MRI 以排除乳突炎。

诊断步骤/外科

- 用软塑料刮勺刮取分泌物或双氧水和清水轻轻冲洗。
- 放置管芯有利于药物治疗。

鉴别诊断

- 坏死性（恶性）外耳道炎。
- 中耳炎。
- 皮脂腺分泌口堵塞引起的毛囊炎。
- 耳内异物。
- 膝状神经节带状疱疹感染。
- 腮腺炎。
- 外周淋巴结炎。
- 乳突炎。
- 牙脓肿。
- 鼻窦炎。
- 扁桃体炎。
- 咽炎。
- 颞下颌关节疼痛。
- 病毒疹。

儿童注意事项

若外耳道疼痛水肿伴有脓性分泌物流出时，应考虑外耳道异物（电池需要迅速拆卸）。

治疗

急诊治疗/程序

- 清理外耳道：
  - 用软的刮勺和棉签去除炎性分泌物。
  - 有时可用 Frazier 吸管处理分泌物。
- 当外耳道水肿严重时，可在外耳道清洁后用 10～12 mm 棉花或纱布条进行填塞。
- 外耳道炎的治疗重点在于减轻疼痛，去除感染灶，预防复发。

药物治疗

- 多数患者对局部治疗效果良好。
  - 消毒清洗并外用滴耳可以杀灭病原微生物，有助于快速治愈。
  - 丙酮酸溶液，如碱式醋酸铝（2%丙酮酸）：4～6 滴，q4～6 h。
  - Corticosporin 混悬液（1%氢化可的松、多黏菌素＋新霉素）：4 滴，每日 4 次（怀疑有鼓膜穿孔时用混悬剂而不用溶液）。
  - 氧氟沙星：5 滴，每日 2 次。
- 口服抗生素：
  - 面部或颈部蜂窝织炎、外耳道严重水肿、并发中耳炎或鼓膜不能看清。
  - 糖尿病和免疫功能低下患者或有疑似恶性外耳道炎可口服环丙沙星。
  - 阿莫西林：500 mg［儿童：40 mg/(kg · d)］，口服，每日 3 次。
  - 环丙沙星：500 mg，口服，每日 2 次。
- 坏死性外耳道炎、严重蜂窝织炎或脓毒症表现患者可予以静脉用抗生素。
• 抗真菌药物：
- 1%克霉唑滴耳液。
• 预防：
- 涂抹乙醇或2%乙酸以保持外耳道干燥防止感染再发。
• 使用对乙酰氨基酚或非甾体抗炎药用于止痛。
• 剧烈疼痛时可以使用阿片类药物。
• 坏死性外耳道炎需通过外科清创术对肉芽组织及碎骨进行清除，并做好必要的引流。

并发症

• 乳突炎。
• 耳郭软骨炎。
• 坏死性外耳道炎。
• 颅底骨髓炎。
• 中枢神经系统感染。

随访

进一步处理

入院指征

• 坏死性外耳炎。
• 耳郭明显受累。
• 系统性疾病的征兆。

出院指征

• 大多数患者。
• 外耳炎高危患者的密切随访。
• 患者说明：
- 避免游泳，保持耳完全干燥3～4周。
- 按指导使用药物。
- 如果出现更严重的疼痛、发热、听力损失，或者精神或神经状态有任何变化，及时回来就诊。
- 如果症状在2～3日没有改善，则进行随访。

转诊问题

耳鼻喉随访：
• 穿孔。
• 症状恶化。
• 传导性听力损失。
• 初始诊疗不佳。

预防

• 避免自伤。
• 避免潮湿。
• 预防性滴耳液：2∶1异丙醇/乙酸。

随访建议

随访初级保健医生或在2～3日回访急诊室，以移除或如果症状更严重。

要点和误区

• 急性外耳道炎和中耳炎常常混淆的原因是急性外耳道炎发病时鼓膜上常有红斑。
• 鼓膜完整的情况下才使用外耳道灌洗。
• 所有的局部治疗方案都必须确保清除外耳道一切堵塞物，并使药物渗入皮下。
• 通过给患者必要的解释和建议，尽量保持外耳道干燥，避免不必要创伤，减少外耳道皮肤不必要的刺激防止接触性皮炎，这都能大大降低外耳道炎的复发率。
• 免疫功能低下人群和糖尿病患者若伴有严重耳痛、化脓性耳漏、外耳道有肉芽组织或暴露的骨组织，那么高度怀疑坏死性外耳道。

外耳道异物 Foreign Body, Ear

Zachary A. Certa · Charles V. Pollack, Jr. 万健 译

W

基础知识

描述

• 异物存留于外耳道内。
• 外耳道：
- 由软骨和骨构成的通道，表面为管膜和皮肤。
- 成人2.5 cm长。
- 内管膜非常敏感，取异物过程中疼痛明显：
◦ 幼小儿童可能需要在全身麻醉下取出异物。
◦ 异物常造成外耳道内端管膜部分或峡部的损伤。
◦ 受面神经、舌咽神经和迷走神经支配。
• 无生命的异物通常不会立即引起不适症状：
- 儿童常因害怕受到惩罚而延迟告知。
- 儿童常于耳部检查时偶然发现异物。
• 物理检查所见可因异物存留时间长短而发生改变。
• 耳垢堆积或异食癖的儿童容易罹患本病。
• 通常发生在右外耳道，缘于右利手者居多。
• 儿童和精神病患者可能将任何较小的物体塞入外耳道。
• 多见于8岁以下儿童。
• 并发症：
- 外耳道撕裂伤：
◦ 多见于反复尝试取出难以抓取的异物。
- 鼓膜穿孔：
◦ 取异物过程造成的鼓膜穿孔似乎更为多见。
- 外耳炎。
- 可因昆虫叮咬或抓括引起鼓膜或外耳道受伤。
- 钮扣电池因其强电流和电压可引起严重损伤。
- 少见原因：
◦ 因侵蚀到颞下颌关节而出现咬合不正。
◦ 咽旁脓肿。
◦ 乳突炎。
◦ 脑膜炎。
◦ 脑脓肿。
◦ 已有面神经和听小骨损伤的报道。
• 外耳道异物取出后数日内症状消失。

病因

• 儿童：
- 石头。
- 小珠子。
- 纸。
- 玩具。
- 种子和爆米花。
- 豆子、食物和其他有机物。
- 纽扣电池：
◦ 造成坏死的风险远高于其他异物。
• 成人：
- 卷棉签头。
- 耳塞。

- 昆虫：
  ◦ 美国最多见的是蟑螂。
- 藏纳违禁药物。

诊断

症状和体征

- 听力下降。
- 婴幼儿过度哭闹。
- 单侧耳痛。
- 耳内充塞感。
- 强噪声。
- 嗡嗡声（活昆虫）。
- 恶心。
- 头晕。
- 同侧溢泪。
- 外耳道内脓性分泌物溢出。
- 耳内瘙痒。
- 出血。

病史

- 旅行、露营或生活环境恶劣，昆虫趁机进入外耳道。
- 询问之前是否曾试图从外耳道中取出异物，以及是否有与之相关的损伤。
- 询问以前做过耳外科手术或是否有鼓膜管。

基本检查

在取异物前后均应行耳镜检查：

- 对双侧外耳道进行检查，特别是儿童和精神病患者。充分检视对侧外耳道内是否存有"静止"的异物。
- 尽量看清鼓膜情况，评估破裂的可能性。
- 评估外耳炎。
- 明确异物类型以决定移除方式：
  - 纽扣电池。
  - 活昆虫。
  - 植物。
  - 无生命异物。
  - 大小。
  - 遇水后膨胀风险。
- 取出后，评估是否有残留碎片、鼓膜破裂、管腔擦伤或裂伤。
- 出现显著疼痛、眩晕或共济失调、眼球震颤、听力损失、耳溢液或面神经麻痹等征象时，均应请耳鼻喉专科会诊。

基本检查

仔细地进行耳镜检查：

- 尽可能减少疼痛。
- 获取患者的信任。
- 在试图取出异物前先明确异物的类型。

诊断检查与说明

实验室检查

没有特别需要。

影像学检查

怀疑感染或腐蚀性损伤时可行 CT 扫描。

诊断步骤/外科

显微耳镜：

- 若常规急诊室设备检查失利或急诊团队易于获得时可以使用。

鉴别诊断

- 耵聍堵塞。
- 肉芽肿。
- 出血。
- 损伤-磨损或撕裂。
- 外耳道炎。
- 鼓膜穿孔。
- 自行取出异物后遗留外耳炎。
- 肿瘤。
- 胆脂瘤。

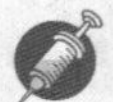

治疗

院前

- 注意事项：
  - 出现严重耳痛、感觉异物活动、响亮的嗡嗡声：
    ◦ 缓慢滴入温利多卡因或液状石蜡至患耳以杀死昆虫。
- 争议：
  - 以下情况下不要试图取出异物：
    ◦ 缺乏适合的设备。
    ◦ 首次异物取出失败将可能使后续取物变得更加困难。

初步稳定/治疗

患者可能因外耳道内进入活昆虫而非常紧张：

- 在尝试移除之前，通过注入以下其中一种方法淹死或固定昆虫：
  - 2%利多卡因温溶液。
  - 温乙醇。
  - 温矿物油。
- 避免使用冷液体，以免引起眩晕。

急诊治疗/程序

- 考虑耳鼻喉科转诊的适应证，而不是在急诊室尝试切除：
  - 鼓膜穿孔的证据。
  - 异物似乎被楔入鼓膜。
  - 锋利的物体。
  - 急诊多次尝试。
- 器械和患者准备：
  - 强光源。
    ◦ 耳镜。
    ◦ 前照灯和鼻镜。
    ◦ 0 号米勒视频喉镜。
    ◦ 如果可行，使用手术显微镜。
  - 妥善固定患者头部。
  - 将患者耳部向后牵拉使外耳道变直以便观察。
- 止痛：
  - 利多卡因局部麻醉：
    ◦ 首先 2%利多卡因黏性溶液。
    ◦ 鼓膜破裂禁忌证。
  - 利多卡因浸润野阻滞。
    ◦ 1%～2%利多卡因，含或不含肾上腺素。
    ◦ 在 4 个象限中的每个象限，在耳道外部注射 0.5 ml 利多卡因。
  - 如果在取出过程中需要进行肠外镇痛，可考虑静脉注射芬太尼。
- 镇静：
  - 适用于儿童和不能配合的成人。
  - 应在取异物前使用，因为取物失败可导致出血、水肿或鼓膜损伤。
- 取异物方法选择：
  - 灌洗法：
    ◦ 将装有温水的 30～60 ml 注射器连接至 18G 血管导管或蝶形装置的导管（切断针头装置）。
    ◦ 将血管导管或导管置于异物和管路之上，或最好在异物和管路的远端。
    ◦ 重复上述步骤，直到异物冲洗干净。
    ◦ 当异物是纽扣式电池时，切勿尝试通过冲洗清除。
    ◦ 鼓膜破裂禁忌证。
  - 机械拆卸选项：
    ◦ 宫颈刮匙或环。
    ◦ 钝直角钩子穿过异物，旋转 90°，与异物一起移除。
    ◦ 鳄鱼钳。
  - 吸引管：
    ◦ 最好用小号。
    ◦ 使用 100～140 mmHg 的负压。
    ◦ 这种方法会让病人大吃一惊。
  - Fogarty 导管：
    ◦ 小心地将导管置于异物后方，充气后回

撤；如有疏忽此方法可能造成鼓膜损伤。
- Cyanoacrylate 胶（一种强力胶），将胶水涂在一钝性探头顶端：
◦ 在尝试此方法之前，确保异物干燥。
◦ 将探头与异物接触 30 s，然后拉出（异物）。
◦ 胶水可能污染到外耳道，此方法也被发现与鼓膜撕裂有关。
- 丙酮：
◦ 用来溶解泡沫聚苯乙烯异物或松解强力胶。
- 显微耳镜：
◦ 虽然报道称急诊室内使用有益处，但通常在手术室进行。
• 特定对象移除技术。
- 植物类异物：
◦ 应以器械法取出。
◦ 钳子常用来取出可钳夹的异物。
◦ 应当对异物与外耳道有炎症的组织的边界十分清楚。
- 避免灌洗异物以防遇水膨胀。
- 非植物类无生命的异物：
◦ 若易于抓取，可用钳子试取。
◦ 若不易夹取，可试用灌洗法。
- 抛光或光滑的异物取：
◦ 看清异物。
◦ 直接吸引。
◦ 直角钝头探针。
◦ Fogarty 导管法。
◦ Cyanoacrylate 胶法。
- 昆虫取出：
- 将 12%利多卡因、矿物油或乙醇注入耳，杀死昆虫。
◦ 待昆虫死亡后用钳子夹出或灌洗冲出。
◦ 再次检查确认昆虫所有身体部分均已清除。
- 尖锐异物：
◦ 在显微外科手术下取出。
◦ 若有创伤证据或患者不能配合时，可考虑转诊到耳鼻喉专科治疗。
• 术后护理：
- 确认没有残留的 FB 碎片。
- 检查鼓膜是否有破裂迹象。
◦ 如果破裂，开始用氧氟沙星或环丙沙星和地塞米松滴剂或口服抗生素如阿莫西林，并咨询耳鼻喉科。
- 是否所有耳道手术患者都应使用类固醇悬浮液预防性使用耳用抗生素，以避免外耳炎的发生。
◦ 许多人建议，如果有外伤的证据或患者处于高风险状态，如糖尿病患者或免疫功能受损患者，则应给予该药。

■ 药物治疗

一线用药

• 利多卡因溶液（1%或 2%）：渗透剂最多 4 mg/kg 用于局部镇痛或滴注 5 ml 用于局部镇痛。
• 氧氟沙星耳用：每次 5 滴，持续 35 日。
• 环丙沙星/地塞米松（环丙沙星）耳用：4 滴入耳，每日 2 次，持续 7 日。

二线用药

• 芬太尼：1 μg/kg，静脉注射。
• 阿莫西林：500 mg，口服［儿童：80～90 mg/(kg·24 h)］，每日 1 次，7～10 日。
• 新霉素/多黏菌素 B/氢化可的松（皮质类固醇）耳用：每日 4 滴，持续 57 日（鼓膜穿孔禁忌证）。

随访

■ 进一步处理

入院指征

异物为钮扣电池且难以取出时需入院治疗。

出院指征

• 异物已取出。
• FB 仍然存在，但患者能够在耳鼻喉科门诊随访：
- 不包括纽扣电池。

转诊问题

耳鼻喉门诊专科随访。
• 异物未能成功取出。
• 有外耳炎的免疫功能下降的患者。
• 鼓膜破裂。

■ 随访建议

• 告诫患者不要将任何物体放入外耳道。
• 创伤性外耳道异物取出后短时应用止痛药。
• 外耳炎应给予预防措施。
• 鼓膜穿孔：
- 抗生素和类固醇滴剂。
- 如果有中度污染的迹象，如灌洗，考虑口服抗生素。
- 耳鼻喉专科随访。
• 若有创伤或感染表现，避免外耳道进水。

要点和误区

• 对不能配合或异物预期取出困难的患者务必使用镇静剂。
• 不要对异物为钮扣电池者使用灌洗法，以免电流或电池内容物造成组织损伤坏死。
• 在将液体注入耳之前，确认鼓膜是完整的。
• 当冲洗或向耳内注入液体时，确保液体加热到体温，以避免热量反应。
• 除了纽扣式电池，耳异物不是真正的紧急情况，可随访耳鼻喉科，尤其是在高风险的医源性损伤。

W

外耳软骨炎/脓肿 External Ear Chondritis/Abscess

Assaad J. Sayah　单怡 译

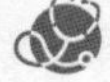

基础知识

■ 描述

炎症和/或耳郭感染。

■ 病因

• 机制：
- 外耳软骨易于损伤的原因：
◦ 缺少覆盖的皮下组织。
◦ 血管相对少。
◦ 处于暴露部位。
- 软骨炎：
◦ 通常继发于创伤或烧伤。
◦ 症状通常隐匿，甚至可能至表面愈合了才表现出来。
• 由于软骨继发性的缺血性坏死，处理不当可能导致耳郭变形：
- 轻者耳郭皱缩，成菜花样，严重者外耳缺失，甚至可能导致耳道狭窄。
• 在老年患者及意识改变患者中常易漏诊。
• 病因：

- 化学性烧伤或热力烫伤。
- 冻伤。
- 血肿形成。
- 创伤。
- 人、昆虫咬伤。
- 深度擦伤。
- 外耳炎。
- 耳垂刺伤，特别是技术、卫生条件和护理条件较差的时候。

• 致病菌：
- 铜绿假单胞菌。
- 葡萄球菌。
- 变形杆菌。

诊断

症状和体征

• 初始为钝痛，渐进性加重。
• 发热。
• 寒战。

病史

• 耳创伤。
• 耳刺伤。

体格检查

• 耳郭：
- 疼痛。
- 痛觉过敏。
- 红肿。
- 皮温升高。
- 小叶水肿致轮廓消失。
- 颅耳沟加深。

• 波动感形成后出现破溃和流脓。

基本检查

临床诊断：
• 典型的体征及以上提及的病因。

诊断检查与说明

实验室检查

仅在感染出现全身反应时。
• 血细胞计数。
• 血培养。
• 脓肿和引流物培养。

鉴别诊断

• 过敏反应。
• 乳突炎。
• 皮炎。
• 血肿。

治疗

急诊治疗/程序

损伤后常规防护性措施：
• 最重要的是防止软骨炎：
- 一旦出现难以处理，且有变形可能。

• 避免压迫损伤后的外耳。
• 焦痂及血痂清创最小化。
• 每日抗菌肥皂水温和冲洗 2 次，完全干燥后局部应用抗生素。
• 头发避免覆盖耳郭。
• 小部分早期耳垂炎症病例可口服抗生素。
• 软骨炎患者早期施行手术引流术、静脉输注抗生素。

药物治疗

• 环丙沙星：500 mg，口服，每日 2 次(成人)。
• 头孢氨苄：500 mg[儿童：50 mg/(kg·d)]，口服，每日 4 次。
• 双氯西林：500 mg[儿童：25 mg/(kg·d)]，口服，每日 4 次。
• 皮肤屏障受损时局部应用抗生素。

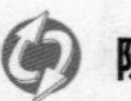

随访

进一步处理

入院指征

• 水肿、红斑及严重的外耳压痛。
• 有发热和寒战中毒症状的患者。
• 免疫功能不全的患者。

出院指征

无全身症状的稳定患者，且有耳鼻咽喉科密切随访。

转诊问题

耳鼻咽喉科会诊：
• 累及软骨的炎症、脓肿和坏死。
• 炎症和脓肿早期手术引流。

要点和误区

• 抗生素抗菌谱需覆盖铜绿假单胞菌。
• 早期侵入性治疗可能预防大范围耳郭变形。
• 对老年患者及存在意识改变患者应彻底完善检查。

腕骨骨折 Carpal Fractures

Kelly K. DiLorenzo · Stephen R. Hayden　彭沪 译

基础知识

描述

• 腕骨组成腕部的 8 根骨，位于近端桡骨和尺骨之间，而远端则位于掌骨之间：
- 腕骨近端：舟骨、月骨、三角骨、豌豆骨。
- 远端：大多角骨、小多角骨、头状骨、钩骨。

• 腕骨是上肢最常见的受伤部位。
- 最常见的腕骨骨折部位是舟骨(68%)和三角骨(18%)。
- 大多角骨，钩骨，头状骨和小多角骨的骨折患病率较高(2%~4%)。

• 腕骨骨折通常合并其他腕部损伤：
- 90%的舟骨骨折是孤立的，而其他所有腕骨骨折中很大一部分涉及多个腕骨。
- 头状骨骨折常合并舟骨骨折(Scaphocapitate 综合征)，有时会合并月骨周围脱位
- 月牙和三尖瓣骨折也与月周畸形相关。
- 钩骨骨折常合并第 4 和第 5 腕掌关节及掌骨损伤并发桡骨远端骨折。

病因

• 伸展位跌倒(FOOSH)时手腕过伸或过曲。
• 所有骨折的损伤机制通常包括 FOOSH。
• 舟骨骨折：
- 摔落在伸直且径向偏离的手腕上。

• 月牙骨折：
- 通常会掉在手腕上。

• 腰带骨折：
- 分为撕脱性骨折(93%)和身体骨折。
- 过度伸展→背侧撕脱骨折。
- 过度屈曲→掌侧撕脱骨折。
- 身体骨折：通常是由于直接打击和高能量导致的。
  ◦ 12%~25% a/w 周轮状错位梯形骨折：
- 通常会掉在手腕上。

• 头状骨折：
- 握紧拳头。
• 斜方肌骨折：
- 第二掌骨的轴向负荷。
• 梨形骨折：
- 直接冲击坚硬的表面。

诊断

症状和体征

病史

• FOOSH 或直接打击：
- 过度屈曲→背侧撕脱骨折。
- 过伸→掌侧撕脱骨折。
• 钩骨骨折：
- 伴有有力的挥拍或挥杆动作。

体格检查

• 疼痛，肿胀，关节活动受限。
• 个体腕骨的触诊有可能与手腕的正确定位有关。
• 舟骨骨折：
- 鼻烟壶背面压痛。
- 舟骨结节压痛。
- 抵抗内旋疼痛。
- 舟骨压缩试验（拇指轴向负荷会引起疼痛）。
• 月牙骨折：
- 腕部背部疼痛。
- 触诊月牙背侧或第三掌骨时轴向负荷加剧。
• 腰带骨折：
- 尺骨茎突远端的腕背压痛。
- 运动检查很重要，因为尺神经深支紧贴在三角骨附近，并可能导致运动障碍。
• 梯形骨折：
- 肿胀最小。
- 患者可能比其他腕骨骨折的疼痛要严重得多。
• 头状骨折：
- 疼痛和手背肿胀。
- 刚好在第三个掌骨基部的背面背压。
• 梯形骨折：
- 通常会出现肿胀。
- 刚好靠近第二掌骨底部的手背压痛。
• 梨形骨折：
- 腕部抵抗屈曲加剧了尺侧腕部疼痛。
- 握力不足。
• 钩骨骨折：
- 感觉异常的第四和第五位数字。
- 降低握力。
- 汗液拉力测试钩：当患者屈伸第四和第五位 DIP 时，手握尺侧偏斜。屈肌腱作为骨折部位的变形力，阳性试验会引起疼痛。

基本检查

• 整个上肢和肩胛带的系统的体格检查。
- 评估合并伤。
• 神经血管检查是必不可少的。
• 钩骨骨折可与尺神经或血管损伤相关。

诊断检查与说明

影像学检查

• 手和手腕的前-后位、侧位、斜位摄片。
• 体格检查怀疑腕骨骨折的大部分都需要特殊摄片（如舟骨摄片）。
- 舟骨视图：腕关节的 PA 视图，尺骨最大偏斜。
- 腕管视图有助于诊断钩状骨折。
- 侧面侧视图使背三角骨远离其他腕骨，有助于可视化骨折。
- Betts 视图：具有 20 度内旋的 AP 视图可用于识别梯形骨折。
- 如果怀疑肩骨不稳定，PA 握紧拳头。
- 腕骨之间的间距＞3 mm，提示韧带破裂，特里·托马斯征。
• CT 扫描对骨折具有极高的灵敏度。
• MRI 可诊断韧带损伤。

鉴别诊断

• 掌骨根部骨折。
• 桡骨远端或尺骨骨折。
• 月骨或月骨周围脱位。

儿科注意事项

警惕桡骨远端骨骺损伤：儿童单纯的扭伤或腕部骨折较为少见。
• ＜10 岁的儿童很少发生腕骨骨折。
• 1/3 的舟骨骨折儿科患者最初会出现慢性骨不连。

治疗

院前

• 防止任何伤口区域叠加污染。
• 手腕或手肿胀或显著疼痛的患者：
- 抬高下肢和冰敷。
- 取下珠宝首饰、手表。
- 带衬垫的护腕固定肢体末端进一步减少损伤。

初步稳定/治疗

正如任何创伤，必须评估是否存在更严重的损伤。

急诊治疗/程序

• 孤立的腕骨骨折可以用夹板进行初始处理：
- 目标是获取和维持正常姿势。
• 拇指人字形绷带：
- 舟骨和梯形骨折。
- 使手腕保持在稍伸展的姿势。
- 将夹板放在前臂侧面，将拇指包裹到 DIP 上，并在肘部下方延伸。
- 多达 20%的裂缝会出现初始负片，因此怀疑骨折需要夹板并进行随访以在 7～14 日重复成像。
• 糖钳夹板：
- 头状骨骨折与月骨骨折。
- 从掌指关节的背侧开始，左右肘缠绕，在掌中折皱终止。
- 手腕保持直立。
• 手掌夹板：
- 三角骨、豌豆骨、小多角骨、钩骨骨折。
- 从掌中折皱到肘部以下伸展。
- 手腕略微延伸。
- 在体格检查的基础上，即使 X 线片阴性，夹板固定可疑骨折（特别是舟骨）。
• 开放性腕骨骨折：
- 需要大量的高压冲洗。
- 在三级开放性骨折（涉及显著的软组织损伤）中，注射抗生素针对金黄色葡萄球菌并覆盖革兰阴性菌。
- 监控神经血管状态。
- 预防破伤风。
- 立即骨科会诊。

药物治疗

• 口服轻度镇痛药、麻醉药品、NSAIDs 以减轻患者痛苦。
• 适当的夹板会减轻这些伤害带来的大部分的痛苦。

随访

进一步处理

入院指征

• 开放性骨折收住入院以早期手术清洗和清创。
• 需要手术治疗（切开复位，不稳定移位骨折）的创伤患者有时收住入院以接受早期干预。

出院指征

• 腕骨骨折经过适当夹板固定后闭合、无移

W

位即可出院，7～10 日后骨科随访。

随访建议

• 确诊的骨折由骨科最终处理，并进一步治疗。
• 几天内紧急转诊给手外科医生的适应证：
- 由于 AVN 高风险，舟骨近端 1/5 处骨折。
- 骨折位移超过 1 mm。
- 考虑到骨不连的高风险，导致急性骨折的延迟呈报（超过 3 周）。
- 与月骨畸形脱位相关的骨折。
- 腕骨不稳定。
- 提早恢复工作/运动时舟骨腰部的无移位骨折很重要，并且患者愿意接受手术。
- 固定疼痛严重的未经授权的任何损伤，并在 7～10 日或更长时间的影像学检查（CT/MRI）中重复进行 X 线摄影。
• 骨折未接或夹板固定不当可能导致长期的并发症和残疾：
- 未经处理的舟骨、头状骨和月骨骨折导致骨折不愈合和股骨头缺血性坏死率很高。
- 夹板是长期功能和运动能力恢复的关键。
- 有显著疼痛的任何伤害均需固定，并考虑 7～10 日复查 X 线片或更先进的影像学检查（CT 或 MRI）。

要点和误区

• 腕骨骨折可能无法在早期的 X 线片显影，如果治疗不当可能导致长期功能残疾。
• 急诊或门诊所有怀疑骨折的患者均需夹板治疗，并考虑复查 X 线片或考虑 CT 检查。
• 大多数（90%）舟骨骨折是孤立的损伤：
- 所有其他腕骨骨折更易合并手腕或手部损伤。
• 适当的治疗包括功能位的夹板固定和最终的固定和治疗转诊。

腕管综合征 Carpal Tunnel Syndrome

Rahul V. Nene · Radhika Sundararajan 彭沪 译

基础知识

描述

• 腕管综合征是由正中神经穿过腕管被压迫引起的。
• 穿过腕管时受压引起的。
• 导致疼痛，感觉异常，有时甚至导致手无力。
• 腕管是由腕骨和腕横韧带包绕的区域。
• 正中神经、指深屈肌、指浅屈肌（FDS）和拇长屈肌均位于腕管。
• 腕管综合征分为急性和慢性。
• 患病率：1%～5%；女>男。

W

病因

• 急性：
- 创伤（尤其是 distal 骨远端和腕骨骨折）。
- 感染（蜂窝织炎、败血性关节炎、病毒综合征）。
- 炎症（痛风、类风湿关节炎）。
- 出血。
- 高压注射伤。
• 慢性：
- 职业/过度使用综合征——高冲击、重复动作。
- 妊娠，避孕药。
- 肉芽肿疾病：结核病、结节病。
- 肿块与正中神经受压。
- 骨赘。
- 淀粉样变。
- 多发性骨髓瘤。
- 类风湿关节炎。
- 内分泌失调：甲状腺功能低下、糖尿病、肢端肥大症。
- 慢性血液透析。
- 特发性。

儿科注意事项

儿童特发性原因较为罕见；大部分病例有一个可纠正的原因，包括：
• 创伤。
• 黏多糖症。
• 正中神经错构瘤。

诊断

症状和体征

病史

• 急性或慢性起病。
• 麻木/感觉异常的正中神经分布：
- 拇指、示指、中指和环骨的手掌部分。
• 手腕和手部疼痛和感觉异常，有时放射到肘部、前臂或肩膀。
• 重复的腕部运动会加剧症状，尤其是在腕部弯曲和振动的情况。
• 通常在晚上恶化，可以从睡眠中唤醒。
• 患者可能抱怨掉落东西或运动控制能力下降。

体格检查

• 手的正中神经分布的运动和感觉缺陷，应保留近端。
• 应保留对鼻尖隆起的感觉（腕管前的感觉神经分支）。
• 高度特异性的发现是迟发的两点歧视和鱼际肌萎缩。
• 缺乏运动或感觉发现不排除。

基本检查

• 特有的夜间疼痛史和正中神经分布区感觉异常。
• 肌肉无力和大鱼际萎缩都是后续出现。
• 挑衅测试：
- 敏感性和特异性总体较差。
- 腕挤压测试：
  ◦ 腕关节屈曲 60 s 在正中神经分布区产生麻木或刺痛。
- Tinel 征：
  ◦ 轻轻敲击正中神经腕关节处，在正中神经分布区的手指产生刺痛。
- 腕部压迫检查：
  ◦ 在近侧腕关节韧带施加直接压力 30 s，正中神经分布区的手指产生刺痛。
- 止血带测试：
  ◦ BP 袖带充气至略高于患者的收缩压 2 mm，正中神经分布区产生麻木。

诊断检查与说明

实验室检查

• 在大多数情况下未标明。
• 甲状腺功能，如果病史和体检检查提示也需检查类风湿因子和免疫功能。

影像学检查

• 如果疑似外伤或退行性关节炎需检查手腕 X 线片。

• 可以选择行 CT 检查(不是常规)：

- 可显示腕管侵犯。

• MRI 对软组织显影很好，但不推荐常规诊断。

- 结果：经腕韧带掌曲，正中神经扁平，正中神经或关节肿胀，腕管积液，正中神经信号异常。

• 超声诊断：

- 灵敏度 44%～95%；特异性 57%～100%。

- 结果：正中神经近端肿胀，正中神经远端压扁，经腕韧带弯曲。

诊断步骤/外科

神经传导检查和肌电图是一种标准规范检测。

鉴别诊断

• 颈神经根受压：

- 正中神经起源于第 6 和第 7 颈椎根。

- 症状因直立的姿势和颈部运动加剧。

• 手臂振动综合征：

- 其特点是当暴露在寒冷或振动时出现雷诺、麻木和尺神经和正中神经分布的刺痛、抓力减弱和上肢肌肉痛。

- 伴有长时间振动。

• 胸廓出口梗阻。

• 第 1 腕掌关节骨性关节炎。

• 肱神经丛炎。

• 一般的神经病变。

• 脊髓空洞症。

• 多发性硬化症。

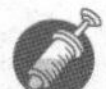

治疗

初步稳定/治疗

无必要。

急诊治疗/程序

• 急性：

- 手外科会诊，通过开放或腔镜技术手术松解腕横韧带。

• 慢性：

- 止痛药。

- 口服皮质类固醇。

- 局部注射糖皮质激素。

- 避免重复手腕动作。

- 手腕夹板固定在中间位置(0)。

◦ 夜间使用，直到出院。

- 瑜伽。

- 推荐：

◦ 初级护理师。

◦ 如果由于重复运动、肌腱滑翔运动、神经滑动或腕骨动员练习造成需进行职业医师人体功率学测试。

◦ 手外科医师评估是否需要手术干预。

药物

• 镇痛药：

- 有很多选择。

- NSAIDs 未被证实可以改善长期预后。

• 口服皮质类固醇激素，可以获得短期获益：

- 泼尼松：每日 20 mg×7 日，每日 10 mg×7 日。

- 泼尼松龙：20～25 mg/d，2～4 周后逐渐减量。

• 局部注射糖皮质激素，瞬间缓解 2/3 患者症状(许多不同的方案)：

- 氢化可的松：20 mg。

- 甲泼尼龙：15～40 mg。

- 曲安奈德：20 mg。

- 一般联合 2%利多卡因 0.15～0.5 mg。

随访

进一步处理

入院指征

急性腕管综合征，需要手术减压。

出院指征

慢性腕管综合征经过充分的疼痛控制。

随访建议

在 1～2 周随访初级护理师或直接专业职业医师或手外科医师。

危险物暴露所致损伤

Thomas W. Engel II　刘雪峰 译

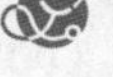

基础知识

描述

• 是指暴露于危险物品所引起的局部或全身中毒反应。

• 病理生理：

- 酸性危险物引起伴焦痂的凝固性坏死，通常对深部组织渗透有限。

- 碱性危险物引起液化坏死，溶解的复合物对深部组织有很强的渗透性。

- 损伤也可由氧化反应、蛋白质变性、细胞脱水、局部组织缺血、新陈代谢加速/抑制所致。

病因

• 危险物在家庭、工厂、农场、运输事故，以及犯罪/恐怖活动等场合都可遇到。

• 物品的毒性与它们所含的特殊物质及其作用有关。

诊断

症状和体征

• 皮肤：

- 化学烧伤，初起看似轻微。

- 皮肤上沾有液体和粉状物。

- 通过皮肤吸收导致全身症状。

• 黏膜(眼睛、鼻咽部及角膜烧伤)：

- 范围包括黏膜的刺激症状到严重的黏膜烧伤。

- 潜在的气道损伤。

• 肺：

- 咳嗽。

- 胸膜性胸痛。

- 支气管痉挛。

- 呼吸困难。

- 速发/迟发性肺水肿。

• 全身症状(因皮肤或肺对毒物吸收所致)：

- 精神状态的改变。

- 抽搐。

- 快速/缓慢性心律失常。

- 低血压。
- 消化道症状。
- 电解质紊乱。
- 碳氧血红蛋白血症与高铁血红蛋白血症。
- 氰化物中毒。
- 胆碱能综合征(详见化学武器中毒、神经毒剂)。

病史

毒物类型、现场环境、数量及暴露时间。

基本检查

• 通过院前供应商、化学品安全说明书、化学品运输紧急事故中心识别毒物性质。
• 化学品安全说明书:
- 识别化学品。
- 区分吸入或接触中毒。
- 是否需要净化毒物。
- 确定治疗方案。
• 确定暴露的时间。
• 封闭空间多产生吸入性损伤。
• 通过毒物管理系统、计算机数据库(如美国毒理通报或毒理学数据网)或标准的毒理学试验确定毒性。
• 观察全身毒性反应。

诊断检查与说明

实验室检查

• 取决于具体毒物。
• 电解质、血尿素氮、肌酐和血糖浓度。
• 肝功能。
• 钙浓度。
• 镁浓度。
• 磷浓度。
• 动脉血气分析:
- 代谢性酸中毒。
- 碳氧血红蛋白血症与高铁血红蛋白血症。
- 呼吸衰竭。

影像学检查

• 胸部放射线检查可辅助诊断肺水肿。
• 鼻咽镜检查以减少气道受累。

鉴别诊断

• 皮肤:
- 过敏性反应。
- 热灼伤。
• 肺:
- 肺炎。
- 肺栓塞。
- 过敏性反应。
• 全身:
- 癫痫持续状态。
- 药物过量。
- 精神疾病。
- 心肌梗死。

治疗

院前

• 识别危险物的状况:
- 工业、农业场所意外。
- 危险物运输意外。
- 怀疑恐怖主义事件。
- 胆碱能综合征。
- 黏膜刺激症状。
- 化学烧伤。
• 保护自身安全:
- 从上风向进入。
- 在确定安全之前不要进入。
- 在安全不确定的状况下使用A级防护装置。
- 能正常运动和说话的人所受污染较轻。
- 防止其他人在无保护的情况下进入污染区。
• 个人化学防护装备:
- A级:正压自给呼吸器、完全封闭式化学防护服、双层化学防护手套、化学防护靴,以及提供衣服、手套与靴子之间的气密性。
- B级:自给呼吸器、非封闭式化学服、双侧手套与靴子。
- C级:空气净化装置、衣服、手套及靴子。
- D级:普通工作服。
- 确定物质:
◦ 运输部公告、化学品安全说明书、货运票据及危险标记。
◦ 联系化学品运输紧急应变中心确定物质与毒性。
◦ 危险物团队可做化学测试。
• 确定毒性以及是否需要去污净化:
- 毒物管理。
- 化学品运输紧急应变中心。
• 去污净化:
- 危险物团队。
- 指导轻微污染患者进行自我净化。
• 治疗:
- 提供基础及高级生命支持。
- 通常支持的清单仅包括高温类现场。
- 立即冲洗皮肤及可见的烧伤部位,并持续至抵达医院。

初步稳定/治疗

• 保护急救人员:
- 继发沾染可由皮肤接触或吸入挥发性气体与颗粒导致。
- 尽早启动医院灾难政策。
• 在洗消前将患者安置在隔离区之外。
• 不确定的情况下按照洗消处理。
• 患者通过紧急医学处置后或使用私人车辆送。
• 若在洗消前或洗消中需要提供治疗:
- 安排采用适当防护的人员,人少为宜。
- 治疗仅需聚焦于生命维持及肢体保存。
• 洗消:
- 保证隔离带的安全性。
- 移动,标记,双袋衣服(包括隐形眼镜)。
- 使用肥皂和清水大量持续冲洗10～15 min,特别需要注意明显的暴露部位、伤口及眼睛。
- 回收洗消后的水以防引起继发污染:
◦ 紧急状况以及群体性事故中,允许废水进入下水道。
- 水治疗法:
◦ 化学烧伤的主要治疗手段。
◦ 禁止用于钾钠元素烧伤。
- 患者可自我洗消或由专业队伍洗消。
- 在监护人的陪同下对于儿童、无法独立的老年人、精神/身体障碍的人及轮椅之类电动用具进行洗消。
- 手套、口罩、护目镜,以及一次性长外衣,都可以提供一定程度上的保护。
- 更换绷带、止血带、人工气道、静滴套装。
- 洗消后再次检伤分类。
- 防止消毒引起的低温。
- 去污后回收。

急诊治疗/程序

• 提供必需的支持。
• 确定解毒剂的效果。
• 危险物容易引起极端的恐慌:
- 期待受伤人员从精神过度紧张中恢复。
- 毒物理论有助于排除患者是否沾染。
• 即使空气中毒物浓度低于中毒剂量,急救人员仍有可能出现症状,需要送至新鲜空气场所。
• 化学烧伤:
- 尽早洗消,对于强碱所致烧伤可能需要数小时的持续冲洗。
- 第一个24 h按照每1%烧伤面积需要2～4 ml/kg的乳酸林格液进行积极地液体复苏,其中一半的液体量需要在第一个8 h内输注完成。
- 止痛。

- 肺部症状：
  - 支气管扩张剂，吸氧，气管插管，以及机械通气。
- 特殊处理：
  - 氢氟酸烧伤：
    - 葡萄糖酸钙局部皮肤涂抹、皮下注射或动脉注射。
    - 全身毒性：静脉滴注葡萄糖酸钙和镁。
  - 石炭酸烧伤：
    - 使用聚乙二醇或异丙醇清除皮肤上的石炭酸。
  - 硝酸盐：
    - 吞入或者广泛的烧伤可以引起高铁血红蛋白症。
    - 高流量吸氧，静脉滴注亚甲蓝。
  - 氰化物中毒。
    - 羟钴胺。
  - 有机磷农药（见化学武器中毒）。

药物治疗

- 沙丁胺醇：2.5～5.0 mg 吸入。
- 葡萄糖酸钙：10%溶液 10 ml 外用。咨询毒物中心。
- 镁：2 g，静脉滴注，持续 20 min。
- 亚甲蓝：1～2 mg/kg 缓慢静滴（儿童：6 岁以下儿童不推荐，6 岁以上 1 mg/kg 静脉滴注或肌内注射，持续 5 min）。
- 羟钴胺：5 mg 静脉注射维持 5 min，必要时可重复 1 次。

随访

进一步处理

入院指征

- 气道损伤，呼吸困难（低氧血症）。
- 严重的全身症状。
- 化学烧伤患者可收入烧伤中心。

出院指征

- 一段时间观察后恢复良好并通过毒物管理中心会诊。
- 弱酸/碱所致的表浅化学烧伤不合并潜在的全身毒性反应。

随访建议

遭受化学恐怖袭击的伤者推荐有精神科医师或社工进行随访。

要点和误区

- 原地洗消。
- 通过个人防护装备保护医疗急救人员。
- 确定毒物后给予特效解毒剂。
- 可正常活动伤员的沾染剂量较低。

围生期心肌病 yopathy，Peripartum

Shamai A. Grossman · Christie L. Fritz 彭沪 王毅鑫 译

基础知识

概述

- 妊娠最后 1 个月至分娩后 5 个月发生的扩张型心肌病。
- 诊断标准（以下需全部满足）：在妊娠最后 1 个月或分娩后 5 个月内发生心肌衰竭；缺乏特定原因；无既往心脏病史。
- 诊断需要严格的超声心动图功能障碍标准：LEVF<45%。
- 发病率：（3～5）/10 000 活产。
  - 因地理位置而异死亡率：18%～56%。
- 50%的病例可自愈。
- 死亡率：18%～56%。
- 危险因素：年长女性（>30 岁）；多胎妇女；多胎妊娠；长期溶胎治疗（>4 周）；肥胖；子痫前期；非洲裔美国人。滥用可待因。
- 与其他形式的心肌病相比，全身症状和肺栓塞发生更加频繁。
- 提示预后不良的因素：产后 6 个月左侧射血分数较低；产后>2 周发病；年龄>30 岁；非洲裔美国人；多胎产。
- 46%～63%多在 6 个月内 LEVF 有所恢复。

病因

多种原因被提出，但仍未得到证实：

- 妊娠期间出现免疫抑制时病毒感染导致心肌炎（最有可能）。
- 对未知母体或胎儿抗原的免疫应答。
- 催乳素异常合成。
- 异常血管生成/血管损伤。
- 对妊娠期血流动力学应激的不适应性反应。
- 应激激活的细胞因子。
- 长时间排卵。
- 硒缺乏。

诊断

症状和体征

- 呼吸困难。
- 头晕。
- 胸痛。
- 端坐呼吸。
- 咳嗽。
- 阵发性夜间呼吸困难。
- 厌食症。
- 疲劳。
- 心律失常。

病史

- 症状发作和持续时间。
- 不明原因持续咳嗽。
- 体重增加 2～4 磅/周及以上（1 磅＝0.45 kg）。
- 先心病。
- 既往妊娠和并发症。

体格检查

- 心悸。
- 颈静脉扩张。
- 奔马律。
- 二尖瓣反流性杂音。
- 第二心音亢进。
- 肺啰音。
- 周围水肿（尤其是快速发作）。
- 肝大。
- 肝颈静脉反流。

基本检查

- X 线表现：肺静脉淤血、心脏肥大（难以与妊娠鉴别）、胸腔积液。
- 心电图表现：非特异性、左心室肥厚、左心房扩大、T 波低平或倒置前 Q 波、心律失常、心室异位（40%）、心房颤动（20%）。

诊断检查与说明

实验室检查

- 电解质：一般正常。
- 尿素氮、肌酐。
- CBC：产后中度贫血可缓解疲劳和呼吸困难，肌酸激酶无活性，伴肌力和脑组织成分。
- B 型钠尿肽：用于区分舒张和收缩功能不全引起的心力衰竭和肺部呼吸困难的病因。BNP>100 pg/ml 诊断心力衰竭的敏感性为 90%，特异性为 76%，预测准确性为 83%。BNP≤50 pg/ml 具有较高的阴性预测值。

影像学检查

- X 线表现：心脏肥大；积液（通常为右侧）；肺部表现的三个阶段[第一阶段：肺再分布至上肺野（头向集中）；第二阶段：Kerley B线间质水肿。第三阶段：肺泡水肿]。双侧合流性肺门周围浸润导致典型的蝴蝶型。可能是不对称的，误认为是肺炎。
- 超声：表现为全心扩张、心壁变薄、射血分数降低；Hibbard 等建立了诊断标准（射血分数<45%或 M 型缩短率<30%；舒张末期内径>2.72 cm/m²）；排除瓣膜病变和心脏压塞。
  - EF<35%的患者存在 LV 血栓风险。
- 心脏 MRI：
  - 在回声成像不清楚时特别有用。
  - 估计左室容积和压力。
  - 晚期增强：预后不良。

诊断步骤/外科

心肌内膜活检：

- 指出 CAD 是否可能导致 HF 心内膜活检：
- 用于评估心肌炎和类固醇治疗。

鉴别诊断

- 扩张型心肌病的其他病因：缺血、梗死、瓣膜破裂或疾病、慢性 HTN、家族史、毒素（乙醇、蒽环类、可卡因、药物过敏）、代谢（硫胺素硒、甲状腺功能减退、甲状腺毒性、低磷血症）、传染性（病毒、寄生虫或立克次体、细菌、真菌）、系统性疾病（硬皮病、系统性红斑狼疮）、嗜酸性心肌炎、神经肌肉营养不良、线粒体心肌病。
- 气短或水肿的其他病因：肺栓塞、肺炎、哮喘、心肌缺血、贫血、甲状腺功能亢进、缩窄性心包炎、心脏压塞、肾病综合征、肝硬化。

治疗

院前

急性反应性气道疾病与肺水肿的鉴别。

初步稳定/治疗

ABC 管理：

- 迅速评估呼吸和血流动力学状态。
- 根据需要控制气道。
- 吸氧。
- 根据需要持续气道正压。
- 减少前后负荷。

急诊治疗/程序

- 产前治疗：硝酸酯类、肼屈嗪、呋塞米、氨氯地平（一种二氢吡啶类钙通道阻滞剂，已被证明能提高非缺血性心肌病患者的存活率）、地高辛控制心房颤动的发生率、卡维地洛（产前非急性失代偿期）、低分子肝素，如果 EF<35%；胎儿监护。
- 不稳定时行有创心脏监护。
- 产后治疗：建议添加 ACEI（依那普利）或 ARB；抗凝治疗通常推荐（用于 30%并发全身或肺栓塞的患者、在妊娠期间，使用皮下或静脉注射肝素而不是华法林，后者会导致出生缺陷）。
- 对于严重症状或对标准治疗缺乏反应的：多巴酚丁胺、多巴胺、硝普钠、辅助装置（主动脉内球囊泵、左心辅助装置、体外膜氧合）（提倡标准药物治疗后 2 周内未能改善的患者使用；泼尼松与环孢素或硫唑嘌呤、免疫球蛋白疗法仍存在争议）。

药物治疗

- 氨氯地平：2.5～10 mg/d，口服。
- 布美奈德：0.5～2 mg，静脉注射。
- 地高辛：0.5 mg，静脉注射；0.25 mg，静脉注射，二次给药；0.125～0.375 mg/d，口服。
- 米力农：50 μg/kg，超过 10 min。
- 多巴酚丁胺：2～10 μg/（kg · min），静脉注射。
- 多巴胺：2～20 μg/（kg · min），静脉注射。
- 依那普利：0.625～1.25 mg，静脉注射；2.5～20 mg/d，口服。
- 呋塞米：20～100 mg，静脉注射。
- 美托洛尔：12.5 mg，口服，每日 2 次。
- 硫酸吗啡：2～4 mg，静脉注射，q5 min。
- 硝酸甘油：0.4 mg，舌下；1～2 in 甘油糊：5～20 μg/min，静脉注射，最大剂量 100～200 μg/min，静脉注射，使用非 PVC 管。
- 硝普鲁司苷：0.5～10 μg/（kg · min），静脉滴注。

随访

进一步处理

入院指征

- 肺水肿、心源性休克或有缺血迹象的患者应住进 ICU。
- 所有有症状的新发围生期心肌病患者均应入院。

出院指征

- 轻度左心室功能不全。
- 明确的围生期心肌病病史（因盐摄入过多而导致的轻度液体超负荷，急诊治疗后症状完全缓解，无心肌缺血迹象，密切随访）。

转诊问题

与心脏病医师密切随访。

随访建议

- 每日喝 6～8 杯水。
- 限制盐的摄入量。
- 避免饮酒，因为可能加重心肌病。
- 支撑袜可以帮助减少腿部肿胀，防止血栓形成。
- 每日体重：体重增加可能是体内液体过多的迹象；如一日内增重>2 磅，请打电话给医师。
- 如出现呼吸急促、感觉昏厥、心悸症状，请及时入院治疗。

要点和误区

- 牢记妊娠和围生期心肌病的血栓栓塞率很高。
- 利用多学科方法进行心脏病学和产科咨询。

胃肠出血 Gastrointestinal Bleeding

Czarina E. Sánchez 祝各亮 译

基础知识

描述

- 源于消化道的出血。
  - 上消化道：屈氏韧带以上。
  - 下消化道：屈氏韧带以下至肛门。
- 死亡率：
  - 总死亡率为10%，儿童死亡率<5%，70岁以上老人死亡率为25%。
  - 上消化道出血(UGIB)为6%～8%，其中静脉曲张占30%～50%。
  - 下消化道出血(LGIB)为2%～4%。

病因

上消化道出血(UGIB)

- 上消化道溃疡性疾病：
  - 消化性溃疡病(40%)：
    - 幽门螺杆菌感染。
    - 药物诱导(非甾体抗炎药、阿司匹林、糖皮质激素、钾补充剂、铁补充剂)。
  - 胃或食管糜烂(25%)：
    - 反流性食管炎。
    - 感染性食管炎(念珠菌、单纯疱疹病毒、巨细胞病毒)。
    - 药物诱导性食管炎。
    - 食管异物。
  - 胃炎、应激性溃疡：
    - 毒性药物(非甾体抗炎药、酒精、胆汁)。
    - 黏膜缺氧(创伤、烧伤、脓毒症)。
    - 严重的中枢神经系统损伤导致的溃疡。
    - 化疗。
- 门静脉高压：
  - 食管或胃底静脉曲张(10%)。
  - 门静脉高压性胃病。
- 动静脉畸形：
  - 主动脉肠瘘(S/P主髂动脉手术)。
  - 遗传性出血性毛细血管扩张症(Osler-Weber-Rendu综合征)。
  - 杜氏病。
  - 胃窦血管扩张(GAVE或西瓜胃)。
  - 原发性血管瘤。
- 贲门黏膜撕裂综合征。
- 胃和食管肿瘤。
- 胰腺出血。
- 胆道出血。
- 粪类圆线虫感染。

下消化道出血(LGIB)

- 憩室病(33%)。
- 息肉癌(19%)。
- 结肠炎(18%)：
  - 缺血、炎症、感染或辐射。
- 血管：
  - 血管发育不良(8%)。
  - 毛细血管扩张。
  - 动脉结肠瘘。
- 炎症性肠病：
  - 克罗恩病和溃疡性结肠炎。
- 息肉切除术后。
- 肛门直肠(4%)：
  - 痔(内痔和外痔)。
  - 肛裂。
  - 肛门直肠静脉曲张。
  - 直肠溃疡。
  - 异物。

儿科注意事项

梅克尔憩室和肠套叠是儿童中最常见的引起LGIB的原因。

诊断

症状和体征

- UGIB和LGIB都会表现出低血容量的症状和体征。
- UGIB经典表现：
  - 呕血或呕吐咖啡样物。
  - 黑便：黑色柏油样便。
- LGIB经典表现：
  - 便血：鲜红色或栗色便。

> **注意**
>
> 便血是LGIB的经典信号，但是在严重的UGIB中也可出现。

病史

- 呕血和黑便最常见。
- 呕吐咖啡样物。
- 大便松弛。
- 经直肠的鲜红色血。
- 腹痛。
- 虚弱或头晕。
- 晕厥。
- 呼吸困难。
- 呆滞或躁动。

体格检查

- 心动过速。
- 低血压。
- 结膜苍白。
- 黏膜干燥。
- 血性、黑色素性或血红素阳性便。
- 休克。
- 门脉高压症的症状：
  - 脾大。
  - 腹壁侧支血管。
  - 腹水。

基本检查

- 血常规、凝血功能和电解质。
- 执行耳鼻喉检查，鉴别咯血与呕血：
  - 肺源性：
    - 外观鲜艳的红色和泡沫。
    - 痰中混有血像肺源性。
    - pH>7。
  - 消化道源性：
    - 暗红色或棕色的血，伴或不伴胃内容物。
    - 伴有恶心与呕吐。
    - pH<7。
- 考虑鼻胃管洗胃：
  - 可能有助于确定是否有活动性出血，便于内镜检查。
  - 研究未能证明结果是有益的，如果出血部位位于幽门以下会出现假阴性。
- 直肠检查：
  - 检查痔和肛裂。
  - 检查粪便的颜色。
  - 粪便潜血假阳性结果：
    - 生的红肉。
    - 铁补充剂。
    - 水果：哈密瓜、葡萄及无花果。
    - 蔬菜：生的花椰菜及萝卜。
    - 亚甲蓝、叶绿素。
    - 碘、溴。
  - 假阴性隐血结果：
    - 胆汁。
    - 含镁的抗酸剂。
    - 抗坏血酸。
  - 引起黑便，但潜血阴性：
    - 铁。
    - 木炭。
    - 铋类。

◦ 食品染料。
◦ 甜菜。

儿科注意事项

新生儿吐血和血便可能是由于婴儿在分娩或哺乳期间吞咽母体血液引起的。

诊断检查与说明

实验室检查

• 血常规：
- 贫血（慢性失血时平均红细胞体积降低）。
- 血小板减少。
• 电解质、尿素氮、肌酐及葡萄糖。
• 凝血项目。
• 乳酸。
• 肝功能检查，怀疑上消化道出血时要做此检查。
• 血型和交叉配血，活动性出血或生命体征不稳定。
• 尿素氮/肌酐＞36，对于上消化道出血具有高灵敏度和低特异性。

> **注意**
>
> 血细胞比容在急性失血后的一段时间内会保持正常，不会立即出现下降。

影像学检查

• 肛门镜检查：
- 怀疑内痔或肛瘘。
• 食管胃十二指肠镜（EGD）：
- 是诊断性检查，也用于治疗。
• 结肠镜：
- 只是诊断性检查。
- 最好在肠道准备后进行。
• 肠切除术：
- 难治性出血。

鉴别诊断

• 鼻出血。
• 咽部出血。
• 咯血。
• 血尿。
• 阴道出血。
• 内脏损伤。

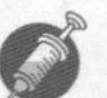

治疗

院前

• 稳定气道：
- 大量上消化道出血的患者，无法保护气道的需要进行插管。
• 建立静脉通道：
- 插入大口径静脉导管（16～18G）和输注晶体保持收缩压＞90 mmHg。
- 尝试建立第二条静脉通路。

初步稳定/治疗

• 建立气道，维持呼吸和循环。
• 生命体征不稳定、大量出血和不能保护气道的患者需要控制气道。
• 建立 2 个大孔静脉通道（16G），放置心电监护。
• 如果不稳定，扩容：
- 补充 1 L 生理盐水（儿童：20 ml/kg），必要时可持续补充。
- 如果存在明显的贫血或输注晶体后生命体征仍不稳定，可输注红细胞：
◦ 如果可行，先进行交叉配血或使用特定类型的血。
◦ 否则，给绝经前的妇女输 O 阴性血，给其他人输注 O 阳性血。
◦ 输血目标血红蛋白 79 g/L。
◦ 提供新鲜冰冻血浆（FFP）和红细胞输血比例为 1∶(2～4)。对于需要大量输血的患者，FFP 与红细胞及血小板的比例为 1∶1∶1。
- 对于凝血病，给药（如果 INR＞2）维生素 K 和凝血酶原复合物浓缩物（PCC），或者如果没有 FFP（15～30 ml/kg）和血小板（如果血小板＜50 000/μl）。

急诊治疗/程序

• 任何的胃肠出血都需咨询胃肠病学专家。
• 大量活动性出血、生命体征不稳定或需要寻找穿孔证据的患者，需进行外科会诊或介入放射检查。
• 放置 Foley 导尿管监测尿量。
• 考虑放置鼻胃管（NGT）。
• 输血指征：
- 显著贫血：
◦ 血红蛋白＜70 g/L。
◦ 血红蛋白＜90 g/L 时缺血性疾病的风险增加（如缺血性心脏病、卒中）。
◦ 终末器官出现缺血的表现。
◦ 胸痛、心电图缺血性改变。
- 输注晶体后生命体征仍不稳定。
- 大出血。

> **注意**
>
> 静脉曲张出血时过度输血会诱发再出血，需避免。
>
> • UGIB 治疗：
> - 静脉输注质子泵抑制剂（PPI，如泮托拉唑）。
> - 活动性出血的 3 个危险因素，占有 2 个称为高危：
> ◦ 鼻胃管引流出鲜红色的血。
> ◦ 血红蛋白＜8 g/dl。
> ◦ 白细胞＞12 000/μl。
> - 急诊内镜。
> - 治疗选择。
> ◦ 烧灼出血的溃疡、血管。
> ◦ 内镜下硬化剂治疗。
> • 对于静脉曲张出血：
> - 奥曲肽。
> - 加压素：
> ◦ 不能降低死亡率。止血的效益在于减少因缺血导致的死亡率。
> ◦ 静脉注射硝酸甘油减少组织缺血。
> - 用布莱克默管进行球囊填塞是治疗静脉曲张的最后手段。
> - 对肝硬化上消化道出血的患者的预防性使用抗生素，可减少细菌感染和所有原因导致的死亡率。
> • LGIB 治疗：
> - 对于大量出血、活动性出血，考虑血管造影并直接注射血管加压素。
> - 大量的难治性出血，考虑肠切除术。

药物治疗

• 维生素 K：10 mg（儿童：1～5 mg），口服、皮下注射或静脉注射，q24 h。
• 泮托拉唑：80 mg（儿童：剂量未统一），静脉推注，接着静脉滴注 8 mg/h，维持 72 h 或间歇推注剂量。
• 奥曲肽：50 μg（儿童：1～2 μg/kg），静脉推注，接着 50 μg/h[儿童：1～2 μg/(kg·h)]，静脉滴注。
• 生长抑素：250 μg（儿童：标准未建立），静脉推注，接着 250～500 μg/h，维持 3～5 日。
• 血管加压素：0.4～1 U/min[儿童：0.002～0.005 U/(kg·min)]，静脉滴注。
• 硝酸甘油：10～50 μg/min（儿童：标准未建立），静脉滴注。
• TXA：1 000 mg 10 min（儿童：20 mg/kg 超过 10 min）。

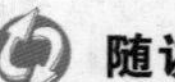

随访

进一步处理

入院指征

• 活动性出血。

- 年龄＞65 岁，或存在其他疾病。
- 凝血功能障碍。
- 血细胞比容下降。
- 任何情况下生命体征不稳定。

出院指征

- 上消化道出血已停止，鼻胃管灌洗和食管胃十二指肠镜未见异常。
- 少量或已停止的下消化道出血。
- 血细胞比容稳定＞30 或血红蛋白＞100 g/L。
- 健康患者。

转诊问题

考虑请消化科会诊行结肠镜或食管胃十二指肠镜检查。

随访建议

- 未收入急诊室的患者应当在 24～36 h 进行密切随访。
- 给予严格的拒收标准，如果出现再出血或其他相关症状（头晕、呼吸困难、胸痛等）需返回医院。
- 上消化道出血患者应携带 PPI 离开医院，并建议避免咖啡因、酒精、烟草、非甾体抗炎药和阿司匹林。

要点和误区

- 10%～15%的 UGIB 患者出现便血。
- 考虑消化道出血患者血容量不足的体征或低血容量性休克。
- 常见的错误：未能利用晶体液和血液制品合适地进行液体复苏。

老年人注意事项

消化性溃疡是老年人消化道出血的主要原因，并且有较高的死亡率。

作者感谢 Leon D. Sanchez 对本章前一版的贡献。

胃肠炎 Gastroenteritis

Isam F. Nasr　祝各亮 译

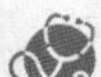

基础知识

描述

伴有腹泻、呕吐的胃和肠道的炎症反应，通常由感染或中毒所致。

病因

感染

- 病毒：
  - 50%～70%的诺如病毒感染病例发生在从墨西哥或印度旅行后。
- 侵入性细菌：
  - 空肠弯曲菌：被污染的食物或水、野外的水、鸟类和动物：
    - 最常见的病因。
    - 在血液中被发现的概率 60%～90%。
  - 沙门菌：被污染水、鸡蛋、禽类或奶制品。
    - 伤寒热：持续的发热、腹痛、玫瑰斑、脾大和心动过缓。
    - 免疫功能低下者敏感。
  - 志贺菌：粪-口途径。
  - 副溶血性弧菌：生肉和未煮熟的海鲜。
  - 鼠疫：受污染的食物（猪肉）、水和牛奶：
    - 可表现为肠系膜淋巴结炎或阑尾炎。
  - 特殊食源传播疾病（食物中毒）：
    - 金黄色葡萄球菌：
      - 最常见的毒素，相关疾病。
      - 症状在摄入食物后 1～6 h 出现。
    - 蜡样芽孢杆菌：
      - 经典的来源是剩饭。
      - 症状在摄入食物后 1～36 h 出现。
  - 霍乱：大量带有黏液的水样便（淘米水样便）。
  - 雪卡毒素：
    - 鱼类毒素。
    - 发病在摄食后 5 min 至 30 h（平均 6 h）。
    - 感觉异常，低血压，外周肌肉乏力。
    - 阿米替林可以治疗。
  - 鲭鱼毒素：
    - 由金枪鱼、长鳍金枪鱼、鲭鱼和鲯鳅等产生。
    - 面红，头痛，红斑，头晕，视力模糊和全身灼烧感。
    - 症状持续＜6 h。
    - 治疗包括抗组胺药。
- 原生动物：
  - 蓝氏贾第鞭毛虫：
    - 高危人群：旅行的人、日间护理的婴儿、男同性恋者和露营的人喝了未经处理的水。

非感染

- 毒物：
  - 锌、铜和镉。
  - 有机化学品：聚氯乙烯。
  - 农药：有机磷农药。
  - 放射性物质。
  - 烷基汞。
- 部分人对特定食品会产生反应（酪胺、谷氨酸钠和色胺）。

儿科注意事项

- 重点评估饮用水状况。
- 大多数是病毒来源并与购买食品相关。
- 轮状病毒占 50%。
- 癫痫发作与志贺菌感染有关。

诊断

症状和体征

病史

- 恶心、呕吐和腹泻。
- 血性、黏液性腹泻。
- 腹部绞痛或疼痛。
- 发热。
- 乏力、肌痛、头痛和食欲不振。
- 低血压、嗜睡及脱水（严重时）。

体格检查

- 黏膜干燥。
- 心动过速。
- 腹部压痛。
- 肛周炎症、肛裂和肛瘘。

基本检查

- 直肠指检以确定是否出血或隐血。
- 粪便白细胞测定：
  - 侵袭性细菌感染时会升高。
  - 原生生物感染、病毒、毒素诱导的食物中毒时不会升高。

诊断检查与说明

实验室检查

- 血常规：

- 明显的血液丢失。
- 全身性中毒。
- 电解质、葡萄糖、尿素氮和肌酐：
- 嗜睡、明显脱水、中毒或精神状态改变。
- 利尿剂的使用，持续腹泻，慢性肝肾疾病。
- 粪便培养：
- 存在粪便白细胞异常。
- 特殊人群（免疫功能低下、旅行、同性恋）。
- 公共卫生（食物处理、日间护工）。
- 血培养：
- 疑似菌血症或全身性感染。
- 需要住院的患者。
- 免疫功能低下者。
- 老年人和婴幼儿。

影像学检查

腹部X线检查有没有价值，除非怀疑肠梗阻或中毒性巨结肠。

儿童

- 实验室检查在大多数病例中并不需要。
- 轮状病毒酶法检测轮状病毒：
- 很少应用于门诊患者。
- 利于住院患者的管理和避免交叉感染。
- 粪便培养：
- 粪便白细胞。
- 中毒。
- 婴儿。
- 免疫功能低下。

W

鉴别诊断

- 胃炎和消化性溃疡。
- 牛奶和食物过敏。
- 阑尾炎。
- 肠易激综合征。
- 溃疡性结肠炎和克罗恩病。
- 先天性中肠扭转不良。
- 梅克尔憩室。
- 药物和毒素：
- 甘露醇。
- 山梨醇。
- 酚酞。
- 含镁的抗酸剂。
- 奎尼丁。
- 秋水仙碱。
- 蘑菇。
- 汞。

治疗

院前

- 严重脱水时建立静脉通道会变得困难。
- 避免接触污染的衣物或身体组织。

初步稳定/治疗

- 心肺复苏。
- 严重脱水时静脉补充生理盐水。

急诊治疗/程序

- 轻度脱水时口服液体（佳得乐/培德赖）：
- 静脉输液：
- 低血压、恶心和呕吐、迟钝、代谢性酸中毒、明显高钠血症或低钠血症。
- 给予生理盐水（成人：500 ml～1 L；儿童：20 ml/kg）液体复苏，然后予以生理盐水或5%葡萄糖 0.45%氯化钠溶液（儿童：5%葡萄糖 0.25%氯化钠溶液）维持适当的尿量。
- 碱式水杨酸铋（佩托比斯摩）：
- 抑酸剂。
- 在没有不良反应的基础上减轻症状。
- 高岭土和果胶制剂（康培特）：
- 减少粪便中的液体丢失。
- 不影响病程。
- 抗动力药[苯乙哌啶（止泻宁）、洛哌丁胺（易蒙停）、帕利高特与可待因]。
- 适用于非感染性腹泻。
- 少量使用可控制感染性腹泻的症状。
- 避免在感染性腹泻中长时间使用，可能会增加发热、腹泻、菌血症的持续时间，可能会引起中毒性巨结肠。
- 抗生素：
- 空肠弯曲菌：喹诺酮类或红霉素。
- 沙门菌：喹诺酮类或甲氧苄氨嘧啶-磺胺甲噁唑（TMP - SMX）。
- 伤寒菌：头孢曲松。
- 志贺菌：喹诺酮类、TMP - SMX 或氨苄西林。
- 副溶血性弧菌：四环素或多西环素。
- 难辨梭状芽孢杆菌：甲硝唑或万古霉素。
- 大肠杆菌：喹诺酮类抗生素或磺胺。
- 蓝氏贾第鞭毛虫：甲硝唑。
- 止吐药：
- 昂丹司琼。
- 丙氯拉嗪。
- 异丙嗪。

药物治疗

- 氨苄西林：500 mg[儿童：20 mg/(kg · 24 h)]，口服或静脉注射，q6 h。
- TMP - SMX（DS）：1 片[儿童：8～10 mgTMP/40～50 mg SMX/(kg · 24 h)]，口服，每日 2 次。
- 头孢曲松钠：1 g[儿童：50～75 mg/(kg · 12 h)]，肌内注射或静脉注射，q12 h。
- 环丙沙星（喹诺酮类）：500 mg，口服；或 400 mg，静脉注射，每日 2 次（>18 岁）。
- 多西环素：100 mg，口服；或 400 mg，静脉注射，每日 2 次。
- 米索前列醇：100～200 μg，口服，每日 4 次。
- 甲硝唑：250 mg[儿童：35 mg/(kg · 24 h)]，口服，每日 3 次（>8 岁）。
- 恩丹西酮：4 mg（儿童：0.1 mg/kg），静脉注射。
- 丙氯拉嗪（氯丙嗪）：5～10 mg，静脉注射，q3～4 h；10 mg，口服，q8 h；25 mg，纳肛，q12 h。
- 异丙嗪（非那根）：25 mg，静脉注射或肌内注射，q4 h；25 mg，口服/纳肛（儿童：0.25～1 mg/kg，口服、纳肛或肌内注射）。
- 四环素：500 mg，口服或静脉注射，每日 4 次。
- 万古霉素：125～500 mg[儿童：40 mg/(kg · 24 h)]，口服，q6 h。

随访

进一步处理

入院指征

- 低血压，静脉补液无法缓解。
- 显著出血。
- 脓毒症或中毒迹象。
- 难治性呕吐或腹痛。
- 严重电解质紊乱。
- 代谢性酸中毒。
- 精神状态改变。
- 儿童出现大于 10%～15%的脱水。

出院指征

- 程度较轻，仅需口服补液。
- 出现脱水，但静脉补液可以缓解。

转诊问题

长期存在症状的患者可向消化科咨询进一步诊治方案。

随访建议

大多数情况下该病都是自限性的，因此随访是可选的。

要点和误区

- 病毒占所有病例的 50%以上。

• 传染性病原体致病的情况下，避免抗动力药物的使用。

• FMP - SMX(DS)、环丙沙星、强力霉素和四环素在妊娠期禁忌使用。甲硝唑可在妊娠晚期内使用。

胃出口梗阻 Gastric Outlet Obstruction

Sean P. Dyer 祝各亮 译

基础知识

描述

• 任何阻碍胃内容物进入十二指肠的过程。

• 不仅可由胃的病理学改变引起，还可由十二指肠及肠腔外病变引起。

• 无论什么原因，胃出口梗阻会导致非胆汁性呕吐。

• 持续性呕吐会导致脱水、电解质紊乱及酸碱平衡失调：

- 慢性症状会导致体重下降、营养不良及发育不良。

- 低钾血症、低氯性代谢性碱中毒也可出现。

病因

• 肿瘤(成人发病最主要的原因)：

- 腔内和腔外肿瘤(胰腺、胃、淋巴结、十二指肠、胆囊肿瘤)、外部肿块可以通过挤压幽门或十二指肠近端引起梗阻。

• 消化性溃疡，随着对幽门螺旋杆菌的治疗及 H_2 受体阻断剂的应用，已不再是成人发病的最主要原因。

• 幽门狭窄(小儿发病的最主要原因)：发病率为 2‰～5‰。

• 术后并发症，特别是胃部手术(如幽门部或十二指肠的水肿、瘢痕形成、狭窄、增生)。

• 机械性原因：胃扭转、息肉、胃石、胃重复囊肿。

• 其他原因造成幽门部或十二指肠的水肿、瘢痕形成、狭窄、增生(如腐蚀性损伤、慢性胰腺炎)。

诊断

症状和体征

病史

• 不完全性梗阻时症状可以是间歇性的。

• 非胆汁性的恶心、呕吐。

• 腹部疼痛：定性与定位不明。

• 早期饱腹感及上腹部肿胀感。

• 呕吐后上腹部不适会减轻。

• 体重下降、发育不良。

体格检查

• 生命体征：

- 可以正常。

- 容量缺失明显时会出现心动过速和低血压。

• 腹部查体：

- 上腹部膨隆。

- 鼓音。

- 餐后 4 h 振水音。

- 直肠检查：隐血。

• 脱水貌：眼、口咽部、皮肤、黏膜改变。

• 营养不良貌：慢性或晚期梗阻时。

• 体重下降：慢性梗阻或恶性肿瘤。

老年患者

• 腹部疼痛、恶心与呕吐：老年人的消化道症状会更加不好把握。

• 尽量多地考虑其他原因(心源性和神经源性)。

儿科注意事项

• 特发性肥厚性幽门狭窄：

- 儿童发病的最主要原因。

- 典型的患者为男性(白种人及美籍亚裔较为多见)。

- 常见于 2～8 周的患者，但也见于 1 周至 3 岁的患者。

- 初始为间歇性的，非喷射性的餐后呕吐，逐渐进展为喷射性非胆汁呕吐。

- 呕吐之前查体可以看见中上腹蠕动波。

- 上腹部“橄榄状”团块可以在 80%～90% 的患者中出现。

基本检查

仔细询问病史和查体。

诊断检查与说明

实验室检查

• 血常规：

- 恶性肿瘤或消化道出血会伴有贫血。

- 高血细胞比容提示红细胞聚集。

• 电解质、血清尿素氮/肌酐、血糖：

- 低钾血症。

- 低氯性代谢性碱中毒。

- 低血糖。

- 氮质血症。

• 尿常规。

• 淀粉酶/脂肪酶。

• 肝功能(如果怀疑恶性肿瘤)。

• 幽门螺旋杆菌(如果怀疑消化性溃疡)。

影像学检查

• 腹部 X 线平片：

- 通常不能诊断。

- 可以看见扩大的胃部以及肠腔中的气体。

• 腹部超声：

- 常用于儿童。

- 没有电离辐射。

- 加长肥大的幽门括约肌。

• 腹部 CT 对于诊断肿瘤及肠腔内外病变具有重要作用：

- 可能是成年人诊断应用最多的方式。

- 辐射量不适合应用于儿童，不适合初步筛查。

诊断步骤/外科

• 上消化道影像学检查：

- 探明梗阻位点及特征。

- 幽门梗阻可见到特异性的“线样征”“双轨征”“鸟嘴征”及“肩样征”。

• 上消化道内镜检查：

- 可视性地检查胃内、胃出口部及近端十二指肠。

鉴别诊断

• 近端肠梗阻。

• 消化性溃疡加重。

• 胃肠炎。

• 胆石症。

• 胆囊炎。

• 急性胰腺炎。

• 糖尿病性胃轻瘫。

• 神经性呕吐。

治疗

院前

- 监测生命体征，稳定气道，供氧，建立静脉通道。
- 如果呕吐、脱水则补液。

初步稳定/治疗

- 如果有显著的容量缺失，静脉补充生理盐水：
  - 成人单次：1 L。
  - 儿童单次：20 mg/kg。
- 纠正电解质紊乱，尤其是低钾血症。

急诊治疗/程序

- 放置鼻胃管。
- 放置导尿管并监测尿量。
- 外科会诊/干预：
  - 良性的狭窄可行内镜下球囊扩张术。
  - 肠道支架置入术（恶性原因）。
  - 胃空肠吻合术（恶性原因）。
  - 迷走神经切断术和胃窦切除术、幽门成形术、胃空肠吻合术等（良性原因）。

药物治疗

- 法莫替丁：成人 20 mg［儿童：0.6～0.8 mg/(kg·24 h)，q6～8 h］，q12 h，静脉注射。
- 雷尼替丁：50 mg［儿童：2～4 mg/(kg·24 h)，q6～8 h］，q8 h，静脉注射。
- 泮托拉唑：成人 40 mg，静脉注射（抗幽门螺旋杆菌治疗同样需要）。

随访

进一步处理

入院指征

大部分胃出口梗阻的患者需要入院进行补液、纠正电解质、外科及消化科评估。

出院指征

很少，考虑以下情况：

- 腹部疼痛、呕吐的症状已经缓解。
- 发病期间外科及消化科评估已经明确病因。
- 实验室检查、影像学检查以及患者容量状态无异常。

转诊问题

外科及消化科会诊。

随访建议

所有没有入院的患者都应进行外科及消化科随访：

- 特别说明症状出现时需回院治疗。

要点和误区

- 不要将胃出口梗阻误诊为胃肠炎。
- 不要因为 X 线平片的限制性而漏诊。
- 对于上腹部疼痛和呕吐的患者，要考虑胃出口梗阻及恶性肿瘤可能。
- 要进行适当的补液治疗，特别是对于老年人及儿童患者。

胃食管反流病 Gastroesophageal Reflux Disease

Yanina Purim-Shem-Tov 祝各亮 译

W

基础知识

描述

- 胃的反流引起的症状以及食管黏膜损伤的病理性改变。
- 反流性食管炎与非糜烂性反流病。
- 北美洲的患病率为 18.1%～27.8%。

病因

感染

- 回流屏障功能不全，导致胃内容物反流到食管的频率与时间增加。
- 食管下括约肌（LES）：
  - 主要的抗反流屏障。
  - 膈脚的附件（膈肌括约肌）。
  - 胃食管交界处的压力屏障。
  - 食管通过蠕动进行酸清除和食管黏膜的抵挡作用是额外的屏障。
  - 大多数健康人存在短暂的反流症状。
- 短暂性食管下括约肌松弛（TLESR）：
  - 胃食管反流病（GERD）患者较易发生。
  - 暴露的食管黏膜酸化并逐渐坏死。
- 造成 LES 功能不全的因素：
  - 吸烟。
  - 食物：酒精（乙醇）、巧克力、洋葱、咖啡和茶。
  - 药物：钙通道阻滞剂、吗啡、哌替啶、巴比妥、茶碱和硝酸盐。
- 胃排空延迟，体重增加，胃扩张有助于回流。
- 食管裂孔疝合并胃食管反流病：
  - 症状因人而异。
  - 大多数食管裂孔疝患者没有明显的胃食管反流病。
- GERD 或非 GERD 患者在胃酸的分泌上是一样的。
- 相关的医疗状况：妊娠、慢性呃逆、脑神经麻痹、唐氏综合征的自身免疫性疾病、糖尿病（OM）、甲状腺功能减退症。

诊断

症状和体征

- 食管表现：
  - 烧心（或胃灼热）。
  - 反流。
  - 吞咽困难。
- 食管外表现：
  - 支气管痉挛。
  - 喉炎。
  - 慢性咳嗽。

病史

- 典型症状和体征：
  - 烧心：
    - 胸骨后烧灼痛。
    - 从腹部通过胸部向颈部和喉部辐射。
  - 吞咽困难：
    - 提示食管痉挛或狭窄。
  - 吞咽疼痛：
    - 提示溃疡性食管炎。
  - 反流。
  - 胃灼热。
  - 嗳气。
  - 食管狭窄，出血。
  - 巴雷特食管（食管癌）。
  - 早饱，恶心，食欲不振，体重减轻。
  - 躺下或屈曲时症状加重。

- 抗酸剂能缓解症状，但只是暂时的。
• 非典型症状和体征：
- 非心源性胸痛。
- 哮喘。
- 持续的咳嗽与呃逆。
- 声音嘶哑。
- 咽、喉溃疡和肿瘤。
- 频繁清喉。
- 复发性肺炎。
- 夜间窒息。
- 上消化道出血。

体格检查

• 无特异性，可能有相同的上腹压痛。
• 患者平躺或头低足高位时症状加重。

儿科注意事项

• 反流在婴儿中很常见，50%的2个月大的婴儿每日反流2次，但1岁时发病率会降至1%。
• 体征：
- 频繁呕吐、烦躁、咳嗽、哭泣和不适。
- 喂养时身体过伸，拒绝喂食。
• 发育不良。
• 不耐受婴儿食品。
• 脓毒症。

基本检查

• 胃食管反流病需与更紧急情况进行鉴别，如缺血性心脏疼痛、食管穿孔或主动脉瓣病变。
• 获取典型病史。
• 进行彻底的体格检查：生命体征、头部、耳、眼睛、鼻、喉（五官）、胸部及腹部检查。

诊断检查与说明

• 没有金标准。
• 有心脏原因行心电图检查。

实验室检查

• 血常规：
- 食管炎所致的慢性贫血。
- 粪便试验为隐匿性出血。

影像学检查

• 无常规影像。
• 胸部X线片：
- 可以找到食管穿孔、食管裂孔疝、主动脉疾病的证据。

诊断步骤/外科

• 抗酸剂的诊断试验：
- 症状持续的患者应该进行内镜检查。
- 90%的胃食管反流病患者对质子泵抑制剂（PPI）治疗有效。
• 突起型吞咽困难可行食管钡餐造影。
• 食管酸碱监测：
- 胃酸反流相关症状。
• 食管测压（敏感性差）：
- 评估LES静息压和食管蠕动收缩。
• 食管胃十二指肠镜（EGD）检测反流性食管炎和并发症（巴特食管、食管裂孔疝、狭窄、溃疡、恶性肿瘤）。

鉴别诊断

• 缺血性心脏病。
• 哮喘。
• 消化性溃疡。
• 胃炎。
• 肝炎和胰腺炎。
• 食管穿孔。
• 食管异物。
• 食管感染。
• 胆囊炎和胆石症。
• 肠系膜缺血。

治疗

院前

• 食管痛可类似于心绞痛。
• 呕吐之后需要积极控制气道。

初步稳定/治疗

• 评估是否需要心肺复苏。
• 大量失血或休克需要进行液体复苏。

急诊治疗/程序

• 缓解症状：
- 抗酸剂。
- 黏性利多卡因抗酸剂。
- 食管痉挛：舌下含服硝酸甘油。
- 止痛药。
• 改变生活方式：
- 避免深夜进食或大量/重油饮食。
- 减少餐后仰卧位时间。
- 抬高床头。
- 减肥。
- 避免吸烟及喝酒。
- 避免刺激物直接刺激食管，如柠檬汁和咖啡。
- 避免降低LES压力的食物，如高脂肪的食物、巧克力和咖啡。
- 避免降低LES压力的药物。
• 质子泵抑制剂（PPI）：
- 比 H_2 受体拮抗剂更强力的长期胃酸抑制剂。
- 比其他药物治疗康复更快。
- 对重度GERD和弗兰克食管炎效果更好。
• H_2 受体拮抗剂：
- 对轻度到中度的疾病有效。
- 对于严重疾病需要用比消化性溃疡病更大的剂量。
• 抗酸药（氢氧化铝、碳酸钙）：
- 治疗轻度和罕见的反流症状。
- 对于食管炎治疗无效。
- 褐藻酸液覆盖于胃内容的表面，提供机械性屏障。
• 硫糖铝：
- 结合损伤黏膜表面暴露的蛋白形成保护屏障。
- 也可能直接刺激黏膜的修复。
• 甲氧氯普胺（促胃肠动力药）：
- 加强蠕动。
- 加速胃排空。
- 增加LES压力。
• 调节短暂性食管下括约肌的药物：
- 巴氯芬。
• 内镜治疗：
- 缝合（折叠）、热损伤和药物注射。
• 抗反流手术（目标：增加LES压力）：
- 慢性反流、年轻患者、不愈合的溃疡、严重出血。
- 在可选择的情况下，胃底折叠术比药物治疗更有效。
- 目前较新的经口咽入路微创术也可考虑。

妊娠注意事项

• 30%～50%的孕妇会出现反流。
• 腹腔压力增加、激素水平波动导致TLESR发生率升高。
• 症状严重者可进行EGD（食管胃十二指肠镜）。
• H_2 受体拮抗剂是首选的治疗方法（有较长的安全记录）。
• PPI：在妊娠期内相对安全。

药物治疗

• 氢氧化铝/镁＋碳酸盐/西甲硅酮：30 ml＋黏性利多卡因10 ml，口服，q6 h。
• 西咪替丁：400 mg，口服，每日2次；300 mg，肌内注射或静脉注射，q6～8 h。
• 埃索美拉唑：20～40 mg，口服，每日1次。
• 法莫替丁：20 mg，口服或静脉注射，每日2次[儿童：0.5～1 mg/(kg·d)，静脉滴注，q8～12 h，最大剂量40 mg/d]。
• 兰索拉唑：15～30 mg，每日1次。
• 甲氧氯普胺：10～15 mg，口服、静脉注射

W

或肌内注射，q6 h，餐前和睡前。

• 尼扎替丁：150 mg，口服，每日 2 次。

• 奥美拉唑：20～40 mg，口服，每日 1 次。

• 泮托拉唑：40 mg，口服或静脉注射，每日 1 次。

• 雷贝拉唑：20 mg，口服，每日 1 次。

• 拉米替丁：150 mg(儿童：5～10 mg/kg，q12 h)，口服，每日 2 次；或 300 mg，口服，睡前。

• 硫糖铝：1 g，口服，餐前 1 h 和睡前。

一线用药

• 改善生活方式：

- 床头抬高。
- 饮食。
- 避免餐后仰卧位。
- 避免紧身的衣服。
- 通过咀嚼口香糖促进唾液分泌。
- 限制饮酒。
- 减少肥胖。

• 抑酸药物：

- PPI 或 H_2 受体拮抗剂。

• 治疗幽门螺旋杆菌感染。

二线用药

• 促动力药(氨甲酰甲胆碱、甲氧氯普胺)。

• 抑制一过性食管下括约肌松弛药物(布洛芬)。

随访

进一步处理

入院指征

• 食管大出血。

• 无控制反应性哮喘。

• 脱水。

• 饥饿和发育不良。

出院指征

• 简单的胃食管反流病：患者转至初级保健医师(PCP)或消化科医师进一步评估。

转诊问题

出现哮喘、喉炎等食管外表现。

随访建议

消化科医师予维持持续性治疗的患者行内镜检查以排除巴雷特食管。

要点和误区

• 胃食管反流病的治疗应包括生活方式的改变。

• 比轻度间歇性 GERD 症状重的患者可进行抑酸治疗。

• 对于 GERD 和中重度食管炎患者，PPI 比 H_2 受体拮抗剂效果更好。

• 慢性治疗失败的患者行内镜检查(至少 8 周)。

• 高剂量 PPI 的患者可行抗反流手术，特别是年轻且可能需要终身治疗的患者。

• 胃食管反流病的并发症：

- 食管炎。
- 消化性狭窄和巴特化生。
- 食管外表现：哮喘、喉炎、反流和咳嗽。

胃炎 Gastritis

Yanina A. Purim-Shem-Tov 祝各亮 译

基础知识

描述

• 炎症反应导致的胃黏膜损伤。

• 3 条胃黏膜的保护机制：

- 黏膜层形成保护性 pH 梯度。
- 表面上皮细胞可以修复小的缺损。
- 后上皮屏障可以中和穿越前两层的酸。

• 陈旧性胃炎与消化不良性胃炎之间没有明确的联系。

• 无相关炎症性的胃上皮细胞损伤称为“胃病”。

病因

• 胃炎的主要病因：感染、自身免疫、药物(如可卡因)、过敏和应激。

• 胃病的主要病因：内源或外源性刺激，如胆汁反流、酒精、非甾体抗炎药、应激及慢性充血。

• 急性胃炎：

- 应激(脓毒症、烧伤和创伤)：
  ◦ 内脏血流量减少导致黏液产生、碳酸氢盐分泌及前列腺素合成减少。
  ◦ 导致黏膜糜烂和出血。
- 酒精(乙醇)：
  ◦ 白三烯的产生减少导致微血管淤滞、充血并增加血管渗透性。
  ◦ 导致出血。
- 非甾体抗炎药，包括阿司匹林：
  ◦ 干扰前列腺素的合成导致与酒精相似的级联反应。
  ◦ 导致黏膜糜烂。
- 类固醇。

• 慢性胃炎：

- 由幽门螺旋杆菌产生。
- 幽门螺旋杆菌的致病机制尚不清楚：
  ◦ 在胃黏膜层发现革兰阳性螺旋菌。
  ◦ 包括脲酶允许它改变微小内环境的 pH。

诊断

症状和体征

• 消化不良。

• 膨隆。

• 恶心与呕吐。

• 呕吐咖啡渣/血液。

• 黑便。

• 厌食。

• 上腹压痛。

• 烧心。

病史

• 消化不良。

• 上腹部疼痛或不适(阵发性或慢性)。

• 膨隆、胃弱、嗳气、胀气和烧心。

• 厌食、恶心与呕吐。

• 呕血、黑便。

体格检查

• 认真查体包括粪便隐血试验以及直立时生命体征。

• 脱水貌、心动过速(呕吐时)。

• 面色苍白(出血性胃炎)。

• 腹部检查。

• 非特异性。

• 上腹部压痛。

基本检查

• 心肺复苏。

• 血细胞比容测定。

• 脱水、休克状态评估。

诊断检查与说明

实验室检查

- 一般胃炎时实验室检查值通常正常。
- 血常规：
  - 急性出血性胃炎时可有贫血。
  - 白细胞增多：感染。
- 电解质、血清尿素氮、肌酐和葡萄糖。
- 淀粉酶/脂肪酶，与胰腺炎鉴别。
- 尿液分析：
  - 评估脱水、酮症(饥饿)。
  - 肝炎时胆红素升高。

诊断步骤/外科

- 心电图：
  - 对于老年患者。
  - 鉴别心肌梗死。
- 内镜检查：
  - 门诊患者存在明显的出血。
  - 可以在直视下找到出血部位，确认黏膜炎症，探测幽门螺旋杆菌。
- 无创性幽门螺旋杆菌检查：
  - ^{13}C、^{14}C 尿素呼气试验。
  - 粪抗原试验。
  - 血清学检测幽门螺旋杆菌抗体。
  - 血清胃蛋白酶同工酶：
    - 血清中胃蛋白酶同工酶Ⅰ和Ⅱ的比例与化生性萎缩性胃炎相关(主要是自身免疫性化生性萎缩性胃炎和恶性贫血)。

鉴别诊断

- 消化性溃疡。
- 非溃疡性消化不良(内镜下看不到溃疡)。
- 胃食管反流。
- 胆绞痛。
- 胆囊炎。
- 胰腺炎。
- 肝炎。
- 腹主动脉瘤。
- 心肌梗死。

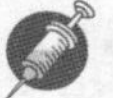

治疗

院前

- 心肺复苏。
- 静脉液体复苏。

初步稳定/治疗

- 严重的糜烂性或出血性胃炎表现出血流动力学不稳定的需要心肺复苏。
- 通过两个大孔导管用乳酸钠林格注射液或生理盐水进行静脉液体复苏。
- 当有呕血史或生命体征不稳定时需插鼻胃管进行胃减压或灌洗。
- 安置 Foley 导管以检测容量。

急诊治疗/程序

- 疼痛控制：
  - 抑酸剂。
  - 胃肠道鸡尾酒疗法：
    - 30 ml 抑酸剂＋10～20 ml 黏性利多卡因。
  - H_2 受体拮抗剂。
  - 质子泵抑制剂(PPI)。
  - 硫糖铝。
  - 避免麻醉药物，会掩盖严重疾病。
- 急性出血性胃炎：
  - 静脉液体复苏。
  - 低血细胞比容时需要输血。
  - 消除诱因(酒精、脓毒血症、非甾体抗炎药、创伤)。
  - 阻止严重疾病时出现急性或糜烂性胃炎：
    - 大量抑酸剂或 PPI 或 H_2 受体拮抗剂。
    - 目标是保持 pH>4。
- 慢性胃炎：幽门螺旋杆菌治疗。
  - 治疗方法：
    - 侵入性或非侵入性试验以确诊感染。
    - 口服抗生素以根除。
  - 对于无症状或非溃疡性的消化不良性胃炎的治疗是有争议的。
- 对于萎缩性胃炎需补充维生素 B_{12}。

药物

- 碱式水杨酸铋：525 mg，2 片，口服，每日 4 次，24 h 内不超过 8 片。
- 西咪替丁(H_2 受体拮抗剂)：800 mg，口服，晚睡前[儿童：20～40 mg/(kg·24 h)]，持续 6～8 周。
- 法莫替丁(H_2 受体拮抗剂)：40 mg，口服，晚睡前(儿童：0.5～0.6 mg/kg，q12 h)，持续 6～8 周。
- 兰索拉唑(PPI)：30 mg，口服，每日 2 次，持续 2 周。
- 氢氧化铝：2～4 片，口服，每日 4 次。
- 米索前列醇：100～200 μg，口服，每日 4 次。
- 碳酸钙：2～4 片，口服，每日 4 次。
- 尼扎替丁(H_2 受体拮抗剂)：300 mg，口服，睡前，持续 6～8 周。
- 奥美拉唑(PPI)：20 mg，口服，每日 2 次(儿童：0.6～0.7 mg/kg，q12～24 h)，持续 2 周。
- 泮托拉唑(PPI)：40 mg，口服/静注，每日 1 次，持续 2 周。
- 雷尼替丁(H_2 受体拮抗剂)：300 mg，口服，晚睡前[儿童：5～10 mg/(kg·24 h)，q12 h]，持续 6～8 周。
- 硫糖铝：1 g，口服，每日 4 次，持续 6～8 周。

一线用药

- 克拉霉素三联疗法：
  - 14 日疗法。
    - 每日 2 次 PPI。
    - 克拉霉素(500 mg)，每日 2 次。
    - 阿莫西林(1 g)，每日 2 次；或甲硝唑(500 mg)，每日 3 次。
- 高发病率地区的序贯 10 日治疗。
  - 双重治疗 5 日：
    - 每日 2 次 PPI。
    - 阿莫西林(1 g)。
  - 随后三联疗法 5 日：
    - 每日 2 次 PPI。
    - 克拉霉素(500 mg)，每日 2 次。
    - 甲硝唑(500 mg)，每日 3 次。
- 铋基四联疗法：
  - PPI(标准剂量)。
  - 次硝酸铋(120～300 mg 或 420 mg)或次水杨酸铋(300 或 524 mg)，每日 4 次。
  - 四环素(500 mg)，每日 4 次。
  - 甲硝唑(500 mg)，每日 3 次。
- 联合治疗 10/14 日。
  - 每日 2 次 PPI。
  - 克拉霉素(500 mg)和阿莫西林(1 g)或甲硝唑(500 mg)，每日 2 次。
- 混合疗法：
  - PPI 每日 2 次加上阿莫西林(1 g)，每日 2 次，持续 5 日，随后：
  - PPI、克拉霉素(500 mg)、阿莫西林(500 mg)加甲硝唑(500 mg)或替硝唑(500 mg)，每日 2 次，共 7 日。
- 左氧氟沙星序贯疗法：
  - PPI 每日 2 次，加上阿莫西林(1 g)每日 2 次，持续 5～7 日，然后：
  - PPI，左氧氟沙星(500 mg)，每日 1 次，阿莫西林(500 mg)每日 2 次，加甲硝唑或替硝唑(500 mg)每日 2 次，共 57 日。
- 抢救性治疗应以药敏试验为基础。

 随访

进一步处理

入院指征

• 急性出血性或糜烂性胃炎表现为上消化道出血、心动过速和低血压。

• 无法控制的疼痛或呕吐。

• 药物或肝脏疾病引起凝血功能障碍。

出院指征

• 体格检查未见明显异常，血细胞计数正常，粪隐血试验阴性。

• 如果上消化道出血患者粪隐血试验阳性，但生命体征稳定，血细胞比容正常，无插鼻胃管指征，则不收治入院。

- 不入院患者需行内镜检查以评估。

转诊问题

• 门诊患者行内镜和幽门螺旋杆菌检查。

• 胃部结构异常和肿瘤患者行病理活检。

随访建议

密切与消化科随访，等待内镜和病理结果回报，以达到诊断目的。

要点和误区

• 胃炎/胃病在急诊室很常见。

• 典型症状为消化不良、恶心和呕吐。

• 急诊室干预措施应当根据患者的临床症状来定，但不能忽视诊断和治疗。

• 治疗性干预包括抗幽门螺旋杆菌治疗。

• 幽门螺旋杆菌对抗生素的耐药性在不断增加。

• 消化科随访以明确病理结果，鉴别胃癌。

喂养问题(儿童) Feeding Problems, Pediatric

Dorka M. Jiménez Almonte · Richard Gabo 万健 译

 基础知识

描述

• "喂养"涉及一种或多种组成要素。

- 食物进入口腔：食欲、觅食行为和摄食。

- 吞咽食物：口咽期。

- 消化和吸收：食物吞咽和胃肠期。

• 营养不良在急性儿科疾病中很常见：

- 感染性，炎症性，阻塞性。

• 慢性进食问题可能由潜在的结构、神经肌肉、心血管、呼吸、胃肠道、行为或环境问题引起：

- 先天性异常、脑瘫、早产、先天性心脏病(CHD)、GERD 避免/限制性食物摄入障碍。

• 轻微的喂养困难可见于 25%～50%的正常儿童。

- 主要有绞痛、呕吐、喂食较慢及拒绝进食。

- 暂时的。不会造成严重后果。

- 经常出现在喂食过渡期(母乳到奶瓶，开始食用固体食物)。

• 较为严重的喂养问题见于 40%～80%的早产儿或合并慢性疾病或合并发育障碍的儿童。

病因

• 一些从病理上可明显区分，但通常有相互重叠。

• 结构异常：

- 鼻咽：

◦ 唇/腭裂。

◦ 后鼻孔闭锁。

◦ 小颌畸形和/或 Pierre-Robin 综合征。

◦ 巨舌症(唐氏综合征、Beckwith-Wiedemann 综合征)。

◦ 舌下肿块。

◦ 扁桃体/腺样体肥大。

- 喉和气管：

◦ 喉裂或囊肿。

◦ 声门下狭窄。

◦ 喉部或气管软化。

◦ 气管食管瘘。

- 食管：

◦ 食管缩小、狭窄或食管蹼。

◦ 血管环或血管悬吊压迫气管食管。

◦ 食管肿块或肿瘤。

◦ 异物。

• 神经病学问题：

- 脑瘫。

- 缺氧性损伤。

- 创伤性脑损伤。

- 脑血管病。

- 颅后窝肿瘤。

- 肌肉萎缩症。

- 线粒体病。

- 重症肌无力。

- 婴儿肉毒中毒。

- 多发性肌炎/皮肌炎。

• 早熟(尤其是那些需要长期的肠外或肠外喂养的人)。

• 免疫功能异常：

- 过敏。

- 嗜酸细胞性食管炎。

- 腹部疾病。

• 胃肠道问题：

- 胃食管反流病。

- 便秘。

- 梗阻。

• 代谢异常：

- 甲状腺功能减退。

- 先天性代谢问题。

• 急性病或急性事件：

- 脓毒症。

- 咽炎、扁桃体炎、扁桃体周围脓肿、咽后脓肿、会厌炎、中枢神经系统感染。

- 口咽/食管病变：牙龈口炎(HSV)、疱疹性咽炎(柯萨奇病毒)、念珠菌、史蒂文森-约翰逊综合征、食管炎、腐蚀性食入。

- 肠套叠、肠扭转。

- 创伤：头部创伤、口咽创伤/烧伤、腹部创伤。

- 异物摄入或吸入。

• 发育问题：

- 普遍发育障碍(包括自闭症谱系障碍)。

- 发育迟缓。

• 行为问题：

- 避免性/限制性食物紊乱(DSM-5)：

◦ 吃得太少。

◦ 限制饮食数量。

◦ 害怕吃东西、恐惧症。

- 反刍(食物反刍后重新消化)。

- 条件性情绪反应。

- 抑郁。

• 环境/父母问题：

- 环境刺激性差。

- 功能失调的儿童喂养互动。

- 贫困(食物不足)。

诊断

症状和体征

• 出现喂养或喂养后的问题。
• 拒食、呕吐、窒息、吞咽困难或反胃。
• 体重增长不良或发育不良。
• 反复或慢性呼吸系统疾病。

病史

• 症状出现的时间。
• 每次喂养时间(经常延长)。
• 挑食或不愿进食。
• 不能独自进食(若>8 个月):
- 神经肌肉问题使摄食能力下降。
• 发育不良或体重增长不良。
• 反复肺部或呼吸道异常:
- 大多数婴儿的误吸不易被发现。
- 反复的肺炎或哮喘可能是慢性误吸的主要表现。
- 慢性肺疾病。
• 反复呕吐或窒息:
- 若有,了解何时发生。
• 腹泻、肠出血。
• 可能导致食欲下降的药物(较大的儿童),如兴奋剂或托吡酯。
• 发育不良/体重增加不良:
- 新生儿在 14 日时应能恢复出生体重。
- 婴儿通常在出生后 3 个月内每月增加 1 kg,从 36 个月大起每月增加 0.5 kg。
- 婴儿 6 个月时出生体重增加 1 倍,1 岁时出生体重增加 3 倍。
• 喂养时间多变,特别是母乳喂养的婴儿,所有年龄常规喂养时间>30 min 都值得注意:
- 足月产婴儿通常每隔 2~3 h 进食 2~3 oz (1 oz 约 30 ml)。
- 母乳喂养的婴儿每隔 2~3 h 哺乳 10~20 min。
- 当孩子长大些,每次喂养时间和频率有所减少。
- 1 个月大的婴儿通常每 4 h 进食 4 oz。

注意

询问看护人如何准备婴儿配方奶粉(通常每 1 勺配方奶粉配 2 oz 水),普通配方奶粉和母乳每盎司含 20 kcal。稀释配方可能导致体重增加不良和低钠血症。患有某些疾病(早产儿、冠心病、FTT)的婴儿可能需要高热量(浓缩)配方奶粉。

体格检查

• 生命体征,包括血氧饱和度。
• 体重、身长和头围:
- 与既往测量值作比较,标记生长曲线。
- 生长速度减慢(身高低于同年龄和同性别的 5%,5 岁后生长<5 cm/年)。
- 营养状况损害。严重病例可出现消瘦、无力、情感淡漠。
• 全身体格检查,特别注意:
- 情感和社会反应。
- 先天性畸形(面部不对称、舌和颌大小等)。
- 耳鼻喉:口咽部炎症、感染或解剖异常。
- 心血管状况(杂音、奔马律、心动过速、股动脉减少/消失、毛细血管充盈)。
- 肺部:呼吸急促、呼吸窘迫、面色改变、干湿啰音、哮鸣音。
- 腹部检查:肠鸣音、膨隆、硬度、肿块、腹膜征。
- 神经系统:音调、协调性、警觉性、力量、发育阶段、脑神经。
- 皮肤:过敏性皮疹或特异反应。
  ◦ 多表现于眼周皮下液体或脂肪丢失,脱水或营养不良的婴儿多出现眼窝"凹陷"。
  ◦ 水肿,但合并蛋白质不足(Kwashiorkor 征)。
• 喂养评估:神经肌肉弹性、姿势,父母的刺激反应,进食模式和功能,进食量不足,发展/运动技能和照顾者反应,以及与孩子的互动:
- 控制唾液的能力。
- 进食节律。
- 吞咽后气道内杂音。
- 喂食时窒息、咳嗽或呕吐。
- 喂食时的血氧饱和度有助于诊断。
- 出现疲乏或易怒。
- 喂食时间。
- 自我喂食技巧。
- 父母喂养技术。

基本检查

• 体格检查正常、近来体重增长良好、无脱水表现的反应良好的孩子,只需要合适的随访,不需要急诊检查。
• 表现为焦虑、脱水、反应不适、呼吸困难或体重增长不良的孩子需要进一步的检查评估。

诊断检查与说明

实验室检查

• 当孩子表现为发育不良或营养不良时给予初步的评估。
- 全血细胞计数、尿常规、电解质、肌酐、血糖、红细胞沉降率和/或 C 反应蛋白、甲状腺功能、肝功能、总蛋白和白蛋白。
• 若考虑感染,行血、尿培养;若考虑脑膜炎,行脑脊液分析和培养。
• 若考虑代谢异常行血清 NH_3、血及尿等相关性先天代谢异常检查。

影像学检查

• 怀疑心肺疾病时行 X 线检查。
• 怀疑心脏疾病时行心电图检查。
• 如果怀疑充血性心力衰竭,床边检查。
• 有指征时转诊或入院行超声及其他影像学检查。可能需要纤维或荧光镜吞咽检查。
• 考虑脑干、颅底或脊髓问题时行 MRI 检查。

诊断步骤/外科

• 根据病因,可能需要多学科评估,可能涉及:语言病理学家、儿科医师、小儿胃肠病学家、儿科营养师、发育儿科医师、儿童心理学家及可能的耳鼻咽喉科医师、整形外科医师或儿科外科医师。
• 特殊病理变化需要手术治疗。
• 喂养过程、亲子互动、儿童行为观察。

鉴别诊断

喂养异常可见于许多疾病。出现特异性表现时应考虑以下病因。
• 喂养时间延长,疲乏:
- 考虑心脏疾病。
• 反复肺炎:
- 考虑慢性误吸。
• 进食时喘鸣:
- 考虑声门或声门下异常。
• 吮吸-吞咽-呼吸协调性:
- 考虑鼻塞、鼻后孔闭塞。
• 呕吐、腹泻、腹痛和绞痛:
- 考虑过敏或胃食管反流。

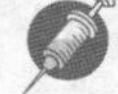

治疗

院前

• 评估生命体征和脱水情况,必要时给予液体复苏。
• 评估并纠正低血糖。

初步稳定/治疗

• 需要时心血管、呼吸、液体复苏。
• 怀疑低血糖时及时评估和治疗。

W

注意

• 某些先天性代谢异常（糖原贮存疾病）可导致难以纠正的低血糖，怀疑上述疾病时如不能口服治疗，应立即给予静脉右旋糖酐。

• 小婴儿呕吐胆汁可能是肠扭转的表现，可导致小肠缺血，需要急诊外科会诊。

■ **急诊治疗/程序**

• 如存在脱水的处理：

- 口服补液。
- 禁忌口服、不能耐受或实施困难时，给予静脉补液。
- 鼻饲补液。

• 急性呕吐给予昂司丹琼治疗。

• 口咽病变、溃疡的疼痛管理。

• 如有呼吸困难的处理：

- 喂食前鼻腔吸引清除分泌物有助于缓解小婴儿的上呼吸道感染、细气管感染症状。
- 需要时给予氧疗和其他措施。

• 怀疑感染时给予治疗。

注意

严重营养不良的患儿有发生脓毒症的风险，并可能出现生理反射迟钝，高度提示感染可能。

■ **药物治疗**

昂司丹琼：一旦出现恶心或呕吐时，0.1 mg/kg 静脉注射或口服，q8 h。最小口服剂量＜15 kg 患儿用 2 mg；＞15 kg 患儿用 4 mg。

• 监测有无 QT 延长的风险。

• 大于 6 个月患儿短期使用（3～5 剂）。

• 反复 QT 延长注意回顾 FDA 的警告。

• 对乙酰氨基酚：10～15 mg/kg，口服，q4～6 h，疼痛时。不超过 4 g/24 h。

• 布洛芬：5～10 mg/kg，口服，q6 h，疼痛时。

随访

■ **进一步处理**

入院指征

• 怀疑全身感染。

• 不能保持正常水平衡。

• 进食时持续低氧、呼吸窘迫。

• 严重的生长困难：

- 尤其是 3 个月以内的婴儿。
- 提供观察喂食的机会。
- 失代偿性心肺疾病。

• 症状性贫血或内分泌功能异常。

• 生活无法自理的患者。

• 监护人疏忽。

出院指征

• 能够经口进食。

• 生长发育不良者体重增加。

• 可靠的监护人和正常的随访。

转诊问题

• 根据问题的原因给予相应的转诊。

• 复杂或慢性喂养问题常需要多学科会诊。

• 行为状况通常需要长期的心理干预和支持。

• 慢性疾病进程可能影响喂食及热量需求：

- 不能口服营养支持的患儿常需要经皮内镜下胃造瘘管饲营养。

■ **随访建议**

• 有条件时一位主治医师是随访最重要的资源。

• 复杂病例常需要多学科会诊，主诊医师是最好的联络协调人。

要点和误区

• 婴儿获得满意的喂养需要复杂的生理因素、发育因素和环境因素间有效的协调统一。

• 几个因素间是相互依赖的，分割其中的一项通常导致其余几项的失调。

- 早产的婴儿吮吸-吞咽的协调性不成熟，给予强行填塞喂养错过吮吸-吞咽反射的重要发展时期，反复的有害刺激可导致患儿产生经口进食的厌恶。

• 反复出现急性的喂养问题可能有明确的病因。

- 口炎、肠胃炎、幽门狭窄、咽炎和脓毒症。

• 有上呼吸症状的婴儿可以在喂养前吸出鼻部分泌物来清理鼻部即可。

• 更多的慢性、长期的喂养问题可能有多因素和/或不易发现的病因。

- 喂养是父母与孩子交流的重要部分之一。
  - 两者关系失调可能是导致喂养问题的原因。

• 医源性的慢性喂养问题即使病因解除后仍可能持续有行为上的喂养困难。

• 吞咽困难和误吸通常比较隐秘。

蚊媒疾病：登革热、基孔肯亚病和西尼罗病毒感染

Mosquito-Borne Diseases: Dengue, Chikungunya, and West Nile Virus

Morgan P. Eutermoser　段立伟 译

基础知识

■ **描述**

• 媒介传播疾病占传染病的 17%。蚊子是最广为人知的媒介。

• 病情严重程度：无症状至致命。

• 尽管采取了控制措施，但蚊媒疾病仍在增加。气候变化、动物迁徙模式、旅行和国际贸易都起到了推动作用。

• 除了疟疾之外，还有几种疾病特别重要：

- 登革热：每年有 3.9 亿登革热感染，1/4 导致临床疾病。在 100 多个国家流行。旅行者发热的第二常见原因。2015 年 320 万例（EHO），存在很多漏报。疾病的范围从轻度疾病［登革热（DF）］到严重症状［登革出血热（DHF）和登革休克综合征（DSS）］不等。
- 基孔肯亚病：2013 年在美洲（加勒比）首次报道。
- 寨卡病毒感染：对孕妇的影响很大（发育中胎儿的严重神经缺陷，特别是小头畸形症）。2015—2018 年，美国报告了 5 635 例有症状的病例（95%的病例是旅行者）。
- 西尼罗病毒（WNV）感染：野生鸟类是主要的宿主。1999 年进入美国。2011 年的一次暴发的死亡率为 4%～5%。在 48 个州报告了病例。

■ **病因**

• 蚊媒病毒由三种蚊子中的一种传播：按蚊（疟疾）、伊蚊（登革热、基孔肯亚病、寨卡

病毒感染)和库蚊(西尼罗热)。

• 疟蚊：
- 夜间叮咬。
- 只传播疟疾。
• 伊蚊属：
- 白天叮咬。
- 埃及伊蚊是主要媒介；白纹伊蚊也能传播疾病。它们在死水中繁殖(轮胎、垃圾桶、水桶、花瓶)。
- 传播情况：
◦ 登革热：热带亚热带地区：亚洲、非洲、中南美洲、加勒比海。4 种血清型：DEN-1、DEN-2、DEN-3、DEN-4。随后被其他血清型感染会增加严重疾病的风险。
◦ 基孔肯亚病：与登革热位于同一地区。
◦ 寨卡病毒感染：太平洋群岛和南美感染负担最重。在北美，墨西哥的病例数量最多；然而，佛罗里达州(2014 年)和得克萨斯州(2015 年)报道了病例。
• 库蚊：
- 夜间叮咬。
- 传播情况：
◦ WNV：1937 年在乌干达首次发现。次于鸟类迁徙模式，特有于欧洲、印度、非洲、亚洲、中东、澳大利亚和北美洲。可以对人类造成风险的马和鸟(鸦)病。
◦ 流行性乙型脑炎和淋巴丝虫病。
• 其他可能的传播方式：母体胎儿传播、性接触、实验室暴露后感染、输血、母乳喂养。
- WNV：固体器官移植。
- 尽管有传播风险，但仍推荐母乳喂养。

诊断

症状和体征

• 总体而言，虫媒病毒感染的症状包括皮疹、发热、关节痛。恶心和呕吐也是常见的症状。
• 登革热：潜伏期 4～10 日。
- 登革热(DF)：流感样疾病。很少会导致死亡。高热、头痛、肌痛、眶后疼痛、淋巴结病、合并的斑丘疹。退热后，可能出现散在的瘀斑。在 50% 的患者中，皮疹与发热不谋而合。症状持续 2～7 日。
- 登革热出血热(DHF)：疾病的三个阶段。发热期：类似 DF 症状。危重期：随着退热，出现腹痛和呕吐。这是一个警告信号。这一阶段持续 24～48 h，也被称为“渗漏期”，原因是腹水、胸腔积液、点状皮疹、鼻出血、毛细血管渗漏和血小板减少导致的整体出血倾向。这可以进展到循环衰竭和死亡，或者进展到第三个恢复阶段。
- 主要体检结果和病史：患者从疫区归来，合并皮疹、发热、关节痛。如果把手放在患者身上，皮疹就会变白，并不会很快褪去。
• 基孔肯亚病：潜伏期 3～7 日。
- 最常见的症状是发热、关节痛、关节肿胀(双侧)、皮疹。
- 大多数人会在 1 周内恢复，但有些人可能会持续几周或几个月的关节疼痛。
- 严重情况：新生儿(垂直传播)、成人≥65 岁和合并其他疾病(高血压、糖尿病)。
• 寨卡病毒感染：潜伏期 3～14 日。
- 18% 的感染患者出现症状。
- 如果有症状，主要为发热、皮疹、头痛、关节痛和结膜炎，持续约 1 周。
- 病毒对发育中的胎儿的影响最大。
- 病毒可能在精液中存在 1 周。
- 吉兰-巴雷综合征。
• 西尼罗病毒感染：潜伏期 2～14 日。
- 疾病的严重程度：
◦ 80% 无症状。
◦ 20% 的轻度流行性感冒表现。
◦ 1/150 累及中枢神经系统。
- 疾病的严重程度与中枢神经系统的受累有关：
◦ 50 岁以上且免疫功能低下者风险增加。

病史

• 诊断更多地基于临床诊断和病史，而不是实验室检查结果。
• 生活在流行区或有旅游史。
• 寨卡病毒感染：前往疫区旅行或与感染者发生无保护措施的性行为。

体格检查

有症状的患者出现典型的皮疹(斑丘疹)、发热和关节痛三联征。
• 登革热：
- 明显的皮疹，尤指在严重病例中。是黄斑皮疹和点状斑点的结合。在严重的情况(DHF 和 DSS)中，可以看到脉压变窄、心动过速、低血压。
- 容易出血。
• 基孔肯亚病：
- 与登革热相似的发现，但没有出血性发现。
- 慢性、持续时间较长的关节痛。
• 寨卡病毒感染：
- 结膜炎。
• 西尼罗热：
- 神经学表现，如精神状态改变、反射亢进、共济失调、瘫痪、癫痫、运动无力和脑膜痉挛。有报告的表明，可能有长期认知问题。

基本检查

• 如有问题，请联系疾病控制和预防中心。
• 提交样品的程序因地区而异。请参阅公共卫生指南。

诊断检查与说明

实验室检查

第 1 周：RT-PCR，培养。第 1 周末：IgM、IgG。Triopex RT-PCR(筛查登革热、基孔肯亚病或寨卡病感染)。
• 登革热：血小板减少、中性粒细胞减少、血细胞比容升高(血浆渗漏)、ARF、低钠血症、INR 延长、APTT 和 PT 延长、D-二聚体升高、纤维蛋白原降低。
• 基孔肯亚病：没有具体的发现。
• 寨卡病毒感染：建议患者接触过寨卡病毒或产科超声检查异常没有症状的孕妇进行检测。
• 西尼罗热：脑脊液中以淋巴细胞为主，蛋白质升高，血糖正常。对西尼罗河病毒最敏感的筛查试验是脑脊液和血清的 IgM 检测。其他实验室异常：白细胞增多(50%)，白细胞减少(15%)，低钠血症。

影像学检查

用于特定疾病的治疗症状，但对特定病毒的诊断没有帮助。
• 登革热：胸部 X 线片可能显示胸腔积液。如果有精神状态改变或由于创伤(出血风险)发生变化，则考虑 CT 头部检查。腹部超声可以显示腹水。
• 基孔肯亚病：没有明确的影像表现。
• 寨卡病毒感染：孕妇可能需要进行多次超声检查，以跟踪胎儿的情况。
• 西尼罗病毒感染：头颅 CT 通常正常。MRI 可显示中枢神经系统炎症，伴有软脑膜和/或脑室周围白质强化，或可模拟脱髓鞘过程。

诊断步骤/外科

• 登革热：止血带试验：将血压袖带充气至血压中值。如果每平方厘米出现 3 个或 3 个以上的瘀点，则检测呈阳性。
• 基孔肯亚病：没有。
• 寨卡病毒感染：没有。
• 西尼罗病毒感染：腰椎穿刺。

W

■ 鉴别诊断

• 感染性疾病：

- 病毒性疾病：非特异性、流感、风疹、斑疹、单核细胞增多症、幼儿急疹。
- 斑疹(见伤寒)。
- 疟疾。
- 钩端螺旋体病。
- 病毒性胃肠炎。
- 梅毒二期。
- HIV。
- 伤寒。
- 中毒性休克综合征。
- 阑尾炎。
- 脑炎(单纯疱疹病毒、巨细胞病毒、EBV、VZV、肠道病毒、其他虫媒病毒)。
- 川崎病。

• Still 病。

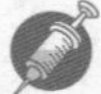

治疗

■ 初步稳定/治疗

• ABC 管理。

• 开通静脉通道、心电监护仪、静脉输液、吸氧。

• 如果考虑存在西尼罗病毒感染，应注意癫痫预防措施。

■ 急诊治疗/程序

• 登革热：治疗支持 DF、DHS、DSS。低血压和脱水的给予静脉输液。退热用的扑热息痛。由于血小板功能障碍，避免使用阿司匹林或非甾体抗炎药。血小板输注对血小板减少症有争议。如果及早诊断并进行适当的治疗，死亡率将从 20% 降至 1% 以下。

• 基孔肯亚病：支持治疗。对乙酰氨基酚仅用于退热，在登革热被排除后停用。

• 寨卡病毒感染：支持治疗。对乙酰氨基酚仅用于退热，在登革热被排除后停用。

• 西尼罗病毒感染：支持治疗。对于有脑膜炎的迹象，在脑脊液结果出来之前使用抗生素/抗病毒药物。可用退热药。目前还没有已知的有效抗病毒疗法或疫苗。没有对照研究证明干扰素 α-2b、利巴韦林、激素、抗惊厥药或渗透剂的有效性。

随访

■ 进一步处理

入院指征

• 登革热：考虑出现 DHS 或 DSS 症状(低血压、DIC、血小板减少、血液浓缩)或随访不良而入院。

• 基孔肯亚病：存在剧烈疼痛，需要静脉用药。

• 寨卡病毒：通常没有入院标准，除非担心吉兰-巴雷综合征。

• 西尼罗病毒感染：神经症状，休克，存在高危因素(高龄，免疫功能低下)。

出院指征

• 登革热：登革热：病情轻微，病情明确，随访密切，疼痛控制，或已耐受。

• 基孔肯亚病：疼痛可控，或已耐受。

• 寨卡病毒感染：神经系统检查正常。

• 西尼罗病毒感染：神经系统检查正常。

■ 随访建议

• 对出现登革热症状的患者进行密切随访，以监测病情是否恶化。

• 在疾病流行区的妇女、到流行区旅行的妇女或与受感染男性或流行区男性有性接触的妇女应接受寨卡病毒风险咨询。如果有上述情况，密切监测产科超声结果。

要点和误区

• 考虑最近到疾病流行区旅行的以发热、皮疹、关节痛为表现的患者中是否存在蚊媒疾病。

• 所有这些都可能被误认为是“流感”。

• 寨卡病毒对发育中的胎儿构成风险。育龄妇女在前往地方病流行地区旅行时，应该得到有关风险、蚊子控制和性接触的建议。

• 为所有前往疫区旅行的患者提供预防性建议：浅色衣服、长袖和裤子。驱虫剂。使用窗纱。

• 疫区蚊子、病媒控制困难。然而，在疫区可以集中在装满水的容器、蚊子繁殖地喷洒杀虫剂。

• 以上所有疾病都是及时上报的传染性疾病。

W

无创呼吸机管理 Ventilation Management, Noninvasive

Stephen M. Carroll 吴昊 李文放 译

基础知识

■ 描述

• 无创通气(NIV)是一种通过正压面罩为呼吸困难和呼吸衰竭的患者输送氧气的方法。

• NIV 几乎可以使任何出现这些症状的患者受益，并且可以避免气管插管。在一些患者群体中，NIV 改善死亡率，尤其是在患者临床病程早期给予 NIV 时。

■ 基础理论：NIV 模式

• NIV 面罩配置：大多数急诊使用全套 NIV 面罩，以及其他可选方案包括仅鼻面罩、覆盖整个面部前部的头戴式面罩和 NIV 头盔。本章将重点介绍全脸面罩 NIV，因为它是大多数美国版最常见的配置。

• NIV 基础模式：连续正压(CPAP)和双层正压(BiPAP)*。

- CPAP 在整个呼吸循环中提供固定的压力支持。
- BiPAP 提供呼气期间和呼吸之间的基础压力，并在吸气周期中增加压力。
- 不管是哪种模式，NIV 都能通过在肺内小气道内植入生理支架来改善呼吸功能。这降低了肺泡水平的肺不张程度。
- 在急性心源性肺水肿(ACPE)患者中，人们普遍错误地认为 NIV 是通过迫使液体排出肺部而起作用的。然而，实际机制是 NIV 增加胸内压，从而降低前负荷和后负荷。
- 注：术语“BiPAP”是特定设备制造商制造的通风模式的专利商标。然而，它被广泛用于指示双水平 NIV。

诊断

症状和体征

- NIV 适应证：
  - 慢性阻塞性肺病加重：
    - 强有力的证据表明 NIV 针对死亡率、插管需求和治疗失败的减少。
    - BiPAP 对 COPD 可能比 CPAP 更有效。
  - 哮喘急性加重：
    - 在这一人群中获益的证据并不一致。
    - BiPAP 是 NIV 的首选治疗模式。
    - NIV 治疗期间，应继续雾化吸入，并使用镁、特布他林和其他药物治疗哮喘。
  - 急性心源性肺水肿：
    - meta 分析的证据显示死亡率及气管插管率降低。
    - 低血压在这些患者中更常见。
    - 一项研究由于担心 NIV 组 MI 发生率较高提前停止。然而，在更大的试验和 meta 分析中并没有发现这一点。
    - ACPE 的治疗包括大剂量的硝酸甘油和利尿剂，应与 NIV 治疗同时进行。
  - 社区获得性肺炎：
    - 在这类患者群体中没有令人信服的益处证据，但可以作为辅助手段来避免气管插管。
- NIV 禁忌证：
  - 绝对禁忌证：
    - 需要立即插管(可用于预充氧)。
    - 分泌物过多和/或呕吐和误吸的高风险。
    - 面部外伤，无法封住面罩。
    - 气胸。
  - 相对禁忌证：
    - 血流动力学不稳定(需要密切监测)。
    - 精神状态不佳(见下文)。
    - 严重缺氧。
    - 患者合作能力差(见后续插管)。
  - 精神状态下降：
    - 根据病情考虑是绝对或相对的禁忌证。
    - 在急诊室或重症监护室，NIV 可用于意识水平下降的患者(尤其是在初始复苏阶段)，前提是要密切监测患者的临床恶化情况。这些患者不应该在没有监控的情况下入院。

病史

- 有重点但全面的病史和体格检查对确定潜在的呼吸困难或急性呼吸衰竭的原因至关重要。
- 从意识障碍患者身上获取病史可能很困难，应重点关注：
  - 相关的既往病史。
  - 使用吸入器和利尿剂等药物。
  - 下肢或腹部水肿增加。

体格检查

检查应重点检查肺部声音(气喘与爆裂声和呼吸深度)以及下肢、腹部或骶前水肿的评估。

诊断检查与说明

实验室检查

- 一般来说，静脉血气(VBG)足以通过 pH 和 $PaCO_2$ 确定患者的通气状态。一旦患者稳定下来，就可以获得动脉血气(ABG)，以评估氧合(PaO_2)：
  - 在急诊室和重症监护室环境下的多项研究表明，pH 和 $PaCO_2$ 在 ABG 和 VBG 结果上具有足够的相关性，可以做出准确的临床决策。
- CBC 和生化将指导进一步的治疗，并可能揭示严重呼吸困难的原因，如严重贫血或急性肾衰竭。
- 肌钙蛋白和脑钠尿肽(BNP)经常出现在呼吸困难患者中，尤其是当怀疑 ACPE 是呼吸困难的原因时。
- 心电图：
  - 所有呼吸困难的患者都应该进行心电图检查，以评估 STEMI 或明显的心脏缺血。
  - 所有呼吸困难的患者都应该进行心电图检查，以评估 STEMI 或明显的心脏缺血。

影像学检查

- 床边超声检查对于确定呼吸困难的常见原因非常有用，包括：
  - ACPE 患者的 B 线。
  - 胸腔积液。
  - 肺炎。
  - 气胸(不应使用 NIV 治疗)。
  - 心输出量总体下降。
  - 有大的肺栓塞迹象。
- 根据不同疾病过程的临床怀疑，根据需要进行胸部 X 线检查或胸部 CT 检查：然而，NIV 患者通常很难耐受仰卧位进行 CT 检查。

鉴别诊断

见上文 NIV 适应证。

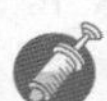

治疗

院前

- 院前使用 NIV 的证据：
  - 一项荟萃分析中死亡率效益和插管需求减少。
- NIV 在院前环境中的应用：
  - 通常通过附在氧气瓶上的布希尼卡面罩完成 CPAP：
    - 该面罩不需要单独的氧气发生器或呼吸机。
    - 除非使用不同的呼吸机设置，否则大多数院前系统通常不提供 BiPAP。
- 患者选择和初始设置：
  - 遵循本地协议，但是一般情况下：
    - 创伤患者通常禁忌证。
    - 在院前环境中尽早应用。
    - 从 10 cmH_2O 的 CPAP 设置开始，并按照方案调整。

初步稳定/治疗

- 静脉通路。
- 心脏监护仪。
- 血压监测。
- 脉搏血氧仪。
- 呼吸末二氧化碳监测(如有)。

急诊治疗/程序

- NIV 使用目标：
  - 在 ED 过程中尽早应用：
    - 在应用 NIV 之前，通常不需要对呼吸困难进行初步诊断。
  - 减少呼吸的工作量。
  - 为需要插管的患者预充氧。
- NIV 初始设置：
  - 压力设置：
    - CPAP：10 cmH_2O，调整至具有治疗效果和舒适适宜。
    - BiPAP：15 cmH_2O 吸气压力和 5 cmH_2O 呼气压力(通常表示为“15/5”)，根据患者的效果和舒适度进行调整。
  - FiO_2：最初设定为 100%，以便最大限度地输送氧气。
  - 如果患者在初始复苏后不需要高浓度的血氧饱和度来维持可接受的动脉血氧饱和度，则应在耐受范围内进行滴定，以避免高氧的负面影响。
  - 面罩泄漏：最初尽可能低，7～15 LPM 长期。
  - 备用呼吸频率：每分钟 10～12 次呼吸：
    - 这需要在患者呼吸暂停的情况下建立起来，并且应该与一个报警器联系起来，提醒治疗临床医生患者的呼吸暂停。
  - 备用潮气量：500～550 ml：
    - 可提供充足的潮气量，同时考虑面罩泄漏和死区。

• 插管前预给氧：

- 因肺炎或急性呼吸窘迫综合征（ACPE）等过程而出现分流和/或缺氧的患者，可在插管前使用 NIV 进行预充氧：

◦ 设置：10 cmH_2O，100% FiO_2 下的 CPAP，向上调整至患者耐受性和可达到的最高血氧饱和度。

• NIV 不耐受：

- 由于 NIV 面罩引起的呼吸困难和/或幽闭恐怖症引起的焦虑，患者可能无法耐受 NIV：

◦ 大多数患者可以通过使用 NIV 的过程得到"指导"，通过是向患者保证这将改善他们的呼吸。

◦ 允许患者将面罩贴在脸上，同时缓慢地使用面罩带可以帮助降低患者的焦虑。

◦ 可以考虑使用抗焦虑药或阿片类药物来帮助患者耐受 NIV，但是应谨慎使用，并密切监测（见药物）。

• 延迟顺序插管：

- 不能耐受 NIV 或插管前任何预充氧尝试的患者，在插管过程中极易发生严重的去饱和。

- 这些患者会因为感到窒息而变得烦躁并摘下 NIV 面罩。

- 对于这些患者，可以考虑延迟顺序插管（DSI），而不是执行快速顺序插管（RSI）：

◦ DSI 是一种程序性镇静剂，用于插管前的预氧。

◦ 所有设备和人员应准备好插管，必要时进行 RSI。

◦ 以缓慢静脉推注的方式给予游离剂量的氯胺酮（1～2 mg/kg 静脉注射），同时保持患者的呼吸动力。

◦ 氯胺酮可使患者配合预氧，通常在 100% FiO_2 条件下至少 3 min。

◦ 像往常一样给患者服用麻醉药物并插管。

◦ 氯胺酮条件下，他们耐受 NIV 后，一些患者可能会显著改善。如果决定不给患者插管，必须密切监视患者是否呕吐和出现反应（氯胺酮的常见副作用）。

• NIV 失败：

- NIV 患者应经常重新评估精神状态、呼吸功能、FiO_2 需求增加和呼吸暂停发作的变化，这些变化可能表明 NIV 未能达到预期效果。

- 分析 VBG/ABG 结果或 $ETCO_2$ 趋势，可能有助于补充临床判断，以确定患者是否正在改善。

- 低氧性呼吸衰竭、急性呼吸窘迫综合征（ARDS）和肺炎的患者可能有更高的 NIV 失败率，应考虑早期插管而不是 NIV 治疗。

- 如果患者没有改善，可以考虑进行气管插管。

• 用于姑息性护理或 DNR/DNI 患者。

- 可提供给登记在临终关怀或有积极的 DNR/DNI 的患者。

- 最适用于慢性阻塞性肺病患者。

- 可以缓解空气饥饿感，并提供一个桥梁，在不违反患者预先指示的情况下，让家人有更多时间探视。

■ 药物治疗

• 患者可能需要镇痛和/或镇静剂来耐受 NIV，但这应谨慎进行，并密切观察呼吸抑制、呼吸暂停和呕吐。

• 吸入药物可以通过 NIV 通路输送，继续治疗哮喘和 COPD。

• 沙丁胺醇：2.5～5 mg/5 ml 生理盐水，q4 h 或持续通过 NIV 面罩。

• 异丙托溴铵：0.5 mg/2.5 ml 生理盐水，q4 h，通过 NIV 面罩。

• 芬太尼：静脉注射 0.5～1.5 μg/kg。小剂量可以提供轻度的焦虑缓解，并且可以在不必进行 DSI 的情况下耐受 NIV。

• 咪达唑仑：成人静脉注射 2～5 mg（0.05～0.1 mg/kg）。滴定抗焦虑作用耐受 NIV，会引起呼吸抑制和低血压。

• 劳拉西泮：成人静脉注射 1～2 mg（0.05～0.1 mg/kg）。副作用类似咪达唑仑。

• 氯胺酮：用于 DSI，剂量 1～2 mg/kg 静脉注射，2～4 mg/kg 肌内注射。维持患者的呼吸功能。应缓慢静推，以避免快速静脉推注时出现短暂性呼吸暂停（通常持续 30～60 s）。轻度支气管扩张剂。当其作用逐渐消失时会引起烦躁不安的出现反应，可以用小剂量的苯二氮䓬类药物治疗。会导致心率和血压升高，但对于呼吸困难的危重患者，一旦药物生效，通常会通过减轻他们的焦虑来缓解。

随访

■ 进一步处理

入院指征

• 大多数在急诊室接受 NIV 治疗的患者都需接受进一步治疗。在极少数情况下，患者的病情会有很大的改善，因此从急诊室安全出院是可能的。

• 在急诊室接受 NIV 治疗的患者应考虑到 ICU 的入院，而在其他监测环境下，可以考虑更稳定的患者。

要点和误区

• 早期应用 NIV 将使几乎所有中重度呼吸困难患者受益，无论其潜在原因是什么。

• BiPAP 与 CPAP 的选择比任何形式的 NIV 都不重要。在 ACPE 中 CPAP 是首选，而 BiPAP 在 COPD 和哮喘中可能更好。

• 假设有足够的患者监护，NIV 的使用几乎没有禁忌证，尤其是在急诊环境下。

• 院前 NIV 已被证明可以降低插管率和死亡率，对于任何呼吸困难的患者（不包括外伤患者），应强烈考虑使用 NIV。

• 大多数患者可以通过指导来忍受 NIV。有些可能需要药物来缓解焦虑。

• 对于对预氧抵抗的患者，应考虑 DSI 与 NIV 相结合。

无力 Weakness

Kathryn A. Volz 吴昊 李文放 译

基础知识

■ 描述

• 被定义为身体力量或能量的减少。

• 患者会用"虚弱"来描述许多不同的症状和表现。

• 可能表现为神经肌肉无力、疲劳、不适、先兆症状或其他症状。

• 病史和体检是帮助缩小诊断和检查范围的关键。

• 通常由多种因素导致的。

• 区分神经肌肉障碍和非神经肌肉障碍。

- 区分局灶性肌无力与双侧或全身性肌无力。
- 神经肌肉疾病类别：
  - 上运动神经元(UMN)病变：
    - 深部腱反射(DTR)亢进。
    - 巴氏征阳性。
    - 肌张力增高。
    - 肌肉萎缩。
  - 下运动神经元(LMN)损伤：
    - 腱反射减弱。
    - 巴氏征阴性。
    - 肌张力减弱。
    - 有肌肉萎缩。
    - 肌束震颤。
  - 神经肌肉接头(NMJ)损伤：
    - 腱反射正常。
    - 病理征正常或缺失。
    - 肌张力减弱。
    - 非神经肌肉病变：
  - 神经性。
  - 感染性。
  - 外伤性/结构性。
  - 内分泌。
  - 代谢性。
  - 心源性。
  - 风湿性。
  - 中毒性。
  - 其他
  - 精神性。

病因

- 神经肌肉疾病：
  - 多发性硬化。
  - 肌萎缩性脊髓侧索硬化症。
  - 横贯性脊髓炎。
  - 吉兰-巴雷综合征。
  - 重症肌无力。
  - Lambert-Eaton 综合征(NMJ)。
  - 周期性瘫痪(可能是家族性的)。
- 神经系统：
  - TIA/脑血管意外。
  - 癫痫发作(托德麻痹)。
  - 恶性肿瘤。
  - 感染/脓毒症：
- 泌尿道感染：
  - 肺炎。
  - 脑膜炎。
  - 单核细胞增多症。
  - HIV 感染。
  - 虫媒病毒。
  - 肉毒杆菌中毒。
  - 硬膜外脓肿(常见于静脉注射药物)。
  - 脊髓灰质炎。
- 外伤性/结构性：
  - 颅内出血。
  - 脊髓损伤/病变。
  - 恶性肿瘤。
  - 马尾综合征。
  - 撞击综合征。
- 内分泌：
  - 甲状腺功能减退。
  - 肾上腺危象。
  - 维生素缺乏。
- 代谢：
  - 脱水。
  - 低血糖。
  - 电解质异常。
- 心脏：
  - 心肌缺血。
  - 心律失常。
  - 先兆症状。
  - 风湿性疾病：
- 系统性红斑狼疮。
  - 风湿性多肌痛。
  - 肌炎。
- 毒理学：
  - 海鲜毒素。
  - 蜱虫麻痹(NMJ)。
  - 氧化碳中毒。
  - 重金属中毒。
  - 滥用药物。
  - 酒精。
  - 有机磷酸盐和氨基甲酸酯(农药接触史)。
- 贫血。
- 妊娠。
- 精神虚弱原因(排除诊断)：
  - 焦虑、抑郁。
  - 依赖性人格。
  - 疑病。
  - 慢性疲劳综合征。
  - 纤维肌痛。
  - 装病。

诊断

症状和体征

- 改变物理强度：
  - 评估肌力：
    - 1：没有收缩。
    - 2：不能抵抗重力。
    - 3：可以对抗重力的主动运动。
    - 4：对抗重力，不能抵抗阻力的主动运动。
    - 5：正常。
  - 肌肉张力的改变：
    - 减弱。
    - 痉挛状态。
    - 强直。
  - 异常肌张力。
  - 异常巴氏征。
  - 肌肉萎缩。
- 系统性的表现：
  - 乏力。
  - 疲劳。
  - 头晕。
  - 麻痹性痴呆。
  - 感觉异常。
  - 声音嘶哑。
  - 吞咽困难。
  - 视觉变化、复视。
  - 上睑下垂。
  - 混乱。
  - 相关症状：
    - 发热。
    - 胸部疼痛。
    - 呼吸困难。
    - 咳嗽、URI 症状。
    - 体重减轻。
    - 皮疹。
    - 排尿困难。
    - 肠道、膀胱失禁。
    - 毒素暴露。
    - 蜱虫暴露。
    - 婴儿摄入蜂蜜(婴儿肉毒杆菌中毒)。

基本检查

- 服药史。
- 指脉血糖。
- 是否接触毒素。
- 完整的病史和体格检查。
- 如果有病史，排除急性脑血管病。
- 通过病史和体格检查指导进一步检查：
  - 广泛＋局灶。
  - 急性和慢性。
  - 近端和远端。
  - 由下往上和由上往下。
  - 对称与不对称。
  - 活动后加重或减轻。
  - 相关症状、暴露。

诊断检查与说明

除非病史和体格检查确定了无力的原因，

否则诊断测试应该是全面的。应根据临床问题选择影像学检查。

实验室检查

- 血清葡萄糖。
- 血常规、电解质、BUN、肌酐。
- β-HCG(排除妊娠)。
- 毒素筛查。
- 尿常规。
- 甲状腺功能测试(排除甲状腺功能减退)。
- 红细胞沉降率(排除风湿病原因)。
- 碳氧血红蛋白(排除一氧化碳中毒)。
- 肌钙蛋白、CK-MB(排除心肌缺血)。

影像学检查

- 心电图[排除急性冠状动脉综合征(ACS),心律失常]。
- 胸部X线平片(排除肺炎)。
- CT或MRI头部(排除颅内病理学)。
- 脊柱MRI(脊髓损伤、硬膜外脓肿)。

诊断步骤/外科

- 床边呼吸功能测定:
  - 用力肺活量、负力吸气、峰值呼气流量。
  - 可以识别那些即将出现的呼吸衰竭的人。
- 腰椎穿刺:
  - 对于疑似吉兰-巴雷综合征:
    - 脑脊液白蛋白细胞学分离(高蛋白,低白细胞)。
- 重症肌无力的Tensilon试验、冰袋试验:
  - 区分肌无力危象和胆碱能危象。
  - 小心使用。

鉴别诊断

- 生理性因素:
  - 单纯性疲劳:
    - 过多的体育活动。
    - 休息不足。
    - 过度或不足的饮食。
    - 妊娠。
- 精神性疲劳:
  - 焦虑、抑郁。
  - 依赖人格。
  - 癔症。
  - 慢性疲劳综合征。
  - 纤维肌痛。
  - 装病。

治疗

针对无力的根本原因进行治疗。

院前

- 吸氧。
- 建立静脉通路。
- 末梢血糖检测。
- 考虑严重呼吸窘迫、无法保护气道的患者气管插管。

初步稳定/治疗

- 吸氧。
- 建立静脉通路。
- 对即将发生的呼吸衰竭建立人工气道。
- 在选择麻醉药物插管时要小心,这个诊断组有许多禁忌证或调整剂量。

急诊治疗/程序

- 当诊断确定后,可以应用针对性治疗方法:
  - 血浆置换和/或原发性球蛋白(IVIG)治疗吉兰-巴雷综合征。
  - 阿托品+磷解磷肟对有机磷的毒性作用。
  - 氢化可的松治疗肾上腺功能不全。
  - 电解质替代低电解质。
  - 葡萄糖治疗低血糖。
  - 抗生素治疗适当的感染病因。
  - 肉毒中毒的特殊解毒剂。
  - 100%氧气或高压氧治疗一氧化碳中毒。
  - 蜱虫麻痹。
  - TPA/血管内治疗CVA符合标准。
  - 神经外科介入治疗某些结构性原因和硬膜外脓肿。

随访

进一步处理

入院指征

- 所有新发神经肌肉疾病或CVA/TIA患者均应入院进行明确诊断。
- 任何即将出现的通气或循环衰竭的患者都应该收治入ICU。

出院指征

- 症状缓解。
- 生命体征稳定。
- 明确诊断和改善症状。

随访建议

- 非神经系统疾病的出院患者应该对他们进行随访。
- 有神经系统疾病的出院患者应该有及时的神经学随访。

要点和误区

- 早期积极治疗因吉兰-巴雷综合征、肉毒杆菌中毒、重症肌无力导致呼吸系统损害的患者。
- 及时发现急性脑卒中并评估适当的治疗方法。
- 确定老年ACS患者或感染表现为虚弱。
- 考虑导致虚弱的内分泌原因,包括肾上腺功能不全和甲状腺功能减退。
- 筛查潜在的毒素暴露。

W

膝关节脱位 Knee Dislocation

Ian R. Grover · Matthew Correia 何超 段立伟 译

基础知识

描述

• 根据胫骨与远端股骨的相对位置定义膝关节脱位：
- 前脱位：
  ◦ 最常见的脱位方式。
  ◦ 由于膝关节过伸造成。
  ◦ 后囊、后交叉韧带（PCL）和前交叉韧带（ACL）断裂。
- 后脱位：
  ◦ 第二常见。
  ◦ 直接对胫骨前的损伤使膝关节屈曲 90°。
- 内侧脱位：
  ◦ 内翻的应力会导致前交叉韧带、后交叉韧带及外侧副韧带的撕裂伤。
- 外侧脱位。
  ◦ 外翻的应力会导致前交叉韧带、后交叉韧带及内侧副韧带的撕裂伤。
  ◦ 旋转。
  ◦ 当胫骨绕股骨旋转时，后交叉韧带保持完整。

• 相关损伤：
- 腘动脉损伤：
  ◦ 40%与错位有关。
  ◦ 由于近端和远端解剖关系导致的动脉破裂率高。
  ◦ 破裂会导致内膜撕裂或横断，通常还会延迟血栓形成。
  ◦ 如果血管修复延迟超过 8 h，致残率非常高。
- 腓神经损伤：
  ◦ 25%与错位有关。
  ◦ 在腓骨颈的下部和远端。
  ◦ 因牵引或横断造成的损伤，通常伴有内侧或旋转脱位。
  ◦ 超过 50%的患者出现永久性足下垂，25%部分恢复。

病因

• 高能量：
- 从高处坠落、机动车碰撞、汽车与行人事故。

• 低能量：
- 运动损伤（通常是足球）、蹦床坠落。

• 超低能量：
- 肥胖。
- 常规行走。

诊断

症状和体征

• 膝关节可能严重变形，也可能处于正常对齐状态，一半的脱位会自发出现。

• 血管损伤：无脉搏、面色苍白、疼痛、温度变化。

• 神经损伤：感觉障碍或感觉异常。

病史

• 损伤机制和时间。

• 减少运动的次数。

• 抗凝剂的使用与血液病病史。

体格检查

• 腘窝：
- 血管损伤的迹象。

• 远端搏动：
- 足背（DP）和胫后（PT）。
- 两侧对比。
- 有温度的肢体和/或完整的脉搏，不能排除动脉损伤的可能性，因为正常的侧支循环通常足以提供一些远端灌注。

• 远端神经功能障碍：
- 第一趾间隙感觉异常。
- 足背屈曲能力减弱。

• 韧带松弛：
- 前抽屉试验（ACL）。
- 后垂度试验（PCL）。
- 外翻、内翻应力（MCL、LCL）。

• 关节囊撕裂后常无肿胀。

基本检查

• 全面而详细的体格检查：
- 动脉搏动：触诊，多普勒超声检查；踝关节-臂指数。
- 神经损伤：足趾的活动障碍和足背屈。

• 超声和双侧的膝关节影像学检查。

• 当尝试进行闭合复位的情况下需要重复检查。

诊断检查和说明

• 双侧膝关节影像学检查：
- 排除合并的骨折。
- 推荐拍摄上下关节以及胫骨、腓骨和股骨全长的非急诊 X 线片。

• 治疗后重复上述步骤，以验证对齐情况。

• 尽快进行 MRI（最好在 1 周内），以确定韧带、半月板和关节损伤。

诊断步骤/外科

• 踝肱指数：
- 当臂指数≥0.9 时提示动脉损伤的可能性较低。
- 在患者平卧时必须执行。
- 必要时用多普勒超声听诊脉搏。
- 敏感性近 100%。

• 正式的血管造影是评估血管损伤（ABI 异常、体检发现不对称或血管损伤迹象）的首选方法。然而：
- 如果时间窗较宽泛，则可以进行 CT 血管造影（CTA）。

鉴别诊断

• 胫骨平台骨折。

• 腓骨头骨折。

• 股骨骨折。

• 韧带或肌腱的撕脱性骨折。

• 韧带损伤。

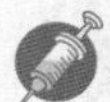

治疗

院前

• 进行急救（ABC 管理）。

• 进行必要的关节动脉搏动和运动功能的记录。

• 存在轻度的旋转脱位时以夹板进行固定以避免动脉的牵拉和受压。

初步稳定/治疗

• 当发生机动车挤压伤或交通事故时进行心肺复苏。

• 液体复苏，低血压能够缓解远端动脉搏动消失或远端肿胀。

• 当存在四肢缺血时立刻进行闭合复位。

• 开放性损伤或高度怀疑动脉损伤时应早期进行外科手术治疗。

急诊治疗/程序

• 必要时持续镇静以减轻疼痛。

• 以纵向股骨牵引进行闭合性复位，但注意不要对腘窝形成压迫。

• 对关节进行相关操作后要进行重复性的血管神经检查。

• 当膝关节存在 15°～20°的旋转脱位时使用夹板固定进行纠正。

X

• 为增加稳定性，尤其是在肥胖人群中，首选膝关节固定器。

• 在脚上敷料处留一个口，这样就可以充分评估血运情况。

• 踝足矫形器如果存在腓总神经损伤，以防止马蹄畸形。

• 急诊操作后，每隔一段时间重复行神经血管检查。

• 静脉镇痛使患者感到舒适。

• 外科会诊(骨科和血管科)：开放性损伤，PA 损伤，或无法复位。

■ 药物治疗

一线用药

• 静脉注射吗啡，每 30 min 静脉注射吗啡 4～6 mg 用于镇痛。

• 静脉注射氢吗啡酮，每 60 min 1 mg 用于镇痛。

• 静脉注射芬太尼，0.05～0.2 mg，每 15 min，必要时用于镇痛。

• 静脉注射头孢唑林，开放性骨折每 8 h 1 g。

• 避免口服药物的使用(因为可能需要进行外科手术治疗)。

随访

■ 进一步处理

入院指征

所有损伤出现下肢的肿胀和腘动脉损伤修复的患者都需要进行住院观察。

转诊注意

韧带损伤的修复：

• 在损伤后的第 3 周进行。

• 损伤后 2 周禁用关节镜手术以预防骨筋膜室综合征的发生。

■ 随访建议

• 进行矫形修复韧带损伤。

• 腘动脉损伤后的血管修复。

要点和误区

• 在损伤后的 6～8 h 腘动脉修复失败的患者约 90% 的概率需要进行截肢。

• 腓神经损伤，预后较差。

• 迟发型的骨筋膜室综合征需要进行预防。

系统性红斑狼疮 Systemic Lupus Erythematosus

Susanne M. Hardy 范浩浩 李文放 译

基础知识

■ 描述

• 慢性自身免疫性疾病，发病高峰期在 15～40 岁；特点是发作和缓解。

• 多系统多临床症状的疾病表现：

- 黏膜皮肤：
  - 最常涉及的系统。
  - 4 种具体皮疹：
- 关节炎。
- 心脏：
  - 心内膜炎。
  - 心肌炎。
  - 慢性心力衰竭。
  - 传导异常。
  - 动脉粥样硬化。
  - 心肌梗死。
- 肾：
  - 肾小球肾炎。
  - 肾衰竭。
- 肺部：
  - 胸腔积液(通常为渗出液)。
  - 肺炎或胸膜炎。
  - 肺出血。
  - 肺栓塞。
  - 肺炎。
  - 肺水肿。
  - 肺动脉高压。
- 神经系统：
  - 狼疮脑炎。
- 血管：
  - 血管炎。
  - 血栓形成。
  - 动脉粥样硬化。
- 消化系统：
  - 腹膜炎。
  - 肠系膜血管炎和局部缺血。
  - 胰腺炎。

儿科注意事项

• 产妇自身抗体穿过胎盘可出现新生儿狼疮：

- 与短暂性贫血和血小板减少症相关。

• 先天性心脏病是最严重的并发症。

老年人注意事项

• 由于动脉粥样硬化导致心肌梗死的风险增加 10 倍。

• 使用类固醇后慢性骨质疏松症的发生率高。

■ 危险因素

遗传学

• 女性比男性更常见(比例为 9∶1)。

• 在育龄妇女中更常见。

• 非洲裔美国人更常见。

• 一级亲属中系统性红斑狼疮(SLE)和其他自身免疫性疾病的发生率较高。

■ 病因

• 细胞质结构和细胞核抗原的产生，导致炎症变化、血管炎和免疫复合物在多个器官系统中沉积。

• 有相当比例的患者有相关的抗磷脂综合征：

- 以抗细胞磷脂成分抗体为特征。
- 复发性血管血栓形成的趋势。

• 狼疮是一种慢性疾病，伴有一些恶化因素：

- 感染。
- 日晒。
- 疲劳。
- 创伤。
- 药物(磺胺类)。
- 压力。
- 饮食。

• 药物引起的狼疮是一种轻微的疾病，一旦药物停药，最终可以缓解，常呈现皮肤和关节表现，肾脏和神经系统受累很少见。

• 常用药物包括：

- 氯丙嗪、甲基多巴、普鲁卡因胺、肼苯哒嗪、异烟肼、奎尼丁、米诺环素。

诊断

• 需要以下列表中的 11 个标准中的 4 个做出诊断：

- 颧骨皮疹。
- 盘状红疹。
- 感光性皮疹。
- 口腔溃疡。
- 关节炎。
- 浆膜炎。
- 神经系统疾病。
- 血液疾病。
- 免疫紊乱。
- 肾脏疾病。
- 抗核抗体。

■ 症状和体征

• 系统性:
- 疲劳。
- 发热。
- 体重减轻。
- 呼吸困难。

• 皮肤:
- 面部红斑。
- 盘状红疹(红色斑块)。
- 感光性皮疹(亚急性皮肤红斑狼疮)。
- 大疱疹(大水疱)。

• 肌肉骨骼:
- 肌痛。
- 关节疼痛。
- 关节炎:
  ◦ 定义为2个或更多外围关节。
  ◦ 多关节炎,对称或游走性。

• 心脏:
- 胸部疼痛。
- 心包摩擦音。
- 杂音。

• 血管:
- 血管炎。
- 血栓形成。
- 动脉粥样硬化。
- 周边血管疾病。

• 肺:
- 呼吸困难。
- 呼吸急促。
- 胸膜摩擦音。
- 啰音。

• 神经系统:
- 精神病及抑郁症。
- 头痛。
- 癫痫发作。
- 周围神经病变。
- 脑卒中或神经缺陷。
- 脑炎。

• 消化系统:
- 无痛性口腔溃疡。
- 腹痛。
- 粪便潜血检测阳性提示肠系膜缺血。

病史

• 症状通常会随着时间反复发作并逐渐累积和恶化,皮疹、关节疼痛和疲劳的病史可能指向该诊断。

• 患者描述关节痛与体格检查的发现不成比例。

• 询问药物应用史(考虑非药物诱发的SLE前应排除是否使用过米诺环素)、阳光暴露史。

体格检查

• 发热。

• 仔细评估皮肤的皮疹和血管炎。

■ 基本检查

• 需要彻底的病史和体格检查,区分主要和次要突发事件。

• 主要突发事件:
- 血常规。
- 电解质、BUN、肌酐、葡萄糖。
- 尿蛋白。
- ESR。
- 胸部X线片、心电图和脉搏血氧仪了解心肺呼吸症状。

■ 诊断检查与说明

实验室检查

• 血常规:
- 白细胞减少症、血小板减少症、正常色素正细胞性贫血。
- 血液异常程度表明程度的疾病活动。

• ESR:
- 在急性加重期间可能会升高。
- 不是活动性疾病的良好指标。

• CRP也可能升高,升高可能是感染的迹象。

• 活化部分凝血活酶时间:
- 狼疮患者抗凝指标可能会升高。

• 尿蛋白:
- 蛋白质(持续蛋白尿>0.5 g/d或+++)。
- 管型尿(红细胞)。
- 血尿。
- 白细胞。

• 补体水平(C3或C4)。
- 过低或过高常提示活动性狼疮,特别是狼疮肾炎。

• 淀粉酶在肠系膜缺血和胰腺炎中升高。

• 如果诊断不明确,进行抗核抗体、类风湿因子(RF)、抗链球菌溶血素O(ASO)滴度。

• 抗Sm和抗dsDNA是具有诊断性的。

• 假阳性性疾病研究实验室(VDRL)测试支持诊断。

• 无需反复检测ANA或其他特异性抗体包括抗双链DNA,因为不大可能随时间变化,且其与病情的活动并不相关。

• 关节吸出物通常显示液体白细胞<3 000。

• 如果怀疑脑膜炎或脑炎,则检测乳酸过氧化酶。

影像学检查

• 胸部X线检查:
- 肺炎。
- 胸腔积液。
- 心脏肥大。

• 心电图/超声心动图。

• 胸部CT:
- 肺栓塞。
- 肺出血。
- 弥漫性肺泡出血。

• 精神状态改变或神经系统发现(狼疮性脑炎是排除诊断)行头部CT。

妊娠注意事项

• 由于自然流产的高风险,在活动性疾病期间不建议怀孕。

• 怀孕对疾病活动的影响是可变的。

■ 鉴别诊断

• 已知狼疮患者的低血压可能是由于一次重大突发事件的冲击,继发于急性类固醇戒断或败血症的结果。

• 其他自身免疫性疾病:
- 风湿热。
- 类风湿关节炎。
- 皮肌炎。
- 重叠综合征。

• 皮肤变化:
- 荨麻疹。
- 多形红斑。

• 特发性血小板减少性紫癜。

• 多发性硬化症。

• 癫痫。

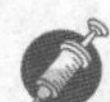

治疗

■ 初步稳定/治疗

基础处理。

■ 急诊治疗/程序

• 主要包括使用NSAIDs、皮质类固醇、抗疟药和免疫抑制药物。

• 必须特别注意中枢神经系统和肾脏受累情况，以及感染情况，这些是发病率的主要决定因素。

• 轻度发作事件：关节痛、肌痛、疲劳和可能出现轻度白细胞减少的皮疹。

- NSAIDs(狼疮肾炎时要小心应用)、乙酰水杨酸(ASA)、皮疹外用类固醇、防晒霜。

- 大多数皮肤表现可以局部使用类固醇。

- 如果不充分，开始使用低剂量泼尼松。

• 中度发作：

- 可能出现胸膜炎性疼痛、关节肿胀和急性期反应物升高。

- 可能需要短期增加或短期使用泼尼松。

• 重度发作事件：生命或器官功能受到威胁：

- 抗凝治疗用于血栓形成，如果需要的话，早期予以血液制品。

- 有神经精神症状的给予精神药物。

- 癫痫发作的给予抗癫痫药。

- 如果反应不佳，在开始使用细胞毒性药物之前咨询风湿病专家。

• 长期治疗：

- 泼尼松逐渐减量。

- NSAIDs。

- 风湿病专家指导治疗：

◦ 抗疟药：奎纳克林、羟氯喹：

▪ 副作用是不可逆的视网膜病变。

- 贝利单抗(FDA 批准用于活跃、自身抗体阳性患者积极治疗，60 岁以下 SLE 治疗的唯一药物)。

- 环磷酰胺。

- 硫唑嘌呤。

- 甲氨蝶呤。

- 环孢素。

- 他克莫司

- 霉酚酸酯

- 利妥昔单抗。

- 激素疗法和自体骨髓干细胞移植正在研究中。

▪ **药物治疗**

• 甲泼尼龙：15 mg/(kg · d)至 1 g 静脉注射；请咨询风湿病专家，以便进行剂量调整。

• 泼尼松：轻微的病情进展可每日口服 5～30 mg(儿童：<0.5 mg/kg)。

• 泼尼松：成人轻微的病情进展可予以 1～2 mg/(kg · d)，口服。

• 布洛芬：800 mg(儿童：5～10 mg/kg)，口服，每日 3 次。

随访

▪ **进一步处理**

入院指征

• 患有终末器官障碍的患者，如肾脏、心脏或中枢神经系统受累。

• 出血、动脉或血栓性血小板减少症、静脉血栓形成。

• 考虑入院时伴有心包炎、心肌炎、胸腔积液或浸润、血管炎证据。

• 严重终末器官或危及生命的患者应入住 ICU。

• 狼疮患者应被视为免疫功能低下，怀疑或诊断为感染的应积极治疗感染。

出院指征

• 患者如果无发热，水分充足，并且没有出现不适，可等情况可在轻微发作的情况下出院回家。

• 不应将 ESR 用作处置标准，在加重缓解之后 ESR 可能会长时间升高。

转诊问题

狼疮是一种慢性疾病，风湿病学家或 ESR 初级保健医师(PCP)必须充分随诊患者。

▪ **随访建议**

初级保健医师必须指导患者有关防晒、免疫、降低动脉粥样硬化风险的知识。

要点和误区

• SLE 的诊断很复杂，实验室检查怀疑 SLE 患者需要一个完整的病史和体格检查支持诊断。

• 慢性类固醇治疗导致免疫抑制。

• 肾脏受累导致预后不良。

• 血清肌酐可能升高，但是不能作为本病的诊断指标(蛋白尿和/或红细胞管型的尿分析更敏感)。

• 所有 SLE 患者均应每年进行一次，季节性流感疫苗接种，并确保肺炎球菌疫苗接种是最新的。

• VDRL 可能是错误的。

• SLE 是冠心病的危险因素。用于预测 SLE 发病最有用的检测是抗双链 DNA 抗体和低补体血症，但特异性不佳。

X

细菌性气管炎 Bacterial Tracheitis

Gary Bubly 宋振举 童朝阳 译

基础知识

▪ **描述**

• 它是一种可能引起急性气道梗阻的气管感染，也被称为细菌性喉头炎、喉气管支气管炎，渗出性气管炎是该疾病中较轻的一种。

• 通常为气管的细菌二次感染，复杂的前驱型病毒感染，混合感染较前两者少见。

• 致死率为 0～20%。

• 气管膜形成，脓液溢出，声门下水肿、糜烂，但会厌无病变。

• 通常表现有与喉头炎相似的前驱症状，随后急剧恶化，并出现通气障碍。

• 平均年龄为 5 岁，成人极少见。

• 在儿童中，该疾病发病率高于会厌炎，可能与对流感嗜血杆菌的免疫有关。

• 8—12 月份多见。

注意

患者在经过一个较为平缓的阶段后，可能会出现病情的急剧恶化，伴有呼吸困难、中毒表现及急性气道梗阻症状。

▪ **病因**

• 葡萄球菌感染(可能有耐甲氧西林葡萄球菌)。

• 卡他莫拉菌。

• 肺炎链球菌。

• A 型链球菌属。

• 假单胞菌。

• B 型流感嗜血杆菌。

• 埃希杆菌。

• 厌氧菌。

• 肺炎克雷伯杆菌。
• 诺卡菌。
• A型流感(包括H1N1)及B型流感、副流感病毒、腺病毒,以及呼吸道合胞病毒(RSV)的联合感染。
• HIV患者的曲霉、生殖器疱疹病毒(HSV)感染。

诊断

症状和体征

病史

通常在疾病急性恶化阶段有前驱病毒感染。

体格检查

• 发热。
• 咳嗽。
• 肌肉痉挛。
• 双相呼吸喘鸣。
• 中毒表现。
• 声嘶。
• 苍白病。
• 鼻翼扑动。
• 咽喉痛、颈部疼痛。
• 流延(非正常流口水)。
• 其他并发症:
- 呼吸系统:
◦ 气道梗阻。
◦ 声门下狭窄。
◦ 肺水肿。
◦ 气胸。
◦ 急性呼吸窘迫综合征(ARDS)。
◦ 气管导管滞留。
- 感染:
◦ 脓毒症休克。
◦ 中毒性休克综合征。
◦ 肺炎。
◦ 咽后蜂窝织炎。
- 心搏骤停。
- 肾衰竭。

基本检查

• 临床辅助通气与管理优先于诊断性检查;安全通气,酌情进手术室控制病情。
• 病情进展之前充分给氧:
- 测定动脉血气。

诊断检查与说明

实验室检查

• 白细胞不同程度升高。
• 血培养通常阴性。
• 需要内镜或手术取气管组织培养。

影像学检查

颈部软组织X线检查。
• 在急诊科开展,持续监测与观察。
• 气道边缘不规则。
• 声门下狭窄。
• 气管气道浸润。
• 不规则气道内密度影。
• 会厌正常。

诊断步骤/外科

• 可屈光导纤维喉镜检查:
- 会厌直接可视化观察。
- 黏膜水肿。
- 声门下水肿,分泌物增多,膜形成。
• 支气管镜检查。
- 气道可视化观察。
- 喉气道炎症与腐蚀。
- 脓性分泌物。
- 膜形成。
- 治疗性膜剥脱。
- 可取材培养。

鉴别诊断

• 感染:
- 格鲁布性喉头炎(对治疗反应不明显,大龄,急性恶化且中毒表现应高度怀疑细菌性气道炎)。
- 会厌炎。
- 扁桃体周脓肿。
- 悬雍垂炎。
- 喉部白喉。
• 血管性水肿。
• 管腔内梗阻:
- 异物吸入。
• 灼烧性狭窄。
• 创伤。

治疗

院前

• 气道/呼吸评估:
- 供氧。
- 若耐受,给予消旋肾上腺素喷雾。
- 安抚患者,避免儿童躁动。
• 呼吸困难时给予面罩给氧。
• 面罩给氧与其他方法均不可行时,进行气管插管。
• 立即转运。
• 要获取急诊科的气道状态。

初步稳定/治疗

气道管理。
• 考虑困难气道。
• 75%(40%~100%)的患者需要插管,年轻患者常更需要。气道通气治疗保证稳定通气、促进吸引。
• 理想化的插管应当是在手术室里,最好有外科通气支持治疗。
• 选择比常规大1~2码的气管内导管(ETT)。
• 细致的插管管理与吸痰。
• 如需面罩通气供氧,选择合适大小的面罩二次密封。
• 提供一定湿度的氧气。

急诊治疗/程序

• 持续监测气道与给氧。
• 必要的情况下静脉补液。
• 若病情进展不迅速,可支气管镜检,留取病原学培养标本:
- 进行必要的插管评估。
- 治疗性膜剥脱。
• 静脉注射覆盖典型病原菌的抗生素:
- 头孢曲松、萘夫西林及万古霉素。
- 青霉素过敏患者采用万古霉素与克林霉素。
- 细菌培养结果将最终指导治疗。
- 考虑皮质醇药物治疗。

药物治疗

• 头孢曲松钠:50 mg/kg静脉注射,最大剂量2 g。
• 萘夫西林:50 mg/kg静脉注射,最大剂量2 g。
• 氨苄西林-舒巴坦:50 mg/kg静脉注射,最大剂量3 g。
• 万古霉素:15 mg/kg静脉注射,最大剂量1 g。
• 克林霉素:10 mg/kg静脉注射,最大剂量1 g。
• 消旋肾上腺素:2.25%溶液1∶8溶于2~4 ml水中,制成喷雾。
• 地塞米松:0.6 mg/kg静脉注射。

一线用药

头孢曲松钠+萘夫西林。

二线用药

万古霉素+克林霉素+左氧氟沙星。
• 如果青霉素过敏,考虑MRSA的区域性流行。

X

随访

进一步处理

入院指征

所有疑似或者证实为细菌性气管炎的：

- 收入 PICU。
- 在 PICU 中住院 3～9 日不等。

出院指征

无。

转诊问题

重症监护，耳鼻喉科专家及肺病专家均需要咨询。

随访建议

一些长期的并发症。

要点和误区

- 患者类似格鲁布性喉头炎但恶化迅速的患者需要考虑本病。
- 由于气管直径较窄，在年轻患者中病情更为严重。

下颌骨骨折

Mandibular Fractures

David W. Munter　王胜云 译

基础知识

描述

- 通常由直接暴力造成。
- 最常见的骨折部位是颌角，其次是髁突和颏区。
- 由于其厚度，下颌骨联合很少发生骨折。
- 由于下颌骨的环状结构，超过 50%的病例可见多发性骨折。
- 双侧下颌骨骨折多由机动车事故造成。
- 开放性骨折是很常见的，包括骨折上覆齿龈的撕裂。

病因

- 下颌骨骨折是仅次于鼻骨骨折和颧骨骨折的第三常见的面部骨折。
- 机动车事故、人际间暴力、身体接触运动或工业事故。
- 患者往往无法给出明确原因。
- 面部、头部撕裂及面部骨折是最常见的合并伤。

X

儿科注意事项

- 下颌骨骨折在 6 岁以下儿童中不常见；如果发生，多为青枝骨折，以食用软食方法处理即可。
- 告知家长，下颌骨骨折可能会使恒牙受损，建议由专业人员后续随访。
- 为儿童患者介绍对儿童生长板和恒牙问题有丰富经验的专家。

诊断

症状和体征

- 下颌骨疼痛。
- 面部不对称、畸形和吞咽困难。
- 咬合不正、颞下颌关节活动度减少、牙关紧闭或耳中有刺耳声。
- 牙龈撕裂，甲下或牙龈血肿。

病史

- 损伤机制。
- 咬合不正，牙痛，合并伤。

体格检查

- 检查颌面部是否有畸形，包括瘀斑或肿胀。
- 咬合不正、牙关紧闭或面部不对称。
- 牙齿松动，骨折或缺失；牙齿排列不齐；牙齿空隙分离；牙根出血；齿间牙龈撕裂；以及口底的瘀斑或血肿。
- 沿下颌骨全长有突然沉降处，有骨质破坏或触诊压痛点。
- 颌突出或横向偏移。
- 正常下颌功能受干扰，包括活动度减少或下颌骨张开有偏移：
  - 检查人员应能在上下颌骨之间插入 3 根手指。
  - 当检查人员拉压舌器时，患者不能保持压舌器水平，或因翻舌损坏压舌器（压舌器测试）。
- 下唇或牙龈的感觉异常说明下牙槽神经受到二次损伤。
- 经外耳道触诊，无法注意到下颌髁突的运动，说明下颌骨骨折。
- 颞下颌关节处髁突压痛。

基本检查

- 下颌骨骨折诊断需要拍摄下颌骨系列或全景 X 线片。
- 全景评估优于除髁突外所有下颌骨的评估。
- 如果怀疑有合并伤，面颊骨 CT 阳性率较低。

诊断检查与说明

实验室检查

仅用于需立即进行手术治疗或为评估其他损伤时。

影像学检查

- 需获得平片或口腔全景 X 线片。
- 需获得包括前后斜肌、双侧斜肌和汤氏位观的平片：
  - 下颌骨照最适合用于评估下颌骨的髁和下颌颈（最常见的骨折部位）。
- 可能需要获得口腔全景 X 线片。
  - 全景 X 线照片最适合评估联合部位和体部（不太常见的骨折部位）。
- 如仍怀疑髁部骨折，且最初的 X 线照片不能发现骨折，则取得冠状面上髁部 CT。
- 如无法找到缺失的牙齿，则必须拍胸片以排除误吸。
- 如果临床上不对颈部清创。
- 如怀疑有其他面部损伤，做面部 CT。

鉴别诊断

- 挫伤。
- 下颌骨脱位：
  - 如果单个髁突脱位，下颌骨会从脱位一侧偏移。
  - 如果骨折，下颌骨会向骨折一侧偏移。
- 独立的牙创伤。

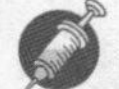

治疗

院前

- 注意：
  - 保护呼吸道。
  - 保护颈椎。

- 保护撕脱牙。

初步稳定/治疗

- 20%～40%下颌骨骨折的患者有合并伤：
- 治疗是针对速发型、可能致命的损伤，如气道阻塞、误吸、大出血、颈椎损伤和颅内损伤。
- 必须保护呼吸道。
- 颈椎防范措施。
- 如果不能进行口腔插管，应进行经鼻插管，除非出现面部合并伤，这种情况下，可能要进行环甲软骨切开术。

急诊治疗/程序

- 除髁突骨折外，许多下颌骨骨折与黏膜、牙龈或齿槽的损伤有关，应考虑为开放性骨折：
- 以抗生素，如青霉素、克林霉素、阿莫西林、阿莫西林-克拉维酸或阿奇霉素，覆盖口腔内厌氧菌。
- 开放性骨折的破伤风预防。
- 镇痛药，如对乙酰氨基酚（扑热息痛）、布洛芬或麻醉药品。
- 确定性救护通常包括用切开复位内固定术将上颌牙和下颌牙以线闭塞，时间为4～6周：
- 裂缝骨折、青枝骨折和无移位骨折可以使用软食方法治疗。
- 如果出现下颌骨脱位，下颌处于开放状态，则抓住下颌骨，在牙下咬合面施加向下的压力：
- 其目的是将髁突从其前位移向隆突处。
- 肌松药（地西泮或咪达唑仑）或咬肌注射麻药可促进切开。
- 需要使用牙垫，或检查人员以纱布包裹手指以防受伤。

药物治疗

- 对乙酰氨基酚（扑热息痛）：500 mg（儿童：10～15 mg/kg，每日不超过 3 次），口服，q4～6 h，每日不超过 4 g。
- 阿莫西林-克拉维酸：500/125～875/125 mg，口服，每日 2 次［儿童：阿莫西林 40 mg/（kg·d），口服，每日 2 次］。
- 阿莫西林：500 mg，口服，每日 3 次（儿童：40 mg/kg，口服，分每日 3 次）。
- 阿奇霉素：首日口服 500 mg，次日至第 4 日每日服 250 mg（儿童：首日服 10 mg/kg，次日至第 4 日每日服 5 mg/kg）。
- 克林霉素：150～450 mg，口服，每日 3 次［儿童：10～20 mg/（kg·24 h）］。
- 地西泮：5～10 mg（儿童：0.1～0.2 mg/kg），静脉注射。
- 布洛芬：600～800 mg［儿童：20～40 mg/（kg·24 h）］，口服，每日 3～4 次。
- 咪达唑仑：2～5 mg（儿童：0.02～0.05 mg/kg，最大剂量 0.4 mg/kg，总量不超过 10 mg）静脉注射超过 2～3 min。
- 青霉素 V 钾：250～500 mg［儿童：25～50 mg/（kg·24 h）］，口服，每日 4 次。

随访

进一步处理

入院指征

- 严重脱位或合并牙创伤，开放性骨折需要紧急专业咨询以安排入院。
- 严重的合并创伤可能需要入院。
- 任何可能呼吸道受损的患者都需要入院。
- 对于不可靠的非移位骨折患者需入院接受固定治疗。
- 在儿科人群中，如果可见伤的损伤机制不明确，需向小儿或儿童保护服务咨询。

出院指征

患无移位性骨折和无创骨折患者可出院，服用镇痛药和软食。

随访建议

对于不复杂的骨折，口腔外科医师或颌面外科医师 2～3 日随访。

要点和误区

- 下颌骨骨折最显著的迹象是咬合不正。
- 没有意识到覆盖在下颌骨骨折上的牙龈撕裂是需要抗生素治疗的开放性骨折。
- 只有一张下颌骨髁突骨折的全景 X 线照片，如果髁突压痛或咬合不正，需拍 X 线平片或做 CT。
- 必须对缺失的牙齿做出解释，如果找不到，需拍胸部 X 线检查以排除误吸。
- 未骨折的下颌骨能将压舌器夹在臼齿间足够紧使其折断。将压舌器在臼齿间转动时不应有痛感。

X

先天性代谢缺陷 Inborn Errors of Metabolism

David H. Rubin · David A. Perlstein 倪沁赟 译

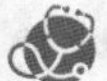

基础知识

描述

- 代谢物的类型、数量和毒性的缺陷，由于酶、辅因子或转运体的代谢途径的遗传缺陷而积累，从而导致各种临床表现；500 种人类疾病是尤先天性代谢异常引起。
- 流行病学：
- 发病率：
  - 出生的儿童中＞1/1000。
- 遗传学：
- 常见遗传性代谢性疾病：
  - 氨基酸紊乱。
  - 尿素循环缺陷。
  - 酸血症。
  - 脂肪酸氧化缺陷。
  - 线粒体脂肪酸缺陷与肉碱转运缺陷。
  - 线粒体病。
  - 碳水化合物（糖类）紊乱。
  - 黏多糖贮积症。
  - 鞘脂类代谢障碍。
  - 过氧化物酶体病。
  - 蛋白质糖基化障碍。
  - 溶酶体障碍。
  - 四肢近端软骨斑点。
- 病理生理学：
- 与代谢途径中的缺陷相关。

病因

不同群体的疾病包括一种中介代谢产物

或膜转运系统的酶的遗传缺陷。

诊断

症状和体征

• 缺陷或障碍可表现为快速失代偿期或者慢性进展期。
• 新生儿的初始临床表现：
- 无症状。
- 低体温(线粒体缺陷)。
- 肌张力低下或肌张力增高(过氧化物酶体病)。
- 呼吸暂停(尿素循环缺陷、有机酸中毒)。
- 癫痫发作(过氧化物酶体病、葡萄糖转运蛋白缺陷)。
- 嗜睡，昏迷(原因较多)。
- 呕吐(原因较多)。
- 喂养差、生长差(原因较多)。
- 黄疸(半乳糖血症、C 型 Niemann-Pick 病)。
- 低血糖(半乳糖血症、枫糖尿病)、肝大、肝衰竭。
- 畸形特征(溶酶体储存障碍、先天性肾上腺增生、Smith-Lemli-Opitz 综合征)。
• 未经治疗的年龄较大的儿童：
- 未能茁壮成长(尿素循环缺陷)。
- 脱水(有机酸中毒)。
- 呕吐(尿素循环缺陷及其他)。
- 腹泻(原因较多)。
- 食物不耐受(脂质缺陷、氨基酸缺陷)。
- 嗜睡(尿素循环缺陷)。
- 共济失调(尿素循环缺陷)。
- 癫痫发作(原因较多)。
- 精神发育迟滞(苯丙酮尿症及其他)。

病史

完整的病史和伴随疾病：
• 新生儿筛查。
• 饮食因素。
• 家庭因素。
• 血缘关系。
• 其他。

体格检查

• 异常气味。
• 精神状态改变。
• 呼吸急促。
• 异常面容。
• 白内障。
• 心肌病。
• 肝大。
• 脾大。
• 皮炎。
• 黄疸。

基本检查

关键是要考虑到鉴别诊断：
• 神经系统状态恶化。
• 生长缓慢无法解释，伴随脱水、持续呕吐或酸中毒。
• 对常规的休克复苏措施反应差。

诊断检查与说明

实验室检查

• 床旁血糖监测。
• 电解质、尿素氮/肌酐、血糖。
• 全血细胞计数。
• 钙水平。
• 肝功能试验、游离胆红素、凝血激活酶时间。
• 动脉或静脉血气分析。
• 乳酸和丙酮酸水平。
• 尿酸。
• 尿液分析：还原性物质、酮类、pH。
• 生化检查，如下：
- 血氨。
- 定量血清氨基酸、酰基碳酸钙。
- 尿液有机酸和氨基酸。
• 培养：
- 血液。
- 脑脊液：包括氨基酸、神经递质。

影像学检查

• 因精神状态改变可行头颅 CT 扫描。
• 胸部 X 线检查。

诊断步骤/外科

腰椎穿刺。

鉴别诊断

• 常常与脓毒症、脱水、生长缓慢、毒物摄入或非意外性创伤混淆诊断。
• 感染：
- 脓毒症。
- 脑膜炎。
- 脑炎。
• 代谢：
- Reye 综合征。
- 肝性脑病。
- 高胰岛素血症。
- 激素异常。
• 肾脏：
- 肾衰竭。
- 肾小管性酸中毒。
• 毒物摄入。
• 中枢神经系统实质性病变。
• 非意外性创伤。

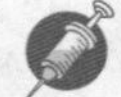

治疗

院前

注意

• ABC 管理。
• 床旁血糖监测。
• 除非休克患者需要进行液体复苏，其余均优先给予葡萄糖液体输注。可以同时进行纠正。
• 避免使用乳酸林格液。
• 保持儿童禁食。

初步稳定/治疗

因精神状态改变，可给予纳洛酮和葡萄糖(理论上在给予血糖检查和维生素 B_1 之后使用)。

急诊治疗/程序

• 评估气道、呼吸和循环。
• 生理盐水 10 ml/kg(新生儿和心力衰竭患者)，20 ml/kg(婴幼儿)；避免乳酸林格和低渗性液体。
• 如果低血糖，新生儿静脉注射葡萄糖 0.25～1.0 g/kg D_{10}，年纪稍大点给予 D_{10} 或 D_{25}；维持 D_{10}～D_{15}，以 8～12 mg/(kg · min)的速度维持血糖水平在 120～170 mg/dl。
• 葡萄糖推注后，在 1～1.5 维持时，在 1/2 生理盐水中加入 D_{10}～D_{15}。
- 如果患者严重低血糖，静脉注射 D_{25}。
• 如果患者低血糖需要再水化：
- 恢复正常的酸碱平衡。
• 如果 pH<7.0，则使用碳酸氢钠和/或乙酸钾：
- 严重酸中毒如果不能很快纠正，需要进行血液透析治疗。
• 增加尿量可以帮助毒素的排出。
• 首先停止所有口服摄入，氨基酸代谢产物可能具有神经毒性。
• 立即行血液透析或使用氨诱导药物治疗严重高血氨症(500～600 mmol/L 及以上)：
- 精氨酸。
- 苯甲酸钠。
- 苯乙酸钠。
- 苯丁酸钠。
- 剂量随疾病而变化，使用前咨询代谢方面的医师。

• 识别并治疗并发或诱发的感染/疾病。

• 当任何儿童出现疑似遗传性代谢性疾病时，请咨询代谢方面的医师。

■ 药物治疗

• 葡萄糖：0.25～1.0 g/kg 静脉注射（新生儿用 D_{10}；其他用 D_{25}）。

• 对于严重代谢性酸中毒：铋钠碳酸盐，0.25～0.50 mmol/(kg·h)高达 1～2 mmol/(kg·h)静脉注射。

• 其他特定疾病的药物，包括吡哆醇和肉碱。

一线用药

葡萄糖：如果低血糖，新生儿静脉注射葡萄糖 0.25～1.0 g/kg D_{10}，如果年龄较大，给予 D_{10} 或 D_{25}。

二线用药

pH<7.0 时使用碳酸氢钠：

• 需要时行血液透析治疗。

随访

■ 进一步处理

入院指征

• 婴儿和儿童新出现疑似遗传性代谢性疾病的表现。

• 尿酮或无法耐受口服摄入。

• ICU：

- 显著精神状态的改变。
- 严重或持续存在的酸中毒。
- 反应迟钝的低血糖。
- 高血氨症。

• 如果需要转至专业儿科中心。

出院指征

• 精神状态正常。

• 正常水合，实验室指标正常。

• 无明显并发症。

• 初级保健医师密切随访。

转诊问题

神经发育：

• 饮食。

• 药物。

■ 随访建议

• 初级保健医师。

• 代谢病专家。

要点和误区

关于脱水：

• 给予生理盐水液体负荷量治疗脱水：

- 密切监测血糖水平，避免发生低血糖。
- 谨慎使用碳酸氢钠，仅在 pH<7.0 时考虑使用。
- 高血氨症的患者可能需要行血液透析治疗。

先天性巨结肠 Hirschsprung Disease

Roger M. Barkin 陈奇通 译

基础知识

■ 描述

• 1886 年哈罗德把先天性巨结肠描述为早期婴儿便秘的原因。

• 先天性巨结肠无神经节细胞症。

• 发病率为 1/5 000。

• 先天性巨结肠的死亡率是 35%～50%。

■ 病因

• 远端肠段的肠神经节缺失。

• 神经节一般来自神经嵴并沿肠道迁移，妊娠 8 周到达近端结肠，妊娠 12 周到达直肠。

• 由于无神经节段与临床疾病，神经嵴细胞没能迁移到麦氏副交感神经（黏膜下层的）和欧氏（Myeneteric）神经节。

• 受累的肠腔在肛门括约肌呈现，累及乙状结肠（75%）。

• 可以延长整个胃肠道长度（通常是致命的）。

• 无神经节段的肠腔长期收缩，造成粪便梗阻，从而导致近端肠腔扩张。

• 肛门的刺激使粪便通畅。

• 遗传及其他原因：

- 家族性自发 RET 原癌基因突变。
- 男女比例为 4∶1：
  ◦ 8%有阳性家族史，5%～12%的兄弟姐妹受影响。
  ◦ 5%～15%存在相关的染色体异常，最常见的 21-三体综合征（唐氏综合征）。
  ◦ 其他先天性异常占 18%，如颅面裂、先天性心脏病、腭裂、先天性耳聋。

诊断

■ 症状和体征

先天性巨结肠患儿通常到 2 岁才诊断。

• 随着年龄的变化有三方面的表现：

- 新生儿：
  ◦ 腹胀。
  ◦ 在出生 48 h 之内，没有排便。
  ◦ 呕吐。
  ◦ 肠炎：腹痛、发热、异味和/或血性腹泻、呕吐，导致脓毒症和潜在的肠穿孔。
  ◦ 脓毒症。
- 婴儿：
  ◦ 便秘。
  ◦ 慢性腹胀。
  ◦ 呕吐。
  ◦ 发育迟缓。
  ◦ 肠炎：腹痛、发热、异味和/或血性腹泻、呕吐，导致脓毒症和潜在的肠穿孔。
  ◦ 中毒性巨结肠。
- 学龄期儿童和成人：
  ◦ 难以用常规方法治疗的慢性便秘伴肠梗阻及尿失禁的少见病例。
  ◦ 肠炎：腹痛、发热、异味和/或血性腹泻、呕吐，导致脓毒症和潜在的肠穿孔。
  ◦ 腹胀。
  ◦ 血便，伴有恶臭的腹泻。
  ◦ 营养不良。

病史

• 脓毒症。

• 排便通常需要直肠刺激或灌肠。

• 大便较细。

• 大便失禁和腹泻较罕见。

• 缺乏与功能性便秘相关的诱因（如肛裂、如厕训练、节食）。

体格检查

左侧可触及结肠。

• 腹胀和肠梗阻征象。

• 因营养不良而导致的发育迟缓。

X

• 直肠检查通常显示为直肠陷窝扩张。

■ 基本检查

腹部X线平片：

• 通常表现为小肠、近端结肠与直肠扩张。
• 过渡区为一个狭窄的直肠乙状结肠段。
• 在新生儿中，一般表现为远端肠梗阻。
• 在患有慢性便秘的儿童中，影像学可能只显示大量粪便。
• 小儿肠炎，可能存在肠壁水肿、肠壁积气可能。

■ 诊断检查与说明

实验室检查

• 血常规、电解质、血糖、尿素氮、肌酐。
• 尿常规。
• 如果有中毒表现，行血培养检查。

影像学检查

消化道钡餐造影：

• 病情平稳时可行，禁忌证是怀疑存在穿孔和小肠结肠炎。
• 扩张的结肠近端黏膜收缩导致不协调的蠕动，狭窄的节段与扩张的正常神经节段之间存在过渡区：
- 由于结肠扩张时间不足或经过直肠检查和灌肠，过渡区可能在新生儿的表现得不明显。
- 可以表现为不平直的直肠，这是先天性巨结肠症的典型标志。
• 延迟排钡。

诊断步骤/外科

• 直肠测压可能有助于诊断，但长期便秘通常是不正常的。
• 直肠活检可发现缺乏神经节细胞：
- 先天性巨结肠的明确诊断依赖于直肠活检。

■ 鉴别诊断

• 新生儿：
- 囊性纤维化致胎粪性肠梗阻或胎粪栓塞综合征。
- 肠闭锁或肛门闭锁或发育不良。
- 旋转不良或重复扭转。
- 坏死性小肠结肠炎。
- 脓毒症。
• 婴儿和儿童：
- 功能性便秘。
- 阿片类药物或抗胆碱能药物中毒。
• 肉毒杆菌感染。
• 获得性结肠黏膜：
- 代谢或内分泌：甲状腺和甲状旁腺功能异常、肾上腺皮质功能不全、电解质异常。
◦ 脊髓缺陷。
• 腹部肿块。

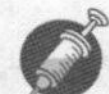

治疗

■ 初步稳定/治疗

• 在必要的情况下，密切监测呼吸道、呼吸情况及循环情况。
• 休克、脱水、脓毒症的早期等渗液体复苏(20 ml/kg)。

■ 急诊治疗/程序

• 婴儿应积极治疗肠梗阻。如果存在呕吐，可能需要插胃管治疗。
• 请小儿外科医师会诊。
- 存在中毒症状或结肠炎的患者需要使用抗生素。
• 不稳定的患者可能需要紧急行结肠造瘘术进行减压：
- 病情稳定的儿童可以做门诊检查。
- 最终的处理方法是切除无神经的肠段，并实现距肛缘1 cm内肠段含有神经节。
• 肠炎可以发生在任何时间，甚至在手术干预后。

■ 药物治疗

• 氨苄西林：50 mg/kg，静脉滴注，q6 h。
• 庆大霉素：2.5 mg/kg，静脉滴注，q12～24 h。
• 甲硝唑：7.5 mg/kg，静脉滴注，q12～48 h。

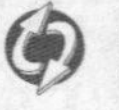

随访

■ 进一步处理

入院指征

• 出现肠梗阻的新生儿及婴儿。
• 小肠结肠炎。
• 新生儿/儿科重症监护室应接纳患病婴儿，并配备儿外科医师。

出院指征

• 充足的水分和口服液。
• 主诉便秘的大龄儿童。
• 负责任的家长。
• 与主治医师保持密切随访。

■ 随访建议

护理应由儿科胃肠病学和/或儿科手术医师指导。通常需要长期营养支持。

要点和误区

• 表达与孩子的年龄不同。
• 从中毒性肠炎到慢性便秘会经过一系列变化。
• 中毒儿童需要镇静，使用抗生素，并紧急行影像学检查和外科干预。

先天性心脏病(发绀型) Congenital Heart Disease, Cyanotic

Lynne M. Palmisciano · William J. Lewander 陈奇通 译

基础知识

■ 描述

• 异常胚胎发育导致不含氧血和含氧血混合并回到外周循环，主要有2个机制：
- 心脏内右向左分流。
- 主动脉根部解剖缺陷。
• 压型：5T、2E和单心室。
- 法洛四联症(TOF)：
◦ 室间隔缺损(VSD)。
◦ 右心室(RV)流出道梗阻。
◦ 主动脉骑跨。
◦ 右心室肥大(RVH)。
- 大动脉转位(TGA)：
◦ 主动脉由右心室发出，肺动脉起自左心室。
- 三尖瓣闭锁：
◦ 右心房无出口进入右心室。
◦ 必然存在心房水平沟通。
- 永久大动脉干：
◦ 外周、肺、颈循环仅有单个动脉干。

- 完全异常肺静脉回流(TAPVR):
  ◦ 肺静脉流入外周静脉循环。
  ◦ 心脏以上、心脏、心脏以下或混合型。
- 三尖瓣 Ebstein 异常:
  ◦ 异常和移位三尖瓣分割右心室,导致右心室功能减退。
- 艾森门格综合征:
  ◦ 持续非发绀的左向右分流的心脏病的并发症。
  ◦ 肺血管阻力高于外周血管阻力水平;右向左分流。
- 单心室生理:
  ◦ 外周和静脉回流完全混合。
- 按肺血流量细分:
  - TOF 和三尖瓣闭锁减少。
  - TGA、动脉干和 TAPVR 增加。

病因

大部分形式、病因未知。

- 遗传原因:DiGeorge 综合征中的 22 号染色体缺失(圆锥动脉干心脏缺陷、法洛四联症,动脉干,还有主动脉缩窄)。
- 环境致畸因素:TGA 在糖尿病母亲的婴儿中更常见。

诊断

- 发绀型先天性心脏病在急诊最常见的临床表现为:
  - 发绀。
  - 充血性心力衰竭。
  - 循环衰竭。
- 先天性心脏病在年龄较大的患者中精神紧张会触发发绀:
  - 肺部疾病。
  - 外周血管阻力降低。
  - 发热。
  - 脱水。

症状和体征

- 中央型发绀:
  - 可见于口唇、甲床、黏膜。
  - 哭泣或激动时加重。
  - 吸入 100%氧气时无明显改变。
- 充血性心力衰竭。
  - 啰音,奔马律、肝大、头皮水肿。
- 重度发绀发作:
  - 烦躁不安和呼吸过度,然后发绀加重,然后晕厥。
  - 以下情况会使已受限的肺部血流进一步降低:
    ◦ 醒来、进食、大哭。
  - 较大的孩子可通过蹲位来代偿。
  - 收缩期喷射杂音在发音时暂时减少或消失。

病史

- 先天性心脏病家族史:
  - 如果父母或兄弟姐妹中存在:先天性心脏病的风险增高。
  - 如果两个亲戚中存在:先天性心脏病的风险增加至 3 倍。
- 胎儿期病史:
  - 畸胎源暴露。
  - 胎儿超声异常。
- 法洛四联症:
  - 常在出生时无症状。
  - 严重的右心室流出道梗阻;新生儿发绀(动脉导管依赖性病灶)。
  - 幼儿学步。
  - 较大的未纠正的患者:
    ◦ 运动后呼吸困难和生长延迟。
- 三尖瓣闭锁:
  - 常在出生时即出现发绀。
  - 喂养困难。
  - 较大的患者表现出活动后呼吸困难和易疲倦。
- Ebstein 异常:
  - 新少年可表现出心律失常。
- 大动脉移位:
  - 在出生后 1 h 至数日出现症状。
- TAPVR:
  - 新生儿表现,严重疾病:
    ◦ 发绀。
    ◦ 机械通气无改善。
  - 婴儿表现,心力衰竭:
    ◦ 轻度发绀。
  - 如果肺静脉回流无梗阻:
    ◦ 无症状或轻度发绀。
    ◦ 频繁肺炎。
    ◦ 生长问题。
- 永存动脉干:
  - 新生儿轻度发绀。
  - 较大的婴儿出现心力衰竭。

体格检查

- 法洛四联症:
  - 胸骨左缘的收缩期杂音(LSB)。
  - 50%收缩性震颤。
  - ±动脉导管未闭持续性续性杂音。
  - 响亮的单一的第二心音(S2)。
  - 右心室明显、膨大。
  - 较大且未纠正的患者:
    ◦ 灰暗泛蓝的皮肤。
    ◦ 杵状指。
    ◦ 视网膜充血。
- 三尖瓣闭锁:
  - 呼吸急促。
  - 因室间隔缺损引起的胸骨左缘反流性杂音。
  - ±持续动脉导管未闭杂音。
  - 单一的第二心音。
  - 明显的左心室搏动。
- Ebstein 异常:
  - 三尖瓣反流引起的全收缩期杂音。
  - 许多有舒张期杂音。
  - 奔马律。
- 大动脉移位:
  - 单一的响亮的第二心音。
  - 严重的低氧血症。
- TAPVR:
  - 新生儿:严重的呼吸增快和发绀。
  - 婴儿:心力衰竭:
    ◦ 心动过速。
    ◦ 胸骨左缘收缩期喷射样杂音。
    ◦ 胸骨左缘下部中度舒张期杂音。
    ◦ 奔马律。
    ◦ 固定分裂的第二心音。
    ◦ 肝大。
- 永存动脉干:
  - 新生儿:
    ◦ 中度发绀。
    ◦ 胸骨左缘舒张期反流性杂音。
    ◦ 单一的第二心音。
- 较大婴儿:心力衰竭:
  - 心前区高动力性。
  - 脉搏跳动。
  - 响亮的单一的第二心音。
  - 收缩期喷射杂音和震颤。
  - 中度舒张期杂音。

基本检查

- 氧饱和度。
- 动脉血气。
- 全血分析、血糖。
- 脓毒症评估。
- 胸部 X 线检查评估肺部血流情况。
- 心电图评估心肌肥大和 QRS 电轴。
- 心脏科医师评估心脏超声。

诊断检查与说明

实验室检查

- 降低的室内氧饱和度。

- 高氧试验:
  - 室内氧和100%氧吸入数分钟情况下的动脉血气。
    - 吸氧时 $PaO_2 > 150$,无心脏内分流。
    - 吸氧时 $PaO_2 < 100$,可能是发绀型先天性心脏病。
- 全血细胞计数:慢性发绀时红细胞增多。

影像学检查

- 胸部X线检查:
  - 肺部血流减少:
    - 法洛四联症(右心室增大)。
    - 三间瓣闭锁(左心室增大)。
    - 单心室生理。
  - 肺部血流增加:
    - 大血管转位(右心室增大)。
    - 完全性异常静脉回流(右心室增大)。
    - 永存动脉瓣(左心室和右心室增大)。
  - 经典胸部X线片描述:
    - 靴型心:法洛四联症;纵隔窄,大血管前/后位。
    - Snowman征:心脏上TAPVR;肺静脉组成上半部。
- 心电图:在所有新的冠心病病例中评估结构,功能和分流。

诊断步骤/外科

心电图:

- 法洛四联症:
  - 电轴右偏(RAD)。
  - 右心室肥大。
- TAPVR:
  - 电轴右偏。
  - 右心室肥大和右心房扩大(RAE)。
- 大血管转位:
  - 电轴右偏。
  - 右心室肥大。
- 三尖瓣闭锁:
  - 电轴偏上。
  - 左心室肥大、右心房扩大和左心房扩大。
- 永存动脉瓣:
  - 右心室肥大、左心室肥大。
- Ebstein异常:
  - 右束支传导阻滞。
  - 常有Wolff-Parkinson-White综合征。

鉴别诊断

- 肺源性:
  - 气胸、血胸。
  - 气质管肺发育不良。
  - 先天性肺发育减退/发育不良。
  - 肺出血。
  - 肺栓塞。
  - 肺动脉高压。
  - 膈疝。
  - 异物、解剖梗阻。
- 心源性:
  - 充血性心力衰竭。
  - 心源性休克。
  - 脓毒症。
- 神经性:
  - 癫痫。
  - 神经肌肉性疾病。
  - 药物所致呼吸抑制。
- 其他:
  - 红细胞增多症。
  - 高铁血红蛋白血症。
  - 脱水。
  - 低血糖。

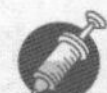

治疗

初步稳定/治疗

- 保暖(寒冷增加氧耗)。
- 治疗低血糖和酸中毒。
- 维持氧合。
- 建立静脉通道。
- 准备气管插管。

> **注意**
> - 高氧分压促进动脉导管的关闭。
> - 所有静脉通路需加装空气滤器以防止通过右向左分流的反常性栓子。

急诊治疗/程序

- 使用前列腺素 E_1 (PGE_1)使动脉导管扩张或重新开放。
  - 0.05～0.1 μg/(kg·min)持续静脉输注。
  - 并发症包括呼吸停止、心动过缓、低血压和癫痫:
    - 通常在转运前插管。
  - 对于梗阻性TAPVR无效:
    - 在等待手术期间可能需要ECMO。
  - 总益处远远超过潜在风险。
- 发绀可逆性原因的评估和处理:
  - 脓毒症检查和经验性抗生素使用。
  - 液体复苏(增加10 ml/kg)。
  - 维持正常血糖。
- 重度发绀的患者:
  - 提供宁静的环境。
  - 将患儿处于膝胸位。
  - 如对患者无刺激时,提供吸氧。
  - 静脉或肌内注射吗啡。
  - 对上述治疗无反应的严重病例:
    - 对于严重酸中毒者静脉使用碳酸氢钠。
    - 静脉使用苯肾上腺素以增加外周血管阻力,以减少右向左分流。
    - 静脉使用普萘洛尔以阻断β受体。
- 已知先天性心脏病的年龄较大患者发生发绀:
  - 如有脱水可能,静脉输注10～20 ml/kg生理盐水。
  - 如怀疑为肺部疾病,则吸氧。
- 先天性心脏病的循环衰竭:
  - 液体复苏。
  - 正性肌力药物:多巴酚丁胺、多巴胺、米力农。

药物治疗

- 对乙酰氨基酚:口服或灌肠15 mg/kg(最大剂量4 g/24 h)。
- 氨苄西林:50 mg/kg,静脉注射。
- 多巴酚丁胺:5～20 μg/(kg·min),静脉注射。
- 多巴胺:5～20 μg/(kg·min),静脉注射。
- 庆大霉素:4 mg/(kg·d),静脉注射。
- 布洛芬:10 mg/kg,口服(>6个月)。
- 米力农:0.25～1 μg/(kg·min),50 μg/kg负荷。
- 硫酸吗啡:0.1 mg/kg,皮下注射、肌内注射或静脉注射。
- 苯肾上腺素:0.5～5 μg/(kg·min),静脉注射。
- 普萘洛尔:0.01～0.2 mg/kg,静脉注射。
- PGE_1:0.05～0.1 μg/(kg·min)。
- 碳酸氢钠:1～2 mmol/kg,静脉注射。

随访

进一步处理

入院指征

- 所有疑似先天性心脏病的新生儿进入重症监护室。
- 先天性心脏病伴发绀急性加重或充血性心力衰竭。
- 先天性心脏病伴有症状的肺炎或呼吸道合胞病毒感染。

出院指征

- 由心脏科医师会诊决定。
- 患者对小的干预治疗有反应(如法洛四联症患者接收无创性治疗)。

- 确保严密随访。

转诊问题

- 责任医师应协调治疗。
- 心脏科医师应负责诊断、药物管理和持续监测。
- 心胸外科医师做手术评估。

随访建议

随访计划需由儿童心脏科医师会诊决定。

要点和误区

- 发绀的视觉表现需要非氧合血红蛋白浓度3～5 mg/dl及以上。
- 动脉导管依赖病灶：
  - 在出生后2～3周时出现临床表现。
  - 突然出现发绀或心血管衰竭。
  - PGE_1治疗：
    - 注意呼吸停止和低血压。

先天性心脏病(无发绀型) Congenital Heart Disease, Acyanotic

Lynne M. Palmisciano · William J. Lewander 陈奇通 译

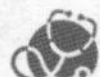

基础知识

描述

出生时即存在的循环系统异常，但是不存在含氧血和非含氧血混合。

- 左向右分流病灶：
  - 室间隔缺损(VSD)。
  - 房间隔缺损(ASD)。
  - 动脉导管未闭(PDA)。
  - 心内肉垫缺损(房室通道)。
- 心室流出道梗阻：
  - 主动脉缩窄(LV)。
  - 主动脉狭窄(LV)。
  - 肺动脉狭窄(RV)。
  - 左心发育不良综合征(HLHS)。
- 导管依赖：动脉导管关闭时出现症状：
  - 主动脉缩窄。
  - 严重主动脉狭窄。
  - 严重肺动脉狭窄。
  - HLHS。

病因

对大部分类型，病因是未知的：

- 基因：Down综合征(房室通道)、Turner综合征(缩窄)。
- 环境：先天性风疹(PDA、AS)。

诊断

症状和体征

病史

- 许多无症状。
- 昏睡，喂养差和成长困难。
- 活动过呼吸困难。
- 反复呼吸系统感染。

体格检查

- 室间隔缺损和房室通道：
  - 色灰暗，肝大。
  - 全收缩期和舒张期杂音＋震颤。
  - 心前区高动力性，PMI替代。
- 房间隔缺损：
  - 固定分裂的第二心音(S2)。
  - 收缩期射血和舒张期杂音。
- 动脉导管未闭：
  - "机械样"杂音和抬举搏动。
- 缩窄：
  - 差异性发绀(仅上1/2呈粉红)。
  - 上肢血压大于下肢血压。
  - 下肢搏动下降或消失。
- 主动脉狭窄：
  - 强烈的收缩期杂音、震颤和主动脉咔哒音。
- 肺动脉狭窄：
  - 收缩性喷射杂音，震颤和肺动脉咔哒音。
  - 宽的第二心音分裂。
  - 颈静脉A波。
- HLHS：
  - 灰暗，倦怠，呼吸急促和脉搏下降。
  - 单心音，收缩期喷射杂音。

基本检查

- 氧饱和度(导管前和导管后)。
- 血气分析、全血分析、基础生化和血糖。
- 脓毒症评估。
- 胸部X线检查以评估肺动脉血流。
- 心电图(电轴、肥大和传导阻滞)。
- 四肢血压。
- 心脏科医师进行心脏超声。

诊断检查与说明

镜像学检查

- 胸部X线检查：
  - 左向右分流病灶全表现为心脏增大(特异的心腔)和肺动脉标记增大。
    - 房间隔缺损(右心房、右心室)、室间隔缺损(右心室、左心房)、动脉导管未闭(左心房、左心室)。
    - 房室通道(全心，所有心腔均增大)。
- 梗阻性病灶：正常到心脏增大。

诊断步骤/外科

心电图：

- 房间隔缺损：电轴向右偏移。
  - 右心室肥大或者右束支传导阻滞。
- 室间隔缺损-左心房肥大、左心室肥大(如果左心室肥大，右心室也有肥大)：
  - P波有切迹或双峰(大的VSD)。
- 动脉导管未闭：双心室肥大(大的PDA)。
- 室通道：电轴向上，左心室肥大、右心室肥大。
  - 右束支传导阻滞和PR间期延长。
- 主动脉狭窄：正常到左心室肥大(严重病例)。
- 肺动脉狭窄：正常到右心室肥大，右心房增大(严重病例)。
  - 右束支传导阻滞。
- 主动脉缩窄：右心室肥大或右束支传导阻滞。
- HLHS：右心房增大，右心室肥大，P波双峰。

鉴别诊断

- 充血性心力衰竭。
- 肥厚型心肌病。
- 心源性休克。
- 主动脉夹层。
- 心肌炎。
- 支气管肺发育不良。
- 肺动脉高压。
- 肺炎、支气管炎。

X

• 低血糖。
• 肾上腺皮质功能不全、CAH。
• 糖原沉积病。
• 脓毒症。
• 休克。

治疗

■ 初步稳定/治疗

• 保暖和吸氧。
• 治疗低血糖和酸中毒。
• 建立静脉通路。
• 准备气管插管。

注意
高氧分压促进导管关闭。

■ 急诊治疗/程序

• 使用前列腺素 E_1 (PGE_1) 以扩张或开放肺动脉导管：
- 持续静脉输注 0.05～0.1 μg/(kg·min)。
- 并发症包括呼吸困难、心动过缓、低血压和癫痫。
• 评估和治疗其他原因的发绀：
- 脓毒症检查和经验性抗生素使用。
- 维持血糖正常。
• 先天性心脏病的循环衰竭：
- 液体复苏(增加 10 ml/kg)。
- 正性肌力药物。
- 积极治疗酸中毒。
• 充血性心力衰竭：
- 地高辛和利尿剂。

■ 药物治疗

• 氨苄西林：50 mg/kg，静脉使用。
• 地高辛的剂量需要高度注意：0.25 mg 静脉注射或口服 q6 h，最大剂量 1.0 mg。
• 多巴酚丁胺：5～20 μg/(kg·min)，静脉使用。
• 多巴胺：2～20 μg/(kg·min)，静脉使用。
• 肾上腺素：0.1～2 μg/(kg·min)，静脉使用。
• 呋塞米：1 mg/kg，静脉使用。
• 庆大霉素：4 mg/(kg·d)，静脉使用。
• 米力农：0.25～1 μg/(kg·min)，50 μg/kg 负荷。
• 前列腺素 E_1：0.05～0.1 μg/(kg·min)。
• 碳酸氢钠：1～2 mmol/kg 静脉使用。

随访

■ 进一步处理

入院指征

• 所有怀疑先天性心脏病的新生儿：
- 收治儿童 ICU。
• 先天性心脏病伴急性发绀加重或充血性心力衰竭。
• 先天性心脏病合并肺炎或支气管炎。

出院指征

由心脏科医师会诊意见决定。

转诊问题

主要负责医师应与心脏科和心胸外科手术的要求相协调。

■ 随访建议

随访计划应与儿童心脏科医师沟通。

要点和误区

• 非发绀性病灶在 2～12 周出现：
- 动脉导管关闭时出现主动脉缩窄。
- 肺血管阻力下降时出现间隔缺损。
• 房室通道经典心电图：QRS 电轴偏前。
• 缩窄经典胸片：肋骨切迹(晚期)。

纤维肌痛 Fibromyalgia

Michael P. Wilson 万健 译

X

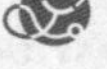

基础知识

■ 描述

• 非关节性、非炎性形式的肌肉痛和关节疼痛，更常见于女性：
- 广泛的疼痛刺激通常不会引起疼痛(触摸痛)。
- 大于 11 个扩散的疼痛点。
- 疲劳。
- 睡眠障碍。
- 肌肉僵硬。
- 注意力、记忆力困难。
- 物理感知受限。

■ 病因

• 发病机制：
- 痛苦的症状被认为是前递质系统的激活信号大于大脑和延髓的镇痛系统所造成的。
• 异常识别机制：
- 增加 P 物质(促进疼痛感)。
- 减少生物胺(去甲肾上腺素、血管收缩素、多巴胺)可促进疼痛效应。
- 减少大脑灰质。
• 遗传学：
- 1/3 纤维肌痛患者存在近亲关系的影响。
- 候选基因包括 5-羟色胺 2A 受体、5-羟色胺转运体、多巴胺 D4 受体等。
- 像许多复杂的疾病一样，心理因素与精神疾病在高发病率中发挥作用。
- 在基因个体倾向中，可能从年龄、创伤、疾病、炎症作为起始的损伤。
• 下丘脑-垂体-肾上腺轴：
- 应激反应功能失调已经表明了纤维肌痛的最新发展。

诊断

■ 症状和体征

腰部以上、腰部以下、身体左侧和身体右侧广泛性疼痛，伴有中轴骨疼痛：
• 大于 3 个月的疼痛病史，症状不能用其他疾病来解释。

病史

• 广泛的肌肉骨骼疼痛和晨僵。
• 虚弱和乏力。
• 睡眠障碍。
• 肌肉痉挛。
• 休息不能缓解的持续疲劳(考虑慢性疲劳综合征)。
• 手臂或腿部麻木和刺痛。
• 受损的注意力和记忆力。
• 恶心和呕吐。

• 腹痛或排便疼痛减轻。
• 耳痛。
• 鼻窦压迫不适（考虑鼻窦炎）。
• 下颌或面部疼痛（考虑颞颌关节功能紊乱）。
• 太阳穴疼痛（考虑颞动脉炎）。
• 骨盆或膀胱不适（考虑间质性膀胱炎）。
• 紧张性头痛或偏头痛（考虑慢性疼痛的原因）。
• 阴道口刺激或瘙痒症状（考虑外阴痛）。

体格检查

检查发现的情况通常比较局限。

基本检查

• 既往史是诊断要点。
• 急诊内容包括从急性疼痛与损伤中区分诊断慢性疾病所致疼痛、哪些需要持续护理和治疗。
• 如果需要诊断纤维肌痛，使用美国风湿病学会（ACR）建立的分类诊断标准确定纤维肌痛。
• 目前认为至少3个月的左右肢体疼痛、腰部上下方痛和轴向骨骼痛，才定义为广泛性疼痛（颈椎前胸部、脊柱胸或腰痛）：
- 18个中的11个具体柔软的小于4 kg/cm压力（小的压力）触诊为普通痛苦指数。
- 位于9个成对敏感点集中如下：
◦ 枕骨部：枕骨下肌肉置入。
◦ 低颈部：前部 $C_5 \sim C_7$ 横突间的空间。
◦ 斜方肌：上缘的中点。
◦ 冈上肌：上方内侧边界的肩胛骨和脊柱。
◦ 第2肋：第2肋软骨的横向连接的上缘。
◦ 外侧上髁：2 cm远端上髁。
◦ 臀肌的：上外象限的臀部。
◦ 大粗隆：转子后突。
◦ 膝盖：医用脂肪垫近端关节线。
- 可以用于诊断疼痛指数≥7和症状反应程度≥5或疼痛指数3～6和症状反应程度≥9者。
- 症状反应程度（0～12）评估疲劳、清醒焦虑和认知症状。
- 过去1周有3个症状达到评估水平：
◦ 0＝没问题。
◦ 1＝轻度到中度问题，一般断断续续的。
◦ 2＝中度的，较大的问题，经常表现为中等程度。
◦ 3＝严重度：广泛的，持续的，影响到生活的困难程度。
- 另外，症状反应程度评分躯体症状等级如下：
◦ 0＝没有症状。
◦ 1＝轻微症状。
◦ 2＝中等症状。
◦ 3＝大量症状。
◦ 躯体症状可被考虑：肌肉痛、肠道易激综合征、疲劳/劳累、思考和记忆问题、肌无力、头痛、腹部疼痛、麻木感、刺痛感、头晕、失眠、忧愁、便秘、上腹痛、恶心、神经紧张、胸痛、视力模糊、发热、腹泻、口干、痒、气喘、雷诺现象、荨麻疹、划痕、耳鸣、呕吐、心痛、口腔溃疡、乏味、癫痫、眼干、气短、食欲不振、皮疹、光敏、听力障碍、易挫伤、掉发、尿频、尿痛、膀胱痉挛。

诊断检查与说明

实验室检查

• 只需要进行评估可替代的诊断或剧烈的疼痛：
- 全血细胞计数。
- 血液生化。
- 红细胞沉降率。
- 血清肌酶。
- 甲状腺功能。
- 尿液分析。
• 没有具体的特异的实验室检查用于纤维肌痛的检查。

影像学检查

没有具体的影像学异常特征。

诊断步骤/外科

只需要评估急性疼痛的原因。

鉴别诊断

• 肌筋膜痛综合征（出现触发点，不是薄弱点）。
• 慢性疲劳综合征。
• 重度抑郁。
• 风湿性多肌痛。
• 莱姆病。
• 甲状腺功能减退。
• 胶原血管病。
• 电解质紊乱。
• 肌肉疾病（新陈代谢和药物诱发）。
• 软骨病。
• 心因性风湿病。
• 嗜酸性粒细胞增多肌痛综合征。
• 泌尿道感染。
• 脊柱关节病。
• 化学物质过敏症。
• 间质性膀胱炎。

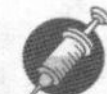

治疗

急诊治疗/程序

• 患者教育、保障及制定护理目标：
- 强调纤维肌痛是没有生命危险的，不减少寿命。
- 功能紊乱不严重但是慢性或变形。
- 目标是管理疼痛和改善功能残疾。
• 患者需要持续的照顾，应该寻求全科医师或疼痛专家的帮助。
• 药物治疗：
- 药物治疗改善疼痛，放松肌肉，改善睡眠治疗，中枢神经系统药物普瑞巴林和加巴喷丁一直是最有效的。
- 阿片类药物对NDMA受体激动剂的慢性疼痛和实际上可能恶化患者的长期痛苦并非一直有效。
- 三环类抗忧郁药（三环类，如阿米替林、去甲阿米替林）可能优于选择性血清素再吸收抑制剂类药物。
- 5-羟色胺去甲肾上腺素再摄取抑制剂（度洛西汀、米那普仑）可能比SSRI类药物更有效，更耐受。
- 曲马多是一个辅助剂。
- 苯二氮䓬类除了在睡眠障碍中起作用，没有任何好处。
- 并没有被证据表明非甾体抗炎药和糖皮质激素是有效的。
- 类固醇或局部麻醉剂注入薄弱点是有争议的。
◦ 没有学术证明是有效的。

药物治疗

• 对乙酰氨基酚：650 mg，4 h口服1次，24 h不超过4 g。
• 阿米替林：25～50 mg，睡前口服。
• 度洛西汀：60 mg，口服，每日1～2次。
• 加巴喷丁：初始每日3次，300 mg，逐步加量至300～1 200 mg。
• 普瑞巴林：初始每日3次，50 mg，逐步加量至每日口服450 mg。
• 曲马多：每日口服，300～400 mg。

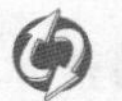

随访

进一步处理

入院指征

• 严重的基础疾病患者、难治性疼痛或免疫功能不全。

• 有自杀倾向的患者。

出院指征

单纯的纤维肌痛患者可以作为门诊患者进行管理。

■ **随访建议**

• 生活方式：
- 应该鼓励体育锻炼。
- 锻炼应该逐步进行，以免过度运动而放弃。
- 有氧运动比简单的伸展更有益。
- 运动停止后效果不能持续。
- 好的睡眠模式也应该被重视。
- 建议保持良好的晚间睡觉习惯。
- 避免在下午或晚上进食含有咖啡因的饮料和食物。
- 鼓励压力管理和应对策略。

• 参与教育计划（如认知行为疗法）：
- 改进经常需要持续几个月。

要点和误区

纤维肌痛患者可以出现急性症状，区分急性和慢性疼痛是至关重要的。

纤维囊性乳腺病 Fibrocystic Breast Changes

Francisco Javier Andrade Jr · David A. Pearson　万健 译

基础知识

■ **描述**

• 广义上是指那些良性的乳房病变为边界不清的。

• 这个疾病在大多数健康女性身上被发现，因此不再将其视为病理性疾病。

• 被视为最常见的良性乳房疾病。

• 变化包括：
- 良性囊肿。
- 乳房疼痛（乳腺痛），这种疼痛可以是周期性的，也可不是。
- 扩散和结节状病灶。
- 明显的纤维肿瘤。
- 乳头溢液，可能是绿色或褐色，不过常有血丝。

• 自发的、持续的溢出需要进一步评估。

• 发生于60%的女性。

• 疼痛症状直到更年期前变得越来越重严重。

• 疼痛通常在经前阶段突出，经期改善。
- 仅有乳房疼痛症状为癌症的病例罕见，只占0.2%～2%。

• 类似的疾病有：腺病、良性的乳房疾病、囊性乳腺病、乳房囊性疾病、纤维腺病、纤维囊肿病乳腺结构不良。

■ **病因**

• 发病机制尚不明确。

• 乳腺组织循环可能增加或扩大生殖激素水平：
- 可能是由于雌激素、孕激素比例失调。
- 雌激素受体敏感性增加。
- 每日可能继发于催乳素分泌增加。

• 最常见于30～50岁女性。

• 疼痛最有可能是由囊肿快速扩张引起的。

• 更年期症状可能持续到激素替代疗法。

• 在口服避孕药的女性中发病率降低。

• 风险因素包括：
- 乳腺纤维囊性改变的家族史。
- 口服避孕药。
- 激素替代疗法。
- 随年龄增加。
- 饮食（高脂肪摄入、咖啡因、甲基黄嘌呤）。

诊断

■ **症状和体征**

病史

• 乳腺痛和乳腺过敏感：
- 持续或间歇性。
- 经常发生在正常月经周期的经前期阶段。
- 通常是双侧的。
- 疼痛可放射到肩膀和手臂。

• 团块和结节：
- 可以是局部的或广泛的。

• 乳腺充血和乳腺密度增加：
- 乳房如同被固定，沉重。
- 形成波动的囊性区。

• 自发的或可挤出的乳头溢液。

• 乳头的感觉异常，如瘙痒。

• 家族史中常见囊肿病史。

体格检查

• 先坐位后卧位，触诊乳腺4个象限。

• 请注意从正常的变化，包括红斑和温度，提示可能的诊断。

• 检查多点区域（腋窝、锁骨等）。

• 纤维囊性的病变时可触及柔软的模糊的结节。

• 结节通常不固定和可移动。

• 通常在上极和外侧象限更为多见。

• 小团的囊肿通常被触诊为如豌豆状。

• 大的囊肿触感似装满水的气球。

• 乳房检查最敏感的是月经后第1日之后的7～9日，此时乳房充血程度最小。

■ **诊断检查与说明**

实验室检查

• 通常没有必要在急诊室完成一个详尽的实验室检查。

• 如果溢乳，检查催乳素和促甲状腺激素可能是有帮助的。

影像学检查

• <30岁建议超声检查。

• >30岁建议乳腺X线片检查。

• 超声检查：
- 可以从固体团块中区分囊性灶。
- 根据发现可分为良性、复杂、复杂三种类型。
- 良性囊肿：
  ◦ 通常都是外观没有不对称和不规则厚度的囊壁。
  ◦ 没有中央回声区。
  ◦ 后壁增强是正常的。
- 深吸气可协助检查触摸不清的囊肿。
- 也用于随访脓肿的大小。
- 应在专门的乳腺中心由受过专门训练的放射科医师进行检查和结果解释。

• 乳腺X线检查：
- 良性的病变可出现假阳性。
- 因组织密度较高，描述30岁以下的女性乳房变得困难。
- 应当在深吸气前后和7～10日后再次检查以避免人为因素干扰。

诊断步骤/外科

• 细针穿刺：

X

- 通常由专科医师进行。
- 对有症状的和大的包块进行治疗。
- 可以区分囊性灶和实质包块。
- 获得恶性肿瘤的细胞学评估。

• 活检：
- 由外科医师进行。
- 当实质包块不能确诊为良性时有必要进行。

鉴别诊断

• 良性的乳房肿块：
- 导管扩张症。
- 炎性囊肿。
- 脂肪坏死。
- 乳腺炎。
- 单发的纤维瘤。
- 孤立的乳头瘤。
- 积液（血肿、浆膜瘤、淋巴囊肿）。

• 恶性的乳房肿块：
- 非典型增生。
- 复杂的纤维瘤。
- 弥漫性乳头状瘤。
- 没有异型性的导管增生。
- 硬化性腺病。

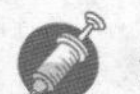

治疗

急诊治疗/程序

• 大部分女性不需要任何医学治疗。

• 保守治疗：
- 合适的胸罩。
- 背心胸罩：
  ◦ 支持以减少乳房韧带的张力。
  ◦ 可以减少炎症反应和水肿。
- 月经前2～3日应用小剂量利尿剂。
- 非甾体抗炎药，对乙酰氨基酚。
- 建议从月经历开始，将乳房疼痛与月经联系起来。

• 床旁超声有助于确定病变的特征。

• 改变饮食习惯，但是尚有争议：
- 限制膳食脂肪总热量（不超过总量的25%）和忌食咖啡因。
- ω-3脂肪酸和维生素E共补充12周对炎症因子和代谢状况有有益影响。
- 报春花油或洋甘菊等草药制剂可以减轻疼痛，但效果并不比安慰剂好。

• 激素治疗：
- 从给予五氯苯酚开始治疗。
- 口服避孕药：
  ◦ 可能会减轻症状，特别是使用1年以后。
- 达那唑（合成雄激素）和他莫昔芬（部分雌激素拮抗剂）：
  ◦ 对治疗严重的周期性乳腺痛有同等疗效。
  ◦ 可能出现副作用（痤疮、多毛症、体重增加、致畸形）。
- 溴隐亭（能抑制催乳素生产）：
  ◦ 使用也受到副作用（疼痛、头晕、恶心、便秘、乏力）限制。

• 手术治疗：
- 如果结节持续存在，无论诊断结果如何，均建议切除。
- 如果一个大囊肿复发2次，应该切除并送病理。

药物治疗

• 溴隐亭：2.5～5 mg/d，每日2次。

• 达那唑：100～400 mg/d，每日2次，持续6个月。

• 他莫昔芬：10～20 mg/d。

• 避孕药（可选）。

随访

进一步处理

出院指征

• 乳腺纤维囊性改变的患者适合放在门诊随访。

• 鼓励患者保持乳房疼痛记录来确定是否循环疼痛。

• 随访的重要性应该强调，确保患者的健康、疾病预防和患者的满意度。

随访建议

• 鼓励定期乳房自检方法，每年1次检查，在适当的时候进行每年1次扫描。

• 所有乳腺癌质量评估需要转诊到家庭医师或专门的乳房诊所。

• 大部分可能是需要在月经期或非月经期进一步检查、摄片和活检。

• 在某些情况下安排普外科医师进行组织活检是必要的。

要点和误区

• 乳腺癌可能与良性乳腺疾病或乳腺纤维囊性改变共存。
- 应考虑所有癌症可能的危险因素。
- 应有确定的随访计划。

• 乳腺炎症患者应该予以抗感染治疗，若已诊断为癌时则不用。

• 纤维囊性的变化通常为双侧的，单侧的改变可能为癌。

• 所有人对乳腺癌都是高度警觉的。
- 以保证纤维囊性的乳房病变在癌变前能被发现。
- 推荐低不适感时及时就诊。

消化性溃疡

Yanina A. Purim-Shem-Tov　赵铭 译

基础知识

描述

• 由胃黏膜或十二指肠黏膜的保护失效造成。

• 酸液的分泌与黏膜的保护之间存在不平衡。

病因

• 幽门螺杆菌：
- 一种生活在黏膜层的革兰阴性螺旋杆菌。
- 与90%～95%的十二指肠溃疡和80%的胃溃疡有关。
- 能增加胃窦胃泌素（促胃液素）的分泌，降低黏膜完整性。

• 非甾体抗炎药。
- 能阻碍前列腺素的合成。
- 导致黏膜破裂。

• 阿司匹林。

• 吸烟。

• 酒精。

• 严重生理压力。

• 分泌过多（不常见）。

• 遗传(>20%有家族病史)。

诊断

■ **症状和体征**

• 上腹疼痛或压痛(80%～90%):
- 灼痛,蚀痛,酸痛。
- 位置:中线,剑突,脐。

• 十二指肠溃疡:
- 饭后 90 min 至 3 h 出现疼痛。
- 使患者在夜间醒来。
- 食物和抗酸药能缓解疼痛。

• 胃溃疡:
- 饭后疼痛加重。
- 恶心,厌食。

• 临床上难以区分胃溃疡和十二指肠溃疡。
• 服用抗酸药可缓解疼痛。
• 粪隐血阳性。
• 消化性溃疡(PUD)的并发症:
- 急性穿孔:
  ◦ 腹部僵硬。
  ◦ 泛发性反跳痛。
  ◦ 疼痛发散至背部或肩部。
- 梗阻:
  ◦ 疼痛和呕吐。
  ◦ 有残留胃内容物的振水音,腹胀。
- 出血:
  ◦ 呕血。
  ◦ 黑粪。
  ◦ 低血压。
  ◦ 心动过速。
  ◦ 皮肤苍白。
  ◦ 直立性变化。

病史

• 非甾体抗炎药,阿司匹林。
• 抽烟。
• 消化性溃疡既往史。
• 胃癌家族病史。
• 腹痛。
• 腹泻。
• 乏力。

体格检查

• 腹痛。
• 贫血迹象。
• 粪隐血阳性。

■ **基本检查**

• 详细体格检查,包括隐血测试和直立体征。
• 病情稳定时,口服胃肠鸡尾酒能缓解疼痛:
- 抗酸药:30 ml。
- 黏性利多卡因:10 ml。

■ **诊断检查与说明**

实验室检查

• 单纯性溃疡的正常实验室值。
• CBC:
- 出血时血细胞比容较低。
- 穿孔、穿透时白细胞增多。
• 淀粉酶、脂肪酶:
- 随穿孔、穿透增高。
- 鉴别诊断胰腺炎。
• 重症患者检查电解质、尿素氮/肌酸酐、葡萄糖。
• 大量失血患者检验血型和交叉配血。
• 幽门螺旋杆菌检测(尿素呼气试验、幽门螺旋杆菌抗体、IgG)。

影像学检查

• 胸/腹部 X 线检查系列:
- 评估穿孔/梗阻。

诊断步骤/外科

• 心电图:
- 高龄患者。
- 鉴别诊断心肌缺血。
• 内镜:
- 优先选择。
- 除出血外皆门诊处理。
- 出现幽门螺旋杆菌时应对胃十二指肠溃疡部位进行活组织检查。
- 检查恶性胃溃疡。
• 上消化道造影:
- 单对比钡诊断率为 70%～80%。
- 双对比诊断率为 90%。
• 胃泌素(促胃液素)水平随佐林格-埃利森综合征升高。

■ **鉴别诊断**

• 胃食管反流。
• 胆绞痛。
• 胆囊炎。
• 胰腺炎。
• 胃炎。
• 腹主动脉瘤。
• 主动脉夹层。
• 心肌梗死。
• 有症状但内镜检查无溃疡称为非溃疡性消化不良。

治疗

■ **院前**

• ABC 管理。
• 为低血压、休克患者静脉注射液体复苏剂。

■ **初步稳定/治疗**

• ABC 管理。
• 鉴定溃疡并发症(出血、穿孔、梗阻)。
• 低血压患者可用两支大口径静脉注射器注射乳酸林格液和生理盐水。
• 尽早确认血型和交叉匹配。
• 用鼻胃管(NGT)进行胃部减压,检查出血。

■ **急诊治疗/程序**

• 用抗酸药(胃肠鸡尾酒)或静脉注射 H_2 受体抗结剂进行疼痛控制。
• 避免麻醉——可能掩盖严重疾病。
• 促进溃疡愈合:
- 抗酸药。
- H_2 受体拮抗剂(西咪替丁、法莫替丁、雷尼替丁):
  ◦ 可持续 2～5 年。
- 质子泵抑制剂(PPI:奥美拉唑、兰索拉唑、泮托拉唑):
  ◦ H_2 受体拮抗剂无效时使用。
- 硫糖铝。
- 前列腺素同系物(米索前列醇)。
- 硫糖铝、H_2 受体抗结剂和质子泵抑制剂不可联用。
• 胃出口梗阻:
- 用鼻胃管进行胃部解压。
- 静脉注射水合物。
• 胃出血:
- 静脉注射液体复苏剂。
- 根据失血量、血细胞比容进行输血。
- 用弗利导管监测出血量。
- 胃肠咨询。
• 穿孔:
- 静脉注射水合剂。
- 用弗利导管监测水合状态。
- 术前抗生素。
- 紧急手术会诊。
• 幽门螺杆菌感染的治疗:
- 侵袭性或非侵袭性检测以确认感染。
- 环丙沙星三联疗法:
  ◦ 14 日 1 个疗程。
  ◦ PPI 类药物,每日 2 次。
  ◦ 环丙沙星(500 mg),每日 2 次。
  ◦ 阿莫西林(1 g),每日 2 次;或者甲硝唑(500 mg),每日 3 次。
- 在高感染率地区进行序贯疗法 10 日:
  ◦ 5 日双联疗法:
    ▪ PPI。

▪ 阿莫西林(1 g)。
◦ 随后 5 日三联疗法：
▪ PPI。
▪ 环丙沙星(500 mg)。
▪ 甲硝唑(500 mg)。
- 铋剂四联疗法：
◦ PPI(标准剂量)。
◦ 柠檬酸铋亚铁盐(120～300 mg 或 420 mg)或水杨酸铋铁盐(300 mg 或 524 mg)，每日 4 次。
◦ 四环素(500 mg)，每日 4 次。
◦ 甲硝唑(500 mg)，每日 3 次。
- 并行治疗 10/14 日：
◦ PPI，每日两次。
◦ 环丙沙星(500 mg)和阿莫西林(1 g)；或者甲硝唑(500 mg)，每日 2 次。
- 混合疗法：
◦ PPI，每日两次，加上阿莫西林(1 g)，每日 2 次，连续 5 日，随后：
◦ PPI、环丙沙星(500 mg)、阿莫西林(500 mg)，加上甲硝唑(500 mg)或硝唑(500 mg)，每日 2 次，连续 7 日。
- 左氧氟沙星序贯疗法：
◦ PPI，每日 2 次，加上阿莫西林(1 g)，每日 2 次，连续 5～7 天，随后：
◦ PPI、左氧氟沙星(500 mg，每日 1 次)、阿莫西林(500 mg，每日 2 次)，加上甲硝唑或替硝唑(500 mg，每日 2 次)，连续 5～7 日。

• 停止非甾体类抗炎药。
• 外科治疗：
- 难治性溃疡。
- 并发症：
◦ 出血。
◦ 穿孔。
◦ 幽门狭窄。

药物治疗

• 次水杨酸铋：口服 2 片，每片含 525 mg。
• 制酸剂 Plus：口服 2～4 片，每日 4 次。
• 米索前列醇：口服 100～200 mg，每日 4 次。
• 碳酸钙制剂Ⅱ：口服 2～4 片，每日 4 次。
• 硫糖铝：口服 1 g，每日 4 次，连续 6～8 周。
• 法莫替丁(H_2 受体阻滞剂)：口服 40 mg，每晚睡前(儿童：0.5～0.6 mg/kg，q12 h)，连续 6～8 周。
• 尼扎替丁(H_2 受体阻滞剂)：口服 300 mg，每晚睡前，连续 6～8 周；口服 20 mg，每日 2 次[儿童：5～10 mg/(kg·24 h)，分 2 次]，连续 2 周。
• 雷尼替丁(H_2 受体阻滞剂)：口服 300 mg，每晚睡前[儿童：5～10 mg/(kg·24 h)4 h，q12 h]，连续 6～8 周。
• 西咪替丁(H_2 受体阻滞剂)：口服 400 mg，每日 2 次，连续 6～8 周。
• 氨氯地平(质子泵抑制剂)：口服 30 mg，每日 2 次，连续 2 周。
• 泮托拉唑(质子泵抑制剂)：口服 40 mg，每日 1 次，连续 2 周。
• 奥美拉唑(质子泵抑制剂)：口服 20 mg，每日 2 次，连续 2 周。
• 雷贝拉唑(质子泵抑制剂)：口服 20 mg，每日 1 次，连续 6 周。
• 埃索美拉唑(质子泵抑制剂)：每日口服 40 mg，连续 4 周。
• 幽门螺杆菌治疗：
- 上述多种选择。

随访

进一步处理

入院指征

• 胃梗阻。
• 穿孔。
• 上消化道出血。
• 黑粪。
• 不受控制的疼痛。
• 贫血，需要输血。

出院指征

• CBC 正常，粪隐血阴性。
• 若为粪隐血阳性，但生命体征稳定，血细胞比容正常，NGT 为阴性，则可以出院。

转诊问题

消化道评估，内镜检查。

随访建议

• 有下列情形的高危患者：
- 出血且血流动力学不稳定。
- 反复咯血或便血。
- 洗胃失败。
- 凝血病。
- 高龄。
- 有需要手术修复的溃疡穿孔或穿透。
• 初步治疗后需进行 2～6 周的随访以评估疗效。
• >55 岁的患者及重症患者需进行内镜检查和幽门螺旋杆菌测试。

要点和误区

• 幽门螺旋杆菌是导致消化性溃疡最常见的原因。
• 非甾体抗炎药诱发的消化性溃疡较隐蔽。
• 消化不良的症状是非特异性的。
• 可用内镜进行诊断，内镜需有幽门螺旋杆菌筛查。
• 治疗中需包含幽门螺旋杆菌的根除以及 H_2 受体阻滞剂或 PPI。
• 并发症有穿孔、出血、贫血等。
• 未能随访可能导致胃癌的误诊。

X

小肠损伤 Small-Bowel Injury

Barry J. Knapp · Michael J. Bono 周健 潘曙明 译

基础知识

描述

两种常见原因：
• 钝性内脏创伤。
• 穿透性：内脏损伤(96%枪伤、50%刺伤)——浆膜撕裂、肠壁血肿、穿孔、肠横断、肠系膜血肿/血管损伤。

病因

• 钝性伤：
- 第三常见损伤(占所有钝器损伤患者的 5%～10%)。

- 机动车事故。
- 非车辆创伤：虐待、殴打、自行车把手、大型动物踢腿。

• 爆炸的受害者。

• 小肠损伤的死亡率为 33%。

• 肠系膜撕裂最初可能无症状：

- 定点减速伤(如 Treitz 韧带)。
- 固定点附近的剪切机构(如回盲肠的结、粘连)。
- 前棘受压。
- 反肠系膜边缘的"井喷"因腔内压力的突然升高而爆裂。

• 相关的伤害：

- 肝、脾损伤；胸、骨盆骨折。
- 安全带综合征：腹壁淤血，小肠损伤，L_1、L_3 的偶发性骨折。

• 渗透：

- 小肠是前腹刺伤中第二常见的损伤器官(32%)。
- 小肠损伤在枪伤中最常见(49%)。

儿科注意事项

• 钝性伤：

- 儿童较少见(1%～8%的儿童钝性伤)。
- 佩戴肩带和膝带的车辆事故中肠道损伤的概率较低。
- 警惕非穿透性损伤：近距离气枪事故(<10 ft)。
- 考虑非意外创伤的可能性。

诊断

症状和体征

• 身体的迹象和症状是不可靠的。

• 诊断延迟是常见的。

• 出现"邻座标志"会使小肠受伤的风险增加 1 倍。

• 最初的表现可能比较温和：

- 患者无一例外地会发展成严重的症状。

• 诊断延误会增加发病率和死亡率：

- 8 h 内诊断的死亡率为 2%，24 h 后诊断的死亡率为 31%。

病史

• 腹部穿透性钝器伤史。

• 必须考虑没有明确外伤史的患病儿童(虐待儿童)。

体格检查

• 在清醒时，警觉的患者寻找：

- 腹部压痛(87%～98%)。
- 腹痛(85%)。
- 腹膜迹象(67%)。

• 许多患者会有：

- 腹壁挫伤(54%)。
- 低血压(38%)。
- 直肠 Guaiac 试验阳性(5%)。

• 小肠损伤最初可能表现为：

- 加剧的腹痛。
- 肠梗阻。
- 尿量减少。
- 心动过速。

基本检查

• 初诊时应注意所有伤口及触痛部位。

• 所有病情稳定的患者均行 CT 检查。

• 对于 CT 阴性但怀疑肠损伤的患者，需要进一步的系列检查。

• 对于医学上不稳定的患者，诊断性腹腔灌洗(DPL)在确定是否存在空洞的内脏损伤方面是最有效的。

诊断检查与说明

实验室检查

• 没有诊断试验被证明对小肠损伤的预测高度敏感。

• 血清淀粉酶、脂肪酶和肝功能检查对急性损伤的敏感性较差。

影像学检查

• 胸部、腹部 X 线平片：

- 对小肠损伤无效。
- X 线平片可见气腹的发生率仅为 8%。

• CT：

- 实体器官损伤和头部创伤的诊断标准，但对空洞的内脏损伤较不敏感。
- 新一代螺旋 CT 扫描的灵敏度为 88%，特异性为 99%。
- 口服造影剂的益处存在争议，仅使用静脉造影剂是可以接受的。
- 冲创伤：

• 用于病情稳定的患者。

• 钝性伤 CT 的适应证包括腹部压痛、低血压、精神状态改变(GCS<14)、肋缘压痛、胸部 X 线检查异常、HCT<30%和血尿。

• 小肠损伤的 CT 特异性征象为气腹(敏感性 50%～75%)和轴位对比(敏感性 12%)。

• 提示小肠损伤的 CT 征象包括不明原因的腹腔内游离液(敏感性 93%)、肠壁增厚>3 mm(敏感性 61%)、肠系膜间液、肠系膜条纹。

- 穿透性：不推荐 CT，因为敏感性仅为 14%，假阴性结果率为 18%。

• 超声：由于肠内空气使观影困难，所以对空性内脏损伤不敏感。

诊断步骤/外科

• DPL：

- 侵入性的，但可能对不稳定的患者或临床可疑但非诊断性的腹部 CT 患者有帮助。
- 对腹腔积血敏感，但对出血源不敏感。
- 红细胞计数为 100 000/mm^3 时为阳性。
- 灌胃淀粉酶>20 U/L 和白细胞计数>500/mm^3(小肠损伤的晚期标志物)。
- 对琥珀酸、植物、粪便的灌洗显微镜检查对小肠损伤有特异性，但不敏感。
- 灌洗碱性磷酸酶(3 U/L)被认为是小肠损伤的一个有用的直接标志物。

• 腹腔镜检查在诊断进展性或症状稳定的小肠损伤中起关键作用。

鉴别诊断

• 由于血管损伤引起的腹膜积血。

• 胃、结肠、直肠穿孔。

• 脊椎损伤和相关肠梗阻。

儿科注意事项

延误诊断 1～2 日是常见的，并增加发病率。

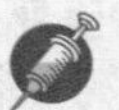

治疗

院前

警报：

• 患者应该被送到最近的创伤中心。

• 不要试图替换取出的腹部内容物，用湿纱布、毯子和运输工具覆盖。

• 不要取出刺穿腹部的物体，用纱布和胶带固定物体后再转运患者。

初步稳定/治疗

• 标准增加的创伤生命支持协议，包括气道、呼吸和循环管理。

• 积极的液体复苏，建议压力输注温静脉液体(乳酸林格液或生理盐水)。

• 用湿纱布覆盖已暴露的小肠，不要除去急诊中穿破的异物。

急诊治疗/程序

• 对于有开腹指征的患者，需要立即转移到：

- 取出内脏。
- 低血压伴腹痛。
- DPL 或腹部 CT 阳性。

• 胸部 X 线检查显示胸腹疝。

- 异物刺入。

X

- 腹部有穿透性枪伤。
- 对于穿透性腹部伤口和需要手术探查的钝性损伤，应给予破伤风和抗生素预防。

• 腹部刺伤的局部探查是安全的。
• 连续腹部检查和观察其他稳定的患者。
• 在确定诊断后，在血压允许的情况下进行适当的镇痛。

▪ 药物治疗

• 头孢替坦(头孢坦)：1～2 g(儿童：20 mg/kg)，静脉滴注，q12 h 或；
• 头孢西丁(mefoxin)：1～2 g(儿童：40 mg/kg)，静脉滴注，q6 h，或；
• Ceftizoxime (cefizox)：1～2 g(儿童：50 mg/kg)，静脉滴注，q8～12 h+；
• 灭滴灵：500 mg(儿童：7.5 mg/kg)，静脉滴注，q6 h。

随访

▪ 进一步处理

入院指征

• 指示的剖腹手术。
• 精神状态异常/腹部损伤中毒。
• 出现腹痛、压痛(即使是阴性的检查)要求入院观察和连续检查。
• 刺伤和枪伤破坏腹部筋膜，诊断性腹腔灌洗(DPL)阳性，或恶化的临床检查结果。

出院指征

• 清醒的患者，检查结果正常，无腹痛，将接受充分的随访，但其机械损伤很小。
• 明确的出院指示，以返回恶化的迹象/症状是重要的，以确定那些与未被怀疑的伤害。
• 穿透性伤口，不侵犯腹部筋膜。

▪ 随访建议

出院患者如有腹部不适，应立即转回急诊室。

要点和误区

• 小肠损伤应考虑任何钝性/穿透性腹部创伤的受害者。
• 小肠损伤患者最初的表现可能并不令人印象深刻。
• 出现“安全带标志”会使小肠受伤的风险增加1倍。
• CT 扫描可能会遗漏相当比例的小肠损伤。
• 观察和系列检查是检测隐匿性损伤的一个重要方面。

哮喘(成人) Asthma, Adult

Melissa H. White · Tyler Giberson 江少伟 潘曙明 译

基础知识

▪ 描述

• 吸气阻力增加：
- 气道炎症。
- 气道痉挛。
- 黏膜水肿。
- 黏液堵塞。
- 平滑肌肥大。

• 结果：
- 气体被密封。
- 气道重建。
- 无效腔增加。
- 肺泡过度膨胀。

• 哮喘持续状态是指在最初的 30～60 min 对治疗无反应。
• 有生命威胁的危险因素：
- 预先插管。
- 入住 ICU。
- 慢性类固醇药物的使用。
- 在最近的几年内因哮喘住院。
- 日常医疗管理的不充分。
- 年龄增加。
- 种族(非裔美国人)。
- 缺少医疗救助。
- 多种合并症。

▪ 病因

• 有证据支持的气道的炎症反应过程，表现为周期及可逆的气道阻塞和气道高反应性，多种细胞及细胞成分参与了病程的进展。
- 中性粒细胞。
- 母细胞。
- 嗜酸性粒细胞。
- 巨噬细胞。
- T 淋巴细胞。
- 上皮细胞。
- 细胞因子。

• 促发因子：
- 花粉。
- 粉尘。
- 真菌。
- 动物的皮屑。
- 其他环境过敏原。
- 上呼吸道病毒感染。
- 职业化学品。
- 烟草。
- 环境改变。
- 冷空气。
- 运动诱发。
- 情感因素。
- 月经相关。
- 药物：
  ◦ 阿司匹林。
  ◦ NSAIDs。
  ◦ β受体阻滞剂。

诊断

▪ 症状和体征

• 气喘。
• 呼吸困难。
• 胸闷。
• 咳嗽。
• 呼吸急促。
• 心动过速。
• 呼吸窘迫：
- 坐立位或前倾位。
- 辅助呼吸肌的使用。
- 没有能力讲整段的对话。
- 出汗。
- 呼吸困难。

• 濒死状态：
- 精神状态的改变。
- 持续恶化的疲劳状态。

• 奇脉，>18 mmHg。

▪ 基本检查

• 首要的临床诊断。

• 测量并动态观察最大呼气流速，判断疾病的严重程度。
• 对潜在疾病的评估。

诊断检查与说明

实验室检查

• 血气分析：
- 对初始评估并没有帮助。
- 气管插管的决定需基于临床诊断标准。
- 轻-中度哮喘：呼吸性碱中毒。
- 严重的气道梗阻和疲劳：呼吸性酸中毒和 $PaCO_2>42$。

• 脉氧饱和度：
- <90%提示严重的呼吸窘迫。
- 对于伴随迫切的呼吸代偿患者，脉氧饱和度仍然可以维持在 90%以上直到突然崩溃。

• 白细胞：
- 中性粒细胞并没有特异性。
- 肺炎。
- 慢性类固醇激素的使用。
- 强调哮喘的恶化。
- 肾上腺素和类固醇激素使用后出现轴抑制。

诊断步骤/外科

• 最大呼气峰流速(PEFR)：
- 评估气道阻塞的程度：
  ◦ 正常成人的流速：400～600 L/min。
  ◦ 100～300 L/min 提示中度气道阻塞。
  ◦ <100 L/min 提示严重的气道阻塞。
  ◦ 连续使用作为对治疗反应的客观监测。

• 用力呼气量(FEV)：
- 比最大呼气峰流速更可靠的测量肺功能的指标。
- 作为筛选工具很难使用。
- 通常在急诊室很难提供。
- 严重气道阻塞：$FEV_1<30\%\sim50\%$。

• 胸部 X 线检查
- 指征：
  ◦ 发热。
  ◦ 怀疑肺炎。
  ◦ 怀疑气胸或纵隔积气。
  ◦ 异物吸入。
  ◦ 哮喘的初始期。
  ◦ 合并有其他疾病，如糖尿病、肾功能不全、慢性心功能不全、艾滋病、肿瘤。
  ◦ 对治疗没有反应。
- 典型的发现：
  ◦ 肺极度膨胀。
  ◦ 散乱的肺不张。

• 心电图：
- 表明患者有心脏疾病的风险：
  ◦ 心律失常。
  ◦ 心肌缺血。
- 重症哮喘患者一过性改变。
  ◦ 电轴右偏。
  ◦ 右束支传导阻滞。
  ◦ 异常 P 波。
  ◦ 非特异性 ST - T 波变化。

鉴别诊断

• 过敏反应。
• 血管神经性水肿。
• 毛细支气管炎。
• 支气管炎。
• 类癌。
• 化学性肺炎。
• 慢性肺心病。
• 慢性阻塞性肺疾病。
• 慢性心功能不全。
• 喉炎。
• 异物吸入。
• 浸泡伤。
• 心肌缺血。
• 肺炎。
• 肺栓塞。
• 烟尘吸入。
• 上气道梗阻。
• 静脉空气栓塞。

治疗

院前

• 认识到“寂静肺”提示呼吸窘迫。
• 补充氧气。
• β受体激动剂的持续雾化。
• 肌内或皮下注射肾上腺素。

初步稳定/治疗

• 即刻β受体激动剂雾化吸入治疗。
• 对极度疲劳和呼吸窘迫患者行气管插管。
• 类固醇激素的使用。

急诊治疗/程序

• 氧气：
- 维持氧饱和度>90%。

• β受体激动剂：
- 选择性β受体激动剂(沙丁胺醇)：
  ◦ 轻-中度哮喘：每 20 min 使用一次。
  ◦ 重度哮喘：持续雾化治疗。
- 皮下注射β受体激动剂(特布他林和肾上腺素)：
  ◦ 严重急性加重。
  ◦ 限制雾化药物的使用。
  ◦ 更多的副作用因为全身吸收。
  ◦ 特布他林，更长效的β受体激动剂伴随气道扩张作用，在急性哮喘的治疗与肾上腺素有等同的作用。
  ◦ 相对禁忌：年龄>40 岁和冠心病患者。

• 皮质类固醇激素：
- 减少气道壁炎症反应。
- 早期使用。
- 从使用开始，效用可持续 4～6 h。
- 可以静脉或口服使用。
- 重症哮喘急性加重时静脉推注甲泼尼龙。
- 轻-中度哮喘加重可以给予泼尼松口服或肌内注射甲泼尼龙。
- 雾化吸入皮质类固醇激素目前不推荐作为初步稳定/治疗。

• 抗胆碱能药：
- 如果初始β受体激动剂使用后无明显作用。
- 严重的气道阻塞。
- 吸入抗胆碱能药可以与β受体激动剂联合使用。

• 硫酸镁：
- 对轻-中度哮喘患者没有益处。
- 在重症哮喘中可能有用。

• 氨茶碱：
- 哮喘急性期很少使用。

• 白三烯：
- 哮喘急性加重过程中目前不被推荐。

• 氦氧混合气：
- 氦气和氧气的混合气(80：20、70：30、60：40)。
- 没有空气稠密。
- 减少气道抵抗。
- 减少呼吸衰竭。
- 常规使用不被推荐。
- 严重哮喘可以考虑使用。

• 无创正压通气：
- CPAP 和 BiPAP。
- 可以改善氧和同时减少呼吸衰竭。
- 仅用于警戒状态的患者。
- 不能取代气管插管。
- 目前不推荐作为常规使用。
- 重症哮喘患者考虑使用。

• 氯胺酮：
- 支气管扩张剂和麻醉剂。
- 在气管插管过程中作为诱导剂有效。

X

- 禁忌证：
  - 高血压。
  - 冠心病。
  - 子癫前期。
  - 颅内压增高。
- 氟烷：
  - 吸入麻醉剂有潜在的支气管扩张作用。
  - 用于气管插管的难治性哮喘。
- 哮喘患者的气管插管：
  - 快速气管插管。
  - 利多卡因减轻气道反应。
  - 依托咪酯和氯胺酮作为麻醉诱导剂。
  - 琥珀胆碱可以被使用作为麻痹作用。
  - 大尺寸气管插管套管直径>7 mm 用来气管插管。
  - 患者需要水化治疗。
  - 允许性高碳酸血症。

■ 药物治疗

- β受体激动剂：
  - 沙丁胺醇：2.5 mg 加入 2.5 ml 生理盐水，q20 min(儿童：每次 0.1～0.15 mg/kg，q20 min，最大剂量 1.25 mg)。
  - 肾上腺素：成人 0.3 mg(1：1 000)，皮下注射，q(0.5～4)h×3(儿童：0.01 mg/kg，最大剂量 0.3 mg，皮下注射)。
  - 特布他林：0.25 mg，皮下注射，q0.5 h。
- 类固醇激素：
  - 甲泼尼龙：60～125 mg，静脉推注(儿童：每次 1～2 mg/kg，静脉注射或口服，q6 h×24 h)。
  - 泼尼松：40～60 mg，口服[儿童：1～2 mg/(kg·d)，单次或分次给药]。
  - Depo-Medrol：160 mg，肌内注射。
- 抗胆碱能药：
  - 异丙托溴铵：0.5 mg 加入 3 ml 生理盐水，q1 h×3。
- 镁剂：2 g，静脉注射大于 20 min(儿童：25～75 mg/kg)。
- 氨茶碱：0.6 mg/(kg·h)输液泵，静脉注射。
- 快速气管插管：
  - 依托咪酯：0.3 mg/kg，静脉注射；或氯胺酮 1～1.5 mg/kg，静脉注射。
  - 利多卡因：1～1.5 mg/kg，静脉注射。
  - 琥珀胆碱：1.5 mg/kg，静脉注射。

随访

■ 进一步处理

入院指征

医疗病房

- 最大呼气流速<40%同时最小的空气流动。
- 持续的呼吸窘迫：
  - 支持住院的因素：
    - 提前的气管插管。
    - 近期的急诊室治疗。
    - 多次的急诊室治疗或住院。
    - 症状超过 1 周。
    - 院外治疗失败。
    - 类固醇激素的使用。
    - 没有足够的随访机制。
    - 精神疾病。

留观部门

- 最大呼气峰流速>40%但是<70%的预计值。
- 患者症状没有得到客观的缓解。
- 患者有持续的喘息症状同时呼吸运动减弱。
- 患者对治疗有适度的反应且没有呼吸窘迫。

出院指征

- 最大呼气峰流速>70%且最大呼气峰流速值>300。
- 患者自我描述症状明显缓解。
- 吸入空气的情况下患者两肺呼吸音清晰。
- 48～72 h 进行充分的随访。

■ 随访建议

鼓励患者在随后的 3～5 日就哮喘有关的问题联系他们自己的私人医师或肺科医师。

要点和误区

- 哮喘患者意识状态的改变等同于通气失败。
- 患者可以正确使用吸入装置或雾化装置。
- 患者出院时携带气流测量计。
- 如果没有脱水的症状和体征，没有证据表明静脉补液有助于清除气道分泌物。
- 抗生素一般推荐用于有脓痰、发热、肺炎或细菌性鼻窦炎的患者。

X

哮喘(儿童) Asthma, Pediatric

Roger M. Barkin · Nathan I. Shapiro 陈凉 王海嵘 潘曙明 译

基础知识

■ 描述

- 全美有 270 万患病儿童(<18 岁)。
- 全美每年有 850 000 人因本病急诊就诊。
- 炎症性因素，通常是病毒感染，导致支气管收缩：
  - 合并有气道高反应性。
  - 炎症因子急剧加重症状。
- 气道梗阻加重气道阻力气体受困：
  - 黏膜水肿。
  - 支气管痉挛。
  - 黏液堵塞。
- 婴儿更容易发生呼吸衰竭：
  - 增加外周阻力。
  - 降低弹性回复伴随早期气道关闭。
  - 胸腔不稳定。
  - 横膈机械活动弱。
- 家族史或过敏史。
- 早期气道损伤的病史(支气管肺发育不良、肺炎、气管插管、哮吼、反流、被动吸烟)、食物药物反应、其他过敏表现。
- 环境暴露，如宠物、烟雾、地毯或灰尘可诱发/加重。

■ 病因

诱因或加重因素

- 感染：
  - 病毒。
  - 细菌。
- 过敏/刺激：
  - 环境：花粉、草地、霉菌、家庭灰尘、螨虫和动物皮屑。
  - 职业性化学物：氯气、氨气——食物和添加剂。
  - 刺激物：烟雾、污染物、气体、气雾剂。

- 运动。
- 寒冷环境。
- 情绪：紧张、恐惧。
- 中毒：β受体阻滞剂、阿司匹林、非甾体抗炎药。

诊断

■ 症状和体征

整体情况

• 疲劳、困倦。
• 出汗、激动。
• 低氧、发绀。
• 心动过速。
• 脱水。
• 奇脉。

呼吸

• 气喘、啰音、鼾音。
• 急性或慢性咳嗽。
• 呼吸急促。
• 胸憋闷。
• 呼吸困难、呼吸短促伴呼气延长。
• 收缩，附属呼吸肌使用，鼻翼扇动。
• 过度膨胀。
• 常有反复发作的病史和慢性限制性疾病。
• 并发症：
- 肺炎反复、支气管炎。
- 肺不张。
- 气胸、纵隔气肿。
- 呼吸困难、衰竭、死亡。

病史

• 诱发事件及已知的触发因素。
• 长期的症状。
• 并发疾病。
• 既往病史：
- 既往因哮喘住院。
- 既往气管插管及重症护理。
- 规则及间歇用药。

体格检查

• 生命体征，包括血氧饱和度和呼吸情况。
• 哮鸣音：未及哮鸣音可能与空气流动严重受损和呼吸音下降有关。
• 缺氧的体征。
• 皮肤和甲床呈蓝色。
• 呼吸疲劳、呼吸窘迫或呼吸衰竭的体征：
- 辅助呼吸肌的运动或三凹征。
- 嗜睡或意识模糊。

■ 基本检查

• 临床诊断主要基于体格检查及病史；通过观察辅助呼吸肌运动及三凹征情况评估通气及换气功能。
• 比较患者此次发病与既往发病时对支气管扩张剂的反应。
• 排除其他诊断。
• 动脉血氧饱和度。
• 初始 SaO_2<91%(海平面水平)提示疾病严重：住院治疗，再发可能，病程延长。
• 能配合的患者(通常>5 岁)，测量峰值流速。
- 50%～70%及以下提示中到重度狭窄。
- 70%～90%及以上提示轻到中度狭窄。
- >90%为正常。

■ 诊断检查与说明

实验室检查

• 除了指脉氧饱和度和体格检查，动脉血气分析(ABG)可以辅助评估通气功能；不是必须或常规检查。
• CBC 可作为感染的标志物。
• 茶碱水平：只在茶碱治疗患者中检测(不推荐)。

影像学检查

下列患者需行胸部 X 线平片检查，尤其要关注有无渗出、气管壁增厚或过度扩张。

<1 岁患者排除异物或肺不张。

• 早期明显哮鸣音(提示要评估慢性疾病，有助于排除其他情况)。
• 呼吸窘迫加重或治疗效果不佳。
• 呼吸窘迫、衰竭。
• 未及哮鸣音，但气促。

诊断步骤/外科

峰值流速检测(详见上文)。

■ 鉴别诊断

• 感染及炎症：
- 细支气管炎：除了年龄及临床病史，临床难以鉴别。
- 肺炎：病毒、细菌、化学物质或高敏性。
- 吸入性。
- 咽后、纵隔的脓肿、肿块。
- 过敏反应。
• 解剖异常：
- 气胸。
- 异物。
• 血管异常：
- 血管异常造成气管压迫。
- 肺栓塞。
- 充血性心力衰竭。
• 先天性疾病：
- 囊性纤维化。
- 气管食管瘘。
- 气管源性囊肿。
- 先天性心脏病。
• 中毒：代谢性酸中毒。
• 肿瘤。
• 声带功能障碍(VCD)。
• 肺水肿——心源性或非心源性。
• 胃食管反流。

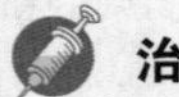

治疗

■ 院前

• 吸氧，监测氧饱和度。
• β受体激动剂雾化吸入：沙丁胺醇。
• 呼吸衰竭或严重呼吸困难时气管插管。
• 有脱水表现时静脉补液。
• 快速转运，并与急诊室良好沟通。

■ 初步治疗

• 保持 SaO_2 在 90%～95%及以上。
• β受体激动剂雾化吸入：沙丁胺醇。
• 呼吸衰竭时气管插管。
• 有脱水表现时，给予总量 20 ml/kg 的生理盐水。

■ 急诊治疗/程序

• 评估患者可能呼吸衰竭的表现：
- 发绀。
- 极度焦虑或易怒。
- 昏睡，嗜睡，疲劳。
- 持续呼吸急促。
- 气道明显狭窄，通气差。
- 严重三凹征。
• 监测氧饱和度：维持血氧饱和度至 SaO_2>95%。
• β受体激动剂雾化吸入：沙丁胺醇。
- 重度哮喘经常或持续应用。
- 左旋沙丁胺醇可能使用频次少，相关副作用少。
• 异丙托溴铵可以作为辅助药物与β受体激动剂联合应用。在中重度患儿中，异丙托溴铵与β受体激动剂 3∶1 联合应用效果最好。
• 激素治疗：
- 能够口服的中度患儿给予口服用药。
- 重度患儿或不能口服的患儿静脉用药。
- 1 剂地塞米松可能等同于传统的激素量。
• 严重或难治性哮喘皮下注射肾上腺素或特布他林(极少使用)。

• 对于严重病例，标准治疗后应用硫酸镁可能有效。

• 呼吸衰竭时气管插管：

- 氯胺酮是有效的诱导药物。

• 如有脱水表现，给予总量20 ml/kg的生理盐水。

• 氦氧混合气(氧气和氦气)可能有效，但研究结果尚不确定。

▪ 药物治疗

• 沙丁胺醇：0.5%溶液或5 mg/ml。

- 雾化：每次0.15 mg/kg，每次最多5 mg，q15～30 min，必要时。

- 定量吸入器(MDI)(有间隔)(90 μg/泡)：2泡q5～10 min，最多10泡。

- 0.083%溶液或2.5 mg/3 ml也可用于雾化。

• 地塞米松：0.3 mg/kg(最多：16 mg)。

• 肾上腺素(1∶1 000)(1 mg/ml)：0.01 mg/kg皮下注射，最多每次0.35 ml，q20 min，共3次。

• 异丙托溴铵：雾化(0.02%吸入溶胶500 μg/2.5 ml)，每次250～500 μg，q6 h。

• 氯胺酮(气管插管用)：作为诱导药物，1～2 mg/kg，静脉注射。

• 左旋沙丁胺醇(0.63 mg和1.25 mg小瓶)：q6～8 h雾化。

• 硫酸镁：每次25 mg/kg静脉应用，超过20 min；最多每次1.2～2 g。

• 甲泼尼龙：每次1～2 mg/kg，静脉应用，q6 h；最多每次125 mg。

• 泼尼松龙：每次1～2 mg/kg，口服，q12 h(剂型为15 mg/5 ml)。

• 泼尼松：每次1～2 mg/kg，口服，q6～12 h；最多每次80 mg。

• 特布他林(剂型1 mg/ml)(0.01%)：每次0.01 ml/kg，皮下注射，q15～20 min；最多每次0.25 ml，q20 min，共2次。

一线用药

• 沙丁胺醇。

• 激素。

• 异丙托溴铵。

二线用药

• 肾上腺素或特布他林。

• 硫酸镁。

随访

▪ 进一步处理

入院指征

• 患儿需要进行客观及主观个性化评估。

• 持续性呼吸困难：

- 持续哮鸣音。

- 呼吸频率加快，呼吸急促。

- 三凹征，辅助呼吸肌应用。

• 不吸氧时，SaO_2<93%(海平面)。

• 呼气峰值流量(PEFR)在50%～70%及以下预测值。

• 不能耐受口服药物或液体。

• 24 h内有急诊就诊史。

• 合并症：

- 先天性心脏病。

- 支气管肺发育不良。

- 囊性纤维化。

- 神经肌肉疾病。

• 伴随疾病：

- 肺炎或严重病毒感染。

入住重症监护室指征

• 重度呼吸窘迫。

• 吸入40%氧气，SaO_2<90%或PaO_2<60 mmHg。

• $PaCO_2$>40 mmHg。

• 严重并发症：

- 气胸。

- 心律失常。

出院指征

• 治疗效果好。最后一次治疗结束后在急诊室观察60 min，然后出院：

- PEFR>70%预测值，根据年龄/身高估算预测值。

- 不吸氧时，SaO_2>93%(海平面)。

- 呼吸频率正常。

- 无三凹征。

- 无或少量哮鸣音。

- 无或轻微呼吸困难。

• 随访及依从性好。减少刺激物(吸烟)或过敏原的暴露。

• 出院后治疗：

- 强化β受体激动剂方案3～5日。

- 中度症状的患儿，需短期(3～5日)激素治疗2 mg/(kg·d)，可以雾化吸入或MDI方式。中重度患儿需要吸入激素1～2个月，如氟替卡松、布地奈德或丙酸倍氯米松。

- 24～72 h随访一次。

- 告知家属如出现呼吸急促应返回医院。

- 对于反复发作、症状持续或活动受限的患儿，应考虑长期治疗。

▪ 随访建议

初级保健医师进行维持治疗，常包括雾化吸入或MDI激素治疗，并进行急救措施的健康教育。

要点和误区

• 快速治疗的同时，持续反复评估病情进展。这点很重要。

• 患儿入院时，确保β受体激动剂的治疗未中断。

蝎蜇伤 Sting, Scorpion

Frank LoVecchio 江伟伟 李文放 译

基础知识

▪ 描述

• 蝎毒有神经毒性：

- 钠通道开放。

- 长时间的神经元放电。

• 自主神经、躯体神经和脑神经兴奋。

• 症状在叮咬后数分钟开始。

• 症状持续1～72 h。

▪ 病因

• 在美国南部、墨西哥、中美洲和加勒比地区的刺尾蝎属物种。

• 亚洲、非洲、以色列、南美洲和中东地区还有许多其他物种。

儿科注意事项

• 可能被误诊为癫痫发作、苯丙胺中毒或脑膜炎。

• 死亡率高和更严重。

X

诊断

症状和体征

- 在几 min 之内发生，在 1～2 h 达到高峰，但可能持续 48～72 h。
- 蝎子种类决定着症状(墨西哥雕像木蝎，又称树皮蝎子，是美国唯一引起症状的物种)。
- 局部组织反应：
  - 无红斑。
  - 疼痛。
  - 感觉过敏。
- 神经反应：
  - 交感神经症状：
    - 心动过速。
    - 高血压。
    - 高热。
    - 肺水肿。
    - 烦躁。
    - 多汗。
  - 副交感神经症状：
    - 低血压。
    - 心动过缓。
    - 过度兴奋。
- 躯体反应：
  - 不自主肌肉收缩。
  - 躁动。
- 脑神经反应：
  - 不自主眼球运动。
  - 视力模糊。
  - 眼球震颤。
  - 舌头麻木。
  - 吞咽困难。

基本检查

- 如果蝎子是美国本土的，则不需要鉴别蝎子物种(见上文)。
- 在流行地区有临床症状需高度怀疑。
- 评估中毒的等级：
  - Ⅰ级：局部疼痛和/或感觉异常。
  - Ⅱ级：较远部位的局部疼痛和/或感觉异常。
  - Ⅲ级：头颅/自主神经或躯体骨骼肌功能障碍。
  - Ⅳ级：颅骨/自主神经和躯体骨骼肌功能障碍。

诊断检查与说明

实验室检查

- Ⅰ级和Ⅱ级：
  - 不需要。
- Ⅲ级和Ⅳ级：
  - 尿素氮，肌酐。
  - 电解质。
  - 尿酸。
  - 血常规。
- 严重躁动的患者：
  - 肌酸激酶。
  - 尿中肌红蛋白。
- 严重呼吸窘迫：
  - 血气分析。

影像学检查

- 呼吸症状行胸部 X 线片。
- 心动过速行心电图。

鉴别诊断

- 蛇、蜘蛛、昆虫蜇伤。
- 破伤风。
- 白喉毒素中毒。
- 肉毒杆菌中毒。
- 肌紧张、肌张力障碍。
- 癫痫发作。
- 感染。

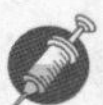

治疗

院前

- 评估气道/通气/循环状态。
- 建立静脉通路。

初步稳定/治疗

- ABC 管理。
- 必要时行气管内插管。
- 建立静脉通路。
- 吸氧。
- 监测生命体征。

急诊治疗/程序

- 轻度蜇伤(Ⅰ和Ⅱ级)：
  - 口服镇痛药。
  - 预防破伤风疫苗。
- 严重蜇伤(Ⅲ和Ⅳ级)：
  - 抗毒素血清，此法昂贵。
  - 预防破伤风疫苗。
  - 高血压急症(罕见)：
    - 标准疗法(如拉贝洛尔)。
  - 低血压：
    - 静脉液体复苏和多巴胺升压治疗。
  - 烦躁不安：
    - 咪达唑仑。
  - 横纹肌溶解症需治疗。

药物治疗

- 抗毒素血清：刺尾蝎属(在 10 min 内静脉注入 3 瓶)；完成输液后监测 60 min，观察症状是否缓解。如果需要，每隔 30～60 min 一次灌注 1 个小瓶。
- 多巴胺：2～5 μg/(kg · min)，静脉注射，根据需要增至 5～10 μg/(kg · min)。
- 咪唑安定：1～2 mg(儿童：0.01～0.05 mg/kg)，静脉注射。
- 拉贝洛尔：20 mg(儿童：0.3～1 mg/kg)，q10 min。
- 芬太尼：50～150 μg(儿童：1～3 μg/kg)，静脉注射。
- 破伤风类毒素：0.5 ml，肌内注射(儿童：相同剂量)。

儿科注意事项

因为剂量是基于毒液负荷的，所以儿童是一样的。

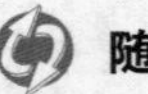

随访

进一步处理

入院指征

- Ⅲ和Ⅳ级的需要入 ICU。
- 如果予以抗毒素血清后，症状消退，如无症状，观察 1～2 h。

出院指征

- Ⅰ级和Ⅱ级在短期观察期(刺伤后 3～4 h)内出现症状进展。
- Ⅲ和Ⅳ级患者给予抗蛇毒血清后，症状改善可出院。
- 如果患者接受了抗毒素血清，则需考虑迟发的症状和体征。
- 讨论刺伤部位持续疼痛和感觉异常的原因。
- 如症状进展，嘱患者继续治疗。

儿科注意事项

幼儿更容易早期危及气道。

随访建议

如果给予抗毒素血清，需密切随访。

要点和误区

当流行地区患者出现典型症状时，高度怀疑该病。

斜颈 Torticollis

Andrew K. Chang · Luke J. Duncan 范浩浩 李文放 译

基础知识

描述

- 斜颈是一种症状，而不是一种疾病。
- "扭曲的脖子"。
- 头部和颈部固定或动态姿势。
- 同义词：颈肌张力障碍，歪脖子。

病因

本地

- 急性斜颈：
  - 在没有外力作用的情况下隔夜进展。
  - 最普遍。
  - 自限，症状在1～2周缓解。
  - 颈椎病。
  - 骨折。
  - 脱位，半脱位。
  - 感染。
  - 椎关节强硬。
  - 肿瘤。
  - 瘢痕组织产生的伤害。
  - 寰枢椎区域的韧带松弛。
- 引起肌肉损伤的炎症性疾病：
  - 肌炎。
  - 淋巴结炎。
  - 结核病。
  - 重症肌无力。
  - 三叉神经颞叶支神经炎。
- 周围软组织感染：
  - 鼻咽脓肿。
  - 咽后脓肿。
  - 颈椎淋巴腺炎。
  - 扁桃体炎。
  - 脑膜炎。
  - 乳突炎。
  - 鼻窦炎。

代偿

- 倾斜头部震颤（患者头部倾斜以抑制震颤）。
- 眼肌麻痹。

中央

- 特发性痉挛性斜颈：
  - 女性＞男性。
  - 31～60岁。
- 肌张力障碍：
  - 扭转肌张力障碍。
  - 广泛性迟发性肌张力障碍。
  - 威尔逊病。
  - 多巴疗法。
  - 急性（精神安定药）。
  - 士的宁中毒。

儿科注意事项

头颈部

- 先天性：
  - 牙齿状发育不全。
  - 半椎体。
  - 脊柱裂。
  - Arnold-Chiari 综合征。
  - 婴儿的假瘤。
  - 肌肉肥大或缺乏颈部肌肉组织。
- 耳鼻喉科：
  - 前庭功能障碍。
  - 中耳炎。
  - 颈椎周围淋巴腺炎。
  - 咽后脓肿。
  - 咽炎。
  - 乳突炎。
  - 食管反流。
  - 脊髓肿瘤的窦道。
- 创伤：
  - 颈椎骨折、脱位。
  - 锁骨骨折。
  - 肺气肿。
- 幼年型类风湿关节炎。

代偿

- 斜视（第四脑神经麻痹）。
- 先天性眼球震颤。
- 颅后窝肿瘤。

中枢神经系统

肌张力障碍：

- 扭转肌张力障碍。
- 药物诱导。
- 脑瘫。

诊断

症状和体征

- 间歇性疼痛性痉挛（SCM），见于胸锁乳突肌、斜方肌和其他颈部肌肉。
- 头部旋转并扭转到单个方向。
- 纯屈曲或伸展情况罕见：
  - 代表肌肉的对称参与。
- 症状通常由于站立、行走或压力的状况而加重。
- 通常不会在睡眠中发生。

病史

- 获得完整的用药病史。
- 大多数抗精神病药物诱导肌张力障碍反应发生在12～23 h。
- 获得完整的创伤史。

体格检查

- 头部旋转并扭转到1个方向。
- 颈部动作从震颤变为流畅。
- 发热的存在支持感染或炎症病因学。
- 如果神经系统检查是局灶性的，考虑脊髓或中枢神经系统疾病。
- 先天形式：
  - 一个固定的、无触痛的大块的SCM肌肉在出生时可见。

基本检查

- 面向诊断以上病因中威胁生命的部分。
- 区分斜颈和其他原因颈部僵硬。
- 颈椎影像学检查评估骨折情况，排除慢性阵发性发作的患者。

诊断检查与说明

实验室检查

没有具体的检查有用。

影像学检查

- 怀疑咽后的脓肿或肿瘤，做颈椎CT或MRI。
- 高频和彩色多普勒超声是诊断先天性肌性斜颈可选择的试验。
- 获得矢状位、侧向和AP视图来评估由创伤引起的斜颈。
- 非创伤性获得性斜颈，行颈部或颈椎CT扫描。

诊断步骤/外科

- 如果怀疑药物诱发的病因考虑给予抗胆碱能药。
- 如果考虑肌无力，请考虑进行Tensilon检测。

鉴别诊断

- 中枢神经系统感染。
- 软组织或骨的肿瘤。
- 基底神经节疾病。
- 颈周腺体脓肿。

- 颈肌肌炎。
- 颈椎间盘病变。
- 重症肌无力。

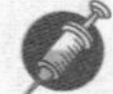

治疗

院前

- 确保气道通畅。
- 有任何创伤史的患者应进行颈椎保护措施。
- 头部支持。

初步稳定/治疗

如果怀疑骨折，颈椎制动。

急诊治疗/程序

- 诱导的药物（如吩噻嗪）：
  - 苯海拉明或苯托品。
- 获得性：
  - 软领衣物和休息。
  - 物理疗法。
  - 按摩。
  - 局部热敷。
  - 镇痛药。

药物治疗

- 苯嘌啶（用于与药物有关的肌张力障碍）：1～2 mg，肌内注射或缓慢静推，接着 3～5 日口服。
- 氯硝西泮（二线药物）：0.5 mg，口服，每日 3 次。
- 苯海拉明（与药物有关的肌张力障碍）：25～50 mg，静脉注射或肌内注射，然后 3～5 日口服，q6～8 h［儿童：5 mg/(kg · 24 h)，q6 h，静脉注射、肌内注射或口服］。
- 苯海索：2～5 mg/d，口服，提高至 30 mg/d。
- 地西泮：2～5 mg，静脉注射；2～10 mg，口服，每日 3 次（儿童：每次 0.1～0.2 mg/kg，静脉注射或口服，q6 h）。
- 肉毒杆菌毒素是治疗非药物诱导的斜颈的一线药物，但事实并非如此，通常在急诊阶段不常用。

随访

进一步处理

入院指征

- 颈椎骨折。
- 有疑问的诊断。
- 传染性原因。
- 中毒表现。
- 无法保持足够的液体摄入量。
- 缺乏支持系统。

转诊问题

一些药物治疗无效的患者可能会受益于手术治疗，如副神消融或深度脑刺激。

随访建议

- 门诊患者转诊给骨科医师、神经科医师或使用肉毒杆菌毒素的神经外科医师。
- 物理治疗并考虑脊椎按摩疗法。
- 出现虚弱或症状恶化，请返回急诊部。

要点和误区

排除感染、炎症、创伤、脊柱和中枢神经系统疾病引起的斜颈。

心包积液/心脏压塞 Effusion/Tamponade

Louisa S. Canham · Carlo L. Rosen　赵铭 译

X

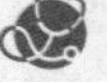

基础知识

描述

- 心包积液：
  - 心包囊中通常含有 15～40 ml 心包液。
  - 过量的心包液聚集即积液。
- 心脏压塞：
  - 心包液聚集使得心包内压力升高，导致心室充盈，心输出量减少。
  - 与积液尺寸和速度有关。
  - 心包液仅增加 80～120 ml 就会导致心包压升高。
  - 约 70%出现于早期压塞，临床情况稳定。
  - 渗透胸部创伤中 2%的患者会出现心脏压塞。

病因

- 医学因素：
  - 心包炎（20%）：
    - 90%为先天性或病毒性。
    - 细菌性、真菌性、寄生性、结核病、HIV。
  - 恶性（13%）：
    - 淋巴瘤、白血病、黑素瘤、胸部、肺部。
    - 转移性疾病、原发性恶性肿瘤、放射后。
  - 心肌梗死后（8%）：
    - 急性：急性心肌梗死（AMI）后 1～3 日。
    - 亚急性（德雷斯勒综合征）：AMI 后数周至数月。
    - 再灌注治疗能降低发病率。
  - 晚期肾脏疾病、尿毒症（6%）。
  - 自身免疫性、胶原血管疾病（5%）：
    - 风湿性关节炎、系统性红斑狼疮、硬皮病。
  - 风湿热。
  - 放射治疗。
  - 黏液性水肿。
  - 充血性心力衰竭（CHF）、心脏瓣膜病。
  - 药物中毒（异烟肼、阿霉素、普鲁卡因酰胺、肼屈嗪、苯妥英）。
  - 先天性。
- 外科因素：
  - 贯穿性胸部创伤。
  - 胸主动脉夹层动脉瘤。
  - 医源性（心导管插入术、心脏术后、中心线定位）。
  - 钝挫伤很少引发心包积液。

诊断

症状和体征

- 贝克三联征——心脏压塞的典型特征：
  - 低血压。
  - 心音低沉。
  - 颈静脉扩张。
- 德雷斯勒综合征：心肌梗死后数周出现的心包炎：
  - 发热。
  - 胸痛。

- 心包摩擦音。

病史

• 重点是既往史：
- 是否有恶性肿瘤病史？
- 近期是否患有病毒性疾病？
- 结缔组织疾病？
- 近期是否有心肌梗死(MI)？

• 现病史：
- 大多数无症状。
- 肺部症状：呼吸困难，咳嗽。
  ◦ 呼吸困难是心包压塞最常见的症状(87%～88%)。
- 胸痛是最主要的症状：
  ◦ 通常为肋膜锐痛，向前倾坐可缓解。
  ◦ 可能涉及肩胛骨。
  ◦ 也可能是钝性的、酸痛、紧缩性的。
- 胃肠症状：恶心，或由肝及内脏充血导致的腹痛，或因食管受压导致的吞咽困难。
- 一般症状：疲劳、萎靡。

体格检查

• 休克或右心力衰竭：
- 心动过速，低血压。
- 颈静脉扩张(若患者血容量低则可能不会出现此症状)。

• 心包摩擦音(100%特征)：
- 尖锐的刮擦声。
- 最好在胸骨左缘听诊。
- 前倾时声音增大。
- 可能是暂时性、间歇性的。

• 奇脉：
- 吸气时收缩压下降>10 mmHg。
- 严重时，可表现为吸气时缺少肱动脉搏或扰动脉搏。
- 灵敏但不特有。

• 通常有低热；一般不超过 38 ℃；若出现则可能是化脓性心包炎(也可能是免疫或结缔组织疾病)。

• 肺部应清净，否则可能是充血性心力衰竭或肺炎。

基本检查

• 心电图。

• 胸部 X 线检查。

• 超声：
- 超声心动描记术，包括主动脉根评估。
- 包括对创伤、主动脉、胸膜积液及气胸的集中评估以排除其他导致低血压的原因。

诊断检查与说明

实验室检查

• CBC。

• ESR、C 蛋白反应：
- 通常随心包炎而升高。

• 心肌酶：
- 若升高则可能为心肌炎。

• 电解质：
- 若怀疑为尿毒症性心包炎可检测尿素氮、肌酸酐。

• 凝血功能检查：
- 特别用于检测肝功能衰竭、抗凝血、创伤。

• 若怀疑有传染源可进行血培养。

影像学检查

• 胸部 X 线平片：
- 心脏肥大 89%可能为心包压塞。
- 若发展迅速，即使有心包积液也可能表现正常。

• 超声波心动描记术：
- 敏感性 97%～100%，特异性 90%～97%。
- 积液：可检测到 20～50 ml 或更多的心包血/液：
  ◦ 小积液只能在后部发现。
  ◦ 前部的脂肪垫可能与积液类似，诊断积液需检查心包腔后部。
- 压塞：
  ◦ 积液过大导致的压塞应是圆的。
  ◦ 右心房或心室弯曲并最终凹陷。
  ◦ 鼻吸试验：吸气时，心包压塞患者的下腔静脉不会凹陷。

• 胸部 CT 以检查心包积血。

• 经食管超声心动图。

• 含钆 MRI(仅限病情稳定患者)。

诊断步骤/外科

• 心电图：
- 低电压。
- 心电交替：QRS 振幅交替变化(通常有大积液时会观察到)。

• 心包穿刺术和液体分析：
- 可治疗心包压塞或症状明显的积液。
- 可诊断细菌性积液(指导抗生素)或恶性水肿。

• 中心静脉压(CVP)测定：
- CVP>15 cmH_2O 表示有压塞，但对于低血容量患者可能表现正常。

鉴别诊断

• 非心源性休克：
- 低血容量性、脓毒性、过敏性、脊髓炎。

• 其他心源性情形：
- 心肌梗死(常见误诊)。
- 心包缩窄(由于心包纤维化)。
- CHF。

• 肺部情况：
- 肺栓塞。
- 张力性气胸。
- 血胸。

• 其他原因：
- 气泡栓塞。
- 主动脉夹层。
- 腹主动脉瘤破裂。

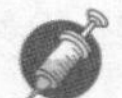

治疗

院前

• 2 根大口径静脉注射管。

• 开始静脉注射液体。

• 补充氧。

初步稳定/治疗

• 继续院前方法。

• 持续心脏监测。

• 对于压塞：
- 静脉注射生理盐水或输血。
- 对于不稳定患者进行心包穿刺术以缓解压塞。

急诊治疗/程序

• 病情不稳定的压塞患者用药：
- 进行心包穿刺术，设置留置导管进行持续引流：
  ◦ 根据最大收集量设置引流部位。
  ◦ 剑突下：剑突向下 2 cm，向左 1 cm，针头与左肩成 30°～45°角。
  ◦ 左侧胸骨旁切口：第 5 肋间隙外侧胸骨，针头垂直扎入皮肤。
  ◦ 根据需要引流。

• 外伤性心包压塞：
- 及时咨询创伤外科医师。
- 最终治疗是胸廓切开术。
- 若病情持续恶化，可选择心包切开术。

• 细菌性心包积液：
- 先用抗生素治疗以除去革兰阴性和厌氧微生物，以及金黄色葡萄球菌。
- 最后可对心包进行局部手术切除。

• 尿毒症性心包积液：
- 安排紧急透析。

• 德雷斯勒综合征及辐照后心包积液：
- 阿司匹林。

X

• 主动脉夹层：
- 及早进行胸心外科会诊以便手术。

▪ 药物治疗

• 布洛芬：800 mg，口服，q8 h。
• 吲哚美辛：75～150 mg，口服，每日 1 次。
• CAD 患者禁用非甾体抗炎药。
• 类固醇：
- 仅限顽固情形（一般为剂量减少后病情反复）。
- 泼尼松：0.2～0.5 mg/kg，至少持续 1 个月，逐步减少。

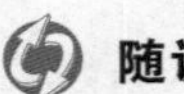

随访

▪ 进一步处理

入院指征

• 急性、症状性心包积液/压塞可进入 ICU。
• 新的心包积液。
• 心包炎且肌钙蛋白升高。

出院指征

• 对于病情稳定患者，已知或偶然发现小的心包积液。
• 年轻、健康的心包炎患者，无压塞迹象，疼痛已用非甾体抗炎药控制。

转诊问题

• 创伤外科：
- 创伤导致的压塞：需进行胸廓切开术。
• 心胸外科：
- 主动脉夹层或其他重要心脏问题导致的压塞、积液。
- 需要开窗术的患者。
- 其他近期做过心脏手术的患者。
• 心脏病学、介入性心脏病学：
- 德雷斯勒综合征。
- 近期经皮介入治疗。
- 任何需要心包穿刺术的患者。

▪ 随访建议

• 出院患者需要初级保健医师随访。
• 医师随访并重复回音以评估积液的清除。

要点和误区

• 心电图变化与心包炎有关，包括 ST 段升高、RP 段降低、T 波倒置。心电图中的 ST 段升高需与 AMI 中 ST 段下降进行对比。
• 如较小的积液迅速发展可倒置压塞（相反的，大的积液若发展缓慢可能为良性）。
• 心输出量可能因压塞而不稳定。
• 处理低血压时（包括创伤）可行超声寻找心包积液及其他压塞症状。
• 若无现成的手术室则不能使用胸廓切开术。

心包炎 Pericarditis

Terrance T. Lee · Shamai A. Grossman 刘静 译

基础知识

▪ 描述

• 包围心脏的心包腔炎症、感染或浸润：
- 心包积液可能存在，也可能不存在。
• 急性心包炎：
- 急骤发生。
- 可能伴随由积液引起的心脏压塞。
• 缩窄性心包炎：
- 由于慢性炎症所导致心包膜增厚，粘连。

▪ 病因

• 先天性（最常见）。
• 病毒性：
- 埃可病毒。
- 柯萨奇病毒。
- 腺病毒。
- 水痘。
- EB 病毒。
- 巨细胞病毒。
- 乙型肝炎。
- 流行性腮腺炎。
- 艾滋病病毒。
• 细菌性：
- 肺结核。
- 金黄色葡萄球菌。
- 链球菌。
- 嗜血杆菌。
- 沙门菌。
- 军团杆菌。
• 真菌性：
- 白色念珠菌。
- 曲霉。
- 组织胞浆菌病。
- 球孢子菌病。
- 芽生菌病。
- 诺卡菌属。
• 寄生虫：
- 变形虫病。
- 弓形虫病。
- 包虫病。
• 肿瘤的：
- 肺癌。
- 乳腺癌。
- 淋巴瘤。
• 尿毒症。
• 心肌梗死：
- 心肌梗死后综合征。
• 结缔组织病：
- 全身性红斑狼疮。
- 风湿性关节炎。
- 硬皮病。
• 辐射。
• 胸部创伤。
• 心包手术后综合征。
• 主动脉夹层。
• 黏液水肿。
• 胰腺炎。
• 炎性肠病。
• 淀粉样变性。
• 药物：
- 普鲁卡因胺。
- 色甘酸钠。
- 肼屈嗪。
- 硝苯呋海因。
- 异烟肼。
- 青霉素（盘尼西林）。
- 阿霉素、柔红霉素。

诊断

▪ 症状和体征

• 胸痛。
• 发热。
• 轻微呼吸困难。

- 咳嗽。
- 声音嘶哑。
- 恶心。
- 厌食。

病史

- 胸痛：
- 由膈神经刺激引起的疼痛扩散至斜方肌隆起线。
- 中央或胸骨下疼痛。
- 突然发作。
- 急剧变化。
- 胸膜炎。
- 平卧时更严重并伴随咳嗽。
- 通过向前倾斜坐着可得到改善。
- 之前发作的心肌炎。
- 发热或感染的病史。
- 恶性肿瘤或自身免疫性疾病的病史。

体格检查

- 呼吸急促。
- 心跳过速。
- 吞咽疼痛。
- 摩擦感：
- 胸骨左缘位置听最佳。
- 非常特殊。
- 三相(triphasic)摩擦最典型。
- 可以有任何这 3 个部分：
- 收缩前期。
- 收缩期。
- 舒张早期。
- 身体前倾导致间歇性和恶化。
- 贝克三体征和心包液的累积：
- 心音低沉。
- 静脉压升高(颈静脉怒张)。
- 体循环动脉压降低(低血压)。
- 尤尔特征：
- 左肩胛骨顶端与脊柱之间支气管呼吸浊音。
- 奇脉：
- 吸气时收缩压过度降低(>10 mmHg)。
- 缩窄性心包炎：
- 右-左侧心力衰竭先兆。
- 肺外周性水肿。
- 腹水。
- 肝淤血。

基本检查

心电图有 4 个典型的阶段。

- 阶段 1：
- 除了 aVR 和 V_1 外 ST 段凹面广泛抬高。
- aVR 升高 PR 部分受到抑制。
- 阶段 2：
- ST 和 PR 部分波形最大化。
- T 波低平。
- 阶段 3：
- T 波反向发散。
- 阶段 4：
- T 波最大化，可能会持续反向。
- 不规则的变化包括局部 ST 升高或 T 波反向。
- 心室内传导阻滞，新的束支传导阻滞或 Q 波暗示心肌损伤。
- 心电交替暗示心包积液。

诊断检查与说明

实验室检查

- CBC：
- 可能出现白细胞增多。
- 红细胞沉降率和 C 反应蛋白：
- 可能会升高，可追查分辨率。
- 心肌酶：
- 有助于从心肌梗死中区分出心肌炎。
- 心肌心包炎可能也会提高。

影像学检查

- 胸部 X 线检查：
- 通常正常。
- 可能显示心脏轮廓扩大或心包钙化。
- 心脏大小不变除非 250 ml 以上的液体累积在心包腔。
- 超声检查：
- 心包液检测的首选诊断方法。
- 可以检测心包腔中至少 15 ml 液体。
- 很好的筛查工具。
- CT 扫描：
- 对检测出心包膜钙化或增厚很有用。
- 有助于排除其他病因。

诊断步骤/外科

心包穿刺术：

- 心包液有助于确定潜在病因。
- 液体用于蛋白质、葡萄糖、培养、细胞学、革兰和抗酸染色、真菌涂片。

鉴别诊断

- 急性心肌梗死。
- 肺栓塞。
- 气胸。
- 主动脉夹层。
- 肺炎。
- 脓胸。
- 胆囊炎。
- 胰腺炎。

治疗

院前

- ABC 管理，建立静脉通道，给氧，监测。
- 如果没有心包破裂，可以考虑弹丸式液体给药。

初步稳定/治疗

- ABC 管理。
- 紧急心包穿刺：
- 血流动力学改变继发于心包压塞。
- 移除少量积液可以产生明显改善。
- 超声引导如果可用。

急诊治疗/程序

- 根据潜在病因治疗。
- 先天的、病毒的、风湿性的、创伤后的：
- 非甾体抗炎药治疗有效。
- 糖皮质激素用于治疗病症顽固不缓解的患者。
- 细菌性：
- 静脉抗生素积极治疗同时引流心包空间。
- 查找感染的主要部位。
- 根据心包液测试发现的病原菌治疗。
- 肿瘤：
- 处理潜在的恶性肿瘤。
- 尿毒症：
- 2～6 周加强透析。
- 如果使用非甾体药物需要小心谨慎。
- 预期的病程/预后：
- 大多数病患 2 周内会对治疗做出反应。
- 大多数患者会症状完全消失。
- 很少反复发作最终发展为缩窄性心包炎或心脏压塞。

药物治疗

一线用药

- 布洛芬：300～800 mg，口服，q6～8 h，疗程 1～2 周，依据严重程度调整服用时间：
- 用 20 mg 奥美拉唑进行胃肠道预防。
- 阿司匹林：口服 800 mg，q6～8 h，持续 7～10 日：
- 3～4 周之后逐渐减量。
- 奥美拉唑用于保护胃肠道。
- 秋水仙碱：每日 2 mg×1 日，然后每日 0.5～1 mg，持续 3 个月。
- 结合阿司匹林能够降低复发率。
- 小剂量可能会有效果。
- 吲哚美辛：25～50 mg，口服，q6 h：

X

- 可能限制冠状动脉血流。

二线用药

• 泼尼松：0.2～0.5 mg/(kg·d)，持续 2～4 周逐渐减少：
- 用于难治性病例。
- 如果阿司匹林或非甾体抗炎药忌服时，可供使用。
- 与复发率的升高有直接关系。
- 对尿毒症和自身免疫性心包炎是有益的。

妊娠注意事项

• 非甾体抗炎药和阿司匹林在妊娠 1～20 周使用不会致畸。
• 妊娠期间可能要使用糖皮质激素。
• 哺乳期间避免使用阿司匹林和高剂量的类固醇。
• 秋水仙碱一般禁服，除非有家族性地中海热。

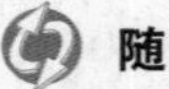

随访

进一步处理

入院指征

• ICU：
- 血流动力学不稳定。
- 心脏压塞。
- 恶性节律障碍。
- 心包穿刺术后状态。
• 遥测单元：
- 怀疑心肌梗死。
- 剧痛。
- 怀疑细菌性病因。
- 任何高风险指征。
• 高风险指征：
- 大量积液(总共>2 cm)。
- 抗凝剂的使用。
- 恶性肿瘤。
- 温度>38 ℃。
- 创伤性心包炎。
- 免疫抑制。
- 奇脉。
- 缓发型。

出院指征

• 没有任何血流动力学改变的症状轻微患者。
• 密切监测。
• 能够耐受口服药物。
• 讨论是否需要心电图评估之前引流的积液。

转诊问题

心脏内科随访。
• 复发的案例。
• 收治的患者。

随访建议

1～2 周安排内科医师随访进行再评估，确认症状缓解没有并发症。

要点和误区

• 经典病史：病毒性疾病前急剧发展，区域性胸痛。
• 摩擦非常特定，但不是总能听见。
• 从急性心肌梗死或其他胸痛的病因中区分心肌炎具有挑战性。
• 主要的治疗方法是非甾体抗炎药。

心房颤动 Atrial Fibrillation

Terrance T. Lee 王丽娜 潘曙明 译

基础知识

描述

• 该节律异常主要表现为快速无序的心房去极化，但缺乏有效的心房收缩。
• 由心房传导的多次折返造成。
• 心房搏动速率为 350～600 次/分。
• 导致心房无序收缩和快速的心室率：
- 心输出量降低。
- 有血栓形成倾向。
• 是临床最常见的心律失常：
- 发病率随年龄升高而增加。
- 男性为更高危的发病因素。

病因

• 系统性疾病：
- 高血压。
- 甲状腺功能亢进。
- 慢性肺源性疾病。
- 感染。
- 肺栓塞。
- 低氧血症。
- 药物(例如，拟交感神经药物)。
- 急性酒精摄入(假日心脏综合征)。
- 肥胖。
- 电解质紊乱。
- 甲状腺疾病。
• 以下心脏疾病：
- 心肌病。
- 冠心病。
- 瓣膜病，尤其是二尖瓣。
- 心包炎。
- 病态窦房结综合征。
- 心肌挫伤。
- 慢性心力衰竭。
- 先天性心脏病。
• 特发性：
- 缺少任何已知发病因素。
- 缺乏心脏疾病的临床或心脏超声证据。

诊断

症状和体征

• 心悸。
• 心输出量降低：
- 虚弱。
- 头晕目眩。
- 晕厥。
- 低血压。
- 心绞痛。
- 肺水肿。
- 意识状态改变。
- 下肢水肿。
- 肝颈静脉回流。
• 血栓形成：
- 急性神经系统损伤。
- 肠系膜血管缺血。

病史

• 起病症状。
• 病程。

• 诱发因素。
• 先前心房颤动发作史。
• 既往心脏疾病史。

体格检查

• 心悸。
• 脉搏绝对不规则。
• 颈静脉搏动A波消失。
• 心室率快时脉搏短绌：
  - 听诊或触诊心尖区搏动快于腕部触诊的搏动。

基本检查

• 病史和体格检查：
  - 评估患者是否稳定，以及是否需要立即电复律。
  - 症状持续时间>48 h或<48 h。
  - 存在全身性疾病或潜在心脏病证据。
• 心电图：充血性心力衰竭体征。
  - P波消失，代之以颤动(f)波，频率为350～600次/分。
  - F波的波幅、形状和间期各异。
  - RR间期绝对不规则。
  - 等电位线消失。
  - 心室率80～150次/分不等：
    ◦ 若心率>200次/分伴宽大畸形的QRS波，则考虑为旁路通道。
  - 心率缓慢提示为房室结传导异常或应用房室结阻滞药物。
  - 通常出现窄QRS复合波，除非：
    ◦ 功能失调。
    ◦ 先前存在的束支。
    ◦ 附加旁路的提前激动。

诊断检查与说明

实验室检查

• 全血细胞计数。
• 电解质。
• 心肌酶谱：如果考虑缺血时。
• 甲状腺功能。
• 地高辛浓度：如果患者正在口服该药物。
• 凝血功能检查。
• 尿液药物筛查。

影像学检查

• 胸部X线平片。
• 心电图。

鉴别诊断

• 心房扑动伴多变的房室传导阻滞。
• 多源性房性心动过速。
• 窦性心律伴频发房性期前收缩。
• 房性心动过速伴多变的房室传导阻滞。

治疗

院前

• 建立静脉通道。
• 心电监测。
• 给氧。
• 心脏复律：
  - 应用于不稳定患者。

初步稳定/治疗

• 建立静脉通路。
• 给氧。
• 心电监测。
• 如果患者不稳定，立即从200 J开始进行同步电复律。

急诊治疗/程序

• 血流动力学不稳定和危及生命：
  - 对药物治疗反应不佳的心肌梗死、肺水肿和心力衰竭患者。
  - 同步电复律：
    ◦ 双相波：从100 J开始，逐步提高至有效能量。
    ◦ 单相波：从200 J开始。
    ◦ 发作持续时间<48 h：考虑肝素提前静脉注射。
    ◦ 发作持续时间>48 h：肝素静脉应用，行经食管超声排除心房血凝块后复律，抗凝治疗4周。不要因为出现致命性心律失常而延误超声检查。
    ◦ 考虑治疗前应用抗心律失常药物，同时电极板的前后放置有利于提高成功复律可能性。
  - 药物复律：
    ◦ 药物的选择依赖于患者是否存在慢性心力衰竭、高血压、左心室肥厚和冠心病病史。
    ◦ 药物可能有致心律失常作用，需谨慎使用。
    ◦ 电复律时，根据发作时间及是否存在血栓需适当应用抗凝药物。
    ◦ 依布利特。
    ◦ 普鲁卡因胺。
    ◦ 氟卡尼。
    ◦ 丙胺苯丙酮。
    ◦ 索他洛尔。
• 血流动力学稳定，症状轻微：
  - 如果可以确定，则积极治疗可能的病因。
  - 如能确定发作时间<48 h，考虑同步心脏复律。
  - 发作时间>48 h，则相较于控制心率，节律的控制并没有使死亡率降低。
  - 对疑似存在旁路传导的稳定患者，可选用普鲁卡因胺治疗。
  - 心率控制：
    ◦ 对于心率<100次/分或自行恢复至窦性心律的患者，不必控制心率。
    ◦ 如果疑似为旁路传导如预激综合征时，房室结传导阻滞剂为禁忌(钙通道阻滞剂、β受体阻滞剂和地高辛)。
    ◦ 钙通道阻滞剂：合并肺部疾病的患者考虑使用。对于失代偿的慢性心力衰竭和二、三度的传导阻滞患者要慎用。
    ◦ β受体阻滞剂：伴冠心病的患者考虑使用。对于失代偿的慢性心力衰竭、二、三度的传导阻滞及肺部疾病的患者要慎用。
    ◦ 地高辛：对原先存在慢性心力衰竭的患者适用。
    ◦ 胺碘酮：对心房颤动复发的患者适用。
  - 心律控制和预防：
    ◦ 包括普鲁卡因胺、索他洛尔、胺碘酮和多非利特。
    ◦ 胺碘酮：有力证据支持可应用于门诊初发患者的唯一药物。
  - 电复律：
    ◦ 复律前3周至复律后4周，口服治疗剂量抗凝药。
  - 尽管推荐电复律治疗，但对于稳定的心房颤动和预激综合征患者可选用普鲁卡因胺或依布利特治疗。
• CHADS2指导的抗凝治疗：
  - 符合以下任一条得1分：
    ◦ 心力衰竭史。
    ◦ 高血压史。
    ◦ 年龄≥75岁。
    ◦ 糖尿病。
  - 有卒中或短暂性脑缺血发作史得2分。
  - 总分0分：
    ◦ 阿司匹林81～325 mg/d。
  - 总分1分：
    ◦ 阿司匹林81～325 mg/d或华法林调整剂量至目标INR为2.5。
  - 总分>1分：
    ◦ 华法林调整剂量至目标INR为2.5(范围2～3)。
  - 校正后的年卒中发生率从CHADS2评分

X

0 分时的 1.9% 到 CHADS2 评分 6 分时的 18.2%。

- 阿司匹林：
  ◦ 有抗凝禁忌证的和不可信的患者。
  ◦ 卒中发生危险性低的患者。

■ 药物治疗

• 美托洛尔：
- 5～10 mg 缓慢静推，每隔 5 min 可重复应用，总量 15 mg。
- 25～100 mg，每日 2 次，口服。

• 地尔硫䓬：
- 0.25 mg/kg 静脉注射 2 min，如未复律，可于 15 min 内以 0.35 mg/kg 重复静脉注射 2 min；继之以 5 mg/h 静脉维持。
- 每日 120～300 mg 口服。

• 地高辛：
- 首剂 0.5 mg 静脉注射，之后每 4 h 静脉注射 0.25 mg 直至显效。

• 艾司洛尔：
- 0.5 mg/kg 静脉注射 1 min，后 4 min 内每分钟静脉输注 0.05 mg/kg。

• 普萘洛尔：
- 以 0.1 mg/kg 等量分次，每隔 2～3 min 静脉注射。

• 维拉帕米：
- 2.5～5 mg 静推 2 min，每 15～30 min 可重复静推 5～10 mg，直至最大剂量达 20 mg。

• 胺碘酮：
- 5～7 mg/kg 静脉注射 30～60 min，之后 1.2～1.8 g/d 持续静脉输注，或者分次口服，直至总量达 10 g。
- 600～800 mg/d 分次应用至总量达 10 g，之后以 200～400 mg/d 维持。

• 普鲁卡因胺：负荷剂量 15～18 mg/kg 缓慢输注 30 min，最大剂量 1 g，之后每分钟 2～6 mg 输注。

• 葡萄糖酸奎尼丁：每 8～12 h 口服 324～648 mg(缓释制剂)。

• 伊布利特：体重大于 60 kg 患者 1 mg 静脉注射；体重小于 60 kg 患者，则以 0.01 mg/kg 静脉输注 10 min；10 min 内如果没有恢复窦性心律可重复一次。

注意

伊布利特给药后，必须对患者进行心电监测，以确定是否有 QT 延长、尖端扭转型室性心动过速和室性心动过速。

• 氟卡尼：2 mg/kg，静脉注射，维持 10 min 后或口服 200～300 mg(用于心脏复苏)。该药不要用于结构性心脏病患者。

• 普罗帕酮：1～2 mg/kg，静脉注射，维持 10 min 或口服 450～600 mg(用于心脏复苏)。

• 索他洛尔：如果 CrCl＞60 ml/min，75 mg 静脉注射，5 h 后给第 2 次。如果 CrCl 40～60 ml/min，给予 1 次。

注意

氟卡尼、普罗帕酮和索他洛尔的静脉注射剂型不被允许在美国使用，必须缓慢输液。

• 肝素：静脉负荷 80 U/kg；维持用量 18 U/(kg · h)。肥胖患者需要调整剂量。

• 低分子量肝素：1 mg/kg，皮下注射，每日 2 次。

• 华法林钠：2.5～5 mg/d，口服，根据 INR 调整剂量。

• 阿司匹林：50～325 mg/d。

• 达比加群：150 mg，口服，每日 2 次，根据肾功能调整剂量。

• 利伐沙班：每日 20 mg，口服，晚上吃饭时服用，根据肾功能调整剂量。

• 阿哌沙班：5 mg 或 2.5 mg，口服，每日 2 次，根据肾功能调整剂量。

随访

■ 进一步处理

入院指征

• 不稳定的心房颤动患者：
- 心率无法控制。

• 卒中风险高：
- 先前心血管事件。
- 慢性心力衰竭。

• 合并导致心房颤动并需住院治疗的疾病。

出院指征

• 症状持续＜48 h 并恢复窦性心律。

• 心室率控制并已抗凝治疗的慢性心房颤动。

• 心率控制并已抗凝治疗的新发心房颤动。

转诊问题

• 心脏专科或电生理学家。

• 评估门诊患者的心脏复律问题。

■ 随访建议

• 应用华法林患者需监测 INR。

• 如果患者出现乏力、头晕、面部及肢体麻木或无力、视物模糊或言语不利，应立即返回急诊。

要点和误区

• 如果血流动力学不稳定或者危及生命，必须行同步心脏复律。

• 稳定心房颤动患者的心率和节律控制需个体化考虑，可用药物包括 β 受体阻滞剂、钙通道阻滞剂或其他抗心律失常药物。

• 不要误把 F 波或 U 波当做 P 波，以至于把心房颤动误诊为窦性心律。

对于由潜在旁路通道引起的心房颤动伴宽复合波的患者，避免使用钙通道阻滞剂、β 受体阻滞剂和地高辛。

心房扑动 Atrial Flutter

Liesl A. Curtis　吴增斌　潘曙明 译

基础知识

■ 描述

• 房性心律失常。

• 每年有 200 000 例新发病例。

• 右心房的大折返环路被认为是其相关的发病机制。

• 多数对心脏复律治疗敏感。

• 很少见于没有器质性心脏病的患者。

• 相对于室上性心动过速(SVT)和心房颤动不常见。

• 典型症状是阵发性发作，持续数秒至数小时。

• 25%～35%的心房颤动患者可同时伴有心房扑动。

X

• 如果未治疗可发展为心肌病。

病因

• 嗜酒。
• 心肌病和心肌炎。
• 慢性心力衰竭。
• 电解质异常。
• 缺血性心脏病。
• 肺栓塞和其他肺部疾病。
• 心脏瓣膜病。
• 心脏手术后(尤其是术后1周)。

儿科注意事项

• 可见于儿童,但通常无症状。
• 新生儿期死亡率最高。
• 可同时伴有:先天性心脏病、感染性疾病(风湿热或心肌炎)。
• 儿童如有新发作的房室传导阻滞须考虑中毒可能。

诊断

症状和体征

• 心悸。
• 晕厥。
• 胸痛。
• 乏力。
• 呼吸困难。
• 运动能力差。
• 心动过速,心率>150次/分。
• 低血压。
• 心力衰竭。

儿科注意事项

• 幼儿不能很好地耐受心房扑动。
• 快速的室性心率可导致休克或心力衰竭。
• 心房扑动可见于没有心脏疾病的婴幼儿。
• 年长的儿童可有相应的心脏疾病,且易复发不易控制。

基本检查

• 心电图:
- 劣质导线的经典锯齿外观。
• 实验室检查。
• 胸部X线检查。

诊断检查与说明

实验室检查

• 电解质和微量元素。
• 心肌酶谱。
• 地高辛水平(适用于使用本药患者)。
• PT、APTT。
• 5-羟色胺。

影像学检查

• 胸部X线检查:
- 可能识别出心肌病或慢性心力衰竭。
• 超声(通常不属于急诊检查的一部分):
- 可能会发现区域性心壁运动异常或瓣膜功能障碍。
• TEE(通常不属于急诊检查的一部分):
- 评估心房血栓。

鉴别诊断

• SVT。
• 窦性心动过速。
• 心房颤动。
• 多灶性房性心动过速。
• 心室颤动。

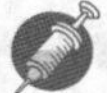

治疗

院前

• 氧气,监测,静脉输液。
• 不稳定患者应该心脏复律:迅速同步心脏复律,以50～100 J开始。

初步稳定/治疗

• 氧气,监测,静脉输液。
• 如果不稳定迅速同步电复律,心房扑动的心脏复律通常需要较少的能量;通常初始能量为50～100 J。从50 J开始并逐步增加剂量。

急诊治疗/程序

• 心率控制:
- 心率控制应早于抗心律失常治疗,以避免1∶1房室传导及血流动力学不稳定。
- 心率控制可能比较困难。
• 抗凝:
- 与心房颤动指南相同:
- 持续性心房扑动患者的血栓栓塞发生率约为每年3%。
- CHA2 DS2-VASc得分:用于评估脑卒中风险。
◦ CHF病史(1分)。
◦ 高血压病史(1分)。
◦ 年龄>75岁(1分)。
◦ 糖尿病病史(1分)。
◦ 脑卒中、TIA病史或血栓栓塞(2分)。
◦ 血管疾病(先前的MI,PAD或主动脉斑块)(1分)。
◦ 65～74岁(1分)。
◦ 女性(1分)。
- 基于共同决策,脑卒中风险评估和患者偏态评估开始抗凝治疗。
◦ 0分和非瓣膜性心房扑动:无抗栓治疗。
◦ 得分1和非瓣膜性心房扑动:无治疗,阿司匹林或口服抗凝药。
◦ 得分2或更高:强烈建议口服抗凝药:
▪ 华法林:
▫ 推荐用于机械瓣膜。
▫ 推荐用于ESRD患者。
▪ 达比加群或阿哌沙班[新型口服抗凝药(NOAC)]:
▫ 与华法林相似的缺血性脑卒中或全身性栓塞风险。
▫ 大出血率明显低于华法林。
▫ 阿哌沙班获准用于ESRD患者:
▪ 利伐沙班(NOAC)。
▫ 缺血性脑卒中或全身性栓塞的风险低于华法林。
▫ 与华法林相当的出血率。
• 抗心律失常药:
- 腺苷:
◦ 不太可能打破心房扑动。
◦ 通过掩盖扑动波可能有助于心房扑动的诊断。
- 胺碘酮:
◦ 无预激性房性心律失常(即WPW)的患者的速率控制。
◦ 对于心功能严重受损的患者,首选抗心律失常药。
◦ 症状超过48 h的患者要小心,因为该药物可能会将其转化为NSR并有血栓栓塞的危险。
- 钙通道阻滞剂:
◦ 控制速率。
◦ 维拉帕米的症状性低血压发生率高于地尔硫䓬。
◦ 维拉帕米仅应用于狭窄型心律失常。
- β受体阻滞剂:
◦ 速率控制。
◦ 为ACS患者增加心脏保护作用的益处。
- 硫酸镁:
◦ 速率控制。
◦ 为ACS患者增加心脏保护作用的益处。
◦ 低水平临床证据。
- 地高辛:
◦ 控制心率。
◦ 三线用药。
◦ 有强心作用,可用于心力衰竭患者。
◦ 起效时间更长。

- 普鲁卡因胺：
  - 控制心律。
  - 具有已知的兴奋前综合征（即 WPW）和心室功能保持正常的患者的首选药物。
  - 注意患者是否 QT 间期延长。
- 索他洛尔：
  - 控制心率。
  - 不是一线药物。
  - 如果心律不齐的持续时间≤48 h，则用于 WPW 和心室功能有保留的患者。
- 依布利特：
  - 控制心率。
  - 使用前纠正钾和镁。
  - 如果 QTc＞440 ms 或患有严重结构性心脏病的患者禁忌使用。
  - 大约 60%的患者成功转换为窦性。
  - 尖端扭转型室性心动过速的发生率是：0.8%。
  - 平均复律时间为 30 min。
  - 给药后观察 4～6 h，观察 QT 情况。
- 多非利特：
  - 仅口服。
  - 前 6 剂需要住院以监测：
    - 非持续性室速。
    - 尖端扭转型室性心动过速突然死亡。
- 心脏电转复：
  - 50～100 J。
  - 尽可能镇静。
  - 恢复窦性心律的最安全、最有效的方法。
- 复律后维持窦性心律：
  - 高复发率：1 年时为 50%；但是，由于数据结合了心房颤动和心房扑动，所以很难确定心率。
  - 胺碘酮疗效确切，但由于其副作用，不适用于长期治疗。
- 经皮导管消融：
  - 急性成功率超过 95%。
  - 并发症发生率低。
  - 适用于：
    - 耐药性心房扑动反复发作。
    - 不耐受药物的患者。
    - 不需要长期药物治疗的患者。

儿科注意事项

- 婴儿和儿童不建议使用维拉帕米，因为可造成心排量下降和严重的心脏损害。
- 地高辛是小儿心房扑动首选的药物。
- 对于新生儿电复律为一线治疗。

■ 药物治疗

- 胺碘酮：在 1 h 内静脉滴注 300 mg，然后在 24 h 内静脉滴注 10～50 mg/h。小儿：在 20～60 min 静脉注射 5 mg/kg[最大剂量 15 mg/(kg・d)]；可能会重复两次，然后维持输注 5～15 μg/(kg・min)。
- 腺苷：静脉注射 6 mg，1 次。如果无电复律，则第二次可在 1～2 min 静脉注射 12 mg。所有剂量均行静脉推注。小儿（体重＜50 kg），初始 0.05～0.1 mg/kg 静脉快速推注（最大 6 mg）；视需要每 1～2 min 以静脉 0.05～0.1 mg/kg 量的增量递增重复；单次最大剂量 0.3 mg/kg。
- 阿替洛尔：10 mg 静脉输注，以 0.5 mg/min 的速度注入 2.5 mg 的等分试样，每等分试样之间间隔 10 min。
- 地高辛：负荷剂量，每 2 h 口服或静脉用 0.25 mg，累计最大 1.5 mg；维持剂量，每日 0.125～0.375 mg 静脉或口服。儿童：口服或静脉用于快速起效，早产儿 15～25 μg/kg；足月儿 20～30 μg/kg；1～24 个月的婴儿 30～50 μg/kg；2～5 岁 25～35 μg/kg；5～10 岁 15～30 μg/kg；＞10 岁 8～12 μg/kg；最初先服用总剂量的一半，然后每 6～8 h 服用总剂量的 1/4，共 2 剂。
- 地尔硫䓬：静脉输注为 0.25 mg/kg 超过 2 min，然后在 15 min 后静脉输注为 0.35 mg/kg 超过 2 min，维持输注 10～15 mg/h 至心率稳定。
- 多非利特：CrCl＞60 ml/min，QTc 为 440 ms 或更短，初始剂量 500 μg 口服每日 2 次；首次给药后 2～3 h 确定 QTc；如果 QTc 增加超过 15%或＞500 ms。

（心室传导异常患者为 550 ms），每日 2 次降低剂量至 250 μg ORALLY；最高剂量 500 μg 口服每日 2 次。

- 艾司洛尔：1 min 内可选的剂量为 500 μg/kg 静脉推注，然后静脉输注 50 μg/(kg・min)；如有必要，可在每次连续提高输注速度之前重复推注；根据心室反应，每 4 min 将输注速率依次提高至 100、150 和 200 μg/(kg・min)；最大 200 μg/(kg・min)；用药时间长达 48 h。
- Flecainide：抗心律失常开始前的单剂 300 mg（体重＞70 kg）和 200 mg（体重＜70 kg），应给予β受体阻滞剂或非二氢吡啶类钙通道阻滞剂，以防止心房房颤快速传导发生颤动。
- 伊布利特：大于 60 kg 的患者在 10 min 内静脉注射 1 mg；对于小于 60 kg 的患者，输注 0.01 mg/kg 静脉 10 min；如果输注后 10 min 内正常窦性心律未恢复，可重复使用一次。
- 硫酸镁：在 5～60 min 内用 D_5W 稀释 1～2 g；如果病情稳定，则可调低速率。
- 美托洛尔：5 mg 静脉输注 5 min，间隔 5 min，总共 15 mg，然后 50 mg 口服每日 4 次持续 48 h。
- 普鲁卡因胺：静脉注射 20 mg/min，直至心律失常得到抑制，低血压，QRS 增加至原来的 50%或总计 17 mg/kg；维持输注速度为 1～4 mg/min。
- 普萘洛尔：1～3 mg 静脉注射（速率不超过 1 mg/min），可在 2 min 后重复；4 h 后可能会再服药。
- 索他洛尔：每日一次或两次，在 5 h 内静脉注射 75 mg；每日 1 次或 2 次，每天 5 h 可增加静脉量至 112.5 mg；每日 2 次最多 150 mg 静脉注射；至少 3 日后可进行剂量滴定。
- 维拉帕米：（静脉）初始，在连续心电和血压监测下至少 2 min 内静脉注射 5～10 mg（0.075～0.15 mg/kg）；如果反应不足，可能会在 30 min 后再给予 10 mg。

随访

入院指征

- 新发作的心房扑动需要抗心律失常，心率控制。
- 有症状（胸痛）。
- CHF。

出院指征

- 新发作的心房扑动符合以下标准：
  - 心率和节律被控制。
  - 找到相关的病因。
  - 已启动抗凝治疗。
  - 安排随访。
- 慢性心房扑动。

■ 随访建议

射频消融治疗目前可作为有症状且没有明确病因的心房扑动的治疗新方法。

要点和误区

- 注意 WPW：不能使用腺苷、β受体阻滞剂、钙通道阻滞剂及地高辛，因为可加速室性心率导致心室颤动。
- 对于不稳定患者及早使用心脏转复。
- 伴有肺部疾病或 CHF，使用β受体阻滞剂应谨慎。
- 4 点主要的治疗相关问题：心率控制；预防栓塞；恢复窦性心律；维持窦性心律。

X

心肌病 Cardiomyopathy

David T. Chiu 彭沪 译

基础知识

描述

心脏功能障碍的心肌疾病：
- 扩张型：
  - 呈特发性，占心力衰竭的25%。
- 肥厚型。
- 限制型。
- 致心律失常性右心室（RV）。
- 未分类的心肌病。
- 特异性心肌病。
  - 心脏肌肉疾病与全身性疾病或疾病相关。

儿科注意事项
- 遗传：20%～30%。
- 获得性。
- 特发性。

病因

- 扩张型：
  - 特发性。
  - 病毒。
  - 遗传、毒性。
  - 免疫。
  - 家族性。
- 肥厚型：
  - 家族性常染色体显性遗传病。
- 限制型：
  - 特发性。
  - 淀粉样蛋白。
- 致心律失常性右心室：
  - 显性和隐性家族性疾病。
- 特异性感染：
  - 莱姆病。
  - 病毒。
  - 南美锥虫病。
  - HIV感染。
- 剧毒药物：
  - 酒精。
  - 化疗药物。
- 围生期。
- 代谢：
  - 甲状腺功能亢进症。
  - 嗜铬细胞瘤。
  - 应激性心肌病（儿茶酚胺）。
- 全身系统疾病：
  - 狼疮。
  - 硬皮病。
  - 神经肌肉疾病。
  - 淀粉样变。

儿科注意事项
- 特发性。
- 遗传性：
  - 先天性代谢缺陷。
  - 畸形综合征。
  - 神经肌肉疾病。
  - 家族性孤立性心肌病。
- 获得性：
  - 维生素、微量矿物质缺乏。
  - 电解质紊乱。
  - 内分泌失调。
  - 毒素。
  - 胶原血管病。
  - 免疫性疾病。
  - 恶病质。
  - 病态肥胖。
  - 心肌炎。
  - 肺疾病。
  - 川崎病。
  - 感染。
  - 辐射。
  - 先天性心脏病。
  - 窒息。

诊断

症状和体征

病史
- 先天性疾病或暴露：
  - 化疗。
  - HIV感染。
  - 莱姆病。
  - 病毒。
- 潜在的系统性疾病：
  - 血色素沉着症。
  - 结节病。
  - 妊娠。
- 药物滥用史。
- 家族史：
  - 家族性猝死。
- 劳力性主诉（晕厥、呼吸困难）。
- 头晕。
- 近晕厥和晕厥。
- 心悸。
- 猝死。
- 室性心律失常。
- 心力衰竭。

儿科注意事项
- 烦躁。
- 肝大。
- 全身肌无力。
- 急性生化危机。
- 低血糖。
- 代谢性酸中毒。
- 高氨血症。
- 发绀。
- 脑病。
- 畸形特征。

妊娠注意事项

参考心肌病，围生期。

体格检查
- 生命体征。
- 心肺功能检查。
- 腹部脏器肿大。
- 水肿。
- 其他。
  - 皮疹。
  - 甲状腺肿。
  - 全身性疾病。

诊断测查与说明

实验室检查
- 血常规。
- 血生化。
- 肝功能检查、甲状腺功能检查。
- 心肌标志物。
- 脑钠肽水平（B型）：>100 pg/ml。
- 血清学：在医院内不用。

影像学检查
- 胸部X线片：
  - 扩张型心肌病：
    - 心脏肥大。
    - 肺充血。
    - 胸腔积液。
  - 肥厚型心肌病（HCM）：
    - 参考肥厚型心肌病。
  - 限制型心肌病：
    - 正常的心脏轮廓。
    - 肺充血。
- 急诊内科医师行经胸超声心动图检查：

X

- 左心室射血分数下降(EF)。
- 排除心脏压塞。
- 正式超声心动图：
- TTE 或 TEE。
- 选择性研究。
- 基础疾病的鉴别。
- 核素显像：
- 当心电图不确定。
- 隔膜和游离壁厚度的测定。
- 超声心动图的替代品。
- CT 和 MRI 区分心包炎和限制型心肌病。
- MRI：
- 心力衰竭的综合评估。
- 评估心肌解剖、区域和整体功能，以及生存能力。
- 可评估灌注和急性组织损伤(水肿和坏死)，以及非缺血性心力衰竭、纤维化、浸润和铁超负荷。

诊断步骤/外科

心电图：

- 肥厚型心肌病：
- 左心室肥厚。
- 青少年异常 Q 波在导联Ⅱ、Ⅲ、AVF、V_5 和 V_6(最常见)表现明显。
- 扩张型心肌病、莱姆病、查加斯病(美洲锥虫病)、病毒性心肌病：
- 心房纤维化。
- 心脏阻滞。
- 传导异常。
- 无冠状动脉疾病患者前壁和下壁存在假性梗死图形与病理 Q 波。

X

注意

应激性心肌病可能和 STEMI(ST 段抬高型心肌梗死)相似。

- 心导管检查。
- 怀疑缺血。
- 治疗系统性疾病。
- 肥厚型心肌病。
- 血流动力学异常的评估。
- 心内膜心肌活检。
- 评估心肌炎或病因。
- 心脏 CT 或 MRI。

儿科注意事项

- 电解质。
- pH。
- 葡萄糖。
- 氨水平。
- 心输出量。
- 畸形的评估。
- 心电图。
- 超声心动图：
- 遗传检查，看个人原因。

鉴别诊断

- 呼吸困难的其他原因：
- 慢性阻塞性肺疾病。
- 贫血。
- 哮喘。
- 间质性肺疾病。
- 肺栓塞。
- 心脏压塞。
- 心脏瓣膜病。
- 缺血性心脏病。
- 甲状腺功能减退症。
- 缩窄性心包炎，通常与限制型心肌病混淆。
- 晕厥的其他原因：
- 低血容量。
- 中暑(热射病)。
- 低血糖。
- 心律失常。
- 心肌缺血。

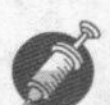

治疗

院前

- 监测。
- 吸氧。
- 怀疑肥厚型心肌病时，避免使用低剂量硝酸甘油。
- 失代偿性心力衰竭：
- 硝酸甘油。
- 无创正压通气。

初步稳定/治疗

ABC 管理：

- 按需控制气道。
- 补充氧气。
- 无创正压通气。

急诊治疗/程序

- 抗凝：
- 扩张型心肌病。
- 标准化治疗心房颤动。
- 全身性栓塞。
- 院内治疗肥厚型心肌病的有限经验：
- 异脉定(维拉帕米)减少梗阻。
- 胺碘酮治疗以维持窦性心律。
- 心力衰竭标准治疗。
- 心律失常的治疗标准。

注意

- 先天性代谢紊乱纠正之前需持续禁食。
- 静脉输液。
- 蛋白质或脂肪酸代谢异常纠正之前需予以 D_{10} 静脉输注。
- 静脉输液需要缓慢和慎重进行，避免快速补液导致水分转移到血管外的空间。

注意

不要给予含乳酸的任何药物避免代谢性酸中毒及乳酸血症。

- 抗氧化剂和维生素辅助因子。
- 左旋肉碱提高线粒体能量代谢。
- 标准治疗充血性心力衰竭。
- 氯乙酸钠(DCA)急性降低线粒体疾病患者的乙酸含量。

药物治疗

- 胺碘酮：5 mg/kg，静脉推注超过 10 min。
- 肉碱：儿童 50～300 mg/(kg·d)，口服或静脉推注。
- Clevidipine：初始剂量：1～2 mg/h，以达到血压目标的间隔 90 s 可以增加 1 倍。当血压接近目标时，剂量可能每 6～10 min 增加不到 1 倍。
- 地高辛：开始 0.125 mg 静脉推注。
- 地尔硫䓬：0.25 mg/kg 实际体重超过 2 min 静脉推注(成人平均剂量：20 mg)；重复剂量(15 min 后反应不明显予以追加)：0.35 mg/kg 实际体重超过 2 min 静脉推注(平均成人剂量：25 mg)；持续静脉滴注 10 mg/h；根据需要量可在 5 mg/h 到 15 mg/h 之间调整。
- 双异丙吡胺：100～200 mg，口服，q6 h。
- 艾司洛尔：负荷剂量：500 μg/kg 超过 1 min；按照 50 μg/(kg·min)静脉输注 4 min；可持续予以 50 μg/(kg·min)静脉输注，如反应不明显，可予以 50 μg/(kg·min)增量(增加不多于 q4 min)直到最大的 200 μg/(kg·min)。
- 呋塞米：20～40 mg 静脉推注，直至最大剂量 200 mg，随后的剂量(儿童：1 mg/kg，静脉注射，q12～24 h)。
- 肝素：负荷量 80 U/kg；然后 18 U/(kg·h)。
- 美托洛尔：2.5～5 mg，q2～5 min(最大总剂量：10～15 min 内予以 15 mg 静脉推注)。
- 米力农：负荷量 50 μg/kg 静脉推注超过 10 min，然后予以 0.375～0.75 μg/(kg·min)

静脉推注。

• 奈西立肽：负荷剂量 2 μg/kg 静脉推注，然后 0.01 μg/(kg·min)静脉推注，最大剂量 0.03 μg/(kg·min)。

• 硝酸甘油：5 μg/min 静脉输注。

老年人注意事项

老年用药剂量要慎重。

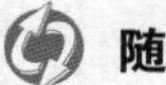

随访

进一步处理

入院指征

• 新的或可疑的心肌病。

• 晕厥、心律失常或肥厚型心肌病是可能的病因。

• 家族性早发性猝死家族史。

• 心源性休克。

出院指征

• 诊断为轻度充血性心力衰竭的心肌病，治疗后改善。

• 限制型心肌病和肥厚型心肌病。

• 咨询心脏病专家。

转诊问题

EF 小于 35%的患者可能需要转诊：

• 单腔植入型心律转复除颤器。

• 心房同步心室起搏。

• 心室辅助装置。

• 心脏移植。

随访建议

• 初级保健医师。

• 心脏病学。

• 基因检测。

要点和误区

• 对存在晕厥或劳力性症状的患者床旁超声心动图是一个有用的工具。

• 怀疑心肌病患者需获得明确的家族史。

心肌挫伤 Myocardial Contusion

Sean Patrick Nordt 伍力学 译

基础知识

描述

• 又称心脏钝性损伤(blunt cardiac injury, BCI)。

• 病理学表现为散在分布的边界清晰的出血灶。

• 常分布于心内膜下。

• 也可表现为锥型透壁性病灶。

• 由于解剖上的毗邻关系，多数情况下可累及右心室和右心房前壁。

病因

• 胸部钝挫伤：
- 高速运动时的减速伤。
- 也可发生在运行速度为 20～35 mph (1 mph=1.6 km/h)的事故中。

• 在自动人行步道行走时发生的损伤。

• 坠落伤。

• 长期行近心部位的胸部按摩。

• 心脏处于胸骨和脊柱之间，易受到压迫。

• 心脏在减速运动时可与胸骨发生碰撞。

• 心脏在腹腔压力增高时可被向上移位的腹腔脏器损伤。

• 震荡伤(如爆炸伤)。

• 相关情况：
- 致命性心律失常。
- 心源性休克、慢性心力衰竭。
- 心包出血、心脏压塞。
- 瓣膜、心脏破裂。
- 心室内血栓。
- 血栓栓塞症。
- 在内膜撕裂或毗邻部位出血，以及少见的水肿等情况下，发生冠状动脉闭塞。

诊断

症状和体征

• 临床表现多样，无特异性：
- 胸痛。
- 心源性休克。
- 无临床症状的心电图改变。

• 最常见的体征是与创伤程度及失血程度不相称的心动过速。

• 少数时候可见局部擦伤。

• 硝酸甘油给药后仍无法缓解的胸骨后疼痛：
- 常持续 24 h 以上。
- 吸氧后有症状有改善。

• 胸部明显创伤的依据：
- 局部淤青、擦伤。
- 明显的捻发音。
- 胸骨骨折伴正常心电图机肌钙蛋白阴性，不代表无心肌钝性损伤。
- 明显的连枷胸。

• 其他损失可能掩盖心肌挫伤的症状和体征。

病史

• 损失机制(如机动车事故、坠落、爆炸、胸部被飞行物撞击)。

• 任何晕厥及意识丧失均提示可能存在心律失常。

• 挤压伤。

老年人注意事项

对于老年人，在心脏钝性损伤后应综合考虑既往心脏疾病及并存的疾病状况。

儿科注意事项

由于儿童胸廓顺应性较好，即便是明显的心脏压迫和损伤也可能只有极小的或根本没有外在的创伤表现。

体格检查

所有创伤患者均应接受全身检查：

• 评估颈静脉扩张情况。

• 心音低钝。

• 额外心音。

• 捻发音。

• 奇脉。

• 胸壁损伤的证据。

基本检查

• 尚无单一的诊断试验(除尸检外)可证实心肌挫伤的存在。

• 心电图：
- 最好的初筛方法。
- 最常见的心律失常是窦性心动过缓(占 70%)。
- 心电图表现正常并不能排除心肌损伤的存在。
- 心电图改变可能是细微的或为非特异性变化，如 ST 段改变、右束支传导阻滞及房性

X

或室性期前收缩。

- 至少复查 1 次心电图以观察有无动态变化。
- 可能发生影响血流动力学的严重心律失常：
  ◦ 心房颤动和心房扑动。
  ◦ 室性心动过速和心室颤动。

• 较之于 CK－MB 检测，目前更推荐肌钙蛋白 I 联合心电图检查以判断病情。

• 对所有心电图有异常变化及肌钙蛋白 I 或肌钙蛋白 T 升高的患者均应行心脏彩超检查。

• 经食管心电图比常规心电图有更高的敏感性，但技术要求较高且耗时较多。

• 多层螺旋 CT 血管成像或 MRI 有资于诊断。

▪ 诊断检查与说明

• 肌钙蛋白 I 是首选实验室指标。

• 肌钙蛋白 T 敏感性低于肌钙蛋白 I：
- 所有疑诊 BCI 的患者均应检查该指标。
- 心肌损伤 6～8 h 后应复查。
- 一旦肌钙蛋白升高则应收治入院。

• 心肌肌钙蛋白较 CK－MB 敏感性更高。

• CK－MB 不再推荐为常规检测指标。

影像学检查

• X 线平片、CT、MRI 监测相关损伤：
- 肺挫伤。
- 肋骨或胸骨骨折。
- 急性肺水肿。
- 心肌挫伤无特异性表现。

• 所有患者均应行快速超声检查以评估心包及腹腔内有无并发损伤。

• 心脏彩超：
- 一般认为是检测心肌挫伤的最佳选择。
- 检测心脏壁异常运动和渗出。
- 可直视心腔和瓣膜运动状况。
- 可能无法看清微小挫伤（可无临床症状）。
- 如患者病情稳定，TEE 较经 TTE 效果更好。
- TTE 还可了解大血管的情况。

• 放射性核素心室造影：
- 随着心脏彩超的广泛应用，该技术已很少使用。

• ^{201}Tl 闪烁扫描（单光子发射 CT，即 SPECT）。
- 对左心室损伤敏感性和特异性较好。
- 但无法评估最常受损伤的右心室。

诊断步骤/外科

• 心包穿刺术：
- 用以治疗心脏压塞，请参考美国指南。

• 开胸术：
- 针对急性心搏骤停或在急诊有急性呼吸困难及心包穿刺不成功者。

▪ 鉴别诊断

• 心脏破裂。

• 心脏压塞。

• 瓣膜受损。

• 其他创伤性胸壁损伤。

• 心绞痛或急性心肌梗死。

治疗

▪ 院前

院前急救人员应向急诊部同事准确报告患者病情信息，包括：

• 损伤发生机制。

• 肇事车情况。

• 方向盘和仪表盘所致损伤。

• 是否使用约束装置。

• 机动车的速度。

• 患者受伤时的体位。

• 营救时间。

• 有无意识障碍。

▪ 初步稳定/治疗

• 畅通气道和复苏。

• 给氧：
- 静脉通路。
- 心电监测。

▪ 急诊治疗/程序

• 心律失常的处理原则同非创伤性心律失常：
- 室上性心动过速：
  ◦ 如患者无低血容量状况，使用腺苷或钙通道阻滞剂。
- 心动过缓：
  ◦ 阿托品。
  ◦ 起搏器。
- 室性心律失常：
  ◦ 电复律。
  ◦ 胺碘酮。
  ◦ 利多卡因。
  ◦ 普鲁卡因胺。
- 心搏骤停：
  ◦ 肾上腺素。
  ◦ 阿托品。
  ◦ 其他恰当的处理措施。
- 快速心房颤动或心房扑动：
  ◦ 如患者无低血压可用地尔硫䓬或地高辛。

• 不推荐预防性抗心律失常治疗。

• 心肌挫伤所致的心源性休克：
- 适度的液体复苏。
- 血管活性药物（多巴胺或多巴酚丁胺）。
- 必要时行主动脉内球囊反搏术。

▪ 药物治疗

• 药物治疗主要是针对继发于心肌损伤的心律失常和血流动力学异常。

• 尚无针对心肌挫伤的原发病治疗方法。

• 腺苷：6 mg（儿童：0.05～0.1 mmg/kg），快速静脉推注，如无效可在 1～2 min 后再推注 12 mg。

• 胺碘酮：以 150 mg 负荷量给药，推注时间 10 min 以上（儿童：5 mg/kg），然后 1 mg/min 的速度滴注 6 h，再续以 0.5 mg/min 维持[儿童：5 μg/（kg · min）]。

• 阿托品：0.5～1 mg（儿童：0.02 mg/kg，0.1 mg/min），静脉或气管内给药（ET）。

• 地高辛：负荷量 0.5 mg（儿童：0.2 mg/kg），静脉给药，然后 0.25 mmg（儿童：0.01 mg/kg）静脉给药，每 6 h 药量加倍递增。

• 地尔硫䓬：均以 0.25 mg/kg（成人和儿童）静脉推注，15 min 后可再次以 0.35 mg/kg 给药。

• 多巴酚丁胺：2～15 μg/（kg · min）（成人或儿童）。

• 多巴胺：2～20 μg/（kg · min）（成人或儿童）。

• 肾上腺素：心搏骤停者，以 1 mg（儿童：0.01 mg/kg）静脉推注或气管内给药（1：10 000 溶液）。

• 利多卡因：以负荷量 1 mg/kg 静脉推注，续以 0.5 mg/kg，q8～10 min 直至极量 3 mg/kg（成人或儿童）。静脉滴注：1～4 mg/min[儿童：20～50 μg/（kg · min）]。

• 普鲁卡因胺：以 3～6 mg/kg 的起始剂量给药，最多不超过 100 mg，给药时间不小于 5 min，最大总负荷剂量为 15 mg/kg。

• 维拉帕米：以 0.1～0.3 mg/kg 静脉推注，给药时间不小于 2 min（儿童禁用）。

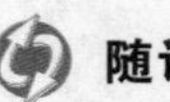

随访

▪ 进一步处理

• 不良事件，尤其是心律失常，并不常见，一般发生在发病后第 1 个 24 h。

• 尚无可以准确地预判患者可从急诊室安

全出院的单一试验或联合检测。

- 所有已诊断该病的患者均应收入监护病区。

入院指征

- 心电图异常。
- 心肌酶异常。
- 血流动力学不稳定。
- 其他检查提示存在心肌挫伤。
- 收入监护病区给予密切观察。

出院指征

心律失常患者不伴心电图异常或心律失常且心肌酶正常者在观察6~8 h后可出院。

转诊问题

以下情形需即刻请外科会诊：

- 怀疑心脏壁破裂。
- 瓣膜或乳突破裂。
- 怀疑心腔间隔破裂。
- 冠状动脉栓塞。
- 心包积液。
- 心脏压塞。

随访建议

出院患者：

- 24 h内应随访。

要点和误区

- 胸壁外伤患者应做心电图。
- 所有患者均应行快速检查以了解心包情况。
- 有胸壁损伤体征者应高度怀疑心脏钝性损伤。
- 儿童患者胸壁创伤后症状甚微。
- 不宜对外伤后出现ST段抬高的患者使用溶栓药物。
- 如肌钙蛋白I及心电图阴性者一般不考虑心脏钝性损伤。

心肌炎 Myocarditis

Liudvikas Jaminas 伍力学 译

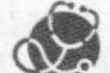

基础知识

描述

- 该病是一种心肌的炎性改变，表现为心肌细胞坏死及继发的心肌损伤。
- 由致病因子造成直接的细胞毒作用后继发免疫反应而引发。
- 由于许多病例无症状，故尚不清楚确切的发病率。
- 尸检结果显示1%~7%的病例有心肌炎征象，其中50%以上为HIV感染者。
- 男性发病多于女性(1.5∶1)。
- 心肌炎平均发病年龄为42岁。
- 该病是40岁以下猝死患者的重要病因(占15%~20%)。

病因

- 病毒：
  - 肠道病毒(柯萨奇病毒B)。
  - 腺病毒。
  - 疱疹病毒[包括巨细胞病毒(CMV)]。
  - 丙型肝炎病毒。
  - 流感病毒。
  - 埃可病毒。
  - 单纯疱疹病毒。
  - 水痘-带状疱疹病毒。
  - EB病毒。
  - 巨细胞病毒。
  - 腮腺炎病毒。
  - 风疹病毒。
  - 天花/牛痘病毒。
  - 黄病毒。
  - 狂犬病。
  - HIV。
- 细菌：
  - 白喉杆菌。
  - 结核杆菌。
  - 布鲁菌。
  - 鹦鹉热。
  - 脑膜炎球菌。
  - 支原体。
  - A型链球菌。
- 原虫：
  - 利什曼原虫。
  - 疟原虫。
  - 弓形虫，见于免疫功能不全患者。
  - 克氏锥虫螺旋体(Chagas病)：
    - 是世界上引起心力衰竭和心肌炎的最常见病原体。
    - 在中南美洲有2000万人感染。
  - 旋毛虫。
  - 锥体虫。
- 螺旋体：
  - 伯氏包柔螺旋体、莱姆病中的螺旋体。
  - 梅毒。
- 立克次体：
  - 斑疹伤寒。
  - 落基山斑疹热。
  - Q热。
- 真菌：
  - 念珠菌病。
  - 曲霉菌病。
  - 隐球菌病。
  - 组织胞浆菌病。
  - 放线菌病。
  - 蠕虫病。
  - 旋毛虫病。
  - 包虫病。
  - 血吸虫病。
  - 囊尾蚴虫病。
- 药物：
  - 对乙酰氨基酚。
  - 氨苄西林。
  - 化学药物(氨茴环素)。
  - 可卡因。
  - 双氢克尿噻(氢氯噻嗪)。
  - 锂盐。
  - 甲基多巴。
  - 青霉素。
  - 磺胺甲噁唑。
  - 磺胺类。
  - 齐多夫定。
  - 放射线。
  - 过敏。
  - 重金属。
  - 碳氢化合物。
  - 一氧化碳。
  - 砒霜。
- 自身免疫紊乱：
  - 系统性红斑狼疮(SLE)。
  - 韦格纳肉芽肿。
  - 川崎病。
  - 巨细胞性动脉炎。

- 类肉状瘤病。
- 围生期心肌病。
- 昆虫叮咬伤：
  - 蝎子。
  - 蛇。
  - "黑寡妇"(毒蜘蛛)。

诊断

症状和体征

心律失常(18%)、呼吸困难(72%)和胸痛(35%)。

病史

- 疲乏。
- 肌痛、关节痛。
- 精神不振。
- 发热。
- 胸痛：
  - 约35%的患者有此症状。
  - 多数表现为心前区肋膜炎样尖刺样锐痛。
- 呼吸困难常见。
- 出现充血性心力衰竭时有端坐呼吸和喘息症状。
- 心悸较常见。
- 局部心肌痉挛、炎症而诱发急性冠状动脉综合征。
- 晕厥：
  - 可能提示严重的主动脉瓣梗阻或有室性心动过速心室颤动而猝死的风险。

体格检查

- 发热。
- 呼吸急促。
- 心动过速：
  - 常与发热不相称。
- 发绀。
- 低血压：
  - 源于左心衰竭。
  - 在急性病程中不常见，一旦出现预后不良。
- 双肺底细湿啰音。
- 水泡音。
- 颈静脉扩张。
- 外周水肿。
- 肝大。
- 腹水。
- 如左右心室均受累则可闻第三心音或奔马律。
- 第一心音减低。
- 二尖瓣或三尖瓣反流杂音。
- 如有心包炎可闻及心包摩擦音。

儿科注意事项

- 该病是平素体健患儿发生心力衰竭的最常见病因。
- 尤其是婴儿，无特异性症状：
  - 发热。
  - 呼吸窘迫。
  - 饮食不良，在部分慢性心力衰竭患儿，在吃饭时甚至大汗淋漓。
  - 新发心脏杂音。
  - 严重者有发绀症状。

基本检查

- 体格检查。
- 心脏彩超。
- 胸部X线检查。

诊断检查与说明

实验室检查

- 脑钠肽(BNP)或脑钠肽前提(pro-BNP)。
- 心肌酶：
  - 肌钙蛋白T：该检测值较低者可排除心肌炎。
  - 肌钙蛋白I：特异性为89%，敏感性为34%。
  - 心肌坏死时肌酸激酶(CK-MB)升高。
- ESR在急性期升高60%。
- 25%的患者有白细胞升高。
- 病毒免疫效价，病毒培养阳性率较低。
- 支原体、抗链球菌溶血素(ASO)、冷凝集试验。
- 肝炎免疫。
- 莱姆病免疫效价。
- 传染性单核细胞增多症检测试验。
- 巨细胞病毒血清学检测。
- 血培养。

影像学检查

- 心电图：
  - 房性心动过速常见。
  - 阵发性、非特异性ST段和T波改变。
  - 心房和心室节律异常。
  - 心脏传导障碍。
    - 20%的患者存在传导延搁。
    - 20%的患者出现左束支传导阻滞。
- 胸部X线片：
  - 心影正常。
  - 肺水肿。
  - 胸膜腔渗出。
- 心脏彩超：
  - 左心室收缩和舒张功能障碍。
  - 心脏壁阶段性运动异常。
  - 射血分数减低。
  - 心包渗出。
  - 15%的患者有心室血栓形成。
- ^{67}Ga和^{111}In标记的肌球蛋白抗体扫描。
- 钆-MRI增强：
  - 可提示心肌炎症和心肌细胞坏死。
- 心脏MRI：
  - 信号异常区域与心肌炎相关。
  - 报道显示敏感性为76%，特异性为96%，诊断准确率为85%。
  - 对诊断不明以及拟行心内膜活检者可行该检查。

诊断步骤/外科

- 右心室心内膜活检：
  - 仅在以下情况发生时才需要：
    - 暴发性心力衰竭。
    - 内科治疗无效的新发心力衰竭伴室性心律失常、二度或三度传导阻滞。
    - 心脏移植受者宜行该检查。
  - 对心内膜下组织行病毒基因组多聚酶链式反应(PCR)扩增。
- 以心包积液或其他部位的体液标本行病毒PCR扩增。

鉴别诊断

- 急性心肌梗死。
- 急性和慢性肺栓塞。
- 主动脉夹层。
- 肾上腺功能减退。
- 环境影响。
- 食管穿孔、破裂、撕裂。
- 高热。
- 低体温。
- 川崎病。
- 肺炎。
- 心包炎。
- 病毒感染。
- 细菌感染。
- 脓毒症。
- 严重的甲减或甲亢。
- 中毒性疾病。

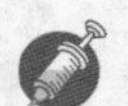

治疗

注意

- 避免使用拟交感和β受体阻滞药物。
- 患者出现莫氏Ⅱ型或完全性心脏传导阻滞需要安装起搏器。

初始/治疗

- ABC管理。

• 吸氧。
• 心电监测。
• 指脉氧监测。
• 建立静脉通路。

■ 急诊治疗/程序

• 处理心律失常。
• 对有症状的心脏传导阻滞予以经胸廓或经静脉起搏。
• 给氧。
• 血管紧张素转换酶抑制剂(卡托普利):
– 减轻后负荷和炎症反应。
• 地高辛:
– 慢性心力衰竭或心房颤动。
• 利尿剂(呋塞米、布美他尼)。
• 大剂量免疫球蛋白冲击疗法治疗巨细胞病毒相关性心肌炎。
• 左心室功能减低或心脏内血栓形成者给予肝肾和华法林治疗。

儿科注意事项

• 静脉应用免疫球蛋白是治疗儿童病毒性心肌炎的有效方法。
• 改善左心功能状况可提高存活率。

■ 药物治疗

• 卡托普利:
– 成人剂量:起始剂量 6.25 mg,可逐步增加至 50 mg。
– 儿童剂量:
◦ 婴儿:0.15～0.3 mmg/kg(极量 6 mg/kg)。
◦ 儿童:0.5～1 mg/(kg · 24 h)。
• 地高辛:
– 成人剂量:负荷量 0.4～0.6 mg,静脉注射,续以 0.1～0.3 mg, q6～8 h。维持剂量:0.125～0.5 mg/d,静脉注射或口服。
– 儿童剂量:
◦ <2 岁:15～20 μg/kg,静脉注射。
◦ 2～10 岁:10～25 μg/kg,静脉注射。
◦ >10 岁:4～5 μg/kg,静脉注射。
• 呋塞米:
– 成人剂量:20～80 mg/d,口服、静脉注射或肌内注射;水肿严重者可逐步增加至 600 mg/d。
– 儿童剂量:1～2 mg/kg 口服;不超过 6 mg/kg;频次不应超过 6 h 1 次,1 mg/kg 在严密监护下缓慢静脉注射或肌内注射,不超过 6 mg/kg。
• 免疫球蛋白静脉注射(如 Gamimune、Gammagard、Gammar-P、Sandoglobulin 等 FDA 批准的免疫球蛋白)。
– 成人剂量:2 g/kg 静脉注射,至少 2～5 日。

随访

■ 进一步处理

入院指征

有症状的心肌炎患者:
• 新发病例。
• 慢性心力衰竭。
• 心律失常。
• 莫氏Ⅱ型或完全性心脏传导阻滞。
• 伴有栓塞事件。
• 心源性休克。

出院指征

无症状且无心律失常或心功能不全证据者。

转诊问题

难治性慢性心力衰竭患者宜行心脏移植术:
• 约 50%的患者在确诊后 5 年内死亡。
• 淋巴细胞性心肌炎预后最佳。

要点和误区

• 任何有不明原因心律失常和心功能不全、肌钙蛋白升高、心肌损伤的心电图改变的患者都需要怀疑心肌炎。
• 通过细致的体检查找慢性心力衰竭和心包炎体征至关重要。
• 拟行心肌炎诊断时应完善心脏彩超检查,尤其儿童患者敏感性更高。
• 有心律失常、慢性心力衰竭或血栓栓塞者应收治入院。

心力衰竭 Heart Failure

Naomi George · Robert A. Partridge 刘雪峰 林兆奋 译

X

基础知识

■ 描述

• 充血性心力衰竭(CHF),现在简称为"心力衰竭"(HF),是一种异质性的临床综合征,由心室充血受损或血液排出引起。
• HF 常导致进行性衰弱,急性失代偿发作。
• 5 年死亡率高(>50%)。
• 影响到约 510 万美国人。
• 据估计,2013 年瑞士用于 CHF 的费用>300 亿美元。
• 领先的医疗保险诊断住院患者≥65 岁。
• 急性失代偿性心力衰竭(ADHF):急性发作新的或恶化的心力衰竭症状(小时-日)。
– 向急诊提交报告的一般理由。
◦ 70%是反复发作的慢性心力衰竭。
◦ 15%是心力衰竭新诊断。
◦ 5%的终端事件。
– ADHF 可能由心脏泵功能恶化,或由前负荷或后负荷变化引起:
◦ 诱发事件包括交感神经张力快速增加,伴随疾病、心律失常、心肌缺血、进展性瓣膜疾病、血管内容量增加。
– 基于灌注充足性(暖与冷)和充血(湿与干)的 4 种常见表型表现。
• 慢性心力衰竭是一种渐进的失效状态(月-年),以结构和功能改变为特征,主要分为两大类:
– 伴有射血分数降低的心力衰竭(HFrEF)。
◦ 收缩力或泵功能受损,导致射血分数下降(EF<40%)。
◦ 估计患病率为 50%。
◦ 许多人同时有舒张功能障碍。
– 保留射血分数(HFpEF)EF>50%的心力衰竭。
◦ 心室舒张和顺应性受损,导致心脏充盈减少。
◦ 常见于老年患者、妇女、高血压(HTN)患者。
• ACCF/AHA 分期:进展期为不可逆心功能障碍。A=危险但无疾病,D=难治性心力衰竭。
• NYHA 分类:功能类Ⅰ～Ⅳ类,其中Ⅰ类对身体能力没有限制,Ⅳ类在休息时有心力衰竭症状。患者可以通过治疗来改善病情。

▪ 病因

潜在原因和急性原因：

• 心力衰竭可由心脏瓣膜、心内膜、心肌、心包及代谢紊乱引起。

• 降低心肌收缩性：
- 缺血性心肌病。
- 非缺血性心肌病。
  ◦ 家族性肥胖糖尿病。
  ◦ 内分泌：甲状腺功能减退，肢端肥大。
  ◦ 妊娠相关扩张 CMP。
  ◦ 毒素相关（酒精、可卡因、化疗）。
  ◦ 炎症：感染性和非感染性心肌炎（病毒性、南美锥虫病、SLE、HIV）。
  ◦ 淀粉样变。
  ◦ 心脏结节病。

• 增加压力状态：
- HTN。
- 瓣膜异常。
- 先天性心脏病。
- 肺动脉高压导致右心衰竭：原发性肺动脉高压、OSA、COPD、CTEPH、IPF 等。
- 肺栓塞。

• 容量负荷过重：
- 饮食不当（钠过量）。
- 导致钠潴留的药物（糖皮质激素、非甾体抗炎药）。
- 输液或静脉输液造成超载。

• 高需求状态：
- 甲状腺功能亢进、甲状腺功能亢进。
- 妊娠。
- 动静脉瘘。
- 脚气病（硫胺素缺乏症）。
- 佩吉特病。
- 严重贫血。
- 主动脉瓣闭锁不全。

• 儿科病因：容量/压力超负荷病变与获得性 HD：
- 前 6 个月：VSD 和 PDA。
- 较大的儿童：瓣膜性主动脉瓣下狭窄。
- 获得性功能障碍：非特定的发病年龄，包括心肌炎、瓣膜病和心肌病、可卡因/兴奋剂滥用的青少年。

诊断

▪ 症状和体征

• 低灌注：
- 疲劳，嗜睡，头昏眼花。
- 心悸或脉搏不规则。
- 呼吸急促。
- 冰冷的四肢。
- 肾功能恶化。
- 肝功能恶化，肠缺血。

• 淤血：
- 呼吸困难。
- 咳嗽。
- 端坐呼吸。
- 阵发性夜间呼吸困难。
- 运动耐受性降低。
- 颈静脉怒张或腹颈反射升高。
- 依赖性水肿（敏感性和特异性差）。
- 啰音或喘息（80%无，由于代偿性淋巴引流导致长期充盈压力升高）。
- 胸腔积液，肺底部暗沉。
- S3 或 S4。
- 侧移位根尖冲量。
- 肝大。

• 血流动力学不稳定的 ADHF：
- 精神混乱、焦虑、晕厥。
- 呼吸急促。
- 心动过速。
- 低血压。
- 四肢冰凉、苍白或发紫。
- 窄脉压或脉轮。
- 潮式呼吸。

▪ 基本检查

诊断往往是具有挑战性的和依赖于测试结果和临床检查。

▪ 诊断检查与说明

没有单一的诊断测试。心力衰竭是一种临床诊断。

实验室检查

• 电解质：
- 开始使用利尿剂或 ACEI 时建立肾功能基线。
- 高钾血症可能伴随低输出量。
- 低钠血症与预后不良有关。

• CBC：
- 贫血会导致或加剧失败。
- 感染可导致或加剧失败。

• 肝功能测试：
- 升高提示肝充血或缺血。

• 甲状腺功能测试：
- 特别是在>65 岁或新的心房纤颤。

• 心肌酶的患者：
- 评估缺血或梗死。
- 常见的轻度肌钙蛋白升高。

• 病毒组：怀疑心肌炎。

• BNP：
- 有助于临床判断和诊断：
  ◦ BNP>500 pg/ml，可能 HF（ppv 90%）。
  ◦ BNP<100 pg/ml，不可能发生 HF（净现值 90%）。
  ◦ 配置 BNP 100～500 pg/ml，不确定。
- BNP 随年龄、心房纤维颤动、心力衰竭、贫血、肾衰竭、睡眠呼吸暂停、败血症、严重烧伤、药物治疗等增高，不应单独使用。
- 急性肺水肿（1～2 h 及以上）和肥胖（BMI>30）患者 BNP 水平可能较低。

• NT - proBNP：
- NT - proBNP>1 000 pg/ml，HF 预测。
- NT - proBNP<300 pg/ml，不可能是 HF。
- 必须使用 NT - proBNP，如果患者是 ARNI。

影像学检查

• 胸部 X 线检查：
- ADHF 的精度不高。
- 心脏肥大不能通过仰卧位片进行评估。
- CHF 的具体症状：
  ◦ 头部穿刺（由于液体过多导致上肺血管突出）。
  ◦ 组织间水肿/Kerley B 线。
  ◦ 肺泡水肿。
- 积液。
- 可能出现症状后 12 h 的滞后。
- 放射线检查结果可能持续数日，尽管临床改善。
- 两侧融合性肺门周围浸润，形成典型的蝴蝶图案：
  ◦ 可能不对称，误认为肺炎。

• 心电图：
- 正常心电图阴性预测值高。
- 潜在心脏缺血。
- 存在心律失常。
- 左心室肥大。
- 心传导阻滞。

• 床旁超声：心、肺、下腔静脉。
- 心脏基础：
  ◦ 预测 EF。
  ◦ 急性瓣膜病理变化。
  ◦ 心脏压塞。
- 心脏高级：
  ◦ EF 测量。
  ◦ 急性瓣膜病理。
  ◦ 心室扩张或肥厚。

X

◦ 区域室壁运动异常。
- IVC：
◦ 2 cm，呼吸变化最小。
- 肺：
◦ Kerley B 线在>2 肋间距双边。
◦ 识别大量积液。

鉴别诊断

• HFpEF、HFrEF 和混合 HF：
- 心律失常。
- 急性冠状动脉综合征。
- 贫血。
- 营养不良。
- 心脏压塞。
- 气胸。
- 胸主动脉夹层。
- 缩窄性心包炎。
- 先天性心脏病（小儿）。
- 脓毒性心肌病。
- 线粒体损伤：
◦ BB 和 CCB 过量。
◦ 氰化物、一氧化碳中毒。
• 右心衰竭：
- 肾衰竭。
- 肝硬化。
- 左心衰竭。
- 静脉淤滞。
- 原发性肺部疾病：
◦ 肺栓塞。
◦ COPD 恶化。
◦ 哮喘恶化。
◦ IPF 恶化。
◦ 有急性呼吸窘迫综合征。
◦ 肺炎。

治疗

院前

• 静脉通道。
• 吸氧。
• 心电监测和脉搏血氧仪。
• 心电图。
• 如果没有低血压，舌下含服硝酸盐。
• 无创通气(NIV)。
• 可能需要气管插管。

初步稳定/治疗

• 静脉通道。
• 吸氧。
• 心电监测和脉搏血氧仪。
• 心电图：急性心肌梗死、心律失常的评估：
- 启动心脏导管实验室，进行可能的再灌注。
• 抬高床头以减少静脉回流。
• 控制气道：
- CPAP 和 BiPAP：
◦ 减少呼吸工作，改善氧合，减少插管的需要，死亡率获益。
- 插管治疗即将发生的呼吸衰竭。
- 治疗潜在疾病。

急诊治疗/步骤

• 灌注充足时淤血：减少前负荷，控制后负荷，考虑限制液体和利尿：
- 减少急性肺水肿的前负荷：
◦ 舌下或静脉给予硝酸甘油。
◦ 硝酸盐（较不可靠，首选静脉）。
◦ 硝普钠：强大的静脉和动脉扩张器，需要动脉通路。
◦ 静脉输入利尿剂（较慢/有效的患者肾灌注不良）：
▫ 考虑从 2 倍的家庭剂量开始。
- 当怀疑病因是主动脉瓣狭窄、HOCM 或肺动脉高压时，避免 ADHF 患者侵略性的前负荷降低。
- HOCM：考虑使用 BB 降低 HR。
• 灌注不良伴低血压：
- 对于心源性休克无一线加压器。
- 去甲肾上腺素：
◦ 推荐多巴胺，但 SOAPⅡ研究人员发现，有增加的不良事件与多巴胺的趋势。
- 多巴胺。
- 多巴酚丁胺：
◦ 肌力增强剂，可引起血管舒张。
- 米力农：
◦ 肌力剂，可能导致血管扩张。
◦ 伴有心律失常。
◦ 配置避免血管扩张药物（硝酸盐、吗啡）。
- 选择收缩术后慎用利尿剂。
• 机械心脏支持(MCS)装置在选择的情况下使用；尽早介入/转到心脏强化治疗或心力衰竭专科医师。
- 非耐久性 MCS 装置（ECMO、LVAD、Impella 心脏泵、球囊泵）在某些情况下和可能恢复或移植时可提供桥接。
• 警告：
- ACEI、ARB、ARNI、BB 和醛固酮拮抗剂。在急诊室中最安全的是避免出现低血压、急性肾衰竭和高钾血症的风险。
- 钙通道阻滞剂抑制收缩性，对心力衰竭处理无作用。

儿科注意事项

• 新生儿（出生后几周）：
- 如果临床 CHF 和氧合状态没有改善，则怀疑导管依赖性心脏病变：
◦ 配置 PGE_1，保持导管。
• 儿童：
- 呋塞米、多巴胺或米力农。
- 静脉注射硝酸甘油治疗肺水肿。

药物治疗

• 如果怀疑 AMI，阿司匹林：325 mg，口服或灌肠。
• 布美他尼：1～3 mg，静脉注射，最大剂量 10 mg/d。
• 多巴酚丁胺：2～10 μg/(kg · min)，静脉注射，最大剂量 40 μg/(kg · min)。
• 多巴胺：2～20 μg/(kg · min)，静脉注射，最大剂量 50 μg/(kg · min)。
• 依那普利：0.625～1.25 mg，静脉注射；2.5～20 mg/d，口服。
• 呋塞米：无前例：40 mg 静脉推注；使用前：24 h 双剂量（静脉注射 80～180 mg）；30 min 无效果：双倍剂量。
• 米力农：50 μg/kg，静脉注射负荷；0.375～0.75 μg/(kg · min)，静脉注射。
• 奈西立肽：2 μg/kg，再滴注 0.01 μg/(kg · min)。
• 硝酸甘油：舌下 0.4 mg；1～2 in 的硝基膏；5～20 μg/min 静脉注射，最多 100～200 μg/min 静脉注射。使用非 PVC 管。
• 硝普钠：0.3～10 μg/(kg · min)，静脉注射（起始剂量），最大剂量 10 μg/(kg · min)。

妊娠注意事项

ACEI 和 ARB 与多种胎儿异常相关，应保持：
• 氧气。
• 硝化甘油。
• 呋喃苯胺酸。

随访

进一步处理

入院指征

• ICU：
- 肺水肿，需要呼吸冷却或 ETT。
- 心源性休克。
- 伴发心肌梗死或缺血。
• 医疗病房：

- 最近诊断为 CHF。
- 急诊治疗未能缓解症状。

出院指征

• 慢性心力衰竭轻度加重：
- 对急诊治疗有反应。
- 没有其他心脏和肺部症状。

• 应安排密切随访，继续使用利尿剂、血管扩张剂或血管紧张素转换酶抑制剂治疗，并对患者进行生活方式教育。

转诊问题

在 HF 考虑 ICD 和/或 BV 起搏器：

• 降低在选定的患者中死亡率和住院率。

随访建议

• 出院后 1 周内密切随访。
• 服药和饮食依从性。
• 经常在家监测体重。
• 长期利尿剂治疗期间监测电解质和肾功能。

要点和误区

• BNP 在 CHF 诊断不确定时可能有用。
• 对于严重的 CHF，NIPPV 可以改善迫在眉睫的呼吸损害。
• 警惕寻找和治疗心力衰竭加重的根本原因（如心肌梗死、肺动脉栓塞、瓣膜病变等）。

心内膜炎 Endocarditis

Michael S. Murphy 单怡 译

基础知识

描述

一种心脏内膜表面的感染。

• 可包括心脏的很多结构：
- 自体心脏瓣膜（最常见）。
- 人工心脏瓣膜。
- 室间隔。
- 腱索。
- 心壁内膜。
- 心脏内装置。

• 以赘生物形成为特点（微生物聚集形成血栓）：
- 细菌定植在由纤维蛋白和血小板形成的无菌性赘生物上。
- 细菌繁殖使赘生物扩大，进一步阻碍血流和刺激炎症反应。
- 炎症通过全身的栓子进行传播。

• 大多数总是继发于细菌感染。
• 非感染性的病因较少：
- 非细菌性血栓性心内膜炎或消耗性心内膜炎：
  ◦ 通常由于血液高凝导致。
  ◦ 小的无菌性赘生物。
- 利布曼-萨克斯心内膜炎：
  ◦ 继发于系统性红斑狼疮。
  ◦ 由于免疫复合物沉积引起炎症反应。
  ◦ 小的疣状赘生物。

流行病学

• 大多为男性：
- 发生率为（3～7）/（10 万人 · 年）。
- 是第三常见的危及生命的感染性疾病。

• 危险因素：
- 高龄。
- 口腔卫生差。
- 合并症：
  ◦ 风湿性心脏病及先天性心脏病。
  ◦ 人工瓣膜和心脏内植入装置。
  ◦ 血液透析和留置静脉导管。
  ◦ 糖尿病及免疫抑制。
- 滥用静脉注射药物（IVDA）：
  ◦ 比风湿性心脏病或人工心脏瓣膜的风险更大。
  ◦ 多侵犯右侧心瓣膜。

• 脓毒症性栓塞：
- 脑部并发症：
  ◦ 脑栓塞。
  ◦ 颅内出血。
  ◦ 脑脓肿。
- 脑外栓塞事件：
  ◦ 肺。
  ◦ 脾。
  ◦ 肾。
  ◦ 细菌性动脉瘤（主动脉、肾动脉脾动脉、肝动脉、肠系膜动脉）。
  ◦ 肝。
  ◦ 冠状动脉。

• 复发性心内膜炎的危险因素：
- 由于心脏内血流的改变，心脏的结构性病变是常见的赘生物形成部位：
  ◦ 二尖瓣脱垂。
  ◦ 主动脉瓣功能障碍。
- 儿童多为先天性心脏病：
  ◦ 法络四联症。
  ◦ 主动脉狭窄。
  ◦ 动脉导管未闭。
  ◦ 室间隔缺损。
  ◦ 主动脉缩窄。
- 人工心脏瓣膜。
- 心脏导管。
- 任何心脏内装置都可以作为微生物侵入或附着的"门户"。

病因

• 主要分类：
- 细菌性心内膜炎。
- 人工瓣膜性心内膜炎。
- 非细菌栓子性心内膜炎：
  ◦ 恶性肿瘤。
  ◦ 尿毒症。
  ◦ 烧伤。
  ◦ 系统性红斑狼疮。

• 常见微生物：
- 金黄色葡萄球菌（最常见的病原体）：
  ◦ 可见于所有患者，尤其是经静脉注射药物依赖者和吸毒者。
  ◦ 起病急，感染性强。
  ◦ 时有转移灶。
- 草绿色链球菌：
  ◦ 口咽部可见，是自体瓣膜心内膜炎的主要病原。
- 牛链球菌：
  ◦ 与结肠息肉或胃肠道恶性肿瘤有关。
- 肺炎链球菌：
  ◦ 造成急性瓣膜破坏、脓肿、急性心力衰竭。
  ◦ 危险因素：酗酒。
- 表皮葡萄球菌。
- 肠球菌：
  ◦ 见于年轻女性及老年男性在器械操作或感染后。
- 假丝酵母和曲霉：

X

    - 见于静脉注射药物依赖、人工瓣膜或免疫功能不全患者。
  - HACEK(嗜血杆菌属),增殖缓慢。
  - 培养阴性的心内膜炎(Q热、鹦鹉热、巴尔通体属、布鲁菌病)。

诊断

症状和体征

- 发热：
  - 86%的患者有发热。
  - 下列情况可无发热：
    - 高龄。
    - 慢性心力衰竭。
    - 极度虚弱。
    - 慢性肾衰竭。
    - 流感样症状。
    - 寒战。
    - 盗汗。
    - 不适。
- 头、眼、耳、鼻和咽喉：
  - 视网膜出血或罗式斑。
- 呼吸系统：
  - 呼吸困难。
  - 咳嗽。
  - 心力衰竭。
- 心脏：
  - 在80%～85%的患者中有新出现杂音或杂音改变。
- 腹部：
  - 腹部或后背疼痛。
  - 脾大(15%～50%)。
- 四肢：
  - 肌痛。
  - 关节痛。
  - 杵状指。
- 神经系统：
  - 意识状态改变。
  - 败血症性栓塞(脑卒中或真菌性动脉瘤)。
- 皮肤：
  - 皮肤血管病变：
    - 黏膜或结膜瘀斑。
    - 出血点。
    - Osler结节：有疼痛的红色硬结节。
    - Janeway损害：手掌足底小出血点。

既往史

- 发热持续时间和热型。
- 危险因素：
  - 既往有心脏病史。
  - 菌血症来源：
    - 留置血管内导管。
    - 静脉用药。
    - 口腔卫生差。

体格检查

- 心肺功能检查：
  - 新出现的心脏反流性杂音。
  - 心力衰竭。
  - 脾大的评估。
- 脓毒症性血栓的评估：
  - 眼底、皮肤和甲床。
  - 细致的神经系统检查小的局灶性神经功能缺损。

基本检查

- 明确不明原因发热患者有无感染性心内膜炎的危险因素。
- 血培养。
- 确诊需要心电图检查。

诊断检查与说明

实验室检查

- 全血细胞计数：
  - 贫血(有时候溶血)。
  - 白细胞增多(粒细胞核增多和杆状核粒细胞增多)。
- 血培养：
  - 使用抗生素前多部位(3次)培养：
    - 5%～10%的心内膜炎培养阴性。
    - 应行导管的病原学培养。
- 红细胞沉降率(血沉)和C反应蛋白升高(缺乏特异性)。
- 尿液分析：
  - 镜下血尿。

影像学检查

- 胸部X线检查：
  - 慢性心力衰竭。
  - 右侧心内膜炎可见到脓毒症性肺栓塞。
- 心电图：
  - 心律不齐、新发的心脏传导阻滞。
- 超声心动图：
  - 急性瓣膜损伤。
  - 脓肿。
  - 赘生物。
  - 经食管心脏超声更敏感。
- CT扫描：
  - 可提供综合信息和发现主动脉根和瓣膜异常。
  - 可以检测到瓣膜周围扩张/瘘管。

鉴别诊断

- 风湿热。
- 心房黏液瘤。
- 急性心包炎。
- 心肌梗死。
- 主动脉夹层伴瓣膜反流。
- 血小板减少性紫癜。
- 系统性红斑狼疮。
- 隐匿性肿瘤转移。
- 败血症。
- 棉花热。

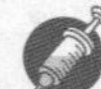

治疗

初步稳定/治疗

- 有心力衰竭症状者需要监测。
- 有以下情况行手术修复：
  - 严重瓣膜功能障碍导致心力衰竭。
  - 不稳定的人造瓣膜。
  - 心脏内脓肿引起瓣环扩大。
  - 抗生素治疗失败。
  - 大的或真菌性赘生物。
- 抗生素治疗：
  - 血培养结果出来前根据经验静脉内使用杀菌性抗生素。
  - 自体瓣膜或先天性异常：
    - 头孢曲松＋庆大霉素(PCN可疑)。
    - 万古霉素＋庆大霉素。
  - 人工瓣膜或既往有IVDA史：
    - 万古霉素＋庆大霉素＋利福平(如果不怀疑甲氧西林耐药的MRSA)。
    - 如果MRSA万古霉素无效或不耐受可考虑达帕霉素或奎奴普丁-达福普汀。
    - 万古霉素耐药。
    - 肠球菌：青霉素＋庆大霉素；万古霉素＋庆大霉素。
    - 肠球菌(庆大霉素耐药)：青霉素＋链霉素。
  - 真菌：
    - 两性霉素B。
  - 巴尔通体属：
    - 头孢曲松钠。

药物治疗

- 两性霉素B：
  - 试验剂量0.1 mg/kg至1 mg,缓慢静脉注射。
  - 等待2～4 h。
  - 如果能忍受,开始0.25 mg/kg直到0.6 mg/kg,静脉注射,3次/日。
  - 每日最大剂量不超过1.5 mg/kg。
- 头孢曲松钠：2 g/d,静脉注射[儿童：100 mg/(kg·24 h)]。

• 达托霉素：4 mg/(kg·d)，静脉注射。
• 庆大霉素：1 mg/kg，静脉注射，q8 h。
• 萘夫西林：2 g，静脉注射，q4 h。
• 青霉素：400 U，静脉注射，q4 h。
• 奎奴普丁-达福普汀：7.5 mg/kg，静脉注射，q8 h。
• 利福平：600 mg，口服，每日 4 次。
• 链霉素：15 mg/(kg·24 h)，静脉注射/肌内注射。
• 万古霉素：15 mg/kg，静脉注射，q12 h。

随访

进一步处理

入院指征

• 有危险因素的患者出现病原菌感染的证据或临床表现。
• 所有的静脉用药者伴发热。
• 心血管病情不稳定患者入住 ICU 或有监护设备的病房。

出院指征

无。

随访

• 病程：
- 大多数患者在 1 周内退热。
• 并发症：
- 心脏：慢性心力衰竭、瓣膜脓肿、心包炎、瓣周漏。
- 神经系统：脑栓塞、脑脓肿、脑出血。
- 栓塞：中枢神经系统、肺部、四肢缺血。
- 细菌性动脉瘤：脑内或全身性。
- 肾脏：梗死、肾炎、脓肿。
- 转移性脓肿：肾脏、脾脏、组织。

要点和误区

• 心内膜炎患者查体可闻及新发或变化的杂音。
• 50%的患者并没有已知的瓣膜疾病史。
• 近期的治疗史、医疗设备接触史应该被认为是危险因素。
• 常见的并发症：脑卒中(中风)、栓塞、心力衰竭、心内脓肿及细菌性动脉瘤破裂。
• 静脉注射药物依赖患者出现发热需排除心内膜炎，除非表现为典型的纺织热热型。
• 急性病程，在不同静脉穿刺部位采血 2～3 次做血培养后，给予经验性治疗。

心室颤动 Ventricular Fibrillation

Marie-France Petchy 周秋香 毛恩强 译

基础知识

描述

• 心室颤动(VF，简称室颤)是心肌完全无组织去极化和小面积的收缩，完全没有有效的心输出量。
• 心脏监护仪显示快速、严重不规则的电活动，心电图波形的长度、形态和振幅都是可变的；心室率通常大于 300 bpm。没有可识别的 P 波、QRS 波群或 T 波。

X

病因

• 损伤的心肌创建新的电活动起点：
- 心肌损伤可能由多种因素引起，包括缺血、坏死、再灌注、愈合和瘢痕形成。
• 最常见的是严重心肌缺血的结果：
- 约 50%存活至住院的 VF－OHCA 患者有 AMI 的证据。
• 心肌病的并发症：
- 结构性心脏病患者出现持续性室颤和室颤的风险更高。
• 室性心动过速的非缺血性病因可能演变为室颤：
- 药物毒性(环状抗抑郁药、洋地黄类)。
- 电解质酸碱异常。
- 先天性和获得性长 QT 综合征。
- 短 QT 综合征。
- Brugada 综合征。
• 具有 R－on－T 现象的室性期前收缩(PVC)。
• 室颤的其他不常见原因：
- 电刑。
- 缺氧。
- 低温。
- 胸部钝挫伤。
- 医源性心脏起搏器安置或肺动脉导管刺激。
• 特发性室颤。

儿科注意事项

• 原发性室性心律失常在儿童中极为罕见。
• 室颤通常是由呼吸停止、低潮或接近溺水引起的。

诊断

症状和体征

• 意识丧失。
• 发作。
• 暂时喘气，然后是呼吸暂停。
• 缺少脉搏和心音。
• 如果室颤仍未得到处理将会死亡：
- 室颤是 5%～70%的院前心脏猝死患者的原因。

基本检查

• AED 或手动除颤器来确认和治疗一个震撼的节奏。
• 心脏监视器。

诊断检查与说明

实验室检查

• 实验室测试在复苏过程中无用。
• 自主循环恢复后(ROSC)：电解质包括钙和镁、BUN、肌酐、肌钙蛋白、ABG、乳酸水平和毒理学筛选。

影像学检查

• 在 ROSC 之后。
• 识别室颤的原因：
- 心电图。
- 心脏超声。
- 胸部 X 线检查，也用于监测气管内导管(ETT)的位置。

鉴别诊断

• 心搏停止：
- 精细的室颤可能会模仿一种单一的铅。
- 检查其他人的节奏是否有细微的颤动。

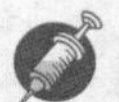

治疗

注意

• 室颤的早期除颤是生存的最重要决定因素，每迟 1 min 除颤，生存率降低 7%～10%。

- 目前制造的手动和自动外部除颤器是双相的。建议使用双相除颤器。如果没有双相除颤器，可以使用单相除颤器。
- 单次电击除颤策略是目前标准治疗。
- 无脉的室上性心动过速或室性心动过速，如果没用同步除颤可能会转化为室颤。
- 在伴有室颤的低温心跳骤停中，在复温患者的同时遵循标准的除颤策略。
- 不要为任何有意识的患者进行除颤。
- 血管加压素在心搏骤停中作为肾上腺素的替代品没有优势，也不再包含在 AHA 指南中。

争议

- 一些研究提出了关于肾上腺素在心搏骤停中的益处的问题。
- 心搏骤停后心肺复苏使用胺碘酮或利多卡因的益处尚不确定。
- 普鲁卡因胺作为二线抗心律失常的心搏骤停疗效仍有争议。
- 对于心搏骤停后 ROSC 患者，任何特定的血糖控制目标范围的益处都是不确定的。

院前

- 及时发现心搏骤停。
- 遵循最初的稳定/治疗措施。
- 理想情况下，运输到最近的设施提供全面的心搏骤停后治疗。

初步稳定/治疗

- 尽快使用 AED 或手动除纤颤器。
- 从胸部按压开始进行早期 CPR，直到除颤器准备就绪。
- 除颤器确认了震颤的节奏。
- 启动 SCREAM 首字母缩略词。
- 休克：
  - 立即 1 次电除颤。
  - 双相能级：
    - 按照制造商的建议（如 120～200 J）进行第一次冲击；如果不知道，请使用最大可用。
    - 下一次除颤的冲击能量相同或更高。
  - 第一次和随后的冲击为 360 J 单相。
  - 2 min 后可重复除颤。
- CPR：
  - 每次休克后立即行心肺复苏 2 min，从胸部按压开始。
  - 30：2 按压通气比。
  - 每分钟 100～120 次按压。
  - 尽量减少心肺复苏中断。
  - 在最初的心肺复苏术中，持续胸外按压可采用正压通气，每 6 s 换气 1 次，直到插入高级气道。
- 心脏复苏每 2 min 后进行心律检查。
- 边复苏边查找潜在病因。
- 建立静脉通道。
- 如果除颤不成功可加用肾上腺素：
  - 第二次冲击后开始。
  - 可以重复隔 3～5 min。
- 抗心律失常药物：
  - 第三次冲击后开始。
  - 胺碘酮。
  - 如果胺碘酮不可用，用利多卡因。
  - 尖端扭转型室速可用镁。
  - 可以考虑持续输注与 ROSC 相关的抗心律失常药。
- 高级气道管理：
  - 应该和 CPR 和除颤同步。
  - 心肺复苏时连续胸部按压 100～120 次/分和正压通气每 6 s 换气 1 次。
  - 使用二氧化碳分析仪监测 ETT 的位置，优化 CPR，并检测 ROSC。

儿科注意事项

- 除颤（双相或单相）：第一次电击 2 J/kg，第二次电击 4 J/kg，后续电击≥4 J/kg，最大 10 J/kg 或成人剂量。
- 心肺复苏术：1 名抢救者为 30：2，2 名抢救者为 15：2。

急诊治疗/程序

- 心搏骤停后护理。
- 识别和治疗室颤的原因，认识到最可能的原因是急性心肌梗死：
  - 指示时提供经皮冠状动脉介入治疗。
- 保持 SpO_2 ≥94% 和 35～40 mmHg 的 $PETCO_2$。
- 治疗 SBP<90 mmHg，MAP<65 mmHg。
- 保持体温在 32～34 ℃≥24 h。
- 评估 ROSC 患者，但随后进展为死亡或脑死亡的器官捐献患者。

药物治疗

- 肾上腺素：1 mg，静脉或骨髓腔推注，可重复给药 q3～5 min。
- 加压素：40 U，静脉或骨髓腔注射单次剂量。
- 胺碘酮：静脉或骨髓腔推注 300 mg，可重复 150 mg 静脉或骨髓腔推注一次：
  - ROSC 后输注胺碘酮：第 1 个 6 h 后 1 mg/min，然后 0.5 mg/min 持续 18 h。最大剂量 2.2 g/24 h。
- 利多卡因：1～1.5 mg/kg，静脉或骨髓腔推注，可重复 0.5～0.75 mg/kg 静脉推注 q5～10 min；最多 3 次。最大剂量 3 mg/kg：
  - 心肺复苏后注射利多卡因：1～4 mg/min [30～50 μg/(kg·min)]。
- 硫酸镁：1～2 g 药加入 10 ml D_5W，静脉或骨髓腔推注。
- 使用每个药物之前用 20 ml 生理盐水冲洗。
- 如无静脉/骨髓腔注射通路，可采用气管内路径注射肾上腺素和利多卡因，剂量为 2～2.5 静脉注射（溶于 5～10 ml 生理盐水）。

儿科注意事项

- 肾上腺素：0.01 mg/kg，静脉注射或骨髓腔注射，可重复 q3～5 min；最大剂量 1 mg。如果没有静脉/静脉注射通道，气管内给药剂量 0.1 mg/kg（溶于 3～5 ml 溶液中）。
- 胺碘酮：5 mg/kg，静脉注射或骨髓腔注射，可重复 5 mg/kg；最大剂量 15 mg/(kg·d)。
- 利多卡因：1 mg/kg，静脉注射或骨髓腔注射。
  - 利多卡因输注 20～50 μg/(kg·min)。
- 硫酸镁：25～50 mg/kg，静脉注射或骨髓腔注射至 2 g。
- 使用每个药物之前，3～5 ml 的生理盐水冲洗药物。

随访

进一步处理

入院指征

所有患者都需要入住 ICU 或 CCU。

出院指征

室颤的患者都需要电除颤。

转诊问题

发生室颤后 48 h 以上发生室颤的患者可能需要参考电生理检查。

要点和误区

ACC/AHA 指南建议，急性心肌梗死患者的血钾应保持在 4 mmol/L 以上，预防室性心律失常。

X

心室停搏

David F. M. Brown · Hiren Patel 于洋 潘曙明 译

基础知识

描述

心室电活动停止。

病因

- 终末期心律，常由以下心律恶化进展而来：
  - 长时间心动过缓。
  - 长时间心室颤动。
  - 长时间无脉电活动。
- 院外发生心室停搏的患者存活概率极小：
  - 最高约有 40%的患者能够恢复自主循环并收治入院，但<15%的患者能存活出院。
  - 室性心动过速/心室颤动电除颤后出现的心室停搏患者预后同样很差，<10%的患者能存活出院。
- 潜在可逆病因包括：
  - 低氧血症。
  - 低血容量(失血)。
  - 酸中毒。
  - 高钾血症。
  - 低钾血症。
  - 药物过量。
  - 低体温。
  - 肺栓塞。
  - 心肌梗死。
  - 张力性气胸。
  - 心脏压塞。

诊断

症状和体征

- 患者无反应。
- 无脉搏。
- 无自主呼吸或濒死呼吸。

检查要点

- 至少 2 个肢体导联确定心室停搏，排除心室颤动。
- 确定导联和电线连接正常。
- 确定监护仪电源开启。
- 确定监护仪增益合适。
- 识别心室停搏可逆病因(见上)。

诊断检查与说明

实验室检查

动脉血气(血钾和血红蛋白)。

影像学检查

心脏超声检查排除心脏压塞。

鉴别诊断

细颤(可误诊为心室停搏)。

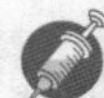

治疗

院前

- 如果患者已签署有效的放弃复苏(DNR)的文件，则不进行心肺复苏。
- 如果能确定患者已死亡，则不进行心肺复苏：
  - 尸僵。
  - 尸斑。
  - 无生命迹象的严重创伤(如断头)。

初步稳定/治疗

- 启动 CPR，重点是不间断、高质量的胸外按压。
- 心电监测确认心室停搏。
- 放置气道辅助装置(气管内插管首选，球囊面罩亦可接受)，确定插管位置，吸入 100%纯氧，缓慢的通气频率(6～12 次/分)，插管时尽量少中断胸外按压。
- 建立静脉或骨髓内通路。
- 使用连续 CO_2 波形监测以优化胸外按压质量(CPR 时 $PETCO_2$ 与心输出量和心肌血流灌注呈正相关)。
- 每 3～5 min 给予肾上腺素。
- 寻找并处理潜在可逆性病因(见上)。
- 如果怀疑有高钾血症或药物过量，给予碳酸氢钠。
- 不推荐经验性给予单次电除颤。
- 不推荐电起搏治疗。
- 如果患者发生心室颤动/室性心动过速，立即给予除颤。

急诊治疗/程序

- 对恢复自主循环的昏迷患者开始诱导性低温治疗。
- 如果下列情况都已满足，则考虑终止复苏：
  - 高质量的胸外按压已进行了一段时间。
  - 已气管插管确保正常氧合。
  - 已排除细颤。
  - 可逆性病因已纠正或排除。
  - 床旁超声检查已排除心包积液。
  - 无张力性气胸的临床证据。

药物治疗

- 肾上腺素：1 mg(儿童：0.01 mg/kg)静脉注射/3～5 min。
- 碳酸氢钠：1 mmol/kg 静脉注射，如果有下列情况：
  - 之前存在酸中毒。
  - 高钾血症。
  - 怀疑三环类抗抑郁药过量。

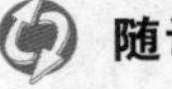

随访

进一步处理

入院指征

所有恢复自主循环的患者。

出院指征

无。所有恢复自主循环的患者都需要收入 ICU 进行复苏后治疗。

随访建议

如果心室停搏是由原发性心脏传导阻滞引起，可考虑安装永久起搏器。

患者监护

适时转运患者至 ICU 进行心电监测和诱导性低温治疗。

要点和误区

- 关键是高质量、不间断的胸外按压，同时寻找心室停搏的可逆病因。
- 只有找到可逆病因并给以纠正才有可能复苏成功。

心源性休克 Cardiogenic Shock

Rodolfo Loureiro · Shamai A. Grossman 彭沪 译

基础知识

描述

• 在血管内容量充足和左心室充盈压正常情况下,因心功能不全所致持续性低血压和组织灌注不足。
• 是住院急性心肌梗死患者中最常见的死亡原因。
• 在急性心肌梗死中的潜在机制:
- 泵衰竭:
◦ 大于40%左心室梗死。
◦ 存在左心室功能障碍的心肌梗死。
◦ 再梗死。
- 机械性并发症:
◦ 急性二尖瓣关闭不全。
◦ 室间隔缺损。
◦ 左心室破裂。
◦ 心脏压塞。
- 右室心肌梗死。
• 5%～8%的ST段抬高型心肌梗死患者会发展成心源性休克。

病理

• 急性心肌梗死。
• 脓毒症。
• 心肌炎。
• 心肌挫伤。
• 心脏瓣膜病。
• 心肌病。
• 左心房黏液瘤。
• 药物毒性:
- β受体阻滞剂。
- 钙通道阻滞剂。
- 阿霉素。

诊断

症状和体征

• 需行ABC程序的重要标志:
- 气道通畅(早期)。
- 呼吸费力和呼吸困难(早期),呼吸衰竭(晚期)。
- 低氧血症。
- 低血压:
◦ 收缩压小于90 mmHg。血压下降至少低于基础水平30 mmHg。
- 心动过速。
- 脉搏微弱。
• 一般表现:
- 青紫。
- 苍白。
- 大汗。
- 感觉减弱。
- 体温下降。
- 尿量小于20 ml/h。
• 颈部:
- 颈静脉怒张。
• 心脏:
- 缺血性胸痛。
- 收缩性心尖部杂音。
- 奔马律:
◦ 第三心音奔马律反映严重的心肌功能障碍。
◦ 有80%窦性心律心肌梗死患者存在第四心音奔马律。
- 收缩期喀哒音:
◦ 提示腱索断裂。
- 腹部体征:
◦ 上腹痛。
◦ 恶心和呕吐。
- 神经系统:
◦ 反应迟钝。

病史

• 从患者的家庭或环境中获取病史,以寻找可能的病因。
• 药物史。

体格检查

• 进行快速检查和稳定的生命体征。
• 颈静脉怒张、四肢凉用以区分分配性休克和低血容量性休克。
• 心肺检查。

基本检查

辅助研究进一步定义心脏损伤的类型和程度,并确定紧急插管或手术干预的适应证。

诊断测查与说明

心电图:
• 正常心电图不能除外心肌梗死。
• 寻找急性心肌梗死证据(2个或多个相邻导联ST段抬高)。
• 可能发生在非ST段抬高型急性冠状动脉综合征。
• 心律失常。
• 左心室肥厚。

实验室检查

• B型利钠肽(BNP):
- 诊断和判断预后均有价值。
• 肌酸激酶、CK-MB、肌钙蛋白。
• 电解质及肾功能:
- 急性肾衰竭预测着死亡率大大提高。
• 血常规:
- 明确是否存在贫血及白细胞升高。
• 乳酸:
- 缺乏通关与更高的死亡风险相关。
• 药物水平(例如,地高辛)。

影像学检查

• 胸部X线检查:
- 肺淤血。
- 胸腔积液。
- 心脏肥大。
- 肺炎。
- 气胸。
- 心包积液。
• 急诊超声心动图:
- 彩色多普勒经胸超声心动图(TTE)。
- 左心室收缩性判断心脏运动迟缓、无运动或运动障碍。
- 急性二尖瓣关闭不全或室间隔缺损。
- 右心室扩张、三尖瓣关闭不全、高肺动脉和右心室压力表明肺栓塞。
- 右心室运动功能减退或消失、右心室扩张、肺动脉压正常显示右心室梗死。
- 心包积液、右心房或右心室舒张期功能障碍表明心脏压塞。

鉴别诊断

• 梗阻性休克:
- 张力性气胸。
- 心脏压塞。
- 肺栓塞。
- 自发性食管破裂。
- 空气栓塞。
• 分布性休克:
- 脓毒症。
- 过敏反应。
- 肾上腺皮质危象。
- 神经源性休克。

X

• 低血容量性休克：
- 出血。
- 胃肠损失。
- 脱水。
- 烧伤。

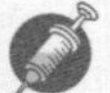

治疗

院前

• ABC 管理，建立静脉通道，吸氧，监测。
• 不考虑心脏破裂可给予液体。
• 阿司匹林。
• 没有低血压时，硝酸甘油或硫酸吗啡用于控制胸痛。
• 将心肌梗死患者送往 24 h 内有血管重建及再通能力的机构。

初步稳定/治疗

• 心肺复苏 ABC 程序。
• 建立两条外周大血管通路。
• 心脏监测。
• 气道损伤患者行气管插管。
- 考虑依托咪酯诱导（对血压影响最小）。
• 在没有肺淤血情况下，可给予液体（100～250 ml 生理盐水）。
• 导尿，监测尿量。

急诊治疗/程序

• 急性心肌梗死：
- 阿司匹林。
- 肝素。
- 无条件行经皮冠状动脉造影或搭桥手术时予以溶栓治疗。
- 在经皮冠状动脉介入术前予以 GP Ⅱb/Ⅲa 抑制剂。
- 氯吡格雷：通常在血运重建后才用，这在需要紧急旁路的患者中可能是禁忌的。
• 低血压：
- 去甲肾上腺素作为一线升压药使用。
- 在没有去甲肾上腺素的情况下考虑多巴胺。
• 血压正常：
- 多巴酚丁胺可与去甲肾上腺素及多巴胺合用，在急性二尖瓣关闭不全患者中可合用硝普钠。
- 米力农可与多巴酚丁胺或多巴胺合用。
• 肺水肿：
- 血压正常患者予以硝普钠或呋塞米治疗。
• 请心内科专业医师会诊明确是否需要如下治疗：
- IABP 在独立性经验型中心研究中证实可提高生存率。
- 评估 VAD 和 ECMO 在难治性心源性休克病例中的作用。
- 早期血管再通及重建是最重要的提高生存率手段。

药物治疗

• 比伐卢定：0.75 mg/kg 静脉推注，然后 1.75 mg/(kg · h)静脉注入。
• 氯吡格雷：600 mg，口服。
• 多巴酚丁胺：3～5 μg/(kg · min)，需要时滴定至 20～50 μg/(kg · min)静脉推注。
• 多巴胺：3～5 μg/(kg · min)，需要时滴定至 20～50 μg/(kg · min)静脉推注。
• 呋塞米：40～80 mg/d(1 mg/kg 静脉推注或肌内注射，不能超过 6 mg/kg)。
• 米力农：50 μg/kg 负荷量，0.375～0.75 μg/(kg · min)持续静脉注入。
• 硝酸甘油：10～20 μg/min[0.1～1 μg/(kg · min)，静脉使用]，不要使用 PVC 管。
• 硝普钠：0.3 μg/(kg · min)，滴定至不超过 10 μg/(kg · min)，静脉使用。
• 去甲肾上腺素：2 μg/min，需要时静脉滴定使用。

随访

进一步处理

入院指征

所有心源性休克患者均需入住监护室治疗。

要点和误区

• 在急性心肌梗死患者中，心源性休克是主要死亡原因。
• 早期识别休克前期至关重要。
• 早期血管重建预后尚可。

心脏瓣膜病 Valvular Heart Disease

Liudvikas Jagminas　周秋香　毛恩强 译

基础知识

描述

• 二尖瓣狭窄：
- 阻碍心舒期血流进入左心室。
• 二尖瓣回流：
- 瓣膜关闭不全至血液反流至左心房。
- 急性：左心房和肺静脉压力负荷过高至急性肺水肿。
- 慢性：左心室容量负荷过大至右心室扩张肥大，使右心室扩大。
• 主动脉瓣狭窄：
- 左心室射出血流受阻伴随收缩梯度的上升。
- 递增的左心室收缩压和心室肌向心性肥大。
• 主动脉瓣反流：
- 急性的左心室压力和容量负荷升高至左心衰竭和肺水肿。
- 慢性的容量负荷增加伴左心室扩张和肥大。

妊娠注意事项

孕妇常伴有严重的血流动力学改变会加重瓣膜病，从而增加血栓栓塞的风险。

儿科注意事项

• 退行性心瓣膜病很常见（主动脉狭窄和二尖瓣反流）。
• 瓣膜置换术是常用的外科手术。

病因

• 二尖瓣狭窄：
- 风湿热。
- 心脏肿瘤。
- 风湿性疾病（狼疮、类风湿关节炎）。
- 黏液瘤。
- 先天性缺陷：降落伞型瓣膜。
• 二尖瓣反流（急性）：
- 乳头状肌破裂（梗死、创伤）。
- 乳头状功能紊乱（缺血）。
- 腱索破裂（创伤、心内膜炎、黏液瘤）。
- 瓣膜穿孔（心内膜炎）。
- 减肥药（氯苯丙胺、氟拉明）。

- 主动脉狭窄：
  - 先天性心脏病：男性>女性(4∶1)。
  - 先天性二尖瓣(1%～2%)。
  - 风湿性主动脉狭窄。
  - 钙化性主动脉狭窄。
- 主动脉瓣反流：
  - 感染性心内膜炎。
  - 瓦氏窦房节破裂。
  - 急性主动脉夹层。
  - 胸痛。
  - 瓣膜术后。
  - 二叶主动脉瓣。
  - 风湿热。
  - 减肥药(氯苯丙胺、氟拉明)。
  - 胶原血管病或结缔组织病。
  - 系统性红斑狼疮。
  - 马方综合征。
  - 弹性假黄瘤。
  - 强直性脊柱炎。
  - 埃勒斯-当洛斯综合征。
  - 多肌痛。

诊断

症状和体征

- 二尖瓣狭窄：
  - 颧颊潮红(“二尖瓣面容”)。
  - 明显的颈静脉A波。
  - 右心室上移。
  - 第一心音(S1)声变强。
  - 开放性锐声。
  - 低沉的心脏舒张期隆隆声。
  - 劳力性呼吸困难。
  - 疲劳。
  - 心悸。
  - 夜间阵发性呼吸困难。
  - 端坐呼吸。
  - 咳血。
  - 系统性栓塞。
  - 肺动脉水肿。
- 二尖瓣回流(急性)：
  - 急性肺动脉水肿。
  - 静脉压表现为“大炮”性A波和巨大的V波。
  - 心间区尖锐的心音由渐弱到渐强，向腋窝发散。
  - 心尖区明显感到震颤。
  - 第三心音(S3)和第四心音(S4)。
  - 心悸。
  - 心房颤动。
  - 呼吸困难。
  - 端坐呼吸。
  - 夜间阵发性呼吸困难。
  - 外周性水肿。
  - 系统性栓塞。
  - 正常的颈静脉压。
  - 左心室肥大。
  - 心间部尖锐高调的全收缩期杂音。
  - 减轻或被遮盖的S1。
  - 分裂的第二心音(S2)。
  - S3。
- 主动脉狭窄：
  - 劳累性心绞痛。
  - 晕厥(运动时)。
  - 慢性心功能不全(先是舒张期，再是收缩期)。
  - 室颤所致猝死。
  - 尖锐的由渐弱到渐强的收缩期杂音，由主动脉区向颈动脉区发散。
  - 大动脉区S2缺失。
  - 外周脉搏的延迟脉冲。
  - S4奔马律。
  - 喷射性咔嗒音。
- 主动脉瓣流：
  - 易疲劳。
  - 劳力性呼吸困难。
  - 夜间阵发性呼吸困难。
  - 端坐呼吸。
  - 晕厥。
  - 急性肺动脉水肿。
  - 尖锐渐弱的舒张期杂音在大动脉区。
  - 加重的主动脉瓣第二心音(A2)。
  - 脉压变大。
  - 水冲脉。
  - 杜氏征。
  - De Musse征。
  - Quincke脉冲。
  - Austin Flint杂音。

基本检查

- 病史和体征。
- 是否有心内膜炎。
- 心电图。

诊断检查与说明

实验室检查

- 全血细胞计数。
  - 贫血。

影像学检查

- 胸部X线检查：
  - 二尖瓣狭窄：
    - 左心房扩大。
    - 肺血管聚集(柯雷B线)。
    - 突出的肺动脉。
  - 二尖瓣反流：
    - 慢性患者左心房和左心室扩大。
    - 急性患者肺动脉水肿左心房和左心室大小正常。
  - 主动脉狭窄：
    - 左心室肥大。
    - 大动脉钙化。
    - 扩张的升主动脉。
    - 肺淤血心脏肥大。
  - 主动脉瓣反流：
    - 急性：正常的心脏轮廓和肺水肿。
    - 慢性：扩大的右心室和扩张的主动脉。
- 心电图：
  - 评估瓣膜结构。
  - 评估流过瓣膜的血流。
  - 识别回流。
  - 心室扩张或肥大。
- 螺旋CT扫描：
  - 当有急性动脉回流时用于排除主动脉夹层。

诊断步骤/外科

心电图：

- 二尖瓣狭窄：
  - 左心房扩大(宽大的P波)。
  - 右心室肥大。
  - 右轴偏离。
  - 心房颤动。
  - 急性二尖瓣反流。
  - 左心房扩大。
  - 左心室肥大。
  - 左轴偏离。
- 主动脉狭窄：
  - 左心室肥大最常见。
  - 心房颤动。
  - 右轴偏离。
  - 室间传导延迟。
  - 完全房室传导阻滞。
- 主动脉瓣反流。
  - 急性：左心室负荷增加。
  - 慢性：左心室肥大负荷增加。

鉴别诊断

见病因。

X

治疗

院前

初步稳定/治疗

• ABC 管理。
• 给氧。
• 静脉补液。

急诊治疗/程序

• 二尖瓣狭窄：
- 慢性心力衰竭的对症治疗。
- 若有心房颤动要控制心室率。
- 地高辛。
- β受体阻滞剂。
- 肝素（如果是新发的心房颤动）。
- 利尿剂。
- 预防心内膜炎。

• 二尖瓣反流：
- 急性：
  ◦ 降低后负荷（硝酸甘油、吗啡或硝普钠）。
  ◦ 利尿剂。
  ◦ 主动脉球囊扩张（暂时措施）。
- 慢性：
  ◦ 硝酸盐类。
  ◦ 利尿剂。
  ◦ 肼屈嗪。
  ◦ ACEI。
  ◦ β受体阻滞剂（心室率控制）。
  ◦ 钙通道阻滞剂。
  ◦ 肝素（如果有心房颤动）。
  ◦ 预防心内膜炎。

• 主动脉狭窄：
- 若有心力衰竭适度利尿。
- 如果有低血压又没有心力衰竭可适度水化。
- 避免使用硝酸盐类后负荷减轻药。
- 地高辛。
- 主动脉球囊扩张（暂时措施）。
- 预防心内膜炎。

• 主动脉瓣反流：
- 慢性：
  ◦ 减轻前后负荷。
  ◦ 利尿剂。
  ◦ 地高辛。
  ◦ 预防心内膜炎。
- 急性：
  ◦ 减轻前后负荷。
  ◦ 主动脉球囊扩张。
  ◦ 急诊手术。

药物治疗

• 阿替洛尔：0.3～2 mg/(kg · d)，口服，最大剂量 2 mg/(kg · d)［推荐剂量 1～2 mg/(kg · d)］。

• 地高辛：0.5 mg，静脉推注；0.25～1 mg，静脉注射，q2 h；0.125～0.375 mg/d，口服。

• 地尔硫䓬：0.25 mg/kg，静脉注射，时间超过 2 min（15 min 后重复使用 0.35 mg/kg）。

• 依那普利：1.25 mg，静脉注射，q6 h；2.5～5 mg，口服，每日 2 次。

• 艾司洛尔：500 μg，静脉推注；50～300 μg/(kg · min) 维持。

• 呋塞米：20～80 mg/d，口服、肌内注射或静脉注射；严重水肿患者最大量至 600 mg/d。

• 肝素：80 U/kg，静脉推注，后以 18 U/(kg · h) 维持，将部分凝血活酶时间控制在 1.5～2 倍正常值（INR 2～3）。

• 肼屈嗪：10～25 mg，静脉注射，q2～4 h（0.1～0.5 mg/kg，肌内注射或静脉注射，q4～6 h；最大剂量 20 mg/剂）。

• 美托洛尔：5 mg，静脉注射，q2 min×3 剂；50 mg，口服 q6 h×48 h。

• 硝酸甘油：从 20 μg/min 开始至起效（3 000 μg/min）；最大剂量 20 μg/(kg · min)。

• 酚妥拉明：5 mg，静脉推注，然后 1～2 mg/min，静脉注射。

• 普萘洛尔：静脉注射，1～3 mg，1 mg/min。

• 硝普钠：静脉注射，0.5 μg/(kg · min)；增加到 1 μg/(kg/min)，5～10 min 后至 10 μg/(kg · min)。

• 阿莫西林：2 g，术前 1 h 口服；或 3 g，术前 1 h 口服；6 h 后再口服 1.5 g。
- 儿童剂量：50 mg/kg，术前 1 h 口服。

• 青霉素：2 g，术前 30 min 静脉注射或肌内注射（50 mg/kg 术前 30 min）。

• 克林霉素：600 mg，术前 1 h 口服（20 mg/kg，术前 1 h，不超 600 mg）。

随访

进一步处理

入院指征

• 新发的心房颤动。
• 慢性心力衰竭、肺水肿。
• 血流动力学不稳定。
• 急性二尖瓣、主动脉瓣反流。
• 心肌缺血。
• 心绞痛。
• 晕厥。
• 心律失常。

出院指征

• 血流动力学稳定。
• 心电图没有异常改变。
• 利尿剂可以控制慢性心力衰竭的症状。
• 慢性二尖瓣反流。

转诊问题

• 门诊的瓣膜病患者需要心内科医师评估瓣膜病情严重程度是否需要手术。
• 教育患者患瓣膜病的一些风险，必要时需要抗生素预防口腔科疾病。

要点和误区

主动脉瓣狭窄引起的胸痛，禁用硝酸甘油。

心脏检查 Cardiac Testing

Steve R. Grosse · Shamai A. Grossman　彭沪 译

基础知识

描述

• 心脏检测可表明急诊患者在心力衰竭（HF）或急性冠状动脉综合征（ACS）的风险。

• 这些病症可能被认为是一个范围：不稳定型心绞痛可以演变成心肌梗死，这反过来又会导致心力衰竭：
- 急诊医疗事故索赔中有 20% 是由于 ACS 的漏诊。
- 约 2% 的 ACS 患者没达到出院标准而

出院。

- 病史、体格检查、心电图是诊断胸痛和ACS/HF的重要手段。
- 尽管如此，病史、体格检查、心电图仍然会漏诊1%～4%的心脏病。
- 胸痛患者也普遍使用各种影像学检查方法，并有帮助。

病因

ACS是动脉粥样硬化引起的冠状血管狭窄或冠状动脉血管痉挛。

妊娠注意事项

在有胸痛和心电图缺血性改变的妊娠患者，同样要考虑自发性冠状动脉夹层的可能。

诊断

症状和体征

病史

- 心绞痛症状通常由身体的应力产生，包括劳力和情感活动通常休息后可缓解。
- ACS时不太可能在触诊时重复出现胸部尖锐疼痛、刺伤、肋膜炎，但仍有13%被诊断为胸膜炎性胸痛，7%的胸痛有触诊疼痛。
- 硝酸甘油可缓解心肌缺血，但也可以缓解胃肠道及主动脉病变。
- 一种包括利多卡因和氢氧化铝的“胃肠道鸡尾酒”疗法，或质子泵抑制剂如奥美拉唑，可以缓解胃肠的病理改变，还能减轻心肌缺血。
- 心绞痛症状常持续＜20 min但＞5 min。

体格检查

往往不被重视。

基本检查

心电图：

- 根据ACC/AHA指南，患者应该在胸部疼痛发生10 min内到达急诊行12导联心电图。
- 仅仅靠单一的心电图将漏诊50%的急性心肌梗死。
- 超急性期的T波（高高的、广泛的，特别是在前壁导联）可能是急性心肌梗死最早和唯一的标志。
- 在心肌梗死的病程中，心电图可能动态发展。连续心电图监测可以识别另外的16%的最初没有明显改变的急性心肌梗死，如果没有连续的心电监测。
- 考虑初始心电图15～60 min后再次复查心电图。
- 如果有新的ST段改变或T波倒置高度怀疑存在缺血。
- 缺血的特点是ST段压低1 mm；或者，有时可以是升高的，所以要检查其他的导联。
- ST段抬高型心肌梗死（STEMI）：在≥2个相邻的导联出现ST段抬高＞1～2 mm。
- 新的左束支传导阻滞（LBBB）提示心肌梗死。
- 陈旧性LBBB会使AMI诊断困难：应用斯加尔博萨诊断标准：如果左束支传导阻滞和ST段抬高＞1 mm方向与QRS波群一致或在V_1、V_2或V_3导联上ST段压低＞1 mm，有急性心肌梗死的可能。
- 目前ACCF/AHA指南建议发生时间不明确的孤立的LBBB不是诊断AMI的标准，应进一步利用血清标志物水平和直接的心脏检查手段（如心脏超声和有创血管造影）来辅助诊断。
- 附加导联心电图：标准12导联常常遗漏在后部、右侧、高侧壁的梗死：
  - 右侧心电图：
    - 移动V_4导联到右锁骨中线第5肋间，重复做心电图，可以捕捉到右心室的梗死。
    - 右侧心电图，往往是在下壁导联（Ⅱ、Ⅲ、AVF）出现为类似ST抬高性心肌梗死（STEMI）的表现，诊断右心室（RV）梗死。
  - 后心电图：
    - V_7、V_8、V_9导联放置后胸部沿第5肋间腋后线：V_7在腋后线，V_8在肩胛下角，V_9椎旁。
    - 表现在下或侧壁心肌梗死；或如果ST在V_1～V_3导联压低可诊断侧支或左回旋支梗死。
- 心电图在诊断其他原因的胸痛是有帮助的：
  - 广泛ST段抬高伴T波倒置、PR压低考虑为心包炎。
- 肺栓塞会表现为不明原因的心动过速、右心衰竭表现（右心室肥大、右束支传导阻滞、肺性P波）、新发心房颤动，或很少有S1、Q3、T3模式。

诊断检查与说明

实验室检查

- 心脏生物标志物：
  - 如果病史明确可考虑ACS。
  - 稳定型心绞痛不会升高，不稳定型心绞痛也可能是正常的。
- 肌钙蛋白T和I：ACS胸痛发作后2～3 h开始上升，在8～12 h达高峰。并持续升高7～14日：
  - 单一的肌钙蛋白对ACS诊断的灵敏度低（一项关于低危胸痛患者初始肌钙蛋白阴性的研究中，30日内有2.3%的AMI发病率和1%的死亡率）。
  - 生物标志物检测的时机是至关重要的：美国急救医师协会（ACEP）赞同“适度的临床确定性”。如果发病后8～12 h单一肌钙蛋白阴性可以排除AMI。然而，在症状发作的时间不能确定、不可靠的病史和梗死前心绞痛可能仍会利用首次肌钙蛋白作为参考。新的、更敏感的检测手段在未来可能会出现，可以减少复测肌钙蛋白。
  - 轻微的肌钙蛋白升高可能与肾脏发生、结构性心脏病、充血性心力衰竭（急性或慢性）、心脏起搏、肺栓塞、败血症、休克等疾病有关。
  - 标准化检测的缺乏（特别是肌钙蛋白I）是指从一个实验室得到的结果往往总是不能与其他实验室的结果简单地相比较。
- 高敏感性肌钙蛋白现已在美国上市：
  - 非常敏感。
  - 可能允许更快更早地识别出MI。
  - 可能有助于更迅速的治疗。
  - 特定于心肌坏死。
  - MI的适当阈值水平仍有争议。
- CK/CK-MB：比肌钙蛋白敏感率低，发病后上升速度慢。通过肌酸激酶和肌钙蛋白检测所获得的信息较少，肌酸激酶升高有以下可能：
  - 肾衰竭存在（TN不准确）。
  - 最近的心肌梗死。
- 肌红蛋白：上升的速度比标准的肌钙蛋白指标快，从而能够更快的识别AMI，但它的最大敏感性也只有70%。
- B型钠尿肽（BNP）：
  - 心室舒张末期弹力素的释放与合成。
  - 用于检测心力衰竭。
  - 检查结果＞100 pg/ml时诊断心力衰竭的敏感性为90%，特异性为76%。
  - 在诊断明确的ACS患者中BNP的升高意义不大。
- HEART分数是急诊室常用的经过验证的决策工具，可对患者进行分层风险并确定适合急诊室出院的患者。在0和3 h测量肌钙蛋白以识别患者。

影像学检查

- 胸部X线检查：
  - 通常正常。

X

- 可显示心脏肥大。
- 可显示肺水肿。
- 可以识别其他原因的胸痛，如肺炎或加宽主动脉夹层的纵隔。

• 越来越多的数据表明，压力测试在急诊患者的危险分层中应用有限，特别是在 ACS 可能性低的患者中。

• 静息超声心动图：
- 可以识别 ACS 或根据患者室壁运动异常来诊断 AMI，还可以检测泵衰竭和瓣膜异常。
- 静息超声对于 ACS 患者诊断灵敏性为 70%，特异性为 87%。
- 静息超声对急性心肌梗死的敏感性为 93%，特异性为 66%。

• ^{99m}Tc 核素检查：
- 放射性静脉染料作用于心肌，用单光子发射 CT 检测成像（SPECT，又称为心肌灌注显像）。
- 可以在静息时成像并检测到低或无血流区域的心肌，也可以在运动或药物应激后成像。
- 在 2009 年 ACC/AHA 指南中指出，可以作为中高危患者筛查的储备检查。
- 对于 ACS 检查的特异性为 81%，敏感性为 73%。
- 对于 AMI 检查的特异性为 92%，敏感性为 67%。

• CT 冠状动脉造影（CTCA）：
- 评估冠状动脉狭窄和钙沉积的程度。
- 预测值准确性在 97%～100%、精度堪比运动负荷试验。
- 最近 *NEJM* 的文章表明 CTCA 虽然减少了患者在急诊停留时间，但是增加了进一步的检查和辐射暴露，同时并没有降低医疗费用。

• 运动负荷试验（ETT）：
- 可以帮助建立诊断心绞痛，提供预后信息。
- 在 3 次连续的心跳和 2 个相邻导联 ST 段压低 1 mm 的是心肌缺血的特点。
- 早期积极（3 min）的运动负荷试验，对不稳定型心绞痛是弊大于利的。
- 标准 Bruce 负荷超声心动图 6 min 提示预后良好。
- 运动负荷试验与单一的心电图检查敏感性为 68%，特异性为 77%。
- 运动负荷试验与超声检查的敏感性为 85%，特异性为 77%。
- 运动负荷试验与 ^{99m}Tc 核素检查的敏感性为 87%，特异性为 64%。
- 40 岁以下的患者进行心脏压力测试的用途有限。

• 心导管：
- 评估冠状动脉的金标准。
- 最近的心脏造影的检查阴性并不能完全排除急性心肌梗死，如在血管痉挛或使用可卡因的情况下。

诊断步骤/外科

心电图、心肌酶、心脏超声、压力负荷试验。

■ 鉴别诊断

见急性冠状动脉综合征词条。

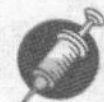

治疗

■ 院前

• 心脏监测。

• 根据医院的心电图：
- 单独对 ACS 的敏感性为 76%，特异性为 88%。
- 单独对急性心肌梗死的敏感性为 68%，特异性为 97%。

■ 初步稳定/治疗

• 心电监测。

• 血氧饱和度。

■ 急诊治疗/程序

• 见"急性冠状动脉综合征：稳定型心绞痛""急性冠状动脉综合征：不稳定型心绞痛""急性冠状动脉综合征：心肌梗死"，有更详细的介绍。

• 心脏检测指南。

• 病史可以提示 ACS：
- 心电图检查和首次肌钙蛋白检查（或其他心脏生物标志物）。

• 心电图或第一肌钙蛋白异常：
- 收住院；心血管病专科咨询。

• 持续胸痛或胸闷：
- 进一步同位素检查或超声检查。
- 考虑连续性心电图监测。

• 同位素、连续心电图或超声异常：
- 收住院或心血管病专科咨询。

• 复测肌钙蛋白（或其他心脏生物标志物）异常：
- 收住院，心血管病专科咨询。

• 辅助测试：
- 对于低到中度风险的患者：标准运动试验（ETT）。
  ◦ 如果低风险的患者有良好的随访性，ACC/AHA 指南允许门诊在 72 h 之内进行运动负荷试验。
  ◦ 2007 年 AHA/ACC 指南提出 CTCA"合理选择"运动负荷试验。
- 对于异常的或不可解释的心电图：负荷超声、核素。
- 患者无法自我管理：药理 ETT（即多巴酚丁胺或双嘧达莫司他比）。
- 辅助测试异常：
  ◦ 心内科咨询或收住院。

■ 药物治疗

患者应该在新的抗心绞痛前进行压力测试。

随访

■ 进一步处理

入院指征

• 病史提示源于心脏病因的胸痛和急诊无法获得的一系列检查。

• 异常或改变的心电图和急诊不能获得的观察指标。

• 心脏生物标志物指标阳性。

• 静息成像阳性。

• 如果诊断不清，住院或急诊观察可以连续检测心脏生物标志物，心电图是非常有用的，并完善进一步辅助检查。

• 早期正应力试验：
- 如果患者负荷试验阳性，办理入院手续应与初级保健医师或心脏病医师联系。

出院指征

• 符合下列标准的患者安全出院：

• 病史提示并非心脏病因的胸部疼痛。

• 正常心电图。

• 心脏检测正常。

■ 随访建议

• 异常运动负荷试验将需要心脏内科或 PCP 密切随访。

• 未明确的 CP，应急诊进行运动负荷试验，除非有明确的后续治疗。

要点和误区

• 正常心电图或酶不能排除 CAD。

• 重复心电图检查或添加心电图导联可以使急性心肌梗死检出灵敏度提高。

• 大多数未明确病因的胸部疼痛的急诊患者需要一些额外的检查。

心脏起搏器 Cardiac Pacemakers

SusanP·Torrey·Ashley L. Deutsch 彭沪 译

基础知识

描述

- 它是一种用足够的电脉冲来收缩心脏肌肉的装置。
- 心脏起搏的方法：
  - 经皮起搏：
    - 2个导联放在患者胸部的前外侧或后下位置。
    - 起搏电流逐渐增加，直至电捕获发生一次脉冲。
    - 作为一种应急治疗直到后续静脉起搏或其他治疗的应用。
  - 经静脉临时起搏：
    - 起搏器导线通过中心静脉进入右心房或右心室(RY)和连接到身体之外的外部发生器。
    - 作为一种过渡，直到永久性心脏起搏器可以放置或病情稳定不再需要一个起搏器。
- 永久性植入心脏起搏器有3个组成部分：
  - 一个电池，提供能源：
    - 锂电池持续7～10年。
  - 起搏器：
    - 一台具有许多可编程参数的精密计算机。
  - 连接到RV/RA的导线：
    - 通常感知心脏的固有电活动并按需带动心肌收缩。
- 心脏起搏器程控：
  - 程控仪放在心脏起搏器脉冲发生器上。
  - 把起搏器调成一固定频率，无论心脏的原始活动如何，该模式都会恢复为恒定的预定速率。
  - 如果看不到有效起搏钉，说明患者自身心率超过了起搏心率。
  - 如果电池耗尽时会导致起搏频率下降约10%。

心脏起搏器术语

- 固定模式：
  - 无论患者的内在的节律如何，起搏器的设置始终为自身固定的发射频率。
  - 很少见到。
- 需求模式：
  - 只有在必要时起搏器才启动。
  - 它可以检测到患者内在的节律。
  - 如果患者内在的节率检测不到或低于一个设定的速度，那它就只有一种节律。
- 传感：
  - 心脏起搏器的一种作用是用来确定心脏是否有自身内在的节律。
- 所有起搏器都可以用5种代码来描述它们的功能。
- 作为急诊治疗的目的，3个字母中只有第一个字母的代码是必要的：
  - 第1个字母代表起搏的心脏。
    - A：为起搏心房。
    - V：为起搏心室。
    - D：为心房心室双腔起搏。
  - 第2个字母代表起搏器能感知的心腔。
    - A：感知心房的激动。
    - V：感知心室的激动。
    - D：心房和心室双腔均感知。
  - 第3个字母表示起搏器感知心脏自身电活动后的反应方式。
    - T：为触发型，即感知心脏自身激动后释放一个刺激脉冲。
    - I：为抑制型，即感知心脏自身激动后起搏器工作受到抑制暂不发放脉冲刺激。
    - D：(或T/I)为既有触发反应又有抑制反应。
    - 0：为无此项功能。
  - 最常见的心脏起搏器VVI(单导)和DDD(两根导线)。
- MRI条件起搏器：
  - 在某些特定条件下显示无已知危害的设备被美国FDA标记为“MRI有条件”。
  - 对于非MRI条件许可的植入性装置，最近显示不经胸的1.5 T MRI具有很宽广的安全范围(即引起金属性植入装置的移位风险)。

病因

- 起搏器相关感染：
  - 心脏起搏器组件的感染常合并感染性心内膜炎。
  - 表皮葡萄球菌感染和金黄色葡萄球菌感染占90%。
  - 食管超声是首选的诊断方法。
- 静脉血栓形成：
  - 非常常见(发生率为30%～50%)。
  - 有症状，急性梗阻少见(3%)。
  - 肺栓塞是少见的。
- 心脏起搏器放电故障：
  - 组件故障是罕见的。
  - 在例行检查中电池耗尽是比较罕见的，一般不会突然发生。
  - 导线断裂或接触不良。
  - 过度感知肌肉活动或外部电气干扰。
- 心脏起搏器未能带动心肌收缩：
  - 导线脱位是常见的。
  - 旋转综合征：
    - 意外操作起搏器造成导线脱出心肌。
  - 心肌阈值升高：
    - 高钾血症。
    - 缺血。
- 心脏(QRS)形态的变化。
- 起搏器介导的心动过速：
  - 发生在双腔起搏器。
  - 使用起搏器和内在的传导系统重新进入另一个节奏。
  - 由于内置保障装置，心率最快通常为140次。
- 起搏器失控：
  - 罕见的，由电池耗尽或组件故障引发。
  - 通常出现快速率(>200次/分)并伴有血流动力学不稳定。

诊断

症状和体征

- 起搏器故障：
  - 心动过缓。
  - 晕厥。
  - 低血压，渐进的冲击和血流动力学崩溃。
  - 疲乏无力。
  - 心力衰竭引起的劳力性呼吸困难或呼吸短促。
  - 缺血性胸痛。
  - 意识水平改变。
- 起搏器引起的心动过速：
  - 呼吸困难。
  - 缺血性胸痛。
  - 头昏。
  - 晕厥。
- 起搏器综合征：
- 非同步心室收缩综合征(典型的VVI起搏器)。
  - 头昏。
  - 呼吸困难。

X

- 心悸。
- 无力或运动耐受。
- 晕厥。

病史

- 安置心脏起搏器的日期。
- 定期随访(电池检查)。
- 起搏器的类型。

体格检查

一般心脏检查:

- 心脏杂音检查。
- 心力衰竭时的肺部检查。
- 胸壁脉冲发射器的检查。

基本检查

- 12 导联心电图可以找到明显的证据来评估起搏器是否有故障。
- 代谢检查以确定所获取的医学症状是否导致心脏阈值的升高。
- 心电图与起搏器程控:
  - 评估程控器频率。
  - 当心电图基线看不到起搏钉时特别有用。
  - 程控器激活异步起搏模式。
  - 按照起搏器预设的速率产生起搏钉,无论患者是否存在自主心率。
  - 如果程控率等于预编程设定速度,说明植入起搏器是好的。
  - 如果程控速率比植入时慢>10%时,说明电池耗尽。
  - 如果没有起搏器的尖峰,有显著起搏器故障。

诊断检查与说明

实验室检查

- 血钾。
- ABG。
- 抗心律失常药物血药浓度。

影像学检查

X线平片:

- 评估起搏器导线的完整性和位置。
- 导线断裂。
- 以下情况可能导致脱落:
  - 中隔穿孔。
  - 导线尖端移动(如在肺动脉)。

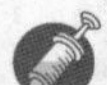

治疗

院前

记录节律条以便分析。

初步稳定/治疗

- 吸氧。
- 必要时给予气管插管。
- 建立静脉通路。
- 高级心脏生命支持药物按通常的治疗方案(尤其是心动过缓)。
- 除颤:避免放置在起搏器上。
- 在起搏器衰竭的患者出现血流动力学不稳定的情况要给予经皮起搏。

急诊治疗/程序

- 起搏器故障:
  - 经皮起搏器。
  - 经静脉临时心脏起搏器:
    - 使用撕开鞘作为中央静脉通路(右锁骨下优先)。
    - 如果可能的话在X线透视下进行操作。
    - 将脉冲发生器设置为异步模式。
    - 调整用所有的方式输出拨号。
    - 通过中心静脉导管推进导管进入心脏直到在监护仪上看见一个QRS波群。
    - 检查股动脉搏动。
    - 如果你发送一个脉冲并可以看到一个QRS波群,那么说明起搏器将其"捕获"。
    - 慢慢将心率下调,直到失去QRS波群(捕获阈值)。
    - 将输出调高至捕获阈值2~3倍。
    - 连续心电图监测有助于将起搏器电极放置在正确位置。
- 高钾血症的治疗(见"高钾血症")。
- 起搏器失控。
  - 房室结阻断或重编程。
  - 在极端的情况,可能需要通过外科手段断开起搏器导线。

药物治疗

腺苷:6 mg,静脉推注。

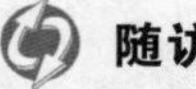

随访

进一步处理

入院指征

- 永久起搏器衰竭或故障。
- 怀疑感染涉及心脏起搏器组件。

出院指征

- 无症状的起搏器故障。
- 心脏专家已经对起搏器进行了校准。

随访建议

涉及心脏病和/或起搏器门诊。

要点和误区

- 总是将心功能失代偿、心动过缓或晕厥作为判断起搏器失效的指标。
- 利用起搏程控器来评估其功能。

心脏停搏

Michael W. Donnino · Brandon Gilerson · Michael N. Cocchi 李家晨 译

基础知识

注意

- 提示:以下信息是根据2015加强心脏生命支持(ACLS)指南(简称2015 ACLS指南)制定的,后续美国心脏协会也并未再做出其他修订。
- 2015 ACLS主要修改内容包括:
  - 从成人心脏停搏算法中去除血管加压素。
  - 潮气末二氧化碳($ETCO_2$)可用于评估心肺复苏质量并检测自发循环(ROSC)。
  - 压缩速率上限为120次/分,压缩深度上限为6 cm(2.4 in),以改善舒张期充盈。
  - 尽管超声的用途尚未得到很好的证实,但如果它不干扰标准ACLS,则可以考虑使用超声。
  - 继续重视心脏停搏后综合征的护理,尤其是实施目标温度管理(TTM)。

描述

• 心脏停搏具有以下特征：
- 呼之不应。
- 脉搏消失。
- 微弱的自主呼吸。
• 影响存活的因素：
- 初始心律。
- 总的"无流量"和"低流量"(CPR)时间。
- 高质量 CPR 的时间。
- 有效除颤的时机(根据迹象)。
- 基础生命支持干预措施的时机。

病因

心搏骤停的潜在可逆原因("5 Hs 和 Ts")：
• 血容量减少。
• 缺氧。
• H^+ 离子(酸中毒)。
• 低钾血症或者高钾血症。
• 体温过低。
• 毒素，包括：
- 钙通道阻滞剂、β受体阻滞剂、地高辛。
- 三环抗抑郁药。
- 阿片类、可卡因。
• 心脏压塞。
• 张力性气胸。
• 血栓形成。
• 创伤。

儿科注意事项

• 儿童的突发心脏停搏往往是呼吸相关的而不是心脏病因。
• 根据目前 ACLS 指南关于儿科心脏停搏、成人与儿童的措施区别包括：
- 儿童的心脏按压深度应该是胸部深度的1/3～1/2。
- 在两个人进行心肺复苏时建议 15∶2 的按压呼吸比。
- 婴儿应使用两指环绕手法进行心肺复苏。
- 药物剂量的区别见用药章节。

妊娠注意事项

根据目前 ACLS 指南关于心脏停搏的孕妇的措施：
• 注意气道开放是相对困难的。
• 胸外按压应当比传统心肺复苏位置更高，要略高于胸骨的中心。
• 根据成人的 ACLS 指南实行除颤。
• 在心搏骤停之前或者之后，应当保持左侧卧位；在心脏停搏时手动使子宫向左偏移。
• 为了确保最好的胎儿预后，所有的治疗都必须有利于母亲的生存。
• 紧急情况下预先准备。
- 假设没有产妇的 ROSC，应在逮捕后 4 min 考虑采用此程序，以优化产妇和胎儿的预后。

诊断

症状和体征

• 呼之不应。
• 脉搏消失。
• 呼吸变浅，喘息样呼吸可能会持续数分钟。
• 偶尔心脏停搏之前会有：
- 胸痛。
- 呼吸困难。
- 心悸。
- 癫痫发作。
• 在心脏停搏之前即刻存在：
- 休克或者低血压。
- 不良的心理状态。

基本检查

• 评估循环、气道、呼吸。
• 依据指南判断可电击复律心律或不可电击复律心律，以及相应的治疗措施。

诊断检查与说明

监测

• 心脏监测和除颤器电极，可立即评估心律。
• 潮气末二氧化碳/波形二氧化碳图。
- $ETCO_2>10$ mmHg 表示高质量的心肺复苏。
- $ETCO_2>30$ mmHg 与 ROSC 有关。
- 在 20 min 时 $ETCO_2<10$ mmHg 是一个不良的预后因素，可以作为终止努力的一个因素。

实验室检查

需要指出的是，仅仅当自主循环恢复时才可以进行。
• 电解质、尿素氮/肌酐。
• 肌酸激酶和同工酶、肌钙蛋白。
• 动脉血气。
• 全血。
• 治疗药物水平。
• 毒物测定。
• 乳酸水平。

影像学检查

• 心电图：急性冠状动脉综合征或 ST 段抬高心肌梗死。
• 胸部 X 线片：
- 气管插管位置。
- 气胸。
- 肺源性心脏停搏。
• 超声心动图：
- 心包积液。
- 急性心包积液导致右心衰竭。
- 异常的室壁运动。
- 瓣膜功能障碍。
• 头颅 CT 扫描(复苏后)：
- 排除出血/神经因素。

诊断步骤/外科

• 可能的心脏病因：
- 心导管检查。
- 可能增加心输出量装置的安装。
• 脑电图(复苏后)：
- 鉴别和治疗癫痫。

鉴别诊断

突然出现的动脉压力持续降低。
• 晕厥。
• 癫痫。
• 脑卒中(中风)。
• 低血糖。
• 急性呼吸道梗阻。
• 头颅创伤。
• 中毒。

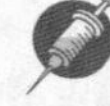

治疗

院前

• 立刻进行标准的心肺复苏。
• 确认不明确的心律。
• 室速或室颤的早期电除颤。
• 保证气道通畅及提供足够的呼吸，如果所处地点会打断基础生命支持治疗，高级别气道开放可以被延后。
• 如果可能发生阿片类药物中毒，可以考虑经验性使用纳洛酮。
• 打开呼吸道并提供足够的呼吸。如果放置中断基础生命支持措施，则应推迟开放气道。
• 复苏后治疗：
- 确认停搏病因。
- 12 导联心电图。
- 心电监测。
- 循环药物和/或低血压时使用升压药物。
• 转运至最近的能够处理复苏后病患的医疗机构。

- 考虑转运到具有心脏介入治疗和特殊复苏后治疗的医疗中心。
- 儿童应当去儿科重症监护室。

初步稳定/治疗

• 高级生命支持。
• 只要脉搏完全不能触及，进行高质量的心肺复苏。
- 医疗救援系统激活启动后立即开始心肺复苏。
- 每分钟 100～120 次胸外按压。
- 至少 2 in(5 cm)的深度。
- 两次按压之间保证胸壁完全回弹。
- 除非进行除颤和心律/脉搏检查，否则切勿停止心肺复苏，这些检查措施的时间应少于 10 s。
- 在可能的情况下，在每次心律检查之前更换按压者，以免按压者疲劳。
- 如果可用，电子反馈设备有助于提供高质量的心肺复苏。
- 在机械心肺复苏设备可能是有限医护人员条件下合理的辅助手段，但不应视为常规救治流程。
• 保证气道通畅。
• 获得静脉/骨髓腔通路。
- 如果预计难以建立静脉通路，立即开设骨髓腔通路；否则应在两次静脉尝试之后立即建立骨髓腔通路。
• 心电监测和连续 $ETCO_2$。
- 根据 ACLS 协议，根据当时的心脏节律进行。
• 对于具有机械循环支持的患者(心室辅助设备，VAD)。
- 通知患者的 VAD 临床医师，并根据需要计划转诊。
- 评估是否有足够的灌注；如果灌注不足：
  ◦ 确认 VAD 是否正常运行；如果 VAD 无法正常运行，请重新启动或启动标准 CPR 和 ACLS(包括通过胸前区除颤电极的电除颤)。
  ◦ 如果 VAD 功能正常但灌注不足，评估 MAP 和 $ETCO_2$。
    ▪ 如果 MAP＞50 或 $ETCO_2$＞20 mmHg，立即开始高级生命支持而无需心肺复苏。
    ▪ 如果 MAP≤50 或 $ETCO_2$≤20 mmHg，立即开始包括心肺复苏在内的高级生命支持。

急诊治疗/程序

• 无脉的室速或者室颤。
- 立即予以电除颤。
  ◦ 电能选择根据电除颤的类型来选择双相(未知选择 200 J)或单相 360 J。
  ◦ 第二次和以后的剂量应该相等，可以考虑使用更高的剂量。
- 如果电除颤未成功，持续心肺复苏 2 min 后重新评估心律。当静脉通路建立后及第二次心律检查后需要考虑：
  ◦ 肾上腺素。
  ◦ 如果对除颤和肾上腺素难治，请考虑：胺碘酮。
  ◦ 用于治疗尖端扭转性心律失常的镁剂。
• 心脏停搏：
- 确认依据≥2 条线索。
- 肾上腺素。
- 针对可逆原因进行治疗。
• 无动脉性电活动：
- 肾上腺素。
- 治疗可逆性原因导致的无动脉搏动的电活动/心脏停搏。
• 复苏后：
- 治疗潜在病因导致的骤停。
- 心电图监测急性冠状动脉综合征。
  ◦ 立即介入治疗 ST 段抬高心肌梗死。
  ◦ 对于可疑的没有 STEMI 的心脏疾病可以考虑介入治疗。
- 机械通气。
- 纠正电解质紊乱。
- 启动容量复苏，以及提供根据需要使用血管加压及调节肌力药物。
- 对于合适患者予以有针对性的体温管理。
- 持续的脑电图来排除癫痫。

药物治疗

给药过程中不应中断心肺复苏。
• 胺碘酮：300 mg(儿童：5 mg/kg 至最大剂量 15 mg/kg)，静脉推注。
• 肾上腺素：1 mg(儿童：0.01 mg/kg)，静脉推注，q3～5 min。
• 利多卡因：在儿童患者只推荐 1 mg/kg 静脉推注，然后 20～50 μg/min 静脉滴注。
• 镁剂：1～2 g(儿童：25～50 mg/kg，最大剂量 2 g)，静脉慢推。
• 碳酸氢钠：1 mmol/kg(儿童：1 mmol/kg)，静脉慢推。

随访

进一步处理

入院指征

自主循环恢复：
• 重症监护室。
• 复苏后监护。
• 潜在骤停病因的治疗。

出院指征

无。

转诊问题

可以考虑转往地区心搏骤停急救中心。

随访建议

进入监护室。

要点和误区

• 在骤停后昏迷患者提供有效的体温管理。
• 预料可能反复发作的心搏骤停及提供近期监测和适当的复苏后治疗，包括液体和血管加压。
• 获得心脏介入治疗结论来决定患者是否是心脏介入候选者。

X

心脏移植术后并发症 Cardiac Transplantation Complications

Jarrod Mosier · Samuel M. Keim 彭沪 译

 基础知识

▪ 描述

• 心脏移植患者是一类独特的人群，他们罹患心肌缺血、心脏衰竭的风险可以等同于免疫力低下患者。

• 在美国每年有 1 900～2 300 人进行心脏移植。

• 1 年生存率为 85%～90%，5 年生存率约为 75%。

• 2004—2015 年，小儿移植数量增加了 37%。

• 典型的免疫抑制疗法是一种"三联疗法"，通常包括类固醇。

• 拒绝评估：

- 最初使用频繁的活检。
- 经常在儿童中使用的超声心动图。

• 并发症最常发生在心脏移植术后 1～6 周。

老年人注意事项

• 老年患者在等待移植的比例，以及接受移植的比例都在增加。

• 由于免疫系统的变化，随着年龄的增长，老年移植受者出现危及生命的感染和急性排斥反应的风险增加。

妊娠注意事项

• 心脏移植后妊娠是越来越普遍。在 1988—2010 年，有 63 名妇女接受心脏或心肺移植。有 108 人妊娠，所有的都是活产婴儿。

• 最常见的并发症包括高血压、先兆子痫和排斥反应。

• 心脏移植的患者由于妊娠引起的生理变化并不增加心力衰竭的发生。

• 特别应注意的是，这些患者的排斥反应和感染使机体产生免疫抑制。

▪ 病因

• 排斥反应：

- 超急性排斥反应。
  - ◦ 发生在刚移植几分钟内。
  - ◦ 罕见的，由于 ABO 血型或受体/供体，其他主要的不相容性。
  - ◦ 反应强烈和立即致命的移植。
- 急性排斥反应：
  - ◦ 淋巴细胞浸润及心肌细胞的破坏。
  - ◦ 在最初 1～6 周最常见。
  - ◦ 随时可能发生。
  - ◦ 移植后第 1 年的发病率为 23%。
- 慢性排斥反应：
  - ◦ 肝纤维化与移植物血管病。
  - ◦ 长期并发症。
  - ◦ 不能完全解释的病因。
  - ◦ 没有有效的治疗。

• 移植心脏血管病：

- 等同于增加了心脏冠状动脉疾病的发生。
- 限制长期生存率，引起死亡的主要原因多发生在移植 1 年后。

• 免疫介导的动脉粥样硬化。

- 慢性排斥的形式。

• 感染：

- 第 1 个月。
  - ◦ 在这个高风险的时间段细菌感染是最常见的死亡原因。
  - ◦ 肺炎(假单胞菌、军团菌肺炎、其他革兰阴性菌)。
  - ◦ 纵隔炎。
  - ◦ 伤口感染。
  - ◦ 尿路感染。
- 第 1 年。
  - ◦ 机会和传统的感染。
  - ◦ 巨细胞病毒(巨细胞病毒)感染。
  - ◦ 单纯疱疹病毒(HSV)感染。
  - ◦ 军团菌感染。
  - ◦ 真菌感染。
  - ◦ 肺孢子菌感染。

• 药物毒性：

- 环孢素、新山地明(第二代环孢素、他克莫司)：
  - ◦ 肾毒性(发病率为 30%)。
  - ◦ 肝毒性。
  - ◦ 神经毒性。
  - ◦ 高脂血症、糖尿病。
- 硫唑嘌呤、霉酚酸酯：
  - ◦ 骨髓抑制。
  - ◦ 白细胞减少症。
- 西罗莫司：
  - ◦ 高脂血症。
  - ◦ 创伤愈合。
- 类固醇：
  - ◦ 骨质疏松症。
  - ◦ 库欣病。

• 肿瘤：

- 辅助免疫抑制。
- 比普通人群多 10～100 倍。
- 皮肤癌和唇癌。
- 淋巴瘤。
- 卡波西肉瘤。
- 实体器官肿瘤。

儿科注意事项

• 如果患者没有使用类固醇，败血症的风险类似于一般人群。

• 肺炎的发生率高。

• 患者对类固醇可能不会显示脑膜刺激征。

诊断

▪ 症状和体征

• 急性排斥反应：

- 以非特异性症状为主，因为心脏通常为失神经支配。
- 乏力。
- 呼吸困难。
- 低热。
- 恶心。
- 呕吐。
- 可能是难以区分的感染和急性排斥反应。

• 心力衰竭：

- 呼吸急促。
- 啰音。
- 缺氧。
- S3。
- 杂音。
- 水肿。

• 同种异体移植血管病变：

- 最早出现在移植后 3 个月(5 年后的发生率为 20%～50%)。
- 失神经支配的心脏心中不会出现典型的心绞痛。
- 潜在发作。
  - ◦ 乏力。
  - ◦ 咳嗽。
  - ◦ 呼吸困难。
- 急性发作。
  - ◦ 心力衰竭。
  - ◦ 猝死。
  - ◦ 梗死。

• 感染(机会感染和常规感染)：

- 发热。

X

- 皮肤损伤(带状疱疹)。
- 巨细胞病毒。
  ◦ 轻度(流感样病例)。
  ◦ 发热。
  ◦ 恶心。
  ◦ 不适。
  ◦ 肺炎(13%～50%的死亡率)。
  ◦ 肝炎。
  ◦ 胃肠炎。
  ◦ 严重的白细胞减少症。

儿科注意事项

• 对于移植后淋巴组织增生性疾病与 EB 病毒血清学转换的风险更高。

• 像成人一样,存在移植血管病变及其相关的心肌缺血风险。

基本检查

• 评估排斥反应、心脏功能障碍、梗死的迹象:
- 心电图。
- 心肌酶。
- 胸部 X 线检查。
- 超声心动图。

• 如果出现排斥需要活检,咨询移植团队。

儿科注意事项

正常监测体温+胸部 X 线检查和心电图;如果使用类固醇,LP 检查。

诊断检查与说明

实验室检查

• 电解质:
- 环孢素效应:
  ◦ 增加血尿素氮、肌酐水平。
  ◦ 高钾血症。
  ◦ 代谢性酸中毒。
  ◦ 低钠血症。

• 全血细胞计数:
- 相关的嗜酸性粒细胞增多可能抑制感染。

• 若发热行血培养与尿培养。

• 如果发作癫痫、精神状态改变或严重的头痛行腰椎穿刺检查。

• BNP(预计水平较高)。

• 巨细胞病毒抗体滴度。

• 尿抗原测试。

• 环孢素谷浓度。

影像学检查

• 心电图:
- 心动过速。
- 心电总电压降低 20%(不敏感)。
- 注意失神经心脏正常窦性节律为 90～110 次/分。
- 根据移植的手术技术,可以看到 2 个 P 波(受体和供体心脏):
- 受体心脏的 P 波不符合伪随机信号。

• 胸部 X 线片:
- 心脏肿大。
- 肺水肿。
- 胸腔积液。
- 与既往比较(健康的供体心脏可能出现大的心脏移植到小的受体中)。

• 超声心动图:
- 减少二尖瓣减速时间。
- 初始舒张功能障碍。
- 双心室扩大。
- 二尖瓣、三尖瓣反流。

鉴别诊断

• 抑制。
• 感染。
• 缺血的影响。
• 巨细胞病毒(CMV)。
• 病毒性疾病。
• 恶性肿瘤。
• 环孢素毒性。

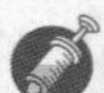

治疗

院前

那些心脏移植的患者不应该使用腺苷,它的影响可能是长期和不可预知的。

初步稳定/治疗

• 开通静脉通路。
• 吸氧。
• 心电监测。
• 气管插管。
• 除颤和起搏。
• 升压药的使用。
• 心律失常:
- 高级生命支持。
- 阿托品对心动过缓无明显效果,应该使用异丙肾上腺素。

急诊治疗/程序

• 血流动力学显著抑制情况下:
- 甲泼尼龙。
- 可能还需要 OKT3 或其他抗 T 细胞抗体治疗。

• 梗死性血管病变:
- 阿司匹林。
- 肝素。
- 可能的血管成形术。
- 很可能需要再次移植。

• 巨细胞病毒:
- 经验性静脉使用更昔洛韦。

• 单纯疱疹病毒。
- 口服或静脉注射阿昔洛韦。

• 腹泻:
- 血清学培养查找巨细胞病毒感染。

• 没有来源的发热:
- 咨询传染病或移植团队。

• 头痛。
- 扫描和腰椎穿刺的阈值应为低(脑膜炎、脓肿)。

• 重病、创伤、手术:
- 类固醇作用暴发。
- 限制非甾体抗炎药的使用是为降低环孢素和他克莫司的引起的肾功能不全的风险。

药物治疗

• 阿昔洛韦:5～10 mg/kg,静脉注射,q8 h,计算剂量根据理想体重;生殖器疱疹:400 mg,口服,每日 3 次,持续 7～10 日;水痘:20 mg/kg,最大剂量 800 mg,口服,每日 4 次,持续 5 日。

• 头孢曲松钠:50 mg/kg,静脉注射,q12～24 h。

• 环孢素、他克莫司、西罗莫司、硫唑嘌呤、霉酚酸酯:每个移植团队不同。

• 更昔洛韦 5 mg/kg,静脉推注,每日 2 次,持续 2～3 周(根据肾功能调整)。

• 异丙肾上腺素:1～4 μg/min,根据病情调整滴率;最大剂量 10 μg/min。

• 甲泼尼龙:1 g,静脉注射;儿童:10 mg/kg。

• OKT3、达利珠单抗或其他抗体治疗:每个移植团队可能有所不同。

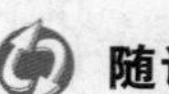

随访

进一步处理

入院指征

• 血流动力学明显排斥反应。
• 血管病变缺血。
• 新节律紊乱。
• 控制不佳的高血压。
• 充血性心力衰竭。
• 呼吸困难。
• 缺氧。
• 成人或儿童使用类固醇的温度>38 ℃。

• 疑似巨细胞病毒（不明原因的发热、肠胃炎或间质性肺炎）。
• 不能耐受口服药物。
• 晕厥。

出院指征

• 轻度排斥反应。
• 与移植团队协商。
• 非毒性儿童的发热：
- 不要给儿童使用应激剂量的类固醇。

心脏杂音 Heart Murmur

Matthew R. Babineau 刘雪峰 译

基础知识

描述

• 心脏瓣膜或血管异常引起的心音异常。
• 收缩期杂音常见于成人（15%～44%）和儿童（80%～96%）。
• 狭窄性病变：
- 房室肥厚：多因瓣膜狭窄致房室收缩阻力增加而产生适应性变化。
• 反流性病变：
- 房室扩张：多因瓣膜关闭不全而出现血液反流导致容量负荷增加所致。
• 遗传性疾病：
- 心脏先天性病变：多引起反常的心脏内血液流动。

病因

• 主动脉瓣狭窄：
- 风湿性心脏病。
- 钙化。
- 人工瓣膜。
• 主动脉瓣关闭不全：
- 风湿性心脏病。
- 心内膜炎。
- 主动脉夹层。
- 人工瓣膜。
• 二尖瓣狭窄：
- 风湿性心脏病。
- 风湿病（系统性红斑狼疮）。
- 钙化。
- 心脏占位病变（心房黏液瘤）。
- 先天性病变。
- 人工瓣膜。
• 急性二尖瓣反流：
- 心内膜炎。
- 乳头肌破裂。
- 腱索断裂。
- 人工瓣膜。
• 慢性二尖瓣反流：
- 风湿性心脏病。
- 二尖瓣脱垂。
- 结缔组织病（马方综合征）。
• 二尖瓣脱垂：
- 先天性病变。
- 结缔组织病。
• 三尖瓣狭窄：
- 风湿性心脏病。
• 三尖瓣反流：
- 风湿性心脏病。
- 心内膜炎。
- 肺动脉高压。
• 心包摩擦音：
- 心包炎。
- 心包积液。
• 室间隔缺损：
- 先天性。
- 创伤性。
- 梗死后。
• 心室辅助装置：
- 植入泵辅助或替代心室功能。

儿科注意事项

• 肺动脉狭窄：
- 先天性。
- 母体中感染风疹。
- 风湿性心脏病。
• 肺动脉反流：
- 先天性。
- 风湿性心脏病。
- 肺动脉高压。
• 房间隔缺损：
- 先天性。
• 动脉导管未闭：
- 先天性。
- 早产儿。
- 母体中感染风疹。
• 主动脉狭窄：
- 先天性。
- 特纳综合征。
• 肥厚型心肌病与特发性主动脉瓣下狭窄：
- 先天性。
- 遗传因素。

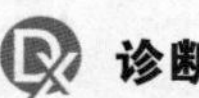

诊断

症状和体征

• 主动脉瓣狭窄：
- 心脏收缩期向颈动脉传导的递增递减型杂音。
- 颈动脉可触及抬举样搏动。
- 心绞痛。
- 劳力性呼吸困难。
- 运动性晕厥。
• 主动脉瓣关闭不全：
- 胸骨左缘可闻及舒张期吹风样杂音。
- 肺水肿。
- 呼吸困难。
- 心动过速。
- 胸痛。
- 脉压增大。
- Austin-Flint 杂音：舒张期隆隆样杂音。
- 水冲脉：按压桡动脉呈现骤起骤落的搏动。
- 毛细血管搏动征：加压于甲床可见毛细血管搏动。
- 点头征：头部随着颈动脉搏动而摆动。
• 二尖瓣狭窄：
- 舒张期隆隆样杂音。
- 第一心音亢进和开瓣音。
- 呼吸困难。
- 端坐呼吸。
- 咯血。
- 肺水肿。
- 体循环栓塞。
- 心房颤动。
• 急性二尖瓣反流：
- 收缩期粗糙的递增递减型杂音。
- 肺水肿。
• 慢性二尖瓣反流：
- 向腋窝放射的全收缩期杂音。
- 劳力性呼吸困难。

X

- 乏力。
- 心房颤动。
• 二尖瓣脱垂：
- 早期可闻及收缩中期喀喇音，之后紧跟收缩期杂音。
- 心悸。
- 胸痛。
• 三尖瓣狭窄：
- 舒张期高调杂音。
- 外周性水肿。
- 肝脾大。
- 腹水。
- 乏力。
- 心房颤动。
- 巨大的颈静脉 A 波。
• 三尖瓣反流：
- 胸骨左缘全收缩期吹风样杂音。
- 外周性水肿。
- 肝脾大。
- 腹水。
- 心房颤动。
- 巨大的颈静脉 V 波。
• 动脉导管未闭：
- 连续性机械样杂音。
- 充血性心力衰竭。
• 心包摩擦音：
- 断断续续的杂音。
- 心脏收缩期和/或舒张期可闻及。
• 室间隔缺损：
- 粗糙的全收缩期杂音，胸骨左下缘最为明显。
• 心室辅助装置：
- 心尖部机械杂音。
- 连续性或脉冲性。
- 在保证灌注的情况下可能出现脉搏和血压无法测量。

儿科注意事项

• 肺动脉狭窄：
- 胸骨左上缘收缩期递增-递减型喷射样杂音。
- 严重者可触及震颤。
- 第二心音分裂。
- 病情严重时出现呼吸困难。
- 可有右心衰竭体征。
• 肺动脉反流：
- 舒张早期高调的递减的杂音。
- 第二心音分裂。
- 可关联肺动脉高压的 Graham-Steel 杂音（舒张早期的高调杂音）。
- 可有右心衰竭表现。
• 房间隔缺损：
- 与缺损大小有关的收缩期喷射样杂音。
- 与肺动脉高压有关。
- 第二心音固定分裂。
- 卵圆孔未闭无杂音。
• 动脉导管未闭：
- 胸骨左上缘连续性机器样杂音，伴有收缩期震颤。
- 发绀。
- 周围血管搏动增强。
- 呼吸急促。
• 主动脉瓣狭窄：
- 连续性或收缩晚期杂音。
- 杂音可能与二叶式主动脉瓣有关。
- 上下肢动脉波动强弱不同。
• 肥厚型心肌病与特发性主动脉瓣下狭窄：
- 胸骨左缘可闻及收缩期递增-递减型杂音。
- 做 Valsalva 动作时杂音增强。
- 呼吸困难。
- 胸痛。
- 运动性晕厥。
- 猝死。

体格检查

• 体格检查对心脏瓣膜病的检测具有较高的敏感性（70%）和特异性（98%）。
• 心肺听诊。
• 对杂音应进行评估：音量最大的位置、级别、时间、持续时间、辐射和有无刺激。
• 等级由Ⅰ级（几乎听不见）至Ⅳ级（用听诊器从胸部取下也可听见）。
• 外周动脉搏动及灌注、组织水肿。

基本检查

更多细节详见心脏瓣膜病、二尖瓣脱垂、先天性心脏病、动脉导管未闭、心包炎、心包积液/心脏压塞。

诊断检查与说明

影像学检查

• 心电图。
• X 线胸片。
• 超声：
- 评估瓣膜、腔室、流量。
- 经训练的医务人员使用时，床旁 Ecrlo 具有很高的灵敏度。
- Ecrlo 应保留给那些有相关心肺症状或高度怀疑有结构性心脏病的人。
• CT：
- 排除主动脉夹层。

诊断步骤/外科

急性反流性病变：心导管检查。

鉴别诊断

• 功能性杂音：
- 收缩期杂音，无明显瓣膜或其他心脏结构疾病。
- 强度和持续时间有助于与病理杂音区分。

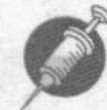

治疗

院前

• 静脉输液：
- 重度主动脉瓣狭窄患者对液体治疗的反应非常敏感，需注意补液量。
• 吸氧。

初步稳定/治疗

• 吸氧。
• 建立静脉通道。
• 心电监护。
• 对症治疗（充血性心力衰竭、心律异常）。
• 对于主动脉瓣狭窄患者的液体和药物治疗需要谨慎。

急诊治疗/程序

更多细节详见心内膜炎、心脏瓣膜病、二尖瓣脱垂、先天性心脏病、动脉导管未闭、心包炎、心包积液/心脏压塞。

药物治疗

• 地高辛：0.5 mg，静脉注射，6～12 h 后可再次予 0.25 mg 静脉滴注。
• 地尔硫䓬（恬尔心）：
- 0.25 mg/kg，静脉注射，持续时间 2 min 以上。
- 15 min 后予以 0.35 mg/kg，静脉滴注。
- 初始输注速度为 5～15 mg/h。
• 呋塞米（速尿）：
- 20～80 mg，静脉注射，如果必要可再增加剂量。
- 24 h 最大剂量为 600 mg。
• 肝素：
- 80 U/kg，静脉注射，之后 18 U/(kg · h) 滴注。
- 监测部分凝血活酶时间。
• 美托洛尔：5 mg，静脉注射，如患者可耐受，必要时可给予总共使用 3 次。
• 硝酸甘油：
- 10～20 μg/min，静脉注射。

- 按照血压调节滴速。
- 最大剂量为300 μg/min。
• 硝普钠：
- 0.3 g/(kg·min)，静脉注射。
- 按照血压调节滴速。
- 最大剂量为10 μg/(kg·min)。
- 避光输注。
- 长时间使用会导致患者体内硫氰酸堆积引起中毒。
• 普萘洛尔：
- 1～3 mg，静脉注射，2～5 min推注完毕，累计剂量不超过5 mg。
- 症状缓解或达到最大剂量后4 h内不宜再次使用。

随访

进一步处理

入院指征

• 心肌缺血症状。
• 晕厥。
• 肺水肿。
• 血流动力学不稳定。
• 心内膜炎。
• 心律不齐。

出院指征

• 临床症状消失。
• 血流动力学稳定。

转诊问题

新发心脏杂音的患者应告知家庭医师或心脏科医师。

随访建议

• 患者应告知家庭医师或口腔医师自身的心脏杂音。
• 避免感染心内膜炎，在洁牙之类的治疗前可给予抗生素。

要点和误区

新发心脏杂音并伴有发热的患者需要考虑心内膜炎。

心脏再灌注治疗 Reperfusion Therapy，Cardiac

Adam S. Kaye · Shamai A. Grossman 袁晓伟 童朝阳 译

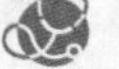

基础知识

描述

• 心脏再灌注治疗适用于ST段抬高型心肌梗死(STEM)患者。
• 对于不稳定型心绞痛(UA)/非ST段抬高型心肌梗死(NSTEMI)可采用经皮冠状动脉介入疗法而非纤溶剂。
• 纤维蛋白溶解疗法：
- 无法在＜120 min内进行PCI的STEMI患者可行此方法，降低发病率和致死率。
- 纤溶药开始得越早，挽救的心肌就越多。
- 在无施行PCI条件或延误＞120 min时采用纤维蛋白溶解疗法的诊疗时间为30 min。
• PCI：
- 导管室中可经气囊膨胀、支架放置、血栓移除来牵张血管壁，部分除去血管内、中、外膜，使管腔及异常血管扩张，恢复心脏外膜冠状动脉血流。
- STEMI初诊PCI诊疗时间为90 min，如果在非PCI中心应＜120 min。
- 经皮腔内冠状动脉成形术(PTCA)中支架放置降低了早期及晚期管腔直径的减小程度。
- 相比纤溶剂，PCI更能促使心肌梗死患者冠状动脉通畅和溶栓，降低死亡率和致病率。
- 相比纤溶剂有更低的出血风险。
- PCI不仅具有诊断性，同时具有治疗性。
- NSTEMI后第一个48 h内强烈建议与心内科医师会诊后进行PCI。
• 糖蛋白Ⅱb/Ⅲa抑制剂：
- 抗血小板药物与血小板受体糖蛋白Ⅱb/Ⅲa结合来抑制血小板聚集。
- 降低PCI术后死亡率和梗死再发率，在初步施行PCI时合理使用。
- STEMI患者不能使用，除非即将进行PCI。
• 普通肝素(UFH)和低分子量肝素(LMWH)：
- 合并阿司匹林、氯吡格雷、纤溶剂、糖蛋白Ⅱb/Ⅲa抑制剂和PCI的附加治疗。
- STEMI(使用PCI或纤溶剂)或UA/NSTEMI患者均可使用UFH或LMWH进行抗凝治疗。
• 无论是否进行PCI或再灌注治疗，氯吡格雷或普拉格雷应作为标准疗法。
• 他汀类药物治疗可降低有稳定型冠状动脉疾病患者的发病率。它也可应用于急性冠状动脉缺血的患者。
• 心搏骤停后患者在进行PCI之前或PCI过程中进行亚低温治疗。

病因

• 由心外膜冠状动脉血管阻塞造成的STEMI通常是由血栓形成导致的。
• UA/NSTEMI是由冠状动脉部分阻塞造成的，同样由血栓导致。

诊断

症状和体征

• 胸痛、沉重或压迫感。
• 呼吸急促。
• 手臂、颈部、背部疼痛。
• 乏力、疲劳。
• 恶心、呕吐。
• 出汗。
• 心悸。
• 头晕或晕厥。
• STEMI心电图。

基本检查

• 评估施行纤溶或PCI的治疗窗时病史很重要。
• 心电图：
- 50%是正常的。
- 如果可以，应与既往记录相对比，可能短时间内变化，应反复做心电图。
- 在至少2个相邻导联中有新ST段在J点抬高，V_2～V_3导联＞2 mm(男)或＞1.5 mm(女)和/或在其他相邻胸导联或肢体导联抬高＞1 mm(0.1 mV)并排除左心室肥大或左束支传导阻滞(LBBB)。
- 既往新发或可能新发的左束支传导阻滞等同于STEMI。很多病例就诊时有LBBB，但“不一定是陈旧的”，因为无法与既往心电图相比较。

X

- 新发或可能新发的 LBBB 在就诊时发作频繁，可能干扰 ST 段分析，如果没有 ACS 临床表现时不能仅仅因此诊断为急性心肌梗死（MI）。推荐使用 Sgarbossa 标准来明确诊断。

- 除了 LBBB 以外的心电图基线异常（如起搏节律、左心房肥大、Brugada 综合征）可能影响诊断。

- 新发的 ST 段改变或 T 波倒置可能是 UA 或非 Q 波型梗死。

- ST 段压低 1 mm，J 点升高 80 ms，是 UA 或非 Q 波型梗死的特征性改变。

• 胸部 X 线检查：可能有助于评估其他诊断，包括主动脉夹层或气胸，但不是必要性的。

• 粪隐血试验：有助于诊断，应早期抗凝治疗。

诊断检查与说明

实验室检查

• 首选心肌酶、肌钙蛋白。

• 初步检查应包括肌酐、血细胞比容和凝血功能。

鉴别诊断

• 主动脉夹层。
• 胆绞痛。
• 冠状动脉瘤。
• 肋软骨炎。
• 食管痉挛。
• 食管反流。
• 食管裂孔疝。
• 高钾血症。
• 精神症状。
• 心包炎。
• 肺炎。
• 肺栓塞。
• 室壁瘤。

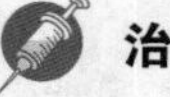

治疗

院前

• 建立静脉通路。

• 心电监测。

• 阿司匹林 162 mg 或 325 mg。

• 如果缺氧，给予吸氧。

• 除非低血压、右心室梗死或者近期 PDE-5 抑制剂，如 sildenafil 或 tadalafil，舌下含服硝酸甘油缓解症状。

• 当地 EMS 系统和医院系统应优先把 STEMI 患者送往能做 PCI 的医院。

• 争议：

- 是否允许 EMS 主动置管及使用纤溶剂。

> **注意**
>
> • 所有的胸痛均应经治疗或作为可能威胁生命的紧急事件送医。
>
> • 纤溶剂和糖蛋白Ⅱb/Ⅲa 抑制剂目前不是标准治疗方法。

初步稳定/治疗

• 静脉置管。
• 吸氧。
• 心电监测。
• 氧饱和度。
• 持续血压脉搏血氧监测。
• 硝酸盐。
• 心脏停搏后亚低温治疗。

急诊治疗/程序

• 阿司匹林。

• 氯吡格雷。

• 纤溶剂治疗 STEMI。

- 除非有禁忌证。

- 如果 120 min 内无法进行 PCI。

• PCI 是首选的，因为它都是诊断的，并提供了更好的治疗方法，用于 STEMI 和 UA/NSTEM。

• PCI 和纤溶治疗需联合 UFH 或 LMWH，如依诺肝素或比伐卢定。

• LMWH：

- 药物动力学可知。

- 无需监测。

- 低出血率。

- 在治疗急性冠状动员脉综合征时至少和 UFH 有同样疗效。

• 糖蛋白Ⅱb/Ⅲa 抑制剂。

• 抗凝血酶类：

- 如果有肝素诱发的血小板减少症病史则使用比伐卢定。

药物治疗

• 阿司匹林：162～325 mg，口服，非肠溶包衣。

• 氯吡格雷（波立维）：300～600 mg，口服；75 mg，口服，每日 1 次。

• 普拉格雷：60 mg 口服负载，10 mg，口服，每日 1 次。

- 有 TIA/卒中病史者禁用。

• 替格雷洛：180 mg 口服；90 mg，口服，每日 2 次。

• 糖蛋白Ⅱb/Ⅲa 抑制剂：

- 阿昔单抗（reoPro）：仅用于 PCI 前；0.25 mg/kg 静脉注射；0.125 μg/(kg · min)，至多 10 μg/min 持续 12 h。

- 依替巴肽(integrilin)：180 μg/kg 于 1～2 min 内静脉注射，随后持续以 2 μg/(kg · min)（最大剂量 15 mg/h）速度静脉滴注，至多 72 h。

- tirofiban (aggrastat)：0.4 μg/(kg · min) 持续 30 min，随后 0.1 μg/(kg · min) 持续 48～108 h。

• 肝素 60 U/kg 静脉注射注入（最大剂量 4 000 U），然后 12 U/(kg · h)（最大剂量 1 000 U/h）必须调整目标 APTT。

• 伊诺肝素（lovenox）：（如果 STEMI 患者年龄<75 岁，给予 30 mg 静脉注射）1 mg/kg 皮下注射 q12 h，请参阅额外的老年患者和肾功能障碍的指导指南。

• 比伐芦定：UA/NSTEMI 患者 0.1 mg/kg 推注随后 0.25 mg/(kg · h)；STEMI 患者 0.75 mg/kg 推注，随后 1.75 mg/(kg · h) 或者 UA/NSTEMI 早期 PCI 后。

β受体阻滞剂

• 美托洛尔：5 mg 静脉注射，q5 min 3 次，仅用于患有高血压的 STEMI 患者中，或有持续缺血的禁忌证。除非出现心源性休克迹象，对于 STEMI 患者 24 h 内美托洛尔 25～50 mg 口服 q6～12 h 初始可耐受剂量（β受体阻滞剂禁用于可卡因胸痛中）。

• 纤维蛋白溶解药物：

- 链激酶：150 万 U 持续 60 min；患者也可使用甲泼尼龙 250 mg 静脉注射。

- 阿替普酶：15 mg 静脉注射，然后 0.75 mg/kg（最大剂量 50 mg）超过 30 min，然后 0.5 mg/kg（最大剂量 35 mg）超过 60 min；患者也应接受肝素。

- 替奈普酶：体重决定剂量，单次给予 30～50 mg 给药时间 5 s；静脉注射，给药时间为 5 s。

- 禁忌证：

◦ 活跃的内出血。
◦ 最近 6 个月有脑血管意外。
◦ 出血性脑血管病史。
◦ 最近（2 个月内）有颅内、脊柱手术或创伤。
◦ 脑肿瘤、动静脉畸形或动脉瘤。
◦ 近 2 周内可导致内部脏器出血的外伤或手术。
◦ 相对禁忌证。
◦ 已知的出血体质。
◦ 严重、未控制的高血压。

◦ 妊娠。
◦ 最近 1 个月内头部创伤。

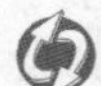

随访

进一步处理

入院指征

• 所有考虑进行再灌注治疗的患者应送入导管室或 PCI 中心或病床、ICU。

出院指征

不需要进行再灌注治疗的患者应从急诊室出院。

要点和误区

• 再灌注治疗目标为首次就医的 90 min 内进行 PCI。治疗窗未过时，送至可行 PCI 的医院或运输时间>120 min 时行溶栓治疗。
• 如果 PCI 不能进行或将延误时，纤溶治疗的目标为诊疗时间不超过 30 min。
• STEMI 患者再灌注的主要目标是行纤溶或 PCI。
• 所有心脏停搏后患者应考虑 PCI 治疗。

新生儿复苏 Resuscitation, Neonate

Erica Lash · Neha Raukar 何融冰 译

基础知识

描述

• 每年全世界有超过 100 万新生儿因出生窒息死亡，10%的新生儿出生时需要辅助。1%的新生儿需要复苏治疗。
• APGAR 评分(活动、脉搏、鬼脸、表情、呼吸)用于评估所有婴儿在 1 岁和 5 min 的生命情况。
- APGAR 评分是一种用于量化婴儿临床状况的工具。它不应该被用来预测结果或指导复苏。
- 5 个类别，得分为 0、1 分或 2 分，评估 1 min 和 5 min。
- 在开始复苏前，不要等待分配 APGAR 得分。
- 复苏 10 min 后，APGAR 评分仍为 0，说明进一步的复苏不太可能成功，这可能是决定何时停止护理的有用工具。
• 卫生保健提供者和高危新生儿的父母必须讨论复苏措施的适当性。这最好在分娩前完成：
- 孕周<23 周或低于 400 g 的新生儿。
- 无脑畸形。
- 婴儿确诊为 13 三体或 18 三体综合征。
- 医生在伦理上或法律上不应执行徒劳或潜在的有害干预，或者在父母的要求下拒绝接受有效的治疗。
• 心率(HR)：0，听不到；1 分，<100 次/分；2 分，>100 次/分。
• 呼吸：0，无呼吸；1 分，缓慢，不规律；2 分，规律，哭泣。
• 肌张力：0，松弛；1 分，稍弯曲；2 分，主动运动。
• 对刺激反射：0，无反应；1 分，皱眉；2 分，咳嗽，喷嚏，哭泣。
• 颜色：0，青紫色或苍白；1 分，躯干粉红色，四肢末梢青紫；2 分，全身粉红色。

病因

• 通过两个从右到左的分流促进了胎儿和母亲的气体交换：
- 动脉导管：缺氧的血液从肺动脉分流至降主动脉，绕过颈动脉。
- 卵圆孔：含氧血从胎盘流出，经胎儿血管进入右心房，再经卵圆孔分流至左心房和主动脉，绕过胎儿肺。
• 婴儿第一次自主呼吸会引发一连串的生理变化，包括肺泡内液体的清除、肺扩张、肺血管阻力的降低和左右分流的关闭。
• 任何呼吸功能、气道或肺功能的问题都预示着向宫外生活过渡的问题，从而导致新生儿缺氧和需要复苏。缺氧最初可能引起呼吸急促，然后是原发性呼吸暂停。
• 需要复苏相关的产前危险因素包括：
- 妊娠糖尿病。
- 妊娠期高血压或慢性高血压。
- 贫血。
- 早产或新生儿死亡。
- 妊娠中后期出血。
- 母体感染。
- 母体心脏、肾、肺、甲状腺或精神方面疾病。
- 羊水过多或羊水过少。
- 羊膜早破。
- 过期妊娠。
- 多胎妊娠。
- 大小与妊娠期不符。
- 药物治疗。
- 母亲药物滥用。
- 胎儿畸形。
- 胎儿活动减弱。
- 无产前保健。
- 生产年龄<16 岁或>35 岁。
• 需复苏的分娩时危险因素：
- 紧急剖宫产。
- 产钳、吸引器助产。
- 臀产式或其他不正常产式。
- 早产。
- 促发临产。
- 绒毛膜羊膜炎。
- 胎膜破裂。
- 第二产程延长。
- 胎儿心动过缓。
- 胎儿心率异常。
- 全身麻醉。
- 子宫强直收缩。
• 4 h 内对母亲应用麻醉药物：
- 胎粪污染羊水。
- 脐带脱垂。
- 胎盘早期剥离。
- 前置胎盘。

诊断

症状和体征

缺乏免疫力需要复苏的新生儿表现如下：
• 肌张力下降。
• 呼吸动力低下。
• 心动过缓。
• 低血压。
• 气促。
• 发绀。

病史

需要行复苏的危险因素同上。

体格检查

- 呼吸：频率和效应。
- 心率：通过听诊或触诊脐带获得。
- 颜色。
- 肌张力，活动，面色。

基本检查

- 三个基本问题指导检查和治疗。
  - 婴儿足月了吗？
  - 婴儿是否有呼吸和/或哭泣。
  - 婴儿的哭声是否好？
- 如果三个问题的答案都是肯定的，那么就刺激、干燥和温暖婴儿，并进行常规护理。
- 如果任何一个问题的答案是否定的，干燥和温暖的婴儿，并继续复苏。刺激可使呼吸恢复。

诊断检查与说明

实验室检查

- 床旁血糖检测。
- 血气，血氧测定。

影像学检查

胸部X线检查。

诊断步骤/外科

- 气管内插管术：
  - 直柄 Miller 1 用于足月产，Miller 0 用于早产儿。
  - 气管内导管(ETT)：
    - 2.5 号用于＜1000 g 或＜28 周。
    - 3 号用于 1000～2000 g 或 28～34 周。
    - 3.5 号用于 2000～3000 g 或 34～38 周。
    - 4 号用于＞3000 g 或＞38 周。
  - 管心针、潮气末二氧化碳、吸引器、胶带，做好抽吸胎粪准备。
- 脐静脉置管：
  - 脐带基底部加压扎紧。
  - 充满液体的注射器连接于脐部导管(3.5F 或 5F)。
  - 钳夹切断脐带。
  - 识别脐静脉(大、粗且单独)。
  - 将导管沿头端置入脐静脉。
  - 前移 2～4 cm 直至血自动流入注射器。
  - 用脐带或荷包缝合固定导管。
  - X线平片检查位置。
  - 注射合适的药物或液体。

治疗

院前

- 院前人员应开始复苏。
- 备好新生儿复苏装置，需提前做好准备。
- 要特别注意散热，保持较低的温度阈值。

初步稳定/治疗

2015 年 AHA/AAP/ILCOR 指南推荐逐步复苏的方法。最初的步骤应该在最初的 60 s 内完成("黄金 1 分钟")。

- 最初的步骤包括：温暖，干燥，通畅气道，刺激。
- 保暖、干燥：维持温度以降低氧和代谢需求。干燥、包裹合适、使用加热器增加辐射热增加室温气道温度。
- 清理气道：卷毛毯或毛巾在肩胛骨下提供轻微的颈部伸展和对齐后咽、喉、气管。先用球囊注射器吸口，如果仍然阻塞气道，再吸鼻。
- 刺激：用干燥、吸力、轻弹脚底、揉搓背部等方式刺激触觉。
- 热疗、干燥、清理气道和刺激后发现呼吸暂停或心率＜100 次/分，复苏应通过呼吸支持、胸部按压和其他必要的辅助措施进行。

- 呼吸支持：氧气和通气支持。
  - 对于足月婴儿，室内空气复苏可能有利于避免氧过多。
  - 对于早产儿，混合氧并密切监测氧饱和度是合适的。
  - 对于缺氧的婴儿，允许 100%的氧气以达到目标范围内的血氧饱和度：
    - 出生后 1 min 动脉血氧饱和度为 65%，5 min 为 90%，出生后 15 min 血氧饱和度为 95%。
    - 对于早产儿，混合氧并密切监测氧饱和度是合适的。
  - 100%氧气正压通气。
  - 自喷或自喷(麻醉型)袋。
  - 合适的面罩。
  - 第一次呼吸可能需要高压(必须关闭"弹出"阀)。
  - 频率：40～60 次/分。
  - 压力：30～40 cmH_2O。
  - 如果需要长时间的通气或胸外按压，则需要气管内插管和放置鼻胃管。
- 循环：在正压通气 30 s 后开始胸外按压，达到心率＞60 次/分。
  - 胸外按压应尽可能通过双拇指技术(双手环绕躯干)而不是 2 指法。
  - 挤压胸部前后径(约 1/3)，然后放松。
  - 推荐的按压通气比为 3∶1，按压通气比约为 90/分，呼吸次数 30 次/分。
- 如果按压 30 s 后心率仍＜60 bpm，继续静脉注射肾上腺素，扩容。对于胎粪如下：
  - 胎粪吸入的风险随着产后的增加而增加。
  - 常规插管以及新生儿胎粪污染羊水抽吸术不再被推荐。
  - 在这种情况下，出现呼吸窘迫或呼吸暂停的婴儿应按照与羊水清澈的婴儿相同的复苏算法进行处理。

急诊治疗/程序

- 如果血液丢失或复苏无效，进行扩容治疗。
  - 生理盐水、乳酸林格液、O型阴性血(如果时间允许进行交叉配血)。
- 如果证明或怀疑有严重代谢性酸中毒：
  - 保证适量通气。
  - 应用碳酸氢钠。
- 如果证明或怀疑有低血糖，静脉注入葡萄糖。
- 不建议常规使用纳洛酮。
  - 对麻醉剂有瘾或使用过美沙酮的母亲来说，是禁用的：会诱发癫痫。
- 持续呼吸窘迫可能表明有气胸。
- 已知或怀疑有膈肌疝时应立刻气管内插管并放置 NG 管。
- 如果心脏停搏 10 min 可考虑停止复苏。

药物治疗

- 葡萄糖：2～4 ml/kg D_{10}W 通过静脉(脐静脉)给药。
- 肾上腺素：0.1～0.3 ml/kg 1∶10 000 溶液，可通过静脉或 ETT(0.3～1 ml/kg，如果通过 ETT 给药)。
- 碳酸氢钠：2 mmol/kg(4 ml/kg，4.2%溶液)(0.5 mmol/ml)，通过静脉缓慢给药(脐静脉)。
- 扩容：生理盐水、乳酸林格液、血液。起始剂量为 10 ml/kg，可以重复使用，均通过静脉(脐静脉)给药。
- 其他药品根据新生儿基本情况应用。

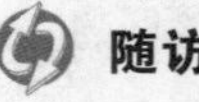

随访

进一步处理

入院指征

- 所有新生儿均需住院。
- 如果需要有效复苏，收入 NICU。

要点和误区

- 低出生体重新生儿的复苏和治疗可能会

引起以下并发症：
- 温度调节困难。
- 脑室内出血。
- 慢性肺疾病。
- 早产儿视网膜病变。
• 氧气与极低出生体重婴儿(VLBW)：
- VLBW婴儿：定义为出生体重<1500 g。
- VLBW婴儿：氧化应激和损伤发生的风险增加，包括早产儿视网膜病变。
- 一些研究表明使用<100%氧气甚至21%氧气(室内空气)进行复苏可以避免氧化应激和损伤。

新生儿黄疸 Neonatal Jaundice

Michele M. Chetham 伍力学 译

 基础知识

• 胆红素产生与清除的不平衡造成的。
• 新生儿红细胞质量大而寿命短，胆红素的产生比成人多。
• 新生儿，尤其是早产儿，在肝脏结合和胆道排泄胆红素方面存在速率限制，肠肝循环增加，胆红素结合白蛋白和胆红素结合蛋白减少。

描述

大多数的新生儿，存在以下表现时，即代表生理性黄疸而非病理性黄疸。
- 正常情况下由脐带血的胆红素水平为1.5 mg/dl，到出生后第3日时增长到6.5 mg/dl水平，而后逐渐下降，到出生后10～12日时，下降到<1.5 mg/dl水平。
• 血清胆红素水平可能升至超过神经保护机制所防御的含量，导致胆红素结合在基底神经节、海马、脑干核和小脑组织：
- 胆红素诱导的神经功能障碍(BIND)是由严重的高胆红素血症引起的，从轻度功能障碍到急性胆红素脑病(ABE)和胆红素脑病(核黄疸)。
◦ ABE：出生后第1周所表现的急性胆红素毒性表现。
◦ 核黄疸：BIND的慢性形式，具有很高的死亡率和永久性的后遗症，如舞蹈症样脑瘫、凝视异常、听力丧失、牙齿发育不良。
- BIND疾病进展速率依赖于血清胆红素的升高速率、高胆红素血症的持续时间、结合白蛋白的储量、非结合胆红素水平、宿主易感性和共患病状态。
- 呼吸衰竭，进行性昏迷和顽固性抽搐是导致的死亡的主要原因。
• 严重高胆红素血症的危险因素：
- 在出生后第一个24 h内观察到黄疸。
- 出院前的总血清胆红素水平(TSB)或经皮胆红素(TCB)水平处于高度危险或中高度危险区间内。
- 低胎龄：35～38周。
- 纯母乳喂养，尤其是当喂养不足导致过多的体重下降时。
- 自身免疫或其他溶血性疾病。
- 同胞的婴儿存在新生儿黄疸。
- 头颅血肿或过度青紫。
- 种族：东亚人群。
- 母体肥胖、初产。
- SGA(小于胎龄)、LGA(大于胎龄)。
• 与严重的高胆红素血症相关的围生期因素：低出生体重、糖尿病孕妇所产的巨大儿、感染、红细胞增多症。
• 高胆红素血症神经毒性的危险因素：
- 自身免疫溶血病。
- G-6-PD缺乏。
- 窒息。
- 脓毒症。
- 酸中毒。
- 白蛋白<3 mg/dl。
• 光疗后(POST-PT)胆红素可能会反弹到令人关注的胆红素水平。
- 高风险患儿：妊娠<32周的新生儿、溶血性疾病患儿、治疗<22 h的患儿。

病因

• 非结合高胆红素血症：
- 生理性黄疸。
- 母乳喂养婴儿黄疸：
◦ 母乳喂养不良性黄疸：出生后第1周，由于哺乳量不足导致的生理性黄疸加重。新生儿脱水。
◦ 母乳性黄疸：出生后3～5日开始，在第2周达到顶峰，可持续到第8周，由于母乳中的β-葡萄糖醛酸酶增多导致的。
◦ 20%～30%的以母乳喂养为主的新生儿可能在3～4周大时出现黄疸；其中30%～40%的婴儿胆红素水平可能为≥5 mg/dl。
◦ 可因脱水而加重。
- 特殊的溶血因素：
◦ ABO、Rh和次要血型不合导致的溶血，其中ABO不合最常见，Rh不合不常见(RhoGAM阻滞)。
◦ 红细胞酶的缺陷：G-6-PD不足。
◦ 红细胞膜的缺陷：遗传性球形红细胞增多症和遗传性椭圆形红细胞增多症。
- 败血症：细菌、病毒、原虫。
- 产伤：
◦ 头颅血肿和瘀斑导致的血红素负荷增加。
- 红细胞增多症：
◦ 母胎输血引起。
◦ 胎儿间输血。
◦ 糖尿病母亲的婴儿。
- 先天性甲状腺功能低下。
- 肝脏结合障碍：
◦ 吉尔伯特综合征(Gilbert综合征)(家族性葡萄糖醛酸转移酶活性部分缺损)是良性的。
◦ 克里格勒-纳贾尔综合征(Crigler-Najjar综合征)(先天性葡萄糖醛酸转移酶缺乏)，表现为终身性未结合高胆红素血症。
- 肠道阻塞：如肠梗阻，功能性或解剖性，增加了肝肠循环。
• 结合性高胆红素血症：
- 肝分泌结合性胆红素障碍。
- 由新生儿肝炎、先天性胆道闭锁、肝外胆道梗阻、新生儿窒息导致肝休克、新生儿含铁血黄素沉着症引起的。

诊断

症状和体征

病史

• 可能有嗜睡、少食、尿少等表现。
• 早期ABE：
- 由于吮吸无力导致的进食困难，尿量减少。
- 哭闹、烦躁不安、肌张力低下。

X

- 出现异于正常睡眠-觉醒模式的昏睡。
• 中度 ABE：
- 高亢的哭喊、烦躁。
- 颈部向后拱起(颈后倾)和躯干向后拱起(角弓反张)增加音调，并伴有肌张力下降。
- 发热。
• 晚期 ABE 体征：
- 颈后倾及角弓反张式发音。
- 半昏迷，抽搐。
- 脚踏车式运动。

体格检查

• 由于胆红素沉积导致皮肤、巩膜及全身黄染。表示血清胆红素水平升高。
• 脱水证据：色斑，毛细血管再充盈时间延长，尿量减少。
• 胆红素水平升高可以从头到足的方向影响皮肤颜色：
- 布兰克皮肤数字压力指数可反映潜在的肤色状况。
- 面部：胆红素水平>6～8 mg/dl。
- 脚部：胆红素水平>12～15 mg/dl。
- 凭视觉诊断黄疸是不可靠的，特别是对于存在暗色素的婴儿。
• 神经功能障碍可由异常的音调来进行识别：张力减退、亢进或可变性、落日征：在上眼睑下方、巩膜可见。
• 其他有助于诊断的体征：
- 出现问题：可能是脓毒症或新陈代谢。
- 胆道闭锁，早期看起来很好，然后是生长障碍(FTT)、腹壁突出静脉、HSM、腹水。

基本检查

• 临床诊断考虑危险因素。
• 任何怀疑或是明显的黄疸婴儿都要强制进行 TSB 检测。
• TSB 应当分为间接(非结合)胆红素和直接(结合)胆红素的检测。

诊断检查与说明

实验室检查

• 依据婴儿的出生的小时时间计算，而非出生日数来解释 TSB，从而来评估风险和治疗需要。
• 确定 TSB 或 TCB 水平。
• 如果都可以进行检测，TCB 与 TSB 相关性好。
• 下列新生儿黄疸应进一步评估：
- 发生在出生后的第一个 24 h。
- 持续时间超过 1 周。
- TSB 达到需要强化 PT 治疗的水平。
- 结合胆红素>10%或>2 mg/dl。
- 出现任何 ABE 征象。
• 血清白蛋白、电解质、尿素氮、肌酐、钙。
• CBC 分类和红细胞形态。
• 网织红细胞计数。
• 母婴血型。
• 脐血的直接 Coombs 试验：
- 不同医院条例不同：有的医院将对所有 O 型母亲的新生儿进行测试。
- 如果没有可用的标本，可利用婴儿血液进行直接 Coombs 测试。
• 对病态表现的婴幼儿进行败血症评估。
• 住院后针对直接怀疑的病因进行的检测：
- 红细胞酶测定：G-6-PD。
- 肝功能检测。
- 尿还原物质检测。
- 代谢或内分泌检测。

影像学检查

• 评估阻塞性肝病(高直接胆红素血症)：从超声开始。
• MRI 扫描显示大脑苍白球信号异常提示核黄疸，并非提示需要紧急处理。

鉴别诊断

• 请参阅“病因”。
• 非结合胆红素血症和结合胆红素血症的鉴别。

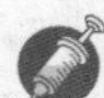

治疗

注意

• 因结局与暴露的持续时间相关，对于严重的新生儿高胆红素血症并伴有脑病征象的需要立即治疗。
• 当 TSB 超过阈值水平(基于年龄-小时和风险因素)，应立即启动 PT 治疗。

初步稳定/治疗

存在脱水体征的应给予生理盐水(20 ml/kg)治疗。

急诊治疗/程序

• 胎龄>35 周患儿治疗指南[基于以出生时间(h)进行危险度分组的 TSB 值]。
• 高危组：35～37 6/7 周+危险因素的患儿。
• 中危组：≥38 周+危险因素，或 35～37 6/7 周+无危险因素。
• 低危组：≥38 周+无危险因素。
• 危险因素：自身免疫性溶血性疾病、G-6-PD 缺乏症、窒息、显著嗜睡、体温不稳定、败血症、酸中毒、白蛋白<3 g/dl(30 g/L)。
• 根据不同的高危人群，需住院进行强化 PT 治疗的 TSB(mg/dl)界值如下：

出生时间(h)	高度	中度	低度
12	6	7.5	9
24	7.5	9.5	11.5
36	9.5	11.5	13
48	11	13	15
60	12.5	14.5	16.5
72	13.5	15	18
96	14.5	17	20
5～7 日	15	18	21

• BiliTool 是一个进行危险分层的在线计算器(http://bilitool.org/)，可提供多种智能手机应用程序。
• 强化 PT 治疗是利用高水平的照射源使婴儿尽可能多的表面积得到照射(顶置光源和下置 Bili 毛毯)每个光源制造商。眼睛一定要进行遮蔽。
• 强化 PT 治疗降低 TSB 的速率应>0.5 mg/(dl·h)，应尽快开始。
• 如果入院/转院有任何延误，在急诊室开始强化治疗。
• PT 相关的不良反应很少，如果已知或怀疑患有先天性卟啉病，请勿使用；如果患者有胆汁淤积，皮肤会出现棕褐色；延长的 PT 可能会增加氧化应激、脂质过氧化、维生素 B_2 缺乏症，可能与皮肤中的 DNA 损伤有关，从而导致恶性肿瘤。
• 换血治疗(ET)的指征应在咨询新生儿科专家后，由患儿的出生时间、危险度分层和 PT 治疗缺少反应来综合决定。换血时需要对血液进行照射和输注白蛋白。
• 当婴幼儿存在 ABE 的迹象时，无论 TSB 水平多少，推荐进行 ET 治疗，并进入新生儿重症监护病房进行监测。
• 与内皮素相关的副作用很严重，如感染、凝血病、移植物与宿主的对抗、坏死性小肠结肠炎、门静脉血栓形成、电解质异常。
• 如果考虑自身免疫溶血性疾病，但 TSB 水平接近换血指征时，应静脉给予免疫球蛋白 0.5～1 g/kg，注射时长超过 2 h。
• 治疗共患疾病(败血症、肝功能异常、红细胞增多症、甲状腺功能减退)。
• 鼓励增多母乳或配方奶的饲喂次数，补充葡萄糖水是没有用的，可能需要肠内补充。没有证据表明静脉输液会影响需要静脉输

X

液的健康足月新生儿的临床结果。只有在容量不足的情况下才需要静脉补液。

• 母乳喂养不良和母乳性黄疸：
- 大多数婴儿可以继续哺乳。
- 在出生后的最初几日，鼓励母亲每日至少护理婴儿8～12次。
- 补充配方奶和/或暂时性的需要静脉输液。
- 母乳性黄疸的婴儿对PT治疗无反应时，推荐停止母乳喂养2～3日。
- 在暂停喂养期间，鼓励母亲通过使用吸奶器或手动方式来维持泌乳。

• 生理性黄疸：再次确认并安排适当的随访。

药物治疗

一线用药

如果患有自身免疫溶血性疾病患儿的TSB水平接近换血治疗的标准并对强化PT治疗无反应时，应该给予静脉注射免疫球蛋白0.5～1 g/kg治疗，持续时间超过2 h。

二线用药

• 苯巴比妥增加胆红素结合和延迟排泄；可能对认知发展产生不利影响，不常规使用。

• 熊去氧胆酸增加胆汁流动，在治疗胆汁淤积性黄疸时是有效的。

 随访

进一步处理

入院指征

• 需要进行密集PT或ET治疗的患儿。

• 存在显著贫血、败血症、脱水或阻塞性肝脏疾病的证据，需要住院诊断评估和治疗。

• 快速转诊到新生儿重症监护病房；如果转诊时间＞30 min，应在转诊期间实行PT治疗。

• 依从性差或无法安排家庭PT。

出院指征

• 稳定的婴儿高胆红素血症不需要PT治疗。

• 没有危险因素的单纯性非溶血性高胆红素血症的稳定足月儿，TSB水平在2～3 mg/dl，低于强化PT治疗的指征，在随访期间，能保证安排及时适当的居家PT治疗的患儿。口服量必须足够。

• 能与初级保健人员和新生儿顾问进行直接沟通者，以确保随访。

转诊问题

• 母乳喂养不良：很多医院都有哺乳顾问。保持水分，直到母乳喂养成功。

• 新生儿科医师：需要进行强化PT或ET。

随访建议

在初级保健人员处进行随访：

• 12 h内：不需要PT治疗和没有危险因素存在高胆红素血症的稳定婴幼儿。

• 8 h内：有家庭PT治疗安排的单纯性非溶血性高胆红素血症的稳定婴幼儿。

要点和误区

• TSB必须根据新生儿的小时出生时间而非日龄进行解释，对于存在严重高胆红素血症患儿，要与风险因素对应。

• TSB超过阈值水平时要进行PT治疗。

• 须对婴儿的喂养情况和脱水情况进行评估和纠正。

• 保险和后勤问题可能会使家庭治疗难以安排。

新生儿脓毒症 Neonatal Sepsis

Lazaro Lezcano 伍力学 译

 基础知识

描述

机制

• 该病为发生在新生儿的致命性感染，＞3月龄的婴儿则很少发生。

• 几乎均为细菌感染：
- 很少为病毒或真菌感染。
- 通常是存在于母体会阴部的菌群。

• 发生率：(3～5)/1000个存活新生儿。

• 危险因素：
- 围生期：
  ◦ 近期发热史(＞37.5℃)。
  ◦ 尿路感染。
  ◦ 绒毛膜羊膜炎。
  ◦ 胎膜破裂时间延长(＞18 h)。
  ◦ 恶露。
  ◦ 子宫压痛。
  ◦ 产时窒息。
- 新生儿：
  ◦ 早产。
  ◦ 胎儿心动过速(＞180次/分)。
  ◦ 男性。
  ◦ 双胞胎(特别是第2次双胞胎)。
  ◦ 发育或先天性免疫缺陷。
  ◦ 肌内注射铁剂治疗。
  ◦ 半乳糖血症。
  ◦ 先天性异常(尿道、无脾、脊髓脊膜膨出、窦道)。
  ◦ 脐炎。

病因

脓毒症

• 细菌：
- B组链球菌。
- 大肠埃希菌。
- 李斯特菌。
- 凝固酶阴性葡萄球菌。
- 梅毒螺旋体。

• 病毒：
- 单纯疱疹病毒是常见的病毒病因。
- 肠道病毒。
- 腺病毒。

• 真菌：
- 念珠菌脓毒症。

• 原生动物：
- 疟原虫。
- 疏螺旋体。

脑膜炎

• 细菌：
- B组链球菌。
- K1型大肠杆菌。
- 单核细胞增生李斯特菌。
- 其他链球菌。
- 不可分型流感嗜血杆菌。
- 凝固酶阳性或阴性葡萄球菌。
- 不常见的：克雷伯菌属、肠杆菌。
- 铜绿假单胞菌、梅毒螺旋体和分枝结核杆菌。
- 异型枸橼酸杆菌(导致脑脓肿的重要

X

原因)。
- 人型支原体和解脲支原体。
• 病毒:
- 肠道病毒。
- 单纯疱疹病毒(2 型更常见)。
- 巨细胞病毒。
- 弓形虫。
- 风疹病毒。
- HIV。
• 弓形虫。
• 真菌:
- 白念珠菌和其他真菌。

诊断

症状和体征

病史

• 非特殊病史:
- 表现异常。
- 食欲不振。
- 烦躁或嗜睡。
• 一般情况:
- 毒性表现。
- 精神状态改变:烦躁或嗜睡。
- 呼吸暂停或心动过缓。
- 皮肤色斑、灰白色、发绀或皮温降低。

体格检查

• 重要体征:
- 高热、低体温。
- 呼吸急促。
- 心动过速。
- 毛细血管再充盈时间延长。
• 腹胀。
• 黄疸。
• 瘀青或出血时间延长。
• 新生儿脓毒症:
- 脓毒性休克。
- 低血糖。
- 癫痫发作。
- 弥散性血管内凝血(DIC)。
- 如不治疗,可致心血管功能衰竭和死亡。

基本检查

• 经验性抗生素治疗与支持治疗后对脓毒症进行评估。
• 确定感染源。
• 识别代谢异常。

诊断检查与说明

实验室检查

• 床旁血糖测定。
• 全血细胞计数(CBC):
- 白细胞升高或抑制。
- 核左移。
- 血小板减少。
• C 反应蛋白(CRP)。
• 尿液分析。
• 诊断后立即进行培养检测:
- 血液、脑脊液、插管或耻骨上的尿液、粪便。
• 腰椎穿刺:
- 血流动力学不稳定时可能需要延迟进行。
- 细胞计数、蛋白质、葡萄糖、培养、革兰染色。
• 血清葡萄糖检测排除低血糖。
• 动脉血气和血氧饱和度检测。
- 代谢性酸中毒常见。
• 电解质和钙:
- 低钠血症。
- 低钙血症。
• DIC 检测:
- 凝血功能障碍是一种晚期并发症。
- 监测 PT、APTT 和纤维蛋白原裂解产物。

影像学检查

胸部 X 线检查排除肺炎。

鉴别诊断

• 心脏疾病:
- 左心发育不良综合征。
- 心肌炎。
• 代谢性疾病:
- 低血糖。
- 肾上腺皮质功能不全(先天性肾上腺皮质增生)。
- 有机酸中毒。
- 尿素循环障碍。
• 肠套叠。
• 受虐儿童。
• 中枢神经系统:
- 颅内出血。
- 围生期窒息。
• 新生儿黄疸。
• 血液病急症:
- 新生儿暴发性紫癜。
- 严重贫血。
- 高铁血红蛋白血症。
- 恶性肿瘤(先天性白血病)。

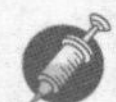

治疗

院前

• 如果存在呼吸抑制、呼吸暂停或呼吸窘迫,应给予通气支持。
• 建立静脉通道。
• 持续监测。

急诊治疗/程序

• 如果临床表现比较符合,特别是存在危险因素的情况下,可以对脓毒症新生儿实施经验性治疗。
• 抗生素使用:
- 氨苄西林和庆大霉素或头孢噻肟。
- 如果患者病情恶化或提示葡萄球菌肺炎,应添加万古霉素。
- 头孢噻肟可以取代庆大霉素。
• 如果存在感染性休克,应给予支持治疗。

药物治疗

• 氨苄西林:如果婴儿出生体重>2 kg,出生年龄>2 周龄,200 mg/(kg · d), q6 h,静脉注射或肌内注射;如果<7 日龄,150 mg/(kg · d), q8 h。
• 头孢噻肟:如果婴儿出生体重>2 kg,出生年龄>1 周龄,150 mg/(kg · d), q6 h,静脉注射或肌内注射;如果出生年龄在 8~28 日,150 mg/(kg · d), q8 h,静脉注射或肌内注射;如果出生年龄在 0~7 日,100 mg/(kg · d), q12 h,静脉注射或肌内注射。
• 庆大霉素:如果妊娠时间>37 周并且出生年龄>7 日龄,每剂 2.5 mg/kg, q8 h,静脉注射或肌内注射;如果<7 日龄,2.5 mg/kg, q12 h。
• 万古霉素:如果妊娠时间>37 周并且出生年龄>7 日龄,每剂 15 mg/kg, q8 h,静脉注射;如果<7 日龄,15 mg/kg, q12 h,静脉注射。

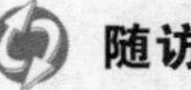

随访

进一步处理

入院指征

• 所有怀疑脓毒症的患儿均应收治入院,给予静脉抗生素和支持治疗,并密切监测。
• 年龄<1 月龄,有发热表现,即便缺乏脓毒症的明确依据,一般应收治入院。年龄大一点的孩子可根据临床表现确定是否收治。

初步治疗

• 如果存在呼吸抑制、呼吸暂停或呼吸窘迫，应给予通气支持。

• 建立静脉通路以便给予液体和升压药治疗。

• 持续监测。

要点和误区

• 那些表现出行为改变的人必须考虑新生儿败血症。

• 发热新生儿必须评估潜在感染。临床表现不足以排除败血症。

• 新生儿必须考虑广泛的差异。

• 在高危新生儿中进行培养前，不应延迟使用抗生素。

新型口服抗凝剂并发症 Novel Oral Anticoagulant Complications

Joanne C. Routsolias 朱妍 译

基础知识

描述

• 在过去的 10 年中，已经开发出几种新型的口服抗凝剂(NOAC)：

- 直接凝血酶抑制剂(达比加群)。
- Ⅹa 因子抑制剂(阿哌沙班、埃多沙班、利伐沙班)。

• 直接凝血酶抑制剂可抑制游离和血纤蛋白结合的凝血酶，以及凝血酶诱导的血小板聚集。

• 凝血因子Ⅹa 抑制剂在内源性和外源性凝血途径中对凝血因子Ⅹa 的选择性和可逆性抑制。

• 所有四种药物都通过肝脏代谢，并被肾脏消除：达比加群＞埃多沙班＞利伐沙班＞阿哌沙班。

• 常用于预防和治疗脑卒中、心肌梗死、瓣膜病和静脉血栓栓塞。

• 通常不需要测量抗凝效果：

- 凝血酶原时间(PT)/国际标准化比值(INR)在衡量抗凝效果方面的效用有限。
- 直接凝血酶抑制剂中抗凝效果的最佳筛选试验是凝血酶时间(TT)和淫羊藿凝血时间(ECT)。
- 凝血因子Ⅹa 抑制剂中抗凝效果的最佳筛选试验是显色抗 FXA 试验。

• 禁忌证包括出血或不良反应风险超过临床益处的任何情况。

- 既往超敏反应。
- 严重肾损害。
- 肝损害。
- 活动性或潜在的胃肠道出血、脑内出血或泌尿生殖道出血。

病因

• 出血发生率：

- 总体主要出血事件少于华法林。
  ◦ 颅内出血发生率低于华法林。
  ◦ 胃肠道出血发生率高于华法林。

• 血栓事件：

- 没有或不能服用处方 NOAC 的患者有发生血栓事件的风险。

诊断

症状和体征

• 表现可能是神秘的，也可能是戏剧性的：

- 需要高度怀疑才能检测到潜在的危及生命的并发症。

• 表现的频谱取决于突破性血栓形成与出血(胃肠道、中枢神经系统、腹膜后)的位置。

• 故意过量。

- 可能是无症状的。

基本检查

• 详尽的历史记录：

- 抗凝原因、最近的剂量变化、最后服用的时间、依从性、任何检查结果、其他处方、非处方药和替代药物。
- 精神状态的细微变化、最近的"轻微跌倒"或出血。

• 评估出血严重程度和血流动力学稳定性：

- 早期失血性休克。
- 高血压和心动过缓可能继发于脑出血的库欣反应。
- 心脏药物通常掩盖生命体征的重要变化。

• 仔细检查：

- 面色苍白、挫伤、擦伤、瘀斑，患肢可触摸到脉搏。
- 检查粪便是否有血液。

诊断检查与说明

• PT、APTT、INR：

- 可用但实用性有限。
- 达比加群延长 APTT＞PT。
- Ⅹa 因子延长 PT＞APTT。

• 如果有检测，考虑达比加群的 ECT 和 TT，以及其他人的抗 FⅩa 水平。

• CBC、电解质、BUN、肌酐、LFT 和葡萄糖：

- BUN 升高可能提示胃肠道的血液。
- 凝集素，如果故意摄入。

• 类型和交叉匹配。

影像学检查

• CT 扫描检测隐匿性但危及生命的出血的低阈值。

• 头颅 CT：

- 钝性脑外伤无意识丧失的次要机制。
- 在症状出现前发现脑出血。

• 腹部 CT：

- 钝性腹部创伤，无明显压痛。
- 腹膜后出血。
- 实质器官或内脏损伤。

鉴别诊断

所有出血原因：

• 胃肠道、腹膜后、中枢神经系统和创伤性。

• 止血缺陷，如血小板紊乱、肝功能损害/衰竭。

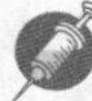

治疗

院前

• ABC 管理。

• 应用 2 条大口径静脉输液和生理盐水输注，治疗低血压。

• 心脏和脉搏血氧饱和度监测。

■ 初步稳定/治疗

• 为低血压建立中心静脉通路，对初始液体推注无反应：
- 仅可压缩部位。
• 尽快补充失血：
- 开始使用O型阴性血，直到有特定类型的血液可用。
- 儿童10 ml/kg推注。
• 对于故意过量：
- 如果在1～2 h发生摄取，则单次服用25～100 g的活性炭。

■ 急诊治疗/程序

• 一般来说，没有一种止血剂是NOAC的真正解毒剂，有血栓形成的风险。
• 具体处理取决于出血情况、抗凝原因和患者的可靠性：
- 新鲜冷冻血浆(FFP)或凝血酶原复合物浓缩液(PCC)取决于容量状态和可用性。
- PCC显示出更快的逆转和止血速度，但是数据仍然有限。
- PCC首选用于脑出血、容量超负荷或大出血的情况。
• 在转移患者之前开始使用逆转剂可带来更好的结果。

■ 药物治疗

• 血液制品：
- FFP，传统上是3～4 U的FFP(1 L)，用于在短期内控制持续出血，而不会有过高的血栓栓塞风险。
- 可能需要额外的设备。
- 副作用：
◦ 液体超载。
◦ 病毒传播：罕见的。
◦ 输血相关的急性肺损伤：罕见的。
◦ 考虑将浓缩红细胞用于严重失血，如果患者血小板减少，则考虑血小板。
• PCC：
- 保质期长，易于重建成高度浓缩的体积(20 ml与1 L/剂)。
- 快速逆转，没有体积过载。
- 副作用：
◦ 血栓形成。
◦ 比脂肪蛋白病毒传播更少。
• 4因子PCC(KCenta)是FFP的分级产品，含有等量的因子Ⅱ、Ⅲ、Ⅸ和Ⅹ：
- 静脉注射50 U/kg，q24 h，最大剂量＝5 000 U。
• 3因子PCC(Bebulin - VH，Profiline - SD)含有极少的因子Ⅶa：
- 服用50 U/kg静脉注射，q24 h。
- 可以补充FFP或rFⅦa。
- 在美国更广泛地提供。
• aPCC (Feiba)。
- 含有激活因子Ⅶa。
- 给予50 U/kg，静脉注射，q6～12 h，最大剂量为200 U/(kg · d)。
- 考虑含有或不含有3因子的重组活化因子Ⅶa(RFⅦa)，这些因子没有因子Ⅶa，但关于其益处的数据有限，并且血栓栓塞并发症的发生率更高。
- 考虑对达比加群进行紧急血液透析。
- 如果有达比加群的解毒剂，idarucizumab(Praxbind)，给5 g静脉注射。
- 对于凝血因子Ⅹa抑制剂，解毒剂正在开发中。

随访

■ 进一步处理

入院指征

• 活动性消化道出血、腹膜后出血或中枢神经系统出血。
• 有活动性出血证据的抗凝创伤患者需要：
- 抗凝和血液置换逆转。
- 手术干预的早期手术会诊。
- 在最初稳定下来后运送到一级创伤中心进行最终护理。

出院指征

• 评估潜在的合并症、出血的总体风险、跌倒的风险、社会状况、可靠性和随访。
• 无症状抗凝患者，创伤小，血红蛋白稳定，影像学检查正常，有可靠的照顾者，密切随访即可出院。

转诊问题

• 患者应在出院后24～48 h至初级保健医师或专科医师随访。
• 因故意服药过量而转诊至精神科。

■ 随访建议

教育患者监测出血过多和/或新的血栓事件的症状和体征。

要点和误区

• 对使用NOAC的创伤患者保持较低的成像门槛。
• 不要服用维生素K来逆转NOAC。
• 4因子PCC或3因子PCC/rFⅦa应用于脑出血、容量超负荷或大出血患者。
• 检查是否有解毒剂，考虑使用。

性病淋巴肉芽肿 Lymphogranuloma Venereum

Joel Kravitz 王胜云 译

基础知识

■ 描述

• 性传播疾病。
• 初级阶段：
- 无痛性丘疹、脓疱或溃疡。
• 第二阶段：
- 蔓延至区域淋巴结。
- 淋巴结炎可为单侧或双侧。
- 腹股沟淋巴结炎。
• 抗生素治疗有效。
• 第三阶段：
- 未经治疗的情况下，可造成组织的显著损伤和破坏。
• 是东南亚、拉丁美洲、部分非洲加勒比地区的地方病。
• 男性同性性行为可显著增高该疾病的发生率。
• 也被称为：
- 瘤状突起。
- 热带性腹股沟淋巴结炎。
- Nicolas-Favre-Durand病。

■ 病因

沙眼衣原体L1、L2、L3血清型。

诊断

症状和体征

病史

- 主要生殖器官病变：
  - 潜伏期：性交病原体暴露后的3～30日。
  - 无痛的生殖器下疳持续2～3日(极少情况下，可出现丘疹和水疱)。
  - 通常出现时间短暂而不被察觉。
  - 可能以直肠炎的形式出现。
- 第二阶段：
  - 系统性症状：
    - 发热、烦躁。
    - 肌痛。
  - 淋巴结炎，通常出现在腹股沟处：
    - 可出现溃疡和排脓。
  - 直肠炎：
    - 肛门出血。
    - 里急后重。
    - 便秘。
- 第三阶段：
  - 症状类似炎性肠病或直肠结肠炎。
  - 橡皮病。
  - 肠道狭窄。

体格检查

- 第一阶段：
  - 无痛性丘疹、脓疱或溃疡。
  - 通常出现在肛门生殖器附近。
- 第二阶段：
  - 轻微的腹股沟淋巴结炎：
    - 在初次暴露1～3周后出现。
    - 约2/3的病例中，腹股沟淋巴结炎为单侧出现。
    - 腹股沟和大腿处出现明显腹股沟淋巴结炎。
    - 凹陷征：瘢痕或合并的腹股沟韧带上下的淋巴结炎肿大，在腹股沟韧带处出现显著线性凹陷(见于30%的病例)。
    - 有肛交接触的患者可发展成为出血性结直肠炎。
    - 直肠周围的淋巴结炎症可导致直肠窦道或狭窄。
- 第三阶段：
  - 慢性结直肠炎：
    - 腹痛。
    - 肛门出血。
  - 生殖器狭窄。
  - 肛门出血。
  - 会阴及肛周窦道形成。
  - 患侧象皮腿。

诊断检查与说明

实验室检查

- 标准衣原体DNA探针不适合对性病淋巴肉芽肿(LGV)进行诊断。
- 实验室诊断(VDRL)的假阳性约为20%。
- 血清学检查和病原体培养是标准方法。
- 滴度>1∶64可考虑患者感染了性病肉芽肿(LGV)。

诊断步骤/外科

腹股沟淋巴结穿刺具有特异性，但是代价太高可行性差。

鉴别诊断

- 生殖器疱疹(LGV中较少出现溃疡)。
- 无痛性梅毒结节，潜伏期更长。
- 软性下疳伴溃疡，不伴有系统性症状。
- 腹股沟转移性肉芽肿瘤，无痛且易出血。

治疗

初步稳定/治疗

症状不危及生命，不需要进行生命维持准备。

急诊治疗/外科

如果腹股沟淋巴结肿块较大，应考虑穿刺抽液或外科切开排除的方式避免或减少瘢痕形成。

药物治疗

一线用药

盐酸强力霉素：100 mg，口服，每日2次，持续3周。

二线用药

- 阿奇霉素：1000 mg，口服，持续3周。
- 红霉素：500 mg，口服，每日4次，持续3周。

妊娠注意事项

妊娠期间和哺乳期间推荐使用红霉素。

随访

进一步处理

入院指征

- 极少情况下需要收入院治疗(如伴有极其严重的系统症状)。

出院指征

免疫功能正常，不存在系统性功能障碍。

转诊问题

- 门诊患者需要进行随访以明确诊断和治疗。
- 直肠感染或需要再次治疗。

随访建议

- 确保患者的性伙伴接受检查和治疗。
- 艾滋病和丙型肝炎随访。
- 同患者60日内有性行为接触的人应当接受检查并进行抗生素治疗。

要点和误区

- 诊断需要基于临床体征、流行病学条件，在排除其他致病原因的前提下进行。
- 该诊断也适用于男性同性性行为的患者。
- 治疗的目的是避免疾病进展到单独使用抗生素无法治疗的第三阶段。
- 抗生素治疗应当超过3周。

X

性侵犯 Sexual Assault

Lauren M. Smith 张溢叟 伍力学 译

基础知识

描述

具体的法律定义因州而异：

- 阴茎和外阴或阴茎和肛门之间未经同意的完全或企图插入。
- 口腔与阴茎、外阴或肛门之间未经同意的接触。
- 手指、手或物体未经同意地插入肛门或生殖器开口。
- 直接或通过衣服非自愿地有意接触生殖器、阴道、肛门、腹股沟、大腿内侧或臀部。

• 该行为在受害者受到身体力量、心理压力等胁逼下或者由于丧失反抗能力或遭受伤害等情形下发生。

• 该行为是在受害者由于年幼或由于存在智能发育障碍等残疾而不具备表达其意愿的能力的情形下发生。

▪ 病因

• 美国人一生中被性侵犯的风险：女性为18%，男性为5%。

• 72%的女性强奸受害者是被认识的人强奸，但是男性主要是被陌生人和熟人强奸及殴打，而不是亲密伴侣。

• 残疾、怀孕或试图离开虐待者的妇女面临亲密伴侣强奸的风险增加。

• 在男性同性恋、双性恋、退伍军人、监狱中的囚犯或寻求精神保健服务的人群中，男性的性侵犯发生率更高。

• 将近25%的女性和7%的男性是被现任或前任伴侣强奸或性侵犯。

诊断

▪ 症状和体征

• 受害者可能不会透露受侵害情况：

- 大多数人仅在回答直接提问时才会透露受侵害情况。

• 心动过速。

• 头痛。

• 恶心。

• 背痛。

• 皮肤改变。

• 月经症状。

• 体重突然变化。

• 睡眠障碍。

• 腹痛。

• 呼吸困难。

• 相关伤害：

- 在受侵害人群中，约有70%的报告未见受伤。
- 会阴裂伤。
- 外阴创伤。
- 阴道壁撕裂（较常见于年轻患者，位于性交部位附近）。
- 多部位挫伤。
- 擦伤。
- 咬伤。
- 肢体撕裂伤或刺伤。
- 烧伤。
- 颅骨凹陷性骨折。

儿科注意事项

女性强奸案中约有54%发生在18岁之前。

• 必须遵守有关虐待儿童的各州法律。

• 儿童性虐待案件中的大多数身体检查都是正常的。

• 在青春期前的孩子中，检查很可能不需要内镜检查。如果需要进行内镜检查，则应在镇静下进行；并考虑让性侵犯审查员参加。

• 在采访孩子时，应提出开放性问题。

• 用玩具、娃娃和图片等让孩子解释发生了什么。

• 早期精神和心理干预是必要的。

妊娠注意事项

孕妇受虐待、殴打的概率较高。

历史

• 即使患者不愿提出指控，也要获取完整的历史记录，包括：

- 受侵害的日期、时间和地点。
- 侵害者的身体特征。
- 侵害者人数。
- 被侵害的部位：阴道、口腔、直肠。
- 如果侵害者有射精：应询问当时侵害者是否使用了安全套。
- 是否发生体液交换。
- 是否使用武力、武器、拘禁、药物或酒精。
- 询问受害者是否记忆力减退或意识丧失。
- 受害者在遭受侵害以后的活动轨迹：
  ◦ 换衣服。
  ◦ 冲洗。
  ◦ 沐浴。
  ◦ 排尿。
  ◦ 排便。
  ◦ 饮食。
  ◦ 使用卫生棉条。
- 完整的妇科病史。
- 最后一次自愿性交时间。
- 精子可在子宫颈中存活最多5日，在阴道中存活12 h。

• 记录所有身体不适主诉。

体格检查

• 即使受害者不确定是否要向警方举报，也要使用证据工具包留取证据。

• 如果由男性医师实施检查，需要有女性助理陪同。

• 如果衣物被污染，应征得患者同意，在脱去衣服之前拍照取证。

• 注意受害者的情绪状态。

• 注意衣物的整体外观：

- 染色。
- 撕裂。
- 泥巴。
- 树叶。
- 树木、种子油渍。
- 让患者站在床单上，然后将所有衣服放在纸袋中。

• 塑料会引起真菌并增加细菌数。

• 只有患者本人可以拿取衣物。

• 给受害者准备换洗衣服。

• 完整的身体检查应着重于：

- 擦伤。
- 撕裂伤。
- 咬伤。
- 抓痕。
- 身体异物。
- 瘀斑。
- 皮肤上的精斑。

• 法证收集：

- 指甲刮屑。
- 头皮或阴毛样本。
- 如果发生口交，请在牙缝之间留取拭子检测酸性磷酸酶（精液分析）和精子。
- 取咽拭子进行淋球菌和衣原体培养。

• 妇科检查：

- 说明所有步骤，并允许患者掌控检查进度。
- 按照当地规程梳理并收集阴毛。
- 用水（不是润滑剂）润滑窥器。
- 对无症状患者中也要查找有无生殖器损伤。
- 可使用甲苯胺蓝查找创伤性性行为造成的盆部裂伤。
  ◦ 最好在阴道口黏膜附近查找。
- 特别注意处女膜是创伤最常见的地方。
- 在阴道口附近的阴道壁裂伤在年轻患者中更常见。
- 收集在阴道后穹隆的分泌物，并放置在无菌容器中，以检查精子和酸性磷酸盐：
  ◦ 如果阴道后穹隆无分泌物，请用棉签擦拭。
  ◦ 留取拭子并在显微镜检查精子和酸性磷酸盐。
- 淋球菌和衣原体的拭子：
  ◦ 有争议，对方可能以此作为受害者存在滥交的证据。
- 阴道镜可以观察到小病变，并可以对发现进行照相（该程序常由性侵犯审查员执行）。
- 进行直肠检查和行淋球菌和衣原体培养，如果阳性提示存在性侵犯或试图性侵犯。

■ 基本检查

• 在进行任何检查、检测或治疗之前，应先取得书面同意。

• 允许患者按其认为舒适的节奏实施检查或暂停检查。

• 在患者的同意下，允许说服或陪同患者前来检查的人在检查期间与患者待在一起。

■ 诊断检查与说明

实验室检查

• 梅毒血清学。

• 乙型和丙型肝炎。

• HIV 检测和咨询。

• 毒物测试（如果受害人是被迫吸毒，其毒物鉴定结果被其他机构获取后，可能被用来作为对受害者不利的证据）。

• 血型。

• 妊娠测试。

• 淋球菌培养。

• 衣原体培养。

• 根据伤情补充其他实验室检查。

影像学检查

依据受伤情况选择。

诊断步骤/外科

依据受伤情况选择。

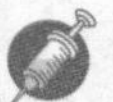

治疗

■ 院前

• 以一种友善的、不带偏见的方式对待患者。

• 有头颈外伤者给予颈椎制动。

■ 初始稳定/治疗

处理威胁生命的损伤。

■ 急诊治疗/程序

• 将患者放置在安静的私人房间中。

• 确保患者姓名和住院原因对来访者保密。

• 确保患者安全。

• 要求所有职员对患者接触时不带偏见。

• 住院期间，应指派熟悉证据收集流程的护理和医务人员开展工作。

• 有条件时应进行 SANE 检查。

• 患者在急诊室期间，请社区或医院内援助人员陪伴患者。

• 提醒医院安全人员可能有攻击者在急诊室出现。

• 如果患者同意或当地法律要求，请联系警方。

• 按前述要求和当地法律收集证据。

• 如果当前未怀孕，则应在药物安全有效的时间窗内向患者提供预防怀孕的方法。

• 进行淋球菌、衣原体、滴虫的预防性治疗。

• 对侵害发生在 72 h 内的受害者，可考虑预防性 HIV 治疗。

• 可对未接种乙肝疫苗者实施预防性治疗或疫苗接种：

– 除非确定侵害者为乙肝感染者，否则受害者无须使用乙肝免疫球蛋白。

• 2015 年的 CDA 指南建议对 9～26 岁的女性和 9～21 岁的男性接种 HPV 疫苗。

• 恰当处理所有软组织或骨骼损伤。

> **注意**
>
> 被性侵犯后怀孕的风险和 HIV 的感染风险未知。
>
> • 下列情况下，HIV 的感染风险增加：
>
> – 男性对男性的性侵犯。
>
> – 肛门侵害。
>
> – 多部位侵害。
>
> – 侵害者或受害者存在创伤、出血及肛门或生殖器损伤。

■ 药物治疗

预防怀孕

• 性侵犯发生在 72 h 内者，给予激素治疗：

– 首选方案：左炔诺孕酮，首剂 0.75 mg，即刻口服，12 h 内重复一次；或左炔诺孕酮 1.5 mg，单剂量口服。

– 次选方案：首剂乙炔雌二醇 100 μg 联合左炔诺孕酮 0.5 mg 即刻口服，12 h 后重复一次（该方案副作用较小，但疗效较差）。

• 如果在 120 h 内进行激素治疗。

– 乌利司他 30 mg，口服。

> **注意**
>
> 所有患者均应预防性传播疾病。

预防性传播疾病

• 头孢曲松：250 mg，肌内注射一次；或头孢克肟 400 mg 单剂量口服（淋球菌）。

• 多西环素：100 mg，口服，每日 2 次，共 7 日；或阿奇霉素 1 g/d，单剂量（衣原体）。

• 甲硝唑（Flagyl）：2 g，单剂量口服（滴虫）。

> **注意**
>
> 如果 PCN 过敏，阿奇霉素 2 g 单次剂量口服治疗淋球菌和衣原体。

预防 HIV 感染

• 恩曲他滨/替诺福韦（truvada）200 mg/300 mg，每日 1 次联合雷格列韦 400 mg，每日 2 次或多洛格韦 50 mg 每日 1 次。

– 如果是高风险暴露源（已知侵害者为 HIV 感染者或者是静脉吸毒者，或者与男性性行为者），推荐多洛格韦方案。

• 如果使用了 HIV 预防性治疗，应完善血常规等常规检验。

• HPV 疫苗：

– 美国只有 9 价（加德西）疫苗。

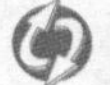

随访

■ 进一步处理

入院标准

严重的外伤。

出院标准

• 对病原学培养和 HIV 检测结果进行医学随访，并监测 HIV 预防药物的副作用。

• 心理科门诊随访。

• 将患者安排到安全住所。

转诊问题

• 心理健康服务与咨询。

• 对于所有儿科病例，应与儿童和家庭服务部联系。

■ 随访建议

应在 6 周、3 个月和 6 个月重复进行 HIV 检测随访。

要点和误区

• 约 70% 的性侵犯受害者不告诉医生或寻求心理保健服务。

• 除非回答直接问题，否则大多数受害者不会透露被侵害情况。

• 在儿童性侵犯案件中，大多数儿童的体格检查并无明显异常（80%～96%）。

• 外生殖器损伤可能比内生殖器和肛门损伤更普遍。

• 美国现有 600 多个 SANE/SART（经过专门培训的法医检查员）计划；如果可能的话，寻求 SANE 项目的帮助可能会改善性侵犯受害者的医疗、法律和心理护理状况。

胸廓出口综合征 Thoracic Outlet Syndrome

Woodrow J. Sams 范浩浩 李文放 译

基础知识

描述

• 胸廓出口综合征(TOS)的症状是通过颈部到腋窝和颈部的通道的臂丛、锁骨下静脉或锁骨下动脉受到压迫。

• 根据不同的主要症状细分为3类:
- 神经源性胸廓出口综合征(NTOS):
  ◦ 90%~98%为成人患者。
  ◦ 女性>男性。
  ◦ 确实存在(1%~3%):有客观症状的人。
  ◦ 有争议(90%):没有或有限的客观症状的人。
- 静脉胸廓出口综合征(VTOS):
  ◦ 2%~4%的患者。
- 动脉胸廓出口综合征(ATOS):
  ◦ 最少见,<1%。
  ◦ 男女发病均等。

• 青少年中血管表现更常见,在>50%的青少年TOS中发生。

• 右下肢更常受到影响。

病因

• 解剖异常:
- 骨性异常包括颈椎肋骨、第1胸椎肋骨或锁骨异常:
  ◦ 颈椎肋骨人群的发生率<1%,约70%在发生女性中,大多数无症状。
  ◦ 锁骨骨折、胸锁关节和肋锁关节外伤更加少见。
- 先天性带状或畸形肌肉。
- 可能在神经和静脉类型中发挥作用,但几乎总是与动脉类型有关。

• 神经源性:
- 常有颈部创伤的病史,比如挥鞭伤(过伸伤)或重复的运动。

• 静脉型:
- 可能与过度活动有关,常见于青少年运动员。
- 由锁骨下静脉急性血栓形成(也称Paget-Schrotter疾病)或静脉损伤引起。

• 动脉:
- 经常自发形成。
- 与创伤或工作无关。
- 可能会出现在负重情况下的跛行。
- 绝大多数患者存在一个完整的颈部肋骨或一个异常第1肋骨。
- 锁骨下动脉瘤或锁骨下动脉、腋动脉撞击所致:
  ◦ 锁骨下动脉瘤附壁血栓形成或锁骨下动脉狭窄引起的远端动脉栓子。

• 上肢带骨下降和肌肉组织下垂也可能倾向于导致TOS:
- 老化。
- 肥胖。
- 乳房过大。

诊断

症状和体征

• 神经源性:
- 大面积,疼痛,手、手臂和肩膀感觉异常和虚弱。
- 也可能会看到鱼际隆起的萎缩,被称为Gilliatt-Sumner手。
- 类似但不像Erb Duchenne综合征那么严重。
- 也可以看到雷诺现象、手冰冷、颜色变化:
  ◦ 不是由缺血引起的,而是由于在臂丛下干范围内的过度活动的交感神经纤维引起的。
  ◦ 在动脉TOS中可以看到类似的症状,两者必须通过评估来区分其他症状和体征来鉴别。

• 静脉型:
- 手臂肿胀和发绀:
  ◦ NTOS和ATOS不会出现手臂肿胀。
- 可能会感到疼痛,手臂疼痛。
- 手感觉异常:
  ◦ 可能由于肿胀而不是神经压缩。

• 动脉型:
- 手指缺血、跛行、苍白、寒冷、感觉异常和手部疼痛。
- 通常肩膀和颈部不受影响。
- 苍白和寒冷是由于缺血而不是雷诺现象。
- 动脉瘤:
  ◦ 无痛的搏动肿块。

病史

• 可能由于重复使用而导致位置或恶化(即超负荷工作)。

• 通常在起病和进展中隐匿。

• 创伤后或突然发生或恶化的急性血肿或肿块。

体格检查

刺激手法可以检查NTOS(只要有病史和症状就可诊断为VTOS和ATOS):

• Roos,亦称手臂抬高压力测试(EAST):
- 手臂外展90°,肘部弯曲90°。
- 肩部稍稍支撑在额平面的后面。
- 拳头放开和握紧3 min。
- 早期有手臂沉重和疲劳的感觉。
- 手部麻木逐渐发作。
- 手臂和肩的顶部的渐进性疼痛。
- 前臂只有疲劳则测试结果为阴性。

• Adson测试:
- 手臂向下,患者向头部旋转,抬起头来,吸气。
- 阳性结果是桡动脉脉搏的变或消除或血压变化。
- 不是一个可靠的测试,因为许多NTOS患者测试结果阴性而许多病情控制的患者测试结果阳性。

• 赖特测试:
- 受影响的手臂过度外展和外旋,同时触诊患侧脉搏。
- 如果出现感觉减退或脉搏减少,则为阳性结果。

• 以上都不是非常敏感或特异。

• 右锁骨下动脉血压差异>20 mmHg的提示临床缓解。

基本检查

• 细致的病史和体格检查。

• 肌酸激酶排除心脏缺血。

实验室检查

考虑静脉或静脉的凝血功能检查。

影像学检查

• 门诊患者排除危及肢体的局部缺血和/或怀疑静脉血栓。

• X线片:
- 评估解剖异常:第1肋骨、颈肋、锁骨畸形:
  ◦ 没有异常,ATOS是不太可能的。
- 肺部疾病。

• 颈椎:
- 骨折。
- 脊柱侧弯。

• 超声可以诊断静脉血栓形成。

• 双面扫描是筛选锁骨下动脉动脉瘤或狭

X

窄的最佳方式，可指导动脉造影。

• 动脉波：

- 通常用于帮助外科医师进行重建计划。

- 适应证包括：

◦ 桡动脉脉搏减弱，血压比对侧肢体低 20 mmHg。

◦ 怀疑锁骨下狭窄。

◦ 锁骨上的异常搏动或杂音或者搏动肿块。

◦ 上肢的外周血管栓子。

• 静脉造影：

- 有水肿、外周性单侧发绀，或胸廓和四肢静脉扩张，则推荐性静脉造影。

• NTOS：

- 没有金标准测试：诊断仍然主要为临床诊断。

- 肌电图和神经传导速度测试通常是正常的。

• 需要评估脊髓疾病、椎间盘突出或评估肺上沟瘤可行 MRI。

鉴别诊断

• 心脏缺血。

• 颈椎病或椎间盘疾病。

• 腕管综合征或神经卡压。

• 肺上沟瘤。

• 其他颈部、纵隔恶性肿瘤。

• 神经炎。

• 肌炎。

• 雷诺病。

• 多发性硬化症或退行性脊髓疾病。

• 肩部炎性疾病：关节炎、旋转、袖带损伤、双肘肌腱炎。

• 动脉粥样硬化或血栓栓塞性疾病。

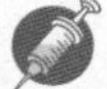

治疗

急诊治疗/程序

• 如果有动脉或静脉血栓形成征象，立即肝素治疗。

• 有缺血的征象则需要向血管外科咨询并按需行导管溶栓治疗：

- 血栓形成患者在抗凝和溶栓随后需要手术减压。

• 初始管理：

- 多数患者保守治疗包括物理治疗和药物治疗后症状缓解。

• 药物治疗失败可行手术：

- 通常需要血管形成术。

- 具有 NTOS 的患者通常在手术干预前需要更广泛的医疗评估与医疗管理。

- 70%～90%的患者达到部分或者完全的术后缓解。

药物治疗

• 环苯偶氮：10 mg，口服，每日 3 次。

• 地西泮：5 mg，口服，每日 3 次。

• 布洛芬：800 mg，口服，每日 3 次。

• 美索巴莫：1 000～1 500 mg，口服，每日 3 次。

• 舒缓搽剂或药膏。

随访

进一步处理

入院指征

• 缺血。

• 静脉血栓形成。

• 动脉血栓形成。

• 动脉瘤或狭窄。

• 难以忍受的痛苦。

出院指征

• 无肢体威胁的神经系统发现。

• 无动脉或静脉血栓形成。

随访建议

根据病情进行血管、神经或骨科咨询。

要点和误区

• 3 种 TOS：神经源性、动脉性和静脉性：

- 神经源性在成人中最常见。

- ATOS 和 VTOS 是儿童和青少年更常见的类型。

• 仅 VTOS 有手臂肿胀和水肿。

• NTOS 和 ATOS 都有手感冷淡和苍白，但出于不同的原因。

• 可能有反复使用或创伤的病史。

• 检查或影像可能会显示先天性颈椎肋骨等结构的异常。

胸腔积液 Pleural Effusion

Sierra Beck · Steven M. Lindsey 瞿金龙 译

基础知识

描述

• 正常情况：

- 胸膜腔有 0.25 ml/kg 清亮、低蛋白质液体，利于肺组织在胸腔内的活动。

- 胸腔积液形成和重吸收受静水压、胶体渗透压影响。

- 通常情况下，这些力量的总和会导致液体从壁层的胸膜毛细血管进入胸膜间隙，而后被内脏表面淋巴管吸收。

• 液体进入和吸收的速率通常是相等的，但在积液过程中会变得混乱。

• 分类：

- 漏出液：

◦ 血浆渗出，以蛋白质低和细胞数低为特征。

◦ 血静水压升高，或者胶体渗透压降低。

◦ 一般不会出现在胸膜腔损伤基础上。

- 渗出液：

◦ 以蛋白质高和细胞数高为特征。

◦ 胸膜损伤导致膜通透性改变或淋巴重吸收异常。

病因

• 漏出液：

- 充血性心力衰竭。

- 腹膜透析。

- 肝硬化腹水。

- 肺栓塞。

- 急性肺不张。

- 肾病综合征。

- 黏液性水肿。

- 低蛋白血症。

- 上腔静脉综合征。

- Megis 综合征：

◦ 腹水三联征、卵巢肿瘤、胸膜腔渗出。

• 渗出液：

- 肺、胸膜腔感染：

◦ 细菌、病毒、真菌、结核、寄生虫。
- 原发性肺部肿瘤。
- 间皮瘤。
- 肿瘤转移(乳腺癌、卵巢癌或淋巴瘤)。
- 心包炎。
- 肺栓塞。
• 腹部疾病:
- 胰腺炎、肝炎、胆囊炎。
- 膈下脓肿。
- 食管破裂。
- 腹膜炎。
- Meigs 综合征。
• 风湿科疾病:
- 系统性红斑狼疮。
- 风湿性关节炎。
- 结节病。
• 创伤:
- 血胸。
- 乳糜胸。
• 药物:
- 药物导致的狼疮。
- 呋喃妥因、美西麦角、丹曲洛林、胺碘酮、溴隐亭。
- 可卡因。

诊断

症状和体征

• 少量渗出一般无症状。
• 呼吸困难、胸痛、伴或不伴有咳嗽。
• 呼吸急促、低氧、呼吸音降低,伴或不伴叩诊浊音。

病史

• 有慢性心力衰竭、肺炎、肺栓塞、胰腺炎等病史,常常并发胸腔积液。
• 静息或活动后呼吸困难。
• 咳嗽。
• 胸膜炎症引起的胸痛。
• 脓胸:发热、乏力、体重减轻。

体格检查

• 呼吸音减低。
• 语音震颤减弱。
• 叩诊浊音。
• 胸膜摩擦音阳性。
• 胸腔积液渗出病因的检查。

基本检查

• 心电监测和指脉氧监测。
• 血细胞、生化、电解质、凝血功能检查。
• 胸部透视。
• 寻找病因方面的检查。

诊断检查与说明

实验室检查

• 血常规。
• 电解质、尿素氮、肌酐、血糖、乳酸脱氢酶(LDH)、血蛋白检查。
• 凝血功能检查。
• 胸腔积液检查,判断是漏出液还是渗出液:
- 胸腔积液蛋白、LDH 水平。
- 渗出液常见重要指标(≥1 项):
◦ 蛋白质和 LDH 水平。
◦ 胸腔积液蛋白/血浆蛋白>0.5。
◦ 胸腔积液 LDH/血 LDH>0.6。
◦ 胸腔积液 LDH>正常的 2/3。
• 漏出液,一般不需特别检查。
• 检查渗出液的病因:
- 常规检验:细胞计数、革兰染色、培养、结核杆菌检查、pH、糖和细胞液检查。
- 基于临床考虑:甘油三酯、淀粉酶、白蛋白、Cr、肿瘤指标等。
- 红细胞计数和血细胞比容:
◦ 5 000~100 000/mm^3 无特别。
◦ >100 000/mm^3 肿瘤转移、创伤或肺栓塞。
◦ 血细胞比容/血浆血细胞比容>0.5,提示血胸可能。
◦ 其他的病因:转移肿瘤,结核、动脉破裂。
◦ 肝素化或凝血功能异常出血,一般细胞学检查能发现。
- 白细胞:
◦ 1 000~10 000/mm^3 无异常。
◦ >100 000/mm^3 肺炎渗出、脓胸、转移肿瘤、结核等。
- 糖:
◦ <60 mg/dl,肺炎渗出或脓胸、转移肿瘤、食管破裂、风湿性疾病。
- 甘油三酯(三酰甘油)。
◦ >100 mg/dl,提示乳糜胸、胸导管破裂。
- 淀粉酶。
◦ >200 U/dl,提示胰腺炎、食管破裂、转移肿瘤、结核或脓胸。
- pH:
◦ 血气检查。
◦ pH<7 提示肺炎渗出或脓胸。
- 细胞学检查肿瘤细胞。

影像学检查

• 胸部 X 线检查:
- 正位片:
◦ 肋膈角变钝。
◦ 200~250 ml 及以上液体。
◦ 胸腔积液常见胃泡和肺组织间间隙增加。
- 侧位片:
◦ 可以鉴别 5~10 ml 的液体。
◦ 可以鉴别分隔液体或肺液间的液体。
• 超声:
- 和侧位片有相同的敏感性,可鉴别 5~10 ml 的液体。
- 能鉴别分隔的液体。
- 提高安全性和减低穿刺并发气胸的风险。
• CT 造影:
- 对检查胸腔积液最敏感,还能区分是否有分隔。
- 检查肺内肿块或胸膜增厚感。

> **注意**
> • 不能解释的胸腔积液,需要考虑肺栓塞。
> • 床旁胸部 X 线和床旁超声检查,可以减少胸腔穿刺术的并发症和误诊的可能性。

诊断步骤/外科

急诊室内诊断和治疗性胸腔穿刺:
• 指征:
- 在老患者中诊断新的渗出。
- 大量渗出引起呼吸困难。
- 诊断性胸腔穿刺可以在入院后实施。
• 没有完全禁忌证。
• 相对禁忌证:
- 血小板<50 000/mm^3。
- PT 和 APTT 超过正常值 2 倍。
- 血 Cr>6。
• 纠正凝血功能异常。
• 位置要求:双上臂交叉胸前,抬高肩胛骨。
• 超声或叩诊确认胸腔积液的边界。
• 肩甲中线或腋后线确定穿刺肋间隙。
• 碘酒消毒,等区域内干燥后操作。
• 2%利多卡因麻醉。
• 在下一个肋骨的上缘进针,边回抽边进针。
• 使用 20G 针头做诊断性穿刺。
• 使用 16~18G 针头做治疗性穿刺。
• 可以在胸腔置入导管。
• 基本的检查至少 100 ml(蛋白质、LDH、细胞计数等)。
• 避免一次抽出>1 500 ml,防止复张性肺水肿。
• 如果在操作中出现胸痛,可能穿破肺组织,有气胸形成可能,立即停止操作并摄片确认。

• 操作完之后，拔除针头，局部压片刻，防止气胸形成，最好能复查胸部 X 线排除气胸。

• 胸腔闭式引流术的指征：
- 分隔的渗出。
- 排脓需要。
- 渗出液 pH<7，或糖<60 mg/dl，胸腔积液培养阳性。
- 血胸。

■ 鉴别诊断

• 实质内的病变鉴别：
- 肺不张。
- 肿块、肿瘤或其他浸润性病变。
- 肺炎。

• 胸腔内的病变鉴别：
- 胸腔外伤后瘢痕形成。
- 间皮瘤或转移肿瘤。

• 其他：
- 膈疝。
- 膈肌麻痹。

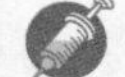

治疗

■ 院前

建立静脉通路，高流量吸氧，心电监测，指脉氧监测。

■ 初步稳定/治疗

• 必要时心肺复苏术。
• 高流量吸氧。
• 必要的紧急呼吸支持。

■ 急诊治疗/程序

• 识别和治疗原发病。
• 如果胸腔积脓，外科会诊行胸腔闭式引流。
• 请介入放射科或呼吸科关于分隔性的胸腔积液。

■ 药物治疗

• 慢性心力衰竭：利尿剂治疗。
• 肺炎渗出：抗生素治疗。
• 肺栓塞：抗凝治疗。
- 血性渗出不是抗凝的禁忌证。
• 风湿性疾病：NSAIDs 治疗。
• 分隔的渗出：可胸腔内注射链激酶或尿激酶治疗。

随访

■ 进一步处理

入院指征

• 呼吸困难。
• 不明原因的胸腔积液。
• 首次查出要求住院治疗。
• 怀疑或考虑肺炎渗出或脓胸。
• 观察 6 h 或收入院，因为胸腔穿刺手术的潜在并发症：
- 气胸。
- 复张性肺水肿。

• ICU 收治指征：严重血流动力学不稳定或需要呼吸支持。

出院指征

• 胸腔积液的性质与来源已经明确。
• 没有呼吸并发症存在。
• 部分原发病治疗后胸腔积液会自行吸收。
• 患者有能力获得电话援助或合适的随访。

转诊问题

能有肿瘤科医师或呼吸肿瘤科医师进行合适的随访。

■ 随访建议

如果患者呼吸困难加重、发热或其他呼吸相关方面的症状加重，必须随时急诊就诊。

要点和误区

• 最常见的胸腔积液原因是慢性心力衰竭、肺炎和恶性肿瘤。
• 鉴别和治疗胸腔积液的原因。
• 超声有助于对渗出液的性质判断和减少胸腔穿刺后出现气胸的风险。
• 常见的致死性胸腔积液病因鉴别包括肺栓塞、食管破裂、血胸。
• 如果大量胸腔积液引起循环和呼吸不稳定，可以适当排放。

胸锁关节损伤 Sternoclavicular Joint Injury

Christopher M. Tedeschi · Wallace A. Carter 江伟伟 李文放 译

基础知识

■ 描述

• 胸锁关节(SCJ)是将上肢连接到躯干的唯一关节。
• 身体中最频繁受伤的关节。
• 最常见的原因是运动或交通事故。
• 先天性或自发性脱位和半脱位罕见。
• SCJ 的稳定性取决于韧带，主要是前后锁骨后韧带、锁骨间韧带和肋锁韧带。
• 需要高度怀疑损伤或脱位的诊断。

■ 病因

• 对 SCJ 的损伤可能来自韧带的扭伤、半脱位或脱位。
• 在扭伤时，韧带囊完好无损。
• 半脱位发生在胸锁乳突韧带断裂而肋锁韧带保持完整时。
• 完全韧带断裂导致脱位。
• SCJ 可以向前或向后脱位，复位需要大力量，将锁骨向后移位需要更大的力量。
• 脱位可能更常见于运动过度综合征的患者，如埃勒斯-当洛斯综合征。
• 脱位的方向取决于肩膀的位置：
- 当肩峰位于胸骨柄后方时，前部脱位的可能性更大。
- 当肩峰位于胸骨柄前方时，后方脱位的可能性更大。

• 前脱位更常见(超过 90%的脱位)：
- 由肩部的前外侧方向的后向力引起。
- 内侧锁骨反向前移。
- 可能与气胸、血胸、肺挫伤和肋骨骨折有关。
- 可能发生半脱位和脱位。

• 后脱位原因：
- 前后击中锁骨内侧。
- 指向同侧肩部外侧的前方力。
- 当受伤的一侧靠在一个不动的物体上时，对侧肩膀受到撞击。

• 后脱位需紧急手术：
- 即刻复位指征：
◦ 压迫或撕裂气管、食管或大血管。

◦ 喉返神经损伤。

儿科注意事项

• 锁骨内侧骨骺生长板最后会骨化，并在22～25岁融合：

- 在融合之前，生长板是关节中最薄弱的部分。

• 内侧骨骺的骨折与SCJ脱位相仿：

- 最常见的是Salter-Harris Ⅰ型或Ⅱ型骨折。

- 由于强韧带，SCJ的真正脱位在儿童中极为罕见。

诊断

症状和体征

• 疼痛和肿胀以适当机制局限于锁骨内侧和SCJ。

• 对侧手臂通过胸部影响手臂支撑。

• 无法外展或外部旋转手臂。

• 如果半脱位或扭伤，SCJ在直接触诊和肩部运动时无力：

- 没有畸形。

• 如果SCJ脱臼，肩膀会缩短：

- 由于胸锁乳突肌痉挛，头部向受伤侧倾斜。

• 在前方脱位时，锁骨内侧端明显突出并可触及。

• 在后脱位时，SCJ区域可能有一个沟，通过该沟可以触摸胸骨柄的外侧边界：

- 脱臼可能被通过SCI的显著肿胀所掩盖，并可能与前脱位相似。

• 后部脱位可伴有血管损害或纵隔结构损伤的体征：

- 休克的迹象。

- 呼吸困难或说话。

- 上肢疼痛或神经症状。

病史

• 高强度撞击，最常见于运动损伤或车辆碰撞。

• 扭伤和半脱位可能与肩胛带的其他损伤有关。

体格检查

• 扭伤和半脱位时无力和肿胀。

• 在前脱位，内侧锁骨突出。

• 对于任何后脱位，评估气道或神经血管损伤的体征：

- 吞咽困难或呼吸窘迫可能意味着气管或食管受压或破裂。

- 评估上肢疼痛。

- 声音嘶哑表示喉返神经损伤。

- 运动或感觉缺陷表明臂丛神经损伤。

- 评估上肢端静脉回流情况：

◦ 静脉压迫可导致上肢静脉充血或静脉血栓形成。

基本检查

• 对其他危及生命的伤害进行全面的创伤评估和复苏。

• 特别注意呼吸、神经和血管状态。

• 后脱位易导致多种损伤机制，必须排除其他危及生命的伤害。

• 患者适当的镇痛。

诊断检查与说明

影像学检查

• 常规X线片难以评估SCJ：

- 可能表现出SCJ与对侧相比的不对称性。

- 评估合并骨、肺和纵隔损伤更有用。

- 胸部X线片可能正常，如果高度怀疑，则需要进一步的检查。

• 超声可以可靠地证明SCJ脱位：

- 可能有助于初步评估不稳定的胸部创伤患者。

- 使用高频率线性探测器。

- 在前方脱位时，与对侧相比，内侧锁骨在胸骨柄前方。

• CT能最好地评估SCJ：

- X线平片无法确定时很有用。

- 准确区分脱位和骨折。

- 看到锁骨的位置。

- 显示胸腔出口和纵隔的详细解剖结构。

- 对比CT可显示相关血管损伤，是首选的影像学检查方法。

• MRI可用于显示韧带和软组织SCJ损伤：

- 在SCJ损伤中，关节盘是最脆弱的软组织。

- 在关节半脱位的情况下可以表现出特定的韧带损伤。

- 在最初的诊断和治疗阶段后更合适。

- 在儿童物理损伤中，可以帮助区分真正的脱位。

鉴别诊断

• 胸锁扭伤、半脱位或脱位。

• 内侧锁骨骨折。

• 化脓性关节炎。

• 锁骨内侧骨髓炎。

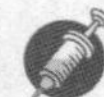

治疗

院前

• 注意气道和生命体征，以及受累肢体的神经血管状态。

• 运送到急诊科之前，受影响的胳膊应该在舒适的位置。

初步稳定/治疗

• 气管插管适用于气道损伤或需插管的创伤患者。

• 紧急SCJ情况：

- 气道不稳定或受损。

- 休克的迹象。

- 脉搏细弱。

- 嘶哑。

- 吞咽困难。

- 神经血管损害：

◦ 上肢无力。

◦ 感觉异常。

急诊治疗/程序

• 扭伤和半脱位可用冰、NSAIDs、吊带固定和后续矫形等对症处理。

• 急诊中前部脱位复位：

- 镇静，充分控制疼痛和肌肉放松。

- 仰卧位，卷曲的毛巾放在肩胛骨之间：

◦ 纵向牵引伸展手臂，肩部外展90°。

◦ 辅助应用温和的压力在锁骨的移动端。

◦ 减少后，用填充良好的“8”字形敷料固定。

- 复位后许多前部脱位依然不稳定。

- 手术很少显示，因为畸形需整形。

• 在全身麻醉下，后部脱位需要紧急减压：

- 整形外科和胸部手术咨询。

- 封闭式复位优选（并且通常是成功的），但在受损>48 h可能不可行。

- 如果没有外科医师，可能需要急诊复位：

◦ 缓解严重的气道、神经系统或血管损伤。

◦ 适当的镇静和止痛是基本的。

◦ 仰卧位，卷曲的毛巾放在肩胛骨之间。

◦ 受影响的手臂被外展，长度延长。

◦ 手臂外展后，纵向牵引。

◦ 如果不成功，则使用无菌毛巾夹固定内侧锁骨头并施加轻微的前牵引。

药物治疗

镇静：

• 依托咪酯：0.1 mg/kg 微量泵。

• 芬太尼：1～2 μg/kg 微量泵。

X

• 氯胺酮：1 mg/kg 微量泵，最多添加 2 次 0.5 mg/kg。

• 咪达唑仑：0.01 mg/kg（儿童 0.05～0.1 mg/kg）静推，q2～3 min。

• 丙泊酚：根据需要静脉注射 1 mg/kg，然后 0.5 mg/kg，q3 min（成人和儿童）。

随访

进一步处理

入院指征

• SCJ 的后部脱位需要入院才能复位或评估潜在并发症。

• 同时存在其他的伤害，需住院治疗。

出院指征

• SCJ 扭伤。

• SCJ 的前部脱位无神经血管损害或其他显著损伤。

• 安排适当的骨科门诊随访。

转诊问题

对于任何显著的 SCJ 损伤，建议患者骨科门诊随访。

随访建议

• 闭合复位脱位后难以达到长期稳定性，因此建议进行整形外科随访。

• 扭伤患者需简单的吊带固定。

• 更严重的伤害需“8”字形敷料固定。

• 重复 MRI 或 CT 检查可能是有益的。

• 即使轻度扭伤和半脱位，也应避免长达 3 个月的高风险活动。

要点和误区

• 由于 SCJ 伤害很少，所以在急诊评估和救治期间这可能是潜在危及生命的伤害，可能会错过治疗。

• 后部脱位要求早期心胸外科会诊。

• 由于关节明显肿胀，后脱位可能被误认为前脱位。

• 在儿科人群中，Salter-Harris 骨折可能与脱位相伤。

胸痛 Chest Pain

Josh W. Joseph 庄育刚 译

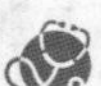

基础知识

描述

• 急诊最常见的主诉。

• 这个主要症状经常反映一种高危的疾病：

- 急性冠状动脉综合征。
- 肺栓塞。
- 主动脉夹层。

• 容易被假设为危及生命的疾病直到明确诊断为其他疾病。

• 虽然分类可能会提示潜在的病因，但胸部疼痛的主诉，可以是非常多变和表述不清的。

• 胸廓痛：

- 可能包括心肌、心包、升主动脉、肺动脉、纵隔和食管。
- 疼痛是深部的、内脏的和特别局限。
- 表现多样从严重压榨痛到轻微痛、烧灼感或消化不良。

• 剑突下痛：

- 可能包括降主动脉、膈肌、胆囊、胰腺和胃。
- 疼痛一般指向剑突和后背。

• 胸膜痛：

- 肋骨、肋软骨、肋间肌、神经、胸膜或心包的炎症或创伤。
- 疼痛随着呼吸、大笑、咳嗽、喷嚏加重。
- 轻轻触诊即可表现疼痛。
- 膈胸膜炎：
  ◦ 上腹部的刺痛、胸廓运动后引起较低位置的胸骨或肩膀疼痛加剧。

• 胸壁痛：

- 皮肤炎症和 SC 结构胸壁。
- 出现下列情况，疼痛会再次发生：
  ◦ 触诊。
  ◦ 手臂的水平弯曲。
  ◦ 颈部伸展。
  ◦ 给予头部纵向压力。

病因

• 胸廓：

- 急性冠状动脉综合征。
- 心包炎。
- 心肌炎。
- 压力诱导的心肌病。
- 微循环缺血。
- 兴奋剂的使用。
- 胸部的主动脉夹层。
- 急性食管炎。
- 食管痉挛。
- 胃食管反流。
- 食管的痛觉过敏。
- 异常运动模式、贲门失弛缓症。
- 食管破裂和纵隔炎。

• 上腹部：

- 降主动脉破裂。
- 消化性溃疡。
- 胰腺炎。
- 胆囊炎。
- 脾破裂。
- 肝损伤。
- 膈下脓肿。

• 胸膜痛：

- 肺栓塞。
- 气胸。
- 肺炎。
- 肋软骨炎。

• 膈胸膜炎：

- 脾破裂。
- 肝损伤。
- 膈下脓肿。

• 食管破裂。

• 肋间肌炎。

• 肋间神经痛。

• 胸小肌紧张。

• 心包炎。

• 胸膜炎。

• 肺炎。

• 肋骨骨折。

• 急性镰刀状细胞胸廓综合征。

• 胸壁刺痛综合征。

- 早期短期发作的尖锐的刺痛持续 30 s 至 3 min，深呼吸症状加重和浅慢呼吸缓解。

• 胸壁痛：

- 胸壁血肿。
- 胸壁外伤。
- 带状疱疹。

X

- 胸腹壁血栓性静脉炎。
- 剑突关节炎。
- 痛性肥胖症。
- 乳腺脓肿、纤维囊性乳腺炎、乳腺癌。

诊断

症状和体征

• 冠状动脉疾病：
- 压力。
- 挤压痛。
- 放射到手臂和下颌。
- 呼吸急促。
- 出汗。
- 晕厥。
- 呕吐。
- 乏力。
- 疲乏，尤其是妇女和老年人表现更明显。
- 冠心病的表现。
- 焦虑。

• 主动脉夹层：
- 突发疼痛，早期十分剧烈。
- 剧痛。
- 放射到后背伴或不伴侧面痛。
- 高血压。
- 主动脉关闭不全引起舒张期杂音。
- 上肢脉搏波动差异。
- 晕厥。
- 眩晕。
- 呕吐。
- 伴随神经系统的改变（如视力的变化）。

• 肺栓塞：
- 胸膜痛。
- 呼吸短促。
- 焦虑。
- 出汗。
- 气促。
- 心悸。
- 低热。
- 晕厥。
- 局限的啰音。
- 哮鸣音。

• 急性心包炎：
- 胸骨下疼痛。
- 呼吸变化。
- 向前倾斜。
- 焦虑。
- 厌食症。
- 发热。
- 心包摩擦音。

• 气胸：
- 胸膜痛。
- 短促呼吸。
- 焦虑。
- 呼吸急促。
- 单侧呼吸音减低。
- 自发性（年轻人）或与外伤有关的继发性（多发生于老年人）。

病史

• 病史是区分不同病因之间的最重要的工具。
• 患者准确地描述病史特征：
- 持续时间。
- 疼痛部位：
  ◦ 胸骨后。
  ◦ 剑突下。
  ◦ 弥漫性。
- 频率：
  ◦ 经常性。
  ◦ 间歇性。
  ◦ 突发或延迟发作。
- 诱因：
  ◦ 用力。
  ◦ 压力。
  ◦ 呼吸。
  ◦ 运动。
- 时间：
  ◦ 发作的时间（如休息、劳累性）。
  ◦ 持续时间。
- 性质：
  ◦ 烧灼样痛。
  ◦ 压榨性痛。
  ◦ 钝痛。
  ◦ 尖锐痛。
  ◦ 撕裂样痛。
  ◦ 沉重痛。
- 伴随症状：
  ◦ 呼吸急促。
  ◦ 大汗。
  ◦ 恶心。
  ◦ 呕吐。
  ◦ 下颌痛。
  ◦ 后背痛。
  ◦ 放射痛。
  ◦ 心悸。
  ◦ 晕厥。
  ◦ 发热。
  ◦ 虚弱：全身或局部性的。
  ◦ 疲乏。

体格检查

• 心脏检查：是否存在杂音、摩擦音，心音是否减低，是否有额外的心音。
• 胸部检查：是否有呼吸音减低，是否有啰音、哮鸣音。
• 肢体检查：是否存在脉搏、奇脉。
• 皮肤检查：是否有皮肤缺损，是否有带状疱疹。
• 腹部检查：检查腹部是否有压痛、反跳痛、肌卫。

诊断检查与说明

心电图：
• 便利和经济的。
• 10 min 内可以得到结果。
• 在诸如急性冠状动脉综合征和最初心电图阴性结果患者，需要高度关注的患者可以给予连续的监测。
• V_7～V_9 导联可能会在最初无法诊断出心电图的高危患者中显示后梗死。
• 得到明确病因。

实验室检查

• 实验室检查应该根据患者的个体情况及威胁生命的潜在的危险来检查。
• 见“心脏检查”。
• D-二聚体：
- 高敏感但低特异性。
- 可以提示低风险的患者如果存在这个指标可以排除肺栓塞。
- 年龄超过 50 岁的患者可以调整阈值。
- 作为主动脉夹层筛查试验的作用有限。

影像学检查

• X 线片：
- 气胸。
- 肺炎。
- 心力衰竭。
- 主动脉夹层。
  ◦ 纵隔增宽见于 55%～62% 的患者。
  ◦ 胸腔积液在 20% 的患者中可发现。
  ◦ 肺尖。
  ◦ 主动脉球消失。
  ◦ 有 12%～15% 患者的 X 线胸片是正常的。
- 急性心包炎：
  ◦ 通常 X 线胸片是正常的，除非心包大量积液使心影增大。
- 食管破裂：
  ◦ 通常显示纵隔积气。
  ◦ 可以存在左侧胸膜积液。
• 螺旋 CT：
- 肺栓塞。
- 对主动脉夹层较敏感。

X

• 通气/灌注影像：
- 用在肺栓塞的患者。
- 必须要查常规 X 线胸片。
• 血管造影：
- 肺栓塞，但是很少做。
- 用在分析患者，特别是稳定的患者。
• 超声：
- 用于检查心包和瓣膜疾病。
- 经食管超声可以用于诊断主动脉夹层，特别是在生命体征不稳定的患者和不能耐受检查的患者。
- 右心室扩张和运动功能减弱可以提示肺栓塞并且可以指导下一步治疗。
- 床旁经胸壁超声可以快速发现有意义的心包积液、气胸和胸腔积液。

■ 鉴别诊断

见病因。

 治疗

■ 院前

• 治疗措施应该根据患者的表现、危险因素和既往史来定。
• 如果一个有心脏病的患者应给予以下治疗：
- 开通静脉通路。
- 心电监测。
- 心电图。
- 吸氧。
- 小剂量阿司匹林或全量阿司匹林。
- 疼痛控制。
◦ 硝酸酯类药物。
◦ 吗啡。

■ 初步稳定/治疗

根据患者的临床表现指导治疗：
• ABC 管理。
• 静脉注射。
• 吸氧。
• 心电监护。

■ 急诊治疗/程序

• 开通静脉通路、吸氧和监测。
• 心电图。
• 基于可疑病因的多重治疗。

■ 药物治疗

基于病因的治疗。

 随访

■ 进一步处理

入院指征

根据危害生命的心脏病的危险程度来决定。

出院指征

如果患者的胸痛是安全的低危险的胸痛。

转诊问题

初级保健医师跟踪随访评估门诊低风险的胸痛。

■ 随访建议

患者有以下情况请返回医院：
• 胸部不适持续>5 min。
• 任何时候的胸部不适加重。
• 通过常规药物治疗不能缓解的心绞痛和胸部不适。
• 气促、大汗、眩晕、呕吐或恶心伴随胸痛或胸部不适。
• 胸部不适放射至手臂、颈部、后背、下颌或胃。

要点和误区

• 慎重处理仅有一个生物标志物的病例，除非疼痛长期没有改变或消失。
• 患者对药物的敏感性也可以作为诊断的工具。
• 不使用怀疑 ACS 患者的连续的心电图或当患者再次发生胸痛时的心电图。
• 与呼吸困难或恶心等相关症状相比，女性描述胸痛的可能性较小。

胸外伤，穿通伤 Chest Trauma，Penetrating

Ioan Belovarski · Jorge Fernandez 庄育刚 译

X

 基础知识

■ 描述

• 刺破胸腔的损伤必须及时发现并解决。
• 如果不纠正，会迅速导致休克甚至死亡。

■ 病因

原因很多，包括：
• 枪伤刺伤。
• 意外损失。
• 钝伤导致复合性肋骨骨折。

 诊断

■ 症状和体征

详尽的病史和身体状况可能揭示：
• 胸痛、呼吸困难或焦虑症的主诉。
• 血流动力学不稳定：
- 心动过速、低血压、呼吸急促、缺氧急性呼吸窘迫。
• 精神状态、焦虑或躁动。
• 呼吸音缺失或减弱。
• 胸部吸气性创伤。
• 胸壁运动不规则或不对称性颈静脉扩张。
• 明显的物体刺入胸腔。
• 胸腔伤口有无出血。
• 颈部或腹部Ⅰ区的伤口：
- 可能与胸部交流。

■ 基本检查

• 评估气道、呼吸和循环。
• 二次创伤调查：
- 去除胸部遮盖物。
- 检查所有表面和褶皱。
- 识别并轻轻检查任何皮肤损伤，不要探测胸部伤口。
- 在活动性出血部位直接施加压力和/或压力敷料。
- 胸部吸气性创伤使用三侧闭塞敷料。
• 关键检查：
- 包括精神状态在内的一般外部特征。
- 呼吸频率和呼吸是否费力。
- 横膈膜上升和下降。
- 呼吸音和心音。
- 胸壁、锁骨上捻发音。
- 颈静脉扩张。

• 床旁 E－FAST 超声可以快速识别气胸、心包积液、填塞物等。
• 直立位胸部 X 线检查（CXR）还可以识别气胸，以及通过膈膜进入腹膜：
－在脊柱预防措施的情况下，仰卧位 CXR 可以代替常规直立位 CXR，但敏感性较低。
• 频繁的生命体征，包括连续指脉氧监测。
• 心电图。
• ABG。
• 床旁血红蛋白。
• 血型和交叉配血试验类型和交叉。
• 全血细胞计数。
• 凝血功能（PT、INR、APTT）、血清乳酸。
• 如果患者稳定，则需进行对比（±血管造影）CT。

■ 诊断检查与说明

实验室检查

一旦患者稳定下来，上述实验室对于任何穿透性损伤，心电图、基本床旁成像和先进的成像方式都至关重要。

影像学检查

• E－FAST 超声应该立即执行：
－评估肺部以确认完整的胸膜滑动运动（M 模式特别有用）。
－评估心包中是否有游离液或明显的壁运动异常（即填塞迹象）：
◦ 在心前区和心包腔大的刺伤时，早期心包积血可减压成血胸，因此在初始的心脏超声检查时是阴性表现。
◦ 血胸行闭式引流减压后，复查心包腔超声。
◦ 任何残留的血胸可能代表心包损伤或心脏撕裂伤。

• 如果患者稳定，CT/CTA 至关重要。
• CT 枪击伤或周围刺伤（如下胸部、上胸部/背部）附近的身体部位（即腹部、骨盆、颈部）。
• 如果怀疑血管严重损伤（尤其是患者持续或严重的血流动力学不稳定），应获取动脉造影。
• 胃泌素吞咽研究或内镜检查可用于识别的食管穿孔（怀疑是子宫颈、锁骨上、纵隔捻发音）。
• 支气管镜检查可评估气管支气管损伤。

■ 鉴别诊断

• 单纯性气胸。
• 张力性气胸。
• 开放性气胸。
• 血胸。
• 肋骨骨折。
• 连枷胸。
• 肺挫伤。
• 心脏挫伤。
• 心脏破裂。
• 心脏压塞。
• 外伤性主动脉破裂。
• 食管损伤。
• 大血管损伤。
• 气管支气管损伤。
• 膈肌损伤。
• 腹腔内损伤。
• 脊髓损伤。

治疗

■ 院前

• 警示：
－院前急救人员明确存在生命体征的患者需送往急救创伤中心救治。
－怀疑脊髓损伤患者需行脊髓固定。
－不要移除胸口的致伤物以防进一步大量出血。
－如果怀疑有张力性气胸，可能需要快速减压。
◦ 单侧无呼吸音，低血压，颈静脉扩张。
－如果存在大的开放性气胸，需行三头带包扎固定。
◦ 完全的胸壁包扎固定可能导致张力性气胸。
• 争议：
－不要为了获取静脉通路延误运送到医院。可在运送途中建立静脉通路。
－如果建立静脉通路失败，可迅速放置骨髓腔通路。任何药物或血液制品均可通过骨髓腔进行管理。
－不要对没有明显脊柱损伤临床症状的患者进行完全的脊柱固定治疗，以免延误运送到医院。

■ 初步稳定/治疗

• ABC 管理：管理呼吸道、呼吸和循环，通过非再呼吸面罩提供氧气。
• 在开始关键干预措施（例如，胸腔穿刺术）之前，请勿等待 CXR。
• E－FAST 超声在诊断气胸方面已显示出比 CXR 更高的敏感性。
• 对于张力性气胸，在放置胸管之前进行胸腔穿刺术。
• 建立静脉通路，必要时需予以两条大的外周静脉（＞18G）行液体复苏。
－限制性液体复苏与住院时间短、总死亡率降低有关。
－在穿透性主动脉损伤，允许性低血压使收缩压在 90 mmHg，直至最终的手术控制，防止再出血。
• 对张力性气胸，需立即进行针引流及放置胸管。
• 不要等到得到 CXR 结果。
• 声像图诊断气胸较 CXR 具有更高的灵敏性。
• 心脏压塞患者需行紧急心包穿刺术。
－需紧急运送到手术室行心包开创手术。
• 如怀疑脊髓损伤可能，需行脊髓固定。

■ 急诊治疗/程序

• 通知创伤科手术医师患者的到来。
• 如果张力性气胸，需要胸腔闭式引流管。
• 如果是少量气胸，可留置尾巴导管或深静脉导管引流。
• 胸腔镜开胸术，如果血胸±气胸：
－通常，成人使用 36F 胸管，但最近文献表明 28F 导管可能是足够的：
－在儿童中，使用肋间空间可容纳的最大导管。
• 大量复苏对于失血性休克至关重要：
－血液产品应是用于复苏的主要液体，以保持足够的凝血和载氧能力。
－考虑使用柠檬酸盐通过导管自动输血。
－挫伤的肺实质会出现毛细血管床渗漏，并且积极的晶体复苏可能会加剧呼吸窘迫。
• 乳头下或肩胛骨下端有进出口的伤口，要考虑到腹内脏器损伤可能性：
－诊断性腹腔灌洗治疗（DPL）、超声、CT 扫描或剖腹探查术、腹腔镜检查协助诊断。
－诊断性腹腔灌洗治疗阳性需输注 5 000 ml 红细胞。
• 准确描述伤口的性质：
－保留子弹碎片、衣服或从伤口中取出的组织。
• 胸壁探查是禁忌，因其可能导致气胸或出血进一步加重。
• 只有在手术室才可以拔除刺伤器物。
• 在穿透性躯干创伤中，当 CPR 不超过 10～15 min 且现场可提供创伤手术后援时，急诊复苏性开胸手术可提高生存率：
－交叉钳住降主动脉并控制活动性出血后，有心脏活动的患者应去手术室。
• 初次插入时从胸管引流的血液＞1 000～

1 500 ml，或>200 ml/h，表明需要进行开胸手术。

• 如果有指示，请务必提供破伤风加强剂。

■ 药物治疗

• 镇痛药：

- 氯胺酮：0.1～0.3 mg/kg，静脉注射。

- 芬太尼（短效）：0.25～2 μg/kg，静脉注射。

- 吗啡（中间作用）：0.1 mg/kg，静脉注射。

- 利多卡因（胸管局部使用）：<6 mg/kg，皮下注射。

• 镇静剂：

- 氯胺酮：1～3 mg/kg，静脉注射。

- 依托咪酯：0.3 mg/kg，静脉注射。

- 咪达唑仑：0.05 mg/kg，静脉注射。

• 抗生素（仅在伤口受到严重污染的情况下）：

- 头孢氨苄：1～2 g（儿童：50～100 mg/kg），静脉注射，q8 h。

• 其他。

- 氨甲环酸：出血控制，在 10 min 内静脉注射 1 g（15 mg/kg），然后在 8 h 内注入 1 g [2 mg/(kg · h)，持续 8 h]。

- 柠檬酸磷酸葡萄糖：用于自体输血的抗凝剂，根据采集的血量进行调整，每 500 ml 血液 70 ml。

随访

■ 进一步处理

入院指征

• 血流动力学不稳定的患者应在初次急诊稳定后立即转移到手术室。

• 任何胸腔穿刺的患者均应放置胸管，并应接受监测。

• 胸管后持续大量漏气的患者通常需要手术修复。

• 老年多肋骨骨折患者应入院，考虑放置硬膜外导管以控制疼痛和肺部抽水。

出院指征

• 存在独立微小胸部损伤或 CXR 正常患者可在急诊室观察 3 h 后复查影像学检查，如果没有胸部穿通伤证据，可放患者出院。

• 如果怀疑没有胸腔穿刺，则可以出院。

• 如果没有胸部穿通伤证据，胸部 CT 检查可代替 CXR 检查，如无异常，可不必复查影像学检查直接出院。

• 可能是 CXR 的替代方法（这些患者无需再次进行 X 线摄影即可出院）。

胸外伤，钝器伤 Thoracic Trauma, Blunt

Benjamin I. Liotta · Christopher J. Coyne　庄育刚 译

基础知识

■ 描述

• 在美国有较高的发生率和死亡率。

• 每日 100 万人中有 12 个胸部外伤受害者。

• 在这些外伤患者中有 33%需要进一步医院内治疗。

• 死亡患者中有 20%～25%死于该种创伤。

• 在死于其他创伤的患者中有 25%合并胸外伤。

■ 病因

• 常规机械性损伤：

- 机动车碰撞（占 70%～80%）。

- 摩托车碰撞。

- 行人被机动车碰撞。

- 高空坠落。

- 人为攻击。

- 爆炸伤。

- 运动相关性损伤。

• 损伤直接来自对胸部的钝力或来自快速减速所带来的冲击力。

诊断

■ 症状和体征

• 明显的胸壁挫伤、创口或胸壁缺损。

• 胸壁的反向性运动，提示连枷胸（通常合并其他部位的损伤）。

• 低血压。

• 有些患者存在严重的胸腔损伤，比如外伤性主动脉破裂就没有明显的外部体征。

病史

• 损伤时间。

• 损伤机制。

• 机动车事故（MVA）对速度和减速度的估计。

• 存在意识丧失。

• 胸痛。

• 深吸气或咳嗽痛。

• 呼吸困难。

体格检查

• 单侧肺呼吸音消失。

• 胸壁皮下捻发音或皮下气肿。

• 呼吸音减弱或消失。

• 胸壁压痛明显。

• 颈静脉扩张。

• 气管中线移位。

• 患侧语音共振增强。

■ 基本检查

• 检查患者气道、呼吸及循环情况，以明确患者生命体征是否平稳。

• 胸部重要检查：

- 呼吸力度及呼吸频率。

- 胸壁偏移度及捻发音。

- 皮下积气。

- 呼吸音及心音。

- 颈静脉扩张表现。

- 应进行 FAST 检查以评估心包积液的证据。

- 考虑使用超声来检测小型气胸，尤其是考虑到仰卧位 CXR 在检测此类气胸中的敏感性较差时。

• 立即拍摄仰卧位 CXR，尽量避免行直立位 CXR 以防存在其他潜在损伤（尤其是脊髓损伤）。

• 心电图及监测心肌缺血及心律失常。

■ 诊断检查与说明

实验室检查

• 基础血红蛋白。

• 脉搏血氧饱和度。

• 动脉血气分析。

X

• 血乳酸水平。
• 交叉配血及血型鉴定。
• 凝血全套。
• 必要时需查心肌酶。
• 患者行充分液体复苏时需进行外周血生化检查。

影像学检查

• CXR 是最基础的影像学选择。
- 如果 CXR 显示纵隔增宽，在患者血流动力学稳定的前提下，需行直立位摄片。
• 在气胸、肺挫伤及隐匿性肺损伤时胸部 CT 更加实用。
• 胸部增强 CT 或主动脉造影，有助于识别主动脉和大血管损伤。
• 考虑在稳定，清醒，未醉的患者中使用 NEXUS 胸部 CT 标准。如果没有所有标准，则可能不需要胸部 CT：
- CXR 异常。
- 分散注意力。
- 胸壁压痛。
- 胸骨压痛。
- 胸椎压痛。
- 肩胛骨压痛。
- 快速减速机制，即 40 mph（1 mph＝1.6 km/h）。
• 机动车碰撞或下降＞20 min（包括快速减速机制会增加敏感性，降低特异性）。
• 胸腔超声可以有效地用于检测气胸和心包损伤。急诊设置中此类损伤的敏感性、特异性和整体准确性＞90%。
• 如果怀疑有食管损伤，可以通过食管镜直接内镜检查。
• 如果食管镜检查阴性，但有食管损伤风险（例如，纵隔），可食管造影（先用水，然后用钡）：
- 依次组合这两个测试可达到接近 100%的灵敏度。
• 如果胸骨存在压痛或心电监测存在异常需行心电图检查。

诊断步骤/外科

• 如果患者的情况不稳定，紧急情况下需行开胸手术修复外伤性主动脉破裂。
• 如果患者有心脏压塞症状，且病情尚稳定，需行紧急超声心动图检查。
- 该项检查也可明确心包积液、室壁运动缺损、主动脉损伤、瓣膜或其他心脏疾病。
• 如果存在心脏压塞且患者病情不稳定，需行紧急心包穿刺术。
• 如果影像学上有主动脉撕裂的迹象，则患者可能需要紧急手术或血管内修复。

• 支气管镜检查常常可诊断可能的上气道损伤（如置入胸管后仍存在持续大量的漏气）。

妊娠注意事项

• 在妊娠的患者中，记得要使用最少的辐射量，并在可能的情况下对子宫进行屏蔽。
• 注意孕妇胸部解剖结构的差异，以及实验值、血管内体积和心血管生理的差异。
• 细节详见妊娠、创伤相关内容。

鉴别诊断

• 单纯性气胸。
• 张力性气胸。
• 血胸。
• 肋骨骨折。
• 连枷胸。
• 胸锁关节骨折/脱位。
• 肺挫伤。
• 心肌挫伤。
• 心脏破裂。
• 心脏压塞。
• 创伤性主动脉破裂。
• 食管损伤。
• 大血管损伤（锁骨下动脉、肺动脉）。
• 气管支气管损伤。
• 膈肌损伤。

儿科注意事项

• 儿童肋骨弹性较好，常常会抵消外力的作用而看不到明显的胸部外伤，不能就此而低估了其发生严重胸内损伤的可能性。
• 回顾性研究已经提出，将儿童创伤中，车辆相关受伤机制或胸部 X 线异常的患者，胸部 CT 检查意义有限。

老年人注意事项

相比年轻人的胸部钝器伤，老年人发生严重呼吸道并发症（包括急性呼吸窘迫综合征和肺部感染）的可能性显著升高，尤其是对大于 85 岁的老年人。

治疗

院前

• 所有仍存在生命体征的患者都应被送往创伤中心。
• 应采用全脊柱预防措施。
• 细针穿刺减压术治疗张力性气胸：
- 单肺呼吸音消失。
- 低血压。
- 颈静脉怒张。
- 胸部叩诊鼓音。
• 如果大的开放性气胸存在，应予以三角巾固定胸壁防止张力性气胸。
• 不要延误运送到医院，建立静脉通路。

初步稳定/治疗

• 插管早期患者如果出现呼吸衰竭、休克或意识状态改变，需进入 ABC 管理进程。
• 只有在有生命体征的患者中，才开始复苏的尝试。
• 开胸手术对创伤性钝器伤致心跳停止患者生存无益，因此不做常规推荐。
• 如果患者的病情不稳定，出现张力性气胸体征，应立即进行针刺引流和放置胸管。
• 不要等待 CXR 结果。
• 如果损伤部位不明显，在损伤侧或双侧放置胸腔引流管。
• 对病情稳定的患者予以非再呼吸面罩吸氧。
• 建立静脉通路，推荐选取 2 条大口径静脉通路。
• 保持脊柱固定。

急诊治疗/程序

• 一旦发现气胸或血胸需立即行胸腔闭式引流术：
- 成人需用 36 号胸腔闭式引流管。
- 在儿童，使用两肋间隔可容纳的最大口径管路。
• 需提供等渗液体或血制品进行复苏：
- 考虑到允许性低血压，对存在严重肺挫伤的患者行过于积极的液体复苏是有害的。
• 行相关的腹内损伤检查（例如，结合腹部超声、腹部 CT 扫描、不常用的诊断性腹腔穿刺）：
- 胸部外伤患者多伴有腹腔内损伤。

药物治疗

• 注射破伤风抗毒素。
• 如果存在脊髓损伤，需予以甲泼尼龙治疗，1 h 内予以 30 mg/kg 速度静脉滴注，剩下 23 h 予以 5.4 mg/(kg · h) 速度持续静脉滴注。

注意

• 这项对患者的处理方案目前存在争议，且越来越不适用，所以要熟悉你所在医院的处理流程。
• 适量予以短效镇痛药物（芬太尼 1～2 μg/kg，或吗啡 0.1 mg/kg 静脉推注）可缓解患者疼痛。

随访

进一步处理

入院指征

• 患者存在传导阻滞、频繁异位心律或心电图提示缺血性改变，需行进一步心电监测设置检查明确可能的心肌挫伤。

• 血流动力学不稳定的患者需紧急进入手术室行开胸或开腹手术。

• 植入胸管后迅速引流出 1 000～1 500 ml 血液者需行开胸手术治疗。

• 持续数小时内胸管引流量大于 200 ml/h 者需行手术干预。

• 存在明显肋骨骨折的患者须予以疼痛控制。

• 在急诊室中失去生命体征的患者应接受快速开胸手术。

出院指征

• 在急诊室患者如果没有明显的临床胸部挫伤，6 h 内站立位 CXR 提示阴性，同时复查影像学未提示气胸、血胸、肺挫伤，患者能深呼吸，临床症状稳定，无明显其他损伤可以排除。

转诊问题

• 对需要积极手术或办理入院的重伤患者，需立即通知创伤科外科医师。

• 急诊手术转诊指征：

- 外伤性开胸术后胸壁完整性丧失。
- 钝性膈肌损伤。
- 胸管插入后漏气明显。
- 大量血胸或胸管持续快速的血液引流量（插入胸管后引流量为 1 500 ml 或每小时引流量为 200～300 ml）。
- 影像学和内镜证实气管、大支气管或食管损伤。
- 消化道内容物覆盖胸管位置。
- 心脏压塞。
- 影像学明确大血管损伤。
- 肺动脉、大血管、心脏血管的血栓或栓塞。

随访建议

• 患者从创伤中心或胸外科出院后应予以密切随访，当然这取决于损伤的程度及所提供治疗的效果。

• 携带胸腔引流管的患者在 48 h 内应予以 CXR 检查及常规伤口护理，以便于去除伤口敷料及重新评估病情。

要点和误区

• 胸部钝器伤占所有创伤死亡的 1/4。

• 创伤患者到达创伤中心后应尽快予以稳定生命体征并运送到相应部门进行处理。

• 开胸手术对因创伤所致心跳呼吸骤停的患者并不能改善其生存率，仅在送到急诊室时存在生命体征的患者中有意义。

• 患者损伤程度与初始临床体征及症状不一定呈正相关，这在儿科患者中尤其常见。

胸主动脉夹层 Aortic Dissection, Thoracic

Jeffrey I. Schneider · Jonathan S. Olshaker 李岩 王瑞兰 译

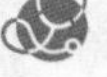

基础知识

描述

• 喷射的血液导致内膜撕裂时会产生主动脉夹层。

• 血液在主动脉收缩压下进入主动脉壁中层。

• 目前认为，高血压是夹层形成过程中的一个重要因素。

• 夹层的位置，近的可以从主动脉根部开始，远的可以累及主动脉的任何或所有分支，如颈动脉、锁骨下动脉。

• 夹层形成过程也可以向近端发展，涉及主动脉、冠状动脉开口及心包。

• 向近端进展的夹层可能导致冠状动脉口闭塞、主动脉瓣关闭不全或心脏压塞。

• 根据累及的主动脉部位分型：

- Stanford 分型：
  - A 型：累及升主动脉。
  - B 型：累及主动脉远端。
- DeBakey 分型：
  - DeBakey Ⅰ型：起源于主动脉弓或根部的内膜撕裂。
  - DeBakey Ⅱ型：起源并局限于升主动脉。
  - DeBakey Ⅲ型：起源于左锁骨下动脉起始部，并向远端扩展。

• 高峰年龄：

- 近端解剖：50～55 岁。
- 远端解剖：60～70 岁。

妊娠注意事项

妊娠时解剖风险增加：

• 在 40 岁以下的女性中，有 50% 的解剖发生在妊娠期间。

病因

任何影响主动脉壁力学性质的过程都可导致夹层：

• 高血压。

• 先天性心脏病（二尖瓣主动脉瓣狭窄）。

• 主动脉壁结缔组织异常（囊性内壁坏死）。

• 结缔组织病（马方综合征、埃勒斯-当洛斯综合征）。

• 妊娠。

• 主动脉的感染性/炎症性疾病（红斑狼疮、梅毒、心内膜炎、巨细胞动脉炎）。

• 先前的心脏手术包括 CABG、主动脉瓣修复。

• 吸烟。

诊断

症状和体征

病史

• 胸痛：

- 约有 15% 的患者不发生。
- A 型主动脉夹层胸骨后疼痛。
- 降主动脉夹层肩胛处疼痛。
- 累及腹主动脉会出现腰痛。
- 突然发生。
- 通常为刀割样剧烈疼痛。
- 刚发病时最严重。

• 背部疼痛：

- 一般肩胛间区或腰部。

• 胸部、背部和腹部混合性疼痛。

• 神经系统症状：

- 视力变化。
- 卒中症状。

• 主动脉夹层可能出现非典型症状，可能导致诊断延迟：

X

- 腹痛。
- 胸部压力。
- 腿痛。
- 晕厥。
- 发热。
- 恶心、呕吐。

老年人注意事项

老年人未经手术许可的可能性较小，死亡率较高。

• 老年人不太可能将疼痛描述为突然发作、脉搏不足或主动脉瓣关闭不全。

体格检查

• 高血压：
- 35%～40%可以正常。

• 脉搏缺失：
- 四肢血压存在差异。
- 通常在上肢。

• 神经/脊髓缺陷。

• 主动脉瓣关闭不全的杂音：
- 最多发生31%的患者。
- 可变强度的音调、振动效果。
- 沿右胸骨边界听效果最好。

• 休克：
- 如果是从解剖到冠状动脉的心包破裂或心肌梗死(MI)。

• 非典型表现：
- 缺血性下肢。
- 精神状态改变。
- 充血性心力衰竭。

基本检查

心电图：

• 对治疗ST段抬高的心肌梗死或缺血有效。

• 夹层可能会累及冠状动脉口并导致心肌梗死：
- 下壁心肌梗死(右冠状动脉病变)较左冠状动脉支配区域更为常见。

• 用于评估左心室肥厚的存在。

• 存在严重的急性发作性胸痛而出现正常心电图，要加强对主动脉夹层的怀疑。

诊断检查与说明

实验室检查

• 白细胞增多。

• 血尿。

• 血肌酐升高。

• 肠缺血后淀粉酶升高。

• 心肌缺血引起的心肌酶升高。

• D-二聚体水平最好用于排除疾病可能性低的患者。

影像学检查

• CXR：
- 用于排除其他病因如气胸、肺炎。
- 若有夹层，可能会出现纵隔增宽或异常的主动脉轮廓。
- 可能存在心包积液(血液)继发心脏扩大。
- 在12%～18%的病例可能完全正常。

• 经胸或经食管超声：
- 经胸：
  ◦ 对主动脉夹层的诊断不是很有帮助。
  ◦ 可能被用于评估已知夹层的并发症，如填塞、瓣膜功能不全或心肌梗死(从开口处闭塞)。
- 经食管：
  ◦ 可在急诊做。
  ◦ 患者可能需要气管插管。
  ◦ 提供有关夹层和并发症的信息。

• CT：
- 在明确夹层的范围中非常有用。
- 也可用于诊断器质性改变，如肺栓塞。
- 对主动脉夹层的诊断具有较高的敏感性，是多个中心选择的诊断方式。

• MRI：
- 高度敏感性和特异性。
- 要求患者在较长的时间内转运出急诊。
- 不能立即获得结果可能是一个问题。
- 肾功能不全或染料过敏的选择性检查。

• 主动脉造影：
- 高度敏感性和特异性。
- 对术前规划有用。
- 在许多中心很难获得。

• 心导管检查：
- 由于与心肌缺血症状重叠，当血管内膜摆动可见时，部分患者可根据心导管术得出诊断。

鉴别诊断

• 心肌梗死/缺血。

• 不稳定型心绞痛。

• 气胸。

• 食管破裂。

• 肺栓塞。

• 心包炎。

• 肺炎。

• 肌肉骨骼疼痛。

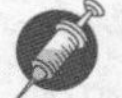

治疗

院前

• 监测。

• 建立静脉通路。

• 给氧。

初步稳定/治疗

• 建立两个静脉通路。

• 连续心电监测。

• 动脉血氧饱和度。

• 给氧。

急诊治疗/程序

• 降低血压来降低主动脉壁的剪切力，以及减缓夹层的形成过程。

• 药物治疗：静脉用β受体阻滞剂和硝普钠。
- 用来控制高血压和心肌收缩力，降低剪切力。
- 艾司洛尔(静脉用)或拉贝洛尔(静脉用)：
  ◦ 禁忌证：心动过缓、COPD、低血压。
- 硝普钠(通常和静脉用β受体阻滞剂合用)。
- 当上述药物一起使用时需注意：为防止剪切力的初始增加，β受体阻滞剂治疗应在加硝普钠治疗前开始。

• 急诊手术：
- A型动脉夹层的治疗选择。
- 用于内科治疗失败的B型动脉夹层。

• 内科治疗：
- 稳定的B型动脉夹层动脉瘤的首选治疗。

> **注意**
>
> 主动脉夹层的症状可能与心脏缺血/梗死及肺栓塞的症状相似。如果存在主动脉夹层，溶栓和抗凝治疗可能是有害的，甚至有潜在的致命性。

药物治疗

• 艾司洛尔：500 μg/kg静脉注射，然后25～50 mg/(kg·min)，滴注。

• 拉贝洛尔：10～20 μg静脉注射，q10～15 min，然后2～4 mg/h，滴注。

• 硝普钠：0.5 μg/(kg·min)静脉注射，滴定至产生预期效果。

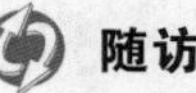

随访

进一步处理

入院指征

• 所有主动脉夹层患者均应入ICU。

• 应紧急心胸外科会诊，尤其是A型主动脉夹层病例。

出院指征

无。

随访建议

心外科和/或心胸外科密切随访至关重要。

要点和误区

• 近75%未经治疗的升主动脉夹层患者预计将在2周内死亡，第一个48 h内每小时的死亡率为1%～3%。

• 大多数患者(84%)存在突然发生的严重程度的疼痛(90%)。

• 虽然最近的一些文献提出了检测D-二聚体的作用，但是还没有足够的证据来支持其作为主动脉夹层的唯一筛选试验。

• 对于胸痛常规治疗(硝酸盐、β受体阻滞剂)无效，以及胸部疼痛伴随其他症状(下肢无力、疼痛、感觉异常腹痛)的患者的诊断应认真考虑。

• 识别风险因素很关键。这些包括：

- 高血压。
- 男性。
- 使用可卡因。
- 高龄。
- 妊娠。
- 结缔组织疾病，如马方综合征或中层囊性坏死。
- 二叶式主动脉瓣。
- Turner综合征。
- 家族史。

休克 Shock

Annette M. Ilg · Nathan I. Shapiro 周健 潘曙明 译

基础知识

描述

• 组织的血液供应不足，无法满足组织的需求。
• 组织氧气需求未得到满足。
• 没有去除有毒代谢物。
• 如果不及时治疗，不可避免地会从灌注不足发展为器官功能障碍，最终死亡。
• 休克的主要类别：
  - 低血容量性休克：
    ◦ 血容量减少。
    ◦ 急性发作时怀疑出血。
    ◦ 如果进行性发作和血细胞比容，BUN和肌酐升高，则严重脱水。
  - 阻塞性(心源性)休克：
    ◦ 心输出量减少和组织缺氧，血管内容积和心肌功能异常。
    ◦ 中心静脉压增高导致静脉充血。
    ◦ SVR的补偿性增加。
    ◦ 可能是由于心脏功能障碍，阻塞心脏血液流入或阻塞心脏血液流出引起的。
  - 败血性休克：
    ◦ 最初的传染性感染使免疫系统不堪重负。
    ◦ 生化信使(细胞因子、白三烯、组胺、前列腺素)引起血管扩张。
    ◦ 毛细血管内皮被破坏，血管泄漏。
    ◦ SVR下降会导致组织灌注不足。
    ◦ 其次，"心动过速导致心输出量减少"，导致冷休克或感染性休克。
  - 神经源性休克：
    ◦ 脊髓损伤破坏了对血管的交感刺激。
    ◦ 交感神经张力降低会引起动脉扩张和血管舒张。
    ◦ T_4附近的病变破坏交感，多余的迷走神经支配引起心动过缓。
  - 过敏性休克：
    ◦ 抗原刺激过敏反应。
    ◦ 肥大细胞脱粒。
    ◦ 组胺的释放，以及自身抗体，会刺激过敏反应的发生。
    ◦ 血管平滑肌松弛。
    ◦ 毛细血管内皮泄漏。
    ◦ SVR下降会导致组织灌注不足。
  - 药物可能会通过平滑肌扩张或心肌抑制而引起休克。

病因

• 低血容量性休克：
  - 腹部外伤，钝器伤或穿透伤。
  - 流产，完全流产、不全流产或难免流产。
  - 贫血，慢性或急性。
  - 动脉瘤，腹部、胸腔、夹层。
  - 主动脉瘘。
  - 动静脉畸形。
  - 钝伤。
  - 烧伤。
  - 糖尿病。
  - 腹泻。
  - 利尿剂。
  - 破裂性异位妊娠。
  - 鼻出血。
  - 骨折(特别是长骨)。
  - 咯血。
  - 出血。
  - Mallory-Weiss征。
  - 穿透创伤。
  - 前置胎盘。
  - 产后出血。
  - 腹膜后出血。
  - 严重腹水。
  - 脾破裂。
• 有毒的表皮坏死溶解：
  - 血管损伤。
  - 呕吐。
• 心源性休克：
  - 心肌病。
  - 传导异常和心律不齐。
  - 心肌梗死。
  - 心肌挫伤。
  - 心肌炎。
  - 心脏压塞。
  - 肺栓塞。
  - 张力性气胸。
  - 瓣膜功能不全。
  - 室间隔缺损。
• 血管源性休克：
  - 急性呼吸窘迫综合征。
  - 细菌感染。
  - 肠穿孔。
  - 蜂窝织炎。
  - 胆管炎。
  - 胆囊炎。
  - 心内膜炎。
  - 子宫内膜炎。
  - 真菌。
  - 被感染的假肢装置。

- 腹腔内感染或脓肿。
- 纵隔炎。
- 脑膜炎。
- 子宫肌炎。
- 盆腔炎。
- 腹膜炎。
- 肾盂肾炎。
- 咽炎。
- 肺炎。
- 化脓性关节炎。
- 血栓性静脉炎。
- 输卵管-卵巢脓肿。

• 过敏性：
- 药物反应（最常见的是对阿司匹林、β-内酰胺类抗生素的反应）。
- 运动（少见）。
- 食物过敏（花生、坚果、贝类、鱼、牛奶、鸡蛋、大豆和小麦占食物相关过敏反应的 90%）。
- 害虫。
- 乳胶。
- 放射线造影剂。
- 合成产品。

• 药理学：
- 降压药。
- 抗抑郁药。
- 苯二氮䓬类药物。
- 胆碱能药。
- 地高辛。
- 麻醉品。
- 硝酸盐。

• 神经源性：
- 脊髓损伤。

诊断

▪ 症状和体征

全身性休克：

• 低血压。
• 外围脉冲减少。
• 心动过速。
• 呼吸急促。
• 尿量减少。
• 发汗。
• 反应迟钝。
• 昏睡。

病史

标准病史，旨在推断休克的病因和重要的诱发因素。

体格检查

• 标准的体格检查有助于确定病因（如伤口、蜂窝织炎和荨麻疹的心脏检查体征等）。
• 有针对性的身体检查，重点放在休克状态的类型上：
- 降血脂（经典症状）：
◦ 颈静脉扁平。
◦ 黏膜干燥。
◦ 四肢很冷。
- 心源性休克（经典症状）：
◦ 存在颈静脉扩张。
◦ 黏膜湿润。
◦ 四肢很冷。
- 败血性休克（经典症状）：
◦ 颈静脉扁平。
◦ 黏膜干燥。
◦ 四肢很温暖。
◦ 在后期休克中，四肢可能会变得寒冷和斑驳。

▪ 基本检查

• 确定存在的休克类型。
• 确定潜在的休克原因。

▪ 诊断检查与说明

实验室检查

• 血红蛋白/血细胞比容。
• 白细胞：
- 高：感染的非特异性标志物。
- 低：中性粒细胞减少症感染。
• 电解质。
• 血糖：
- 高：糖尿病性酮症酸中毒或败血性休克。
- 低：小儿败血症。
• 凝血酶原时间/部分凝血活酶时间。
• 心肌酶。
• 尿液分析。
• β-人绒毛膜促性腺激素。
• 乳酸水平：
- 良好的冲击状态替代指标。

影像学检查

• 胸部 X 线检查。
• 心电图。
• 腹部超声。
• 腹部 CT：
- 要求患者第一要稳定。
- 在腹部创伤的情况下，寻找怀疑有腹部感染的情况。

▪ 诊断步骤/外科

心电图：

• 评估局部缺血和其他心肌疾病。
• 心脏压塞所致电交替或低电压。
• 右心劳损伴肺栓塞。

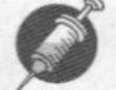

治疗

▪ 院前

• 根据标准方案进行 ABC 管理。
• 根据需要进行液体复苏。

▪ 初始稳定/治疗

• 大口径静脉输液通路：
- 如果可能，进行中心静脉通路输液和监测。
• 非心源性休克患者的液体复苏。
• 采用直接压迫来控制出血。
• 采用悬吊布单或商用装置或外固定器来稳定骨盆骨折。

▪ 急诊治疗/程序

• 低血容量性休克：
- 寻找容量减少的原因。
- 积极的液体复苏，使收缩压（SBP）保持在>100 mmHg，直到确定性治疗。
- 最初使用 2～3 L 晶体液。
- 如果 2～3 L 晶体液不能改善收缩压，使用袋装红细胞悬浮液。
- 确定出血的原因并快速转向确定性治疗。
- 考虑在穿透性躯干创伤的难治性休克中进行开胸和主动脉交叉夹闭。

• 心源性休克：
- 通过插管减少呼吸做功。
- 针对特定损害的治疗（例如，心肌梗死的溶栓疗法、心脏填塞的心包穿刺术）。
- 治疗心律失常。
- 按需使用血管加压药（去甲肾上腺素或多巴胺）。

• 脓毒性休克：
- 积极使用晶体液进行复苏。
- 滴定液体量以维持尿量在每小时>30 ml 和平均动脉压>65 mmHg。
- 输注血制品以维持血细胞比容在 30%～35%。
- 早期使用抗菌药物。
- 根据需要使用正性肌力支持。
- 去甲肾上腺素作为首选的静脉升压药物。

• 过敏性休克：
- 气道不通畅行气管插管。
- 肌内注射 0.3 mg 肾上腺素。
- 在非紧急情况下行皮下注射肾上腺素。
- 对于即刻威胁到生命或难治性低血压，使用静脉滴注。
- H_1 受体阻滞剂(苯海拉明)。
- H_2 受体阻滞剂(西咪替丁)。
- 糖皮质激素(氢化可的松或甲泼尼龙)。
- 对于支气管痉挛,使用 β_2 受体阻滞剂雾化。
- 使用β受体阻滞剂的患者可能更容易出现严重的过敏反应症状。

• 药物源性休克:
- 使用活性炭进行药物过量的解毒。
- 根据需要使用肌力药物。
- 药物特异性解毒剂。

• 神经源性休克:
- 支持性治疗。
- 牵引和骨折固定。
- 糖皮质激素。

■ 药物治疗

• 沙丁胺醇:2.5 mg/2.5 ml,雾化器,必要时。
• 葡萄糖酸钙:100～1 000 mg,静脉输注,0.5～2 ml/min。
• 西咪替丁:300 mg,静脉输注。
• 苯海拉明:3 分钟内静脉注射 50～100 mg。
• 多巴酚丁胺:5～40 μg/(kg · min)静脉内:
- 多巴胺能:1～3 μg/(kg · min),静脉输注。
- β效应:3～10 μg/(kg · min),静脉输注。
- α/β效果:10～20 μg/(kg · min),静脉输注。
- α效应:20 μg/(kg · min),静脉输注。

• 肾上腺素:
- 1～4 μg/min,静脉输注。
- 气管内 1 mg(10 ml 1∶10 000)次,随后进行 5 次快速吹气。
- 将 1 mg 放入 250 ml D_5W=4 μg/ml。

• 胰高血糖素:最初 1～5 mg 静脉推注,然后以 1～20 mg/h 的速度输注。
• 氢化可的松:5～10 mg/kg,静脉输注。
• 甲泼尼龙:1～2 mg/kg,静脉注射。
• 纳洛酮:首次静脉注射 0.01 mg/kg,滴定至有效。
• 去甲肾上腺素:开始 2～4/(μg · min)静脉滴定,直至 1～2 μg/(kg · min),静脉注射。
• 去氧肾上腺素:40～180 μg/min,静脉输注。

随访

■ 进一步处理

入院指征

• 所有休克患者都需要入院。
• ICU 标准:
- 所有持续性休克患者都需要 ICU 监测。

• 休克已明确逆转的患者可以收治于非 ICU 设置的科室。

出院指征

休克的患者不应从急诊科带回家。

转诊建议

创伤失血性休克(低血容量性休克)可能需要收治于创伤中心。

要点和误区

• 使用临床检查和即时超声把休克分类为低血容量性休克。心源性休克或血管性休克。
• 根据休克类型经验性的积极救治,使用静脉输液、输血或血管加压药物治疗(例如,脓毒性休克-液体复苏、失血性休克-输血和过敏性休克-肾上腺素)。

悬雍垂炎 Uvulitis

James P. Brewer 张晟 林兆奋 译

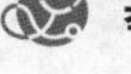

基础知识

■ 描述

炎症反应侵及悬雍垂,可分为两大类:
• 感染:
- 细菌。
- 病毒。
- 念珠菌。

• 外伤或非感染(因素)。

■ 流行病学

发病率和流行性分析

• 因为报道少,确切发病率不明确。
• 以前认为不多,但实际上可能相对普遍(如病毒病因)。
• 儿童(5～15 岁)相对成人更易患此病,多因 A 群链球菌(GAS)感染。
• 成人得此病时非感染因素多于感染因素。

■ 病因

• 感染:
- 细菌。
  ◦ A 群链球菌感染最多见。
  ◦ B 型流感嗜血杆菌。
  ◦ 其他细菌(具核梭杆菌属、中间普氏菌、链球菌肺炎)。
- 病毒。
  ◦ 报道不多,但有轻症、短病程病例。
  ◦ 已知可引起悬雍垂炎,但很少能分离的病毒:
    ▪ 柯萨奇病毒。
    ▪ 单纯疱疹病毒。
    ▪ 水痘-带状疱疹病毒。
    ▪ EB 病毒。
- 念珠菌感染。

• 非感染因素。
- 创伤、操作相关。
- 吸入、吞入化学物品或热刺激物。
- 血管炎。
- 过敏反应。
- 神经性水肿:
  ◦ 遗传(遗传性神经性水肿Ⅰ型和Ⅱ型)。
  ◦ 药物引起(如血管紧张素转化酶抑制剂、血管紧张素受体阻滞剂)。

诊断

■ 症状和体征

依靠病因和累及的部位(咽炎、喉炎、会厌炎等)。

病史

• 通常发病很快(<4～6 h),这取决于病因。
• 类型:
- 异物感。
- 咽喉痛。

X

- 吞咽困难。
- 吞咽痛。
- 呼吸困难。
• 感染：
- 发热。
• 非感染。
- 创伤或者近期接受操作。
- 新药物暴露(ACEI)。
- 摄入腐蚀性或热的东西。
• 可先表现为舌、唇、口的水肿。
• 有神经源性水肿的病史或家族史。
• 儿童人群伴有免疫接种史。
• 合并症引起免疫功能不全。

体格检查

• 程度从轻微肿胀明显肿胀一直到严重肿胀和明显疼痛。
• 通常表现：
- 中毒表现。
- 低沉声音或上气道阻塞的声音。
- 流涎。
- 喘鸣。
- 恶心。
- 呼吸窘迫。
• 五官：
- 悬雍垂苍白或红斑。
- 悬雍垂水肿。
- 分泌物(集中在悬雍垂、舌咽)。
- 颈部淋巴结肿大、喘鸣。
- 咽炎。
• 其他表现：
- 发热。
- 低氧。
- 荨麻疹。
- 喘息。

基本检查

• 按需评估和保证气道通畅。
• 明确感染和非感染因素。
• 起始治疗基于可能的病因(抗生素、激素、抗组胺类药物等)。
• 必要时请耳鼻喉科医师会诊。

诊断检查与说明

实验室检查

• 快速 GAS 抗原检测。
• 黏膜表面细菌培养。
• 全血细胞计数：
- 白细胞增多提示细菌感染。
- 嗜酸性细胞增多提示过敏反应。
• 补充检测：
- C4 水平升高提示酯酶缺乏。
- C1 免疫生化分析。

影像学检查

• 当临床诊断有疑问或者体格检查受限，用于鉴别诊断。
• 颈部侧位 X 线片用于观察和评估悬雍垂或吸除异物。
• CT 造影检查用于评估颈部软组织积液的占位效应，蜂窝织炎及深层次组织的累及程度。

诊断步骤/外科

• 严重的病例需确保有耳鼻喉科医师会诊：
- 纤维鼻咽镜检查。
- 环甲软骨切开术。
- 悬雍垂减压术。
- 悬雍垂切除术。

鉴别诊断

• 咽炎。
• 扁桃体周围脓肿。
• 咽后脓肿。
• 会厌炎。
• 神经性水肿。
• 吸入异物。

治疗

院前

• 快速评估气道，确保气道通畅。
• 氧疗。
• 建立静脉通路。
• 评估患者周围环境，分析可能吞入或吸入的物品。
• 根据实际情况，肌内注射肾上腺素，雾化给予 β 受体激动剂或消旋肾上腺素。
• 快速转运后送。

初步稳定/治疗

• 首先是注意生命体征支持。
• 快速评估气道并做出处置。
• 建立静脉通路。
• 心电监测、血氧饱和度监测。
• 续贯院前治疗或开始呼吸治疗：
- 氧气支持。
- 雾化给予 β 受体激动剂或消旋肾上腺素。
• 气道开放：
- 气管插管：
◦ 紧急插管。
◦ 择期插管。
◦ 纤维喉镜或间接喉镜辅助。
- 严重患者行环甲膜切开术。
• 必要时尽早请耳鼻喉科医师会诊。

急诊治疗/程序

• 基础治疗重点是尽快抑制免疫反应(过敏、神经性水肿)。
• 口服或静脉用药根据病情严重程度。

药物治疗

• 病情严重(气道受限)：
- 肾上腺素(1∶1 000 溶液)：0.3～0.5 mg (0.01 mg/kg)，皮下注射或肌内注射，q30 min，3 次。
- 苯海拉明：25～50 mg(1～2 mg/kg)，静脉注射。
- 甲泼尼龙：125 mg(0.5～1 mg/kg)，静脉注射，q4 h。
• 可疑感染因素：
- 经验性静脉使用抗生素覆盖常见病原体(链球菌和流感嗜血杆菌)。
- 根据患者过敏史选择抗生素：
◦ 头孢曲松钠：1～2 g(50 mg/kg)，静脉注射(最大剂量 2 g/d)。
◦ 克林霉素：300 mg(25～40 mg/kg)，静脉注射，q8 h。
- 经验性口服抗生素：
◦ 青霉素 V：500 mg(＜27 kg 250 mg；＞27 kg 500 mg)，口服，每日 2～3 次，持续 10 日。
◦ 阿莫西林：875 mg[50 mg/(kg · d)]，口服，q8 h，持续 10 日。
◦ 克林霉素：300 mg(25～40 mg/kg)，口服，每日 4 次，持续 10 日。
• 可疑遗传性血管性水肿：
- 合成代谢类固醇：
◦ 达那唑：200 mg 口服，每日 2～3 次。
- 纯化 C1 抑制剂。
◦ 伯力内特：20 U/kg，静脉注射 1 次。
◦ cinyze：1 000 U，静脉注射。
- 选择性缓激肽 $β_2$ 受体阻滞剂：
◦ icabitant：30 mg 皮下注射×1。
- 可逆的血管激肽酶抑制剂。
◦ 艾卡拉肽：30 mg 皮下注射×1。
- 新鲜冷冻血浆：
◦ 一般不用于急性发作。

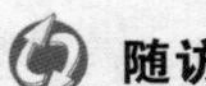

随访

进一步处理

取决于病情严重程度和治疗效果。

入院指征

- 严重的气道梗阻。
- 需要手术处理。
- 提示全身感染需要静脉使用抗生素。
- 病情加重治疗效果不佳：
  - 低氧或需氧疗。
  - 进行性呼吸困难。
  - 无法口服药物。
  - 顽固性疼痛。
- 伴发严重疾病。
- 院外条件有限无法按时门诊诊疗。

出院指征

- 病情迅速好转。
- 急诊观察 4～6 h 症状未复发。
- 没有呼吸困难。
- 可以耐受口服药物。
- 24～48 h 能随访的。
- 能迅速就诊得到治疗。

转诊问题

反复发作的神经性水肿要及时调整药物，并请耳鼻喉科医师会诊。

随访建议

- 严重的细菌感染要医师在 24～48 h 密切随访确保治疗有效。
- 怀疑神经性水肿，要立即停止 ACEI 和 ARB 类药物使用。

血管性水肿

Sean-Xavier Neath 李岩 王瑞兰 译

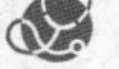

基础知识

描述

- 无瘙痒的、边界清楚的、无凹陷的真皮性水肿。
- 由于炎性介质释放引起的毛细血管和小静脉扩张，以及通透性增加：
  - 肥大细胞介导的。
  - 与来源于缓激肽产生过程和补充来源的介质的激肽相关。
- 除了受影响的组织更深外，与荨麻疹的病理基础相似。
  - 荨麻疹影响浅表组织，引起对表皮肥大细胞和神经的刺激，从而导致强烈的瘙痒。
  - 血管性水肿发生在更深层，此层肥大细胞和神经较少，因此不会引起瘙痒。
  - 血管性水肿会影响皮肤以外的组织，如肠道。
  - 血管性水肿可能与荨麻疹混合出现。
- 遗传性和获得性的病因是 C1 抑制剂(C1 INH)功能不足，而不是超敏反应。
- 遗传性血管性水肿(HAE)：
  - 由 C1 INH 缺乏引起的常染色体显性遗传病。
  - 遗传性血管性水肿的发病率为 1/80 000～1/30 000。
  - C1 INH 在通信、纤溶、凝血途径中起调节作用。
  - 缺乏会导致血管活性介质缓激肽、激肽释放酶、纤维蛋白溶酶非调节性活化。
  - 已经有超过 100 个突变的 C1 INH 基因被报道。
  - 类型 1：C1 INH 的表达下降。
  - 类型 2：C1 INH 的血浆水平正常但蛋白质功能失调。
  - 类型 3：凝血因子Ⅻ突变导致激肽产生增加：
    - 含雌激素的药物会增加症状。
  - 当炎症、外伤或其他因素导致 C1 INH 减少时，3 种类型均会发生症状。
- 获得性血管性水肿：
  - C1 INH 的质量和功能正常。
  - 1 型与淋巴组织增生性疾病有关，并由恶性细胞的 C1 INH 蛋白耗尽所引起。
  - 2 型由抑制 C1 INH 活性的循环抗体所导致的自身免疫引起。
- ACE 抑制剂引起的血管性水肿：
  - 占接受 ACE 抑制剂的所有血管性水肿病例的 20%～30%，占接受 ACE 抑制剂的患者的 0.1%～0.7%。
  - 通常发生在服药的第一个月内，但是第一次事件可能在很多年后自然发生。
  - 与白种人相比，非洲裔美国人罹患 ACE 抑制剂引起的血管性水肿的风险更高。

病因

- 关键点：病史和检查应指导怀疑是缓激肽介导的还是病因介导的组胺药引起的患者的血管性水肿发作。这对于选择对靶向介体有效的疗法非常重要。
- 激肽相关的病因：
  - HAE。
  - 遗传性血管性水肿。
  - 获得性血管性水肿。
    - 淋巴组织增生。
    - 自身免疫。
  - ACE 抑制剂引起。
- 肥大细胞介导的病因：
  - 食物过敏：
    - 添加剂。
    - 坚果。
    - 鸡蛋。
    - 贝类。
    - 大豆。
    - 小麦。
    - 鲜奶。
  - 药物过敏：
    - 阿司匹林。
    - 非甾体抗炎药。
    - 抗高血压药。
    - 毒品。
    - 口服避孕药。
  - 昆虫叮咬。
  - 物理诱导：
    - 冷。
    - 热。
    - 振动。
    - 运动。
    - 创伤。
    - 应激。
    - 紫外线。
- 嗜酸性粒细胞增多综合征(如 Gleich 综合征)。
- 甲状腺自身免疫性疾病。
- 特发性复发性 AE。

诊断

症状和体征

病史

- 家族史或使用特定试剂能使症状复发的病史会对诊断有用。

X

• 腹痛伴恶心、呕吐和腹泻。
• 遗传性血管水肿发作时不伴有荨麻疹。
• 情绪压力或身体创伤可激发疾病的侵袭。

体格检查

• 血管性水肿的病变为较大、肿胀、非凹陷性风团。
• 眼睑和口唇经常受累。
• 咽部和喉部受累可能会导致气道阻塞。
• 病变通常是不对称的，通常不涉及重力依赖性区域。

基本检查

• 诊断是根据非凹陷性、非瘙痒性风团的临床面积所得。
• 不需要家族史的出现来诊断疾病。25%的 HAE 患者具有基因突变，可能没有阳性家族史。

诊断检查与说明

实验室检查

• 可以检测 C4 级水平，但结果通常不可用 STAT。在大多数类型的 HAE 中，C4 低。
• 类胰蛋白酶水平可能有助于从差异中排除组胺介导的过敏反应。
• C1 INH 水平和 C1 INH 活性的测量（急诊室通常不提供）。
- 患有 1 型 HAE 的患者的水平非常低，正常人将有一半正常水平。

诊断步骤/外科

如果有荨麻疹病变，可以考虑进行皮肤活检。

鉴别诊断

• 水肿：
- 上腔静脉综合征。
- 右心衰竭。
- 缩窄性心包炎。
- 肾衰竭。
- 肾病综合征。
• 变应性接触性皮炎。
• 眼睑皮肤松弛症。
• 面部蜂窝织炎。
• 面部淋巴水肿。
• 继发于自身免疫功能障碍的水肿。
- 皮肌炎。
- 狼疮。
- 多肌炎。
- Sjögren 综合征。
• 甲状腺功能减退症。

儿科注意事项

复发性血管性水肿在青春期出现时应高度怀疑遗传性血管性水肿。

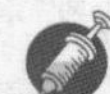

治疗

院前

• 建立静脉通路。
• 由于喉肿胀发展迅速，早期插管可能是必要的。
• 如果条件允许，给予 H_1 受体阻滞剂。
• 肾上腺素被认为可治疗喉头水肿，特别是怀疑瘙痒或肥大细胞病因及其他组胺释放的其他征兆。

初始稳定/治疗

• 积极的气道管理和支持治疗是急诊治疗的主要目的。
• 在严重的情况下，插管可能是必要的：
- 由于喉水肿、痉挛或软组织肿胀，经口气管插管是首选，但是可能很难。
- 考虑先进的气道辅助技术如弹性树胶探条协助以确保气管内导管放置。
- 如果软组织肿胀阻碍经口的术式，采取经鼻气管盲插。
- 经气管喷射通气或环甲膜切开术可有效控制气道。
• 给予肾上腺素、抗组胺药和阻塞性气道肿胀的类固醇，但是患者的反应是不同的。

急诊治疗/程序

• 伴Ⅰ型超敏反应特点的急性血管神经性水肿：
- H_1、H_2 受体阻滞剂和糖皮质激素治疗过敏性反应。
- 对于难治性病例给予肾上腺素，其益处大于风险。
- 对于腹部的受损，考虑增加肠外疼痛的治疗、止吐药和静脉注射补液。
• 遗传性和获得性血管性水肿：
- C1 INH。
- 新鲜冰冻血浆（FFP）可以作为 C1 INH 的替代剂。
- 激肽释放酶抑制剂在 2009 年被批准用于 HAE 的急性发作。
- 氨甲环酸（止血环酸）、抗纤维蛋白溶解剂，尽管也用但对于急性发作效果不明显。

注意

• 建议谨慎地使用 FFP（作为未纯化的 C1 INH 的来源）进行治疗，因为它可能由于补体成分浓度高而使某些攻击变得反常。当纯化产品不易获得时可以考虑。
• 抗纤维蛋白溶解剂和减毒雄激素，如促性腺激素抑制剂达那唑，通常用于长期预防性治疗。在急性环境中，它们可能在 24～48 h 没有任何作用。
• 在喉头水肿和血管性水肿中，具有过敏性气道控制和肾上腺素的使用是关键的初始治疗方式。

药物治疗

药物治疗的一般原则基于可疑的潜在原因。有两大类：怀疑的 HAE 或非 HAE。所用药物的详细信息如下：

• 疑似 HAE：
- C1 酯酶抑制剂替代蛋白（C1 INHRP）。
- 激肽释放酶抑制剂。
- 缓激肽 β_2 受体阻滞剂。
• 非 HAE：
- H_1 受体阻滞剂。
- H_2 受体阻滞剂。
- 皮质类固醇。
• ACE 抑制剂诱导的 AE：
- 一线建议是非 HAE 药物。
- 在异常或难治性情况下可以考虑使用 HAE 药物。已经报道了各种实用程序。
• C1 INHRP：
- 血浆衍生产品仍被认为是一线治疗：
  ◦ cinryze：20 U/kg 静脉缓慢输注。
  ◦ berinert：如果在 2 h 内无改善，则以 20 U/kg 的速度缓慢进行静脉输注，并附加剂量，如果恶化或出现喉部症状则更快。
  ◦ ruconest：也可以使用来自轻度转基因兔的重组 C1 INHRP，剂量为 50 U/kg 缓慢静脉输注。
- 西咪替丁（H_2 受体阻滞剂）：300 mg 静脉注射。
- 苯海拉明：50 mg 静脉注射；儿童：1～2 mg/kg 缓慢静脉注射。
- ecallantide（激肽释放酶抑制剂，仅在美国销售）：30 mg 皮下注射，分 3 次注射（每次从解剖学上距离 AE 受累区域约 1 ml）。
- 肾上腺素：0.3～0.5 mg（皮下注射途径使用 1∶1 000 稀释，静脉注射途径使用 1∶10 000）；儿童：0.01 mg/kg，皮下注射/静脉注射。
- 外消旋肾上腺素：2.25%溶液（将 0.5 ml 置于雾化器中的 2.5 ml 生理盐水中）。
- FFP（如果不提供 C1 INH）：成人 2 U。
- 氢化可的松：500 mg 静脉注射；儿童：4～8 mg/kg，静脉注射。

- 伊卡替班(firazyr)：缓激肽 $β_2$ 受体阻滞剂：由于体积大(3 ml)，一次缓慢 30 mg 皮下注射。
- 甲泼尼龙：125 mg，静脉注射；儿童：1～2 mg/kg，静脉注射。
- 泼尼松：60 mg，口服；儿童：1 mg/kg，口服。
- 雷尼替丁：成人 50 mg，静脉注射。
- 氨甲环酸：必要时，1 g，口服，q3～4 h，长达 48 h。

儿科注意事项

在儿童和青少年中，HAE 治疗剂的安全性和功效尚未得到广泛研究。在撰写本文时，berinert 已获得 FDA 的儿科批准，cinryze 在青少年中有适应证。kalbitor 被批准用于 12 岁及以上的患者。ruconest 已获成人和青少年批准。

随访

进一步处理

入院指征

• 系统性症状没有完全缓解的患者需要住院观察。
• 气道受累的患者推荐使用监测床。

出院指征

• 经观察 4～6 h 血管性水肿症状轻微无进展的患者可以安全出院回家进行短疗程的类固醇和抗组胺药治疗。
• 应该给患者配备预装肾上腺素的自动注射器及其使用说明。

转诊问题

患者初步治疗后应该经变态反应学家和免疫学家进行评估，特别是有家族史的血管性水肿，或者血管性水肿伴有腹痛，或由创伤引发的患者。

随访建议

没有系统性症状病情稳定的患者应该在出院几日内于门诊随访。

要点和误区

• 应及早采取措施来维持患者的气道。
• 考虑给遗传性血管性水肿的患者使用最新药物(如 C1 INH 和胰激肽原酶抑制剂)。

血管性血友病 Von Willebrand Disease

Ryan A. Stroder · Connor A. Cohick 吴昊 李文放 译

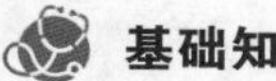

基础知识

描述

• 由于血友病因子(vWF)缺乏或功能障碍导致的凝血功能障碍。
• vWF 功能：
- 介导血小板内皮细胞黏附。
- Ⅷ因子的载体蛋白。
• 在一般人群中患病率高达 1%～2%。
• 遗传学：
- 大多数病例是遗传的——多基因缺陷。
- 1 型：vWF 因子的数量缺乏。
◦ 占 75%的病例。
◦ 常染色体显性遗传。
◦ vWF 的缺乏是由于合成的减少及蛋白质清除能力增加。
• 表现从无症状到中度出血：
- 2 型：vWF 的功能缺陷：
◦ 占 10%～20%的病例。
◦ 分为 2A、2B、2M、2N。
◦ 2A(10%～15%的病例)和 2M 为常染色体显性或隐性遗传。
◦ 2B(5%的病例)是常染色体显性遗传。
◦ 2N 是常染色体隐性遗传。
◦ 2A、2B 和 2M 降低了高分子量多聚体，降低了 vWF 活性。
◦ 2N - vWF 活性正常，多聚体电泳正常，与因子Ⅷ结合减少。
◦ 导致因子Ⅷ的下降(5%～15%)，继而引起更严重的凝血障碍。
- 3 型：缺乏或严重缺乏 vWF 因子。
◦ 罕见病：1/100 万。
◦ 常染色体隐性。
◦ 严重凝血病。
- vWD 因子与镰状细胞病、血友病 A、因子Ⅻ缺乏、遗传性出血性毛细血管扩张和血小板减少症有关。

病因

• 除了遗传因素外，还存在各种形式。
• 多因素：
- vWF 抗体生成。
- 合成减少。
- 蛋白质水解。
- 增加了与肿瘤细胞结合的清除率。
• 与以下内容相关：
- 恶性肿瘤：
◦ 肿瘤。
◦ 多发性骨髓瘤。
◦ 慢性淋巴细胞白血病。
◦ 非霍奇金淋巴瘤。
◦ 慢性粒细胞性白血病。
◦ Waldenstrom 巨球蛋白血症。
◦ 不明原因的单克隆丙种球蛋白病。
- 免疫相关：
◦ 系统性红斑狼疮。
◦ 类风湿关节炎。
- 药物诱导：
◦ 丙戊酸。
◦ 环丙沙星。
◦ 羟乙基淀粉。
◦ 灰黄霉素。
- 其他：
- vWF 是一种急性期反应物，在肾上腺素能刺激、兴奋和运动期间水平升高：
◦ 甲状腺功能减退降低血浆 vWF 水平。
◦ 尿毒症。
◦ 血红蛋白病。
◦ 肝硬化。
◦ 先天性心脏病。
◦ 弥散性血管内凝血。

诊断

症状和体征

• 症状因疾病类型而异。
• 很多 1 型和 2 型都是无症状的，严重的 2 型和 3 型有症状：
- 容易擦伤。
- 月经过多。
- 复发性鼻出血。
- 牙龈出血。
- 胃肠道出血。
- 软组织出血和关节积血。

X

- 长期或过度的出血。
- 术后出血。

病史

• 通常在儿童和青少年时期被诊断。

• 家族史。

• 轻微、中度复发性黏膜出血是最常见的可疑病史。

• 月经量过多。

体格检查

• 大多数正常。

• 多发性瘀伤。

• 深层血肿、关节积血。

妊娠注意事项

• 妊娠中期和晚期导致 1 型和 2 型疾病患者 vWF 水平升高(2～3 倍)。

• 妊娠和分娩通常不受影响。

• vWF 在分娩后迅速下降:

- 患者可能会在分娩后 10～28 日出现产后出血。

儿科注意事项

通常需要鉴别非意外伤害的婴儿或儿童出现瘀伤或出血的原因。

基本检查

• 结合患者病史＋体格检查，筛查并予以相关检查。

• 对于 1 型诊断，患者必须有明确的黏膜出血、实验室检查，以及 1 型疾病家族史。

诊断检查和说明

实验室检查

• CBC：血小板计数和形态正常，2B 型除外，可能有轻度血小板减少症(100 000～140 000/mm^3)。

• PT：正常。

• APTT:

- 适度延长 50%以内。
- Ⅷ因子降低或相关因子缺乏。

• 对 vWF 水平和活性的测量:

- vWF 利托菌素的共因子活性(vWF：RCo):

• 用血小板凝集法测定 vWF 功能:

- vWF 抗原(vWF：Ag)：使用免抗体测试血清中的 vWF 水平。
- 降低(vWF：RCo)到(vWF：Ag)2A、2B、2M 型。

• 如有异常，可采用多聚体凝胶电泳或瑞斯托西汀诱导血小板聚集(RIPA)进行专门检测。

• 出血时间:

- 在 1 型(50%)中可能是正常的。2 型和 3 型时间延迟。
- 非特异性，难以重复；已经不用于诊断。

鉴别诊断

• 血友病 A、B。

• 血小板的缺陷。

• 使用抗血小板药物：NSAIDs。

• 血小板型 vWD。

• Bernard-SouIier 综合征。

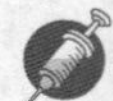

治疗

院前

直接压迫以控制出血。

初步稳定/治疗

必要时用晶体和红细胞悬液进行复苏。

急诊治疗/程序

• 如同所有严重出血一样，直接加压止血。

• 3 种治疗策略:

- 增加内源性 vWF。
- vWF 置换。
- 通常给予促进止血的药物，但不改变 vWF 的水平。

• 醋酸去氨加压素(DDAVP):

- 促进 vWF 从内皮细胞中释放，增加因子Ⅷ水平。
- 30～60 min 达到最高血药浓度，持续时间为 6～8 h。
- 对 1 型有效；2 型的可能有效；对 3 型不明确。
- 患者可在月经前或小手术前在家中使用鼻内喷剂。
- 在月经期或小手术前，患者可在家中使用鼻喷雾剂。
- 妊娠时应谨慎，理论上可能会引发子宫收缩。
- 高危心血管患者和 CVA 疾病可能会加剧血栓栓塞并发症。

• vWF 替代疗法:

- 重组血管性血友病因子 rvWF、vonicog-alfa、vonvendi 的有限证据。
- 适用于 1 型、2 型和 3 型 vWD，以及轻微、中度和严重出血。
- 含 vWF 的 Humate-P 因子Ⅷ浓缩液:
  ◦ 治疗以降低病毒传播风险。
  ◦ 剂量及治疗时间取决于出血的严重程度。
  ◦ 低温沉淀不推荐使用，因为它携带着病毒传播的风险。但如果没有其他的治疗方法并且患者有危及生命的出血，它可以被使用。

• 纤溶治疗:

- 氨基苯丙酸(阿米巴酸)和环己酸(氨甲环酸)。
- 阻止血纤维蛋白溶酶，以防止凝块降解。

• 局部药物——直接应用于出血点:

- 在外科手术中，运用凝胶泡沫或浸泡在凝血酶中。
- 微粉化胶原蛋白。
- 纤维蛋白原。

• 避免抗血小板药物。

一线用药

• 轻微出血(鼻出血、口咽、软组织):

- 静脉注射或鼻内去氨加压素。

• 大量出血(颅内、腹膜后):

- vWF 置换和因子Ⅷ，维持活性至少是 100 U/dl。

二线用药

• 小出血:

- vWF 浓度:
  ◦ 如去氨加压素无效，补充 vWF 因子。
  ◦ 联系血液科会诊。
- 氨基苯丙酸或环己酸：用于轻度黏膜出血。

药物治疗

• 氨基苯丙酸：50～60 mg/kg，口服或静脉，q4～6 h。

• 低温沉淀：10～12 U 初始剂量或 2～4 U/10 kg。

• 去氨加压素(DDAVP):

- 0.3 μg/kg，静脉，最大剂量 20 μg。
- 0.3 μg/kg，腹腔，最大剂量 20 μg。
- 300 μg(每鼻孔喷一次)鼻内。
- 儿童：(＜50 kg) 150 mg(每个鼻孔里喷洒)鼻内。

• 抗血友病因子/vWF 复合体：20～40 U/kg 静脉给药。

• 氨甲环酸：10 mg/kg，口服或静脉，q8 h。

• 新鲜冷冻血浆(FFP)：10～20 ml/kg，静脉给药。

• rvWF、vonicog-alpha、vonvendi：40～50 U/kg(轻微出血)，50～80 U/kg(严重出血)。

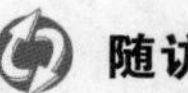

随访

进一步处理

入院指征

• 严重出血的患者需要进一步的静脉医疗管理。

• Ⅱ型和Ⅲ型的创伤性患者创伤后观察。

• 对于考虑将有重大出血事件的患者建议转移到综合性中心，该中心有包括一名血液学家和一名熟练管理出血性疾病的外科医师在内的护理团队。

出院指征

• 出血控制。

• 适当的随访，并且能够获得医疗治疗。

■ 随访建议

血液学：

• 管理严重出血。

• 优先行择期或限期手术。

• 疑似病例的进行明确诊断。

要点和误区

• 患者可能并不知道他们的血友病类型。

• 在创伤或出血的背景下，患有未知类型血友病的患者考虑 FFP。

血管炎 Vasculitis

Richard S. Klasco 周秋香 毛恩强 译

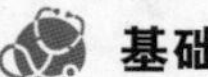

基础知识

■ 描述

• 炎症引起的血管壁损伤：
- 缺血和坏死。
- 动脉瘤和出血。
- 免疫病理机制：
  ◦ 循环抗原-抗体复合物的沉积和补体固定。
  ◦ 细胞调节机制过度。
  ◦ 持续炎症和上皮样巨细胞形成的肉芽肿组织反应。

• 血管炎代表了一大组疾病：
- 具有体质症状和炎性实验室指标的多系统疾病。
- 继发于另一种原因不明但以血管炎为主要特征。
- 决定介绍的因素有多种：
  ◦ 受影响血管的大小。
  ◦ 炎症的具体分布、严重程度和持续时间。

• 2000 名成人中有 1 人患有某种形式的血管炎。

■ 病因

• 大血管血管炎：
- 颞(巨细胞)动脉炎：
  ◦ 主动脉的肉芽肿性动脉炎及其主要分支通常涉及颞动脉。
  ◦ 患者>50 岁。
- 大动脉炎：
  ◦ 主动脉及其主要分支的肉芽肿性炎症。
  ◦ 通常在<50 岁的住院患者中发生。

• 中血管炎：
- 结节性多动脉炎(PAN)：
  ◦ 中小动脉炎。
  ◦ 常见分布包括代谢肌肉、关节、肠、神经、肾和皮肤的血管。
  ◦ 在中年人最常见。
- 川崎病(皮肤黏膜淋巴综合征)：
  ◦ 常常累及冠状动脉，涉及大、中、小型动脉。
  ◦ 通常发生在儿童中。

• 小血管血管炎：
- 多血症肉芽肿病(韦格纳肉芽肿病)：
  ◦ 坏死性血管炎影响小到中型血管。
  ◦ 上呼吸道和下呼吸道的肉芽肿性炎症和肾小球性肾炎。
- 显微镜下多血管炎：
  ◦ 小血管坏死。
  ◦ 肾小球肾炎非常常见。
  ◦ 经常发生肺毛细血管炎。
- 嗜酸性肉芽肿伴多发性血管炎(Churg-Strauss 综合征)：
  ◦ 累及小型和中型动脉，主要是肺、胃肠道和神经。
  ◦ 还可以影响心脏、皮肤和肾脏。

• 小血管：
- 过敏性紫癜：
  ◦ 大多数患者<20 岁。
- 伯格病(血栓闭塞性脉管炎)：
- 冷球蛋白性血管炎。
- 抗肾小球基底膜病(肾炎综合征)。
- 红斑狼疮血管炎、类风湿关节炎、Sjogren 综合征。
- 药物性血管炎。

• 大小不一的动脉和静脉。
- 白塞病。
- 复发性多软骨炎。

• 继发性血管炎：
- 细菌感染：
  ◦ 链球菌、结核、葡萄球菌、莱姆病、麻风病。
- 病毒感染：
  ◦ 乙型肝炎或丙型肝炎、巨细胞病毒、单纯疱疹病毒、艾滋病病毒或立克次体感染。
- 立克次体感染。
- 毛细胞白血病。
- 淋巴瘤。
- 血清病。

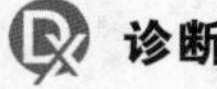

诊断

■ 症状和体征

• 在发生血管相关并发症之前，系统性疾病在血管炎的早期表现中很常见：
- 发热，疲劳，体重减轻，弥漫性疼痛。

• 动脉供血不足的迹象：
- 缺血性疼痛：
  ◦ 心绞痛、腹绞痛、跛行、下颌运动障碍。
- 神经系统缺血：
  ◦ 头痛、TIA、脑卒中、视觉和感觉神经性听力损失、幻觉、神经病变、视力减退。
- 肾缺血：
  ◦ 严重或耐药性。
- 皮肤缺血：
  ◦ 经典的皮肤表现包括可触及的紫癜。
  ◦ 也可以看到结节性病变、溃疡、网状细菌和缺血性缺血。
- 少关节炎。
- 眼局部缺血：
  ◦ 复视、视网膜出血、巩膜炎和巩膜外层炎。
- 呼吸道：
  ◦ 鼻窦炎、鼻出血、鼻腔和口腔溃疡、草莓舌。
- 胃肠缺血：
  ◦ 便血、黑便、呕血、腹膜炎、肝炎。
- 心脏：
  ◦ 冠状动脉瘤、心肌炎、心包炎、瓣膜病、慢性心功能不全。
- 黏膜：草莓牙龈炎、口腔溃疡。

病史

• 怀疑伴有一般系统和动脉供血不足的血管炎：

- 年轻人患有跛行、心绞痛、腹绞痛或 TIA。
- 长期系统性疾病伴多器官功能障碍。
- 肾小球肾炎史、周围神经病变或自身免疫性疾病。

• 诊断线索的病因：

- 年龄、性别、种族、旅行史。
- 涉及的血管和器官大小。
- 最近的感染。
- 结缔组织疾病。
- 可能导致血管炎的药物：
  ◦ 左旋咪唑(作为可卡因掺杂物)、苯妥英、卡马鲁嗪、异烟肼、甲巯咪唑、米诺环素、青霉胺、丙基硫氧嘧啶、柳氮磺吡啶。

体格检查

血管炎分类：

• 大动脉：

- 脉搏减弱，大动脉有血管杂音。
- 左右肢之间血压差异>10 mmHg。
- 左右肢之间脉压>30 mmHg。
- 由于跛行和溃疡而使肢体皮温低。

• 中小动脉：

- 可触及性紫癜(结节、溃疡、真性丘疹)。
- 皮肤溃疡。
- 数字缺血。

▪ 基本检查

• 病史和体格检查。

• CBC、ESR、CRP、尿分析、BUN、肌酐。

实验室检查

X

• CBC：

- 白细胞增多。
- 嗜酸性粒细胞增多。
- 贫血。

• 肌酐。

• LFT。

• CRP。

• ESR。

• ANA。

• ANCA。

• 补体。

• CPK。

• 尿液检查：

- 蛋白尿和血尿。

影像学检查

• CXR：

- X 线平片上通常具有不明显的斑片状肺泡浸润。

• CT 扫描：

- 鼻窦 CT 平扫疑似肉芽肿性多血管炎(Wegener)。

• CTA：

- 川崎病冠状动脉瘤。

• 超声心动图：

- 川崎病冠状动脉瘤。

• MRI 和 MRA：

- 对疑似大动脉炎和川崎病做 PET 扫描。

• 心电图：

- 提示：发现大动脉炎和川崎病。

• 超声：

- 颞动脉超声发现巨细胞动脉炎。
- 使用预测概率来解释结果。

• 动脉造影。

诊断步骤/外科

• 心电图：

- 心包炎，传导障碍。

• 胃肠道受累的内镜检查、乙状结肠镜检查和结肠镜检查。

• 组织活检。

▪ 鉴别诊断

• 心内膜炎。

• 药物不良反应。

• 病毒感染(如肠道病毒)。

• 猩红热。

• 葡萄球菌皮肤感染。

• 毒性休克综合征。

• 史蒂文斯-约翰综合征。

• 钩端螺旋体病。

• 抗磷脂抗体综合征。

• 弥散性血管内凝血。

• 胆固醇栓。

• 钙化。

治疗

▪ 初步稳定/治疗

稳定脑血管并发症。

▪ 急诊治疗/程序

• 血管炎的治疗由潜在的原因或特定的疾病决定，最好参照风湿病学治疗。

• 川崎病：阿司匹林、IVIG。

• 巨细胞动脉炎：皮质类固醇。

• 嗜酸性肉芽肿伴多发性血管炎：美泊利单抗。

• 白塞病：阿普斯特。

• ANCA 相关性血管炎：利妥昔单抗。

• PAN：类固醇、环磷酰胺。

• 大动脉炎：皮质类固醇、甲氨蝶呤、硫唑嘌呤、环磷酰胺。

• Wegner 肉芽肿病：

- 皮质类固醇。
- 环磷酰胺。
- 硫唑嘌呤。
- 严重疾病血浆置换。

▪ 药物治疗

• 硫唑嘌呤：2 mg/(kg・d)，口服。

• 环磷酰胺：

- 静脉注射：0.5～1 mg/m^2。
- 口服：2 mg/(kg・d)(最大剂量 4 mg/kg)(儿童：根据顾问的剂量)。

• IVIG：0.1～2 g/kg，静脉注射。

• 甲泼尼龙：0.25～1 mg/d，静脉注射。

• 甲氨蝶呤：每周 7.5～15 mg，口服。

• 泼尼松龙：1 mg/(kg・d)，口服。

• 泼尼松：40～60 mg/d[儿童：1～2 mg/(kg・d)]，口服。

随访

▪ 进一步处理

入院指征

• 应该接受有严重疾病和终末器官功能障碍的患者。

• 需要恢复缺血性器官供血。

出院指征

症状较轻且患者没有器官受累。

转诊问题

• 任何疑似血管炎并作为门诊患者进行治疗的患者都应尽快向风湿科医师提供明确的诊断和治疗。

• 根据最终器官损伤的严重程度咨询专科医师。

▪ 随访建议

强调需要密切随访，早期确认诊断并开始治疗，这将极大改善患者预后。

要点和误区

• 药物治疗可能有毒，需咨询专科医师。

• 患者可能会免疫抑制，并有机会致病的风险。

• 不要将细菌性心内膜炎视为血管炎。

• 50 岁以前不会发生颞动脉(巨细胞)动脉炎。

• 结节性病变是最有可能诊断为血管炎的皮肤变化。

血尿和蛋白尿 Hematuria/Proteinuria

Philip Shayne 刘雪峰 译

基础知识

描述

- 镜下血尿：3份合格尿液标本中2份尿液每高倍镜下≥3RBC。
- 肉眼血尿：尿液标本中可见血液。
- 蛋白尿：尿蛋白量>150 mg/d。
- 无症状蛋白尿的危险因素：
  - 糖尿病。
  - 高血压。
  - 非甾体抗炎药滥用。
  - 吸毒(海洛因)。
- 无症状血尿的危险因素：
  - 吸烟。
  - 苯、芳香胺、燃料等暴露史。
  - 肉眼血尿病史。
  - >40岁。
  - 泌尿系统疾病史。
  - 排尿疼痛的病史。
  - 泌尿系统感染的病史。
  - 止痛药滥用。
  - 盆腔放疗病史。

病因

- 蛋白尿。
  - 肾小球性：
    - 肾性(感染后、IgA、狼疮、血管炎)。
    - 肾病性(微小病变、糖尿病、先兆子痫)。
  - 肾小管性。
  - 溢出(溶血反应、横纹肌溶解、多发性骨髓瘤)。
  - 肾后性蛋白尿。
- 血尿：
  - 尿路感染。
  - 结石(肾、膀胱)。
  - 前列腺良性增生。
  - 膀胱、肾脏、前列腺等肿瘤。
  - 原因不明的短暂血尿。
  - 急性肾小球肾炎。

诊断

症状和体征

- 排尿困难。
- 血尿。
- 发热。
- 侧腹部疼痛。
- 侧腹部瘀斑。
- 初始血尿(前尿路病变)。
- 终末血尿(后尿道、膀胱、膀胱三角区)。
- 循环血尿(子宫内膜异位症、尿路)。
- 近期上呼吸道感染(10～21日前)。
- 近期皮肤感染(10～21日前)。
- 失明(奥尔波特综合征)。
- 外周性水肿。
- 充血性心力衰竭。
- 咯血(肺出血-肾炎综合征)。
- 月经。
- 睾丸、附睾及前列腺的创伤。
- 后尿道缺损。
- 前列腺增生。
- 阴茎、阴囊血肿。
- 心房颤动：
  - 肾动脉栓塞。
- 器官肿大,可触及包块。
- 妊娠原因器官肿大。
- 头痛。
- 高血压,血压>140/90 mmHg。
- 右上腹疼痛。

病史

- 疾病的特点(开始,持续时间)。
- 关联症状(近期疾病)。
- 既往病史(糖尿病、高血压、孕产史)。
- 药物治疗(肾毒性药物、抗凝药物、抗生素)。

体格检查

- 详细检查,需要特别注意：
  - 水肿,包括眼眶周围。
  - 彻底的泌尿生殖系统检查,包括前列腺：
  - 皮疹。
  - 侧腹部(瘀斑、触痛)。

基本检查

- 尿液分析。
- 显微镜观察尿液标本。
- 尿培养。
- 尿素氮水平。
- 血清肌酐水平。
- 全血细胞计数。
- 妊娠的考虑。
- 肝功能。
- 血小板计数。
- 凝血功能。

诊断检查与说明

实验室检查

- 尿：
  - 培养。
  - 细胞学检查。
  - 24 h尿蛋白和肌酐水平。
  - 尿蛋白肌酐比值。
  - 尿蛋白与渗透压梯度比值。
  - 尿蛋白电泳。
- 血清：
  - 凝血功能。
  - 蛋白电泳。

影像学检查

- 螺旋CT。
- 肾脏超声。

诊断步骤/外科

- 膀胱尿道镜检查。
- 泌尿系统造影。
- 膀胱造影。
- 逆行肾盂造影。
- 静脉肾盂造影。

鉴别诊断

- 肾小球性血尿：
  - IgA肾病。
  - 感染后肾小球肾炎。
  - 膜性增生性肾小球肾炎。
  - 局灶性肾小球硬化。
  - 狼疮肾炎。
  - 韦格纳肉芽肿。
  - 结节性多动脉炎。
  - 过敏性紫癜综合征。
- 血栓性血小板减少性紫癜：
  - 溶血性尿毒症综合征。
  - Alport综合征。
  - Goodpasture病。
- 肾性血尿：
  - 感染(肾盂肾炎、结核、血吸虫病)。
  - 炎症反应(药物、放疗)。
  - 尿路上皮肿瘤。
  - 肾及肾外肿瘤。
  - 间质性肾炎。
  - 肾乳头坏死。
  - 多囊肾病。

- 髓质海绵肾。
- 肾动脉栓塞/血栓。
- 肾静脉血栓。
- 镰状细胞病。
- 恶性高血压。
- 高尿钙症。
- 高尿酸症。
- 尿石症。
- 尿道狭窄。
- 子宫内膜异位症。
- 异物。
- 良性前列腺肥大。
- 凝血功能障碍/出血性疾病。
- 创伤(肾蒂损伤、尿道损伤、膀胱破裂)。
- 近期创伤性操作检查。
- 频繁性交或性交突然中断。
- 人为性的。

• 肾小球性蛋白尿(>2 g/d):
- 肾小球微小病变。
- 膜性肾小球肾炎。
- 局灶性节段性肾小球肾炎。
- 糖尿病。
- 胶原血管病。
- 淀粉样变性。
- 先兆子痫。
- 感染(HIV 感染、乙型肝炎、丙型肝炎、链球菌、梅毒)。
- 淋巴瘤。
- 慢性移植肾排异。
- 吸毒。
- 青霉胺。

• 肾小管性蛋白尿:
- 高血压性肾硬化。
- 尿酸性肾病。
- 急性过敏性间质性肾炎。
- 范科尼综合征。
- 镰状细胞病。

• 溢出性蛋白尿:
- 单克隆丙球蛋白病。
- 白血病。

• 蛋白尿其他病因:
- 脱水。
- 应激。
- 发热。
- 灼伤。
- 炎性过程。
- 直立性蛋白尿。

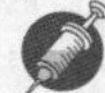

治疗

院前

• 急救 ABC 管理。
• 控制其他创伤。

初步稳定治疗

• 急救 ABC 管理。
• 首先治疗影响血流动力学稳定的损伤。
• 初步的实验室检查(显微镜下尿液分析、肌酐、尿素氮、电解质)。

妊娠注意事项

如考虑到先兆子痫:
• 积极控制血压。
• 硫酸镁。
• 妇产科会诊。

急诊治疗/程序

• 无并发症的泌尿道感染:
- 抗生素(详见尿路感染,成人/儿童)。

• 肾盂肾炎:
- 抗生素(详见尿路感染,成人/儿童)。
- 镇痛药。
- 解热药。

• 急进型肾小球肾炎:
- 类固醇疗法。
- 肾脏科会诊。

• 急性肾衰竭:
- 血液透析。
- 肾脏超声。
- 尿电解质。
- 肾脏科会诊。

• 肾绞痛:
- 液体治疗。
- 镇痛药。
- 如果是首发症状,无须 CT 检查。

• 肉眼血尿:
- 使用三腔导尿管行膀胱冲洗,以防血凝块堵塞尿道引起尿潴留。

药物治疗

• 尿路感染推荐的抗生素已经在相关章节叙述。
• 和肾内科医师讨论决定激素在急进性肾小球肾病中的使用。

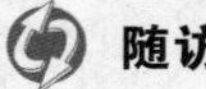

随访

进一步处理

入院指征

• 急性肾衰竭。
• 氮质血症、尿毒症、高血钾。
• 血流动力学不稳定。
• 创伤性血尿。
• 导致全身性感染或肾衰竭的输尿管结石。
• 高血压急症。
• 少尿、无尿。
• 合并先兆子痫、肾盂肾炎、阻塞性肾结石的孕妇。
• 顽固性疼痛。
• 无法口服药物治疗。

出院指征

• 血流动力学稳定且不伴有威胁生命的问题。
• 无肾衰竭或尿路阻塞的尿路结石感染。
• 无肾衰竭的轻度血尿或蛋白尿。

• 血尿:
- 肉眼血尿需泌尿科随访,证实尿路感染的青年女性除外。
- 镜下血尿需复检,将来可能需要泌尿科、肾内科随访复诊。
- 伴有感染症状的孕妇患者需要密切随访治疗效果。

• 蛋白尿:
- 轻症患者需初级保健医师门诊进行病情的随诊。
- 肾病蛋白尿合并肾衰竭的患者需要立即到肾病专科就诊。

要点和误区

• 对于急性肾小球肾炎的患儿,无论是误诊泌尿系统感染,还是漏诊不同点,都是医疗缺陷。
• 随机尿蛋白/肌酐与 24 h 尿蛋白有关。
• 眼眶水肿不仅仅是过敏反应的结果,还是肾病综合征的一种体征。
• 无症状血尿未能确保随访,对患者来讲,尤其是 40 岁以上的,是一个医疗缺陷。

血清病 Serum Sickness

Anika Backster · Martine Lory Camille 周健 潘曙明 译

基础知识

描述

- Ⅲ型过敏反应。
- 当外来蛋白或药物(抗原)被注射时,机体的免疫系统会对外来物质产生抗体,然后形成抗原、抗体和补体组成的复合物。
- 这些复合物随后沉积在组织中,引发炎症反应:
  - C3a 和 C5a 作为过敏性反应蛋白。
  - C5a 对中性粒细胞具有强的趋化作用。
  - 中性粒细胞在免疫复合物沉积和释放酶的部位浸润血管壁,如胶原酶和弹性蛋白酶,损伤血管壁。
- 一般来说,初次接触抗原后 6～21 日出现症状。
- 如果最初接触过疫苗,症状可在接触后 1～4 日出现。
- 症状通常持续 1～2 周后才会自动消退。

病因

- 血清病:
  - 含有外来蛋白或血清的疫苗,如肺炎球菌疫苗或狂犬病疫苗。
  - 用马或羊蛋白制成的抗蛇毒和破伤风接种。
  - 单克隆抗体。
- 血清病样反应:
  - 非蛋白药物引起,主要是抗生素:
    - 青霉素、阿莫西林。
    - 头孢菌素(氯氨苄西林)。
    - 磺胺类药(即复方新诺明)。
    - 利尿剂。
    - 金硫脲嘧啶。
    - 乙内酰脲。
    - 苯基丁氮酮。
    - 链霉素阿司匹林。

诊断

症状和体征

典型表现为发热、皮疹、关节痛和淋巴结肿大。

病史

- 发热。
- 皮疹(荨麻疹、麻疹、猩红热)。
- 关节痛。
- 肌痛。
- 淋巴结病。
- 面部和颈部水肿。
- 胸痛。
- 气短。

体格检查

- 发热。
- 皮疹。
- 淋巴结病。
- 关节炎。
- 水肿。
- 脾大。
- 周围神经炎。
- 心肌炎和心包炎。
- 速发型过敏反应。

基本检查

- 在出现症状前 6～21 日,有可能发生侵犯行为的病史和时间过程。
- 体格检查显示出皮疹,以及关节、肌肉、心脏、神经或肾损伤。

诊断检查与说明

- 降低补体水平。
- 白细胞,嗜伊红细胞过多。
- ESR 升高。
- 高丙种球蛋白血症。
- 尿中含有蛋白尿或血尿。

影像学检查

考虑胸部 X 线检查。

诊断步骤/外科

活检是唯一确定诊断的方法。

鉴别诊断

- 血管炎(如多动脉炎、多动脉炎、韦氏肉芽肿病)。
- 皮疹(如多形性红斑、有毒表皮坏死溶解)。
- 免疫学(如系统性红斑狼疮、多发性肌炎、过敏反应)。
- 传染性(如蜱传播疾病、落基山斑疹热、单核细胞增多症)。

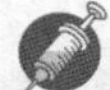

治疗

院前

- ABC 管理。
- 过敏反应治疗。

初步稳定/治疗

如果出现严重的全身反应,则使用 ABC 管理。

急诊治疗/程序

症状缓解,直至疾病在 1～13 个月自动消退。

- 抗组胺药。
- 退热药。
- 非甾体抗炎药。
- 泼尼松是有争议的。

药物治疗

- 醋氨酚:325～650 mg,口服或灌肠(儿童:q4～6 h,10～15 mg/kg)。
- 苯海拉明:50～100 mg[儿童:5 mg/(kg · d),div];50 mg/剂或 300 mg/24 h,q6～8 h。
- 羟嗪:25～50 mg(儿童:0.5 mg/kg),q6～8 h。
- 布洛芬:200～800 mg,口服(儿童:>6 个月,q6～8 h,5～10 mg/kg)。
- 泼尼松:5～60 mg/d,口服[儿童:0.5～2 mg/(kg · d)],2 周 Taper。

随访

进一步处理

入院指征

- 气道介入。
- 初期使用类固醇后症状和体征复发。
- 免疫抑制。
- 伴随严重的疾病。
- 注意事项。

出院指征

稳定的,大多数情况下是自限性。

转诊问题

对外源性抗血清进行皮肤测试,以避免对未来的异种血清进行过敏反应。

X

■ 随访建议

初级保健医师随访。

要点和误区

• 在治疗血清疾病时，发现并停止抗原是至关重要的。

• 显著的发病率来自在未考虑血清病的情况下无法诊断。

血栓性血小板减少性紫癜 Thrombotic Thrombocytopenic Purpura

Hariy Y. Atallah　范浩浩　李文放 译

基础知识

■ 描述

• 血栓性血小板减少性紫癜（TTP）是严重的影响多器官系统的凝血障碍疾病。

• 经典的五大特征：

- 血小板减少症。
- 溶血性贫血。
- 轻度肾功能不全。
- 神经系统体征。
- 发热。

• 1 名患者表现出全部 5 项特征不常见到；如果出现，严重的器官损害或缺血可能已经发生。

• 血小板减少症和溶血性贫血是最常见的特征。

• 与后天或先天血浆 von Willebrand 因子切割蛋白酶（vWFcp）不足有关。

• 患有严重神经系统疾病的患者伴急性肾衰竭异常最好由综合术语 TTP - HUS 描述。

典型病程

• 急性起病。

• 持续几日到几个月的急性起病。

• 未经治疗是几乎总是致命的：

- 未经治疗时有>90%的死亡率。
- 经历现代治疗，生存率逆转到>90%。

• 临床表现包括：

- 特发性。
- 家族性，慢性或复发。
- 药物诱导：
  ◦ 过敏或免疫介导的（奎宁、噻氯匹定、dopidogrel）。
  ◦ 剂量相关毒性（丝裂霉素 C、环孢素）。
- 妊娠，产后相关：
  ◦ 见于 10%～25%的孕妇。
- 骨髓移植相关。
- 感染。

• 30～60 岁更为常见。

• 在儿童或老年人群中罕见。

• 女性发病率是男性的 2 倍。

■ 病因

• 未知的初级启动因子，可能系统性内皮细胞损伤导致凝血途径失活。

• 发生血小板聚集和纤维蛋白沉积在小动脉和毛细血管中导致微血栓并阻碍血流。

• 血小板聚集导致：

- 血小板的消耗。
- 广泛的微血管透明血栓形成。

• 血小板聚集致微血管阻塞然后导致：

- 红细胞溶血。
- 血红素分解产物的积累。
- 贫血。

• 终末器官缺血导致小血管内弥散性血栓形成：

- 常见于心脏、脑、肾脏、胰腺和肾上腺。

• vWFcp 的缺失导致凝血途径的控制失败。

■ 风险因素

遗传学

• 有些病例是遗传/家族性的。

• vWFcp 最近被确定为 ADAMTS 家族新的成员，被指定为 *ADAMTS*13。

• *ADAMTS*13 基因突变导致常染色体隐形异常的慢性复发性 TTP。

诊断

■ 症状和体征

经典五大特点。

• 血小板减少症：

- 血小板计数<20 000/mm^3。

• 微血管病和溶血性贫血：

- 血红蛋白<100 g/L（40%的病例中<60 g/L）。

• 神经症状：

- 60%的病例出现并发症，90%的病例出现症状。
- 典型波动。
- 头痛。
- 神志改变（混乱、昏迷、昏迷）。
- 行为或人格变化。
- 焦点感觉或运动障碍或失语。
- 癫痫。
- 自发性颅内出血。

• 肾功能不全：

- 通常轻微。
- 肌酐<3 mg/dl。

• 发热：

- 发生在急性发作和前驱综合征。
- 发热是最不常见的特点。

• 在同一个患者身上出现五大典型症状，这种情况很少见。

病史

• 一般：

- 虚弱。
- 疲劳。
- 发热。
- 不适。

• 出血：

- 容易瘀伤。
- 鼻出血。
- 月经过多。
- 胃肠道出血。
- 视力丧失或改变。

• 胃肠道并发症：

- 厌食症。
- 腹泻。
- 腹部疼痛。

• 神经系统：

- 头痛。
- 混乱。
- 癫痫。
- 行为或人格变化。
- 焦点感觉或运动障碍或失语。

体格检查

• 紫癜。

• 胃肠道出血。

- 鼻出血。
- 黄疸。
- 休克。
- 精神状态改变。
- 局灶性感觉或运动障碍。
- 肺部浸润和水肿。
- 视力改变,视网膜出血、脱离。
- 心脏传导异常。

基本检查

临床诊断

- 由于成功的治疗基于以下诊断:
  - 确定2个主要发现:
    - 血小板减少症。
    - 微血管病性溶血性贫血。
  - 排除其他主要鉴别诊断。
- 全面的病史和体格检查并进行确定性的实验室检查。
- 确定可能的药物相关疾病并避免再次暴露。

诊断检查与说明

实验室检查

- CBC、血小板计数、网织红细胞计数:
  - 贫血:血红蛋白<100 g/L。
  - 血小板减少<20 000/mm^3。
  - 网织红细胞计数增加。
- 凝血研究:
  - 正常。
- 外周血涂片:
  - 大血管的改变。
  - 裂红细胞。
  - 头盔细胞。
  - 有核红细胞。
- Coombs试验:
  - 直接Coombs试验阴性。
- 电解质、BUN、肌酐、葡萄糖:
  - BUN、肌酐轻度升高。
  - 由于红细胞溶解导致的高钾血症。
- 乳酸脱氢酶(LDH):
  - 由于溶血和组织缺血而升高5~10倍。
- 胆红素:
  - 非结合胆红素增加。
- 尿液分析:
  - 血尿(镜下血尿至肉眼血尿)。
- *ADAMTS*13分析可用于区分慢性复发性TTP,继发于*ADAMTS* 13抑制剂的TTP和溶血性尿毒症综合征(HUS):
  - *ADAMTS*13缺陷不能检测到所有可能会对血浆交换做出反应的患者。

影像学检查

- 头部CT:
  - 排除颅内出血。

诊断步骤/外科

- 活组织检查:
  - 确诊。
  - 在小血管中显示透明病变。
  - 暴发性起病时禁忌(出血风险)。
- 脑电图:
  - 预测是否需要抗惊厥疗法。

鉴别诊断

- 溶血性尿毒症综合征:
  - 血小板减少症三联征、裂红细胞症和肾功能不全。
  - 神经症状不常见。
  - 常以传染性先兆和腹泻为先驱症状。
- 弥散性血管内凝血(DIC):
  - 引起微血管中纤维蛋白的沉积,而不是透明血栓。
  - 凝血研究异常。
- 特发性血小板减少性紫癜(ITP):
  - 没有溶血证据。
  - LDH和胆红素正常。
- 妊娠相关血小板减少症:
  - 先兆子痫、子痫。
  - 妊娠相关的溶血。
  - HELLP(溶血、肝酶升高、低血小板)。
- Evans综合征:
  - 自身免疫性溶血性贫血。
  - 突出微粒细胞而不是裂细胞。
  - 直接阳性Coombs试验。
- 恶性高血压。
- 细菌败血症。
- 亚急性细菌性心内膜炎。
- 自身免疫性疾病[如系统性红斑狼疮(SLE)]。
- 弥漫性恶性肿瘤。
- 肝素相关血小板减少症。
- 人工瓣膜或严重主动脉瓣钙化狭窄。

治疗

院前

- 检查气道、呼吸、循环。
- 评估神志改变的其他可能原因(低血糖、高血糖)。

初步稳定/治疗

- 检查气道、呼吸、循环。
- 生理盐水(NS)静脉输入液体复苏治疗休克或胃肠道出血。
- 红细胞输血:
  - 对于显著的贫血或出血并发症。
- 血小板输血:
  - 预防危及生命的出血(例如,CNS出血)或需要侵入性操作。
  - 可能会加重血栓形成,微血管阻塞的过程并使末端器官缺血恶化并引起休克。

急诊治疗/程序

- 新鲜冷冻血浆(FFP)或新鲜未冷冻血浆:
  - 在明确TTP诊断的基础上开始,作为过渡到血浆置换的桥梁。
  - 成功率接近64%。
  - 没有提供血小板抗凝聚因子或在患者自身血清中减少。
  - 在慢性复发型预防性使用,以防止复发。
- 血浆置换:
  - 治疗的最重要组成部分。
  - 血浆置换和FFP输注的组合。
  - 血浆除去法:
    - 导致内皮损伤和开启TTP过程的免疫复合物。
    - 促进循环集成因素可促进血小板聚集。
  - 每日执行,直至:
    - 血小板计数正常化。
    - 神经症状改善。
    - LDH正常化。
  - 肾功能改善可能滞后于其他发现。
  - 基于疗效的经验判断的完成频率;如果发生复发,可能需要重新开始。
  - 并发症包括:
    - 过敏或血清病。
    - 继发感染。
    - 低血压。
- 皮质类固醇:
  - 临床获益未经证实。
  - 可能会限制免疫介导的内皮细胞损害和减少脾破坏血小板和损伤红细胞。
  - 如果通过出血或局部缺血致肾上腺受损,可以受益于支持疗法。
- 抗血小板或免疫抑制药物:
  - 最常用的阿司匹林和双嘧达莫。
  - 磺胺吡嗪、葡聚糖和长春新碱的用法已被报道。
  - 疗效会发生变化。
  - 会加重出血并发症。
- 脾切除术:
  - 曾经被推荐。

- 疗效不确定。
• 透析：
- 用于肾衰竭。

▪ **药物治疗**

• 阿司匹林：325～650 mg，口服，q4～6 h。
• 双嘧达莫：75～100 mg，口服，每日 4 次。
• FFP：
- 血浆输注：30 ml/(kg·d)，75～100 ml/h。
- 血浆置换：3～4 L/d。
• 甲泼尼龙：0.75 mg/kg，q12 h。
• 泼尼松：1～2 mg/(kg·d)，最大剂量至 200 mg/d。
• 利妥昔单抗：375 mg/m^2，静脉输注，每周 1 次，4～8 次。
• 长春新碱：每周 1 次，1.4 mg/m^2，静脉输注。

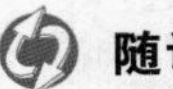

随访

▪ **进一步处理**

入院指征

• 新诊断的严重血小板疾病，特别是出血并发症或精神状态改变或肾功能障碍。
• 入住 ICU 时 TTP 有活动性出血或神经系统发现：
- 适当运送到配备专科护理设施三级护理中心。

▪ **随访建议**

血液科医师应随访已发现疾病且稳定的患者。

要点和误区

• 在妊娠的女性，TTP 可能与 HELLP 综合征混淆。
• 由于未经处理的 TTP 具有很高的死亡率，对疾病的识别和启动治疗是关键。

血胸 Hemothorax

Anthony C. Salazar 陈奇通 李文放 译

基础知识

▪ **描述**

• 胸腔积血是由于钝性/穿透性胸部创伤或其他非创伤性病因所导致的胸壁、胸膜或胸腔内脏器的组织/血管破裂出血。
- 导致肺活量减少、缺氧和呼吸系统损害。
- 大血管损伤导致血流动力学不稳定和出血性休克。
- 大量血胸可导致胸腔内压升高，导致静脉回流障碍和心输出量降低。
• 胸腔积血在钝性损伤中很少单独出现：
- 通常与气胸（25%的病例）、胸外损伤（73%的病例）和肺挫伤同时出现。
• 大量的胸腔积血会导致一些抗凝物质释放，并加重胸腔内持续出血。
• 如果未进行治疗，可导致脓胸和纤维胸（粘连导致肺不张）。

▪ **病因**

• 大血管损伤（包括医源性）：
- 与胸腔出血有关的常见血管，包括肋间动脉、乳内动脉、肺动脉、肺静脉、主动脉、腔静脉和心脏。
• 创伤性肺实质损伤：
- 由于肺内的低压和高浓度的凝血活酶，出血通常能自行停止。
- 通常合并气胸。
• 非创伤性或自发性血胸：
- 非常少见。
- 考虑凝血功能障碍、恶性肿瘤、原发性血管事件（如主动脉夹层、动脉瘤破裂）、肺栓塞合并梗死、感染（结核）、大疱性肺气肿、肺动脉畸形、肺叶隔离。
• 自发性气胸或胸腔闭式引流并发胸膜粘连撕裂。

诊断

▪ **症状和体征**

• 少量胸腔积血（<400 ml）：患者外表、生命体征或体格检查很少或没有变化。
• 大量胸腔积血（>1 000 ml）：躁动、焦虑、面色苍白、胸膜炎疼痛、咯血、呼吸困难或呼吸窘迫：
- 失血量>30%（1 500～2 000 ml）的休克表现。
- 心动过速、呼吸困难、低血压。
• 起病隐匿（如恶性肿瘤）：因为失血通常较缓慢，不会产生明显的血流动力学改变，所以呼吸困难是最常见的症状。

病史

• 胸部受到严重的钝性损伤或穿透性创伤。
• 近期发生肋骨骨折或连枷胸。
• 在胸部 X 线片上没有胸腔内病理的初步证据时，延迟性血胸可发生在数小时至数日后；可能与活动时胸壁血肿破裂或肋骨骨折边缘损伤肋间血管有关。
• 恶性肿瘤或转移性疾病。
• 近期外科操作：胸腔穿刺术、胸腔闭式引流等。

体格检查

• 生命体征：根据严重程度和时间进展，可能出现缺氧、呼吸困难、心动过速和低血压。
• 颈部：胸腔内压增高致颈静脉怒张，气管偏斜。
• 胸部检查：不对称扩张，严重畸形，胸廓反常运动，擦伤，血肿和挫伤。
• 胸部触诊：肋骨、锁骨、肩胛骨或胸骨压痛或骨擦音；肺气肿，叩诊浊音。
• 听诊：同侧呼吸音减弱或消失（适用于直立体位）。

▪ **基本检查**

• 胸部 X 线片是理想的诊断工具。
• 对于血流动力学稳定的患者，吸气后屏气直立后前位（PA）投影最佳。
- 200～300 ml 及以上的液体通常可以在直立位或卧位胸部 X 线片上观察到。
- 在正常无瘢痕的胸膜腔内，液体会显示为弯月形/液体平面，使肋膈角变钝。
• 在仰卧前后位（AP）X 线片（便携式）中，多达 1 000 ml 的血液也可能不是很明显。
- 在受累的半侧胸腔内可能仅可见轻微的模糊影。
• 看胸片时寻找相关损伤（气胸、肋骨骨折、肺挫伤、纵隔增宽等）。

X

诊断检查与说明

实验室检查

- 如果血细胞比容在系列检查中下降或变化，则有助于诊断。
- 血型和交叉配血试验。
- 脉搏血氧饱和度。
- 胸腔积液抽出后其血细胞比容应大于血液血细胞比容的50%。

影像学检查

- 超声诊断成像是评估胸腔积液的重要手段。
  - 扩展FAST扫描可以诊断血胸，其灵敏度高于便携式胸部X线片。
- CT可检测出X线片上看不到的少量胸腔积液。

鉴别诊断

- 血气胸。
- 气胸。
- 肺挫伤。
- 胸腔积液。
- 脓胸或肺炎。

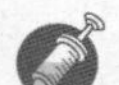

治疗

院前

- 评估生命体征和脉搏血氧饱和度：吸氧并开放静脉通道。
- 低血压时需要进行液体复苏。
- 注意事项：
  - 血胸与气胸临床鉴别困难：
    - 所有患者均可出现呼吸困难、胸膜炎性胸痛、呼吸音减低和血流动力学不稳定。
    - 一些线索有助于诊断，如气胸的肺气肿和血胸的叩诊浊音。
  - 如果患者血流动力学不稳定，进行针式胸腔闭式引流术治疗潜在的张力性气胸。

初步稳定/治疗

- 管理气道、呼吸、循环：
  - 根据需要控制气道；为即将发生呼吸衰竭的患者进行气管插管。
  - 吸氧。
  - 2个大口径静脉输液通道和液体复苏恢复循环血容量。
  - 对于血流动力学不稳定的患者，除非胸部闭式引流套件立即可用，否则应行针式胸腔闭式引流术。
- 除非有禁忌证，患者应保持坐姿直立。

急诊治疗/程序

- 尽快进行直立位胸部X线片，如果患者病情不稳定，不应等待针对性的治疗。
- 血胸的治疗方法是抽出胸膜腔内积聚的血液。
- 胸腔闭式引流术能排出血液，使肺部恢复扩张，并持续监测是否有失血。
- 胸腔闭式引流术：
  - 用大口径胸导管(36～40F)。
  - 在腋中线第4～5肋间，向后上方插入。
  - 然后将胸导管连接到水下密封引流和抽吸(20～30 ml H_2O)。
  - 通过胸部X线片确认导管位置和充分引流。
- 如果条件允许，应进行自体输血。
- 开胸手术适应证：
  - 初次引流>20 ml/kg血液(或成人引流1 000 ml)。
  - 持续出血速度>7 ml/(kg·h)(或200 ml/h，持续出血4 h)。
  - 胸部X线片显示血胸增加。
  - 充分补充血容量并排除其他部位出血后，患者仍保持低血压。
  - 初始复苏后患者失代偿。
  - 穿透伤：
    - 外伤发生于急诊或10 min内到达急诊。
    - 严重休克伴心脏压塞的临床症状。
  - 钝性损伤：外伤发生于急诊创伤中心或外科医师生可于10 min内到达。

药物治疗

- 清醒、有意识的患者行胸腔闭式引流术术前局部皮肤麻醉。
- 程序性镇静(咪达唑仑)和镇痛(芬太尼)可用于行胸腔闭式引流术的病情稳定、清醒的患者。
  - 芬太尼：成人和儿童，2～5 μg/kg。
  - 咪达唑仑：成人和儿童，0.02～0.04 mg/kg。
  - 可以考虑使用其他镇静剂。

随访

进一步处理

入院指征

血胸患者需要进行胸腔闭式引流术，应接受创伤科、心胸外科或普通外科的监护和胸腔引流管护理。入院单位应具有管理胸腔引流管装置的经验。

出院指征

- 孤立性小范围血胸患者(在超声或CT检查中偶然发现)，在观察4～6 h后如果没有持续性出血的证据，并且患者没有缺氧及其他症状，应予以出院。
- 无症状的钝性胸部创伤和首次胸部X线片正常的患者在出院前不需要重复摄片。

要点和误区

- 因为平均70 kg体重的男性的胸膜腔可以容纳超过4 L的血液，所以发生出血时可能没有任何外部失血的表现。
- 仰卧位创伤合并大量血胸的患者可能由于血液沿整个胸膜间隙后方的分布而导致听诊和叩击的结果不准确。
- 没有明确的外伤史时，胸部X线片可能被误诊为肺炎。
- 如果同时有膈肌损伤，血胸可能源于腹腔脏器损伤。
- 尽早做好自体输血的准备，因为大部分失血发生在首次插入胸腔引流管时。
- 对于仰卧位外伤患者，一个常见的错误是胸腔引流管插入位置过于偏前上方，导致引流困难。
- 确保所有的胸腔引流管的开口都在胸腔内。
- 实施胸腔闭式引流术的患者预防性使用抗生素并不能降低肺炎或脓胸的风险。

血友病 Hemophilia

Steven H. Bowman 陈奇通 译

基础知识

描述

- 由缺乏凝血因子Ⅷ或Ⅸ引起。
- 功能因子缺乏引起局部灭活凝血和止血功能障碍。
- 两型：
  - 血友病 A：凝血因子Ⅷ缺乏。
  - 血友病 B(Christmas disease)：凝血因子Ⅸ缺乏。
- 症状由功能因子的活性决定：
  - 因子活性为 5%～30%(轻度血友病)：
    - 主要有创伤或手术后出血。
  - 因子活性为 1%～5%(中度血友病)：
    - 中度的创伤或手术后出血。
    - 偶尔自发关节血肿(<1 次/月)。
  - 因子活性<1%(重度血友病)：
    - 婴儿期自发性出血。
    - 可能出血频率达到 1 周 1～2 次，经常需要因子置换。
- 并发症：
  - 出血甚至死亡。
  - 反复关节出血导致关节破坏和功能丧失。
  - 输血导致的感染(风险降低与血液净化技术有关)。
  - 能够防止出血的抑制剂开发(抗因子的 IgG 抗体)。

病因

遗传学

- X 染色体隐性遗传，有 1/3 的自发突变可能。
- 罕见病。
  - 血友病 A 发生率：1/(5000～7000)男性。
  - 血友病 B 发生率：1/30000 男性。
- 抑制剂的发病率：20%的严重血友病 A 和<5%的严重血友病 B。

诊断

症状和体征

- 出血。
  - 关节出血(最常见)：
    - 膝关节>肘关节>踝关节>肩关节>腕关节。
  - 肌肉出血。
  - 软组织伤口出血。
  - 拔牙或口腔黏膜出血。
  - 鼻出血(仅见于严重病例)。
  - 血尿。
  - 颅内出血。
  - 胃肠道出血。
  - 假瘤(血性囊肿)。

基本检查

全面的病史采集和体格检查。

诊断检查与说明

实验室检查

- 血小板计数：正常。
- 出血时间：正常。
- 凝血酶原时间：正常。
- 凝血酶原时间测定：延长。
- 尿液分析：无症状血尿(经常)。
- 特定因子测定：
  - 因子Ⅷ：抗体(剂量)降低。
  - 因子Ⅷ：C(活性)降低。
  - vWF：Ag 和 vWF 正常。

影像学检查

影像学检查一般在特定情况下使用：

- 头颅 CT：评估颅内出血。
- 肾脏超声和膀胱镜：发现大量血尿或肾脏损伤。
- 腹部 CT：了解及发现腹膜后出血。

鉴别诊断

- 血管性血友病。
- 抗凝药物。
- 抗血小板药物。
- 血小板减少症。
- 肝功能失代偿。

治疗

初步稳定/治疗

- 尽量控制出血。
- 建立静脉通道，进行血型鉴定和抗体筛查。
- 考虑输注浓缩红细胞。

急诊治疗/程序

常规

- 患者一般会了解自己的用药剂量、疾病分型，以及他们是否有用抑制剂。当出现任一症状，可降低因子替代治疗的使用门槛。
- 协调急诊室力量与血液科专家。
- 尽快实施因子替代治疗，甚至可以在影像学检查和咨询之前。

因子替代治疗

- 1 U 在 1 ml 普通血浆中看作凝血因子活性 100%。
- 没有血友病的人因子活性水平在 60%～150%。
- 第一步：以出血的位置/系统为基础来决定因子活性。
  - 低到中度出血：需要 30%～50%的活性。
    - 软组织挫伤/撕裂伤。
    - 关节或肌肉出血(除了髂腰肌)。
  - 中度到重度出血：需要 50%～100%的活性。
    - 胃肠道或胃溃疡出血。
    - 大的肌群出血(髂腰肌)。
  - 重度到危及生命的出血：需要 100%的活性。
    - 中枢神经系统损伤/颅内出血。
    - 外伤或手术后出血。
    - 腹腔内/腹膜后出血。
    - 喉部/颈部影响气道的出血。

第二步：计算所需活动水平的因子剂量。

- 因子Ⅷ需要量(单位 U)＝体重(kg)×0.5×(所需因子活动水平%)。1 U/kg 可以增长 2%活性。每 12 h 用药，持续 1～2 日。
- 因子Ⅺ需要量(单位 U)＝体重(kg)×1×(所需因子活动水平%)。1 U/kg 可以增长 1%活性。每 24 h 用药，持续 1～2 日。
- 输注因子时静脉推注 1～2 min 及以上。

具体管理的注意事项

- 关节血肿：
  - 夹板，血管紧张素转化酶，冰敷。
  - 关节穿刺很少使用。
- 肌肉出血：
  - 前臂和小腿：考虑筋膜室综合征。
  - 腰大肌：腹股沟疼痛，股神经感觉异常。
- 拔牙或口腔黏膜出血：
  - 局部胶原海绵治疗(avitene)或其他止血剂。
  - 严重的话使用因子替代治疗。
  - 氨基己酸(amicar)或氨甲环酸(cyklokapron)可能有用。
- 血尿(一般轻度)：

- 补液。
- 避免使用氨基己酸和冷沉淀。
• 颅内出血：
- 所有头部受伤应尤为重视，特别是在儿童。
- 不要延误头颅CT检查。
• 消化道出血：
- 继发溃疡、息肉、痔：因子替代治疗优先于内镜检查。

药物治疗

计算重组和血浆因子Ⅷ和Ⅸ浓缩物的剂量请参考前文因子替代治疗。

无抑制剂的患者

• 首选：重组人凝血因子。
- 重组凝血因子Ⅷ的选择：recombinate、kogenate、advate、helixate FS、xyntha。
- 重组凝血因子Ⅸ的选择：beneFⅨ。
• 次选：血浆衍生因子。
- 血浆衍生Ⅷ因子高纯度浓缩液：monodate-P、hemofil-M、koate DVI、alphanate。
- 血浆衍生Ⅷ因子中等纯度浓缩液：humate。
◦ 只在之前选项不可用情况下使用。
- 血浆衍生Ⅸ因子高纯度浓缩液：alphaNine、mononine。
• 其他选择：
- 冷沉淀(仅对A型血友病有效)：
◦ 从新鲜冰冻血浆在4℃解冻后获得。
◦ 包含凝血因子Ⅷ、vWF、纤维蛋白原。
◦ 在1U冷沉淀中有80～100U凝血因子Ⅷ。
◦ 最初给10包，儿童用量为1包/6kg。
◦ 只有在因子Ⅷ浓缩液不可用时使用。
- 新鲜冰冻血浆(包含凝血因子Ⅶ和Ⅸ)：
◦ 1U新鲜冰冻血浆包含200～300U凝血因子Ⅶ和Ⅸ。
◦ 1U新鲜冰冻血浆可使体重60kg的患者凝血因子活性提高5%～10%。
◦ 在大部分的急诊室可以立即使用，可用于因不可获得特殊因子而耽误治疗的大出血患者。
- 因子疗法的辅助治疗：DDAVP(仅针对A型血友病)。
◦ 提高因子Ⅷ水平2～3倍(只可用于轻型血友病以及轻度出血的患者)。
◦ 副作用：轻度面红、头痛、心动过速、低血压、低钠血症。
◦ 将DDAVP按0.3μg/kg的剂量加入50ml生理盐水中，通过静脉或皮下注射给药时间超过15～30min(体重超过50kg的患者可鼻内给予stimate，每个鼻孔1喷)。
◦ 不可用于1岁以下儿童。
- 因子疗法的辅助治疗：抗纤维蛋白溶解药(适用于轻度出血)。
◦ 抑制纤溶酶活性，防止血凝块溶解。
◦ 只适用于黏膜、口腔、牙齿出血。
◦ 儿童禁用。
◦ 示例：氨基己酸按75mg/kg剂量每6h最大可使用4g，氨甲环酸按25mg/kg剂量每8h使用1次。
- 因子疗法的辅助治疗：局部凝血酶。
◦ 用于局部控制浅表组织撕裂导致的出血。

有抑制剂的患者

• 首先：重组因子Ⅶa(novoSeven)。
- 每2～3h给予90～120μg/kg。
- 在未充分止血的情况下最大剂量300μg/kg可能会促进凝血酶形成和稳定纤维蛋白凝块。
- 绕过凝血级联反应，减少凝血系统风险。
- 安全性强，最小风险的抑制剂开发，昂贵。
• 其次：活化凝血酶原复合物(APCC)。
- 示例：FEIBA和Autoplex-T。
- 剂量：每8～12h按75～100U/kg给予。
- 包含因子Ⅶa、Ⅸa和Ⅹa。
- 绕过凝血级联反应。
- 大剂量使用可导致血栓栓塞性事件：DVT、PE、AMI和DIC。
• 其他选择：
- 在那些有低抗体滴度(低反应)者可以使用高剂量重组因子或血浆源性因子浓缩物(2～3倍的正常值范围)。
- 猪凝血因子Ⅷ目前使用较普及。

注意

• 所有的凝血因子浓缩物禁止肌内注射使用。
• 禁止使用阿司匹林或含有阿司匹林成分的制品。
• 在任何影像学检查、会诊、侵入性手术或转院前使用因子替代疗法。

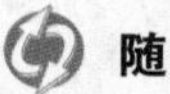

随访

进一步处理

入院指征

• 收入院要求低。
• 包括所有的关节/肌肉出血、内出血、严重出血。
• 出血以至于需要多次输血。
• 严重并发症或者任何颅脑损伤。

出院指征

较小的软组织出血，出血已控制的浅表组织撕裂伤。

转诊问题

血液病学所有出血。

随访建议

• 血液科门诊。
• 复发出血须返回急诊室。

要点和误区

• 对于有颅脑损伤的患者不要因为头颅CT而耽误治疗措施干预。
• 对于不清楚凝血因子水平的可疑出血急诊患者，假定凝血因子水平为0并按严重出血处理。
• 熟悉不同因子替代疗法对患者有无抑制剂的影响。
• 急诊治疗中应向血液科专家咨询关于适当的剂量、疗程的长短及有无抑制剂的治疗方法。
• 收入院治疗的门槛低。

荨麻疹 Urticaria

Fred A. Severyn 张晟 林兆奋 译

基础知识

描述

• 皮肤肥大细胞和嗜碱性细胞释放炎症介质，主要是组胺：
- 引起血管通透性增高和瘙痒。
• 表皮、真皮的上中层水肿：
- 多见于儿童和年轻人。
- 多见于女性。
- 多见于过敏体质人群。
• 40%的荨麻疹出现血管神经性水肿：
- 主要影响更深的真皮下和/或黏膜下层。

儿科注意事项

• 荨麻疹常因食物或感染引起：
- 特别是病毒性上呼吸道感染(URI)。
• 四肢水肿、发绀多见于婴儿。
• 腿、臀部可见水疱。

病因

急性

• 可能性找到怀疑的诱因，但大多是特发性的。
• 急性荨麻疹的病程为 6 周。
- 75%为特发性的。
- 自身免疫性疾病范畴。
- 免疫复合物引起。
- 通常是一种无法识别的反复出现的全身性荨麻疹。
- 可能由于隐蔽性或亚临床感染或全身性疾病(引起)。

诊断

症状和体征

病史

• 既往有荨麻疹病史。
• 有神经性水肿的家族史。
• 减轻和加重的因素。
• 疾病活动期的关注程度，以及对生活质量的影响。
• 病变持续时间和演变：
- 标记病变，有助于记录其持续时间。
- 发热和全身症状。
- 关节痛和肌肉痛。
- 体重减轻和淋巴结肿大。
- 低血压、面部发红、头痛。
- 黏膜水肿。
- 呼吸窘迫或气道受阻表现：
◦ 可能也是过敏反应的一部分。

体格检查

• 重点关注全身性过敏反应和感染。
• 气道：血管神经性水肿，气道受阻，无法排出分泌物，发声异常，喘鸣。
• 呼吸：喘息，支气管痉挛。
• 循环：过敏反应全身表现，如低血压。
• 腰部：肝脾大，妊娠。
• 皮肤：相关的水肿、淤斑、红斑。
- 广泛的、短暂的、瘙痒的、边界清楚的皮疹。
- 可以包括手掌和足底。
- 包括大疱和紫癜。
- 皮损大小、形态各异，分布不规则，可合并。
- 风团常在 3～4 h 消失。
- 随着旧的皮疹消失，新的皮疹会出现。
• 淋巴结肿大。
• 皮肤划痕症：
- 用压舌板划过皮肤，观察划痕。
• 类胆碱：
- 剧烈运动去提高体温和诱发出汗。
• 暴露于阳光下。
• 低温诱导：
- 皮肤上放一块冰块持续 5 min。
• 水源性：
- 使用不同温度的自来水。
• 严重的黏膜水肿：
- 可疑的血管神经性水肿。
- 严重低血压反应。
- 可疑的全身过敏反应。
• 持续时间长，疼痛、未变白的病灶：
- 怀疑是荨麻疹性血管炎。

基本检查

• 完整的病史和体格检查。
• 皮损的表现、位置、出现和持续时间。
• 确认是急性还是慢性。
• 相关症状，诱发因素。
• 合并症、过敏史、药物使用史。
• 分析感染源和系统性疾病体征。

诊断检查与说明

实验室检查

• 急性荨麻疹：不需要实验室检查。
• 慢性荨麻疹：
- 分析感染和系统性疾病：
◦ 全血细胞计数、红细胞沉降率、C 反应蛋白。
◦ 促甲状腺素和甲状腺功能。
◦ 尿常规，肝功能。
• 如果怀疑荨麻疹性血管炎可以做皮肤活检。

影像学检查

• 急性不需要。
• 慢性。
- 目的在寻找潜在感染源。

诊断步骤/外科

对于慢性荨麻疹和荨麻疹性血管炎行皮肤活检。

鉴别诊断

• 神经性水肿：
- 可能有生命危险。
- 可以有腹部症状。
- 遗传或后天获得。
• 皮肤性血管炎。
• 血清病。
• 多形性红斑。
• 大疱性类天疱疮。
• 幼年性类风湿关节炎。
• 环形红斑。
• 疱疹样皮炎。
• 全身性肥大细胞增多症。
• 过敏性紫癜。

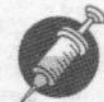

治疗

院前

• 注意：
- 全身过敏反应如果不早期给予肾上腺素，可能进展迅速。
• 严重反应：
- 气道管理，给氧。
- 肌内注射肾上腺素。
- 吸入 β 受体激动剂缓解支气管痉挛。
- 必要时静脉滴注晶体液和升压药。

初步稳定/治疗

尽可能去除致病原。

急诊治疗/程序

• 主要对症治疗，除非有严重的全身反应。

• 治疗主要针对刺激源、效应细胞、炎症介质和目标受体。

• β受体激动剂(静脉或吸入)：

- 严重的荨麻疹、神经性水肿、全身性症状。

• H_1 受体阻滞剂(第一代或第二代)：

- 主要治疗手段。

• H_2 受体阻滞剂：

- 当单独使用 H_1 受体阻滞剂效果不佳时，可以起协同作用。

• 糖皮质激素(口服)：

- 严重或难治病例。

• 避免使用非甾体消炎药和阿片类药物：

- 会使病情恶化。

• 同时使用酮康唑和大环内酯类药物会改变肝脏对抗组胺药的代谢，需引起注意。

■ 药物治疗

• β受体激动剂：

- 肾上腺素(1∶1000 溶液)：0.1～0.5 mg，肌内注射，q10～15 min，必要时(儿童：0.01 mg/kg，最大单次剂量不超过 0.3 mg，q15 min，必要时)。

- 静脉滴注肾上腺素：0.1～0.25 mg(1∶10000 溶液)，时间超过 5～10 min，q5～15 min，然后按 1～4 μg/min 静滴，仅用于过敏性休克患者。

- 沙丁胺醇(0.5% 溶液)：0.5 ml 雾化，q20 min，必要时(儿童：0.01～0.05 ml/kg，最大剂量 0.5 ml，雾化 q20 min，必要时，缓解支气管痉挛)。

- 特布他林：0.25 mg，皮下注射，q15～30 min，必要时(最大剂量 0.5 mg/q4 h，儿童大于 6 周)。

要点和误区

• 如果表现很严重，经常会出现双相病程。

• 反弹可能出现在 4～6 h。

• 慢性荨麻疹常有全身性的因素。

X

牙痛 Toothache

Franklin D. Friedman 范浩浩 李文放 译

基础知识

描述

• 牙痛是由位于牙髓组织的根神经受刺激引起的：

- 牙髓是牙齿的中心和神经血管供应。

• 其他病因，无论是在口中还是口腔相关，可能会导致牙痛。

病因

• 口腔科：

- 龋齿（细菌使坚硬的结构去盐化）。
- 牙髓炎（继发于感染的发炎的牙髓）。
- 可逆性牙髓炎是由龋齿侵入引起轻微的牙髓炎症。
- 不可逆的牙髓炎是未经治疗的龋坏病变引起严重的牙髓炎症、牙髓严重、持续性、弥散的不适。
- 根尖周脓肿（坏死牙髓及随后的脓肿）。
- 拔牙后疼痛（干牙槽，感染）。
- 破牙综合征（疼痛，冷敏感，损坏不直观）。

• 牙周疾病：

- 牙龈炎和牙周炎（伴有牙周韧带附件损失的牙龈炎）。
- 牙周脓肿（齿龈溃疡）。
- 冠周炎（因牙齿错位引起的牙龈炎）。
- 急性坏死性溃疡性牙龈炎（牙龈疼痛，有/无假膜的溃疡）。
- 义齿口腔炎。
- 疱疹性牙龈炎。
- 阿弗他溃疡（口疮）。
- 创伤性溃疡。

诊断

症状和体征

病史

• 牙痛：

- 可能牵涉下颌、耳、面部、眼睛和颈部（第5脑神经的感觉分布区）。
- 通常与咀嚼有关的疼痛、温度改变和斜卧。

• 恶臭的气味。

• 发热和发冷。

• 口腔味觉不好。

• 相关症状。

• 症状持续时间。

• 已经尝试过的治疗。

体格检查

• 牙齿腐烂。

• 面部肿胀或红斑。

• 牙关紧闭症：

- 最大张口程度减小（正常开放，35～50 mm）。

• 检查和触诊唇、唾液腺、口腔底部、颈部淋巴结。

• 评估发音更改。

• 确定牙周脓肿。

• 评估深部感染。

• 检查面部肿胀、发红、柔软度和是否发热。

• 检查颈部腺体和颈项强直。

• 轻叩牙齿查看硬度和活动度。

• 应检查牙齿是否断裂和有无缺失。

• 成人使用的口腔科数字系统：

- 上颌骨：从右至左 1～16；下颌：从左到右 17～32（儿童：A～J 和 K～T）。
- 或者通过牙齿位置识别牙齿也是合适的（即左后方、上磨牙）。

基本检查

• 获取适当的医疗和口腔科病史。

• 询问药物过敏，尤其是抗生素、止痛药和目前的药物。

• 评估对预先采用的口腔科抗生素预防用药的需求：

- 风湿热。
- 心脏瓣膜置换。
- 矫形关节置换。
- 二尖瓣脱垂或瓣膜心脏病。

• 如果体格检查与患者的病史冲突且口腔内疼痛的来源并不明显，考虑其他疼痛来源：

- 疼痛的非牙源性病因。
- 人为的痛苦、寻求药物阵痛的行为。

诊断检查与说明

实验室检查

• 除有全身中毒症状和那些可察觉的深部感染患者外，不需要进行实验室检查。

• 与任何其他全身中毒感染症状一样，考虑全血细胞检查、血培养、炎症标志物（如 ESR 或 CRP）。

影像学检查

• 如果怀疑存在牙齿感染性病变或断裂，进行全景和根尖片 X 线查看。

• CT 或 MRI 评估更深层的感染。

诊断步骤/外科

有时可能局部或区域的神经阻滞为治疗和诊断提供益处。

鉴别诊断

• 鼻窦炎。

• 中耳炎。

• 咽炎。

• 扁桃体脓肿。

• 颞下颌关节综合征：

- 通常在耳周围出现疼痛。

• 三叉神经痛。

• 血管性头痛。

• 带状疱疹。

• 心脏缺血。

儿科注意事项

• 小孩或婴儿出现牙齿断裂可能导致牙痛、烦躁、低热、腹泻和食物摄入减少。

• 面部肿胀伴发热和白细胞>15 000/mm^3提示非牙源性。

• 儿童最多有 20 颗乳牙，10 颗在上部和 10 颗在下部。

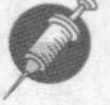

治疗

院前

• 对严重面部肿胀或张口困难的患者保持专用气道。

• 如果可能，患者应该保持坐姿。

初步稳定/治疗

• 深部感染和气道阻塞进行呼吸道管理。

• 按照指示进行早期疼痛管理。

急诊治疗/程序

• 适当的镇痛。

• 非甾体抗炎药（NSAIDs）用于无并发症牙痛的一线治疗。

• 阿片类止痛剂是一种替代疗法。

• 口腔科麻醉区域神经阻滞：

- 沿受影响牙齿的颊面注射。
- 多颗牙齿的特殊神经阻滞。
- 长效麻醉剂（如布比卡因）。

• 如果存在牙齿感染，则使用抗生素：

- 如果患者不过敏，青霉素是可选择的抗生素。

- 克林霉素适用于青霉素过敏或以厌氧菌感染为主的患者。

• 局部根尖周炎和牙周脓肿应切开，引流和药物灌注：

- 引流管可放置 24 h。

• 在家中每日盐水洗 4 次，并在 24 h 内转诊至口腔科治疗。

■ 药物治疗

• 抗生素：

- 氨苄西林-舒巴坦：1.5～3 g，肌内注射或静脉注射，q6 h[儿童：300～600 mg/(kg · d)，最大剂量 3 g，分 4 次用药，q6 h]。

- 克林霉素：150～450 mg，口服，q6 h[儿童：15～30 mg/(kg · 24 h)，最大剂量 2 g，q6 h]：

◦ 静脉剂量 300～900 mg[儿童：25～40 mg/(kg · 24 h)]，div，q8 h。

- 青霉素 V 钾：500 mg，口服，q6 h[儿童：25～50 mg/(kg · 24 h)，最大剂量 3 g，q6 h]。

- 青霉素 G 钾：4 mU，肌内注射或静脉注射，q4 h[儿童：250 000～400 000 U/(kg · d)，肌内注射或静脉注射，div，q4～6 h，最大剂量 24 mU/d]。

• 镇痛药：

- 对乙酰氨基酚：500 mg，口服或灌肠，q4～6 h(儿童：每次 10～15 mg/kg；不超过 5 次/24 h)；不要超过 4 g/24 h。

- 对乙酰氨基酚和可待因：1～2 片，口服，q4～6 h(儿童：酏剂-可待因 12 mg/5 ml)。

- 羟考酮 5 mg 与对乙酰氨基酚 325 mg：1 或 2 片，口服，q6 h[儿童：0.05～0.15 mg/kg(羟考酮)/剂量，最大剂量 5 mg]；不可用于液体制剂。

- 布洛芬：400～800 mg，口服，q8 h(儿童：10 mg/kg，口服，q6 h)。

- 酮咯酸：30 mg 静脉注射，30～60 mg，肌内注射，q6 h(儿童：每次 1 mg/kg，肌内注射或静脉注射)。

- 硫酸吗啡：2～8 mg，皮下注射、肌内注射或静脉注射，q2 h(儿童：0.1 mg/kg，皮下注射、肌内注射或静脉注射，q2 h)。

儿科注意事项

出牙的婴儿可能会受益于非处方的局部麻醉剂和口服镇痛药。

随访

■ 进一步处理

入院指征

• 怀疑深部感染(例如，急性坏死性口底蜂窝织炎、咽后脓肿)。

• 眼睛附近的面部蜂窝织炎。

• 严重张口困难。

• 无法维持营养和水分。

• 全身中毒的证据。

出院指征

牙痛和局部牙齿感染性病变的患者可以从急诊部出院。

转诊问题

在急诊室接受治疗的患者应请口腔科医师及时会诊。

■ 随访建议

定期和例行的口腔科评估。

要点和误区

• 误诊深部感染为局部感染。

• 未能确定口腔牵涉痛的来源。

牙外伤 Dental Trauma

Brian N. Corwell · Natalie L. Davis 许磊 郭东风 译

基础知识

■ 描述

• 乳牙：共 20 颗。

- 6～10 个月开始萌出，30 个月左右长齐。

- 常常是对称性萌出。

• 恒牙：共 32 颗。

- 5～6 岁开始萌出。

- 共 32 颗(4 颗中切牙、4 颗侧切牙、4 颗犬齿、8 颗前磨牙和 12 颗磨牙)。

- 恒牙从右上第三磨牙(1)至左上第三磨牙(16)和左下第三磨牙(17)至右下第三磨牙(32)。

- 用解剖来命名可以更好更简单地描述累及的牙齿。

• 最常见的受伤牙齿：

- 上颌中切牙、上颌侧切牙和下颌切牙。

• 牙齿骨折：

- 牙齿骨折分为简单骨折(只涉及釉质或釉质和牙本质)和复杂骨折(涉及神经、血管)。

- 骨折可以根据受伤的深度或 Ellis 分类系统进行分类。

- Ⅰ类骨折(简单骨折)：

◦ 只涉及表面的牙釉质。

◦ 骨折线出现白垩色。

◦ 对温度、空气、打击无痛感。

- Ⅱ类骨折(简单骨折)：

◦ 包括牙釉质和牙本质。

◦ 骨折线将出现乳白色或淡黄色。

◦ 对热、冷或空气更敏感。

◦ 不稳定。

- Ⅲ类骨折(复杂骨折)：

◦ 真正的口腔科急诊。

◦ 伤及牙釉质、牙本质、牙髓。

◦ 牙髓可呈粉红色、红色和肉色。

◦ 擦拭牙齿表面后出现出血或发红，表示牙髓损伤。

◦ 可能明显疼痛或麻木(由相关的神经与血管的损伤所致)。

• 损伤分类：

- 震荡过的牙齿：

◦ 不管是松动还是移位。

◦ 对咀嚼或碰撞敏感。

- 半脱位：

◦ 牙齿松动，但没有移位。

◦ 可能存在牙龈出血。

◦ 咀嚼或冲击的时候更敏感。

◦ 牙周韧带损伤。

• 脱位受伤：

- 牙齿可以在任何方位发生位移：

◦ 涉及支持结构，包括牙周韧带(PDL)和牙槽损伤。

- 侵入性脱位：

◦ 牙齿嵌入组织。

◦ 牙槽受损。

◦ 牙周韧带压缩。

- 侧向脱位：

◦ 牙齿的非轴对称位移。
◦ 牙周韧带损伤。
◦ 与潜在的牙槽骨折相关。
- 喷出脱位：
◦ 牙齿变长或过度移位。
◦ 部分从牙槽窝中心脱出。
◦ 牙周韧带损伤。
- 撕脱牙：
◦ 真正的口腔科急诊。
◦ 牙齿从牙槽完全移位。
◦ 牙周韧带断裂。
• 牙槽骨骨折：
- 下颌骨或上颌骨的牙齿支撑部分骨折。
- 牙齿咬合错位，咀嚼疼痛，整块牙齿松动。
- 根据临床或影像学诊断。

■ **病因**

• 近 50% 的儿童会出现牙外伤。
• 好发年龄：
- 幼儿（跌倒和故意致伤）。
- 适龄儿童和青春期（跌倒、自行车和游乐场事故）。
- 青少年（田径、打闹、机动车碰撞）：
◦ 牙套使用大大减少了运动相关的牙齿受伤。
• 殴打、家庭暴力或多发性创伤。
• 机动车、摩托车、自行车事故。
• 虐待儿童、故意致伤：
- 经常合并有颜面部损伤。
• 喉镜。
• 某些诱发解剖因素导致风险增加：
- 前覆＞4 mm 使牙外伤的风险增加 2～3 倍。
- 短或不完全覆盖的上唇、张口呼吸、身体残疾，采用固定矫治器。

Y

诊断

■ **症状和体征**

病史

• 牙齿不稳定、撕脱或松弛。
• 牙齿咬合畸形或牙关紧闭。
• 加重疼痛的因素（可能预示牙髓损伤或牙周韧带损伤）：
- 咀嚼、饮水或温度骤变。
- 触痛。
• 机制：
- 通过评估多发伤和相关损伤支持外伤发生的机制（如颌骨骨折）。
• 受伤的确切时间：
- 会影响治疗及预后。
• 使用的存储媒介和存储时间。
• 识别牙齿是乳牙还是恒牙。

体格检查

• 检查口腔黏膜是否有撕裂或外伤。
• 检查所有牙齿有无外伤或骨折。
• 检查每个牙面是否有损伤，叩诊移动性或用舌片测试敏感性。
• 检查受伤牙齿的牙髓是否暴露：
• 用纱布擦干牙齿，观察有无活动性出血或面色潮红。
• 评估咬合不正和中部稳定性，记录所有缺失的牙齿：
- 牙齿碎片和假体可能被吞食、吸入、嵌入邻近软组织或嵌入牙槽。
• 仔细检查口腔：
- 邻近软组织或骨外伤。
- 怀疑下颌骨骨折而那些无法张口＞5 cm 或咬压舌板测试阳性的患者。
- 合并伤：
◦ 唾液腺、导管、血管、脑神经和眶下神经。

■ **基本检查**

• 全面的体格检查。
• 必要的影像学检查。
• 稳定病情和正确的转诊。

■ **诊断检查与说明**

影像学检查

• 普通口腔科 X 线检查：
- 复合牙外伤。
- 关注侵入性损伤或牙齿移位至周围软组织。
• 全景牙片适应证：
- 异物。
- 牙位移。
- 牙槽嵴或下颌骨骨折。
- 考虑是否有做 CT 的条件。
• CT 适应证：
- 创伤与咬合不正或牙关紧闭。
- 疑似牙槽或下颌骨骨折。
• 胸部 X 线检查：
- 提示牙齿或片段缺失：
◦ 膈下不需要移动即可看见牙齿。
• 支气管镜检查：
- 提示需要取出吸入的牙齿。

■ **鉴别诊断**

排除其他显著的并发面部或全身外伤。

治疗

■ **院前**

• 气道保护。
• 处理及保存撕脱的牙齿或碎片：
- 现场即时再植是最好的治疗方法。
- 在没有误吸风险的情况下，最有能力的人应尝试将恒齿移植至牙槽窝：
◦ 在牙冠旁，而不是牙齿根部处理牙齿。
◦ 用冷水或生理盐水简单冲洗牙齿（最多 10 s），以清除牙齿碎片：时间就是牙齿：牙齿脱位每增加 1 min，牙齿的活力会降低 1%。
  ▪ 成功的最好的机会，在 15 min 完成重植。
  ▪ 如果撕脱＞1 h 牙齿几乎没有活力。
  ▪ 一旦牙齿复位，咬紧手帕以保持牙齿的位置。
- 如果不能做到或者不成功，将牙齿放进存储运输溶液中。
◦ Hanks 平衡盐溶液（HBSS）：
  ▪ 市售的 Save - A - Tooth 平衡 pH 培养基。
  ▪ 撕脱后几小时仍有效。
• 冷牛奶：
- 最好的备用存储介质。
- 将牙齿放入盛有牛奶的容器中，然后用冰填充（阻止稀释）。
• 唾液：
- 储存在装有唾液的容器中。
- 切勿使用自来水或干运输。

■ **初步稳定/治疗**

• 确保气道通畅。
• 让患者咬上纱布以压迫止血。
• 记录脱落的所有牙齿和牙齿碎片。
• 立即重植撕脱齿。

■ **急诊治疗/程序**

• 一般处理：
- 夹板到达前试图行裂伤修补术。
- 重新复位或活动的牙齿通常需要夹板固定。
- 咬合始终是矫正牙齿位置的最佳目标。
- 口腔面神经阻滞可以提供良好的镇痛，以协助适当的检查和裂伤修复。
- 建议使用鼻或口腔抗焦虑药来帮助焦虑的儿童患者。
- 所有牙齿外伤的患者应进 1 日的流质饮

食,避免使用吸管,接下来进 1～2 周的饮食。
- 每顿饭后用软毛刷轻柔地刷牙。
- 破伤风的预防措施:
◦ 考虑为非破伤风多发伤。
◦ 表示为污染的伤口、深裂伤、脱位牙、侵入伤及骨折。
- 应用抗生素的适应证:
◦ 开放性牙槽骨骨折。
◦ 继发感染的治疗。
◦ 再植的撕脱牙。
◦ 未提示的感染预防。
• Ellis Ⅰ级:
- 化学损伤。
- 没有急救指征。
- 锉刀/挫甲板光滑锐利的边缘:
◦ 防止进一步损伤软组织。
- 转诊口腔科进一步美容修复。
• Ellis Ⅱ级:
- 治疗目标是防止细菌从暴露的牙本质污染牙髓。
- 暴露伤口表面用氢氧化钙或类似的阻隔剂覆盖。
- 覆盖之前擦干净牙齿表面。
- 如果没有上述阻隔剂,可使用氰基丙烯酸酯组织黏合剂。
- 疼痛控制。
- 在 24～48 h 转诊口腔科。
• Ellis Ⅲ级:
- 立即转诊到牙医/牙髓病专家。
- 对于活动性出血患者,嘱患者咬住浸泡过表面麻醉剂和肾上腺素的纱布。
- 如果没有口腔医师/口腔外科医师:
◦ 像 Ellis Ⅱ级一样覆盖牙齿表面。
◦ 疼痛控制。
• 不稳定牙齿:
- 不需要夹板。
- 根据需要决定是否转诊口腔科。
• 牙齿半脱位:
- 夹板固定仅适用于牙齿过度或严重松弛。
◦ 考虑患者的舒适度。
- 洗必泰冲洗。
- 口腔科随访。
• 挤压伤:
- 数字压力重新定位。
- 夹板固定 2 周。
- 随访口腔科。
• 侧向脱位:
- 可能因为外力、创伤需要重新定位。
◦ 可能需要从骨锁脱开。
- 可能需要局部麻醉。
- 使用 2 指技术:
◦ 第 1 个手指放在顶点下面和后面,而第 2 个手指重新定位牙冠。
- 洗必泰冲洗。
- 通常需要夹板固定。
- 口腔科随访。
• 侧向脱位:
- 不要操作。
- 疼痛控制。
- 24 h 内口腔科随访。
• 牙齿部分撕脱:
- 可能需要局部麻醉剂。
- 仔细降低到正常位置。
- 考虑徒手清除神经损伤的极度松弛的牙齿,以防止误吸。
• 撕脱牙:
- 切勿拔出撕脱乳牙。
- 尝试再植可能存活的所有恒牙。
- 只能夹持牙冠:
◦ 忌夹持牙根。
- 用生理盐水轻轻漂洗,清除杂物。
- 不要擦拭、打磨或尝试清除牙齿。
- 局部麻醉要控制,除非需要。
- 轻轻浇灌或抽吸血栓。
- 使用时注意不要损坏牙槽壁。
- 牙齿重植时要用力而不是轻轻用力。
- 牙齿到位时发出"咔嗒"。
- 一旦牙齿重植,让患者轻轻地咬上折叠的纱布垫,以帮助牙齿自动到合适的位置。
- 咬合是断牙后正确选择牙位的最佳指南。
- 可能需要夹板:
◦ 夹板可用材料,如牙周膏或自愈复合材料。
◦ 适用于撕脱牙齿/牙龈的前后表面和相邻的 2 颗牙齿的两侧。
◦ 避免用于咬合面。
◦ 保持牙龈和牙釉质完全干燥。
- 24 h 内由口腔医师彻底固定。
- 使用抗生素或洗必泰漱口水。
• 如果院前牙齿重新植入:
- 确保正确的位置和排列。
• 牙槽骨骨折:
- 口腔外科/牙医再植和/或固定(拱板)。
- 疼痛控制。
- 预防性应用抗生素。

■ 药物治疗

• 布洛芬:600～800 mg,口服,每日 3 次(10 mg/kg 口服,每日 4 次)。
• 对乙酰氨基酚与羟考酮:1～2 片,口服,q4～6 h,必要时;羟考酮 0.05～0.15 mg/kg(最大剂量 5 mg/次),口服,q4～6 h;24 h 内不超过 12 片。
• 青霉素 V:250～500 mg,口服,q6 h;50 mg/(kg·24 h),最大剂量 3 g,口服,q6 h,持续 1 周。
• 强力霉素:100 mg,口服,每日 2 次,持续 1 周(儿童)。
• 葡萄糖酸氯己定:0.12% 漱口液,每日 2 次,持续 1 周。
• 破伤风:0.5 ml,肌内注射。

注意

对乙酰氨基酚或含对乙酰氨基酚的所有药物中含量不能超过 4 g/24 h。

随访

■ 进一步处理

入院指征

• 合并其他相关的外伤。
• 怀疑虐待儿童或与老人,以及没有安全环境的人。

出院指征

不伴有其他外伤、无法控制的疼痛或严重牙关紧闭不能口服给药等的血流动力学稳定的牙损伤患者。

转诊问题

• Ellis Ⅲ级患者:立即转诊口腔科。
• 牙齿松动、偏移或缺牙。
• 建议并安排远期口腔科护理。

■ 随访建议

所有撕脱和 Ellis Ⅱ级患者均应该在 24 h 内口腔科随访,Ellis Ⅲ级患者应立即口腔科会诊。

要点和误区

• 恒牙撕脱后应尽快再植。
• 撕脱的牙齿不能在干燥的介质或自来水中运输。
• 解释清楚所有牙齿缺失的原因。
• 不要把内缩脱位误认为撕脱伤。
• 脱位牙不应该在干燥介质中或在自来水转运。
• 闭塞是再植后矫正牙齿位置的最佳方法。
• 警惕牙齿骨吸收、颜色的变化、潜在牙齿脱落的风险和/或以后需要根管治疗的牙外伤患者。

Y

牙周脓肿 Periodontal Abscess

John E. Sullivan 刘静 译

基础知识

描述

• 脓液聚集在牙齿支撑结构：
- 牙周韧带。
- 牙槽骨。

• 牙周袋是由于牙周病的进展和由此导致的骨丢失造成的：
- 食物和碎片积累在牙周袋。
- 冠状上皮组织能重新接上牙齿，但细菌和食物碎片仍受困于牙周袋，影响引流。
- 食物和碎片会感染受损的引流环境。

• 并发症：
- 骨髓炎。
- 肠外瘘。
- 海绵窦血栓。
- 咽峡炎。
- 上颌窦炎。
- 纵隔炎。
- 牙缺失。
- 败血症。

儿科注意事项

• 牙周脓肿在儿童中很罕见。
• 根尖脓肿比较常见：
- 起源于髓。
- 与龋有关。

病因

• 厌氧的革兰阴性菌。
• 消化链球菌属。
• 草绿色链球菌。
• 奈瑟菌属。
• 一般是多种微生物。

诊断

症状和体征

牙周脓肿属于临床诊断。

病史

• 牙痛。
• 心神不安。
• 发热。
• 面部肿胀。

体格检查

• 面部肿大或牙龈松动。
• 触痛。
• 牙齿松动度增加。
• 龈脓肿：
- 像疙瘩一样的病变出现在齿龈，提示窦道晚期问题。
- 可能出现慢性脓肿。
• 来自窦道的脓液表现形式。
• 热敏性。
• 淋巴结病变。
• 牙关紧闭症通常不会存在，除非感染蔓延至咀嚼肌。

基本检查

临床诊断：

• 图像和实验室数据在诊断中不是必需的。

诊断检查与说明

实验室检查

脓液的厌氧培养：

• 并发性脓肿。
• 免疫受损患者。

影像学检查

• 全景的、根尖的或咬合的射线照片。
• 床旁超声可能有助于确诊。
• CT 有助于可视化脓肿扩展至相邻的结构。
• 图像检查可以确定和有助于明确肿胀的程度，但是对诊断来说不是必需的。

诊断步骤/外科

电活力测试：

• 由口腔科咨询顾问来验证牙齿的可行性。
• 口腔科医师随访期间执行。

鉴别诊断

• 根尖脓肿。
• 上颌窦炎。
• 口疮性溃疡。
• 口腔疱疹。
• 唾液腺肿瘤。
• 流行性腮腺炎。
• 由唾液腺炎或脱水引起的唾液腺阻塞。
• 由口腔感染引起的局域性肿大。
• 面部蜂窝织炎。
• 急性中耳炎。
• 牙周脓肿。

儿童考虑：根尖脓肿。

• 对于无症状的龈脓肿：
- 纤维瘤。
- 化脓性的或外周骨化的肉芽肿瘤。
- 卡波西肉瘤。

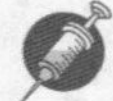

治疗

院前

儿乎很少与呼吸道急症有关，但是目前如果出现呼吸道损害的症状：

• 身边配有气管插管的医疗设备。
• 坐式体位运送。
• 辅助供氧。
• 需要时吸痰。

初步稳定/治疗

• 评估呼吸道是否通畅。
• 在下列情况下通过气管插管术或气管造口术建立明确的呼吸道：
- 呼吸困难。
- 不能够处理分泌物。
- 口咽组织肿胀，损害或压迫呼吸道。

急诊治疗/程序

• 需要用非甾体抗炎药或镇静剂止痛。
• 切口引流：
- 用 2%利多卡因麻醉齿龈，用 1∶100 000 肾上腺素直至黄化现象发生。
- 用解剖刀片对牙槽骨划出 1 cm 的切口。
- 用蚊式止血钳进行钝性分离。
- 用生理盐水冲洗腔。
- 如果脓肿腔足够大，放置的 1/4 的碘仿纱条引流或窗状 Penrose 引流 24～48 h：
  ◦ 为了防止吸入，使用安全的纱布或消耗缝合丝线。
• 抗生素：
- 表明如果脓肿广泛或出现身体症状。
- 考虑青霉素作为首要的经验疗法。
- 红霉素、阿奇霉素、克林霉素针对青霉素过敏的患者。
- 克林霉素针对青霉素过敏的患者或对没有反应的患者。
- 氨苄西林-舒巴坦针对严重感染。
• 清醒时用温盐水每小时冲洗一次，持续 24～48 h。

■ 药物治疗

一线用药

• 青霉素 V 钾：250～500 mg 口服，q6 h[儿童：25～50 mg/(kg · d)，口服，div，q6 h]。

• 阿奇霉素：500 mg(儿童：10 mg/kg)，口服，每日 1 次，然后 250 mg(儿童：5 mg/kg)，口服，每日 1 次×4 日(针对青霉素过敏的患者)。

• 克林霉素 150～450 mg，口服，q6 h[儿童：10～25 mg/(kg · d)div，口服，q6 h]。

• 克林霉素 300～900 mg，静脉注射，q8 h[儿童：15～25 mg/(kg · d)，静脉注射，div，q8 h]。

• 红霉素 250～500 mg，口服，q6～8 h(儿童：30～50 mg/d，口服，div，q6 h)。

二线用药

• 氨苄西林-舒巴坦：1.5～3 g，静脉注射，q6 h[>1 岁，<40 kg 的儿童：300 mg/(kg · d)静脉注射，div，q6 h]。

• 阿莫西林-克拉维酸：875 mg，口服，q12 h[儿童：25～45 mg/(kg · d)，div，q12 h]。

• 莫西沙星：400 mg，口服或静脉注射，每日 1 次(通常不推荐给儿童使用)。

随访

■ 进一步处理

入院指征

• 严重感染或并发症需要肠外应用抗生素。

• 坏死或蜂窝织炎涉及的部位有潜在的呼吸道损害。

• 海绵窦血栓形成。

• 骨髓炎。

• 门诊治疗失败。

• 免疫功能不全的患者：

- 中性粒细胞减少症。
- 不受控制的白血病。
- 晚期的艾滋病。
- 化疗的癌症患者。

• 咽峡炎。

• 身体系统严重缺水。

• 不能处理分泌物的患者。

• 在家不能控制感染的患者，因为生理、精神障碍或社会心理因素。

出院指征

• 不复杂的病例。

• 24～48 h 时可以进行口腔科随访。

转诊问题

• 口腔科随访用于：

- 受影响的牙齿活力。
- 拔牙。
- 根管治疗。
- Penrose 引流术或阻断法移除。

■ 随访建议

在 24～48 h 进行口腔科随访：

• 不到位的口腔科随访，在 24～48 h 患者应该有选择性地随访在疾病护理的过程中(口腔外科医师、急诊室、急救护理、初级治疗)。

要点和误区

上颌窦炎没有进行充分的口腔检查时，可能会被错误诊断：

• 口腔科随访是必需的，对于症状短期缓解、牙齿的长期生存能力和口腔卫生问题。

咽后脓肿

Tyler J. Berliner · Maria E. Moreira 袁晓伟 童朝阳 译

基础知识

■ 描述

• 咽后间隙深部组织感染：

- 潜在间隙前部是：颊咽筋膜，后部为翼状筋膜，上部是颅底，下部是 T_2 筋膜层融合而成。
- 间隙正中线为舌背，成链状淋巴结延伸至各边。
- 翼状筋膜薄弱可导致咽后感染蔓延至"危险"间隙和后纵隔。

• 起初是发生于儿童的一种疾病，但后来在成人中频繁发生：

- 3～5 岁发病率最高，此时咽后结节最突出。

• 如能迅速诊断，积极行静脉输注抗生素和/或外科引流治疗后预后良好。

• 肿块影响、破裂或播散导致的并发症是发病的主要原因，包括：

- 呼吸道损伤。
- 由于脓肿破裂导致的吸入性肺炎。
- 脓毒症。
- 自发性穿孔。
- 坏死性筋膜炎。
- 纵隔炎。
- 颈内静脉血栓形成。
- 化脓性血栓性静脉炎(Lemierre 综合征)。
- 侵蚀主动脉(主要发生于成人)。
- 韧带侵蚀导致的寰枢椎脱位。
- 颅内神经疾病(特别是Ⅸ～Ⅻ)。
- 硬膜外脓肿。
- 脓肿再发(1%～5%)。

■ 病因

• 原因：

- 经常由鼻咽、鼻旁窦或中耳炎症引起。
- 感染扩散至咽后壁和翼筋膜之间的淋巴结。
- 创伤、异物和医源性器械检查也是常见病因，尤其是成年患者。
- 糖尿病和其他免疫力低下状态容易感染。

• 细菌性：占优势的有多种微生物包括厌氧菌和需氧菌。

• 最常见的病原菌有：

- 酿脓链球菌和草绿色链球菌。
- 金黄色葡萄球菌(包括 MRSA)。
- 呼吸道厌氧菌(包括梭杆菌属和韦荣球菌属)。

• 少见的致病菌：

- 嗜血菌属。
- 抗酸杆菌。
- 肺炎克雷伯菌。
- 大肠埃希菌。
- 结核分枝杆菌。
- 曲霉菌属。
- 假丝酵母属。

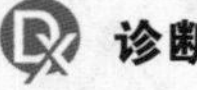

诊断

■ 症状和体征

病史

• 最常见：

- 咽部疼痛。

Y

- 颈部疼痛、僵直。
- 吞咽痛。
- 吞咽困难。
- 发热。

• 附加临床症状：
- 喘鸣。
- 呼吸困难。
- 声音低沉。
- 牙关紧闭。

儿科注意事项

幼龄儿童可能仅表现为：
• 进食少。
• 昏睡或易怒。
• 咳嗽。

体格检查

• 成人：
- 咽后壁水肿。
- 颈背僵硬。
- 颈腺病。
- 发热(67%)。
- 流涎。
- 喘鸣。
- 发声困难(cri du canard)。
- 气管"rock"征：移动喉和气管从一边向另一边时有压痛。

• 儿童和新生儿：
- 颈腺病。
- 发热。
- 伸颈时常受限僵直。
- 咽后部膨出。
- 牙关紧闭。
- 斜颈。
- 多涎。
- 焦虑。
- 呼吸窘迫。

基本检查

快速评估气道和呼吸状态：
• 一般检查不能排除诊断。
• 实验室检查不能做出诊断。
• 怀疑此病时应行颈外侧 X 线或静脉注射造影剂 CT。

诊断检查与说明

实验室检查

• 全血细胞计数(91%的儿童白细胞>12000)：
- 非特异性。
• 血培养(厌氧和需氧)。
• 咽喉培养。

影像学检查

• 如果关注气道损伤最适合使用可搬运式摄片。
• 外侧颈 X 线片：
- 颈稍伸直在吸气时摄片。
- 如果由于疼痛或年幼不能恰当伸颈可能不会良好暴露软组织。
- 加深怀疑如果：
  ◦ 喉后间隙距 C_2 之前距离>7 cm 或是椎体直径的 2 倍(敏感度 90%)。
  ◦ 学龄前儿童间隙距 C_6>14 mm，成人为 22 mm。
  ◦ 正常颈椎前凸消失。
• 胸部 X 线检查：
- 当脓肿明确需要评估感染下方扩散程度和/或脓肿破裂误吸时。
- 纵隔增宽提示有纵隔炎或脓肿破裂的可能性。
• 颈部超声：
- 低敏感度。
- 不推荐。
• 静脉注射造影剂的颈部 CT：
- 目前推荐的影像学检查模式。
- 当 X 线未诊断或需要确定 X 线片上脓肿的确切大小和位置时使用。
- 脓肿表现为喉后间隙中伴有周围增强环的低密度灶。
- 敏感度：64%～100%。
- 精确度：45%～88%。
- 可协助手术计划，揭示脓肿在喉后、旁间隙的侵袭范围。
- 是否能可靠辨别其与蜂窝织炎、淋巴结炎还不确定。
- 由于射线暴露和需要镇静，CT 只能在 X 线无法诊断时应用于幼儿。
• MRI：
- 比 CT 更敏感。
- 也应用于检查血管灶，如血栓性颈静脉炎。

诊断步骤/外科

• 外科引流、穿刺抽吸需要在手术室进行。
- 出现脓肿是诊断金标准。
- 脓肿应彻底排空。
- 脓液需送检行革兰染色和培养。
• 无需行鼻咽喉镜检查。

鉴别诊断

• 扁桃体咽炎。
• 会厌炎。
• 扁桃体周脓肿。
• 化脓性腮腺炎。
• 下颌下间隙感染(路德维希心绞痛)。
• 急性颈长肌钙化性肌腱炎。
• 哮喘。
• 异物。
• 气管炎。
• 脑膜炎。
• 咽后出血。
• 肌张力障碍。
• 颈部骨髓炎。
• 牙齿炎症。
• 单核细胞增多症。
• 硬膜外脓肿。
• 其他颈部深间隙感染。

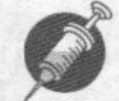

治疗

院前

• 使儿童在舒适体位：
- 迫使儿童端坐或曲颈可能阻塞呼吸道。
• 指脉氧，心电监护。
• 补充氧气。
• 足量液体。
• 抽吸、气管插管、环甲切除术(年龄 10～12 岁及以下患者或针式环甲切除术)准备好进行潜在的紧急插管。
• 需要控制呼吸道：
- 气道损伤。
- 长途运送前。

初步稳定/治疗

• 评估控制呼吸道。
• 提供充足氧气。
• 静脉置管：
- 如果有气道损伤体征时应用。

急诊治疗/程序

• 呼吸道窘迫或即将阻塞的患者应尽早行气管内插管或气管切开：
- 诱导时必须谨慎，因为镇静药物可以使气道肌肉放松从而导致彻底阻塞。
- 可使用喉罩等急救气道设备。
- 咽部肿胀可能使插管困难。
- 如果上呼吸道阻塞则需要行环甲膜切开术。
• 外科会诊(耳鼻喉科)。
• 尽早静脉使用抗生素。

药物治疗

静脉经验性使用抗生素覆盖 A 组链球菌

属、金黄色葡萄球菌(包括 MRSA)、呼吸道厌氧菌：

• 根据局部偏好和敏感性使用抗生素。

• 当培养和药敏结果回复后覆盖面将缩窄。

• 皮质类固醇应用有争议，只有在请耳鼻喉科会诊后才推荐使用。

• 免疫功能低下、糖尿病、静脉药物滥用者、福利机构患者、幼儿(＜1 岁)等 MRSA 高风险人群。

一线用药

口腔或牙源性感染：

• 氨苄西林-舒巴坦：3 g，静脉输注，q6 h(儿童：50 mg/kg)。

• 青霉素：200 万～400 万 U，静脉输注，q4～6 h＋甲硝唑 500 mg，静脉输注，q6～8 h。

• 克林霉素：600～900 mg(儿童：15 mg/kg)静脉输注，q8 h(最大剂量 4.8 g/d)。

鼻源或耳源性感染：

• 氨苄西林-舒巴坦：3 g，静脉输注，q6 h。

• 头孢曲松：1 g，静脉输注，q24 h＋甲硝唑 500 mg，静脉输注，q6～8 h。

• 强力霉素：100 mg，静脉输注 2 次/日；疑似牙源性感染(如有牙源性感染)：

• 莫西沙星：400 mg/d。

二线用药

如果患者对药物无反应或考虑有 MRSA：

• 万古霉素：15～20 mg/kg[儿童：40～60 mg/(kg·24 h)，静脉注射，q6～8 h]，静脉注射，q12 h。

• 利奈唑胺：600 mg[0～11 岁：30 mg/(kg·24 h)，q8 h；＞12 岁：成人剂量]，静脉注射或口服，q12 h。

• 头孢吡肟：2 g，静脉滴注＋甲硝唑 500 mg，静脉滴注，q6～8 h。

• 亚胺培南：500 mg，静脉注射，q6 h。

• 美罗培南：1 g，静脉注射，q8 h。

• 哌拉西林-他唑巴坦：4.5 g，静脉注射，q6 h。

随访

进一步处理

入院指征

• 所有患喉后脓肿的患者应该住院经静脉使用抗生素治疗，必要时进行外科引流。

• 外科引流标准：

- 气道损伤或其他威胁生命的并发症。
- 大(CT 显示＞2 cm 低密度灶)。
- 非口服抗生素治疗无效。

• 需要送入 ICU 的患者：

- 呼吸道损伤。
- 脓毒症。
- 精神状态改变。
- 血流动力学不稳定。
- 婴幼儿和中毒表现的儿童。
- 较严重并发疾病。

出院指征

患有喉后脓肿的患者不能出院。

转诊问题

如果没有引流设备的话应考虑转诊。

• 转运前应稳定呼吸道。

要点和误区

• 所有有发热、颈部僵直或吞咽困难的儿童应考虑此诊断。

- 对儿童应保持高度临床怀疑，因为他们临床症状和体征不典型。

• 成人经常在有基础疾病的情况下，最近有口腔内手术、颈部外伤或头部、颈部感染。

• 当影像学检查无法诊断且临床上高度怀疑时，应请外科会诊。

• 早期外科会诊和静脉应用抗生素治疗对于防止并发症(如气道损伤及感染蔓延至纵隔组织中)很重要。

咽峡炎 Ludwig Angina

Paul Blackburn · Chelsea C. Bonfiglio 王胜云 段立伟 译

基础知识

描述

• 以德国医师路德维希(Ludwig)的名字命名，其在 1836 年首次描述了此以颈部及舌下坏死性筋膜炎、坏疽性蜂窝织炎为表现，进展迅速的症状。

• 坏疽是组织坏死后因继发腐败菌的感染和其他因素的影响而呈现黑色、暗绿色等特殊形态改变：

- 持续进展可能导致气道及纵隔受压。
- 紧急介入情况较少运用手术或引流技术。

• 大多数死亡因为气道狭窄和阻塞引起的窒息：

- 抗生素问世前死亡率高达 50%，目前死亡率＜8%。

病因

• 成年患者 90%以上为牙源性起病，多为第二、三下磨牙。

• 少见原因：下颌骨骨折、口唇裂伤、感染、药物注射部位错误、舌穿刺等。

• 微生物：溶血链球菌、消化链球菌属、阴性杆菌。

- 微生物培养分析可以指导治疗。

发病率和死亡率增加的因素

• 同时合并其他疾病。

• 糖尿病：表现为独立增加危及生命的并发症高于其他合并症。

• 妊娠。

• 体型偏大。

• 累及多个颈部间隙。

• 前内脏间隙受累(舌骨→上纵隔间隙)。

儿科注意事项

通常病因不明或找不到感染源。

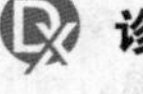

诊断

症状和体征

病史

• 非特异性症状：发热、焦虑、不适。

• 疼痛：舌、咽喉、下颌、胸部、颈部等。

• 吞咽困难、发音障碍。

• 牙齿日常护理欠佳。

体格检查

• 发热、中毒症状。

• 喘鸣。

• 眼耳鼻咽喉：

- 舌偏离中线。
- 气道可能受阻。

Y

- 流涎、唾液失禁。
- 牙关闭合受阻。

• 头颈部之外的检查通常无意义。

■ 基本检查

• 诊断主要基于临床症状。

• 未做气道开放保护准备是非常危险的。

• 开放气道优先。

■ 诊断检查与说明

实验室检查

• 无特异性诊断检测，评估病情及直接治疗。

影像学检查

• 增强 CT：
- 颈部增强 CT 是首选：
  ◦ 从颅底到主动脉弓的标准横断面影像。
  ◦ 能较好地评估纵隔、深部感染及气道受累情况。
  ◦ 异常发现包括脂肪坏死、腺体病变、脓腔形成等。
  ◦ 潜在缺陷：患者需仰卧接受扫描。

• X 线平片：
- 软组织可能正常结构改变，尤其是上呼吸道。
- 胸部 X 线意义不大，主要观察纵隔情况。

• 增强 MRI：
- 与增强 CT 相似：
  ◦ 潜在缺陷：与 CT 相同。

• 超声：
- 检测组织中气体、脓肿及淋巴结病变。
- 可能可以定位颈前肿胀组织病变部位。
- 脓肿穿刺引流定位。
- 评估气道受累程度，测量声门开口大小。
- 气道操作前后准确标记环甲膜位置。

诊断步骤/外科

尚无手术或侵入性方法能明确诊断、评估严重程度或直接治疗。

■ 鉴别诊断

• 感染：蜂窝织炎、会厌炎、气管炎、扁桃体炎。

• 外伤：贯通伤、舌下血肿、软组织伤。

• 血管神经性水肿。

• 肿瘤。

治疗

■ 院前

• 保持舒适体位转运。
- 允许成人保持三角“嗅探”姿势以利于分泌物排出。
- 允许儿童在母亲膝部上轻柔转运。

• 最大化氧气供应：
- 氧浓度 100%。
- 使用鼻导管、面罩吸氧。

• 射流加压给氧：
- 潜在缺陷：使用经验不足。
- 新方法更易使用从而被替代。

儿科注意事项

• 尽量使患儿平静：
- 在父母的怀抱中转运。
- 评估介入措施的必要性：静脉通路、氧气、监护设施等。
- 病情复杂患儿尽可能转运到设施完善的医疗机构。

■ 初步稳定/治疗

• 最大化吸氧。

• 保持舒适体位。

• 为气道支持准备物品。

• 详见“气道管理”。

血管通路

• 血管通路：提供快速、可滴定的药物输注。

• 第二条通路：为抢救做准备，同时方便药物输注。

■ 急诊治疗/程序

• 优先保证气道通畅然后开始药物治疗，减少急诊手术介入，除非气道受累。

• 少见可治疗性脓肿形成。

气道管理

• 由于解剖变异、破伤风、气道分泌物多等原因开放气道方法可能比较困难实施。

• 避免盲插以减少喉痉挛、医源性损伤、出血等风险。

• 考虑使用超声来评估气道受累情况，标记环甲膜位置，测量声门直径以选择正确的插管大小，并增加第一次成功率。

• 设备情况：
- 小的 ET 管。
- 预先凝胶润滑导管。
- 使用带探针或探条的导管。
- 将远端管弯曲成“曲棍球棒”形状。
- 纤维鼻气管镜插管。
- 使用电子喉镜。

• 快速气管插管可能会导致肌肉、气道受损。

• 患者出现喘鸣、声音改变、牙关紧闭等情况要注意呼吸衰竭的可能。

明确标准

• 传统手术金标准：局麻下气管切开术。
- 潜在难点：外科手术医师、手术设备是否具备。

• 传统非手术金标准：纤维支气管镜引导下气管插管：
- 可以在不损害患者气道保护的情况下尝试插管。
- 潜在困难：
  ◦ 产品舒适度。
  ◦ 短视镜通常缺少抽吸口或注射口。
  ◦ 视野容易受干扰。

• 最佳选择双重准备。
- 患者置于可以手术的地方以备气管切开。
- 尝试无创性介入方式。
- 如果不成功立即外科介入。

■ 药物治疗

• 抗生素：经验性应用广谱抗生素进行治疗，待培养结果明确后进一步调整治疗方案：
- 氨苄西林：1.5～3 g，静脉注射，q6 h。
- 先锋霉素：1～2 g，静脉注射，q6～8 h。
- 林可霉素：600～900 mg，静脉注射，q8 h。
- 哌拉西林-他唑巴坦：3.375 g，静脉注射，q8 h。
- 维生素 B_1。

• 镇痛剂：疼痛控制应首要考虑。

• 止吐剂：可预防性应用。

• 类固醇：经验性使用，用于减轻：
- 水肿。
- 炎症反应。

• 高压氧：合并纵隔感染或坏死时可考虑。

随访

■ 进一步处理

入院指征

• 所有患者均应入院：
- 气道受累情况随时可能出现并进展。

• 有气道受累症状者应进入 ICU 或密切监测。

转诊问题

• 咽峡炎只是临床诊断，伴有不可预期的疾病进展情况：
- 早期仔细询问病史非常必要，尽早发现有无气道问题。

• 如当地医疗水平及设施不足，尽早转运至上级医院诊治。

妊娠注意事项

• 孕妇受影响及并发症情况与非孕妇一样。

• 焦点：气道管理，氧气供应，如有感染及时抗感染治疗。

• 转到产科进行胎儿监护，必要时紧急分娩。

老年注意事项

患者合并慢性疾病、长期用药等情况会使临床表现及治疗更复杂。

并发症

• 窒息。
• 累及胸腔：
- 脓胸。
- 纵隔炎症。
- 肺脓肿。
• 心包炎。
• 颈内静脉血栓形成。
• 颈动脉受累。
• 脓毒血症。
• 膈下脓肿。

要点和误区

• 及时做好气道管理准备。
• 为困难气道的患者准备多种设备选择和双重准备。
• 尽快请相关科室会诊，做好转运或就地治疗双重准备。
• 可视喉镜使用方便，可提高插管成功率。
• 未充分预见到气道损伤。
• 未充分预见病情的进展速度。
• 未充分认识到合并症，尤其是导致糖尿病患者发病率和死亡率的增加。
• 诊断性检测及影像学检查不应耽误气道管理准备。

咽炎 Pharyngitis

Daniel B. Gingold · Brian J. Browne 瞿金龙 林兆奋 译

基础知识

描述

• 咽部炎症/感染。
• 第三大最常见的就诊主诉。
• 每年确诊 3 000 万例。
• A 组乙型溶血性链球菌(GAS)：
- 化脓性链球菌。
- <3 岁的儿童中不常见。
- 导致 20%～30%的儿童产生咽炎。
- 双峰发病，5～7 岁及 12～13 岁高发。
- 导致 5%～15%的成年人产生咽炎。
- 高峰月：1 月到 5 月，包括学校开学初期。

病因

• 病毒(最常见的感染原因)：
- 鼻病毒(20%)。
- 冠状病毒(>5%)。
- 腺病毒(5%)。
- 单纯疱疹病毒(4%)。
- 副流感病毒(2%)。
- 流感病毒(2%)。
- 柯萨奇病毒(<1%)。
- EB 病毒(<1%)。
- 人类免疫缺陷病毒(HIV)急性感染。
• 细菌：
- A 组乙型溶血性链球菌[化脓性链球菌(15%～30%)]。
- 坏死梭形杆菌(10%)。
- C 组和乙型溶血性链球菌(5%)。
- 奈瑟淋病球菌(<1%)。
- 白喉棒状杆菌(<1%)。
- 溶血隐秘杆菌(<1%)。
- 肺炎衣原体。
- 肺炎支原体(<1%)。
- 梅毒。
- 肺结核。
• 真菌：
- 念珠菌(鹅口疮)。
• 化学灼伤。
• 异物。
• 吸入剂。
• 后鼻漏。
• 肿瘤。
• 胃食管反流疾病。

诊断

症状和体征

病史

• 病毒：
- 咳嗽。
- 鼻漏。
- 通常紧接着咽喉痛。
- 治疗但仍存在持续性咽炎的高危患者，要高度怀疑 HIV 急性感染。
• 细菌：
- 突发的咽喉痛，通常先于其他症状。
- 吞咽痛。
- 发热。
- 头痛。
- 腹痛。
- 恶心和呕吐。
- 非典型症状：
◦ 鼻炎。
◦ 声音嘶哑。
◦ 腹泻。

体格检查

• 咽炎严重并发症的高危特点：
- 喘鸣，呼吸窘迫。
- 流口水。
- 发声困难。
- 明显的颈部肿胀。
- 神经功能障碍。
• 病毒：
- 咳嗽。
- 鼻炎。
- 鼻漏。
- 咽部水肿。
- 龈口炎。
• A 组乙型溶血性链球菌：
- 扁桃体咽红斑、渗出。
- 软腭瘀斑。
- 结实的红、肿小舌。
- 颈前淋巴结肿大。
- 猩红热样疹。
- 非典型症状：
◦ 结膜炎。
◦ 前部口炎。
◦ 离散性溃疡性病变。
• 单核细胞增多症：
- 由于症状相似而被误认为是 A 组乙型溶血性链球菌。
◦ 渗出性咽炎。
◦ 颈部淋巴结肿大疼痛。
◦ 发热。

◦ 出疹。
- 其他可能的诊断结果：
◦ 肝脾大。
◦ 黄疸。
• 白喉：
- 考虑未接种疫苗的患者。
- 气道威胁性灰咽膜。
- 心肌炎(2/3 的患者)，临床上明显的心功能不全(10%～25%)。
- 脑神经及周围神经病变(5%)。
• 淋菌性咽炎：
- 可能无症状。
- 总是评估遭性侵犯的儿童。
- 咽炎复发性发作。

■ 基本检查

A 组乙型溶血性链球菌咽炎诊断的修正中心准则(应用最广泛的决策规则)：
• 准则(要点)：
- 无咳嗽(+1 分)。
- 扁桃体分泌物或肿胀(+1 分)。
- 颈前淋巴结肿大和疼痛(+1 分)。
- 体温>38 ℃(+1 分)。
- 不同年龄：
◦ 3～14 岁(+1 分)。
◦ 15～44 岁(0 分)。
◦ >45 岁(+1 分)。
• 打分：
- <1 分：可不用检测和治疗。
- 3 分：风险为 28%～35%。
- >4 分：风险为 51%～53%。
• 达到 3 分标准的患者应该接受快速抗原检测测试(RADT)。
• 如果没有检测而进行治疗会导致 50%的病例使用抗生素不当。
• 有些人建议>4 分的患者应该进行以经验为主的治疗而不用做 RADT。

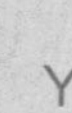

■ 诊断检查与说明

实验室检查

• 咽喉细菌检查：
- 金标准。
- 等待检测结果需 24～48 h，可能会延误治疗。
- 需要与患者及其家庭接触。
- 发现疑是淋病球菌时可确诊。
• A 组乙型溶血性链球菌的 RADT：
- 30 min 内可得测试结果。
- 对所有 RADT 结果呈阳性的患者进行治疗。
- 技术：用拭子拭抹扁桃体或后咽。
◦ 避免接触舌、口腔黏膜及唇。
- 灵敏度为 85%～95%。
- 特异性为 96%～99%：
◦ 证实在儿童、青少年的传统咽喉细菌检查中，RADT 结果呈阴性。
◦ 光学免疫分析方法非常准确，阴性结果不需要验证性检测。
• 传染性单核细胞增多症检测试剂盒：
- 异嗜性抗体的检测：
◦ 灵敏度：
▪ <2 岁：<30%。
▪ 2～4 岁：75%。
▪ >5 岁：90%。
- CBC 和外周血涂片：50%淋巴细胞，10%非典型淋巴细胞。
- 如果发现疑是 HIV 则获得快速病毒载量。

影像学检查

• 侧颈部 X 线摄片提示会厌炎、咽后脓肿或异物。
• 颈部的声学造影 CT 用于识别并发症，如扁桃体周脓肿和咽后壁脓肿。

■ 鉴别诊断

• 会厌炎。
• 扁桃体周或咽后壁脓肿。
• 白喉。
• 单核细胞增多症。
• Lemierre 病。
• 路德维希(Ludwig)咽峡炎。
• 念珠菌感染。
• 淋病。
• HIV 急性感染。
• 急性白血病、淋巴瘤。
• 口腔癌。
• 异物。
• 吸入剂和化学烧伤。
• 后鼻漏。
• 胃食管反流疾病。

治疗

■ 院前

• 做好呼吸道管理，预防呼吸窘迫。
• 用常规生理盐水对低血压及脱水患者进行补水。

■ 初步稳定/治疗

• 基本体征。
• 输液：1 L 常规生理盐水药剂（儿童：20 ml/kg)用于有血容不足迹象，或者患者无法忍受口服药物。

■ 急诊治疗/程序

• 退热剂和止痛剂：
- 醋氨酚。
- 布洛芬。
- 局部止痛剂(如本品喷)。
• GAS 感染：
- 通常温和及自我限制的：
◦ 抗生素治疗加速症状(发热和疼痛)在 1～2 日缓解。
- 抗生素治疗的目的是降低急性风湿热、症状和化脓性并发症的发生率。
• 抗生素：
- 青霉素 V：GAS 咽炎的首选抗生素。
- 头孢菌素类或大环内酯类抗生素：是对治疗无效和青霉素过敏患者的可以接受的替代治疗。
• 皮质甾类：
- 与抗生素、皮质甾类等联用：可使症状在 24 h 内缓解的可能性增加 3 倍。
- 需要治疗的病例数：3.3～3.7。
- 避免对糖尿病患者和免疫功能低下的患者使用。
• 潜在的念球菌感染并发症：
- 化脓性并发症：
◦ 扁桃体、咽后脓肿。
◦ Lemierre 病。
◦ 中耳炎、乳突炎。
- 非化脓性并发症：
◦ 急性风湿热：
▪ 在工业化国家很少见，但在 50 岁内仍是导致心脏死亡的主要原因。
▪ GAS 后遗症：在相关的 C 组或 G 组中未获得证实。
◦ 急性链球菌感染后肾小球肾炎。
◦ 西德纳姆(Sydenham)舞蹈病。
◦ 反应性关节炎。
◦ PANDAS：与链球菌感染相关的小儿自身免疫性神经精神病。
▪ 类似于强迫症的突然症状，强迫性障碍。
▪ 由影响基底神经节的自身免疫反应所致。
▪ 罕见并有争议。
• 白喉：
- 治疗目标：
◦ 预防气道阻塞。
◦ 治疗感染。
- 青霉素或大环内酯类抗生素。
- 并发症：
◦ 毒素介导的心肌炎、神经炎(脑神经病变)。

• 淋菌性咽炎：
- 若同时引起衣原体感染，可用第三代头孢菌素加大环内酯类抗生素来联合治疗。

■ 药物治疗

一线用药
• 青霉素：
- <27 kg：苄星青霉素(比西林 LA)：60 万 U，肌内注射×1。
- >27 kg：苄星青霉素(比西林 LA)：120 万 U，肌内注射×1。
• 青霉素 V：
- <12 岁：25～50 mg/(kg·d)，口服，div，q6～8 h×10 日。
- >12 岁：250～500 mg，口服，q6～8 h×10 日。
• 阿莫西林：
- 50 mg/kg，口服，每日 1 次，(最大剂量 1 g)×10 日。

二线用药
• 大环内酯类：
- 阿奇霉素：20 mg/(kg·d)×3 日(每剂最大剂量：500 mg)。
- 红霉素：40～50 mg/kg，口服，div，q6 h×10 日(每剂最大剂量：500 mg)。
• 口服头孢菌素：
- 头孢氨苄：20 mg/(kg·d)，口服，每日 2 次×5 日(每剂最大剂量：500 mg)。
• 类固醇：
- 地塞米松：0.6 mg/kg，肌内注射或口服×1(最大剂量 10 mg)。
- 泼尼松：40～60 mg，口服×1。
• 特殊条件：
- 怀疑淋菌性咽炎时：
◦ 头孢曲松：125～250 mg，肌内注射×1。

 随访

■ 进一步处理

入院指征
• 气道损伤。
• 严重脱水。
• 怀疑虐待儿童。

出院指征
能经口进食。

■ 随访建议
• 如果症状在 72 h 内没有得到改善。
• 经过 24 h 抗生素治疗后患者不再具有传染性。
• 单核细胞增多症的患者应避免接触性运动。

要点和误区
• 使用修改后的新标准来决定测试 GAS 咽炎。
• 儿童 RADT 测试呈阴性时需要做进一步的喉细菌检测。
• 在非工业化的国家，急性风湿热是 GAS 咽炎的一个非常普遍的并发症。
• 对细菌性咽炎的高危并发症进行评估(如扁桃体周脓肿、咽后脓肿、Lemierre 病)。

烟雾吸入 Smoke Inhalation

Trevonne M. Thompson 周健 潘曙明 译

 基础知识

■ 描述
• 在封闭空间内或有失聪史的人发生火灾时，可吸入可疑烟雾。
• 可能对上颌窦道结构造成严重损伤。
• 可使下呼吸道结构发生化学刺激反应。
• 可因吸入物质而引起全身性紧张症。

■ 病因
• 来自被加热气体的直接热损伤：
- 限制在声门上结构，因为上部空气的散热性能。
• 系统性毒性来自吸入细胞毒素：
- 碳。
- 氰化氢。

> **注意**
> 吸入蒸汽可能很快致命：
> • 蒸汽的热容大约是热空气的 4 000 倍。
> • 可迅速引起梗阻性声门水肿、热性气管炎及支气管黏膜血水肿。

诊断

■ 症状和体征

病史
• 暴露在烟雾中。
• 通常是在有限的空间里。
• 保持高度警惕，有意识丧失史。

体格检查
• 可能有一个正常的身体检查与症状发展期间 24 h 间隔暴露。
• 上呼吸道：
- 鼻咽刺激。
- 声音沙哑。
- 喘鸣。
- 咳嗽。
• 下呼吸道：
- 胸部不适。
- 咳血。
- 支气管痉挛。
- 支气管。
• 可能有一氧化碳和氯化物中毒的症状和体征。

> **警报**
> 这些起落的迹象表明是吸入性损伤。
> • 面部及上颈部烧伤。
> • 含碳质的痰。
> • 烧焦的眉毛和鼻。

■ 基本检查
• 脉搏。
- 在一氧化碳暴露的情况下，可能错误地升高。
• ABG：
- 缺氧。
- 一氧化碳或氰化氢引起的代谢性酸中毒。
• 胸部 X 线摄片：
- 初始 X 线片显示正常。
- 可能在接下来的 24 h 内出现肺损伤的迹象。

■ 诊断检查与说明

实验室检查
• 电解质、BUN、肌酐、葡萄糖。

• CBC。
• 凝固酶。
• 显示肌酸磷酸激酶。
• 一氧化碳血红蛋白评估潜在一氧化碳暴露。
• 氰化物水平：
- 在疑似氰化物接触的病例中，在开始治疗前不要接触氰化物。
- 可将乳酸水平作为氰化物毒性标志物。
• 妊娠检查。

诊断步骤/外科

• 心电图。
• 呼气流量峰值：
- 低峰值血流减少与更严重的损伤。
- 随着呼吸衰竭的发展，初始复苏后的比值<300。

■ 鉴别诊断

• 气体接触。
• 窒息性气体暴露。
• 心源性肺水肿。
• 慢性阻塞性肺疾病恶化。
• 哮喘恶化。
• 肺炎。

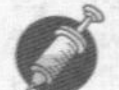

治疗

■ 院前

• 面罩100%氧气。
• 呼吸困难患者插管。
• 有哮喘者快速运送至急诊室。
- 可能需要高级气道管理。
• 沙丁胺醇美布利泽治疗支气管痉挛。

■ 初步稳定/治疗

• 面罩100%氧气。
• 插管：
- 呼吸窘迫。
- 流口水。
- 耳鸣。
- 再缺氧。
- 中枢神经系统抑制。
- 显著面部、上呼吸道烧伤。
• 建立静脉通路。

■ 急诊治疗/程序

• 吸入或雾化沙丁胺醇需要支气管痉挛。
• 有哮喘或慢性阻塞性肺病病史的患者需要使用糖皮质激素。
• 插管患者：
- 气管内插管袖带压力低。
◦ 频繁抽吸。
◦ 呼气末正压通气。
• 如果有，治疗一氧化碳中毒：
- 高压氧在适当情况下可用。
• 如果有指示，处理氰化物中毒：
◦ 100%氧气。
◦ 羟钴胺素(首选)。
◦ 只有含亚硝酸盐氰化物解药包可用。
◦ 应该小心使用亚硝酸钠在重大的情况下一氧化碳暴露。
- 硫代硫酸钠与一氧化碳暴露在一起使用是安全的。

■ 药物治疗

• 沙丁胺醇雾化吸入：2.5～5 mg/2.5 ml 生理盐水，q20 min：
- 或者，15 mg 喷雾器处理持续超过1 h。
• 甲泼尼龙 40 mg，静脉输注(儿童：1～2 mg/kg)。
• 泼尼松：40～60 mg，口服(儿童：1～2 mg/kg)。
• 硫代硫酸钠：12.5 g(50 ml 25%溶液)慢速静脉滴注(儿童：412.5 mg/kg 或 1.65 ml/kg 25%溶液)。
• 羟钴胺素：5 g 静脉注射15 min以上(儿童：70 mg/kg)。

随访

■ 进一步处理

入院指征

• 气管插管。
• 显著相关的烧伤。
• 持续性呼吸困难、声音嘶哑、吞咽困难、含碳的痰。
• 持续咳嗽。
• 哮喘或慢性阻塞性肺疾病和支气管痉挛。
• 大量接触一氧化碳或氰化物。
• 合并症。

出院指征

• 最小接触史。
• 无症状。
• 有明显的接触史，无症状。
• 4～6 h观察。

转诊问题

• 如果出现严重的烧伤相关损伤，应酌情转移到烧伤处理。
• 在一氧化碳中毒严重的情况下，转移到高压氧。

■ 随访建议

对合并烧伤的患者进行烧伤随访。

要点和误区

• 对于疑似氰化物暴露的病例，在开始治疗前不要等到氰化物水平。
• 通过碳氧血红蛋白评估潜在的一氧化碳暴露。

炎症性肠病 Inflammatory Bowel Disease

Dhara P. Amin 倪沁赟 译

基础知识

■ 描述

• 特发性、慢性肠道炎症性疾病，也可能涉及肠外器官。
• 溃疡性结肠炎和克罗恩病之间的区别并不总是明确的，中间形式的炎症性肠病(IBD)是存在的。
• 可能表现为初发疾病或现有疾病加重。
• 因克罗恩病频繁的微妙的改变，对该疾病需要保持高度的怀疑。
• 儿科患者的考虑：
- 可发生在生命的最初几年。
- 可能以肠外表现为主。
• 克罗恩病和溃疡性结肠炎之间的区别：
- 溃疡性结肠炎总是以直肠病变为主，表现为近端持续性炎症。
- 溃疡性结肠炎无小肠病变。

- 克罗恩病可发生在从口到肛门的任何部位,病变部位之间有正常的胃肠道黏膜。
- 克罗恩病是透壁性炎症,而溃疡性结肠炎则局限于黏膜下层。
• 克罗恩病和溃疡性结肠炎之间的相似之处:
- 病程>10 年,结肠癌发病率高。
- 双峰年龄分布,第一高峰在青少年和 30 岁出头之间,第二高峰在 60 岁左右。
• 克罗恩病的临床类型:
- 回盲部:约 40%。
- 小肠:约 30%。
- 结肠:约 25%。
- 其他:约 5%。
• 溃疡性结肠炎的临床类型:
- 全结肠炎:30%。
◦ 大部分临床表现严重。
• 直肠炎或乙状结肠炎:30%。
- 轻度临床表现。
• 左侧结肠炎(至脾曲):40%。
- 中度临床表现。

病因

• 不明。
• 克罗恩病和溃疡性结肠炎是各自独立的,具有共同的遗传倾向。
• 有家族史是非常普遍的。
• 多种因素起病,各因素之间相互作用:
- 遗传。
- 环境。
- 免疫。
• 发病机制:
- 肠壁无法下调免疫反应,最终导致慢性炎症的发生。
• 具有致病作用的传染媒介目前尚无确切的证据。
• 心理因素可能导致某些临床症状的加重。

诊断

症状和体征

• 克罗恩病可以表现为任何临床相关的慢性炎症、纤维狭窄或瘘管形成。
• 溃疡性结肠炎可隐匿起病或起病非常凶险。
• 全身症状、胃肠道及肠外表现,两者相似。

病史

• 全身症状:
- 克罗恩病:
◦ 低热。
◦ 盗汗。
◦ 体重下降。
◦ 疲劳。
◦ 儿科患者:生长或青春期延迟。
- 溃疡性结肠炎:
◦ 通常只在暴发性疾病时出现发热。
◦ 体重下降,疲劳。
• 胃肠道:
- 腹部疼痛/压痛:克罗恩病。
◦ 发作性。
◦ 脐周,可定位于右下腹回肠疾病。
◦ 全身弥漫性肠受累。
◦ 可定位于腹腔脓肿区域或瘘管。
◦ 压痛和腹胀考虑肠梗阻或中毒性巨结肠。
- 腹部疼痛/压痛:溃疡性结肠炎。
◦ 较克罗恩病更加广泛。
◦ 往往局限在排便前阶段。
◦ 压痛伴肠道扩张考虑毒性肠腔扩张。
• 粪便:
- 克罗恩病:
◦ 轻度、软条状粪便,很少>5 日。
◦ 约 50%带血性。
- 溃疡性结肠炎:
◦ 腹泻多见,可非常严重。
◦ 大部分为血便,有时严重出血。
◦ 黏液。
◦ 里急后重和紧迫感常见。
• 恶心和呕吐:
- 克罗恩病:
◦ 回结肠疾病梗阻常见。
- 溃疡性结肠炎:
◦ 梗阻少见。
◦ 伴毒性肠腔扩张的肠鸣音减少。
• 肝脏:
- 硬化性胆管炎可见。
- 35%~60%的克罗恩病患者可见胆囊结石。
• 肾脏:
- 肾结石。
- 梗阻性肾积水。
• 肌肉骨骼:
- 外周关节炎或关节痛:伴随疾病活动出现。
- 儿科患者:可能与幼年型类风湿性关节炎、特发性生长障碍、神经性厌食症混淆。

体格检查

• 肛周:
- 克罗恩病:
◦ 肛周脓肿。
◦ 肛裂:特征性无痛。
◦ 肛瘘:可见于 50%的克罗恩病患者。
◦ 可见于其他临床症状之前。
- 溃疡性结肠炎:
◦ 无肛周脓肿。
• 右下腹疼痛/压痛常被误认为胰腺炎。
• 严重毒性/腹部疼痛:必须排除中毒性巨结肠。
• 肠外:
- 眼睛:
◦ 葡萄膜炎。
◦ 巩膜炎。
◦ 角膜炎。
- 口腔:
◦ 口疮性口炎。
- 皮肤:
◦ 结节性红斑。
◦ 坏疽性脓皮病。

基本检查

• 可表现为初发疾病或现有疾病的加速恶化。
• 因克罗恩病频繁的微妙的改变,对该疾病需要保持高度的怀疑。

诊断检查与说明

实验室检查

• 无诊断性检查。
• 全血细胞计数:
- 贫血继发于慢性或急性血液丢失。
• 电解质、尿素氮/肌酐、血糖。
• 粪便检查:
- 隐血。
- 难辨梭状芽孢杆菌。
- 粪便白细胞阳性。
- 培养用于排除因肠炎引起的感染。
• 红细胞沉降率(血沉)通常升高。
• 新的研究中的血清学试验可用于辅助诊断艾滋病、作为筛选试验或预测治疗。

影像学检查

• 辐射剂量是可累积的,而炎症性肠病患者需要反复暴露于射线。如果可以的情况下考虑 MRI。
• 站立的胸部和腹部 X 线:
- 中毒性巨结肠(扩张>6 cm)。
- 肠梗阻。
- 结肠壁空气(可能预示即将发生穿孔)。
- 穿孔:膈下积气或肝脏或胆囊周围游离气体。
• 腹部 CT/MRI:
- 区别克罗恩病的局部炎症肿块和脓肿。

Y

• 行结肠镜检查明确诊断溃疡性结肠炎或克罗恩病：
- 因穿孔风险，严重症状可能被掩盖。
• 小肠造影，尤其是回肠末端的造影，可用于确诊克罗恩病。
• MRI可用于克罗恩病肛周疾病，且避免电离辐射。

鉴别诊断

• 感染性肠炎。
• 假膜性结肠炎。
• 阑尾炎。
• 憩室炎。
• 憩室。
• 功能性肠道疾病。
• 恶性淋巴瘤。
• 缺血性结肠炎。
• 淋病或衣原体直肠炎。
• 艾滋病。
• 结肠癌。
• 血管炎。
• 淀粉样变性。

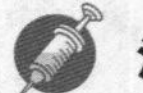

治疗

院前

基础生命支持(BLS)维持生命体征稳定。

初步稳定/治疗

• 如果存在脱水表现，给予生理盐水复苏治疗。
• 如果有显著血液丢失，给予输血治疗。

急诊治疗/程序

• 如果怀疑梗阻或毒性肠腔扩张行胃肠减压。
• 暴发性溃疡性结肠炎或怀疑穿孔给予广谱抗生素治疗。
• 考虑激素替代治疗，如果近期有口服激素，需要给予负荷剂量。
• 手术评估指征：
- 穿孔。
- 肠梗阻。
- 大量的、迟发性出血。
- 毒性扩张：
◦ 不是手术治疗的绝对指征。
◦ 使用小肠减压、闭合射线监测和外科会诊加强疾病管理。
• 脓肿壁穿孔：
- 通常不是急诊手术的指征。
- 严密观察腹膜炎体征。
• 药物治疗：
- 除非诊断已经明确，一般不会开始药物治疗。
- 在已知疾病的患者中，重新使用或重新开始药物治疗。
- 急诊会诊医疗方案应该个体化，并强烈建议胃肠病学专家。
◦ 氨基水杨酸(柳氮磺胺嘧啶/美沙拉嗪)适用于轻度至中度病例。
◦ 可使用止泻药物(复方地芬诺酯)，可能会掩盖严重疾病或疑似中毒性巨结肠。
◦ 类固醇激素(泼尼松、布地奈德或氢化可的松灌肠、ACTH)适用于中度至重度病例。
◦ 抗生素[甲硝唑和/或环丙沙星]用于克罗恩病结肠/会阴联合治疗的辅助治疗。
◦ 免疫抑制药物(硫唑嘌呤、甲氨蝶呤)用于严重病例。
◦ 单克隆抗体中和细胞因子肿瘤坏死因子-α和肿瘤坏死因子-α受体抑制剂[英夫利昔单抗(类克)]。用于对其他治疗方式反应差的肠外治疗。不是急诊治疗药物，需要注意潜在的严重不良反应、输液反应、自身免疫性疾病和感染。

儿科注意事项

如果怀疑是非意外性创伤，及时转诊可进行医学治疗的合适的儿童保护机构。

药物治疗

• 环丙沙星：500 mg(儿童：10～20 mg/kg，q12 h)，口服，q12 h。
• 氢化可的松灌肠剂：60 mg 直肠。
• 美沙拉嗪灌肠剂：1～4 g，保留灌肠，保留过夜(成人)。
• 美沙拉嗪直肠栓剂：500 mg，直肠，2次/日(成人)。
• 美沙拉嗪片：
- 亚沙可：800 mg，口服，3次/日。
- 颇得斯安：1 000 mg，口服，4次/日。
• 甲泼尼龙：125～250 mg，静脉注射负荷量(儿童：2 mg/kg，静脉注射负荷量，维持剂量同成人)，然后 0.5～1 mg/kg，q6 h，维持5日。
• 甲硝唑：250～500 mg[儿童：30 mg/(kg·24 h)]，口服，3次/日。
• 泼尼松：40～60 mg(儿童：1～2 mg/kg)，口服，1次/日。
• 柳氮磺胺嘧啶(SASP)：500 mg(儿童：30 mg/kg)，口服，4次/日。

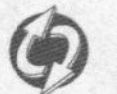

随访

进一步处理

入院指征

• 手术指征：
- 大量、迟发性出血。
- 穿孔。
- 中毒性肠腔扩张。
- 梗阻。
• 疾病严重发作：
- 电解质紊乱。
- 严重脱水。
- 严重疼痛。
- 高热。
- 显著出血。

出院指征

• 首发表现为腹泻、轻度疼痛，无中毒症状，需要密切随访。
• 原有疾病的轻度至中度加重，无梗阻、严重出血、严重疼痛、脱水，需要密切随访，重新治疗或增加类固醇治疗。

转诊问题

肠外表现：
• 眼。
• 皮肤。

随访建议

胃肠病专家或可提供外科治疗意见的初级保健医师。

要点和误区

• 疾病严重发作，需要排除中毒性巨结肠。
• 儿童生长/发育延误需要考虑克罗恩病。
• 肛周疾病需要考虑克罗恩病。
• 疾病严重发作时排除艰难梭菌感染，炎症性肠病合并艰难梭菌感染的发生率增加。
• 严重溃疡性结肠炎患者避免使用止泻/痉挛性药物。

眼球破裂 Globe Rupture

Alexander T. Limkakeng Jr · Brandon T. Ruderman 祝各亮 译

基础知识

描述

- 外伤造成的全层角膜或巩膜损伤。
- 钝性创伤和眼球破裂：
  - 突然导致眼内压弥漫性升高。
  - 随后眼球在冲击点的对侧或最薄弱的点出现破裂：
    - 眼外肌附着点。
    - 角巩膜缘。
    - 边缘是巩膜最薄弱的地方。
- 穿透伤和挫裂伤：
  - 尖锐物体或子弹直接损伤眼前部或巩膜。
  - 最常见的损伤位于角膜及其前部，眼球的侧方和后方有骨性眼眶的保护。
  - 后部损伤可来自眼眶骨折或眼睑和眉部的贯穿伤。
- 出现下列情况愈合较差：
  - 大的撕裂伤。
  - 眼直肌后损伤。
  - 钝伤。
  - 眼内异物，特别是用有机材料制成。
  - 玻璃体挤出。
  - 晶状体损伤。
  - 前房积血。
  - 视网膜脱离。
  - 出现严重视力下降。
  - 瞳孔传入障碍。
  - 未及时手术。

病因

- 坠落，冲击伤。
- 运动相关性损伤(如肘击、球的冲击、箭伤等)。
- 间接震荡伤(爆炸)。
- 锐器伤和刺伤，意外或故意的。
- 高速弹丸伤害(枪支、BB弹、爆炸的弹片玻璃等)。

诊断

症状和体征

- 疼痛，外伤后发红、流泪。
- 局部淤血和肿胀。
- 巩膜或角膜裂伤。
- 眼内内容物挤压。
- 视力明显下降。
- 前房积血。
- 严重的结膜下出血、水肿，尤其在结膜周围血性水肿时。
- 异常深或浅前房。
- 低眼压：
  - 注意：如果怀疑眼球破裂，不要进行眼压测量。
- 瞳孔不规则(朝向损伤部位)。
- 晶状体半脱位。
- 视网膜震荡，视网膜变为灰白色。

病史

- 损伤时间和机制：
  - 眼内是否存在残留异物，不要取出突出的异物。
- 眼球手术史。
- 伤前视力。
- 破伤风接种情况。
- 口服药摄入情况。

体格检查

- 手电筒或裂隙灯检查眼球破裂的体征。
- 如果诊断为眼球破裂，则在手术修复前延迟进一步的眼科检查。
  - 避免在眼球上施加任何压力，从而增加挤出眼球内容物的风险。
- 如果初始检查没有眼球破裂的证据，则进行全面的眼科检查。
  - 视力(艾滋病预后)。
  - 眼球运动。
  - 裂隙灯检查：角膜、前房、虹膜、巩膜、眼底、视网膜。
  - 传入性瞳孔缺损提示后路损伤。
- 赛德尔试验：观察荧光素是否远离(黄绿色)，从而明确破裂处有无渗漏。
- 测眼内压：
  - 只有在无眼球破裂表现时进行。
- 超声(当不怀疑破裂时)。
- 明确是否有并发症。

基本检查

完成上述眼部检查：

- 一旦诊断为眼球破裂或怀疑眼球破裂，则在修复前延迟进一步的眼科检查。

诊断检查与说明

实验室检查

术前实验室检查：

- 血常规。
- 电解质。
- 凝血功能。

影像学检查

- 眼眶X线片(正/侧位)以探测眼内金属异物。
- 眼球B超。
- 眼眶CT扫描比MRI更能识别骨折和异物(敏感性只有56%～75%)。考虑是否有必要进行脑部或颈椎成像。

诊断步骤/外科

- 裂隙灯。
- 荧光素。

鉴别诊断

- 眼内异物。
- 前房积血。
- 严重的结膜下出血和水肿。
- 部分角膜和巩膜撕裂伤。
- 面部/眼眶骨折。
- 球后出血。

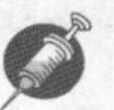

治疗

院前

- 在眼球外放置一个无压力的护罩。
- 如果没有护罩可用塑料杯代替。

初步稳定/治疗

如果怀疑眼球破裂，要尽量控制眼球不动。防止任何会引起眼压升高的活动，如牵拉、咳嗽或呕吐。抬高头部。

急诊治疗/程序

- 为明确的手术治疗做准备：
  - 紧急的眼科会诊。
  - 彻底的体格检查，以明确并发的损伤。
  - 术前相关的实验室检查及心电图检查。
  - 禁食，禁水。
- 降低眼内压以减少进一步的损伤：
  - 使用止吐药防止恶心与呕吐。
  - 疼痛控制。
  - 必要时使用镇咳药。
  - 抬高床头。
  - 保护性眼罩(本身无压力)。
- 接种破伤风疫苗。
- 预防性应用抗生素。
  - 皮肤致病菌(金黄色葡萄球菌、链球菌)最常见。眼内炎的风险为2.6%～30%。
  - 万古霉素和氟喹诺酮(莫西沙星或左氧氟沙

Y

星)或头孢他啶。氟喹诺酮首选玻璃体穿透伤。

- 琥珀胆碱是相对禁忌的:
  - 然而在一定剂量的非极化肌松药和充分的麻醉情况下,它是可以使用的。

儿科注意事项

- 考虑非意外性创伤。
- 由于存在挤压眼内内容物的风险,应避免牵拉或哭,试着让他们开心。

药物治疗

- 头孢他啶:1～2 g(儿童:30～50 mg/kg),静脉注射,q8 h。
- 克林霉素:450 mg(儿童:8～12 mg/kg),静脉注射,q8 h。
- 左氧氟沙星:750 mg(儿童:10 mg/kg),静脉注射,q24 h。
- 莫西沙星:400 mg(儿童:10 mg/kg),静脉注射,q24 h。
- 昂丹司琼(枢复宁):4 mg,静脉注射。
- 丙氯拉嗪(甲哌氯丙嗪):5～10 mg,静脉注射或肌内注射。
- 妥布霉素:2 mg/kg(儿童:2 mg/kg),静脉注射,q8 h。
- 万古霉素:15 mg/kg,静脉注射,q8～12 h(儿童:10 mg/kg,静脉注射,q6 h)。

随访

进一步处理

入院指征

- 所有眼球破裂、渗漏的患者。
- 对于严重的损伤尽早行眼球摘除术。

出院指征

排除眼球渗漏的患者。

转诊问题

- 由于检查的复杂性以及尽量减少在眼部的操作,急诊眼科会诊是需要的,以排除眼球破裂的可能。
- 手术修复时间的延长会增加感染风险,速度是非常重要的。
- 如果合适的话,应建议患者使用防护眼罩,防止再次损伤。

随访建议

术后进行眼科随访。

要点和误区

- 如果确诊或怀疑眼球破裂,不要在眼部做操作:
  - 放置一个眼罩覆盖受累的眼。
- 使用止吐药控制恶心和呕吐,以防止眼内压升高和眼球内容物挤出。
- 防治破伤风。
- 根据临床情况进行经验性抗生素治疗。

摇头丸中毒 MDMA Poisoning

Mark B. Mycyk　段立伟 译

基础知识

描述

- MDMA:3,4-甲基苯丙胺(迷幻药,又称摇头丸)。
- 非法生产的药品。
- 用来取乐:
  - 狂欢派对。
  - 舞蹈俱乐部。
  - 大学校园。
- 发病时间:服用后 15～30 min。
- 持续时间:2～6 h。
- 药片通常含有污染物:
  - 咖啡因。
  - 麻黄素。
  - 右美沙芬。
  - 氯胺酮。
  - 相关的甲基化苯丙胺:
    - 3,4-亚甲二氧基苯丙胺(MDA)。
    - 3,4-亚甲二氧基-N-己基苯丙胺(MDEA)。
    - 3,4-亚甲二氧基-N-丁基苯丙胺(MDBA)。
    - 对甲氧基苯丙胺(PMA)。
- 病理生理学:
  - 苯丙胺样结构刺激儿茶酚胺释放。
  - 酶斯卡灵样环状结构提高血清素和多巴胺活性。

病因

故意或意外摄入摇头丸。

诊断

症状和体征

- 过量:
  - 精神状态改变。
  - 严重神经系统症状。
- 中枢神经系统:
  - 激动。
  - 昏迷。
  - 癫痫发作。
  - 脑水肿。
- 心血管:
  - 高血压(早期)。
  - 低血压(晚期)。
  - 心悸。
  - 室上性心动过速和异位。
- 肺:
  - 肺水肿。
- 代谢:
  - 低钠血症。
  - 低血糖。
  - 抗利尿激素分泌异常综合征。
- 肌肉骨骼:
  - 磨牙症。
  - 躁动。
  - 强直。
- 肾:
  - 横纹肌溶解。
- 肝脏:
  - 黄疸。
  - 肝炎。
- 血液:
  - 弥散性血管内凝血(DIC)。
- 胃肠道:
  - 呕吐。
  - 腹泻。
  - 腹部绞痛。
- 精神:
  - 兴奋。
  - 思维奔逸。
  - 精神错乱/幻觉。
- 其他:
  - 高热。
  - 瞳孔散大。
  - 眼球震颤。

基本检查

- 诊断基于临床表现和准确的病史。

• 获得核心体温。
• 排除有毒污染物。

诊断检查与说明

实验室检查

• 电解质、尿素氮、肌酐和血糖水平。
• 凝血酶原时间、部分凝血活酶时间、国际标准化比值。
• 尿液中血液和肌红蛋白。
• 如果怀疑横纹肌溶解时检查肌酸激酶水平。
• 明显过量或怀疑肝炎时检查肝功能。
• 尿液毒理学筛查排除污染物:
- 可能导致苯丙胺阳性和甲苯丙胺筛查。
• 定量 MDMA 水平很少有帮助。

影像学检查

• 如果怀疑吸入性肺炎行胸部 X 线检查。
• 如果怀疑颅内出血行头颅 CT 检查。

诊断步骤/外科

心电图:
• 窦性心动过速(最常见)。
• 心律失常,传导障碍。

鉴别诊断

• 可卡因过量。
• 苯丙胺过量。
• 抗胆碱能药物过量。
• 卡西酮过量(如浴盐)。
• 羟色胺综合征。
• 隐匿性头部损伤。
• 脓毒症。
• 甲状腺危象。
• 嗜铬细胞瘤。

治疗

院前

• 在急诊室检查装有药物的瓶子是否过量。
• 注意 MDMA 用具:
- 奶嘴。
- 发光棒。
- 外科口罩。

初步稳定/治疗

ABC 管理:
• 气道控制是本质。
• 供氧。
• 如果需要给予气管插管。
• 建立静脉通道。
• 如果有精神状态改变,给予纳洛酮、硫胺素、葡萄糖。

急诊治疗/程序

• 支持治疗。
• 监测核心体温和心脏节律至少 6 h。
• 使用生理盐水静脉注射水化。
• 高血压:
- 硝普钠。
- 酚妥拉明。
- 艾司洛尔。
• 低血压:
- 给予生理盐水负荷量。
- 头低足高位。
- 压缩机滴定调节血压。
• 焦虑、躁动、不安:
- 需要时使用地西泮或劳拉西泮。
• 癫痫发作:
- 首先给予苯二氮䓬类药物治疗。
- 持续性癫痫发作给予苯巴比妥。
• 横纹肌溶解:
- 给予生理盐水积极水化。
- 考虑给予碳酸氢钠。
- 如肾衰竭给予血液透析。
• 高热:
- 标准降温治疗。
- 使用地西泮治疗焦虑。

药物治疗

• 地西泮(安定):5～10 mg(儿童:0.2～0.5 mg/kg),静脉注射,q10～15 min。
• 艾司洛尔:500 μg/kg 静脉注射负荷量,然后 50 μg/(kg·min)静脉注射。
• 劳拉西泮:2～6 mg(儿童:0.05～0.1 mg/kg),静脉注射,q10～15 min。
• 纳洛酮:0.4～2 mg(儿童:0.1 mg/kg;新生儿:10～30 mg/kg),静脉注射或肌内注射。
• 硝普钠:0.3 mg/(kg·min)至最大剂量 10 μg/(kg·min)。
• 苯巴比妥:10～20 mg/kg,静脉注射(负荷剂量)。
• 酚妥拉明:1～5 mg(儿童:0.02～0.1 mg/kg),静脉注射,q5～10 min。

随访

进一步处理

入院指征

• 精神状态改变。
• 癫痫发作。
• 持续心血管状态不稳定。
• 横纹肌溶解。
• 行为失控。
• 弥散性血管内凝血。

出院指征

过量口服后无症状 6 h。

随访建议

• 娱乐性药物滥用患者转诊。
• 意外中毒患者需要毒物预防咨询。
• 故意中毒(如自杀)患者需要接受精神评估。

要点和误区

• 始终监测核心体温。
• 医院常规的药物筛查中可能没有伴随的娱乐性药物。
• 对于持续性精神状态改变,评估有无低钠血症。
• 考虑引起精神状态改变的非毒性因素。

Y

咬伤(人) Bite, Hum

Daniel T. Wu 宋振举 童朝阳 译

基础知识

描述

• 第三常见的咬伤(前两种分别是犬咬伤和猫咬伤)。
• 多数咬伤(约 75%)出现在打斗行为中。
• 15%～20%与性行为有关。
• 两种类型的咬伤:
- 闭塞性咬伤:受影响的部位出现撕裂伤或挤压伤,出现在牙齿咬伤皮肤时,与动物咬伤相比更容易引发感染。
- 握拳性损伤(更严重的类型):优势手的

掌指关节处出现小伤口，常见于握拳时袭击其他人口齿时。

• 放松受伤的关节可引起：厌氧环境中的口腔细菌接种到受伤关节，细菌通过肌腱被接种到手部深层部位感染，增加其他严重感染的概率。

病因

• 需氧菌和厌氧菌：
- 最常见：
  ◦ 链球菌。
  ◦ 金黄色葡萄球菌。
- 其他：
  ◦ 侵蚀艾肯菌。
  ◦ 流感嗜血杆菌。
  ◦ 消化链球菌属。
  ◦ 棒状杆菌。
  ◦ 侵蚀艾肯菌与链球菌、金黄色葡萄球菌、拟杆菌、革兰阴性菌有协同作用。
- 尽管病毒(肝炎病毒、HIV及疱疹病毒)经咬伤传播少见，但仍有报道。

诊断

症状和体征

• 部位：
- 上肢(60%～75%)。
- 头颈部(15%～20%)。
- 躯干(10%～20%)。
- 下肢(5%)。

• 常见并发症：
- 蜂窝织炎。
- 严重深层感染(浓度性关节炎和骨髓炎)。
- 骨折和肌腱损伤。
- 手咬伤具有最高的感染风险。

病史

• 受伤时间。
• 患者的过敏原。
• 相关用药史(免疫状态)。
• 上一次注射破伤风疫苗的时间。
• 咬人者是否携带HIV、乙肝病毒。

体格检查

• 记录所有伤口的部位和程度。
• 记录每一处肿胀、擦伤及失活组织。
• 注意受伤部位影响区域的运动范围。
• 注意肌腱和神经功能。
• 记录任何感染征象，包括局部腺瘤。
• 记录所涉及的每个关节和骨骼。

基本检查

对受伤部位的深部结构和外部组织进行详细的检查：

• 针对握拳性损伤，应将手指伸展到最大运动范围，对深层部位进行检测，并注意有无肌腱裂伤和关节损伤。

诊断检查与说明

实验室检查

• 咬伤后感染部位的需氧菌和厌氧菌培养。
• 如果没有临床感染征象可不进行培养。
• 如果怀疑感染，应检测CBC、C反应蛋白(CRP)、红细胞沉降率(ESR)。
• 糖尿病患者及患者要检查电解质、血糖、肌酐、尿素氮。

影像学检查

• 通常来说对诊治的意义不大。
• X线摄片。
- 骨折。
- 怀疑其他部位损伤，如牙齿。
- 如果有骨骼和关节深处的损伤可摄X线片以对骨髓炎进行评估。
- 有靠近骨骼和关节的感染时。
• 超声可以协助鉴别脓肿和蜂窝织炎。

鉴别诊断

其他动物咬伤：

• 尖锐的牙齿更容易导致刺伤撕裂伤，而人的牙齿一般引起挤压伤。

其他

• 怀疑存在性虐待：
- 检查是否有皮肤挫伤及吸吮后的唇印。
• 手足表面的线性损伤及挫伤是咬伤的重要提示标志。
• 尖牙间距离大于3 cm提示处于恒牙期(袭击者年龄大于8岁)。
• 如果怀疑存在虐待：
- 在受伤部位用生理盐水湿润过的拭子采集唾液然后进行后续分析。
- 拍摄图片。
- 通知相关部门。

治疗

院前

按压止血。

初步稳定/治疗

保证气道通畅及充足的外周灌注。

急诊治疗/程序

• 伤口灌洗：
- 用1号针或塑料导管加足量的生理盐水进行灌洗。
- 注意不要将液体注射到组织中。
• 清创：
- 清除任何外源物、坏死皮肤和失活组织。
- 对刺伤不要进行清创。
- 清除焦痂使潜在脓液呈现出来以进行清创。
• 握拳性损伤：
- 固定伤口。
- 固定位置，要保持关节的功能位。
- 应用厚敷料。
- 咨询手外科医师是否需要手术灌洗和伤口探查。
- 抬高患肢数日，直到血肿减轻。
- 门诊患者可用吊带固定。
- 住院患者可用松紧绷带将手置于静脉输液架上。
- 应用抗生素。
• 对撕裂伤患者不要进行初始修复。
• 伤口缝合：
- 伤口缝合增加了感染概率，因此要对保持伤口开放使其自然愈合还是进行缝合进行权衡。
- 不要缝合感染部位或受伤24 h仍未处理的伤口。
- 对咬伤后大于8 h的伤口进行缝合与否争议。
- 面部咬伤24 h候的伤口仍需缝合，但要提醒患者有感染的风险。
- 感染部位和受伤24 h后的伤口不要进行缝合。
- 尽可能第一次无菌缝合在接近伤口边缘。
- 不要缝合闭合性伤口。
• 对低感染风险部位预防性应用抗生素存在争议。
• 下述情况可应用抗生素：
- 合并挤压伤或血肿的中到重度损伤。
- 骨骼或关节受损。
- 手部被咬伤。
- 伤口靠近人工关节。
- 合并其他疾病或能够增加严重感染风险的疾病，如糖尿病、脾切除术前或免疫抑制状态。
• 预防破伤风。
• HIV感染的检查或随访。

药物治疗

一线用药

• 阿莫西林-克拉维酸：500/15 mg[儿童：

40 mg/(kg · 24 h)],q8 h,口服。

• 氨苄西林：3 g，q6 h,静脉给药。

• 哌拉西林-三唑巴坦：4.5 g，q8 h，静脉给药。

• 羟基噻吩青霉素：3.1 g，q4 h,静脉给药。

• 头孢曲松钠：1 g/d 加甲硝唑钠 500 mg，q8 h。

二线用药

• 二联药物治疗：以下药物中的一种外加一种能够覆盖需氧菌的药物。

- 甲氧苄啶-磺胺甲噁唑：1 片，q12 h(儿童：8 mg/kg 甲氧苄啶和 40 mg/kg 磺胺甲噁唑)，口服。

- 青霉素：500 mg[儿童：50 mg/(kg · 24 h)]，口服，q6 h。

- 环丙沙星：500～750 mg，q12 h，口服；或 400 mg，q12 h，静脉。

- 脱氧土霉素：100 mg，口服，每日 2 次。

• 加能够覆盖需氧菌的药物：

- 克林霉素：150～450 mg[儿童：8～20 mg/(kg · 24 h)]，口服，6 h；或 600～900 mg[儿童：20～40 m/(kg · 24 h)]，静脉，q8 h。

- 甲硝唑：500 mg，口服，每日 3 次(儿童：10 mg/kg，每日 3 次)。

随访

进一步处理

入院指征

• 出现感染伤口。

• 严重的或进展性的蜂窝织炎或骨髓炎。

• 系统性感染征象。

• 门诊服用抗生素无效的感染伤口。

出院指征

• 存在局限性感染的健康患者：予以抗生素治疗并随访 24 h。

• 未感染的患者随访 48 h。

老年人注意事项

• 较少出现的人咬伤痕迹，有感染性伤口征象。

• 存在虐待可能。

儿科注意事项

• 较少出现的人咬伤痕迹，有感染性伤口征象。

• 牙间隔＞3 cm，可能是来自成人的咬伤，并考虑存在虐待。

推荐问题

怀疑存在儿童虐待行为的随访建议。

随访建议

• 存在手部感染时要有手外科专科的随访。

• 存在局限性感染的健康患者：予以抗生素治疗并随访 24 h。

• 未感染的患者随访 48 h。

要点和误区

• 握拳性损伤要检查受伤部位的最深处，并保持关节的功能位，以检查肌腱和关节有无损伤。

• 低于存在高感染风险的握拳性损伤患者，都要对手外科进行咨询是否需要手术清洗。

• 对于牙间隔大于 3 cm 的伤口提示处于恒牙期(袭击者年龄大于 8 岁)。

药物戒断 Withdrawal

Treronne M. Thompson 吴昊 李文放 译

基础知识

描述

• 神经兴奋是苯二氮䓬类、巴比妥类和阿片类药物戒断的标志。

• 苯二氮䓬类及巴比妥类药物戒断症状，可能危及生命。

• 阿片戒断症状通常会极度不适，但通常不会危及生命。

• 可卡因和苯丙胺的戒断症状同样不会威胁生命。

病因

• 慢性接触某些药物会导致中枢神经系统的适应性变化。

• 当药物的持续存在被移除或减少并且适应性变化持续时，就会出现戒断症状。

• 当需要增加数量的药物来达到特定的反应时，就会产生耐受性。

• 戒断和耐受是截然不同的。

诊断

症状和体征

• 苯二氮䓬类、巴比妥类药物：

- 焦虑。
- 激惹。
- 易怒。
- 震颤。
- 睡眠障碍。
- 心动过速。
- 高血压。
- 高热。
- 自主神经不稳定。
- 癫痫。

• 阿片类药物：

- 不安。
- 激惹。
- 药物渴望。
- 打呵欠。
- 立毛。
- 瞳孔放大。
- 恶心。
- 呕吐。
- 腹泻。
- 腹痛。
- 心动过速。
- 血压升高。

• 可卡因：

- 抑郁情绪。
- 疲劳。
- 多梦。
- 睡眠障碍。
- 精神运动迟缓或激动。

• 苯丙胺：

- 疲劳。
- 易怒。
- 睡眠障碍。
- 焦虑。

病史

• 药物滥用史：

Y

- 最后使用药物的时间。
- 既往的戒断病史。

体格检查

彻底的身体检查是必要的。

基本检查

彻底的病史和身体检查注意生命体征。

诊断检查与说明

实验室检查

- 电解质、BUN、肌酐、葡萄糖。
- 血常规。
- 尿液药物筛选很少改变管理。

影像学检查

如果临床情况不明确，可根据临床表现选择中枢神经系统或 X 线平片影像学检查。

鉴别诊断

- 酒精戒断。
- 脑内出血。
- 中枢神经系统感染。
- 脑病变。
- 低血糖症。
- 甲状腺功能亢进。
- 脓毒症。
- 精神病。
- 电解质紊乱。
- 药物中毒。

治疗

院前

- 评估生命体征。
- 评估末梢葡萄糖。

初步稳定/治疗

- ABC 管理。
- 建立静脉通路。
- 静脉液体管理。
- 心肺功能监测。

急诊治疗/程序

- 苯二氮䓬类和巴比妥类药物戒断治疗。
  - 积极治疗。
  - 开始一种可引起戒断作用的同一类长效药物。
- 阿片类药物戒断治疗：
  - 支持性护理。
  - 止吐剂治疗恶心和呕吐。
  - 如果戒断使其他疾病复杂化，则采用阿片类药物治疗。
- 可卡因和苯丙胺戒断治疗：
  - 支持性护理。

药物治疗

- 地西泮：5～20 mg 口服用于轻度症状和体征；必要时，5～10 mg 重复剂量静脉滴注用于严重的症状和体征。
- 氯拉西泮：轻度症状和体征时用 1～2 mg 口服；严重的症状和体征时用重复剂量 2 mg 静脉滴注。
- 苯巴比妥：轻度症状和体征时用 30～60 mg 口服；对于严重症状或癫痫持续状态，可缓缓地静脉滴注 15～20 mg/kg。
- 昂丹司琼：4～8 mg，口服或静脉滴注。

随访

进一步处理

入院指征

- 中重度戒断症状。
- 持续的戒断症状。
- 精神性戒断症状。
- 自主神经不稳定者。
- 伴随而来的医疗状况可能使戒断复杂化。
- 自杀倾向或精神不稳定。

出院指征

- 对治疗有轻微反应的症状。
- 精神状态稳定。

随访建议

转诊至解毒项目或中心。

要点和误区

- 误诊为戒断综合征。
- 对戒断综合征与合并症的关系存在误解。
- 在苯二氮䓬类药物戒断状态下，给患者服用足够数量的苯二氮䓬类药物是非常重要的。

一氧化碳中毒 Monoxide Poisoning

Trevonne M. Thompson 高婷 译

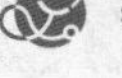

基础知识

描述

- 一氧化碳为一种无色、无味、无刺激性的气体。
- 其可与血红蛋白结合形成碳氧血红蛋白：
  - 减少血红蛋白携带氧量。
- 具有直接的细胞毒作用。
- 损伤细胞对氧的摄取。

病因

- 内源性：
  - 源于正常代谢。
- 未完全燃烧的含碳燃料：
  - 内燃机。
  - 天然气。
  - 加热器。
  - 室内烤架。
  - 壁炉。
  - 炉。
  - 意外火灾。
  - 香烟烟雾。
- 二氯甲烷：
  - 存在于用于除油漆的溶剂。
  - 人体暴露后可在体内转化为一氧化碳。
  - 暴露后体内碳化血红蛋白浓度峰值延迟。
  - 其形成的碳化血红蛋白半衰期为吸入一氧化碳所致者的 2 倍。

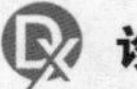

诊断

症状和体征

病史

- 中枢神经系统：
  - 头痛。
  - 头晕。
  - 共济失调。
  - 意识模糊。
  - 晕厥。

- 癫痫发作。
- 消化道：
  - 恶心。
  - 呕吐。
- 心血管：
  - 胸痛。
  - 心悸。
- 呼吸系统：
  - 呼吸困难。

体格检查

- 中枢神经系统：
  - 急性脑病。
  - 癫痫发作。
  - 昏迷。
- 心血管：
  - 心动过速。
  - 各种心律失常。
  - 心肌缺血或梗死。
- 呼吸：
  - 呼吸急促。
  - 非心源性肺水肿。
- 其他：
  - 呼吸性碱中毒。
  - 横纹肌溶解。
  - 乳酸性酸中毒。

基本检查

- 病史：
  - 保持高度怀疑。
  - 症状可能较轻或不典型。
  - 需询问：
    - 有相同症状的家庭其他成员。
    - 炉故障。
    - 使用空间加热器，打开烤箱用于补充热量。
    - 患病的宠物。
- 动脉血气：
  - 正常动脉氧分压。
  - 正常血氧饱和度。
  - 低血氧饱和度。
  - 在重症患者中可出现代谢性酸中毒。
- 碳氧血红蛋白浓度：
  - 尽快测量。
  - 其浓度不能反映病情严重程度。
  - 在病情危重的患者中，血碳氧血红蛋白浓度可无显著升高。
  - 如果暴露后错过最佳检测时间，血中碳氧血红蛋白浓度可不高。
  - 碳氧血红蛋白正常范围为0～3%（在吸烟者中可高达10%）。

诊断检查与说明

实验室检查

- 脉搏血氧饱和度监测：
  - 假性高血氧饱和度。
  - 脉搏血氧饱和度不能区分氧合血红蛋白及碳氧血红蛋白。
- 电解质：
  - 代谢性酸中毒及阴离子间隙升高，其与临床严重程度相关。
- 心肌酶检测：
  - 当怀疑存在心肌缺血或梗死时。
- 妊娠检查。
- 心电图：
  - 一氧化碳可促发心肌缺血或梗死。
  - 心律失常。
  - 非特异性ST段改变或T波异常。

影像学检查

- X线平片：
  - 肺水肿。
- 头颅CT检查：
  - 当出现意识状态改变时用于评估颅内是否有其他病变。
  - 在诊断不明确的患者中，双侧苍白球低密度灶可能为一氧化碳中毒的诊断提供线索。

鉴别诊断

- 病毒性疾病或病毒性综合征。
- 脑膜炎或脑炎。
- 颅内出血。
- 胃肠炎。
- 偏头痛。
- 紧张性头痛。
- 酒精（乙醇）中毒。
- 镇静剂过量。
- 氰化物中毒。
- 水杨酸类药物过量。
- 有毒醇类暴露。

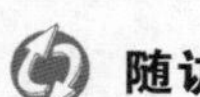

治疗

院前

吸纯氧。

初步稳定/治疗

- ABC管理。
- 开放静脉通路。
- 氧气吸入（100%吸入氧浓度）。
- 心电监测。

急诊治疗/程序

- 氧疗：
  - 吸入100%氧浓度的常压氧：
    - 经面罩或气管插管。
  - 持续氧疗直至血碳氧血红蛋白浓度<10%。
  - 碳氧血红蛋白有长半衰期：
    - 吸入空气时其半衰期约为300 min。
    - 吸入常压纯氧时其半衰期约为90 min。
    - 吸入3个大气压的高压纯氧时其半衰期约为20 min。
- 高压氧疗：
  - 剂量：
    - 3个大气压的高压纯氧。
    - 可以重复治疗。
  - 益处：
    - 可减少迟发性神经系统后遗症。
    - 可缩短碳氧血红蛋白半衰期。
  - 潜在的副作用：
    - 鼓膜破裂。
    - 气胸。
    - 癫痫发作。
    - 减压病。
    - 肺水肿。
  - 使用高压氧治疗尚存在争议。
  - 上级会诊指征：
    - 意识状态改变或昏迷。
    - 局灶性神经功能缺损。
    - 癫痫发作。
    - 心血管损害（梗死或持续性心律失常）。
    - 持续代谢性酸中毒。
    - 碳氧血红蛋白浓度>25%。
    - 妊娠合并碳氧血红蛋白浓度>10%。

妊娠注意事项

- 胎儿血红蛋白对一氧化碳亲和力高于成人血红蛋白。
- 胎儿碳氧血红蛋白浓度较产妇高10%～15%。
- 胎儿碳氧血红蛋白清除较产妇延迟。

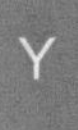

Y

随访

进一步处理

入院指征

- 在吸入纯氧治疗后4 h出现症状的患者。
- 有证据表明存在心肌缺血或心脏功能不稳定的患者。
- 癫痫发作。
- 持续代谢性酸中毒。

• 晕厥。

出院指征

• 观察 4 h 无症状者。

• 无前述入院指征者。

• 有自杀倾向而精神症状恢复者。

转诊问题

需要高压氧治疗者。

随访建议

与当地消防部门联系，以防一氧化碳家庭暴露。

要点和误区

• 当使用家用加热器的患者出现头痛时，需怀疑一氧化碳中毒。

• 当在同一密闭空间生活的家庭成员出现相似症状时，需怀疑一氧化碳中毒。

• 在治疗上需吸入纯氧，对于符合上述指征患者需给予高压氧治疗。

胰腺创伤 Pancreatic Trauma

Vaishal M. Tolia 王虑 译

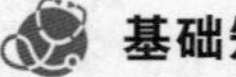

基础知识

描述

• 直接的上腹部撞击致胰腺撞击脊柱致钝挫伤。

• 胰腺被异物穿透致伤。

儿科注意事项

• 和成人相比，儿童在创伤时会致身体更大比例受伤，导致多系统伤。

• 儿童更缺少肌肉和胃肠组织的保护。

• 年龄小的儿童还应考虑安全带使用不当和虐待等原因。

• 儿童低血压表现较少见。

病因

• 穿刺伤为最常见病因。

• 钝挫伤：胰腺位置较深，需要巨大的冲击力才会受伤。

- 方向盘、安全带和自行车把手撞击腹部。

- 儿童还应考虑非意外创伤。

常见相关情况

90%的胰腺损伤会连带伤及附近的组织器官：

• 肝、胃。

• 主要动静脉。

• 脾、肾。

• 十二指肠、结肠、小肠。

• 胆总管、胆囊。

• 脊柱：机会骨折。

诊断

注意

胰腺伤波及范围要比表面上看起来得大。

症状和体征

• 腹痛：

- 弥漫性或上腹部。

- 体格检查发现的重要体征。

• 上腹部软组织挫伤。

• 伤及低位肋骨或肋软骨。

• 急腹症常伴有腹腔内损伤。

• 伴随脾损伤表现出背痛。

• 低血压。

• 格雷特纳征：

- 侧腹瘀斑。

• 库伦征：

- 脐周瘀斑。

病史

简洁，尤其重要的是钝性伤的细节。

体格检查

• 对擦伤、挫伤、穿刺伤进行检查：

- 必须对患者进行详细全面的体查并记录。

- 检查安全带相关性损伤。

• 听诊肠鸣音存在与否。

• 触诊腹痛的位置和程度，有无肌紧张、反跳痛。

• 直肠检查是否有隐匿出血、阴道或阴茎检查。

• 对未确认的伤情需进行持续的体格检查，重要体征持续观察。

注意

胰腺损伤中的血管伤是患者致死的首要原因。如果怀疑应立即评估必要时手术探查。

基本检查

• 病情检查工作的进度应根据患者的实际情况和其他伤情决定。

• 腹部增强 CT 是评估胰腺损伤必需的检查。

• 磁共振胰胆管成像能更好地评估胰管损伤，越来越多在临床应用。

诊断检查与说明

实验室检查

• 血型检查和交叉配血试验。

• 血细胞比容、红细胞分型。

• 淀粉酶：

- 不是提示胰腺损伤的可靠指标。

- 持续的增高可以增加敏感性，但特异性仍不高。

- 淀粉酶增高可以作为潜在胰腺损伤的指标。

- 淀粉酶正常不能完全排除胰腺损伤。

- 如果腹腔灌洗液发现淀粉酶增高，则敏感性特异性更高。

• 脂肪酶：

- 不是胰腺损伤的特异性指标。

• 尿液分析。

• 妊娠检查。

• 必要时酒精和药物检测。

• 凝血酶原时间测定和部分凝血酶原时间测定、尿素氮和肌酐。

影像学检查

• 要注意所有的影像学检查方法都可能漏诊胰腺损伤。

• 所有钝性伤患者都应行脊柱骨盆、胸部 X 线检查。

• 还包括超声快速检查。

• CT 增强扫描，多排螺旋 CT 扫描：

- 增强扫描能比平扫更好地显示胰腺组织。

- 多排螺旋 CT 尤其适合儿童患者。

• 磁共振胰胆管成像：

- 非侵袭性检查胰管。

• 内镜逆行胰胆管造影：

- 适用于持续高淀粉酶血症的患者。

- 无法解释的腹部体征。
- 有人认为早期使用可减轻并发症。

• 手术探查术中胆管造影仍然是理想的诊断方法，尤其是对不稳定的患者。

诊断步骤/外科

诊断性腹腔灌洗可协助诊断腹腔损伤：

• 分析腹腔灌洗液淀粉酶水平。

• 有可能漏诊严重胰腺损伤。

鉴别诊断

其他或伴随的腹部损伤。

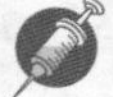

治疗

院前

转运至最近的创伤中心。

初步稳定/治疗

• 气道管理和复苏，补充晶体液、胶体液或血制品。

• 鼻胃管负压吸引对胰腺损伤有益。

一般措施

按照腹部创伤的治疗原则进行：

• 穿刺伤：
- 破伤风抗毒素和广谱抗生素治疗。

• 腹部伤需要剖腹探查的：
- 广谱抗生素治疗。

• 必需覆盖到肠道菌群：
- 需氧菌：大肠埃希菌、肠杆菌、克雷伯杆菌、肠球菌。
- 厌氧菌：拟杆菌、梭菌、消化链球菌。

急诊治疗/程序

按照创伤治疗的原则治疗，在急救外科医师指导下复苏生命体征不稳定的患者迅速转运至创伤急救中心：

• 评估腹部伴随损伤的严重程度。

• 使用影像学方法快速评估(CT或磁共振胰胆管成像)。

• 早期明确胰管损伤证实可以减低发病率和死亡率。

• 手术：胰十二指肠切除术、远端胰腺切除、内镜支架置入(有争议)、引流/负压吸引。

• 2009年美国东部创伤外科学会创伤指南。

• Ⅲ级证据：Ⅰ级和Ⅱ级损伤，引流；Ⅲ级和Ⅳ级损伤，切除加引流。

药物治疗

• 成人：
- 哌拉西林-他唑巴坦：3.375 g，静脉注射。
- 头孢替坦：2 g，静脉注射＋庆大霉素2 mg/kg，静脉注射。
- 头孢西丁：2 g，静脉注射＋庆大霉素2 mg/kg，静脉注射。
- 头孢曲松钠：1～2 g，静脉注射＋甲硝唑15 mg/kg，静脉注射。
- 克林霉素：2 mg，静脉注射＋庆大霉素2 mg/kg，静脉注射。

• 儿童：
- 头孢替坦：20 mg/kg，静脉注射＋庆大霉素2 mg/kg，静脉注射。
- 头孢西丁：40 mg/kg，静脉注射＋庆大霉素2 mg/kg，静脉注射。
- 头孢曲松钠：50 mg/kg单位剂量，静脉注射＋甲硝唑15 mg/kg，静脉注射。

一线用药

头孢曲松钠庆大霉素或哌拉西林-他唑巴坦或碳青霉烯：

• 目标是选取全面覆盖需氧菌和厌氧菌的抗生素，特别是针对肠道革兰阴性菌。

二线用药

联合氨基糖苷抗生素，因为它在碱性环境有较好的活性。

• 特别适用于在使用广谱肠道革兰阴性菌抗生素情况下，体征仍不稳定的患者。

协助治疗

还没有充分的证据支持使用奥曲肽，它的益处和副作用仍有争议。

随访

进一步处理

入院指征

• 所有可能患有胰腺损伤的患者。

• 钝性伤导致的腹痛需要持续性检查并观察24～72 h。

• 醉酒创伤患者需收入院，持续性检查排查一些不确定伤情。

出院指征

仅限于伤很轻可以排除胰腺和腹部其他损伤的患者，还需要合适的随访安排和预防措施。

转诊问题

• 经手术后放置引流或有并发症瘘管形成的患者需再次手术，并提高护理等级。

• 大部分患者需密切监测并随访1周。

随访建议

延迟发作的胰腺损伤比较少见，但并发症会出现，需引起重视：

• 胰腺炎、假性囊肿、血管动脉瘤(脾动脉)。

• 内分泌和外分泌功能失调较少见，除非胰腺大部分被切除或毁损：
- 评估糖耐量和消化功能异常情况。

要点和误区

• 钝挫伤和穿刺伤出现腹部背部疼痛，应考虑是否有胰腺伤。

• 考虑附近可能的血管损伤。

• 评估并发的损伤。

• 以最快的速度行影像学检查协助诊断。

• 穿刺伤和生命体征不稳定患者需迅速准备剖腹探查。

胰腺炎 Pancreatitis

Trevor Lewis　王虑 译

基础知识

描述

• 因激活作用，间质释放和腺体被自己释放酶的消化作用所致的胰腺炎症反应。

• 急性胰腺炎：
- 腺体的内分泌和外分泌功能损坏数周到数月。
- 胰腺功能可以恢复正常。

• 慢性胰腺炎：
- 腺体的内分泌和外分泌功能渐渐损害，伴有脂肪泄和吸收障碍。
- 腺体功能逐渐损害不可恢复。

• 胰腺假性囊肿：
- 由缺乏上皮组织的纤维构成囊壁，囊内充满的液体富含胰腺酶。

- 囊肿局限于胰腺实质组织内或毗邻胰腺(极少腹膜囊)。
- 自急性胰腺炎发病来4～6周形成。

病因

• 胆结石和酗酒是急性胰腺炎最常见的病因(75%～80%)。

• 酗酒占慢性胰腺炎致病因素的70%～80%。

• 急性:
- 胆管疾病。
- 慢性酒精中毒。
- 胰管阻塞。
- 缺血。
- 药物。
- 感染。
- 手术后。
- ERCP术后。
- 代谢性疾病。
- 创伤。
- 蝎毒。
- 消化系统溃疡穿孔。
- 遗传。

• 慢性:
- 慢性酒精中毒。
- 胰管阻塞。
- 热带地区。
- 遗传。
- Shwachman综合征。
- 酶缺乏。
- 特发性。
- 高脂血症。
- 高钙血症。

• 胰腺假性囊肿:
- 胰腺炎的并发症,5%～16%的急性胰腺炎患者、20%～40%的慢性胰腺炎患者可能并发。

儿科注意事项

患病原因主要是病毒、创伤和代谢。

诊断

症状和体征

• 常见表现:
- 腹痛:95%～100%。
- 上腹部肌紧张:95%～100%。
- 恶心和呕吐:70%～90%。
- 低热:70%～85%。
- 低血压:20%～40%。
- 黄疸:30%。
- 格雷特纳征和库伦征:<5%。

• 消化系统:
- 持续剧烈的上腹痛并向背部发散:
  ◦ 绞痛或反跳痛提示非胰腺引起。
  ◦ 仰卧疼痛加重。
- 恶心、呕吐和食欲不振。
- 肠鸣音减少,甚至缺失。
- 严重的消化系统出血同时伴急性胰腺炎并不常见。
- 库伦征:
  ◦ 脐周出现蓝色瘀斑,继发于出血性胰腺炎。
- 格雷特纳征:
  ◦ 侧腹出现蓝色瘀斑,继发于出血性胰腺炎。

• 呼吸系统:
- 胸膜炎性胸痛。
- 呼吸困难。
- 肺部检查:
  ◦ 左侧胸腔积液(最常见)。
  ◦ 肺不张。
  ◦ 肺水肿。
- 低氧血症(30%)

• 心血管系统:
- 心律不齐。
- 低血压。
- 休克。

• 神经系统:
- 易激。
- 混乱。
- 昏迷。
- 面神经征(Hvostek征)和低钙束臂征(Trousseau征)较少见,除了实验室检查有明显低钙血症。

Ranson标准

• 发病率和死亡率的指标:
- 符合0～2条标准:2%死亡率。
- 符合3条或4条标准:15%死亡率。
- 符合5条或6条标准:40%死亡率。
- 符合7条或8条标准:100%死亡率。

• 入院标准:
- 年龄>55岁。
- 红细胞计数>16000/mm^3。
- 血糖>200 mg/dl。
- 血清乳酸脱氢酶>350 U/L。
- 谷草转氨酶>250 U/L。

• 48 h标准:
- 血细胞比容下降>10%。
- 尿素氮上升>5 mg/dl。
- 血清钙<8 mg/dl。
- 动脉氧分压<60 mmHg。
- 碱缺失>4 mmol/L。
- 估计体液隔离>6 L。

基本检查

实验室检查以明确胰腺炎的诊断。

诊断检查与说明

实验室检查

• 脂肪酶:
- 疼痛出现4～8 h上升。
- 比淀粉酶更加可靠的诊断胰腺炎指标。

• 淀粉酶:
- 疼痛出现6 h内上升。
- >3倍正常值提示有胰腺炎。
- >1000 U提示胆源性胰腺炎。
- 在炎症急性期淀粉酶水平可能正常,因为胰腺被严重毁损。
- 除了胰腺其他一些脏器也能释放。

• 电解质、尿素氮、肌酐、血糖:
- 体液流失过多致低血钾。
- 高糖血症。

• 全血细胞计数:
- 血细胞比容增加伴液体丢失。
- 血细胞比容>47%,胰腺有坏死可能。
- 血细胞比容下降提示伴有腹膜后出血。
- 异常红细胞计数>12000。

• 钙/镁:
- 低血钾提示严重的胰腺炎症。
- 低血镁见于酗酒胰腺炎患者。

• 肝功能测试。
- 若怀疑胆源性胰腺炎可作为预测预后指标。

• CRP:
- 可用于胰腺炎症状出现24～48 h评估病情严重程度。

• 妊娠检测。

• 动脉血气:
- 是否有低氧血症(PO_2)酸中毒(剩余碱)。

• 心电图:
- 电解质是否平衡,心肌有无缺血。

影像学检查

• 腹部X线片:
- 排去气体。
- 胰腺有无钙化灶。
- 经常能发现胰腺旁独立膨胀的肠腔。

• 胸部X线片:
- 胸腔积液。
- 肺不张。
- 肺浸润。

- 超声：
- 对诊断胆源性胰腺炎很有帮助。
- 腹部 CT：
- 高风险胰腺炎（>3 条 Ranson 标准）。
- 出血性胰腺炎。
- 怀疑胰腺假性囊肿。
- 诊断不明。

诊断步骤/外科

内镜下逆行胰胆管造影术（ERCP）：

- 用于严重胰腺炎伴有胆管炎或胆管阻塞的患者。

鉴别诊断

- 肠系膜缺血/梗死。
- 心肌梗死。
- 胆绞痛。
- 肠梗阻。
- 溃疡穿孔。
- 肺炎。
- 动脉瘤破裂。
- 宫外孕。

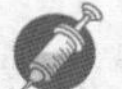

治疗

院前

- 患者的配合应立即建立静脉通道。
- 心电监测。

初步稳定/治疗

- 生命体征支持。
- 吸氧。
- 心电监测。
- 静脉补液。

急诊治疗/程序

- 气道管理：
- 肺动脉需要充足氧供。
- 对于急性呼吸窘迫综合征和脑病患者需紧急气管插管。
- 液体复苏：
- 大量补液（第一个 24 h 达到 5～6 L）补充丢失的体液。
- 持续监测生命体征、尿量、电解质，确保快速大量液体补充。
- 纠正电解质紊乱：
- 低钙血症（葡萄糖酸钙）。
- 大量体液丢失致低钾血症。
- 低血镁见于酒精性胰腺炎患者。
- 血制品：
- 出血性胰腺炎患者输血使血细胞比容保持在 30%水平。
- 如果有凝血功能障碍和出血可以输冰冻血浆和血小板。
- 止痛：
- 阿片类药物止痛。
- 鼻胃管吸引：
- 轻度胰腺炎效果不大。
- 对于重症胰腺炎和顽固呕吐患者效果好。
- 止吐药。
- 抗生素：
- 若腹部 CT 示胰腺坏死灶>30%。

老年人注意事项

为防止液体负荷过重可予以监测中心静脉压。

药物治疗

一线用药

镇痛药和抗生素：

- 吗啡：2～4 mg，静脉注射。
- 二氢吗啡酮（盐酸二氢吗啡酮）：1 mg，静脉注射或肌内注射。
- 昂丹司琼：4 mg，静脉注射、肌内注射或口服。

二线用药

电解质和抗生素：

- 氯化钾：10 mmol/h，静脉注射，时间要长于 1 h。
- 10%葡萄糖酸钙：10 ml，静脉注射，时间要长于 15～20 min。
- 硫酸镁：2 g，静脉注射。
- 亚胺培南：500 mg，静脉注射，q6 h。

随访

进一步处理

入院指征

- 急性胰腺炎患者伴有严重腹痛、恶心、呕吐。
- 出血性胰腺炎和坏死性胰腺炎是 ICU 纳入的标准。
- 醉酒创伤患者需收入院，持续性检查排查一些不确定伤情。

出院指征

- 轻型胰腺炎并没有胆道疾病可以口服补液的患者。
- 慢性胰腺炎伴有轻微腹痛可以口服补液的患者。

转诊问题

- 外科和消化科医师就重症胰腺炎合并胆管炎或胆道堵塞患者行内镜下逆行胰胆管造影术（ERCP）治疗的问题。
- 急诊外科医师认为一旦出现假性囊肿破裂或破裂出血，剖腹手术是唯一确定有效治疗手段。

随访建议

所有出院的轻度胰腺炎患者需 24～48 h 行随访。

要点和误区

- 胆结石和酒精占急性胰腺炎发病因素的 75%～80%。
- 早期积极补液体治疗是大量体液丢失患者必需的治疗手段。
- 鼻胃管吸引治疗对轻型胰腺炎并无多大益处。
- 但诊断不能明确或患者 Ranson 标准≥3 条时，需尽快行腹部 CT 检查。

Y

移植排斥 Transplant Rejection

Brooks L. Moore · Erika Phindile Chowa 张晟 林兆奋 译

基础知识

描述

针对移植物基因异种抗原的免疫反应引起了移植器官排斥反应：

- HLA 不相容：
- 排斥的最常见原因。
- 实体器官的排斥反应。
- 血型不相容：
- 相比于 HLA 不相容，移植物存活风险低。
- 可能引起带血管移植物超急性排斥反应（肾脏和心脏）。

- 排斥的 3 个阶段：
- 超急性期：
  - 术后即刻。
  - 抗体针对红细胞或 HLA 抗原。
  - 内皮损伤。
  - 血小板聚集，发生血栓、组织坏死。
  - 供受体配型吻合时罕见。
- 急性期：
- 术后 3 个月内。
- 停用免疫抑制剂（IS）后。
- T 细胞依赖的过程，炎症细胞浸润同种异体移植物，释放细胞因子，破坏移植物。
- 表现为移植器官功能不全的全身症状或体征。
- 慢性期：
- 多年后发病。
- 导致慢性器官衰竭。

■ 流行病学

发病率和患病率估计

- 实体器官移植：
- 每年移植的器官超过 3 万个。
- 最常见的移植器官：肾脏、肝脏、心脏、肺、肠、胰腺。
- 就诊急诊最常见的诊断：感染、胃肠道疾病、脱水、电解质紊乱、心血管及肺部疾病、损伤、排斥反应。
- 高达 75% 的人需要住院治疗。

■ 病因

- 减量或不服从药物治疗：
- 与环孢素、他克莫司和西罗莫司相互作用的药物治疗：
  - 苯巴比妥、苯妥英钠、卡马西平、利福平、异烟肼。
- 肾脏移植排斥：
- T 细胞、B 细胞引起早期排异，攻击微血管和损害移植物灌注；体积损耗，低血压，感染。
- 感染、进行性肾血管硬化引起的慢性排斥反应。
- 肝移植排斥：
- 急性：6 周内 48%，1 年内 65%。
  - 常常伴随 IS 方案降低。
- 慢性：<5%。
  - 经验表明 MC 范围为 1 周到 6 个月。
- 心脏移植排斥：
- 急性排斥：
  - 75%～85% 的患者在首个 3～6 个月发生，由于 T 细胞介导的免疫反应。
- 慢性排斥：
  - 动脉硬化加速是标志。
  - 与 IS 疗法中的改变有关。
- 肺移植排斥：
- 急性排斥反应早期发生：
  - 在第 1 年内可发生频率高达 6 次。
- 慢性排斥：
  - 25%～40% 的术后患者。
  - 术后第 2 年内死亡 MCC。
  - 内皮、血管和淋巴细胞炎症引起排异，复发性急性排异。
- 骨髓移植排斥：
- 急性移植物抗宿主疾病：
  - 供体骨髓针对肺组织的免疫攻击。
- 慢性移植物抗宿主病：
  - 25%～50% 的患者。
- 骨髓排斥：
  - 患有再生障碍性贫血且未接受全身放疗的患者，或患者接受配型不吻合的移植物。

诊断

■ 症状和体征

- 肾移植排斥：
- 系统性高血压。
- 尿量减少。
- 肿胀、发热和触痛。
- IS 治疗不耐受。
- 肝移植排斥：
- 发热、上腹部疼痛、黄疸。
- 心脏移植排斥：
- 发热、呼吸困难、胸痛、低血压或高血压、心悸、恶心、呕吐、晕厥、猝死。
- 可能无症状。
- 肺移植排斥：
- 咳嗽、呼吸困难、发热、干湿啰音。
- 骨髓移植排斥：
- 发热、消瘦、黏膜炎、角膜炎、吞咽困难、组织缺氧、胸痛、腹痛、腹泻、黄疸、皮疹、脑病、癫痫。

■ 诊断检查与说明

实验室检查

- CBC。
- IS 药物水平：
- 如果患者在急诊前服用药物，水平可能不代表低谷。
- 血培养。
- 怀疑脓毒症时测血清乳酸水平。
- 肾移植排斥：
- 电解质、BUN、肌酐、CRP。
- 微量尿液分析：
  - 蛋白尿可能标志存在早期排斥，排斥或感染时可见到白细胞。
  - FENa 有助于鉴别排斥和医源性因素。
- 肝移植排斥：
- 凝血功能、脂肪酶、微生物培养（血、尿、腹水）、肝功能检查。
- 晚期急性排斥表现为胆红素升高和转氨酶升高。
- 心脏移植排斥：
- 心脏肌钙蛋白。
- 肺移植排斥：
- ABG、电解质、肾功能、CRP、肝功能、胆红素、LDH、CPK、EBV、CMV、环孢素水平。
- 骨髓移植排斥：
- ABG、肝功能测试。

影像学检查

- CXR：
- 急性肺排斥：
  - 弥漫性浸润早期可见。
  - 移植后 1 个月以上可正常。
- 骨髓移植排斥：
  - 间质浸润、胸腔积液、肺水肿。
- 超声：
- 上腹部：在肝移植排斥反应中的适应证。
- 肾：疑似肾移植排斥反应。
  - 肾积水表明是梗阻性肾病，可能需要紧急行经皮肾穿刺造口术。
- CT：
- 胸部：肺移植。
- 腹部：用于肝和肾移植。
- 超声心动图：
- 心脏移植。
  - 评估心输出量的改变。
- MRI：
- 肾移植：
  - 有无造影均可。
  - 造影前咨询移植团队。

诊断步骤/外科

- 肝移植排斥：
- ERCP 胆道造影。
- 心脏移植排斥：
- 心电图：
  - 由于原本窦节点备用，通常表现为 2P 波。
  - 心房颤动是最常见的心律失常。
- 肺移植排斥：
- FEV_1 峰值流量减少。

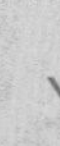
Y

– 早期支气管镜和活检可鉴别排斥反应和感染。

▪ 基本检查

• 考虑排斥的同时考虑药物毒性和感染。
• 询问药物剂量和依从性更改。
• 有轻微的症状或体征，及时行影像学和实验室检查。

▪ 鉴别诊断

• 感染：
– 多种细菌、结核分枝杆菌、真菌、病毒、寄生虫引起移植患者的机会性感染。
• IS 中毒。
• 药物与 IS 的互相作用。
• 肾移植排斥：
– 任何影响原肾脏的因素均可发生在移植肾脏上。
– 医源性肾毒性：环孢素、他克莫司、其他药物治疗。
– 尿路感染/肾盂肾炎：
◦ 原肾脏感染的经典微生物。
◦ BK：多瘤病毒引起的小管间质性肾炎(发生率为 3%～5%)。
– 移植肾脏动脉或静脉的急性堵塞：
◦ 急性堵塞通常发生于移植后第 1 周(发生率为 0.5%～8%)，造成少尿和急性肾衰竭。
– 移植前血肿。
– 漏尿。
– 梗阻性尿路疾病。
– 移植肾脏活检后出血。
• 肝移植排斥：
– 上行性胆管炎：
◦ 可能来源于术后胆管支架。
– 硫唑嘌呤引起的胆汁淤积型肝炎。
– 甲氨蝶呤诱导的肝毒性。
• 肺移植排斥：
– 肺部 MC 细菌感染、巨细胞病毒肺炎。
– MC 真菌感染、曲霉感染。
– 上呼吸道感染或支气管感染：
◦ 模拟慢性肺部感染。
– 药物引发的肺炎。

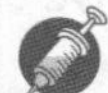

治疗

▪ 院前

避免积极的液体复苏。

▪ 初步稳定/治疗

• ABC 管理。
• 休克阶段使用静脉补液治疗及升压药物。
• 像处理其他高血压急症一样处理高血压危象。避免钙通道阻滞剂，因为它们与 IS 药物相互作用。

▪ 急诊治疗/程序

注意

尽量早期与移植服务部门讨论，尤其是在增加或更换药物时，除非患者病情不稳定。

注意

慎用 NSAIDs，移植患者可能有多种相关的并发症。

• 肾、心脏、肺及肝移植排斥：
– 使用高剂量类固醇激素。
– 应激剂量糖皮质激素的覆盖范围也适用于任何精神不佳的移植患者。尽早咨询移植服务。
– 避免输血，因为此类操作需特殊筛查以避免疾病传播。
• 心脏移植排斥：
– 移植心脏需照常使用升压药和强心剂。
– 阿托品对于心动过缓无效，因为无迷走神经支配。
– 如有典型的心动过缓，使用多巴胺、肾上腺素或体内起搏器来加快心率。
– 静脉注射甲泼尼龙：持续 3 日，1 mg/d。
• 肺移植：
– 治疗排异和感染。
– 静脉注射甲泼尼龙：持续 3 日，15 mg/(kg・d)。
• 移植物抗宿主病：
– 口服或静脉注射糖皮质激素 1～2 mg/(kg・d)。
– 慢性时，可能需要调整 IS 疗法。
• 普通的 IS 方案为环孢素、泼尼松和硫唑嘌呤，或他克莫司和泼尼松。

▪ 药物治疗

由移植团队指导。

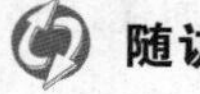

随访

▪ 进一步处理

入院指征

• 允许有发热、呼吸急促、排斥反应、腹痛或其他器官感染、气胸和呼吸衰竭症状的移植受者入院。
• ICU 收入有脓毒血症、急性肾衰竭或心肺功能不全的患者。

出院指征

已被排除排斥或严重感染的无毒患者可保持密切随访出院，同时要咨询其移植服务。

转诊问题

治疗意见应与患者的肿瘤学家、移植外科医师或器官专家商议后决定。

▪ 随访建议

• 患者的移植团队应积极参与到随访计划中。
• 当患者在急诊室出现任何暗示有排斥反应的症状时，应尝试与覆盖的移植医师进行口头沟通。

要点和误区

• 移植患者表现为轻微抱怨时有高排斥风险，需要与其移植团队联合在急诊内进行深度评估。
• 有移植排斥可能症状的患者同样需要考虑感染和药物毒性。
• 有很高比例需要收入院。

乙烯乙二醇中毒 Ethylene Glycol Poisoning

Kirk L. Cumpston 单怡 译

基础知识

描述

- 血清浓度高峰在 1～4 h。
- 半衰期为 2.5～4.5 h。
- ＜20%以原形方式由肾脏排出。
- 病理生理学：
  - 经肝乙醇脱氢酶及醛脱氢酶代谢最终生成草酸。
  - 生成醛及酸代谢产物。
  - 直接造成中枢系统、心脏及肾脏毒性。
  - 乙烯乙二醇代谢：
    - 第 1 步：乙烯乙二醇由乙醇脱氢酶转化成乙醇醛。
    - 第 2 步：乙醇醛由醛脱氢酶转换成羟基乙酸。
    - 第 3 步：羟基乙酸由乳酸脱氢酶转换成乙醛酸。
    - 第 4 步：乙醛酸转换成草酸。

病因

- 含乙烯乙二醇的物品：
  - 防冻液。
  - 有机溶剂。
- 据报道浓度 100%的乙烯乙二醇最小致死剂量为 30 ml。

诊断

症状和体征

- 心血管系统：
  - 心动过速。
  - 低血压。
- 中枢神经系统：
  - 醉酒样状态、易怒。
  - 共济失调。
  - 感觉迟钝。
  - 脑神经功能异常。
- 胃肠道：
  - 恶心、呕吐。
  - 腹痛。
- 肺：
  - 过度通气、呼吸急促、Kussmaul 呼吸。
  - 肺水肿。
- 肾脏：
  - 急性肾衰竭。
  - 结晶尿。

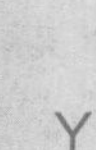

病史

- 蓄意或误食乙烯乙二醇。
- 无相关病史但患者存在阴离子间隙增加的代谢性酸中毒。
- 无法解释的渗透压升高。

体格检查

- 呼吸急促。
- 精神状态的改变。

基本检查

- 所有摄入食物的病史。
- 同时检测：
  - 动脉血气。
  - 血清乙烯乙二醇、甲醇、异丙醇及乙醇浓度。
  - 血电解质、尿素氮、肌酐、血糖。
  - 测量血浆渗透压（通过冰点降低法）。
  - 血钙、磷、镁浓度。

诊断检查与说明

实验室检查

- 测定阴离子间隙。
  - 阴离子间隙 ＝ $Na^{+}-(Cl^{-}+HCO_3^{-})$。
  - 正常阴离子间隙：8～12。
- 测定渗透压差：
  - 实际测得的摩尔渗透压浓度-理论值。
  - 渗透压差增加＞10 mmol/L。
  - 理论渗透压浓度＝2 Na^{+} ＋血糖/18＋尿素氮/2.8＋乙醇(mg/dl)/4.6。
  - 通过计算甄别乙烯乙二醇的摄入，因为大多数临床实验室无法及时有效地测定乙醇的中毒浓度。
  - 有助于早期识别乙烯乙二醇中毒或伴有乙醇摄入的情况。
  - 在同时伴有乙醇中毒时，相对较少的乙烯乙二醇转化生成酸性代谢产物，因此渗透压差将趋向增大，而酸中毒将趋向减轻。
  - 渗透压差正常不能排除乙烯乙二醇摄入。
  - 乙烯乙二醇摄入后迟发表现可仅有阴离子间隙升高，而无明显的渗透压差异。
- 乙烯乙二醇、甲醇、异丙醇血清浓度。
- 乙醇血清浓度：
  - 有助于判定共同摄入乙醇(100 m/dl)疗效并评估如何影响渗透压。
- 尿液分析：
  - 信封状草酸结晶：不敏感但特异性强。
  - 尿中未检出草酸钙结晶不能排除乙烯乙二醇的暴露史。
  - 酮体可能来源于异丙醇摄入、饥饿或糖尿病酮症酸中毒。

诊断步骤/外科

伍德灯检测尿或胃内容物：

- 检测到荧光素，一种常见的防冻添加剂。
- 防冻液摄入非敏感和非特异性的标志物。
- 尿液中缺乏荧光素不能排除乙烯二乙醇的暴露史。

鉴别诊断

- 渗透压差增大：
  - 甲醇。
  - 乙醇。
  - 利尿剂（甘露醇、甘油、丙二醇、山梨醇）。
  - 异丙醇。
  - 乙烯乙二醇。
  - 丙酮氨。
  - 山梨糖醇。
- 阴离子间隙增大的代谢性酸中毒：A CAT MUDPILES。
  - 酒精性酮症酸中毒。
  - 氰化物、CO、H_2S 及其他。
  - 对乙酰氨基酚。
  - 抗反转录病毒药物(NRTI)。
  - 甲苯。
  - 甲醇、二甲双胍。
  - 尿毒症。
  - 糖尿病酮症酸中毒。
  - 三聚乙醛、苯乙双胍（降糖灵）、丙二醇。
  - 铁剂、异烟肼。
  - 乳酸性酸中毒。
  - 乙烯乙二醇。
  - 水杨酸盐、乙酰水杨酸(ASA，阿司匹林)、饥饿性酮症。

治疗

院前

- 带上所有含可疑摄入物的容器。
- 气道管理，中枢神经系统抑制。
- 除去污染的衣物、首饰，并用肥皂及清水冲洗以去除沾染于皮肤的乙烯乙二醇。

初步稳定/治疗

- ABC 管理。

• 氧疗，心电监测，用生理盐水维持静脉通路。

• 50%葡萄糖溶液（或 Accu-Check）、纳洛酮及维生素 B_1 治疗精神异常。

急诊治疗/程序

• 防止乙烯乙二醇的进一步吸收：
- 通过鼻胃管洗胃：
  ◦ 用于摄入时间小于 1 h，患者处于昏迷或者大量摄入者。
- 首剂给予活性炭吸附潜在的共同摄入物，但对于单纯的乙烯乙二醇摄入可能无明显作用：
  ◦ 活性炭只能吸收少量乙烯乙二醇。

• 应用甲吡唑防止乙烯乙二醇转化为有毒的代谢产物，一种乙醇脱氢酶的竞争性抑制剂：
- 甲吡唑(4-MP，抗发酵剂)：
  ◦ 如意外摄入超过一小口，蓄意摄入或出现精神异常伴随无法解释的渗透压差、阴离子间隙增大的酸中毒，pH<7.3 或肾衰竭时，需在血清中乙烯乙二醇浓聚之前即开始使用。
  ◦ 血清乙二醇浓度>20 mg/dl。
- 缺点：
  ◦ 短暂的肝功能异常。
- 优点：
  ◦ 易给药。
  ◦ 无需持续给药。
  ◦ 无宿醉或中枢神经系统抑制。
  ◦ 无低血糖、低钠血症及高渗性改变。
  ◦ 无需检查血清乙二醇浓度。
  ◦ 降低护理及监测等级。
  ◦ 无需收至 ICU。

• 乙醇治疗：
- 无法获取甲吡唑时解毒剂的第二选择。
- FDA 未批准用于治疗乙烯乙二醇中毒。
- 如果怀疑潜在的毒物摄入，在血清中出现乙烯乙二醇之前即开始使用。
- 乙醇：比乙烯乙二醇更易与乙醇脱氢酶结合。
  ◦ 延迟转化为有毒代谢产物。
- 适应证：
  ◦ 意外摄入超过一小口或蓄意摄入乙烯乙二醇的病史。
  ◦ 精神异常伴无法解释的渗透压差增加、阴离子间隙增大的酸中毒。
- 目标：血清乙醇浓度在 100～150 mg/dl。
- 持续乙醇治疗直到乙烯乙二醇血清浓度<20 mg/dl。

• 给予维生素 B_1、B_6 及镁剂：
- 乙烯乙二醇代谢的辅酶，可能促进其转化为无毒代谢产物。
- 目前尚无临床数据支持此理论。

• 血液透析：
- 缩短乙烯乙二醇的清除半衰期，清除毒性代谢产物。
- 适应证：
  ◦ 代谢性酸中毒碳酸氢根浓度<20 mmol/L 且 pH<7.3。
  ◦ 升高的渗透压差>10 mmol/L。
  ◦ 肾损伤+代谢性酸中毒。
  ◦ 血清乙二醇浓度>50 mg/dl。
- 持续血液透析直至乙烯乙二醇血清浓度<20 mg/dl 及代谢性酸中毒纠正。

• 继发异常症状的处治：
- 通过静脉输液确保足够的尿量。
- pH<7.3 时给予碳酸氢钠纠正酸中毒：
  ◦ 目标是维持 pH 在正常范围内（pH 7.35～7.45）。

• 监测并调节血钙：
- 钙沉积于组织后可导致低钙血症。

妊娠注意事项

• 甲吡唑对孕妇分级为 C 级。

• 乙醇不能应用于孕妇，分级为 D/X。

儿科注意事项

儿童摄入乙醇可导致严重的中枢神经系统抑制和低血糖。

药物治疗

• 活性炭：1 g/kg，口服。

• 葡萄糖：1 安瓿 50%葡萄糖溶液：50 ml 或 25 g（儿童：25%葡萄糖溶液，2～4 ml/kg），静脉注射。

• 乙醇：
- 口服：50%乙醇溶液（50%酒精）胃管注入：
  ◦ 负荷剂量：1.5 ml/kg。
  ◦ 维持剂量：0.2～0.4 ml/(kg·h)。
  ◦ 血液透析时的维持剂量：0.4～0.8 ml/(kg·h)。
- 静脉注射：10%乙醇加入 5%葡萄糖溶液：
  ◦ 负荷剂量：8 ml/kg 持续 30～60 min 输注。
  ◦ 维持剂量：1～2 ml/(kg·h)。
  ◦ 血液透析时的维持剂量：2～4 ml/(kg·h)。

• 甲吡唑：
- 负荷剂量：15 ml/kg，缓慢输注超过 30～60 min。
- 维持剂量：10 mg/kg 每 12 h 给 4 剂，再 15 mg/kg 每 12 h 给 1 次直至血清乙烯乙二醇浓度<20 mg/dl。
- 血液透析时的剂量：
  ◦ 若上一次给药<6 h，在透析开始时不用给药。
  ◦ 若上一次给药>6 h，在透析开始时给予下一剂量。
  ◦ 透析时每 4 h 给药一次。
  ◦ 若上一次给药距透析结束时间<1 h，下一时间点不用再次给药。
  ◦ 若上一次给药距透析结束时间在 1～3 h，下一时间点给予 1/2 剂量。
  ◦ 若上一次给药距透析结束时间>3 h，下一时间点给予完整剂量。

• 镁剂：25～50 mg/kg 静脉注射一剂直至最高 2 g。

• 纳洛酮：起始剂量 2 mg（儿童：0.1 mg/kg）静脉注射或肌内注射。

• 维生素 B_6：100 mg/d，连续 2 日。

• 碳酸氢钠：1～2 mmol/kg 加入 5%葡萄糖溶液中静脉注射。

• 维生素 B_1：100 mg（儿童：50 mg），静脉注射或肌内注射，每日 1 次，连续 2 日。

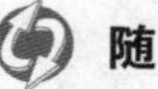

随访

进一步处理

入院指征

• 所有摄入乙烯乙二醇的患者，即使最初无临床症状。

• 生命体征或精神状态不稳定患者收入 ICU。ICU 可能需要行紧急血透来纠正代谢性酸中毒或肾衰竭。

• 如果需要血流透析或甲吡唑治疗而目前医疗机构不能获得，则转至其他有条件的机构。

出院指征

单纯摄入乙烯乙二醇后无症状的患者，若血清乙烯乙二醇浓度<20 mg/dl 且无代谢性酸中毒。

随访建议

自杀患者转至精神科专科医师。

要点和误区

• 渗透压差<10 mmol/L 不能排除乙烯乙二醇接触史。

• 对于阴离子间隙增大和乙烯乙二醇接触的患者，在鉴别诊断时通过血清浓度确认接触史，并立即给予甲吡唑。

·如果无法明确乙烯乙二醇接触史，或者无法全天行血液透析，或者无解毒剂，则将患者转运至具有上述条件的医院。

·并非所有患者均会出现渗透压差及阴离子间隙增大，早期表现可仅有渗透压差变化，后期表现可能仅有阴离子间隙变化。

·尿中无结晶或无荧光素不能排除乙烯乙二醇接触史。

·使用碳酸氢钠纠正代谢性酸中毒、维持pH浓度于正常范围（7.35～7.45）可能有效。

异丙醇中毒 Isopropanol Poisoning

Paul Kolecki 何超 译

 基础知识

描述

·异丙醇对中枢的抑制性作用是乙醇的2～3倍。

·许多物质同时含有异丙醇、甲醇、乙二醇和乙醇。

·经口摄入时吸收迅速。

·会在体内转化为酮，但不会造成酸中毒。

·经乙醇脱氢酶代谢转化为丙酮（一种中枢抑制剂）。

- 和乙醇同时摄入时会使异丙醇的半衰期加倍，但并不影响丙酮。
- 丙酮后经由肺、肾脏排泄。

·致死剂量：250 ml。

·Vd：0.45～0.55 L/kg。

·半衰期：

- 异丙醇：3～6 h。
- 丙酮：7.5～26 h。

病因

·异丙醇：透明、无色，有令人眩晕气味的易挥发液体，味苦。

·在70%左右的外用乙醇溶液中含有异丙醇：

- 一般会添加蓝色的染料进行提示。

·包含于：

- 各种各样的化妆品。
- 消毒剂。
- 玻璃清洁剂。
- 脱漆剂。
- 各种溶剂。
- 珠宝清洁剂。
- 清洁剂。
- 防冻剂。
- 洗手液。

·成年患者：长期大量饮酒但在近期突然停止饮酒。

·皮肤、直肠对异丙醇的吸收会造成全身毒性。

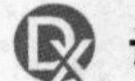 诊断

症状和体征

·一般会在接触后30～60 min出现症状。

·神经毒性：

- 昏睡。
- 虚弱。
- 头痛。
- 醉酒症状。
- 眩晕。
- 共济失调。
- 窒息。
- 昏迷。
- 摄入乙醇后初期的神经兴奋症状一般不会出现在异丙醇中毒患者中。

·消化系统症状：

- 恶心、呕吐。
- 腹痛。
- 胃肠炎。
- 咯血。

·心血管系统症状：

- 低血压。
- 心动过速。
- 心肌抑制。
- 周围血管扩张。

·呼吸系统症状：

- 呼吸抑制。
- 出血性支气管炎。

·皮肤症状：

- 皮肤刺激症状、烧伤。

·眼部症状：

- 刺激感。
- 流泪。

基本检查

·接触史。

·患者呼吸中有异丙醇或丙酮的气味。

诊断检查与说明

实验室检查

·电解质、尿素、肌酐、血糖：

- 常有低血糖发生。
- 如果不伴有终末器官的低灌注一般不会出现代谢性酸中毒。
- 丙酮会带来血清肌酐的假性升高：
  - 当丙酮>40 mg/dl时，每100 mg/dl的丙酮会带来肌酐升高1 mg左右。
  - 一旦丙酮代谢消耗后，肌酐水平恢复正常。

·全血细胞计数：

- 当出现消化道出血时会出现血红胞比容的降低。

·动脉血气：

- 除了出现器官低灌注，一般不会出现代谢性酸中毒。

·尿液分析：

- 尿酮体阳性。

·出现酮血症。

·异丙醇的血液浓度：

- 出现昏迷时异丙醇浓度>150 mg/dl。

·血清渗透压：

- 渗透压间隙：测量和计算的渗透压梯度之间的差异。
- 计算的是渗透压梯度＝2Na＋BUN/2.8＋血糖/18＋乙醇/4.6。
- 当测量的渗透压梯度高于计算的渗透压梯度10以上时，才考虑存在渗透压间隙。

影像学检查

·胸部X线摄片：对于意识障碍和呕吐严重的患者排查吸入性肺炎。

·头颅CT：合并头部外伤时检查。

鉴别诊断

·针对中枢抑制和渗透压间隙增大需要与以下鉴别：

- 乙醇。

Y

- 乙二醇。
- 甲醇。
- 丙三醇。
- 甘露醇。

治疗

院前

怀疑患者存在用药过量导致中毒时，需要收集患者所用药物和药瓶。

初步稳定/治疗

• ABC 管理：
- 必要情况下保持呼吸道通畅和良好的通气。

• 低血压：
- 首先静脉使用大量的生理盐水。
- 持续性低血压时使用多巴胺或去甲肾上腺素。
- 存在消化道出血的患者需要持续监测红细胞计数。

• 咯血患者需要放置胃管并进行冲洗。
• 当患者出现意识障碍时可使用纳洛酮、硫胺素和葡萄糖。

急诊治疗/程序

• 基础生命支持治疗。
• 皮肤和角膜污染的患者需要进行皮肤和眼部的冲洗。
• 活性炭洗胃：
- 对于摄入者。

• 不输注乙醇或 4-甲基吡唑。
• 血液透析。
- 能够有效地清除异丙醇和丙酮。
- 指征：
  ○ 充分的液体复苏和血管活性药物的使用后仍存在血流动力学不稳定。
  ○ 异丙醇＞400 mg/dl，并且合并低血压和持续性昏迷。

用药

• 活性炭悬浮液：1～2 g/kg，最大剂量 90 g 口服。
• 葡萄糖：50 ml 或 25 g。
• 多巴胺：2～20 mg/(kg · min)，静脉用药。
• 纳洛酮：2 mg，静脉用药或肌内注射。
• 硫胺素：100 mg，静脉用药或肌内注射。

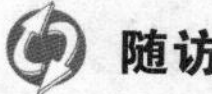

随访

进一步处理

入院指征

中度或重度异丙醇重度（意识障碍、低血压）。

出院指征

• 摄入 2～4 h 后患者无明显症状。
• 轻度中毒，并完全治疗后 4～6 h。

转诊问题

对于近期有消化道出血的患者推荐消化道内镜检查。

随访建议

存在酒精依赖或精神异常的患者反复摄入异丙醇中毒。

要点和误区

• 最基本的治疗是对患者密切的监测和生命支持。
• 不输注乙醇或 4-甲基吡唑。

异常子宫出血 Uterine Bleeding, Abnormal

Andrew J. French · Jamal J. Taha 张晟 林兆奋 译

基础知识

描述

• 以前称为功能失调性子宫出血。
• 异常子宫出血是指正常月经的规律性、频率、持续时间或量的改变：
- 正常月经期间出血量为 30～80 ml。
- 月经间隔正常 28(±7)日。

• 2 种分类：
- 异常子宫出血(AUB)：
  ○ 激素相关。
  ○ 无排卵和排卵类别。
  ○ 非器质性或医源性原因。
  ○ 排除诊断。
- 器质性子宫出血：
  ○ 与全身疾病或生殖道疾病有关的出血。

病因

• 无排卵(最常见)：
- 无拮抗的雌激素刺激增殖期子宫内膜。
- 雌激素戒断引起的出血。
- 由以下原因引起的神经内分泌功能改变：
  ○ 多囊卵巢综合征(PCOS)。
  ○ 极低热量饮食、快速体重变化、剧烈运动、神经性厌食症。
  ○ 心理应激。
  ○ 肥胖。
  ○ 药物，包括口服避孕药。
  ○ 麻醉剂。
  ○ 甲状腺功能减退。
  ○ 原发性下丘脑功能障碍。

• 排卵：
- 子宫 $PGF_{2\alpha}$ 不足：
  ○ 增加子宫收缩力。
- 子宫前列环素过多：
  ○ 降低血小板功能，增加子宫血管扩张。

• 如果出现以下情况，应怀疑有出血性疾病：
- 家族史。
- 自幼月经过多。
- 其他出血或瘀伤。

儿科注意事项

青春期常见的无排卵性出血，原因是下丘脑-垂体-卵巢轴发育不成熟。

诊断

症状和体征

病史

• 无全身性或结构性疾病的异常子宫出血。
• 最常见于子痫前期、围绝经期妇女。
• 通常无痛。
• 无排卵表现：
- 子宫出血：
  ○ 经期间不规则出血。
- 月经过多：

• 有规律的月经过多(＞80 ml)或出血＞7 日。

- 月经过少：
  ◦ 月经周期>35 日。
- 月经过多。
  ◦ 月经期间或月经之间过度出血。

体格检查

• 痤疮、多毛症、肥胖提示多囊卵巢综合征的前兆。

• 盆腔检查有轻度至中度出血。

• 面色苍白、心动过速、低血压、立位严重病例。

• 评估外伤、异物。

> **注意**
>
> 继发于 AUB 的血流动力学不稳定是罕见的；如果存在这种不稳定，应考虑异位妊娠(宫外孕)或其他导致月经过多的原因。

基本检查

尿妊娠试验(UPT)。

诊断检查与说明

实验室检查

• 妊娠试验、血细胞计数、PT、APTT、分型/筛查。

• 可将铁质检查、促甲状腺激素(TSH)、促黄体生成素(LH)、卵泡刺激素(FSH)、催乳素(PRL)、宫颈培养送基层医师(PMD)/妇科进行常规随访。

影像学检查

盆腔超声可显示子宫、输卵管或卵巢异常，鉴别诊断时可能需要排除其他器质性或医源性原因。

诊断步骤/外科

• 对于对其他干预措施无效的大出血，可能需要扩张和刮宫。

• 如果年龄>35 岁，请参考子宫内膜活检。

鉴别诊断

器质性/医源性

• 妊娠并发症：
- 先兆、不完全或自然流产。
- 异位妊娠。
- 葡萄胎妊娠。

• 感染性：
- 阴道炎。
- 宫颈炎。
- 盆腔炎(PID)。

• 凝血系统疾病：
- 血友病。
- 特发性血小板减少性紫癜。
- 遗传性血小板缺陷。
- 地中海贫血珠蛋白生成障碍性贫血。

• 药物：
- 阿司匹林。
- 抗精神病药。
- 皮质类固醇。
- 口服避孕药。
- 选择性 5-羟色胺再摄取抑制剂。
- 三环类抗抑郁药。
- 华法林。

• 系统性疾病：
- 肾上腺、肝脏、肾脏或甲状腺功能障碍、糖尿病、其他内分泌疾病。

• 解剖病变：
- 子宫内膜异位症。
- 子宫内膜增生。
- 子宫肌瘤。
- 息肉。
- 肿瘤。

• 宫内节育器。

• 创伤。

激素相关

请参考无排卵和排卵病因。

治疗

院前

静脉滴注晶体液以治疗大出血导致的低血压和心动过速。

初步稳定/治疗

ABC 管理：

• 对晶体类药物无反应的大量出血应输注红细胞悬液。

急诊治疗/程序

• 如果轻度出血，通常先充分观察。

• 静脉输注晶体液、红细胞悬液以防止继续出血或血流动力学不稳定。

• 如果出血严重且对晶体液及药物治疗无反应请妇科会诊：
- 血流动力学不稳定可能需要 D&C。
- 对其他治疗无反应的持续大出血可行子宫内膜消融或子宫切除术。

药物治疗

• 联合雌激素(倍美力)治疗大出血、血流动力学不稳定：
- 2.5 mg，口服，q6 h。
- 25 mg，静脉注射，如果需要，在 3 h 内重复使用。

• 布洛芬 400～800 mg，口服，q8 h(减少前列腺素合成)。

• 静脉注射剂量并不优于口服方法：
- 当出血减少时加入醋酸甲羟孕酮 5～10 mg/d，口服。

• 口服避孕药：
- 乙炔雌二醇 35 μg 和炔诺酮 1 mg，口服，每日 4 次，疗程 1 周。

• 抗纤溶药物：
- 氨甲环酸(TXA)：1 300 mg 口服或 10 mg/kg 静脉给药 q8 h×5 日。
- 可能与 OCP 联合使用。
- 因胃肠道反应、过敏、血栓病史限制使用。

• 在没有已知或怀疑出血的情况下，激素治疗被认为是 AUB 的一线药物治疗。

• 轻度病例可以推迟药物治疗，转诊到妇科。

• 透皮或长效雌激素是其他选择。

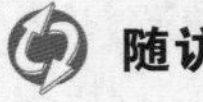

随访

进一步处理

入院指征

• 失血所致症状性贫血。

• 持续出血。

• 血流动力学不稳定需要积极复苏和/或手术干预。

出院指征

一旦出血得到控制且患者血流动力学稳定，大多数患者可以转诊至妇科后出院。

转诊问题

35 岁时子宫内膜活检：

• 患有 AUB 的患者需要与妇科医师或初级保健医师进行随访。

• 必须评估持续的失血或潜在的恶性肿瘤可能。

要点和误区

• AUB 为排除性诊断。

• 只有 2%的子宫内膜癌发生在 40 岁之前。

• 如果血流动力学不稳定，诊断 AUB 的可能性不大。

异位妊娠 Ectopic Pregnancy

Ivette Motola · Patricia De Melo Panakos 姜颢 译

基础知识

描述

- 受精卵在子宫外着床:
- 最常见于输卵管(93%~97%)。
- 腹腔和腹膜着床:
- 与高发病率相关。
- 诊断困难。
- 出血倾向。
- 发生在2%以内的孕妇。
- 引发的死亡占所有孕产妇死亡的6%(早期妊娠相关死亡的首要原因)。
- 60%的异位妊娠妇女随后能正常妊娠。

病因

- 危险因素包括:
- 35岁以上的女性。
- 非洲裔美国人。
- 既往感染所致输卵管损伤,如盆腔炎(PID)。
- 既往输卵管手术(即输卵管结扎术)。
- 既往异位妊娠。
- 宫内节育器(IUD)的使用:
- 25%~50%官内节育器者妊娠是异位的。
- 己烯雌酚(DES)暴露。
- 体外受精。
- 正在吸烟者。
- 超过一半的异位妊娠妇女无危险因素。

诊断

症状与体征

典型的三联征(闭经、阴道出血、腹痛)只存在于15%的异位妊娠妇女:

- 闭经(75%~95%)。
- 腹痛(80%~100%):
- 经常单侧。
- 异常阴道出血(50%~80%)。
- 妊娠症状(10%~25%)。
- 体位性低血压、头晕、晕厥(5%~35%)。
- 腹部压痛(有55%~95%)。
- 附件压痛(75%~90%)。
- 附件包块(35%~50%)。
- 宫颈摇摆痛(43%)。

病史

- 末次月经(LMP):
- 大多数的异位妊娠出现在末次月经后5~8周。
- 孕产史。
- 阴道出血。
- 疼痛的部位、性质和严重程度。
- 盆腔手术史、异位妊娠史和宫内节育器(IUD)。
- 生育治疗史。
- 性病史。

体格检查

- 评估腹膜刺激征。
- 盆腔检查:
- 注意子宫大小。
- 附件大小,肿块。
- 附件压痛。
- 阴道穹窿组织的存在。
- 宫颈运动触痛。
- 宫颈口开放或闭合。

基本检查

- 妊娠试验:
- 在育龄期的妇女阴道出血或腹痛,必须行尿或血清妊娠试验。
- 包括测试有近期人工流产或自然流产史、输卵管结扎史或宫内节育器使用史的患者。
- 定性试验阳性的患者行β人绒毛膜促性腺激素(β-HCG)定量试验。
- 生命体征不稳定:
- 2条大口径静脉注射。
- 血型和交叉配血,血红蛋白(Hg)/血细胞比容(HCT)。
- 如果立即可用,复苏的同时行床边超声(US)(经阴道优先)。
- 产科/妇科(OB/GYN)会诊,准备即刻手术治疗。
- 生命体征稳定:
- 快速测定Hg/HCT。
- 血型及Rh。
- 超声(经阴道首选)。

诊断检查与说明

实验室检查

- 尿妊娠试验可检测β-HCG水平为25~50 mU/L。
- 血清可检测β-HCG水平为25 mU/L。
- 定量血清β-HCG用于诊断和随访:
- 在正常妊娠早期每2日加倍(妊娠早期β-HCG<10 000 mU/L,8日至7周)。
- β-HCG在异位妊娠时增加较少。
- 与阴道超声关联会增加预测价值。
- 使用甲氨蝶呤治疗前的额外检查。
- 血常规。
- 肝功能。
- 血肌酐。

影像学检查

- 宫内妊娠的超声证据使异位妊娠的可能性更小:
- 异位妊娠是可能的。
- 双环孕囊、卵黄囊或胎极,以及子宫可见心跳,表明阳性宫内妊娠。
- 经阴道超声:4周时孕囊显示,5.5周时心脏搏动。
- 腹部超声:5~6周时孕囊显示,8周时心脏搏动。
- 22%的异位妊娠可看到复杂附件包块和盲管内液体,当它们存在时有94%的阳性预测值。
- 妊娠试验阳性伴没有确认的宫内妊娠和盆腔内的液体、异位妊娠出血的高风险。

诊断步骤/外科

- 超声连同β-HCG定量。
- β-HCG水平>6 500 mU/L的患者,超声上未见宫内孕囊者100%有异位妊娠的可能。
- β-HCG水平>6 500 mU/L的患者,宫内孕囊存在者94%有正常妊娠的可能。
- β-HCG水平<2 000 mU/L的患者,因太早以至于经腹部超声不能看见孕囊,故不能排除异位妊娠。
- β-HCG水平>2 000且<6 500 mU/L的患者,经阴道超声应见到宫内妊娠;如没有宫内妊娠应怀疑异位妊娠:
- 经阴道超声的HCG判别值在1 500~3 000 mU/L。
- 如果超声不可用,行后穹窿穿刺以评估腹腔积血。

鉴别诊断

- 妊娠试验阳性伴阴道出血:
- 自然流产。
- 宫颈炎。
- 创伤。
- 妊娠试验阳性,无宫内妊娠的证据:

- 完全流产。
- 早期先兆流产。
- 妊娠试验阳性，伴宫内妊娠的证据、腹痛或附件压痛：
- 感染性流产。
- 先兆流产。
- 破裂的黄体或卵巢囊肿。
- 卵巢扭转。
- 尿路感染。
- 肾结石。
- 胃肠炎。
- 阑尾炎。
- 异位妊娠(宫内妊娠＋异位)。
- 盆腔炎。

治疗

院前

警告：育龄女患者出现休克，可能有未确认的异位妊娠破裂。

初步稳定/治疗

- 生命体征不稳定：
- 气道管理，必要时行复苏。
- 经2条大口径静脉补液治疗，氧气，监测。
- 最初液体输注后仍低血压，予以特定型或O型血。
- 妇科会诊，立即转运至手术室行手术。
- 生命体征平稳：
- 超声上异位妊娠的证据：
  - 妇产科手术评估对比门诊甲氨蝶呤治疗。
  - 对于渴望未来生育的患者，甲氨蝶呤是最好的选择，否则手术仍是确定性治疗。
- 无异位妊娠证据[不明位置妊娠(PUL)：早期宫内妊娠对比早期异位妊娠]：
  - 理想妊娠：稳定、可靠的患者每48h连续的β-HCG，与妇产科医师协同。
  - 意外妊娠：扩张术和刮宫术，确定妊娠产物的存在。

急诊治疗/程序

甲氨蝶呤：仅在结合产科咨询和密切随访时才开始。

- 未破裂异位妊娠<3.5 cm的可靠患者。
- β-HCG水平<5 000 mU。
- 禁忌证：
- 血流动力学不稳定。
- 母乳喂养。
- 免疫缺陷。
- 已有血液病。
- 临床显著性贫血。
- 已知对甲氨蝶呤敏感。
- 活动性肺疾病。
- 消化性溃疡。
- 肝功能不全。
- 肾功能不全。
- 酒精中毒。
- 酒精性肝病。
- 相对禁忌证。
  - 异位肿块>4 cm。
  - β-HCG水平>5 000 mU。
  - 超声提示胎心搏动活跃。
  - 拒绝接受输血。
  - 无法随访。
- 最常见的剂量，单次剂量(50 mg/m^2)；在2、4和7日连续测β-HCG：
- 如果从第1日注射开始β-HCG下降<25%，则给予第二次剂量。
- 多剂量治疗与治疗失败的减少有关。
- 常见的副作用：
- 腹痛加重。
- 恶心、呕吐和腹泻。
- 腹痛加重通常发生在甲氨蝶呤开始后3～7日：
- 这些通常是输卵管流产。
- 排除异位破裂必须随访超声。
- 最常见的并发症，输卵管破裂占4%。
- 与甲氨蝶呤治疗失败相关的因素：
- 初始HCG>5 000 mU(5 000～9 999 mU/ml失败率达13%，>15 000 mU/ml失败率高达32%)。
- 超声上中等至大量的游离腹腔积液。
- 存在胎心活动。
- 预先处理使血清HCG水平在48h增加超过50%。

药物治疗

- 甲氨喋呤：50 mg/m^2，肌内注射或静脉推注×1。
- Rh阴性妇女使用罗加姆蛋白：
- 妊娠≤12周者：50 μg，肌内注射。
- 妊娠>12周者：300 μg，肌内注射。

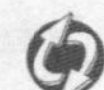

随访

进一步处理

入院指征

- 任何确诊的血流动力学不稳定的异位妊娠患者。
- 风险因素增加的不可靠患者，没有可用的超声，β-HCG>6 500 mU，无宫内妊娠证据应入院观察并进行连续的β-HCG测试。

出院指征

- 协同妇产科做出门诊处理的决定。
- 血流动力学稳定且可靠的患者，检查不能排除异位妊娠：
- 每2日严格随访β-HCG系列测试。
- 应在日志上记录患者电话号码以保证随访。
- 异位预警：下列情况患者应立即返回急诊室：
- 腹痛加剧。
- 阴道出血。
- 晕厥或头晕。
- 在安全排除异位妊娠前患者不能独处。
- 家人和朋友也应被指导异位妊娠破裂/出血的预警症状与体征。

转诊问题

当排除可能的异位妊娠时，电话咨询(至少)妇产科是必要的。

随访建议

所有妊娠试验阳性的患者和未经证实的宫内妊娠必须在妇产科随访。

要点和误区

- 育龄期妇女应经常行妊娠试验。
- 所有妊娠试验阳性妇女伴腹痛或阴道出血应查血清HCG和阴道超声。
- 确认异位妊娠的可能性，特别是在接受生育治疗的妇女。
- 被鉴定为异位妊娠并出院的患者，确保密切随访。

异烟肼中毒 Isoniazid Poisoning

Sean M. Bryant 何超 译

基础知识

描述

- 能够与5-硫酸吡哆醛(吡哆醇也就是维生素 B_6 的活性形式)相互作用并使其失去活性。
- 抑制吡哆醇磷酸激酶的活性，从而阻碍吡哆醇转化成其活性状态。
- 减少γ氨基丁酸(GABA)的产生。
  - 抑制由于GABA引起的中枢神经的兴奋和癫痫。
- 抑制乳酸脱氢酶，减少乳酸向丙酸的转化。
  - 影响离子通道，造成代谢性酸中毒。
- 慢性毒性：
  - 干扰烟酸的合成。
  - 在数月的治疗后会引起一种与糙皮病相类似的综合征(烟酸缺乏症)。
- 某些生物学行为与单胺氧化酶抑制剂类似：
  - 但躁狂、发汗、抑郁、分神的发生率较低。
- 药代动力学：
  - 吸收快速，吸收高峰在1～2 h。
  - 分布容积0.6 L/kg，同时蛋白结合经肾脏排泄。
  - 快速乙酰化酶的作用下半衰期<1 h，在某些肝脏乙酰化作用较慢的个体内半衰期为2～4 h。

病因

- 高危群体：
  - 移民。
  - 流浪者。
  - HIV感染者。
  - 嗜酒者。
  - 社会经济地位较低的群体。
- 慢乙酰化个体(60%的美洲人和20%的亚洲人)更容易形成慢性毒性。
- 半致死量在80～150 mg/kg。
- 摄入量<1.5 g会导致轻度中毒，摄入量≥10 g会导致死亡。

诊断

症状和体征

- 急性中毒：
  - 神经症状：
    - 意识状态改变。
    - 对于标准治疗方案无效的癫痫发作。
    - 情绪激动。
    - 昏迷。
    - 头晕。
    - 共济失调。
    - 反射亢进。
    - 口齿不清。
    - 出现幻觉。
    - 精神错乱。
  - 消化系统症状：
    - 恶心。
    - 呕吐。
  - 肾性症状：
    - 少尿。
    - 无尿。
  - 心血管症状：
    - 低血压。
    - 心动过速。
    - 休克。
    - 发绀。
  - 代谢症状：
    - 体温过高。
    - 离子通道异常所引起的代谢性酸中毒。
- 慢性中毒。
  - 神经系统症状：
    - 周围神经病变。
    - 视神经炎和视神经萎缩。
    - 精神错乱。
    - 失眠。
    - 眩晕。
    - 糙皮病。
- 胃肠型肝炎。
  - 肝衰竭、肝炎。
  - 恶心、呕吐、便秘。
  - 厌食。

诊断检查与说明

实验室检查

- 动脉血气分析。
  - 严重的代谢性酸中毒。
- 电解质、尿素、肌酐、葡萄糖。
  - 高阴离子间隙酸中毒。
  - 高血糖状态。
- 全血细胞计数。
  - 急性中毒。
    - 白细胞增多。
    - 嗜酸性粒细胞增多。
  - 慢性中毒。
    - 粒细胞缺乏。
    - 嗜酸性粒细胞增多。
    - 血细胞溶解。
    - 贫血。

影像学检查

- 胸部X线平片：
  - 肺部发现结核病灶时可怀疑异烟肼中毒。
  - 评估是否存在吸入性肺炎。
- 对于病史可疑的患者可进行CT或腰椎穿刺排查。

鉴别诊断

- 中毒：
  - 三环类抗抑郁药物。
  - 阿司匹林。
  - 茶碱。
  - 甲醇、乙二醇。
  - 锂。
  - 一氧化碳。
  - 氰化物。
  - 引起代谢性酸中毒的其他物质。
- 中枢神经系统：
  - 脑血管意外。
  - 颅内出血、肿物、创伤、脓肿。
- 低血糖。
- 尿毒症。
- 甲状腺功能亢进。

治疗

院前

收集患者服用的药物和药瓶以进行进一步的确认。

初步稳定/治疗

- ABC管理：
  - 充足的供氧。
  - 必要时进行气管插管。
  - 开放静脉通路。
  - 心电监测。
  - 输注生理盐水。
- 当患者发生意识障碍时输注纳洛酮、维生素 B_1，监测血糖。

急诊治疗/程序

- 维生素 B_6：

- 异烟肼中毒的特异性解毒剂。
- 目标：每 1 g 维生素 B_6 对抗 1 g 异烟肼（2～3 min 给予 1 g）。
- 对于未知剂量的异烟肼中毒给予 5 g 维生素 B_6。
- 对于持续性的昏迷和反复性惊厥，每 20 min 重复给药。

• 控制惊厥：
- 维生素 B_6 能够扭转 GABA 的缺乏。
- 苯二氮䓬类药物能够与维生素 B_6 产生协同作用。
- 苯妥英钠对疾病没有作用。

• 病情稳定后进行洗胃：
- 仅仅在患者拥有充分的气道保护并且 1 h 内出现危及生命的中毒症状时考虑洗胃。
- 活性炭与药物按 10 : 1 混合。

• 血液净化：
- 充分治疗后症状无好转。
- 患者症状持续同时出现肾衰竭。

• 碳酸氢钠：
- 惊厥控制后酸中毒通常会自动好转。

随访

进一步处理

入院指征

• 对于反复发作惊厥、严重酸中毒、昏迷、意识改变的患者收入 ICU 治疗。

• 难以控制的恶心、呕吐、消化系统溃疡病史或有自杀倾向的患者。

• 遵循当地毒物中心的规定。

出院指征

6 h 后无症状的患者。

随访建议

对于有自杀倾向或反复超剂量的患者进行精神科的干预随访。

要点和误区

• 对异烟肼中毒的不重视和治疗不充分：
- 标准治疗方案后的反复惊厥是异烟肼中毒的一个重要原因。
- 高乳酸引起的严重酸中毒会使惊厥患者病情恶化。

• 对于一个被捆绑住的患者不要忽略心电监测。

• 维生素 B_6 治疗的目标是等质量对抗异烟肼。

• 获得足够的静脉注射吡哆醇是一项挑战。

• 报道了用 NG 管成功地给药粉碎的吡哆醇。

• 使用维生素 B_6 治疗惊厥后患者仍昏迷，可适当增大剂量。

抑郁症 Depression

Jonathan Florman 谭美春 译

基础知识

描述

重性抑郁症：

• 情绪抑郁和相关体征和症状持续超过 2 周。

• 显著的患病率和死亡率，包括自杀风险。

• 通常和其他内科疾病共存。

病因

• 生物学疾病，它和一些神经递质系统紊乱有关，包括 5-羟色胺、去甲肾上腺素和多巴胺。

• 成因：
- 遗传因素。
- 内科疾病。
- 药物影响。
- 心理社会应激：抑郁通常伴随着不良生活事件、创伤、重要亲属或生活角色的丧失。

• 在妇女中有较高的患病率。

诊断

症状和体征

• 5 个或以上的症状至少持续 2 周：
- 情绪抑郁。
- 兴趣或乐趣减弱。
- 食欲变化，体重减少或增加。
- 睡眠障碍。
- 疲乏或能量损失。
- 专注力减弱。
- 感觉无价值或内疚。
- 反复的死亡或自杀的想法。
- 精神运动性激越或阻滞。
- 其中一个症状必须是情绪低落或兴趣或乐趣的缺失。

• 亚型：精神病特征，抑郁型，紧张性精神症，非典型，产后型，季节性。

• 可以是焦虑、激动或沉默寡言。

• 躯体相关症状：
- 虚弱，心神不安。
- 体重减少。
- 头痛及背痛。

病史

• 病程，严重程度，应激来源。

• 回顾抑郁症状（见前）。

• 既往病史（包括过去的治疗、住院史及自杀企图）。

• 过去精神病史。

• 药物（处方的和非处方的）。

• 药品滥用。

• 家族史。

• 社会和职业史；损失、转变、创伤和其他主要生活事件。

• 安全评定：
- 自杀风险。
- 评估自理能力与营养状况。

• 来自家庭或门诊医师的担保。

• 文化和语言的不同可能使评估复杂化，适当的时候用翻译人员。

体格检查

• 生命体征。

• 神经系统功能检查：
- 运动测试。
- 认知测试。

• 精神状态检查：情感和情绪、思维方式和内容。

老年人注意事项

• 注意医疗条件、药物的相互作用和副作用。

• 排除低活动性谵妄、早期痴呆。

儿科注意事项

• 在儿童和青少年，对抑郁的诊断可能是不同的。

• 在儿童，主要的抑郁症指标可能包括：
- 在学校、家里和社交能力的改变。

Y

- 睡眠的改变。
- 不合群。
- 躯体症状。
- 咨询儿童精神病学家。

注意

排除双相情感障碍：可能需要情绪稳定剂、抗精神病药，在双相情感障碍患者应用抗抑郁药也可能导致躁狂。

基本检查

- 确定重性抑郁的症状和体征。
- 排除相关的或并存的精神疾病，以及医疗状况和药物滥用。
- 安全评估。

诊断检查与说明

实验室检查

- 首选：
  - 全血细胞计数，化学检查包括电解质、尿素氮/肌酐、葡萄糖、钙、肝功能检查。
  - 尿液分析。
  - 血清和尿毒理学检查。
  - 甲状腺功能检验。
  - 维生素 B_{12} 和叶酸。
- 进一步检查，由病史和最初的检查结果指导：
  - HIV 测试、梅毒快速血清反应素实验、莱姆病。
  - ESR、CRP、ANA。

影像学检查

- 头颅 CT：推荐用于不典型表现或有局灶的神经学发现时。
- 检测肿瘤、脑卒中、白质病变时，脑 MRI 优于 CT。

鉴别诊断

- 精神疾病：
  - 情绪障碍。
  - 适应障碍。
  - 双相型障碍。
  - 焦虑性障碍
  - 急性应激反应、创伤后应激障碍。
  - 精神分裂症，分裂情感性障碍。
  - 人格障碍。
  - 饮食失调。
  - 药物诱发型情绪障碍。
- 可能引起或者表现为抑郁的医疗状况：
  - 药物引发：
    - 降压药。
    - 口服避孕药。
    - 类固醇。
    - 镇静催眠药。
    - 阿片类药物。
    - β受体阻滞剂。
  - 内分泌疾病：
    - 甲状腺功能减退。
    - 肾上腺皮质功能不全。
    - 性腺功能减退。
    - 产后、围绝经期和经前综合征。
  - 肿瘤：
    - 胰腺。
    - 肺。
    - 脑。
  - 神经系统疾病：
    - 痴呆（早期阶段或额叶型）。
    - 癫痫。
    - 帕金森病。
    - 多发性硬化。
    - 亨廷顿病。
    - 中风（脑卒中）。
    - 头部创伤、硬脑膜下血肿。
    - 正常压力脑积水。
  - 传染病：
    - 尿路感染。
    - HIV 感染。
    - 单核细胞增多症。
    - 莱姆螺旋体病
  - 营养性疾病：
    - 叶酸缺乏。
    - 糙皮病。
    - 维生素 B_{12} 缺乏。
  - 电解质紊乱。
  - 终末期肾脏、肝、肺和心血管疾病。
  - 阻塞性睡眠呼吸暂停。
  - 慢性疼痛综合征。

治疗

院前

- 确保患者和供养者安全。
- 了解当地关于强制性入院的法律。

初步稳定/治疗

- 安全：自杀的风险评估，暴力。
- 一般医学评估。
- 管理：
  - 适当时候一对一观察和防范自杀。
  - 处理潜在医学原因。

急诊治疗/程序

- 心理管理：
  - 富有同理心地倾听以及了解背景故事及相关压力。
  - 安慰和教育（举例来说，抑郁症是一种可治疗的情况）。
- 初始治疗措施：
  - 抗抑郁药物治疗可以开始用于一些已明确诊断和建立随访的患者。
  - 通常需要应用几周的抗抑郁治疗解决重性抑郁。
  - 小剂量苯二氮䓬类药物或精神安定剂可以用于相关的激动、失眠或精神错乱。
- 药物的选择基于：
  - 适应证、功效、既往用药反应。
  - 副作用和风险。
  - 便利、费用、有效性。
- 抗抑郁药可能应在几周内滴定：
  - 可能需要几周来充分反应。

一线治疗

- 选择性 5-羟色胺再吸收抑制剂（SSRI：氟西汀、帕罗西汀、舍曲林、西酞普兰、艾司西酞普兰）：
  - 耐受良好。
  - 不良反应可能包括：
    - 轻度恶心。
    - 头痛。
    - 焦虑，坐立不安，失眠。
    - 嗜睡。
    - 性功能障碍。
    - 体重增加。
  - 最小的药物过量风险。
- 多巴胺和去甲肾上腺素再吸收抑制剂（安非他酮）：
  - 可能导致激动，震颤，失眠。
  - 减少癫痫发作阈值。
  - 耐受良好，没有性功能不良反应。
- 去甲肾上腺素和 5-羟色胺调节剂（米氮平）：
  - 体重增加。
  - 镇静。
  - 静态平衡位。
  - 便秘。

二线治疗

- 5-羟色胺和去甲肾上腺素再吸收抑制剂（SNRI：文拉法辛、度洛西汀、去甲文拉法辛、左旋体米那普仑）：

Y

- 耐受良好。
- 可能对一些疼痛综合征患者有益。
- 不良反应与 SSRI 相似。

• 5-羟色胺调节剂(伏替西汀、维拉唑酮)。

- 恶心。
- 腹泻。
- 性功能副作用。

• 三环类抗抑郁剂(阿米替林、丙米嗪、去甲替林、氯米帕明):

- 抗胆碱作用。
- 体重增加。
- 体位性低血压(直立性低血压)。
- 镇静。
- 减少癫痫发作阈值。
- 心脏危险,药物过量风险。
- 去甲替林和去郁敏耐受性最好。

• 单胺氧化酶抑制剂(苯乙肼、强内心百乐明、司立吉林):

- 饮食和其他药物的限制来避免高血压危象和5-羟色胺综合征。
- 药物过量的危险。

老年人注意事项

• 老年人可能需要低剂量,小心留意潜在的药物交互作用。

• 警惕直立性低血压和胆碱能阻滞。

儿科注意事项

FDA 黑框警告:在一些有抑郁症的儿童、青少年或是年轻人中,抗抑郁剂可能增加自杀想法和行为的风险。

妊娠注意事项

在妊娠或哺乳期妇女要特别注意药物治疗的风险和益处,考虑咨询围生期精神病学专家。

注意

• 停药综合征:可发生在抗抑郁药物,特别是 SSRI 或 SNRI 中断、减少剂量或停药后。

• 可能包括流感样症状、失眠、恶心、失衡、感觉障碍。

随访

进一步处理

入院指征

• 自杀倾向或自杀高风险患者。参见自杀,风险评估。

• 极少或无法依靠社会支持。

• 症状严重需要持续观察或护理支持。

• 精神病特征。

• 如果患者拒绝治疗,并有伤害自身和他人风险,精神患者民事强制入院是必要的。

出院指征

• 低自杀风险。

• 充足的社会支持。

• 有效的密切随访。

转诊问题

• 门诊精神健康预约和/或未入院患者提供部分(日间)病房服务。

• 许多患者将受益于药物和心理联合治疗,或考虑认知行为疗法(CBT)。

• 在急诊科的个案处理或社会服务有助于问题的处理。

• 和其他服务提供者(包括初级保健医师)沟通协调。

随访建议

随访取决于疾病和风险的严重程度:

• 如果未入院,有显著症状的患者应该在1~2周随访。

• 当药物治疗开始,应该在1~2周随访中探视患者。

• 比较稳定的患者或那些较轻症状患者可以减少随访次数。

要点和误区

• 经历重大发病的抑郁症患者,可能有自残风险。

• 考虑其他表现为抑郁的疾病、同时共存的精神疾病和医疗状况、精神药滥用。

• 了解你的地区入院和强制收治的标准。

阴道出血 Vaginal Bleeding

Carla C. Valentine 张晟 林兆奋 译

基础知识

描述

• 通常出现在急诊。

• 多数患者病因良好。

• 一些患者有潜在性的致命病因。

• 关键是对阴道出血妇女做出合适的评估。

- 任何有生育能力的妇女阴道流血可能是妊娠。
- 月经和性生活史不能排除妊娠。

病因

妊娠相关

• 早孕:

- 宫外孕(异位妊娠)。
  ◦ 妊娠女性发生率为2%。
- 流产。
  ◦ 先兆流产、不完全流产、完全流产、稽留流产、难免流产、脓毒症。
- 葡萄胎妊娠。
- 创伤。

• 晚期妊娠:

- 前置胎盘。
- 胎盘早剥。
- 葡萄胎。
- 劳累。
- 创伤。

• 产后:

- 产后出血。
- 子宫外翻。
- 胎盘滞留。
- 子宫内膜炎。

非妊娠患者

• 异常子宫出血(以前是功能失调性子宫出血)。

• 功能失调性子宫出血。

• 解剖结构异常:

- 子宫平滑肌瘤。
- 子宫内膜息肉。
- 骨盆肿瘤。

• 子宫内膜萎缩:

- 最常见的绝经后妇女出血原因。

• 全身性疾病:

- 血管血友病。
- 特发性血小板减少性紫癜。

• 创伤。

• 异物。

• 感染。

诊断

症状和体征

病史

• 轻度头痛。
• 疲劳。
• 虚弱。
• 口干。
• 持续出血。
• 出血量：
- 卫生棉吸纳 5 ml。
- 棉垫能吸纳 5～15 ml。
• 轻度头痛。
• 疲劳。
• 虚弱。
• 口干。
• 末次月经日期。
• 家庭妊娠测试。
• 先前有宫外孕史。
• 血块。
• 月经史。
• 家族史。
• 血块。

体格检查

• 重要体征。
• 心肺检查。
• 腹部检查(妊娠子宫、肿块)。
• 骨盆检查。
- 出血源。
- 创伤证据。
- 子宫颈口是否开放。
• 若有神志改变说明出血量大有低血压。

基本检查

• 妊娠定性试验：
- 床旁尿妊娠检查为首选。
• 盆腔检查：
- 所有阴道出血患者都需要做。
- 子宫颈口是否开放。
- 妊娠后期需依靠超声。
◦ 是否存在前置胎盘。
- 如果患者有胎膜破裂，可以推后检查。
• 对所有适龄女性必须完成妊娠检查。
• 早孕：
- 血型 Rh。
- 超声检查。
- HCG 检查。
- 血细胞比容。
- 血型交叉配血。
◦ 宫外孕。
◦ 低血细胞比容。
◦ 血流动力学不稳定。
• 妊娠晚期：
- 血型 Rh。
- 胎心。
- 超声：
◦ 没有胎心。
◦ 没有宫内妊娠征象。
◦ 胎盘线不清。
- 如果出血量大要查血细胞比容。
- 行血型交叉配血，如果有前置胎盘和流产征象或血细胞比容低。
- 若胎盘早剥行 DIC 检测：
◦ 血小板、PT、APTT、纤维蛋白原、纤维蛋白原产物。
• 产后早期：
- 超声检查看是否有子宫残留组织。
- 血细胞比容。
- 考虑有子宫残留可行 β-HCG 检查。

诊断与说明

实验室检查

• HCG 定性定量检测。
• 如果出血量大要查血细胞比容。
• 血型 Rh。
• 考虑血小板减少可行血小板计数。
• 凝血功能障碍查 PT、APTT。
• 送组织血块行病理检查。

影像学检查

• 超声检查明确妊娠状况和其他情况。
• 超声分辨区：
- 经腹部超声：
◦ 检测妊娠囊 HCG＞6 500 mU/ml。
- 经阴道声。
◦ 检测妊娠囊 HCG 1 000～1 500 mU/ml 及以上。

鉴别诊断

• 异常子宫出血(AUB)。
• 宫外孕。
• 月经过多。
• 外因引起流产。
• 胎盘早剥。
• 前置胎盘。
• 产后出血。
• 平滑肌瘤。
• 盆腔肿块或肿瘤。
• 性交后出血。
• 外伤出血。
• 甲状腺功能不全。
• 出血性疾病。

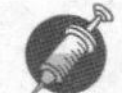

治疗

院前

• 当有大量出血或血压低时，静脉输注 1～2 L 生理盐水。
• 不稳定或孕妇高流量给氧。
• 妊娠晚期：
- 让患者取左侧卧位。

初步稳定/治疗

• 稳定生命体征，畅通气道。
• 心电监测。
• 不稳定或孕妇：给氧气支持。
• 低血压患者：建立两路静脉通道补充液体(1～2 L)。
• 血型交叉配血：
- 如果持续液体复苏血压仍低则输血。
- 对于难治的月经过多可以使用结合雌激素，25 mg 缓慢静滴 10～15 min，q4～6 h：
◦ 不要超过 4 次。

急诊治疗/程序

• 如果没有手术条件，要尽快安排患者转运。
• 对于阴道流血、妊娠和 Rh 阴性母亲可以使用免疫球蛋白。

妊娠早期

• 如果 B 超发现是宫外孕：
- 甲氨蝶呤按照标准使用。
- 但根本治疗手段还是手术。
• 如果 B 超发现是宫内孕：
- 将患者转移至产科，严密观察防止流产。
• 如果 B 超无法分辨是宫内孕还是宫外孕，并且 β-HCG 超过基准值：
- 不能排除宫外孕。
- 如果出血量不多血流动力学稳定，可以复查 β-HCG，并且门诊产科密切随诊 48 h。
- 严格的返回参数。
• 如果 B 超无法分辨是宫内孕还是宫外孕，并且 β-HCG 小于基准值：
- 患者稳定基本宫外孕可能性小，可出院。
- 复查 β-HCG，并且产科密切观察 48 h。
- 患者仍然有宫外孕可能。
• 完全性流产。
- 如果患者稳定且没有进行性出血，可以

出院。

• 不完全流产：

- 需要产科医师意见。
- 清宫术和待产管理。

• 过期流产：

- 待产管理。

• 感染性流产：

- 静脉使用抗生素。

• 葡萄胎：

- 化疗。

妊娠晚期

• 前置胎盘：

- 产科意见是否入院。

• 胎盘剥离：

- 引产。
- 可能引起胎儿死亡。
- 必要时可剖宫产术。

• 子宫脱出：

- 常后避免用力拖拉脐带。
- 迅速给子宫复位。
- 偶尔需要手术处理。

• 产后出血：

- 如果有胎盘残留将其取出。
- 如果出血严重危及生命可将子宫摘除。
- 偶尔需要手术处理。

早期产后出血

• 残留组织：

- 清宫刮宫术。

• 子宫内膜炎：

- 静脉用抗生素。

非妊娠

• 月经：

- 非甾体抗炎药和护理。

• 异常子宫出血：

- 35～40 岁及以下。
  ◦ 如果是无卵性异常子宫出血。
  ◦ 甲羟孕酮。
  ◦ 口服避孕药 7 日。
- 35～40 岁及以上。
  ◦ 超声检查并仔细触诊。
  ◦ 产科医师意见。
  ◦ 激素治疗前行子宫抽样。
  ◦ 子宫内膜癌也不能排除。

结构异常

• 子宫涂片活检是否有宫颈病变。

• 超声排除盆腔异物。

• 子宫肌瘤或子宫其他肿瘤。

• 保守治疗或子宫切除术。

■ 药物治疗

• 结合雌激素，25 mg 缓慢静滴 10～15 min，q4～6 h，直至出血停止：

- 如果无反应可以重复使用 1～2 次。

• 无卵性异常子宫出血：

- 甲羟孕酮：10 mg 口服，每日 1 次，在月经周期前 10 日服用。
- 炔诺酮或炔雌醇 1/35：每日 2 次×7 日。

• 丙种球蛋白：50 μg，肌内注射，妊娠<12 周。

• 丙种球蛋白：300 μg，肌内注射，妊娠>12 周。

 随访

■ 进一步处理

入院指征

• 宫外孕。

• 子宫脱出。

• 脓毒性流产。

• 胎盘早剥。

• 产后出血。

• 子宫内膜炎。

• 不稳定异常子宫出血

• 新诊断的葡萄胎。

出院指征

• 生命体征稳定。

• 确定的宫内孕。

• 宫外孕符合甲氨蝶呤出院标准。

• 孕妇但宫外孕风险低：

- 超声无发现。
- β-HCG 水平低于标准。

• 非孕妇的阴道出血但血流动力学稳定。

转诊问题

妇科和产科医师会诊。

■ 随访建议

妊娠 3 个月以内的出血又无明确宫内孕证据的需要产科医师 48 h 内随诊。

■ 患者教育

• 异位妊娠的预防措施：

- 迅速出现的不断加剧的腹部疼痛，阴道出血致卫生棉 1 h 浸透，持续 3～4 h，体温高于 100.4 ℉(38 ℃)，头晕或晕厥。
- 患者不能让其独处直到宫外孕能被排除为止。
- 家人与朋友也应当被告知宫外孕出现的一些表现。

要点和误区

• 妊娠试验适合于一切适龄女性。

• 如果是妊娠 3 个月以内的出血，分析是否存在宫外孕。

Y

阴道分泌物/阴道炎 Vaginal Discharge/Vaginitis

Elizabeth M. Foley · Carrie D. Tibbles 周秋香 毛恩强 译

 基础知识

■ 描述

• 阴道炎是外阴炎症反应并可伴有分泌物。

- 通常表现：痒、灼热感、刺激性、疼痛。
- 异常分泌物是指分泌物量增加，颜色改变。

• 一些患者的阴道分泌物正常：

- 子宫颈的腺体分泌清亮黏液，当暴露于空气时会变白或黄色。

■ 病因

• 细菌性阴道炎(BV)：

- 最常见的原因。
- 正常乳酸杆菌缺失(抗生素)。
- 无法维持阴道正常的酸碱度。
- 阴道正常菌群过度生长，如阴道加德纳菌、阴道支原体、动弯杆菌、普氏菌属、链球菌。

• 细菌感染：

- 滴虫性阴道炎。
- A 型链球菌。
- 金黄色葡萄球菌。

• 真菌感染：

- 假丝酵母菌(最常见)。
- 多有潜在的免疫功能缺陷:
  - 糖尿病。
  - HIV 感染。
- 化学刺激物。
- 异物。
- 萎缩性阴道炎:
  - 雌性激素缺乏。
- 过敏症。
- 胶原血管病。
- 单纯性疱疹病毒(HSV):
  - 外阴阴道炎。
  - 子宫颈炎。
- 硬化性苔藓。
- 瘘。

诊断

症状和体征

- 反常阴道分泌物。
- 阴道或外阴刺激。
- 局限疼痛。
- 性交疼痛。
- 皮肤红斑。
- 水肿。
- 排尿困难。
- 蜕皮。
- 异位。
- 可以无症状。

病史

- 症状的描述和持续时间。
- 分泌物的描述。
- 月经周期。
- 患者和性伴侣的性交史。
- 性生活的频率。
- 避孕药和抗生素用药史。
- 是否妊娠。
- 其他症状(如腹痛,需排除盆腔炎症疾病)。

体格检查

- 腹部触诊。
- 检查外阴、阴道口、阴道。
- 窥阴器检查。

基本检查

- 骨盆检查。
- 盐水和氢氧化钾预湿阴道分泌物。

诊断检查与说明

实验室检查

- β- HCG。
- 硝嗪试纸检测分泌物酸碱度:
  - 绝经期妇女 pH＜4.5。
  - pH＞4.5 提示细菌性阴道炎,滴虫阴道炎。
  - 念珠菌感染 pH 正常。
- 盐水预湿阴道分泌物:
  - 线索细胞:细菌性阴道炎。
  - 带鞭毛的微生物:滴虫性阴道炎。
  - 有多形核白细胞。
- 氢氧化钾预湿阴道分泌物:
  - 假菌丝、出芽酵母、念珠菌。
- 氢氧化钾预湿阴道分泌物测试:
  - 胺或其他异味提示细菌性阴道炎、滴虫性阴道炎。
- 毛滴虫快速检测:
  - 点对点检测。
  - 量油尺免疫层析法。
- 细菌脉冲测试:
  - 点对点检测。
  - 检测脯氨酸胺肽酶。
- 核酸探测检测,滴虫、阴道加德纳菌、白色念珠菌。
- 革兰染色:
  - 大的革兰阳性杆菌:乳酸杆菌。
  - 小的、变化的革兰球杆菌和弯曲杆菌:加德纳菌、普氏菌、克氏动弯菌。
- 阴道分泌物培养:
  - 加德纳菌不常规推荐。
  - 假丝酵母:对复发患者可做培养。
  - 动弯杆菌:金标准。
- 子宫颈棉拭子检测淋病。
- 单纯疱疹病毒,DFA 做病毒培养,Tzanck 涂片检测多形巨核细胞。
- 排尿困难时可做尿液检查/尿培养。
- 排除性传播感染:
  - GC 衣原体检测。
  - RPR 检测排除梅毒。
  - HIV 检测。

影像学检查

怀疑有瘘管形成时做检查。

鉴别诊断

- 尿路感染。
- 盆腔炎。
- 皮炎。
- 子宫颈炎的分泌物可被误认为阴道炎。
- 沙眼衣原体。
- 淋球菌。

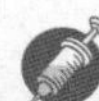

治疗

急诊治疗/程序

- 细菌性阴道炎:
  - 甲硝唑阴道凝胶剂:每日 1 次×5 日。
  - 甲硝唑:口服 500 mg,每日 2 次×7 日。
  - 克林霉素阴道乳膏:×7 日。
  - 克林霉素霜:每日 1 次×3 日。
  - 经妇产科医师诊治后开出处方。
  - 建议在使用甲硝唑治疗 24 h 内不接触含酒精饮料。
  - 患者的性伴侣不需要常规治疗。
  - 乳酸菌并不比安慰剂治疗效果好。
- 念珠菌病:
  - 单剂口服氟康唑。
  - 阴道塞咪唑类药物:×7 日。
  - 患者的性伴侣不需要常规治疗。
- 化学刺激物:
  - 避免刺激。
  - 坐浴,穿棉内裤。
- 异物:
  - 将异物移除。
  - 移除时需要适度镇静。
  - 如有感染存在给予适量抗生素。
- 衣原体性子宫颈炎:
  - 阿奇霉素口服 1 g。
  - 或使用 7 日多西环素、氧氟沙星、左旋氧氟沙星、红霉素。
  - 若合并淋球菌感染要一并治疗。
  - 患者的性伴侣需要常规治疗。
- 淋球菌性子宫颈炎:
  - 头孢曲松 250 mg 肌内注射×1 日,阿奇霉素口服 1 g×1 日,多西环素口服每日 2 次 100 mg×7 日。
  - 并不推荐口服头孢菌素。
  - 治疗合并的衣原体感染。
  - 患者的性伴侣需要常规治疗。
- 单纯疱疹病毒感染:
  - 对于初次感染,服用阿昔洛韦、法昔洛韦、伐昔洛韦 7～10 日,再次感染服用 5 日。
  - 利多卡因胶冻剂:缓解局部症状。
  - 排除其他原因致外阴溃疡,行 RPR、HIV 检测。
  - 患者的性伴侣常规治疗:
- 苔藓硬化:
  - 请妇产科医师会诊,使用雌激素药膏。
- 滴虫性阴道炎:
  - 灭滴灵:口服 2 g×1 次。
  - 替硝唑:口服 2 g×1 次。

Y

- 灭滴灵口服 500 mg，每日 2 次×7 日。
- 患者的性伴侣需要常规治疗。

• 性传播疾病：
- 建议患者禁止密切接触同伴，直至治愈。
- 进行性病、安全性行为、HIV、肝炎疫苗的有关教育。

妊娠注意事项

• 细菌性阴道炎：
- 用甲硝唑和克林霉素治疗有症状的孕妇。
- 对无症状的孕妇，找到患病依据再治疗。

• 念珠菌病：
- 仅推荐局部使用唑类药膏，不口服氟康唑。

• 衣原体性子宫颈炎：
- 阿奇霉素是一线用药。
- 不使用多西环素、氧氟沙星、左旋氧氟沙星。

• 滴虫性阴道炎：
- 妊娠早期用灭滴灵治疗，增加早产风险。
- 妊娠 37 周后使用甲硝唑口服 2 g×1 次。

儿科注意事项

• 考虑一些刺激物：泡沫剂、香皂、洗衣液。
• 考虑是否有性侵犯/性虐待。

药物治疗

• 阿昔洛韦：200 mg，口服，5 次/日×10 日，400 mg，每日 3 次×10 日（初次患病）；200 mg，口服，5 次/日×5 日，400 mg，每日 3 次×5 日（复发）。
• 阿奇霉素：1 g，口服×1。
• 2％布康唑霜：5 g，外用患处×3 日。
• 头孢曲松：125 mg 或 250 mg，肌内注射×1 次。
• 环丙沙星：500 mg，口服×1 次。
• 2％克林霉素霜：1 外用患处，睡前×7 日。
• 克林霉素霜 300 mg，口服，每日 2 次×7 日。
• 1％克霉素霜：5 g，外用患处×（7～14）日。
• 克霉素：100 mg，口服×7 日。
• 多西环素：100 mg，口服，每日 2 次×7 日。
• 琥珀酸盐乙烯红霉素：800 mg，口服，每日 4 次×7 日。
• 红霉素：500 mg，口服，每日 4 次×7 日。
• 法昔洛韦：250 mg，口服，每日 3 次×（7～10）日（初次患病）；125 mg，口服，每日 3 次×7 日（复发）。
• 氟康唑：150 mg，口服×1 日。
• 左氧氟沙星：500 mg，口服，每日 1 次×7 日。
• 甲硝唑：500 mg，口服，每日 2 次×7 日。
• 0.75％甲硝唑胶：外用患处×每日 1 次×5 日。
• 咪康唑：1 200 mg，外用患处×1。
• 制霉菌素：100 000 U：每晚用×14 日。
• 0.8％特康唑霜：5 g，外用患处×3 日。
• 0.4％特康唑霜：5 g，外用患处×7 日。
• 替硝唑：2 g，口服×1 日。
• 6.5％噻康唑霜：5 g，外用患处×1 日。
• 伐昔洛韦：1 g，口服，每日 2 次×（7～10）日（初次患病）；500 mg，口服，每日 2 次×（3～5）日；或 1 g，口服，每日 1 次×5 日（复发）。

随访

进一步处理

入院指征

• 播散性淋球菌感染。
• 因异物所致脓毒症。
• 盆腔炎有全身炎症反应。
• 因疼痛无法正常排便或排尿。

出院指征

大多都能出院，建议 1 周后随访。

转诊问题

• 阴道分泌物和阴道炎都可以在门诊经内科或妇科医师处理好。
- 建议 1 周后随访。

随访建议

• 保持良好的卫生习惯。
• 有下列情况建议患者找医师或到急诊就诊。
- 症状 3～5 日未见缓解。
- 出现腹部痛。
- 发热或寒战。
- 性交时出现疼痛。
- 下腰部或侧腹部疼痛。
- 排尿困难或尿频。

要点和误区

• 细菌性阴道炎 pH＞4.5。
• 念珠菌性阴道炎常发生在月经前，且使用抗生素、糖尿病、免疫功能低下者易患。
• 滴虫性阴道炎常发生在月经后，风险因素和性传播疾病相同，如性伴侣多性生活频繁。
• 需要同时治疗性伴侣的是淋球菌感染、衣原体感染和滴虫病。

阴茎持续勃起 Priapism

David Barlus　郑金浩　毛恩强 译

基础知识

描述

• 在没有性刺激时阴茎勃起（海绵体充血）持续时间很长，并且经常出现此现象，非常痛苦。
• 低血流性阴茎持续勃起：
- 最常见的发病机制。
- 静脉回流受阻。
- 常伴有疼痛。
- 缺血和血栓引起血流受阻，之后数小时内可出现低氧血症。
- 后遗症为阴茎纤维化和勃起功能障碍。

• 高血流性阴茎持续勃起：
- 少见。
- 阴茎动脉撕裂引起动脉血不受控制，流入阴茎海绵体。
- 往往无疼痛。
- 往往比低血流阴茎勃起的患者就诊晚。
- 阴茎缺血和勃起功能障碍后遗症不常见。

病因

• 先天性。

• 药物因素：
- 海绵体内注射治疗勃起功能障碍：
◦ 前列腺素 E_1。
◦ 罂粟碱。
◦ 酚妥拉明。
- 精神药物：
◦ 哈嗪嗪。
◦ 丁酰苯。
◦ 曲唑酮。
◦ 镇静催眠药。
◦ 选择性 5-羟色胺摄取抑制剂。
- 抗高血压药物：
◦ 哌唑嗪。
◦ 肼屈嗪。
◦ 酚苄明。
◦ 胍乙啶。
- 少数有关的药物：
◦ 磷酸二酯酶抑制剂：西地那非(伟哥)、他达拉非(西力士)、伐地他非(艾力达)。
◦ 抗凝剂。
◦ 可卡因。
◦ 大麻。
◦ 乙醇。
◦ 雄烯二酮。
- 毒素(黑寡妇、蝎子)。
• 血液系统疾病治疗引起的淤血：
- 镰状细胞性贫血(最常见的原因)。
- 白血病。
- 多发性骨髓瘤。
- 红细胞增多症。
• 阴茎或会阴部外伤(动脉撕裂及高血流性阴茎持续勃起)。
• 脊髓外伤(对肾上腺素能受体的抑制作用丧失)。
• 少见的病因：
- 骨盆肿瘤及感染。
- 浸润性疾病(如淀粉样变)。
- 透析。
- 含有脂肪乳的肠外营养。

儿科注意事项

镰刀状细胞贫血是引起阴茎持续勃起的最常见原因。

诊断

症状与体征

病史

• 详细了解病史，可能有助于分析持续阴茎勃起。
• 低血流性的持续阴茎勃起症：
- 疼痛。
- 有诱发条件或诱发药物使用史。
• 高血流性持续阴茎勃起症：
- 无疼痛。
- 阴茎外伤。

体格检查

• 通过临床表现进行诊断
• 检查阴茎血液灌注。
• 评估外伤伤势(如尿道损伤、直肠损伤)。
• 尿潴留。

基本检查

首要请泌尿外科会诊进行确诊，其次进行实验室检查及影像学检查。

诊断检查与说明

实验室检查

• 血常规。
• 凝血常规。
• 镰状细胞贫血对诊断有重要价值。

影像学检查

• 多普勒超声可以确诊高血流性阴茎持续勃起，定位动脉撕裂处。
• 血管造影可以定位栓塞破损的动脉。

诊断步骤/外科

对于分型困难的患者，海绵体血气分析有助于持续阴茎勃起的分型。
• 因为阴茎动脉有损伤的可能性，诊断需要泌尿外科医师协助。
• 高血流性阴茎持续勃起：结果基本正常。
• 低血流性阴茎持续勃起：低氧，偏酸($pH<7.25$，$O_2<30$ Torr)。

鉴别诊断

• 性兴奋引起的阴茎勃起无疼痛，持续时间短。
• 阴茎填充物是引起持续阴茎勃起的良性疾病。

治疗

院前

• 静脉用药。
• 吸氧。
• 止痛。

初步稳定/治疗

• 镇静镇痛。
• 静脉滴注液体。

急诊治疗/程序

• 泌尿外科急会诊。
• 下面是特殊病因以及相对应的治疗：
- 镰刀红细胞性贫血：
◦ 采集红细胞分离回输。
◦ 如果其他治疗均无效，可行高压氧治疗。
- 白血病：
◦ 化疗。
- 动脉破损：
◦ 可选择性的实施标准化治疗。
◦ 通过介入进行血管造影确定破损部位并栓塞治疗。
• 特布他林(β受体激动剂)：
- 可能有助于起始治疗低血流性阴茎持续勃起，但是单独使用没有效果。
• 以下为低血流性阴茎持续勃起的治疗方法，但经常需要海绵体内注射：
- 最好泌尿外科医师行海绵体内注射，若泌尿外科医师不能及时到达进行处理，可以按以下过程操作：
◦ 无菌准备区域。
◦ 注意麻醉镇静。
◦ 行局麻或阴茎神经阻滞麻醉(在阴茎根部注射利多卡因)。
◦ 至患者右方用左手握住患者阴茎。
◦ 用带有 19G 蝶翼型针头的注射器在 2 点钟或 10 点钟方向以 45°角穿刺海绵体，避免损伤腹侧尿道和背侧神经血管束。
◦ 一边挤压阴茎一边缓慢抽取血液直至抽到动脉血，一般抽取 30～50 ml。临床上常需要生理盐水冲洗。
◦ 不需要两侧海绵体都进行抽液，因为两侧海绵体相通。
◦ 如果阴茎出现肿胀，可能需要通过蝶翼型针注射苯肾上腺素(尽量减少对全身的作用)或肾上腺素。使用上述药物后注意监测心率和血压，防止心血管和脑血管疾病。它们可以抑制单胺氧化酶，但是有引起高血压甚至高血压危象的风险。
◦ 隔 45～55 min 可以重复注射。
◦ 以上处理均无效可能需要实施分流手术(如海绵体分流)。

药物治疗

一线用药

• 特布他林：0.25～0.5 mg 皮下注射(可能 15 min 需要重复一次)或 5 mg 口服。
• 苯肾上腺素：用 100 ml 生理盐水稀释 1 mg 苯肾上腺素，取 10 ml 阴茎海绵体内注射。

二线用药

肾上腺素：用 100 ml 生理盐水稀释 1 mg 苯肾上腺素，抽取 1～3 ml(最大剂量为 10 ml)进行阴茎海绵体内注射。

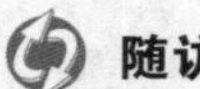

随访

进一步处理

入院指征

- 未经侵入性治疗而持续阴茎勃起的患者。
- 严重的基础疾病(镰刀状红细胞贫血、白血病)。

出院指征

- 阴茎完全消肿，经过观察数小时后不再复发。
- 经泌尿外科会诊同意出院。

转诊问题

单独安排 1 名泌尿外科医师对于所有阴茎持续勃起的患者进行随访。

随访建议

- 确定患有引起阴茎持续勃起的基础疾病。
- 停止使用药物。
- 建议患者再次出现阴茎持续勃起及时就诊。

要点和误区

- 在持续勃起的海绵体内注射血管活性药物，增加全身不良反应。
- 应及时进行持续勃起标准化治疗，以减少后续勃起障碍并发症。
- 应该告知患者即使得到及时成功的治疗，仍有后续完全性阴茎勃起障碍的可能。

阴茎折断 Penile Shaft Fracture

Ian R. Grover 赵铭 译

基础知识

描述

- 阴茎海绵体及白膜的外伤性破裂。
- 可能涉及尿道海绵体和尿道。
- 折断部位出现血肿。
- 损伤一般为单侧的、横向的。
- 折断部位大多位于阴茎近端。
- 勃起时，阴茎海绵体内压力接近动脉压，海绵体体积达到最大，使得白膜变薄，容易破裂。
- 阴茎勃起时海绵体拉伸至极限，纵向活动受限，仅能侧向活动。这导致阴茎底部发生弯曲，使其易受到侧向损伤以及海绵体折断。
- 25%～30%伴随部分或完全的尿道损伤。
- 发生于下列情形中阴茎勃起时的钝性挫伤。
  - 性行为。
  - 推拿。
  - 外物跌落。
  - 衣物缠结。
  - "Taghaandan"——中东地区的一种做法，通过弯曲勃起的阴茎来使其疲软。

病因

- 阴茎纤维性海绵体炎。
- 尿道炎。
- 由海绵体手术或创伤导致的薄弱瘢痕组织。

诊断

症状和体征

- 受伤时听到"啪"或"嘎吱"的响声。
- 迅速疲软。
- 阴茎剧痛。
- 损伤部位阴茎错位。
- 阴茎肿胀并有瘀斑。
- 如果有尿道损伤，尿道口可能会出血。
- 可能导致排尿困难，无法排尿，或排尿时因尿外渗而导致肿胀扩大。

病史

- 由受伤导致。
- 性行为时或性行为结束后突感疼痛。
- 性行为后尿道口出血。
- 勃起不良。
- 勃起时阴茎错位。
- 尿潴留或尿线无力。

体格检查

- 阴茎的肿胀或蓝黑变色，通常为单侧。
- 阴囊上可能会有瘀斑。
- 阴茎疲软、水肿，撕裂处有折角。
- 阴茎撕裂处有明显的缺损。
- 阴茎前端出血或血尿表明可能有尿道损伤。
- 晚期并发症可能出现尿道海绵体或尿道皮肤瘘。

基本检查

- 尿液分析。
- PT、APTT。
- 若怀疑有尿道损伤，则进行逆行性尿道造影。

诊断检查与说明

实验室检查

尿液分析结果：

- 可能有血或镜下血尿。
- 若患者正在使用香豆素或有出血性疾病，则进行 PT、APTT 检测。

影像学检查

- 对于所有疑似尿道损伤的情形都建议使用逆行性尿道造影：
  - 须在导尿前进行，注射时保持低压。
- 可能需要阴茎海绵体造影术和 MRI 以确认诊断及撕裂部位。
- 可用超声检查以确认疑似撕裂部位。

诊断步骤/外科

若阴茎海绵体造影术为阴性，但临床上折断的疑似程度很高，建议做诊断探查。

鉴别诊断

- 阴茎蜂窝织炎。
- 阴茎挫伤。
- 阴茎淋巴管炎。
- 阴茎肿瘤。
- 嵌顿包茎。
- 由缩窄环或其他结构导致的创伤。
- 尿道损伤。
- 血管破裂，尤其是背深静脉、背浅静脉或背动脉破裂。

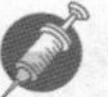

治疗

院前

- 优先处理其他外伤。
- 局部治疗：冰敷阴茎，用压舌板固定阴茎。
- 垫高损伤部位以减少肿胀。

初步稳定/治疗

- 疼痛控制。
- 若患者有尿道损伤或膀胱充盈，使用耻骨上膀胱造口术以减少不适。

急诊治疗/程序

- 急诊医师和泌尿科医师共同治疗，以恢复受损阴茎的外形及性功能和排尿功能。
- 急诊治疗主要针对止血，以防止进一步的并发症。
- 无需使用预防性抗生素。
- 除尿道损伤外都可采用导尿术。
- 泌尿系统评估和早期手术治疗能有效阻止勃起功能障碍、阳痿、阴茎畸形、尿道狭窄等并发症。
- 所有疑似或确诊病例都须有早期泌尿系统评估。

药物治疗

- 地西泮（安定）：2～5 mg，静脉注射，q1～6 h，焦虑时使用。
- 芬太尼：0.05～0.2 mg，静脉注射，q1 h，疼痛时使用。
- 氢吗啡酮：0.5～1 mg，静脉注射，q1～2 h，疼痛时使用。
- 劳拉西泮：0.5～1 mg，静脉注射，q1～6 h，焦虑时使用。
- 硫酸吗啡：0.1 mg/kg，静脉注射，q1 h，疼痛时使用。

随访

入院指征

注意

所有阴茎折断患者都必须住院并及时手术。

转诊问题

如不能及时诊断和治疗，达到转诊标准的患者需在初步稳定后转至适当的医院。

随访建议

与泌尿科医师随访以确保患者完全康复并恢复性功能及排尿功能。

要点和误区

- 阴茎断裂并不罕见。
- 性交和阴茎推拿是最主要的原因。
- 治疗延误是导致功能不健全的主要原因。
- 主要临床诊断：
  - 阴茎海绵体造影术、MRI、超声可用于确诊。
  - 早期手术修复很重要。

银屑病 Psoriasis

Allison Tadros · Erica B. Shaver 郑金浩 毛恩强 译

基础知识

描述

- 慢性、非接触传染、皮肤炎性病变。
- 增生性疾病。
- 近来归于自身免疫性疾病。
- 表现主要为红斑和银屑。
- 大部分侵袭肘部、膝盖、腰部、臀裂和阴茎头。
- 多达 1/3 的患者与关节炎相关，10%的患者有眼部表现。
- 发展情况无法预测，随着时间的推移可能看到病情的缓解情况。
- 确切的病因不明：可通过感染、压力、药物、外伤触发。
- 在夏季往往可以得到改善，可以与紫外线暴露有关。
- 和代谢综合征相关。
- 白种人和遗传性过敏性疾病的患者易感。
- 2 个发病高峰：年龄在 20～30 岁及 50～60 岁。
- 患者占美国总人口的 2.2%，女性比男性略多。
- 很少导致死亡，但在美国每年至少 100 人死于病情严重或治疗药物的不良反应。
- 部分临床表现：
  - 板块型银屑病（寻常性银屑病）。
    - 为最常见的类型（75%～80%）伴红斑、丘疹，边界清楚，常分布在头皮、后背、肘和膝的伸肌肌群侧。
  - 点滴型银屑病。
    - 突然出现大量分离的鲑鱼色点滴样的小丘疹，患者先前并没有银屑病病史。
    - 好发于鼻和近端肢体。
    - 常发于链球菌感染前，很快自行消失。
  - 脓疱型银屑病。
    - 呈现为广泛分布的红斑、鳞屑、浅薄的脓疱糜烂，偶尔单发于手掌和足掌。
    - 患者可出现中毒症状以及其他全身症状，如精神差、发热、腹泻。
    - 若全身分布，有潜在的病情加重甚至威胁生命，需收入院治疗。
  - 红皮病型银屑病：
    - 广泛分布的红斑、瘙痒伴细小鳞屑。
    - 增加感染、脱水的风险。
    - 常常需收住院治疗。
  - 指甲银屑病：
    - 在甲板上有凹痕，或者甲床出现改变。
    - 有超过 50%的患者有指甲的改变。
  - 屈侧银屑病。
    - 病变在屈侧引起损伤并且在皮褶处，由于皮褶处比较潮湿故并无鳞屑附着。
  - HIV 相关性银屑病：
    - 可能是 AIDS 的首发表现，在 HIV 感染人群中常见并且表现严重。
- 遗传学：
  - 有遗传倾向并且已经证实的遗传基因位置。
  - 40%的银屑病患者在一代亲属中有家族史。

病因

- 以往研究表明，红斑和银屑是由表皮干细胞和角化细胞过度增生、细胞周期减短、炎性浸润、血管病变引起的。

• 引发因素包括：
- 药物因素：
  ◦ 锂离子。
  ◦ β受体阻滞剂。
  ◦ 抗疟药物。
  ◦ 类固醇激素的减退。
  ◦ 非甾体抗炎药。
  ◦ 酒精。
  ◦ 碘化钾。
- 感染因素：
  ◦ 链球菌性咽炎。
  ◦ HIV感染。
  ◦ 葡萄球菌。
- 局部外伤：
  ◦ 冻疮。
  ◦ 晒伤。
  ◦ 近期皮肤外伤(同形反应)。
- 压力：情绪和身体。
- 冬天：
  ◦ 低阳光暴露。
  ◦ 气候干燥。
- 吸烟。
- 体重增加。

诊断

症状和体征

病史

• 长期有红斑银屑。
• 可能前期有诊断为银屑病的病史。
• 轻度瘙痒。
• 可能与以上引发因素有关。
• 特殊部位皮损。
• 有家族史。
• 日光暴露后缓解，或者如果复发，先发的皮损好转。
• 全身症状，如发热、关节疼痛。

体格检查

• 典型的皮肤红斑为圆形红色斑点，中央有银屑，白色银屑出现在伸肌表面。
• 红斑和银屑在脐、肘部应高度怀疑为银屑病。
• 奥斯皮茨征阳性：
- 刮除银屑时会有红斑和点状出血。
• 在黑种人中红斑皮损可能为灰白色。
• 头皮皮损可能被皮脂腺隐藏：
- 皮损扩展到头发边界外可提示银屑病。
• 指甲和甲剥离处粗糙毁损：
- 缠绕指甲的黄色或棕色带有助于区分银屑病和甲真菌病。
• 患有斑块状银屑病的患者可能伴有银屑病关节炎：
- 常常影响上肢和下肢的远端关节。
• 不对称的少关节型关节炎：
- 银屑病患者中有70%的发病率。
- 关节旁组织肿胀。
- 受侵犯的手指、足趾呈“香肠状”。

基本检查

• 诊断为临床诊断。
• 没有检验指标可以确诊或排除其他疾病。

诊断检查与说明

实验室检查

• 没有实验室检查可以确诊。
• 红皮病型和脓疱型银屑病的红细胞沉降率升高。
• 链球菌培养阳性，根据效价考虑为滴状银屑病。
• 低钙血症和白细胞增多常见于脓疱型银屑病。
• 风湿免疫指标。
• 尿酸水平可能有所升高。
• 开始药物治疗前应进行血细胞、肝功能、肾功能结核等基本情况筛查。

影像学检查

• 银屑病关节炎上下肢X线片可能有异常。
• X线片可能显示患有骶髂关节炎和强直性脊柱炎。

鉴别诊断

根据发病部位认真鉴别：
• 头皮：皮脂溢出。
• 弯曲皮皱处：
- 念珠菌病。
- 摩擦疹。
- 湿疹。
• 指甲：甲真菌病。
• 躯干和四肢：
- 钱币状湿疹。
- 毛发红糠疹或红色毛发角化病。
- 癣。
- 系统性红斑狼疮。
- 梅毒。
- 神经性皮炎。
- 过敏性药疹。
- 蕈样肉芽肿病。
- 鳞状细胞癌。

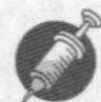

治疗

院前

• 维持常规的预防措施。
• 建立静脉通路，控制疼痛。

初步稳定/治疗

• 常规液体复苏的目的为纠正脱水和电解质紊乱。
• 治疗脓毒症：
- 血、尿、皮损培养。
• 避免全身使用糖皮质激素，全身使用糖皮质激素可能引起严重并发症。

急诊治疗/程序

• 告知患者银屑病的慢性病程，没有治愈方法。
• 治疗费用可能比较昂贵，患者依从性差。
• 在轻症患者可以暂缓治疗。
• 银屑病患者有以下3种治疗类型：
- 局部治疗。
- 全身治疗。
- 光疗。
• 局部治疗是急诊诊疗过程中最常用的治疗方式。
• 全身治疗往往在局部治疗和光疗无效的情况下使用，请皮肤科医师会诊。
• 以下为全身治疗的禁忌证：
- 泛发性脓疱型银屑病。
- 非常活跃的银屑病关节炎。
- 考虑可严重致残的银屑病。
• 光疗不是急诊治疗的方式。
• 在病情严重的病例需皮肤科会诊。

药物治疗

• 轻中度患者：
- 通常只局部治疗。
- 没有单独的药物可以对所有患者有效。
- 润肤剂：
  ◦ 对斑状银屑病效果好。
  ◦ 油脂效果最好，但部分患者不能耐受。
- 局部激素：
  ◦ 控制此种疾病发展的主要治疗方式。
  ◦ 可以单一使用，每日1～2次，或者和润肤剂共同使用。
  ◦ 一旦有效可考虑减量使用。
  ◦ 可能需要更换药物。
  ◦ 封闭敷料可以提高疗效。
- 水杨酸：

◦ 局部使用角质解离剂。
◦ 若全身使用阿司匹林要引起注意。
- 煤焦油制剂：
◦ 需要和局部激素联合使用。
◦ 新剂型杂质更少。
- 维生素D类似物：
◦ 卡泊三醇和骨化三醇。
- 他佐罗汀：
◦ 外用0.1%维生素A乳霜。
◦ 妊娠级用药。
- 他克莫司：
◦ 局部治疗用于皮皱褶银屑病或面部皮损。
◦ 可降低类固醇并减轻激素引起的萎缩。
• 中重症患者：
- 以上治疗药物可以和光疗及全身用药联合使用。
- 光疗。
◦ 紫外线照射用于抗增殖抗炎性反应。
◦ 户外紫外线(UVB)往往联合1种以上局部用药，有效率在80%以上。
◦ 在滴状银屑病患者可以单独应用户外紫外线。
◦ 补骨脂素长波紫外线(PUVA)治疗联合全身药物(补骨脂素)效果更佳。
◦ 每周治疗2~3次。
- 全身药物：可能与以上药物有各种组合方式联合使用：
◦ 皮肤科会诊后使用。
◦ 甲氨蝶呤(免疫抑制剂)：肝肾功能和造血功能正常后使用，孕妇禁用。
◦ 维生素A：可能引起皮肤干燥症、皲缩变红变柔软。
◦ 全身性糖皮质激素：不良反应为医源性库欣综合征；红皮病型银屑病患者病情危重的时候考虑使用。
◦ 环孢素：与皮肤科医师协商使用。
- 注射免疫抑制剂：依那西普和阿来法塞。

随访

进一步处理

入院指征

> **注意**
>
> 上面提到急性红皮病型银屑病和急性脓疱型银屑病，依据准条件进行支持治疗和系统治疗。

出院指征

• 提醒患者此病没有传染性。
• 告诫患者避免皮肤外伤和暴晒。
• 向患者宣教避免使用引起银屑病发病的药物。
• 推荐患者访问 www. psoriasis. org。

儿科注意事项

• 有10%~15%的患者发生在10岁以下。
• 常见的发病位置包括面部和皮肤皱褶处；脓疱疮型和红皮病型不常见。
• 许多患儿有重要的心理因素影响疾病发生。

妊娠注意事项

许多用于治疗银屑病的药物对妊娠期妇女禁忌使用。

转诊问题

• 大多数银屑病患者都愿意转至皮肤科。
• 银屑病患者可能需要家庭医师或精神科医师治疗影响生活质量的症状。

随访建议

后续家庭医师或皮肤科医师评估治疗效果。

要点和误区

• 脓疱型银屑病患者有引起全身严重疾病的风险。
• 红皮病型银屑病有脱水风险，治疗可能与重度烧伤患者相似。
• 治疗在几日内没有作用，往往需要数周见效。

婴儿猝死 Sudden Infant Death Syndrome (SIDS)

Kristine Knuti Rodrigues · Genie E. Roosevelt 江伟伟 李文放 译

基础知识

描述

• 1岁以下的婴儿意外死亡，通常在入睡前无异常。
• 在彻底调查尸检、死亡现场检查、情况调查和家庭及婴儿病史回顾后，死亡仍然无法解释。
• 婴儿1个月至1岁的主要死亡原因。自1994年启动了“仰卧位睡眠运动”计划以来，发病率显著下降：
- 1992年：120人死亡/10万正常出生(美国)。
- 2001年：56人死亡/10万正常出生(美国)。
- 2001—2006年没有变化。
• 1~4月龄是发生SIDS的高峰期：
- 90%发生在<6个月的婴儿。
- 2%发生在>10个月的婴儿。
• 种族差异：2006年每10万名新生儿中的死亡人数，在所有人中为54.5；非洲西班牙裔白色人种中为55.6；非西班牙裔黑色人种中为103.8；美洲印第安人/阿拉斯加原住民中为119.4；亚洲裔美国人或太平洋岛民中为22.8；西班牙裔中为27。
• 仰卧位明显降低发病率(“仰卧位睡眠运动”)。在婴儿中做仰卧位处理最初在欧洲开始，然后在美国开始应用。

病因

• 最有可能是多元化的。
• SIDS婴儿可能有易感因素，这些因素很容易受外在和内在压力因素影响。
• 潜在的压力因素包括贫血、先天性疾病、心律失常、电解质异常、遗传缺陷、感染、代谢紊乱、神经系统事件、窒息、外伤、上呼吸道阻塞。
• 产妇和产前风险因素：
- 酒精和非法药物使用。
- 宫内生长受限。
- 较低的社会经济地位。
- 产前护理不佳。
- 之前兄弟姐妹有SIDS。
- 妊娠间隔较短。
- 抽烟。
- 年龄较小。
• 婴儿危险因素：
- 共用床位。
- 暴露于环境吸烟。
- 胃食管反流(GER)。

- 高热。
- 出生体重低，早产。
- 男性。
- 软床铺，床面软。
- 最近有发热。

• 仰卧睡姿、哺乳和奶嘴的使用都是保护性的。

• 没有证据表明家庭监测能够阻止 SIDS。

诊断

体征和症状

病史

• 没有显著的预先存在的体征或症状来提醒看护人员。

• 不可预料的。

• 大多数婴儿在放到床上前看起来很正常。

• 在睡觉时发生死亡。

• 通常情况下，死亡是安静的，没有任何的挣扎。

• 没有死亡的临床或病理解释。

• 生命威胁事件（ALTE）是一个令看护者害怕的急性事件：
- 表现为呼吸暂停（中枢或阻塞性）引起皮肤颜色变化（发绀、苍白）或伴有软弱、窒息和/或恶心。
- 应将婴儿运送到医院进行评估和监测。
- 从 ALTE 恢复后，由临床医师进行评估时表现良好。
- 与 SIDS 风险增加有关。

体格检查

• 在此之前，婴儿看起来健康并且表现出色，发育良好，并且营养良好。

• 如果事件是短暂的并且是自限的，那么事件发生后评估良好。

• 存活婴儿的潜在并发症包括肺水肿、吸入性肺炎和继发于缺氧的神经系统后遗症，包括癫痫发作。

基本检查

• SIDS 是排除性诊断，因此需要进行评估以确定主要和/或次要的状况。

• 彻底调查死亡现场：
- 环境隐患（温度、表面、床上用品、床位共享）。
- 婴儿睡觉的位置。
- 父母、家人和照顾者的采访。
- 从死亡现场检查可能相关的物品。
- 保持对家庭的敏感性，因为调查可能对他们来说很困难。

• 回顾婴儿和家庭的既往史：
- 产前、围生期和产后婴儿病史。
- 家庭医学和社会史学，特别是母亲。

• 调查家庭的影响：
- 调查期间，家庭非常脆弱。
- 可以帮助他们渡过悲伤期。

诊断检查与说明

实验室检查

• 反映发作性质和患者状况的选择性研究。

• 动脉/静脉血气。

• 血培养和其他败血症检查。

• 血常规。

• 心电图。

• 评估家族性心律失常，如长 QT 综合征，包括家族成员。

• 脑电图。

• 电解质包括钙、镁和磷和肝功能。

• 毒物鉴定。

• 尿酸和培养。

影像学检查

• 胸部 X 线片评估心肺状态。

• 骨骼调查评估是否有儿童虐待（可由病理学家进行）。

• 如果儿童存活，评估颅内病变，行头颅 CT。

• 上消化道胃酸评估胃食管反流。

诊断步骤/外科

• 尸检：
- 美国大多数州要求对潜在的 SIDS 患者进行尸体解剖。
- 尸检是重要的，因为 SIDS 是排除性的诊断。
- 包括组织样本及总体检查，对重要器官的详细的检查。
- SIDS 患者尸检发现其病性可能与以下有关：
  ◦ 先天性心肌病。
  ◦ 心脏横纹肌瘤。
  ◦ 结节性硬化症。
  ◦ 罕见的遗传/代谢疾病。
  ◦ 病毒性心肌炎。
  ◦ 颅内动静脉畸形。

鉴别诊断

• 心血管系统：
- 冠状动脉异常。
- 主动脉瓣狭窄。
- 心肌病。
- 心律失常。
- 心肌炎。

• 呼吸系统：
- 误吸。
- 窒息。

• 感染：
- 肉毒杆菌中毒。
- 细支气管炎和呼吸道合胞病毒。
- 脑炎。
- 脑膜炎。
- 百日咳。
- 脓毒血症。

• 中枢系统：
- 动静脉畸形。
- 中枢通气不足。
- 神经肌肉疾病。
- 癫痫发作。
- 结节性硬化症。

• 消化系统：
- 胃食管反流。
- 腹泻。
- 胰腺炎。
- 肠扭转。

• 内分泌系统：
- 肉碱缺乏。
- 先天性肾上腺皮质增生。
- 糖原贮积病。
- 长链或中链酰基辅酶 A 缺乏症。
- 尿素循环缺陷。

• 全身表现：
- 虐待儿童。
- 脱水。
- 中毒。
- 高热。

治疗

• 在现场进行复苏，并在转运途中维持复苏。

• 少数情况下，婴儿在现场发声，综合社会因素和临床情况。在医疗指导下，可中止复苏。

院前

• 家庭复苏。

• 评估环境，确定有无虐待。

初步稳定/治疗

• 评估并维持生命体征（床旁）。

• 如果无法建立静脉通路，可通过气管给药（阿托品、肾上腺素、利多卡因和纳洛酮）。

• 监测生命体征：连续监测血压、心率、呼吸和氧饱和度。

• 进行彻底的体格检查，寻找意外伤害和故意伤害。

Y

• 评估现场、家庭成员和其他照顾者。

急诊治疗/程序

• 按照程序，院前人员对患儿进行复苏：

- 鼓励医疗人员培训家庭成员复苏，以进行现场复苏。

• 如果复苏失败并且未明确诊断，则不应告知双亲死因是SIDS：

- 在与父母交谈时，提及死因可能是SIDS。
- 直到完成尸体解剖、死亡现场调查、询问婴儿和家庭的病史后才能做出诊断。

• 家庭支持：

- 如果复苏不成功，那么关注点应该集中在家庭上。如果正在进行复苏，家庭的沟通和支持至关重要。
- 所有家庭成员和看护人都受到影响，他们经历了悲伤、内疚、失败和不满。
- 一些父母希望在复苏失败后，安静地陪着婴儿。
- 家庭在不同文化中有不同的定义，急诊应该尝试满足家庭的文化需求和期望。

• 急诊人员支持：

- 对所有参与婴幼儿护理的员工（包括急诊人员）应进行急诊报告。重要的是，让人们表达自己的感受，在支持的环境中自由地处理事件。

随访

进一步处理

入院指征

• 在首次复苏和稳定后，对ALTE的婴儿进行评估和监测。

• 大多数高危婴儿有以下1个情况：明显需要入院，有明显的病史，24 h内>1次ALTE。

出院指征

通常有观察和监测记录患者的家庭发作和支持情况。

转诊问题

• 所有存活的婴儿都应该进行儿科会诊。

• 需要家庭支持。

要点和误区

SIDS或ALTE的婴儿应适当地复苏。尸检对于诊断至关重要，应被视为强制性要求。

婴儿烦躁 Irritable Infant

David H. Rubin　何超 译

基础知识

描述

• 在白天某些特定的时期内，经常是接近傍晚的时间内，大多数婴儿会表现为易激惹：

- 正常婴儿的哭声在6周龄时为3 h/d，逐渐减少直到16周龄时。
- 在婴儿出生后的第一个6个月内，1个月的婴儿最容易出现啼哭。

• 我们所说的刺激性婴儿是基于与婴儿的正常行为特征的比较。

• 腹痛或不明原因的婴儿过度哭闹，是婴儿哭闹的最常见原因，在健康婴儿中的发生率占25%：

- 突发剧烈的尖叫伴随出现阵发的肠腔过气感。
- 通常在婴儿2～3周的时候开始出现，持续12周的时间，每日持续3 h。
- 需要进行排除性诊断。

病因

• 咬伤：蜘蛛或昆虫的咬伤。

• 烫伤。

• 心源性因素：室上性心动过速、充血性心力衰竭、左冠状动脉畸形、主动脉狭窄、心内膜炎、心肌炎。

• 对儿童的虐待。

• 角膜擦伤或眼内异物。

• 尿布带来的不适。

• 白喉、百日咳、破伤风（百白破）或其他疫苗带来的反应。

• 内分泌或代谢性因素：先天性代谢异常、代谢性酸中毒、高钠血症、低血糖、低钙血症或由母体甲状腺激素经胎盘传给婴儿刺激甲状腺球蛋白所引起的甲亢。

• 骨折或异物刺激：毛发对于阴茎或足趾的刺激。

• 胃肠道因素：胃肠炎、疝气、胃食管反流、食管炎、肠扭转、便秘、牛乳蛋白的不耐受、肛裂、肛瘘、阑尾炎。

• 泌尿生殖因素：嵌顿性疝、睾丸扭转、尿潴留。

• 感染：系统性的。

• 缺铁或贫血。

• 药物性或毒性因素：阿司匹林、抗组胺类药物、阿托品、肾上腺素、某些偏方、水银（汞）中毒。

• 脑膜炎。

• 少数急性炎症：上呼吸道感染、中耳炎、鹅口疮、龈口炎。

• 神经因素：颅内压增高、脑积水、颅内出血、硬膜下或硬膜外血肿、颅骨骨折。

• 骨髓炎。

• 父母的焦虑。

• 肺炎。

• 镰状细胞危象。

• 严重营养不良。

• 牙齿因素。

• 创伤。

• 泌尿道感染。

• 血管因素。

诊断

症状和体征

病史

完整的病史特点：包括出生时的病史、日常的喂养信息和啼哭特点。

体格检查

• 测量重要的体征包括肛温和指脉氧饱和度。

• 测量身高、体重和头围。

• 将婴儿脱尽衣物进行全面的体格检查。

基本检查

根据对病史的理解和体格检查的发现选择检查项目，这需要一定的专科知识。

实验室检查

• 全血细胞计数、尿液分析、生化检查，根据病史及体格检查结果选择细菌培养。

• 必要时监测血糖。

• 当存在消化体统症状或体征时检查粪便血细胞计数。

影像学检查

• 胸部 X 线检查排除心肺疾病。

• 必要时进行骨骼 X 线片。

• 根据病史及体格检查选择进行头部或胸部 CT。

• 钡灌肠造影成像。

诊断步骤/外科

• 荧光素眼部检查。

• 心电图。

鉴别诊断

根据病因的介绍，这需要将良性或自限性疾病与威胁生命的疾病鉴别。

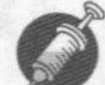

治疗

院前

依据病史、体格检查和实验室检查决定。

初步稳定/治疗

• 维持基础生命体征：稳定气道、呼吸和循环。

• 立即清除碎片或止血带的压迫。

急诊治疗/程序

• 对于婴儿最初的病情评估要注意婴儿与家长的沟通反应和基本的生命体征。

• 当肠绞痛发作时要对婴儿进行充分的安抚，避免如咖啡、可乐的刺激，减少白天的睡眠时间：

- 食用大豆或易于水解的婴儿乳酪食品会使病情有所缓解。
- 家长需要适当舒缓紧张的情绪。
- 尚无非常有效的药物治疗方案。
- 服用益生菌会有一定帮助。

• 对患者要给予一定的精神支持、心理安慰和密切的随访。

• 对患儿可以适当延长随访观察的周期。

药物治疗

依据潜在病因而定。

一线用药

依据潜在病因而定。

二线用药

依据潜在病因而定。

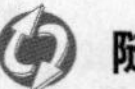

随访

进一步处理

入院指征

• 存在威胁生命的潜在风险。

• 由于婴儿的啼哭所带来的父母的精神极度紧张。

出院指征

• 无严重的病情。

• 患者家属要求。

• 需要一定的后续随访，重视患者父母的担心和忧虑。

随访建议

推荐长期的随访。

要点和误区

• 引起婴儿刺激性啼哭的威胁生命的病因：

- 心血管因素：室上性心动过速、充血性心力衰竭、心内膜炎或心肌炎。
- 神经性因素：硬膜下或硬膜外出血、脑膜炎、颅内出血、颅内压增高、颅骨骨折。
- 消化性因素：肠扭转、肠套叠、阑尾炎、腹膜炎。
- 代谢性因素：代谢性酸中毒、电解质紊乱。
- 泌尿性因素：泌尿道感染、睾丸扭转、嵌顿性疝。
- 感染：全身或局部的。
- 呼吸性因素：异物阻塞、肺炎、气胸。
- 皮肤性因素：绞窄性痔。
- 中毒性因素：摄入毒性物质及毒性物质所引起的机体免疫反应。
- 创伤。
- 眼科性因素：角膜擦伤、青光眼。
- 其他因素：虐待儿童，母体经由胎盘传给婴儿各种药物都可能引起婴儿烦躁。

• 对于患病婴儿在开具实验室检查和影像学检查之前需要进行详细的病史的询问和完整的体格检查。

硬膜外脓肿 Epidural Abscess

Richard S. Krause　单怡 译

Y

基础知识

描述

• 硬膜外间隙少见的化脓性感染：

- 发生率为(2～25)/10 万。

• 胸椎最常见，其次为腰椎和颈椎。

病因

• 主要由一个感染灶经血行播散(约 50%)或直接蔓延造成：

- 1/3 不能明确感染灶。

• 最常见的感染源是皮肤感染：

- 任何化脓感染均可能成为感染源。

• 金黄色葡萄球菌感染占 50%以上：

- 最常见的是 MRSA。
- 其次为链球菌。

• 流感嗜血杆菌、革兰阴性杆菌、分枝杆菌、厌氧菌、凝固酶阴性葡萄球菌、真菌及混合感染也可引起。

• 硬膜外导管或脊柱手术的并发症。

• 腰椎穿刺的少见并发症(多见于反复穿刺)。

儿科注意事项

• 和成人表现相似，可表现为后背痛、发热、神经系统症状及非特异性全身症状。

• 婴儿可能仅表现为发热、易激惹及脑膜炎表现。

• 括约肌功能障碍较常见。

• 常继发于血行播散。

• 感染部位和致病菌与成人类似。

诊断

症状和体征

• 发热和严重的后背痛“红旗症”提示病情严重：

- 如有神经性痛或神经功能紊乱，硬膜外脓肿可能性大。

• 典型表现：

- 严重的进展性后背痛(多为神经痛)。
- 发热。
- 神经功能障碍:
  - 肌力下降及瘫痪。
  - 感觉障碍。
  - 括约肌功能障碍。
  - 可有脓毒症表现,但不伴明显后背痛。
- 发生于包括婴幼儿在内的任何年龄段:
  - 发病高峰是60～70岁。
- 多数患者有高危因素:
  - 静脉药物滥用。
  - 糖尿病。
  - 恶性肿瘤。
  - 长期使用糖皮质激素。
  - 慢性酒精中毒。
  - 置管或脊髓手术。
  - 留置硬膜外导管或硬膜外注射。
  - 留置血管内导管。
- 无明确诱因时亦可发生。

既往史

- 后背痛。
- 发热。
- 神经功能障碍:
  - 肌无力。
  - 感觉异常。
  - 失禁。

体格检查

- 发热。
- 脊柱局部压痛和红斑。
- 神经功能障碍。
- 静脉滥用药物或其他诱因。

基本检查

- 怀疑该诊断时病史应询问诱因。
- 体格检查(感染源、局部脊柱压痛及神经系统表现):
  - 括约肌张力减弱。
  - 鞍区感觉缺失。
  - 下肢无力。
- 残余尿量或超声检查:
  - 年轻人残余尿量应<50 ml。
  - 老年人残余尿量应<100 ml。
- 红细胞沉降率(ESR)。
- MRI平扫或增强均可用于诊断:
  - 若无MRI,可行增强CT或脊髓造影。
  - 怀疑硬膜外脓肿时需紧急行影像学检查。

诊断检查与说明

实验室检查

- 大多数常有ESR增快(约100%),但无特异性。
  - ESR正常提示诊断可能性小。
- CRP多升高。
- 血培养多为阳性(60%)。
- 白细胞增多伴核左移多见(70%)。
- CSF多异常,但无诊断价值,怀疑该诊断时应避免常规腰椎穿刺(可能会导致脑膜炎)。

影像学检查

- MRI平扫或增强敏感度高(90%):
  - 在 T_2 加权像显示高信号病灶。
- 无MRI或脊髓造影时可行增强CT。
- 脊髓造影敏感,但有播散的风险。
- X线平片多有异常,但非特异。

鉴别诊断

- 因发病率低及表现不典型,诊断较困难:
  - 诊断前多科会诊。
  - 大多初步诊断为良性的肌肉骨骼病变:肌肉或韧带疼痛、退行性关节炎、压缩性骨折、椎间盘性疼痛。
- 后背痛、伴发热及全身表现:
  - 脊髓炎。
  - 脊柱肿瘤。
  - 脑膜炎(与颈椎硬膜下脓肿相似,但细菌性脑膜炎多伴有异常的精神状态)。
  - 椎间盘炎。
  - 肾盂肾炎。
- 伴有神经系统症状的后背痛:
  - 脊髓受压。
  - 脊髓缺血。
  - 椎间盘突出。

儿科注意事项

发热、后背痛,怀疑硬膜下脓肿时应紧急行MRI。

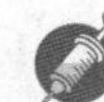

治疗

院前

若怀疑创伤或骨折,脊髓制动。

初步稳定/治疗

尽早静脉应用广谱抗生素。

- 必须覆盖金黄色葡萄球菌、链球菌和革兰阴性杆菌。
- 万古霉素(预防MRSA)和第三代头孢菌素(革兰阴性杆菌)可作为初始抗生素选择。
- 若静脉滥用毒品,覆盖假单胞菌。
- 一线用药包括万古霉素、头孢他啶和甲硝唑(厌氧菌)。

急诊治疗/程序

- 考虑该诊断时需紧急行影像学检查。
- 未能及时治疗的预后较差。
- 若体格检查不能明确病变部位,考虑行全脊柱影像学检查。
- 明确诊断后,神经外科急会诊或转至神经外科行最终治疗(手术减压)。
  - 保守治疗(延长至6周的抗生素治疗)可能有效。

药物治疗

- 头孢他啶:2 g(儿童:50 mg/kg)。
- 万古霉素:15 mg/kg,静脉负荷剂量(儿童:10～15 mg/kg,q6～8 h),q12 h。
- 甲硝唑:500 mg,静脉注射。

一线药物

- 头孢他啶。
- 万古霉素。
- 甲硝唑。

随访

进一步处理

入院指征

硬膜下脓肿患者需入院,需紧急行MRI检查,必要时可转运患者。

出院指征

明确或高度怀疑硬膜下脓肿患者不应出院。

转诊问题

硬膜下脓肿患者需转至有神经外科医院:

- 若无神经外科医师或无法行MRI则需转院。
  - 给予抗生素治疗并在给药前行血培养(阳性率～60%)。

要点和误区

- 硬膜下脓肿治愈后可能复发,尤其在免疫力低下时。
- 细菌感染,尤其葡萄球菌感染且有后背痛或神经系统症状体征的患者需考虑硬膜下脓肿。
- 在使用抗生素前优先行血培养。
- 不能明确检查部位时需检查。
  - 仔细检查脊柱压痛区域及神经异常水平有助于避免这种情况。
    - 怀疑后背中部病变时同时行胸椎和腰椎检查,后背上部和颈部病变行颈椎和胸椎检查。
    - 若不能定位病变部位,检查全部脊柱。

Y

硬膜外血肿 Epidural Hematoma

Colleen J. Campbell · Stephen R. Hayden 单怡 译

基础知识

描述

• 直接的头颅创伤。
• 颅盖内弯使硬脑膜与头颅分离时可导致出血：
– 50%以上为中脑膜动脉出血。
– 1/3 为脑膜静脉出血。
• 75%有颅脑骨折，儿童少见。
• 大于 50%闭合性脑外伤有硬膜外血肿：
– 多同时有硬膜下血肿和颅脑损伤。
• 典型 CT 表现为双凸镜形、新月形，多位于颞区。
• 多不越过缝合线，但可能越过中线。

病因

• 占脑外伤(TBI)的 1.5%。
• 男女发病率之比为 3∶1。
• 发病高峰在 20～30 岁。
• 交通事故、斗殴和坠落是最常见病因：
– 所有钝性伤中，斗殴最可能合并颅内损伤，需神经外科介入治疗。
• 低龄儿童(<5 岁)或老年人少见。
• 成人死亡率为 10%，通常低于儿童死亡率且与术前情况相关。
• GCS 评分较低、瞳孔反射异常、老年患者、手术前颅内压升高、CT 见中线偏移>10 mm、混合密度病变灶、存在合并颅内损伤，以及出血量>30 ml 患者预后较差。

儿科注意事项

• 脑外伤是最常见的死亡原因，可导致儿童残疾。
• PECARN 原则可能有助于风险分层：
– 存在下列因素之一的儿童风险较低且不需要行头颅 CT 检查：
◦ LOC≥5 s。
◦ 呕吐(2 岁以上)。
◦ 剧烈头痛(2 岁以上)。
◦ 对待父母态度异常。
◦ 病情严重。
◦ 精神状态异常。
◦ GCS 评分<15 分。
◦ 头皮血肿，鼻额部。
• 坠落、自行车事故是常见病因：
– 儿童大多数严重的脑外伤由交通事故导致。
– 常需考虑非事故外伤的可能。
• <50%有意识障碍：
– CT 检查有利于鉴别诊断。
• 出血多为静脉出血。
• <5 岁儿童 95%预后较好。

诊断

症状和体征

病史

• 意识障碍。
• 85%在病程中有意识障碍：
– 仅 11%～30%有中间清醒期。
• 40%有恶心、呕吐症状。

儿科注意事项

• 在婴儿大多时候仅表现为血细胞比容下降 40%。
• 囟门突出伴呕吐、癫痫、昏睡提示硬膜外出血。
• <50%儿童在受伤时有意识障碍。
• 儿童摔倒后导致的颅后窝损伤多见。

体格检查

• 20%～40%瞳孔扩大：
– 多见于损伤同侧(90%)。
• 偏瘫>1/3：
– 多见于损伤对侧(80%)。

基本检查

头颅影像学检查(具体见以下说明)。

诊断检查与说明

实验室检查

• 动脉血气分析、全血细胞计数、凝血时间及活化的凝血酶原时间。
• 酌情行血液酒精和药物筛查。

影像学检查

• 头颅 CT 平扫：
– 入院时 CT 检查有助于判断预后。
– 可见双凸形、边缘清晰的病灶。
– 不会超过缝合处。
– 可能越过中线。
– 混合密度病变可能暗示有活动性出血。
– 常见于颞顶叶区。
– CT 的骨窗用于检查颅骨骨折；MRI 通常比 CT 更敏感，尤其在头顶部。
– T_2 加权像中的急性团块状低密度影常由脱氧血红蛋白所致。
– 新型快速 MRI 已经在一些中心应用。
• 脊髓检查。
• 进一步检查其他创伤。

儿科注意事项

囟门未闭婴儿可用超声检查其颅内结构。

鉴别诊断

• 近期脑损伤病史：
– 婴幼儿脑损伤可能较轻。
• 考虑其他疾病：
– 硬膜下血肿。
– 脑震荡。
– 脑出血。
– 弥漫性轴索损伤。
– 硬膜下囊瘤。
– 摇晃婴儿综合征。
– 中毒、代谢性或感染性因素。

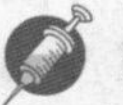

治疗

院前

• 送至区域性创伤中心的脑外伤患者的病死率可降低 25%。
• 必须脊柱固定。
• 转运过程中保证足够的氧合：
– 可能需要气管插管和气道保护。

初步稳定/治疗

• 避免缺氧和低血压：
– 一旦出现颅内压(ICP)的升高或恶化立即气管插管。
– 控制性通气维持 PCO_2 35～40 mmHg。
– 除非出现脑疝的表现，否则避免过度通气。
– 避免可能升高颅内压的麻醉诱导剂(如氯胺酮)。
• 足量的液体复苏后抬高床头 20°～30°。
• 进行快速的神经系统评估：
– Glasgow 昏迷评分：
• 14～15 分，轻度颅脑损伤。
• 9～13 分，中度颅脑损伤。
• <8 分，重度颅脑损伤。
– 反射：瞳孔对光反射、角膜反射、吞咽反射、脑干反射。
• 二次评估有>50%的概率发现同时存在

的损伤。

急诊治疗/程序

• 硬膜外血肿的昏迷患者早期的手术干预(<4 h)可改善平均生存率：
- 在骨折部位或者瞳孔散大的同侧头颅钻孔。
- 如果头颅钻孔侧出血不能控制，有时需要做快速的颅骨切除术。
• 保守治疗的无临床症状的患者病情恶化的比例很高，>30%需要手术干预。
• 保证等渗溶液的液体量。
• 持续的呼气末 CO_2 监测：
- 动脉置管严密监测 MAP、PO_2、PCO_2。
- 导尿管监测出入量(I/O)。
• 控制 ICP：
- 避免疼痛、僵直及呼吸作功增加：
◦ 使用苯二氮䓬镇静。
◦ 气管插管患者使用维库溴铵或罗库溴铵进行神经肌肉阻滞。
◦ 依托咪酯是较好的诱导剂。
◦ 神经外科 ICU 难治性的 ICP 过高可给予巴比妥药物昏迷治疗。
- 高渗盐水(3%)比甘露醇在降低 ICP 上显示了更长效的作用。
- 甘露醇可用于保持液体量平衡：
◦ 提高 MAP 以增加冠状动脉灌注压(CPP)和脑血流量(CBF)，同时降低颅内压(ICP)。
◦ 保持渗透压在 295～310 mmol/L。
• 处理高血压：
- 使用拉贝洛尔或肼屈嗪。
• 处理高血糖：
- 与颅脑创伤患者的血乳酸增加和死亡率增高有关。
• 处理和避免抽搐：
- 使用地西泮(安定)和苯妥英钠。
• 处理持续性出血以及改善凝血异常：
- TXA 1 g 静推不少于 10 min，然后 1 g 静滴维持 1 h，在伤后 3 h 内给药。
• 并无益处的处理：
- 激素治疗。
- 预防性应用抗生素。
- 脑疝时过度通气。
- 限制液体量。
- 钙通道阻滞剂。
• 预后不良的因素：
- 年龄>40 岁。
- 入院时碱剩余升高。
- 快速扩大的大血肿(CT 表现为混合密度损伤)。
- 中线显著移位>10 mm。
- 入院时低 GCS 评分 9 分或出现昏迷。
- 术后 ICP>3。
- 持续的瞳孔不等大。
- 脑实质损伤或合并其他创伤。

儿科注意事项

头皮撕裂和帽状腱膜下出血可导致大量失血：应当压迫控制出血。

药物治疗

• 地西泮(安定)：5～10 mg(儿童：0.1～0.2 mg/kg)，静脉注射。
• 苯妥英钠：成人/儿童，以 25～50 mg/min 的速度达到负荷量 18 mg/kg。
• 依托咪酯：0.3 mg/kg，静脉注射。
• 芬太尼：2～4 Ug/kg，静脉注射。
• 肼屈嗪：10 mg/h，静脉注射[儿童：0.4～1 mg/(kg · h)持续静脉注射，最大剂量 3 mg/(kg · h)]。
• 左乙拉西坦：1 500 mg，静脉注射或口服，q12 h。
• 利多卡因：诱导前剂量，1.5 mg/kg，静脉注射。
• 甘露醇：成人/儿童，0.25～1 g/kg，静脉注射，q4 h。
• 咪达唑仑：1～2 mg(儿童：0.15 mg/kg，静脉注射 1 次)，静脉注射，必要时 q10 min。
• 戊巴比妥：1～5 mg，静脉注射，q6 h。
• 凝血酶原复合物：50 U/kg，静脉注射。
• 罗库溴铵：1.2 mg/kg，静脉注射。
• 琥珀酰胆碱：诱导剂 20 mg/kg，静脉注射。
• 硫喷妥钠：诱导剂，20 mg/kg，静脉注射。
• 氨甲环酸：1 g 静脉注射不少于 10 min，之后 1 g 静脉持续输注维持 60 min 以上。

儿科注意事项

• 一些儿科研究提示高渗溶液对儿童患者有益(1.7%～3%)。
• 3%氯化钠：2～6 ml/kg，静脉注射，0.1～1 ml/(kg · h)，静脉滴注。

随访

进一步处理

入院指征

• 所有 CT 异常或意识状态改变的患者都需要入住 ICU 进行重复的神经系统评估。
• 12～24 h 后复查 CT，或当临床症状恶化时随时复查 CT。
• 快速出血、颅骨骨折、低 GCS 评分或神经系统功能障碍时提示病情恶化的风险较高。

出院指征

所有硬膜外血肿的患者都必须住院治疗。

Y

硬膜下血肿 Subdural Hematoma

Colleen J. Campbell 江伟伟 李文放 译

基础知识

描述

• 硬膜下血肿分类(SDH)：
- 急性：1～3 日。
- 亚急性：3 日至 3 周。
- 慢性：3 周后。
• CT 表现：
- 很少穿过中线。
- 交叉缝合线。
- 内缘往往被认为是不规则的。
• 急性：
- 最常见的原因是加速后突然减速，而不是直接创伤。
- 头部的矢状运动引起旁矢状静脉桥的延伸。
- 其他出血部位包括：
◦ 硬脑膜裂伤。
◦ 静脉窦损伤。
◦ 皮质动脉。
◦ 非外伤性损伤：手术后脑膜破裂、动静脉畸形、凝血功能紊乱、高血压、药物或酒精滥用。
• 慢性：

- 包膜血肿很可能是由于桥静脉反复出血造成的。

病因

- 急性:
- 颅内血肿最常见的类型(66%~70%)。
- 最常见大脑>大脑镰>小脑幕。
- 发病高峰在15~24岁,第二高峰为>75岁。
- 钝性脑外伤的发生率为26%~63%。
- 机动车辆碰撞(MVC)是最常见的原因。
- 与MVC(24%)相比,摔倒和殴打更常见导致SDH分离(72%)。
- 老年患者和癫痫患者风险增加。
- 死亡率与体征、症状及合并症有关:
  - 70岁以上的死亡率为50%。
  - 少于1/2表现为轴外血肿(22%的死亡率)。
  - 40%的患者会出现复杂的SDH:实质裂伤或脑内血肿(死亡率>50%)。
  - 与挫伤相关的排第三(死亡率30%,功能恢复20%)。
- 凝血功能障碍:INR>2增加了出血的风险,INR>3与开始出血量大和扩张明显相关。
- 慢性:
- 最常见于婴儿或有萎缩症的老年人:
  - 与脑梗死相关。
- 75%的患者>50岁。
- <50%有创伤史。
- 50%发生于酒后。
- 癫痫和分流手术。

儿科注意事项

- 可能会继发于创伤分娩。
- 非意外创伤更常见。

诊断

症状和体征

- 急性:
- 1/5在尸检时诊断。
- 最常被误诊为中毒或脑血管意外(CVA)。
- 头痛和精神状态改变:
  - 50%在发现时无意识。
- 亚急性/慢性:
- 头痛、恶心、呕吐和癫痫发作是常见的症状。
- 不同表现。
  - 不同意识状态。
  - 行走不稳。
  - 缺陷逐渐进展。

儿科注意事项

影像学检查对于持续呕吐、新发作、嗜睡、烦躁、肿胀的婴儿是必要的。

体格检查

- 急性:
- 头痛和精神状态改变。
- 最常见的临床体征是轻偏瘫或偏瘫:
  - 40%~65%。
  - SDH对侧运动缺陷在60%~85%。
- 瞳孔异常28%~79%。
  - 70%~90% SDH的瞳孔异常的在同一侧。
- 癫痫发作最初可能在10%以内。
- 视乳头水肿<1/3。
- 慢性:
- 表现多样,其他疾病相似。

基本检查

获取有针对性的既往史:

- 损伤机制。
- 神经状态:基线和现场。
- 相关因素:
- 既往史、药物史。
- 过敏史、吸毒史。
- 快速神经功能评估:
- 格拉斯哥昏迷评分(液体复苏后GCS评分最重要)。
- 脑干反射:
- 瞳孔不等。
- 瞳孔对光反射。
- 角膜反射、眼前庭反射。
- 头部影像学。

诊断检查与说明

实验室检查

- 血气分析、血常规、葡萄糖、电解质、PT、APTT。
- 血乙醇、药物检测。

影像学检查

- 与其他创伤一样,头部行CT。
- 急性:
- 特征性CT表现是新月形凝块覆盖半球形凸面。
- 血肿内侧边界可能不规则。
- MRI对颅内出血(ICH)和小的硬膜下血肿更为敏感。
- 对幕下血肿更为敏感。
- 混合密度的血块可能代表活动性出血。
- 大多数(60%)与其他颅内病变相关。
- 血肿颅内体积>2%预示预后不良。
- 慢性:
- MRI是一个更好的选择,因为2~3周后CT上的病变可能会变成等密度。
- 弥散加权成像的MRI容积与Rankin功能障碍评分相关。
- 3周后CT可能显示低密度病灶。
- 脊柱X线片。

儿科注意事项

如果囟门是暴露的话,可以行超声检查来可视化大脑结构。

鉴别诊断

- 急性:
- 弥漫性轴索损伤。
- 脑挫裂伤。
- 脑内出血。
- 硬膜下水囊瘤。
- 硬膜外血肿。
- 婴儿摇晃综合征、受虐儿童综合征。
- 慢性:
- 假瘤脑。
- 脑肿瘤。
- 痴呆。
- 脑膜炎。
- CVA/短暂性脑缺血发作。
- 脑动脉粥样硬化。
- 中毒、代谢、呼吸系统或循环系统疾病。

治疗

初步稳定/治疗

- 呼吸道管理和复苏:
- 缺氧是可预料的结果。
- 保持SaO_2>95%。
- 快速插管(RSI)用于GCS<9分或颅内压增高(ICP)的患者。
- RSI用于$PaCO_2$>45 mmHg、瞳孔不等大、GCS下降3分、窒息、颈椎脊髓损伤。
- 由于脑灌注压降低,不再推荐常规过度通气。
- 控制通气使PCO_2维持在35~40 mmHg:
- 生理盐水补液维持平均动脉压(MAP)100~110 mmHg是必要的:
  - 收缩压<90 mmHg与预后不良有关。
- 脊椎预防措施。
- 床抬高20°~30°(只有在充分的液体复苏后避免脑血流减少)。
- 不被认为有用:
- 类固醇。

- 预防抗生素。
- 过度换气(除非疝气即将出现)。
- 液体限制。
- 钙通道阻滞剂。
- 低温未被证实。
- 3%氯化钠尚未被证实有用。

急诊治疗/程序

• 紧急处理。

• 昏迷患者早期神经外科干预(<4 h)显示降低死亡率:

- 对于病情恶化的患者,可使用颅骨钻孔作为临时措施。
- 针对 CT 异常的已插管患者,应行颅内压监测。
- 硬膜下脑室引流系统已被证明对于硬膜下血肿急性治疗与颅骨钻孔具有同等效果。

• 对于小的硬膜下血肿,非手术治疗可能是有指征的:

- 血液量<20 ml,直径<1 cm,中线移位<5 mm,无占位效应,无神经功能缺陷。
- 需要频繁对患者进行神经功能再评估。
- 10%的患者最终需要手术干预。

• 保持等容状态并使用等渗液体:

- 动脉插管用于监测平均动脉压、动脉血氧分压和二氧化碳分压。
- 导尿管用于监测液体入/出量情况。

• 控制颅内压:

- 预防疼痛、姿态异常和呼吸努力增加:
  ◦ 用苯二氮䓬类药物镇静。
  ◦ 对于已插管患者,使用琥珀胆碱或罗库溴铵进行神经肌肉阻滞。
  ◦ 依托咪酯是一种良好的诱导剂。
  ◦ 3%高渗盐水已被证明比甘露醇更长时间地降低颅内压。
- 等容状态下可以使用甘露醇:
  ◦ 显示能提高平均动脉压>脑灌注压和脑血流量,同时降低颅内压。
- 保持血浆渗透压在 295~310 mOsm/kg。
- 治疗高血压:
  ◦ 拉贝洛尔、尼卡地平或硝苯地平。
- 治疗凝血功能障碍。
- 考虑使用氨甲环酸 1 g 静脉注射,随后 1 h 内静脉输注 1 g。
- 使用新鲜冰冻血浆 4 U。
- 使用凝血酶原复合物。
- 治疗高血糖:
  ◦ 与创伤性脑损伤的死亡率增加有关。
- 治疗和预防癫痫:
  ◦ 地西泮和苯妥英钠、左乙拉西坦:不需要预防性使用抗惊厥药物。

药物治疗

• 地西泮:5~10 mg(儿童:0.2~0.3 mg/kg),静脉注射或肌内注射,q10~15 min;最大剂量 30 mg(儿童:10 mg)。

• 苯妥英:成人和儿童以 25~50 mg/min 至 18 mg/kg。

• 依托咪酯:0.3 mg/kg 静脉注射用于诱导 RSI。

• 芬太尼:2~4 μg/kg。

• 肼屈嗪:10~20 mg(儿童:0.1~0.5 mg/kg 静脉输注),q2~4 h。

• 拉贝洛尔:20 mg 静脉推注,然后 40~80 mg q10 min;最大剂量 300 mg;随后连续输注。0.5~2 mg/min[儿童:0.4~1 mg/(kg · h)连续输注;最多 3 mg/(kg · h)]。

• 呋塞米:成人和儿童 0.5 mg/kg,静脉注射。

• 左乙拉西坦:1 500 mg,口服或静脉注射,q12 h。

• 利多卡因:1.5 mg/kg,静脉注射。

• 甘露醇:成人和儿童:0.25~0.5 g/kg,静脉注射,q4 h。

• 咪达唑仑:1~2 mg(儿童:0.15 mg/kg,静脉)静脉注射,q10 min,必要时。

• 尼卡地平:静脉滴注 5~15 mg/h(儿童:未建立安全性)。

• 戊巴比妥:1~5 mg,静脉注射,q6 h。

• 凝血酶原复合物:50 U/kg,静脉注射。

• 罗库溴铵:1 mg/kg 诱导。

• 硫喷妥钠:作为诱导剂,20 mg/kg,静脉注射。

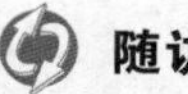

随访

进一步处理

入院指征

• 急性 SDH 患者应通过神经外科入手术室或重症监护室。

• 监测亚急性硬膜下血肿。

出院指征

患有慢性 SDH 的患者通常可以门诊神经外科随访,有充足的家庭资源及适当的随访管理。

转诊问题

所有患者都需要立即进行神经外科评估。

要点和误区

以下因素预测预后:

• 入院 GCS 评分。
• 治疗时间。
• 瞳孔异常。
• CT 血肿体积和中线偏移。
• 中线移位>血肿体积。

Y

幽门狭窄 Pyloric Stenosis

Roger M. Barkin 郑金浩 毛恩强 译

基础知识

描述

• 产后幽门处圆形平滑肌细胞增生肥大,引起幽门窦壁增厚,进而导致胃流出道进行性梗阻。

• 神经元型一氧化氮合酶(NOS-1)可能是遗传性易感因素。

• 婴幼儿在出生后 2 周内使用红霉素可能增加肥厚性幽门狭窄的风险。

• 黄疸由葡萄糖醛酸转移酶缺乏引起。

• 成人:由消化性溃疡引起。

病因

• 婴幼儿最常见的幽门梗阻的病因;发生率为 1/150 男婴和 1/750 女婴(平均为 3/1 000 存活婴儿)。

• 男性的发病率为女性的 5 倍,第一个出生的孩子最常见。

• 女性,15%:

- 父母患有此疾病,孩子的发病率升高至 7%。
- 随后复发的风险在男孩为 10%,女孩为 2%。

诊断

症状和体征

病史

- 呕吐：
  - 慢性起病，常发生在出生后 3～6 周，很少发生在 1 岁以后。
  - 逐渐加重，常会发展为喷射状呕吐。
  - 呕吐物无胆汁。
  - 可能呕吐物中带血(比食管炎、胃炎、胃溃疡少见)。
  - 逐渐加重。
  - 出现在进食后。
- 有幽门肥厚的表现：
  - 确诊。
- 便秘或大便减少。
- 婴儿早期表现为消瘦，易饿；后期出现脱水，不愿进食。
- 基于症状持续的时间可以出现脱水和消瘦。
- 8%的儿童伴黄疸。
- 成人表现为呕吐、厌食、早饱、胃痛。

体格检查

- 腹部松弛，其他均正常。
- 常常呕吐后在右上腹腹直肌外侧缘可能触及橄榄状肿块(80%的患者)：
  - 扩张的胃体覆盖在幽门，当呕吐后或吸空胃内容物后立刻好转。
  - 幽门肥厚表现：
    - 协助诊断。
    - 蠕动波从左边的左上腹移到右边，喂养后呕吐前更容易观察到。

基本检查

如果出现“橄榄状”肿块，可不需进一步诊断，但要考虑到请外科会诊。若没有“橄榄状”肿块，需进一步影像学检查。

诊断检查与说明

实验室检查

- 电解质、肌酐、尿素氮、葡萄糖：
  - 低钾低氯代谢性碱中毒。
  - 电解质正常不能作为排除诊断的依据。
- 胆红素升高，常表现为非结合胆红素。
- 若呕吐物中带血，需查血细胞计数。
- 水化治疗。

影像学检查

- 腹部超声：
  - 选择性检查。
  - 超声诊断依赖于幽门肌层的鉴定和测量(幽门或肌肉长 1.5 cm，环的厚度为 3 mm，幽门直径为 10～14 mm)，并能观察到液体经过幽门的表现。
  - 阳性预测值接近 100%，假阴性为 19%。
  - 对于可疑或阴性患者复查超声。
- 上消化道造影：
  - 造影剂呈线状影像通过狭窄的胃出口。
  - 准确性 95%。
  - 检查结束后去除胃中的造影剂，防止误吸。
- 仰卧位腹部 X 线平片：
  - 没有诊断价值，很少有所帮助。
  - 扩张型胃和幽门的远端没有空气。
  - 对于其他医师评估腹部其他病变时有很大用处。

鉴别诊断

- 胃肠道解剖或功能性疾病：
  - 胃食管反流。
  - 食管裂孔疝。
  - 梗阻或闭锁。
  - 胃或十二指肠网膜缠绕。
- 感染：
  - 胃炎。
  - 尿路感染。
  - 脓毒症。
- 代谢：
  - 肾上腺功能不全症。
  - 遗传性代谢缺陷。
- 饮食问题：
  - 心理相关因素：母婴互动不良或压力大。
  - 贲门食管松弛症。
  - 配方奶不耐受。
  - 暴饮暴食。
  - 撤药反应。
- 颅内压增高。

治疗

院前

如果有容量不足的表现进行液体复苏。

初步稳定/治疗

- 建立静脉通道。
- 迅速行床旁葡萄糖负荷试验，排除低血糖因素。
- 以 20 ml/kg 的剂量使用生理盐水进行静脉补液，可以重复进行。

急诊治疗/程序

- 纠正电解质紊乱。
- 液体复苏 1～1.5 倍后使用葡萄糖溶液：
  - 确定尿量正常后补钾。
- 留置胃管，进行胃肠减压。
- 禁食水。
- 请儿科医师会诊，评估幽环肌切开术的指征。
- 成人：质子泵抑制剂(兰索拉唑或奥美拉唑)。

药物治疗

成人

- 兰索拉唑：30 mg，口服，每日 1 次。
- 奥美拉唑：20 mg，口服，每日 1 次。

随访

进一步处理

入院指征

- 所有的儿童患者应住院进行纠正脱水和手术矫正，手术可选经脐带幽门环肌切开术或腹腔镜幽门环肌切开术。
- 成人患者：如果质子泵抑制剂治疗失败不能改善症状，入院进行补液，择期行幽门环肌切开术。

出院指征

无。

转诊问题

外科会诊，协助治疗脱水和电解质紊乱的并发症。

随访建议

遵从术后随访计划。

要点和误区

临床表现结合实验室检查结果，考虑行上消化道成像，并纠正电解质紊乱。

疣 Warts

Gary M. Vilke · Rahul V. Nene 吴昊 李文放 译

基础知识

描述

- 疣是由人乳头瘤病毒(HPV)引起的。
- 机制：局部细胞增殖和血管生长导致皮肤损害的发展，典型的疣状和角化过度。
- 病变是典型的疣状和角化病。
- 在大多数情况下，病变可自愈：
  - 30%在6个月内自愈。
  - 60%～70%在2年内自愈。
  - 90%在5年内自愈。
- 皮肤疣的类型：
  - 寻常疣(常见疣)：
    - 常见于：手背、手指、毗邻的指甲。
    - 通常无症状。
  - 跖疣：
    - 足底的承重部分：足跟、跖骨头。
    - 通常有症状和伴有疼痛。
    - 在青少年和年轻人中更常见。
  - 扁平(或幼年)疣：
    - 主要在暴露部位：头、脸、颈部、腿、手背。
    - 面积小。
    - 数量从几到数百不等。
- 肛门-生殖器疣：
  - 尖锐湿疣或性病疣。
  - 大多数是无症状的，容易被忽略。
  - HPV6 和 HPV11，占肛门生殖器疣的90%。
- HPV16 和 HPV18 占子宫颈癌的 70%。

病因

- 人乳头病毒是人类特有的：
  - 引起上皮组织和黏膜的感染。
  - 感染皮肤或黏膜的基底层。
- 有上百种 HPV 病毒可以感染不同的身体部位(如 HPV1 容易感染足底)。
- 人乳头状瘤病毒传播：
  - 直接传播：皮肤到皮肤，黏膜到皮肤等。
  - 间接间接：受污染的表面到皮肤。
  - 自体接种：抓挠、吸吮(特别是在幼儿中)。
- 潜伏期从数周到1年不等，然而，最常见的范围是2～6个月。

儿科注意事项

- 10%～20%的儿童会有疣。
- 12～16岁是发病率高峰。
- 婴儿出生时接触病毒可能导致喉部乳头瘤病。
- 必须考虑对患有肛门生殖器疣的儿童可能存在性虐待。

诊断

症状和体征

病史

- 重要组成部分包括：
  - 完整的性病史。
  - 既往疣和治疗史。
  - 特应性皮炎病史。
  - HIV 状况和/或细胞免疫功能下降史。
    - 易感患者，使初始治疗失败的可能性更大。
- 皮肤疣的症状和体征：
  - 共同的特点：
    - 通常是无症状的，除非病变在受力点。
    - 可能表现出继发于创伤后的出血。
  - 足底疣的症状和体征：
    - 常伴有负重的疼痛。
  - 扁平(或幼年)疣：
    - 在暴露的皮肤区域。
    - 可以通过剃须的脸、颈部、腿来传播。
- 肛门-生殖器疣：
  - 在男性中，通常是在阴蒂头、阴茎、阴囊或肛门。
  - 在女性中，在阴唇、阴道、子宫颈或肛门。
  - 可以延伸到尿道、膀胱或直肠：
    - 排尿困难。
    - 疼痛、瘙痒和/或肠蠕动出血。
  - 如果口交时，可能有口腔或喉的症状。

体格检查

- 皮肤疣：容易掩盖正常的皮肤纹理：
  - 共同的特点：
    - 硬的、粗糙的、凸起的、穹状的病变。
    - 血管增生，可能会因轻微的创伤而流血。
  - 足底疣：
    - 与普通人相似，但通常较大，见于足底。
    - 血管增生，可能会随着轻微的刮擦而流血。
  - 扁平(或幼年)疣：
    - 肉色。
    - 平顶和光滑。
    - 小：从一个点到橡皮擦大小。
- 肛门-生殖器疣：
  - 菜花状生长。
  - 病变是软的，通常呈多发。
  - 肉色，略带色素或红色。

基本检查

由特征外观特征诊断。

诊断检查与说明

实验室检查

- 女性妊娠试验。
- 典型病变不推荐活检和病毒分型。
- 如果难以鉴别，将醋酸添加到可疑区域，这将导致受感染区域变白，变得更加明显。
- 其他性传播疾病的筛查。

诊断步骤/外科

如果治疗失败，患者免疫系统受损，或疣有色素、硬化、固定或溃疡，进行活检。

鉴别诊断

- 皮肤疣：
  - 常见的疣：
    - 胼胝，不会流血。
    - 拇外翻。
    - 黑色爪(不会破坏皮肤标记)。
    - 痣、肤赘、扁平苔藓。
    - 脂溢性角化病(常粘连，色素沉着)。
    - 恶性肿瘤(无色素细胞黑色素瘤、鳞状细胞癌)。
- 肛门-生殖器疣：
  - 硬脂瘤(继发性梅毒)。
  - 单纯疱疹。
  - 阴茎头周围突出的腺体。
  - 良性或恶性肿瘤。
  - 接触传染性软疣。

治疗

初步稳定/治疗

没有要求。

急诊治疗/程序

- 皮肤疣：
  - 水杨酸：
    - 一线治疗是局部水杨酸和液氮冷冻疗法；手部疣的最佳证据，对足底/足部病变的疗效较差。
    - 价格便宜，副作用轻微，使用方便，患者使

Y

用，无痛。
◦ OTC 强度为 17％水杨酸，处方强度高达 70％。
◦ 在温水中浸泡疣 10～20 min。
◦ 夜间持续应用水杨酸。
◦ 早晨温和地清除。
◦ 贴剂也可以。
◦ 治疗需要数周到数月的时间。
◦ 可能结合冷冻疗法更有效。
- 用银胶带进行周期性闭塞；然而，影响疗效的证据：
◦ 损伤小。
◦ 在疣上保留银胶带 6 日。
◦ 在第 7 日用浮石或指甲油轻轻清创，重复 7 日周期。
◦ 对幼儿有益。
◦ 也可以加强其他局部治疗。
- 肛门生殖器疣：
◦ 没有一种疗法对所有病例都是最好的。
◦ 最常见的一线，患者应用的治疗包括局部咪喹莫特、普达非洛(鬼臼毒素)或儿茶素软膏。
◦ 最常见的一线，治疗的疗法包括冷冻疗法、切除术和三氯乙酸(TCA)/二氯乙酸(BCA)。
◦ 不干预可能是儿童的最佳治疗方案，因为治疗还没有得到很好的研究，疣可能会自行消退。
• 替代疗法：
- 液态氮或干冰的冷冻疗法。
- 电烙术。
- 激光疗法。
- 手术切除。
- 在专家指导下使用适当干扰素。
• 为门诊随访提供适当的转诊。

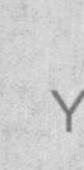

妊娠注意事项

• 尽管有可见病变的患者在阴道分娩时有向新生儿垂直传播的风险，但除非病变阻碍了产道，否则不应仅为防止传播而进行剖宫产。
• 如果可能的话，应在怀孕后治疗疣。
• 水杨酸、咪喹莫特、鬼臼毒素和 TCA/BCA 不得用于妊娠。
• 冷冻和手术是首选。

药物治疗

• 皮肤疣和肛门生殖器的一线治疗：局部用药(患者应用)：
- 17％～40％水杨酸最常用于成人和儿童：
- 每日 1 次；用温水浸泡 5 min，彻底干燥，敷于整个疣体表面。
- 每 48 h 1 次；用温水浸泡疣体，彻底干燥，用新的软垫牢固覆盖疣体。
- 未经临床医师随访，不得超过 12 周。
- 妊娠危险因素 C(不建议在妊娠期间使用)。
• 肛门生殖器疣的首选治疗方法：局部用药(患者应用)。
- 3.75％乳霜：每日睡前使用，涂抹在皮肤上保持 8～10 h，然后用肥皂和水洗净。可重复 8 周。
- 5％乳霜：睡前每周 3 次，涂抹在皮肤上保持 6～10 h，然后用肥皂和水清洗。可重复 16 周。
- 注意：可能会削弱隔膜和避孕套。
- 妊娠危险因素 C(不建议在妊娠期间使用)。
• 二线和其他替代方案：
- 使用液氮或低温探头进行冷冻治疗：
◦ 每隔 1～2 周重复一次(由医师完成)。
- 0.5％鬼臼毒素凝胶或成人溶液(患者使用)：
◦ 每日 2 次连续使用 3 日，然后停用 4 日，重复 4 个周期。
◦ 不要在肛周、直肠、尿道或阴道病变上使用。
- 15％儿茶素软膏(患者使用)：
◦ 可以用来治疗生殖器疣。
◦ 每日 3 次，不洗脸，持续 16 周。
- 80％～90％ TCA/BCA(医师局部应用)。
◦ 常用于掌跖疣。
◦ 每周应用，持续 6～10 周。
◦ 使用过程中避免灼伤皮肤。
• 疫苗：
- 加德西(Gardasil)：针对 HPV6、HPV11、HPV16、HPV18：
◦ 推荐给 9～25 岁女性。
◦ 三次给药连续 6 个月。
◦ 预防宫颈癌、外阴癌和阴道癌、生殖器疣，以及其他轻度宫颈病变。
- 希瑞适(Cervarix)：针对 HPV16、HPV18 致癌型，不包括最常见的导致疣状病毒的 HPV 类型：
◦ 在发展中国家，普及疫苗接种可显著降低宫颈癌的发病率，而无需进行完善的筛查。
◦ 两种疫苗的有效率都是 96％。
◦ 在日常使用和接受方面仍然存在争议。
◦ 一些研究表明给年轻男性接种疫苗也有好处。

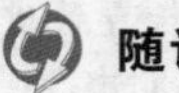

随访

进一步处理

入院指征

免疫缺陷患者的传播性病例可能需要入院。

出院指征

大多数患者可以被当作门诊患者来治疗。

转诊问题

• 所有基于药物的治疗都需要初级健康保健医师或皮肤科随访和后续剂量。除非能保证随访，否则不应开始治疗。
• 对于治疗失败，应转诊至 PMD 或皮肤病学进行其他治疗方案。
• 将性活跃的少女介绍给儿科医师或初级保健，以进行 HPV 疫苗接种。

随访建议

• 若出现疼痛、灼烧感、发红或其他症状的变化需要立即重新评估。
• 安排适当的医师进行随访：儿科医师、妇科医师、皮肤科医师、初级保健医师。
• 对于外阴受累的免疫功能低下的女性患者，建议活检，因为疣状病变可能掩盖高级别瘤样病变。
• 建议专家随访。

要点和误区

• 在进行医学治疗之前必须进行妊娠检查。
• HPV 疫苗不能保护所有形式的 HPV 病毒，只是那些最常与子宫颈癌还有生殖器疣相关的。
• 必须考虑对患有肛门生殖器疣的儿童可能存在性虐待。
• 临床上根除疣并不意味着患者没有 HPV。
• 专家随访活检以评估免疫功能低下患者的肿瘤。

有机磷中毒 Organophosphorus Poisoning

Vinodinee L. Dissanayake　朱妍 译

基础知识

描述

- 有机磷酸酯(杀虫剂和神经毒剂)不可逆结合并使胆碱酯酶失活,包括乙酰胆碱酯酶。
- 乙酰胆碱在神经突触积聚导致中枢和周围神经胆碱能递质超载。
- 主要影响(毒蕈碱样、烟碱样、中枢神经)可多样化和重叠。
- 死亡率仅次于呼吸衰竭:
  - 呼吸肌无力。
  - 气道分泌物和支气管梗阻。
  - 抑制呼吸驱动中枢。

儿科注意事项

- 症状在幼儿中很难鉴别。
- 常见症状:瞳孔缩小、流涎、肌无力。
- 儿科病例有25%出现癫痫:
  - 成人中仅为3%。

病因

- 接触杀虫剂(有机磷化合物)。
- 接触化学神经毒剂(沙林、梭曼、塔崩、VX)。
- 尤其是易于被肺、消化道、皮肤、黏膜、眼吸收。

诊断

症状和体征

- 典型表现:胆碱能中毒征。
  - DUMBELS:
    - 腹泻、发汗。
    - 排尿。
    - 瞳孔缩小、肌束震颤。
    - 心动过缓、气道分泌物、气道痉挛。
    - 呕吐。
    - 流泪。
    - 流涎。
  - 可能有大蒜味。
- 慢性间歇性中毒,非特异症状:
  - 无力。
  - 虚弱。
  - 萎靡。
  - 厌食。
- 轻度中毒:
  - CNS:
    - 头痛。
    - 头晕。
    - 舌和眼睑震颤。
    - 无力。
  - 消化道:
    - 厌食。
- 中度中毒:
  - CNS:
    - 肌束震颤而后迟缓性瘫痪。
    - 呼吸肌无力。
    - 运动共济失调。
    - 激动。
    - 震颤。
    - 意识混乱。
  - 视觉:
    - 瞳孔针尖样无对光反应。
  - 呼吸:
    - 呼吸肌无力。
    - 气道分泌物。
  - 心血管:
    - 心动过缓。
  - 消化道:
    - 恶心、呕吐。
    - 腹部痉挛。
  - 外分泌腺:
    - 流涎。
    - 流泪。
- 重度中毒:
  - CNS:
    - 惊厥。
    - 昏迷。
    - 中枢性呼吸抑制。
  - 呼吸:
    - 呼吸道梗阻。
    - 哮喘。
    - 呼吸困难。
    - 气管分泌物增多。
  - 心血管:
    - 心动过缓(肺水肿和低氧血症可导致心动过速)。
    - 心脏传导阻滞。
    - 发绀。
  - 消化道:
    - 恶心、呕吐。
    - 腹痛。
    - 腹泻、大便失禁。
  - 外分泌腺:
    - 发汗。
    - 流涎。
    - 流泪。
  - 膀胱:
    - 尿频。
    - 尿失禁。
    - 烟碱样表现。

基本检查

询问可能的接触史、职业、近期家中杀虫、贴错标签或保存不当的杀虫剂。

- 若是自杀,获取原始容器。
- 寻找副交感神经和中枢神经体征,如肌无力或瘫痪。

诊断检查与说明

实验室检查

- 红细胞和血浆胆碱酯酶水平确诊:
  - 评估突触抑制首选红细胞(真)胆碱酯酶水平(外送实验室)。
  - 血浆(假)胆碱酯酶水平不可靠但更及时:
    - 它们是中毒标志物。
    - 这些指标的水平会根据毒物和患者不同而发生变化。
  - 胆碱酯酶水平:
    - 隐性中毒:>50%正常值。
    - 轻度中毒:20%～50%正常值。
    - 中度中毒:10%～20%正常值。
    - 重度中毒:<10%正常值。
  - 在胆碱酯酶结果出来前就应进行治疗。
- 血细胞计数、电解质、血糖、尿素氮、肌酐。
- 当有呼吸系统症状时检查动脉血气。

影像学检查

- 如果出现呼吸困难或怀疑肺水肿行胸部X线检查:
  - 吸入性肺炎。
- 心电图:
  - 心律不齐(心房颤动、室性心动过速、尖端扭转性室速、QT延长)。
  - 心动过缓。
  - 心脏传导阻滞。
  - ST-T波形异常。
- 当引起精神状态异常的诊断不确定时行头颅CT扫描检查。

■ 鉴别诊断

• 轻度至中度中毒：
- 胃肠炎。
- 哮喘。
- 有毒节肢动物咬伤（黑寡妇、蝎子）。
- 进展性周围神经病变（吉兰-巴雷综合征）。
- 一氧化碳中毒。
• 重度中毒：
- 麻醉药过量。
- 昏迷和瞳孔缩小：
◦ PCP、氨甲丙二酯、非诺地平、可乐定。
◦ 含毒蕈碱的蘑菇，胆碱能危象不伴烟碱样症状。
◦ 烟碱中毒。
- 代谢性疾病和感染：
◦ 酮症酸中毒、脓毒症、脑膜炎、脑炎。
◦ 低血糖。
◦ Reye 综合征。
- 神经科：
◦ 脑血管意外。
◦ 硬膜下或硬膜外血肿。
◦ 癫痫发作后状态。

治疗

■ 院前

• 首先要尽快清除毒物：
- DABC：清除毒物、气道、呼吸、循环。
- 去除所有衣物和储存毒物的垃圾（二次污染）。
• 医务人员的防护是至关重要的：
- 毒物不能透过的手套（氯丁橡胶、腈类）、长袍、护眼。
• 使用香皂和水清除皮肤毒物：
- 最好淋浴或轻微刷洗后再进急诊室。
• 维持气道通畅和吸氧。
• 静脉通道和进行心电监测。

■ 初步稳定/治疗

• DABL：
- 去除毒物并保护工作人员。
• 维持气道通畅和吸氧：
- 不稳定气道行插管，机械通气。
- 静脉输注 5%葡萄糖溶液和生理盐水。
• 精神状态改变：应用硫胺素、葡萄糖和纳洛酮。

■ 急诊治疗/程序

• 阿托品：
- 阻断乙酰胆碱在 M 受体位点结合。
- 对烟碱受体无影响。
- 1～4 min 起效，8 min 达到峰值。
- 治疗目标/终点：
◦ 气管支气管分泌物减少至干燥。
- 使用试验剂量 1～2 mg，静脉注射或肌内注射：
◦ 临床无反应：剂量每 5 min 加倍，直到胆碱能作用消退。
- 剂量：1～4 mg，静注每 5 min（儿童：0.05～0.2 mg/kg）。
- 治疗中常见误区：
◦ 阿托品没有足量。
◦ 将瞳孔变化（瞳孔散大）作为治疗终点。
◦ 误把散大的瞳孔或心动过速作为阿托品的禁忌证。
• 解磷定（2-PAM）：
- 通过逆转酶磷酸化重新活化胆碱酯酶。
- 与阿托品协同作用，毒蕈碱样症状和体征将于 10～40 min 缓解。
- 副作用：快速输注导致神经肌肉阻滞、呼吸抑制、高血压、恶心、呕吐、头晕、视物模糊。
- 治疗终点是肌无力和肌颤缓解。
- 在酶老化（胆碱酯酶永久失活）前起效。
- 不同毒物致酶老化开始的时间不同。
- 即使 24～48 h 过去后仍无使用限制。
• 支持性治疗：
- 皮肤消毒：去除衣物，用水冲洗皮肤。
- 洗胃（早期表现为重度中毒者）：
◦ 通过鼻胃管持续抽吸清除胃内容物。
◦ 小心处理胃内容物：避免直接接触，防止个人中毒。
- 呼吸困难：
◦ 频繁口咽吸引。
◦ 使用阿托品缓解气道痉挛，而不是支气管扩张剂。
◦ 心动过速可能由低氧血症引起（肺分泌物和气道痉挛）。
◦ 阿托品可清除分泌物，反而降低心率。
◦ 必要时插管、机械通气。
◦ 避免使用琥珀胆碱，被胆碱酯酶代谢的时间延长。

■ 药物治疗

• 阿托品：1～2 mg（儿童：0.05～0.2 mg/kg），静脉注射，q5 min（详见急诊治疗）。
• 葡萄糖：50%葡萄糖，1 支（25 g）50%葡萄糖（儿童：2～4 ml/kg 25%葡萄糖），静脉推注。
• 纳洛酮：2 mg（儿童：0.1 mg/kg），静脉注射或肌内注射。
• 解磷定：1～2 g（儿童：25～50 mg/kg）溶解于生理盐水，静脉注射超过 30 min；必要时 1 h 内重复，以后每 6 h 按需使用：
- 有一些建议持续输注（500 mg/h）来维持血浆浓度 4 mg/L。

随访

■ 进一步处理

入院指征

• ICU 收治对阿托品有反应的各种程度的中毒患者。
• 一些有症状的患者需留观。
• 避免阿片类、吩噻嗪类和抗组胺类药物使用，它们可能增强有机磷的毒性。

出院指征

• 中毒后 6～12 h 无症状。
• 患者回家前评估应保证可给予密切可靠的随访和特效治疗药物。

转诊问题

重度中毒需要重复使用阿托品的患者需联系毒理学家或毒物中心。

■ 随访建议

故意摄入者需请精神科会诊。

要点和误区

• 治疗失败多由于阿托品给药不足。
• 识别烟碱样临床表现（心动过速、癫痫）。

幼儿皮疹 Rash, Pediatric

Roger M. Barkin · Bruce Webster 袁晓伟 童朝阳 译

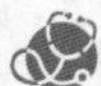

基础知识

描述

• 病变形态：

- 斑疹：局部无触诊颜色变化。紫癜或瘀斑(触诊不褪色)。
- 斑丘疹：以微隆起为特点的局部皮肤改变。
- 丘疹：实性，隆起，直径<5 mm；角化病(表面粗糙的病灶)；非角化(光滑病变)；可触及紫癜(触诊不褪色)。
- 斑块：实性，隆起，直径>5 mm；通常由丘疹汇合而成。
- 结节：实性，隆起，病灶深入真皮或皮下组织，直径 5 mm。
- 风团：圆形不规则病灶，呈红色或苍白色。
- 囊泡：直径<5 mm，充满液体的透明病灶。
- 大泡：透明充满液体的病灶直径>5 mm。
- 脓疱：脓性病变。

• 继发性病变：

- 鳞屑：干燥的角质化上皮薄片，部分与表皮分离。
- 苔藓样变：使皮肤产生皱纹的干燥斑块。
- 糜烂：由于水疱或大疱破裂而暴露的潮湿表面。
- 表皮脱落：因外伤造成的皮肤线性脱落。
- 溃疡：皮肤深部脱落，不同程度累及表皮、真皮和皮下组织。

• 形状：

- 圆形或弧形。
- 锯齿状(匍匐或蠕虫状)。
- 虹膜样(牛眼外观)。
- 不规则。
- 带状疱疹样。
- 线性。
- 网状。

• 皮肤颜色(由于一些物质导致病灶或整个皮肤的颜色改变)。

- 红色或红棕色病灶是红细胞中的氧和血红蛋白引起的。
- 病毒疹的黄斑性红斑病变通常表现为表皮血管扩张。
- 紫癜和瘀斑是由于红细胞从血管腔泄漏造成的。
- 色素沉着或色素过度是炎症后黑色素生成增加或减少的表现。
- 脱色是指由于自身免疫作用(白癜风)或先天性疾病(白化病)引起的色素完全丧失。
- 一致性。
- 病变的感觉可能有帮助。
- 鳞屑表现为表皮细胞翻转的增殖障碍。

病因

• 鳞屑性丘疹：

- 感染：病毒、细菌、立克次体或真菌。
- 过敏反应。
- 自身免疫性疾病。

• 紫癜和瘀斑：

- 凝血或血小板紊乱。
- 血管疾病的脆弱性。
- 血管炎。
- 严重感染。

• 水疱：

- 感染。
- 药物反应。
- 自身免疫性疾病。

• 溃疡：

- 感染。
- 血管功能不全。

诊断

体征和症状

• 发热(考虑感染性皮疹)。
• 瘙痒。
• 关节疼痛。
• 腹部疼痛。
• 心脏杂音。

病史(获取详细的病史)

• 年龄组：条件、分布、外观可能随年龄而异。
• 皮疹的发展、进展、模式和持续时间。
• 病变部位同步或异步。
• 相关症状。
• 前驱症状：咳嗽、鼻漏、咽炎、发热、脑膜炎症状、瘙痒。
• 家族史、接触史、免疫接种史。
• 最近旅行史。
• 昆虫或节肢动物咬伤史。
• 药物，特别是新药；近期治疗及反应。
• 常见的皮肤病。
• 特应性皮炎、牛皮癣。

体格检查

• 心脏杂音、摩擦音。
• 肺脏：爆破音、喘息声。
• 腹部：紧张度、肝脾大。
• 皮肤：见基本检查。

基本检查

根据原发病灶对皮疹进行分类：丘疹鳞状、大疱、紫癜。

诊断检查与说明

实验室检查

• 紫色皮疹：

- CBC 及血小板计数。
- 出血筛查：凝血酶原试验、部分凝血活酶时间、出血时间、弥散性血管内凝血(DIC)筛查。

• 发热：

- CBC、电解质、BUN、肌酐，评估脱水和猩红热皮疹(不包括肾小球肾炎)。
- 病毒培养和可疑的皮疹滴度。
- 疑似脓毒症、菌血症患者查乳酸和血培养。
- 如怀疑脑膜炎或脑炎，行腰椎穿刺。

影像学检查

怀疑合并肺部感染行胸部 X 线片。

诊断步骤/外科

• 氢氧化钾(KOH)制剂：用于皮肤病与麻木湿疹、玫瑰糠疹的鉴别。
• 用手术刀或玻璃片边缘从皮肤上取下的病灶活跃边缘的浅表鳞屑样本放置在幻灯片上，加入 1 滴 10%氢氧化钾，盖上盖子，慢慢加热，不要沸腾，静置几分钟，扫描菌丝。
• Wood 灯：用于皮肤病和红斑。
• 疥疮制剂：

- 螨虫主要分布在手和足上。
- 在患处滴一滴矿物油，用 15 号刀片制作血涂片。
- 在低功率下灯下检查螨、卵、幼虫的粪便。

• 皮肤镜：需要培训才能运用。

鉴别诊断

斑丘疹的皮疹

• 固体、皮肤颜色或黄色：

Y

- 角化病。
- 疣。
- 肉刺或胼胝。
- 非角化病。
- 接触传染性软疣。
- 皮脂囊肿。
- 基底细胞癌和鳞状细胞癌。
- 痣。
• 固体，棕色：
- 咖啡牛奶斑。
- 痣。
- 雀斑。
- 黑素瘤。
- 光致敏/光毒性药疹。
- 手掌黑癣色素沉着。
• 固体，红色，非隆起性：
- 非紫癜性的。
- 皮疹。
- 红疹、风疹或蔷薇疹。
- 猩红热。
- 产生毒素的葡萄球菌或链球菌疾病。
- 传染性红斑（"第五病"）。
- 风疹样皮疹（埃可病毒、柯萨奇 A 组病毒）。
- 水痘（早期表现）。
- 天花（早期表现）。
- EB 病毒。
- 肠道病毒和腺病毒。
- 支原体。
- 川崎病。
- 多形性红斑。
- 局限性痒疹。
- 昆虫叮咬，疥疮。
- 过敏性或刺激性接触性皮炎。
- 紫癜。
- 菌血性脓毒症。
- 脑膜炎球菌血症、肺炎球菌血症、淋病球菌血症、流感嗜血杆菌血症。
- 心内膜炎。
- 鼠疫。
- DIC。
- 落基山斑疹热（RMSF）。
- 过敏性紫癜。
- 特发性血小板减少性紫癜。
- 白血病。
- 潜在凝血障碍。
- 坏死性脓疮。
- 罕见，玫瑰糠疹。

• 固体、红色、鳞屑：
- 无上皮破坏：
◦ 体癣、足或下腿部。
◦ 玫瑰糠疹。
◦ 二期梅毒。
◦ 红斑狼疮。
- 上皮破坏：
◦ 丘疹性荨麻疹。
◦ 湿疹。
◦ 脂溢性皮炎、尿布性皮炎、接触性皮炎。
◦ 脓疱性皮炎。
◦ 念珠菌病。
◦ 体癣、头皮炎、足部癣或小腿癣。
◦ 水疱性皮疹。
◦ 疱疹病毒：水痘、天花。
◦ 单纯疱疹、带状疱疹。
◦ 手足口病。
◦ 疥疮。
◦ 药物过敏、中毒性表皮坏死松解症。
◦ 葡萄球菌烫伤皮肤综合征。
◦ 脓疱病、大疱性脓疱。
◦ 擦伤疾病。
◦ 疱疹样皮炎。
◦ 湿疹。
◦ 多形性红斑。
◦ 扁平苔藓。

脓疱

• 痤疮。
• 毛囊炎。
• 念珠菌病。
• 淋球菌血症。
• 脑膜炎球菌血症。
• 目前发热，考虑感染、药物反应、全身性炎性疾病（少年类风湿关节炎、系统性狼疮等）。

治疗

院前

当出现生命体征不稳定迹象时，就需要进行现场救治。

• 采取预防措施，避免接触呼吸道分泌物；建立静脉通路。
• 确认伴有潜在的威胁生命的皮疹或需要特殊隔离。

初步稳定/治疗

• 对伴有发烧或生命体征不稳定的紫癜性皮疹的儿童进行积极、经验性的治疗：
- 气道支持、静脉输液、液体复苏、心血管衰竭时使用升压药。
- 对于可疑的感染应给予静脉抗生素。

急诊治疗/程序

• 针对潜在病因给予特异性急诊治疗。
• 怀疑过敏反应时应使用苯海拉明。

药物治疗

• 对乙酰氨基酚：10～15 mg/kg，口服或灌肠，q4～6 h，不超过 5 剂/24 h。
• 头孢噻肟：50 mg/kg，静脉注射，q6 h，最大剂量 12 g/24 h。
• 头孢曲松：50 mg/kg，静脉注射，q12 h，最大剂量 4 g/24 h。
• 苯海拉明：1.25 mg/kg，口服、肌内注射或静脉注射，q6 h。

随访

进一步处理

入院指征

• 入院由疾病本身决定。
• 伴有系统性疾病或潜在恶化风险，如 SSS、红疹、水痘，以及其他疾病，可能需要住院治疗。

出院指征

出院指导应以潜在的疾病为依据。

转诊问题

对于生命体征稳定的自限性的皮疹应安排与初级保健医师或皮肤科医师进行随访。

随访建议

对于任何迅速蔓延的皮疹、皮疹形态的改变、瘀点或出血、新发发热或颈部僵硬，患者应及时急诊随访。

要点和误区

• 注意皮疹最先出现的部位及其传播方式。
• 明确对先前疗法的反应。
• 注意相关的体征和症状，它们通常是危重疾病的关键。
• 在任何皮疹瘀点或紫癜伴有发热，需要考虑脑膜炎球菌血症。

幼年型特发性关节炎 Arthritis, Juvenile Idiopathic

Kathleen A. Kerrigan · Sulynn Walker 汤璐佳 潘曙明 译

 基础知识

描述

• 旧称幼年型类风湿性关节炎。

• 不明原因的持续性关节炎，持续 6 周以上，发病年龄小于 17 岁，影响生长发育。

• 发病率约为 1/1000。

• 女性发病率高于男性。

• 分为 7 个亚型：全身发病型、RF 阴性型、RF 阳性型、少关节型、银屑病型、与附着点炎症反应相关型和未分类型。

• 根据受累关节的位置、数量、对称性、发病症状、皮肤症状、家族史、实验室检查分类。

• 约 20% 的患者为未分类型或符合多种类型。

• 亚型不同病程的转归也不同（孕妇病程较特殊），不到一半的患者可完全康复。

• 成年发病患者病程可有反复。

病因

由于某种感染及环境因素的影响，因遗传易感性个体发生自身免疫反应而导致。

诊断

亚型

• 全身性（SJIA）（以前称为"斯蒂尔病"）：

- 4%～15% 的病例，发病率男女相等，年龄可能在 1 岁以下。

- 伴发热和关节炎：

◦ 发热＞39 ℃ 超过 2 周，持续 3 日以上的"quotidian"发热（恢复到基线的峰值），孩子在生病时出现不适。

◦ 关节炎：＞6 周可能会累及任何数量的关节，可能仅在发热后几周到几个月出现。

- 至少以下之一：

◦ 躯干和腋窝有斑丘疹，鲑鱼色皮疹。

◦ 淋巴结肿大。

◦ 肝脾大。

◦ 浆膜炎。

- 起病最急、症状最重的亚型。

- 破坏性关节炎、小颌、颈椎融合等常见并发症经治疗后减少。

- 可能患有严重的贫血。

- 经常与感染或恶性肿瘤混淆。

注意

• 系统性发作的 JIA 患者有巨噬细胞活化综合征（MAS）的风险。

• MAS 是具有细胞因子释放的巨噬细胞增殖，引起类似 DIC 的图像，从而导致发热、黏膜出血、神经系统改变和多器官衰竭，这可能是致命的，死亡率为 8%～22%。

• 需要立即治疗。

• MAS 中的 ESR 可能正常。

• 寡关节：

- 30%～60%JIA。

- 3∶1 女孩，最高发病年龄为 2～4 岁。

- 隐匿性发作。

- 6 个月内涉及≤4 个关节：

◦ 不对称涉及较大的关节（89% 膝关节），髋部很少受影响。

◦ 关节肿胀，轻度压痛，无红斑，活动度（ROM）减少，可能有腿长不等。

◦ 6 岁以上男孩无 HLA-B27。

◦ 无肠炎。

- 葡萄膜炎约占 20%；如果 ANA 阳性，则风险增加；没有其他全身性症状。

- 分组：6 个月后受累关节数（1～4）；扩展（＞4）则不良预后。

• 多关节：

- 20%～30% 的病例，女孩多于男孩，双峰高峰在 2～5 岁和 10～14 岁。

- 根据 RF（−）和 RF（+）分类，RF（−）多于 RF（+）。

- 在 6 个月内涉及 4 个关节：

◦ 关节炎通常是对称性，大小关节均可受累，通常是膝、手腕和踝。

◦ 颈腰椎和颞下颌关节（TMJ）的活动度减少。

- 除疲劳和贫血外，全身性累及在射频中很少。

- 患有 RF（+）的大龄女孩经常继续发展成典型的成人类风湿关节炎（RA），并被置于单独的亚型中。

• 银屑病型：

- 关节症状：非对称性，下肢及背部大关节多见。

- 按关节炎和银屑病皮疹或关节炎含以下至少两项进行分类：趾炎、指甲凹陷、甲床分离（指甲与甲床分离）或一级亲属存在银屑病皮疹。

- 肌腱骨止点炎症（肌肉或肌腱起止处发炎）有关。

- 发病双峰。

- 可能只影响 1 个关节，80%＜5 个关节。

- 骶髂（SI）关节疼痛。

- 腰椎屈曲受限。

- 葡萄膜炎占 10%～15%。

- 经常出现 FH。

• 肠炎相关关节炎（ERA）：

- 按关节炎或肌腱骨止点炎症和以下至少两种分类：骶髂部压痛，HLA-B27，或前葡萄膜炎（FH+），脊椎病或 IBD。

- 大小关节均可受累，多个关节。

- 对称轴向参与。

- 既往可能被诊断为脊椎关节炎。

- 男性＞6 岁。

• 其他：

- 不能完全满足上述任何类别或不适合多个类别的关节炎。

病史

• 不同亚型病史不同。

• 典型症状为隐袭性关节炎，上午症状明显可出现一段时间关节固定，后进展为关节受限。

• 部分亚型起病症状较重，患者常就诊于急诊，大多数亚型起病较隐袭。

提醒

• 幼年型特发性关节炎不常伴随严重关节红、肿、热、痛。

• 快速进展累及多关节非幼年型特发性关节炎典型症状，应排除感染性疾病或反应性关节炎。

• 应注意使用免疫抑制药物者发生的隐匿性感染。

体格检查

• 如患儿全身系统症状较重，应注意体温、皮疹或其他非关节症状。

• 检查评估关节症状，清点累及关节，注意是否存在关节红、肿、热、痛，是否合并关节受限。

基本检查

• 排除炎症性疾病及恶性骨肿瘤。

• 排除其他原因造成的关节炎症。

• 排除长期药物治疗引起的并发症。

Y

■ 诊断检查与说明

实验室检查

• 全血细胞计数、红细胞沉降率，必要时血培养。
• 怀疑特殊亚型应进行必要的实验室检查：类风湿因子、抗核抗体、HLA-B27、肝功能：
- 全身发病型：常伴随红细胞沉降率、白细胞、血小板升高，贫血，轻度 AST/ALT 升高，类风湿因子及抗核抗体阳性少见，巨噬细胞活化综合征常合并肝功能异常及凝血功能异常而红细胞沉降率正常。
- 少关节型：年轻女性抗核抗体多为阳性；其他实验室检查多正常；贫血及红细胞沉降率升高多提示伸展性亚型。
- 多关节型：可伴有贫血，如类风湿因子阳性可进展为成人风湿性关节炎，红细胞沉降率可升高。
- 肠炎型：HLA 多为阳性；如类风湿因子或抗核抗体阳性可排除此型。
- 银屑型关节炎：类风湿因子常为血清反应阴性。
• 急性感染也可以引起类风湿因子与红细胞沉降率升高。

> **注意**
> 如患者来自莱姆关节病疫区发生关节肿大应考虑增加莱姆滴度检查。

影像学检查

• 关节 X 线摄片：
- 早期表现：软组织水肿，关节渗出。
- 晚期表现：骨质疏松、关节破坏、生长板提前关闭。
• 超声检查：
- 用于评估少量渗出，小关节首选。

诊断步骤/外科

如果考虑到败血性关节炎，则进行关节穿刺术：WBC 5 000～8 000/mm^3，革兰染色阴性，JIA 典型培养。

■ 鉴别诊断

• 外伤。
• 感染：
- 化脓性关节炎、病毒感染（尤其是肠炎病毒）、莱姆病、风湿热、结核、亚急性心内膜炎、疟疾、淋球菌感染。
• 其他风湿免疫结缔组织疾病：
- 系统性红斑狼疮、结节性动脉炎、过敏性紫癜、结节病。
- 雷卡佩病/股骨头骨骺滑脱。
• 赘生物：
- 当患儿表现为明显的骨中段疼痛应怀疑赘生物可能。
• 血液系统疾病：
- 镰状细胞疾病、血友病。
• 药物因素。

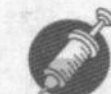

治疗

■ 初步稳定/治疗

全身毒性症状患儿：开放静脉通路，吸氧。

■ 急诊治疗/方法

• 排除感染及其他因素引起的关节炎。
• 如患儿已确诊为幼年型特发性关节炎，当患儿症状出现急性加重应联系儿童风湿免疫专家协调患儿诊治方案。

■ 药物治疗

• 确诊幼年型特发性关节炎的患儿的治疗目的为减轻疾病活动期临床症状、最大限度地保护关节功能、维护患儿生长发育（慢性炎症可影响四肢发育）。
• 药物有效性取决于疾病亚型与疾病严重程度。
• 非甾体抗炎药及关节腔注射对大多数少关节型患儿有效；多关节型及全身发病型常需要根据疾病针对性使用抗风湿病程改善药物和/或抗生素。
• 关节腔感染时应考虑使用抗生素。

> **注意**
> 目前认为，早期的充足积极治疗对于预防部分幼年型特发性关节炎的并发症有效，因此推荐患儿在病程早期即开始使用抗风湿病程改善药物与抗生素。当然，这些药物可能存在潜在的副作用：
> • 免疫抑制。
> • 疫苗作用减弱（禁止使用活性疫苗）。
> • 结核病激活：儿童应首先进行潜在结核病检测，如果存在风险，应改为中度或重度。
> • 肿瘤潜在风险增加。
> • 非甾体抗炎药：
> - 所使用的非甾体抗炎药亚型不同效果也不同。
> - 轻度幼年型特发性关节炎患者可单独或联合其他药物使用。
> - 布洛芬：30～45 mg/kg，每日 3～4 次。
> - 萘普生：10～20 mg/kg，每日 2 次，每日最大剂量 1 000 mg。
> - 吲哚美辛：1～2 mg/(kg·d)分 2～4 次服用。
> - 副作用：胃肠道不适、肝肾功能损害、头痛、皮炎。
> - 关节内使用类固醇：曲安奈德，1 ml/mg 溶解在 20 mg/ml 盐水中。
> - 可长期缓解症状(6～18 个月)，如果＜4 个月考虑升级治疗。
> • 全身性皮质类固醇：
> - 糖皮质激素：少见，可用于严重多关节疾病或全身性 JIA 合并 MAS、心肌炎或浆膜炎患者的短期桥接治疗。
> - 泼尼松：0.5～2 mg/kg，口服。
> - 甲泼尼龙：30 mg/kg，静脉注射，持续 1～5 日，每日 1 g 的高剂量冲击治疗。
> - 副作用：胃肠道不适、肾上腺功能抑制、骨质疏松、Cushing 综合征、感染。
> • DMARD
> - 甲氨蝶呤：5～15 mg/m^2，皮下注射、口服或肌内注射，每周 1 次。
> ◦ 为抗风湿病程改善药物一线用药。
> ◦ 通常 6～8 周改善。
> ◦ 副作用：胃溃疡、呕吐、肝毒性、致畸。
> - 来氟米特：前 1、2 或 3 日予以 100 mg，然后根据体重予以 10 mg 或 20 mg。用于对甲氨蝶呤不耐受的轻度疾病患者（未获 FDA 批准）。
> • 副作用：胃溃疡、皮疹、厌食。
> • 生物制剂：
> - 靶特异性细胞因子——用于对 DMARD 失败或不耐受的患者。
> - TNF-α 抑制剂；在 MTX＞3 个月且疾病活动中等至高度时使用。
> - 依那西普：0.4 mg/kg 皮下注射，每周 2 次或 0.8 mg/kg 皮下注射，每周一次。
> - 阿达木单抗：＜30 kg：20 mg；＞30 kg：40 mg，每隔一周皮下注射。
> ◦ 副作用：感染、注射部位反应，抑制 T 细胞活化。
> - 阿巴西普：10 mg/kg，静脉注射，每 4 周一次。
> ◦ 选择性 T 细胞共刺激阻断剂。
> ◦ 副作用：输注反应、头痛、咳嗽、恶心、感染。
> - 妥珠单抗：每 4 周 8～12 mg/kg，静脉注射（或每 2 周 8 mg/kg 静脉注射，用于系统性青少年特发性关节炎）。
> ◦ IL-6 受体拮抗剂。
> ◦ 副作用：感染、代谢、肝功能。
> - 阿那白滞素：2 mg/kg，每日皮下注射。
> ◦ IL-1 受体拮抗剂。

◦ 用于具有难治性系统特征的患者。
◦ 副作用：感染、抗体产生、头痛、呕吐。
◦ 未获得 FDA 批准。
- 卡那奴单抗：每 4 周 4 mg/kg；用于系统性青少年特发性关节炎。
◦ IL-1 受体拮抗剂。
◦ 副作用：感染、注射部位反应、体重增加、腹泻。
• 干细胞移植很少用于对医学治疗无效的严重病例：
- MAS 的治疗并未标准化，但可能包括高剂量的类固醇、环孢素或静脉免疫球蛋白。
• 对药物治疗无效的严重病例可考虑骨髓移植：
- 巨噬细胞活化综合征无标准化治疗方案，可考虑使用大剂量类固醇、环孢素、环磷酰胺，或静脉使用免疫球蛋白。

随访

进一步处理

入院指征

诊断不明的危重患儿或继发关节感染。

出院指征

• 无化脓性关节炎、全身感染或药物引起器官衰竭症状。
• 患者无不适主诉。
• 已妥当安排定期随访。

转诊问题

• 如怀疑化脓性关节炎应考虑骨科就诊。
• 必要时请风湿科专家会诊。

随访推荐

• 患儿应在风湿科长期随访。
• 确诊为幼年型特发性关节炎患儿应定期进行眼科检查排除葡萄膜炎（初期症状可不明显，但可造成永久性损伤）。

要点和误区

• 应排除急性关节感染（如有疫区接触史应考虑莱姆病）。
• 如患儿表现为抗生素无效的日间发热应考虑为全身发病型。
• 如全身发病型患儿出现脓毒症应考虑巨噬细胞活化综合征。
• 反复评估患者使用药物确认潜在副作用及免疫抑制可能。

浴盐——合成卡西酮中毒 Bath Salts — Synthetic Cathinones Poisoning

Alexander J. M. Ruby · Jenny J. Lu 宋振举 童朝阳 译

基础知识

描述

浴盐：
• 化合类药物包括合成卡西酮。
- 3,4-亚甲基二氧吡咯戊酮在美国很常见。
◦ 还有美沙酮、醋酸甲泼尼龙等。
• 销售时，它有许多名字，例如：
- Aura、Bliss、Bolivian Bath、Bromo-Dragonfly、Cloud 9、Ivory Snow、Ivory Wave、Meow-Meow、Vanilla Sky、White Dove、White Rush：
◦ 它们都标签“不供人类消费”，从而规避管理控制。
◦ 有时被错误地当作植物的化肥、驱虫剂、浴盐。
◦ 在化学上与泻盐（硫酸镁）或浴盐无关。
• 这些物质可能是粉末状、药片状，或者是结晶状。
◦ 颜色有白色、黄色、棕色、灰色。
• 可能是口服、喷雾吸入、烟雾、静脉注射。
• 它会使中枢神经系统兴奋，并且具有高度成瘾性，还有致幻效应。
- 它可能与可卡因、麻黄碱有相似的效应，使人入迷。
- 有报道称它可以使人精神错乱、有暴力倾向、MODS、DIC、心肌梗死、脑卒中（中风），甚至死亡。

流行病学

事件及流行状况估计

• 2010 年这类物质首次在美国使用：
- 2004 年 3,4-亚甲基二氧吡咯戊酮和美沙酮在欧洲有记录。
• 2011 年被称为“美国新药问题”。
- 毒品控制中心在全国范围内报道了数以千计的案例。
• 作为 DEA 计划的临时分类。
• 仍然可以在网上或者店铺买到这类物质。

病因

• MDPV 是一类与卡西酮结构类似的物质，它是从阿拉伯茶中提取的一种生物碱。
• 结构上属于苯乙胺的衍生物，常见的药物包括多巴胺、去甲肾上腺素、苯丙胺、合成卡西酮等。
• 药物化学配方改变使其逃避了检测、化合物的鉴定，从而将其分类为“非法物品”。
• 主要的毒性来源于多巴胺、去甲肾上腺素、5-羟色胺受体。
• 其效应来自现在的掺杂物及污染物。

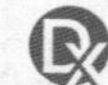

诊断

症状和体征

病史

• 通常是含糊不清或者难以获得的：
- 朋友、家人、旁观者可能会提供关于患者的行为。
- 但症状和体征出现难以符合要求的解释时要高度怀疑。

体格检查

• 没有病理性的症状和体征。
• 拟交感神经兴奋症状：
- 发热。
- 心动过速。
- 高血压。
- 心律失常。
- 大汗。
- 瞳孔散大。
- 横纹肌溶解。
- 呼吸困难。
- 反射亢进。
- 癫痫。
• 心理状态及行为效应：
- 精神亢奋。
- 产生幻觉。

Y

- 攻击性。
- 精神错乱。
- 妄想症。
- 谵妄。
- 自杀倾向。
- 惊恐发作。
- 失眠。

■ 基本检查

最基本的就是关注中毒的严重程度，排除其他药物及毒物导致的精神状态异常。

■ 诊断检查与说明

• 在急诊中目前没有方法去检测 MDPV：
- 摄取物、血清、尿液的样本可以送去实验室检测。
◦ 在急诊机构，结果是无法获取的。

• 实验室检测：
- 尿液、血清中的 MDPV 可以被检测到。
- 血常规、骨形成蛋白、肝功能、PT、APTT。
- 乳酸、pH。
- CK 测定。
- 如果有感染证据，可以行血、尿培养。

• 心电图：
- 评估 QT/QRS 间期，以及心脏的节律。

• 影像学检查：
- 根据病情考虑是否行头颅 CT 检查（如排除外伤）。

■ 鉴别诊断

• 其他中毒疾病。
- 可卡因。
- 苯丙胺。
- 抗胆碱能药物。
- 乙醇。

• 急性精神错乱。
• 血清素综合征。
• 感染或者代谢引发精神错乱。

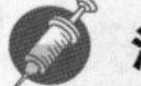

治疗

■ 院前

• 稳定气道。
• 生命体征。
• 建立静脉通路。
• 测指尖血糖。
• 需要时供氧。

■ 初步稳定/治疗

• 稳定气道，建立静脉通路，监测生命体征，心电监测。
• 苯二氮䓬类镇静剂是一线用药。
• 在必要的情况下采取肢体约束，预防患者及工作人员受伤。

■ 急诊治疗/流程

• 支持治疗是持续心脏和温度监测治疗的基础：
- 液体复苏。
- 氧气供应。
- 苯二氮䓬类镇静剂是一线用药。

• 发热时积极降温措施：
- 冰箱、凉水雾化、风扇、冷却毯、静脉输低温液体。

• 在极少数情况下，可能需要气管插管。
• 谨慎使用可能降低癫痫发作阈值的抗精神病药物，引起锥体外系症状和心律失常。
• 赛庚啶只作为苯二氮䓬类药物的佐剂使用。
• 毒物控制中心/毒理学指导。

■ 药物治疗

• 劳拉西泮：2～4 mg 递增，肌内注射或静脉注射。
• 地西泮（安定）：10～30 mg 递增，肌内注射或静脉注射。

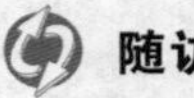

随访

■ 进一步处理

入院指征

• 所有有症状的患者均应入院接受监测。
• 包括无法控制的高血压、精神状态改变、心血管不稳定和高热在内的严重症状需要 ICU 监测。

出院指征

只有无症状的患者在适当的观察期后仍然无症状（MDPV 的半衰期估计为 1.88 h，持续作用 6～8 h）可以出院；每种情况下确切的时间会有所不同（请咨询毒物控制中心）。

■ 随访建议

出院后进行初级保健医师随访。

要点和误区

• 谵妄、精神病拟交感神经中毒综合征应怀疑“浴盐”中毒。
• 应积极控制高热。
• 将苯二氮䓬类作为初步稳定/治疗时，应将支持治疗作为基础。

Y

预激综合征 Wolff-Parkinson-White (WPW) Syndrome

Daniel Beslin Walk 吴昊 李文放 译

基础知识

■ 描述

• 由于在心房和心室之间绕过房室结（肯特束）的异常（附属）通路而引起。
• 心电图上的 WPW 模式，定义为由一个短的 PR 间期和一个提前下传（预激发）的 Δ 波：
- 在 0.1%～0.3%的人群中存在旁路。

• WPW 综合征需要心电图提供旁路及心动过速的证据。
• 旁路：
- 发育过程中未能分离的小条状组织：
◦ 左侧（游离壁）旁路：最常见。
◦ 房室结后区域：第二常见的位置。
◦ 游离右侧壁。
◦ 前间壁。

• WPW 中的传导可能是顺行的，也可能是逆行的，或者两者兼有。
• 最常见的是直传性再折返型心动过速（70%）：
- 冲动顺向从心房沿房室结点向下到心室，然后沿旁路通路逆行。
- 这种折返型心动过速是一种少见的复杂节律，除非存在束支阻滞或心室传导延迟。

• 逆行性较不常见（30%）：

- 脉冲沿着旁路顺行，从房室结折返，产生宽大的随机的(QRS)复合波。

• 已知的心室预激患者中，猝死率为1/100。

■ 病因

• 特发性：
- 大多数机制尚不清楚，具有家族性倾向。
• 很少作为常染色体显性遗传。
• 罕见病例伴有家族性肥厚性心肌病。

诊断

■ 症状和体征

病史

• 无症状的。
• 心悸：
- 快速或不规则。
• 胸痛。
• 呼吸困难。
• 头晕。
• 出汗。
• 晕厥。
• 猝死(罕见)。

体格检查

• 心动过速：
- 快速和有规律：
◦ 室上性心动过速。
◦ 心房扑动。
- 不规则的：
◦ 心房纤颤。
• 不稳定的迹象：
- 胸痛。
- 低血压。
- 精神状态改变。
- 啰音。
- 发绀。

■ 基本检查

• 在所有心律失常病例中，WPW 综合征应被视为潜在的病因。
• 诊断应以特征性心电图表现为依据。

■ 诊断检查与说明

实验室检查

• 只有在出现心肌缺血迹象时检测心肌酶。
• 考虑电解质和甲状腺疾病。

影像学检查

• 心电图。
• 预激：
- 短 PR 间期，<0.12 s。
- Δ 波：QRS 波群开始时的轻微上抬表现。
- QRS 群延长>0.10 s，形态可变，与特定旁路相关。
• 左外侧通路：
- 正向 Δ 波。
- 在 V_1 和下壁导联上提示带负向等电偏转的 Q 波。
◦ 可能提示既往高侧壁 MI 和电轴右偏。
• 左后间隔的旁路途径：
- 负向偏转 Δ 波。
- 提前出现的 QRS 波群：
◦ 常被误认为是下壁心肌梗死前期。
• 心动过速：
- 房室折返性心动过速(OAVRT)：
◦ 将冲动传导到心室的通路是房室结/希氏束系统。
◦ 窄 QRS 复合波心动过速。
◦ 在预先存在或者心率相关的功能性束支阻滞存在的情况下，可能会表现为宽大的 QRS 波群。
◦ QRS 波群后的 P 波。
◦ 速率在 150～250 次/分。
◦ 窦性心律时的 Δ 波消失，考虑顺行传导不是通过旁路进行的。
- 逆向的房室折返性心动过速。
◦ 常见的。
◦ 宽 QRS 波群。
◦ 前壁是常见的旁路。
- 心房纤颤：
◦ 不规则的。
◦ 宽大畸形的 QRS 波群。

■ 鉴别诊断

• 预激：
- 下壁心肌梗死。
• 无附属通路的狭窄复杂室上心动过速：
- 房室结折返性心动过速(AVNRT)。
• 广泛复杂的心动过速：
- 房颤伴心室传导延迟。
- 室性心动过速。

治疗

■ 院前

• 吸氧并进行监测。
• 迷走神经运动(Valsalva)：颈动脉窦按摩、面部冰敷。
• 同步复律法：
- 生命体征不稳定(低血压、AMS 等)。
- 房颤伴 WPW、广泛复杂的心动过速。
• 院前应用腺苷：
- 稳定患者：无需紧急复律。
- 不稳定患者：需要心脏复律，而不是腺苷。

■ 初步稳定/治疗

• 不稳定的患者：
- 同步电复律(100 J 开始)。
- 逐渐增加直到恢复窦性心律(200 J，然后 360 J)。
• 广泛性复杂心动过速稳定患者：
- 胺碘酮。
- 普鲁卡因胺。
- 在广泛性复杂心动过速和疑似 WPW 患者中禁用：利多卡因、钙通道阻滞剂、β 受体阻滞剂、地高辛。

■ 急诊治疗/程序

• 稳定的患者：
- 刺激迷走神经：Valsalva 和颈动脉窦按摩：
◦ 右侧颈动脉窦按摩不得超过 10 s。
◦ 主动脉听诊区有杂音，禁止此操作。
- 如果患者有轻度低血压，补液和特伦德伦伯卧位。
- 如果颈动脉窦按摩失败，可进行药物复率。
• 顺行(通常是窄波)AVRT：
- 腺苷或维拉帕米。
• 逆向(通常是宽波)AVRT：
- 普鲁卡因酰胺是首选药物。
- 确诊时可以使用维拉帕米和 β 受体阻滞剂，但因其很难与室性心动过速和 WPW 合并房颤相鉴别，故具有危险性。
• 不规则宽大心动过速：
- WPW 综合征合并心房颤动。
- 胺碘酮或普鲁卡因酰胺。

儿科注意事项

• 儿童可能发展到心室率高达 320 次/分，此种情况难以耐受。
• 不稳定儿童电复律 0.5～2 J/kg。
• 迷走神经运动和腺苷在稳定的儿童中是安全的。

■ 药物治疗

• 腺苷：6 mg 快速静脉注射 1～2 s 或以上。如果无效，重复使用 12 mg(儿童：0.1 mg/kg

快速静脉推压，重复使用 0.2 mg/kg)。

- 胺碘酮：150 mg 静脉超过 10 min，360 mg 超过 6 h(60 mg/h)。
- 镁：2 g 静脉快推注。
- 普鲁卡因酰胺：6～13 mg/kg 静脉在 0.2～0.5 mg/(kg·min)，直到心律失常得到控制，QRS 扩大 50%，或低血压，然后 2～6 mg/min，最大剂量 1 000 mg。

一线用药

- 胺碘酮用于宽大复杂心动过速。
- 腺苷用于狭窄复杂的心动过速。

二线用药

- 普鲁卡因酰胺用于复杂的心动过速。
- 维拉帕米 5～10 mg，静脉普鲁卡因酰胺，地尔硫䓬 10～20 mg，或艾司洛尔可被认为是常规狭窄复杂心动过速的 WPW 患者的二线药物。

随访

进一步处理

入院指征

- 不稳定的表现和/或晕厥的病史。
- 门诊连续药物控制或消融治疗失败。

出院指征

- 大多数患者病情稳定，一旦转为窦性心律，即可出院。
- 应安排心脏病专家进行随访。

转诊问题

可在门诊进行评估射频消融术或手术的电生理学研究。

随访建议

如出现任何提示心跳过速的症状(心悸、头晕、胸部疼痛、感到头晕或晕厥)应及时至急诊就诊。

要点和误区

有心房颤动或广泛性复杂心动过速的预激患者禁用钙通道阻滞剂、β受体阻滞剂或地高辛：

- 这些药物延长了房室结的不应期，增加了通过旁路的概率，可能导致致命的室性心律失常。
- 如果症状持续＞48 h，抗凝必须在心脏复律前处理，因为 1%～3%的患者会发生栓塞事件。应当考虑使用经食管超声来清除左心房血栓。

月骨脱位 Lunate Dislocation

Stephen R. Hayden　王胜云 译

基础知识

描述

- 月骨脱位多与掌骨中的腕骨活动半径相关，多为掌侧脱位，背侧较少。
- 通常为手腕尺骨偏离过度造成。

病因

- 韧带受损。
- 腕管中正中神经损伤。
- 桡骨茎突、舟状骨、头状骨、三角骨等常见骨折时应考虑合并韧带损伤脱位的可能。

诊断

症状和体征

腕部疼痛、肿胀。

病史

- 高处坠落或车辆事故。
- 疼痛伴手腕处压痛。

体格检查

- 手腕处肿胀(掌侧或背侧)。
- 肿胀可能会掩盖手腕处的严重畸形。
- 可有正中神经受损表现。

基本检查

- 临床检查通常不是诊断性的。
- 评估皮肤完整性及血管神经功能。
- X 线平片检查见以下描述。

诊断检查与说明

影像学检查

- 腕部 X 线平片检查包括 3 个位置。
- 侧位 X 线平片最有价值：
  - 通过桡骨、月骨和头状骨中心的正常纵向线的破坏，发现脱位或半脱位。
  - 在掌侧脱位中，月骨经常倾斜，“杯子”的开口朝向手掌(茶杯溢出征)。
- 后前位 X 线平片：
  - 与“通常”的“四边形”相反，呈三角形。
  - 桡腕骨行形成的平滑连续的弧线中断表明月骨脱位。
- 如果 X 线平片上看不到可疑骨折，则考虑 CT 扫描。

儿科注意事项

除非完全骨化，否则影像学很难解释。

老年人注意事项

其他骨折也很常见。

鉴别诊断

- 月骨骨折。
- 环月状骨脱位。
- 舟月骨脱位。
- 舟状骨骨折。

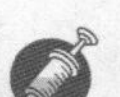

治疗

院前

- 包扎伤处。
- 固定受伤中间位置。

初步稳定/治疗

夹板固定。

急诊治疗/程序

- 明确伤情。
- 联系手外科，必要时手术。
- 闭合复位术可能较困难且不稳定。
- 开放复位术应用较多。

儿科注意事项

儿科严重受伤情况不常见，但是对于有手腕部疼痛的患者应及时明确检查，排除骨折。

药物治疗

一线用药

止痛剂：

- 吗啡：
  - 儿童：0.05～0.20 mk/kg，最高 1.5 mg。

- 成人：4～8 mg。
• 对乙酰氨基酚与氢可酮：
- 儿童（＞12 岁）：对乙酰氨基酚 2.5～10 mg，q4～6 h，最大剂量 60 mg/24 h；或氢可酮 4 g/24 h。
- 成人：对乙酰氨基酚 5～10 mg，q4～6 h，最大剂量 60 mg/24 h；或氢可酮 4 g/24 h。
• 对乙酰氨基酚与可待因：
- 儿童：对乙酰氨基酚 0.5～1 mg/kg（基于可待因每 4～6 h 口服的基础上），24 h 不超过 10～15 mg/kg。
- 成人：30～60 mg，q4～6 h，对乙酰氨基酚 24 h 不超过 4 g。

二线用药

非甾体类：
• 布洛芬：
- 儿童：5～10 mg/kg，q6～8 h，最大剂量 40 mg/(kg·d)。
- 成人：600 mg，口服，q6 h。
• 萘普生：
- 儿童（＞2 岁）：2.5 mg/(kg·d)，口服，每日 2 次[最大剂量不超过 10 mg/(kg·d)]。
- 成人：250～500 mg，口服，每日 2 次。

随访

进一步处理

入院指征

开放性骨折、多发伤及其他严重外伤患者。

出院指征

在急诊已经处理、固定且无需手术的患者同时后期有整形科医师随访。

随访建议

• 有夹板固定患者建议整形科医师随访。
• 未完全治愈前不宜重复导致受伤的活动。

要点和误区

• 注意手腕脱位的漏诊。
• 中枢神经系统损伤的漏诊。
• 月骨缺血性坏死。
• 退行性病变。

月骨周围脱位 Perilunate Dislocation

Cameron S. Smyres · Ian R. Grover　刘静 译

 基础知识

描述

• 月骨仍然位于半径但是远侧腕骨向背侧移位（～95%的情况下）或者向掌侧移位（～5%的情况下）。
• 建议进行早期的外科治疗。
• 这种损伤有很高的创伤后关节炎发病率。

病因

• 损伤机制：一般是腕关节过度伸展和向尺骨端偏移。
• 下列为高能量损伤：
- 高空坠落。
- 机动车事故。
- 工伤事故。
- 运动事故。

> **注意**
> 腕舟状骨骨折常伴有月骨周围脱位。

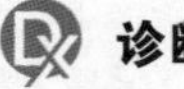 诊断

症状和体征

• 手腕严重疼痛。
• 手腕肿胀。
• 手腕触痛扩散。
• 正中神经分布感觉异常。

病史

• 高能量损伤病史。
• 任何合并伤。
• 腕关节疼痛。
• 可能主诉正中神经分布感觉异常。

体格检查

• 腕关节肿胀。
• 腕关节可能畸形。
• 腕关节运动范围减少。
• 正中神经分布感觉可能减少。
• 应该特别注意皮肤的完整性，因为开放性骨折很常见。
• 应该密切监测神经与血管的状态，包括两点阈。
• 密切检查合并伤，尤其是上肢。

> **注意**
> 临床检查经常漏诊。

基本检查

腕关节 X 线。

诊断检查与说明

影像学检查

• X 线图包括腕关节的 3 个位置。
• 月骨周围脱位在侧位片中最直观：
- 远侧腕骨，尤其是头状骨，可以看到相对于月骨向背侧移位（95%）或向掌侧移位（5%）。
- 月骨位于桡骨线内。
• CT 扫描和 MRI 一般不用于诊断，但是一些骨科医师进行术前计划时可能要求进行这方面的检查。

儿科注意事项

• 儿童很少会出现腕关节扭伤。
• 在儿科患者中腕关节 X 线很难表现出来。
• 与对侧腕关节比较可能会有帮助。

鉴别诊断

• 月骨骨折。
• 月骨移位。
- 在月骨和远端桡骨之间发生移位。
• 舟月骨分离和其他类似韧带断裂。
• 桡骨远端骨折。

儿科注意事项

考虑非意外创伤。

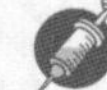 治疗

> **注意**
> 关注合并的、更严重的损伤。

院前

• 评估其他损伤。

Y

• 固定。
• 止痛。
• 抬高。

■ **初始稳定/治疗**

• 识别出其他更严重的合并伤。
• 固定。
• 抬高。
• 冰敷。

■ **急诊治疗/程序**

• 止痛。
• 闭合复位术进行镇静：
- 甲苄咪酯：0.1～0.15 mg/kg 静脉注射。
- 巴比妥：1～1.5 mg/kg 静脉注射。
- 丙泊酚(异丙酚)：40 mg/10 s 静脉注射直至诱导期。
• 应立即对脱位进行闭合复位：
- 胳膊用 10～15 磅(4.5～6.8 kg)平衡重牵引悬挂 10 min 并且套住手指。
- 手指从圈中移除后，继续进行徒手牵引。
- 医师的一个拇指放在月骨掌侧，然后通过手腕的伸展来恢复损伤。
- 持续牵引腕关节，然后缓慢弯曲腕关节，这样可以固定远端腕骨。
• 需要手术固定来减少损伤并保持腕关节稳定性。
• 用夹板将腕关节固定在中间位置，以便后期 X 线检查。

儿科注意事项

尽管月骨周围脱位在儿童患者中不常见，儿童腕关节疼痛应当用夹板固定而且交给少儿手外科医师处理。

■ **药物治疗**

• 地西泮(安定)：焦虑时 2～5 mg，静脉注射，q2～4 h(儿童：最大剂量是 0.25 mg/kg q4 h)。
• 芬太尼：疼痛时服用 0.05～0.2 mg，静脉注射，qh。
• 氢化吗啡酮：疼痛时 0.5～1 mg，静脉注射，q4～6 h(儿童：0.015 mg/kg 的剂量 q4～6 h)。
• 劳拉西泮(氯羟去甲安定)：疼痛时 0.5～1 mg，静脉注射，q1～6 h(儿童：0.044 mg/kg，q4～6 h)。
• 硫酸吗啡碱：疼痛时 0.1 mg/kg，静脉注射，qh。

随访

■ **进一步处理**

入院指征

• 开放性脱位，存在多处创伤，或者其他更严重的损伤。
• 无法减少移位。
• 神经与血管的状态。

出院指征

• 损伤闭合。
• 适当减少移位。
• 不涉及神经与血管。
• 2～3 周骨科随访。

转诊问题

所有月骨周围移位的病患应该进行外科手术稳定和韧带修复手术。

■ **随访建议**

• 所有月骨移位的患者必须进行外科手术稳定和韧带修复的随访。
• 应当在 2～3 周进行随访。

要点和误区

• 多达 25%的损伤没有早期发现。
• 对于腕关节疼痛、肿胀、活动受限的患者，取得腕关节的 X 线照片很重要，通过侧面的腕关节 X 线确保月状骨和头状骨位于其凹窝中。
• 这些损伤的延迟出现会导致很坏的结果，经常需要补救性手术。
• 并发症包括正中神经损伤、肌腱问题、疼痛综合征、腕关节不稳定，以及创伤性关节炎。
• 即使适当的治疗，创伤性关节炎的发病率也很高而且丧失握力。

晕厥 Syncope

Jarrod Mosier · Samuel M. Keim 江伟伟 李文放 译

Y

基础知识

■ **描述**

• 与丧失姿势张力有关的瞬间意识丧失。
• 脑干网状上行激活系统缺氧，导致意识和姿势张力的丧失。
• 最常见的原因是心输出量下降。
• 通过自主调节和由事件导致的躺卧姿势重新建立脑灌注。
• 占急诊患者数的 3%。

妊娠注意事项

• 妊娠的患者经常遇到来自各种原因的晕厥。5%的患者在妊娠期间经历过晕厥，28%的患者经历过呕吐。
• 胎盘作为 AV 畸形，导致 SVR 降低，从而加重直立症状。
• 胎儿压迫 IVC 可能导致神经源性和低血容量性晕厥。
• 妊娠患者深静脉血栓形成(DVT)、肺动脉栓塞(PE)、尿路感染(UTI)、癫痫发作(先兆子痫)、瓣膜功能不全的风险较高，急诊评估时应排除这些诊断。

老年人注意事项

• 老年人的发病率最高，随年龄增加发病率升高。
• >1/3 的患者会有多个潜在的原因。

■ **病因**

• 神经源性晕厥：
- 反射性反应引起血管舒张和心动过缓伴脑血流灌注不足。
- 血管迷走神经(常见晕厥)：
◦ 常因疼痛或恐惧而发作。
◦ 通常有前驱症状。
◦ 通常持续<20 s。
◦ 直立倾斜试验是诊断的金标准。
- 颈动脉窦晕厥：
◦ 咳嗽，打喷嚏。
◦ 胃肠道刺激(如排便)。
◦ 排尿。
• 体位性晕厥：
- 位置改变导致静脉回流到心脏突然下降。
- 血容量不足：
◦ 严重脱水(如呕吐、腹泻、利尿剂)。
- 出血(见“失血性休克”)。

• 自主神经衰竭：
- 糖尿病或淀粉样神经病。
- 帕金森综合征。
- 药物(如β受体阻滞剂)和酒精。

• 心律失常：
- 通常突然并且没有前驱症状。
- 快速心律失常或缓慢性心律失常。
- 遗传病(如长QT综合征、Brugada综合征)。
- 起搏器/植入心脏除颤器故障。

• 结构性心脏或心肺疾病：
- 瓣膜疾病(特别是主动脉瓣狭窄)。
- 肥厚型心肌病。
- 急性心肌梗死。
- 主动脉夹层。
- 心脏压塞。

• 肺栓塞。

• 神经源性：
- 颅内压的瞬时峰值超过脑灌注压。
- 晕厥后头痛很普遍。
- 可能会出现蛛网膜下腔出血。

• 脑血管盗血综合征。

诊断

症状和体征

病史

• 前驱症状：
- 头晕。
- 大汗。
- 视物模糊。
- 恶心。
- 乏力。

• 存在以下情况有潜在的生命威胁：
- 突发事件没有警告。
- 胸痛或心悸。

• 6种晕厥史：
- 1. 前驱活动。
- 2. 前驱症状：视觉症状、恶心。
- 3. 诱发因素：年龄、慢性病、家族猝死史。
- 4. 发病因素：压力、姿势。
- 5. 路人证人：他们看到了什么？
- 6. 发作后阶段(如果有的话)：癫痫发作。

体格检查

• 评估创伤。

• 体位性生命体征。

• 检查双臂血压，如果存在差异提示主动脉夹层或锁骨下动脉盗血综合征。

• 心血管检查，包括杂音和心律失常。

• 直肠检查检查消化道出血。

• 妊娠期女性的尿妊娠试验。

• 神经系统检查。

儿科注意事项

• 有以下症状，提示严重潜在疾病：
- 运动时发生晕厥。
- 大声喧哗、惊慌、极度压力下晕厥。
- 晕厥时仰卧。
- 家族年轻人猝死史(<30岁)。

基本检查

• 在到达时立即检查心电图：
- 心肌缺血。
- 心律失常。
- 传导阻滞。
- 长QT间期。
- Brugada综合征。
- WPW综合征。

• 详细的病史和体检将决定最终获得诊断的患者中85%的诊断。

诊断测查与说明

实验室检查

• 受既往史和体格检查影响。

• 怀疑出血时行血常规。

• 血清碳酸氢钠：
- 大多数晕厥患者是正常的。
- 事件发生后<1 h标记的碳酸氢盐减少：
  ◦ 提示癫痫大发作而非晕厥。
  ◦ 如果是癫痫发作，应该在事件发生后1 h给予治疗。

• 怀疑局部缺血时行心肌酶谱。

• 妊娠期女性行妊娠试验。

• 严重脱水或使用利尿剂的患者检查电解质。

• 血肌酐升高与30日病情恶化风险相关。

影像学检查

• 心电图监测，直到排除心脏原因。

• 如充血性心力衰竭(CHF)、夹层或怀疑大面积肺栓塞，行胸部影像±CT血管造影。

• 如果出现异常神经系统检查或暂时性缺血性表现行头部CT。

• 如果考虑心脏结构缺陷行超声心动图。

鉴别诊断

• 癫痫最常被误认为晕厥：
- 关键的区分因素是癫痫发作后精神错乱。
- 晕厥可能出现短暂的强直运动和尿失禁。

• 代谢紊乱(如低氧血症、过度换气、低血糖)。

• 中毒。

• 休克。

• 精神性晕厥。

• 装病。

• 小儿屏气发作(哭泣、晕厥)。

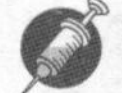

治疗

院前

• 吸氧。

• 心电图。

• 建立静脉通路。

初步稳定/治疗

• 针对不稳定患者行高级心脏生命支持(ACLS)。

• 吸氧。

• 心电监测。

• 怀疑低血容量则静脉输液。

• 考虑昏迷“鸡尾酒”：持续精神状态改变者予以葡萄糖、硫胺素和纳洛酮。

急诊治疗/程序

• ACLS在治疗心律失常方面的应用。

• 急性心肌梗死的标准治疗方案。

• 控制蛛网膜下腔出血和主动脉夹层患者的血压。

• 考虑肺栓塞的溶栓剂。

药物治疗

• 葡萄糖：D_{50} W 1安瓿(50 ml或25 g)，静脉注射(儿童：D_{25} W 2～4 mg/kg静脉注射)。

• 纳洛酮：2 mg，静脉注射或肌内注射(儿童：0.1 mg/kg)。

• 硫胺素：100 mg，静脉注射或肌内注射(儿童：50 mg)。

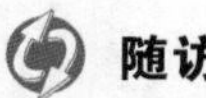

随访

进一步处理

入院指征

• 旧金山晕厥指南确定了严重短期后果的高危患者(“CHESS”)：
- CHF的既往史。
- 血细胞比容<30%。
- 心电图异常。
- 患者抱怨呼吸急促。
- 收缩压<90 mmHg。

• 其他建议：
- 怀疑心源性晕厥必须入院监测。

- 消化道出血考虑进入重症监护室。
- 老年人患有晕厥。
- 血肌酐升高、慢性心衰病史、入急诊时出现低血压、心律失常病史、肌钙蛋白异常都与 30 日的严重不良事件相关。
- 存在短期临床不良事件高风险者应在急诊接受全面的检查。

出院指征

• 如果患者是可靠的并且具有良好的社会结构，则可以在门诊基础上密切随访，评估原因不明的晕厥或直立性晕厥。
• 限制驾驶，直到治愈。

要点和误区

• 使用旧金山晕厥指南等标准可防止不必要的患者入院。
• 不要认为血管迷走神经引起的晕厥与头痛或胸痛有关。

孕妇外伤 Pregnancy, Trauma in

Kyle Roedersheimer · Bryant K. Allen　郑金浩　毛恩强 译

基础知识

▪ 描述

• 妊娠前 3 个月，胎儿和孕妇外伤：
- 增加流产的风险，但不会增加孕妇的死亡率。
• 胎儿外伤可能随着孕妇外伤增加。
• 妊娠后生理性血容量增加，可能导致预估出血量偏少：
- 孕妇失血 30% 以上才出现休克的临床表现。
• 腹部体征在孕妇患者人群中不明显。
• 孕妇轻微的颅脑损伤也会导致胎儿的外伤（在妊娠异常中占 50%）。
• 创伤严重程度评分＞9 分的患者与预后有关。
• 消化道损伤频率降低。
• 大多数腹膜后出血是由于盆腔器官血管损伤引起的。
• 骨盆和子宫充血将增加盆腔出血的发病率和死亡率。
• 胎儿或子宫外伤包括：
- 胎盘早剥。
- 胎母输血综合征（FMH）。
- 早产。
- 子宫挫伤破裂。
- 新生儿脑病。
- 羊膜早破早产。
- 胎儿缺氧性或结构上损伤（颅骨骨折）。
• 流产率在孕妇严重颅脑损伤中高达 60%，在轻微颅脑损伤中占 1%～5%。
- 高达总数的 50%。
- 可能并没有出血（20%）。
- 发生在妊娠 16 周以后。
- 可以表现为腹部绞痛或阴道出血。
- 特点为出现宫缩。
• 子宫破裂：
- 常发生在瘢痕子宫的孕妇。
- 接近通常死亡率。
- 孕妇死亡率占 10%。
• 骨盆骨折：
- 可以作为胎儿死亡的独立预测因素。
- 对胎儿致命的打击可以在所有妊娠时期出现。
- 10% 的胎儿死于孕妇轻伤。
• 严重外伤中有＞30% 出现胎儿或子宫出血：
- Rh 阴性的同种免疫孕妇（出血量最少为 0.03 ml 即会出现）。
• 穿透性创伤可以导致胎儿直接外伤、孕妇休克及早产。
• 约 1/4 的孕妇会出现滑倒或跌倒，可能会引起：
- 早产的发生率提高 4.4 倍。
- 胎盘早剥的发生率提高 8 倍。
- 胎儿窘迫综合征的发病率提高 2.1 倍。
- 胎儿宫内缺氧的发生率提高 2.9 倍。
• 烧伤：如果烧伤面积＞40%，胎儿死亡率几乎为 100%。
• 故意伤害或家暴使早产的发生率提高 2.7 倍，低出生体重的发生率升高 5.3 倍。
• 触电是引起胎儿死亡的重要原因。

▪ 病因

• 孕妇发生外伤的概率约为 7%。
• 外伤为孕妇非产科发病和死亡最常见的原因。
• 流产率为 3.4%～38%。
• 机动车事故占 48%～84%。
• 家庭暴力。
• 跌倒。
• 直接腹部外伤。
• 贯穿伤（刺伤或枪伤）。
• 触电或烧伤。
• 年轻女性更易发生。
• 机动车事故和家庭暴力常伴有药物滥用。
• 自杀和接触毒物。

诊断

▪ 症状和体征

病史

• 机械损伤。
• 末次月经的时间。
• 腹部疼痛。
• 宫缩。
• 阴道流血或流液。
• 既往妊娠、剖宫产。
• 滥用药物。

体格检查

• 如果查体需要可以让患者取左侧卧位。
• 初步评估。
• 再次评估。
• 最终评估。
• 胎盘早剥：
- 子宫压痛。
• 子宫破裂：
- 子宫压痛和形态改变。
- 可触及胎儿部位。
• 依据妊娠的年龄评估生育能力：
- 获取末次月经时间。
- 妊娠月份＝宫高（宫高：妊娠 16 周后宫高为耻骨到子宫底的距离）。
• 经阴道检查获取：
- 流血。
- 羊水。
- 宫颈扩张度和成熟度。

▪ 基本检查

• 脊柱制动。

Y

• 首先确定产妇的情况：
- 如果需要进行开放气道和复苏。
• 确定妊娠月份，预估保胎可行性：
- 孕周：与妊娠16周后宫高相关。
- 多普勒超声探测胎儿心音。
- 超声(可能漏诊轻微胎盘早剥)。
• 胎儿/孕妇监测4～6 h：
- 仅监测有成活希望的胎儿(一般要求妊娠24周以上)。
- 在1～4 h监测过程中，如果宫缩消失继续监测。
- 如果每h宫缩>8次，持续4 h表示预后不好。
- 如果每10 min至少有一次宫缩，流产的概率高达20%。
- 出现心动过缓，NST无反应型，或二型晚期减速预示着胎儿窘迫。
- 心电监测异常对于预测胎儿不良结局有62%的敏感性和49%的特异性。
- 心电监测和查体都正常并没有预后的评估价值。

诊断检查与说明

实验室检查

• 血常规和尿常规。
• 血气分析和电解质。
• 血型及特异性抗体筛查。
• 胎儿血红蛋白酸洗脱试验：
- 确定阴道中的FMH是液体还是血液。
- 确定FMH的性质很重要。

影像学检查

• 在获得必需的影像学结果的同时尽可能保护子宫免受辐射。
• 告知孕妇有关射线暴露的潜在风险。
• 并没有X线引起先天畸形或胎死宫中的确切证据。
• 射线引起肿瘤也颇受争议。
• 射线量在<1rad范围内认为没有任何风险。
• 射线量在5～10rad胎儿畸形的风险增加。
• 以下情况有必要进行影像学检查：
- 胸部X线(正侧位)：最小射线剂量。
- 骨盆(前后位)：1rad。
- 颈椎X线：最小剂量。
- 胸椎X线：最小剂量。
- 腰椎X线：0.031～4.9rad。
- 头颅CT：<0.05rad。
- 胸部CT：0.01～0.59rad。
- 腹部CT：2.8～4.6rad。
- 骨盆CT：1.94～5rad。
• 超声：
- 用超声检查重点评估创伤。
- 评估实质性器官的损伤以及腹腔积血。
- 胎儿心脏活动。
- 胎龄。
- 羊水量(羊水指数)。
- 漏诊50%～80%的胎盘早剥。
• 二硝基苯基偶氮萘酚二黄酸钠试纸(变蓝)检测阴道液体。
- 检测出羊水提示羊膜可能破裂。
• 穿透性创伤，特别是刺伤，推荐使用三维CT。

诊断步骤/外科

创伤性损伤。

鉴别诊断

诊断范围很广，应该仔细检查以防漏诊。

治疗

院前

• 保持脊柱位置固定。
• 妊娠中后期患者应该送至创伤救治中心。
• 通知创伤中心妊娠早期和EGA以便于调动适当的医疗资源。
• 患者保持左侧卧位(在背板上)避免仰卧位低血压(妊娠20周以上或多胎妊娠)。
• 腹部禁用抗休克裤。

初步稳定/治疗

• 由于处于妊娠期，孕妇外伤需即刻开始治疗。
- 首要开放气道和复苏。
- 心电监测。
• 左侧倾斜患者或靠板15°～30°(或手动移动子宫偏向左侧)。

急诊治疗/程序

• 乳酸林格液更适合配伍：
- 大量生理盐水可能引起高氯性酸中毒。
• 预估失血量按3∶1进行输血：
- 如果血液配型配不上使用O型血浓缩红细胞替代。
• 如果发生严重出血，按照冰冻血浆、红细胞悬液、血小板1∶1∶1的比例输注减少凝血功能障碍的发生，也可能改善预后。
• 输注2 000 ml晶体液后仍然考虑血容量不足，或估计失血量1 000 ml以上均应依靠输血治疗。
• 鼻胃管减压(孕妇患者误吸的风险更高)。
• 通过放置导尿管，评估尿量。
• 胸腔穿刺术。
- 增加1～2个肋间，避免损伤横膈膜。
• 按照顺序快速置管：
- 以安全和方便为前提。
- 避免误吸及缺氧。
• 必要时进行诊断性腹膜灌洗，使用脐上开口技术建立通道。
• 仅对于血流动力学稳定的孕妇进行保胎治疗：
- 宫颈口直径>4 cm或胎母输血综合征或流产物未能排除干净均为禁忌证。
- 只有在每小时8次以上宫缩持续4 h才进行保胎治疗。
• 可能在心脏呼吸骤停后4～5 min内施行Perimortem剖宫产。参考紧急剖宫产章节。
• 妊娠20周以后轻微的颅脑外伤，在产房最好进行胎儿和孕妇心电监护。
• 如果烧伤面积>50%并且胎儿在妊娠中期或晚期考虑分娩。
• 对所有Rh阴性的孕妇72 h内输注免疫球蛋白。
• 孕周<12周的肌内注射50 μg>12周的肌内注射300 μg。
• 24 h内复查正在进行的胎儿红细胞入母体的血量：
• 必要时复查Rh免疫球蛋白(胎儿入母体血量>30 ml)。
• 使用保胎药：硫酸镁4 g静脉注射。
• 尽量避免使用阿司匹林、镇静催眠药物、非甾体抗炎药、升压药。

随访

进一步处理

入院指征

• 阴道流血或胎膜早破。
• 胎母输血综合征。
• 腹痛。
• 不规律宫缩。
• 具有胎儿窘迫的依据。
• 胎盘早剥。
• 腹腔出血或内脏及实质脏器的损伤。
• 24周(9.9%)以上的胎儿才有成活的可能：
- 比较有价值的成活在26周(54.7%)以上的胎儿。

Y

出院指征

- 以下标准应全部具备：
  - 使用子宫分娩力计 4 h 内不显示宫缩。
  - 没有胎儿窘迫的依据。
  - 没有阴道流血或羊膜早破。
  - 没有腹痛及压痛。
  - 定期产检。
- 详细向患者说明以上情况，若有出现需再次入院。
- 只有在产科医师评估后方可出院。

随访建议

孕妇外伤经过产科医师详细地了解评估病情方可出院。

要点和误区

- 轻微的外伤可以导致孕妇和/或胎儿的死亡。
- 优先维持孕妇病情平稳。
- 1 500～2 000 ml 的失血量可能不会出现母亲妊娠期应激。

谵妄 Delirium

LoriA. Stolz · Arthur B. Sanders 许磊 译

基础知识

描述

• 谵妄是一种临床综合征，表现为意识、认知和感知的急性变化，并伴随漫长的过程。
• 谵妄通常继发于潜在急性疾病。
• 病理生理学未知：
- 弥漫性脑功能障碍。
- 脑乙酰胆碱的紊乱。
- 中枢神经系统多巴胺、γ-氨基丁酸和5-羟色胺可能参与。
• 经常被急诊医师漏诊。
• 与住院患者死亡率增加有关，并增加住院时间。

病因

• 神经：
- 脑膜炎或脑炎。
- 癫痫发作。
- Wenicke脑病。
- 缺氧和脑血流灌注不足。
- 颅内出血或肿块。
- 脑卒中症状。
• 肺：
- 肺炎。
- 缺氧或高碳酸血症的其他肺部病因。
• 心血管：
- 高血压危象。
- 急性冠状动脉综合征。
- 心律失常。
• 消化道：
- 肝性脑病。
- 脱水。
• 泌尿系统：
- 尿路感染。
- 急性肾衰竭。
• 内分泌：
- 低血糖。
- 高血糖。
- 甲减。
• 风湿病：
- 胶原血管疾病。
• 毒理学：
- 环境毒素。
- 药物或营养品。
- 撤巴比妥类或酒精。
• 其他：
- 电解质异常。
- 维生素缺乏。
- 低温。
- 热疗。
- 创伤。
- 手术。

老年注意事项

• 中老年急诊患者常见的表现。
• 年龄较大的急诊患者中高达10%的可能有谵妄。
• 许多患者都会有轻微的症状介绍和模糊的主诉：
- 失落、头晕或不舒服。
• 长期的症状。
• 已知痴呆的患者容易从急性疾病状态发展至谵妄。
• 危及生命的情况。

诊断

症状和体征

• 意识混乱：
- 高警觉：
◦ 好斗。
◦ 躁动。
- 活动减退：
◦ 嗜睡。
◦ 昏睡。
◦ 昏迷。
- 可以混有高警觉和活动减少状态并具有快速摆动。
- 活动减少状态未被充分认识。
• 认知变化：
- 迷失。
- 记忆受损。
- 思维和语言杂乱。
- 错觉、幻觉、妄想和幻觉。
• 周围环境认识不清。
• 注意力不集中：
- 注意力、移动、保持状态困难。
- 躁动。
- 分心。
- 不稳。

病史

• 监护人提供的病史对于确定病程及症状变化是必不可少的。
• 时间过程：
- 数小时至数日。
- 躁动过程。
• 药物：
- 处方，过度的非处方和非法药物。
- 剂量。
- 最近添加药物。
- 最近停止药物。
• 相关症状、体征、既往史、摔倒或创伤，将表明潜在的病因。

体格检查

• 利用体格检查来明确可能的潜在疾病并针对性的进一步检查，尤其是有感染和脓毒症来源的时候。
• 生命体征。
• 完整的神经系统检查：
- 详细的精神状态检查。
- 颅神经、运动和协调性。
- 局灶性神经功能缺损。
- 幻觉或妄想。
• 精神病学的检查。
• 心血管、呼吸、消化道系统和全身皮肤检查。
• 使用体格检查，以确定潜在的可能的医学疾病和进一步处理，尤其是感染和败血症的病因。
• 几种筛选工具可用于评估谵妄：
- 大多数谵妄评估工具没有在急诊室得到验证。
- 谵妄的评估方法由4个关键特点：
◦ 1：急性发作或波动的过程。
◦ 2：注意力不集中。
◦ 3：思维紊乱。
◦ 4：意识水平改变。
◦ 做出诊断时的特点1和2是前提并有3或4。
- 简易精神状态检查：
◦ 可连续检查，并会出现波动；因依赖于患者的合作正确的认知评估可能难以完成。

基本检查

• 谵妄意识综合征是关键。
• 病情的检查应该是全面的，以确定潜在的器质性病变。
• 辅助研究由病史检查、体格检查和初始检查决定。

■ 诊断检查与说明

实验室检查

• 初步测试：
- 电解质、钙、镁、磷。
- 肾功能。
- 肝功能。
- 葡萄糖。
- 全血细胞计数。
- 尿培养及药物敏感试验。
- 促甲状腺激素。
- 毒理学测试。

• 根据症状和体征进一步研究：
- 动脉血气。
- 心肌酶。

影像学检查

• 心电图。
• 头颅 CT/MRI。
• 胸部 X 线。
• 其他成像根据病史、体格检查和可能的病因。

■ 诊断步骤/程序

• 潜在病因。
• 腰椎穿刺，如果有指征。
• 脑电图可以区分谵妄和非惊厥发作的持续性癫痫。

■ 鉴别诊断

• 其他疾病的过程应该与谵妄鉴别，包括：
- 精神疾病：
  ◦ 症状没有波动的过程。
  ◦ 通常没有意识水平的变化。
  ◦ 与幻觉和幻听的精神疾病有关。
- 老年痴呆症：
  ◦ 谵妄具有起效快，而老年痴呆症缓慢渐进的，潜在过程中没有症状波动。
  ◦ 老年痴呆症在意识方面没有急性的变化。

• 一旦确定为谵妄，根本原因的区别是相当广泛的。

Z

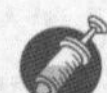

治疗

■ 院前

• 建立静脉通路：
- 脉搏血氧饱和度监测呼吸状态：
  ◦ 血糖监测。
  ◦ 心电监测。

• 如果呼吸功能不全，可使用纳洛酮。
• 监测患者：
- 高级生命支持(ALS)，使用药物治疗。

• 寻找一个根本原因的症状：
- 药物。
- 医疗警报链。

• 基本神经系统检查记录：
- 格拉斯哥昏迷量表评分。
- 瞳孔。
- 肢体动作。

■ 急诊治疗/程序

• 治疗应该以基本的医疗条件为目标。
• 建立静脉通路。
• 吸氧。
• 心律、脉搏血氧饱和度和血压监测。
• 硫胺素应给予酒精中毒和营养不良的患者。
• 非药物的方法是预防和治疗谵妄的有效方法：
- 早期运动。
- 适应。
- 补液。
- 视觉及听觉辅助器。
- 补充睡眠。

■ 药物治疗

• 谵妄的治疗应针对潜在的病因。
• 避免使用引起谵妄的药物。
• 药物治疗不大可能改变谵妄的病程、严重程度及降低死亡率。
• 药物治疗应该用于那些可能给自己或别人造成伤害或因严重躁动而中断或延迟其他治疗和干预的患者。
• 苯二氮䓬类应该是治疗酒精或苯二氮䓬药物减量患者的首选药物。
• 其他原因引起谵妄者应该避免使用苯二氮䓬类。

一线用药

• 使用抗精神病药物前评估患者有无 QT 间期延长综合征。
- 氟哌啶醇：5～10 mg，静脉注射和肌内注射。
- 低剂量(0.5～2 mg)适合老年患者。
- 研究表明，非典型抗精神病药物和典型抗精神病药物可以是同样有效的。

• 利培酮：0.25～0.50 mg，更少的锥体外系副作用。
• 硫胺素：100 mg，静脉注射、肌内注射或口服。

二线用药

• 阿普唑仑：0.25～0.5 mg，口服。
• 劳拉西泮：0.5～2 mg，静脉注射、肌内注射或口服。

随访

■ 进一步处理

入院指征

• 病因不清。
• 谵妄一直没有解决。
• 出院时谵妄原因不明的患者死亡率高。

出院指征

• 可治疗的原因被发现，并得到处理。
• 精神状态清晰在急诊。
• 可靠的护理人员。
• 确保随诊。

■ 随访建议

• 随访根据基本条件来进行。
• 当谵妄已在急诊室内解决，接下来的随访有初级保健者提供，最好是在 2 日内。
• 患者和护理人员应告知随访有关的注意事项：
- 谵妄复发，应及时送到急诊。
- 谵妄可以是威胁生命的。

要点和误区

• 找出根本原因。
• 谵妄往往有急诊内科医师误诊，谵妄的意识状态作为一种综合征是至关重要的。

掌骨损伤 Metacarpal Injuries

Stephen R. Hayden 段立伟 译

基础知识

描述

- 多由直接暴力如打击、挤压伤或烧伤造成。
- 最常见的是拳击手远端第 5 掌骨颈骨折。

诊断

症状和体征

- 损伤部位疼痛和肿胀。
- 损伤部位畸形。
- 骨折有旋转或侧方成角畸形。
- 每个手指单独屈曲时指尖均指向舟骨结节。
- 患肢处于限制体位。
- 多发闭合性掌骨骨折导致骨筋膜室综合征。

> 注意
>
> 有"战斗痕"(手打击人类牙齿形成的齿痕)的患者需高度怀疑掌骨损伤。

- 伸肌鞘、掌指关节(MCP)继发感染口腔内细菌。

病史

不是所有患者都能如实告知受伤的原因。

基本检查

检查时应该特别注意皮肤的完整性和指骨屈伸的一致性。

诊断检查与说明

影像学检查

- 手部 X 线提示骨折和/或排除异物。
- CT 未提示明显骨折时刻可行三维成像检查。

鉴别诊断

掌骨骨折可能伴随着相邻指骨或腕骨错位。

治疗

院前

- 不需要将掌骨损伤患者快速送医。
- 注意事项:
- 掌骨伤害应该用夹板固定住在舒适的位置。

初步稳定/治疗

- 其他更严重伤害应该首先治疗。
- 妥善固定等待评估。
- 伤口应尽快清洗,应该考虑异物的可能性。
- 烧伤早期镇痛治疗。

急诊治疗/程序

- 患肢高位、休息和间歇性冰敷在第一个 24 h 对所有手部外伤都有必要。
- 拳击手的骨折远段通常有一些掌屈。
- 尽可能减少掌曲至 40°或更多。
- 第 4 和第 5 掌骨骨折稳定,没有明显的旋转可以用软垫或夹板固定避免过度液体复苏,这会导致出血增加。
- 骨折的示指和中指掌骨较难固定。
- 径向沟形夹板和早期骨科转诊。
- 拇指掌骨骨折复杂,应尽早骨科转诊。
- 拇指夹板。
- 用夹板固定后避免错位,掌骨脱位罕见,通常需要固定。
- 掌指关节妥善夹板固定,或者"眼镜蛇"(超过腕关节的 20%~30%):
- 掌指关节尽可能接近 90°弯曲。
- 涵盖近侧指间关节和远侧指间关节。
- 为任何开放性掌骨骨折,可疑牙齿损伤尽早使用抗生素,必要时需在手术室行清创引流术。
- 单纯性环面(扣)骨折可采用夹板固定,并进行随访。

药物治疗

- 破伤风皮试接种破伤风疫苗。
- 烧伤患者可使用烧伤宁软膏或杆菌肽软膏外敷。
- 必要时止痛:非甾体类止痛药或氢可酮。
- 对人类咬伤或污染伤口,可使用阿莫西林-克拉维酸钾(安灭菌),或非口服途径给予头孢菌素或其他耐青霉素酶类抗生素。

随访

进一步处理

入院指征

- 开放性骨折或脱臼需要紧急手术治疗。
- 所有拇指掌骨骨折或脱位应骨科转诊。
- 咬伤后感染需要骨科会诊清洗伤口,清创,静脉注射抗生素。

出院指征

- 横向或斜裂缝稳定且已行早期夹板固定患者可出院随访。
- 掌指关节脱位通常不需要手术,即便需要也不是立即手术。
- 如果掌骨骨折产生损害范围较大或手指功能受损,为择期手术。

随访建议

骨骺损伤应骨科转诊。

要点和误区

所有掌骨损伤保证适当的复位。

针刺伤 Needlestick

Gordon S. Chew · Stephen R. Hayden 伍力学 译

基础知识

描述

- 潜在暴露于 HIV、乙型肝炎(HBV)或丙型肝炎(HCV),定义为暴露于感染性体液和入口处(经皮、黏膜、不完整皮肤)。
- 感染性体液:
- 血液。
- 精液、阴道液。
- 羊水、母乳。
- 心包、腹膜、胸腔。
- 滑液、CSF。

- 请注意，唾液、尿液、呕吐物、粪便、汗液、泪液、分泌物除非明显带有血色，否则不被视为接触。

• 一般预防：
- 常规注意事项。
- 避免重新盖针帽。
- 戴手套：可使血液暴露的概率降低 50%。
- 戴双层手套。
- 遵循身体物质隔离规则。
- 乙肝疫苗接种。

• 危险因素：
- 未免疫接种人群因一次针头暴露导致的感染风险。
  ◦ HBV：37%～62%来自 HBsAg 阳性合并 HBeAg 阳性的患者，23%～37%来自 HBsAg 阳性合并 HBeAg 阴性的患者。
  ◦ HCV：1.8%。
  ◦ HIV：血液 0.3%，黏膜 0.09%。
- 各种体液导致的 HIV 感染：
  ◦ 血浆和血清：10～5 000 ppm。
  ◦ 脑脊液：10～1 000 ppm。
  ◦ 精液：10～50 ppm。
  ◦ 阴道分泌液、尿液、唾液、泪液、乳汁：<1 ppm。
- 影响风险的因素：
  ◦ 病毒载量。
  ◦ 实际注入体液量。
  ◦ 针头的类型和尺寸。
  ◦ 刺入方式（刺入的深度）。
  ◦ 接触的持续时间。
  ◦ 所接触患者的疾病状况。
  ◦ 宿主易感性。
  ◦ 屏障（如手套）。

诊断

症状和体征

病史

血液或体液暴露：

• 日期、时间、环境、暴露细节、暴露来源。

• 免疫接种情况。

诊断检查与说明

体液暴露的女性在考虑进行抗病毒治疗前要进行血液或尿液的妊娠试验检测。

实验室检查

如果有条件，应在具备专业医疗卫生条件下进行。

• 接触者：HIV（酶免疫分析，Western blot）、HBV、HCV（抗- HCV）、丙氨酸氨基转移酶（ALT）的基线血清学。评估乙型肝炎病毒疫苗接种的充分性：
- HIV-Ab、HCV-Ab、HBsAg、HBsAb 滴度。
- CBC、ALT、肌酐。

• 暴露源患者首选 HIV（考虑快速 HIV 抗体筛查）、HBV、HCV（抗- HCV）的检测。
- HIV-Ab、HCV-Ab、HBsAg。

影像学检查

除非考虑有外源组织遗留体内，一般不进行影像学检查。

鉴别诊断

主要考虑 HBV、HCV 和 HIV 感染。

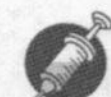

治疗

院前

> **注意**
>
> • 启动 PEP 的最佳时间是在暴露后几小时，而不是几日；越快越好，理想情况是<72 h。
>
> • 院前人员应始终保持普遍的预防措施，以防止针头或其他体液暴露。

初步稳定/治疗

• 充分清洗，伤口保护，眼部或黏膜冲洗。

• 条件允许时，直接或间接的求助专业卫生人员，以确保实验室检测和治疗的可信度。

• 在急诊室，针头暴露的患者具有优先权，暴露后早期快速给予预防性药物治疗是十分必要的。

急诊治疗/程序

• 如果不能向专业卫生人员求助，或非职业性暴露，应该在急诊室立即给予预防性药物治疗。

• 如果有必要，应给予破伤风预防措施。

• HIV：
- 建议对所有需要治疗的暴露进行 3 种药物方案治疗。
- 指南不再要求评估暴露的严重程度，但是不建议对微不足道的暴露使用 PEP（暴露于来源尿液、鼻分泌物、唾液、汗水或泪水，如果没有明显的血液污染）。
- 暴露源的未知艾滋病病毒状态：根据具体情况进行治疗，考虑提供 PEP。
- 对于不明来源状态，最好开始 PEP，如果发现暴露源为阴性，则停止。
- 治疗持续时间为 28 日。
- 3 种药物方案：
  ◦ Truvada（替诺福韦 DF[tdf]＋恩曲他滨[FTC]）；加：
  ◦ 拉替格列韦；或：
  ◦ 度鲁特韦。
  ◦ 如果过敏或可获得性排除了上述方案，请联系当地传染病或艾滋病顾问以获得替代方案，或访问加州大学旧金山分校的 PEP 快速指南。
- 指导预防二次感染：
  ◦ 安全的性行为。
  ◦ 避免妊娠。
  ◦ 禁止捐献血液/组织。
  ◦ 禁止哺乳。

• HBV：
- 暴露于已知 HBsAg 阳性暴露源：
  ◦ 依据抗体滴度确定为完全免疫者：无需治疗。
  ◦ 未免疫者：乙肝病毒免疫球蛋白 ASAP，开始乙肝病毒疫苗接种。
  ◦ 对疫苗无反应性者：乙肝病毒免疫球蛋白 ASAP，30 日内重复一次，考虑给予 3 倍剂量的乙肝病毒疫苗接种。
  ◦ 因抗体滴度不达标而不能明确疫苗反应性者：乙肝病毒免疫球蛋白 ASAP，接种疫苗增强剂。
- 已知 HBsAg 阴性暴露源暴露：
  ◦ 已免疫者：不用给予治疗。
  ◦ 未免疫者：提供乙肝病毒疫苗接种。
- 未知暴露源：
  ◦ 依据抗体滴度确定为完全免疫者：无需采取行动。
  ◦ 未免疫者：开始接种乙肝疫苗，如果为高危暴露，考虑给予乙肝病毒免疫球蛋白 ASAP。
  ◦ 对疫苗无反应性：乙肝病毒免疫球蛋白 ASAP，并给予 3 倍剂量的乙肝病毒疫苗接种，如果为高危暴露，免疫球蛋白在 30 日内重复 1 次。
  ◦ 因抗体滴度不达标而不能明确疫苗反应性：疫苗增强剂，并在 1～2 个月检测抗体滴度。
- HCV：
  ◦ 给予免疫球蛋白或抗病毒药物（干扰素、利巴韦林）作为预防性用药，当存在感染证据时，早期用药可能使患者获益；遵循当地的指南。

• 妊娠期间使用的药物：
- 基于有限的数据，妊娠期间使用抗逆转录病毒药物（Arv）似乎不会增加出生缺陷的风险，但多洛替格列韦可能会增加神经管缺陷的风险。

- 当益处超过婴儿和母亲使用抗逆转录病毒药物的风险时，大多数 PEP 药物都是合理的。

药物治疗

• HIV：特鲁瓦达(恩曲他滨加替诺福韦)：
- 恩曲他滨：
  ◦ 200 mg/d，口服×28 日。
  ◦ 副作用：皮疹、色素沉着。
- 替诺福韦：
  ◦ 300 mg/d，口服×28 日。
  ◦ 副作用：胃肠道症状、头痛、疲乏、神经病变、头晕。
- 雷特格韦：
  ◦ 400 mg，每日 2 次，口服×28 日。
  ◦ 副作用：史蒂文斯-约翰逊综合征、皮疹、中性粒细胞减少、睡眠障碍、头晕、恶心、精神问题、肝脏问题。
- 度鲁特韦：
  ◦ 50 mg/d，口服×28 日。
  ◦ 副作用：中性粒细胞减少、肝功能受损、睡眠障碍、头痛、高血糖。
- 一些抗反转录病毒药物的致癌和致畸作用未知。
- NRTI 和 NtRTIS 类药物会导致乳酸性酸中毒与肝脂肪变性。
- 所有药物都可能有严重的药物相互作用从而导致伤害或死亡。

• 乙型肝炎：
- 乙肝免疫球蛋白：0.06 ml/kg，肌内注射，暴露后 24 h 内，最多 7 日；如果拒绝接种疫苗或无应答，在 1 个月内重复注射。
- 乙肝疫苗：＜20 岁 0.5 ml，肌内注射；＞20 岁 1 ml，肌内注射。

随访

进一步处理

入院指征

无需入院治疗。

出院指征

按门诊病例处理，并在专业医疗机构随访。

镇静药中毒 Neuroleptic Poisoning

Theresa Kim · Steven E. Aks 朱妍 译

基础知识

描述

• 镇静药物(抗精神病药)用于多种情况：
- 精神分裂症和其他精神障碍。
- 严重抑郁。
- 创伤后应激障碍。
- 躁动。
- 老年痴呆症的老年人。
- 注意缺陷多动障碍。
- 孤独症和儿童行为问题。
- 饮食失调。
- 镇吐。
- 偏头痛。

• 最广泛使用的分类系统将它们分为典型或非典型抗精神病药物。

• 急性过量：
- 症状通常为轻度至中度。
- 以中枢神经系统和心血管系统症状为主。

• 治疗剂量也可能出现毒性，表现为锥体外系综合征：
- 根据症状的不同症状，发作时间从几小时到几年不等。
- 急性肌张力障碍。
- 静坐不能。
- 帕金森病。
- 抗精神病药物恶性综合征(NMS)。
- 迟发性运动障碍。
- 其中 NMS 最严重的。

病因

• 主要作用机制是不同程度的多巴胺拮抗，以及潜在的 5-羟色胺能、组胺能、毒鼠碱和 α 肾上腺素能阻滞。

• 也可能阻滞钠和钾通道。

• 经典抗精神病药(吩噻嗪类、丁酰苯类)强效抗多巴胺受体，其中包括：
- 氟哌啶醇(好度)。
- 氯丙嗪(可乐静)。
- 丙氯拉嗪(甲哌氯丙嗪)。
- 硫利达嗪(甲硫哒嗪)。
- 氟奋乃静(氟非那嗪)。
- 异丙嗪(非那根)。
- 氟哌利多(氟哌啶)。
- 羟嗪(安泰乐)。

• 非经典抗精神病药有较弱的抗多巴胺能和适中的抗血清素作用，其中包括：
- 阿塞那平。
- 阿立哌唑(安律凡)。
- 氯氮平。
- 利培酮(维思通)。
- 舍吲哚。
- 奥氮平(再普乐)。
- 喹硫平(思瑞康)。
- 齐拉西酮(卓乐定)。

诊断

症状和体征

• 急性过量：
- 症状通常在 6 h 内出现。
- 使用缓释制剂或如果抗胆碱能症状占主导地位，可能会推迟症状出现。
- 中枢神经系统：
  ◦ 程度：从轻度镇静到昏迷。
  ◦ 抗胆碱能药致谵妄。
  ◦ 锥体外系症状。
  ◦ 癫痫发作。
- 心血管系统：
  ◦ 心动过速。
  ◦ 心肌抑制。
  ◦ 低血压。
  ◦ 心电图间期异常。
  ◦ 尖端扭转(罕见)。
- 呼吸系统：
  ◦ 呼吸抑制。
  ◦ 呼吸道反射消失。
- 胃肠道：
  ◦ 便秘。
  ◦ 口干。
- 泌尿生殖系统：
  ◦ 尿潴留。
- 眼科：

◦ 视力模糊。
◦ 散瞳。
- 皮肤：
◦ 干性皮肤。
◦ 皮肤血管扩张。
• 急性肌张力障碍：
- 最常见的不良反应。
- 可在任何时候发生，通常在开始服药后48 h内。
- 面部、颈部、背部和四肢的非随意肌肉痉挛。
- 戏剧性外观。
- 喉部肌张力障碍是一种罕见的形式，可能导致颤音和呼吸困难。
• 静坐不能：
- 发病数小时到数日。
- 以运动不安、不安和需要不断地调步或移动为特征。
• NMS：
- 发生于<1%的患者，30%的死亡率。
- 特殊的危及生命的事件。
- 随时都可能发生，但最常见的是服药过量。
- 严重过高热。
- 骨骼肌强直。
- 意识状态改变。
- 自主神经功能紊乱。
- 电解质紊乱。
- 横纹肌溶解。
• 迟发性运动障碍：
- 通常在服用抗精神病药物多年后影响患者的运动障碍。
- 无意识的舞蹈动作，特别是嘴唇和面部的动作，如做鬼脸、伸舌或拍打嘴唇。
• 粒细胞缺乏症：
- 见于氯氮平和奥氮平。
- 长期治疗时发生。
• 内分泌系统：
- 随着抗精神病药的应用，高血糖、新发糖尿病和酮症酸中毒都被报道过。

基本检查

• 大量用药后监测生命体征。
• 心电监测。
• 血脉氧仪。
• 过高热时监测核心体温。

诊断检查与说明

实验室检查

• 电解质、尿素氮、肌酐、血糖、肝功能检查。
• 氯氮平过量查血常规、白细胞可能升高。
• 如果疑似NMS、情绪激动或长期制动，检测肌酸磷酸激酶(CPK)水平。
• 根据共同的用药史进行血清药物筛选与药物水平检查：
- 阿司匹林。
- 对乙酰氨基酚。
- 锂。
- 丙戊酸钠。
- 苯妥英钠。
- 苯巴比妥。
• 尿毒理学筛选：很少有用，假阴性和假阳性有可能带来误导。
• 定量水平：很少使用，而且对急性治疗没有帮助。

影像学检查

• 心电图：
- QRS波群增宽。
- QT间期延长。
- 尖端扭转。
- 非特异性ST段改变。
• 头颅CT：
- 用于明确显著的意识状态变化。

鉴别诊断

• 5-羟色胺综合征。
• 恶性高热(如果近期麻醉)。
• 抗抑郁药物过量。
• 抗胆碱危象。
• 拟交感神经药物过量。
• 阿片类药物过量。
• 隐匿性颅脑损伤。
• 内分泌紊乱。
• 脓毒症。
• 中暑。

治疗

院前

运送患者到医院的时候带上药瓶。

初步稳定/治疗

气道、呼吸和循环管理(基础支持)：
• 给予补充氧气。
• 精神状态改变考虑纳洛酮、维生素B_1、50%葡萄糖(或检查血糖)。
• 如果呼吸抑制行气管插管。

急诊治疗/程序

• 支持治疗是最主要的治疗。
• 咨询当地毒物控制部门或毒理学家。
• 去污：
- 在摄入后1 h内使用单剂量活性炭。
- 无呼吸道保护的患者不用木炭。
- 只有仅仅当患者没有插管时才通过鼻胃管使用木炭。
- 如果大量缓释制剂摄入，建议灌洗整个肠道。
- 由于蛋白结合率高，血液透析疗效差。
- 考虑脂肪乳剂治疗心力衰竭。
• 低血压：
- 生理盐水(NS)静脉注射。
- 使用去甲肾上腺素或去氧肾上腺素治疗顽固性低血压。
- 多巴胺可能无效。
• 室性心律失常：
- ⅠA、ⅠB和Ⅲ类抗心律失常药能增加心脏毒性。
- 镁可用于QT间期延长或尖端扭转性心动过速。
- 如果不稳定建议电复律。
- 建议脂肪乳(20%脂肪乳)用于循环衰竭。
- 对于无症状的QTc间期延长，补充钾、钙和镁到正常水平。
- QRS波群延长(>0.12 s)应用碳酸氢钠治疗。
• 肌张力障碍：
- 使用抗胆碱药物，如苯海拉明或甲磺酸苯并托品和苯二氮䓬类药物。
- 治疗应持续3日，以防复发。
• NMS：
- 识别和停用精神抗病药至关重要。
- 过高热时积极退热。
- 躁动时积极使用苯二氮䓬。
- 建议气管插管和神经肌肉阻滞剂。
- 重症患者可能需要溴隐亭或金刚烷胺(多巴胺激动剂)或丹曲林(直接的肌肉松弛剂)。
• 癫痫发作：
- 苯二氮䓬类药物是一线药物。
- 持续性发作用苯巴比妥。
- 像苯妥英这样的抗癫痫药物并没有被证明是有效的，而且可能会加重毒性。
• 抗胆碱能药物致谵妄：
- 苯二氮䓬是首选药物。
- 毒扁豆碱可慎用。
◦ 节律不齐或心电图间期异常的患者禁忌。

药物治疗

• 活性炭：1~2 g/kg，口服或每克摄入药物的比例为 10∶1。

- 苯甲托品甲磺酸：1～2 mg，静脉注射或口服。
- 溴隐亭：2.5～10 mg，q8 h，口服。
- 丹曲林：2～3 mg/(kg·d)持续注射(最大量 10 mg/kg)。
- 地西泮：5～10 mg，静脉注射，q10～15 min。
- 苯海拉明：25～50 mg，静脉注射(1 mg/kg)。
- 利多卡因：1～1.5 mg/kg 随后静滴。
- 脂质乳剂(20%)：1.5 ml/kg 静推，之后 0.25 ml/(kg·min)持续输液 30～60 min，可反复静推维持血流动力学稳定。
- 劳拉西泮：2～4 mg(儿童：0.03～0.05 mg/kg)，静脉注射，q10～15 min。
- 硫酸镁：1～2 g，静脉注射超过 5～15 min。
- 去甲肾上腺素：1～2 μg/(kg·min)，静脉注射维持血压。
- 苯巴比妥：10～20 mg/kg(负荷剂量)，监测呼吸抑制。
- 毒扁豆碱：0.5 mg，静脉注射，q3～5 min。

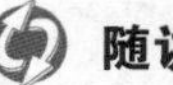

随访

进一步处理

入院指征

- 过量使用致中枢神经系统抑制、躁动、心律失常，或生命体征异常者需要监测床或 ICU。
- NMS 需要 ICU 级别的监护。
- 新发糖尿病(继发于使用抗精神病药)并有严重的高血糖和/或酮症酸中毒。

出院指征

- 观察 6 h 无症状。
- 服用阿立哌唑和缓释制剂需要更长的时间观察。

转诊问题

- 无意(意外)中毒的患者需要毒药预防咨询。
- 患者故意(如自杀)中毒需要精神鉴定。
- 新发糖尿病，需要社区医院、内分泌科随访。

随访建议

- 故意服用药物过量转诊至精神科。
- 意外服药需社区医院随访或监测药物副作用。

要点和误区

- 抗精神病药代表一组有不同适应证和不同程度毒性的药物。
- 药物过量大部分是轻症，且中枢神经系统抑制占多数。
- 肌张力障碍反应是安定药最常见的副作用。虽然很容易治疗，但表现很严重。
- NMS 是一种潜在的致命副作用，可以在镇静药的急性或长期用药过程中出现。
- 较新的抗精神病药可以延迟起病长达 24 h。
- 联系毒物控制中心或毒理学服务中心进行进一步的指导。

支气管炎 Bronchitis

Robin R. Hemphill 张晓彬 译

基础知识

描述

- 这是一自限性的肺内气道炎症，而非肺炎。
- 充血和黏膜水肿。
- 产生黏液及脓性分泌物。
- 纤毛、淋巴管和吞噬细胞的再生性功能障碍。
- 气道因以下原因阻塞：
  - 水肿。
  - 分泌物。
  - 支气管肌肉痉挛。

病因

- 病毒性感染是支气管炎的主要原因。
  - 副流感病毒。
  - 甲型、乙型流感病毒。
  - 呼吸道合胞病毒。
  - 人偏肺病毒。
  - 埃可病毒。
  - 冠状病毒。
  - 腺病毒。
  - 柯萨奇病毒。
  - 鼻病毒。
  - 麻疹和疱疹病毒(可以引起严重病毒性支气管炎)。
- 特别严重或长期持久的支气管炎。
  - 支原体肺炎。
  - 衣原体肺炎。
  - 百日咳。
    - 百日咳的发病率持续上升，甚至在完全免疫的人中发病(疫苗在 10 年后仍有少量保护效果)。
- 其他尚未证明引起支气管炎的细菌(引起慢性肺疾病的除外)。

诊断

症状和体征

病史

上呼吸道感染(上呼吸道感染)的可能症状：

- 萎靡不振。
- 畏寒。
- 肌痛。
- 鼻炎。
- 咽喉痛。
- 出现上呼吸道感染症状：
  - 轻度呼吸困难。
  - 咳嗽，最初为干咳，无痰。
  - 咳嗽，出现黏液或脓性黏液。
  - 咳嗽引发胸部疼痛或刺痛。
  - 最初的症状改善后 3～5 日，与 1～3 周的残咳和不适。

体格检查

- 发热，通常不高于 102 ℉(38.5 ℃)。
- 呼吸急促。
- 轻度咯血。
- 干啰音(喘息)。
- 无啰音(噼啪声)或自鸣音。
- 脓性咳嗽并不意味着细菌感染。

基本检查

- 对需要治疗或上报的患者检测甲型、乙型流感病毒。
- 百日咳检查：

- 急性咳嗽病持续 14 日及以上,伴有阵发性咳嗽、咳后呕吐或呼吸困难的人。
- 剧烈咳嗽 14 日及以上。

■ 诊断测查与说明

实验室检查

• 通过检测甲型、乙型流感病毒可立即确诊。

• 在大多数情况下,并没有可以立即确诊的特定的测试。

• 病毒或细菌培养很少用。

• CBC 可能显示白细胞增多,但是其为非特异性方法。

• 可通过 PCR 试验确诊百日咳,但将延误诊断时间。

影像学检查

CXR:一般不需要行影像学检查。

• 没有确切的证据。

• 适应证:
- 呼吸急促。
- 缺氧。
- 胸部疼痛。
- 心率>100 次/分。
- 呼吸速率呼吸≥24 次/分。
- 温度≥38 ℃。
- 胸部检查有明显结果。
- 有多个并发症的老年患者。
- 缺氧。
- 14 日以上的咳嗽。

■ 诊断步骤/外科

肺功能检查结果异常。

■ 鉴别诊断

• 急性和亚急性小于 8 周:
- 肺炎。
- 反应性呼吸道疾病。
- 误吸。
- 急性鼻窦炎。
- 细菌性气管炎。
- 职业病。

• 慢性大于 8 周:
- 哮喘。
- 胃食管反流。
- 慢性支气管炎。
- 支气管扩张症。
- 使用 ACEI。
- 原发性支气管肺癌。
- 癌症。
- 结节病。
- 左心室衰竭。
- 吸入综合征。
- 心理因素或习惯。

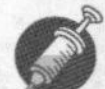

治疗

■ 院前

• 充足供氧。

• 如果有喘息症状,使用支气管扩张剂。

■ 初步稳定/治疗

这些患者很少需要激进的初步治疗。

• 如果患者是缺氧,控制供氧。

• 如果患者脱水,补充水分。

■ 急诊治疗/程序

• 支气管炎通常是病毒性的,也有可能是细菌性的,并没有实际的测试可以区分。
- 因为这通常为病毒性,针对症状进行治疗:
  ◦ 考虑使用镇咳药。
  ◦ 为气道阻塞的患者提供 β 肾上腺素。

• 金刚烷胺可用于治疗 A 型流感,虽然其局部治疗原理仍未知。

• 考虑使用奥司他韦(达菲)和扎那米韦(乐感清)治疗近期发作的甲型流感患者。

• 抗生素:
- 一般来说,不推荐使用抗生素(甚至当分泌物为化脓性的时候)。
- 对于没有潜在肺病的患者,抗生素可能会帮助其更快更好地恢复健康,但考虑到它对大多数人没有效果,还有成本、副作用和耐药性的因素,抗生素不推荐使用。
- 考虑对那些症状减轻且再次发热的患者使用抗生素。

• 使用退热药和镇痛药控制症状。

• 虽然应鼓励患者戒烟,但除非患者有肺气肿病史,否则灭菌烟草不是抗生素的指征。

> **注意**
>
> 呼吸道病毒可以造成免疫力下降进而导致重大疾病,患者和护理应讨论其初级护理。

老年人注意事项

• 特征性的体征和症状。

• 在没有影像学检查的情况下诊断急性支气管炎时须格外谨慎。

儿科注意事项

• 患者很少需要激进的初始管理。

• 如果患者是缺氧,予以供氧。

• 如果患者脱水,补充水分。

• 反复发作的儿童应进行完整的呼吸道感染检查。

■ 药物治疗

• 呼吸阻塞的患者使用沙丁胺醇吸入器。

• 金刚烷胺:100 mg/d,口服,在出现症状的 48 h 内使用。

• 奥司他韦(达菲)和扎那米韦(乐感清):在出现流感相关支气管炎症状的 48 h 内使用。
- 扎那米韦:100 mg,吸入,q12 h(儿童:>7 岁,10 mg;或 2 次吸入,q12 h),用 5 日。
- 奥司他韦:75 mg,口服,每日 2 次(儿童:2 mg/kg),用 5 日。

• 红霉素应给予已经证实的百日咳患者和其接触人员。

• 应鼓励在卫生保健系统服务人员和高危人口(老年人、免疫功能低下、慢性肺部疾病)每年接种流感疫苗。

老年人注意事项

• 使用对乙酰氨基酚,而不是用阿司匹林镇痛。

• 抗生素使用方式与成人相同。

随访

■ 进一步处理

入院指征

• 潜在的显著的心肺功能减退。

• 显著缺氧。

• 诊断不明确的患者。

出院指征

• 已没有肺功能减退。

• 指导患者,特别是高危患者,如果症状没有改善或进一步恶化应及时返回医院。

• 卧床休息。

• 补液。

• 阿司匹林和对乙酰氨基酚。

■ 随访建议

• 不需要随访已改善的那些患者。

• 应告知患者如果出现呼吸急促及时回到急诊室,如果 2～3 周症状没有改善必须就医。

要点和误区

• 高热或肺部症状明显的患者应评估是否存在肺炎。

• 老年患者可能肺炎表现往往更不明显,故在诊断支气管炎之前要考虑行更多的诊断性检查。

脂溢性皮炎 Seborrheic dermatitis

Ian Glen Ferguson · Maia Alexandra Mosse 周健 潘曙明 译

基础知识

描述

• 这是一种常见的慢性丘疹鳞状炎症性皮肤疾病。

• 影响所有年龄人群，表现可以从轻度头皮屑到广泛的黏附鳞屑。

• 存在于皮脂腺聚集的部位和腺体周围。

• 病变区域呈现黄色、红色或棕色的油性结垢或结皮斑块/斑块，与周围皮肤分布清楚。

• 在成人，病情缓解期和恶化期频繁交替。

病因

• 确切的发病机制尚未完全了解。

• 与环境、遗传、激素免疫、微生物和营养等多种因素相关。

• 与马拉色菌有很强的相关性。

• 复杂的生理反应：

- 免疫。
- 炎性增生。
- 过度增殖。

• 疾病暴发与身体和情绪压力或疾病有关。

• 诱发患者发生脂溢性皮炎和更严重或顽固性疾病的因素：

- 帕金森病。
- 瘫痪。
- HIV/AIDS。
- 情绪障碍包括抑郁症。
- 充血性心力衰竭。
- 早产儿免疫抑制。

• 已知诱发或加重脂溢性皮炎的药物包括：

- 砷。
- 奥兰诺芬。
- 葡萄糖。
- 丁螺环酮。
- 卡马西平。
- 氯丙嗪。
- 西咪替丁。
- 乙酰胺。
- 黄金。
- 灰黄霉素。
- 氟哌啶醇。
- 干扰素 α。
- 锂。
- 甲氧沙林。
- 甲基多巴。
- 吩噻嗪类。
- 苯妥英钠。
- 普里米酮。
- 补骨脂素。
- 司他洛尔。
- 硫噻吩。
- 三氧化二砷。

诊断

症状和体征

婴儿

• 起病为出生的第 1 周，通常是自限性的，1 岁后可缓解。

• 可并发特应性皮炎。

• 皮肤褶皱部位受累可表现为尿布相关性皮炎：

- 可能发生细菌或真菌的混合感染。

• “摇篮帽”：

- 油脂肥厚，附着于头皮顶点的鳞屑。
- 在出生后的前 3 个月，可影响多达 70% 的新生儿。
- 可能伴有炎症或继发感染。

婴幼儿

• 睑缘炎：

- 白色鳞屑黏附于睫毛和眼睑边缘，有红斑。
- 具有耐药性和持久性。
- 可导致眼睑结膜炎。

青少年和成年人

• 典型的脂溢性皮炎：

- 轻微瘙痒、可见油腻、细腻、干燥、白色鳞屑覆盖红色、发炎的皮肤上。

• 不清洗可导致恶化。

• 通常是双侧的、对称的，好发于以下区域：

- 头皮、前额、眉毛、眼睑。
- 面部有毛发的区域。
- 外耳道。
- 鼻唇和耳后皱褶。
- 后颈部。
- 胸骨前、脐和身体褶皱处：
  ◦ 腋窝和乳房下区域。
  ◦ 腹股沟和肛门生殖器区域。

• 可能会导致深色皮肤的人出现色素减退。

基本检查

诊断主要基于临床病史和体检。

诊断检查与说明

• 皮肤碎屑性氢氧化钾实验可提示是否存在酵母菌感染。

• 真菌培养作为可选择的诊断方法，有助于排除皮肤真菌病。

影像学检查

不需要。

诊断步骤/外科

皮肤活检（很少使用）：

• 可能有助于排除其他诊断。

• 如果诊断仍然不清楚，或者病情对治疗没有反应，可考虑皮肤活检。

鉴别诊断

• 特应性皮炎：

- 婴儿发病较晚（通常为＞3 月龄）。
- 在成人，可特征性影响前肘窝和腘窝。
- 存在瘙痒、局部渗出和啼哭支持特应性皮炎的诊断。
- 有过敏性皮炎的家族病史（哮喘和变应性鼻炎）有利于过敏性皮炎的诊断，腋窝受累有利于皮脂溢性皮炎的诊断。

• 接触性皮炎：

- 表现为多形性红斑、水肿和小疱。
- 皮肤皱褶处不易受累。
- 可能使脂溢性皮炎变得复杂，成为治疗药物的不良反应。

• 皮肤念珠菌病：

- 由念珠菌引起的皮肤原发性或继发性感染。
- 可影响任何身体部位。
- 瘙痒、红斑、轻微的脱皮和偶尔的起疱。
- 通常与糖尿病、肥胖或其他疾病有关。
- 常见于婴儿。
- 在氢氧化钾细胞学检查中发现假菌丝并不排除脂溢性皮炎。

• 皮肤真菌病：

- 一般分布不对称。
- 头癣（头皮）、体癣（身体）、股癣（腹股沟）、巴巴多斯癣（面部毛发）、面部癣（面部）。
- 很难与脂溢性皮炎区别。
- 氢氧化钾细胞学检查的菌丝提示有足癣。

• 朗格汉斯细胞组织细胞病：

- 全身体征（如发热、腺病）。
- 受影响的婴儿可能出现鳞屑。

- 红棕色丘疹或小疱。
- 伴有脾大。
- 紫癜性病变。

• 莱纳病：
- 女性婴儿多见。
- 出生后2～4个月迅速发病。
- 补体C3、C5降低。
- 严重全身性、剥脱性、红皮病样溢性皮炎。
- 有发热、贫血、腹泻、呕吐、体重减轻、发育不良。

• 红斑狼疮：
- 鼻和颧骨隆起的红斑性颧骨皮疹。
- 慢性或盘状红斑狼疮：
  ◦ 离散的红斑丘疹或斑块。
  ◦ 有厚鳞屑附着。
  ◦ 去除后显示"地毯钉"外观。

• 银屑病：
- 较厚的有银白色鳞屑样斑块。
- 不太可能局限于头皮。

• 红斑痤疮：
- 通常伴有面部中央红斑或前额受累。

• 花斑藓(糠疹)：
- 慢性浅表真菌疾病，通常位于颈部、上臂和躯干。
- 特征为细的、鳞屑状、凝聚的、低色素或色素沉着的斑点。
- 患者通常无症状。
- 也与马拉色菌有关：
  ◦ 不属于皮肤真菌病。
- 短的，厚的孢子、菌丝。
  ◦ (意大利面样和肉丸样改变)可见于氢氧化钾细胞学检查。

儿科注意事项

有脂溢性皮炎和"摇篮帽"的婴儿可以并发特应性皮炎。

> **注意**
>
> • 脂溢性皮炎是导致红皮病(广义去角质皮炎)的原因之一。
> - 严重结垢红斑性皮炎可累及身体的90%或更多。

治疗

院前

无需特殊处理。

初步稳定/治疗

无需特殊处理。

急诊治疗/程序

• 脂溢性皮炎是一种慢性疾病：
- 不需要紧急治疗，除非存在继发性感染或红皮病。

药物治疗

• 药物选择和用药方式较多。

• 治疗的目的是减少亲脂性酵母菌和支持其生长的皮脂的残留，从而减少炎症，改善卫生状况。

• 严重的病例可能需要去除鳞屑和角质化的无活性上皮细胞，以便进一步处理。

• 使用矿物油可软化鳞屑(如有必要，可在过夜前清洗)。

• 清洗后用软刷(牙刷)或用细齿梳子去除顽固的病变。

• 患者教育：
- 病情发作时的早期治疗。
- 注意卫生，及时清理鳞屑病灶。
- 中等强度(UVA/UVB)阳光照射可能有助于抑制马拉色菌的生长。
- 避免使用喷发剂和发胶。

• 成人脂溢性皮炎：
- 治疗的目的主要是控制症状而非治愈该病。

• 婴儿脂溢性皮炎：
- 可能对洗发水、润肤剂有反应，可局部使用类固醇激素。
- 剧烈的去角质方式或机械去除可造成进一步的炎症。

• 婴儿"摇篮帽"：
- 外用橄榄油(用作润肤剂)。
- 局事业咪唑类药物(酮康唑)。
- 使用低效常规类固醇激素。

• 睑缘炎：
- 对受影响地区进行暖到热的压缩。
- 用婴儿洗发水和棉签尖轻柔清洗厚鳞屑。

• 咪唑类：
- 抑制真菌细胞膜的麦角甾醇合成。
- 针对马拉色拉菌：
  ◦ 2%酮康唑。
  ◦ 尼佐拉。

• 局部皮质类固醇：
- 长期使用可能会出现皮肤萎缩、皱纹、色素减退和毛细血管扩张。
- 高效药物仅适用于难治性患者。
- 只能短暂使用，因为频繁使用可能会促进病情复发和反弹。
- 在皮肤较薄的部位(如皮肤皱褶、颈部、面部)使用低效制剂：
  ◦ 2.5%氢化可的松。
- 仅在皮肤较厚的区域(如躯干、头皮)使用中等至高效力的药剂：
  ◦ 氟轻松丙酮。
  ◦ 氟羟强的松龙。
  ◦ 倍他米松二丙酸盐。
  ◦ 丙酸氯倍他索。

一线用药

• 面部(成人)：
- 2%酮康唑乳膏和2.5%氢化可的松乳膏。至少2周。

• 头皮(成人)：
- 每周2%酮康唑洗发3次，0.05%氟轻松醋酸酯洗发，每日2次。
  ◦ 洗发水必须在2～3 min清除。
  ◦ 超出每周3次的有效使用。
  ◦ 洗澡后应用类固醇。
  ◦ 氟轻松：儿童低剂量使用。

• 儿童和成人的身体有表现：
- 局部抗真菌及皮质类固醇治疗。

• 有褶皱、裂缝或分泌物。
- 考虑启动抗菌等头孢菌素(如头孢氨苄)。
- 参考随访建议。
- 如果症状持续建议咨询皮肤科医师。

二线用药

• 面部：
- 局部钙调神经磷酸酶抑制剂：
  ◦ 抗炎和抗真菌特性。
  ◦ 非长效皮质类固醇的长期作用。
  ◦ 关于恶性肿瘤的黑盒警告：
  ◦ 1%吡美莫司。
  ◦ 0.1%他克莫司。

• 头皮：可将酮康唑洗发水(每周使用3日以上)与其他外用洗发水混合使用：
- 吡硫酮锌(头部和肩部)：
  ◦ 减少表皮细胞生长周期。
  ◦ 抗真菌和抗菌作用。
- 硫化硒(赛尔孙蓝)：
  ◦ 减少表皮和滤泡角质细胞。
  ◦ 抗真菌作用。
- 煤焦油/液态碳清洁剂(LCD)(露得清T/凝胶或T/Sal)：
  ◦ 抑制有丝分裂细胞分裂。
  ◦ 止痒、防腐作用。
  ◦ 减少表皮厚度。
  ◦ 避免面部损伤、皮肤变形或增殖。
- 硫/磺胺化合物(Denorex)联合使用：
  ◦ 通过抑制二氢蝶酸合酶(PABA)阻止对氨基苯甲酸向叶酸转化。
  ◦ 卡梅尔头皮治疗。

- 水杨酸：
    - 促角质分离。
    - 适用于有明显鳞屑化和过度角化症状者。
- 环磷酰胺。
- 氟轻松头皮油：
    - 抗炎。
    - 保留过夜。

随访

进一步处理

入院指征

除非病情严重，否则不必住院。

出院指征

可依从用药和随访建议者，可安排出院。

转诊问题

- 在考虑潜在疾病或合并症时，应将患者推荐给初级保健医师。
- 当诊断仍不明确或治疗无效时，考虑转介给专业的皮肤科医师。包括诊断仍然难以确定，病情难以治疗，或需要二线药物等情形。

随访建议

- 症状可能在2周内改善，但可能需要数月才能完全康复，并且可能复发。
- 青春期和成年患者可能持续存在慢性皮炎持续症状。
- 对有继发性细菌或真菌感染的征象者应提供防范措施和建议：
    - 如有发热、红斑、压痛或溃疡者。

要点和误区

- 严重和突发的脂溢性皮炎可能是免疫缺陷患者(如艾滋病)的最初表现。
- 入院后可能需要对潜在的疾病进一步评估。

蜘蛛咬伤(黑寡妇) Spider Bite, Black Widow

Tarlan Hedayati 范浩浩 李文放 译

基础知识

描述

- 黑蜘蛛咬伤致中毒综合征。
- 毒性的机制：
    - 母蛛致病。
    - 毒液含有强效神经毒素曲霉毒素：
        - 导致阳离子通道提前开放结果增加神经递质释放突触和神经肌肉接头。
        - 增加神经递质释放及对自身影响。
- 发病率和死亡率与剂量有关。
- 中毒的严重程度取决于：
    - 受害人的病前健康：
        - 高血压或心血管疾病风险增加。
    - 受害人的人数和年龄：
        - 儿童(即在特定剂量的毒液中，体型较小的儿童)具有更高的发病率和死亡风险。
    - 咬伤次数。
    - 咬伤的位置。
    - 蜘蛛的大小和状况。
- 很少致命。

病因

黑寡妇蜘蛛特点：

- 外观：
    - 有光泽的黑色，带有红色斑点，形状像一个沙漏，或在球状腹部的腹侧有一对斑点。
    - 女性有25～50 mm的腿跨度和15 mm长的身体。
- 发现于北美各地，除了法诺斯和阿拉斯加。
- 喜欢阴暗的隐蔽的地方，如车库、谷仓、户外小屋、木桩和低矮的树叶。
- 大多数的叮咬发生在温暖的月份，那时蜘蛛正在保卫它们的网和卵。

诊断

症状和体征

病史

- 蜘蛛咬伤的历史非常不可靠，而且物种通常不被识别。
- 咬伤分3个等级。
- 1级：
    - 如果有感觉，描述为针刺或夹痛。
- 2级：
    - 叮咬局部烧灼感。
    - 叮咬局部和躯干肌肉疼痛。
- 3级(毒蛛中毒)(15～60 min)：
    - 心脏：
        - 心悸。
        - 胸痛和紧张。
    - 肺：
        - 气短。
        - 咳嗽。
    - 神经肌肉：
        - 头痛。
        - 头晕。
        - 疼痛区域肌肉痉挛和抽搐。
        - 抽筋，可能累及大肌肉群。
        - 胳膊叮咬可能导致手臂、胸部肌肉紧张和呼吸困难。
        - 腿部叮咬可能导致腹痛和腿部痉挛。
        - 单纯感觉迟钝，感觉过敏。
        - 局部或弥漫性发汗。
    - 胃肠道：
        - 恶心，呕吐。
        - 腹部疼痛。
    - 泌尿生殖器：
        - 痛苦的持续勃起。
    - 妇科：
        - 妊娠患者可能产生子宫收缩和早产。
    - 皮肤：
        - 瘙痒症。
    - 精神：
        - 焦虑。
        - 濒死感。

体格检查

- 生命体征可能异常：
    - 高血压或低血压。
    - 心动过速或心动过缓。
    - 热。
    - 呼吸急促。
- 心脏：
    - 心律失常。
    - 心肌炎。
- 肺：
    - 支气管黏液溢。
    - 肺水肿。
    - 呼吸衰竭：

◦ 一般由于呼吸肌肉无力。
- 腹部：
- 腹肌紧张。
- 泌尿生殖器：
- 阴茎异常勃起。
- 神经系统发现：
- 四肢强直性收缩、束状或震颤。
- 大肌肉群的痉挛和僵直。
- 自主神经不稳定。
- 癫痫。
- 皮肤：
- 局部。
◦ 出现 2 个蜘蛛毒牙刺痛。
◦ 皮肤变白（"晕"）。
◦ 周围有红斑（"目标病灶"）。
◦ 肿胀。
◦ 局部发汗。
- 弥漫性：
◦ 荨麻疹。
◦ 毛发直立。
◦ 广泛性发汗。
- 精神病学：
- 急性中毒性精神病。
- 烦躁不安。

基本检查

诊断依据：
- 临床表现。
- 仔细询问蜘蛛咬伤史。
- 蜘蛛的鉴别。

诊断检查与说明

实验室检查

- 没有针对黑寡妇蜘蛛毒液的特定血液测试。
- CBC：
- 白细胞可能轻度升高。
- 电解质、钙。
- 尿酸，肌酐。
- 脂肪酶，肝功能。
- 肌酸激酶：
- 明显肌肉痉挛患者升高。
- 心肌酶。
- 妊娠检查。
- 尿分析：
- 可表现为蛋白尿。
- 肺水肿的罕见病例。
- 心电图和心脏监测：
- 已知患有心脏病的患者。
- 胸痛、生命体征不稳定或心律失常患者。
- 可短暂显示洋地黄效果。

影像学检查

- 呼吸系统疾病的 CXR。
- 腹部成像排除其他原因的疼痛。

鉴别诊断

- 急腹症（如阑尾炎、胆囊炎、胰腺炎、AAA）。
- 输尿管结石/肾结石。
- 拟交感神经（如可卡因、苯丙胺）。
- 低钙血症。
- 破伤风。
- 肌肉损伤或劳损。
- 高血压紧急。
- 心肌梗死/急性冠状动脉综合征。
- 焦虑性障碍。
- 过敏反应。
- 妊娠患者的早产。

治疗

院前

- ABC 管理/ACLS。
- 固定伤口部位，在送往医院的过程中使用冷敷布或冰以获得舒适。
- 有全身症状的患者可能需要支持措施（镇痛药、抗焦虑药）。
- 负压毒液提取装置还没有被推荐用于黑寡妇蜘蛛咬伤。
- 看护者应尽一切努力在现场找到并带回致病的蜘蛛进行识别。

初步稳定/治疗

- ABC 管理。
- 根据需要 ACLS。
- 孕妇胎儿监护。

急诊治疗/程序

- 彻底清洁咬痕。
- 破伤风预防。
- 止吐药。
- 止痛剂。
- 抗组胺药。
- 用于治疗躁动和不安的苯二氮䓬类药物。
- 肌肉痉挛/痉挛疗法：
- 苯二氮䓬类。
- 麻醉药物。
◦ 症状性高血压的降压药。
◦ 抗蛇毒血清。
- 对马血清过敏或有马血清过敏史。
- 适应证：
◦ 对症措施没有反应的中度至重度症状。
◦ 重度高血压。
◦ 呼吸窘迫。
◦ 妊娠的症状。
◦ 阴茎异常勃起。
◦ 严重的横纹肌溶解。
◦ 筋膜室综合征。
◦ 癫痫发作。
- 在抗蛇毒血清注射前，对马血清进行皮肤敏感性试验（抗蛇毒血清包中包含检测试剂盒）。
- 观察第 1 型超敏反应前 20 min：
- 发生率达 25%。
- 考虑使用抗组胺药或皮下注射肾上腺素 1∶1 000 预处理。
- 用类固醇、抗组胺药、肾上腺素和心肺支持治疗过敏反应。
- 由于使用了少量的抗蛇毒血清，如果发生血清病反应，通常是轻微的。
- 疗效通常在第一次治疗后 2 h 内明显，很少需要重复剂量。
- 抗蛇毒血清可能有助于预防持续性神经病症状。

药物治疗

- 抗蛇毒血清：1 安瓿（2.5 ml）稀释成 50～100 ml 的 D_5W 或生理盐水（儿童：相同剂量），静置 1 h 以上。
- 苯海拉明：10～50 mg 静脉注射或肌内注射 q6～8 h[儿童：5 mg/(kg · d) div，每日 4 次]。
- 劳扎泮：1～2 mg 静脉注射或肌内注射（儿童：0.01 mg/kg 静脉注射或肌内注射）。
- 硫酸吗啡：2～10 mg（儿童：0.1 mg/kg）。
- 硝普钠：舒张压＞120 mmHg 时 5～10 μg/(kg · min)。
- 破伤风预防。

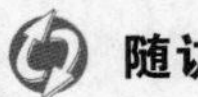

随访

进一步处理

入院指征

- 儿科、老年人、孕妇或有症状的患者。
- 显著的心血管症状和体征，或重度高血压，特别是有心脏病史或慢性高血压。
- 呼吸窘迫或肺水肿。
- 症状持续存在对积极的管理和特定的抗蛇毒血清没有反应。

出院指征

- 无症状且没有阳性发现的黑寡妇蜘蛛患者在观察 1～2 h 后即可出院。

Z

• 无合并症且明确辨认黑寡妇蜘蛛的无症状患者应观察至少 4～6 h，如果病情没有改变就出院。
• 所有出院患者均须留意下列病征，并寻求适当跟进：
- 血尿。
- 皮疹。
- 关节疼痛。
- 淋巴结病。
- 呼吸急促。
- 感染的迹象。
• 应指示接受抗蛇毒血清的出院患者注意血清病的迹象：
- Ⅲ型迟发超敏性。
- 不常见的。
- 治疗后第 5 日至 3 周发生。
- 用抗组胺药和类固醇治疗。

转诊问题

毒理学咨询需要入院或抗蛇毒血清的患者。

随访建议

• 在大多数未经治疗的患者中，症状在 2～3 h 后达到顶峰，然后开始消退，在接下来的几日中，偶尔会出现周期性发作。
• 在其他健康的成人中，症状在 2～3 日完全消失。
• 如果持续的神经症状持续数周至数月，神经病学随访包括：
- 疲劳。
- 全身无力或肌痛。
- 感觉异常。
- 头痛。
- 失眠。
- 阳痿。
- 多神经炎。

要点和误区

• 婴儿黑寡妇蜘蛛咬伤可表现为顽固性哭泣。
• 高热和白细胞计数应促使考虑蜘蛛咬伤的替代方法(如感染)。

蜘蛛咬伤(棕色隐士) Spider Bite, Brown Recluse

Tarlan Hedayati 江伟伟 李文放 译

基础知识

描述

局部或全身疾病引起的棕色隐士蜘蛛咬中毒。

病因

• 棕色隐士蜘蛛(也被称为 fiddleback 蜘蛛)的特点：
- 外观：
◦ 精致的身体和腿跨度 10～25 mm。
◦ 棕褐色到深褐色，头部上部可见较深的小提琴状斑纹。
◦ 3 双眼睛。
- 分布在美国中南部。
- 生存环境：通常在温暖干燥的地方，室内或室外，如木桩、成捆的破布、地窖、岩石下或阁楼。
- 咬是典型的防御行为。
• 毒性的机制：
- Benom 是一种复杂的酶和肽的混合物：
◦ 与红细胞结合并引起溶血。
◦ 引起前列腺素释放，激活补体级联。
◦ 导致脂肪分解和组织坏死。
◦ 引发血小板聚集和血栓形成。
◦ 虎蛇对毒液抗原的过敏反应。
◦ 可能导致休克和 DIC 的罕见病例。
- 毒性与以下相关：
◦ 毒液与患者体重相关。
◦ 毒液在身体上的部位。

儿科注意事项

• 儿童比健康的成年人更容易受到一定量的毒液的伤害。
• 严重的血管内溶血在儿童中更常见。

诊断

症状和体征

诊断不仅基于临床表现，而且基于可靠的蜘蛛咬伤史。

病史

• 孤立的皮肤病变是最常见的表现。
• 咬伤部位通常位于蜘蛛被衣服和皮肤夹住的地方。
• 局部伤口症状：
- 咬伤通常无症状，但 1～24 h 后可出现灼烧感或刺痛感，患者可出现局部疼痛或瘙痒。
• 综合表现：
- 罕见的并发症。
- 儿童比成人更常见。
- 显影时间为 1～3 日。
◦ 患者可能主诉：
◦ 发热、发冷。
◦ 无力、倦怠。
◦ 恶心、呕吐、腹泻。
◦ 呼吸困难。
◦ 肌痛、肌肉痉挛、关节痛。
◦ 黄疸。
◦ 有瘀点的或有荨麻疹的皮疹。
◦ 广泛痒的皮疹。
◦ 血尿或深色尿。

体格检查

• 咬伤：
- 通常在 1～3 日检查是看不到的。
- 可能有针刺损伤、局部变白、硬化或红斑。
- 咬伤部位可能出现组织损伤：
◦ 最初咬痕可能被水肿包围。
◦ 接下来，红斑边界将围绕一个紫色中心发展，在两者之间有一个薄的缺血环。
◦ 24～72 h 后可在中心形成浆液性或出血性大疱。
◦ 在 3～4 日，随着皮肤的发展、痂化和皮下组织坏死，水泡会逐渐变大、变暗。
◦ 焦痂脱落 2～5 周后在其位置留下溃疡。
◦ 皮下脂肪最多的部位坏死最广泛。
◦ 重力作用下，下肢水疱可向远处扩散。
◦ 局部反应并不依赖于中毒的程度，也不能用来预测随后全身疾病的可能性或严重程度。
• 皮肤：
- 黄疸。
- 瘀斑。
- 荨麻疹。
- 广泛黄斑皮疹。

基本检查

• 需要仔细调查，以引出蜘蛛咬伤的病史。

• 除非出现全身毒性,否则无需进行常规实验室检测。

■ 诊断检查与说明

实验室检查

• 蜘蛛毒液可以在皮肤损伤处检测到,但目前还没有广泛的临床试验。
• 全血细胞计数:
- 溶血性贫血。
- 血小板减少,特别是 DIC。
- 白细胞增多。
• 电解质:
- 高钾血症或肾衰酸中毒。
• 尿素氮、肌酐。
• 肌酸激酶在横纹肌溶解时可能升高。
• 凝血酶原时间/部分凝血活酶试验在 DIC 中可延长。
• D-二聚体和纤维蛋白降解产物在 DIC 中可能升高。
• 纤维蛋白原在 DIC 可降低。
• 尿分析:
- 血红蛋白尿。
- 蛋白尿。

影像学检查

• 全身毒性的 CXR。
• 咬伤部位软组织 X 线片。

■ 鉴别诊断

• 血管性水肿。
• 细菌性软组织感染,耐甲氧西林金黄色葡萄球菌。
• 皮肤灼伤。
• 皮肤炭疽。
• 糖尿病溃疡。
• 压疮性溃疡。
• 结节性红斑。
• 真菌感染。
• 淋球菌的出血性病变。
• 单纯疱疹。
• 静脉吸毒或"皮肤爆裂"。
• 血管功能不全伴继发性溃疡。
• 莱姆病。
• 肿瘤病变。
• 其他的蛛形纲动物表面变质。
• 毒葛。
• 脓皮病,坏疽。
• 孢子丝菌病。
• 史蒂文斯-约翰逊综合征。
• 血栓形成。
• 血管炎。
• 华法林抗凝剂使用。

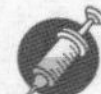

治疗

■ 院前

• 松散固定伤口。
• 抬高受影响的肢体。
• 冷敷伤处。
• 当患者出现症状时立即送往医院。
• 系统性症状患者的支持性措施。

> **注意**
> 护理人员在现场应尽一切努力寻找并将致病的蜘蛛带进来进行识别。

■ 初步治疗/稳定

静脉输液、吸氧、心电监测如果患者出现全身衰竭的迹象。

■ 急诊治疗/程序

• 彻底清理咬痕部位。
• 破伤风预防。
• 止痛剂。
• 抗生素:
- 如果伤口出现感染,则适当使用。
- 预防性。
- 一种葡萄球菌。
• 氨苯砜:
- 有争议的:考虑严重的毒性。
- 在接受治疗时,要对 G-6-PD 缺乏症进行监测。
- 监测是否有可能出现脑出血、溶血和白细胞增多症。
• 坏死伤口切除:
- 在前 8 周不推荐,因为可能导致更严重的溃疡形成。
• 血红蛋白尿:
- 经静脉输液和碱化处理,监测肾脏、液体、电解质状态。
• 肾衰竭予以透析。
• 休克状态时用升压药。
• 严重溶血、DIC 时使用血液制品。
• 抗蛇毒素:
- 没有在商业上使用。
- 没有 FDA 批准。
• 需要进一步研究的治疗方法:
- 局部或全身性类固醇(可预防肾衰竭和溶血)。
- 高压氧治疗(已证实可降低动物模型的伤口大小)。
- 局部硝酸甘油可能增加全身副作用的风险。
- 负压伤口治疗或真空辅助闭合。

■ 药物治疗

• 抗生素:
- 克林霉素:150~300 mg,口服,q6 h[儿童:8~16 mg/(kg·d),口服,分区,每日 4 次]。
- 严重的皮肤感染:
○ 万古霉素:1 g,静脉注射,q12 h(儿童:10 mg/kg,q6 h)。
• 氨苯砜:50~200 mg/d 的渐进式剂量[儿童:2 mg/(kg·24 h),口服]。
• 甲泼尼龙:125 mg,静脉推注,泼尼松 30~50 mg/d,持续 5 日(儿童:甲泼尼龙 1~2 mg/kg,静脉推注,泼尼松 1~2 mg/kg,口服)。
• 硫酸吗啡:2~10 mg(儿童:0.1 mg/kg),静脉注射或肌内注射,必要时。

儿科注意事项

只有在严重的情况下才使用氨苯砜,因为增加了副作用风险,如肝炎、高铁血红蛋白症、溶血性贫血、白细胞减少症。

随访

入院指征

• 明显的局部反应或全身毒性的迹象。
• 降低儿童、重度合并球病患者的阈值。

出院指征

• 无全身毒性或局部伤口坏死严重进展的证据。
• 每日由初级医师重新评估,包括血液检查,直到 3~4 日后评估全身毒性。
• 应建议患者延长皮肤愈合疗程,并在 8 周后考虑手术切除。
• 患者应被告知广泛的瘢痕、感染和复发性溃疡的可能性。

儿科注意事项

• 较长的观察期或入院时间。
• 这个人群的死亡率更高。

转诊问题

• 用于伤口管理的一般手术或整形手术。
• 创伤管理高压氧专家。
• 毒理学家。
• 肾衰竭的肾病学家。
• 休克或 DIC 的情况。

■ 随访建议

• 继续评估伤口的初级护理医师。
• 综合外科或整形外科治疗复杂伤口。

Z

• 负责伤口管理的高压氧专家。

要点和误区

• 请记住，棕色隐遁的蜘蛛的范围有限，以及罕见的蛛形纲动物导致皮肤坏死。

• 在没有史上可靠的蜘蛛咬伤的情况下，必须仔细寻找并排除其他诊断。

• 确保 G-6-PD 缺陷/引起高铁血红蛋白症和溶血的患者接受氨苯砜。

• 对儿科患者、有全身症状的成人或有严重、疼痛或感染伤口的人有较低的准入门槛。

直肠创伤 Rectal Trauma

Elaine M. Sapiro 何融冰 译

基础知识

描述

• 直肠黏膜损伤。

• 简单挫伤到扩大至腹膜或会阴的全层撕裂伤。

• 2/3 的直肠在腹膜外。

病因

• 穿透伤：
- 枪伤：80%穿透直肠创伤。
- 刀伤。
- 刺穿伤。

• 钝挫伤：
- 机动车事故。
- 滑水运动和船只事故。
  ○ 静水压损伤。
- 骨盆骨折：
  ○ 骨折碎片穿透直肠。

• 异物：
- 自体性行为。
- 肛交。
- 袭击。
- 摄入尖锐物品。

• 医源性创伤：直肠损伤最常见原因。
- 钡剂灌肠：
  ○ 0.04%的患者发生穿孔。
  ○ 死亡率为 35%。
- 结肠镜检查：
  ○ 穿孔率为 0.2%。
  ○ 息肉切除术增加风险。
- 痔切除术。
- 泌尿科和妇产科手术：
  ○ 外阴切开术。

儿科注意事项

• 温度计插入不当可导致直肠损伤。

• 任何幼儿直肠外伤应该提高对非偶然性创伤的怀疑。

诊断

症状和体征

• 会阴、肛门或下腹部疼痛。

• 穿孔或腹膜炎体征：
- 肌紧张。
- 反跳痛。
- 发热。

• 直肠出血。

• 顽固性便秘。

• 存在骨盆骨折。

• 有肛门操作、异物插入、性虐待史。

病史

• 受伤时间和机制。

• 所有躯干、臀部、会阴部、大腿根部受到枪伤、刺伤或刺穿伤的患者应怀疑直肠损伤。

• 考虑任何主诉下腹部或盆腔疼痛的有肛门操作史的患者。

体格检查

• 彻底视诊及触诊臀部、肛门和会阴。

• 如果是贯穿伤应确认伤口出入口。

• 进行直肠指检：
- 评估全血或粪便隐血试验阳性。
- 注意前列腺的位置。

• 评估会阴完整性：
- 所有女性患者：窥器及双合诊检查。
- 所有男性患者：泌尿生殖器检查，包括前列腺检查。

基本检查

• 实验室检查：全血计数和尿液分析。

• 急腹系列。

• 钝挫伤做腹部骨盆 CT。

• 乙状结肠镜检查：取出异物后。

• 证据性检查：性侵犯案例中要求。

诊断检查与说明

• 全血细胞计数：
- 失血量。
- 白细胞增多、杆状核粒细胞增多提示腹膜炎。

• 类型与筛查：
- 如需出血证据。

• 尿液分析。

• 粪便物评估。

影像学检查

• 仰卧位、立位腹部 X 线平片，骨盆 X 线片：
- 观察提示穿孔的气腹或腹膜外直肠外密度影。
- 确定异物的位置、大小及形状。
- 识别骨盆骨折或耻骨联合分离可能伴随的直肠损伤。

• 腹部及盆腔 CT：
- 根据临床情况静脉注射、口服或造影剂灌肠（泛影葡胺）。

诊断步骤/外科

• 如直肠检查发现高位前列腺应行逆行尿道造影。

• 肠道造影，只有在穿孔不明确的情况下有用：
- 水溶性造影剂（如泛影葡胺）。

鉴别诊断

• 结肠损伤。

• 泌尿生殖器损伤。

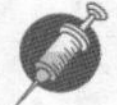

治疗

院前

• ABC 管理。

• 钝挫伤的脊髓保护。

• 对失血、低血压进行液体复苏。

• 不要试图去除直肠异物。

• 控制出血。

Z

■ **初步稳定/治疗**

腹部贯穿伤或钝挫伤遵循创伤治疗方案：
- 初步检查。
- 复苏。
- 再次检查。
- 治疗。

■ **急诊治疗/程序**

- 如需则采用破伤风预防。
- 如果重要黏膜破坏或出现腹膜炎体征，用广谱抗生素。
- Foley 导尿管（排除尿道损伤后）。
- 急诊室中直肠异物移除。
  - 取决于异物位置和类型。
  - 镇静：
    - 尽可能避免镇静；理想情况下，患者可在过程中屏气用力来协助异物取出。
    - 如果不能处理异物，则考虑程序性镇静以优化放松括约肌。
  - 患者取截石位：
    - 局部麻醉最大限度放松肛门括约肌——利多卡因皮下注射在 6 点钟和 12 点钟位置，然后避开直肠黏膜，向四象限更深层浸润。
    - 温和地用手指扩张括约肌。
    - 用产科的环，或活检钳、钩，或用抽吸装置来辅助取出。
    - 患者做 Valsalva 动作。
  - Foley 导尿管：
    - 通过异物上方，气囊充气，轻柔牵拉来抽吸并协助异物取出。
    - 用 3 根导尿管，经过异物旁，充气，并轻拉（使异物平滑或在 Foley 导尿管不能通过异物上方的情况下）。
  - 移除异物后，通过乙状结肠镜评估黏膜损伤。
- 外科会诊：
  - 腹膜炎。
  - 所有创伤性直肠黏膜撕裂伤。
  - 异物距肛外缘>10 cm。
  - 移动时可能引发黏膜损伤的尖锐物体。
  - 不能在急诊室中移除异物。

■ **药物治疗**

- 覆盖革兰阴性及厌氧微生物：
  - 氨苄西林-舒巴坦：
    - 成人：3 g，q6 h，静脉注射（儿童：50 mg/kg，静脉注射）。
  - 哌拉西林-他唑巴坦：
    - 成人：3.375 g，静脉注射（儿童：75 mg/kg，静脉注射）。
  - 头孢替坦：
    - 成人：2 g，q12 h，静脉注射（儿童：40 mg/kg，静脉注射）。
  - 头孢西丁：
    - 成人：2 g，q6 h，静脉注射（儿童：80 mg/kg，q6 h）。
- 额外厌氧菌覆盖：
  - 克林霉素：
    - 成人：600～900 mg，静脉注射（儿童：10 mg/kg，静脉注射）。
  - 甲硝唑：
    - 成人：1 g，静脉注射（儿童：15 mg/kg，静脉注射）。
- 联合治疗：
  - 成人：氨苄西林 500 mg，静脉注射，q6 h；庆大霉素，1～1.7 mg/kg，静脉注射；甲硝唑，1 g，静脉注射。
  - 儿童：氨苄西林 50 mg/kg，静脉注射，q6 h；庆大霉素，1～1.7 mg/kg，静脉注射；甲硝唑，15 mg/kg，静脉注射。
- 镇静和止痛：
  - 芬太尼：2～3 μg/kg，静脉注射（成人和儿童）。
  - 咪达唑仑：0.01～0.2 mg/kg，静脉注射（成人和儿童）。
  - 丙泊酚：
    - 成人：2～2.5 mg/kg，静脉注射（老人和儿童：1 mg/kg，静脉注射）。
    - 氯胺酮：1～2 mg/kg，静脉注射；2～4 mg/kg，肌内注射（老人和儿童）。
  - 利多卡因：局部或注射。

■ **手术/其他方法**

- 穿孔。
- 括约肌撕裂。
- 异物：
  - 移除高位或尖锐物体需要全身麻醉。
  - 经肛门微创手术（TAMIS）。
  - 剖腹手术是最后的手段。

随访

■ **进一步处理**

入院指征
- 穿孔。
- 严重出血。
- 生命体征不稳定。
- 腹痛。
- 肛门括约肌撕裂。
- 需要在手术室取出的异物。

出院指征
- 生命体征稳定。
- 无腹痛。
- 乙状结肠镜检查、肛门镜检查正常。
- 备选方案：观察穿孔体征和症状（最长 12 h），提供 12～24 h 的重复检查，密切回访注意事项。

■ **随访建议**

- 12～24 h 反复腹部检查。
- 返回急诊室：
  - 腹痛。
  - 呕吐。
  - 发热。

要点和误区

- 低位胃肠道或泌尿生殖系统手术后腹痛的所有患者应考虑直肠损伤。
- 仔细的病史和检查是必要的，因为许多直肠异物患者可能会感到尴尬，掩盖导致其腹部和直肠不适的原因。
- 60%的异物可以在急诊室中移除。
- 取出异物后未能识别穿孔。
- 创造力和想象力有助于成功在急诊室中取出异物。

直肠脱垂 Rectal Prolapse

Marilyn M. Hallock 何融冰 译

基础知识

描述

• 直肠壁全层外翻至肛门外。
• 3 种类型的直肠脱垂：
- 全层脱垂：
◦ 直肠壁通过肛管的突出物，最常见。
- 部分层或黏膜脱垂：
◦ 只有黏膜层经肛门突出。
- 隐性(内部)脱垂或直肠套叠：
◦ 直肠壁脱垂未见经肛门突出物。
◦ 可能很难诊断。

病因

• 原因尚不明确且多因素化：
- 慢性便秘、过度紧张。
- 括约肌松弛：
◦ 骨盆底创伤、薄弱，分娩。
◦ 神经系统疾病。
• 在女性中更为常见，70 岁以上。

儿科注意事项

• 4 岁后非常罕见。
• 完全直肠脱垂在儿童中很少见，更可能是部分或肠套叠。
• 考虑慢性腹泻、寄生虫、囊性纤维化(CF)、营养不良为致病因素。

诊断

症状和体征

• 暗红色块状物脱出于直肠。
• 可能有黏液性或血性分泌物。
• 直肠肿块感。
• 里急后重。
• 便秘或失禁。

病史

• 病史重点在于肠梗阻和脱垂持续时间。
• 起初为自行缓解的脱垂，症状通常随着时间加重。

体格检查

• 直肠检查须将脱垂与息肉、痔、肠套叠区分。
• 完全脱垂可见深红色肿物在肛外缘伴或不伴黏液；脱出直肠结实的黏膜形成环状皱襞。
• 黏膜脱垂的突出物很少超过几厘米，不包含环状的肌肉层皱襞。
• 内痔通过如车轮辐条般放射状黏膜皱襞鉴别。
• 脱垂的息肉和痔未涉及全部直肠黏膜，中心没有洞。
• 肠套叠以间歇、严重腹痛的主诉，可能表现得更严重。
• 检查者的手指可以通过脱垂肠管的顶段和肛门括约肌之间，直肠脱垂时突出的黏膜与肛周皮肤是连续的。

基本检查

仔细身体检查。

诊断检查与说明

• 单纯脱垂无需实验室检查。
• 嵌顿直肠脱垂的术前检测，准备手术。

影像学检查

单纯脱垂无需影像学检查。

鉴别诊断

• 内痔脱出。
• 直肠息肉脱垂。
• 肠套叠。
• 其他肠道肿物。

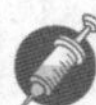

治疗

院前

• 舒适体位。
• 用潮湿纱布防止黏膜干燥。
• 预防黏膜创伤。

初步稳定/治疗

• 单纯脱垂一般无需治疗。
• 嵌顿或缺血性脱垂：
- 禁食。
- 静脉补液。
- 术前准备。

急诊治疗/程序

手法复位直肠脱垂。
• 位于膝胸位。
• 持续轻压 5～15 min。
• 使黏膜从远端进入肠腔。
• 根据需要可镇静放松括约肌。
• 手指可入直肠以引导脱垂翻转。
• 脱垂很大或缓解困难：
- 用 1/2～1 杯糖减轻肿胀，协助手法复位。
• 回纳后脱垂立刻再发：
- 用润滑剂、纱布、绷带加压包扎，臀部可粘贴在一起达数小时。
• 如果脱垂出现嵌顿或缺血，人工回纳失败或脱垂频繁复发：
- 入院紧急外科矫治。

> **注意**
> • 肛门括约肌收缩引起的直肠血流减少可能会导致缺血、静脉阻塞和血栓形成、全层坏死及肠损失。
> • 及时回纳，降低危险。
> • 缺血黏膜需外科干预。
> • 自发或人工还纳最常见并发症：
> - 局部疼痛。
> - 自限性黏膜出血。

药物治疗

镇静止痛药物治疗仅限于需要时。

随访

进一步处理

入院指征

• 坏死或缺血黏膜。
• 未能还纳的严重脱垂或频繁复发。

出院指征

• 直肠脱垂已还纳。
• 术后稳定可耐受。
• 治疗根本病因。
- 纠正便秘：
◦ 软便剂。
◦ 增加液体摄入。
◦ 增加膳食纤维。
• 避免久坐或压力。

出院指征

诊断检查参考包括：
• 检查主要损害。
• 复发脱垂建议外科修补。
• 儿童检测 CF。

随访建议

结直肠随访。

Z

要点和误区

进行详细体检鉴别息肉与直肠脱垂、痔、肠套叠。

• 脱垂很大或还纳困难时用 1/2～1 杯糖，减轻肿胀，协助手法复位。

直肠异物 Foreign Body, Rectal

Joanna W. Davidson　万健 译

基础知识

描述

• 自行插入物(自体性行为)：
- 由患者或伙伴插入的阴茎替代物。
- 多见于 20～40 岁男性，男女比例为 20∶1。

• 异物卡顿于直肠：
- 鸡骨。
- 鱼刺。
- 牙签。

• 医源性事故：
- 体温计。
- 灌肠剂接头。
- 用于清除嵌塞粪便的异物(FB)。

• 袭击：
- 强行插入的小刀或管子。
- 重伤常见，穿孔的概率高。

• 隐匿物：
- 体内藏毒，“mules”非法转运毒品。

诊断

症状与体征

• 主诉有直肠异物。
• 直肠充满状态。
• 直肠疼痛。
• 直肠周围脓肿(由埋入的骨头、牙签所致)。
• 异物的直肠检查：
- 高位的异物处于接近直肠乙状结肠交界处故，直肠检查时难以触及。
- 低位的异物通常处于直肠壶腹部，在直肠检查时可触及。

• 有些患者可能不会马上报告病史。
• 表现出腹部疼痛或不适的模糊症状。
• 表现出肠穿孔腹膜炎症状。
• 常于异物置入直肠数小时或数日后且反复尝试去除异物失败后延迟就诊。
• 直肠损伤程度(由美国创伤外科协会推荐)：
- 第Ⅰ级：血肿。挫伤或血肿，不伴血供阻断。
  ◦ 大部分直肠异物损伤属于第Ⅰ级。
- 第Ⅱ级：50%周长的肠管撕裂。
- 第Ⅲ级：>50%周长的肠管撕裂。
- 第Ⅳ级：全层撕裂扩展到会阴。
- 第Ⅴ级：肠段血运阻断。

基本检查

• 确定异物的数量、类型、留置时间和插入机制。
• 体格检查重点放在腹部和直肠检查：
- 以直肠乙状结肠连接处为界划分高位或低位。

• 腹部 X 线平片可确定异物的数量和尺寸。

诊断检查与说明

实验室检查

• 血常规：
- 判断出血和腹膜炎。

• 尿液分析：
- 判断尿道、膀胱损伤。

影像学检查

• X 线平片：
- 考虑做肾脏、尿道、膀胱(KUB)摄片应优先于直肠检查，先排除异物对检查者来说是否存在危险性。
- 明确和定位异物。
- 评估异物引起的并发症，包括肠穿孔和肠梗阻。
- 可以连续跟踪异物的位置。

• CT 扫描腹部和骨盆：
- 排除肠穿孔和脓肿。

鉴别诊断

• 假伪异物：
- 患者强调有直肠异物，但经 X 线检查、直肠检查、直肠镜检查未发现异物。

• 直肠周围脓肿。
• 痔。

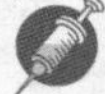

治疗

院前

注意：

• 患者通常已尝试去除异物，未成功。
• 进一步尝试去除异物将徒劳且可能导致穿孔。

初步稳定/治疗

• 肠穿孔合并腹膜炎及脓毒症：
- 生理盐水 500 ml，静脉输注。
- 使用广谱抗生素(覆盖厌氧菌和革兰阴性菌)：
  ◦ 头孢西丁、头孢替坦、替卡西林(羧噻吩青霉素)-克拉维酸、氨苄西林-舒巴坦、亚胺培南、美罗培南及厄他培南。
  ◦ 甲硝唑、克林霉素＋氨基糖苷类、第三代头孢菌素、氟喹诺酮、氨曲南。
- 紧急外科会诊。

• 给予高级创伤生命支持(ATLS)若合并其他创伤的证据。

急诊治疗/程序

• 适当的镇静和镇痛治疗对减轻肠道痉挛和水肿是很重要的。
• 避免应用灌肠和塞肛剂。
• 低位较小、非易碎或尖锐的异物可在急诊去除：
- 用手或钳子控制异物。
- 轻柔地移除异物并持续牵引克服肛门括约肌阻力。
- 因结肠黏膜紧密附着在异物的远端而产生真空状态会阻碍异物的脱出。
  ◦ 利用 Foley 导管越过异物消除真空状态取出异物。
- 清醒并配合的患者能协助更容易地取出异物利用瓦尔萨尔法(Valsalva 法)。
- 可通过器械协助取出异物，如产钳、持钩、环钳、吸引器。
- 在适当的镇静下 60%的直肠异物可在急诊部被取出。
- 随着异物取出，必须评估肛门直肠发生隐匿性损伤的可能。

• 高位的直肠异物：

- 不能立即从直肠取出。
- 通常需要消化科、外科会诊。
- 可尝试通过施以轻柔的腹部压力将异物从高位降至低位。
- 避免盲目地经肛门取异物。
- 用润滑的可视化的肛镜（以局部麻醉阻滞括约肌和会阴部神经）。
- 确认并观察异物的自行下降（通过连续的X线片）。
- 当其他方法都失败或已存在确凿的穿孔证据时行剖腹手术是必要的。

• 当碰到复杂异物时请外科、消化科会诊：
- 异物体积较大。
- 异物留置时间>24 h并出现水肿。
- 异物存在锋利的边缘。
- 异物取出后行直肠镜、乙状结肠镜检查结肠黏膜。

• 体内运毒者：
- 如果藏于体内的毒品包裹破裂将可引发全身中毒、肠坏死，甚至死亡。
- 禁用锐性的器械取异物，且在用其他器械取异物的过程中必须十分地谨慎。

■ 药物治疗

• 氨苄西林-舒巴坦（优立新）：3 g，静脉输注，q6 h[儿童：100～2 mg/(kg · d)div，q6 h]。

• 头孢菌素（头孢曲松）：1～2 g，静脉输注，q12 h（儿童：50～75 mg/kg，静脉输注，每日1次）。

• 环丙沙星（盐酸环丙氟沙星制剂）：400 mg，静脉输注，q8～12 h。

• 克林霉素：600～900 mg[儿童：20～40 mg/(kg · 24 h)]，静脉输注，q8 h。

• 左氧氟沙星：500 mg，静脉输注，q24 h。

• 甲硝唑：15 mg/kg，静脉输注，每日1次；之后7.5 mg/kg，静脉输注，q6 h。

• 哌拉西林-三唑巴坦（特治星）：3.75 g，静脉输注，q6 h；或4.5 g，静脉输注，q8 h[儿童：240～400 mg/(kg · d)div，q6～8 h]。

儿科注意事项

• 对于年龄太小难以配合的儿童在施以全身麻醉的情况下取出异物。

• 如果异物是除灌肠剂接头、温度计之外的物体的话，很可能患儿受到了虐待。

随访

■ 进一步处理

入院指征

• 在急诊部取异物失败后需要在手术室由外科干预。

• 直肠镜检查发现有黏膜撕裂需要观察24 h（无使用抗生素指征）。

• 当尖锐的异物取出后出现直肠疼痛的症状，提示可能存在小的穿孔甚至发展成脓肿，此时需在麻醉下进行检查。

出院指征

• 患者以保护性的方式插入异物且直肠异物已被取出。

• 遵嘱患者若出现直肠疼痛、腹痛、发热、大量直肠出血的情况应及时复诊。

转诊问题

若在急诊部不能取出异物请消化科或外科会诊。

■ 随访建议

推荐在取出异物后用可屈性乙状结肠镜或刚性直肠镜检查评估肠黏膜的损伤。

要点和误区

• 利用Foley导管越过异物消除真空状态取出异物。

• 试图在急诊取出异物时应给予患者足够的镇静或麻醉。

直肠周围脓肿 Perirectal Abscess

James A. Nelson · Scott A. Miller 钱斌斌 译

基础知识

■ 描述

肛门或直肠附近局部感染和脓性物质堆积。

■ 病因

• 肛腺感染，扩散到由肌肉和筋膜分隔的相邻区域：
- 肛周：
  ◦ 最常见。
  ◦ 经常在肛门附近有红色隆起。
- 坐骨直肠区域：
  ◦ 潜在空间大。
  ◦ 在确诊前可能变得非常大。
  ◦ 可以扩散后与其他部分形成"马蹄形"脓肿。
- 肛门内括约肌：
  ◦ 包含在内外括约肌之间起源的原发部位。
- 上提肌：
  ◦ 肛提肌上面很深。
  ◦ 需要在全麻下进行清创手术。
  ◦ 在诊断之前经常有全身性症状。

• 细菌原因通常是粪便病原体的混合：

• 相关疾病：
- 糖尿病。
- 炎症性肠道疾病。
- 恶性肿瘤。
- 免疫功能低下的宿主。

诊断

■ 症状和体征

• 疼痛：肛周、直肠或骨盆。

• 肿胀，波动性，引流，发热。

病史

• 肛周疼痛：
- 排便，坐下和咳嗽时加重。

• 缓慢的深部盆腔或直肠疼痛：
- 如果在齿状线以上（坐骨直肠和上提肌）出现会减少疼痛。

• 直肠或直肠周围渗液。

• 发热或发冷。

• 便秘。

体格检查

• 肛周肿胀，红斑，硬结，波动性，柔软。

• 臀部脓肿内裂，危险信号。
- 直肠脓肿可以追踪到臀部。

• 直肠检查是最重要的诊断介入：
- 直肠肿胀或柔软。
- 瘘可以探查，或触诊为脐带。

■ 基本检查

• 注意病史和配合直肠检查的体格检查，对于诊断结果是极其重要的。

• 对于持续的直肠周围疼痛应保持高度怀疑。

诊断检查与说明

没有实验室和影像学常规指示。

实验室检查

• 全血细胞计数：白细胞增多症伴核左移。
• 伤口培养：不是常规指标。
• 血液培养：主要用于脓毒症。

影像学检查

• CT(静脉造影±口服造影剂)。
• MRI(有助于检测瘘)。
• 有时使用超声检查。

诊断步骤/外科

切开与引流是明确的操作。

鉴别诊断

• 肛裂。
• 在臀部中线或后中线有前哨痔。
• 血栓或痔发炎。
• 肛门溃疡(即 HIV)。
• 直肠炎(即淋球菌)。
• 肛门直肠肿瘤。

治疗

初步稳定/治疗

止痛药物。

急诊治疗/程序

• 延迟引流可能引起恶化。
• 临床引流：
- 只有局部的肛周脓肿。
◦ 排除更深层次的地方。
- 切口靠近肛门边缘。
- 探索腔洞，击碎小腔。
- 优先冲洗。
- 48 h 内拆线。
• 全麻下清创术：
- 不适合局部麻醉，或者严重脓肿。
• 抗生素很少需要：
- 广泛的蜂窝织炎。
- 免疫抑制。
- 心脏瓣膜疾病。
- 全身性感染。
- 假体装置。
- 口服：
◦ 阿莫西林-克拉维酸或氟喹诺酮。
◦ 考虑耐甲氧西林金黄色葡萄球菌感染。
- 静脉注射：
◦ 头孢西丁。
◦ 氨苄西林-舒巴坦。
◦ 与氨苄西林、庆大霉素和克林霉素或甲硝唑联合治疗。
• 术后护理：
- 切开与引流 24 h 后坐浴，每日 3 次。
- 高纤维饮食或松软食品。
- 止痛剂。

药物

• 阿莫西林-克拉维酸：875 mg，口服，q12 h；或者 500 mg，口服，q8 h。
• 氨苄西林-舒巴坦：1.5～3 g，静脉注射，q6 h。
• 头孢西丁：1～2 g，静脉注射，q6～8 h。
• 克林霉素：每日 600～900 mg，静脉注射，q8 h。
• 庆大霉素：每日 3～6 mg/kg，静脉注射，q8 h。
• 甲硝唑：7.5 mg/kg，静脉注射，q6 h。

随访

进一步处理

入院指征

• 需要引流手术。
• 全身毒性、脓毒症。

出院指征

完成适合的切开与引流。

转诊问题

在 24～48 h 都应该听外科医师的指导。

随访建议

外科医师在 24～48 h 应评估瘘。
• 瘘形成在 25%～50%的肛门直肠脓肿中。

要点和误区

• 一定程度上的脓肿：
- 通过直肠检查和探测是必要的。
- 影像学检查来观察那些不易发现的深部区域。
• 在齿状线上面的深度脓肿有较少疼痛，并且出现单独的发热。

植入式除颤器 Defibrillators, Implantable

Robert D. Sidman · Lawrence S. Rosenthal 许磊 译

基础知识

Z

描述

• 一种可植入的心脏设备(ICD)，是一个小的由电池供电的电脉冲发生器，被植入患心律失常有心搏骤停风险的患者皮下。
• 引线通过回流心脏的静脉放置：
- 心内膜(右心房和右心室)。
- 心外膜(左心室经冠状静脉窦)。
• 腋窝中部定位通过皮下放置：
- 消除对循环系统的暴露(S-ICD)。
• 在植入式除颤器和右心室内的线圈(单线圈)和上腔静脉与右心房交界处(双线圈)之间。该设备能够检测并通过电除颤转换室性和房性心律失常为窦性心律。
• 植入的方法类似起搏器。
• 在美国每年有 450 000 人突发心脏病死亡：
- 每年在美国植入>100 000 设备。
- 在患有左心室功能不全的患者中，除颤器在降低死亡率上要比抗心律失常药物的治疗更有效：
◦ 2 年内死亡率绝对风险降低 7%。
◦ 抗心律失常药物治疗有效性上被限于患者的射血分数<35%。
- 有效降低肥厚型心肌病的死亡率。
- 在安装植入式除颤器后，缺血性和非缺血性扩张型心肌病患者表现出生存获益。
• 植入时并发症：
- 气胸。
- 血管穿孔。
- 急性引线移位。
• 合适的电击：
- 5%，每年用于一级预防。
- 20%，每年用于二级预防。
• 电击：

- ≥2 次合适的冲击，24 h 内送达。
• 不适当的电击：
- 10%～20%接受植入式除颤器的患者。
- 感知过度。
- 分类不当：室上性心动过速（阵发性室上速、房颤）。
• 设备感染：
- 1%～12%的患者。
- 急性 1～30 日，金黄色葡萄球菌。
- 亚急性 30 日，表皮葡萄球菌感染或革兰阴性。
- 31%～65%的死亡率，如果该装置被留在原处。
- 传染可能涉及皮肤、电池、除颤口袋或引线。
- 凝固酶阴性葡萄球菌（42%）。
- 甲氧西林敏感的金黄色葡萄球菌（25%）。
- 耐甲氧西林金黄色葡萄球菌（4%）。
- 革兰阴性杆菌（9%）。
• 血肿不吸收。
• 血管闭塞。

病因

• 电击（≥2 次合适的电击，24 h 内送达）：
- 未知。
- 心脏代偿功能衰竭。
- 急性缺血。
- 代谢紊乱。
- 致心律失常药。
- 甲状腺毒症。
- 发热伴扩张型心肌病。
- 遗传离子通道，Brugada 综合征，QT 间期延长，儿茶酚胺引起多形性室性心动过速。
- 致心律失常性右心室心肌病。
- 心脏术后。
• 不适当的电击：
- 过度感知：
◦ QRF、T 波、P 波、肌电、电磁干扰（EMI）。
◦ 频繁的短阵性室性心律失常。
◦ 引线断裂。
◦ 固定螺丝松动。
◦ 导线之间连接的问题。
◦ 头端（设备电路）的问题。
- 快速分类不当：
◦ 室上性心动过速。
◦ 心房颤动。
◦ 窦性心动过速。
◦ 心房扑动。
◦ 其他室上性心动过速（SVT）。
• 设备、位置相关：
- 伤口感染：
◦ 金黄色葡萄球菌（最具侵略性和可见性）。
◦ 表皮（更慢性和延后）。
◦ 大肠埃希菌、假单胞菌属和链球菌种（较少见）。
- 袋状血肿。
- 血管（静脉血栓、栓塞继发到静脉血流的阻抗由 ICD 引线引起）。

诊断

症状和体征

• 电击之前感觉不适和电击之后感觉舒适：适当的治疗。
• 电击之前舒适和电击之后感觉不适：可能不当的治疗。
• 在电击之前和之后症状很好：考虑持续存在的心律失常、缺血性或慢性心力衰竭。
• 合适的电击：
- 晕厥或接近晕厥。
- 头昏或眩晕。
- 呼吸急促。
- 心悸（非 SVT）。
- 胸部不适或疼痛。
- 发汗。
• 不适当的电击：
- 心悸（SVT）。
- 无自觉症状（引线有关的断裂、不合适的感应）。
• 设备感染：
- 发热。
- 寒战。
- 萎靡不振。
- 厌食症。
- 恶心。
- 发汗。
- 低血压。
- 心脏杂音。
• 伤口感染：
- 疼痛。
- 红斑。
- 脓肿引流。
- 温暖。
- 波动感。
- 皮肤糜烂。
- 血肿在插入位点位置（袋状血肿）：
- 疼痛（轻度）。
- 肿胀。
• 血管（血栓现象）：
- 在上肢单侧肿胀。
- 浅表静脉曲张。

病史

• 治疗相关：
- 近期心绞痛、心力衰竭。
• 设备相关的：
- 近期植入（<14 日）。
- 皮肤外伤或者伤口。
- 导丝相关的：
◦ 重复性手臂动作。
◦ 金德勒综合征（设备操作失误或导线脱出）。
- 血管：
◦ 近期植入。
◦ 多导丝。

体格检查

• 重要指征。
• 心脏衰竭、急性冠状动脉综合征的证据：
- 心尖搏动点移位。
- 左心室增大。
- 一个 S3 或 S4 的存在。
- 基底啰音的出现。
- 浊音。
- 对颈静脉压测定。
- 肝颈静脉反射。
- 周围水肿。
• 设备/位置相关：
- 伤口检查：
◦ 袋状线（红斑）。
◦ 脓肿引流。
◦ 受影响上肢的检查。

基本检查

• 以下 ICD 治疗：
- ICD 检查将决定治疗是否是适当的，如果存在的话，可以确定导丝断裂。
- 心电图（在电击后，暂时性的 ST 段改变和心肌酶升高可以看到，并不一定表明心肌损伤）。
- X 线胸片可能诊断导丝断裂。
• 设备/位置相关：
- 体征和局部症状与全身感染。
- 上肢肿胀表明静脉血栓形成。

诊断检查与说明

实验室检查

• 治疗相关：
- 12 导联心电图。

- 心肌酶。
• 设备相关的：
- CBC+白细胞分类。
- 血培养。
- 不要吸除血肿。

影像学检查

• PA和横向X线胸片：
- 导丝断裂。
- 电极导管错位。
• 上肢血管B超。
• MRI绝对禁忌，除非明确表明MRI是安全的。
- 磁场可能会损坏心脏除颤器及引起加热导丝尖端。

■ 诊断步骤/手术

• 治疗相关：
- 由电生理学家/心脏病专家进行调试，如果除颤仪配置有遥控处理功能也可以遥控。
- 磁体的应用抑制心动过速治疗（不影响布雷迪支持起搏）。
• 设备/位置相关（袋状血肿/感染）：
- 转入外科医师或电生理学家。
- 有编程或电磁应用程序。
• 胸外除颤是安全的，但避免直接在ICD上除颤（见下文）。

■ 鉴别诊断

• 适当的治疗：
- 单冲击下心动过速或者心室起搏波段以恢复正常的节奏。
• 不适当的治疗：
- 通常是由于室上性心动过速，导丝断裂，或者EMI。
• 幻影冲击：
- 从睡梦中惊醒被感知的患者。

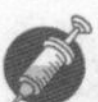

治疗

■ 院前

ICD放电：
• 静脉通路。
• 连续心电图监测。
• 高级心脏生命支持（ACLS）协议。

■ 初步稳定/治疗

• ACLS协议。
• 应用电磁抑制ICD治疗。
• 设备相关的：
- 疼痛管理。
- 抬高患肢（上肢的血栓形成）。

■ 急诊治疗/程序

• 佩戴设备的患者应当接受治疗，根据标准ACLS协议。
• 电刺激可能需要静脉抗心律失常药，如胺碘酮。
• 不适当的治疗：
- 室上性心律失常的治疗可以预防ICD电击与β受体阻滞剂或钙通道阻滞剂。
• 导丝相关的问题可能需要进一步的手术干预或设备重新编程：电磁应用程序将抑制快速心律失常疗法。
• 设备感染：
- 广谱抗生素。
- 首先获得血培养。

■ 药物治疗

• 胺碘酮150 mg或300 mg静脉推注后以1 mg/min输注，然后降低到0.5 mg/min。通常需要150 mg的负荷剂量。
• 美托洛尔：根据需要控制心率，5 mg，静脉点滴。
• 地尔硫䓬：5～20 mg静脉再维持点滴，控制心率。
• 头孢唑林：1 g静滴，q2 h。
• 万古霉素：1 g静滴，q12 h。
• 头孢氨苄：500 mg，口服，每日3次。
• 华法林：明确的静脉栓塞，国际标准化比值2～3，维持3～6个月。
• 利伐沙班（拜瑞妥）：20 mg，每日1次，3～6个月。
• 阿哌沙班（艾乐妥）：5 mg，每日2次，3～6个月。
• 达比加群酯（泰必全）：注射用药5日后，150 mg，每日2次，持续3～6个月。
• 伊多沙班：注射用药5～10日后，60 mg，1次/日3～6个。

随访

■ 进一步处理

入院指征

• 治疗相关：
- 正在进行/怀疑心肌缺血或心力衰竭。
- 多个ICD电击和启动抗心律失常药物的室颤/室速或者其他室上性心律失常。
- 基本治疗程序，并咨询电生理学家，确定是否需要立即干预。
• 设备/位置相关：
- 皮肤糜烂。
- 伤口裂开。
- 全身感染、心内膜炎。
- 需要改进导线。
- 扩大袋状血肿。
- 上肢血栓形成。

出院指征

• 治疗相关：
- 如果患者血流动力学稳定无缺血或心脏衰竭的迹象，通常无需干预：
◦ 单冲击，适当的治疗。
◦ 咨询电生理学家和安排适当的随访。
- 设备重新编程，以避免不当治疗。
• 设备/位置相关：
- 局部感染。
- 无皮肤糜烂的迹象。
- 袋状血肿没有扩张：
◦ 预防性应用抗生素不表示有袋状血肿。
• 稳定的伤口。

■ 随访建议

• 治疗相关：
- 心脏病医师或电生理学家。
• 设备相关：
- 外科医师或心脏病专家、电生理学家。

要点和误区

• 不建议设备袋状植入。
• 提供外部冲击时，应注意不直接在该装置上，因为它可能会分流能量远离心脏。

植物中毒 Plant Poisoning

Patrick M. Lank　瞿金龙 译

基础知识

描述

• 植物暴露是接触中毒的一个重要原因。

• <6 岁的儿童，大部分是因为无意识的摄入。

病因

如果有条件应区分摄入植物的种类。

具有抗胆碱类药物特性的植物

• 颠茄属、曼陀罗属的植物、天仙子属、甲茛菪属。

• 常见的抗胆碱药包括曼陀罗叶、龙葵属植物、天仙子、当归属。

• 与乙酰胆碱竞争与乙酰胆碱受体结合。

具有心脏毒性的植物

• 包括洋地黄、夹竹桃属、黄花夹竹桃属和嚏根草属。

• 常见心脏毒性的植物包括指顶花、夹竹桃、山谷的百合花、菟葵。

• 抑制 Na^{+} - K^{+} - ATP 酶的活性：可以参考地高辛中毒。

含有烟碱样生物碱类植物

• 主要包括烟草属、红毛七属和毒人参属植物。

• 包括烟草、蓝籽类叶牡丹和有毒铁杉。

• 主要起到激活烟碱样乙酰胆碱受体的作用。

含有生氰的化合物类植物

• 主要包括八仙花属、苹果属、李属、接骨木属等。

• 常见的植物包括杏子、樱桃树、李树、桃树、木薯、苹果树、接骨木等。

• 氰化物主要干扰电子链的传递导致细胞中毒。

含有草酸钙类植物

• 主要包括海芋属、花叶万年青属植物、喜林芋属等。

• 常见的植物包括热带海芋属植物等。

• 主要表现为细胞内草酸钙的释放：

- 局部组织暴露在草酸钙结晶引起炎症反应。

含有吡咯啶生物碱类

• 主要包括猪屎豆属、天芥菜属、千里光属和田菁等。

• 常见的有蝎子的尾巴、刘寄奴属植物、野百合。

• 机制主要包括肝毒性，导致肝脏血管增殖和肝静脉血管慢性闭塞疾病。

具有 Na^{+} 通道活性类

• 主要包括乌头属、翠雀(草)属、木藜芦属、南烛属等。

• 常见的有：乌头碱、藜芦属、生物碱类、棋盘花辛碱，Na^{+} 通道开启器有乌头、藜芦属、棋盘花辛碱。

• 参见的具有灰安毒素的植物，有不同的作用在 Na^{+} 通道上，包括杜鹃花等。

• 不同的 Na^{+} 通道影响主要在于毒素的作用，一般延长 Na^{+} 通道的开放。

含有毒白蛋白

• 主要包括相思子属、麻风树属、穗花桑寄生属等。

• 常见的植物名称：相思子、槲寄生和蓖麻子。

• 主要影响核糖体的功能。

诊断

症状和体征

抗胆碱能药

• 皮肤干暖，皮肤潮红。

• 肠鸣音消失。

• 尿潴留。

• 精神错乱。

心脏毒性的类固醇类

• 地高辛样中毒。

• 腹痛、恶心、呕吐。

• 多种心脏反应，包括心率快、室性心动过速和心室扑动。

• 高钾血症。

烟碱类生物碱

• 高血压。

• 心率快。

• 出汗。

• 流涎症。

• 呕吐。

• 肌束震颤。

• 肌力减弱。

氰类化合物

• 潜在延迟，跟氰气不一样。

• 起始症状：

- 腹痛、恶心、呕吐。
- 昏睡。
- 发汗。

• 进而出现：

- 神志改变。
- 乳酸中毒。
- 牙关紧闭。
- 心律失常。
- MODS。

草酸钙结晶

• 口咽部烧灼样痛和肿大。

• 眼睛暴露引起角膜结膜炎。

• 皮肤接触后刺激明显。

吡咯啶类生物碱

• 引起急性肝炎。

• 慢性暴露引起肝静脉血管闭塞疾病。

Na^{+} 通道激活剂

• 腹痛、恶心、呕吐。

• 中枢神经系统：神志改变、呼吸抑制昏迷。

• 心血管系统：窦缓或房室阻滞。

毒蛋白

• 对机体的影响主要看植物的种类(槲寄生等毒性少)和暴露的时间。

• 胃肠炎、腹泻或腹痛。

• 如果吸入可能对肺有影响。

• 如果注射了可能出现多器官功能不全。

儿科注意事项

• 一般有唇、舌口咽部的刺激。

• 主要是接触种子、叶子和浆果等。

• 烟碱类：1～2 根烟可能致命。

• 曼陀罗叶：

- 叶子高度蓄积。
- 100 片相当于 6 mg 阿托品。
- 4～5 g 叶子能致命。

• 黄色夹竹桃：

- 2 片叶子可致 12.5 kg 以下小孩死亡。

基本检查

区分摄入的物种。

诊断检查与说明

实验室检查

• 电解质、BUN、肌酐、糖、肝功能。

• ABG/VBG、pH。

- 地高辛的浓度。
- 生氰的乳酸的水平。

影像学检查

- ECG。
- CXR。

鉴别诊断

- 意识改变：
  - 药物的使用。
  - 癫痫。
  - 创伤。
  - 脑血管意外。
  - 低血糖。
- 地高辛中毒。
- 胃肠炎。
- 代谢性酸中毒的物质。
- 心脏方面的用药。

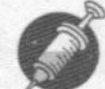

治疗

院前

- 常见的无毒的室内植物：
  - 非洲紫罗兰。
  - 极乐鸟。
  - 无花果属。
  - 栀子。
  - 葡萄。
  - 兰花。
  - 猩猩木(尽管声誉不佳)。
  - 蛛状吊兰。
  - 吊竹梅。
  - 橡胶树。
  - 蜡。
  - 斑叶竹芋。
- 收集种子、叶子、孢子等。
- 请教当地的植物学家。
- 不建议用吐根的叶汁。

初步稳定/治疗

- ABC 管理。
- 生理盐水静脉滴注：
  - 对于脱水和低血压患者可以容量复苏。
  - 如果低血压患者容量复苏效果不好，必要时加用血管活性药物。
- 心电监测。
- 支持治疗。

急诊治疗/程序

- 支持治疗。
- 很少有植物有解毒药物。

抗胆碱能药

- 烦躁时可给予苯二氮䓬类。
- 严重的精神错乱可以考虑毒扁豆碱治疗。

刺激心脏的甾类药物

地高辛：

- 心动过缓。
- 快速心律失常。
- 高钾血症。

类尼古丁样生物碱类

- 使用短暂的抗高血压药活性(如硝普钠)治疗高血压危象。
- 与苯二氮䓬类药物结合。

生氰类化合物

- 纠正电解质异常。
- 使用羟钴胺或者氰类解毒药，对于严重的酸中毒或者循环不稳定。

草酸钙结晶

- 轻症患者局部可冰敷。
- 对于严重的患者，给予利多卡因和镇痛药。
- 对于表皮的局部暴露，可予以局部清洗。

吡咯啶生物碱类

- 支持治疗。
- 源头阻断。
- 请肝脏科医师会诊。

钠通道激活剂

- 阿托品可以治疗窦性心动过缓。
- 对于低血压患者给予生理盐水快速静注，必要时使用血管活性药物。

毒白蛋白

根据临床症状采用支持治疗：补液，补充电解质。

药物治疗

- 阿托品：0.5 mg(儿童：0.02 mg/kg)静脉注射，0.5～1 mg 静脉注射重复。
- 氰化物解毒药：
  - 吸入戊基亚硝酸盐每分钟吸入半分钟，然后加入亚硝酸钠。
  - 亚硝酸钠：3% 10 ml 溶液，或者 300 mg，静脉注射超过 3～5 min 输完(儿童：0.15～0.33 ml/kg)。
    - 监测高铁血红蛋白<30%。
  - 硫代硫酸钠：25% 50 ml 溶液，静脉注射或 12.5 g(儿童：1.65 ml/kg)。
- 地高辛：经验性治疗，5～10 安瓿。
- 羟钴胺：成人 5 g，静脉注射，70 mg/kg，最多不超过 5 g(对于儿童)。
- 镁：2～4 g，静脉注射。
- 毒扁豆碱：0.2～2 mg，静脉注射。
- 碳酸氢钠：8.4% 1 安瓿静脉注射，直到 QRS 波群变窄。

随访

进一步处理

入院指征

- 心电监测提示心律失常。
- 顽固性呕吐。
- 顽固性低血压。
- 器官功能损伤。
- 神志改变。

出院指征

- 生命体征稳定。
- 可以口服液体。
- 心电活动正常。
- 没有发生延迟性毒物作用。

儿科注意事项

收治指征比成人低：

- 吃了更多的植物汁。
- 低的致死剂量。
- 症状不典型。

随访建议

可以与内科毒理学医师或内科医师保持随访。

要点和误区

- 一般很少因为偶然的植物暴露致死。
- 植物暴露后，过度的治疗或不正确的治疗可能致死。
- 如果患者摄入有毒植物，与当地的毒物中心联系。

Z

致幻剂中毒 Hallucinogen Poisoning

Joanne C. Routsolias　祝各亮　译

基础知识

描述

• 主要改变患者的感知、认知和情绪。
• 所有的致幻剂能够增强神经递质的释放或直接与受体结合：
- 血清素(5-羟色胺，5-HT)：许多致幻剂是5-HT受体亚型的激动剂或拮抗剂。
- 去甲肾上腺素、多巴胺及N-甲基-D-天冬氨酸(NMDA)。

病因

• 大多数致幻剂中毒是人为的。
• 常见的致幻剂：
- 吲哚胺：
◦ 麦角酸二乙酰胺(LSD，持续时间为6～12 h)。
◦ 牵牛花(牵牛属)。
- 色胺：
◦ 裸头草碱(迷幻蘑菇)，常掺入LSD中使用。
◦ 二甲基色胺(DMT)、5-甲氧基DMT("狡猾的甲氧基")和其他的色胺的同系物。
- 苯乙胺(致幻性苯丙胺)：
◦ 甲基/烯二氧苯丙胺(MDA)。
◦ 甲基/烯二氧甲基苯丙胺(MDEA)。
◦ 甲基/烯二氧甲基苯丙胺(MDMA，"狂欢"，持续8～12 h)。
◦ 对甲基氧苯丙胺。
◦ 二甲基氧苯丙胺。
◦ 麦司卡林(皮约特仙人掌)，常掺入LSD中使用(持续6～12 h)。
- 烷基/环烷基胺：
◦ 苯环己哌啶(PCP，根据报告可持续11～96 h)。
◦ 氯胺酮(时间长短取决于摄入方式，为30～120 min)。
- 抗胆碱能药物：
◦ 颠茄。
◦ 曼陀罗。
- 其他：
◦ 哌嗪类：苄基哌嗪(BZP)和三氟甲基苯基哌嗪(TFMPP)。
◦ 右美沙芬(DXM，持续3～6 h)。
◦ 大麻。
◦ Kratom(持续4～6 h)。

诊断

症状和体征

• 个体差异较大；根据药剂和剂量的不同，效果可以持续4～12 h或长达96 h。
• 以交感神经兴奋症状为特点。
• 即使存在妄想，行为通常有目的性，能够询问出接触的病史。
• 初始症状：
- 恶心、面红、发冷及震颤。
• 神经症状：
- 摄入后早期出现烦躁与头晕。
- 发笑(尤其是裸头草碱)。
- 焦虑、绝望、无助与恐惧。
- 知觉强化，视觉扭曲/强化。
- 触觉扭曲(特别是麦司卡林)。
- 通感(感觉模式的混合，如看到声音)。
- 宗教或神秘的经历。
- 睡眠中断。
• 神经体征：
- 反常/奇异行为。
- 言语中断。
- 瞳孔散大。
- 立毛。
- 反射亢进。
- 接触大剂量药剂会导致昏迷。
- 抽搐：
◦ 致幻性苯丙胺。
◦ 儿童食用迷幻蘑菇后发热。
• 肺部：
- 轻度呼吸急促。
- 呼吸骤停(大量接触)。
• 心血管系统：
- 心动过速。
- 高血压(致幻性苯丙胺)。
- 心律失常(致幻性苯丙胺)。
- 自发性脑出血(致幻性苯丙胺)。
• 消化道：
- 恶心与呕吐(尤其是麦司卡林)。
• 代谢：
- 高热：
◦ 特别是在"狂欢"俱乐部使用MDMA。
◦ 接着可能出现肝功能衰竭、肾衰竭和弥散性血管内凝血。
◦ 可能会致死。
- 低钠血症：有MDMA使用导致的报道。
• 造血：
- 大剂量时会破坏血小板中5-羟色胺的功能，出现凝血功能障碍和出血。

病史

了解致幻剂及使用情况：
• 使用的方法。
• 剂量。
• 接触时间。
• 接触部位。

体格检查

• 获得准确的生命体征，包括温度。
• 进行详细的神经系统和精神科检查。

基本检查

• 核心温度测量和其他生命体征。
• 心电监测。
• 对横纹肌溶解的风险测定：
- 肌酸激酶水平。
- 尿液试纸或肌红蛋白水平。

诊断检查与说明

实验室检查

• 电解质、尿素氮、肌酐、血糖水平、凝血功能、动静脉血气。
• 尿液毒物筛查：
- 很少能够明确。
- 对于区分致幻剂种类是没有价值的。
- 大多数致幻性物质不作为常规药物进行筛查。
- 致幻性苯丙胺(如MDMA)筛查通常是阴性的。

影像学检查

• 如果需寻找主动脉夹层、肺吸入物或创伤相关性损伤，考虑胸部X线检查。
• 如果需寻找颅内出血或损伤，考虑头颅CT。
• 如果怀疑摄入药物包，考虑腹部X线检查。

鉴别诊断

• 低血糖。
• 脑膜炎，脑炎。
• 脓毒症。
• 颅内出血或病变。
• 戒断反应(乙醇、镇静催眠药、巴氯芬)。
• 5-羟色胺综合征(尤其是血清素类药物)。

• 精神疾病：
- LSD 相关的长期类似精神病的分裂情感障碍。
- 慢性苯丙胺、可卡因滥用。
- 激素。

• 在高热儿童中出现感染性/热性惊厥。

儿科注意事项

评估亲子关系以判断忽视或虐待的可能性。

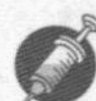

治疗

院前

• 有争议的：
- 镇静：苯二氮䓬类或氟哌啶醇类或躯体约束。
  ◦ 通常更倾向于苯二氮䓬类。
  ◦ 镇静剂常常会掩盖症状，可能会限制病史的采集。

• 注意事项：
- 镇静或约束患者以确保安全的转运。
- 对于高热的患者：
  ◦ 更倾向于用镇静剂而不是躯体约束。
  ◦ 采取降温手段。

初步稳定/治疗

• 急救 ABC 管理。

• 如果有高热进行积极降温处理。

• 如果有显著的液体丢失或横纹肌溶解证据，静脉补充等渗性液体。

• 如果患者精神状态改变，需测血糖，补充纳洛酮、葡萄糖和硫胺素。

急诊治疗/程序

• 降温措施：
- 冷雾和风扇。
- 如果躁动不安，使用苯二氮䓬类药物。
- 如果呼吸肌麻痹，进行气管插管。

• 对躁动或自主体征进行镇静：
- 苯二氮䓬类。
- 很少用抗精神病药物：
  ◦ 可能加剧致幻效果。
  ◦ 可能会较低癫痫发作的阈值。

• 由于吸收迅速和症状延迟出现，活性炭(AC)是对于大多数致幻剂是无效的。
- 对于在完整保护性气道反射下口服摄入致幻剂 2～3 h 的患者，可考虑使用活性炭，尤其是对于抗胆碱能药等延迟胃肠运动/吸收的药物。

• 将患者放置在安静的环境中。

• 保持 2～3 ml/(kg · h)的尿量并考虑碱化尿液治疗横纹肌溶解。

药物治疗

• 苯二氮䓬类(地西泮)：5～10 mg，静脉注射(儿童：0.2～0.5 mg/kg，静脉注射)；或劳拉西泮：1～4 mg，静脉注射/肌内注射(儿童：0.02～0.05 mg/kg，静脉注射或肌内注射)，需要时可重复。

• 低血糖补充 50%葡萄糖：25 g/50 ml(儿童：25%葡萄糖 0.5～1 g/kg 或 2～4 ml/kg)，静脉注射，需要时可重复。

• 氟哌啶醇：2.5～5 mg，静脉注射或肌内注射，每 30～60 min 可重复一次直到镇静为止，通常最大剂量为 10～20 mg；不推荐用于儿童。

• 纳洛酮：初始剂量 2 mg(儿童：0.01～0.1 mg/kg)，静脉注射或肌内注射，需要时可重复。

• 横纹肌溶解时输注碳酸氢钠：3 安瓿瓶溶于 1 L 5%葡萄糖溶液，1.5～2 倍剂量进行维持(保持尿液 pH>7.5)。

• 硫胺素(维生素 B_1)：100 mg(儿童：25 mg)，静脉注射或肌内注射。

随访

进一步处理

入院指征

• 严重中毒。

• 非典型表现。

• 延迟性症状(接触>12 h 发作)。

• 长期的躁动和高热：
- 横纹肌溶解或器官损害的风险。

出院指征

接受支持治疗和观察后，无症状的患者可以出院。

儿科注意事项

如果怀疑有儿童虐待或忽视的案例，需向儿童保护性机构咨询。

随访建议

出院的患者应当与他们的家庭医师、心理医师或药物咨询机构进行随访。

要点和误区

• 不要延误高热的诊断和治疗，一旦出现高热需积极降低躯体温度。

• 使用适当的物理或化学镇静方法来控制暴力躁动的患者，以防止患者及医护人员受伤。

• 进行连续的查体和生命体征监测(特别是体温)，不要因为躁动患者的一过性平静就认为已经康复，患者可能会进展为更严重的疾病。

痔 Hemorrhoid

Julia H. Sone 陈奇通 译

Z

基础知识

描述

• 通常：
- 直肠远端和近端肛管的静脉窦正常。
- 肛管的正常血管垫能够有助于肛门自制。
- 动静脉短路系统存在于不同程度的内痔中，是导致经直肠出血的主要原因。

• 当出现相关症状时，说明痔在进展。

• 一般不会产生疼痛，除非是出现血栓和绞窄。

• 在独立的厚黏膜下层中包含：
- 血管。
- 平滑肌。
- 弹性组织与结缔组织。

• 部分肛管黏膜向下移位。

• 外痔：
- 血管处于齿状线下方。
- 被皮肤或者肛膜覆盖。
- 汇入髂内静脉。

• 内痔：
- 黏膜下层血管位于齿状线上方。
- 汇入门静脉系统。
- 通常在左侧壁、右后外侧壁、右前外侧壁等位置。

- 1 度：无痛，出血。
- 2 度：排便时脱出，可自发还原。
- 3 度：排便时脱出，需人工还纳。
- 4 度：长期脱垂，不可还纳。

病因

- 具体原因不明。
- 重力和腹腔压力导致血窦膨胀。
- 与痛性牵动和不规律的排便习惯有关：
  - 巨大坚硬的粪便或者腹泻可以引起里急后重/痛性牵动。
  - 促进肛管血管垫脱出肛管。
  - 薄弱的黏膜下组织引起脱垂。
- 较高的肛门静息压力：
  - 直立姿势。
- 遗传：
  - 缺乏静脉瓣。
- 与腹腔内压力增高有关：
  - 腹水。
  - 妊娠。
- 门静脉高压。

诊断

症状和体征

- 排便时伴随无痛、直肠出血。
- 血液在粪便或手纸表面。
- 鲜红色的血滴进便池。
- 直肠不适或者腹腔压力大。
- 以下情况可能引起剧烈疼痛：
  - 内痔脱垂和绞窄。
  - 外痔形成血栓。
- 肛门瘙痒症。
- 有可能存在肛裂。

病史

- 出血的时间。
- 相关的疼痛。
- 直肠新生肿块或包块。
- 粪便性状：成形或呈液体。
- 既往存在直肠相关问题。
- 粪便改变。

体格检查

- 肛周检查：
  - 轻柔地将臀部展开。
  - 被皮肤覆盖的独立、深蓝色、柔软组织：血栓性外痔。
    - 可能有内部构造。
    - 通常与增大的血栓性外痔有关。
  - 肿块被略带紫色的黏膜覆盖：脱垂，绞窄性内痔。
  - 需要患者肛门用力使劲才能检查脱垂的内痔。
  - 直肠指检可以排除恶性肿瘤。
- 肛门镜检查能将肛管显现：
  - 识别出血性内痔。

基本检查

通过彻底的肛门直肠检查了解详细病史。

诊断检查与说明

实验室检查

- 如果病史中有明显的失血，行 CBC 检查。
  - 血红蛋白与血细胞比容。
- 血小板计数。
- 如果患者在使用抗凝药物或者处于重病中可查 PT、APTT、INR。

鉴别诊断

- 直肠脱垂。
- 肛裂。
- 肛周脓肿与肛瘘。
- 尖锐湿疣。
- 恶性上皮肿瘤或黑色素瘤。

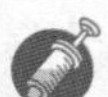

治疗

院前

严重出血时须尽快建立静脉通道。

初步稳定/治疗

指压法压迫止血。

急诊治疗/程序

- 适用于全部患者的保守治疗：
  - 每日 3 次和排便后行热水坐浴 15 min。
  - 高纤维饮食：30 g/d。
    - 进食大量新鲜水果和蔬菜。
    - 增加麸皮摄入。
  - 每日饮水 10～12 杯。
  - 大便软化剂。
  - 大便成形剂。
- NSAIDs：镇痛和抗感染效果。
- 剧痛须排除外痔形成血栓，＜5 日陈旧血块未分解。
  - 遵循保守治疗。
  - 将患者摆放成折刀状卧位或者左侧卧位，并将臀部分开。
  - 渗入周围皮肤和皮下的凝块，使用含肾上腺素的利多卡因 27G 针。
  - 使用椭圆形切口去除凝块与皮肤。
  - 可以使用硝酸银棒止血。
  - 将一小片明胶海绵和/或纱布覆盖在伤口表面。
  - 移除敷料，第一次坐浴时间约 6 h。
  - 镇痛药：
    - NSAIDs。
    - 对乙酰氨基酚。
    - 5%利多卡因药膏外用：表面麻醉剂减轻疼痛。
    - 局部 0.2%硝酸甘油药膏外用，通过抑制肛门括约肌痉挛止痛。
- 人工操作减少非血栓、脱垂内痔：
  - 遵循保守治疗。
  - 可以使用表面麻醉剂或者通过局部麻醉阻滞肛门括约肌。
  - 可以使用 2.5%鱼肝油酸钠或者 3%高渗盐水使出血内痔硬化。
  - 可以使用橡皮圈结扎内痔。
    - 避免免疫功能低下患者出现会阴感染导致的脓毒症。
- 不可还纳的内痔：
  - 非绞窄型：保守治疗和外科手术治疗。
  - 绞窄型：立即手术切除。

妊娠注意事项

- 通常在第 3 个月出现症状，可以保守治疗。
- 禁止使用 AnalpramHC(C 级)。

药物治疗

- 对乙酰氨基酚：325～650 mg（儿童：15 mg/kg）和可待因 15～30 mg（儿童：0.5 mg/kg）口服，q4 h，必要时。成人对乙酰氨基酚不超过 4 g/24 h，儿童不超过 75 mg/(kg. 24 h)。
- 麸皮/纤维素：20 g，口服，每日 1 次。
- 多库酯钠：50～200 mg（儿童：＜3 岁，10～40 mg/d；3～6 岁，20～60 mg/d；＞6～12 岁，40～150 mg/d），口服，q12 h。
- 5%利多卡因乳膏：疼痛时涂于肛周，q4 h，必要时（儿童：＜12 岁禁止使用）。注意：少量使用，100 g 乳膏中含 5 g 利多卡因，容易被吸收。
- 氢化可的松/普莫卡因外用（AnalpramHC）1%/1%乳膏、2.5%/1%乳膏/洗剂（儿童：同样的剂量）涂于局部，每日 3～4 次。
- 氢化可的松/利多卡因外用（AnaMantle HC）0.5%/3%乳膏、2.5%/3%凝胶（儿童：未表示）涂于肛管，每日 2 次。
- 布洛芬（Motrin）：400～600 mg［儿童：40 mg/(kg · d)］，口服，q6 h。

• 0.2%硝酸甘油药膏：棉签蘸取局部外用，每日 3 次。

• 车前子胶：1～2 tsp(儿童：0.25～1 tsp/d)，口服，q24 h。

随访

进一步处理

入院指征

• 4 度绞窄型内痔：

- 对于脱垂、形成血栓的内痔请外科会诊。

• 因痔出血导致贫血。

• 行抗凝治疗和门静脉高压的严重出血痔患者。

出院指征

大部分患者将出院回家。

转诊问题

手术治疗指征：

• 3 度或 4 度内痔。

• 可疑的肛门直肠或结肠肿瘤、炎症性肠病、凝血功能障碍、妊娠或免疫功能低下。

随访建议

• 结直肠外科治疗术后对 3 度或 4 度内痔或者可疑肿瘤患者进行随访。

• 非复杂的痔进行初始治疗随访。

注意

所有经直肠出现鲜红色出血的患者应考虑胃肠道或结直肠外科手术，以及恶性肿瘤。

要点和误区

痔不是肛门直肠疼痛和出血的唯一原因。应全面考虑其他病因。

中毒 Poisoning

Mark B. Mycyk　瞿金龙 译

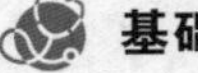

基础知识

描述

• 中毒可能是故意或无意的。

• 症状有变化的没有去除病因的患者，可能考虑其他的诊断。

病因学

• 故意：

- 抑郁症。
- 自杀。
- 他杀。
- 娱乐精神类药物滥用，或过量。

• 无意：

- 一般发生在小孩。
- 治疗错误。
- 精神类药物试验。

儿科注意事项

• 偶尔误服，尤其小孩(1～5 岁)。

• 如果有无意或怀疑的病史，因该考虑诊断。

诊断

症状和体征

• 神经症状：

- 昏睡。
- 过激。
- 昏迷。
- 幻觉。
- 强直。

• 呼吸情况。

- 呼吸困难，不能呼吸。
- 没有保护气道的能力。

• 心血管：

- 心律失常。
- 传导阻滞。

• 生命体征：

- 主要依赖于毒性物质。
- 体温过高或过低。
- 心率过快或过慢。
- 低血压或高血压。

中毒综合征

• 抗胆碱能药：

- 神志改变(意识模糊、错乱、昏睡)。
- 皮肤黏膜干燥。
- 扩大的瞳孔。
- 心动过速。
- 高热。
- 面色潮红。
- 尿潴留。

• 胆碱能药：

- 过度分泌(流涎症、流泪)。
- 瞳孔缩小。
- 支气管痉挛，哮鸣音。

• 阿片类：

- 中枢神经和呼吸抑制。
- 瞳孔缩小。

• 拟交感神经药：

- 中枢兴奋。
- 攻击性。
- 心动过速。
- 高血压。
- 出汗。

基本检查

• 生命体征包括体温。

• 体格检查，包括眼睛、皮肤、呼吸气味。

诊断检查与说明

实验室检查

• 电解质、BUN、Cr、血糖。

• 预测阴离子间隙：$Na^{+}(Cl^{-}+HCO_3^{-})$：

- 正常阴离子间隙(8～12)。
- 评估酸中毒：
  ◦ 酒精性酮症酸中毒。
  ◦ 氰化物、一氧化碳。
  ◦ 阿司匹林、水杨酸。
  ◦ 甲苯。
  ◦ 甲醇、二甲双胍。
  ◦ 尿毒症。
  ◦ 糖尿病酮症酸中毒。
  ◦ 副醛、苯乙双胍。
  ◦ 铁、异烟肼。
  ◦ 乳酸酸中毒。
  ◦ 乙烯乙二醇。
  ◦ 绝食后酮症。

• 血浆渗透压：

- 如果潜在有毒酒精引起的阴离子间隙升高性酸中毒，则计算渗透压间隙。
- 早期中毒敏感。
- 正常的血浆渗透压不能完全排除酒精的摄入。

Z

- 可算渗透压＝2(Na^+)＋血糖/18＋BUN/2.8＋乙醇(mg/dl)/6。
- 渗透压间隙＝测得渗透压－计算的渗透压。
- 当渗透压间隙＞10：
  ◦ 甲醇。
  ◦ 乙醇。
  ◦ 利尿药。
  ◦ 异丙基乙醇。
  ◦ 乙烯乙二醇。
  ◦ 丙酮。
• 妊娠试验。
• 自杀的患者醋氨酚水平。
• 毒物检测。

影像学检查

• 心电图：心律失常，或者 QRS/QT 变化。
• 神志改变不明确的需行头颅 CT 检查。
• CXR 检查，如果有误吸或肺炎。

鉴别诊断

• 神志改变。
• 头颅肿块或出血。
• 感染、脓毒症。
• 内分泌异常。
• 低氧。
• 低体温。
• 代谢异常。
• 心理因素。

治疗

院前

• 现场寻找毒物的证据。
- 胶囊等瓶子。
- 药物的储存器械。
- 证人。
- 把所有的药物和瓶子做鉴定。
• 对于不配合治疗的患者，给予一定的约束。
• 考虑合并疾病：
- 创伤。
- 内科疾病。
- 环境暴露。
• 可以在院前给予活性炭，减少毒物的吸收。

初步稳定/治疗

• ABC 管理：
- 必要时气道保护、气管插管、机械通气治疗低氧。
- 对于低氧患者给予吸氧。
- 指脉氧监测。
- 心电监测。
- 建立静脉通路。
• 低血压：
- 生理盐水静脉滴注。
- Trendelenburg(头低足高)卧位。
- 必要时血管加压药。
• 如果神志改变，摄入就过量：硫胺素、D_{50}W、纳洛酮等。

急诊治疗/程序

• 去污：
- 清除胃内污物。
- 减少毒素的吸收。
• 口胃灌洗：
- 如果不知道毒物，可以 1 h 洗胃。
- 必要时保护气道。
• 活性炭：
- 很多毒素在数小时内出现最大的反应。
- 保护气道和防止并发症。
- 很多不结合活性炭的：金属(硼酸盐、溴化物、铁等)。
• 全肠灌洗：
- 聚乙二醇(Colyte, Golytly)排空肠道，不会引起电解质紊乱。
- 不能被木炭(如铁和锂)很好吸附的毒素，如身体包装器/填充物缓慢释放毒素摄入时可考虑应用。
- 如果存在肠梗阻、穿孔或低血压，则禁忌。
• 增强清除功能：
- 增强对全身已吸收毒素的清除。
• 多剂量活性炭：
- 茶碱。
- 酰胺咪嗪。
- 苯巴比妥。
• 碱化尿液：
- 水杨酸盐类。
- 苯巴比妥。
• 血液透析、血液灌流：
- 锂。
- 水杨酸盐。
- 茶碱。
- 酒精中毒。
- 丙戊酸盐。
• 抽搐：
- 开始予地西泮或劳拉西泮等治疗。
- 持续抽搐，给予苯巴比妥。
- 苯妥英钠，非中毒性抽搐。
  ◦ 继发于原发性癫痫、创伤后或癫痫持续状态。
• 解毒药：
- 醋氨酚：N-乙酰半胱氨酸。
- 抗胆碱能药：毒扁豆碱。
- 苯二氮䓬类：氟马西尼。
- 美托洛尔(倍他乐克)：胰高血糖素。
- 钙通道阻滞剂：氯化钙/葡萄糖酸钙、胰岛素。
- 一氧化碳：氧气、高压氧。
- 华法林：维生素 K_1。
- 氰化物：氯化物 1 套、羟钴胺。
- 地高辛：羊地高辛抗体 Fab 片段。
- 乙烯：乙二醇、甲基吡唑。
- 铁：去铁胺。
- 异烟肼：维生素 B_6。
- 甲醇、乙醇、甲基吡唑。
- 高铁血红蛋白血症：亚甲蓝。
- 阿片剂：纳洛酮。
- 有机磷：阿托品、解磷定。
- 抗忧郁药：$NaHCO_3$。

药物治疗

• 活性炭：1～2 g/kg，口服。
• 葡萄糖：D_{50}W 1 安瓿：50 ml 或 25 g。
• 地西泮：5～10 mg，静脉注射，q10～15 min。
• 劳拉西泮：2～6 mg，静脉注射，q10～15 min。
• 纳洛酮：0.2～2 mg，静脉注射，起始剂量。
• 维生素 B_1：100 mg，静脉注射或肌内注射。

随访

进一步处理

入院指征

• 生命体征改变。
• 心肺不稳定。
• 自杀。
• 实验室检查异常。
• 可能因为不能及时的药物治疗，出现自身失代偿。

出院指征

• 排除精神病。
• 已经解毒。
• 血流动力学稳定。

转诊问题

• 无意中毒要求毒物保护咨询。
• 有意中毒可能要求精神科评估。
• 建议药物不能滥用。

妊娠注意事项

对于孕妇的治疗也是对胎儿最好的治疗。

■ 随访建议

• 建议患者不能过量服用药物。
• 无意中毒要求毒物保护咨询。
• 有意中毒可能要求精神科评估。

要点和误区

• 对生命体征变化的患者不要忘了考虑非中毒的因素。
• 不能靠尿检来确定药物的诊断，除非有限的药物种类。
• 可以请毒理学专家协助诊断。

中毒性表皮坏死松解症 Toxic Epidermal Necrolysis

Andrew K. Chang · Jessica M. Noonan　范浩浩　李文放 译

 基础知识

■ 描述

• 皮肤病中最具暴发性和潜在致命的一种。
• 真皮-表皮界面皮肤脱落，相当于二度烧伤。
• 可以影响身体表面总面积(BSA)的100%。
• 可能涉及以下方面：
- 肠道黏膜。
- 呼吸道黏膜。
- 泌尿生殖/肾上皮组织。
• 机制不明确，研究表明免疫学、细胞毒性、迟发性超敏反应及遗传易感性可能与此相关。
• 现行分类系统在史蒂文斯-约翰逊综合征(SJS)和中毒性表皮坏死溶解(TEN)的范围内提出3种类型，不同于来自多形红斑的主体和基于BSA总量的百分比。
- SJS：<10%的BSA。
- SJS - TEN重叠综合征：10%～30%的BSA。
- TEN：>30%的BSA，可以影响高达100%的BSA。
• 在老年患者和免疫力低下的患者中更常见。
• 死亡率约为30%，通常是继发于金黄色葡萄球菌和铜绿假单胞菌败血症。
• 同义词：
- 莱尔综合征。
- 固定药物的坏死溶解。
- 表皮坏死梭菌。
- 大疱性表皮松解症。

■ 病因

• 剂量无关的药物反应是常见TEN的原因：
- 在前1～3周使用的药物是最可能的原因。
- 经常涉及的药物包括：
◦ 磺胺和PCN抗生素。
◦ 抗惊厥药(卡马西平、苯妥英、苯巴比妥、拉莫三嗪)。
◦ NSAIDs(昔康类、吡唑类、舒林酸)。
◦ 别嘌醇。
◦ 皮质类固醇。
◦ 抗反转录病毒药物。
• 其他罕见原因：感染、移植物抗宿主病、疫苗接种、特发病例(合并<4%)。

诊断

■ 症状和体征

病史

• 前驱症状：像流感一样，一到几日的发热，不适，瘙痒，皮肤压痛，红斑，厌食，肌痛，关节痛。
• 出现皮肤损伤前，黏膜通常受到1～3日的影响(口咽、眼睛、生殖器、肛门、食管和肠黏膜、呼吸道上皮)，导致结膜炎、食管炎、咽炎、胃肠道出血、呕吐、腹泻、排尿困难、咳嗽、呼吸困难。

体格检查

• 皮肤：
- 皮疹通常从面部开始(头皮通常幸免于难)和躯干为红斑斑块，不规则靶状大疱，或弥漫性、疾病相关的红斑；最初可能会让局部痛苦不堪，难以忍受。
- 广泛的表皮溶解，表皮剥脱，松弛大疱和片状脱落的表皮一般在3～4日发生，但是可以在数小时内迅速进展。
- 尼氏征：给侧向压力，皮肤从表皮和真皮交界分离脱落和脱落。
• 黏膜病变见于90%以上病例，初始肿胀和红斑，然后起疱和溃疡。
• 眼部病变(伪膜、粘连、角膜炎、角膜糜烂)。

■ 基本检查

• 临床诊断：
- 根据病史和特征皮肤和黏膜病变诊断。

■ 诊断检查与说明

实验室检查

• 不存在确诊性实验室检查。
• CBC：正常细胞性贫血、白细胞增多症、淋巴细胞减少症/中性粒细胞减少症、血小板减少症可能存在。
• 由于系统性炎症，ESR可能会升高。
• 血清化学：电解质紊乱如果大量的流体损失：
- 肾前性氮质血症。
- 血清碳酸氢盐<20可能导致死亡率升高超过40倍。
• LFT：转氨酶升高，总蛋白和白蛋白降低。
• UA可能出现血尿(尿道黏膜糜烂、肾小球肾炎)或管型(急性肾小管坏死)。
• 伤口/皮肤培养和血培养。
• 血清颗粒溶素(一种牵连的细胞毒素)。

影像学检查

应拍摄胸部X线片。

诊断步骤/外科

• TEN(SCORTEN)的疾病严重程度评分：每项风险因素获得1分，更高的分数意味着预后更差：
- 年龄>40岁。
- 恶性肿瘤。
- 心动过速>120次/分。
- 表皮分离的初始百分比>10%。
- BUN>27 mg/dl。
- 血糖水平>252 mg/dl。
- 血清碳酸氢盐水平<20 mmol/L。
• 活检可以通过会诊进行。皮肤科医师排除自身免疫性大疱疾病、葡萄球菌烫伤样皮肤综合征和其他诊断：
- 急诊医师无法立即获得结果。

■ 鉴别诊断

• 史蒂文斯-约翰逊综合征(SJS)。
• 多形性红斑(EMM)：

Z

- 从 EMM 区分 SJS/TEN：
- 免疫病理学不同。
- 病因：SJS/TEN 主要是药物诱导的，机制不确定；EMM 既可因感染又可经药物诱导，或由Ⅳ型超敏反应引起。
- 病变：
  ◦ TEN：广泛分布，主要在躯干和面部，非特异性的靶标样病变往往相互融合，数不胜数，然后脱屑。
- • EMM：数量有限，对称性和肢端分布，典型的靶型（至少 3 个同心环）带或不带水疱。
- 预后：EMM 通常是良性的，疾病复发很常见（30%）。

• 葡萄球菌烫伤样皮肤综合征（SSSS）：
- TEN 与 SSSS 的鉴别诊断。
- 年龄：TEN 主要是成人（但可能见于儿童），SSSS 主要影响儿童。
- 病因学：
  ◦ TEN 通常代表一种特殊的，药物诱导的，剂量依赖性反应，并且不需要用抗生素进行治疗。
  ◦ SSSS 由感染引起并且需要抗生素。
- 疼痛：TEN，疼痛；SSSS，无痛。
- 黏膜：TEN 时涉及黏膜病变；SSSS 则幸免。
- 皮肤分离：TEN 中的皮肤-表皮连接处分离；SSSS 中的表皮内分离（均可产生阳性尼氏征）。

• 自身免疫性大疱性疾病（天疱疮，大疱性类天疱疮）。
• 猩红热。
• 中毒性休克综合征。
• 化学性或热性烫伤。
• 过敏性血管炎。
• 川崎综合征。

治疗

院前

• 运送到有烧伤中心的机构。
• 运输过程中的护理应温和避免皮肤创伤。
• 如果出现短途运输，血流动力学稳定，应避免使用静脉导管（在急诊部更多保证无菌条件）。
• 避免使用黏性材料。

初步稳定/治疗

• 如果需要插管或鼻胃管，操作温柔以减少黏膜损伤。
• 细致的无菌技术。
• 为降低脓毒症的风险，外周静脉通路优于中心静脉。
• 心脏监护仪，脉搏血氧仪，鼻胃管，导尿管。

急诊治疗/程序

• 确定并停止任何致病药物。
• 像烧伤护理一样地（Parkland 配方）积极的液体复苏和电解质管理：
- 尿量应该以一定的速度为目标 0.5～1 ml/（kg · h）。

• 保温措施和频繁的核心温度评估很重要。
• 如果可以的话，用生物敷料覆盖（例如，生物膜）：
- 减少疼痛，减少热量消耗和蒸发损失，并促进愈合。

• 抗生素滴眼液。
• 应用唇膏。
• 预防消化性应激性溃疡。
• 外用抗生素，包括硝酸银，未经证实，但可能除外磺胺嘧啶银（磺酰胺衍生物）。
• 及时入院烧伤单位/ICU。
• 眼睛需要眼科会诊（评估和清除假膜和粘连）。

药物治疗

没有确定的治疗方案，但是有几个建议的指导方针：

• 疼痛应该用静脉注射阿片类药物来控制。
• 诊断明确的败血症存在或临床情况突然恶化时应使用抗生素，覆盖面应该包括革兰阳性、革兰阴性（包括铜绿假单胞菌）和好氧细菌。
• 抗组胺药可用于瘙痒症。
• 患者应考虑抗凝治疗来预防血栓栓塞事件。
• 全身性皮质类固醇继续存在争议：
- 回顾性研究显示没有益处且提示感染导致死亡的风险增加。

• IVIG 应在大疱形成后 48～72 h 开始，但在 72 h 后可能有用。
• 下面的实验疗法正在研究阶段：
- 血浆置换。
- 环孢素。
- 环磷酰胺。
- N-乙酰半胱氨酸。
- 抗 TNF-α 抗体（即英夫利昔单抗），但是沙利度胺禁忌（显示有害）。

随访

进一步处理

入院指征

所有疑似 TEN 的患者都应该入院进入烧伤单元（如果烧伤单元不可用并且不可能转运，进入 ICU 治疗）。

转诊问题

• 转入有烧伤单元的医院可改善患者预后。
• 应协同皮肤科帮助确诊。
• 找眼科医师评估和预防角膜溃疡和粘连。
• 手术或整形手术应评估伤口清创需求。
• 在肺部黏膜脱落的情况下，呼吸治疗应启动肺部抽吸。

要点和误区

• 烧伤单位和 ICU 提供最佳管理。
• 记住要教育患者使用药物（包括组合、药物和结构类似的药物）。
• 积极的补液是必不可少的。

中毒性滑膜炎 Synovitis, Toxic

Daniel A. Popa · Ian R. Grover　范浩浩　李文放 译

基础知识

描述

• 儿童滑膜非特异性炎症和肥大的伴有髋关节积液。
• 它会影响任何关节，但最常见的是影响臀部。
• 疾病过程是自限性的。
• 3～10 岁的儿童急性髋关节疼痛和跛行的最常见原因。
• 也被称为急性短暂性滑膜炎和易激惹综合征。

• 受影响最严重的年龄组为 3～6 岁。

• 男性＞女性(2∶1)。

• 右侧臀＞左侧。

病因

• 中毒性滑膜炎的病因未知。

• 怀疑传染性病因,因为约 50%的病例有上呼吸道感染,先于短暂性滑膜炎症状。

诊断

症状和体征

• 单侧臀部疼痛。

• 大腿前内侧和膝盖疼痛。

• 承重疼痛。

• 跛行。

• 低热。

• 受影响的髋关节活动范围缩小(ROM)。

• 患有髋关节疼痛。

病史

• 急性发作单侧髋关节疼痛。

• 无创伤史。

• 走路疼痛。

• 最近上呼吸道感染。

体格检查

• 低热,通常＜38.5 ℃(101.3 ℉)。

• 高热更加怀疑化脓性关节炎。

• 检查双臀。

• 无毒性出现。

• 由于疼痛导致髋关节活动度有限。

• 髋部通常保持在屈曲和外展外旋的位置以获得最大舒适度。

基本检查

• 髋部 X 线片。

• 骨盆。

• 血常规、C 反应蛋白(CRP)、红细胞沉降率(ESR),如果怀疑化脓性关节炎。

诊断检查与说明

实验室检查

血常规、CRP、ESR:

• 可能正常或升高。

• 单独使用白细胞(WBC)计数、CRP 或 ESR 升高,不能区分中毒性滑膜炎化脓性关节炎或骨髓炎。

• 如果 WBC 计数、CRP 和 ESR 正常,则髋关节疼痛的严重原因不太可能。

• 如果 CRP＜2 mg/dl 并且能够承受更重的体重可能是中毒性滑膜炎。

影像学检查

• 臀部 X 线平片(正位和蛙腿视图):

- 通常正常。

- 可能检测到积液或其他髋部疼痛原因。

• 超声排除关节积液并可在必要情况下进行引导下行髋关节穿刺。

• MRI(罕见):

- 对诊断股骨头缺血性坏死(LCP)非常有用。

• 骨骼扫描:

- 用于区分 LCP 疾病与中毒性滑膜炎。

- 可以检测骨髓炎。

- 对于复发病例或仍然存在疑问的病例,辐射通常会累积。

诊断步骤/外科

关节吸引术:

• 如果患者无法正常发热,则不需要白细胞计数、CRP 和 ESR。

• 关节液分析异常提示 SA(见化脓性关节炎)。

• 送检关节液,行白细胞计数检测和培养,同时可考虑行血培养及核酸测序以排查金氏杆菌。

鉴别诊断

• 化脓性关节炎。

• 骨髓炎。

• 软组织感染。

• 股骨头缺血性坏死疾病。

• 股骨头骨骺滑脱。

• 幼年型类风湿关节炎。

• 风湿热。

• 软骨分解。

• 戈谢病。

• 骨肉瘤。

• 尤因肉瘤。

• 骨样骨瘤。

• 白血病。

• 髋关节结核。

• 骨折。

• 莱姆病。

• 腰大肌脓肿。

• 镰状细胞危机。

儿科注意事项

• 4%～17%的儿童反复发作。

• 10%的复发病例可能是慢性炎症的特征。

• 2%～10%的患有中毒性滑膜炎的患者后来发展为 LCP 疾病:

- 建议中毒性滑膜炎可能代表 LCP 疾病的早期阶段。

治疗

院前

• 保持腿部舒适。

• NSAIDs。

急诊治疗/程序

• 保守治疗。

• 卧床休息舒适:屈曲和外展外旋。

• 启动 NSAIDs 治疗。

• 给患病部位加热。

• 考虑行超声和引流液检查。

• 不推荐抗生素和类固醇。

• 一些学者建议正常髋关节功能改善和恢复后 7～10 日不要承重,防止复发。

• 密切随访至关重要,由于与 LCP 相关,需要重复 X 线片。

药物治疗

一线用药

• 布洛芬:200～600 mg(儿童＞6 个月:5～10 mg/kg),口服,q6 h,必要时。

• 萘普生:250～500 mg(儿童＞6 个月:5～10 mg/kg),口服,每日 2 次,必要时。

二线用药

对乙酰氨基酚:500 mg(谷物:10～15 mg/kg,不超过 5 次/24 h),口服或灌肠,q4～6 h,不超过 4 g/24 h。

随访

进一步处理

入院指征

严重关节疼痛或大量积液的患者可能需要住院治疗,卧床休息和使用镇痛药。

出院指征

所有患者在已经排除较严重的髋关节疼痛原因,并已被诊断为中毒性滑膜炎的,可以在良好的后续处置出院。

转诊问题

• 若超声提示存在积液,可能需要手术抽除积液。

• 在 1～2 周接受骨科医师随访重复评估。

随访建议

• 臀部疼痛或发热立即返回急诊室以缓解疼痛。

• 1～2 周随访儿科骨科医师进行重复评估。

• 患者应该在 6 个月后重复进行 X 线检查

排除 LCP 疾病。

要点和误区

• 大多数病例是通过病史和身体确诊的，以发热和负重为主要就诊原因。

• 约 50%的儿童先前有病毒感染疾病史。

• NSAIDs 帮助治疗疼痛并缩短疾病的病程。

• 几乎所有的儿童都可以 2 周内从中毒性滑膜炎中恢复过来并且没有后遗症。

• 毒性滑膜炎的患儿有 2%～10%发展为 LCP 疾病。

中毒性休克综合征

Shock Syndrome

Michelle J. Sergei · Kenneth Young 范浩浩 李文放 译

基础知识

描述

• 中毒性休克综合征（TSS）是一种严重急性威胁生命的疾病。

• 病原体：

- 金黄色葡萄球菌，更常见（TSS）。
- A 族链球菌（GAS），不太常见（链球菌 TSS 或 STSS）。

• 这两种生物体都会产生毒素（SAgs）来上调免疫反应。

• 金黄色葡萄球菌产生结构相似的毒素：

- 中毒性休克综合征毒素（TSST-1）。
- 肠毒素 A～E，I（SEA～SEE，SEI）。

• GAS 产生 M 蛋白，导致多种致病因子。

- 产生充当超抗原的外毒素（SPE）。
- 与纤维蛋白原形成复合物，激活中性粒细胞并诱导炎症反应。
- 干扰补体途径，避免吞噬。

• SAgs 充当超抗原致压倒性免疫反应：

- 大量的细胞因子产生（细胞因子风暴）。
- 直接作用于下丘脑引起发热或间接通过白细胞介素-1（IL-1）和肿瘤坏死因子（TNF）引起发热。
- 增强迟发性超敏反应。
- 抑制中性粒细胞迁移和免疫球蛋白。
- 直接作用于组织部位，引起额外的局部反应。

• 发生大规模血管舒张：

- 血清蛋白质和液体转移导致低血压。

病因

• 最初的病例来自月经期间使用高吸水性卫生棉条的年轻健康女性群体。

- 改变卫生棉条成分以减少发病率。

• 约有一半 TSS 病例的报道是非月经期：

- 手术伤口。
- 产后伤口感染。
- 乳腺炎。
- 鼻中隔鼻成形术。
- 鼻窦炎。
- 骨髓炎。
- 关节炎。
- 烧伤。
- 鼻腔填塞止血术（鼻腔填塞）。
- 皮肤和皮下病变。

• 非月经期病例主要是由于金黄色葡萄球菌产生的 SEB 和 SEC。

• 30%～50%的健康成人和儿童携带 MRSA，见于鼻腔前庭、阴道、直肠内和/或皮肤上。

• GAS 感染通常在轻微创伤的部位伤后 24～72 h 开始，常常在皮肤没有明显证据。

• 尽管耐甲氧西林的金黄色葡萄球菌感染致发病率增加，最近的一项研究报道，金黄色葡萄球菌（MRSA）感染仅占病例的 7%。

• 严重流感暴发和随后的金黄色葡萄球菌感染具有相关性。

诊断

症状和体征

TSS 诊断标准

• CDC 病例定义：

- 发热＞38.9℃（102℉）。
- 低血压（收缩压＜90 mmHg），小于 16 岁儿童血压低于 5 个百分位数。
- 弥散性，非瘙痒性黄斑，红皮疹。
- 发病后 1～2 周脱屑（尤其是手掌和足底）。
- 多系统参与，至少应具备以下 3 项：
  - 消化系统：发作时腹泻或呕吐。
  - 肌肉骨骼：严重肌痛或肌酸磷酸激酶（CPK）增加 2 倍以上。
  - 黏膜炎症：结膜、阴道或咽部充血。
  - 肾：BUN 或肌酐增加＞2 倍正常值上限或无尿路感染证据的脓尿。
  - 肝脏：总胆红素或转氨酶＞正常值上限 2 倍。
  - 血液学：血小板减少症，＜100 000/mm³。
  - 中枢神经系统：当发热和低血压消失时，无方向感，神志不清或幻觉。
- 如果获得对以下项目的结果，测试结果为阴性：咽喉或脑脊液培养、落基山斑疹热（RMSF）、钩端螺旋体病或麻疹的滴度升高。

链球菌 TSS（STSS）标准诊断

• CDC 病例定义：

- 从正常无菌部位分离 A 族溶血性链球菌。
- 低血压
- 以下两项或多项：
  - 肾损害（肌酐＞2 倍正常值上限）。
  - 凝血病。
  - 肝脏受累（转氨酶或胆红素＞2 倍正常值上限）。
  - ARDS。
  - 红斑性黄斑疹，可能脱落。
  - 软组织坏死。

其他

• 频发心动过速。

• 可以迅速进入多系统功能障碍（ARDS 或 DIC）。

• STSS 通常表现弥漫性或局部性疼痛，突然发作且严重。

• 疼痛先于体检发现。

• 近 80%的 STSS 患者有临床症状的软组织感染。

• STSS 的死亡率明显高于 TSS（5%～50%）。

• 发展中国家 STSS 的疾病负担显著增加。

基本检查

• 没有其他归因疾病时使用诊断标准进行临床诊断。

• 全面地询问病史和体格检查。

诊断检查与说明

实验室检查

• CBC：

- 白细胞增多或白血球减少症，显著的杆状核粒细胞增多症常见。
• 电解质、BUN、肌酐、葡萄糖：
- 常见 BUN 和肌酐升高。
• 钙，镁：
- 低钙血症/低镁血症经常出现。
• 尿液分析：
- 正常或无菌脓尿，没有感染的证据。
• CPK：
- 增加 2 倍。
• 肝功能：
- 总胆红素升高，AST、ALT 升高。
• PT、APTT、血小板。
- 血小板减少症，$<100\,000/mm^3$。
• 尽可能损伤/感染部位培养。
• 所示的血液、尿液、咽喉和脑脊液培养物：金黄色葡萄球菌的病例确诊不需要血培养阳性，链球菌确诊需要血培养阳性。
• RMSF、麻疹和钩端螺旋体病的血清学检查。
• 乙型肝炎表面抗原。

影像学检查

• 胸部 X 线：排除其他来源系统性疾病。
• 如果局部疼痛考虑与脓肿或坏死性感染相关，请考虑进行 X 线或 CT 扫描。

▪ 鉴别诊断

• 葡萄球菌性烫伤样皮肤综合征：
- 年龄<5 岁的儿童。
- 最初的黄斑疹随后形成界限不清的大疱，大疱擦掉后显示有光泽，湿润的表皮(尼氏征阳性)。
• 猩红热：
- 前驱链球菌咽炎。
- 皮疹从上胸部、颈部和背部开始传播到躯干的其余部分，除了手掌和足底。
- 不发生低血压。
• 川崎病：
- 发热、结膜充血和黏膜红斑。
- 与肾衰竭、低血压、血小板减少症无关。
• 史蒂文斯-约翰逊综合征：
- 严重的多系统受累。
- 口腔、结膜、阴道、肛门和尿道口黏膜受累。
- 通常与药物有关。
• 钩端螺旋体病：
- 通过接触感染动物传播。
- 发热、头痛、严重肌痛和结膜弥漫性皮疹。
- 仅在儿童中出现躯干皮疹。
• RMSF：
- 皮疹是粉红色和黄斑，从手腕、手掌、踝和足掌开始，扩展到躯干和面部。
- 4 日后出现瘀点。
• 脑膜炎球菌血症：
- 脑膜炎的表现。
- 皮疹是瘀点。

治疗

▪ 院前

• 检查气道、呼吸、循环。
• 建立静脉通路。
• 循环休克的积极治疗。

▪ 初步稳定/治疗

• 再次检查气道、呼吸、循环。
• 积极管理休克：
- 静脉输液。
- 升压药。

▪ 急诊治疗/程序

低血压

• 积极补液：
- 第一个 24 h 可能需要 4～20 L 晶体和/或新鲜冰冻血浆(胶体)。
- 警告：大量静脉输液和升压药用于治疗顽固性低血压可导致起病急骤的肺水肿。
- 升压药(多巴胺/去甲肾上腺素)，如果液体复苏不能恢复正常的动脉压。

感染管理

• 寻找并治疗感染的关键点。
• 移除感染源(如卫生棉条、鼻腔或伤口敷料)。
• 如果感染部位需要引流或清创，请及早进行手术/妇科会诊。
• 葡萄球菌 TSS 的抗生素治疗：
- 推荐用于减少复发，但没有显示出可以改变最初感染的进程。
- 克林霉素和利奈唑胺是有效细菌毒素合成抑制剂。
- 克林霉素或利奈唑胺＋万古霉素用于治疗 TSS。
- 利奈唑胺＋万古霉素用于 TSS 广泛感染型。
- 如果 TSS 是由于已知的甲氧西林敏感金黄色葡萄球菌所致，用克林霉素＋苯唑西林或萘夫西林。
- 克林霉素＋亚胺培南或美罗培南或替卡西林-克拉维酸或哌拉西林-他唑巴坦治疗 STSS。
• 链球菌 TSS 的抗生素治疗：
- 克林霉素＋亚胺培南或美罗培南或克林霉素＋替卡西林-克拉维酸或哌拉西林-他唑巴坦。
• 静脉免疫球蛋白(IVIG)治疗。
- 几项研究支持链球菌中毒性休克的有效性，但仅有零星证据表明对葡萄球菌 TSS 有效。
- 如果对液体，升压药和抗生素无反应的肺水肿和低血压的患者，可能使用 IVIG。

▪ 药物治疗

• 克林霉素：600～900 mg(儿童：20～40 mg/(kg·24 h)，静脉滴注，q6～8 h。
• 多巴胺：2～20 μg/(kg·min)，静脉滴注，至血压正常。
• 利奈唑胺：600 mg[儿童：10 mg/(kg·12 h)]，静脉滴注，q12 h。
• 美罗培南：1 g，静脉滴注，q8 h。
• 萘夫西林：1.5 g[儿童：100 mg/(kg·24 h)]，静脉滴注，q4 h。
• 去甲肾上腺素：0.01～3 μg/(kg·min)，静脉滴注，至血压正常。
• 苯唑西林：1～2 g[儿童：50～100 mg/(kg·24 h)]，静脉注射，q4 h。
• 哌拉西林他唑巴坦：4.5 g，q6 h。
• 替卡西林-克拉维酸盐：3.1 g，q4 h。
• 万古霉素：30 mg/kg，静脉滴注，每日 1 次 div。以 2 个剂量(儿童：40 mg/kg 每日 1 次，静脉滴注 div，以 4 个剂量)。
• 葡萄球菌 TSS：IVIG，400 mg/kg 数小时以上。
• 第 1 日，链球菌 TSS：IVIG 1 g/kg，第 2 日和第 3 日 0.5 g/kg。

随访

▪ 进一步处理

入院指征

• 情况危急，需要住院。
• 重症或休克患者入住 ICU。
• 菌血症患者接受最少 14 日治疗：
- 取决于临床过程。
- 从最后一次培养阳性后继续治疗 14 日。
• 金黄色葡萄球菌鼻腔携带的筛查及莫匹罗星根除携带状态。

出院指征

无。

转诊问题

需要引流或清创的早期外科/妇科会诊。

要点和误区

• 对葡萄球菌 TSS 和 GAS TSS 诊断的思考。

• 确保对 TSS 中的低血压患者给予足够的支持性护理。液体管理可能需要通过升压药进行补充。

• 对疑似深部感染的迅速和积极的探查和清创。

• 推荐经验性广谱抗生素，包括克林霉素或利奈唑胺。

中毒与解毒 Poisons and Antidotes

Suzan S. Mazor 瞿金龙 译

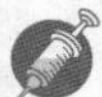

治疗方法

N-乙酰半胱氨酸(NAC)

• 指征：醋氨酚过量。

• 提醒：

- 味道不适、恶心、呕吐。
- 前 8 h 内给药一般效果最好。

• 剂量：

- 口服：140 mg/kg，然后 70 mg/kg，q4 h 维持 17 个剂量。
- 静脉注射：150 mg/kg 配置 200 ml D_5W 超过 60 min，然后 50 mg/kg 500 ml D_5W 超过 4 h，最后 100 mg/kg 1 000 ml D_5W 超过 16 h。

儿科注意事项

D_5W 必须减少避免液体过多和低钠血症。

阿托品

• 指征：

- 药物引起的心动过缓。
- 有机磷酸盐中毒。

• 提醒：

- 慎用于重症肌无力、窄角型青光眼、高血压、冠状动脉缺血和输尿管梗阻患者。

• 剂量：

- 成人：1～2 mg，静脉注射。
- 儿童：0.02 mg/kg，静脉注射。
- 有机磷中毒可重复大剂量。

苯扎托品

• 指征：急性肌张力障碍反应。

• 提醒：慎用于氨基甲酸酯、肌无力、窄角型青光眼、高血压、冠状动脉缺血和输尿管梗阻患者。

• 剂量：

- 成人：1～2 mg，静脉注射或口服。
- 儿科：0.02 mg/kg，静脉注射或口服。

苯二氮䓬类

• 指征：烦躁、兴奋等。

• 提醒：呼吸和中枢抑制。

• 剂量：

- 咪达唑仑：
  - 成人：1 mg，静脉注射或肌内注射，2～3 min，必要时。
  - 儿童：0.1 mg/kg，静脉注射或肌内注射。
- 地西泮：
  - 成人：2～5 mg，静脉注射或肌内注射，10～15 min，必要时。
  - 儿童：0.1 mg/kg，静脉注射或肌内注射。

碳酸氢盐或碳酸氢钠

• 指征：抗抑郁药中毒、代谢性酸中毒、肾性碱性。

• 提醒：可能引起心力衰竭、碱中毒和低钾血症。

• 剂量：

- 酸中毒：
  - 1 mmol/kg，IVP。
- 肾性：
  - 100～150 mmol/L DW 2～3 ml/(kg · h) 静脉注射，目标至尿液 pH 7～8。

黑寡妇毒蜘蛛抗毒血清

• 指征：严重的高血压、肌肉痉挛持续不缓解，肌松剂效果不好。尤其对于＜5 岁和＞65 岁患者、先兆流产妊娠妇女。

• 提醒：

- 马抗毒血清：高敏感性，1～14 日。
- 如果对马抗毒血清过敏，更换或脱敏注射。

• 剂量：1～2 安瓿肌内注射或静脉注射，持续 15～30 min，50 ml 生理盐水稀释 1 安瓿静滴。

肉毒杆菌毒素抗毒素三价 A、B、E

• 指征：肉毒中毒，先兆麻痹。

• 提醒：

- 结合游离的毒素。
- 不能用于婴儿食物中毒。
- 马抗毒血清：高敏感性，持续 10～14 日。
- 如果对马抗毒血清过敏，更换或脱敏注射。
- 静脉慢推。

• 剂量：1～2 安瓿，静脉推注，q4 h，4～5 个治疗剂量。或者 2 ml 稀释 1 安瓿 0.5 ml/(kg · h)，静脉推注。如果无效，可以 15 min 后速度加倍。

钙

• 指征：

- 高钾血症可能伴有心脏毒性。
- 氢氟酸阻滞剂过量。
- 钙通道阻滞剂过量。
- 柠檬酸盐、草酸盐、磷酸盐中毒。

• 提醒：

- 地高辛中毒、高钙血症慎用。
- $CaCl_2$ 可腐蚀皮肤等组织。
- 有特性的溶液一起静脉使用有禁忌。
- 缓慢静脉推注。

• 剂量：

- 成人：$CaCl_2$ 5～10 ml，或 10～20 ml 10% 葡萄糖酸钙。
- 儿童：$CaCl_2$ 0.1～0.2 ml/kg，或 0.2～0.3 m/kg 10% 葡萄糖酸钙。

依地酸钙钠

• 指征：金属铬、镍、锰、锌中毒。

• 提醒：恶心、呕吐、畏寒、肾毒性、高钙血症。

• 剂量：1 g/(m^2 · d)，静脉输注，持续 8～12 h×5 日，2～4 日后再重复，监测金属浓度。

银环蛇抗毒素

• 指征：东部和 Taxas 银环蛇。

• 提醒：
- 马抗毒血清：高敏感性，持续 10～14 日。
- 如果对马抗毒血清过敏，更换或脱敏注射。
• 剂量：4～10 安瓿缓慢静脉注射 15～30 min。

■ **氰化物中毒解毒药**

• 指征：氰化物中毒。
• 提醒：低血压、高铁血红蛋白血症。
• 剂量：
- 亚硝酸异戊酯：1～2 安瓿吸入。
◦ 吸入，直到静脉途径建立。
- 亚硝酸钠：
◦ 成人：300 mg 稀释 10 ml，静脉注射 5 min 以上。
◦ 儿童：0.3 ml/kg 3%溶液，静脉注射。
- 硫代硫酸钠：
◦ 成人：12.5 g，静脉注射，1 h 后重复。
◦ 儿童：50 mg/kg，静脉注射。

■ **羟钴胺**

• 指征：氰化物中毒。
• 提醒：红斑、高血压。
• 剂量：
- 成人：5 g 静脉注射 15 min 以上，根据临床情况和严重程度是否行第二个 5 g 重复，最大剂量 10 g。再次 2.5 g 稀释 100 ml 生理盐水静脉注射。
- 儿童：没有有效性和安全性相关资料，推荐起始剂量：70 mg/kg，静脉注射。

■ **丹曲林**

• 指征：
- 恶性高热。
- 神经阻滞剂恶性综合征。
- 血清素综合征。
- 肌肉强直。
• 提醒：肌力减弱、呼吸抑制、肝炎。
• 剂量：1～2 mg/kg，静脉注射，q10～15 min 重复，最大剂量 10 mg/kg。

■ **去铁胺**

• 指征：铁中毒。
• 提醒：
- 治疗抢在 24 h 之内，否则容易出现 ARDS。
- ＞15 mg/(kg・h)，出现低血压、面部潮红、荨麻疹。
• 剂量：10～15 mg/(kg・h)静脉注射，在严重的铁中毒可能有效果。

■ **地高辛抗体**

• 指征：地高辛中毒。
• 提醒：
- 使用地高辛后，浓度高于正常值。
- CHF 和心房颤动发作。
• 剂量：
- 1 安瓿(40 mg)＋0.6 mg 地高辛。
- 安瓿的数量＝地高辛浓度(ng/ml)×体重(kg)/100。
- 剂量估算：急性最多 10～20 安瓿，慢性 4～6 安瓿。

■ **二巯丙醇**

• 指征：砷、金、汞、铅等导致的脑病。
• 提醒：肾毒性、发热、恶心、呕吐、荨麻疹、胆碱能药物综合征。
• 剂量：
- 3 mg/kg 深部肌内注射 q4 h×2 日后，改 q12 h×7 日，随访神志情况。
- 如果铅浓度＞100 μg/dl，可以联合 EDTA。

■ **苯海拉明**

• 指征：抗组织胺药，急性张力障碍反应。
• 提醒：镇静作用，儿童可能出现兴奋作用。
• 剂量：
- 成人：25～50 mg，静脉注射、肌内注射或口服，q4～6 h。
- 儿童：0.5～1 mg/kg，静脉注射、肌内注射或口服，q4～6 h。

■ **二巯基丁二酸**

• 指征：儿童铅中毒。
• 提醒：
- 肾功能损伤，经泌尿系统代谢。
- 恶心、呕吐和腹泻。
• 剂量：10 mg/kg 口服 q8 h×5 日后改 q12 h×14 日，监测血铅水平。

■ **肾上腺素**

• 指征：血管性水肿、过敏、哮喘急性发作、脊髓休克、β受体阻滞剂过量。
• 提醒：心律失常、高血压、震颤、焦虑。
• 剂量：
- 低血压和休克。
- 成人：1～4 μg/min，静脉注射。
- 儿童：开始 0.1 μg/(kg・min)。
- 过敏：
◦ 成人：0.3～0.5 mg，肌内注射或皮下注射。
◦ 儿童：0.01 mg，肌内注射或皮下注射。

■ **乙醇**

• 指征：甲醇、乙烯、乙二醇中毒。
• 提醒：
- 双硫仑反应，中枢系统镇静作用。
- 儿童可能出现低血糖。
- 慢性酒精中毒，在透析治疗中需要增加剂量。
• 剂量：
- 静脉注射：10 ml/kg 负荷量，10%浓度的溶液持续 1 h 后，1 ml/(kg・h)持续维持。
- 口服：1.5 ml/kg 100 Proof 溶液后，0.3 ml/(kg・h)持续维持。
- 目标：乙醇水平 100～150 mg/dl。

■ **氟马西尼**

• 指征：苯二氮䓬类药物过量。
• 提醒：
- 三环抗抑郁药物过量是禁忌。
- 可能引起苯二氮䓬类戒断综合征。
• 剂量：
- 成人：0.2 mg 缓慢静脉注射，q2～3 min 重复，最大剂量 1 mg。
- 儿童：0.01～0.05 mg/kg 静脉滴注 30 min 至 1 h。

■ **甲吡唑**

• 指征：甲醇、乙烯、乙二醇中毒。
• 提醒：呕吐、眩晕、头痛。
• 剂量：15 mg/kg 静脉注射负荷量，10 mg/kg q12 h 四个量后，15 mg/kg q12 h。

■ **胰高血糖素**

• 指征：
- β受体阻滞剂或钙通道阻滞剂过量引起的心动过缓和低血压。
- 低血糖。
• 提醒：
- 恶心、呕吐和高血糖。
- 稀释性低血压(苯酚常含有)。
• 剂量：
- β受体阻滞剂或钙通道阻滞剂过量：
◦ 成人：5～10 mg，静脉注射，超过 1 min。
◦ 儿童：0.15 mg/kg，静脉注射，超过 1 min。
- 低血糖：
◦ 成人：0.5～1 mg，肌内注射、静脉注射或皮下注射。
◦ 儿童：0.025～0.1 mg/kg，肌内注射、静脉注射或皮下注射(每次不超过1 mg)。

胰岛素/糖

• 指征：
- 钙通道阻滞剂过量合并严重的低血压、症状性的心动过缓，其他治疗不耐受。
- 高钾血症。
• 提醒：
- 实验性治疗：请毒理学专家会诊。
- 第一次治疗后或提高治疗剂量后监测15 min到1 h后血糖，后面1 h监测一次。
• 剂量：
- 推注负荷量：0.5～1 U/kg 正规胰岛素后，25 g糖。
- 维持量：
◦ 胰岛素 0.5 U/(kg·h)，逐步增加到 1 U/(kg·h)。
◦ 10%葡萄糖开始 100 ml/h(10 g/h)逐步增加保持血糖≥100 mg/dl。

英脱利匹特

• 指征：麻醉致心跳骤停，可能由布比卡因引起，可能对其他脂溶性药物有效。
• 提醒：实验性治疗，请毒理学专家会诊。
• 剂量：
- 20%英脱利匹特负荷量：1.5 ml/kg＞1 min后，0.25 ml/(kg·min)维持。
- 如果循环不稳定，可以 3～5 min 一次负荷量。

亚甲蓝

• 指征：高铁血红蛋白血症＞25%或伴有呼吸困难。
• 提醒：G-6-PD缺陷。
• 剂量：1%溶液 1～2 mg/kg 缓慢静脉注射，1 h后重复。

纳洛酮

• 指征：
- 阿片类药物中毒、昏迷的经验性治疗。
• 提醒：
- 急性阿片类药物截断综合征、严重的烦躁焦虑。
• 剂量：
- 成人：0.4～2 mg，静脉注射或肌内注射，重复到10 mg。
- 儿童：0.1 mg/kg，静脉注射或肌内注射。

奥曲肽

• 指征：磺酰脲过量伴有低血糖。
• 提醒：糖尿病患者使用需注意。
• 剂量：
- 成人：50 μg，皮下注射，q6 h。
- 儿童：4～5 μg/(kg·d)，皮下注射，div. q6 h。

高压氧

• 指征：CO中毒。
• 提醒：
- 鼓膜穿孔、氧毒性。
- 监测患者困难。
• 剂量：2～3 安瓿的 100%纯氧。

青霉胺

• 指征：砒霜、铜、铅、水银(汞)，伴 BAL、EDTA。
• 提醒：肾功能不全相对禁忌。
• 剂量：
- 铅：
◦ 成人：250～500 mg，口服，q8～12 h。
◦ 儿童：20～40 mg/(kg·d)，口服分 3 次。
- 砒霜：100 mg/(kg·d)，口服分 4 次×5日，最大剂量 1 g/d。
- 水银(汞)：
◦ 成人：250 mg，口服，每日 2 次。
◦ 儿童：20～30 mg/(kg·d)，口服，分 4 次。

酚妥拉明

• 指征：
高血压急诊：兴奋、拟效感神经药、MAO-酪胺反应、升压药物外渗。
• 提醒：高血压，心动过速，心律失常。
• 剂量：
- 高血压：
◦ 成人：1～5 mg，静脉注射负荷量。
◦ 儿童：0.02～0.1 mg/kg，静脉注射负荷量。
- 升压药物外渗：
◦ 成人：5 mg 稀释 10～15 ml，皮下注射。
◦ 儿童：0.1 mg/kg 稀释 10～15 ml，皮下注射。

毒扁豆碱

• 指征：严重的抗胆碱能药综合征。
• 提醒：TCA 过量时出现药物蓄积。
• 剂量：
- 成人：0.1～1 mg，静脉注射，必要时 10 min 后可以重复。
- 儿童：0.02 mg/kg，静脉注射，必要时 10 min 后可以重复。

解磷定

• 指征：
- 有机磷中毒。
- 烟碱的副作用。
- 激活酶。
- 阿托品合用。
• 提醒：
- 重症肌无力患者发生肌无力危象。
- 恶心、头痛、眩晕，喉头痉挛、肌肉强直。
• 剂量：
- 成人：1～2 g，静脉滴注，稀释 100 ml 静滴 15 min 以上，必要时 1 h 后重复，如果烟碱样反应再次出现，可以 6 h 内再次重复。
- 儿童：25～50 mg/kg，静脉滴注，15 min 以上，必要时 1 h 后重复，如果烟碱样反应再次出现，可以 6 h 内再次重复。

鱼精蛋白

• 指征：肝素抗凝的副作用。
• 提醒：
- 对鱼过敏。
- 对于婴儿避免苯甲基乙醇稀释。
• 剂量：每 100 U 肝素 1 mg 鱼精蛋白，30～60 min 1/2 的剂量，肝素使用 2 h 后，予以 1/4 的剂量；25～50 mg 静脉注射，慢推 15 min，开始剂量不要超过 50 mg。

维生素 B_6

• 指征：
- 异烟肼诱导发作。
- 鹿花菌属香菇引起。
• 提醒：无毒副作用。
• 剂量：
- 异烟肼诱导发作：
◦ 摄入剂量不明：5 g(成人)，1 g(儿童)。
◦ 剂量(mg)＝摄入异烟肼的剂量(mg)。
◦ 鹿花菌属：25 mg/kg 静脉滴注持续 30 min 至 1 h。

响尾蛇抗毒素

• 指征：响尾蛇类咬中毒作用，包括响尾蛇、毒水蛇、水蛇、凹纹头毒蛇。
• 提醒：
- 羊抗毒血清：立即给予，高敏感性，10～14 日。
- 如果过敏，可以先使用药物脱敏。

Z

• 剂量：羊抗毒血清。
- 4～6 安瓿，如果中毒反应没有得到控制可以重复 4～6 安瓿，之后予以 2 安瓿 q6 h，直到 3 个剂量。
- 可以每安瓿消毒水稀释 25 ml，稀释到 250 ml 生理盐水给药 1 h 以上。

■ 维生素 K

• 指征：华法林抗凝过量。
• 提醒：静脉给药高敏感性。
• 剂量：
- 2～10 mg，皮下注射/慢静脉，8 h 后可以重复。
- 2～10 mg，口服，可以 12～48 h 内重复。

中毒与洗胃 Poisoning, Gastric Decontamination

Frank LoVecchio　瞿金龙 译

基础知识

■ 描述

胃内除污的物理疗法。

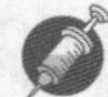

治疗方法

注意

• 催吐相对禁忌。
• 争论：
- 总体来说，不推荐家庭使用催吐药。
- 除非在个别例子里有地区毒物控制中心的会诊咨询。
- 减少活性炭摄入的时间。

■ 初步稳定/治疗

• ABC 管理：
- 神志改变保护气道。
- 建立静脉通路。
- 心电监测。
• 因过量神志改变：
- 纳洛酮。
- 硫胺素(维生素 B_1)。
- 右旋糖。

■ 急诊治疗/程序

• 活性炭：
- 概述：
◦ 加热活性炭，形成大的表面来吸收毒素。
◦ 胃去污的主要办法。
◦ 当活性炭进入小肠起效果。
- 剂量：
◦ 1～2 g/kg，一般和山梨糖醇混合。
◦ 口服或鼻胃管插管。
- 适应证：
◦ 可以是任何毒素的摄入者。
◦ 最好是 1 h 内毒物摄入者。
- 副作用：
◦ 呕吐和便秘。
◦ 活性炭误吸和活性炭肺炎。
- 禁忌证：
◦ 腐蚀性的毒物摄入。
◦ 无保护气道的患者。
◦ 肠梗阻。
- 不被活性炭吸附的药物：
◦ 金属(硼酸盐、溴化物、锂等)。
◦ 酒精。
◦ 钾。
◦ 氰化钾。
◦ 碳化氢。
◦ 腐蚀剂。
- 儿科建议：
◦ 可以与饮料一起，提高患儿的依从性。
- 争论：
◦ 随意双盲研究对比活性炭和无的结果提示，对于无症状患者，活性炭有不好的预后和更高的并发症发生率。
◦ 小部分患者可以在洗胃中获益。
• 大剂量的活性炭：
- 概述：
◦ 用在消化道摄入毒物并且能被活性炭很好的吸收，同时毒物经过肠肝循环。
- 剂量：
◦ 0.5 g/kg，q2～6 h 后 1 g/kg。
◦ 不要使用泻药联合大剂量的活性炭。
- 适应证：
◦ 水杨酸盐。
◦ 茶碱。
◦ 大剂量的活性炭可以降低药物曲线下的面积，如苯巴比妥、苯妥英、卡马西平等，但是并没有能提高预后。
• 泻药：
- 概述：
◦ 一般和活性炭一起使用，减少毒物的吸收和减少消化道内的时间。
◦ 缺少对于联合活性炭是否能减少吸收相关数据。
◦ 泻药单独使用并没有证明有效，应避免。
◦ 不要和大剂量活性炭一起使用。
- 剂量：
◦ 柠檬酸镁：10%溶液：250 ml(4 ml/kg)。
◦ 硫酸镁：15～20 g(250 mg/kg)。
◦ 山梨糖醇：0.5～1 g/kg 到 70%溶液 100 g。
- 副作用：
◦ 脱水。
◦ 高镁血症。
◦ 腹泻。
◦ 腹部不适。
- 禁忌证：
◦ 已经存在的脱水。
◦ 肾功能不全。
◦ 小孩慎用。
- 争论：
◦ 没有证据证明有效，有报道对于少量患者是有害的。
• 全肠灌洗：
- 概述：清洗肠道。
- 适应证：
◦ 不容易被活性炭吸附的毒素，包括锂等金属。
◦ 密封容器不会引起肠道穿孔的毒素。
- 剂量：
◦ 聚乙烯。
◦ 成人 2 L/h 溶液直到排泄物干净。
◦ 可以通过口服、鼻胃管摄入，可以通过持续或弹丸式的方法。
- 副作用：
◦ 胃胀气。
◦ 肠激惹。
◦ 频繁的肠蠕动。
- 争论：
◦ 机械性或药物性肠梗阻。
◦ 肠梗阻。
◦ 低血压。

- 肠穿孔。
- 没有气道保护的患者。
- 口胃灌洗：
  - 概述：
    - 32～36F 导管到胃内清除毒物。
    - 口胃灌洗的有效性取决于毒物摄入的时间、最后一餐的时间和毒物的吸收情况。
    - 必要时保护气道。
  - 适应证：
    - 很少使用。
    - 在没有已知解毒剂的情况下摄入潜在致命性食物后 1 h 内送达。
    - 中毒的插管患者在约 1 h 内送达。
  - 副作用：
    - 插管误入气道。
    - 食管和胃穿孔。
    - 误吸。
    - 患者不适。
  - 禁忌证：
    - 大片剂。
    - 腐蚀性毒素。
    - 碳氢化合物的摄入。
    - 摄入的物质迅速改变神志。
    - 无保护的气道。
  - 儿科建议：
    - 儿科禁用。
    - 小口径口胃管(即 18F)不太可能导致任何临床上有效的二次药丸抽取。
    - 误吸的风险高。
    - 争论：随机对照研究证实口胃灌洗联合活性炭和活性炭单用无明显差别。
- 催吐：
  - 概述：
    - 很少使用。
    - 起源于植物中毒的治疗。
    - 通过直接刺激胃产生催吐。
    - 延迟了活性炭的摄入时间。
    - 对比单用活性炭无优势。
  - 剂量：
    - ＞12 岁：30 ml。
    - 1～12 岁：15 ml。
    - 6 个月～1 岁：5～10 ml＋15 ml 液体。
  - 适应证：
    - 急诊不实用。
  - 副作用：
    - 呕吐可能并发症加重临床表现。
    - 延迟了活性炭和解毒药的摄入。
  - 禁忌证：
    - 腐蚀类毒素。
    - 碳氢化合物的摄入。
    - 很快改变意识的毒素。
    - 患者频繁呕吐。

要点和误区

- 吐根急诊室不实用。
- 对于中毒 1 h 内的患者尽早给予活性炭。
- 不要联合多种剂量的泻药和活性炭。

中毒与中毒综合征 Poisoning, Toxidromes

Mihael S. Wahl 瞿金龙 译

基础知识

描述

- 中毒综合征是指由某种特定的毒物所致的一系列症状和体征。
- 作用机制由于毒物种类及目标器官不同而各异。

诊断

症状和体征

中毒综合征

- 有多种中毒综合征：
  - 抗胆碱能作用。
  - 胆碱能作用。
  - 拟交感作用。
  - 致幻觉作用。
  - 阿片类作用。
  - 镇静催眠作用。
  - 戒断症状。
  - 5-羟色胺综合征。
  - 恶性神经阻滞综合征。
- 抗胆碱能作用：
  - 发热。
  - 干燥，皮肤潮红。
  - 瞳孔扩大。
  - 谵妄。
  - 心动过速。
  - 高血压。
  - 过高热。
  - 尿潴留。
  - 肠鸣音减弱。
  - 抽搐。
  - 精神改变。
  - 嗜睡。
- 胆碱能作用：
  - 蕈毒碱样症状：
    - 腹泻、发汗。
    - 排尿。
    - 瞳孔缩小。
    - 心动过缓、支气管痉挛、痰液过多。
    - 呕吐。
    - 流泪。
    - 流涎。
  - 烟碱样症状：
    - 瞳孔增大。
    - 心动过快。
    - 虚弱。
    - 高血压。
    - 肌束震颤。
- 拟交感作用：除皮肤和肠道症状外，其他与抗胆碱能作用类似。
  - 出汗。
  - 瞳孔增大。
  - 心动过快。
  - 高血压。
  - 发热。
  - 抽搐。
  - 肠蠕动增加。
- 致幻觉作用：与拟交感作用重叠，因为很多拟交感药物都含有致幻觉成分。
  - 定向障碍。
  - 幻觉。
  - 焦虑。
  - 恐慌。
  - 抽搐。
- 阿片类作用：
  - 经典三联征：
    - 瞳孔缩小。
    - 过度通气。
    - 昏迷。
  - 同时会表现为：

Z

◦ 心动过缓。
◦ 低血压。
◦ 低体温。
◦ 肠鸣音减弱。
• 镇静催眠和酒精作用：
- 镇静。
- 精神状态改变(意识模糊、谵妄、幻觉)。
- 视力改变(视觉模糊、复视)。
- 语言模糊。
- 共济失调。
- 眼球震颤。
• 戒断症状(酒精、安定类、巴比妥类)：
- 出汗。
- 瞳孔增大。
- 心动过快。
- 高血压。
- 发热。
- 呼吸增快。
- 肠鸣音增加。
- 震颤。
- 焦虑。
- 烦躁。
- 幻觉。
- 意识模糊。
- 抽搐。
• 戒断症状(阿片类)：
- 恶心。
- 呕吐。
- 腹泻。
- 腹部绞痛。
- 肠鸣音增加。
- 瞳孔增大。
- 竖毛。
- 心动过快。
- 流泪。
- 流涎。
- 高血压。
- 打哈欠。
• 恶性神经阻滞综合征：
- 近期有使用典型或不典型的抗精神类药物治疗：
◦ 通常在开始用药或增加剂量后几小时或几周内发生，也可发生在任何时候。
- 发热。
- 肌紧张。
- 出汗。
- 精神状态改变。
- 高血压或低血压。
- 流涎。
- 震颤。
- 大小便失禁。
- 肌酐磷酸激酶升高。
- 白细胞升高。
- 代谢性酸中毒。
• 5-羟色胺综合征：
- 在增加其他5-羟色胺类药物或剂量后很快发生。
- 症状多样。
- 以下最常见，见于25%～57%的患者：
◦ 精神状态改变(意识模糊、焦虑、催眠、嗜睡)。
◦ 抽搐。
◦ 肌阵挛。
◦ 反射亢进。
◦ 肌紧张。
◦ 震颤。
◦ 眼球震颤。
◦ 发热。
◦ 出汗。
◦ 瞳孔增大。
◦ 心动过快。
◦ 高血压。

体格检查

• 心动过缓：
- α_2 受体激动剂(如可乐定)。
- β受体阻滞剂。
- 钙通道阻滞剂。
- 地高辛类药物。
- 胆碱类药物。
- 阿片类药物。
• 心动过速：
- 拟交感药物。
- 抗胆碱药。
- 茶碱类药物。
- 三环类抗抑郁药。
- 戒断。
- 吩噻嗪类药物。
- 不典型抗精神药。
- α_1 受体阻滞剂伴反射性心动过缓。
- 磷酸二酯酶5阻滞剂(如西地那非)。
• 发热：
- 拟交感药物。
- 抗胆碱药。
- 5-羟色胺综合征。
- 恶性神经阻滞综合征。
- 恶性高热。
- 二硝基酚类。
- 水杨酸类药物。
- 戒断。
• 低体温：
- 二氧化碳。
- 口服降糖药。
- 阿片类药物。
- 酒精。
- 镇静催眠药。
- α_2 受体激动剂。
• 高血压：
- 拟交感药物。
- 抗胆碱药。
- 尼古丁。
- 苯环哌啶。
- 麦角碱。
• 低血压：
- α_2 受体激动剂。
- α_1 受体阻滞剂。
- β受体阻滞剂。
- 钙通道阻滞剂。
- 血管紧张素转化酶抑制剂。
- 胆碱类药物。
- 硝酸酯类。
- 阿片类药物。
- 吩噻嗪类药物。
- 磷酸二酯酶5阻滞剂。
- 镇静催眠药。
- 酒精。
- 三环类抗抑郁药。
- 不典型抗精神药。
• 瞳孔缩小：
- 胆碱类。
- 可乐定。
- 利血平。
- 吩噻嗪类药物。
- 不典型抗精神药。
• 瞳孔增大：
- 拟交感药物。
- 抗胆碱药。
- 戒断(特别是阿片类)。
- 肉毒中毒。
• 抽搐：
- 有机磷酸酯类。
- 三环类抗抑郁药。
- 异烟肼、胰岛素。
- 拟交感药物、水杨酸类药物。
- 樟脑、可卡因、西酞普兰。
- 苯丙胺、抗胆碱药。
- 茶碱类药物、蕈菌、哌替啶。
- 苯环哌啶、丙氧酚、植物(尼古丁、毒芹)。
- 苯二氮䓬类戒断、安非他酮。
- 酒精戒断。
- 锂剂、利多卡因。

Z

- 铅、林丹。
- 出汗：
- 拟交感药物。
- 胆碱类。
- 水杨酸类药物。
- 戒断。
- 5-羟色胺综合征。
- 呼吸过缓：
- 阿片类。
- 镇静催眠药。
- 酒精。
- γ羟基丁酸和同类药物。
- 肉毒中毒。
- 肌肉受体阻滞剂。
- 呼吸急促：
- 百草枯(和其他引起肺炎的药物)。
- 水杨酸类。
- 拟交感神经药。
- 二硝基苯酚导致酸中毒的药物。
- 甲基黄嘌呤。
- 导致酸中毒的药物。

皮肤科

- 米氏线：
- 砷化物。
- 铊中毒。
- 化疗药物。
- 辐射
- 大疱：
- 巴比妥类。
- 一氧化碳。
- 卡托普利。
- 潮红或红色面容：
- 抗胆碱药物。
- 双硫兰反应。
- 烟酸。
- 硼酸。
- 鸡冠花中毒。
- 谷氨酸一纳。
- 一氧化碳(通常是死后)。
- 氰化物(罕见)。
- 万古霉素。
- 蓝色皮肤：
- 麦角胺。
- 高铁血红蛋白血症来自：
  - 亚硝酸盐。
  - 硝酸盐。
  - 氨苯砜。
  - 苯胺染料。
  - 吩唑吡啶。
  - 苯佐卡因。
  - 氯喹。
- 假性青霉病来源于：
  - 氯丙嗪。
  - 胺碘酮。
  - 米诺环素。
  - 银。
  - 金。

基本检查

取决于摄入的物质：

- CBC。
- 电解质、尿素氮、肌酐、葡萄糖。
- 尿液分析。
- 动脉血气,静脉血气。
- 碳氧血红蛋白、高铁血红蛋白水平。
- 毒理学筛查。
- 阿司匹林和对乙酰氨基酚水平。
- 凝血酶原时间。
- 肝功能检查。

诊断检查与说明

- 阴离子间隙酸中毒：助记：*A CAT MUDPILES* (包括有限数量的常见原因)：
  - A 酒精酮症酸中毒。
  - C 一氧化碳、氰化物。
  - A 西氨酚治疗暴发性肝衰竭。
  - T 甲苯。
  - M 甲醇。
  - U 尿毒症。
  - D 糖尿病酮症酸中毒。
  - P 双醛、苯乙双胍/二甲双胍。
  - I 异烟肼、铁。
  - L 乳酸酸中毒。
  - E 乙烯。
  - 水杨酸盐、叠氮化钠、硫化氢。
- 渗透压间隙增大：
  - 甲醇。
  - 乙烯。
  - 异丙醇。
  - 乙醇。
  - 丙酮。
  - 甘油。
  - 甘露醇。
  - 甘氨酸。

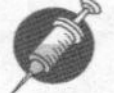

治疗

初步稳定/治疗

ABC 管理。

急诊治疗/程序

取决于摄入的物质(参见中毒与洗胃)。

要点和误区

- 获取适当的实验室测试。
- 识别毒物的体征、症状和实验室证据。

中耳炎 Otitis Media

Assaad J. Sayah　王虑 译

Z

基础知识

描述

- 儿童第二大常见病,仅次于上呼吸道感染(URI)。
- 中耳发生的炎症。
- 最常见于 6～36 个月的儿童。
- 迅速出现的局部和/或全身症状。
- 1/3 或更多的儿童在 7 岁之前会感染超过 5 次。

病因

- 伴咽鼓管(ET)阻塞或功能障碍。
- 通常和上呼吸道感染有关。
- 病毒：
  - 副流感病毒。
  - 呼吸合胞体病毒。
  - 流感病毒。
  - 腺病毒。
  - 鼻病毒。
- 细菌：

- 肺炎链球菌。
- 卡他莫拉菌。
- 流感嗜血杆菌。
- 肺炎支原体。

• 和咽鼓管堵塞有关。

• 易感因素：

- 缺乏黏液纤毛或抗体。
- 插管尤其是经鼻气管插管。
- 北美印第安人和因纽特人。
- 唐氏综合征。
- 腭裂。
- 糖尿病。
- 维生素 A 缺乏。
- HIV 感染。

• 危险因素：

- 家族史。
- 托儿所。
- 父母吸烟。
- 吸奶嘴。
- 奶瓶喂养。

诊断

根据《美国儿科学会指南》。

• 诊断为中耳炎：

- 中重度鼓膜肿胀。
- 耳痛伴中度鼓膜肿胀(无语言能力的儿童出现拽拉揉搓耳)。
- 非外耳道炎引起的耳漏。

• 若没有中耳积液不能诊断为中耳炎(耳镜检查)。

• 复发性中耳炎：

- 6 个月发病 3 次。
- 1 年发作 4 次并且 6 个月内发作过 1 次。

症状和体征

病史

• 耳痛。

• 烦躁。

• 鼻炎。

• 呕吐、腹泻。

• 发热

• 耳有堵塞感。

• 结膜炎。

• 考虑渗出性中耳炎(OME)：

- 听力损失。
- 眩晕，耳鸣。

体格检查

• 鼓膜炎症、肿胀、活动受限。

• 新发耳漏并可以排除外耳道炎。

• 中耳的某些解剖结构看不清。

基本检查

• 排除一些相关的条件。

• 对发热患者充分进行脓毒症相关检查。

• 耳镜检查鼓膜外观和活动性：

- 完全可视。
- 可见血管、红斑、脓。
- 标志物模糊：骨，反光性。
- 耳镜检查：肿、凹陷、活动性下降。

诊断检查与说明

实验室检查

血清检测：如血钙、甲状旁腺素、碱性磷酸酶，有助于该病与其他疾病的鉴别。

影像学检查

• 除非怀疑有并发症，否则不显示。

• CT 扫描可以帮助诊断许多并发症，包括乳突炎、硬膜外脓肿、乙状窦血栓性静脉炎、脑膜炎、脑脓肿和硬膜下脓肿。

诊断步骤/外科

• 鼓膜穿刺：指征如下。

- 严重的疼痛或毒性反应。
- 抗生素治疗无效。
- 疑似有化脓症状。
- 新生儿患病。
- 免疫功能低下患者。

• 对一些不易进行一般体格检查的患者，鼓膜穿刺和耳镜检查对病情的诊断是很有帮助的。

鉴别诊断

• 感染：

- 外耳道炎。
- 乳突炎。
- 牙周脓肿。
- 过敏性鼻炎。
- 胆脂瘤。
- 扁桃体脓肿。
- 鼻窦炎。
- 淋巴结炎。
- 腮腺炎。
- 脑膜炎。

• 创伤：

- 鼓膜穿孔。
- 耳内异物。
- 气压伤。
- 仪器损伤。

• 严重中耳炎或咽鼓管功能不全。

• 耳叮咛的影响。

• 第三磨牙的影响。

• 颞下颌关节功能不全。

治疗

急诊治疗/程序

• 大部分症状较轻的患者无需抗生素就能治愈。

• 抗生素使用指征：

- 所有＜6 个月的婴儿。
- ＜2 岁同时有双耳中耳炎的儿童。
- ＞6 个月的小孩伴有严重感染的[耳痛超过 48 h 或体温高于 102.2 ℉(39 ℃)]。
- ＞6 个月的小孩伴有鼓膜破裂流脓。

• 对于年龄＞6 个月的患者，症状较轻，诊断还不确定的，可以先不使用抗生素，过 2～3 日再对病情进行评估：

- 可以开些口服抗生素给有责任心的患儿家长，若患儿症状加重或病情持续超过 2 日可服用。

• 还需要考虑以下情况，如自发性中耳炎、缺少临床反应、社区性耐药性等。

• 对于＜1 岁伴有发热脓毒症表现或免疫功能低下的患儿需静脉用抗生素。

• 没有证据表明解热镇痛药、类固醇激素、解充血类药对治疗有益。

• 退热药和止痛药十分重要(对于鼓膜穿孔患儿避免使用局部止痛剂)。

药物治疗

• 抗生素：

- 阿莫西林：500～875 mg，口服，q12 h[80～90 mg/(kg · d)，口服，q12 h]，服用 10 日。
- 阿莫西林-克拉维酸：500～875 mg，口服，q12 h[90 mg/(kg · d)，口服，q12 h]，服用 10 日。
- 阿奇霉素：10 mg/kg，口服，每日 1 次；然后 5 mg/kg，口服，每日 1 次，服用 2～5 日。
- 头孢呋辛：500 mg，口服，q6 h[30 mg/(kg · d)，口服，q12 h]。

• 镇痛药：

- 对乙酰氨基酚：500 mg 口服，q6 h[15 mg/(kg · d)，口服或纳肛，q4～6 h]，24 h 不超过 4 g。
- 安替比林/苯佐卡因(5.4%/1.4%溶液)：2～4 滴滴耳，每日 4 次。
- 布洛芬：400～600 mg，口服，q6～8 h[10 mg/(kg · d)，口服，q6 h]。

随访

进一步处理

入院指征

发热脓毒症表现的患儿：

• ＜1 岁，免疫功能低下。
• 中重度脱水。
• 无法经口补液，用药。
• 怀疑严重感染。
• 可疑滥用药物。
• 监护不力。

出院指征

无上述入院指征的患儿。

■ **随访建议**

• 10～14 日后随访确保痊愈。
• 有以下指征随访应提前：
- 患儿在 24～48 h 病情无明显好转。
- 出现任何病情加重的症状和体征。
- 出现新发情况，包括皮疹等。
- 其他新问题出现。

■ **并发症**

• 中耳炎复发：
- 6 个月内发病 3 次。
- 1 年发病 4 次并且最近 6 个月内发病 1 次。
• 鼓膜穿孔。
• 重度中耳炎。
• 听力丧失（传导性和感音性）。
• 面神经受损。
• 乳突炎。
• 胆脂瘤。
• 脑膜炎。
• 硬膜下积液。
• 迷路炎。
• 静脉窦栓塞。
• 脑脓肿。

要点和误区

对于年龄＞6 个月且症状较轻或诊断尚不明确的患者，可以考虑暂不使用抗生素治疗，对病情观察评估 2～3 日后再考虑下一步措施。

肿瘤压迫综合征 Tumor Compression Syndromes

Hany Y. Atallah　张晟　林兆奋 译

基础知识

■ **描述**

• 实体肿瘤压迫神经或血管结构或直接浸润此类结构引起的并发症。
• 脊髓受压迫：
- 每年有超过 20 000 名患者受影响。
- 肿瘤患者的发生率为 5%～14%。
- 超过 90% 的病例是肺癌、乳腺癌、前列腺癌、多发性骨髓瘤、霍奇金淋巴瘤和非霍奇金淋巴瘤的转移。
- 在儿童中，肉瘤和神经母细胞瘤是最常见的病因。
- 脊椎转移瘤远比硬膜外脊髓压迫常见。
- 硬膜外脊髓压迫的病例中，有 20% 的病例表现为恶性肿瘤。
• 其他神经源性的肿瘤压迫：
- 臂丛神经。
- 纵隔淋巴结压迫喉返神经。
• 上腔静脉综合征：
- 由肿瘤压迫、浸润或血栓形成造成的上腔静脉血液回流受阻。
- 上腔静脉引流的区域的静脉高压。
- 在严重的病例，颅内压逐渐升高伴随神志状态的改变甚至昏迷。
• 60%～85% 的上腔静脉综合征是由恶性肿瘤所致。

■ **病因**

• 脊髓压迫：
- 前列腺癌。
- 乳腺癌。
- 肺癌。
- 肾癌。
- 多发性骨髓瘤。
- 黑色素瘤。
- 甲状腺癌。
- 淋巴瘤。
- 肉瘤。
• 臂丛压迫：
- 0.4% 的癌症患者存在臂丛受压迫。
- 2%～5% 接受放疗的患者存在气管臂丛受压迫。
- 肺癌。
- 乳腺癌。
• 肿瘤压迫所致上腔静脉综合征：
- 肺癌（最多见）：主要是肺小细胞癌。
◦ 非小细胞肺癌为主（50%）。
◦ 小细胞肺癌（25%）。
- 非霍奇金淋巴瘤（10%）。
- 用导管和起搏器等血管内装置导致血栓发生率上升。
- 照射后纤维化。
- 淋巴瘤。
- 乳腺癌。
- 睾丸癌。
- 非恶性病因见上腔静脉综合征的“鉴别诊断”。

儿科注意事项

• 在有脊髓受压的小儿患者，较常见的病因是肉瘤、神经母细胞瘤、生殖细胞肿瘤和淋巴瘤。

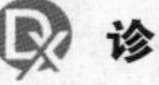

诊断

■ **症状和体征**

病史

• 脊髓受压：
- 恶性肿瘤病史。
- 背痛或颈项痛。
◦ 经久不愈。
◦ 休息后加重。
◦ 最常见影响胸椎。
◦ 诊断通常延迟 2～3 个月，直到确诊。
- 感觉异常。
- 行走困难。
- 便秘。
- 尿潴留。
- 大小便失禁。
- 体重下降。
• 臂丛受压：
- 累及上肢内侧的神经性疼痛。
• 胸内迷走神经受压。
- 患侧耳周面部痛。
• 上腔静脉综合征：
- 端坐呼吸。
- 呼吸困难。
- 口唇发紧。
- 咳嗽。
- 胸痛。

Z

- 头痛。
- 面部肿胀。
- 头发胀。
- 视力模糊。
- 眩晕。
- 昏厥。

体格检查

• 脊髓受压：
- 直肠张力丧失。
- 肛门括约肌功能障碍。
- 60%～85%的患者虚弱。
- 传入神经异常不常见。

• 喉部神经受压：
- 声音嘶哑。
- 声带麻痹。

• 臂丛受压：
- 尺侧感觉异常。
- 手部固有肌肉无力。
- 泛神经丛病变。
- Horner 综合征。

• 上腔静脉综合征：
- 眶周水肿。
- 结膜弥漫性肿胀。
- 面部肿胀。
- 面部胀满。
- 上肢水肿。
- 平卧或弯腰体位时症状加剧。
- 通常在早晨的数小时内症状加重。
- 在严重的病例颅内压会升高：
  ◦ 神志状态改变。
  ◦ 昏迷。
  ◦ 视乳头水肿。

▪ 诊断检查与说明

影像学检查

• 胸部 X 线片(CXR)。
- 脊髓压迫：
  ◦ 可能辨别出一个原发性肺部肿瘤。
  ◦ 有助于排除结核性脊柱炎。
- 上腔静脉受压：
  ◦ 10%的患者有肿块。
  ◦ 25%的病例有胸腔积液。
  ◦ 脊柱 X 线平片。
- 可以显示 85%转移瘤会造成压迫。
- 一个正常的脊柱 X 线平片(或者只显示退行性变的脊柱)并不能排除脊髓受压的可能性。

• 超声：
- 多普勒超声可以诊断锁骨下静脉、腋下静脉和头臂静脉的血栓。

• CT：
- 相比 CT 比 X 线平片敏感性和特异性更高，放射性核素显像应用于脊柱受压综合征良恶性鉴别诊断。
- CT 静脉造影提供更好的血管细节。
- 可识别腔静脉阻塞的病因是肿块压迫还是肿瘤侵犯。

• MRI：
- 明确脊髓压迫方式。
- 适合有背痛或颈项痛的患者，并且：
  ◦ 有癌症史。
  ◦ 肠或膀胱功能障碍。
  ◦ 下肢无力。
  ◦ 感觉缺失。
  ◦ 鞍区麻痹。

诊断步骤/外科

• CT 脊髓造影：
- 适用于脊髓受压但无 MRI 条件或有 MRI 禁忌证(起搏器、金属植入物、严重幽闭恐惧症)时。
- 敏感性和特异度与 MRI 大致相当。
- 仍用来指导放疗。

• 微创技术常被用于上腔静脉阻塞综合征的患者的组织检查。

• 上腔静脉阻塞综合征的患者偶尔需要侵入性手段获取组织活检：
- 支气管镜检查。
- 纵隔镜检查。
- 斜角肌淋巴结活检。
- 限制性开胸手术。
- 胸腔镜手术。

• 放疗可用于缩小肿瘤：
- 放疗应在明确组织诊断后进行，因放疗会使组织界限不清从而确诊困难。

• 血管内支架可比放疗获得更快的缓解效果。

▪ 鉴别诊断

脊髓受压

• 肌萎缩侧索硬化症。
• 动静脉畸形。
• 硬膜外脓肿。
• 椎间盘疾病。
• 多发性硬化。
• 神经系统疾病。
• 脊柱骨质疏松性骨折。
• 原发性骨肿瘤。
• 脊髓梗死。
• 脊髓炎症。
• 脊柱炎
• 横贯性脊髓炎。

上腔静脉综合征

• 心脏压塞。
• 肾病综合征。
• 肺心病。
• 硬化。
• 上腔静脉综合征的非恶性病因：
- 甲状腺肿。
- 心包狭窄。
- 特发性硬化性主动脉炎。
- 纵隔结核。
- 纵隔纤维化。
- 组织胞浆菌病。
- 中心静脉置管。

治疗

▪ 初步稳定/治疗

• 早期诊断和治疗是改善预后的关键。

• 神经元功能障碍的程度是预测脊髓受压预后的关键。

• 若出现上腔静脉阻塞综合征，避免上半身放置静脉置管。

▪ 急诊治疗/程序

脊髓受压

• 糖皮质激素(地塞米松)：
- 在急诊的管理。
- 高剂量可快速缓解疼痛，但研究表明在不同剂量下，括约肌功能和活动能力的变化无明显区别。

• 放疗：
- 最终治疗方法。
- 用麻醉剂(易成瘾药物)止痛。
- 肿瘤科、放疗、神经外科联合会诊进一步管理恶性肿瘤。
- 如果考虑有硬膜外脓肿，在做 MRI 前经验性使用广谱抗生素。

• 紧急神经外科会诊。

上腔静脉受压

• 使用化疗或放疗治疗潜在的恶性肿瘤。
• 抬高床头。
• 补充性给氧。
• 存在呼吸功能障碍时用类固醇药物。
• 合理使用利尿剂可以暂时改善症状，但没有疗效的证据。
• 紧急肿瘤科转诊。
• 血管内支架可快速缓解梗阻。

▪ 药物治疗

• 证明类固醇药物对硬膜外脊髓压迫有益

Z

的证据有限，但常将其作为标准化治疗的一部分。

• 瘫痪或截瘫用大剂量地塞米松：1 mg/kg 载荷剂量，然后每 3 日剂量减半。

• 对于有轻微神经功能障碍的患者，地塞米松 10 mg，随后每日 16 mg，最初分次剂量，一旦进行最终治疗，就逐渐减少。

• 对于上腔静脉综合征，类固醇可以逆转淋巴瘤或胸腺瘤等类固醇反应性恶性肿瘤的症状。

• 正在行放疗的患者，类固醇物质常被用来预防肿胀。

• 呋塞米（速尿）：之前未用过 40 mg 静脉推注；之前用过双倍 24 h 剂量（80～180 mg 静脉注射）。

• 氢可酮/对乙酰氨基酚：5/500 mg，口服，q4～6 h，每日不超过 4 g 对乙酰氨基酚。

• 羟考酮/对乙酰氨基酚：5/500 mg，口服，q4～6 h，每日不超过 4 g 对乙酰氨基酚。

随访

进一步处理

入院指征

• 有肿瘤压迫症状的患者都建议住院治疗。

• 有脊髓压迫的患者有必要转去有神经外科手术能力的中心。

出院指征

无。

转诊问题

• 存在肿瘤压迫症状的患者应咨询肿瘤放疗专家的意见。

• 有脊髓受压者应尽早请神经外科会诊。

要点和误区

• 与恶性肿瘤相关的上腔静脉阻塞综合征患者平均生存期约为 6 个月。

• 肿瘤压迫的表现复杂难辨，已知存在恶性肿瘤且合并难以解释的并发症时要考虑是肿瘤压迫组织引起的。

重症肌无力

Christopher J. Dudley　伍力学　段立伟 译

基础知识

描述

• 该病是一种由自身免疫抗体介导的以无痛性肌肉疲劳无力症状为表现的疾病。

• 眼部或全身受累：

- 眼部（眼睑和眼外）肌肉无力：
  ◦ 大多数的首发症状（60%）。
  ◦ 80%以眼部症状首发的重症肌无力（MG）患者将在 2 年内发展为全身肌无力。
- 全身表现：
  ◦ 常影响近侧肢体，轴向肌群（如颈肌、面肌、延髓肌）。

• 急性或亚急性病程，复发和缓解交替。

• 10%～15%的患者伴有胸腺瘤，60%～70%有胸腺增生。

• 肌无力危象：

- 由于呼吸无力导致呼吸衰竭或无法维持气道通畅所致。
- 诱因：
  ◦ 感染。
  ◦ 手术。
  ◦ 创伤。
  ◦ 妊娠。
  ◦ 药物剂量调整（如激素用量骤减）。
- 较难与因过量使用乙酰胆碱酯酶抑制药物所致的类胆碱能危象鉴别。
  ◦ 除肌无力外，胆碱能危象还可出现毒蕈碱效应，如出汗、流泪、流涎和胃肠道高反应性。
  ◦ 由于治疗性使用乙酰胆碱酯酶抑制剂引起的胆碱能危象是罕见的，通常发生在使用超常规剂量后。

流行病学

• 儿童重症肌无力（Ma）较罕见且具有特征性：

- 先天性重症肌无力：基因缺陷。
- 青少年重症肌无力：自身免疫异常。
- 新生儿暂时性重症肌无力：母体抗体经胎盘进入胎儿所致的分娩后并发症。

• 成人重症肌无力呈双峰型年龄分布特征：

- 第一峰值出现在 20～30 岁的女性。
- 第二峰值出现在 60～70 岁的男性。

• 重症肌无力患者可能有其他自身免疫性疾病（如狼疮、类风湿关节炎、Graves 病等）。

病因

• 作用于 N 型胆碱受体的抗体介导的免疫反应。

• 超过 20%的患者为胆碱受体抗体（AChR Ab）阴性。

• 青霉胺可引发重症肌无力和其他自身免疫状态。

• 许多药物可能加重肌无力：

- 氨基糖苷类、大环内酯类、喹诺酮类抗生素和抗疟疾药。
- 局麻药。
- 抗心律失常药物（普罗帕酮、奎尼丁、普洛卡因胺）。
- β 受体阻滞剂、钙通道阻滞剂。
- 抗惊厥药物（苯妥英钠、卡马西平）。
- 抗精神病药物（吩噻嗪、其他非典型药物）。
- 神经肌肉阻滞药。
- 他汀类药物。
- 含碘造影剂。

• 青霉胺可诱导产生抗 AChR 抗体。

诊断

症状和体征

• 骨骼肌收缩力减弱。

• 肌肉疲倦感，或疲倦但不虚弱，与重症肌无力不一致。

病史

• 活动后症状加重。

- 休息后缓解。

• 眼部无力：

- 复视。
- 在驾驶或阅读时眼睑下垂。

• 延髓肌和面肌无力：

- 咀嚼、说话及吞咽困难。
- 咀嚼后无法下颌无法合拢。
- 发音含糊，鼻音明显。

• 肢体无力：

- 爬楼梯困难，无法从椅子上站起，无力向上攀爬等。

体格检查

• 眼部表现：

- 上睑下垂，复视。

Z

- 有阻力时眼睑无法闭合。
- 瞳孔无缩放变化。
• 延髓肌和面肌表现：
- 让患者数到 100，观察言语改变。
- 面部表情减少。
- 头部下垂。
• 肢体表现：
- 对近侧肢体或手部小肌肉无力情况进行反复检查。
- 神经反射和感觉检查正常。

基本检查

• 评估呼吸受累程度。
• 查找有无继发因素（如感染源）。

诊断检查与说明

实验室检查

• 血常规。
• 电解质。
• 肝功能。
• 甲状腺功能。
• 抗胆碱抗体：
- 90%的全身肌无力症状患者呈阳性。
- 50%的眼部肌无力症状患者呈阳性。
• 有助于初步诊断的其他检查：
- 抗横纹肌抗体。
- 抗核抗体。
- 类风湿因子。
- 红细胞沉降率（血沉）。

影像学检查

• 行头颅 CT 或 MRI 以明确导致脑神经症状的颅内压迫病灶。
• 行胸部增强 CT 明确有无胸腺瘤。
• 行 CXR 检查评估感染灶。

诊断步骤/外科

• 依酚氯铵（腾喜龙）试验：
- 一种短效的 AChE 抑制剂。
- 该试验可快速产生的短时程（2～5 min）肌力增强效应。
- 全身肌无力者敏感性为 95%，眼部肌无力者敏感性为 86%。
- 兰伯特-伊顿综合征、吉兰-巴雷综合征、肉毒梭菌感染等疾病患者可出现假阳性。
- 增强乙酰胆碱的毒蕈碱效应。
◦ 诊治过程中予以持续心电监测。
◦ 床边备阿托品以防突发心动过缓。
◦ 床边备吸引器以防分泌物增多。
◦ 注意：老年人及有心脏病史者慎用。
• 冰块测试：
- 在眼睑上放置冰块维持 2 min。
- 如眼睑下垂好转则提示重症肌无力。
- 敏感性为 80%。

鉴别诊断

• 肌萎缩性脊髓侧索硬化。
• 肉毒中毒。
• 电解质紊乱。
• 吉兰-巴雷综合征。
• 甲状腺功能亢进症。
• 感染性肌病。
• 颅内实性病变。
• 兰伯特-伊顿综合征。
• 多发性硬化。
• 周期性麻痹。
• 蜱瘫痪。

治疗

院前

加强气道管理，保持气道通畅。

初步稳定/治疗

肌无力危象：
• 最重要的是尽早插管和机械通气。
• 即将发生呼吸衰竭的征象：
- 肺活量＜20 ml/kg。
- 吸气负压＞$-30\ cmH_2O$。
- 呼气压＜$40\ cmH_2O$。
• 有麻痹症状患者的注意事项：
- 对去极化药物敏感性减低，需增大药物剂量；琥珀胆碱的剂量可能加倍。
- 非去极化药物可能导致麻痹症状蔓延，可将药量减半。
- 其他药物如咪达唑仑、依托咪酯或硫喷妥钠。

急诊治疗/程序

• 查找并消除诱因：
- 积极处理感染。
- 仔细了解用药史。
• 肌无力危象可能需要行血浆置换或静脉应用免疫球蛋白（IVIG）：
- 血浆置换：以 1～1.5 倍血浆容积的剂量行血浆置换，共 5 次。
- IVIG：0.4 mg/（kg · d）×5 日。
• 初始给予大剂量糖皮质激素。
• 插管后可停用 AChE 抑制剂。
• 应用阿托品以拮抗 AChE 效应（如心动过缓、胃肠道症状、气道和口腔分泌物增加）。

药物治疗

一线用药

• 依酚氯胺（腾喜龙）：2 mg，静脉推注，推注时间在 15～30 s 以上；如无效可在 45 s 后再予以 3 mg 静脉推注。如无反应，最后剂量 5 mg 静脉推注（总剂量 10 mg）。
• 肌无力危可予以泼尼松龙 1 mg/（kg · d）。
• 胆碱能危象可予以阿托品 0.5 mg 静脉推注或肌内注射。

二线用药

• 其他药物应由神经科医师始用：
• 泼尼松、AChE 抑制药、咪唑硫嘌呤、麦考酚吗乙酯、环孢素、他克莫司、利妥昔单抗。

随访

进一步处理

入院指征

• 新发肌无力症状者。
• 诊断尚不明确，但疑诊肌无力者。
• 肌无力患者症状加重的。
• 出现肌无力危象或呼吸状况不明者建议收入 ICU。

出院指征

病情缓解的肌无力患者可请神经科医师会诊后安排出院。

随访建议

所有出院患者均应安排神经科随访。

要点和误区

• 所有送入急诊室的重症肌无力患者均应查找有无肌无力危象表现。
• 对于病情加重的重症肌无力仔细查找有无继发疾病状况。
• 在行腾喜龙试验时应给予心电监测并在床边备好阿托品和负压吸引装置。
• 调整插管时的麻药用量（双琥珀酰胆碱，去极化药减半）。

舟状骨骨折 Scaphoid Fracture

Stephen R. Hayden　周秋香 译

基础知识

描述

- 舟状骨是最常见的腕骨骨折。
- 这根骨是远端和近端腕管之间的稳定器。
- 损伤可能导致关节炎、缺血性坏死或畸形。
- 分类为：
  - 近端 3 日(10%～20%)。
  - 中三(腰部,70%～80%)。
  - 远端第三(结节)结节骨折。
- 在最初的 X 线上有 10%～15%的时间漏诊骨折,延迟诊断大大增加了并发症的风险。
- 舟状骨的血液供应远端进入。
- 骨折越近,越容易发生血管坏死。
- 手腕用力过伸,肩胛骨的掌侧张力下降,背侧压力下降导致骨折。

病因

通常情况下是由于摔倒造成的背屈手(上肢在伸展位跌倒受伤)。

诊断

症状和体征

病史

上肢在伸展位跌倒受伤。

体格检查

- 解剖型鼻烟壶内最大的疼痛和压痛(可通过直接触诊或拇指轴向负荷引起),敏感性为 90%,特异性为 40%。
- 桡骨茎远端手腕背痛、手腕和拇指活动范围减小。
- 很少,轻微的桡神经浅分支损伤会导致感觉改变。
- 通过桡骨偏离腕关节,触诊肩胛骨,触诊肩胛骨结节,敏感性为 87%,特异性为 57%。
- 内翻抗拒疼痛。

儿科注意事项

- 腕关节骨折在儿童(和老年人)中很少见,因为桡骨远端通常在 1 英石以下。
- 如果存在,仔细评估机制。

诊断检查与说明

影像学检查

- 影像学应包括手腕的 3 个视图：PA、侧向、斜向和肩胛骨视图(腕部和尺侧偏移)。
- 请特别注意骨头的中间 1/3 或腰部：70%的损伤发生在这里。
- 超声诊断隐蔽性骨折的灵敏度为 85%,特异性为 83%。
- 骨折可以通过一些细微的发现来确定,如移位的脂肪垫。
- 损伤时 X 线片上 10%～15%的骨折不可见。
- 骨闪烁成像或 MRI 在受伤后 3 日就可以排除骨折的可能性,并允许早期康复：
  - CT 不那么可靠。

诊断步骤/外科

- 如果骨折是开放性的或相关的损伤,需要紧急手术治疗。
- 舟状骨折相关损伤：
  - 舟月骨离解。
  - 远端桡骨骨折。
  - 半月形骨折/脱位。
  - 拇指-桡腕关节脱位。
  - 近端和远端腕关节脱位。

鉴别诊断

- 贝内特骨折。
- 罗兰多骨折。
- 拇指掌骨底部的关节外骨折。
- 猎场看守人的拇指。
- 腱鞘炎腱鞘炎。
- 半月状骨周边脱位。
- 舟月骨离解。
- 月牙骨折或脱位。

治疗

院前

用夹板固定或固定。

初步稳定/治疗

- 评估患者的其他伤害。
- 开放伤应包扎伤口。
- 用拇指固定在中立位置,冰敷,抬高。

急诊治疗/程序

- 评估损伤机制和最大压痛点。
- 特别注意皮肤完整性和神经血管状况的检查。
- 如果鼻烟壶有压痛,放在拇指夹板中。
- 就骨不连(10%)和无血管性坏死风险为患者提供咨询。
- 无影像学证据的临床疑似舟状骨折：
  - 应将其视为一种不间断的舟状骨骨折。
  - 夹板拇指在一个位置,好像患者在拥抱一个酒杯。
  - 在 7～10 日内进行物理/X 线检查。
- 非错位舟状骨骨折：
  - 拇指穗状花序夹板。
- 粉碎性舟状骨骨折：
  - 骨折不愈合率为 50%。
  - 通常是指内固定。

药物治疗

使用非甾体抗炎药或麻醉药进行疼痛控制。

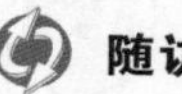

随访

进一步处理

入院指征

开放性骨折或其他较严重的损伤。

出院指征

- 闭合性损伤,术后随访 72 h。
- 如果石膏模型不影响工作或特定运动活动,对于无消除性骨折的夹板患者,可以恢复工作或运动。

转诊问题

- 如果骨折呈角状或移位>1 mm,应立即进行矫形。
- 所有舟状骨或疑似舟状骨损伤都必须考虑到骨科问题。
- 如果在最初的 X 线图上没有发现放射性异常,放置在拇指人字形夹板后,请在 7～10 日使用重复的 X 线片检查骨科或初级护理。

要点和误区

- 远端灌注进入舟状骨。
- 无血管性坏死(尤其对于近端第三骨折),发生于低强度或固定化骨折。
- 出现腕关节扭伤症状的患者必须排除急性舟状骨折的诊断。

周期性呕吐综合征 Vomiting, Cyclic

Rosaural Fernández 吴昊 李文放 译

基础知识

描述

• 腹痛一种特发性疾病，其特征是反复发作，不连续的恶心和呕吐，持续数小时到数日的腹痛，间隔期可无症状。

• 在儿童人群中更常见，但在成人中的认知较高。

• 成人：平均诊断年龄为 31 岁。

- 平均发病年龄为 21 岁。

• 儿童：平均诊断年龄为 9 岁。

• 总体特征：

- 第一阶段：间歇期。

◦ 无症状。

- 第二阶段：前驱症状。

◦ 不同程度的恶心和发汗。

- 第三阶段：催吐阶段。

◦ 剧烈恶心、呕吐、腹痛和嗜睡持续 7 日。

- 第四阶段：恢复阶段。

◦ 恶心改善和可耐受经口摄入。

流行病学

发病率和患病率估计

• 虽然对疾病了解不断深入，但由于有限的数据和研究，成人总发病率和患病率具体不详。

• 有 0.04%～2%儿童中患周期性呕吐综合征，并且以每年新发 3/10 万例增长。

病因

• 病因不明。

• 病理生理学仍在研究中。

- 有限的研究提示疾病由多因素影响：比如主观因素、中枢性因素和环境性因素。

诊断

症状和体征

通常表现为不明原因的恶心、呕吐和腹痛。

病史

• 类似发作史。

• 以前没有确定的诱因，但通常是当被问到具体的问题时可确定。

• 主诉腹部疼痛，以上腹部多见。

• 可能有以下个人病史：

- 偏头痛。

- 抑郁/焦虑。

- 长期服用大麻。

- 肠易激综合征。

- 自主神经功能障碍。

• 触发因素通常包括：

- 压力。

- 感染(URI/鼻窦炎)。

- 晕动病。

- 睡眠不足。

- 月经。

体格检查

• 可能出现阴性检查结果或根据脱水情况有不同临床表现。

• 正常生命体征或异常生命体征。

- 心动过速。

- 低血压(包括直立性低血压)。

- 呼吸急促。

• 四肢湿冷和/或毛细管充盈时间延长(>2 s)提示休克。

• 不同程度的意识改变：

- 警觉、嗜睡、反应迟钝。

• 黏膜干燥：

- 眼窝凹陷。

- 嘴唇干裂。

• 皮肤弹性差。

• 少尿或无尿。

儿科注意事项

拒绝进水进食，哭少泪或哭无泪，前囟凹陷，少尿或者尿。

基本检查

必须排除其他潜在的严重情况(参见鉴别诊断)。

诊断检查与说明

• 对具有相似的表现症状和体征，进行必要的检查和实验室或放射学检查，以排除其他诊断。

• 周期性呕吐综合征没有特定的诊断标准，也没有特定的生化标记。

• 排他性诊断。

• 成人反复呕吐的诊断是基于罗马的诊断标准。

- 典型发病形式的呕吐(急性)和持续时间(<1 周)。

- 年至少发生 3 次，最近 6 个月发生 2 次，间隔至少 1 周。

- 在 1 年里至少有 3 次。

- 发作间无呕吐。

- 缺乏中枢神经系统或胃肠道结构或代谢紊乱。

- 偏头痛的辅助诊断标准包括病史或 FH。

实验室检查

• 血常规。

• 电解质、BUN/Cr、葡萄糖。

• 肝酶、肝功能。

• 脂肪酶。

• 乳酸。

• 尿妊娠试验。

• 毒物筛查/血药浓度：

- 对乙酰氨基酚。

- 水杨酸。

- 酒精：乙醇、异丙醇、甲醇、乙二醇。

- 地高辛。

影像学检查

• 非典型的严重程度或非典型发作应鉴别其他疾病，不能单纯考虑周期性呕吐综合征。

• 影像学表现因人而异。

诊断步骤/外科

应进行门诊胃排空试验排除胃轻瘫或其他导致频繁呕吐的肠道蠕动障碍的疾病。

鉴别诊断

• 感染：

- 阑尾炎。

- 肾盂肾炎。

- 肺炎。

- 胆囊炎。

• 代谢/内分泌：

- 肾衰竭和尿毒症。

- 电解质紊乱。

- 糖尿病酮症酸中毒。

- 甲状腺疾病。

- 肾上腺功能不全。

- 嗜铬细胞瘤。

- 妊娠或妊娠期剧吐。

• 泌尿道/妇产科：

- 输尿管结石。

- 输尿管阻塞/肾盂积水。

- 妊娠。

- 经前期综合征。

• 胃肠道：

Z

- 胃轻瘫。
- 肠阻塞。
- 消化性溃疡。
- 胆石症。
- 胰腺炎。
- 肠扭转。
- 炎症性肠病。

• 中枢神经系统：
- 颅内出血。
- 肿瘤。
- 脑积水。
- 脑血管意外。

• 心血管疾病：
- 心绞痛等同症状。
- STEMI/NSTEMI(冠状动脉综合征)。

• 毒理学：
- 大麻素剧吐。
- 蕈类毒性：
- 急性酒精/有毒酒精摄入：乙醇、异丙醇、甲醇、乙二醇。
- 酒精戒断。
- 海洛因戒断。
- 急性/亚急性摄入：对乙酰氨基酚、水杨酸、地高辛。

• 精神：
- 自我诱导。
- 暴食症。
- 神经性厌食症。
- 焦虑症。

儿科注意事项

孟乔森代理综合征。

治疗

院前

• 气道/呼吸/循环管理。

• 开通静脉通路，吸氧，心电监测。

• 血糖监测。

• 如在出现呕吐和/或生命体征异常时始给予静脉输液。

初步稳定/治疗

• 气道/呼吸/循环管理。

• 继续维持静脉通路/吸氧，心电监测。

• 特别处理异常生命体征：低血压和心动过速。
- 成人：快速输注 500～1 000 ml 生理盐水。
- 儿科：快速输注 20 ml/kg 生理盐水。

急诊治疗/程序

• 急性期的支持性护理。

• 使用止吐药物。

• 静脉给予生理盐水。

• 纠正电解质异常。

• 止痛剂止痛。

• 适当给予胃酸抑制剂：H_2 受体阻滞剂、质子泵抑制剂。

• 曲坦类抗焦虑。

药物治疗

止吐药

• 昂丹司琼：4～8 mg，静脉、口服/口腔崩解片，q4～8 h，必要时。

• 甲氧氯普胺：10 mg，静脉、肌内注射，q2～3 h，必要时；4～8 mg，静脉或口服，q4～8 h，必要时。

• 丙氯哌嗪：5～10 mg，静脉、口服或肌内注射(儿童：每次 0.1 mg/kg，口服、肌内注射或灌肠)，q6～8 h，必要时。

• 氯丙嗪：12.5/25 mg，口服、肌内注射或灌肠，q4～6 h(静脉给药未被批准)(儿童：0.25～1 mg/kg，口服、肌内注射或灌肠，q4～6 h 必要时如果＞2 岁)。

疼痛/镇静

• 酮咯酸：15～30 mg，静脉输注。

• 地西泮：0.5～1 mg，静脉输注、肌内注射或口服。

• 吗啡：0.1 mg，静脉输注。

• 舒马曲坦：4～6 mg，皮下注射，必要时。

胃酸抑制剂

• 西咪替丁(H_2 受体阻滞剂)：800 mg，口服，夜间[儿童：20～40 mg/(kg・24 h)]。

• 法莫替丁：20 mg，静脉输注，q12 h。

• 泮托拉唑：40 mg，静脉输注，q24 h。

• 雷尼替丁：50 mg，肌内注射，q8 h。

随访

进一步处理

入院指征

• 重要的症状/实验室或物理检查结果提示中度至重度脱水。

• 无法耐受口服补液。

出院指征

• 生命体征稳定。

• 停止呕吐和疼痛控制。

• 能够耐受口服补液并维持体液水平。

转诊问题

• 无症状时，门诊进一步随访。

• 考虑转诊至治疗这种综合征的专家处。

随访建议

• 识别和避免诱因：
- 如情感压力，睡眠不足，禁食，疾病、大麻、特殊食物(巧克力、奶酪等)。

• 管理共存的疾病：
- 偏头痛。
- 精神疾病。
- 慢性麻醉和大麻使用。

• 药物(在积极研究中)：
- 三环类抗抑郁药(阿米替林，去甲替林)。
- 抗偏头痛药(舒马曲坦、普萘洛尔)。
- 辅酶 Q10。
- 抗组胺和抗酸剂(法莫替丁、雷尼替丁)。
- 抗焦虑药物(劳拉西泮)。

要点和误区

• 充分获取既往病史及相似点。

• 必要时，管理共存疾病。

• 排除其他具有类似症状(恶心、呕吐、腹痛)的疾病。

周期性瘫痪 Periodic Paralysis

Betty B. Dean 刘静 译

基础知识

描述

• 周期性瘫痪(PP，又称周期麻痹)：肌肉代谢紊乱，通常遗传，导致肢体运动迟缓无力。血钾过多、血钾过少、甲状腺功能亢进(甲亢)都会使症状加剧。

• 原发性：家族性 AD 骨骼肌钙、钠或钾通道突变。

• 继发性：甲状腺毒性、低钾血症、高钾血症。

流行病学

发病率和流行情况

- 低钾性周期性瘫痪麻痹(HypoPP)：
  - MC,发病率为 1/10 万。
  - 1/3 新的 AD 突变。
- 高钾性周期性瘫痪(HyperPP)：
  - 发病率为 1/20 万。
  - 90%突变的人会有临床症状。
- 甲亢性周期性瘫痪(ThyroPP)：
  - 在甲亢患者中有 2%的发病率。
  - 多见于亚洲国家。
  - 低钾性周期性瘫痪的子集,临床上难以辨别。
- Andersen-Tawil 综合征：
  - 低钾性周期性瘫痪的子集。
  - 罕见。
  - 患病率未知。

病因

- 骨骼肌钠通道基因突变：
  - *SCN4A*。
  - 低钾性周期性瘫痪和高钾性周期性瘫痪：
    - AD 遗传。
    - 自然突变。
- 骨骼肌钙通道 *CACN1AS* 基因突变：
  - 低钾性周期性瘫痪。
- *KCNJ*2 基因突变：
  - Andersen-Tawil 综合征。
    - AD 遗传。
    - 50%先天性。
- 男性＞女性。
- 发病年龄：
  - 低钾性周期性瘫痪：
    - 10 年 1 次或 2 次。
  - 高钾性周期性瘫痪：
    - 10 年 1 次。
  - Andersen-Tawil 综合征。
    - 10 年 1 次或 2 次。
  - 甲亢性周期性瘫痪：
    - 10 年 2～5 次。

诊断

症状和体征

病史

- 间歇性无力：
  - 散发性。
  - 起病急骤。
  - 疾病复发及肌无力的反复发作很常见。
  - 经常从单次发作到日常发作。
- 疾病发作类型：
  - 先天性。
  - 晚上或清晨。
  - 继发性：
    - 甲状腺疾病病史。
    - 近期摄入富含碳水化合物(糖类)的食物。
    - 剧烈运动后休息。
    - 患病。
    - 缺少睡眠。
    - 药物：胰岛素、肾上腺素、类固醇、β受体激动剂、利尿剂。
    - 寒冷的环境。
    - 月经。
    - 睡眠减少。
    - 妊娠。
    - 减少甲状腺疾病的药物。
- 疾病发作的时间。
  - 低钾性周期性瘫痪：1 h/d。
  - 高钾性周期性瘫痪：15 min 至 4 h。
  - 甲亢性周期性瘫痪：同低钾性周期性瘫痪。
  - Andersen-Tawil 综合征：时间不定。
- 无力的周期性发作家族史。

体格检查

- 常规：
  - 甲亢性周期性瘫痪：
    - 体温过高。
- 五官：
  - 低钾性周期性瘫痪和高钾性周期性瘫痪：
    - 眼睑迟滞：罕见。
    - 吞咽困难：罕见。
  - 甲亢性周期性瘫痪：
    - 眼球突出。
    - 甲状腺肿。
  - Andersen-Tawil 综合征：
    - 生理缺陷：身材矮小,低位耳,广泛的鼻,小颌畸形。
- 心脏：
  - 低钾性周期性瘫痪和高钾性周期性瘫痪：
    - 可能存在心律失常。
  - 甲亢性周期性瘫痪：
    - 心动过速,心律失常。
  - Andersen-Tawil 综合征：
    - 心律失常。
- 肺：
  - 低钾性周期性瘫痪：
    - 呼吸肌感染：罕见。
    - 严重的血钾过低。
- M/S：
  - 低钾性周期性瘫痪、高钾性周期性瘫痪和甲亢性周期性瘫痪：
    - 对称肌肉在 1 个或更多的肢体上出现无力。
    - 腿＞胳膊。
  - Andersen-Tawil 综合征：
    - 周期性肌肉无力＜1 h。
    - 近侧的＞远侧的。
- 神经系统：
  - 警觉的,有意识的。
  - 感觉正常。
  - DTR 减少或缺失。
  - 骨骼肌无力,对称。
  - 括约肌正常。
- 皮肤：
  - 甲亢性周期性瘫痪：
    - 温热,湿润。

基本检查

实验室检查和心电图。

诊断检查与说明

- 心电图：
  - 低钾性周期性瘫痪：
    - 窦性心动过缓。
    - T 波水平。
    - ST 段压低。
  - 高钾性周期性瘫痪：
    - T 波很少达到顶峰。
  - 甲亢性周期性瘫痪：
    - P 波高、QRS 波群宽、T 波减少、房室传导阻滞、心室颤动或心脏停博。
  - Andersen-Tawil 综合征：
    - QT 间期长,室性心律失常。
    - U 波、T 波延长下坡。
    - 从其他长 QT 综合征中区分出 Andersen 综合征。
- 电解质：
  - 钾：
    - 高钾性周期性瘫痪：正常或增加。
    - 低钾性周期性瘫痪：正常或减少。
    - 甲亢性周期性瘫痪：疾病发作期间减少。
    - Andersen-Tawil 综合征：减少,正常,或增加。
  - 钙：
    - 甲亢性周期性瘫痪：疾病发作期间减少。
  - 磷：

甲亢性周期性瘫痪：疾病发作期间减少。

- 甲状腺研究：
  - 甲亢性周期性瘫痪：
    - TSH：低。
    - T_4：升高。

影像学检查

对诊断来说不是必需的。

诊断步骤/外科

不在急诊部门时专科医师可能要考虑以下几方面。

- 肌电图：
  - 低钾性周期性瘫痪：
    - 无肌强直。
  - 高钾性周期性瘫痪：
    - 肌强直。
  - Andersen-Tawil 综合征。
- 肌肉活组织切片。
- 刺激测试：
  - 高钾性周期性瘫痪：
    - 钾和肾上腺素。
  - 低钾性周期性瘫痪：
    - 胰岛素和葡萄糖。

鉴别诊断

低血钾和高血钾的其他原因。

- 高血钾：
  - 药物：螺内酯、ACEI、非甾体抗炎药、肝素。
  - 遗传：21-羟化酶缺乏症、麦卡德尔病。
  - 胃肠道：
    - 回肠造口术紧密的紧密气孔。
  - 肾：
    - 慢性肾衰竭。
  - 内分泌：
    - 肾上腺皮质功能衰竭。
- 低钾性周期性瘫痪：
  - 药物：
    - 安胎药、两性霉素 B、利尿剂、减少钾的摄入量、恶性高温综合征。
  - 胃肠道：
    - 呕吐。
    - 腹腔和热带口炎性腹泻。
    - 短肠综合征。
  - 肾：
    - Conn 综合征。
    - 巴特综合征。
    - 急性肾小管坏死。
    - 肾小管酸中毒。
  - 神经肌肉：
    - Andersen-Tawil 综合征。
    - 重症肌无力。
  - 内分泌系统：
    - 甲亢。
    - 高醛固酮血症。
    - 糖尿病酮症酸中毒。

治疗

院前

- 支持性措施：
  - ABC 管理，建立静脉通路，给氧，监测生命体征。

初步稳定/治疗

- 支持疗法。
- 高钾性周期性瘫痪：
  - 一些短暂发作不需要治疗。
  - 静脉注射葡萄糖酸钙可能有效。
- 低钾性周期性瘫痪：
  - 钾：
    - 首选：口服液 40 mg。
    - 静脉注射钾 10 mg，只有 1 剂或 2 剂。
    - 注意矫正过度。
    - 静脉注射水合剂能够纠正钾。
- Andersen-Tawil 综合征：
  - 钙变化莫测：
    - 有益于低钾性周期性瘫痪。
- 甲亢性周期性瘫痪：
  - 治疗甲状腺异常：
    - 心跳过速：非选择性 β 受体阻滞剂。
  - 治疗潜在异常：
    - 同低钾性周期性瘫痪。
    - 观察甲亢部分。

注意

低钾性周期性瘫痪应该避免可能造成疾病或恶性高温的挥发性麻醉剂和去极化肌松药。

随访

进一步处理

- 低钾性周期性瘫痪或高钾性周期性瘫痪：
  - 改变生活方式：
    - 避免触发因素：乙醇、持续锻炼、含钾高的食物、斋戒。
- 甲亢性周期性瘫痪：
  - 取决于潜在疾病的严重程度，如果无症状和受控可能要考虑咨询神经科医师和内分泌医师。

入院指征

- 低钾性周期性瘫痪或高钾性周期性瘫痪：
  - 如果血钾过低或过高，而且有症状的，心脏或呼吸道损害时考虑。
- Andersen-Tawil 综合征：
  - 收治，心脏猝死的风险高。

出院指征

- 低钾性周期性瘫痪、高钾性周期性瘫痪和甲亢性周期性瘫痪：
  - 症状得到解决，转诊到神经科，无心脏或呼吸系统危害。

转诊问题

- 神经科。
- 甲状腺内分泌科。
- 基因咨询：
  - 50%风险遗传主要的周期性瘫痪。

随访建议

- 代谢性肌病方面的神经专科医师。
- 遗传学家。

要点和误区

- 收治 Andersen-Tawil 综合征患者和所有仍有症状的周期性瘫痪患者。
- 所有形式的周期性瘫痪患者谨慎使用挥发性麻醉剂和去极化肌松药。

周围神经疾病 Peripheral Neuropathy

Minh V. Le 钱斌斌 译

基础知识

描述

外周神经病是周围神经障碍的总称，它可能影响运动、感觉或血管运动性神经纤维，表现为明显的肌肉无力、萎缩性疼痛和麻木。

病因

多变的，取决于症状表现，参阅鉴别诊断。

诊断

症状和体征

- 感觉神经功能障碍。
  - 麻木。
  - 局部刺痛。
  - 感觉异常。
  - 感觉迟钝。
  - 大纤维神经病变，降低振动和位置感觉。
  - 小纤维神经病变，降低疼痛和温度感觉。
  - 深腱反射降低，促发肢体感觉减退。
- 运动神经功能障碍。
  - 缺点：
    - 末梢＞近端。
    - 偶发肌束震颤。
  - 肌肉萎缩，减弱的健康与长期运动神经受累。
  - 反射损失，促发运动神经传导速度减慢。
- 自主神经障碍。
  - 静态平衡位。
  - 便秘。
  - 尿潴留。
  - 阳痿。

病史

- 症状持续时间。
- 对称或不对称症状。
- 远端或近端症状。
- 运动、感觉相关症状，或者两者混合的。

体格检查

- 彻底的从头到脚的体检。
- 关注神经检查：
  - 运动无力。
  - 感觉通常丧失在手套袜子分布中。

> **注意**
>
> - 在早期情况下，没有反射可能存在脱髓鞘性神经病，如吉兰-巴雷综合征[急性炎症性脱髓鞘综合征(AIDP)]。

基本检查

- 基于神经病变剧烈程度的研究，做出极有可能的诊断。
- 如果有急性重度症状，进行早期神经会诊。

诊断检查与说明

实验室检查

- 基本代谢组。
- 全血细胞计数。
- 肝功能检测。
- 尿液分析。
- 促甲状腺激素。
- 基于个人陈述的 HIV 或维生素 B_{12}。
- 心电图。

影像学检查

- 胸部 X 线片。
- 头部 CT。

诊断步骤/外科

- 肌电图检查、神经传导检查、入院会诊或门诊随访时进行神经活检。
- 腰椎穿刺确认吉兰-巴雷综合征。

鉴别诊断

- 病灶：
  - 压迫。
  - 常见压缩位置：
    - 腕骨、尺骨管。
    - 跗骨管。
    - 腓骨。
  - 黏液性水肿。
  - 类风湿关节炎。
  - 淀粉样变性。
  - 肢端肥大症。
  - 创伤。
  - 缺血性病变。
  - 糖尿病。
  - 血管炎。
  - 麻风病。
  - 结节病。
  - 肿瘤浸润或压迫。
- 多病灶(多数性单神经病)。
  - 糖尿病。
  - 血管炎：
    - 结节性多动脉炎。
    - 全身性红斑狼疮。
    - Sjögren 综合征。
  - 结节病。
  - 麻风病。
  - 恶性肿瘤。
  - HIV/AIDS。
  - 遗传体质的压力麻痹。
- 对称的：
  - 内分泌：
    - 大多数为糖尿病。
    - 甲状腺功能减退症。
  - 药物：
    - 异烟肼。
    - 锂。
    - 甲硝唑。
    - 苯妥英。
    - 西咪替丁。
    - 肼酞嗪。
    - 阿米替林。
    - 胺碘酮。
  - 营养性疾病：
    - 酒精中毒。
    - 维生素 B_{12}、叶酸缺乏。
    - 维生素 B_1。
  - 危重性神经病变。
  - 低磷血症。
  - 吉兰-巴雷综合征。
  - 中毒性神经病：
    - 一氧化碳。
    - 丙烯酰胺。
    - 二硫化碳。
    - 环氧乙烷。
    - 有机磷酸酯。
    - 铅。
- 脊髓型周围神经病变。
- 背部疼痛。
- 脊椎麻木。
- 下肢无力。

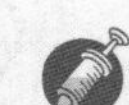

治疗

院前

- 如需要进行疼痛控制。

Z

• 气道保护。

■ 初步稳定/治疗

对于严重急性外周神经病应建立气道保护，如吉兰-巴雷综合征。

■ 急诊治疗/程序

• 根据视力症状的变化。
• 停止违规的毒素或药物。
• 全身性疾病治疗。

■ 药物治疗

• 根据基础诊断变化。
• 阿片类药物。
• 加巴喷丁 300 mg，口服，每日 1 次，然后第 2 日每日 2 次，然后第 3 日每日 3 次；累计到 1 800 mg 后，每日 3 次。
• 卡马西平 100 mg，口服，每日 2 次，针对三叉神经痛。
• 针对吉兰-巴雷综合征，静脉注射免疫球蛋白。

随访

■ 进一步处理

入院指征

• 呼吸窘迫或急性步态障碍。
• 顽固性疼痛。

出院指征

神经疾病康复，根据持续严格的报告。

■ 随访建议

根据病因和症状的严重程度进行初级健康管理或神经疾病康复。

要点和误区

错误诊断为吉兰-巴雷综合征。

周围血管疾病 Peripheral Vascular Disease

Lindsay Taylor • Sally A. Santen 钱斌斌 译

基础知识

■ 描述

• 外周动脉阻塞≥1，栓塞或血栓。
• 动脉粥样硬化或血栓可导致。
• 外周动脉疾病一般都有冠状动脉和脑血管疾病。
• 流行病学：
- 风险因素(可选择)：
◦ 年龄。
◦ 抽烟。
◦ 糖尿病。
◦ 高脂血症。
◦ 高血压。
- 与其他形式的动脉粥样硬化的发病率和死亡率相关(冠心病、脑卒中)。
- 并发症：
◦ 动脉瘤。
◦ 血栓症。
◦ 溃疡。
◦ 肢体损失。
• 慢性动脉供血不足(CAI)：
- 进行性梗阻性动脉粥样硬化性疾病致亚急性缺血和疼痛(跛行)。
- 10%发展到严重的下肢缺血。
• 急性动脉供血不足(AAI)：
- 由 50%的动脉血栓或栓塞造成。
- 导致急性肢体缺血的 6P 征(下述)。
• 动脉栓塞：
- 由动脉粥样硬化斑块破裂或部分破裂造成(主动脉、股动脉、髂骨)。
- 导致胆固醇栓塞，使小动脉网络阻塞。
- 可能由侵入性动脉手术，如心导管等引起。

■ 病因

• 粥样硬化斑块(CAI)。
• 动脉血栓。
• 动脉栓塞：
- 心肌栓塞，继发于心律失常、心脏瓣膜疾病或心肌病(80%)。
- 动脉瘤。
- 感染。
- 肿瘤。
- 血管炎或异物。
- 预先存在的动脉粥样硬化斑块形成血栓。
• 动脉栓塞。

诊断

■ 症状和体征

病史

• CAI：
- 跛行：
◦ 小腿疼痛(股动脉闭塞)或臀部和大腿(主髂动脉区)。
◦ 通过休息或固定体位可产生急性或慢性缓解。
◦ 典型跛行在 1/2 的外周血管疾病患者中会出现。
- 严重疾病在休息时会出现四肢疼痛：
◦ 经常从足开始。
◦ 快速渐进性跛行或溃疡。
• AAI：
- 肢体疼痛：
◦ 突发性。
◦ 严重程度逐渐增加。
◦ 随着时间的推移，远端向近端开始移动。
◦ 一旦缺血的感觉丧失，强度会降低。
• 动脉栓塞：
- 主诉手指或脚趾冰冷疼痛。
- 小动脉粥样硬化血栓可能影响四肢。
- 经常与最近的动脉造影、血管或心脏手术有关。
- 多器官受累常见(肾脏、肠系膜、皮肤等)。

体格检查

> **注意**
>
> 突然性疼痛和四肢苍白有生命危险。
>
> • CAI：
> - 缺失或减少周围脉搏。
> - 寒冷的皮肤延迟毛细管填充。
> - 增加静脉充盈时间。
> - 杂音。
> - 苍白和红肿的腿。
> - 肌肉和皮肤萎缩。
> - 增厚的指甲和背发的损失。
> - 溃疡(特别是足趾或足跟)或严重的坏疽疾病。
>
> • AAI：
> - 6P 征：
> ◦ 疼痛(首先，有时只是征兆)。

◦ 苍白。
◦ 无脉。
◦ 变冷。
◦ 感觉异常(晚发现)。
◦ 麻痹(晚发现)。

- 识别一个可能的栓塞过程源是关键的(心房颤动、心脏肥大)。

• 动脉栓塞:
- 缺血性和痛苦症状。
- "蓝趾综合征"。
- 网状青斑。

■ **基本检查**

• CAL:
- 臂-踝指数(心脏收缩压与上臂收缩压区分开)。
- 临床测试在确认是否存在 CAI。
- 比例<0.9 是异常的,并且 0.4~0.5 或以下表示严重疾病。
- 动脉钙化(糖尿病)可以有 ABI 假阴性或 ABI 升高(>1.3)。

• AAI:
- 物理诊断使用 6P 征。
- 那些有急慢性动脉供血不足、肢体缺血者比没有 CAI 的要好一些,因为形成了良好的侧支流通。

• 动脉栓塞。
- 临床诊断:影响区域疼痛,压痛,并且可能昏暗或坏死。
- 使用多普勒超声、CT 血管造影,心电图检查可以探测栓塞源。

■ **诊断检查与说明**

实验室检查

• 全血细胞计数和血小板。
• 电解质、尿素氮、肌酐、葡萄糖。
• 凝血功能检查。
• 肌酸磷酸激酶测定缺血。
• 对疑似病因进行特殊检测:
- 血液高凝状态检查。
- 沉降率、CRP、检测血管炎。
- 血液培养,检测血管炎。

影像学检查

• 多普勒超声:
- 可视化静脉与动脉系统。
- 确定动脉阻塞水平、血栓和动脉瘤。
- 敏感性和特异性,80%~90%及以上的血管阻塞在腘血管近端。

• 体积描记法/节段压力测量:
- 使用测量血液流速的体积和特性来查明 CAI 的区域。
- 不如超声应用广泛,需要一个有经验的技术员。
- 在敏感性和特异性上接近超声。

• 血管造影:
- 确定解剖学细节,包括阻塞水平、狭窄度和侧支循环。
- 对诊断 AAI 的部位不确定或紧急旁路移植术是有用的。
- 具有在诊断的时候治疗(旋切术、血管成形术或腔内溶栓)的优势。

• CT 血管造影:
- CT 对诊断闭塞性动脉疾病和夹层是有用的。
- 迅速有效和可靠。
- 许多中心已经把 CT 血管造影作为首选的诊断工具。对手术决定和血管造影干预都建立在 CT 血管造影的基础之上。

• MRI:
- 对诊断 CAI 和解剖评估是灵敏的。
- 缺点是磁共振消耗时间,而且价格很贵。

■ **鉴别诊断**

• 急性血栓形成或栓塞。
• 动脉夹层。
• 深部静脉血栓形成。
• 静脉瓣膜功能不全。
• 间隔综合征。
• 血栓闭塞性脉管炎。
• 椎管狭窄。
• 神经病变。
• 滑囊炎。
• 关节炎。
• 反射交感性营养不良。

治疗

■ **院前**

• 补充液体保持血流动力学稳定。
• 允许心电监测。
• 放置缺血肢体在一个可依靠的位置休息。
• 如果低氧气饱和度或肺症状应供应氧气。

■ **初步稳定/治疗**

• 低血压药物静脉推注。
• 心电图、监测仪、脉搏血氧饱和度。
• 辅助供氧。
• 疼痛控制。
• 避免极端体温。

■ **急诊治疗/程序**

• CAI:
- 首选抗血小板治疗,使用阿司匹林 75~325 mg 或氯吡格雷(75 mg/d)。双重疗法虽然可以在其他形式的动脉粥样硬化有效,但这里并没有被证明能改善结果。
- 其他认可的药物:西洛他唑 100 mg,每日 2 次;双嘧达莫 200 mg,每日 2 次;己酮可可碱 400 mg,每日 3 次。
- 根据阻塞的严重程度和位置进行血管重建术:
◦ 球囊血管成形术。
◦ 旋切术。
◦ 旁路移植术。
- 风险因素修正:
◦ 戒烟。
◦ 高血脂、高血压、糖尿病的积极控制。
◦ 运动疗法。

• AAI:
- 用静脉注射肝素限制血栓的进一步发展。
- 不要怀疑抗凝患者有一个动脉切开或症状性动脉瘤。
- 血管外科或介入放射学的紧急会诊:
◦ 决定哪一个诊断研究是最好的结论。
◦ 开始为可能的手术治疗或其他干预进行安排。
◦ 选择手术治疗包括血栓切除术、栓子清除术、血管成形术、局部动脉溶栓、旁路移植术。
◦ 在缺血性症状的发作之后,血液流至患肢的通道必须在 4~6 h 重新建立。
- AAI 的并发症包括:
◦ 间隔综合征。
◦ 不可逆的缺血需要切除。
◦ 横纹肌溶解、肾衰竭。
◦ 电解质紊乱。

• 动脉栓塞。
- 如果数量有限的组织受影响并且肾功能没有明显的损害,采取保守治疗。
- 除了支持伤口护理和镇痛,没有清除治疗缺血性手指与足趾。
- 有些研究尝试糖皮质激素来减少炎症,他汀类药物稳定斑块,阿司匹林或双嘧达莫。
- 对不可逆坏死的足趾进行截肢。
- 12~24 h 血管外科转诊或急诊处理。
- 通过深入调查和对动脉粥样硬化性栓塞源校正来预防进一步血栓活动。

■ **药物治疗**

• 阿司匹林:81~325 mg/d。

Z

• 西洛他唑：100 mg，每日 2 次。
• 氯吡格雷：75 mg/d。
• 肝素：80 U/kg 丸剂，静脉注射；然后 18 U/h，静脉注射。
• 己酮可可碱：100 mg，每日 3 次。

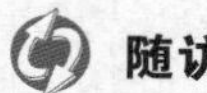

随访

进一步处理

入院指征

• 所有患 AAI 的患者需要得到评估和血管再形成的确认。
• CAI：考虑入院快速渐进性跛行或休息时的缺血性疼痛：
- 经过肝素化和血管造影来排除急性血栓形成。
• 动脉栓塞入院涉及大面积受累、显著疼痛或肾损害。

出院指征

• 动脉栓塞：
- 小的损伤、足够的疼痛控制、没有肾损伤或重复感染的证据，并且在 24 h 内进行随访。
• CAI：
- 没有快速发展、严重的下肢缺血、坏疽或感染的证据。

转诊问题

• CAI 需要紧急转诊到血管手术。
• 动脉栓塞，根据原始栓子源，可以需要转诊到血管手术或心脏病学门诊。

随访建议

CAI 没有急性缺血并且动脉栓塞最小存在，应该密切随访以评估疾病的程度。

肘部损伤 Elbow Injuries

Christian M. Sloane 姜颢 译

基础知识

描述

骨损伤

• 肱骨髁上骨折：
- 最常见于儿童。
- 峰值年龄为 5～10 岁，15 岁以上很少发生。
- 伸展型（98%）：在伸展位跌倒（FOOSH），伴上肢充分伸展或过伸：
◦ 1 型：最小或无位移。
◦ 2 型：轻度移位骨折，后皮质完整。
◦ 3 型：完全移位骨折，后皮质破裂。
- 屈曲型：直接打击屈肘。
◦ 1 型：最小或无位移。
◦ 2 型：轻度移位骨折，前皮质完整。
◦ 3 型：完全移位骨折，前皮质破裂。
• 桡骨头骨折：
- 通常是间接机制（如 FOOSH）。
- 桡骨头嵌入小头。
• 尺骨冠状突骨折：
- 以肱尺关节部分为肘关节提供临界稳定性。
- 骨折常常导致关节不稳定。
- 多数常伴发于其他损伤比如肘关节脱位。
• 危险三角：
- 桡骨头骨折、冠状突骨折及肘关节脱位。
- 治疗困难且预后较差。

软组织损伤

• 肘关节脱位：
- 像大多数关节脱臼一样仅次于肩关节。
- 多数是后脱位（90%）。
• 内/外上髁炎：
- 过劳损伤通常与肘关节的旋转运动有关。
- 伤及手腕到肘关节屈、伸肌群的附着点。
- 水管工、木匠、网球运动员、高尔夫球手。
- 特定肌肉群的抵抗收缩使疼痛加重。

儿科注意事项

• 桡骨头关节半脱位（保姆肘）。
• 20%的上肢损伤发生在儿童。
• 高峰年龄为 1～4 岁，女性比男性更容易发生。
• 前臂旋前时突然受到纵向拉力。

病因

• 机制有助于确定预期的损伤。
• 外伤为主。
• 多数间接性创伤所致肘部损伤是由前臂骨传递的（如 FOOSH）。
• 直接打击很少引起骨折或脱位。

诊断

症状与体征

患者如何支撑手臂可为诊断提供线索。

骨损伤

肱骨髁上骨折：
• 屈曲型：
- 患者用另外的手臂支撑受伤的前臂，肘屈曲 90°。
- 尺骨鹰嘴突损毁。
• 伸展型：
- 患者侧面持臂呈 S 形。

软组织损伤

• 肘关节脱位：
- 后脱位：尺骨鹰嘴突出异常。
- 前脱位：尺骨鹰嘴突出损毁。
• 桡骨头半脱位：
- 肘微屈，前臂旋前，肘部手臂运动抵抗。
• 内/外上髁炎：
- 肘内侧/外侧面涉及前臂的钝性疼痛逐渐发作。
- 抓和扭转运动使疼痛增加。

基本检查

• X 线平片。
• 评估腕和肩的相关损伤。
• 评估肢体神经血管状态（必须在一切操作前进行）。
• 评估皮肤完整性。
• 检查筋膜间隙综合征，它更常见于肱骨髁上骨折。

> **注意**
> • 同侧上肢损伤很常见，尤其是肱骨中段和前臂远端骨折。
> • 评估相关的神经血管损伤（高达 20%）。

诊断检查与说明

实验室检查

肘部损伤无特定指标。

影像学检查

• 如怀疑过劳损伤时通常不必检查。
• 常规前后位（AP）和侧位，评估桡骨头、肱骨远端的轻微损伤需加斜位。
• 脂肪垫征：
- 见于关节内损伤。

- 通常前脂肪垫是肱骨前的一个狭窄透亮带。
- 后脂肪垫通常不可见。
- 当前脂肪垫征被抬高并变得更垂直于前肱骨皮质(航行征),表明有关节积液/损伤。
- 后脂肪垫征表明积液/损伤:
  ◦ 在成人,没有其他明显骨折的后脂肪垫征表明桡骨头骨折。
  ◦ 在儿童这表明肱骨髁上骨折。

儿科注意事项

• 儿童骨折经常发生在未钙化的软骨,使影像难以解读。

• 肱骨前表面的划线在侧位片应始终与肱骨小头交叉。

• 如果X线平片上任何骨间关系出现问题,应做未受损肘部的对照片。

• 如果病史与损伤不符合,应怀疑非意外创伤。

• 骨化中心:首先出现:
- 小头:3～6个月。
- 桡骨头:3～5岁。
- 内上髁:5～7岁。
- 滑车:9～10岁。
- 鹰嘴:9～10岁。
- 外上髁:9～13岁。

鉴别诊断

• 扭伤或劳损。
• 积液。
• 挫伤。
• 滑囊炎。
• 关节炎。

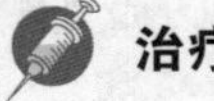

治疗

院前

使用合适的夹板。

初步稳定/治疗

为防进一步损伤,拍摄X线平片前必须固定。

急诊治疗/程序

• 无移位、稳定骨折一般可以夹板固定,骨科随访24～48 h,除此之外建议骨科会诊。

• 通常需要骨科会诊的骨折:
- 经髁、髁间、髁突、髁上骨折。
- 伤及关节面的骨折(如小头或滑车)。

• 肱骨髁上骨折:
- 1型可由急诊医师处理,骨科随访24～48 h。
- 应用后夹板肘部可弯曲和固定。
- 2型和3型需要立即骨科会诊。越来越多的这类型患者被送往各地创伤修复中心(其中24%需要手术治疗)。
- 当骨折与血管损害有关时应在急诊室复位。

• 前脱位:
- 如果血管结构受到损害,应立即复位。
- 然后弯曲至90°,并放置后夹板。

• 后脱位:
- 如果血管结构受到损害,应立即复位。
- 然后弯曲至90°,并放置后夹板。

• 桡骨头骨折:
- 轻度移位的骨折可抽吸以清除血肿,注入布比卡因(麻卡因)并固定。
- 其他类型应请骨科会诊。

• 危险三角部位:
- 尽量快速复位作或避免过多的关节活动度检查以免加重损伤。
- 使用后夹板固定肘关节于90°,前臂屈曲维持休息位。

• 桡骨头半脱位:
- 做1个连续的运动,当轻压桡骨头时旋转和弯曲肘部。
- 旋前复位法可能更有效,当握住患者肘部时,腕部保持旋前直到有明显的咔哒感。
- 复位时通常会有咔哒感。
- 等待并观察儿童患者是否能够恢复正常手臂功能以确保复位是否成功,X线检查无阳性表现。
- 如体检提示骨折而X线平片阴性,行夹板固定,让患者随访24～48 h再评估。

• 内/外上髁炎:
- 严重病例可用夹板固定。
- 休息,加热,抗炎剂。

注意

• 经过肘部的大量组织出现神经血管损伤,包括前骨间神经、尺神经和桡神经、肱动脉。

• Volkmann缺血性肌挛缩是前臂筋膜间隙综合征,通常与髁上骨折相关。

药物治疗

• 要成功复位往往操作时需要镇静,见“清醒镇静”。

• 布洛芬:600～800 mg(儿童:5～10 mg/kg),口服,每日3次。

• 萘普生:250～500 mg(儿童:10～20 mg/kg),口服,每日2次。

• 泰诺与可待因:1片或2片(可待因:儿童0.5～1 mg/kg),口服,q4～6 h;对乙酰氨基酚不超过4 g/24 h。

• 硫酸吗啡:0.1 mg/kg,静推,q2～6 h。

• 氢吗啡酮5 mg/对乙酰氨基酚300 mg。

• 对乙酰氨基酚:不超过4 g/h。

• 氢吗啡酮5 mg/对乙酰氨基酚300 mg:对乙酰氨基酚不超过4 g/24 h。

随访

进一步处理

入院指征

• 血管损伤,开放性骨折。
• 需要手术复位或内固定的骨折。
• 收治所有广泛肿胀或瘀斑患者,整夜观察,抬高以监测骨筋膜室综合征和降低其风险。

出院指征

• 稳定骨折或已复位的脱位,无上述特征。
• 夹板固定,24～48 h后安排骨科随访。
• 无并发症的软组织损伤。

要点和误区

• 未能鉴别后脂肪垫征是不正常的。

• 肘关节损伤时总是检查血管神经损伤,尤其是伴脱位、复位前后。

• 要告诉肱骨髁上骨折儿童的父母关于骨筋膜室综合征的症状与体征。

Z

蛛网膜下腔出血 Subarachnoid Hemorrhage

Thien H. Nguyen · Binh T. Ly　江伟伟　李文放 译

基础知识

描述

- 蛛网膜下腔和脑脊液出血：
- 自发：
◦ 最常见的是脑动脉瘤破裂。
◦ 动脉瘤更可能破裂(>25 mm)。
- 创伤：
◦ 严重的头部受伤。

流行病学

- 发病率是每 10 万人中有 6～16 人。
- 美国每年 21 000 人。
- 30%～50%的死亡率。
- 在 30 岁年之前不常见，发病高峰在 60 岁。

风险因素

- 动脉瘤≥7 mm 时有更大的破裂风险。
- 通过大小和位置校准后，那些纵横比>1.3 和不规则形状的动脉瘤的破裂风险明显增加。
- 有其他动脉瘤，先前破裂的。
- 家族史。
- 高血压。
- 抽烟。
- 滥用酒精。
- 拟交感神经药物：
- 可卡因、甲基苯丙胺和摇头丸。
- 性别(女性：男性为 1.6：1)。

遗传学

- 1 位亲属有蛛网膜下腔出血(SAH)，则风险增加 3～7 倍。
- 2%的 SAH 患者与遗传有密切关系：
- 常染色体多发性硬化症、Ehlers-Danlos Ⅳ型、家族性颅内动脉瘤。

儿科注意事项

- 最常见的原因是儿童动静脉畸形。
- 尽管儿童罕见，但 SAH 是儿童死亡的主要原因。

病因

- "先天性"，囊状或浆状动脉瘤破裂(80%～90%)：
- 发生在主要动脉的分叉处。
- 发病率随着年龄增加。
- 20%～30%的动脉瘤可能是多发性的。
- 非动脉瘤性中脑周围出血(10%)。
- 剩下 5%的原因包括：
- 由梅毒或心内膜炎引起的真菌性(败血性)动脉瘤。
- 动静脉畸形。
- 椎动脉或颈动脉异常。
- 颅内肿瘤。
- 垂体卒中。
- 严重头部闭合性损伤。

诊断

体征和症状

病史

- 典型体征是一个严重、突然的头痛：
- 被描述为"突然的"或"生命中最糟糕的头痛"。
- 头痛往往是枕后或颈部，但可能是单侧的。
- 通常在几秒内发展，在几分钟内达到峰值。
- 与以前的头痛不同。
- 头痛通常在发病时最严重。
- 头痛和少量出血发生在 20%～50%：
- 可能会在临床表现和诊断之前的几日到几周发生。
- 超过 50%的患者出现癫痫、意识丧失或意识水平改变。
- 呕吐发生率为 70%。
- 晕厥、复视和癫痫发作是 SAH 的特别高风险特征。

体格检查

- 局灶性神经缺陷与 33%的患者头痛同时发生：
- 第三脑神经(CN Ⅲ)麻痹发生率为 10%～15%。
- 单独第四神经麻痹或乳头状扩张也可能发生。
- 颈强直的发生率为 25%～70%。
- 昏迷患者是再次出血的线索。

基本检查

- 完成神经系统检查和眼底检查。
- 眼底镜检查可能有帮助。
- 急诊头部 CT 扫描：
- 如果在头痛发作后 6 h 内进行，则灵敏度和特异度可分别达到 97.0～100%和 99.5%～100%。
- 超过 6 h 以后 CT 用来诊断蛛网膜下腔出血依然是准确的，但不应用来排除蛛网膜下腔出血。
- 薄层扫描(3 mm)可提高诊断率。
- 24 h 后 CT 不敏感，血红蛋白<10 g/L。
- 在行腰椎穿刺前，应考虑风险与收益：
- 有 250～15 200 个病例需要行腰椎穿刺来确认是否存在动脉瘤所致的蛛网膜下腔出血，这类患者需要外科的干预，但 6 h 内的 CT 检查往往会漏诊，建议分享诊治策略。

孕妇注意事项

- 妊娠时发病率略有增加。
- 应该包括 CT 和腰椎穿刺。

诊断检查与说明

实验室检查

- 基线血常规和分类。
- 电解质、肾功能测试。
- 凝血功能。
- 心肌酶谱：
- 肌钙蛋白 I 升高 10%～40%。
- 脑脊液检查(见下文)。

影像学检查

- 胸部放射学显示肺水肿：
- 发生率高达 40%，伴有严重的神经功能缺陷。
- 传统的金标准：数字化脑血管造影。
- 螺旋 CT 血管造影：
- 用于手术前检查。
- 对于检测>4 mm 的较小动脉瘤非常敏感。
- MR 血管造影：
- MRI 对出血不太敏感。
- 对于检测>4 mm 的较小动脉瘤非常敏感。
- 经颅多普勒超声：
- 可能有助于检测血管痉挛。

诊断步骤/外科

- 腰椎穿刺：
- CSF 中存在红细胞表示 SAH 或创伤性打击：
◦ 最近的文献显示，SAH 患者腰椎穿刺时，最后一管脑脊液内的而红细胞计数不可能低于 100；而最后一管脑脊液中红细胞

Z

计数大于 10 000 者，是 SAH 的概率将增加 6 倍。
◦ 如果怀疑有头部创伤性打击，LP 应该在更高的腰椎间隙。
◦ 连续管中的红细胞计数减少提示但不能确定头部创伤性打击。
◦ 如果发病 12 h 后脑脊液变黄诊断 SAH。
- 压力升高提示 SAH、脑静脉窦血栓形成或脑肿瘤。
• 心电图：
- Q 波和 QRS 波改变。
- ST 段抬高或压低。
- QT 延长。
- T 波异常。
- 局部缺血或死相似。
- 有症状的心动过速、室性心动过速和心室颤动。

鉴别诊断

• 肿瘤。
• 动脉夹层。
• 动脉瘤(未破裂)。
• 脑动脉血管畸形。
• 偏头痛。
• 假性脑瘤。
• 脑膜炎。
• 脑炎。
• 高血压脑病。
• 高血糖或低血糖。
• 颞动脉炎。
• 急性青光眼。
• 硬膜下血肿。
• 硬膜外血肿。
• 脑出血。
• 血栓栓塞性脑卒中。
• 鼻窦炎。
• 癫痫。
• 脑静脉窦血栓形成。
• 海绵窦血栓形成。

Z

治疗

院前

• 初步评估和病史：
- 意识水平。
- 格拉斯哥昏迷量表评分。
- 运动缺陷。
- 其他缺陷。
• SAH 患者可能因意识水平急剧恶化紧急气管插管。
• 应该建立静脉通路。
• 吸氧。
• 监测心率。
• 应该将患者转运到有急诊 CT 和 ICU 能力的医院。

初步稳定/治疗

• 呼吸道护理，按以下复苏：
- 快速插管。
- 在插管过程中，因钝伤使颅内压升高者，用非去极化肌松剂进行预处理。
- 气管插管前可予利多卡因和芬太尼减少神经刺激。
- 心电监测和脉搏血氧测定。
- 建立适当的静脉通路。
• 神经外科急会诊。

急诊治疗/程序

• 防止再出血：
- 在动脉瘤破裂后的前几小时出血风险最高。
• 控制颅内压：
- 将床头抬高 30°。
- 用止吐药和大便软化剂防止呕吐和排便增加颅内压。
- 实施控制性通气使 $PCO_2=30$。
- Meta 分析结果提示快速给予高渗盐水比应用甘露醇更加有效，但其对长期的临床结局的影响尚未明确。
- 保持尿量＞50 ml/h。
• 血压控制：
- 保持血压在正常水平。
- 防止再出血与脑低灌注。
- 目标平均动脉压 100～120 mmHg，收缩压＜160 mmHg：
◦ 拉贝洛尔、肼屈嗪、硝普钠或尼卡地平片。
- 纠正血容量不足：
◦ 应该在 SAH 96 h 内开始。
◦ 液体复苏低血压。
• 脑血管痉挛：
- SAH 后可能导致继发性缺血和梗死：
- 口服尼莫地平可改善功能结果。
◦ 用药前神经外科医师会诊。
- 经颅多普勒监测。
• 充分止痛。
• 癫痫发作：
- 苯二氮䓬类药物静脉治疗。
- 考虑出血后预防性抗惊厥药。
• 纠正温度、电解质、葡萄糖或 pH 异常。
• 治疗凝血功能障碍、血小板减少症和严重贫血。
• 监测并纠正肺水肿和心律失常。
• 抗纤维蛋白溶解疗法：
- 在开始之前神经外科医师会诊。
- 考虑到再次出血的高危患者动脉瘤破裂后立即给予治疗，并将其与动脉瘤治疗和低血压监测相结合。
• 当患者稳定时，加急转诊到神经外科医院是必需的。

药物治疗

抗痉挛药

• 地西泮：5～10 mg(儿童：0.2～0.3 mg/kg)，静脉注射或肌内注射，q10～1 min，最大剂量 30 mg(儿童：10 mg)。
• 芬太尼：1～3 μg/kg(成人和儿童)，静脉注射，q1～4 h。
• 磷苯妥英：15～20 苯妥英类相当量 PE/kg(成人和儿童)静脉注射；维持量 4～6 mg/(kg・d)静脉注射。
• 肼屈嗪：10～20 mg(儿童：0.1～0.5 mg/kg，静脉注射)，q30 min～4 h。
• 拉贝洛尔：20 mg 静脉推注，然后 40～80 mg q10 min；最大剂量 300 mg；继续静脉注射连续输注 0.5～2 mg/min[儿童：0.4～1 mg/(kg・h)静脉注射连续输注；最多 3 mg/(kg・h)。
• 利多卡因：1～1.5 mg/kg(成人和儿童)。
• 劳拉西泮：2～4 mg(儿童：0.03～0.05 mg/kg；最大剂量 4 mg)，静脉注射，q15 min，必要时。
• 咪达唑仑：1～2 mg(儿童：0.15 mg/kg，静脉×1)，静脉内给药。
• 吗啡：2～10 mg(儿童：0.05～0.2 mg/kg 静脉注射)，q2～4 h，必要时。
• 尼卡地平：静脉滴注，5～15 mg/h(儿童：未建立安全性)。
• 尼莫地平：60 mg，口服或 NGT，q4 h(儿童：未建立安全性)。
• 硝普鲁司德：0.25～10 μg/(kg・min)，静脉注射连续输注(成人和儿童)。
• 昂丹司琼：4～8 mg(儿童：0.1～0.15 mg/kg，最大剂量 4 mg)，口服、肌内注射或静脉注射，每日 3 次。
• 苯妥英：15～20 mg/kg 静脉注射至最大 50 mg/min；最大剂量 1.5 g；维持 4～6 mg/(kg・d)静脉注射(成人和儿童)。
• 异丙嗪：12.5～25 mg(儿童＞2 岁：0.25～1 mg/kg；最大剂量 25 mg)，口服、肌内注射或静脉注射，q4～6 h，必要时。

颅内压(ICP)控制

• 芬太尼：气管插管时予 2～5 μg/kg 控制 ICP；1～3 μg/kg，静脉输注，q1～4 h，必要时。

• 高渗盐水：250 ml 3%（513 mmol/L）或 30 mL 23.4%（4000 mmol/L）经中心静脉给药，给药时间不小于 20 min；血清钠目标范围 145～150 mmol/L；但应避免血钠浓度变化＞12 mmol/24 h，以防渗透性脱髓鞘病变。

• 甘露醇：静注：0.25～1 g/kg；q6～8 h 重复一次，目标渗透压 300～320 mOsm/kg（儿童用量相同）。

手术/其他程序

• 神经外科会诊。

• 早期手术或血管内介入治疗可预防血管痉挛并改善预后。

随访

进一步处理

入院指征

• 所有 SAH 患者都应该入住 ICU。

• CT 检查结果阴性和不明确的 LP 结果的患者应接受观察。

出院指征

• 阴性的 CT 和 LP 结果，症状发作＜2 周的患者。

• 门诊随访头痛治疗和进一步评估。

转诊问题

尽早转到中心医院，神经外科医师和血管内专家诊治。

预后

• 在抵达医院之前，死亡率是 12%。

• 最终死亡率超过 50%。

• 在"少量出血"或早期发现动脉瘤破裂的情况下，采用早期手术或介入方法可改善预后。

要点和误区

• 在急性头痛的鉴别诊断中未考虑 SAH。

• 未能评估以前的头痛治疗是否完整（CT 和 LP）。

• 目前 CT 是确认 SAH 的更为可靠的检查方式。

• 脑脊液颜色变黄可能有助于确认 SAH，但不是用以排除蛛网膜下腔出血的可靠指标。

主动脉闭塞 Arterial Occlusion

David W. Schoenfeld · Christie L. Fritz　赵洁　王海嵘　潘曙明 译

基础知识

描述

外周动脉的突发阻塞导致肢体血供受到即刻严重的危害，甚至可能发生坏死。

• 动脉栓塞：
- 血栓或斑块。
- 源于动脉瘤或动脉粥样硬化损伤。
- 栓子经常嵌顿在动脉急性狭窄部位。
- 75%的栓子涉及四肢脉管系统：
  ◦ 股动脉：28%。
  ◦ 手臂：20%。
  ◦ 腹主动脉与髂动脉系统：17%。
  ◦ 腘动脉：17%。
  ◦ 内脏和其他：9%。

• 血栓形成。

• 动脉夹层。

• 创伤：
- 挤压伤。
- 压迫。
- 动脉挫伤和血栓形成。
- 动脉横断伤。

• 肢体缺血＞6 h 通常会导致功能障碍或肢体丢失：
- 如果是慢性急性发作，则侧支循环可能会使组织保留超过 6 h。
- 远端血流完全取决于侧支循环。

• 由于流量低，血栓随着时间的流逝向近端和远端延伸。

病因

• 栓子：
- 心房颤动。
- 心肌梗死。
- 心脏瓣膜疾病。
- 心内膜炎。
- 心房黏液瘤。
- 动脉瘤。
- 粥样硬化斑块。
- 反常栓塞：
  ◦ 卵圆孔未闭。

• 血栓形成：
- 血管移植。
- 动脉粥样硬化。
- 动脉瘤的血栓形成。
- 挤压综合征。
- 凝血功能异常。
- 低血流状态。
- 肝素诱导的血栓症。

• 动脉夹层：
- 内膜片。
- 夹层。
- 假性动脉瘤。
- 医源性：
  ◦ 导管置入。
  ◦ 动脉造影。
  ◦ 血管成形术。
  ◦ 动脉穿刺并发症。
- 穿透伤：
  ◦ 枪击伤、刺伤、散弹枪、弹片伤。
  ◦ 应用静脉药物。
- 钝器伤：
  ◦ 关节脱位。
  ◦ 骨折。
  ◦ 筋膜室综合征。

诊断

症状和体征

• 突然起病，肢体温度降低，疼痛。

• 6 P 征：
- 疼痛：
  ◦ 渐进性，初期严重程度逐渐加重而后随着进行性感觉丧失疼痛逐渐减轻。
  ◦ 远端向近端发展。
  ◦ 栓塞起病突然。
- 苍白。
- 感觉异常。

Z

- 麻痹。
- 无脉(后期发现)。
- 皮温低。
• 渐进性外周神经功能缺损：
- 早期丧失本体感觉和轻触觉。
- 随后丧失感觉，随后乏力。
• 蓝趾综合征：
- 一个或多个足趾变为蓝色或蓝紫色。
- 患趾常伴有疼痛。
- 发绀初期按压或抬高患肢皮色苍白。
• 严重血管闭塞和预后不良的体征：
- 缺少毛细血管血流。
- 皮肤花斑。
- 远端脉搏消失。
- 肢体麻痹。

病史

• 起病时间。
• 跛行或者抽搐的病史：
- 活动后可再现的特定肌群不适，休息后可缓解。
- 通过用药史鉴别血栓或栓塞的危险因素。

体格检查

• 感觉丧失。
• 肌无力。
• 皮肤颜色改变。
• 脉搏消失。
• 慢性动脉血供不足的体征：
- 毛发缺失。
- 皮肤萎缩。
• 踝臂血压指数测量：
- 用多普勒流量计准确测量上臂收缩压。
- 记录双侧上臂和双侧踝部胫动脉血压值。
- 下肢收缩压和上臂肱动脉收缩压的比值：
◦ 下肢血压测量时将袖带置于踝上方。
◦ 将多普勒置于胫后动脉或足背动脉。
- 慢性 PVD<0.9。
- 急性动脉闭塞<0.5。
• 将肢体温暖部分和低温部分分界估计阻塞水平。

基本检查

> **注意**
> 禁忌抬高患肢，冷敷或冰敷，热敷患肢。

诊断检查与说明

实验室检查

• 电解质/阴离子间隙。
• 血尿素氮。
• 肌酐。
• 全血细胞计数。
• 肌酸磷酸激酶。

影像学检查

• 由于急诊室影像学检查应用受限，大部分临床决策基于临床表现。
• 多普勒超声：
- 为下肢动脉狭窄提供图像。
• CT 血管造影：
- 多探头，成像效果接近血管造影。
- 和血管造影一样，需要静脉注射造影剂和放射线暴露。
• MRI：
- 是血管造影的另一种可行的选择。
- 非侵入性。
- 无需造影物质。
• 血管造影。

分类

• 1类：可逆性。
- 疼痛但无麻痹或感觉缺失。
- 需要关注，但并非即刻危及生命。
• 2类：有威胁，但可挽救。
- 2A：部分感觉缺失，无肢体麻痹，即刻无生命威胁。
- 2B：感觉和运动丧失，需要立即治疗。
• 3类：无法挽回。
- 感觉丧失，麻痹，毛细血管血流缺失，皮肤花斑，动脉多普勒血流缺失。
- 需要截肢。

鉴别诊断

• 腰椎疾病。
• 机械性背痛。
• 晚期的粥样硬化性疾病引起的心输出量减少。
• 冻伤。
• 外周神经病变。
• 腹部动脉瘤。
• 踝部软组织损伤。
• 深静脉血栓症。
• 脓毒性血栓性静脉炎。
• 浅表血栓性静脉炎。
• 创伤，外周血管损伤。

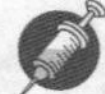

治疗

院前

• 早期识别和快速转运至急诊部。
• 将肢体处于下垂位置。
• 保持肢体温暖。
• 鼻导管给氧。
• 阿司匹林。

急诊治疗/程序

• 血管外科医师会诊。
• 负荷量肝素静脉注射后静脉滴注维持。
• 1类：可逆性。
- 通常由于血栓形成引起。
- 应用动脉内溶栓药物还是手术血管再通或者血管内修复依赖于肢体存活能力。
• 2类：有威胁，但可挽救。
- 立即手术血管再通。
- 有指征的话进行取栓术。
- 术后进行血管造影和口服抗凝药。
• 3类：无法挽回。
- 截肢。
- 临床评估，影像学检查通常不需要。
- 止痛。

药物治疗

肝素：根据体重计算抗凝治疗方案，经典方案为 80 U/kg 负荷量，18 U/(kg · h)，静脉维持。

随访

进一步处理

入院指征

所有临床诊断为急性动脉闭塞或(ABI<0.5)应该在急诊血管外科医师会诊后收住院。

出院指征

• 慢性动脉闭塞性疾病患者，疼痛缓解，ABI 测量结果稳定。
• 无其他急性医疗问题(如新发心房颤动)。
• 确保血管外科随访。
• 健康宣教：患者出现任何症状复发或加重时及时复诊。

随访建议

• PVD 患者病情不严重或非急性，不需要住院治疗的可以出院血管外科随访。
• 各种运动和药物对疾病过程的潜在影响应被讨论。
• 应该考虑宣教关于戒烟、肢体保温和血管收缩药物的应用。

Z

椎基底动脉供血不足 Vertebrobasilar Insufficiency

Andrew K. Chang · Annette M. Grajny 吴昊 李文放 译

基础知识

描述

• 椎基底动脉(VB)血管系统供血脑后部,包括脑干、小脑和内耳。

• 2 个椎动脉(VA)来源于锁骨下动脉,形成脊髓前动脉,然后连接形成基底动脉。

• 支配脑和小脑的动脉在分支到 2 个大脑后动脉(PCA)之前来源于椎基底动脉系统,使得椎基底动脉循环障碍产生多种局灶性神经缺陷。

• 椎基底动脉供血不足(VBI)导致血栓形成,栓塞或低流量状态的椎基底动脉循环灌注不充分。

病因

• 机制:
- 血栓形成:
◦ 由于 VB 动脉粥样硬化和凝块形成引起的 VB 缺血。
- 栓子:
◦ 近端血管血栓栓塞导致的 VB 缺血。
- 低流量状态:
◦ VB 系统的低灌注来自全身性(如心源性休克)或局部(如锁骨下窃取)血流量减少。
- 不太常见的病因:
◦ 肌纤维发育不良。
◦ 高凝状态。

• 导致 VB 不足的缺血机制可导致先兆并导致 VB 区梗死。

• 严重的 VB 低灌注或循环流失可导致:
-"洛克-迪"综合征:
◦ 四肢瘫痪(只有眼睑或眼球运动),意识完好。
-"基底顶部"综合征:
◦ 脑桥和小脑功能障碍的意识水平降低。

诊断

症状和体征

所有的病史和体检都表现为间歇性。

病史

• 头晕、眩晕("轻度","非暴力";可能是孤立的发现)。

• 发病通常是突然和自发的,而不是因姿势引起。

• 可能会在几周内出现一连串症状。

•"掉落攻击"。

• 头痛。

• 恶心、呕吐。

• 轻度瘫痪/感觉异常。

• 发作。

• 昏厥。

• 定位于后循环的神经学症状:
- 视觉变化(复视、视力模糊、失明)。
- 脸或四肢麻木。
- 手臂或腿部虚弱。
- 手臂或腿运动迟缓。
- 意识丧失。
- 讲话困难。
- 吞咽困难。
- 颈部或肩部疼痛。

体格检查

• 脑干:
-"交叉"的发现(即同侧面部和对侧躯干功能缺陷)。
- 精神状态或反应改变的。
- 呼吸力减弱。
- Horner 综合征(眼内炎、眼睑下垂、瞳孔缩小、无汗症)。
- 核间性眼肌麻痹。
- 眼球震颤(特别是无法觉察,垂直/旋转)。
- 麻痹/感觉异常。

• 脑神经:
- 眼外肌麻痹(如复视)。
- 瞳孔异常。
- 感觉异常、面部肌肉麻痹。
- 听觉异常。
- 吞咽困难。
- 构音障碍。

• 大脑皮质(PCA 循环):
- 视觉障碍(如同侧偏盲)。

• 小脑:
- 共济失调。
- 辨距不良。
- 步态异常。

• 心脑血管:
- 颈动脉/椎基底动脉杂音。
- 不规则、不对称、虚弱的脉搏。

基本检查

• 急诊头部 CT(非增强)评估出血(薄壁组织质、蛛网膜下腔、创伤)及大面积急性梗死,优先于病理。

• 彻底的神经和心脏体格检查。

• 神经功能评估。

• 12 导联心电图用于心律失常和心肌缺血。

• CTA 和/或 MRA 用于后循环成像。

诊断检查与说明

实验室检查

• 全血细胞计数:
- 贫血、血小板减少症、红细胞增多症、血小板增多症。

• 凝血研究(PT、APTT):
- 低凝和高凝状态,为是否用抗凝剂和纤维蛋白溶解治疗提供依据。

• 电解质、BUN/肌酸酐、葡萄糖。

• 提示心肌缺血的有关指标。

• 尿液分析。

• ESR 用于系统性血管收缩药检测。

• 快速血浆反应素。

• 甲状腺刺激激素。

• 血脂代谢。

影像学检查

• 急诊头部 CT(非增强)。

• 头颈部 CT 血管造影(CTA)评估后循环和有可能行急性血管介入。

• 胸部 X 线片;心脏和大血管病理学 CTA 检查。

• MRI/MRA 改善缺血性病灶和脑血流循环的表征(如先天性 VB 异常、排除 VA 剥离)。

• 心内膜超声心动图。

• 颈部多普勒超声。

• 经颅多普勒超声。

诊断步骤/外科

• 用于诊断的神经血管造影术。

• 直接动脉内血栓溶解疗法、血管成形术、支架置入、栓子去除术仍在研究中。

鉴别诊断

• 中枢神经系统:
- CVA(出血性或缺血性):
◦ 脑。
◦ 小脑。
◦ 脑干。

Z

- 多发性硬化症。
- 偏头痛综合征。
- 癫痫(病灶)。
- 创伤性损伤/后震颤。
- 瘤。
- 血管畸形出血(动静脉畸形、蛛网膜下腔出血)。
- 脑干疝。
• 外周神经系统:
- 前庭神经炎。
• 耳朵、鼻、喉:
- 桥小脑角肿瘤。
- 耳道病理(异物、肿瘤)。
- 迷路炎/中耳炎。
- 梅尼埃病。
- 良性阵发性位置性眩晕。
• 心血管系统:
- 心律失常。
- 心肌缺血、梗死。
- 动脉瘤/解剖(VA、基底动脉、锁骨下动脉、主动脉)。
- 低血容量。
- 血管炎。
• 内分泌系统:
- 肾上腺功能不全。
- 甲状腺功能减退症。
• 血液系统:
- 贫血。
- 凝血功能障碍、高凝状态。
• 传染性:
- 脑炎、脑膜炎。
- 中耳炎、乳腺炎。
- 感染性休克。
- 梅毒。
• 新陈代谢:
- 低血糖症,高血糖。
- 电解质失衡。
• 毒理学:
- 共济失调:酒精、锂、苯妥英钠。
- 水杨酸中毒。
- 血清素综合征。
- 医源性。

Z

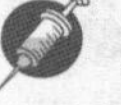

治疗

院前

• ABC 管理。
• 手指末端葡萄糖测量。
• 纳洛酮(如果需要)。
• 通知:
- 如果气道损害或血流动力学不稳定,请紧急与医疗机构联系。
- 考虑激活卒中警报。

初步稳定/治疗

• ABC 管理。
• 补充氧气。
• 心脏监测仪和脉搏血氧仪。
• 用生理盐水建立静脉通路。

急诊治疗/程序

• 脑血管灌注管理:
- 支持性护理。
- 仰卧位。
- 如果没有出血,使用抗血小板药物。
- 抗凝:
○ 如果栓塞源不稳定或进行性缺血症状等重要危险因素需考虑与神经科医师协商。
- 理想的血压目标不明确;将血压保持在患者预期的范围内(考虑慢性高血压)。
• 如果低血压:液体复苏,血管加压素或必要时输血液。
• 如果对于严重高血压(平均动脉压>140 mmHg,收缩压>220 mmHg,舒张压>130 mmHg)或出血、动脉瘤、剥离,心肌或其他器官功能障碍:可静脉用降血压药物。
• 胃肠道:
- NPO(静脉补液水化,维持血糖正常)。
- 止吐。
• 咨询:
- 神经内科。
- 用于神经血管造影的血管介入放射学。

药物治疗

• 阿替普酶:60 min 后 0.9 mg/kg;开始10%的剂量作为静脉推注。
• 阿司匹林:325 mg,口服。
• 氯吡格雷:75 mg,口服。
• 华法林(心房颤动剂量):2~5 mg,口服,负荷剂量。
• 肝素(心房纤维化剂量):50~60 U/kg,静脉推注,然后以 12~18 U/kg,静脉输注,目标是 APTT 50~70 s。
• 拉贝洛尔:2 min 内 20~40 mg,静脉;然后 40~80 mg 静脉,q10 min(最多 300 mg,静脉)。
• 氯苯甲嗪:25 mg,口服,q8~12 h。
• 纳洛酮:0.4~2 mg,肌内注射/静脉,q2~3 min,必要时。
• 硝普钠:0.25~10 μg/(kg·min)静脉输注,最大剂量 10 μg/(kg·min)。
• 昂丹司琼:4 mg,静脉。
• 异丙嗪:12.5~25 mg,口服/PRI/静脉,q6~8 h。
• 噻氯吡啶:250 mg,口服,每日 2 次。

随访

进一步处理

入院指征

• 入 ICU 标准:
- 精神状态改变已影响呼吸。
- 血流动力学不稳定。
- 恶性心律失常。
- 给予阿替普酶。
• 承认医院识别或排除 VB 缺血的病因,并防止复发或进展到 VB 循环血管内血栓事件,特别是在以下人群:
- 老年。
- 无法走动。
- 无法忍受口服摄入。
- 出院后无法安排随访。
- 新的或变化的神经缺陷。
- 持续性头晕。
- 昏厥。
- 血管风险因素。

出院指征

• 考虑在人群中不进行随后的随访,具体如下:
- 都没有以上纳入的条件。
- 症状学的替代解释。

转诊问题

• VB 缺血相关的转诊由急救医师安排/推荐。
• 根据症状学的替代解释,安排与 PCP 或适当专科医师(如神经病学、耳鼻咽喉科、血管外科)进行快速转诊。

随访建议

• VB 缺血相关随访由接诊团队安排/推荐。
• 其他后续行动的紧迫性和性质由替代性的症状学解释决定。

要点和误区

• 总是考虑 VB 不足引起头晕、眩晕、精神状态改变、晕厥和重叠/非典型神经系统表现。
• 早期神经科会诊。

• VBI更有可能发生在伴随神经系统症状并伴有心血管事件风险因素的自发性血管痉挛患者中。

• 由于缺乏禁忌证，VB一开始就抗血栓/抗栓塞治疗。

• 考虑转移到脑卒中中心进行神经血管内治疗。

子宫内膜异位症 Endometriosis

Francis L. Counselman 单怡 译

基础知识

描述

• 子宫内膜组织和腺体出现于子宫外。
• 一种雌激素依赖性的慢性炎症疾病。
• 影响全部人群中的2%～10%，50%的不育女性，50%～60%的妇女/少女盆腔痛。
• 在盆腔、卵巢、子宫韧带(由于月经逆行)和远离子宫的部位，包括肠和肺，出现子宫内膜组织。

病因

未明。

儿科注意事项

不早于初潮前。

危险因素

• 月经流出部位的解剖性梗阻。
• 月经初潮早。
• 月经周期短。
• 遗传疾病，一级亲属中有着7倍以上的流行性。

诊断

症状和体征

既往史

• 痛经(50%～90%)。
• 深部盆腔痛。
• 性交痛。
• 功能性子宫出血。
• 下腹痛。
• 恶心、腹胀。
• 不孕(30%～50%)。

体格检查

• 盆腔检查局部疼痛或压痛。
• 沿宫骶韧带触痛。
• 子宫后倾。
• 直肠阴道结节。
• 盆腔包块。
• 由于子宫内膜位置不同体格检查阳性体征不同。
• 胸部子宫内膜异位，月经期间可出现月经性气胸。

基本检查

• 妊娠试验。
• GC、衣原体检测。
• 根据既往史和体格检查所需的其他检查。
• 很少在急诊室诊断。

诊断检查与说明

实验室检查

• 妊娠试验。
• GC、衣原体检测。
• 如果出血测血细胞比容。
• 如果大量出血，测血型和输血。
• 根据既往史和体格检查所需的其他检查。

影像学检查

• 超声(敏感性11%)。
• 多普勒超声。
• CT扫描(敏感性15%)。
• MRI(敏感性69%，特异性75%)。
• 急诊影像没太大帮助。

诊断步骤/外科

通常需要腹腔镜手术和活检确诊。

鉴别诊断

• 阑尾炎。
• 功能失调性子宫出血。
• 异位妊娠。
• 炎症性肠病。
• 肠易激综合征。
• 经期痉挛、痛经。
• 卵巢囊肿。
• 卵巢扭转。
• 盆腔炎性疾病。
• 输卵管卵巢脓肿。

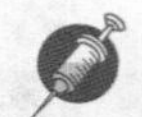

治疗

院前

• 需要时给予镇静。
• 必要时给予镇痛。

初步稳定/治疗

• 等渗液体静脉输注纠正失血后的低血压和心动过速。
• 如果大量出血，可能需要输注红细胞悬液。

急诊治疗/程序

• 镇痛。
• 在妇科医师或初级保健医师指导下口服避孕药(甲羟孕酮酯)或促性腺激素释放激素激动剂(醋酸亮丙瑞林)。
• 大量失血，疼痛或严重的并发症，请妇产科会诊。

药物治疗

• 布洛芬：400～800 mg，口服，q6～8 h(最大剂量3.2 g/d)。
• 对乙酰氨基酚：325～650 mg，口服，q4～6 h(最大剂量4 g/d)。
• 酮洛酸：15～30 mg，静脉注射；或30～60 mg，肌内注射。
• 吗啡：4～8 mg，肌内注射/静脉注射，或等效药物镇痛。

一线用药

• 布洛芬：400～800 mg，口服，q6～8 h(最大剂量3.2 g/d)。
• 对乙酰氨基酚：325～650 mg，口服，q4～6 h(最大剂量4 g/d)。
• 酮洛酸：15～30 mg，静脉注射；或30～60 mg，肌内注射。

随访

进一步处理

入院指征

• 顽固性疼痛。

• 大出血。

• 诊断不明确。

• 需要进一步的检查和处理。

• 腹膜刺激征。

出院指征

大多数疑诊患者疼痛控制后，可以出院，妇科医师随访。

转诊问题

疑诊子宫内膜异位症的患者应请妇产科医师评估和处理。

要点和误区

• 发生于所有人群中的 2%～10%。

• 子宫内膜异位症常引起周期性盆腔疼痛。

• 在急诊室很少被诊断，出现症状多年后才明确诊断。

• 排除其他急诊情况并对症处理。

• 子宫内膜异位症是一种慢性疾病，需要妇科医师或初级保健医师门诊随访。

子痫前期和子痫 Preeclampsia/Eclampsia

Bonnie Kaplan　瞿金龙　林兆奋 译

基础知识

描述

流行病学

• 妊娠合并高血压：

- 妊娠期妇女发病率为 10%。
- 死亡孕产妇的 7.4%。
- 早产的主要原因。

• 妊娠期高血压(GH)：

- 妊娠引起的高血压。
- 分娩后血压恢复正常。
- 妊娠妇女的发病率为 6%～17%。

• 产前子痫前期：

- 生长激素合并蛋白尿或生长激素合并终末器官损害：
  ◦ 血小板减少：血小板＜100 000/μl。
  ◦ 肾功能不全：Cr＞1.1 mg/dl。
  ◦ 肝功能受损：LFT＞2 倍正常水平。
  ◦ 肺水肿。
  ◦ 脑或视觉症状。
- 在所有孕妇中占 4.6%。

• 子痫：

- 子痫前期合并癫痫发作。

• 产后子痫前期：

- 发生在产后 6 周内。
- 无高血压病史。
- 占产后人群的 5%。
- 非洲妇女的发病率高。

• HELLP 综合征：

- 发生在子痫或子痫前期。
- 出现溶血。
- 重点监测肝功能。
- 血小板低。

• 并发先兆子痫前期：

- 慢性高血压合并子痫前期。
- 多胎妊娠妇女合并慢性高血压发病率上升至 25%。
- 危险因素。
  ◦ 非洲裔美国人。
  ◦ 降压药物的使用。

• 慢性高血压：

- 收缩压＞140 mmHg 或舒张压＞90 mmHg。
- 妊娠 20 周内或产后 12 周检测 2 次血压。

病因

• 子痫前期：

- 不完全胎盘植入和再灌注。
- 导致血管生长因子的减少和母体的胎盘循环碎片增多。
- 导致母体血管系统功能障碍增加。

• 子痫：

- 子痫患者中有 1/3 患者并没有高血压病史。

• 危险因素：

- 生育年龄过小或过大。
- 流产。
- 多次妊娠。
- 葡萄胎。
- 吸烟。
- 体质指数增高。
- 糖尿病、胶原血管病。
- 有高血压或肾病病史。
- 有产前子痫前期的病史(增加 7.5%～10%的风险)。
- 子痫的独立危险因素。
  ◦ 未产妇。
  ◦ 孕妇年龄。
  ◦ 妊娠期高血压。

诊断

• 妊娠期高血压：

- 直至妊娠 20 周均无高血压病史。
- 两次测量结果均为收缩压＞140 mmHg 或舒张压＞90 mmHg。
- 重度：收缩压＞160 mmHg 或舒张压＞110 mmHg。

• 子痫前期：

- 妊娠期高血压合并蛋白尿。
- 24 h 尿蛋白＞300 mg。
- 尿蛋白(＋)。
- 轻度。
  ◦ 收缩压＜160 mmHg 或舒张压＜110 mmHg。
  ◦ 血小板正常。
  ◦ 肝功能正常。
  ◦ 无中枢异常。
- 重度。
  ◦ 收缩压＞160 mmHg 或舒张压＞110 mmHg。
  ◦ 24 h 尿蛋白定量 5 g。
  ◦ 两次尿常规显示(＋＋＋)。
  ◦ 少尿。
  ◦ 血小板减少。
  ◦ 右上象限疼痛。
  ◦ 肝功能受损。
  ◦ 出现中枢神经系统症状。
  ◦ 宫内发育迟缓。
  ◦ 视力受损。
  ◦ 肺水肿。

• HELLP 综合征：

- 溶血。
- 肝酶升高。
- 低血小板。
- 可伴以下现象：

◦ 肺水肿。
◦ 肾功能衰竭。
◦ 肝功能衰竭。
◦ 败血症。
◦ 肺部疾病。
◦ 脑卒中(中风)。

注意

在急诊室,如果临床上高度怀疑,不应等待 4 h 再重复测量升高的血压。

症状和体征

• 子痫前期病史。
• 经产数。
• 体重增加。
• 双腿水肿。
• 腹部疼痛。
• 恶心、呕吐。
• 气促。
• 头痛。
• 视觉改变。
• 黄疸。
• 脑卒中(中风)症状。

体格检查

• 连续监测血压。
• 仔细触诊右上腹。
• 注意四肢水肿。
• 神经精神系统检查:
- 深腱反射。
- 精神状态的改变。
- 视敏度。

基本检查

• 连续血压监测。
• 尿常规。
• 血常规、肝功能、肾功能、尿酸。
• B超。
• 胎儿监护。
• 根据胎儿先露的位置决定头颅 CT 的必要性。

诊断检查与说明

实验室检查

• 尿常规:
- 蛋白质>1(+)(30 mg/dl)。
- 蛋白质>1(+)需要进一步检查 24 h 尿蛋白总量。
- 尿沉渣监测寻找红细胞、白细胞、管型。
• 血常规。
• 肝肾功能。
• 尿酸。
• 乳酸脱氢酶。
• D-二聚体。
• 纤维蛋白原水平。
• 凝血功能。

影像学检查

• B超:
- 胎龄。
- 胎儿发育情况以及是否有胎儿窘迫。
- 羊水过少。
• 胎儿监测,无应激试验。
• 头颅 CT:排除坏死出血。

诊断步骤/外科

• 腰椎穿刺:排除感染或蛛网膜下腔出血。
• 尿毒理学检测:排除药物滥用。
- 可卡因。
- 甲氧苯丙胺。

鉴别诊断

• 原发性高血压。
• 肾衰竭或胶原血管病。
• 葡萄胎、胎儿水肿。
• 药物滥用。
• 癫痫。
• 脑炎。
• 脑膜炎。
• 脑病。
• 颅脑肿瘤。
• 颅内出血。

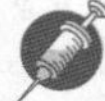

治疗

院外

• ABC 管理。
• 氧疗。
• 左侧卧位。

初步稳定/治疗

• ABC 管理。
• 输纯氧。
• 左侧卧位(减少下腔静脉压,提高心输出量)。
• 孕产妇心电监测,指脉氧监测。
• 使用硫酸镁抗癫痫发作。

急诊治疗/程序

• 准备紧急剖宫产。
• 硫酸镁预防和抗癫痫。
• 肼屈嗪或拉贝洛尔降血压:
- 目标是降血压至起始时血压的75%,然后尽量保持<160/100 mmHg。
• 镁的毒性:
- 低血压。
- 膝跳反射消失。
- 尿量减少。
- 肌酐升高。
- 钙糖酸盐倒置。
• 气管插管以保持呼吸道畅通,防止癫痫持续状态及窒息。
• 分娩力(描记)图和胎心监护。
• OB 转归:
◦ 一旦发病均会经历子痫前期-子痫谱。
- 妊娠<30 周进行子痫的预期处理。
- 紧急处理严重的症状:症状及剖宫产。

药物治疗

一线用药

• 硫酸镁:10 g 肌内注射或 4 g 静脉注射,进而转为 1~2 g/h 维持。
- 硫酸镁最大剂量不超过 1 g/min。
- 血清硫酸镁的目标值为 4~7 mEq/L。
• 肼屈嗪:5~20 mg 静脉注射。
• 拉贝洛尔:起始为 10 mg 静脉注射,继而以 5~10 mg,增量,增加至理想水平。

二线用药

• 地西泮(安定):硫酸镁无效时,5~10 mg 静脉注射。
• 磷苯妥英:相当于 15~20 mg 苯妥英钠静脉注射×1(最大剂量相当于 150 mg/min 苯妥英钠静脉注射)。
• 苯妥英钠:15~18 mg/kg 静脉注射用于癫痫持续状态,不要超过 25~50 mg/min。
• 葡萄糖酸钙:1 g 静脉注射。

随访

进一步处理

入院指征

• 子痫前期。
• 子痫。
• HELLP 综合征。
• 监护室中分娩。

出院指征

• 子痫前期患者高血压引起并发症。
• 无症状。
• 确定停止产科随访。

随访建议

• 随访至分娩。
• 重新随访:

- 头痛。
- 腹痛。
- 腿部水肿。
- 尿量减少。
- 气促。

要点和误区

• 分娩是治疗子痫和子痫前期最有效的手段。

• 血压 130/80 mmHg 的孕妇需要重视，防止子痫。

• 需要注意产后 30 日内仍需要考虑子痫前期/子痫：
- 水肿。
- 气促。
- 头痛。
- 癫痫。

• 子痫前期和子痫的患者需要注意保持呼吸道通畅：
- 减少气道充血引起的狭窄。
- 可能出现气道水肿。
- 使用直径较小的气管导管。
- 如需要使用气管镜引导。
- 风险高。

紫癜 Purpura

Ashley L. Greiner　郑金浩　毛恩强 译

 基础知识

■ 描述

• 血管内的血外渗至皮肤或皮下组织引起的皮损。

• 毛细血管脆性增加、皮肤结构变差、血小板功能异常均可引起紫癜。

• 紫癜受(通过玻璃载玻片压迫时)压力不会完全变白。

• 病变的大小不同而命名有所差异：
- 瘀点(≤4 mm)。
- 紫癜(5～10 mm)。
- 瘀斑(>10 mm)。

• 颜色取决于出血的深度和起始时间：
- 红色：考虑出血在表面并且最近发病。
- 深部出血为紫色。
- 深紫色、褐色、黄色、蓝绿色：后面进一步解释。

• 肺接触性紫癜：
- 单纯性出血或微血管阻塞，缺血性出血。
- 一般由于血小板异常引起：
  ◦ 生成减少。
  ◦ 破坏增多。
  ◦ 分布改变。
  ◦ 功能异常。

• 接触引起的紫癜：
- 一般由于血管病变：
  ◦ 自身免疫性疾病、白细胞破碎相关的小血管炎。
  ◦ 对各种抗原过敏。
  ◦ 形成循环免疫复合物，沉积在毛细血管静脉壁，激活补体，趋化多形核白细胞。
  ◦ 释放酶损伤血管壁，引起血液渗出。
  ◦ 血管炎性病变在免疫力弱的患者中可能并不明显。

■ 病因

• 非接触性紫癜：
- 病毒：
  ◦ 人肠道孤病毒。
  ◦ 柯萨奇病毒。
  ◦ 麻疹病毒。
  ◦ 细小病毒 B19。
- 药物：
  ◦ 对乙酰氨基酚(扑热息痛)。
  ◦ 别嘌醇。
  ◦ 抗凝药物。
  ◦ 阿司匹林。
  ◦ 地高辛。
  ◦ 呋塞米。
  ◦ 金属盐。
  ◦ 甲基多巴。
  ◦ 利多卡因。
  ◦ 非甾体类解热镇痛抗炎药。
  ◦ 青霉素。
  ◦ 保泰松。
  ◦ 奎纳定。
  ◦ 奎宁。
  ◦ 利福平。
  ◦ 甾体化合物。
  ◦ 磺胺类药物。
  ◦ 噻嗪类。
- 营养缺乏：
  ◦ 维生素 K 缺乏。
  ◦ 维生素 C 缺乏(坏血病)。
- 骨髓疾病。
- 脾功能亢进。
- 特发性血小板减少性紫癜(ITP)。
- 弥散性血管内凝血(DIC)。
- 血栓性血小板减少性紫癜。
- 肝或肾功能不全。
- 血小板减少症(<50 000/mm^3)。
- 血小板增多症(>1 000 000/mm^3)。
- 血管内压力出现高峰(分娩、呕吐、阵发性咳嗽)。
- 血友病。
- 日光性紫癜(仅发生在日光暴露的区域)。
- 输血后。

• 接触后紫癜：
- 病毒引起：
  ◦ 人肠道孤病毒。
  ◦ 柯萨奇病毒。
  ◦ 乙型肝炎。
- 链球菌性咽炎。
- 药物。
  ◦ 别嘌醇。
  ◦ 流感疫苗。
  ◦ 头孢类抗生素。
  ◦ 含金元素的药物。
  ◦ 肝素。
  ◦ 肼屈嗪。
  ◦ 碘。
  ◦ 左旋咪唑。
  ◦ 甲氧氯普胺。
  ◦ 青霉素。
  ◦ 保泰松。
  ◦ 苯妥英钠。
  ◦ 奎钠定。
  ◦ 奎宁。
  ◦ 链霉素。
  ◦ 磺胺类药物。
  ◦ 噻嗪类。
  ◦ 抗血小板药物。
- 恶性肿瘤。
- 自身免疫和结缔组织病。

Z

- 淋病。
- 脑膜炎球菌感染。
- 假单胞菌(深脓疱、坏疽)。
- 落基山斑疹热。
- 免疫力低下的患者(念珠菌、曲霉)。
- 由于微生物侵犯血管引起闭塞(一般为免疫力低下的患者)：毛霉病、曲霉病和播散性粪类圆线虫病。
- 由于微血管血小板增加引起闭塞(肝素相关性坏死)。
- 寒冷相关的凝固或凝集(冷球蛋白血症)。
- 局部或全身凝血异常：猩红热、嗜盐弧菌、恶性水痘和出血性麻疹(此两种疾病均罕见)、香豆素坏死。
- 栓塞：胆固醇、晶体、血栓(心房黏液瘤、感染性心内膜炎、多发性骨髓瘤)。

儿科注意事项

• 亨诺-许兰综合征。
• 溶血性尿毒症综合征。
• 川崎病。
• 新生儿：
- 风疹和巨细胞病毒感染情况下，髓外生成红细胞(像蓝莓松饼宝宝)。
- 暴发性紫癜(蛋白C和S缺乏)。
- 产妇特发性血小板减少性紫癜。
- 威斯科特-奥尔德里奇综合征。

诊断

症状和体征

• 可触及或不可触及，非烫伤。
• 大小：
- 瘀点(≤4 mm)。
- 紫癜(5～10 mm)。
- 瘀斑(>10 mm)。
• 形状：
- 圆形病灶：由白细胞破坏形成的栓子引起。
- 不规则(网状)病灶：由感染物的栓子引起。
- 环形或红斑多形性细胞瘤(靶病变)。
• 分布：
- 全身性的：考虑DIC和脑膜炎球菌血症。
- 依从性的：在下肢末端最常见(血管静水压增高)。
- 肢体末端：仅在肢体末端。
- 口唇黏膜：考虑特发性血小板减少性紫癜。
• 低血压。
• 精神状态改变。
• 牙龈出血。
• 鼻出血。
• 血尿。
• 发热。
• 萎靡不振。
• 关节疼痛/关节血肿。
• 肌肉疼痛。
• 暴发性紫癜：
- 大、不规则瘀斑。
- 发热。
- 休克。
- DIC。
• 假单胞菌(深脓疱、坏疽)：
- 以水肿、红色丘疹起始。
- 在环带区水疱形成。
• 散播性淋病感染：
- 经常<10处皮损，紫色丘疹或脓性水疱分布在手伸面足踝和足趾侧。
- 发热。
- 关节疼痛。
• 脑膜炎球菌血症。
- 小面积皮肤梗死引起网状的紫癜。
- 可能出现在包括头、手掌、足底、黏膜、包括关节等地方。
- 发热。
- 头痛。
• 落基山斑疹热。
- 4～7日全身症状后，四肢远端包括手掌和足掌出现红斑，然后出现瘀斑。
- 发热。
- 头痛。
• 亨-希紫癜：
- 出现在下肢的伸肌方面及臀部。
- 约5日消退。
- 发热。
- 关节疼痛。
- 腹部疼痛。
- 血尿。
• 川崎病：
- 很少出现紫癜。
- 发热加以下4条：肢体末端多形性皮疹，双侧结膜炎，嘴唇和嘴巴的改变，单侧颈淋巴结肿大。
• 左旋咪唑掺入可卡因：
- 网状的坏死性紫癜累及耳、面部，可出现在任何地方。
- 中性粒细胞减少。
- 持续滥用的复发症状。

基本检查

• 获得完整病史。
• 之前出血的问题。
• 深静脉血栓、肺梗死提示因子Ⅴ突变引起。
• 脾切除术。
• 酒精和药物滥用。
• 出血性疾病的家族史。
• 高出血风险的药物。

诊断检查与说明

• 血小板计数：血小板数量不正常必须通过外周血涂片的手动检查核实。
• DIC筛选：患者出现中毒症状暗示可能是DIC前期。
• PT、APTT。
• 检验项目包括肝功能。
• 快速链球菌检测。
• 尿常规。
• 门诊患者的管理：
- 出血时间。
- 乙肝、丙肝血清学检查。
- 咽喉链球菌培养或抗链球菌溶血酶O滴度。
- 抗核抗体。
- 冷球蛋白类。
- 血小板功能检测。
- 血清补体。
- 血清蛋白电泳。
- von Willebrand因子缺乏症筛选。

鉴别诊断

• 微血管扩张性疾病：
- 樱桃状血管瘤。
- 遗传性出血性毛细血管扩张。
- 慢性光化性毛细血管扩张。
- 硬皮病。
- CREST综合征。
- 共济失调毛细血管扩张。
- 慢性肝脏疾病。
- 妊娠相关性毛细血管扩张症。
• 卡波西肉瘤和其他血管肉瘤。
• 法布里病。
• 新生儿髓外造血。
• 匐行性血管瘤。

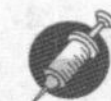

治疗

院前

• 建立静脉通路。
• 检测：
- 发热。

- 低血压。
- 精神状态改变情况。

■ 初步稳定/治疗

• 对于发热、低血压、精神状态改变或全身紫癜：
- 保持气道通畅。
- 静脉通路畅通。
- 液体复苏。
- 尽早静脉注射抗生素。

■ 急诊治疗/程序

• 依据经验对因治疗感染：
- 脑膜炎双球菌：头孢曲松（预防：利福平或环丙沙星）。
- 肺炎链球菌：头孢曲松，可以考虑使用哌拉西林。
- 立克次体：多西环素，孕妇使用氯霉素。

■ 药物治疗

• 头孢曲松：2 g[儿童：100 mg/(kg·24 h)]，静推，每日 2 次。
• 环丙沙星（预防）：500 mg，口服，每日 1 次。
• 氯霉素：75 mg/(kg·24 h)，口服或静推，每日 4 次。
• 多西环素：100 mg[儿童：4 mg/(kg·24 h)]，口服或静推，每日 2 次。
• 哌拉西林 G：400 万 U[儿童：240 000 U/(kg·24 h)]，静推，q4 h。
• 利福平（预防用药）：600 mg，口服，每日 2 次，持续服用 2 日。
• 新生儿败血症：氨苄西林 100 mg/(kg·24 h)，静推，q6 h 和庆大霉素 7.5 mg/(kg·24 h)，静推，q8 h[或头孢噻肟 200 mg/(kg·24 h)，静推，q6 h]。

随访

■ 进一步处理

入院指征

• 生命体征不稳定。
• 精神状态改变。
• 发热。

出院指征

• 危及生命的病因排除。
• 严重的细菌感染。
• 严重血小板减少症。

转诊问题

如果患者没有住院治疗，严重血液系统疾病、风湿病和恶性肿瘤需要在门诊深入评估，在医师检查前不进行接触性运动和服用抗血小板药物。

■ 随访建议

• 提供紧密的随访日程。
• 考虑同时随访皮肤科（皮肤活检）和血液科。

要点和误区

如果考虑患者的潜在感染，经验性使用抗生素抗菌谱覆盖脑膜炎球和落基山斑疹热引起的败血症。

紫外线角膜炎 Ultraviolet Keratitis

Megan Bevis Core · Yasuharu Okuda 张晟 林兆奋 译

基础知识

■ 描述

• 由于直接暴露于紫外线光造成角膜上皮损伤。
• 也被称为光性角膜炎、紫外线结膜炎、雪盲和焊工闪光。

■ 病因

• 工作相关的暴露见于焊接工人、电气师和机械师。
• 娱乐性暴露包括水上运动、雪上运动和日光浴。
• 当角膜吸收 290 nm 光波时发生，这一波长在紫外 B 和紫外 C 之间。
• 紫外线光渗透上皮伤害感受器轴突并摧毁前者从而引发从内皮神经末梢受刺激而产生的疼痛。
• 与暴露强度和持续时间相关。
• 尽管与紫外线角膜炎发作的相关性尚未得到证实，长期紫外线对眼睛的损害可能会导致翼状胬肉和某些形式的角膜变性。

诊断

■ 症状和体征

• 患者出现双眼痛、畏光、红肿和流泪。
• 无化脓性分泌物。
• 可能出现相关的面部水肿、眼睑肿胀、面部红斑和眼睑痉挛。

病史

• 引出在疼痛前暴露于紫外线 6～12 h 的经历。
• 获取其他相关病史，包括接触镜使用情况、过去的眼部病史（如外伤、手术、青光眼）、目前的药物治疗和药物过敏。
• 具体询问异物的风险。
• 除了疼痛，主诉还可能有：
- 畏光。
- 流泪。
- 异物感。

体格检查

• 视敏度可能轻微下降。
• 眼科检查提示球结膜水肿、刺痛、流泪。
• 严重病例可见到弥漫性角膜混浊。
• 眼内压正常。
• 用局部麻醉和荧光素进行裂隙灯检查。
- 多处角膜表面斑点病变或荧光素的弥漫性摄取。
- 可能会注意到保护眼睑的上或下边界有一条界限分明的线。

■ 基本检查

• 准确的病史包括暴露类型、暴露时间和暴露时长。
• 视敏度。
• 完全的眼部检查包括：
- 眼球运动。
- 球结膜、巩膜、角膜荧光素检查。
- 前房细胞和闪光检查。
- 翻转眼睑以查看异物。
- 眼压。

■ 诊断检查与说明

• 实验室检查：血液检查是不必要的，除非有大范围严重的日照烧伤或担心继发感染。

Z

• 影像学检查：详细采集病史可避免做眼周超声、CT、MRI 以寻找异物。

鉴别诊断

• 感染。
- 细菌或病毒性球结膜炎。
- 角膜溃疡。
• 过敏性球结膜炎。
• 角膜磨损。
• 创伤性虹膜炎。
• 异物。
• 酸、碱或热烧伤。
• 急性闭角型青光眼。

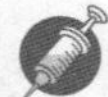

治疗

院前

当诊断确切，闭眼给予适当压力眼贴或轻微压眼睛可能获得暂时缓解。也可口服止痛药。

急诊治疗/程序

• 局部麻醉使裂隙灯检查容易进行。
• 如果必要给足够口服镇痛药。
• 局部应用抗生素软膏。
• 实施短效散瞳。
• 因为眼贴可能会延迟上皮再生，尽管有争议但为了舒适可以使用。
- 温和压力下的软双重修复。
- 如果两只眼睛都受到影响，贴两只眼睛，或贴受影响更严重的眼睛。
- 应该保持 24 h。

药物治疗

• 局部麻醉药剂（仅用于后续阶段）。
- 0.5%盐酸丁卡因滴眼液：1～2 滴滴患眼。
- 0.5%普罗帕卡因：1～2 滴滴患眼。
- 不要给门诊患者开局部麻醉剂，因为这个药可能影响愈合并增加角膜溃疡形成。
• 口服镇痛药。
- 布洛芬：600～800 mg 每日剂量，随餐服用（儿童：10 mg/kg）。
- 对乙酰氨基酚和羟考酮：325 mg/5 mg，q4～6 h 必要时服用（疼痛发作）。
• 局部应用抗生素（常规使用仍有争议）。
- 0.5%红霉素：眼用软膏，涂抹于患眼，每日 4 次。
- 庆大霉素。
• 散瞳剂（有助于缓解反射性睫状肌痉挛的疼痛）。
- 0.25%氢溴酸东莨菪碱眼用溶液：1～2 滴用于患眼，q6～8 h。
- 0.5%～1%盐酸环喷托酯滴眼液：1 或 2 滴于患眼，q6～8 h。

随访

进一步处理

入院指征

在视力严重下降、有继发感染的证据或双侧修补的情况下，考虑入院。

出院指征

• 几乎所有的患者在口服镇痛药、局部抗生素、睫状肌麻痹剂和/或贴剂治疗后都可以结束治疗后出院：
• 伤口应该在 24～48 h 完全愈合。

随访建议

• 在症状完全消除前避免使用隐形眼镜。
• 在 24～48 h 与眼科医生进行随访，以监测愈合情况和症状解决情况。
• 如果无法与眼科医生进行随访，如果症状在 24～48 h 没有解决，则应返回急诊室。

要点和误区

• 提前 6～12 h 确定紫外线暴露是诊断和预防的关键。
- 患者可能没有意识到暴露风险。
• 有职业暴露风险的人必须佩戴紫外线安全护目镜，而不是眼镜或镜片。
• 这是一种非常痛苦但自我限制的伤害，重复暴露的风险没有明确。

自发性细菌性腹膜炎 Spontaneous Bacterial Peritonitis

Alison Foster-Goldman · Christopher T. Richards 江伟伟 李文放 译

基础知识

描述

• 腹腔积液感染，没有明显的腹腔外科治疗原因引起：
- 腹腔积液培养腹水多形核白细胞计数（PMN）>250/ml。
• 必须与继发性细菌性腹膜炎区分开来：
- 非手术治疗继发性细菌性腹膜炎可导致 100%的死亡率。
- 自发性细菌性腹膜炎（SBP）的手术治疗带来 80%的死亡率。
• 腹水患者每年 SBP 发生率高达 30%。

病因

• 机制：
- 门静脉高压引起肠道细菌通过水肿肠黏膜移位至腹膜腔。
- 由于胃肠道和血流之间的屏障受损，静脉曲张出血增加了 SBP 的风险。
- 血清补体低下的暂时性菌血症。
- 抵抗力下降。
- 网状内皮组织吞噬和调理作用受损。
- 也可以通过肠道外感染菌血症产生腹水。
• 通常见于肝硬化的情况：
- 罕见于其他导致腹水的病症（肾炎综合征或 CHF）。
• 主要微生物：
- 63%有氧革兰阴性菌（大肠埃希菌、克雷伯菌等）。
- 15%革兰阳性（链球菌）。
- 6%～10%的肠球菌。
- <1%厌氧。
• 在使用氟喹诺酮类药物预防性治疗的患者中，有 50%的革兰阳性菌。

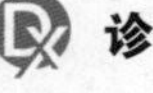

诊断

症状和体征

高达 30%的 SBP 患者没有感染迹象或症状。

病史

• 腹痛：弥漫性，持续性，通常非常轻微。
• 发热，寒战。
• 细菌过度生长引起的腹泻。
• 恶性腹水。
• 精神状态改变。

Z

- 疲劳，肌痛。

体格检查

- 发热是最常见的：
  - 由于基础体温低，肝硬化患者的发热（>37.8 ℃或>100 ℉）一般为低热。
  - 80%的 SBP 患者有发热和寒战。
- 精神状态改变。
- 腹水。
- 腹部压痛：
  - 由于腹水导致内脏和壁层胸膜分离，可能不会有腹壁紧张。
  - 稀便。
  - 麻痹性肠梗阻。

基本检查

- 除非患者有腹膜透析，否则腹腔镜检查是诊断的主要依据。
- 在手术前不必更正凝血酶原（除非血小板<20 000）。
- 程序：
  - 使用超声定位引导。
  - 位置（患者卧位）：
    - 腹直肌外侧，距髂前上棘 3～5 cm。
    - 脐上 2 cm（预先确保膀胱排空）。
  - 抽 40～50 ml，然后换针以避免污染：
    - 每个培养瓶 10 ml。
    - 10 ml 用于细胞计数、生化、革兰染色（肝素管、EDTA 管和无菌容器）。
  - 立即在床边接种腹膜液的培养瓶。

诊断检查与说明

实验室检查

- 常规腹水化验：
  - 细胞计数和分类：
    - 中性粒细胞计数。
  - 总蛋白质。
  - 白蛋白。
  - 培养。
  - 革兰染色。
  - 其他腹水分析：
    - 葡萄糖。
    - LDH。
    - 淀粉酶。
- 与 SBP 一致的腹水特征：
  - PMN>250/mm^3。
  - 诊断包括以下：
    - WBC>1 000/mm^3。
    - WBC>250/mm^3 和>50% PMN。
  - 总蛋白<1 g/dl。
  - pH<7.34。
  - 正常淀粉酶。
  - 培养阳性：
    - 只有 30%～50%的培养阳性，这种阳性率随着床边接种培养瓶的容量增加而增加。
  - 革兰染色阳性结果。
  - 葡萄糖<50 mg/dl。
  - 腹水 LDH>血清 LDH。
  - 乳铁蛋白>242，可作为 SBP 的标志物。
  - 血清腹水白蛋白>1.1 g/dl，符合门静脉高压。
  - 如果出血性腹水（红细胞>10 000/mm^3），在腹水液体判读中每 250 个红细胞/mm^3 减去 1 PMN/mm^3。
- 血液检查（通常反映潜在的疾病）：
  - 白细胞及分类。
  - 生化检测。
  - PT、APTT。
  - LFT（含白蛋白）。
  - 血培养。
  - 培养。

影像学检查

- 腹部超声：
  - 有腹水。
  - 超声引导下腹腔穿刺。
- 胸部 X 线片。
- 腹部 X 线片：平板和直立以评估穿孔或阻塞。
- 如果怀疑继发性细菌性腹膜炎行水溶性 CT 造影。

诊断步骤/外科

如果腹部立卧位有游离气体或 CT 造影液体增多，外科会诊确定是否行探查性剖腹手术。

鉴别诊断

- 继发性细菌性腹膜炎：
  - 由于穿孔或脓肿。
  - 革兰染色示多种细菌感染或以下两条：
    - 腹水总蛋白>1 g/dl。
    - 腹水葡萄糖<50 mg/dl。
    - 腹水 LDH>225 或正常血清 LDH 上限的 1/2。
  - 橙色腹水伴胆红素>6 mg/dl 考虑胆囊破裂。
- 急性肝炎：
  - 发热，白细胞增多，腹痛±腹水。
  - 腹水 PMN<250/mm^3。
- 培养阴性，有中性粒细胞的腹水：
  - 腹水 PMN>250/ml，培养阴性。
- 单核细胞非中性粒细胞芽孢杆菌：
  - 由于 SBP 的定植阶段。
  - 腹水 PMN<250/m^3，培养出单一微生物。
  - 如果有症状，就像 SBP 一样治疗。
- 多细菌性腹水：
  - 由于意外肠穿孔（1/1 000 穿孔）。
  - 腹水 PMN<250/mm^3，培养出多种微生物。
- 胰腺炎：
  - 腹水淀粉酶升高。
- 腹膜癌病或结核性腹膜炎：
  - 以非中性粒细胞为主且无发热的继发性细菌腹膜炎标准。

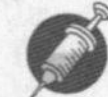

治疗

院前

- 低血压者建立静脉通路补液。
- 血糖引起意识状态改变者，补充糖。
- 呼吸道疾病：吸氧。

初步稳定/治疗

- 基本处理。
- 感染性休克迅速应用抗生素和补液治疗。

急诊治疗/程序

- 只有在血小板计数<20 000/mm^3 时，在穿刺前给予血小板。
- 腹腔穿刺后立即给予经验性抗生素：
  - 腹水 PMN>250/mm^3。
  - 温度>37.8 ℃。
  - 意识状态改变。
  - 腹痛/压痛。
  - 临床特征几乎与 SBP 一致。
- 抗生素选择：
  - 头孢曲松或头孢噻肟。
  - 氨苄西林。
  - 舒巴坦、哌拉西林。
  - 他唑巴坦或氨曲南。
  - 避免氨基糖苷类、氟喹诺酮类。
  - 继发性细菌性腹膜炎加用甲硝唑治疗。
- 静脉输注白蛋白有助于预防 SBP 患者的肾脏损害，降低死亡率。

预后

- 非院内感染死亡率是 20%。
- 可能是肝肾综合征的前兆。
- SBP 发作后 1 个月和 6 个月死亡率分别为 32%和 69%。

■ 药物治疗

一线用药

• 头孢噻肟：2 g，静滴，q8 h。

• 高风险患者的白蛋白：第 1 日 1.5 g/kg，静滴和第 3 日 1 g/kg，静滴。

二线用药

• 头孢曲松：2 g，静滴，q8 h。

• 哌拉西林-他唑巴坦：3.375 g，静滴，q6 h。

• 氨苄西林-舒巴坦：1.5～3 g，静滴，q6 h。

• 氨曲南：0.5～2 g，静滴，q6～12 h。

随访

■ 进一步处理

入院指征

• 需使用静脉抗生素治疗和外科会诊。

• 感染性休克或严重脑病入住 ICU。

出院指征

• 所有疑似或已知 SBP 的患者应予以住院。

• 如果患者拒绝入院，并且没有休克、脑病、氮质血症或消化道出血，则可以考虑静脉注射头孢曲松和口服氟喹诺酮类药物，然后密切随访。

转诊问题

• 转入肝病科或胃肠科治疗。

• 使用诺氟沙星或甲氧苄啶-磺胺甲噁唑预防。

注意

与连续腹膜透析有关的感染：

• 症状：腹膜透析液混浊（90%）、腹痛（80%）和发热（50%）。

• 体征：腹部压痛 70%。

• 诊断：腹膜透析液 WBC＞100/ml、＞50% PMN 和培养阳性：

- 应由专业人员处理腹膜透析液。

• 微生物学：

- ＞50%的病例是由于革兰阳性菌引起，最常见的是葡萄球菌。

- 大肠埃希菌是慢性腹膜透析患者腹膜炎的罕见原因。

• 治疗：

- 通过腹膜内（IP）途径给予抗生素。

- 第一选择：头孢唑林（每日 1 g IP）＋头孢他啶（每日 1 g IP）。

- 万古霉素（每周 2 g IP）是头孢唑林的替代品。

- 阿米卡星 2 mg/(kg · d)(IP)。

■ 随访建议

SBP 患者到胃肠科随访。

要点和误区

• 首先排除继发性细菌性腹膜炎。

• 用血培养瓶接种腹水可提高阳性率。

• 保持对 SBP 的高度怀疑，因为许多患者都没有症状。

自然流产 Abortion，Spontaneous

Ivette Motola · Patricia De Melo Panakos　马林浩　林兆奋 译

基础知识

■ 描述

• 子宫内不足 20 周妊娠的自然终止。

• 同义词：早期妊娠丢失、流产。

• 经确认过的妊娠中有最高 10%～15%会发生流产（早期妊娠最为常见的并发症）。

- 80%出现在妊娠第一阶段。

• 25%的孕妇在妊娠早期的 3 个月内出现阴道流血。

• 概念：

- 先兆流产：阴道流血，子宫颈外口处于关闭，确认的子宫内有活力的妊娠。

◦ 急诊室内 50%先兆流产的妇女将最终流产。

- 难免流产：阴道流血、子宫颈外口处于开放；妊娠产物还未排出。

- 不全流产：阴道流血、子宫颈外口处于开放；妊娠产物部分排出，部分滞留。

- 完全流产：阴道流血、子宫颈外口处于关闭；妊娠产物全部排出，无需外科或者药物干预。

- 稽留流产：胎儿死亡而无子宫排出活动。

- 感染性流产：自然流产并发子宫内感染。

- 习惯性流产：3 次或更多的连续流产。

■ 病因

• 胎儿染色体异常。

• 子宫异常（如平滑肌瘤、子宫粘连、先天异常）。

• 危险因素包括：

- 父亲和母亲的年龄偏大。

- 产次增加。

- 饮酒。

- 抽烟。

- 吸毒。

- 上次分娩 3～6 个月再次受孕。

- 慢性母源性疾病。

◦ 控制不佳的糖尿病。

◦ 自身免疫性疾病。

◦ 腹腔疾病。

- 子宫内装置。

- 母亲 BMI＜18 kg/m² 或＞25 kg/m²。

- 母亲感染：

◦ 细菌性阴道病。

◦ 支原体病。

◦ 单纯疱疹病毒感染。

◦ 弓形虫病。

◦ 李斯特菌病。

◦ 衣原体病/淋病。

◦ 艾滋病。

◦ 梅毒。

◦ 细小病毒 B19 感染。

◦ 疟疾。

◦ 巨细胞病毒感染。

◦ 风疹。

- 药物。

◦ 米索前列醇。

◦ 甲氨蝶呤。

◦ 非甾体抗炎药。

- 多次既往选择性流产。

- 既往早期流产。

- 毒素。

诊断

■ 症状和体征

病史

• 末次月经周期。

• 产科病史：
- 产次。
- 流产危险因素。
- 产前保健。
• 腹痛，痛性痉挛。
• 阴道流血：
- 持续时间。
- 出血量（以用过的卫生巾的量，让患者与正常月经时期相比）。
- 排出的血凝块。
• 眩晕，晕厥。

体格检查

• 确定患者的血流动力学状态：
- 妊娠患者在早期妊娠的第 3 个月期间血容量是增加的。
- 生命体征异常之前可能丢失大量的血液。
• 妇科检查：
- 确定内部的子宫颈外口是开放还是关闭。
- 出血量。
- 妊娠产物的存在。
- 附件区压痛或腹膜刺激征的存在提示存在异位妊娠。
• 双合诊确定子宫的大小：
- 般大小：6～8 周。
- 子宫底位于耻骨联合：12 周。
- 子宫底位于脐：16～20 周。

基本检查

• 妊娠试验。
• 影像学检查。

诊断检查与说明

实验室检查

• 通过尿液或者血清检测确认妊娠：
- 尿妊娠试验：大多在妊娠 1 周时 β - HCG 水平在 25～50 mIU/ml 时为阳性，在分娩或者自然流产后 2～3 周仍然保持阳性。
• 全血细胞计数。
• 快速血红蛋白鉴定：ABO 血型和 Rh 血型。
• 为血细胞比容低或者存在活动性出血征象的妇女进行血型检测和交叉配血。
• β - HCG 水平定量检测。
• 任何的宫内妊娠产物应该送病理检查以确认。

影像学检查

• 经阴道超声（TVS）：
- 妊娠囊可在第 4 周被看见。
- 胎心活动可在第 5.5 周被看见。
• 经腹超声（TAS）：
- 妊娠囊可在第 6 周被看见。
- 胎心活动可在第 8 周被看见。
• 有差别的阈值：β - HCG 水平的具体数值决定何时正常宫内妊娠应该被检出。
- 1 500～2 000 时行经阴道超声。
- 6 500 时行经腹超声。
• 超声结果与流产一致：
- 胎儿头臀长度≥7 mm 且胎心消失。
- 胚囊平均直径≥25 mm 且无胚胎。
- 扫描确认妊娠囊存在而无卵黄囊之后胚胎缺失伴胎心消失≥2 周。
- 扫描确认妊娠囊存在伴卵黄囊之后胚胎缺失伴胎心消失≥11 日。

鉴别诊断

• 妊娠试验阳性伴阴道流血：
- 宫颈炎。
- 异位妊娠。
- 葡萄胎妊娠。
- 未知位置的妊娠。
- 感染性流产。
- 绒毛膜下出血。
- 创伤。
• 妊娠中期和晚期阴道流血：
- 前置胎盘。
- 胎盘破裂。

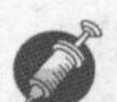

治疗

院前

• 静脉输液，吸氧及心电监测。
• 监测生命体征和转运。
• 注意：
- 自然流产/阴道流血的患者可能存在严重的出血和出现休克，尤其是在妊娠 12 周以后。
- 血压在妊娠中期会下降，平均为 110/70 mmHg。

初步稳定/治疗

• 稳定的患者：
- 静脉输液。
- 妇科检查。
• 不稳定的患者：
- 氧气，通过双腔中心静脉输液，心电监测。
- 如果患者输注 2～3 L 晶体液后仍不稳定输红细胞悬液。
- 立即请产科会诊。
- 缩宫素或甲麦角新碱可能需要被用来控制出血。
- 这些患者有很高的异位妊娠破裂的风险并且可能需要急诊手术干预。

急诊治疗/程序

• 先兆流产：
- 骨盆支架器，密切由产科医师随诊。
- 6 周半以内经阴道超声未发现胎心活动的患者需要检测 β - HCG 水平来评估胎儿的活力和排除异位妊娠。
• 难免流产和不全流产：
- 待产妇的处置：
  ◦ 成功率高达 80%。
  ◦ 与外科处置相比，有更高的非计划外科干预比率和血液丢失。
- 药物处置：
  ◦ 米索前列醇。
  ◦ 成功率高达 80%～93%。
  ◦ 药疗后刮宫术的必要最多可减少 60%。
  ◦ 可短时间完成。
- 外科处置：
  ◦ 膨胀刮除术或泄出术，在子宫颈外口清除妊娠产物从而帮助减少出血量和痛性痉挛。
  ◦ 在急性大出血，血流动力学不稳定，感染迹象时应紧急外科干预。
  ◦ 更少的可能面临非计划中的住院、刮宫术和输血。
  ◦ 成功率为 99%。
  ◦ 妊娠产物由病理科确认以排除异位妊娠。
• 完全流产：
- 如果出血严重，可以用甲麦角新碱或者缩宫素治疗。
- 如果定量 β - HCG 水平小于 1 000 并且超声检查也是阴性的，由产科医师随诊做连续的 β - HCG 水平检测以确认其水平在下降中。
• 稽留流产：
- 这些患者存在弥散性血管内凝血（DIC）的风险，尤其是死胎被保留超过了 4～6 周。
- 获取血常规、凝血酶原时间/部分活化的凝血酶原时间、纤维溶解产物和纤维蛋白原水平。
- 这些患者如果病情稳定、早期确认宫内妊娠并且没有 DIC 的征象，可以门诊密切随访。
- 患者可以选择晚一些再行刮宫术，或在家行药物流产，或不做任何干预。这些决定应该由妇产科医师来做出。

■ 药物治疗

一线用药

• Rh 阴性的妇女 RhO 免疫球蛋白:

- 早于 12 周的先兆流产或完全流产妇女给 50 μg。

- 晚于 12 周的先兆流产或完全流产妇女给 300 μg。

• 需要 RhO 免疫球蛋白的患者需要在 72 h 以内注射以防将来的同种免疫。

• 如果妇产科会诊选择医疗处置,米索前列醇 800 μg 阴道内给药。

• 同样的剂量在 48 h 重复一次。

二线用药

通常由妇产科医师会诊后给药。

• 缩宫素: 20 IU 加至 1 000 ml 生理盐水按照 20 mIU/min 的速度滴定至出血减少;有可能需要重复给药,最大剂量为 40 mIU/min。

• 甲麦角新碱: 对于出血,0.2 mg,肌内注射/口服,每日 4 次。

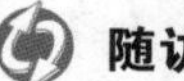

随访

■ 进一步处理

入院指征

• 怀疑不稳定的异位妊娠(见异位妊娠)。

• 血流动力学不稳定的患者存在低血容量或者贫血。

• DIC。

• 感染性流产。

• 怀疑存在妊娠滋养层疾病。

出院指征

• 对于不全和难免流产,刮宫术可以在急诊室进行,并且患者可以在稳定 2~3 h 后出院回家。

• 一些早期的难免流产可以出院并在家完成流产,并不需要行刮宫术。

• 出院时给予镇痛药物和密切的妇产科医师随访。

• 先兆流产的患者应被告知避免剧烈的活动。

• 骨盆休息(如活动性出血期间阴道内避免异物,可能增加感染的风险)。

• 患者应被告知出现任何出血、眩晕或者发热体温大于 38 ℃,应该回到急诊室。

• 患者和她的伴侣应被劝告妊娠早期流产很常见,而且不是任何一方的过错。

■ 随访建议

妊娠试验阳性和阴道流血的患者,无论是否存在腹痛,应该由妇产科医师随诊。

要点和误区

• 认识到异位妊娠的可能性。

• 自然流产的患者可能存在严重的血液丢失。

自杀,危险评估 Suicide, Risk Evaluation

Robyn P. Thom · Helen M. Farrell 江伟伟 李文放 译

基础知识

■ 描述

• 故意结束自己的生命。

• 自杀意念:

- 被动的:有意识地不想活下去。

- 主动的:有意识地要结束自己的生命,无论是否有计划。

• 自残行为:自我伤害并非意在致死(如轻微划伤、香烟烫伤、撞头)。

• 鲁莽行为:不服用处方药、过量服用处方药、冲入交通车辆中。

• 风险与救援比例——计划的致死性与被救援的可能性的比较:

- 高的风险与救援比例表明尝试自杀的严重程度增加。

• 隐匿表现:

- 许多有自杀风险的个体因医学而非行为问题而前往急诊就诊。

- 可能需要改进自杀筛查方法以识别出这一人群。

■ 病因

• 2014 年美国自杀人数为 42 826(美国 CDC,2014)。

• 每一次自杀成功有 12~25 次自杀未遂。

• 男性每 10 万人口中,发生 20.7 例成功自杀(美国 CDC,2014)。

• 女性每 10 万人口中,发生 5.8 例成功自杀(美国 CDC,2014)。

• 普通人群,每 10 万人口中,发生 13.4 例成功自杀(美国 CDC,2014)。

• 每 10 万人口中,有 21 386 例死亡。

• 窒息(每 10 万人口中有 11 407 例死亡)。

• 中毒(每 10 万人口中有 6 808 例死亡)。

• 其他:上吊、跳楼。

流行病学风险因素

• 性别:

- 女性自杀企图的可能性是男性的 3 倍。

- 男性自杀完成的可能性是女性的 3 倍。

• 年龄。

• 民族:白种人或美洲原住民。

• 婚姻状况:丧偶或离婚。

• 单身居住:家中没有孩子。

• 就业:失业,与工作相关的致死手段(如医生)。

• 获得枪支的途径。

与成功自杀相关的诊断

• 超过 90% 的自杀者患有精神疾病,超过 50% 的人在自杀时患有抑郁症。

• 抑郁症(尤其是带有幻觉特征或双相情感障碍)。

• 焦虑症(尤其是惊恐症)。

• 物质使用障碍(尤其是酒精)。

• 精神分裂症。

• 慢性医学疾病(尤其是创伤性脑损伤、癫痫、多发性硬化、亨廷顿病、帕金森病、癌症、艾滋病)。

完成自杀的其他风险群体

• 最近从精神病机构出院。

• 最近去看家庭医师或全科医师。

• 自杀意念或自杀企图的病史。

• 家族中有自杀企图/完成自杀的病史。

• 曾被监禁。

• 边缘化的个体(如无家可归者、失业者、社交孤立者)。

• 受暴力/虐待的受害者。

降低风险的干预措施

• 强化明确定义的支持网络,包括全科医师、行为健康、社会服务和患者管理的全方位关怀团队。

• 情绪障碍患者(严重抑郁症和双相情感障碍)使用锂治疗。

• 严重抑郁症患者使用电休克治疗法,精神分裂症患者使用氯氮平治疗。
• 氯胺酮可能减少自杀倾向,但需要进一步研究证实。
• 没有显示降低自杀率的作用:对严重抑郁症患者使用选择性单胺再摄取抑制剂(SSRIs)治疗。

保护性因素

• 强大的社会支持。
• 家庭的凝聚力。
• 同龄群体关系(如宗教、就业、志愿服务)。
• 良好的应对和解决问题的能力。
• 积极的价值观和信念。
• 寻求和获取帮助的能力。

诊断

▪ 症状和体征

• 抑郁的情绪,没有快乐感。
• 失眠。
• 绝望。
• 无助。
• 严重焦虑,惊恐发作。
• 自我意识、社交脱节。
• 愤怒、攻击性。
• 冲动。
• 解决问题能力差。
• 精神症状(即偏执狂、指令性听觉幻觉)。
• 缺乏社会支持或失去纪念仪式感。
• 对暴力或自残有积极想法。

病史

• 必须获取病史以评估风险。
- 询问自杀病史并不增加自杀风险。
• 自杀想法有多严重:
- 持续时间。
- 频率。
- 强度,想法对患者本人的控制感。
• 是否存在自伤风险:
- 完成计划的手段是否可以获得。
- 启动计划的活动(研究、排练计划,计划自杀的日期)。
- 患者对于计划致死性的预期。
• 意图:自杀的原因/目标。
• 计划的风险与营救比。
• 是否存在死亡准备的行为:
- 自杀信。
- 抛弃随身物品。
- 编写遗嘱。
- 向亲人告别。
• 是否有伤害他人的计划或意图?
• 存在急性诱发因素:
- 最近的亲人去世,缺乏社会支持,学术/工作压力。
• 风险因素(像上面列出的,但包括):
- 过去自杀企图的病史。
- 精神科症状复查:
◦ 抑郁症。
◦ 精神症状。
◦ 恐慌、焦虑。
- 慢性疾病。
- 酗酒或药物滥用。
• 对精神状况的连续评估,反应的一致性。
• 预防自杀的因素:
- 短期和长期的未来规划。
- 使命感、责任感。

体格检查

• 根据需要突出急性医疗问题。
• 寻找受伤的证据和自我忽视的迹象。

评分系统

• 修改后的 SAD PERSONS 评分:
- 性别:男性 1 分。
- 年龄<19 岁或>45 岁 1 分。
- 抑郁或绝望 2 分。
- 先前的自杀企图或精神病治疗 1 分。
- 过度酒精或药物使用 1 分。
- 丧失理性思维 2 分。
- 分居、离婚、丧偶 1 分。
- 有组织的或严重的自杀企图 2 分。
- 没有社会支持 1 分。
- 表达未来实施意图 2 分。
- 数据表明,评分<5 分的患者可以安全地在门诊进行管理。

▪ 基本处理

• 源自门诊诊疗者、家人、朋友的相关信息。
• 安全计划:
- 如果出现自杀意念,患者是否会立即寻求帮助?
- 消除自杀的手段。
- 接触其他自杀的手段。
- 在门诊环境中的支持与指导。
- 推进心理治疗的门诊随访。
- 患者不尝试自杀的投入。
- 辨识生存的原因。
- 安全协议并不能保证个体不会尝试自杀。

▪ 诊断检查与说明

实验室检查

• 血液酒精水平。
• 血清毒理学筛查:阿司匹林、对乙酰氨基酚和其他药物(如锂)。
• 尿液药物筛查:
- 许多精神科机构要求留置患者前进行毒理学筛查。
• 一氧化碳(根据需要)。

影像学检查

不是常规进行。

诊断步骤/外科

心电图:根据需要(如果担心中毒,尤其是三环类抗抑郁药)。

▪ 鉴别诊断

• 正常的沮丧。
• 丧失亲人。
• 调整障碍伴有抑郁情绪。
• 严重的抑郁障碍。
• 双相情感障碍。
• 器质性精神障碍(头部外伤、痴呆、谵妄)。
• 精神分裂症。
• 恐慌和焦虑障碍。
• 酒精或药物滥用。
• 边缘型人格障碍。
• 反社会人格障碍。
• 意外死亡。
• 企图杀人。

儿科注意事项

• 自杀是 15～24 岁年轻人的主要死因。
• 美国每年约有 4 600 个青少年自杀(美国 CDC,2017)。
• 10～14 岁的年轻黑种人男性自杀率迅速增加。
• 青少年自杀与明显的精神疾病有关的证据较少。
• 考虑并检查欺凌。
• 压力:
- 先前的尝试。
- 家庭破裂。
- 精神障碍病史。
- 抑郁。
- 纪律危机。
- 恋情破裂。
- 学校困难。
- 丧失亲人。
- 拒绝。
- 身体或性虐待病史。
• 早期预警信号:
- 逐渐下降的学业成绩。
- 多种身体不适。
- 物质滥用。
- 家庭关系紊乱。

- 放弃社交。
- 无乐趣感。

老年人注意事项

- 年龄>65岁的自杀率最高。
- 完成自杀：83%为男性。
- 风险因素：离婚、丧偶、男性、社交孤立。
- 倾向于使用更致命的方法。
- 尝试与完成的比例较低。

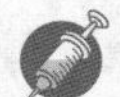

治疗

院前

- 对于拒绝前往治疗场所的潜在危险患者，通知警方并施加限制。
- 医护人员在现场面临枪支或其他武器的风险。
- 了解州和地方法律、移动危机单位的可用性，以及何时让警方介入。

初始稳定/治疗

- 防止逃跑的能力。
- 确保患者安全。
- 移除尖锐物体、皮带、鞋带和其他可能用于自伤的物品。
- 提供安全的环境。
- 适当的监督。

急诊治疗/程序

- 如有可能，与患者的门诊治疗者或医师协商。
- 自愿入住精神科机构。
- 如果患者拒绝自愿入住并且存在高风险(具有意图和手段的高致命性、最近的压力因素、精神障碍症状)，则强制入院。
- 对于低风险患者(必须符合下文中列出的出院标准)，在安全规划中涉及社会支持并安排门诊随访。
- 对于强制性精神科入院，患者必须患有精神障碍并具备以下一种情况：
- 危害自身的风险。
- 危害他人的风险。
- 无法照顾自己。

药物治疗

治疗潜在的精神障碍。

随访

进一步处理

入院指征

- 如果患者表达有自杀意念并且有计划和意图，可能需要入院以确保安全。
- 如果冲动、愤怒或攻击性影响控制行为的能力。

出院指征

- 患者没有自杀意念。
- 患者同意在自杀意念再次出现时立即返回急诊室寻求精神医疗帮助。
- 患者有被动自杀意念但没有计划或意图。
- 患者对恶化情绪和危险行为的预警信号有良好的认识。
- 患者有良好的支持网络或安置在适当的危机居所中。
- 确保适当的门诊精神科后续治疗。
- 在某些情况下，酗酒时表达自杀意念的患者在酒醒后如果不再有自杀意念可能会出院。
- 一些具有边缘型人格障碍和慢性自杀意念的患者经过与长期门诊护理人员协商慎重的精神评估后出院。

随访建议

对于不需要入院的急性疾病患者进行密切的精神科后续随访。

要点和误区

- 仔细的病史询问会确定自杀风险因素。
- 获取关联来源(先前的医疗记录、家人、朋友、治疗提供者)相关患者最近想法和行为的信息。
- 在评估过程中保持患者的安全。
- 如果患者表达自杀意念和计划，则可能需要住院。

纵隔气肿 Pneumomediastinum

Matthew D. Bitner · C. Hunter Matthews 瞿金龙 译

基础知识

描述

- 纵隔存在游离气体。
- 其他可以来源于食管、气管、肺等。
- 可以自发性(原发性纵隔气肿)或继发于创伤、手术或其他原因(继发性纵隔气肿)。
- 自发性纵隔气肿：
- 由胸膜外的气管支气管损伤引起：
  - 增高的肺泡压，低的外周血管压力，或者同时存在。
  - 终末肺泡破裂入肺泡间隙和支气管血管鞘。
  - 气体进入肺门和纵隔。
  - 纵隔气体进入皮下或筋膜内，尤其是颈部组织。
- 剧烈呕吐，合并气管痉挛或吸入药物使用。
- 男性>女性(2∶1)。
- 年轻人(20～30岁)>老年人。
- 儿科患者有两个年龄高峰(<7岁和13～17岁)。
- 发生率低，1/(30 000～50 000)住院患者。

病因

- 原发性或自发性气肿：
- Valsalva法相关：
  - 剧烈呕吐。
  - 剧烈运动。
  - 剧烈排便。
  - 咳嗽、喷嚏。
  - 剧烈尖叫。
  - 分娩。
  - 吹乐器。
  - 肺功能检查。
  - 呼吸系统、胸部和纵隔疾病。
  - 肥胖。
  - 已经存在的肺的疾病(间质性肺病、肺纤维化、肺炎)。
  - 非法吸入药物的使用(印度大麻、可卡因、去氧麻黄碱)。

◦ 烟草滥用。
- 大部分患者无特定的原因。
- 在牙科取出术等很少被描述。
• 继发性纵隔气肿：
- 继发于气压伤。
- 常见的创伤疾病：
◦ 车祸。
◦ 高空坠落伤。
◦ 胸部或颈部创伤。
◦ 近期食管/气管等手术。
- 呼吸机通气的正压伤。
- 食管破裂。
- 空腔脏器引起的纵隔感染。
• 张力性纵隔气肿：
- 很少，但是很严重的疾病。
- 常常发生在机械通气患者。
• 张力性纵隔气肿和张力性气胸常常同时存在。

诊断

症状和体征

• 胸痛：
- 剧烈。
- 尖锐的痛。
- 胸骨后。
- 背部和手臂放射痛。
- 位置比较确定。
• 呼吸困难。
• 颈部疼痛：
- 发生在颈部皮下气肿。
- 常常主述为：颈部肿胀、颈部疼痛、咽喉部疼痛、吞咽困难。
• 肺气肿。
• 吞咽困难、吞咽痛。
• 发声困难、声音嘶哑。
• Hamman 摩擦音：常常在心脏收缩时听见。
- 不常见，但是比较有特征性的标志。
- 在患者左侧卧位时，最能听见。
• Meckler 三联征：呕吐、胸痛和皮下气肿。

病史

• 使用吸入性药物。
• 哮喘加重。
• 已经存在的肺疾病。
• 剧烈呕吐。
• 在紧张的剧烈运动之后。

体格检查

• 肺气肿。
• Hamman 摩擦音。

基本检查

• 包括继发性因素、食管破裂。
• CXR。
• 胸部 CT。

实验室检查

血常规检查。

影像学检查

• CXR：
- 有价值的检查之一。
- 尤其是侧位片，很多患者在后前位时不容易显现。
- 有助于排除气胸和纵隔气肿。
- 用来区分气体胸膜来源或食管来源。
- 阴性率 30%～35%。
- 帆征。
- 肺气肿或者上纵隔气肿。
• 胸部 CT：
- 适用于高度怀疑纵隔气肿但胸片是阴性的患者。
• 食管造影 X 线照片：
- 排除食管破裂。

诊断步骤/外科

• 食管镜检查：
- 作用有限。
- 作为 CT 诊断食管损伤的进一步检查。
• 喉镜检查/支气管镜：
- 作用有限。
- 用来排除气管或喉部损伤。
• 心包穿刺术：
- 用于危重病患者。
• 胸腔闭式引流：
- 仅用于合并气胸患者。

鉴别诊断

• 主动脉夹层。
• 冠状动脉缺血。
• 食管憩室。
• 食管炎。
• 纵隔炎。
• 心肌炎。
• 肺炎。
• 心包积气。
• 气胸、张力性气胸。
• 肺栓塞。
• Schatzki 环。

治疗

院前

• 急危重患者的复苏（合并纵隔炎）。
• 监测和标准护理创伤患者。
• 禁食。
• 评估和送至有条件处理的医院。

初步稳定/治疗

• 建立静脉通路。
• 吸氧。
• 心电监测。
• 指脉氧监测。

急诊治疗/程序

• 自发性纵隔气肿：
- 一般比较轻微和自限性。
- 不需要特殊处理。
- 主要在明确诊断后控制疼痛。
- 高流量吸氧。
- 食管破裂，禁食处理。
- 一般自限性，一般 2～5 日吸收。
• 继发性纵隔气肿：
- 一般诊断明确后，可以行食管镜、气管镜等明确病因。
- 找出原因，对因治疗。

药物治疗

• 对因治疗（如控制哮喘发作）。
• 吸氧 15 L，或无创面罩吸氧。
• 止痛。
• 抗生素的使用需要慎重，如出现纵隔炎，可以使用广谱抗生素包括覆盖耐药菌和假单胞细菌属。
- 万古霉素：10～15 mg/kg，静脉滴注，q12 h。
- 哌拉西林-他唑巴坦：3.75～4.5 g，静脉滴注，q6 h。
- 克林霉素：600～900 mg，静脉滴注，q8 h；或甲硝唑 500 mg，静脉滴注，q8 h。

随访

进一步处理

入院指征

• 继发性纵隔气肿。
• 合并气胸。
• 食管破裂没有排除。
• 生命体征不平稳。
• 危重患者。

• 顽固性疼痛。
• 原发病要求入院(如哮喘、原发性肺疾病等)。
• 可能有并发症出现的患者。
• 高龄或合并妊娠。
• 免疫抑制患者。
• 院外处理失败的患者。

出院指征

• 自发性纵隔气肿。
• 各项指标正常。
• 无合并气胸。
• 急诊处理后明显吸收。

■ 随访建议

• 如患者的症状未见明显好转,需再次评估。
• 反复发作的自发性气胸需心胸外科会诊,明确诊断可能的病因。

要点和误区

• 确定病因。
• 注意患者的症状:胸痛、呼吸困难、颈部胀痛等。
• Hamman 摩擦音是特征性的,但不是每个患者都能看到。

足部骨折 Foot Fractures

Colleen J. Campbel 万健 译

基础知识

■ 描述

跗骨或跖骨损伤,其中包括跟骨、距骨、舟状骨、骰骨和楔状骨。

■ 病因

• 足部损伤最常见于跖骨和趾骨。
• 在跗骨中跟骨最易发生骨折。
• 跟骨骨折:瞬间高速的压力伤作用于足后跟:
- 75%关节内,50%和外伤关联。
◦ 10%脊柱骨折。
◦ 25%与下肢创伤有关。
◦ 9%是双侧的,5%是开放性的。
• 跖骨骨折:分为应力性骨折、扭伤和直接创伤。
- 第 1 跖骨:直接作用力。
- 第 2 和第 3 跖骨通常受累于应力性骨折、扭伤。
- 第 5 跖骨:撕脱性骨折(Dancer 骨折)近端骨突最易受伤。
- Jones 骨折:第 5 跖骨干骺端和骨干间的横断骨折,由足部反转扭伤所致。仅从营养动脉供血可能导致骨不连。
• 距骨:常见于单板滑手,由轴向负重背屈引起。
• 舟状骨:由轴向压力或应力导致的骨折。
• 骰骨和楔状骨骨折较少发生,常合并于跗-跖骨损伤中。
• 跗-跖骨损伤(Lisfranc 损伤)是高能损伤:
- 足底的轴向负荷,后足的暴力翻转。
- 不稳定的前足作用于后足。
- 20%未明原因。
- 3 种类型:会聚型、发散型和不协调型。

儿科注意事项

• 在儿童的足部骨折中跖骨骨折占 90%,通常由于直接的创伤导致。
- 第 1 和第 5 跖骨骨折较第 2~4 跖骨骨折常见。
- 骨后板损伤常发生于第 1 跖骨近端。
• 其他常见的损伤包括趾骨骨折(17%)和舟状骨骨折(5%)。
• 距骨或跟骨的骨折易合并胫骨远端和腓骨骨折(8%)。
• 跟骨骨折较少与脊柱骨折关联。

诊断

■ 症状和体征

病史

• 发病前通常有创伤史。
• 应力性骨折可出现随活动而不断加重的疼痛。

体格检查

• 瘀斑、疼痛、肿胀、足部畸形。
• 负重性疼痛或直接压迫骨骼(即跟骨)。
• 关节不稳定。

■ 基本检查

• 体格检查对评估神经血管状况、皮肤完整性、肿胀程度、畸形及功能障碍是十分必要的。
• 检查疑似跟骨骨折患者的脊柱情况是必要的,有 10%的患者合并脊柱损伤。
• 对所有的足部骨折患者行正侧位和斜位摄片。
• 合并症:
- 筋膜室综合征常见于足部肿胀伴疼痛的患者:
◦ 常见于跟骨骨折和跖骨骨折。
◦ 压力>35 mmHg 时应开放足部主要的筋膜腔。
◦ 足底感觉减退。
◦ 足趾弯曲无力。
◦ 后期出现爪状趾畸形。
- 距骨颈骨折因为末梢血供不足常发生骨不连和缺血性坏死。
- 跟骨骨折可能出现腓肠神经损伤,沿足外侧检查感觉变。

■ 诊断检查与说明

• 如果患者在受伤时无法行走 4 步,舟骨疼痛,或第 5 跖骨头疼痛,则进行影像学检查。
• 某些骨折需要特殊的摄片摆位。
• 跖跗关节骨折会出现因负重引起的受压征象,需行 MRI 评估韧带的稳定性。当临床疑似时需行 CT 排除细微骨折。
• 斑点征:特殊病理征,韧带从 2MT 底部至的楔状骨中部撕裂。
• 距骨骨折需 45°内斜位,需行 CT 检查。
• 舟骨骨折需要 CT 检查,如果怀疑只有 33%在 X 线平片上看到。
• 中足骨折需外斜位。
• 跟骨骨折需要轴位并需做 CT:
- Bohler 角<28°提示跟骨压缩性骨折。
- 行腰骶部摄片对所有的跟骨骨折患者来说都是必要的。
• 应力性骨折需 2 周后拍摄 X 线平片,骨扫描或者 CT 可用于鉴别疑似骨折。

■ 鉴别诊断

• 跟骨前段骨折和距骨圆顶部骨折需与踝

扭伤鉴别。

• 足挫伤。

• Freiberg 病：第 2 跖骨头骨软骨病易误诊为应力性骨折。

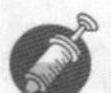

治疗

■ 院前

• 患侧足部和踝关节用冰袋冰敷。

• 所有疑似跟骨骨折的患者均应采取脊柱固定，通常按＞6 ft(1.8 m)的高处坠落伤处理。

■ 初步稳定/治疗

按指示同时对创伤进行处理。

■ 急诊治疗/程序

• 气道、呼吸和循环的管理。

• 对骨折处相关的神经血管进行评估。

• 尽可能快地进行神经血管评估并降低脱位的发生率：

- 过程中通常需要镇静。

• 制动，冰块和夹板固定：

- 环扎固定应在肿胀消退后应用。

- 减少跖骨骨折复位大于 4 mm 或成角 10%。

• 用拐杖。

• 疼痛管理：

- 如果随着足趾活动后出现大面积的肿胀和疼痛，应警惕筋膜室综合征。

- 超声引导下麻醉可用于减少疼痛。

• 骨科专科早期行骨折复位：

- 较多骨折需在 6 h 内复位以预防因肿胀因素而延迟 6～10 日切开复位内固定。

■ 药物治疗

• 头孢唑林：1 g，静脉或肌内注射(儿童：25 mg/kg，静脉或肌内注射)。

• 丙泊酚(异丙酚)：40 mg，静脉输注，q10 s 至镇静。

• 依托咪酯：0.1～0.2 mg/kg，静脉输注。

• 芬太尼：50～250 μg，静脉输注，滴定(儿童：2 μg/kg，静脉输注)。

• 氢化吗啡酮：0.5～2 mg，静脉输注，q2 h(儿童：0.15 mg/kg，静脉输注，q4～6 h)。

• 布洛芬：800 mg，口服(儿童：10 mg/kg，口服)。

• 1%利多卡因＋肾上腺素：10 cc 用于神经阻滞。

• 哌替啶：25～100 mg，静脉或肌内注射，滴定(儿童：1～1.75 mg/kg，静脉或肌内注射)。

• 美索比妥：1～1.5 mg/kg，静脉输注。

• 吗啡：2～10 mg，静脉或肌内注射，滴定(儿童：0.1 mg/kg，静脉输注)。

随访

■ 进一步处理

入院指征

• 开放性骨折。

• 确诊筋膜室综合征或神经血管受损。

• 需要尽快行切开复位内固定术。

出院指征

• 大部分的跖骨骨折患者经骨科后续治疗后均能出院。

• 足趾骨折累及踇趾应转为骨科随访。

转诊问题

所有未成功复位的开放性骨折、中足/跖跗关节损伤、位移性骨折患者应在急诊室转由骨科专家处理。

足趾骨受伤 Phalangeal Injuries, Foot

Megan Tresenriter · Christanne H. Coffey 马林浩 译

基础知识

■ 描述

• 足趾骨容易受伤。

• 第 5 趾(小趾)受伤最常见。

■ 病因

• 通常由直接创伤导致。

• 踩到足趾、踢到硬表面或重物砸在足趾上，是最常见的受伤机制。

诊断

■ 症状和体征

病史

病史可用来预计所受伤的类别，这些类别应该包括：

• 受伤时间。

• 受伤机制。

• 既往创伤史。

• 破伤风免疫状态(如果出现撕裂伤的话)。

体格检查

• 压痛、肿胀、关节捻发音及受影响足趾淤青。

• 经常出现指甲下血肿。

• 撕裂伤或粉碎型伤口。

• 受影响足趾的神经血管状态检查，做好记录。

■ 基本检查

所伤到足趾的 X 线检查。

■ 诊断检查与说明

影像学检查

• 所伤到足趾的 X 线检查。

• 侧面观是最灵敏的。

■ 鉴别诊断

• 骨折。

• 挫伤。

• 磨损或撕裂。

• 脱臼。

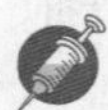

治疗

■ 院前

• 所伤足趾冰块冷敷。

• 直接静液压法，伤口包扎。

■ 初步稳定/治疗

• 所伤足趾冰块冷敷。

• 直接静液压法及伤口包扎。

■ 急诊治疗/程序

• 骨折涉及踇趾的近趾端和指节间(IP)关节：

- 无移位骨折、无关节内骨折的可打上带有趾延长的短肢行走管型石膏，以便行走舒适。
- 有移位骨折、无关节内骨折的：
• 带有足趾阻滞麻醉的闭合复位术。
• 纵向牵引。
• 打上带有趾延长的短肢行走管型石膏：
- 如涉及跗趾关节内骨折最好咨询整形外科的意见：
◦ 频繁地进行切开复位术和内固定处理。
• 骨折涉及小趾的近趾端和指节间关节：
- 很少造成长期残疾。
• 无移位骨折：
- 通过打夹板或石蜡膜带固定。
- 在包扎的足趾间垫上纱布垫，防止皮肤破裂。
• 移位骨折：
- 带有足趾阻滞麻醉的闭合复位术。
- 纵向牵引。
- 打石蜡膜或夹板固定。
- 穿硬底鞋，耐受承重。
- 口服止痛药止痛。
- 通常 2～3 周后不再疼痛。
• 指节间关节脱臼：
- 带有足趾阻滞麻醉的闭合复位术。
- 纵向牵引，并对远节趾骨进行轻柔的向下按压。
- 给邻近的足趾打石蜡膜带。
- 不稳定的或不成功的复位术要咨询整形外科。
- 口服止痛药止痛。
• 远趾端粉碎性骨折：
- 甲下血肿必须要清除。
- 甲床撕裂修复可能有必要。
- 给邻近的足趾打石蜡膜带。
- 穿耐受承重的鞋。
- 口服止痛药。
- 通常 2～3 周后不再疼痛。
• 开放性骨折：
- 咨询整形外科。
- 预防性抗生素。

■ 药物治疗

• 非类固醇抗炎药在治疗急性疼痛方面有效果：
- 布洛芬 800 mg（儿童按体重用量：5～10 mg/kg），口服，每日 3 次。
• 对于严重疼痛可能会要求使用麻醉性止痛剂。
• 对于开放性伤口考虑使用抗生素：
- 头孢唑林：对于开放性骨折，急诊室治疗采用肌内注射或静脉注射，用量 1 g（儿童按体重用量：5～100 mg/kg，急诊室治疗采用肌内注射或静脉注射）。
- 头孢氨苄：对于污染伤口，口服 500 mg，每日 4 次［儿童按体重日用量：25～50 mg/(kg·d)，剂量分开］，服用 7 日。

随访

■ 进一步处理

入院指征

• 不稳定的闭锁性脱臼。
• 急诊开放性骨折且要咨询整形外科。

出院指征

所有其他骨折在 2～3 周的整形外科随访且评估愈合情况后方可出院。

转诊问题

患者所拍的任何 X 线照片副本可方便尽早的随访。

■ 随访建议

• 涉及跗趾近趾端的关节内骨折迫切要求整形外科或足与踝关节外科医师的随访。
• 简单的小趾无移位骨折通常可以由初级医师随访。

要点和误区

开放性的、位移的或关节内骨折，尤其是涉及跗趾的，应咨询整形外科。

左心室装置急诊 Left Ventricular Device Emergencies

Tarlan Hedayati　段立伟 译

基础知识

■ 描述

左心室辅助装置（LVAD）：
• 心力衰竭患者的便携式机械泵。
• 组件：
- 左心室流入管。
- 主动脉流出管。
- 泵：连续流动。
◦ 轴向或离心式。
◦ 由于左心室持续的血流，患者没有可触及的脉搏。
- 经皮传动系统：连接泵和系统控制。
- 系统控制器：
◦ 调节电机功率和速度。
◦ 进行诊断监视。
◦ 报警显示。
◦ 存储数据以供下载。
- 电池：电源系统控制和维持泵运转。
- 电源基本单元：为电池充电，并为控制器和泵供电。
• VAD 治疗的目的：
- 移植支持（BTT）：在心脏移植前支持心脏功能。
- 目的性治疗（DT）：在患者的余生中支持心脏功能。
- 恢复支持（BTR）：暂时支持心脏功能，给予心脏恢复时间。

■ 流行病学

• 全球有 2 300 万心力衰竭患者。
• 美国有 510 万心力衰竭患者。
• 高达 150 000 名严重心力衰竭患者，当其他治疗失败时，心脏移植是首选治疗方法。
• 美国每年进行的心脏移植手术<3 000 例。
• 由于 LVAD 作为 BTT，等待心脏移植的患者的年死亡率从 2001 年的 17% 持续下降。

■ 病因

常见的与 LVAD 有关的紧急情况：
• 贫血（0.5%～18%的患者）。
- 由于红细胞的异变导致的 2A 型血管性血友病。
- 使用抗凝剂。
• 出血。
- 颅内出血（ICH）（11%）。
- 胃肠道（22%～40%）。
◦ 动静脉畸形。
◦ 血管发育不良。
- 血尿。

Z

- 鼻出血。
• 感染(30%～50%的患者)。
- 传动系统：最常见(17%～30%)。
- 泵腔(2%～10%)。
- 套管或装置(0.6%)。
- 血流(20%～27%)。
• 血栓形成(35%)。
- 泵血栓可导致泵/设备故障。

诊断

症状和体征

病史

• 头晕,乏力。
• 胸痛。
• 心悸。
• 气急。
• 咯血。
• 便血。
• 黑便。
• 晕厥。
• 癫痫。
• 局灶性神经功能缺损。
• 头痛。
• 传动系统或手术部位疼痛、发红或渗出。

体格检查

• 肱动脉多普勒血压测定及手动袖带血压测定。
- 当有可听动脉血流时,压力读数代表平均动脉压(MAP)。
- 目标 MAP 为：60～90 mmHg。
• 颈部。
- 颈静脉扩张。
• 肺部。
- 啰音。
• 腹部。
- 手术部位疼痛、红斑或脓性渗液。
- 听到泵位"嗡嗡"声：正常。
- 直肠检查：血常规或粪潜血试验阳性。
• 四肢及末梢。
- 花斑样改变或肢体厥冷。
- 水肿。
• 神经系统损害。
- 意识改变。
- 运动和/或感觉异常。
- 癫痫。
- 脑血管意外。
• 皮肤。
- 传动系统部位皮肤疼痛、红斑或脓性渗液。

基本检查

实验室检查

• 血常规。
• BMP。
• 乳酸脱氢酶、胆红素、直接胆红素、间接胆红素。
• 尿常规。
• 肌钙蛋白。
• 凝血：治疗期间 INR 2～3.5。
• 血培养。
• 血型和交叉配血。
• 血气分析评估血氧饱和度。
• 心电图用于心率评估、心肌缺血和/或心律失常。

影像学检查

• 胸片。
• 腹部 X 线平片。
• CT 胸部检查：评估泵或套管血栓形成。
• 腹部/盆腔 CT：评估 LVAD 相关性感染或脓肿、血尿。
• 床边超声心动图：评估心脏压塞、左心室和右心室大小、下腔静脉宽度。

鉴别诊断

• 胸痛。
- 局部缺血。
- 心肌炎。
- 主动脉夹层。
- 气胸。
- 纵隔气肿。
• 胃肠道。
- 溃疡。
- 胃、十二指肠、结肠动静脉畸形。
- 憩室病、憩室炎。
- 胃窦血管扩张综合征。
• 低血压
- 低血容量。
- 出血。
- 脓毒症。
- 吸力变化。
◦ LVAD 向下吸附在左心室壁。
- 心脏压塞。

治疗

院前

• 病情稳定的患者应被送往最近的 LVAD 中心。
• 心搏骤停或危急的病人应送往最近的医院。
• 院前医务人员应随身携带所有与 LVAD 相关的设备,包括额外的电池和电源底座。
• 院前医务人员应向 LVAD 患者提供标准的 ACLS,包括胸外按压、除颤和药物治疗。

初步稳定/治疗

• 呼叫 VAD 中心进行转接。
• 评估控制器上的正常 VAD 参数。
- Flow 4～6 LPM。
- 电源 Power 4～6 W。
- 速率 8 000～10 000 RPM。
- 泵上可听到正常"嗡嗡"声。
◦ 没有"嗡嗡"声代表泵已损坏。
- 触诊控制器：应感觉温暖,不冷不热。
• 心律失常：通常耐受性良好。
- 稳定：药物复律。
- 不稳定：电性复律或除颤。
◦ 在复率/除颤期间,断开系统控制器。

急诊治疗/程序

• 降压药：VAD 对后负荷敏感；MAP 目标<90 mmHg。
• 抗感染：广谱抗生素或抗真菌药。
• 补液：取决于 VAD。
• 危及生命的出血
- 凝血酶原复合物浓缩物或新鲜冷冻血浆。
- 凝血药物。
- 维生素 K。
• 泵血栓形成
- 心胸外科或心脏介入科会诊。
- 肝素。
- 如处于危急状态,使用组织纤溶酶原激活剂(TPA)。

随访

进一步处理

将所有需要入院的 VAD 患者转移到 VAD 中心。

要点和误区

• LVAD 患者需要抗生素预防才能进行手术。
• 电池失效。
- 一次换一块电池,千万不要同时换。

坐骨神经痛/椎间盘突出 Sciatica/Herniated Disc

Matthew Michael Nolan · Leslie C. Oyama 周健 潘曙明 译

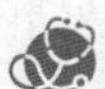

基础知识

描述

• 疼痛从背部辐射至臀部、下肢远至膝盖，有无感觉或运动障碍：
- 95%敏感性和 88%特异性：椎间盘突出(HD)。
- 第 4～5 个 10 年高峰。
- 2%～10%的腰痛。
- 95% L_5 或 S_1 神经根。
- 90%通过保守治疗改善神经根症状通常在 6 周内消失，其中 5%～10%需要手术。

病因

• 胶体凝胶(髓核)突出通过薄弱的周围纤维囊(环纤维化)。
• 风险因素：
- 吸烟。
- 重复的起重/扭。
- 车辆、机械振动。
- 肥胖。
- 久坐不动的生活方式。

诊断

症状和体征

病史

• 腰痛先于腿痛。
• 腿痛主要是随着时间的推移而产生的。
• 尖锐，定位良好，向膝远端辐射。
• 通过增加椎间盘内压力的活动而加剧。
- Valsalva 动作。
- 咳嗽。
- 神经根紧张(坐直，抬腿)。
• 通过降低压力/张力缓解：
- 仰卧。
- 行走。
• 感觉异常是最常见的感觉症状。

体格检查

• 神经系统检查(运动、感觉、深腱反射)。
• L_4 根/L_3～L_4 盘：
- 膝伸展/髋关节内收。
- 前内侧腿、膝、内侧踝。
- 膝反射。
• L_5 根/L_4～L_5 盘。
- 跗趾和足背屈。
- 背体内侧/第一虎口。
- 无反射。
• S_1 根/L_5～S_1 盘：
- 足跖屈。
- 后肢/外侧踝/背外侧足。
- 跟腱反射。
- 直肠检查(张力)。
• 直腿抬高试验：
- 将同侧腿抬高 30°～60°，足背屈或不屈足。
- 80%敏感。
• 交叉直腿抬高试验(病理形态学)：
- 抬高对侧的腿。
- 患侧腿出现疼痛。
- 不太敏感，但对 HD 非常特殊。
- 足背屈曲疼痛增加。
• 如果检查发现或有马尾病史，则指直肠检查的敏感性增加。

基本检查

• 完成病史和体格检查。
• 检测指标见下文。

诊断检查与说明

实验室检查

• 如果临床怀疑有鉴别诊断(DDX)，针对<10 年患者，以下临界值更低：CBC、ESR、CRP。

影像学检查

PA/LS 脊柱侧

• 有助于排除一些 DDX。
• 适应证：
- 年龄界限(<20 岁或>55 岁)。
- 未解决的背痛(超过 4～6 周)，尽管保守治疗。

MRI(标准)

• 适应证：
- 急性，严重的神经功能缺陷(来自急诊科)。
- 怀疑感染性腰痛病因：
◦ 硬膜外脓肿。
◦ 骨髓炎。
◦ 脊髓受压。
- 6 周失败保守治疗(门诊随访)。
- 椎间盘疾病(>25%)：
◦ 偶然发现无症状患者的 MRI。
◦ 突出程度和症状程度没有关系。
- 病史和体检上的危险信号：
◦ 创伤。
◦ 不明症状(发热、不明原因的体重减轻、倦怠)。
◦ 癌症。
◦ 免疫缺陷。
◦ 既往静脉药物滥用。
◦ 近期细菌感染。
◦ 夜间病情加重/患者从睡眠中醒来。
◦ 发热。
◦ 中枢神经系统病变。

诊断步骤/外科

• 排尿残余(PVR)。
- 溢出性尿失禁：PVR>100 ml(疑似马尾综合征)。

鉴别诊断

• 腰骶的拉伤。
• 退行性关节疾病。
• 脊椎前移。
• 髋关节、骶髂关节(感染、骨折、滑囊炎)。
• 肺炎、肺栓塞。
• 肾盂肾炎、肾结石。
• 异位妊娠、盆腔炎性疾病。
• 腹主动脉瘤(AAA)。
• 外周血管疾病(跛行)。
• 带状疱疹。
• 心理：功能性或继发性病变(寻找药物、残疾)。
• 影响腰骶神经路径上任何地方的刺激性病变：
- 大脑：
◦ 脊髓(脊髓病变)：
◦ 椎管狭窄、肿瘤、血肿、感染(硬膜外脓肿、椎间盘炎、骨髓炎)。
- 根(神经根病)：
◦ 硬膜内的：肿瘤、感染。
◦ 硬膜外的：HD、腰椎/孔的狭窄(椎间狭窄)、脊椎前移、囊肿、肿瘤。
- 感染神经丛(神经丛疾病)：
◦ 肿瘤、感染(髂腰肌脓肿)、血肿(腹膜后)。
- 外围神经(神经病)：
◦ 有毒代谢/营养、感染、创伤、缺血、渗透、压缩、截留。

Z

儿科注意事项

• 通常继发于创伤或严重的潜在疾病(如白血病);考虑完成检查。

• <10 岁:

- 感染。
- 肿瘤。
- 动静脉畸形。

• >10 岁:

- 创伤性 HD。
- 脊椎前移。
- Scheuermann 病。
- 肿瘤。

妊娠注意事项

• 异位妊娠。

• 分娩。

• 肾盂肾炎。

• 肌肉骨骼。

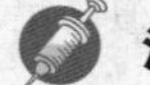

治疗

院前

为创伤受害者提供完整的脊椎预防措施。

初步稳定/治疗

评估神经外科急救。

急诊治疗/程序

缓解疼痛:

• 非甾体抗炎药。

• 肌肉松弛剂,急性期需要的阿片类药物。

药物治疗

• 非甾体抗炎药:

- 布洛芬(motrin, advil):600~800 mg(儿童:5~10 mg/kg),口服,每日 3~4 次。
- 萘普生(naprosyn, aleve):500 mg,口服,每日 2 次。

• 肌肉松弛剂(短期):

- 环苯扎林(flexeril):5~10 mg,每日 3 次。
- 地西泮(安定):2~10 mg(儿童:每次 0.1 mg/kg),口服,每日 3~4 次。
- 美索巴莫(robaxin):1 000~1 500 mg,口服,每日 4 次。
- 替扎尼定(zanaflex):α_2 受体激动剂;2 mg,口服,每日 3 次。

• 神经疾病:

- 加巴喷丁(neurontin):合成的 GABA;400~1 200 mg,口服。
- 普雷巴林(lyrica):调节中枢神经末梢的钙内流;75~150 mg/d(尽管 RCT 没有明显的疼痛减轻)。

• 阿片类药物(短期内):

- 氢吗啡酮(dilaudid):2~4 mg,口服;0.5~2 mg,肌内注射或静脉注射,q4~6 h,必要时。
- 硫酸吗啡:2~10 mg(儿童:0.1 mg/kg/剂量),肌内注射或静脉注射,q2~4 h,必要时。
- 可待因 30 mg+醋氨酚 300 mg,不要超过对乙酰氨基酚 4 g/24 h。
- 氢可酮 5 mg+对乙酰氨基酚 300 mg,不超过对乙酰氨基酚 4 g/24 h。

随访

进一步处理

入院指征

• 严重的神经系统缺陷(马尾综合征,不能行走)。

• 进行性神经功能缺陷。

• 涉及多个根。

• 不稳定的骨折、感染、肿瘤。

• 无法作为门诊患者(社会状况/痛苦)管理。

出院指征

患者能走动,听从指示,有可靠的家庭情况和计划的随访。

转诊问题

不需要立即承认的异常检查。何时何地取决于结果(大的 DDX)。

随访建议

• 骨科脊柱外科医师或神经外科医师随访或 PCP 在 1 周内。

• 保守治疗(4~6 周):

- 药物如前所述。
- 避免完全卧床休息,最多 2 日。
- 急性期活动受限,但在可接受的情况下逐渐增加活动量/锻炼量。
- 避免下腰或加重疼痛的运动:
  ◦ 重体力活、扭转、弯曲、弯着腰、身体的振动。

• 未被证明有效的治疗方法:

- 硬膜外类固醇注射(轻度短期疗效,但 3 个月时残疾无显著差异)。
- 按摩保健。
- 经皮电神经刺激。
- 牵引。
- 背带、束腹。
- 超声。
- 动脉粥样硬化。
- 针灸、按摩。
- 全身糖皮质激素。

• 外科干预(椎间盘切除术):

- 对于>持续 6 周的坐骨神经痛患者 3 个月缓解。
- 2 年后差异不大。

Z

附　录

急诊用药

药物	成人	儿童(儿童用药剂量通常不应超过成人)
阿昔单抗(ReoPro)	0.25 mg/kg，IV，随后 0.125 μg/min 输注直至最大剂量 10 μg/min 维持 12 h	N/A
腺苷(3 mg/ml)	6 mg IV(快速，1～2 s) 如果 1～2 min 无反应，予以 12 mg IV；如果 2 min 后仍无反应，必要时重复 12 mg IV	0.1 mg/kg，IV(快速)；如果 2 min 后无反应则予 0.2 mg/kg，IV，最大单次剂量不应超过 0.3 mg/kg
沙丁胺醇(0.5%溶液：5 mg/ml)	2.5 mg(0.5%溶液中的 0.5 mg)加入 2.5 ml 生理盐水雾化吸入；可重复给药；必要时定量雾化吸入器(MDI)	0.03 ml(0.15 mg)/kg 通过雾化吸入给予最大至 0.5 ml/剂；可重复或持续性给药；必要时定量雾化吸入器(带鼻-口两用雾化器)
阿替普酶(rt-PA)	缺血性卒中：0.9 mg/kg(最大剂量 30 mg)，静脉给予总量的 10%超过 1 min，随后剩余部分给药超过 1 h 肺栓塞：100 mg，IV，超过 2 h	N/A
胺碘酮	心搏骤停：300 mg，IV/IO。如果没有脉搏，或超过 10 min，可在初始剂量后迅速给予 150 mg 一次，以避免低血压宽 QRS 波群心动过速：150 mg，IV，超过 10 min(15 mg/min)，然后 1 mg/min，IV，6 h；接着 0.5 mg/min，IV，18 h。最高 2.2 g/24 h	心搏骤停：5 mg/kg，IV/IO。可重复高达 15 mg/kg，最大剂量 300 mg 宽 QRS 波群心动过速：5 mg/kg，IV，20～60 min 及以上，最大剂量 300 mg
氨力农	0.75 mg/kg，IV，10～15 min 及以上 维持：5～10 μg/(kg·min)，IV，每日总剂量不应超过 10 mg/(kg·24 h)	0.75 mg/kg，IV，10～15 min 及以上 维持：婴儿及儿童：5～10 μg/(kg·min)，IV，新生儿：3～5 μg/(kg·min)，IV，每日总剂量不应超过 10 mg/(kg·24 h)
阿替洛尔	5 mg，IV，超过 5 min；然后随后 10 min 5 mg，IV，总剂量为 10 mg	N/A
阿托品	0.5～1.0 mg，IV/ET 注意：有机磷中毒的剂量要高得多。详见中毒治疗	0.02 mg/kg，IV/ET，q5 min，根据需要 2～3 剂(最小剂量 0.1 mg/剂) 注意：有机磷中毒的剂量要高得多。详见中毒治疗
碳酸氢钠(44 mEq/50 ml，50 mEq/50 ml)	代谢性酸中毒：1 mEg/kg，IV，q10 min 必要时(根据动脉血气)；稀释：1∶1 稀释于 5%葡萄糖溶液中 注意：治疗中毒时剂量可能更高。详见中毒治疗	代谢性酸中毒：1 mEq/kg，IV，q10 min，必要时(根据动脉血气) 注意：治疗中毒时，剂量可能会更高。详见中毒治疗
氯化钙(10%溶液：100 mg/ml，1.36 mEq Ca/ml) 20 mg/kg，缓慢静滴 q10 min，必要时	500 mg/kg，缓慢静滴 q10 min，必要时 高钾血症：1～2 g，IV，5～10 min 及以上	20 mg/kg，缓慢静滴 q10 min，必要时
晶体液(生理盐水)	补液：1～2 L，IV，20～30 min 及以上，必要时重复	补液：20 ml/kg，IV，20～30 min 及以上，必要时重复
除颤	200 J；后续剂量加倍；同步：50～100 J	200 J；后续剂量加倍；同步：50～100 J
地塞米松(4 mg/ml，24 mg/ml)	5～10 mg，IM/IV	0.15～0.60 mg/kg，IM/IV
葡萄糖溶液	25～50 g，IV (50%：25 g/510 ml)	0.5～1.0 g(2～4 ml 5%葡萄糖)/kg，IV (25%葡萄糖溶液：6.25 g/25 ml)
地西泮(5 mg/ml)	5～10 mg，IV 注意：静脉和灌肠准备可能含有丙二醇、乙醇、苯甲酸钠和苯甲醇	0.2～0.3 mg/kg，IV q2～5 min 缓慢 对于>30 日至 5 岁儿童，最大剂量 5 mg 对于>5 岁儿童，最大剂量 10 mg 0.2～0.5 mg/kg，灌肠，q5 min
地高辛抗体(40 mg 剂量，拮抗 0.6 mg 地高辛或洋地黄毒苷)	3～5 瓶治疗慢性药物过量；10～20 剂治疗急性药物过量	剂量(瓶)＝地高辛浓度(ng/ml)×体重(kg)/100
地高辛	负荷：初始 0.5 mg，IV，随后 0.25 mg，q6 h×2 将终末期肾脏疾病的负荷剂量减少 50%	初始静脉负荷剂量： <2 岁：15～25 μg/kg 2～5 岁：10～15 μg/kg 5～10 岁：7～15 μg/kg
地尔硫䓬	15～20 mg(0.25 mg/kg)，IV，2 min 以上； 可在 15 min 内重复 IV：25～30 mg(0.35 mg/kg)，IV，2 min 以上 输液：5～15 mg/h，最多 24 h	N/A

（续表）

药物	成人	儿童（儿童用药剂量通常不应超过成人）
多巴酚丁胺（250 mg/20 ml）	2～20 μg/（kg·min），静脉滴注；最大剂量 40 μg/（kg·min）	2～15 μg/（kg·min），静脉滴注；最大剂量 40 μg/（kg·min）
多巴胺（40 mg/ml，80 mg/ml，160 mg/ml）	5～20 μg/（kg·min），静脉输注	5～20 μg/（kg·min），静脉输注
依那普利	1.25 mg，IV，5 min 以上，然后 1.25～5 mg，IV，q6 h	N/A
依诺肝素	1 mg/kg，SC，q12 h	N/A
肾上腺素	心搏停止： 静脉输注：0.5～1 mg（5～10 ml 1∶10 000），q3～5 min 气道内给药：1 mg（10 ml 1∶10 000），然后 5 次快速吹气 速发型过敏反应/过敏： 皮下给药：0.3 mg（0.3 ml 1∶1 000），q15～20 min，必要时	心搏停止： IV/IO：0.01 mg/kg（0.1 ml/kg 1∶10 000），q3～5 min，必要时，最大剂量 1 mg ET：1 mg/kg（0.1 ml/kg 1∶1 000），q3～5 min，必要时，最大剂量 2.5 mg 速发型敏反应/过敏： 皮下给药：0.01 mg/kg（0.01 ml/kg 1∶1 000），q15～20 min，必要时，不超过 0.5 mg
肾上腺素 2.25%溶液	0.5～0.75 ml/剂，加入 3 ml 生理盐水雾化；可重复	0.25～0.75 ml/剂，加入 3 ml 生理盐水雾化；可重复
依替巴肽	180 μg/kg（最大剂量：22.6 mg）静脉推注，然后 2 μg/（kg·min）（最大剂量 15 mg/h）输注维持 72 h	N/A
艾司洛尔	负荷：500 μg/kg，IV，1 min 以上 维持：50～200 μg/（kg·min）至 300 μg/（kg·min）（最大 300 mg 总剂量），IV 注意：该维持剂量可能用于血压控制，而不是快速心律失常	负荷：100～500 μg/kg，IV，1 min 以上 维持：25～200 μg/（kg·min），IV，最大剂量 1 000 μg/（kg·min）
甲磺酸非诺多泮 针对高血压危象	0.01～0.3 μg/（kg·min）持续输注；可每 15 min 或更长时间增加 0.05～0.1 μg/（kg·min），直到达到目标血压。最大剂量：1.6 μg/（kg·min）治疗持续时间：维持输注可持续 48 h	少于 1 个月（至少 2 kg 或足月）至 12 岁：0.2 μg/（kg·min）连续输注；每 20～30 min 可增加 0.3～0.5 μg/（kg·min）至最大剂量，最大剂量：0.8 μg/（kg·min） 治疗时间：维持性输液可持续 4 h
芬太尼（50 μg/ml）	0.5～1 μg/kg，慢静脉注射，可达 50～100 μg/剂。小心地滴定到所需的效果	1～2 μg/kg，慢静脉注射，可达 4 μg/kg。小心地滴定到所需的效果
氟马西尼	在 15 s 内注射 0.2 mg，然后每分钟注射 0.2 mg 直到意识达到所需水平或总剂量为 1 mg	0.01 mg/kg，IV，超过 15 s 至最大一次性剂量 0.2 mg，IV，总累积剂量不应超过 1 mg
磷苯妥英	15～20 mg 苯妥英当量（PE）/kg，IV，30 min 以上，也可肌内注射 静脉输液速率不应超过 50 PE/min	15～20 mg 苯妥英当量（PE）/kg，IV，30 min 以上，或肌内注射 静脉输液速率不应超过 50 PE/min
呋塞米（10 mg/ml）	10～20 mg，静脉滴注，1～2 min 及以上	1 mg/kg，静脉滴注，1～2 min 及以上
胰高血糖素	静脉滴注 1 mg，IV/IM/SC，q5 min；最大 5 mg（用于低血糖）	0.03～0.1 mg/kg，IV/IM/SC，q5～20 min，最大 1 mg（用于低血糖）
肝素钠 不同浓度无数的肝素钠产品（避免药物治疗错误）	60～80 U/kg，IV，随后 15～18 U/（kg·h） 调整肥胖患者静脉给药剂量为：瘦体重＋0.4×（实际体重－瘦体重）	50～75 U/kg，IV，随后 15～25 U/（kg·h） 使用不含防腐剂（不含苯甲醇）肝素在新生儿和婴儿中的应用
肼屈嗪（20 mg/ml）	10～20 mg，IV/IM	0.1～0.2 mg/kg，IV/IM；最大剂量 20 mg/剂
胰岛素，常规	酮症酸中毒：静脉注射 2～10 U，然后静脉输注 0.1 U/（kg·h）	酮症酸中毒：0.05～0.2 U/（kg·h），静脉输注
异丙肾上腺素（200 μg/ml）	0.5～5 μg/min，IV	0.05～2 μg/（kg·min），静脉滴注
拉贝洛尔（5 mg/ml）	负荷：20 mg/剂，IV，2 min 以上，q10 min，直至最高总剂量 300 mg 维持：0.5～2 mg/min，静脉滴注	负荷：0.25～1.0 mg/kg，静注 2 min 以上；必要时每 q10 min 重复。最大剂量 20 mg/剂，静脉注射 维持：0.4～1 mg/（kg·h），静脉输注，最大 3 mg/（kg·h）
利多卡因（10 mg/ml，20 mg/ml）	负荷：1～1.5 mg/kg，IV，IO。可重复 0.5～0.75 mg/kg，q5～10 min 必要时；最大总剂量：3 mg/kg 当静脉通路无法建立时，可以使用气管内给药 维持：静脉滴注 1～4 mg/min	负荷：1 mg/kg，IV/IO。最大剂量 100 mg/剂 如果维持输注出现延迟，可以重复 0.5～1 mg/kg，IV 当静脉通路无法建立时，可以使用气道内给药。注射 2～3 mg/kg，用 5 ml 生理盐水冲洗，然后进行 5 次人工辅助通气。维持：20 μg/（kg·min）静脉滴注

（续表）

药物	成人	儿童（儿童用药剂量通常不应超过成人）
劳拉西泮（2 mg/ml，4 mg/ml）	0.5～2 mg，IV/IM/PO，可达 5 mg	0.05～0.1 mg/kg，IV 注意：注射剂型含有苯甲醇、聚乙二醇、丙二醇
硫酸镁	重度哮喘：1～2 g，IV，20 min 以上 先兆子痫：4 g，IV，20 min 以上	25～50 mg/kg，IV，超过 20 min
甘露醇（200 mg/ml，250 mg/ml）	负荷：0.25～1 g/kg，IV，超过 30 min 维持：0.25～0.5 g/kg	负荷：0.5～1 g/kg，IV，超过 30 min 维持：0.25～0.5 g/kg，IV
美托洛尔	5 mg，IV，q5 min，分 3 次服用。最大剂量 15 mg	N/A
米达唑仑（1 mg/ml）	1～2.5 mg，IV，超过 2～3 min，最大剂量 2.5～5 mg	6 个月至 5 岁：0.05～0.1 mg/kg，IV，2～3 min 及以上；0.3 mg/kg，IV 年龄较大的儿童服用的剂量较低。使用理想的 IBW 来计算肥胖患者的剂量
吗啡（0.5～25 mg/ml）	0.1～0.2 mg/kg，IV/IM。最大剂量 15 mg	0.05～0.2 mg/kg，IV/IM。最大剂量 15 mg。使用不含防腐剂的配方
纳洛酮（0.4 mg/ml，1 mg/ml）	1～2 mg 静脉滴注，IM，SC 或滴鼻	0.1 mg/kg，IV，IO，ET。由于吸收减少，ET 剂量应比 IV 剂量大 2～3 倍
尼卡地平（按 2.5 mg/ml 提供，混匀静脉注射）	开始注射 2.5～5 mg/h，IV，可能增加 2.5 mg/h，q10～15 min 至最大 15 mg/h	
硝酸甘油（浓缩液：5 mg/ml。预混袋：100 μg/ml、200 μg/ml、400 μg/ml）	5 μg/min，IV，每 3～5 min 先滴入 5 μg/min，直到 300 μg/min。使用非聚氯乙烯通路	0.25～0.5 μg/(kg · min)，静脉滴注。每 3～5 min 必要时增加 0.5～0.1 μg/(kg · min)，达到 5 μg/(kg · min)。使用非聚氯乙烯通路
硝普钠	0.1 μg/(kg · min)，静脉输注直至 10 μg/(kg · min) 0.5～1 μg/min，静脉输注直至 30 μg/min	0.01 μg/(kg · min)，静脉输注，直至 5.0 μg/(kg · min)
去甲肾上腺素		0.05～0.1 μg/(kg · min)静脉滴注。滴定最高可达 1～2 μg/(kg · min)
潘库溴铵（1 mg/ml，2 mg/ml）	0.04～0.1 mg/kg，IV。额外剂量为 0.01 mg/kg，IV，每隔 25～60 min 给药一次	0.04～0.1 mg/kg，IV。额外剂量为 0.01 mg/kg，IV，每隔 25～60 min 给药一次
苯巴比妥 （30 mg/ml，60 mg/ml，65 mg/ml，130 mg/ml）	负荷：15～20 mg/kg，静脉输注（5～50 mg/min 及以下）。需检测呼吸抑制情况	负荷：15～20 mg/kg，静脉输注，<1 mg/(kg · min)。需检测呼吸抑制情况
苯妥英（50 mg/ml）	癫痫负荷：10～15 mg/kg，静脉输注（<40 mg/min）至 1 000 mg。如果使用苯妥英钠，则在加载剂量前获得苯妥英钠血清水平（参见苯妥英钠）	癫痫负荷：10～20 mg/kg，静脉输注，<0.5 mg/(kg · min)。如果使用苯妥英钠（参见苯妥英），在负荷剂量之前，获得血清苯妥英素水平
普鲁卡因酰胺	负荷：15～18 mg/kg，IV，超过 30 min 维持：1～4 mg/min。心脏或肾脏损害患者的剂量减少	负荷：2～6 mg/kg，超过 5 min（最大剂量 100 mg）；每 5～10 min 重复给药一次，最大剂量 15 mg/kg 维持：20～80 μg/(kg · min)持续输注，最大剂量 2 g/d
普萘洛尔（1 mg/ml）	1 mg，IV，超过 10 min，总剂量 5 mg	0.01～0.1 mg/kg IV 超过 10 min；最大剂量 1 mg
瑞替普酶	10 U，IV，2 min 以上，除非发生严重出血，否则 30 min 内重复	N/A
琥珀酰胆碱 （针剂：20 mg/ml，100 mg/ml） （注射剂：500 mg，1 g）	1～1.5 mg/kg，IV，10～30 s 及以上，可达 150 mg	1～1.5 mg/kg，IV，超过 10～30 s。小于 6 岁的患者可能需要更高的剂量 每毫升琥珀胆碱含 10 mg 苯甲醇
替奈普酶（TNKase）	静脉滴注 5 s 以上： <60 kg：30 mg 60～70 kg：35 mg 70～80 kg：40 mg 80～90 kg：45 mg 90 kg 及以上：50 mg	N/A
特布他林	0.25 mg 皮下注射，可重复 15～30 min 一次	N/A
替罗非班	0.4 μg/(kg · min)，30 min；0.1 μg/(kg · min)，12～24 h	无脉 VT/VF：40 U 加入 20 ml 生理盐水静脉注射。如无自发性循环，可重复 3 min
血管加压素	无脉 VT/VF：40 U 加入 20 ml 生理盐水静脉注射。如无自发性循环，可重复 3 min	0.08～0.1 mg/kg，快速 IV，在 7 周至 1 岁的患者中使用低剂量，可在 1～9 岁的患者中使用高剂量

（续表）

药物	成人	儿童(儿童用药剂量通常不应超过成人)
维库溴铵	0.08～0.1 mg/kg,快速静脉注射	0.08～0.1 mg/kg 快速静脉输注,在 7 周至 1 岁的患者中使用低剂量,可在 1～9 岁的患者中使用高剂量
维拉帕米	2.5～5.0 mg IV 超过 2 min;老年患者心率较慢(>3 min);如果 15～30 min 无反应,然后静脉注射 5～10 mg,最大剂量为 20 mg	N/A

注:ET,气管内给药;N/A,不适用;IM,肌内注射;IO,骨髓腔输注;IV,静脉注射;SC,皮下注射。

快速序列插管(RSI)

1. 用 100%氧气预充氧。
2. 应用环状压力。
3. 诱导：依托咪酯(0.3 mg/kg)、异丙酚(0.5～2 mg/kg)或氯胺酮(2 mg/kg)静脉推注。
4. 神经肌肉阻滞：琥珀胆碱 1.5 mg/kg 静脉推注。
5. 等待 30～45 s。
6. 当条件达到最佳时插管。

如果担心加重颅内压或重度高血压,考虑使用芬太尼(1～2 μg/kg)静脉推药(1～2 min 或以上)和利多卡因(1.5 mg/kg)静脉推药进行预处理。

如果涉及颅内压升高,应考虑去肌颤剂量的肌松药物(见下表)。

阿托品：0.02 mg/kg 静脉推注(用于 1 岁以下的儿童)。

神经肌肉阻断剂

药剂	RSI 剂量(麻醉肌松)	剂量(抗肌颤*)	开始时间	维持时间
琥珀酰胆碱	RSI：1～2 mg/kg		30～60 s	4～6 min
罗库溴铵	RSI：0.6～1.2 mg/kg	0.06 mg/kg	2 min	30 min
维库溴铵	RSI：0.015～0.25 mg/kg	0.01 mg/kg	2.5～5 min	25～40 min

注：* 约束剂量,肌颤预防/去肌颤剂量。

镇静和诱导剂

药剂	剂量	开始时间	维持时间
依托咪酯	0.2～0.3 mg/kg	60 s	3～5 min
芬太尼	诱导：2～10 μg/kg 镇静：0.5～1 μg/kg	60 s	30～60 min
氯胺酮	2 mg/kg 缓慢 IVP[<0.5 mg/(kg·min)]	30～60 s	15 min
咪达唑仑	诱导：0.07～0.3 mg/kg 镇静：0.02～0.04 mg/kg	2 min	1～2 h
丙泊酚	0.5～2 mg/kg IVP	30 s	3～10 min
硫喷妥钠	3～4 mg/kg	20～40 s	5～10 min

儿科生命体征和复苏设备尺寸

项目	年龄	6 个月	1 岁	2 岁	5 岁	10 岁
近似体重	2～4 kg	8 kg	10 kg	13 kg	20 kg	35 kg
生命体征						
血压	60±10	89±29	96±30	99±25	99±20	112±19
心率	125	130	125	115	100	75
呼吸频率	40±10	38±10	39±11	28±4	27±6	21±4
复苏						
除颤	8 J	16 J	20 J	26 J	40 J	70 J
复律	2～4 J	4～8 J	5～10 J	7～13 J	20～40 J	25～70 J
吸痰管	8F	8～10F	8～10F	10F	10F	12F
气道						
喉镜窥视片	1(st)	1～2(st)	1～2(st)	2(st/c)	2(st/c)	2～3(st/c)
气管内导管(mm)	3.0～3.5	3.5～4.0	4.0～4.5	4.5	5.0～5.5	6.5
气管长度(mm)	10.5	12	12	13.5	16.5	19.5
管子						
鼻胃管	5/6	8	10	10	10～12	12
尿管	5 Fr	5～8 Fr	8 Fr	10 Foley	10 Foley	10 Foley
胸腔引流管(Fr)	10～12	14～20	16～20	14～24	20～28	28～32

温度换算：摄氏度↔华氏度

摄氏度(℃)	华氏度(℉)	摄氏度(℃)	华氏度(℉)
34.2	93.6	38.6	101.4
34.6	94.3	39.0	102.2
35.0	95.0	39.4	102.9
35.4	95.7	39.8	103.6
35.8	96.4	40.2	104.3
36.2	97.1	40.6	105.1
36.6	97.8	41.0	105.8
37.0	98.6	41.4	106.5
37.4	99.3	41.8	107.2
37.8	100.0	42.2	108.0
38.2	100.7	42.6	108.7

注：℉=9/5×℃+32。

重量换算：磅(lb)↔千克(kg)

lb	kg	lb	kg
10 lb	4.53 kg	110 lb	49.89 kg
20 lb	9.07 kg	120 lb	54.43 kg
30 lb	13.60 kg	130 lb	58.96 kg
40 lb	18.14 kg	140 lb	63.50 kg
50 lb	22.68 kg	150 lb	68.04 kg
60 lb	27.21 kg	160 lb	72.57 kg
70 lb	31.75 kg	170 lb	77.11 kg
80 lb	36.28 kg	180 lb	81.64 kg
90 lb	40.82 kg	190 lb	86.18 kg
100 lb	45.36 kg	200 lb	90.72 kg

注：kg=lb×2.2。

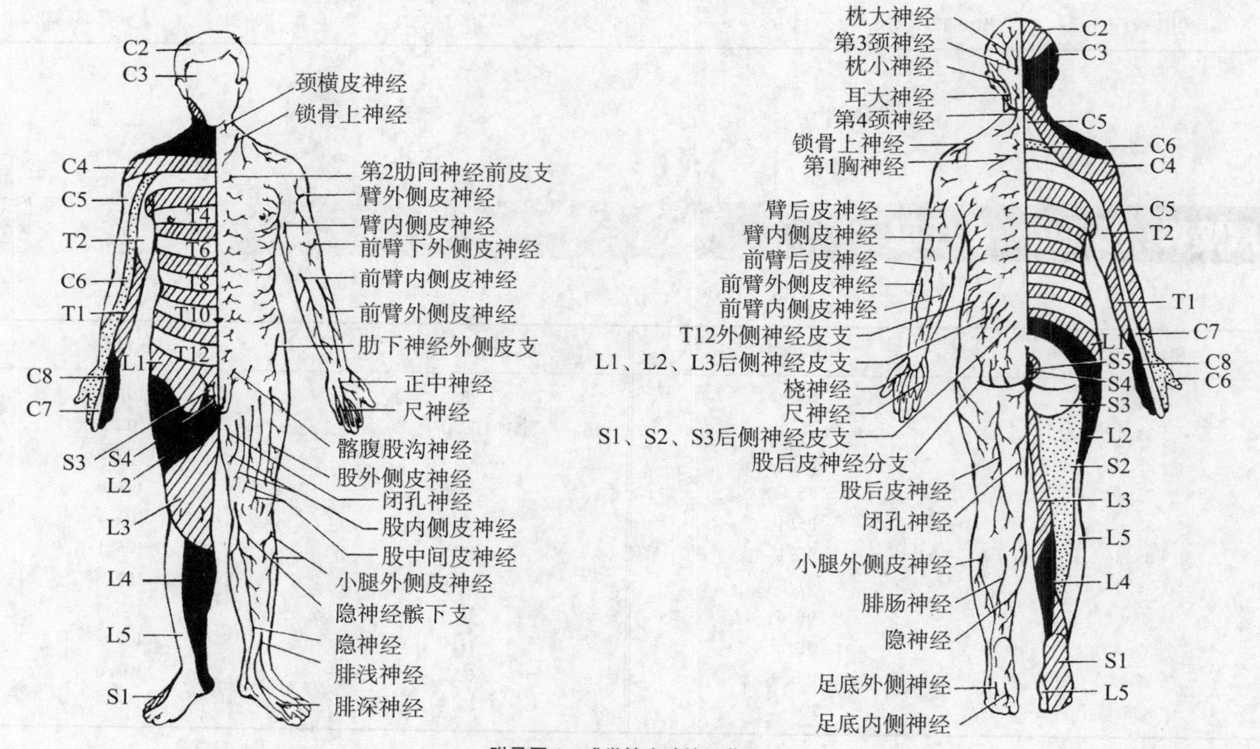

附录图 1 感觉性皮肤神经节段